MELMON AND MORRELLI'S

# CLINICAL PHARMACOLOGY

ADEGBOYEGA Q. ADIGUN MD
DIVISION of CLINICAL PHARMACOLOGY
DEPARTMENT of MEDICINE
Indiana University Medical School
IUPUI
MARCH 2001.
(Gift from the Dept.)

## NOTICE

MELMON AND MORRELLI'S

# CLINICAL PHARMACOLOGY

## BASIC PRINCIPLES IN THERAPEUTICS

FOURTH EDITION


**EDITORS**

**S. GEORGE CARRUTHERS, M.D.**

Richard Ivey Professor and Chair, Department of Medicine, Professor, Department of Pharmacology and Toxicology, London Health Sciences Centre and University of Western Ontario, London, Ontario, Canada

**BRIAN B. HOFFMAN, M.D., F.R.C.P.(C)**

Professor of Medicine and Molecular Pharmacology, Stanford University and Veterans Affairs Palo Alto Health Care System, Palo Alto, California

**KENNETH L. MELMON, M.D.**

Professor of Medicine and Molecular Pharmacology, Associate Dean for Postgraduate Medical Education, Stanford University, Stanford, California

**DAVID W. NIERENBERG, M.D.**

Edward Tulloh Krumm Professor of Medicine and Pharmacology/Toxicology, Chief, Division of Clinical Pharmacology, Associate Dean for Medical Education, Dartmouth Medical School, Hanover, New Hampshire



**McGRAW-HILL**

**MEDICAL PUBLISHING DIVISION**

New York / St. Louis / San Francisco / Auckland / Bogotá / Caracas / Lisbon / Madrid / Mexico City / Milan / Montreal / New Delhi / San Juan / Singapore / Sydney / Tokyo / Toronto

McGraw-Hill

A Division of The McGraw-Hill Companies

**Melmon and Morrelli's Clinical Pharmacology**



ISBN 0-07-105406-5

1234567890 DOWDOW 09876543210

This book was set in Times Roman by York Graphic Services, Inc.
The editors were John J. Dolan, Mariapaz Ramos Englis, and Lester A. Sheinis.
The production supervisor was Richard C. Ruzycka.
The text designer was Marsha Cohen / Parallelogram.
The cover designer was Edward Smith
The indexer was Irving Condé Tullar.
R. R. Donnelley and Sons Company was printer and binder.

This book is printed on acid-free paper.

**Library of Congress cataloging-in-publication data for this title are on file with the Library of Congress.**

*In 1932 Albert Einstein said "The scientist finds his reward in what Henri Poincaré calls the joy of comprehension, and not in the possibilities of application to which any discovery may lead." (Albert Einstein from the Epilogue to Planck,* "Where Is Science Going?" *1932, p 211.) Our editors concur but add that the thoughtful physician has the advantage over the basic scientist in that he or she can experience the joy of comprehension in both the discovery and application phases of rational therapeutics.*

*This book is dedicated to the recognition that scientific achievement applicable to people requires the output of many collaborating and working in sequence often in silence, often without tangible reward. This book is dedicated to the proposition that ordinarily little can be accomplished by one. In this instance, the editors note that the task of succeeding editions has become increasingly and remarkably more complex. The first edition compiled the work of 19 authors; each edition has needed more and this edition required 89 contributors.*

*This book is dedicated to those who tenaciously and effectively collaborate in order to develop and to pass on wisdom.*

*This book is dedicated in gratitude to those in biology and therapeutics*
*Who are of the past,*
*Who are involved in the present,*
*And who are invested in any way in the future of human health.*

# Contents

# Contributors

**John A. Abisheganaden, M.R.C.P. (UK)** Associate Consultant, Department of Respiratory Medicine, Tan Tock Seng Hospital, Singapore
Chapter 2

**Moira L. Aitken, M.D., F.R.C.P.** Associate Professor of Medicine, Division of Pulmonary and Critical Care Medicine, Department of Medicine, University of Washington School of Medicine, Seattle, Washington
Chapter 2

**J. Malcolm O. Arnold, M.D.** Professor of Medicine, Pharmacology and Toxicology, University of Western Ontario, Division of Cardiology, London Health Sciences Centre, Victoria Campus, London, Ontario, Canada
Chapter 1

**Christopher M. Barnard, M.D.** Clinical Assistant Professor of Dermatology, Stanford University School of Medicine, Monterey, California
Chapter 11

**David W. Bates, M.D.** Associate Professor of Medicine, Harvard Medical School, Chief, Division of General Medicine, Brigham and Women's Hospital, Boston, Massachusetts
Chapter 24

**Neal L. Benowitz, M.D.** Professor of Medicine, Psychiatry and Biopharmaceutical Sciences, Division of Clinical Pharmacology and Experimental Therapeutics, University of California, San Francisco, California
Chapter 17

**Joseph R. Bertino, M.D.** Chairman, Program of Molecular Pharmacology and Therapeutics, American Cancer Society Professor of Medicine and Pharmacology, Memorial-Sloan Kettering Cancer Center, New York, New York
Chapter 13

**Brian G. Birdwell, M.D.** Clinical Assistant Professor of Medicine, University of Oklahoma Health Sciences Center, Oklahoma City, Oklahoma
Chapter 1

**Terrence F. Blaschke, M.D.** Professor of Medicine and Molecular Pharmacology, Chief, Division of Clinical Pharmacology, Stanford University School of Medicine, Stanford, California
Chapter 26

**Homer A. Boushey, M.D.** Chief, Asthma Clinical Research Center and the Division of Allergy and Immunology, Professor of Medicine, Department of Medicine, University of California, San Francisco, California
Chapter 2

**D. Craig Brater, M.D.** Professor of Medicine, Chairman, Department of Medicine, Director, Division of Clinical Pharmacology, Indiana University School of Medicine, Indianapolis, Indiana
Chapter 6

**Peter Brooks, M.D.** Professor and Executive Dean (Health Sciences), The University of Queensland Royal Brisbane Hospital, Herston, Queensland, Australia
Chapter 10

**Christopher P. Cannon, M.D.** Associate Physician, Cardiovascular Division, Brigham and Women's Hospital, Assistant Professor of Medicine, Harvard Medical School, Boston, Massachusetts
Chapter 1

**S. George Carruthers, M.D.** Richard Ivey Professor and Chair, Department of Medicine, Professor Department of Pharmacology and Toxicology, London Health Sciences Centre and University of Western Ontario, London, Ontario, Canada
Chapter 1

**David Coffey, M.D.** Associate Professor of Medicine (Neurology) and Psychiatry, Section of Neurology, Dartmouth-Hitchcock Medical Center, Lebanon, New Hampshire
Chapter 7

**Paul E. Cooper, M.D., F.R.C.P.C.** Associate Professor of Medicine, University of Western Ontario, Chief, Clinical Neurological Sciences, St. Joseph's Health Centre, London, Ontario, Canada
Chapter 7

**Richard Day, M.D., F.R.A.C.P.** Professor of Clinical Pharmacology, University of New South Wales, Director Clinical Pharmacology and Toxicology, St. Vincent's Hospital, Darlinghurst, New South Wales, Australia
Chapter 10

**B. M. Demaerschalk, M.D.** Fellow, Stroke Service, Department of Clinical Neurological Sciences, University of Western Ontario, University Campus, London Health Sciences Centre, London, Ontario, Canada
Chapter 7

**George C. Ebers, M.D.** Professor, Department of Clinical Neurology, University of Oxford, Radcliffe Infirmary, Oxford, England
Chapter 7

**Kevin R. Forward, M.D.** Associate Professor, Chief, Division of Microbiology, Dalhousie University, Halifax, Nova Scotia, Canada
Chapter 14

**Raymond R. Gaeta, M.D.** Associate Professor of Anesthesiology, Director, Pain Management Service, Stanford University Medical Center, Stanford University School of Medicine, Stanford, California
Chapter 15

**Sean P. Gaine, M.D.** Assistant Professor of Medicine, Director, Pulmonary Hypertension Center, Division of Pulmonary and Critical Care Medicine, Johns Hopkins Hospital, Baltimore, Maryland
Chapter 2

**Gabriel Garcia, M.D.** Associate Professor of Medicine, Stanford University School of Medicine, Stanford, California
Chapters 3, 4

**Lewis R. Goldfrank, M.D.** Associate Professor of Clinical Medicine, New York University School of Medicine, Director, Emergency Medicine, Bellevue Hospital Center/New York University Medical Center, New York, New York
Chapter 18

**Marc E. Goldyne, M.D., Ph.D.** Clinical Professor of Dermatology, Department of Dermatology, University of California, San Francisco, California
Chapter 11

**Jerry H. Gurwitz, M.D.** The Dr. John Meyers Professor of Primary Care Medicine, University of Massachusetts Medical School, Executive Director, Meyers Primary Care Institute, Fallon Healthcare System and University of Massachusetts Medical School, Worcester, Massachusetts
Chapter 21

**Gordon Guyatt, M.D., M.Sc.** Professor of Medicine and Clinical Epidemiology and Biostatistics, McMaster University, Hamilton, Ontario, Canada
Chapter 29

**Vladimir Hachinski, M.D., F.R.C.P.C., M.Sc., D.Sc.** Richard and Beryl Ivey Professor and Chair, Chief, Department of Clinical Neurological Sciences, London Health Sciences Centre, University Campus, London, Ontario, Canada
Chapter 7

**Malcolm Handel, M.D.** Arthritis and Inflammation Program, Garvan Institute of Medical Research and University of New South Wales, Darlinghurst, New South Wales, Australia
Chapter 10

**Andrew R. Hoffman, M.D.** Professor of Medicine and Molecular and Cellular Physiology, Stanford University School of Medicine, Chief, Medical Service, VA Palo Alto Health Care System, Palo Alto, California
Chapter 9

**Brian B. Hoffman, M.D.** Professor of Medicine and Molecular Pharmacology, Stanford University and VA Palo Alto Health Care System, Palo Alto, California
Chapter 1

**Paul Hoffman, Ph.D.** Professor of Microbiology, Dalhousie University, Halifax, Nova Scotia, Canada
Chapter 14

**Leo E. Hollister, M.D.** Clinical Professor of Medicine, Research Director, Harris County Psychiatric Center, University of Texas Medical School, Houston, Texas
Chapter 8

**Zhuo Wei Hu, M.D., Ph.D.** Senior Research Pharmacologist, Stanford University School of Medicine, Division of Endocrinology/Gerontology and Metabolism, Department of Medicine, Palo Alto, California
Chapter 12

**John C. Hunter, Ph.D.** Head, Department of Analgesia, Neurobiology Unit, Roche Bioscience, Palo Alto, California
Chapter 15

**Lawrence R. Jenkyn, M.D.** Associate Professor of Neurology and Psychiatry, Department of Neurology, Dartmouth-Hitchcock Medical Center, Lebanon, New Hampshire
Chapter 7

**B. Lynn Johnston, M.D.** Associate Professor, Infectious Diseases, Dalhousie University, Halifax, Nova Scotia, Canada
Chapter 14

**Lori D. Karan, M.D.** Assistant Professor of Medicine, Division of Clinical Pharmacology and Experimental Therapeutics, University of California, San Francisco, California
Chapter 17

**Gideon Koren, M.D., F.A.C.C.T., F.R.C.P.C.** Head, Population Health Science Program, Director, Division of Clinical Pharmacology/Toxicology, Professor of Pediatrics, Pharmacology, Pharmacy Medicine, and Medical Genetics, The CIBC World Market Children's Miracle Foundation, Chair in Child Health Research, University of Toronto, Toronto, Ontario, Canada
Chapter 20

**Fredric B. Kraemer, M.D.** Chief of Endocrinology, VA Palo Alto Health Care System, Associate Professor of Medicine, Stanford University, Division of Endocrinology, Stanford, California
Chapter 9

**Lucian Leape, M.D.** Adjunct Professor of Health Policy, Department of Health Policy and Management, Harvard School of Public Health, Boston, Massachusetts
Chapter 24

**Spencer Lee, Ph.D.** Professor of Microbiology, Dalhousie University, Halifax, Nova Scotia, Canada
Chapter 14

**Steven A. Lieberman, M.D.** Associate Professor, Division of Endocrinology, Department of Internal Medicine, The University of Texas Medical Branch, Galveston, Texas
Chapter 9

**David J. Liepert, M.D.** Clinical Assistant Professor of Anesthesiology, University of Calgary College of Medicine, Calgary, Alberta, Canada
Chapter 16

**Richard Lin, M.D.** Assistant Professor of Medicine, Division of Clinical Pharmacology, Department of Pharmacology and Medicine, University of Texas Health Sciences Center, San Antonio, Texas
Chapter 12

**Ronen Loebstein, M.D.** Division of Clinical Pharmacology and Toxicology and Department of Medicine A, The Chaim Sheba Medical Center, Hashomer, Israel
Chapter 20

**Richard D. Mamelok, M.D.** Internist-Clinical Pharmacologist, Consultant to Industry, Palo Alto, California
Chapter 27

**Robert Marcus, M.D.** Professor of Medicine, Stanford University School of Medicine, VA Palo Alto Health Care System, Palo Alto, California
Chapter 10

**Thomas J. Marrie, M.D.** Professor and Chair, Department of Medicine, University of Alberta, Edmonton, Alberta, Canada
Chapter 14

**Mervyn Maze, M.D., Ch.B., F.R.C.P., F.R.C.A.** Sir Ivan Magill Department of Anaesthetics, Imperial College School of Medicine, Chelsea and Westminster Hospital, London, England
Chapter 15

**Richard S. McLachlan, M.D.** Professor, Departments of Clinical Neurological Sciences, Medicine, and Physiology, University of Western Ontario, Neurologist, London Health Sciences Centre University Campus, London, Ontario, Canada
Chapter 7

**Kenneth L. Melmon, M.D.** Professor of Medicine and Molecular Pharmacology, Associate Dean for Postgraduate Medical Education, Stanford University, Stanford, California
Part 1

**Naseema B. Merchant, M.D.** Pulmonary Fellow, Division of Pulmonary and Critical Care Medicine, Yale University School of Medicine, West Haven, Connecticut
Chapter 2

**Urs A. Meyer, M.D.** Professor of Pharmacology, Chairman, Department of Pharmacology, Biozentrum, University of Basel, Basel, Switzerland
Chapter 22

**Thomas Michel, Ph.D., M.D.** Associate Professor of Medicine, Harvard Medical School, Chief, Cardiology Section, West Roxbury VA Medical Center, Physician, Brigham and Women's Hospital, Boston, Massachusetts
Chapter 1

**Jeffrey Wells Miller, M.D.** Senior Clinical Pharmacologist, Lilly Laboratory for Clinical Research, Eli Lilly & Co., Inc., Indiana University Hospital and Outpatient Center, Indianapolis, Indiana
Chapter 9

**Stanley Nattel, M.D.** Director, Research Center, Montreal Heart Institute, Professor of Medicine, University of Montreal, Montreal, Quebec, Canada
Chapter 1

**Lewis S. Nelson, M.D.** Assistant Professor of Clinical Surgery (Emergency Medicine), New York University School of Medicine, Fellowship Director, New York City Poison Control Center, New York, New York
Chapter 18

**Michael W. Nicolle, M.D., F.R.C.P.C., D. Phil.** Assistant Professor of Medicine, University of Western Ontario, Director, Myasthenia Gravis Clinic, Department of Clinical Neurological Sciences, London Health Sciences Centre, University Campus, London, Ontario, Canada
Chapter 7

**Michael S. Niederman, M.D., F.A.C.P., F.C.C.P., F.C.C.M.** Chief, Department of Medicine, Winthrop University Hospital, Mineola, New York
Chapter 2

**David W. Nierenberg, M.D.** Edward Tulloh Krumm Professor of Medicine and Pharmacology/Toxicology, Chief, Division of Clinical Pharmacology, Associate Dean for Medical Education, Dartmouth Medical School, Hanover, New Hampshire
Part 1

**Paul W. Noble, M.D.** Associate Professor of Medicine, Yale School of Medicine, Pulmonary Section Chief, VA Connecticut Healthcare System, West Haven, Connecticut
Chapter 2

**Owen A. O'Connor, M.D., Ph.D.** Clinical Assistant Attending Physician, Department of Medicine, Memorial-Sloan Kettering Cancer Center, New York, New York
Chapter 13

**Ronald G. Pearl, M.D., Ph.D.** Chairman and Professor of Anesthesia, Department of Anesthesia, Stanford University School of Medicine, Stanford, California
Chapter 16

**David Quinn, M.B.B.S., F.R.A.C.P.** Director of Clinical Training and Lecturer, Department of Clinical Pharmacology and Toxicology, University of New South Wales and St. Vincent's Hospital, Darlinghurst, New South Wales, Australia
Chapter 10

**Stephen I. Rennard, M.D.** Larson Professor of Medicine, Pulmonary and Critical Care Medicine, Department of Internal Medicine, University of Nebraska Medical Center, Omaha, Nebraska
Chapter 2

**G. P. A. Rice, M.D.** Professor, Department of Clinical Neurological Sciences, London Health Sciences Centre, University Campus, London, Ontario, Canada
Chapter 7

**David Robertson, M.D.** Elton Yates Professor of Medicine, Pharmacology and Neurology, Autonomic Dysfunction Center, Vanderbilt University, Nashville, Tennessee
Chapter 1

**Dan M. Roden, M.D.** Professor of Medicine and Pharmacology, Director, Division of Clinical Pharmacology, Vanderbilt University, Nashville, Tennessee
Chapter 1

**Irwin H. Rosenberg, M.D.** Professor of Nutrition and Medicine, Director, USDA Human Nutrition Research Center on Aging, Tufts University, Boston, Massachusetts
Chapter 5

**Elizabeth M. Ross, M.D.** Assistant Professor, Tufts University School of Medicine, Assistant Physician, Divisions of Clinical Nutrition and General Internal Medicine, New England Medical Center Hospital, Boston, Massachusetts
Chapter 5

**Peter C. Rubin, M.D.** Department of Medicine, University Hospital, Queens Medical Centre, Nottingham, England
Chapter 19

**Jane M. Rutherford, D.M., M.R.C.O.G.** Department of Feto-Maternal Medicine, Queens Medical Centre, Nottingham, England
Chapter 19

**David L. Sackett, F.R.S.C., M.D.** Trount Research and Education Centre at Irish Lake, Markdale, Ontario, Canada
Chapter 29

**Daniel S. Sitar, Ph.D.** Professor and Head, Department of Pharmacology and Therapeutics, Professor, Department of Internal Medicine (Clinical Pharmacology Section), Professor, Department of Pediatrics and Child Health, University of Manitoba, Winnipeg, Manitoba, Canada
Chapter 23

**Kathryn L. Slayter, Pharm. D.** Infectious Diseases Pharmacist, Queen E II Health Sciences Centre, Halifax, Nova Scotia, Canada
Chapter 14

**Peter H. Stone, M.D.** Associate Professor of Medicine, Cardiovascular Division, Brigham and Women's Hospital, Harvard Medical School, Boston, Massachusetts
Chapter 1

**Brian Strom, M.D., M.P.H.** Professor of Biostatistics and Epidemiology, Medicine, and Pharmacology, Chair, Department of Biostatistics and Epidemiology, Director, Center for Clinical Epidemiology and Biostatistics, University of Pennsylvania School of Medicine, Philadelphia, Pennsylvania
Chapter 30

**Arturo Tamayo, M.D.** Clinical Stroke Fellow, Department of Clinical Neurological Sciences, University of Western Ontario, London, Ontario, Canada
Chapter 7

**Mark R. Tonelli, M.D., M.A.** Assistant Professor of Medicine, Division of Pulmonary and Critical Care Medicine, University of Washington, Seattle, Washington
Chapter 2

**Claire Touchie, M.D.** Assistant Professor, Infectious Diseases and Microbiology, Dalhousie University, Halifax, Nova Scotia, Canada
Chapter 14

**John Urquhart, M.D., F.R.C.P. (Edin)** Professor of Pharmacoepidemiology, Department of Epidemiology Maastricht University, Maastricht, Netherlands
Chapter 28

**Robert E. Vestal, M.D.** Senior Medical Director, Early Clinical Development, Covance Inc., Walnut Creek, California
Chapter 21

**Sunita Vohra, M.D., F.R.C.P.C., M.Sc.** Clinical Epidemiologist, Population Health Sciences, The Hospital for Sick Children Research Institute, Scientific Consultant, Division of Clinical Pharmacology and Toxicology, The Hospital for Sick Children, Assistant Professor of Pediatrics, University of Toronto, Toronto, Ontario, Canada
Chapter 20

**Thomas N. Ward, M.D.** Associate Professor of Medicine (Neurology), Dartmouth-Hitchcock Medical Center, Lebanon, New Hampshire
Chapter 7

**Mark S. Weinfeld, M.D.** Assistant Professor of Medicine, Washington University School of Medicine, Washington University Cardiology Consultants, St. Louis, Misssouri
Chapter 1

**Thomas L. Whitsett, M.D.** Professor of Medicine and Pharmacology, Department of Medicine, Cardiovascular Section, University of Oklahoma Health Sciences Center, Oklahoma City, Oklahoma
Chapter 1

**Kenneth Williams, B.Sc. (Hons), Ph.D.** Associate Professor, Deputy Director, Department of Clinical Pharmacology and Toxicology, St. Vincent's Hospital and University of New South Wales, New South Wales, Sydney, Australia
Chapter 10

**James M. Wright, Ph.D.** Associate Professor, Department of Medicine and Department of Pharmacology, University Hospital, University of British Columbia, Vancouver, British Columbia, Canada
Chapter 25

# Preface to the Fourth Edition

The prompt and accurate diagnosis of many diseases has been facilitated in recent years by technological advances in medical imaging and clinical chemistry. At the same time, the clinician's ability to treat disease has also been enhanced by the development of many useful new medications; the conduct, publication and widespread communication of major clinical trials; the development of useful clinical guidelines and critical paths; and the ready access to other sources of information: MEDLINE, Web sites, professional societies, and many others.

Despite these advances in diagnostic capabilities and availability of information, prescribing drugs optimally has not become correspondingly easier. Modern health-care management has often increased expectations that primary-care physicians will assume more direct responsibility for the comprehensive medical management of patients with a wider range of diseases. Access to prompt consultation with subspecialists is sometimes restricted.

There has been a proliferation of new drugs within established drug classes and discovery of new classes of drugs as well. These newer agents often exhibit greater efficacy or reduced toxicity. However, they sometimes are accompanied by new (even unknown) adverse effects; and they are often extremely expensive. Many new drug-drug interactions (involving new drugs and older agents) are also important to consider. Under these circumstances, it might be anticipated that "information overload" could challenge the physician's ability to select an optimal drug, dose, and duration of treatment for the individual patient.

Consequently, a major focus of the fourth edition of this text is to provide a solid foundation of information and skills useful for physicians interested in optimizing their use of drugs over a broad range of common and important therapeutic problems. In this edition, the editors and contributors have tried to tie recommendations for pharmacotherapeutic decisions in common major diseases to the best available evidence, as presented in such primary forms as clinical trials, meta-analyses, or structural reviews. Such evidence is often very reliable and is rooted in the careful assessment of experience in hundreds or thousands of patients with a specific disease. While it is true that personal experience and anecdotal information sometimes may have an important role in pharmacotherapy, especially when good evidence is not available, we as a profession have learned that it is a serious mistake to use such impressions instead of objective observations. A major theme of this book is that difficult therapeutic decisions are most likely to succeed when they are generally based on the results of well-planned and well-performed clinical trials.

This edition emphasizes at the same time that it is important to recognize that the best available evidence is often derived from studies conducted in groups of patients who do not completely resemble the specific (really unique) patient sitting before the physician. For example, there may be extensive evidence that may suggest an optimal approach to the drug choice in the management of a serious staphylococcal infection in a group of otherwise healthy patients or to the management of essential primary hypertension in otherwise healthy adults. However, the careful physician may need to modify these recommendations after considering the factors that make his or her patient unique. Some examples of these patient-specific factors discussed in this book are patient gender, age, renal function, hepatic function, prior history of adverse drug reactions or drug allergies, pregnancy or desire to breast feed, genetic predisposition to alterations in drug clearance or drug action, use of concomitant medications, or the presence of other medical problems. This book has been created to help emphasize therapeutic principles so that the careful, thoughtful physician can adapt the "best available evidence" to suit the specific needs of each individual patient.

Physicians are becoming increasingly aware that judging the quality of their therapeutic decisions requires them to consider more clinical endpoints than merely "Did the drug work?" We need to consider a number of clinical outcomes on at least four "axes," including asking the following questions:

1. How has this treatment improved the patient's functional status (e.g., ameliorated the headache, epistaxis, and shortness of breath associated with hypertension)?
2. How has the treatment altered the course of the disease (e.g., controlled the blood pressure, improved renal function, lessened LVH, lowered overall mortality etc.)?

3. What are the direct and indirect costs of the treatment chosen (e.g., cost of medication, cost of monitoring, cost of adverse reactions, cost of doctor visits, etc.)?
4. What is the level of the patient's overall satisfaction with the treatment provided (e.g., the patient is delighted that his blood pressue has been lowered, but his drug-induced erectile dysfunction or depression is just not worth the benefit obtained)?

The editors hope that the approaches described in the book will help the prescriber (whether medical student, resident house officer, or experienced physician) practice clinical pharmacology in a manner that delivers greater overall quality of care to patients. We also have the conviction that personal efforts aimed at understanding the principles of rational drug therapy will help physicians to maintain competence in a rapidly changing and advancing medical environment, as well as making therapeutic decisions more reliable and decision-making more interesting.

We are grateful to all the contributors to this fourth edition for their hard work in elaborating the important themes outlined above in preparing chapters aimed at meeting these goals. We acknowledge the patience and support of Ms. Barbara Ordway, our editorial consultant, and the staff of McGraw-Hill for their ongoing support.

S. George Carruthers
Brian B. Hoffman
Kenneth L. Melmon
David W. Nierenberg

# Preface to the Third Edition

The goals and objectives for revising this book were not only to update material previously covered, but also to deliberately shift emphasis to deal with most of the therapeutic decisions commonly made by practicing physicians. We hope that this edition attracts the student and practitioner into wanting to learn core facts, skills, and the most basic principles of clinical pharmacology by drawing them into the subject via discussions of routine as well as difficult therapeutic decisions encountered in the practice of medicine. We have tried to avoid the Charybdis of cookbook practicality and the Scylla of excessive dry theory.

We present what we believe is mandatory to know about decisions about drugs in brief introductory form in the first chapter. The rest of the first section of the book builds on these principles in specific clinical settings to ensure that most common therapeutic problems are discussed. To learn what the most common decisions were, we reviewed the list of 100 most used drugs and 100 most common diagnoses for which prescriptions were written in North America and Western Europe. The list for the United States was obtained from IMS America. It probably covers about 80% or more of the volume of prescription drugs used in North America and Europe today. Individual authors were assigned to cover each of those diagnoses and the drugs used to treat them. All are covered in the first section of the book as minimum subject matter. Thus, this section should be more useful as a reference text to clinicians than were the previous editions. For heuristic purposes, essential principles are highlighted throughout the text as they have been in previous editions.

Section II contains the basic subject material that is the core of clinical pharmacology without reference to specific diseases. Chapters in Section I consistently refer to chapters in Section II as the basis of most therapeutic decisions. This book continues to be a supplement to, not a substitute for, the basic textbooks of medicine and pharmacology.

The editors are very grateful for the editorial and secretarial assistance, patience, and dedication of Wallace Waterfall and Dana O'Neill.

Kenneth L. Melmon
Howard F. Morrelli
Brian B. Hoffman
David W. Nierenberg

# Preface to the Second Edition

The objectives of this book have not changed since the first edition. *Clinical Pharmacology: Basic Principles in Therapeutics* is designed to illustrate a consistency of approach to qualitative and quantitative decision making in therapeutics. Its use should allow the therapist to distinguish drug-related events from spontaneous alterations in disease and provide general knowledge about objective therapeutics that will allow him/her to individualize therapy. The text is written with medical, osteopathy, pharmacy, and allied health students uppermost in mind; such students are the best candidates to evolve therapeutics from an "art" to a rational and objective science.

Readers might legitimately ask why a textbook of "principles" requires revision, since true principles remain constant. In short, the editors are students in a rapidly evolving and novel discipline. Although a number of useful principles were identified in the first edition, some that were designated as principles were not fundamental concepts and, because the field of clinical pharmacology has grown rapidly in recent years, a number of new principles have evolved. Many factors that now impact on therapeutic decisions were not known in 1972, nor were data related to the psychology of the doctor-patient "therapeutic contract" necessarily widely available or easily summarized (Chapter 4). The science of pharmacokinetics was not as aggressively applied to man as it has been in the last 5 to 10 years. Furthermore, the mathematical concepts necessary to make precise and therefore biologically useful decisions during use of high-risk drugs had not been tested in therapeutic settings (Chapters 2 and 3). Clinical pharmacologists had not developed a useful, defensible, and systematic approach about placebos, about how to make therapeutic decisions in circumstances of uncertainty, or about the economic factors that overtly or covertly influence therapeutic decisions and the epidemiology of drug use (Chapters 24 to 26). Only in the last few years has consideration been given to therapeutic decisions affecting women of child-bearing age, pregnant women, the fetus, and the neonate (Chapter 5). Patients with dermatologic disorders can be rationally as well as empirically approached (Chapter 19). The therapeutics of some hepatic, respiratory, endocrine, and inflammatory disorders have become much more specific and effective, and this has allowed the description of new "principles."

The organization of this second edition is similar to that of the first edition. Unit I presents general principles that apply to all therapeutic decisions; Unit II emphasizes the specific factors about a disease and a drug that justify the setting of therapeutic objectives in their coordination; and Unit III stresses the obvious and less overt factors that impact on therapeutic decisions and the observations that can be made and attributed to the drug per se. Unit IV has been deleted from this revision; although the programmed cases were popular, they were too individualized in some respects to justify the space they occupied.

As in the first edition, successful use of this book requires knowledge of both pharmacology and medicine. It should serve as a supplement to, rather than a replacement of, the basic textbooks of medicine and pharmacology. We hope that *Clinical Pharmacology: Basic Principles in Therapeutics* will not foster dogma, recipes, or folklore about drugs, but will help to stimulate scholarly and rational thought about therapeutics that is applicable to individualized settings.

We deeply appreciate the persistent, imaginative, and sometimes exciting writing of our contributors as well as the assistance of our editors, Elyce Melmon and Emma Ponick. We also gratefully asknowledge the thoughtful suggestions made by our fellows and students and the secretarial help of Ms. Vivian Abe.

KENNETH L. MELMON
HOWARD F. MORRELLI

# Preface to the First Edition

Even in medicine, though it is easy to know what honey, wine and hellebore, cautery and surgery are, to know how and to whom and when to apply them so as to effect a cure is no less an undertaking than to be a physician.

Aristotle, *Nicomachean Ethics*, Vol. IX

Detailed pharmacologic knowledge stands alone as a basic science, but successful therapeutics requires application of this information to disease-induced abnormalities in individual patients. Aristotle did not claim that physicians were successful, only that they attempted to be. There is abundant information that physicians generally are poor therapists, despite their detailed knowledge of the pathogenesis of disease and the pharmacology of specific drugs that can alter a disease. The consequences of poor therapy include both toxic reactions to drugs and unchecked or even exacerbated disease. No longer can it be said, "The diagnosis is always more important than the treatment." Therapeutics must not continue to lag so far behind pharmacology, physiology, biochemistry, and pathophysiology, which serve as its foundation. Much information must be applied to clinical settings to allow major improvements in the management of disease and decreases in the incidence, morbidity, and mortality of drug toxicity.

This textbook was written (1) to help medical students understand how to approach the problems of administration of drugs to man, and (2) to show house staff and practicing physicians who learned therapeutics in a "hand-me-down" fashion that this instructional approach at best fosters mediocrity in therapeutics and should be replaced by a more efficacious and satisfying method. A consistent approach to therapeutic settings is possible, and the organization of the book generally describes the rationale for therapeutic decisions. An underlying principle herein is that the pathophysiology of disease and basic facts of pharmacology must be interdigitated in order to select drugs and establish therapeutic objectives. Once a category of drug is considered, the therapist must recall and use the basic principles of drug administration (Unit I); then the specific factors of disease and drug that justify bringing them together must be contemplated, so that the dynamics of pharmacology and pathophysiology can be put into perspective in the therapeutic plan (Unit II). Once the therapeutic objectives have been set, a plan must be made and implemented to observe, recognize, and evaluate the effects of drug administration (Unit III). The student may then evaluate his ability to recognize and apply principles in programmed problem-solving situations, taken from actual cases of the clinical pharmacology consultation service, University of California Medical Center, San Francisco (Unit IV).

Successful use of this book requires knowledge of both pharmacology and medicine. It does not replace the basic textbook in either discipline; rather, it is a supplement to both. Unit II does not include all, or even most, of the important diseases or drugs tht might be discussed. The approach described in each chapter—physiology, pathophysiology, pharmacology, and, finally, the integration of these subjects—is consistent, can be applied at the bedside, and constitutes what the editors consider to be active clinical pharmacology. Such an approach can be subdivided into guidelines (principles), and some clinical states lend themselves more readily than others to illustration of principles that can be applied broadly. We hope the reader will find that principles applicable to one disease also apply to other disorders, for that is what makes them principles. They should help to stimulate thought rather than to propagate dogma or provide further recipes for therapeutics.

The contributors have demonstrated extraordinary diligence and patience in writing this innovative textbook. The editors thank their colleagues, fellows, house staff, and students for encouragement, criticism, and help during the long gestation period. They are greatly indebted for the thoughtful criticism and suggestions made by Arthur P. Grollman, Jr., M.D., associate professor of pharmacology and medicine, Albert Einstein College of Medicine, Bronx, New York. They are also indebted to Peggy Langston for editorial assistance in preparing the final manuscript.

Kenneth L. Melmon
Howard F. Morrelli

# PART 1 INTRODUCTION

# INTRODUCTION TO CLINICAL PHARMACOLOGY AND RATIONAL THERAPEUTICS

David W. Nierenberg, Kenneth L. Melmon

*Chapter Outline*



## HISTORICAL PERSPECTIVE ON CURRENT PROBLEMS WITH THERAPEUTICS

Successful clinical decisions, like most human decisions, are "complex creatures" (Mulrow et al. 1997). Factors contributing to the decision process include validated medical/scientific evidence (such as clinical trials), patient factors (e.g., personal beliefs or special physiologic features), physician factors (e.g., personal values and experience), and constraints (systems of reimbursement, etc.). "Evidence-based medicine," with its emphasis on making sound decisions informed by the best data available, is an important theme in medical education. The laudable goal of trying to make clinical and therapeutic decisions based on the best available evidence, however, can be frustrated by limitations in the quality, scope, and applicability of such evidence. The best evidence available may not apply to a particular patient with a particular and, possibly, unique set of characteristics, for example, a combination of concomitant conditions, pregnancy, or previous drug allergies (Feinstein and Horwitz 1997).

This increased complexity in making medical decisions is reflected in the need for an increasingly sophisticated way of looking at the process of medical care and of assessing the value of its outcomes. The concept of the "value compass" to track the various outcomes of care is gaining increasing acceptance as an important tool to help doctors understand what they are doing. This general way of looking at the process of medical care is illustrated in Figure 1 (modified from the work of Nelson, Mohr, et al. 1996 and Nelson, Splaine, et al. 1996).

The scheme shown in Figure 1 applies to the process of medical care in general. Pharmacotherapeutic decisions are one subtype of medical care, with their own set of patient expectations, process issues, and outcomes. The application of the value compass to the process of rational therapeutics is illustrated in Figure 2. Note that we can now try to evaluate the quality of our therapeutic decisions by including assessment of outcomes along four major axes. For example, an uncomplicated patient with moderate essential hypertension treated with propranolol and hydrochlorothiazide might have results including clinical outcomes (decline in blood pressure, decline in heart rate, slightly decreased exercise tolerance, more frequent nocturia, improved prognosis for less morbidity and mortality), functional outcomes (fewer headaches, less anxiety about future, greater ease in obtaining health insurance, some frustration with nocturia), overall satisfaction (glad

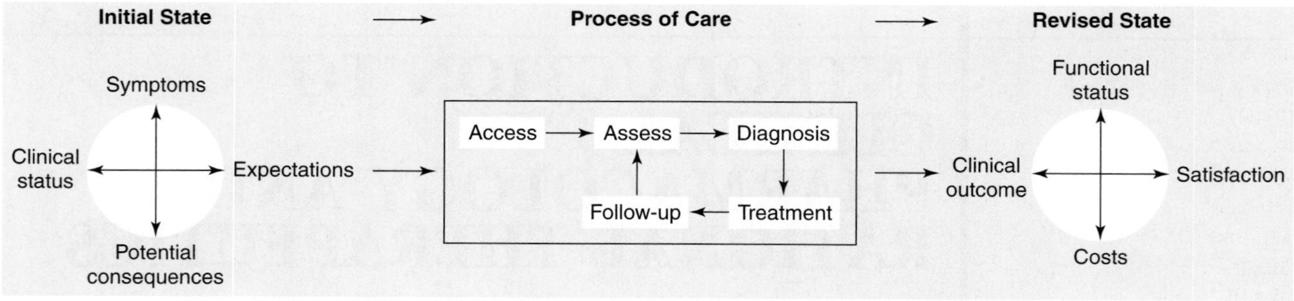

FIGURE 1 **Patient presentation, process of care, and patient outcomes as a general model for medical care. (adapted from Nelson, Mohr, et al. 1996; Nelson, Splaine, et al. 1996.)**

that his hypertension could be treated easily and inexpensively with minimal wasted time and expense, but would like to avoid nocturia if possible), and cost (small direct costs of several visits to physician; checking blood urea nitrogen [BUN], creatinine, and ECG; small yearly drug cost; minimal indirect costs of several hours of missed work).

Therapeutic decisions are becoming more complex and difficult daily, and these tougher decisions are being made more and more regularly by primary care providers. For some diseases and indications, groups of experts review clinical evidence carefully and are able to generate practice guidelines or protocols that can produce measurable improvements in clinical outcomes, cost, and functional status (McFadden et al. 1995). In other situations, however, individual practitioners are left "on their own" to develop optimal therapeutic plans based on their knowledge, careful review of quality clinical trials and reviews, personal experience, and recommendations from textbooks. There is no shortcut to the practitioner's arrival at a sound pharmacotherapeutic decision for a particular patient.

**SUMMARY**

**The quality of a therapeutic decision (outcome) can be measured by**

- **Clinical outcomes (efficacy, toxicity, allergy, etc.)**
- **Functional status (and change in status) of patient**
- **Overall patient satisfaction**
- **Costs (direct and indirect)**

Ironically, as we improve our diagnostic capabilities, there seems to be little concomitant improvement in therapeutic decisions. The latter still seems to rest too often on personal impression or bias, tradition, sentiment, or uncritical acceptance of advertising claims. Relative inattention to therapy and the therapeutic decision process is not new. In 1903, a clinical pharmacologist observed

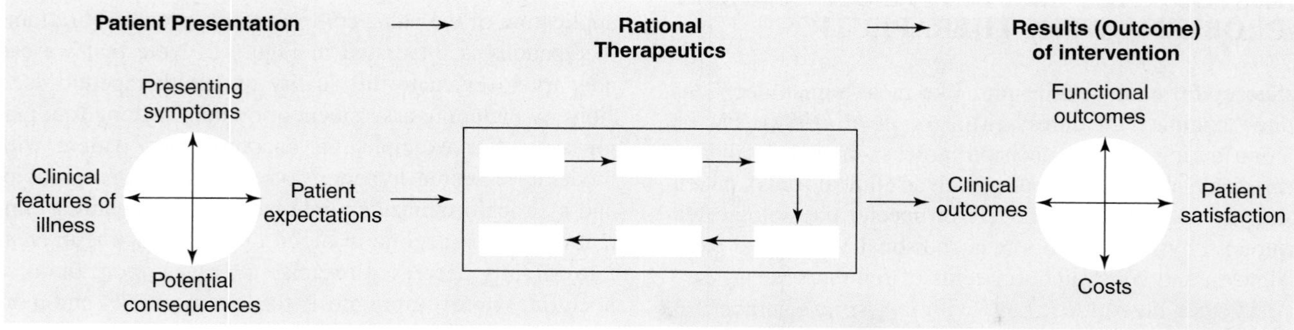


FIGURE 2 **Patient presentation, process of care, and patient outcomes as focused on the process of rational drug therapy.**

that "... the day has come when something more is demanded of the practitioner or physician-consultant than a diagnosis. A mere diagnosis is not sufficient;... Our obligation will not be satisfied until general principles have been fitted to the particular patient. The *what* may be the easiest determined; the *how much,* the *when* and *in what form* and *under what precautions,* must be fully stated" (Wilcox 1903). In 1905, the President of the American Therapeutic Society recommended that "... every medical school should have a special chair of applied therapeutics, held by a clinical man who is a specialist in internal medicine" (Osborne 1905). Yet, medical students and residents continue to be undermotivated to, and have inadequate opportunity to, develop their therapeutic skills, since "... most teachers of clinical medicine, though brilliant in diagnosis and learned in pathology, glide over the therapy of disease" (Osborne 1916).

These early concerns about instruction in rational therapeutics remain appropriate. Melmon and Morrelli observed that the clinical pharmacologist "... must teach students at all levels the basic concepts of an approach to rational therapeutics. Although new specific therapeutic agents will be discovered, the new agents will be used properly only if the student has developed a critical approach to the choice and use of drugs" (Melmon and Morrelli 1969). Other arguments for the importance of teaching rational therapeutics were summarized in a commentary pointing out the need for instruction in clinical pharmacology for all medical students (Nierenberg 1986). But despite those calls to action, only a few countries (mostly in Europe) have established obligatory courses in clinical pharmacology (Anglo-American Workshop 1986).

The medical community has not yet fully accepted the challenge to improve therapeutics. One reason may be that, fortunately, most patients appear to improve while taking drugs, perhaps because most drugs have a large margin of safety; many conditions are self-limiting; and, problems caused by drugs often can be attributed to the disease for which they are prescribed. Nevertheless, depending on homeostatic mechanisms to protect the patient from the effects of poor therapeutic decisions is no way to practice medicine. If improving decisions about therapy would improve patient response and outcome, why not use and enjoy the principles of therapeutics and the rewards of philosophically sound decisions? Suboptimal therapeutics have begun to receive attention. Pharmacists have been active in highlighting the extent of therapeutic misadventures (Manasse 1989; Lesar et al. 1997). Both the American College of Physicians and the federal government have agreed that corrective measures to address the widespread problem of poor prescribing by physicians are urgently needed (Meyer 1988; Kusserow 1989).

Consider the following bits of data concerning overall drug use in the United States alone.

- Many entirely new classes of drugs have been introduced during the last 15 years.
- The US Food and Drug Administration (FDA) approves over 30 new drugs each year.
- Most physicians prescribe medications that were not discovered at the time the physicians graduated from medical school.
- Between 1974 and 1986, the total retail cost of prescription drugs increased from \$5.7 billion to \$18.9 billion per year (Office of Technology Assessment 1987).
- In 1987, about \$30 billion was spent on prescription drugs and another \$8 billion on nonprescription products. In 1988, the estimates were about \$160 per capita for prescription drugs.
- Over 1.5 billion outpatient prescriptions (6 prescriptions per person per year in the United States) are filled annually (Manasse 1989).
- The elderly make up only about 12% of the population, but they receive about 30% of prescription drugs and purchase about 40% of nonprescription drugs.
- Hospitalized patients receive an average of 15 drug administrations per day, costing about \$5 billion per year.
- About two-thirds of all physician visits lead to a prescription.
- Although antibiotics have little or no benefit for colds, upper respiratory tract infections, or bronchitis, they are frequently prescribed by office-based physicians across the country. More than half of patients with these complaints received prescriptions for antibiotics, which accounted for 21% of all antibiotic prescriptions to adults in 1992 (Gonzales et al. 1997).
- More than 50 million antibiotic prescriptions a year are written for colds and other viral infections. This massively inappropriate use of antibiotics has contributed to a sharp increase in strains of *Streptococcus pneumoniae* that have become resistant to penicillin G (up to 30%), erythromycin, cotrimoxazole, or tetracycline (Jellin 1997).
- In a recent study of geriatric nursing home patients, more than two-thirds of the patients studied experienced one or more adverse drug reactions (ADRs) (Cooper 1996).
- In one recent study of adverse drug events in hospitalized patients, ADEs occurred in 6.5% of admis-

sions; of these, 28% were judged to be preventable. On average, each ADE was associated with about 2.2 days in additional length of stay, and the increase in cost was about $3244 for each patient affected (Bates et al. 1997).

- Serious ADRs occur in about 6.7% of hospital patients and fatal ADRs in about 0.32%, making these reactions between the fourth and sixth leading causes of death (Lazarov et al. 1998).
- A systems approach to ADEs can be useful. ADEs in hospitalized patients are measurable, potentially dangerous, and expensive (Avorn 1997).
- Doctors make errors in prescribing drugs in hospitals about 4 times per 1000 orders. The most common reasons for errors were failure to recognize abnormal renal or hepatic function; patients with a history of allergy to the same medication class; or the use of the wrong drug name, dosage form, or abbreviation, or incorrect dosage calculations (Lesar et al. 1997).
- A recent assessment of 112 physicians by means of standardized patients revealed that unnecessary prescribing of nonsteroidal anti-inflammatory drugs (NSAIDs), and suboptimal management of NSAID-related side effects, were quite common (47 and 23% of these test visits, respectively) and raised questions about the appropriateness of NSAID use in geriatric patients (Tamblyn et al. 1997).
- Since the publication of national consensus guidelines for optimal evaluation and treatment of hypertension in 1993, the prescribing of the recommended first-line drug classes for most patients declined. Between 1992 and 1995, prescriptions for $\beta$-adrenergic antagonists (beta-blockers) dropped from 18 to 11% of all antihypertensive prescriptions, while diuretics dropped from 16 to 8% of all antihypertensive prescriptions. The percentage of prescriptions written for calcium antagonists and angiotensin-converting enzyme (ACE) inhibitors rose during this period. This shift in prescribing patterns, running counter to national consensus guidelines published in 1993, has enormous cost implications (Siegel and Lopez 1997).

**SUMMARY**
**Adverse drug events are**

- **Common (occur in about 6.5% of hospital admissions)**
- **Often preventable (about 28% are)**
- **Add significantly to length of stay (about 2.2 days on average)**
- **Add significantly to the cost of hospitalization (about $3244 for the average patient)**
- **May be a relatively frequent cause of death in hospital patients**

To comprehend fully the meaning of the summary statements for the practice of medicine, we need more information based on studies than we have today—systematic studies of patterns of use and the effects of marketed drugs. To correct the deficiencies in patterns of prescribing described, we need better education about rational therapeutics than we are providing today.

**WARNING** Physician errors in drug prescribing are most commonly related to

- Failing to compensate for abnormal renal or hepatic function
- Failing to determine prior history of drug allergy
- Using the wrong drug name
- Using the wrong dosage form
- Using misunderstood abbreviations
- Calculating doses incorrectly

Physicians often learn about new drugs from colleagues, advertisements, drug sales representatives, or other sources that may lack scientific data and balance (Avorn et al. 1982). In 1985, only 14% of U.S. medical schools offered formal courses in clinical pharmacology (Nierenberg 1986), compared with 100% of medical schools in the United Kingdom. Consequently, at least in the United States, medical students become physicians without being exposed to (much less mastering) an acceptable standard of rational therapeutics. Medical students in the United States have rarely been exposed to the challenge and satisfaction of considering each drug prescription a therapeutic experiment.

This book is dedicated to a deliberate, thoughtful approach to drug therapy as a base for rational therapeutics. Rational therapeutics means prescribing drugs in a manner that maximizes clinical effect (maximizing efficacy and minimizing toxicity), functional status, and overall patient satisfaction, at the lowest possible total cost. Rational therapeutics strives to individualize the therapeutic plan to match the needs of a particular patient by drawing upon the scientific principles of medicine and pharmacology. The core of information needed to practice rational therapeutics is *introduced* in Part 1, this Introduction. The principles of rational therapeutics will be illustrated in specific settings, but the challenge to both the authors and the student is to test the validity of these principles by making them live in a host of settings illustrated in this book and encountered in clinical practice.

**PRINCIPLE The outcomes of a therapeutic decision (clinical effects, functional status, patient satisfaction, and cost) are most likely to be optimized when the decision takes into account the factors that make each patient different, and often unique.**

## AN APPROACH TO RATIONAL THERAPEUTICS

What are the key components of a rational approach to medical therapeutics that can be applied to most situations? Consider a case gone awry and try to envision the important steps that could have been taken to make this patient's management rational and effective.

**CASE HISTORY** *A 60-year-old diabetic woman developed new-onset, mild-to-moderate, seropositive rheumatoid arthritis. Her symptoms were not relieved by the ingestion of 8 aspirin tablets per day. Oral gold had been tried, but was discontinued because of side effects. Noting her failure to respond to aspirin and her inability to continue oral gold, her physician prescribed a drug recently approved for the treatment of rheumatoid arthritis, oral methotrexate 7.5 mg given orally each week.*

*This regimen worked well for several months until the physician prescribed oral probenecid to treat her asymptomatic hyperuricemia. The next dose of methotrexate therapy was associated with profound pancytopenia and sepsis. The probenecid was discontinued; the patient recovered, methotrexate was successfully continued for several more months with clear clinical benefit without clinical toxicity. The patient, however, began to complain of fevers, dyspnea on exertion, and a dry nonproductive cough. Her physical examination was remarkable only for dry rales throughout both lung fields, and her chest film showed a bilateral and symmetric interstitial infiltrate. The physician treated her presumed mild congestive heart failure with furosemide, and her methotrexate was continued.*

*The next week her symptoms were worse, and, as an outpatient, she was given cefalexin orally to treat a possible pneumonia. Her other medications were continued. Finally, her symptoms became so severe that she required hospitalization. All of her medications were discontinued. Her laboratory studies confirmed severe hypoxemia, hyperventilation, and bilateral and symmetric interstitial pneumonitis. She received folinic acid to treat a possible methotrexate-induced interstitial pneumonitis. Lung biopsy was performed, but the patient deteriorated rapidly and required intubation. The lung biopsy results were consistent with the diagnosis of methotrexate-induced interstitial pneumonitis. Corticosteroids were begun, but the patient died several days later.*

**Discussion** *This patient's case illustrates a number of ways in which irrational therapeutics can insidiously creep into medical decisions. Sometimes the results can be severe and irreversible. Initially, the diagnosis of rheumatoid arthritis was made. As the physician clinched his diagnosis, he considered the pathophysiology of the disease, and the drugs that are available to interrupt or palliate it. Aspirin was appropriately chosen as a first-line drug. It is relatively safe and efficacious, has minimal toxicity, and is not costly. The drug, however, was used suboptimally. If a target effect had been chosen and followed, and if a therapeutic concentration of salicylate in blood had been established, the efficacy/toxicity profile of the drug could have been optimized. Instead, the physician prematurely concluded that aspirin was not useful. Use of one of the available NSAIDs would also represent an excellent first-line option, since these drugs have an excellent balance of efficacy, safety, and cost. Oral gold was prescribed next, perhaps prematurely, but unfortunately could not be continued because of adverse effects. The optimal point in a patient's disease to prescribe methotrexate, a powerful but frequently toxic drug newly approved for this indication, is still a matter of some controversy. In most cases, this drug is reserved for more severe disease that is refractory to maximally tolerated doses of more common anti-inflammatory drugs.*

**PRINCIPLE Set the legitimately expected clinical effects of therapy (endpoints demonstrating efficacy and lower limits of toxicity) before starting therapy. Use those objectives to monitor drug effects and to signal the need for qualitative or quantitative changes in therapy.**

*The physician proceeded to prescribe methotrexate without fully understanding its pharmacokinetics or profile of adverse reactions. When he (inappropriately) treated the patient's asymptomatic mild hyperuricemia with probenecid, he unwittingly caused a well-known and well-defined, but not frequently anticipated, drug–drug interaction. Probenecid is a potent inhibitor of the renal tubular secretion of weak organic acids. It can similarly inhibit the tubular secretion (and thereby the renal clearance) of methotrexate. The decreased clearance of methotrexate was associated with persistent concentrations of the drug in plasma (so-called increased area under the concentration-versus-time curve), thereby leading to systemic toxicity. Fortunately, the physician recognized this mistake, and the patient recovered from the near-fatal episode of methotrexate-induced pancytopenia.*

*The patient developed an unusual but by no means rare idiosyncratic reaction to methotrexate, an inflammatory interstitial pneumonitis. Because the possibility of such an adverse drug reaction was not considered seriously, both "congestive heart failure" and "pneumonia" were "treated." By the time the correct drug-induced problem was recognized, the condition was irreversible, and the patient died.*

*Finally, whereas methotrexate-induced lung injury in patients with rheumatoid arthritis has been thought to be an "idiosyncratic" and unpredictable adverse reaction, newer evidence suggests that this particular patient was at greater relative risk for this ADR given her age, the presence of diabetes, and previous treatment with a disease-modifying agent (Alarcon et al. 1997). Thus, new medical evidence can modify estimates of drug efficacy or toxicity, and lead to different therapeutic decisions.*

**PRINCIPLE New information about a drug's efficacy or toxicity leads to the necessity of continuously reestimating the risk–benefit analysis for the use of any drug in any specific patient.**

## Six Key Steps When Practicing Pharmacotherapeutics

Drug therapy can be logically approached. Such logic results in rational prescribing of even the most common or "trivial" medications. Steps required in therapy that are rational include the following: 1) making a diagnosis with reasonable certainty; 2) understanding the pathophysiology of the disease and the opportunities for drug intervention; 3) understanding the pharmacology of the drugs that could be used to treat the disease; 4) selecting the drug and dose that are likely to be optimal for the specific patient; 5) selecting appropriate endpoints of efficacy and toxicity to follow; and 6) developing a therapeutic alliance with the patient, and maintaining it.

In retrospect, the physician's failure in each of these steps, sometimes more than once, is easy to spot. Even a seemingly trivial decision such as how to administer aspirin to a patient with arthritis, or deciding to treat a patient with asymptomatic mild hyperuricemia, can have important implications.

**SUMMARY**
**Six key steps to a rational therapeutic decision are**

- **Making an accurate diagnosis**
- **Understanding the pathophysiology of disease**
- **Reviewing the menu of pharmacotherapeutic options**
- **Selecting patient-specific drug and dose**
- **Selecting endpoints to follow**
- **Maintaining a therapeutic alliance with the patient**

Now that we understand these six key steps to a rational therapeutic decision, it is useful to return to the figure illustrating the presentation of the patient, the results of interventions, and the important process of rational therapeutics. We are now in a position to fill in the details of the "black box" corresponding to the process of rational therapeutics shown in Figure 2. A more detailed model is shown in Figure 3.

Case histories in this Introduction will reinforce the value of the fundamental steps that should be considered whenever you prescribe a medication, use a device, or perform a procedure. The steps can be applied with adequate knowledge of the core of clinical pharmacology. Do you understand how the body handles drugs (pharmacokinetics) and how drugs affect the body (pharmacodynamics)? Do you understand that many patients require special consideration when drugs are prescribed? For example, patients with renal or hepatic disease, the very young, the very old, pregnant or nursing women should not receive the "usual" medications in the "standard" doses. Do you know how to distinguish symptoms due to drug toxicity from symptoms due to disease? Can you recognize, or better yet predict, which drugs are likely to interact adversely with others? Do you understand the important legal rules and regulations that govern prescribing, and are you aware of the complex and perhaps subconscious forces that are at work when you write a prescription?

All of these factors will be introduced in Part 1 and discussed more fully in Part 3. Mastery of the information in this Introduction is important in order to practice rational therapeutics. Understanding the material in Part 3 is necessary to help perfect your practice of rational therapeutics. The chapters in Part 2 will illustrate how these principles of rational therapeutics can and should be applied to the treatment of common, serious diseases.

# AN OVERVIEW OF DRUG ACTION

## Sites of Drug Action

Most medications given to patients have a direct effect on a particular and often specific molecule or class of molecules. These molecules are likely to be proteins serving

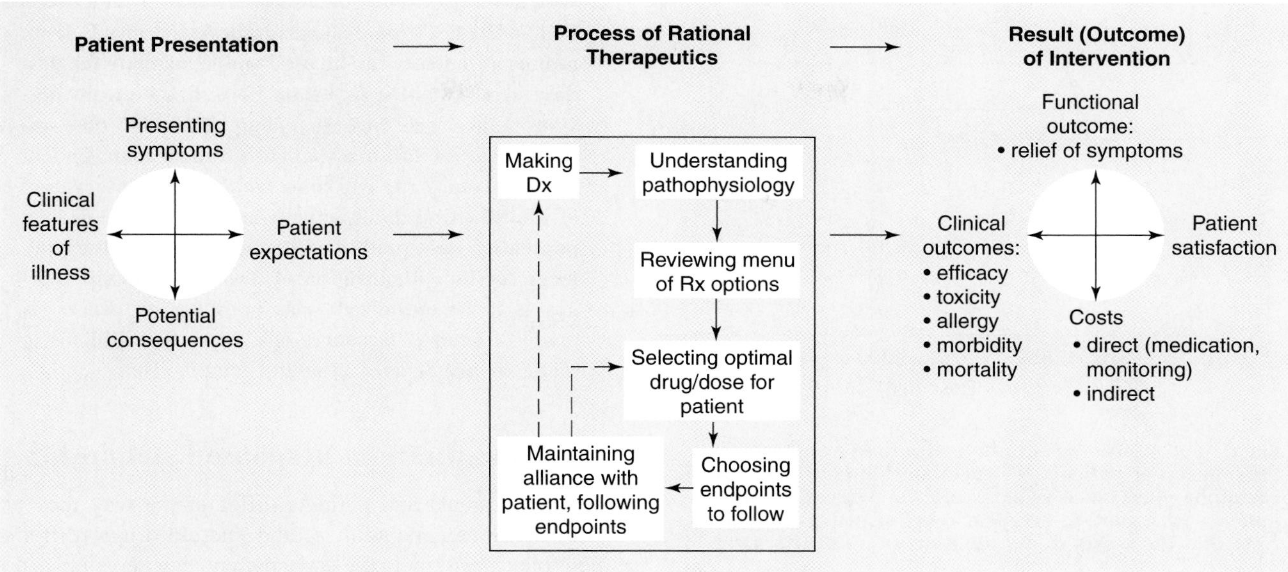


FIGURE 3 **More details about the process of care, as focused on the process of rational drug therapy.**

as enzymes to catalyze chemical reactions, or as receptors, ion channels, or transport molecules. Other common sites of action include direct binding to nucleic acids. Some useful medications have less "interesting" sites of action, especially those drugs that do not enter the body. For example, sun-blocking creams stay on the surface of the skin to physically block UV rays in sunlight and have no specific molecular site of action. Antacid tablets (e.g., magnesium hydroxide or calcium carbonate) chemically buffer the HCl acid in the stomach, but could just as easily buffer other acids; this is hardly a specific molecular target of action.

Once a drug interacts with its target molecule, however, its pharmacologic effects then can become obvious at other levels. Interaction of a drug with its molecular target then has effects on the cell, subsequently on a tissue, eventually on an organ system, and ultimately, on the intact organism (or patient in clinical pharmacology). In fact, a further level of action might be on the patient's community. For example, the use of vancomycin in one hospitalized patient can have an effect on the broader hospital community by helping to increase the development of *Staphylococci* resistant to vancomycin within that hospital environment.

Thus the question "What does terazosin do?" might be answered by saying that the drug acts as an antagonist of alpha-1 adrenoceptors (at the molecular level), thereby decreasing the influx of calcium into smooth muscle cells; thereby relaxing the smooth muscle tissue at the bladder neck and prostate; thereby facilitating bladder emptying and increasing rate of urine flow (at the system level); and thereby decreasing complaints of poor urine flow, frequency, dribbling, or nocturia (at the level of the 68-year-old man with bladder outlet obstruction due to benign prostatic hyperplasia with some component of reversibility). When treating patients with drugs, it is important to keep all of these levels of drug action in mind.

**SUMMARY**
**Most drugs act at several important levels including the following**

- **Molecular target**
- **Cell**
- **Tissue**
- **Organ/system**
- **Intact animal or patient**
- **Larger community of patients (for some drugs)**

## The Dose–Response Relationship

Nearly all drugs exhibit a characteristic relationship between dose given and pharmacologic effect that is characteristic, whether the drug is given to a single patient or a group of patients. This relationship with illustrative data for a drug commonly used for headache, acetaminophen, is depicted in Figure 4.

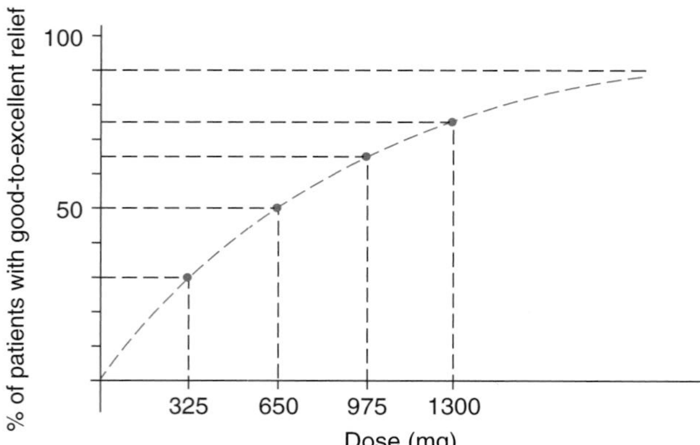


FIGURE 4 **An example of a dose–response curve for a group of patients. The relationship between dose of acetaminophen taken (*x*-axis) and the percentage of patients with good-to-excellent relief of headache (*y*-axis). Note that the *x*-axis shows the dose on a linear scale.**

A low drug dose produces a small effect, larger doses produce greater effect, until a "ceiling" or maximal effect is reached. In other words, even greater doses produce little or eventually no additional pharmacologic effects. Figure 4 shows this relationship when an oral analgesic such as acetaminophen is given to a group of patients experiencing moderately severe pain from headache. A dose of 325 mg provides adequate analgesia for few adults (about 30% in this example); 650 mg provides adequate analgesia for many adults (about 50%); even more adults (about 65%) will respond when the dose is increased to three tablets (975 mg); but there is little if any additional benefit (about 75% of patients find adequate relief) in taking four tablets (1300 mg). Note the ceiling effect as well; even at higher doses (and remember that doses greater than 4 g/day can become hepatotoxic), only about 90% of patients will report adequate analgesia from acetaminophen for the headache pain.

When the same data are plotted on a logarithmic scale (in Figure 5), note the abscissa is now log dose rather than dose, the dose–response curve tends to take on a characteristic sigmoid-shaped curve. Such a curve makes it relatively easy to estimate an $ED_{50}$ for the drug: namely, the dose that is associated with a specific pharmacologic effect (e.g., analgesia) in 50% of patients who respond. Other dose–response relationships can be estimated as well, such as a $TD_{50}$ (dose associated with a toxic effect in 50% of patients), or $LD_{50}$ (dose associated with lethal effect in 50% of test animals), and so on. In this example, the $ED_{50}$ appears to be about 650 mg; in other words, that dose would provide adequate analgesia in this pain model to about 50% of subjects (patients).

**PRINCIPLE Dose–response curves derived from groups of patients can be used to approximate the first dose in a patient with whom there has been no previous experience with the drug. The best dose–response curves for that patient's future management with the same drug will come from careful observation of what the first doses actually accomplish. Even when population data predict individual responses, the challenge for individualization of dosing remains if therapy is to be optimized. This optimization process is made difficult if measures of efficacy are difficult to make, or are delayed after the drug is given.**

## The Concentration–Response Relationship

Because animals and patients differ in the way they absorb, distribute, metabolize, and excrete drugs (differ in their pharmacokinetics), each patient can develop a different and sometimes unique concentration of drug even when the same dose has been administered. This is one reason why the dose–response relationship tends to be less predictable than the concentration–response relationship. That is, the pharmacologic effects of a drug relate better to the drug's concentration in plasma than to the dose that was administered. Although there is still some patient-to-patient variation in the concentration–response relationship, the variation tends to be less than occurs in the dose–response relationship.

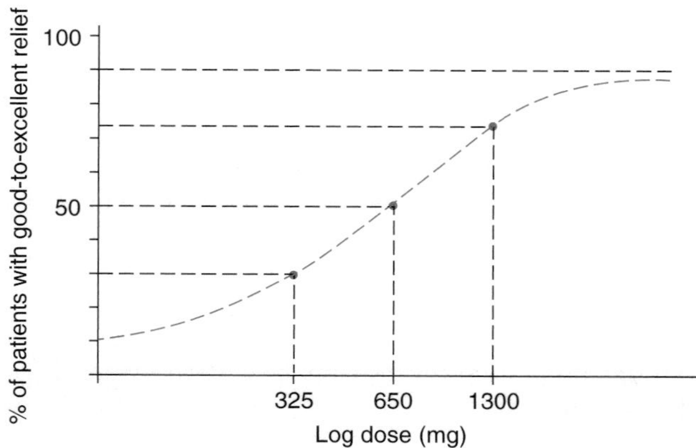


FIGURE 5 **An example of the same dose–response curve as seen in Figure 4 for a group of patients taking acetaminophen for headache but this time, the *x*-axis (dose of acetaminophen) is presented on a logarithmic scale. Note the characteristic shape of the dose–response curve, with an $ED_{50}$ (650 mg) and a ceiling effect (at best, only 90% of patients receive good-to-excellent relief of their headache pain, even at very high doses of the analgesic).**

A possible concentration–response relationship for 100 patients experiencing some relief of pain of rheumatoid arthritis with aspirin is shown in Figure 6. As was apparent in the dose–response curve for the drug, a few patients achieve adequate analgesia at low plasma concentrations of salicylate (<100 mg/L), most require an intermediate concentration (100–250 mg/L), and a few patients require very high concentrations in plasma to achieve good pain relief (>250 mg/L). Some patients fail to achieve adequate analgesia despite high concentrations. A "therapeutic range" in which most patients achieve therapeutic effect (it is hoped without excessive drug toxicity) begins to become apparent, and physicians may aim to achieve a therapeutic and safe salicylate concentration of between 100 and 250 mg/L. Eventually, however, a ceiling effect is reached such that even higher concentrations offer little if any additional analgesia to this group of patients, but will increase the risk of drug-related toxicity (e.g., tinnitus or gastric irritation).

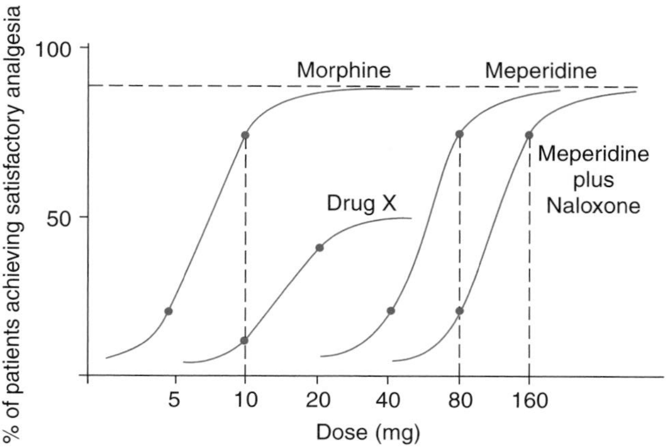


**FIGURE 7 A series of dose–response curves for a population of patients with postoperative pain receiving three different parenteral opioid analgesics. Note the log scale for the *x*-axis (dose), the characteristic shape of the curves, and the ceiling effect. Note also that morphine and meperidine have similar ceiling effects but different values of $ED_{75}$ (10 mg vs. 80 mg); the opioid antagonist naloxone shifts the dose–response curve of meperidine to the right ($ED_{75}$) shifts from 80 to 160 mg); and drug X has a lower ceiling effect than either morphine or meperidine.**

## Agonists and Antagonists

Typical dose–response relationships for three different opioid analgesics [morphine, meperidine, and a hypothetical new drug (X)] are illustrated in Figure 7. Note that the ceiling effect for morphine and meperidine is about the same: they are equally effective, and about 90% of patients will achieve adequate postoperative analgesia from either of them. The $ED_{75}$, however, is about 80 mg for meperidine and 10 mg for morphine (when given parenterally). Drugs that have similar ceiling effects (overall efficacy) but differ in $ED_{50}$ (or $ED_{75}$), are said to differ in potency, with morphine being more potent than meperidine. (Other opioids not shown in the figure such as hydromorphone and fentanyl are even more potent.) Potency usually is not an important quality that can be used to select between drugs used for the same clinical indication. Similar effects can be obtained with less potent drugs simply by giving a larger dose. Pharmaceutical companies sometimes make advertising claims about drug potency, however, when a more important property is efficacy.

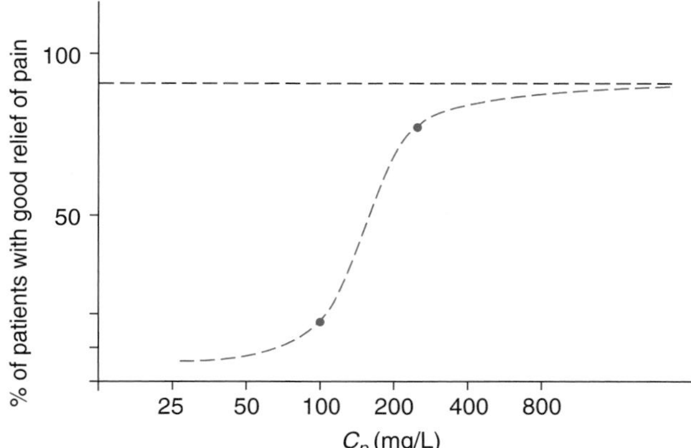


**FIGURE 6 An example of a concentration–response curve, demonstrating the percentage of patients with arthritis who achieve good relief of their pain (*y*-axis) as a function of the concentration of salicylate in plasma ($C_p$, *x*-axis). Note that the *x*-axis is drawn on a logarithmic scale, that the curve has a characteristic shape, the ceiling effect, and that most patients who achieve good pain relief do so at concentrations between 100 and 250 mg/L (referred to as the therapeutic range).**

Drug X illustrates properties that suggest that it is a "weak" agonist (i.e., qualitatively, its efficacy is similar to the others, but it has a considerably lower ceiling effect (less absolute efficacy) than the other two drugs). Such an agonist is termed a "partial agonist."

Finally, in Figure 7, we see a dose–response curve for meperidine in the absence and presence of naloxone, a drug that has no direct effects of its own, but that shifts an agonist drug's concentration–response curve to the right, and is called an antagonist. In this case, naloxone would be termed a reversible antagonist since higher doses of meperidine will eventually produce an unchanged ceiling. Higher than usual drug concentrations will be needed to attain that ceiling.

## IMPORTANCE OF INTERPATIENT VARIATION

Many medical students, physicians, and patients believe that most patients are more similar than individualistic in their response to drugs. Physician therapeutic behaviors often result in the same dose of a drug being given for the same medical problem in all patients with the expectation of similar or the same results in all. For many drugs, particularly those with a wide margin of safety (wide therapeutic index), this behavior appears to be valid. Thus, "Take two aspirin for a headache," "Take two acetaminophen tablets for a toothache," "Take ampicillin four times a day for 3 days for your urinary tract infection (UTI)," or "Take one sleeping pill for difficulty sleeping" may sound like sound advice, and often works.

But even in these "simple" situations, "cookbook" dosing (which is done on the assumption that all patients are similar and will react similarly to the same medications) fails upon even the briefest inspection when judged even by the simplest yardsticks of efficacy and safety. Two acetaminophen tablets taken several times for the headache can be a toxic dose for a malnourished, alcoholic patient with hepatic disease. Two aspirin can be too many in the patient already receiving warfarin, or in the patient with asthma and nasal polyps who develops hives and wheezing on exposure to aspirin. Ampicillin can be ineffective in the patient with a hospital-acquired, ampicillin-resistant, gram-negative bacillus as urinary pathogen, and can be fatal in the patient with a prior history of allergy to penicillin. Finally, even the single OTC or prescription hypnotic can be excessive in the patient with hepatic encephalopathy, or the patient taking other drugs with CNS depressant effects.

Patients are different, and each patient can present unique challenges in therapeutic decisions. In fact, it might be wise to assume this until proven otherwise. It is essential to consider all of the factors that make each patient different when planning a course of rational drug therapy for a patient.

**PRINCIPLE Each patient is unique in response to particular drugs; therefore, each patient poses unique challenges to the physician attempting to practice rational pharmacotherapeutics.**

### Sources of Interpatient Variation

What are the most common factors that vary from patient to patient and are key determinants of response to drug? Which factors must be considered when planning a rational course of pharmacotherapeutics? Patients differ with respect to their pharmacokinetics. They differ in the way they "handle" drugs, that is, the way they absorb, distribute, metabolize, or excrete drugs. Each determinant will be discussed more fully in the next section.

Patients also differ in the way they react to drugs: they differ with respect to their pharmacodynamics. Although a few patients may demonstrate totally unexpected and unpredictable reactions to drugs (so-called idiosyncratic reactions), in most cases, a patient's response to challenge by a dose of drug showing altered pharmacokinetics or pharmacodynamics becomes predictable. These patients often are members of groups with well-defined causes of the alteration.

Many patient groups that most commonly demonstrate altered pharmacokinetics or pharmacodynamics have now been fairly well studied and described. Many are left to be discovered. Patients at extremes of age often differ from young adults in both their pharmacokinetics (e.g., neonates and premature infants have immature systems of hepatic biotransformation) or pharmacodynamics (e.g., elderly men are more likely to develop urinary retention when receiving diphenhydramine than are young men). Patients who are pregnant or breast-feeding pose special concerns for adjustment of pharmacotherapy. In these settings, a drug may affect two people rather than one. Patients differ with respect to their genotype and phenotype for properties that determine how a patient will "handle" a drug (e.g., slow acetylator phenotype) or how a patient will "react" to a drug (e.g., patients deficient in the enzyme glucose-6-phosphate dehydrogenase [G6PD] are more likely to develop hemolysis when treated with an oxidant drug such as dapsone than will others without the deficiency). Patients with renal or hepatic disease can differ not only in the way they handle drugs (e.g., slowed renal excretion or hepatic biotransformation), but also in the way they react to drugs (e.g., greater likelihood of developing drug-induced nephro- or hepatotoxicity). Patients receiving multiple medications pose a large number of possible drug–drug interactions, some of which may be useful and some detrimental. Likewise, patients with different concomitant illnesses pose increasing potential for drug–disease interactions (some useful, some harmful, most neutral).

One other common way in which patients differ is their history of prior experiences with drugs and medications. If a patient truly has had an adverse drug reaction (e.g., prior episode of deafness related to gentamicin) or allergy to a drug (e.g., anaphylaxis related to penicillin), then the prescriber gains very important warnings about future consequences of administering the drug, or a chemically similar drug, even if it is not being used for the same indication. These potential sources of between-patient variation are explored briefly in the rest of Part 1 and in more detail in the chapters in Part 3 of this book. These differences often call for careful individualization of dosages and intervals between doses of any given drug.

**SUMMARY**

**Patients differ from one another with respect to their**

- **Pharmacokinetics**
- **Pharmacodynamics**
- **Age**
- **Gender**
- **Pregnancy or breast-feeding**
- **Pharmacogenetic phenotype**
- **Renal function**
- **Hepatic function**
- **Concurrent drugs**
- **Concurrent diseases**
- **Prior adverse drug reactions or drug allergies**

## PHARMACOKINETIC AND PHARMACODYNAMIC VARIATION

### Overview of Pharmacokinetics

A detailed discussion of pharmacokinetics can be found in Chapter 23; however, a brief introduction to the subject is helpful to the student trying to understand pharmacokinetics as a clinically important source of interpatient variation in requirement for drugs.

A simplified model of the pharmacokinetics of a typical drug following oral administration is shown in Figure 8. After systemic administration, a drug achieves a certain concentration in the blood (or plasma) that changes over time. We usually determine the concentration of drug in plasma $(C_p)$ rather than in whole blood. The concentration of drug in plasma ultimately determines and is in equilibrium with the concentration of drug at its site of action. The relationship between the dose of the drug given and its concentration in plasma is described by the pharmacokinetics of the drug.

The pharmacokinetics of a drug describes what the body does to the drug. Once a drug is administered, a number of processes make up the body's handling of the drug, and each can have substantial impact on the concentration of the drug in plasma at any given time.

We briefly describe the 14 steps outlined in Figure 8. First, a dose of the drug is prescribed. Next (step 2), that dose or a different dose is ingested. Whether the prescribed dose is actually taken as directed relates to the patient's compliance, which in turn depends on how well the prescriber has communicated the importance of drug therapy to the patient. Other factors such as the cost of the drug and the understanding by the patient of why the drug and dose are justified are obviously involved in determining compliance.

Next (step 3), the tablet or capsule disintegrates in the stomach or small bowel, and dissolves so that it can be absorbed into the portal venous system (step 5). Of course, if the drug fails to disintegrate or dissolve, it can pass completely through the GI tract and be excreted in the stool unabsorbed (step 4). When drugs such as neomycin or polyethylene glycol are administered, $<1\%$ is absorbed. Consequently, when administered by mouth, they are designed to be used as drugs that act within the GI tract alone.

The drug in the portal venous system must traverse the liver (step 6) before reaching the central compartment of the arterial-venous circulation (step 7). The theoretical central compartment (remember that models make it easier to understand what is actually happening, but do not necessarily reflect specific reality) is composed of the blood, plasma, and well-perfused organs such as the heart and brain. Some drugs are well-absorbed (step 5), but are extensively removed or metabolized by the liver or gut mucosal cells to metabolites (step 6), such that relatively little of the drug makes it to the central circulation as unmodified drug (step 7). Such drugs are said to have low oral bioavailability due to a high first-pass (through the liver) effect. Orally administered drugs such as lidocaine, propranolol, nitroglycerin, and morphine have oral bioavailabilities that are less than 30% due to their extensive first-pass metabolism by the liver to (inactive) metabolites.

The free active drug (D) that reaches the central compartment (step 7) is in a dynamic equilibrium with bound drug in the central compartment (step 7), as well as with free drug in a larger peripheral compartment (step 8), and the effect compartment (step 9). The last-mentioned (step 9) is the critical area that the drug must reach to have its beneficial or toxic pharmacologic effects. As drug equilibrates from its central to its peripheral compartment, the drug is redistributed. Even as a drug is distributed to the central compartment, and redistributed to one or more pe-

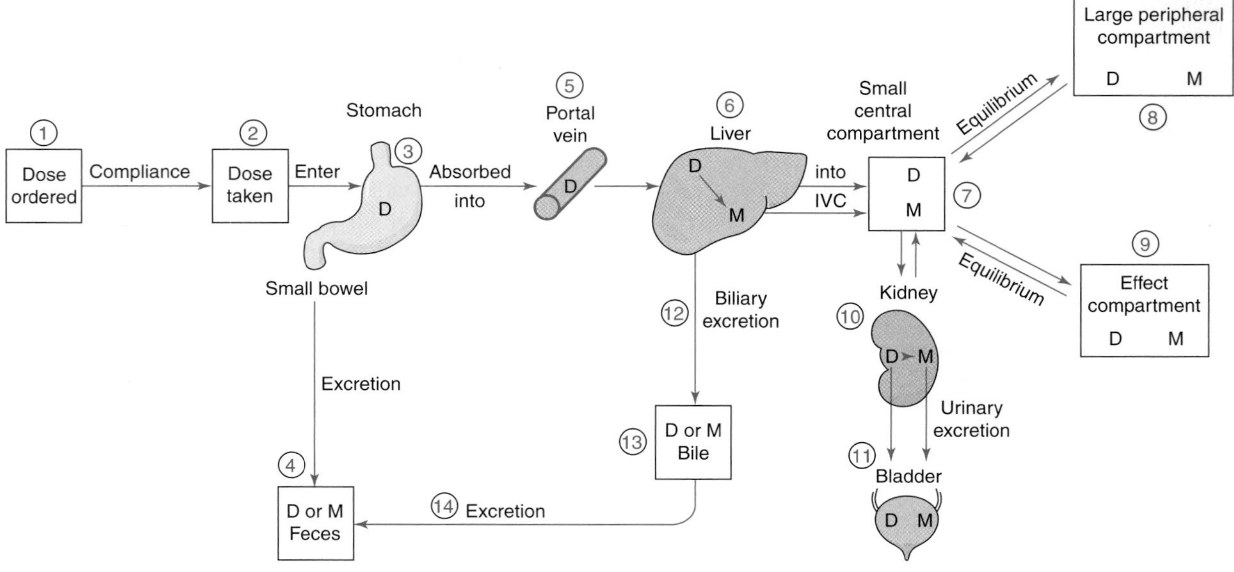


**FIGURE 8** **A summary of the processes involved in drug absorption, distribution, redistribution, biotransformation, and elimination. D, drug; M, metabolite (product of biotransformation).**

ripheral compartments, other processes of drug biotransformation or excretion are occurring simultaneously.

Step 10 illustrates that the kidneys receive about one-fourth of the cardiac output or about 1250 mL/min of blood flow. The kidneys are well-suited to excrete small, hydrophilic drugs (D) or metabolites (M) into the urine (step 11) by glomerular filtration, active tubular secretion, or a combination of these processes. In a healthy adult, maximal renal plasma flow is about 720 mL/min. Therefore, the upper limit of renal clearance of a drug is about 720 mL/min (if all the plasma is "cleared" of drug during each pass through the kidney). The maximal rate of glomerular filtration is only about 125 mL/min, since only about one-sixth of the plasma actually is filtered by the glomerulus. (The small arrow drawn within the kidney indicates that for some drugs, the kidney is also capable of metabolizing the drug [D] to a metabolite [M], although certainly the kidney is more commonly involved in drug excretion rather than drug metabolism.)

Although the kidney excretes hydrophilic drug or metabolite molecules, the liver, with its blood flow of about 1500 mL/min (step 12), metabolizes or transforms drug molecules to active or inactive metabolites (M), which are usually more hydrophilic than the parent drug molecules (D). Metabolite molecules either can return to the central circulation via the hepatic vein (step 7), or can be excreted into the bile (step 13), and thereby excreted in the stool (step 14).

Figure 8 is a very simplified schematic of the pharmacokinetics of an orally administered drug.

**SUMMARY**
**Key pharmacokinetic steps include the following**

- **Absorption of drug**
- **First pass through the liver (for drugs given orally)**
- **Overall bioavailability**
- **Drug distribution and redistribution**
- **Urinary excretion (and sometimes metabolism)**
- **Hepatic biotransformation (and sometimes excretion)**

## More About Drug Absorption and Bioavailability

Drugs are variably absorbed from different sites of administration, however, all routes of administration do not allow equivalent access of the drug to the systemic circulation. The physician should deliberately make a choice among the oral, transdermal, intravenous, intra-arterial, intramuscular, and rectal routes to assure himself or herself of the drug's absorption into the body as a whole. Sometimes, we attempt to prevent entry of the drug into the systemic circulation by administering it locally as in eye drops (e.g., sulfacetamide), nose sprays (phenylephrine), or topical creams (vaginal estrogens). Although these maneuvers can maximize the percentage of the dose that focuses its concentration and effects on a desired target organ, they rarely prevent at least a portion of the dose from entering the systemic circulation and producing some drug effects distant from the target tissue. For example, timolol eye drops can cause a systemic reaction of asthma or worsening of congestive heart failure; whereas skin creams or sprays (e.g., Solarcaine) can sensitize the body, producing a systemic allergy to local anesthetics.

Absorption of the drug from the site of administration is dependent on properties of the drug, the vehicle in which it is administered, and local conditions, for example, adiposity, rates of blood flow, and temperature of the tissue in question. For drugs administered orally, the rate of absorption often can be deliberately controlled by altering the pharmaceutical properties of the tablet or capsule itself.

The rate of absorption of drug is reflected in the time it takes to achieve the maximal concentration of drug in plasma. These variables are referred to as the $T_{max}$ (time) and $C_{max}$ (concentration), respectively. A rapid-release formulation produces a higher peak concentration ($C_{max}$) in a shorter time ($T_{max}$) than a slow-release formulation. The sustained-release formulation produces a lower peak that is reached considerably later than that of the progenitor preparation. Theophylline, morphine, and procainamide are three of many drugs prepared in sustained-release formulations. These products enable the patient to take the drug fewer times per day, at longer intervals between doses. The fewer doses of drug needed per day, the better the compliance (for most patients) with a therapeutic regimen.

**PRINCIPLE Sometimes sustained-release formulations of a drug can make an important difference in a drug's profile of convenience, efficacy, and safety.**

Patient factors also are important in determining the rate and extent of absorption of some drugs. Patients in shock have decreased blood flow to subcutaneous tissues and highly variable rates of flow through skeletal muscle. Therefore, these sites should not be relied on for prompt or reliable absorption of drug. For example, a patient in anaphylactic shock may need epinephrine but its administration via the subcutaneous route (routinely used in the treatment of patients with asthma) would not be advisable. The immunogenicity of hepatitis B vaccine is different when it is given IM in the deltoid muscle as compared with the gluteal muscle. (Perhaps the latter injection was often made into fat tissue rather than muscle.)

**PRINCIPLE Absorption of drugs is a complex process that depends on factors related to the drug itself, the vehicle of administration, the site of administration, and the state of the patient. The choice of a route or site of administration of a drug should be made deliberately as part of a well-planned therapeutic program.**

When a drug is given by direct intravenous injection or infusion, 100% is delivered to the systemic circulation in most situations (barring inactivation of the drug by light, or adsorption of the drug to the plastic tubing). Drugs delivered via any other route can result in less than 100% bioavailability (i.e., $<$100% of the administered dose is delivered to the systemic circulation in its original form).

**PRINCIPLE When drugs are given by any route other than the intravenous route, the extent of absorption and bioavailability must be understood in order for one to prescribe it rationally and to make appropriate quantitative adjustments as to whether the route of administration needs to be changed.**

## More About Drug Distribution

After a drug has been absorbed and reaches the systemic circulation, the process of distribution begins. Usually, the drug appears to be mixed rapidly in the intravascular space and comes to a rapid equilibrium with other tissues in the body. Drugs that are tightly bound to plasma proteins, or drugs that have very high molecular weight (large proteins, dextrans, etc.), are confined to the intravascular space (about 5 L). Most drugs are sufficiently small and lipid soluble that much or even most of the dose is distributed to tissues outside the vascular space.

After an intravenous dose of most drugs, a concentration-of-drug-versus-time curve similar to that illustrated in Figure 9A is observed. In this example, a 500-mg dose of a drug was injected intravenously, and very rapidly achieved a concentration in plasma ($C_p$) of 20 mg/L. The drug appeared to be distributed promptly throughout the

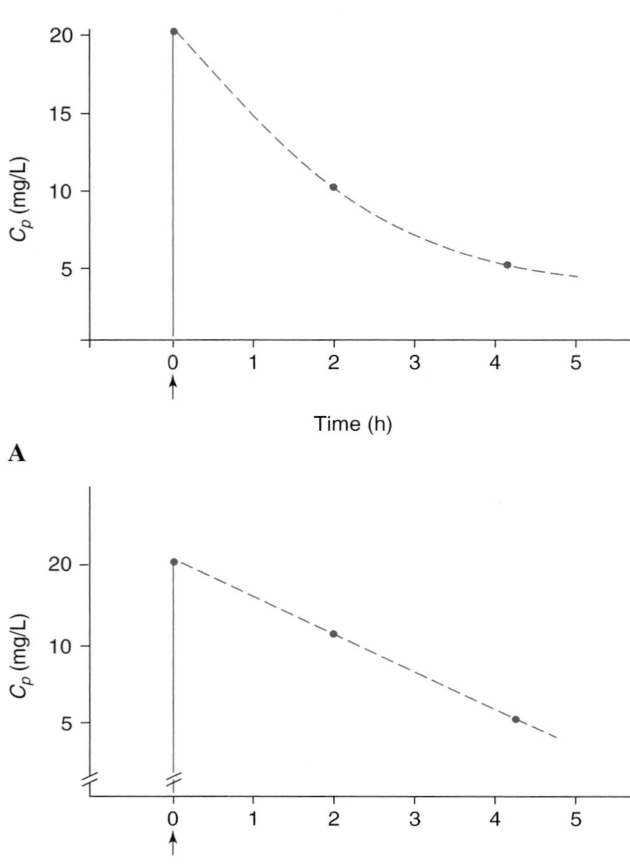


**FIGURE 9 (A) A typical drug-concentration-versus-time curve, with $C_p$ displayed on the *y*-axis with a linear scale. A rapid peak is seen following the intravenous bolus injection (arrow at time zero) and then a characteristic exponential decay in $C_p$ as the drug is cleared from the plasma. A half-life of 2 hours is apparent from the figure. (B) The same drug-concentration-versus-time data, but this time with $C_p$ displayed on the *y*-axis on a logarithmic scale. The straight line on this scale also represents exponential decay (or first-order drug elimination). Once again, the drug's half-life of 2 hours is obvious from the figure.**

body into an "apparent" space (compartment) with a volume of 25 L. In other words, the 500 mg of drug was promptly distributed throughout a space (compartment) of about 25 L in volume, with a resultant concentration of 20 mg/L. The characteristic decline of $C_p$ over time seen in Figure 9A is typical of exponential decay characteristic of the clearance of most drugs (so-called first-order elimination). That is, the rate of elimination of a drug is proportional to the drug's concentration in plasma (to the first power). There is no real 25-L compartment in the human body. The term *apparent* volume of distribution is a useful way to think about how drugs appear to be distributed.

The same concept is shown in Figure 9B but displayed on a semilog plot. Note that the *y*-axis is displayed using a log scale for $C_p$, and that the same exponential decay of $C_p$ over time appears to be a straight line when displayed in this manner. Since $C_p$ declines by 50% every 2 hours in this example, the drug is said to have a half-life of elimination of 2 hours.

Most drugs appear to be distributed rapidly into a compartment that actually includes the blood volume plus other tissues. The apparent volume of distribution ($V_d$) is dependent on a number of factors intrinsic to the drug. Properties of molecular weight, lipophilicity, affinity for binding to plasma and tissue proteins, and active transport into target tissues are all factors that help determine a drug's apparent $V_d$. Patient factors also are important determinants of $V_d$. Patients show interpatient variation in apparent $V_d$ depending on their body build (fat or lean), extent of perfusion of different types of tissue, the presence or absence of large pleural or peritoneal effusions, and so on.

Some drugs, such as diazepam and thiopental, demonstrate more complex concentration-of-drug-in-plasma-versus-time curves. Figure 10 illustrates what such a curve can look like in a 70-kg patient receiving a 10-mg intravenous dose of diazepam. On this semilog plot, the decline in concentration of drug over time has two phases. The initial phase lasts several hours, during which the concentration of drug in plasma declines relatively rapidly. This is followed by a more prolonged phase of gradual decline in $C_p$ that lasts for days.

The initial phase is called the alpha phase of drug distribution. The rapid decline in $C_p$ is predominantly caused by the prompt distribution of drug from the small central compartment of well-perfused tissues (that includes the blood, brain, and heart) into a much larger peripheral compartment of more poorly perfused tissues (e.g., fat, muscle, and other tissues). The second phase is called the beta phase. In this phase, the decline in $C_p$ is predominantly caused by the gradual clearance (removal) of diazepam from the plasma, in this case accomplished by hepatic biotransformation.

**SUMMARY**
**Drug distribution**

- **For most drugs, is characterized by rapid mixing into one compartment**

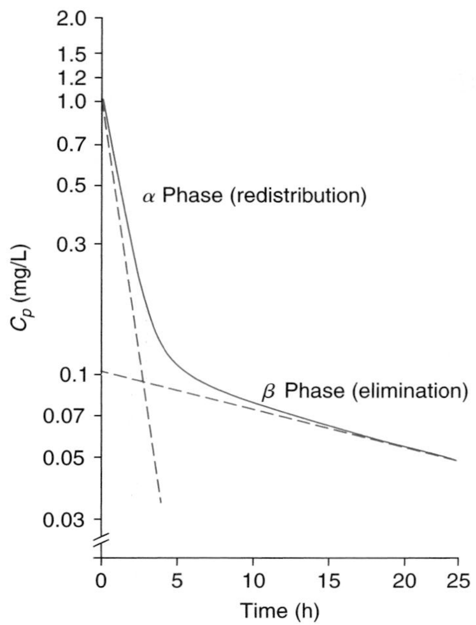


**FIGURE 10 An idealized plot of plasma concentration of diazepam over time following a rapid IV injection of 10 mg. Note that the ordinate ($C_p$) has a logarithmic scale. The decay curve (dashed line) is the sum of two straight dashed lines, each representing a different exponential process (redistribution and elimination).**

- **For a few drugs (like thiopental), is better characterized by rapid distribution from a small central compartment into a larger peripheral compartment**
- **Has some between-patient variation**

Concentrations of diazepam in plasma following an injection closely resemble data displayed in Figure 10 (Greenblatt et al. 1989). Diazepam works quickly to suppress grand mal seizures because the small central compartment includes the blood and brain. Consequently, a high concentration of drug is achieved quickly in the brain (usually within a few seconds of an intravenous injection), and the seizures usually are rapidly controlled. The seizures can recur, however, after 15–60 minutes, not because the drug is metabolized and then eliminated from the body (this actually takes many hours to occur), but because the drug is rapidly distributed from the small central compartment into the larger peripheral compartment. When this happens, $C_p$ falls to a concentration that is subtherapeutic for controlling seizures. As a consequence, acute management of grand mal seizures usually consists of rapidly controlling the seizures with intravenous diazepam, and then "loading" the patient with a second drug such as phenytoin or phenobarbital. Although a loading dose of phenytoin can take 30 minutes to administer, it should start to work as the beneficial effects of diazepam are waning.

This rapid distribution of diazepam helps explain why this drug is such an excellent first-line agent for urgent termination of grand mal seizures but is not used for chronic prevention of such seizures. Rapid distribution of intravenous boluses of diazepam (half-life of redistribution about 1 hour) helps to lower $C_p$ quickly, terminating both its beneficial effects (e.g., termination of seizure activity) and also its adverse effects (e.g., CNS depression). If repeated oral dosing of diazepam were used to "build up" plasma concentration to a therapeutic level, however, then distribution would no longer be an important consideration. High and persisting plasma concentrations (half-life of elimination 24–36 hours) would produce suppression of seizure activity and profound somnolence or even coma. Clearly, other antiseizure medications are preferable for the chronic management of awake and alert outpatients with seizure disorders.

Other commonly used drugs that exhibit such prominent, rapid, and clinically important distribution from central to peripheral compartments include midazolam and thiopental. These drugs exhibit the same property: their clinical effects decline much more rapidly than can be accounted for by their elimination from the body. In these cases, (re)distribution rather than elimination is responsible for the dominant pharmacodynamic effects of these drugs when given as intravenous injections for indications such as induction of general anesthesia (e.g., thiopental), termination of seizures (e.g., diazepam), or inducing conscious sedation (e.g., midazolam).

Not surprisingly, patients show considerable patient-to-patient variation in both drug distribution and redistribution. Patients' body structures, their relative proportions of muscle (high water content) to fat (low water content), and other features are predictably associated with patient-to-patient differences in values for apparent $V_d$ on the order of 30%. The really large patient-to-patient variation in pharmacokinetics, however, comes in the area of clearance of drugs from plasma, where patients can vary by 80-fold or more (e.g., see the beta-blocker, propranolol).

## More About Drug Clearance

Clearance, in its simplest terms, is the body's ability to rid itself of a drug, xenobiotic (foreign substance), or waste product (such as creatinine). This process is referred to both as drug clearance from the body and as clearance of the drug from plasma. Perhaps the most clinically useful term to use for purposes of calculations of dosages and intervals of administration in therapeutics is clearance of the drug from plasma. This is often referred to as "drug clearance" or "plasma clearance." A drug's rate of clearance is important in determining that drug's maintenance dose.

The main organs responsible for drug clearance are the kidneys (usually responsible for excretion of drug or metabolites into urine via transport mechanisms or filtration, but occasionally also responsible for important drug metabolism) and the liver (usually responsible for drug metabolism or biotransformation, but sometimes contributing to drug excretion directly into bile by transport). Although these concepts are discussed in more depth in Chapter 23, the general concept is that small, water-soluble drugs (e.g., lithium, salicylate, gentamicin) can be cleared by simple renal excretion. Larger or more lipid-soluble drugs (e.g., diazepam, propranolol) cannot be filtered by the glomerulus, or are extensively reabsorbed from urine if they are present in the tubular urine. Consequently, before they can be excreted in urine, such lipophilic drugs must first be metabolized in the liver to more hydrophilic (i.e., less lipophilic) metabolites. Patients differ substantially in their abilities to clear drugs via renal excretion and hepatic biotransformation. Units of drug clearance usually are expressed as milliliters/minute or liters/hour. Upper limits of such values in healthy adults are shown in Table 1.

Why do patients differ so widely in their ability to clear drugs? Each aspect of drug clearance (primarily renal excretion and hepatic biotransformation) is influenced by a number of variables including inherited genotype, concurrent illnesses, previous damage to the organ responsible for clearance, concomitant use of drugs that can either enhance or diminish drug clearance, and so on. These independent determinants of clearance lead to very large potential patient-to-patient variations in drug clearance. Thus even as much as 100-fold differences in clearance can be seen between patients using the same drug.

Many drugs undergo both renal and hepatic clearance. Some drugs are cleared from plasma by other routes as well, such as via exhalation (halothane), renal metabolism (imipenem), excretion in the feces (charcoal), metabolism by plasma enzymes (succinylcholine), and so on. As discussed previously, the total plasma clearance of a drug equals the sum of each clearance term contributed by each organ of biotransformation (most often the liver) or elimination (most often the kidney). For example, the total plasma clearance of procainamide in a healthy adult is about 500 mL/min, of which about one-third is contributed by hepatic biotransformation and the rest by renal filtration and secretion.

There are many different types of reactions involved in hepatic biotransformation. The hepatic microsomal enzymatically mediated reactions include oxidation, reduction, hydrolysis, hydroxylation, and *N*-dealkylation. Many of these reactions are mediated by a class of enzymes called the mixed-function monooxygenase system, also known as the cytochrome P450 system. The metabolites of drugs that undergo these types of reactions (also called phase I or nonsynthetic reactions) are more hydrophilic than their progenitor drugs and, therefore, are more likely than the progenitor to be cleared by the kidneys.

**PRINCIPLE Analysis of the chemical characteristics of drugs can aid in choices between chemical entities used for the same indication. If inspection of a molecule's structure (or known pharmacokinetic data) allows sensible estimates of hepatic versus renal clearance of a drug, make a point of using this information in your therapeutic decisions. Basic pharmacology texts infrequently make this analysis for you.**

In addition, since these types of phase I changes to the drug often are sterically small (e.g., removal of a methyl group, addition of a hydroxyl group), the metabolites frequently are pharmacologically active. Moreover, the pharmacologic profile of an active metabolite can be very different from that of its progenitor.

The amount and activity of the drug-metabolizing enzymes in the liver can be markedly determined by pharmacogenetic factors (see Chapter 22) and increased (induced) by a variety of conditions, including smoking or

Table 1 **Maximal Contributions to Total Plasma Clearance by the Liver and Kidneys**

| Organ | Total blood flow (mL/min) | Total plasma flow (mL/min) | Maximal plasma clearance (mL/min) |
|---|---|---|---|
| Liver | 1500 | 900 | 900 |
| Kidney | 1250 | 720 | 720 |

previous administration of some enzyme-inducing drugs such as phenytoin, phenobarbital, or rifampin. The enzyme activity also can be inhibited or diminished because of hepatic disease (cirrhosis, hepatitis) or coadministration of inhibitory drugs such as cimetidine or ketoconazole. The large potential for drug–drug interactions at the hepatic drug-metabolizing enzyme level is described in Chapter 4, Hepatic Disorders and the Influence of Liver Function on Drug Disposition; Chapter 22, Pharmacogenetics; Chapter 25, Drug Interactions.

Many drugs are cleared by both the liver and kidneys, with variable total plasma clearance. For example, phenobarbital is cleared by both the liver (75% of total clearance) and the kidney (25%), but the total clearance of the drug is only 6 mL/min. Such a low rate of clearance from plasma is less than 1% of the rate of plasma flow to these organs, implying a very low efficiency of these organs with respect to clearance of phenobarbital. The importance of both hepatic and renal clearance also is illustrated when drugs are first transformed to active metabolites that are themselves cleared by the kidney. This type of arrangement can lead to interesting consequences, as in the following case.

**CASE HISTORY** *A 68-year-old woman with metastatic breast cancer was admitted to the hospital for radiation therapy of painful bone metastases. She was given large doses of meperidine, up to 100 mg every 2 hours, to control her pain. Due to unrecognized prerenal azotemia and hypercalcemia, she developed progressive renal failure, and her creatinine increased from 1.4 mg/dL on admission to 4.2 mg/dL 4 days later. On her fifth hospital day, she had severe myoclonic jerking movements of her extremities. By the next day, she had severe and refractory grand mal seizures.*

**Discussion** *The intense pain of bone metastases can be difficult to control. Opioids may be needed. In this patient, meperidine was a poor choice of analgesic for several reasons. Meperidine is cleared predominantly (about 85%) by hepatic biotransformation to normeperidine, a phase I (nonsynthetic) demethylation reaction. Normeperidine is not very active as an analgesic, but it stimulates CNS activity and can result in myoclonus and even seizures. Normally, this metabolite is readily excreted by the kidneys. In patients receiving high doses of meperidine who develop renal dysfunction, however, large amounts of normeperidine will be formed in the liver but slowly cleared by the kidneys. The resultant accumulation of this metabolite can lead to severe seizures, as occurred in this patient. Another disadvantage to using meperidine is the fact that because the drug is rapidly transformed and has a short half-life, it has to be given every 2 to 3 hours.*

**PRINCIPLE The balance of hepatic and renal clearance of both the parent drug and any active metabolites must be understood to prescribe a drug wisely.**

## More About the Half-Life of Elimination

The concept of half-life of elimination of a drug was indirectly evident in both panels of Figure 6. A certain percentage of the drug is eliminated from the body per unit time. For most drugs, there is a time interval during which an "average" patient eliminates half the drug from the body (or clears half the drug from plasma, or reduces the concentration of drug in plasma by 50%). This period is known as a drug's elimination half-life.

The half-life of elimination is very drug-dependent. The average half-life of elimination of penicillin G is about 30 minutes. Diazepam has an elimination half-life of more than 24 hours, thyroxine about 7 days, and amiodarone more than 1 month. There also is potential for wide patient-to-patient variation of the elimination of the same drug. The elimination half-life for a drug is not determined by its route of clearance. It can be long or short whether it is cleared by the kidney, liver, or lung.

The half-life of elimination of any drug is determined by its volume of distribution, and its clearance, in a specific patient. The half-life is directly proportional to the drug's volume of distribution ($V_d$) and inversely proportional to the drug's clearance (CL). Since both $V_d$ and CL vary widely from patient to patient, it is not surprising that the half-life of a drug will also vary widely from patient to patient.

**SUMMARY**
**The half-life of drug elimination**

- **Is directly proportional to $V_d$**
- **Is inversely proportional to CL**
- **Varies greatly from patient to patient**

## Variation in Pharmacodynamics

Pharmacokinetic variation can explain why different patients achieve very different steady-state plasma concentrations of a drug after chronic dosing at the same daily dose, or even at the same dose in milligrams per kilogram (of body weight). A different phenomenon, however, explains why different patients receiving the same drug, and with doses carefully adjusted to produce deliberately similar values of $C_p$, can still demonstrate different pharmacologic reactions to drugs. Why will two patients, who develop comparable plasma concentrations while receiving ampicillin to treat a UTI, demonstrate a clinical cure in one patient and resistant infection in another, no adverse effects in one patient, and anaphylaxis in the second? Why will timolol eye drops improve one patient's glaucoma, yet worsen asthma or congestive heart failure in a second patient, both with low and similar plasma concentrations?

Pharmacokinetic variation cannot explain these observations. Pharmacodynamics is the term that explains what the drug does to the patient, and patients also demonstrate a great deal of variation in the way they react to comparable concentrations of drugs in plasma—in their pharmacodynamics. To improve a physician's ability to practice rational therapeutics individualized to specific patients, the thoughtful doctor must anticipate and understand the common causes for variation in both pharmacokinetics and pharmacodynamics between patients.

Certain subsets of patients demonstrate predictable pharmacokinetic and pharmacodynamic differences. In fact, it is just this predictability that the thoughtful physician uses to optimize pharmacotherapeutic plans. The next section focuses on several of these patient subsets and how they account for important patient variation in both pharmacokinetics and pharmacodynamics.

**PRINCIPLE The thoughtful prescriber will anticipate, and compensate for, likely and predictable pharmacokinetic and pharmacodynamic differences in his or her patients. The prescriber will also seek these abnormalities as explanation of unexpected effects of efficacy or toxicity appearing at doses that usually do not cause such events. Lack of attention to these sources of interpatient variation will result in diminished probability of therapeutic success and greater likelihood of adverse reactions.**

## SPECIAL PATIENT GROUPS

Although each patient is unique with respect to his or her pharmacodynamics and pharmacokinetics, several variables such as patient gender, age, the state of organ function, and the concomitant use of other medications present predictable perturbances of each and thereby, anticipated challenges to the optimal use of many medications. Whereas important perturbers of pharmacokinetics and dynamics are detailed and referenced in Part 3, the introductory material that follows is meant to convince the reader that understanding more about these patient subsets will improve the quality of his or her rational therapeutic decisions.

### Pediatric Patients

The physician should not treat premature infants, neonates, children, and adolescents as small adults. Not only are their diseases and hence their treatments often different from those of and for adults (e.g., recombinant human surfactant for respiratory distress syndrome or the use of specific antibiotics to treat necrotizing enterocolitis), but each age from premature neonate to adolescent may exhibit substantially altered pharmacokinetics and pharmacodynamics when compared with adults. Healthy neonates exhibit a rapidly changing ability to clear drugs via the liver and kidney. This seems due to rapidly changing drug pharmacokinetics as the patient progresses from the neonate to the infant to the toddler. In addition, the premature infant may distribute or clear drugs differently from the neonate born at term. For many drugs, FDA approval was obtained after there was sufficient data concerning efficacy, toxicity, and pharmacokinetics in healthy adults, but little or no experience with the drug in neonates, infants, and children. For all of these reasons, rational drug treatment of infants and children can be as difficult or even more difficult to achieve than rational drug treatment of mature adults (Roberts 1984).

**SUMMARY**
**Special features of pediatric pharmacotherapeutics include the following.**

- **Immature and changing routes of drug clearance**
- **Pharmacodynamics different from what occurs in adult patients**
- **Less data available from manufacturer at time of FDA approval**
- **Less clinical experience with many drugs in pediatric patients**

#### *Differences in pharmacokinetics*

It is difficult to generalize about changes in drug pharmacokinetics in pediatric patients, since between-patient variations are so large. Whereas absorption of most drugs in the healthy neonate is often similar to that in the adult, premature neonates can secrete relatively small quantities of bile into the gut, thus decreasing the absorption of highly lipid-soluble drugs such as vitamins A, D, E, and K. Drug distribution can change rapidly as the percent of body weight present as water rapidly drops from 85% in premature infants, to 75% in full-term infants, to 60% in the adult. Total body fat content in the premature infant can be as low as 1%, contrasted to 15% in the normal full-term neonate. The implications of these differences for the distribution of water-soluble and lipid-soluble drugs are substantial. In addition, drug binding to plasma proteins can be much less in the fetus and neonate than in the adult, thereby increasing the free fraction of total drug in plasma (percent unbound) for many drugs.

Hepatic biotransformation, enzyme activity for many pathways is substantially reduced in early neonatal stages. Decreased hepatic clearance (leading to increased steady-state plasma concentrations and prolonged half-life of elimination) has been observed for a wide variety of drugs that undergo hepatic biotransformation, including acetaminophen, diazepam, tolbutamide, phenobarbital, theophylline, and many others. Perhaps the most widely publicized example in which such decreased hepatic biotransformation has led to neonatal drug toxicity was the case with chloramphenicol. This older antibiotic, which is still in use because of several clinically important properties (penetrates the blood–brain barrier, covers ampicillin-resistant *Haemophilus influenzae*, covers many anaerobes, covers rickettsial species, etc.), can still be used in pediatric settings but not without appropriate adjustment of dosage and/or dosage intervals.

**CASE HISTORY** *A 1-week-old, 4-kg infant develops neonatal septicemia and meningitis. A broad-spectrum antibiotic that penetrates the CSF is desired. Chloramphenicol (100 mg/kg/day) is chosen since it meets both criteria. After about 4 days, the baby develops listlessness, refusal to suckle, abdominal distention, and irregular and rapid respiration. This syndrome progresses to periods of cynanosis, flaccidity, hypothermia, and the baby develops an ashen gray color. The antibiotic is stopped, and the infant recovers. What happened?*

**Discussion** *This syndrome is now known as the "gray syndrome" or the "gray baby syndrome." It was first recognized in 1959, and by 1963, it was known that when this antibiotic was given in conventional doses (on the basis of milligrams/kilogram of body weight) to neonates, especially premature babies, the antibiotic accumulated, and the drug reached extremely high plasma concentrations by about the fourth day of treatment. (Since the half-life of elimination was prolonged, it took several days for the steady-state plasma concentration to be achieved.) It appears that neonates display altered pharmacokinetics of this drug for two reasons. First, their livers have inadequate glucuronyl transferase activity (a phase II biotransformation enzyme) for the first 3–4 weeks of life leading to a diminished rate of drug metabolism. Second, the immature kidney demonstrates inadequate renal excretion of both the unconjugated drug and the glucuronide conjugate as well. Elimination half-life in infants less than 1 week old is as long as 26 hours, compared with 4 hours in older children. It is best to avoid this drug during the first 4 weeks of life, or to use it in reduced doses (e.g., 25 mg/kg/day). In situations in which the drug must be used, close clinical monitoring of efficacy and toxicity and measurement of plasma concentrations are recommended.*

Renal function in the premature and full-term neonate, both glomerular filtration and tubular secretion, is significantly reduced in comparison with function in older children. Drugs such as penicillin G exhibit clearance rates only 7% as great as that of adults when compared on the basis of body surface area. Other drugs cleared by either tubular secretion or glomerular filtration, such as aminoglycosides, salicylate, and digoxin, exhibit decreased renal clearance in neonates.

Practical pharmaceutical problems can be seen in infants and other pediatric patients that are not seen in adults. Oral liquid suspensions and elixirs may be refused or expectorated, but tablets and capsules are impractical for the young. The small muscle mass of the neonate can make intramuscular (IM) injections difficult. Limits on the acceptable volume of intravenous fluid may require drugs to be prepared in more concentrated solutions than would be needed in adults. Flow rates through intravenous lines may need to be so slow (several milliliters per hour) that an intravenous dose of a drug delivered via "piggyback" can take hours to be infused.

#### *Pharmacodynamic changes*

Drugs can produce different pharmacodynamic effects in children than in adults. Amphetamine-like drugs usually produce CNS stimulation and excitement in an adult, but can be useful in treating hyperactive (hyperkinetic) children with attention disorders. Glucocorticoids can be more likely to produce psychotic reactions in adults (this is not entirely clear), but they are obviously more likely to produce problems with bone growth and epiphyseal maturation in children. Most differences in pharmacodynamics are probably due to the fact that certain diseases such as infant respiratory distress syndrome, necrotizing enterocolitis, and kernicterus occur predominantly or exclusively in neonates and infants, and drugs used in their treatment (e.g., human surfactant) are not used for similar diseases in adults.

In short, while the problems encountered in treating pediatric patients may seem new and different when compared with those encountered treating adults, the same principles of rational therapeutics apply. Close attention to the scientific basis of treatment and deliberate attempts to individualize therapy will result in increased drug efficacy and decreased drug toxicity.

## Elderly Patients

***Overview of the problem***

The elderly (often defined as patients older than 65 years) are more likely to receive medications and to develop problems while taking medications. The increasing number of review articles in this area (Lamy 1986; Everitt and Avorn 1986; Montamat et al. 1989; Beers and Ouslander 1989) suggests that the special problems of elderly patients are beginning to be more widely appreciated and disseminated. Recent statistics suggest that although Americans age 60 years or greater comprise only about 17% of our population, they may account for 39% of all hospitalizations for and 51% of deaths from drug reactions. Although those over age 65 years constitute less than 12% of the population, they purchase 25% of all drug prescriptions. Even as ambulatory patients, elderly patients may take an average of three to six prescription drugs, and another three over-the-counter products.

Recent data obtained from a case–control study of 4108 admissions to medical and surgical units in two tertiary-care hospitals (mean patient age 56 years) reveal that 190 adverse drug events (ADEs) occurred over this 6-month period (4.6% of admissions), of which 60 were preventable without compromise of the efficacy for which the drugs were given. The average additional length of stay associated with an ADE was 2.2 days, at an average increase in cost of $3244 (Bates et al. 1997).

**WARNING** Elderly patients

- Purchase a disproportionate percentage of all drug prescriptions
- Account for a disproportionate percentage of total and fatal adverse drug reactions
- Experience significantly increased length of stay and expense when adverse drug reactions occur in hospital

In 1985, perhaps as many as 243,000 older adults were hospitalized because of adverse drug reactions. In fact, a government report noted that "A growing body of evidence accumulated over the past 10 years indicates that mismedication of the elderly has become a critical health care issue" (Kusserow 1989). Such mismedication can include the prescription of higher doses when lower doses would be equally effective and less toxic; prescription of more dangerous drugs when less dangerous drugs would be equally effective; prescription of drugs that are unnecessary; or use of drug combinations that lead to interactions that produce adverse effects. In addition, the elderly patient's understanding of instructions can be dulled, and compliance problems (over- and under-use of medications) can ensue. The importance of noncompliance has been addressed (Stewart and Caranasos 1989). Perhaps 14 to 21% of patients never fill their original prescriptions; in 50% of patients, drugs may not have their desired effects because of improper use. Compliance with drug regimens can be especially poor in the elderly because of their poor vision or hearing; cognitive decline; complicated drug regimens with large numbers of medications; or even difficulty opening childproof containers. Additionally, because of financial concerns, elderly patients may not be able to afford to purchase their prescription medications.

Other factors make the elderly patient more likely to receive medications and to develop associated adverse effects. A review of geriatric medicine features discussion of a large number of syndromes that are present either predominantly or uniquely in the elderly. These include orthostatic hypotension, stroke, dementing illness, urinary incontinence, osteoporosis, constipation, and poor nutrition (Bender and Caranasos 1989). The presence of these problems can lead to the prescription of types of drugs rarely used in younger patients and thereby to drug-induced toxicity not encountered in younger patients. The following case illustrates this double jeopardy that is risked the elderly patient.

**CASE HISTORY** *A 70-year-old man was living in a nursing home because of chronic Alzheimer's disease, mild urethral obstruction, and congestive heart failure. With the death of a roommate, his room was changed and he became disoriented, especially at night. He was prescribed thioridazine to help control his agitated behavior in the evenings. During the next several weeks, he developed increasing symptoms of slow and diminished movement, tremor, and stiffness. A diagnosis of parkinsonism was made, and the drug benztropine was added to his regimen. During the next several days, the patient had a progressive downhill course, marked by difficulty with his vision, dry skin, fever, constipation, difficulty voiding, and increasing confusion and agitation. He was transferred to the hospital for management of an episode of acute urinary retention.*

**Discussion** *The patient's initial episodes of disorientation late in the day (sundowning) is a common problem, especially in patients who have recent provocations leading to the disorder (loss of a roommate or change in rooms and nurses, etc.). Prescribing a neuroleptic agent may have been* *overly aggressive in such a patient, since the likelihood of drug toxicity often outweighs the minimal benefit expected. Studies have demonstrated the overuse of neuroleptics in this setting and have revealed the relationship between the use of a neuroleptic and the risk of hip fracture. In this case, one could anticipate toxicities such as increased sedation, or side effects related to the anticholinergic or antidopaminergic properties of thioridazine. Drug-induced pseudoparkinsonism is one such common effect that was not recognized as a drug-induced effect in this patient. So what could have been cured by simple withdrawal of the drug was instead protracted and treated with another drug, benztropine. This anticholinergic agent was deliberately prescribed to treat the parkinsonism that was not attributed to the original drug therapy.*

*Many physicians are not aware of the anticholinergic effects of a large variety of drugs commonly prescribed to the elderly. In addition to the antiparkinsonian drug benztropine, tricyclic antidepressants (e.g., amitriptyline), antiemetics (e.g., promethazine), bronchodilators (as ipratropium), antipsychotics (thioridazine), antiarrhythmics (disopyramide), and drugs for dizziness (meclizine) all have anticholinergic properties in addition to their intended pharmacologic effects (Peters 1989). Anticholinergic adverse effects (atropinism) can present in a spectrum of manifestations. They can be easily remembered by recalling the saying, "Dry as a bone, red as a beet, mad as a hatter, blind as a bat, and hot as a pistol." The elderly can be especially vulnerable to the side effects of constipation, difficulty with vision (pupillary dilation, cycloplegia), decreased bladder tone, and confusion caused by such drugs. The episode of acute urinary retention in this patient was likely precipitated by the two drugs with anticholinergic properties superimposed on the patient's underlying symptoms of benign prostatic hypertrophy.*

**PRINCIPLE The elderly patient is at risk of entering a vicious cycle in which the patient is more likely to receive drugs, more likely to develop adverse drug reactions, and potentially more likely to receive even more drugs to treat the unrecognized adverse drug effect.**

### *Altered pharmacokinetics in the elderly*

Although elderly patients can show altered pharmacodynamic responses to a few classes of medications (see the discussion that follows), they more commonly exhibit altered drug pharmacokinetics. This is often a "surprise" to physicians, but remember that during the development of most drugs, their pharmacokinetics are investigated in younger volunteers or patients. Only recently has the FDA begun to require that new drugs that will be prescribed for elderly patients (e.g., NSAIDs for patients with arthritis) have their kinetics and dynamics evaluated in a number of elderly patients before approval.

Age-related changes in drug pharmacokinetics are complex and often difficult to predict. Age-related changes in drug bioavailability, distribution, hepatic biotransformation, and renal clearance are discussed in detail in Chapter 21. Although general conclusions valid for all drugs are difficult to make, it is clear that the physiologic changes that occur in most elderly patients can predict pharmacokinetic changes.

Although changes in GI function occur in the elderly, this usually does not translate into altered oral bioavailability, even though the rate of drug absorption may be slowed. For some drugs with large first-pass effects, decreased hepatic function can reduce the extent of the first-pass effect and thereby increase the apparent oral bioavailability of the native drug.

More age-related changes are seen with respect to drug distribution. The tendency to decrease total body water and to increase total body fat with increasing age, along with a fall in plasma concentration of albumin, lead to alterations in the volume of distribution of many drugs (decreased $V_d$ for water-soluble drugs, such as ethanol and lithium, and increased $V_d$ for lipid soluble drugs, such as diazepam).

Decreased cardiac output, decreased blood flow to the liver (with decreased activity of some phase I enzymes), and decreased blood flow to the kidney (with decreased renal plasma flow, glomerular filtration, and tubular secretion) are associated with decreased drug clearance for some drugs cleared by the liver (lidocaine, theophylline, diazepam, but not lorazepam) and most drugs cleared by the kidney (e.g., gentamicin, lithium). Remember that the between-patient differences in organ function of the elderly are often large and make it difficult to offer general statements as to appropriate doses of drug based solely on age of the patient. Some elderly patients have well-preserved renal function into old age. "Average" patients, however, do experience a predictable decrease in renal function with increasing age. Measure these functions in the elderly if you need to reach relatively narrow target ranges of drug in plasma of any individual patient.

Changes in drug distribution and drug clearance described previsously can combine to cause large changes in elimination half-life for certain drugs. For example, the elimination half-life of diazepam can be prolonged from 24 hours in a young man to 96 hours in an octogenarian, because of the combination of an increased volume of distribution and decreased hepatic clearance (remember, half-life is directly proportional to $V_d$ and inversely proportional to CL).

**SUMMARY**
**With respect to changing pharmacokinetics with age**

- **Hepatic biotransformation can decline for some drugs**
- **Renal clearance declines for most renally excreted drugs**
- **It is unusual for either route of clearance to increase**
- **Therefore, the maintenance dose for many drugs decreases**

### *Altered pharmacodynamics in the elderly*

Even when medications are not overprescribed or misused in this population, elderly patients experience changes in their physiology that are partially responsible for altered pharmacodynamic responses to some medications.

**CASE HISTORY** *An 83-year-old man had been in good health until he suffered a compression fracture of his thoracic spine. The nocturnal pain had made it difficult for him to fall asleep. His physician prescribed chlorpromazine 50 mg* per os *before bed to help him sleep. Over the next few days, he noted increasing faintness when he stood up, increasing difficulty urinating, and he fell twice, injuring his right hip and wrist.*

**Discussion** *There are many important issues hidden in this very brief case history. Although the cause of the compression fracture could be simple osteoporosis, other causes such as boney metastatic disease need to be considered. The difficulty falling asleep was probably caused by pain, and therefore, if a drug were needed, an analgesic probably makes more sense than a hypnotic. If a hypnotic were prescribed, it almost certainly should not be a phenothiazine such as chlorpromazine, but a more effective and less toxic hypnotic one, such as one from the benzodiazepine class.*

*The phenothiazines can cause adverse reactions in any patient but in the elderly, the wide spectrum of varied pharmacologic actions that phenothiazines have over and above their sedating effects can cause special problems. The alpha-adrenergic receptor blocking effects cause increased orthostatic hypotension, sometimes leading to faintness, presyncope, or even syncope. Their anticholinergic effects can cause acute urinary retention, especially in an elderly man with underlying prostatic hyperplasia and mild to moderate urethral obstruction. Epidemiologic studies have shown that the phenothiazines, like other drugs with CNS depressant properties, dramatically increase the risk of falling and hip fractures in the elderly. In addition, a spectrum of acute and chronic extrapyramidal neurologic adverse reactions can develop, some of which (e.g., pseudo-parkinsonism or neuroleptic malignant syndrome) are more common in elderly patients than in young adults.*

**PRINCIPLE The elderly patient can exhibit increased or different pharmacodynamic effects of medications when compared with the effects observed in younger and healthier patients.**

Clearly documented examples of such pharmacodynamic changes with age are only recently being described. Other examples of pharmacodynamic changes in the elderly include greater anticoagulation in response to similar plasma concentrations of warfarin, increased risk of bleeding while receiving therapeutic concentrations of heparin, increased analgesic effects from opioids, increased sedation from longer-acting benzodiazepines (and paradoxical agitation from shorter-acting agents), and decreased tachycardia in response to $\beta$-adrenergic agonists. More detailed discussion of these and other pharmacodynamic changes in the elderly is presented in Chapter 21.

The mechanisms for such changes in pharmacodynamic responses to drugs are often not fully understood, but can include alterations in receptor number or affinity, altered second-messenger function or production, or altered cellular response to second messengers.

### *Adverse drug reactions and drug interactions*

The elderly experience an excessive number of adverse drug reactions and drug interactions, however, age per se may not be an independent variable in this equation. Rather, the presence of increased number of diseases, increased severity of disease, and increased number of total medications, all act together to increase the probability of an ADR. Similarly, the increased number of total medications increases the chances of an unintended drug interaction. In addition, since elderly patients are more likely to receive digoxin and quinidine, they are more likely to experience the common interaction of quinidine increasing the steady-state plasma level of digoxin. Other drug pairs often prescribed to elderly patients, with a resultant risk of an interaction, include diuretics with digoxin (hypokalemia increasing the risk of digoxin toxicity), a tricyclic antidepressant with guanethidine (decreased control of blood pressure), or oral hypoglycemic agents with beta-blockers (more prolonged and therefore more severe episodes of hypoglycemia, etc.).

Some authors believe that certain drugs have such excessive risk profiles when given to the elderly that they should rarely, if ever, be prescribed. For example, it has been proposed that drugs such as amitriptyline (excessive anticholinergic effects), older antipsychotics (movement disorders), chlorpropamide (long half-life with risk of prolonged hypoglycemia), disopyramide (highly anticholinergic), or long-acting benzodiazepines (confusion, sedation, falls, and even increased risk of hip fracture) are all relatively contraindicated in this age group, as equally effective and safer alternatives are available (Beers and Ouslander 1989).

***Summary***

A balanced approach to prescribing for the elderly patient is difficult to achieve. Data concerning dosing and adverse reactions in elderly patients can be lacking for many drugs, especially recently approved drugs, which may not have been given to many elderly patients during phase II and III testing. It is equally important to avoid the extreme positions of inappropriate therapeutic fear (depriving patients of helpful medications) and cavalier and unthinking prescribing of unnecessary medications (predisposing to increased adverse drug reactions and drug interactions without the possibility of efficacy).

Although our knowledge base in the area of geriatric clinical pharmacology is incomplete, it is adequate to suggest that a few general principles should be applied to drug use in elderly patients. The principles of rational therapeutics outlined near the beginning of this Introduction should serve the practitioner well when he or she is prescribing for any patient, including an elderly one. Additional principles of special relevance to prescribing for the elderly are listed as follows.

1. *Make extra efforts to establish a diagnosis.* Since drugs are more likely to produce adverse effects in the elderly, empiric therapy is less likely to result in a favorable benefit/risk ratio than it would in younger patients. Therapeutic drug use is more likely to result in toxicity due to drug–disease interactions. Establishing a firm, working diagnosis is important before treating any patient, but perhaps is especially important when approaching the elderly.
2. *Obtain a detailed drug history.* The elderly are more likely to be taking prescription medications, OTC drugs, and topical agents (e.g., eye drops) with systemic effects. It is essential to know all the agents a patient is receiving in order to assess the possibility of an ADRs occurring or being present and to plan the rational introduction of a new agent.
3. *Make extra efforts to know the clinical pharmacology of drugs prescribed.* Understand both the intended and unintended pharmacologic actions of drugs. For example, a neuroleptic drug may not only act as a "major tranquilizer," but can cause unacceptable toxicity because of its tendency to cause orthostatic hypotension, anticholinergic effects, sedation, ataxia, or extrapyramidal syndromes. Neuroleptics differ widely in these unintended pharmacologic properties.
4. *Reevaluate drug use at frequent intervals.* Most physicians feel it is "easier" to begin a new drug than to discontinue a chronically used medication. Drugs can and should be discontinued when no longer necessary. Antihypertensives, antiseizure medications, sedative-hypnotics, neuroleptics, and digoxin can all be safely discontinued in certain types of patients—especially those receiving the drugs inappropriately to begin with. Since the number of medications taken is a major determinant of drug toxicity by drug interactions, reducing the number of medications is an important goal.
5. *Understand nonpharmacologic as well as pharmacologic approaches to treating diseases.* Many of the problems of the elderly may respond to nonpharmacologic treatments. Examples include exercise to help relieve leg claudication, exercise to help relieve constipation, weight loss to help lower blood pressure and hyperglycemia, and so on. Usually, such nonpharmacologic interventions are safer than drug use or may permit the use of lower doses of drugs when drug therapy becomes necessary.
6. *Make extra efforts to individualize treatment.* It is essential to individualize treatment in the elderly patient based on knowledge of what other drugs the patient is taking, other diseases the patient may have, and altered pharmacokinetics or pharmacodynamics of the drug in the elderly. The loading dose, or especially the maintenance dose, may need to be reduced in the elderly patient. Each of these factors is more likely to be a relevant concern in the elderly compared with the younger adult patient.
7. *Pick endpoints to follow carefully.* More or different endpoints to follow can be required in treating an elderly patient. As mentioned in paragraph 3, the use of a drug such as a neuroleptic can require the physician to inquire about and follow endpoints of dizziness on standing, sedation, falling, ataxia, constipation, urinary retention, stiffness or difficulty moving, and so forth. Many of these endpoints would be less necessary when giving the same drug to a younger patient.
8. *Emphasize the alliance with the patient.* The physician must take extra steps to assure compliance with his or her prescription. The fewer the drugs and the simpler the drug regimen, the more likely the patient will be to take all drugs correctly. Clear labeling on prescriptions and supplying accompanying patient information inserts can be especially important for patients with

poor hearing, vision, or memory. Instruction may have to be given to a spouse, relative, or friend in addition to the patient. A medication schedule or calendar, or weekly drug administration aids (such as boxes or plastic containers), may be necessary. The patient must be encouraged to call the physician and to report problems that might be drug-related. Finally, the physician must keep close track of all medications being taken and must reassess the need for each at regular intervals.

## Pharmacogenetic Factors

Patients differ in both their genotype and phenotype. Often, the genetic differences have a direct impact on a patient's pharmacokinetic or pharmacodynamic response to a certain medication. Although we expect to see interpatient differences in drug pharmacokinetics and pharmacodynamic responses to drugs, occasionally, a patient will react in a manner so qualitatively or quantitatively different from the "average" patient that the reaction is termed "idiosyncratic." As more is learned about pharmacogenetic influences on drug kinetics and dynamics, more examples of "idiosyncrasy" become explainable.

Most commonly, pharmacogenetic anomalies are caused by inheritance of an abnormal gene that leads to synthesis of an abnormal protein, or absence of a gene with resultant decreased synthesis of a normal protein. In most cases, the protein affected is an enzyme, although inherited abnormalities in quality or quantity of proteins that function as receptors, transport carrier proteins, or hemoglobin have been reported.

Inheritance of such genes often will lead to one of three scenarios: 1) the patient will exhibit altered drug pharmacokinetics, such as enhanced or diminished clearance of the drug; 2) the patient will exhibit altered pharmacodynamics, with a usual pharmacologic effect being enhanced or diminished; 3) the patient will exhibit a novel pharmacologic response to the drug that was not seen or anticipated in previous "average" patients without the same genotype.

A recently described example of the first two possibilities was the observation that a small minority of patients receiving conventional doses of azathioprine as an immunosuppressive agent experienced acute and prolonged bone marrow toxicity during short courses of low-dose therapy. This occurred despite the presence of normal renal and hepatic function. When compared with control patients who tolerated standard doses of azathioprine without such problems, the patients with "hypersensitivity" to the drug all demonstrated substantially reduced activities of the enzyme thiopurine methyltransferase (TPMT). This enzyme plays an important role in azathioprine metabolism. Reduced activities of this enzyme led to higher concentrations in plasma of 6-mercaptopurine, that in turn led to higher concentrations of the drug in tissues, leading to higher levels of 6-thioguanine nucleotides in tissues as well. This later led to increased myelosuppression (Lennard et al. 1989). We now know that about 1 in every 300 patients will have an increased susceptibility to the bone-marrow depressant effects of azathioprine, caused by this inherited marked decreased activity of an enzyme important in the drug's catabolism.

Heterozygous patients for TPMT, or homozygous wild-type patients with low-normal activities of TPMT, also may be more likely to experience certain drug–drug interactions. For example, one recent report described a patient in whom a derivative of 5-aminosalicylic acid was found to inhibit low-normal activities of TPMT, thereby leading to unexpected bone marrow suppression from azathioprine, but only when azathioprine was given with the inhibitory drug at the same time (Lewis et al. 1997).

Pharmacogenetic factors also can lead to novel reactions to drugs. One common example of this type of pharmacogenetic condition is seen in the X-linked genetic trait of a deficiency in the red-cell enzyme G6PD (glucose-6-phosphate dehydrogenase). Such patients can develop drug-induced hemolytic anemia when exposed to any of a wide variety of drugs that tend to oxidize red cell membranes. Normally, red cells protect themselves from oxidizing stresses and injury by maintaining adequate stores of reduced glutathione. For the red cell to maintain adequate cellular concentrations of reduced glutathione, however, the cell must generate adequate amounts of NADPH (the reduced form of NADP). Cells deficient in G6PD activity are deficient in their ability to generate adequate amounts of NADPH when needed during periods of oxidizing stress. These patients can feel fine until confronted with drugs such as antimalarial agents (e.g., primaquine), sulfonamides (sulfisoxazole), sulfones (dapsone), nitrofurans (nitrofurantoin), or analgesics (aspirin), after which the oxidant stress on their red blood cells causes disruption of their membranes and hemolysis. The degree of hemolysis can range from mild to severe and life-threatening.

**SUMMARY**

**Pharmacogenetic abnormalities can lead to**

- **Unexpected drug toxicity even when low doses of drug are being administered**
- **Unexpected drug–drug interactions**
- **Novel drug effects not seen in "average" patients**

An increasing number of pharmacogenetic conditions have been identified, leading to the three types of problems outlined in the summary box. These conditions are discussed in more detail in Chapter 22. The importance of these pharmacogenetic conditions to the practice of rational therapeutics is illustrated in the following case histories.

---

**CASE HISTORY** *During a busy day at a large hospital, three previously healthy college athletes are scheduled to undergo abdominal or orthopedic surgery. In each case, the anesthesiologist plans an induction with intravenous thiopental; initial muscle relaxation with succinylcholine to facilitate endotracheal intubation; maintenance anesthesia and relaxation with oxygen, halothane, and pancuronium; and extubation assisted by neostigmine and glycopyrrolate. In the first case, everything seems to go smoothly. In the second case, no pancuronium is needed since the patient seems to remain flaccid and paralyzed after receiving only succinylcholine. In fact, as the patient awakes from the halothane, he remains paralyzed and requires mechanical ventilation for a further 12 hours after his surgery. The third case proceeds smoothly for the first 45 minutes, until the anesthesiologist notices the patient has developed tachycardia and cyanosis. Further examination reveals that the patient has a core temperature of 41°C and a profound metabolic acidosis. The surgery and anesthesia are abruptly terminated, the patient is actively cooled, and an antidote is administered. What happened to the second and third patients?*

**Discussion** *The first patient behaved as a so-called average patient would, with an uneventful anesthetic induction, surgical course, and reversal. The second patient demonstrated an exaggerated or prolonged response to his first muscle relaxant. Succinylcholine, a depolarizing muscle relaxant, worked well but continued to cause paralysis for 12 hours; its normal duration of action is only about 10–15 minutes. This abnormally prolonged response to this drug was caused by a pharmacogenetically determined inability in this patient to metabolize the drug succinylcholine. Succinylcholine is structurally quite similar to the natural neurotransmitter acetylcholine and is metabolized by the plasma cholinesterase enzyme. In a small number of patients, this plasma enzyme is qualitatively abnormal or absent. Such patients will appear normal until challenged with succinylcholine, at which point, they experience normal onset of drug effect and dramatically prolonged elimination half-life of the drug with consequent prolonged and pronounced pharmacodynamic effects. As long as such a prolonged response is recognized promptly, the patient can be supported (with mechanical ventilation) until the drug is cleared and the patient regains motor strength.*

*The third patient also experienced an unusual or "idiosyncratic" reaction to his anesthetic agents. Likely the succinylcholine or the halothane were culprits. This bizarre and life-threatening reaction that can include extreme hyperthermia, acidosis, shock, arrhythmia, and even death is known as malignant hyperthermia. It too can be caused by an inherited abnormal protein, in this case thought to be located in the sarcoplasmic reticulum of the skeletal muscle cells. As a result of this pharmacogenetic defect, when skeletal muscle cells are exposed to a variety of anesthetic agents they develop an unusually massive accumulation of intracellular calcium, leading to severe tetany, which in turn is responsible for the dramatic increase in heat production.*

*Although the two pharmacogenetic conditions described in this case are not common, they are not rare and are seen each year in most hospitals. More important, they dramatize the necessity of understanding and recognizing abnormal responses to common medications, since many such responses are predictable (on the basis of a good family history); treatable if recognized, even if not predictable; or preventable. Other important examples of such pharmacogenetic conditions are discussed in Chapter 22.*

---

## Patients with Renal Disease

A variety of disease states alters both the pharmacokinetics and pharmacodynamics of a drug. Renal disease is especially likely to alter these parameters since so many drugs (or their active metabolites) are cleared via renal excretion.

### *The presence of unsuspected renal compromise*

Note that glomerular filtration and active tubular secretion decline progressively with age. This decline in renal function may not be apparent, however, since muscle mass declines with age as well. Therefore, plasma creatinine which represents a steady-state concentration determined by creatinine production (from skeletal muscle) and clearance (via the kidneys) can be "normal," masking both a decline in production and a decline in renal clearance. The trap of assuming that renal function in an elderly patient is normal if the creatinine is normal is illustrated by the following case.

---

**CASE HISTORY** *An 80-year-old woman was admitted to the hospital with a fractured hip. On admission, her BUN was 25 mg/dL, and her creatinine was 1.5 mg/dL, both at the upper limits of "normal." She was assumed to have normal kidney function. She underwent open reduction and internal fixation of her femur and did well for several days. A Foley catheter was placed at the time of surgery.*

**Discussion** *When the physician learned that the creatinine was "normal," she mistakenly concluded that the patient's creatinine clearance (an indirect measure of glomerular filtration rate) was normal as well. We now know* *that we can estimate or approximate the patient's GFR using a number of nomograms or equations. One of the easiest to use is the following:*

$$\mathrm{GFR} = \frac{[114 - 0.8 \times \mathrm{age}]}{Ccr} \times (1.0 \text{ or } 0.85)$$

*where GFR is in mL/min,* $C_{Cr}$ *represents the serum creatinine concentration, and a correction factor of 1.0 or 0.85 is assigned for men and women, respectively (Paladino et al. 1986). For this woman, we can calculate her GFR to be*

$$\mathrm{GFR} = \frac{[114 - 0.8 \times 80]}{1.5} \times (0.85) = (33)(0.85) = 28 \text{ mL/min}$$

*If we assume a "normal" GFR to be 85–100 mL/min for a healthy young woman, this woman's GFR is only about one-third of normal.*

**PRINCIPLE When a number such as a plasma creatinine concentration represents a dynamic balance between two simultaneous processes (e.g., input and clearance), knowledge of the concentration alone may not be sufficient to understand the status of important underlying physiologic processes such as glomerular filtration.**

***The effects of renal disease on drug pharmacokinetics***

The presence of renal insufficiency can alter any aspect of drug pharmacokinetics. Although drug absorption and bioavailability do not seem to be predictably altered in the presence of renal disease, drug distribution is sometimes altered to an important degree. For example, the free fraction of an acidic drug such as phenytoin is about 10% in healthy patients (i.e., 90% is bound to albumin, 10% is free). In the presence of severe azotemia, the free fraction can double to 20%, owing to a decline in serum albumin concentration (especially in a patient with nephrosis) and the presence of nondialyzable acidic substances that displace phenytoin from its protein binding site. This increase in free fraction means that at any total concentration of the drug in plasma (as measured by a clinical laboratory), twice as much free drug is present than is usually the case. The "therapeutic range" for the drug, measured in terms of total concentration of drug (bound plus free), drops from 10–20 mg/L to 5–10 mg/L. This shift in the therapeutic range and appropriate target concentrations must be recognized if the drug is to be used rationally.

Distribution of a drug also can be altered by the presence of edema, pleural effusions, or ascites in patients with liver, renal, or cardiac disease. For example, the presence of a pleural effusion increases the volume of distribution of a water-soluble drug such as methotrexate. The half-life of elimination of this drug can be prolonged in patients with renal failure and pleural effusions, partly because the renal clearance of the drug is reduced and partly because the volume of distribution is increased.

The most frequent and worrisome effect of the presence of renal insufficiency on drug pharmacokinetics is the effect on its clearance. This becomes clinically important in patients in whom the drug of interest is cleared predominantly by the kidneys and has a narrow therapeutic index. Commonly prescribed drugs that share these properties include aspirin, methotrexate, vancomycin, and the aminoglycosides. The presence of renal insufficiency would *not* be expected to significantly alter the use or safety of drugs such as lorazepam (cleared almost entirely by the liver) or low-dose penicillin G (eliminated almost completely by the kidneys, but with a large therapeutic index).

WARNING Renal insufficiency is most likely to alter drug clearance to a clinically important degree for drugs that are predominantly cleared by the kidney (>50%) and that have a narrow therapeutic range (index).

Returning to the case introduced previously, we can see how the presence of renal insufficiency alters the safety profile of a drug such as gentamicin.

CASE HISTORY *On the fifth postoperative day, the patient appeared septic. Urinalysis obtained through a Foley catheter revealed many leukocytes and gram-negative bacilli. A presumptive diagnosis of gram-negative bacillary urosepsis was made, most probably due to* E. coli. *Her physician prescribed the "usual" loading dose of gentamicin (2 mg/kg) and the "usual" maintenance dose (1.5 mg/kg every 8 hours). Peak and trough concentrations of drug were determined the next day after the fourth dose. They were both excessively high, well into the toxic range.*

**Discussion** *In a patient with urosepsis, the first dose of antibiotic should be administered quickly to promptly achieve a therapeutic concentration in plasma. The loading dose of a drug is* not *affected by its clearance rate. It would be affected if the disease or circumstances changed the volume of distribution, as would be the case of patients in congestive heart failure receiving lidocaine. Thus, if the physician had decided to select gentamicin as the antibiotic of choice, the usual loading dose of gentamicin could have* *been given right away, even before the physician knew the plasma creatinine concentration. To prescribe a loading dose, the physician only needed to know the patient's weight (in kilograms), the drug's volume of distribution (in liters/kilogram), and the target concentration for gentamicin. Using information about the volume of distribution ($V_d$=0.25 L/kg), and aiming for a target concentration of 8 mg/L, an appropriate loading dose would be 2 mg/kg as was given*

$$[LD = V_d \times C_{target} = (0.25 \text{ L/kg}) \times (8 \text{ mg/L}) = 2 \text{ mg/kg}]$$

*Since this drug is almost entirely (>95%) cleared by the kidneys, however, the maintenance dose is determined by the target concentration selected and the renal clearance of the drug. The drug's clearance parallels the creatinine clearance. Since her renal function (creatinine clearance) is only about one-third normal, her maintenance dose of gentamicin should be only about one-third normal (e.g., about 1.5 mg/kg every 24 hours instead of every 8 hours). Since the maintenance dose of gentamicin was not reduced in this case, toxic concentrations were achieved at steady-state, raising the risk of causing ototoxicity, nephrotoxicity, or both.*

*In general, the decline in a drug's renal clearance closely parallels the decline in renal function per se, whether the drug is eliminated by glomerular filtration or tubular secretion. Thus to the extent that creatinine clearance can act as a marker of overall renal function, it can act as a marker for changes in clearance of drug as well. A more detailed approach to adjusting maintenance doses of drugs in patients with renal insufficiency is presented in Chapter 7 and Chapter 23.*

**PRINCIPLE The renal function of a patient must be known to prescribe some drugs wisely. For some of those drugs, dosing is not affected; for others, the maintenance dose of the drug must be reduced; and for yet others, the presence of renal insufficiency is a relative contraindication to using the drug at all.**

Even when the pharmacokinetics of a drug itself are not altered by renal disease, the pharmacokinetics of an active drug metabolite can be altered. This interesting and not uncommon permutation is illustrated in the following case.

CASE HISTORY *A 75-year-old woman with a creatinine of 2.4 mg/dL was admitted to the hospital complaining of severe bone pain caused by widely metastatic breast cancer. She received meperidine up to 100 mg every 2–3 hours to control her pain. On her third hospital day, she began to exhibit myoclonic jerks, which progressed to severe and refractory grand mal seizures.*

**Discussion** *Meperidine is cleared almost entirely by the liver and is initially demethylated to form normeperidine. This metabolite has minimal analgesic properties, but is much more likely than the parent drug to cause myoclonus and seizures. As is true of many drug metabolites, normeperidine is cleared primarily by renal excretion. In this patient, high doses of meperidine resulted in rapid production of normeperidine. Because of the patient's renal insufficiency, however, the concentration of normeperidine in plasma steadily increased until it reached a level sufficiently toxic to cause the CNS effects. Thus, drug metabolites primarily eliminated by the kidneys will accumulate in patients with renal insufficiency.*

Other drugs that have active or toxic metabolites that can accumulate in the presence of renal insufficiency include procainamide (*N*-acetylprocainamide), nitroprusside (thiocyanate), and allopurinol (oxypurinol).

**PRINCIPLE Understand a drug's route of clearance, as well as the route of clearance of any active or toxic metabolites, before prescribing it.**

### *Drugs with altered pharmacodynamics*

A number of different classes of drugs exhibit altered drug action in patients with renal insufficiency. Potassium salts, potassium-sparing diuretics, NSAIDs, and ACE inhibitors are all more likely to cause hyperkalemia in patients with preexisting renal disease than in patients with normal renal function. Diuretics can be less effective, or produce a slower or more delayed diuresis, in patients with renal disease. Nonsteroidal anti-inflammatory drugs can be more likely to cause GI bleeding from gastritis or ulcer disease in patients with underlying renal disease, possibly because such patients are already at higher risk for these problems and possibly because of the qualitative platelet defect in patients with uremia. Renal insufficiency is a relatively strong contraindication to the use of methotrexate. The toxicity of this drug is determined more by the drug's duration of action than by the peak concentration in plasma. Since the elimination half-life of the drug and its duration of action are altered by the presence of renal disease, the drug's ratio of benefit to risk is also significantly altered.

**PRINCIPLE Renal disease induced alteration of a drug's pharmacodynamic effects of both efficacy and toxicity can significantly alter the benefit/risk ratio of the drug.**

***Drug-induced nephrotoxicity***

As is discussed in Chapter 7, the kidneys receive a large portion (about one-quarter) of the total resting cardiac output (approximately 5000 mL/min), extract a high percentage of their oxygen supply, and actively concentrate drugs and metabolites in tubular fluid and parenchymal cells. Perhaps for these reasons, the kidneys are quite vulnerable to drug-induced toxicity. Essentially any anatomic area of the kidney can be adversely affected by drug-induced disease. Prerenal azotemia related to drug-induced hypovolemia or low-output states, renal parenchymal disease (glomerulonephritis, interstitial nephritis, tubular necrosis), and postrenal disease (ureteral obstruction, bladder outlet obstruction) are all frequent manifestations of drug-induced renal disease. Rare but serious syndromes have also been described such as retroperitoneal fibrosis compressing the ureters induced by methysergide, or acute renal failure and hemolysis induced by mitomycin C. Although certain drugs are notorious for commonly causing nephrotoxicity (e.g., aminoglycosides causing tubular necrosis, methicillin causing interstitial nephritis, older sulfonamides causing obstruction), many drugs have a lower but still significant incidence of renal toxicity.

A variety of fluid and electrolyte abnormalities mediated by the kidneys also can be caused by drugs. Fluid retention (NSAIDs), nephrogenic diabetes insipidus (lithium), a syndrome of inappropriate secretion of ADH (chlorpropamide), potassium depletion (thiazide diuretics, amphotericin), hyperkalemia (NSAIDs, potassium-sparing diuretics), metabolic acidosis (acetazolamide), and metabolic alkalosis (loop diuretics) are all frequently drug-related.

**PRINCIPLE Since underlying renal disease can drastically alter the pharmacokinetics and pharmacodynamics of many drugs and lead to changes in the choice of drugs themselves, insist on knowing a patient's renal status before planning therapeutic decisions.**

## Patients with Hepatic Disease

Many of the concerns for patients with renal disease apply to those with hepatic disease (chronic active hepatitis, acute hepatitis, cirrhosis, etc.). Such patients may handle drugs differently than the average patient, especially when given those drugs that are predominantly cleared by the liver (altered pharmacokinetics). Those with liver disease also can respond to drugs differently than the average by virtue of altered pharmacodynamics. In addition, drugs that can cause hepatic disease may be more likely to do so in patients with preexisting disease. Some of these issues are illustrated in the following case history.

**CASE HISTORY** *A 38-year-old alcoholic man was admitted to the hospital for treatment of gastritis and alcohol detoxification. He was known to have severe cirrhosis and, in addition, was found to have acute alcoholic hepatitis on admission. He received prophylactic thiamine and acetaminophen 650 mg q4h (every 4 hours) p.r.n. (as the occasion arises) for pain from a painful abscess on his arm. As he began to experience alcohol withdrawal and hallucinations, he received increasing doses of oral diazepam. Over the next 24 hours, he received a total of 650 mg of diazepam, which induced a state of obtundation. His diazepam was discontinued. Over the next 6 days, he very slowly regained consciousness, and his hepatitis dramatically worsened.*

**Discussion** *This "simple" case conceals several important points. First, the patient required relatively high doses of diazepam to treat his alcohol withdrawal because of his high tolerance to ethanol and cross-tolerance to benzodiazepines (both examples of altered pharmacodynamics). His slow recovery from the obtundation induced by diazepam was due to the slow clearance of that drug (an example of altered pharmacokinetics). In a healthy young adult, diazepam has a half-life of about 24 hours. The presence of both cirrhosis and active hepatitis, however, can reduce the activity of microsomal (P450) enzymes responsible for the first two steps of diazepam metabolism. Thus in this patient, the prolonged half-life of diazepam was probably caused by the effects of his liver disease on the hepatic clearance of the drug (Klotz et al. 1975). For this reason, such patients are often given lorazepam instead of diazepam. Lorazepam is cleared by the liver by a conjugation (phase II) reaction to form a glucuronide. Conjugation reactions are less likely to be compromised in patients with hepatic disease.*

Generalization about the effects of hepatic disease on the pharmacokinetics of all drugs predominantly cleared by the liver can be misleading. Although clearance of some drugs such as meperidine and lidocaine may be impaired (Thomson et al. 1973; Klotz et al. 1974), liver disease can also be associated with hypoalbuminemia, leading to decreased binding of drug to plasma proteins and thereby both increased hepatic extraction and higher fractions of free pharmacologically active drug will result.

For example, the presence of acute viral hepatitis does not appear to alter the clearance of phenytoin (Blaschke et al. 1975). Other drugs such as enalapril can exhibit altered pharmacokinetics (bioactivation of enalapril to enalaprilat is impaired in patients with cirrhosis), but the pharmacodynamic effects do not appear to be blunted in those patients (Ohnishi et al. 1989).

**PRINCIPLE Because liver disease produces so many alterations in physiology, it is difficult to accurately predict the effects of liver disease on a particular drug's pharmacokinetics. Close attention to the individual patient when initiating therapy in patients with liver disease is still a fundamental.**

This same patient also illustrates two other important points related to altered pharmacodynamics. First, he had an abnormal response to the usual dose of acetaminophen. Such a low dose of the drug (approximately 3.9 g/day) rarely causes hepatotoxicity in healthy patients, although acute severe hepatitis is a well-known toxic reaction in patients taking large overdoses. This alcoholic patient was particularly sensitive to the hepatotoxic effects of acetaminophen. Some metabolites of acetaminophen produced in the liver appear to be toxic. Their detoxification is via conjugation in the liver with glutathione. Patients with preexistent liver disease or those with severe nutritional deficiencies (this patient had both) have decreased liver stores of glutathione and are therefore more susceptible to the hepatotoxic effects of acetaminophen. This patient had an altered pharmacodynamic response to acetaminophen: he was much more susceptible to the toxic effects of the drug itself. Similarly, patients with liver disease can be more sensitive to toxic effects of aspirin, developing hepatitis, prolonged prothrombin times, gastritis and ulcers with upper gastrointestinal hemorrhage, and more.

Finally, this patient again reminds us that almost every type of liver disease can be caused by medications. Acute fulminant hepatitis, chronic active hepatitis, cholestasis, hepatitis and cholestasis, fatty changes in the liver, and prolongation of the prothrombin time all can be caused by drugs, as discussed in Chapter 4. As was true of the kidney, the liver is also especially prone to the toxic effects of medications. It receives a high blood flow (1.5 L/min), and drugs given orally first pass through the liver in the portal venous blood. Some drugs are so predictably toxic to an already diseased liver that they are relatively contraindicated in patients with preexistent liver disease. Halothane, isoniazid, rifampin, erythromycin, tetracycline, and high doses of acetaminophen should not be prescribed to patients with moderate or severe liver disease unless the potential benefits clearly outweigh the increased risks.

**PRINCIPLE The presence of an underlying disease can change the relative contraindications to the use of a drug, or convert a relative contraindication to an absolute one. Calculation of benefits and risks of drug administration is a dynamic process, which will change from patient to patient and also will change for a given patient as his or her condition improves or deteriorates.**

## Pregnant Women

The pregnant woman poses a set of therapeutic problems that must be considered before prescribing medications. She can exhibit altered pharmacokinetic or pharmacodynamic responses to a number of medications because she is subject to diseases unique to pregnancy (e.g., eclampsia). Perhaps most importantly, all drugs administered to the pregnant woman have the potential to cross the placenta and to cause a variety of pharmacologic and teratogenic effects in the fetus. Many drugs have known potential for causing teratogenesis during the first trimester and other problems if given later, especially just before term. When needing to use newer drugs that have never been formally tested or evaluated in pregnant women, the therapist should be particularly vigilant for immediate and delayed effects not able to be anticipated.

**PRINCIPLE Drug therapy for pregnant women is especially difficult because of the real likelihood of altered drug pharmacokinetics and pharmacodynamics; the possibility of drug-induced fetal toxicity; and the likelihood that for many drugs, precise estimates of fetal risk are not available. The very concerns about drug safety during drug development and clinical testing increase the chances that at the time of formal FDA approval, little human data will be available concerning safety issues during pregnancy.**

### *Placental transfer of drugs*

The ability of medications to cross the placenta from the maternal to the fetal circulation is dependent on several factors. Drugs that are small, uncharged at physiologic pH, and highly lipid soluble (such as thiopental) cross the placenta rapidly. Charged drugs such as heparin and succinylcholine, both of which are weak acids that are highly ionized at physiologic pH, diffuse across the placenta much more slowly. When there are large maternal-to-fetal concentration gradients, however, even highly polar compounds can cross the placenta. The molecular weight of the drug, and the extent to which it is bound to maternal plasma proteins, will also significantly influence the extent to which drugs will diffuse across the placenta.

***Altered pharmacokinetics and pharmacodynamics***

During pregnancy, the mother's cardiac output increases up to 40%, renal blood flow and glomerular filtration and plasma volume increase, and plasma albumin concentration decreases. These physiologic changes can result in altered pharmacokinetics or pharmacodynamics for some drugs. For example, intravenous terbutaline can be administered as a tocolytic agent in women presenting with premature labor. This pharmacologic effect would of course only be noted in pregnant women. However, a dangerous syndrome of chest pain, pulmonary edema, tachycardia, ischemic changes on the ECG, and even myocardial infarction have been reported in some women receiving this drug. Such toxicity is more likely to occur when using excessive infusion rates, but the underlying hyperdynamic state of the cardiovascular system can also predispose pregnant women to such toxicity.

***Risks to the fetus***

There are few situations in which it is more important to weigh potential benefits and risks of drug administration than when prescribing for a pregnant woman. In fact, in terms of risk to the fetus, the classification of drugs that engender risk to the fetus is based on assessments in animal preclinical research and, much less frequently, clinical studies or reports. Human data often are scanty or incomplete, since most drugs are approved by the FDA before the drug has ever been administered to a pregnant woman (preclinical animal studies in several species are required before FDA approval).

Risk/benefit analysis of drug use in pregnant women is summarized in a 5-point scale. This scale and supporting references are described in several excellent reference texts (Berkowitz et al. 1986; Briggs et al. 1990). The five categories of drug risk are as follows.

**Category A.** When there are considerable data available concerning use in pregnant women, and risk of fetal harm appears to be remote. This is the category in which drugs are the safest for use during pregnancy.

**Category B.** Either animal studies have shown no risk and there is little human data, or animal studies showed some risk, but human data did not confirm that risk.

**Category C.** Either studies in animals revealed risk and there are no human studies, or there are no animal or human studies.

**Category D.** There is evidence of human fetal risk, but benefits of the drug may still outweigh risks in certain situations.

**Category X.** There is animal or human experience that shows risk to the fetus, and this risk clearly outweighs any potential benefit to the mother. Drugs in this category pose definite and high risk if used during pregnancy.

---

WARNING When prescribing any medication to a pregnant woman, or a woman who could become pregnant, be sure to be aware of the drug's fetal toxicity rating (from category A to X).

---

In short, no drugs should be prescribed for the pregnant woman unless careful consideration leads to the conclusion that potential benefits from the drug either to mother or fetus outweigh potential risks to both. Although much of the previous discussion focused on the teratogenic risk of drugs administered during the first trimester or pregnancy, drugs can be toxic to the fetus if given just before delivery. Narcotics given to the mother can cause CNS depression, apnea, and low Apgar scores. Beta-blockers can cause fetal bradycardia and hypoglycemia. These harmful effects are usually classic pharmacologic effects, as opposed to the teratogenic effects outlined above.

Drugs of abuse such as ethanol and cocaine can cause both teratogenic effects and toxic effects at birth, as well as withdrawal syndromes in the newborn infant. Recent work has elegantly laid out the syndrome of abnormalities we now refer to as the fetal alcohol syndrome, and the fetal toxicity of other drugs of abuse is becoming increasingly well-described.

***Choosing the best drug when therapy is indicated***

Finally, there are several diseases that occur commonly during pregnancy that have specific drug treatments that are either more effective, less toxic, or better studied than alternative treatments in the pregnant woman. For example, consider Table 2, which shows diseases and recommended treatments for pregnant women. Each of these topics is considered in Chapter 19, however, recognize that pregnancy is a condition that distinctly alters the patient's pharmacokinetic and pharmacodynamic response to medications. In addition, the whole new element of fetal toxicity makes prescribing during pregnancy an especially challenging task.

**Table 2 Diseases and Recommended Treatments for Pregnant Women**

| DISEASE | RECOMMENDED TREATMENT | NOT RECOMMENDED |
|---|---|---|
| Diabetes | Tight control with insulin | Sulfonylureas |
| Hypertension | Methyldopa, hydralazine | Beta-blockers, diuretics, ACE inhibitors |
| Urinary infections | Ampicillin, cephalosporins | Sulfonamides (late), ciprofloxacin |
| Thrombophlebitis | Heparin | Warfarin (first and third trimesters) |
| Hyperthyroidism | 6-Propylthiouracil (PTU) | Surgery, radioactive iodine |

## Breast-Feeding Mothers

Prescribing medications for a mother who is breast-feeding is common and almost as complicated as prescribing for a pregnant woman. In 1930, about 80% of women breast-fed their children. As recently as 1970, only about 28% of American mothers chose to breast-feed. By 1985, this figure had risen to about 50%. Although the nursing mother is less likely to have altered drug pharmacokinetics, she still poses the added factor that many drugs can be excreted into breast milk. As in the case of the patient who is pregnant, the nursing mother poses the additional problem that treatment of the mother exposes a second patient, the nursing baby, to risks from the medications.

***Secretion of drug into breast milk***

Most drugs are secreted into breast milk, however, the rate of secretion into milk, and the relative concentrations of drug in milk and maternal plasma, are determined by a variety of factors. The most important include the size (molecular weight), lipophilicity, charge at physiologic pH, and concentration of the drug in maternal plasma. Since the mother produces approximately 600 mL of milk per day, the nursing infant could ingest significant amounts of drug if it were present in breast milk in high concentration.

In theory, nursing infants might be at high risk for drug toxicity since their renal and hepatic pathways of drug excretion and biotransformation will likely be immature at birth. Fortunately, many drugs are well-tolerated by both the mother and the nursing baby. We do, however, have to pay careful attention to certain drugs that are toxic to the nursing infant.

These drugs usually are secreted into breast milk quite actively and are well-absorbed by the infant but have low therapeutic indices. Some of the better described examples are listed in Table 3.

***Approach to drug treatment in nursing women***

The indications for the use of any drug in this situation should be evaluated with knowledge of potential or known risk of infant toxicity (see, for example, Briggs et al. 1990). As in analogous situations, close attention to risk and benefit can produce different "right" answers for similar patients. For example, continuation of phenobarbital in a woman with well-controlled epilepsy would be beneficial to the mother, and the mild sedation seen in the infant would probably be acceptable. Continuation of phenobarbital or diazepam in a woman who takes it only for intermittent difficulty falling asleep would likely lead to a different analysis of risk and benefit, and a different conclusion.

If the physician and patient agree that both drug treatment and continued breast-feeding are indicated, there are several strategies that can be followed to minimize the potential for drug toxicity to the infant. First, milk can be expressed from the breasts and discarded during the period immediately following the administration of a toxic drug. For example, if a technetium-containing radionuclide must be administered, the mother can discontinue breast-feeding for several days, since that radionuclide has a relatively short decay half-life. Second, drugs can be taken as far apart from breast-feeding as possible. Third, if more than one drug alternative is possible, the drug with the fewest effects on the infant should be chosen. Despite

**Table 3 Drugs to Be Avoided during Breast-Feeding**

| | |
|---|---|
| Endocrine drugs: | Propylthiouracil, methimazole, iodine |
| Radiopharmaceuticals: | Technetium, iodine, gallium |
| Cytotoxic agents: | Methotrexate, cyclophosphamide |
| Antibiotics: | Sulfonamides, isoniazid, chloramphenicol |
| Hormones: | Estrogens, androgens |
| Psychoactive: | Lithium, ethanol, barbiturates |
| Opioids: | Morphine, heroin |

all these "tricks," it can occasionally be necessary to continue drug therapy in the mother, but recommend that she discontinue breast-feeding if the risks to the infant are too great.

## Patients with Drug–Disease Interactions

Patients can have two or more medical conditions that require pharmacotherapy at the same time. Although the first illness may be treatable by a large number of therapeutic options, the presence of the second disease can dramatically alter the rank ordering of those options. Some drugs become more useful in treating both conditions and other drugs become strongly contraindicated because of the presence of the second condition.

One of the more interesting examples of this way of thinking about rational drug therapy is the treatment of the hypertensive patient. As hypertensive patients age, they are at increasing risks to develop one or several concomitant conditions. Table 4 lists some common concomitant conditions and gives examples of antihypertensive drugs that may be relatively indicated or contraindicated given the presence of a second condition. In fact, recent guidelines for the treatment of hypertension (Joint National Committee on Prevention, Detection, Evaluation, and Treatment of High Blood Pressure IV, as discussed in Kaplan 1997) emphasize the need to individualize therapy of hypertension according to patients' risk and presence of other conditions.

In short, because patients differ so widely with respect to their concomitant conditions, recommendations for "optimal treatment" of a group of patients with specific conditions often may need to be individualized. Since many patients are unique in terms of their particular combinations of indications for and contraindications to specific medications, presence of other conditions, presence of drug allergies, and so on, it is often a real challenge to apply the "best available evidence" from published trials to a particular patient with his or her unique characteristics (Feinstein and Horwitz 1997).

**PRINCIPLE Although practicing evidence-based medicine is an important goal of rational therapeutics, remember that results obtained from studying a certain group of similar subjects may not apply perfectly to your particular patient, even a patient with the same indication for drug therapy.**

## Patients with Drug–Drug Interactions

Elderly ambulatory outpatients may take an average of two or three prescription medications (often from several doctors), plus eye drops, skin creams, and over-the-counter nonprescription but pharmacologically active and important medications. Elderly patients who are residents of nursing homes or chronic care facilities may average four or five prescription medications. Medical inpatients often receive nine or more prescription drugs during their admissions and it is not unusual for patients in an ICU to receive 15–20 prescription medications during their stay.

Any patient receiving two or more medications is at risk for a drug interaction, which is simply a response to both drugs given together that would not be expected to be seen if either drug were given in the same dose alone. Drug interactions can be beneficial or harmful, deliberate or unexpected. For example, the prescription of probenecid before a dose of penicillin (given to inhibit the tubular secretion of penicillin and thereby prolong its half-life) is an example of a deliberate, beneficial drug interaction. The administration of penicillin plus gentamicin to treat enterococci, or the administration of hydrochlorothiazide plus propranolol to treat hypertension, are

Table 4 **Antihypertensive Drugs Indicated or Contraindicated by the Presence of a Concomitant Condition**

| Concomitant condition | Drug indicated | Drug contraindicated |
|---|---|---|
| Angina | Propranolol, verapamil | Hydralazine |
| Myocardial infarction | Propranolol, enalapril | Hydralazine |
| Systolic dysfunction | Enalapril, diuretic | Propranolol |
| Diastolic dysfunction | Verapamil | — |
| Asthma | — | Propranolol |
| Diabetes | Enalapril | Propranolol |
| Peripheral vascular disease | — | Propranolol |
| Prostatic hypertrophy | Terazosin | — |
| Pregnancy | Methyldopa | Enalapril, propranolol |

other examples of beneficial drug interactions deliberately prescribed.

Harmful drug interactions are most likely to occur when the physician does not anticipate their significance, and does not plan for them. On the other hand, thoughtful prescribers will try to anticipate drug–drug interactions that have been reported previously, and even those that are likely that may not have been reported or observed yet (Melmon and Nierenberg 1981).

**PRINCIPLE When drug interactions are anticipated in advance, they can be deliberately used to advantage, or their negative impact can be reduced. Dangerous drug interactions usually occur when the prescribing physician does not recognize or anticipate their occurrence.**

Several examples illustrate the potential harm of such unplanned and unexpected drug interactions.

### *Pharmaceutical drug interactions*

CASE HISTORY *A 59-year-old man suffered a massive anterior wall acute myocardial infarction. In the CCU, he developed cardiac arrest secondary to electromechanical dissociation. Through the patient's subclavian catheter the patient first received 0.5 mg (5 mL) epinephrine 1:10,000. He next received 50 mEq (50 mL) of 8.4% sodium bicarbonate. Finally, the resident began to "push" 0.5 g (5 mL) calcium chloride 10% through the same intravenous line. During this last maneuver, the resident noted that the intravenous catheter had become occluded. No fluids would run through the line. The transparent catheter seemed to contain an opaque white material that had not been present earlier. With a firm push, the resident was able to inject 10 mL normal saline and clear the line of the occluding material.*

**Discussion** *This brief report actually includes not one but two unintended and unrecognized adverse drug interactions. First, epinephrine is packaged in vials that are buffered to a pH of between 2 and 3. The drug is stable at acidic pH, but quite unstable at alkaline pH. The epinephrine administered was present in a small volume (5 mL) and was immediately followed by 50 mL of a concentrated and very alkaline solution of sodium bicarbonate. It is very likely that much of the epinephrine already in the intravenous tubing was inactivated by the large following dose of alkaline sodium bicarbonate. Such a drug interaction would deprive the patient of his most important drug—pharmacologically active epinephrine.*

*A second unrecognized drug interaction occurred just seconds later. The sodium bicarbonate solution was followed immediately by the calcium chloride solution. When these two solutions intermixed, a chemical reaction occurred as follows:*

$$CaCl_2 + NaHCO_3 \rightarrow CaCO_3 + NaCl + HCl$$

*The white material occluding the catheter lumen was $CaCO_3$, better known as calcium carbonate or chalk. By pushing 10 mL of normal saline to clear the line, the resident actually forced this chalk to embolize to the lungs.*

*Once again, the main problems with such drug interactions are that the physician did not anticipate that they might occur and/or failed to recognize them when they did occur. If the interactions had been anticipated, they easily could have been avoided by flushing the intravenous catheter with a solution such as 5% dextrose in water ($D_5W$) between drugs. If the interactions had been recognized, then steps could have been taken to be sure that appropriate doses of the drugs were given through separate lines.*

The two interactions discussed in this case are examples of pharmaceutical drug interactions—those that occur because of known physicochemical properties of both drugs. They often occur outside the patient. Other common examples of such pharmaceutical drug interactions include the incompatibility of calcium chloride and potassium phosphate in hyperalimentation solutions, and the inactivation of penicillin and gentamicin when they are mixed in the same infusion device.

### *Pharmacokinetic drug interactions*

Drug interactions more commonly occur because of two other mechanisms, pharmacokinetic interactions and pharmacodynamic interactions. (In one sense, the pharmaceutical interactions described previously could also be viewed as pharmacokinetic drug interactions that served to reduce the bioavailability of the drugs in question.)

**SUMMARY**

**The three major mechanisms of drug interactions are**

- **Pharmaceutical**
- **Pharmacokinetic**
- **Pharmacodynamic**

Pharmacokinetic drug interactions can be most clearly illustrated with a case study.

CASE HISTORY *A 23-year-old nurse was involved in the care of an infant with meningococcal meningitis. The hospital infection control nurse recommended that all health care workers closely involved in the patient's care receive 4 days of oral rifampin, to reduce their chances of carrying or developing meningococcal disease. The nurse was married and used a "low-dose" oral contraceptive (containing ethinyl estradiol estrogen and a progestin) for birth control. Although the nurse had used this method of birth control successfully for 4 years, she became pregnant during her next cycle of ovulation, even though her compliance with the pill remained excellent.*

**Discussion** *Over the years, both the estrogen and the progestin component of the oral contraceptive pill have been reduced to minimize the toxic effects of the drug. The current "low-dose" formulations contain one of several estrogens, but in a dose as low as 35 μg per day of ethinyl estradiol. At this low dose, there is little margin for error, and a few missed doses can result in ovulation and pregnancy. In addition, most of the estrogens are metabolized in the liver by the cytochrome P450 (microsomal) enzyme system. This enzyme system is inducible by a number of environmental factors (e.g., smoking) and drugs (e.g., phenobarbital or phenytoin). One of the most potent enzyme inducers is the drug rifampin. In this case, the administration of only 4 days of oral rifampin caused an induction of the nurse's hepatic P450 drug-metabolizing enzymes, which developed over several days and can persist for several weeks. The induced enzymes led to enhanced clearance of the estrogens contained in the low-dose pill and loss of efficacy—hence, the unexpected and undesired pregnancy. This is an example of a pharmacokinetic type of drug interaction in which one drug alters the pharmacokinetic behavior of a second drug. Other examples of this type of interaction are listed in Table 5. Such pharmacokinetic interactions are quite common and can alter any aspect of a drug's pharmacokinetics, including absorption, distribution, protein binding, biotransformation, and/or excretion. These interactions are discussed in much greater depth in Chapter* 30.

### *Pharmacodynamic drug interactions*

The third type of drug interaction is the most common, the pharmacodynamic interaction. These interactions result in two drugs combining their known pharmacologic effects in a predictable fashion that either increases or diminishes their total pharmacodynamic effects. Drugs may affect the same receptor, tissue, or organ system to produce enhanced effects or antagonistic effects. There are many common examples of such pharmacodynamic interactions and many can be used to clinical advantage (e.g., treatment of hypertension with a diuretic plus a beta-blocker). Other examples are listed in Table 6.

Physicians should try to avoid adverse drug interactions or prevent them from occurring in the first place. The two simplest ways of avoiding adverse drug interactions are straightforward but not often considered. First, keep the number of medications that the patient receives to the minimum required because the frequency of drug interactions rises almost exponentially in relation to the total number of drugs simultaneously administered. Thus, the physician should strive to discontinue unnecessary medications, reduce doses of drugs whenever feasible, and should begin treatment with new agents only after weighing the benefits against the risks.

Second, before adding a new drug to a patient's regimen, carefully review the drugs the patient is already receiving. If there are doubts about whether the new drug might interact with an agent already "on board," consult one of the several excellent reference sources (Tatro 1997). Remember that even excellent reference sources cannot list all drug–drug interactions, especially those that have not been reported yet (Melmon and Nierenberg 1981). If the drug is absolutely required, be willing to monitor for both unusual gains and toxic events and to consider attribution of the unexpected to an interaction. Serious adverse drug interactions will most likely occur with drugs having a narrow therapeutic index, as discussed in Chapter 29.

**PRINCIPLE The best treatment for unwanted adverse drug interactions is prevention.**

## Patients with Previous Adverse Drug Reactions

### *Definition of an adverse drug reaction*

The broadest definition of an adverse drug reaction (ADR) might be any unwanted consequence of drug administration, even administration of the wrong drug to the wrong

**Table 5 Common Examples of Pharmacokinetic Drug Interactions**

| DRUG A | DRUG B | EFFECT OF DRUG B ON DRUG A |
|---|---|---|
| Estrogens | Rifampin | Increased hepatic metabolism of estrogens |
| Phenytoin | Cimetidine | Decreased hepatic metabolism of phenytoin |
| Salicylate | $NaHCO_3$ | Increased renal excretion of salicylate in alkaline urine |
| Penicillin | Probenecid | Decreased tubular secretion of penicillin |
| Digoxin | Quinidine | Decreased renal and nonrenal clearance of digoxin and decreased $V_d$ of digoxin |

Table 6 **Common Examples of Pharmacodynamic Drug Interactions**

| Drug A | Drug B | Interaction (site of interaction) |
|---|---|---|
| Ethanol | Benzodiazepines | Increased CNS depression (organ) |
| Phenothiazines | Opioids | Increased CNS depression (organ) |
| Scopolamine | Diphenhydramine | Increased anticholinergic effects (receptors) |
| Atropine | Physostigmine | Decreased anticholinergic effect (receptors) |
| KCl | Triamterene | Increased risk of hyperkalemia (tissues) |
| Thiazides | Amphotericin | Increased risk of hypokalemia (organ) |
| Morphine | Naloxone | Decreased pain relief, sedation (receptor) |
| Propranolol | Nitroglycerin | Increased relief of angina pectoris (organ) |
| Midazolam | Fentanyl | Increased efficacy of intravenous conscious sedation (organ) |
| Prochlorperazine | Dexamethasone | Increased efficacy of antiemetic action (organ) |

patient (often termed a medication error or incident in hospital jargon), in the wrong dosage, at the wrong time, or for the wrong disease. Any of these errors can cause an adverse reaction in a patient.

Although these scenarios are, unfortunately, common, a narrower definition of an ADR may be more useful. Most physicians assume that the "right" drug is being given to the "right" patient, although errors in this category are frequent. In addition, failure of a patient to improve while receiving a drug is unfortunate, but is not usually viewed as an ADR. A more acceptable definition of an ADR might be "any response to a drug that is noxious, unintended, and unwanted and that occurs at doses usually given for prophylaxis, diagnosis, or therapy" (Karch and Lasagna 1975). Many recent studies of the incidence of ADRs use definitions similar to this one, although exact definitions differ, and some studies try to distinguish "acceptable" ADRs (e.g., neutropenia caused by chemotherapy) from unintended and usually unexpected ADRs (e.g., penicillin-induced anaphylaxis).

***Dimensions of the problem***

Adverse drug reactions are a major problem throughout medical care. These unintended, adverse drug-induced events are frequent and, at times, severe. Exact rates of incidence and prevalence are nearly impossible to estimate. Approximate rates have been reported in a number of studies for outpatients, for hospital inpatients on various services, and in nursing homes. Some observers believe that the rate of occurrence is increasing, possibly related to the increasing average number of drugs taken per patient, increasing number of drugs available, and the increasing toxicity of both prescription and nonprescription medications.

Multiple epidemiologic studies suggest that up to 30% of hospitalized patients will experience one or more ADRs while they are in the hospital. On the order of 6.7% of hospital patients experience a severe ADR (that requires hospitalization, produces permanent disability, or leads to death), and about 0.3% of patients will die as a result of an ADR (Lazarov et al. 1998). In addition, approximately 5% of admissions to the medical service of many hospitals will be caused by the development of an ADR in an outpatient (Lakshmanan et al. 1986). One recent study of a cohort of 4108 admissions to 11 medical and surgical units in two tertiary-care hospitals revealed that there were 247 adverse drug events (rate about 5 per 100 admissions). Although this figure sounds low and reassuring, further analysis of evaluable ADEs revealed that about 32% of the ADEs were preventable, that on average an ADE was associated with an increased length of stay of 2.2 days, and that the average increase in hospital cost per ADE was $3244 (Bates et al. 1997).

Although ADRs are a problem in patients of all ages, they are an especially large problem in the elderly. As outlined in several reports (Meyer 1988; Kusserow 1989), although the elderly (greater than age 65) make up only about 12% of the population, they receive about 30% of prescription drugs and purchase about 40% of nonprescription drugs. In 1985, as many as 243,000 older adults apparently were hospitalized because of ADRs. Furthermore, since elderly patients constitute a large subset of hospitalized patients, they are most at risk for the ADRs that are known to occur during the course of hospitalization. As mentioned earlier, the largest risk factor for developing an adverse drug interaction is the number of drugs being taken by the patient.

While it is difficult to separate avoidable from unavoidable ADRs (e.g., neutropenia following appropriate doses of cancer chemotherapeutic agents) in epidemiologic studies of ADRs, clearly drug-induced adverse reactions cause significant morbidity and mortality, in both inpatients and outpatients, and are a frequent cause of hospital admissions. It is also likely that we detect only a fraction of the ADRs that truly occur, since many ADRs are missed completely, whereas others are attributed to the natural progress of the patient's disease or on a new illness altogether.

***"Blaming" an innocent drug***

Although detection of an ADR when it occurs is important, equal importance is attached to not attributing an ADR to a drug if it is not the cause. Were this to occur during the treatment of some diseases, the best or most effective drug might be unjustly denied. A case illustrates this potential problem.

**CASE HISTORY** *A 65-year-old man developed enterococcal endocarditis on his prosthetic mitral valve. Because of a prior anaphylactic reaction to penicillin, he was treated with vancomycin and gentamicin. Appropriate target concentrations were chosen, and doses of both drugs were adjusted to keep the plasma concentrations (peak and trough) in the desired range. He required valve replacement after several days when his first prosthetic valve failed, and this open heart surgery was technically difficult with significant intraoperative and postoperative blood loss. His physicians planned to administer vancomycin and gentamicin for 6 weeks from the date of the surgery. Approximately 3 weeks postoperatively, the patient complained of anorexia and nausea, and occasional vomiting. Several days later the housestaff checked his BUN and creatinine, which had climbed from 25 mg/dL and 1.2 mg/dL 1 week earlier to 80 mg/dL and 2.4 mg/dL, respectively. His physicians concluded that he was experiencing progressive renal dysfunction caused by the combination of gentamicin and vancomycin. Both drugs were discontinued, but there were no clear alternative drugs.*

**Discussion** *In this case, his physicians incorrectly attributed the patient's progressive azotemia to use of vancomycin and gentamicin. When the patient was interviewed and examined more carefully, his anorexia and nausea had been preceded and accompanied by mild right upper quadrant abdominal pain and slight jaundice, with decreased oral intake of both liquids and solids. Laboratory studies revealed a moderately severe hepatitis with a pattern suggesting viral infection; urinary sediment, specific gravity, and sodium suggested the presence of prerenal azotemia and the absence of acute tubular necrosis. The timing was classical for a transfusion-acquired, non-A non-B viral hepatitis. The patient was given intravenous replacement and maintenance fluids, and the vancomycin and gentamicin were later reinstituted (at a reduced dose). Within 24 hours, the patient's BUN, creatinine, and specific gravity were back to normal, and he began to develop an appetite for both solids and liquids. Both antibiotics were continued uneventfully for the last 3 weeks. "Blaming" the azotemia on his two antibiotics would have deprived him of the best drugs for treating bacterial prosthetic valve endocarditis, postponed appropriate treatment of the prerenal azotemia, and perhaps, resulted in failure to clear the serious infection from his new prosthetic valve, with catastrophic results.*

**PRINCIPLE Attributing an adverse reaction to an "innocent drug" may deprive the patient of a useful drug, or even a medication that is potentially life-saving.**

***Failure to detect true adverse drug reactions when they are present***

"Justice" with respect to ADRs requires that "innocent" drugs be cleared of suspicion, whereas "guilty" drugs must be identified and discontinued. Failure to recognize the presence of a true ADR can lead to continued administration of a drug and worsening of the problem, as in the next case.

**CASE HISTORY** *A 48-year-old woman had mild rheumatoid arthritis. It was easily controlled with moderate doses of naproxen that was started about 4 months earlier. Her other medications included propranolol for treatment of hypertension and an oral antacid when needed for "heartburn." Her annual physical examination was unremarkable, but her physician ordered a chemistry panel "just to check on things." Electrolytes, BUN, and creatinine were all normal, but her liver function tests revealed a picture of moderate elevation of transaminases, with the AST and ALT levels about three times normal, and a slight elevation of her bilirubin. Further questioning revealed that she was totally asymptomatic. The physician pursued this biochemical abnormality with a liver-spleen scan (normal), and an ultrasound of the liver (common bile duct upper limits of normal, or perhaps slightly dilated; head of pancreas not visualized). The patient was transferred to a university hospital where a 4-day admission yielded a normal CT scan of the abdomen and a normal ERCP (endoscopic retrograde cannulation of the pancreatic duct) study. At this point in her work-up, her medical student added to the differential diagnosis the possibility that her abnormal liver function tests might be caused by one of her medications.*

**Discussion** *Review of the literature revealed that this pattern of mild-to-moderate asymptomatic biochemical hepatitis is common during treatment with NSAIDs, including naproxen. Propranolol appeared to be less likely to cause such a syndrome. The timing of such a reaction, should it occur, is usually weeks or months into therapy. Although rare cases of fatal hepatotoxicity have been reported, most patients improve over several weeks after the drug is discontinued. A tentative diagnosis of drug-induced hepatitis was made, and the patient was discharged on the fifth hos-*

*pital day, with naproxen discontinued. Over the next 4 weeks, her liver function tests returned to normal. She remained asymptomatic.*

*In this patient, the failure to recognize the possibility of an ADR caused by naproxen resulted in added morbidity and inconvenience, not to mention the expense of a work-up costing more than $3000, including one uncomfortable procedure. In this asymptomatic patient, a more rational strategy would have been to consider the possibility of an ADR in the first instance, and to discontinue the most likely potentially offending drug(s). If the problem improved, then the probability of a drug-induced syndrome would be increased, and no further work-up would be necessary. If the problem did not improve, then an appropriate work-up could continue with little downside risk to an otherwise asymptomatic patient.*

### *How to evaluate potential adverse drug reactions*

The two cases we have described illustrate the importance of a rational approach to evaluating a patient who has a syndrome that might be caused by adverse effects of a drug. The literature on this subject is voluminous and contains algorithms that can be used and that have been formally evaluated and tested (see chapter 24, Adverse Drug Reactions.)

The practicing physician needs to remember a simple sequence of questions. The answers will aid in identifying true ADRs. The responses to the questions can be set from 0 (clearly no), to 1 (equivocal response), to 2 (clearly yes). Total point scores can help to sort possible ADRs into those that appear to be very likely (10–12 points), probable (7–9 points), possible (4–6 points), or highly unlikely (0–3 points).

1. Has this drug ever caused this type of reaction as reported in the literature?
2. Is the timing of the patient's response to the drug typical of previous reports?
3. Are other likely reasons or causes for the patient's syndrome absent?
4. Has the patient ever had a similar response to this drug?
5. If the drug is stopped, does the patient improve (dechallenge)?
6. If the drug is restarted, does the syndrome recur (so called rechallenge)?

**SUMMARY**

**Key points to consider for evaluating a possible adverse drug reaction—**

- **Previous reports in literature**
- **Timing of onset after starting the drug**
- **Other possible etiologies absent**
- **Previous similar response in the patient**
- **Improvement with dechallenge**
- **Recurrence with rechallenge**

Application of these questions to the two patients discussed generate a more thoughtful approach than simply blaming vancomycin and gentamicin for the first patient's renal compromise, or not thinking of the contribution of naproxen to the second patient's hepatitis. In the first case, the key points discovered were that vancomycin and gentamicin do not cause prerenal azotemia, that there was another likely cause for the azotemia (dehydration), and that correction of the azotemia resulted in improvement in renal function (2 total points). For the second case, the key points included the recognition that naproxen can cause this type of hepatic dysfunction, that the timing was typical of such an ADR, that there were no other likely etiologies in an asymptomatic patient, and that drug dechallenge resulted in prompt improvement (8 total points).

### *Uncertainty concerning adverse drug reactions*

There are several important sources for uncertainty concerning our knowledge of whether a particular patient is experiencing an adverse drug reaction. Clearly if the physician does not suspect the possibility of an ADR, then he or she is unlikely to attribute symptoms to the drug. In several studies in hospitalized patients, the harder the investigators searched for the presence of an ADR (often using specially trained nurses or pharmacists), the more true ADRs were identified. The key issue in evaluating these reports is whether the adverse reactions could have been prevented without compromising the legitimate efficacy of the drugs. Only if the answer is yes are we dealing with important and preventable adverse reactions.

Other less obvious sources of uncertainty need mention. Rare ADRs may not occur or be identified during clinical phases of drug testing required before a drug is released, or a true incidence rate may not be apparent (see Chapter 23). For example, during the past few years, two NSAIDs were recalled after the drugs were on the market because they unexpectedly were found to produce a high incidence of anaphylactic reactions (Zomax) or hepatic and renal failure (Oraflex). More recently, the incidence of intracranial hemorrhage in patients receiving tissue plasminogen activator for coronary thrombolysis has been found to be higher than original premarket studies indicated (Kase et al. 1990).

Pharmacoepidemiologic studies while the drug is on the market are required to reveal previously unknown ADRs that are literally inevitably going to occur. For example, postmarketing studies have suggested that sedatives with long half-lives, tricyclic antidepressants, and antipsychotic agents are all associated with increased risk of hip fractures in the elderly (Ray et al. 1987). What all of this amounts to is that the physician should realize that he or she is in an excellent position to be the first to spot a drug-induced adverse effect. The mental set is to believe what he or she sees and act accordingly.

As experience with new drugs develops, so does the recognition of new ADRs. For example, when cisplatin was initially released, the most feared dose-limiting toxicity was renal failure. Careful clinical observation proved that close attention to adequately hydrating patients could dramatically reduce the incidence and severity of this ADR. It then became apparent that drug-induced peripheral neuropathy was replacing nephrotoxicity as a dose-limiting toxicity. Recent studies with an adrenocorticotropic hormone (ACTH) analog have suggested that larger doses of cisplatin can now be given before the onset of neurotoxicity, thereby allowing greater chance of cure for equal toxicity (effectively altering the risk/benefit ratio for the use of cisplatin) (Mollman 1990).

***Mechanisms and prevention of adverse drug reactions***

Multiple studies have suggested that most ADRs (70 to 80%) are caused by known pharmacologic effects of the drugs themselves. Fewer ADRs are caused by mechanisms that make them unpredictable (e.g., penicillin-induced anaphylaxis), abnormal pharmacogenetic factors causing predisposition (e.g., G6PD deficiency), or idiosyncratic reactions (e.g., anaphylactoid reaction to intravenous contrast agents). The physician should recognize that patients at highest risk for ADRs appear be those receiving many drugs, those receiving high doses of drugs, those who have renal insufficiency, and those who are more than 60 years old. A detailed drug history can detect patients at risk for the "unpredictable" types of reactions as well. Many ADRs can be prevented by considering the particular patient and drug carefully before initiating a new drug regimen.

**PRINCIPLE Reducing the incidence of adverse drug reactions requires that physicians have a sound knowledge of the pharmacology of the drugs they prescribe, that they repeatedly evaluate the changing risk/benefit ratio of each drug, and that they have interest in relating new clinical events to the possibility that an ADR has occurred.**

When a true ADR is identified, it can be important to stop the drug and to initiate appropriate treatment if necessary. Record the event in the patient's chart and report the event to the hospital's pharmacy and therapeutics committee, particularly if the event produced significant morbidity, required treatment, or required discontinuing the drug. Inform the manufacturer or the FDA (using their Medwatch reporting system) if the event was clinically important, novel, or severe; thoroughly inform the patient of the event; and, if appropriate, arrange for an alert bracelet or necklace with a medical warning.

**PRINCIPLE Adequate documentation that an adverse drug reaction occurred is essential for the care of the patient and to further our knowledge of the true incidence and severity of ADRs in general.**

## Patients with Drug Allergies

***Definition and features***

Allergy to medications is a subset of adverse drug reactions. Perhaps the clearest definition of drug allergies is "adverse reactions resulting from immunologic responses to drugs or their metabolites" (deShazo and Kemp 1997). Understanding the pathophysiology and presenting symptoms of such reactions is essential to recognizing and avoiding them. As mentioned in the previous section, 80% or more of all adverse drug reactions are caused by undesired, dose-dependent, pharmacologic responses to drugs. Drug allergies, however, are fundamentally different. They are adverse effects mediated by immunologic mechanisms, either humoral or cell-mediated. They are never intended or desired, since deliberate effects mediated by immunologic mechanisms would be termed vaccination (e.g., active immunity with tetanus toxoid) or treatment (e.g., passive immunity with tetanus antiserum). Drugs that stimulate the immune system in a benign or beneficial way are usually referred to as immunogens, whereas drugs that cause allergic reactions are referred to as allergens.

Drug allergies have been termed "hypersensitivity reactions." This reference is poor since "hypersensitivity" implies an individual has developed a pharmacologic response to a drug at the lower end of the dose–response curve. To make matters more confusing, some adverse reactions to drugs mimic drug allergy closely, even though there is no evidence that the immune system is involved at all.

Some distinctive features of drug allergies that aid in their identification include the following. The allergy has no relation to the intended or adverse pharmacological properties of a drug. The allergic reaction is not dose related. The result is a predictable pattern of organ-specific or systemic toxicity. The drug allergy often, but not always, recurs on subsequent exposure to the same drug (Parker 1975; Assem 1985; deShazo and Kemp 1997). Microgram quantities of a drug can trigger a drug allergy, whereas most drugs are administered in milligram or gram amounts to achieve their intended pharmacologic effect. For example, the development of systemic lupus following exposure to procainamide has no relation to that drug's properties as an antiarrhythmic agent.

Drug allergy is sometimes associated with symptoms typical of other allergies, such as a maculopapular rash, itching, hives, or eosinophilia. Usually, there is a delay after the initial exposure to the drug, during which the immune system prepares its response to the agent. Reexposure to the drug, even with a lower dose given for a shorter period, can quickly trigger a more severe reaction. Drug allergies usually will disappear on cessation of drug therapy. In some cases, deliberate desensitization is necessary and possible. Since desensitization is an inherently risky procedure, however, this dangerous and time-consuming procedure should be undertaken only when the benefits of the drug clearly outweigh the risks (for details see Condemi 1986). For instance, desensitization might be appropriate in a patient who was allergic to penicillin, but who developed an infection that would likely be fatal if penicillin could not be given.

**SUMMARY**
**Key features of drug allergy include**

- **No relationship to usual or toxic pharmacologic effects**
- **Not dose related**
- **Common patterns of organ or systemic toxicity**
- **Appearance usually delayed after first exposure to drug**
- **Are uncommon and first episode is unpredictable**
- **Reexposure often but not always results in allergy again**
- **Allergy on reexposure may appear more quickly, or be more severe**
- **Desensitization is sometimes possible, but risky**

Allergies to drugs can present at various times after exposure to the drug. Reactions that occur less than one hour following exposure usually are called immediate reactions. Those developing 1–72 hours following exposure are termed accelerated reactions, and those developing more than 3 days following exposure are termed late reactions. Drug allergies can present in trivial or life-threatening forms and can involve essentially any part of the body (Assem 1985; deShazo and Kemp 1997). Minor reactions such as macular rashes and asymptomatic eosinophilia represent the benign end of the spectrum. Reactions with more pronounced toxicity, such as major skin eruptions, serum sickness, immune cytopenias, hectic fever, hepatitis, or nephritis represent more severe reactions. Drug allergy can be life-threatening when it is related to development of acute renal failure, acute hepatitis, acute pulmonary infiltrates, vasculitis, or anaphylaxis.

**PRINCIPLE A wide variety of reactions caused by drug allergies are possible. They range from acute to chronic, trivial to life-threatening, restricted to one organ system or involving the entire body.**

Because drug allergies are often unpredictable, the physician needs to understand their pathophysiology and become vigilant in settings where these pathways are likely to be operating. If an allergy-based reaction has occurred before, it will likely recur with rechallenge to the same drug. For such patients, drug allergies can be averted by obtaining a careful drug history. A patient exposed to streptokinase a few weeks before is more likely to develop an acute allergic reaction to rechallenge than a patient who is receiving the drug for the first time. A patient with a previous history of an anaphylactic reaction to penicillin is more likely to have a similar reaction on reexposure, even though the chances of this recurring are considerably less than 100% (Saxon et al. 1987; Condemi 1986). For a few drugs such as penicillin, the predictive value of positive or negative skin tests before readministration of drug has been fairly well established, thus making it somewhat easier to interpret the implications of a prior allergic reaction to the drug (Saxon et al. 1987; Condemi 1986). Skin tests have not proven useful for identifying patients at high risk for acute allergic reactions to other drugs (VanArsdel and Larson 1989). For a few drugs such as sulfonamide, in vitro tests identifying patients with decreased ability to detoxify reactive metabolites can help identify those at risk for developing allergic reactions (Rieder et al. 1989).

Knowledge of a prior anaphylactic reaction to penicillin should lead to selection of an alternate family of antibiotics when one is required. For reasons that are not at all clear, however, patients with a prior history of allergy to penicillin are at increased risk for developing allergic reactions to other drugs, even though these drugs bear little or no chemical similarity to the major and minor immune determinants of penicillin (Saxon et al. 1987). In addition, some cross-reactivity of antipenicillin antibodies with drugs from the cephalosporin and carbapenem classes exists (Saxon et al. 1987).

**PRINCIPLE A detailed drug history is the best strategy for reducing the risk of repeated drug allergic reactions. For a few drugs, appropriate skin testing can further reduce the risk of drug administration. This risk, however, can only be minimized. Given our current state of knowledge of drug allergy, it is difficult to eliminate this risk completely by taking a good history and appropriate use of challenge tests.**

### *Mechanisms of allergic reactions*

What leads a chemical to allergic propensity is not fully understood, but there is considerable evidence that the size of the drug is an important factor. Some drugs or their metabolites are allergenic only when complexed to large molecules such as proteins. These drugs are called haptens. The property of conjugation is utilized when penicilloyl-polylysine (PPL) is used to perform skin tests for penicillin allergy. This commercially available diagnostic agent is a penicillin metabolite complexed to a polypeptide that mimics one of the important haptens in patients receiving benzylpenicillin, but does not in itself constitute an immunogen. So it can be used to detect circulating antibodies but will not contribute to further antibody production.

The patient may not be aware of prior exposure to a drug or immunogen. In the case of antibiotics, perhaps the patient was exposed to the antibiotic as a child, or perhaps the antibiotic was present in beef or poultry meat without the patient's knowledge. In the case of streptokinase, a prior streptococcal infection may have exposed the patient to this bacterial enzyme. Insulin-requiring diabetics receiving protamine-insulin (such as NPH) are at increased risk of serious allergic reactions when intravenous protamine is administered to reverse heparin anticoagulation in patients undergoing coronary catheterization or bypass surgery (Weiss et al. 1989). Patients with an "allergic" or atopic history appear to be more likely to develop drug allergies, whereas the presence of kidney or liver disease does not appear to predispose the patient to drug allergies.

There are four basic mechanisms of drug allergies. Most allergic reactions can be readily explained by one of these four mechanisms. Important decisions about avoiding and treating allergic reactions are based on the knowledge of their pathogenesis.

**SUMMARY**
**Four basic types of drug allergies are**

- **IgE-mediated, acute, or anaphylactic allergy (type I)**
- **Cytotoxic reactions (type II)**
- **Immune-complex disease or serum sickness (type III)**
- **Cell-mediated or delayed-hypersensitivity reactions (type IV)**

**TYPE I (ACUTE, ANAPHYLACTIC) REACTIONS** Perhaps the most feared allergies to drugs fall under the classification of type I, or acute allergic reactions. These can be manifest by anaphylaxis as the most extreme example of allergic effects. Other less severe clinical manifestations of type I reactions include hives or urticaria, angioedema, bronchospasm, and laryngospasm. These reactions develop quickly (immediate reactions usually in minutes, but accelerated reactions may occur in up to 72 hours) after reexposure to the drug. The reaction is mediated by the release of a variety of vasoactive substances (kinins, leukotrienes, histamine, serotonin) from mast cells that are coated with immunoglobulin E or IgE (and sometimes IgG) antibody molecules. There must be more than one antibody molecule per cell, and they must be bridged by an antigen (allergen) having at least two haptens. Inhibition of the crosslinking of two IgE molecules can be attempted by administration of monovalent hapten, and deliberate desensitization can be initiated by administration of small but increasing doses of the drug. Treatment of the reaction is determined primarily by the severity of the reaction and ranges from simple observation and the passage of time (mild hives), to use of diphenhydramine to counteract moderate hives or mild bronchospasm, to an all-out effort at countering the event by using epinephrine, diphenhydramine, intravenous fluids, and possibly, corticosteroids (Assem 1985). The importance of preventing such reactions if at all possible is illustrated by the following case history.

**CASE HISTORY** *A 75-year-old man with severe angina was scheduled to undergo elective coronary artery bypass graft surgery. Several years earlier he had received oral penicillin for a local cellulitis and had developed mild anaphylaxis. Knowing this, the surgical team avoided prophylactic nafcillin before surgery and prescribed a cephalosporin in the induction room to prevent sternal wound infection. Within 4 minutes of beginning the rapid infusion, the patient developed hives, angioedema, bronchospasm, hypotension,* *and angina. Epinephrine and diphenhydramine were given promptly in appropriate doses, but the patient's hypotension persisted and resulted in ischemic changes shown by his ECG. He continued to complain of chest pain, then became unconscious and profoundly hypotensive. Despite his dire situation and the inability to stabilize his condition, the decision was made to proceed with his bypass surgery. He underwent general anesthesia, was placed on cardiopulmonary bypass, and completed a triple bypass. During the surgery, he required more than 20 liters of crystalloid to maintain his intravascular volume. His lungs became markedly edematous and stiff, and he developed profound diffuse edema. He could not be weaned off bypass at the end of the case, and died. At autopsy a large acute myocardial infarction (several hours old) was found.*

**Discussion** *There are several important and intriguing aspects to this case. First, the team did well to take a complete drug history and discover the patient's prior type I (acute, anaphylactic) reaction to penicillin. Such a history implies that the patient is at a greater than usual risk of developing a severe anaphylactic reaction if challenged again with penicillin. In patients with no prior history of such an allergic reaction, about 1:10,000 will develop a systemic type I reaction; this will be fatal in about 10% of cases (overall about 1:100,000). Mild urticarial reactions will occur in about 5% of patients who have no prior history of penicillin allergy, while about 10% of such patients will develop a morbilliform rash from ampicillin (Saxon et al. 1987). The occurrence rate of all of these changes are increased considerably (exact risk unknown) in patients who report a previous history of a type I reaction to penicillin.*

Since prior history of an allergic reaction to penicillin also increases the chances of subsequent allergic reactions to other drugs, and since cephalosporins are structurally similar to penicillins, such patients are at increased risk for developing type I reactions to cephalosporins as well. In this patient, if prophylactic antibiotics were to be used at all, an antistaphylococcal drug that is structurally different from penicillin, such as vancomycin, would have been preferable.

Two other points are important in this case. First, the danger from an anaphylactic reaction in this patient was greater than it would be in a younger, healthier patient. Although the proper drug therapy was initiated immediately after the reaction occurred by a skilled anesthesiologist, the initial episode of severe hypotension led to a large and ultimately fatal myocardial infarction. Second, consider why this patient developed such extensive angioedema. The lungs are an important organ in clearing autacoids from the blood. When the patient went on heart–lung bypass, blood flow to the lungs was greatly diminished. Hence, the vasoactive substances released during the anaphylactic reaction may not have been adequately cleared from the blood and may have contributed to the enormous extravasation of fluid during the surgical procedure.

For drugs such as streptokinase or penicillin, skin tests can help identify which patients are at higher risk for developing such reactions. For example, in patients who reported previous allergic reactions to penicillins, between 9 and 63% will develop positive reactions to skin tests with benzylpenicillin or the metabolite penicilloyl-polylysine. Of those who are skin-test negative, less than 1% will develop a systemic type I reaction on reexposure to penicillin within 24–72 hours. Of those patients with a positive reaction, perhaps two-thirds will develop a systemic acute reaction if reexposed (Saxon et al. 1987; Condemi 1986). For this drug, results of skin testing have useful positive and negative predictive values. Unfortunately, the utility of skin testing for other drugs has not been as well-established (VanArsdel and Larson 1989).

**TYPE II (CYTOTOXIC, AUTOIMMUNE) REACTIONS** In type II reactions, the drug (or drug hapten) induces the development of antibodies directed against the drug, a similar antigen on a cell, or an unrelated antigen in the patient. The antibody–allergen complex can recruit complement, leading to cell lysis and death. A common example of the first type is the hemolytic reaction induced in some patients by penicillin. The penicillin is bound to the erythrocyte membrane; antibodies then bind to the membrane-bound penicillin, recruit complement, and the "innocent" erythrocyte is harmed in the process. Since penicillin is essential for antibody binding and complement activation, hemolysis ceases as soon as the penicillin is cleared from the blood.

A slightly different reaction is seen with methyldopa-induced positive Coombs' reaction or hemolytic anemia. In this case, the drug "tricks" the body into developing antibodies against an antigen on the erythrocyte membrane. Although a positive Coombs' test is a relatively common occurrence (perhaps 30% of patients develop this while taking methyldopa), clinically significant hemolytic reactions are fortunately relatively rare (developing in less than 1% of patients receiving the drug). In this situation, the binding of antibody to antigen on the surface of the red blood cell can continue, even after all the methyldopa is cleared from the body.

Drug-induced systemic lupus erythematosus also appears to be a type II reaction. For some drugs such as hydralazine or procainamide, the chances of developing this drug allergy are increased in individuals with slow acetylation phenotype. Perhaps other subtle defects in the metabolism of the parent drug or a toxic metabolite eventually will be shown to be responsible for the development of this form of drug allergy, as seems to be true in patients with allergic responses to sulfa derivatives (Rieder et al. 1989).

**TYPE III (SERUM SICKNESS, IMMUNE COMPLEX) REACTIONS** These reactions were first observed years ago when horse serum containing horse antibodies (antiserum) was administered to patients with an infectious disease such as diphtheria. Since the horse serum contained foreign (horse) proteins, it was not surprising that many patients developed human antibodies to the horse proteins. The sickness that developed 7–14 days after the initial exposure to horse antiserum is known as serum sickness. Reexposure to the allergen resulted in onset of disease in just a few days because of an anamnestic response.

Serum sickness consists of a combination of general malaise, fever, rash, arthralgias, lymphadenopathy, hepatitis, and a peculiar serpiginous petechial rash, which develops along the lateral aspects of the palms and feet. The reaction develops as immune complexes between foreign proteins and human antibodies are formed in the circulation and then deposited in various tissues leading to end-organ damage. Other examples of this type of reaction appear to include drug-induced vasculitis and penicillin-induced serum sickness. Other names for this reaction include an Arthus reaction and immune-complex disease.

Serum sickness usually will gradually improve over several days as long as the offending drug is discontinued. In such situations, no other specific treatment is needed. Recognize the existence of this syndrome to administer appropriate therapy, as demonstrated in the following case.

**CASE HISTORY** *A 45-year-old man underwent elective open repair of a poorly healed tibial fracture. While recovering nicely at home 3 weeks after surgery, he developed classical symptoms of deep venous thrombophlebitis and pulmonary thromboembolism. He was admitted to his local hospital, where studies confirmed the presence of two segmental pulmonary emboli and an extensive clot in the deep venous system of his injured leg. His physicians elected to treat the patient over 48 hours with streptokinase, followed by intravenous heparin. All went well, and on the 4th day of heparin therapy (day 6 after admission), oral warfarin was begun. His heparin was discontinued on the 10th hospital day when his prothrombin time was controlled by warfarin. Plans were made for discharge on the 11th hospital day.*

*On the day of planned discharge, he developed fever, malaise, arthralgias, a macular rash, mild hepatitis, and a peculiar petechial rash on the lateral aspect of his feet and palms. Fearing an unusual reaction to warfarin, his physicians stopped that drug, reinstituted his heparin infusion, and transferred the patient to a university hospital. At the university hospital, his heparin was continued, and he was evaluated for placement of an inferior vena caval "umbrella" to prevent further episodes of pulmonary embolism, given his adverse reaction to his most recent drug, warfarin.*

**Discussion** *Although both warfarin and heparin can cause side effects other than simple bleeding (e.g., blue toes syndrome or thrombocytopenia, respectively), the reaction described in this patient is a classic case of serum sickness. This reaction had not been previously described following administration of either heparin or warfarin. Although the full syndrome had not been described following administration of streptokinase, each of the elements of the reaction had been described. In addition, streptokinase was a foreign protein given 11 days before the reaction occurred. Heparin seemed not to be involved since it had been restarted without worsening of the patient's syndrome. The decision was made to warn the patient not to use streptokinase again and to continue using heparin while reintroducing warfarin. This was done uneventfully, and the patient was able to be discharged home several days later. Interruption of the inferior vena cava was avoided by the prompt recognition of this drug allergy. No other specific treatment was indicated.*

**PRINCIPLE Sometimes the value of recognizing an adverse drug reaction or drug allergy is not that it leads to specific treatment, but that inappropriate, more toxic, or risky therapeutic procedures can be avoided.**

**TYPE IV (DELAYED-HYPERSENSITIVITY, CELL-MEDIATED) REACTIONS** The delay in onset of these immune-mediated reactions is related to the fact that they are mediated by sensitized lymphocytes rather than humoral antibodies. This is the type of reaction that is evaluated when certain intradermal skin tests are placed (e.g., mumps, candida, PPD [purified protein derivative of tuberculin]), or when a patient develops a delayed reaction to topical exposure to poison ivy. Drugs that can cause this type of delayed reaction include ethylenediamine (a solubilizing agent for drugs such as in aminophylline preparations) or its closely related derivative, ethylenediaminetetraacetic acid (EDTA), a preservative used in many topical and ophthalmic preparations.

**REACTIONS MIMICKING DRUG ALLERGY** Many reactions to drugs appear to be "allergic" in nature, but no firm evidence of involvement of the immune system has been uncovered. Skin rashes of various types ranging from a benign macular eruption to toxic epidermal necrolysis or erythema multiforme major can be caused by this type of reaction. Drug fevers are assumed to be caused by drug allergy, since they usually develop after days or weeks of therapy, develop almost immediately upon reexposure, are not dose-related, and are occasionally accompanied by eosinophilia. Direct involvement of the immune system, however, has not been documented (Mackowiak and LeMaistre 1987).

Drugs such as vancomycin and morphine can cause sudden itching and hypotension, probably caused by a direct release of histamine rather than drug allergy. Intravenous contrast agents, especially the ionic variety, can cause a reaction mimicking an anaphylactic reaction. Although these are called anaphylactoid reactions, they can be quite severe and are treated in the same fashion as true IgE-mediated anaphylactic reactions. Aspirin appears to cause an "allergic" reaction associated with hypotension and bronchospasm, particularly in patients with nasal polyposis and asthma. All of the NSAID agents can cause a similar reaction, apparently mediated by their shared ability to inhibit cyclooxygenase.

Many drug-induced cytopenias are mediated by drug-induced antibody formation against circulating cells or bone marrow precursors, whereas other similar reactions have not been linked to the development of specific antibodies. Drug-induced liver or renal disease can sometimes have the appearance of a drug allergy and can include peripheral eosinophilia, even though direct involvement of the immune system is hard or impossible to demonstrate. Phenothiazine- and halothane-induced hepatitis and methicillin-induced interstitial nephritis appear to be allergic reactions, although debate continues on this point. A variety of drug-induced interstitial pneumonitides, such as that caused by methotrexate, produce similar controversy.

In summary, allergies to medications represent a small percentage of total adverse drug reactions. Because they are not dose-dependent and not related to the pharmacologic effects of their respective drugs, they are viewed as being "idiosyncratic" or unpredictable. Nevertheless, a detailed drug history often will enable the physician to identify patients with known previous drug allergies or with an atopic history, making drug allergy in general more likely. Some allergic reactions can be avoided by taking a detailed history or using appropriate skin testing. Even when a drug allergy cannot be avoided, prompt recognition is essential to minimize its consequences and to avoid a new round of treatments for the "new disease."

**PRINCIPLE Rare events become important when they contribute to patient morbidity and mortality. Lack of predictability of occurrence does not lead to lack of responsibility for prompt recognition and management.**

## FACTORS THAT INHIBIT THE PRACTICE OF RATIONAL THERAPEUTICS

The approach to rational therapeutics outlined in the beginning of this Introduction should appear simple, reasonable, straightforward, and even self-evident! Nevertheless, it is clear that many therapeutic decisions are suboptimal and sometimes dangerous. What are the reasons for our failure as a profession to achieve optimal performance in the area of therapeutics?

One white paper concluded that mismedication of the elderly had become a critical health care issue (Kusserow 1989). The author described four ways in which mismedication could occur: 1) prescribing higher doses of a medication when lower doses would be equally effective and less toxic; 2) using more dangerous drugs when less toxic ones could achieve equivalent efficacy; 3) using a drug that was unnecessary; and 4) prescribing two or more medications that produce an unintended drug interaction. These errors can be compounded by an even more basic problem. Even if a house officer or attending physician has chosen an appropriate drug to prescribe, he or she frequently lacks the ability to write a coherent and complete prescription (Walson et al. 1981).

**SUMMARY**
**Common problems in drug prescribing include**

- **Prescribing an excessively high dose**
- **Prescribing more toxic drug than necessary**
- **Prescribing a drug that is unnecessary**
- **Prescribing a drug that produces a drug–drug interaction**
- **Prescription itself flawed or illegible**

These errors appear to be straightforward and avoidable. Most physicians probably feel that they rarely make such basic and fundamental errors in prescribing. We believe that there are a large number of additional factors that influence prescribers, both consciously and subconsciously, and thereby promote a situation in which irrational therapeutic decisions can become almost inevitable. An editorial discussing the problem of polypharmacy discussed several subtle causes of irrational prescribing leading to inappropriate polypharmacy (Kroenke 1985). These included patients with multiple complaints; multiple physicians prescribing without full knowledge of one another's behavior; prescribing by a physician to keep up with the latest fad; prescribing an older medicine out of habit; prescribing to satisfy the expectation of the patient; falsely generalizing the conclusions of a study; and salesmanship (external pressure) exerted by forces such as pharmaceutical companies (via drug detailing), by other physicians, or by the media. Others have commented on internal pressures or conflicts of interest experienced by physicians trying to conduct unbiased research (Healy et al. 1989). Similar types of conflicts of interest can interfere with the ability of physicians to prescribe in a scientific and unbiased fashion.

It might be useful to take another look at the six steps we presented earlier as the foundation of an approach to rational therapeutics. For each step, we will consider some of the more subtle factors that can work to prevent physicians from achieving their goal of practicing rational, objective, medically and scientifically sound therapeutics.

## 1. Knowing the Diagnosis with Reasonable Certainty

### *Problems encountered with empiric therapy*

Making a correct diagnosis seems logical and simple enough as the first step toward rational therapeutic decision making. Yet problems can be encountered even in responding to such a self-evident requirement. Consider the febrile leukemic patient, now neutropenic from chemotherapy, who is appropriately started on broad-spectrum antibiotics. Because the risks of not treating a real infection in such patients are so great, nearly all such patients are begun empirically on antibiotics, even though it is acknowledged that only a minority (perhaps as low as 37%) have a documentable infection during the course of their fever and neutropenia. Yet the very fact that definitive culture results usually are not available before treatment is started means that persistent or intermittent fever without diagnostic culture results would be the most likely course for such a patient. Such uncertainty in diagnosis creates strong pressure on the physician to broaden the spectrum of coverage, to use more antibiotics, and to use more expensive antibiotics (O'Hanley et al. 1989). In this study, an average of 4.9 antimicrobials were employed per course of treatment, with analysis indicating that the number of antibiotics employed correlated with apparent increased toxicity (especially renal and hepatic toxicity). Those patients who developed renal or hepatic toxicity from their antibiotics had a higher mortality rate than patients who did not develop such toxicity (39 vs. 7.5%).

Efforts to establish a firm diagnosis can also be more difficult than expected. For example, in the management of acute stroke, intracranial hemorrhage must be excluded by CT scan before administration of thrombolytic agents. In one recent study, however, only 17% of emergency physicians, 40% of neurologists, and 52% of radiologists achieved 100% sensitivity for identification of hemorrhage when asked to read a variety of CT scans. The authors of the study concluded that this level of sensitivity in identifying intracerebral hemorrhage by these physicians was not sufficient to permit safe selection of candidates for thrombolytic therapy (Schriger et al 1998).

**PRINCIPLE Failure (or inability) to establish a firm diagnosis makes therapeutic plans difficult, especially in critically ill patients. When empiric drug treatment (treatment initiated without a firm diagnosis) is necessary, it is even more important that data be carefully gathered and form the basis of sound therapeutic decisions.**

### *Inappropriate acceptance of empiric treatment*

The "rules" for treatment of febrile immunosuppressed patients (treat early, treat before a pathogen is identified, treat with multiple agents, use broad-spectrum coverage) often are generalized and applied to other populations of patients who do not have cancer, have not received chemotherapy, are not immunosuppressed, and are not neutropenic. The overuse of antibiotics for irrational indications has been documented repeatedly and appears to be an international problem (Moss and McNicol 1983). In fact, the causes of spiraling empiricism in the use of antibiotics, with its allure and perils, have been specifically addressed (Kim and Gallis 1989). Commonly, a surgical patient recovering nicely from an operation develops a low-grade temperature. Even before a thorough fever work-up is completed, antibiotics appropriate for the febrile neutropenic patient often are empirically begun. In fact, even though indicated, a rigorous fever work-up itself may not be attempted, since physicians have become so used to obtaining unrevealing cultures in the febrile neutropenic patient. This unreasonable analogy between treating different groups of patients with unrelated disease as if they were the same makes no sense at all. On the one hand, the danger is too great to withhold therapy from a neutropenic immunosuppressed febrile patient. But treating an otherwise normal postsurgical patient with modest fever and no neutropenia without the benefit of a diagnostic work-up (e.g., urinalysis, urine Gram stain, wound inspection, or chest x-ray), is to deny all knowledge of pathogenesis and toxicity of the misuse of antibiotics.

The necessity for initiating empiric treatment in neutropenic, febrile cancer patients has conditioned physicians to accept empiric therapy when it may be inappropriate. "Empiric" in this setting means using a drug within the setting of an uncertain diagnosis that, if it were correct, would be expected to produce efficacy. Empiric decisions like these can be tested for their validity by carefully describing the patient population that is considered for treatment, finding these patients, randomizing them into two groups, and giving one group the active drug. Thus, empiric therapeutic decisions can and should be subjected to our usual standards of "best available evidence."

Another example can help to demonstrate the efforts to employ best available evidence when making empiric decisions. Consider an immunosuppressed patient (perhaps receiving methotrexate) who develops a new cough, hypoxemia, and pulmonary infiltrates. The differential diagnosis (and possible empiric treatments) is long and includes drug reactions (possibly benefiting from steroids), typical bacterial pneumonia (requiring several antibiotics), atypical bacterial pneumonia (requiring erythromycin), mycobacterial pneumonia (requiring two antimycobacterial drugs), viral pneumonia (requiring acyclovir), pneumocystis pneumonia (requiring co-trimoxizole), fungal pneumonia (requiring amphotericin), interstitial pneumonitis, and so on. The physician may speak of employing a "shotgun" approach to empiric treatment when sputum samples have been nondiagnostic. Indeed, for nonneutropenic cancer patients with diffuse infiltrates, there is evidence that empiric treatment with co-trimoxizole plus erythromycin can be successful in up to 71% of such patients (Rubin et al. 1988). Neutropenic patients pose a larger problem, however, and for patients who fail to improve, an "adequate shotgun" can require ten barrels! In such a situation, the physician is likely to overestimate the risks of a diagnostic procedure (such as bronchial aspirate or lavage with transbronchial biopsy, or even open lung biopsy) and to underestimate the frequent success of bronchoscopy and open lung biopsy in providing a definitive diagnosis (Greenman et al. 1975; Masur et al. 1985; Stover et al. 1984; Cockerill et al. 1985). This error is compounded when the physician underestimates the risks of drug toxicity resulting from such an approach to empiric treatment.

**PRINCIPLE Even when an appropriate diagnostic test is available with acceptably low morbidity and mortality, empiric treatment may be chosen inappropriately because of the physician's failure to weigh adequately risks and benefits of alternative treatment strategies.**

### *Excessive fear of a trial of empiric treatment*

Although "empiricism" can provoke misgivings, the therapist should realize that data must be examined carefully to determine their value and that many therapeutic decisions will need to match specific clinical demands, even when pathogenesis and definitive diagnosis are not available. As was discussed earlier, the best available evidence from formal, clinical trials can cover well-defined patient groups, but perhaps not the specific patient sitting in the physician's office, with his or her specific features relating to age, gender, pregnancy, concomitant medical conditions, medications, previous ADRs or allergies, presence of renal compromise, and so on (Feinstein and Horwitz 1997).

Equally difficult can be the physician's decision as to when empiric treatment, absent a firm diagnosis, is the most appropriate route to take. Recall the patient presented earlier in the discussion of adverse drug reactions. This woman with rheumatoid arthritis developed totally asymptomatic and mild chemical hepatitis while receiving several drugs that can cause this syndrome. The diagnosis of a drug-induced hepatitis was not considered, and she underwent an aggressive, expensive, invasive, and unnecessary work-up to find out "what was really going on." Only after this work-up was completed was a diagnosis of drug-induced hepatitis entertained. For this patient, an early tentative diagnosis of an ADR would have led to the "empiric treatment" of drug withdrawal. The improvement of the hepatitis after discontinuing medications would have served to confirm that diagnosis. Thus, the desire to obtain a "real" diagnosis and to avoid empiric treatment actually worked to this patient's disadvantage.

**PRINCIPLE Aggressive, early, broad-spectrum empiric treatment before a diagnosis is made may be ei-**

**ther essential or foolish. Aggressive, invasive, and thorough efforts to establish a firm diagnosis before beginning treatment may be essential or foolish. The physician must consciously balance the risks and benefits of treatment and diagnostic studies in the dynamic state posed by the patient's disease and the unique interaction of features in each patient.**

## 2. Understanding the Pathophysiology of the Patient's Disease

### *Confusion between syndrome and disease*

Once the patient's disease is tentatively identified or established beyond a reasonable doubt, the physician should move directly to a relatively complete understanding of the pathophysiology of the disease process itself and thereby to an understanding of the possibilities for therapeutic intervention. One situation in which failure to understand the disease process leads to poor therapeutic decisions occurs when the disease diagnosed is really a syndrome that can result from several different pathophysiologic mechanisms.

Consider four patients with severe hyponatremia. The first patient with hyponatremia secondary to psychogenic polydipsia may respond best to treatment of the underlying psychiatric disorder plus restriction of excessive intake of free water. A second patient with a known bronchogenic carcinoma and hyponatremia secondary to inappropriate secretion of antidiuretic hormone (ADH) may respond best to simple fluid restriction, treatment of the underlying malignancy, or administration of a drug to block the effects of ADH on the kidney. A third patient with hyponatremia resulting from severe losses of salt and water, with some oral replacement with free water, may respond best to therapy with intravenous solutions of isotonic and hypertonic saline, as well as treatment of the underlying condition causing such losses. A fourth patient with adrenal insufficiency may require administration of salt and water, plus glucocorticoids and mineralocorticoids. In such hyponatremic patients, the understanding of the pathophysiology of the observed state of hyponatremia is paramount in selecting the most appropriate therapeutic option.

### *Being misled by a name*

Sometimes the name or presentation of the disease itself can fool the physician into misunderstanding both the underlying pathophysiology of the disease and the optimal therapeutic plan. A patient with systemic lupus erythematosus and a circulating "lupus anticoagulant" can present with a slightly prolonged prothrombin time. The name *lupus anticoagulant* and the abnormal prothrombin time can blind the physician to the fact that such patients are actually in a hypercoagulable state and therefore at increased risk for thromboembolic events. Thus the introduction of prophylactic, empiric, or therapeutic courses of heparin or warfarin can be delayed even when the clinical situation warrants their use.

### *Further advantages of understanding the disease*

At times, the proper understanding of the disease not only leads to appropriate therapeutic plans but also to appropriate preventive measures as well. For example, one of our hospitals recently experienced a cluster of patients with urinary tract infections caused by *Pseudomonas aeruginosa.* In this cluster of cases, the patients were all on the orthopedic service recovering from hip surgery. They had all had unremarkable urinalyses the day before surgery. The positive urine cultures were obtained on the fourth postoperative day as the Foley catheter was being removed. In each case, the resident correctly deduced that the infection was related to the presence of the Foley catheter and prescribed an appropriate oral antibiotic with excellent coverage of the pathogen.

A more rigorous consideration of the etiology of these cases, however, brought to light the fact that urinary catheters increase the risk of developing cystitis by facilitating entry of pathogens into the bladder along or through the catheter itself. *Pseudomonas aeruginosa* is a relatively uncommon pathogen for such infections, and the cluster of cases in time and space suggested a common vector. This more sophisticated approach to the disease eventually led to the discovery that one of the nurses on the ward responsible for catheter care was not washing her hands between patients and was spreading the organism from one patient to the next. In this situation, understanding the disease led to the most appropriate therapeutic response: a conference for the ward nurses, increased emphasis on hand-washing, and improved catheter care. Postoperative bladder infections in patients on the orthopedic service rapidly decreased with this therapeutic intervention. The few that did occur were caused mostly by *E. coli,* the usual pathogen in this situation.

**PRINCIPLE We should not be fooled into thinking that if we know the name of the patient's condition or disease, we fully understand its pathophysiology. A little time spent rigorously defining the most likely**

**pathophysiologic sequence in each patient will pay dividends in a more sophisticated and accurate approach to planning optimal therapeutic interventions.**

## 3. Understanding the Pharmacology of Possible Drugs

### *Drugs that lack scientific evidence of efficacy*

Drugs that can be used to treat a given disease should be determined by the pathophysiology of the disease process, as well as by solid and compelling data derived from rigorous clinical trials. For example, one could hypothesize that senile dementia or peripheral arterial insufficiency might improve if treated with cerebral or peripheral vasodilators, respectively. Although this might appear to be an attractive hypothesis, clinical studies have firmly established that such drugs are not useful for treatment of these two conditions. In the usual doses employed, such drugs have negligible ability to effect vasodilation in vessels fixed and narrowed by atherosclerosis. To the extent that they lower mean arterial pressure, vasodilators can even reduce flow to ischemic areas (Avorn et al. 1982).

The irrational prescribing of cerebral and peripheral vasodilators for such patients was examined more closely (Avorn et al. 1982). In a study of primary care physicians picked at random in the greater Boston area, 71% of the physicians believed that "impaired cerebral blood flow is a major cause of senile dementia," and 32% said that they found "cerebral vasodilators useful in managing confused geriatric patients." The most likely source of such misinformation was drug advertisements and pharmaceutical representatives, but not scientific papers. However, only 4% of these same physicians felt that drug advertisements were very important in influencing their prescribing, 20% felt that pharmaceutical detailing was very important, and 62% felt that scientific papers were very important. The authors of the study concluded that these data demonstrated a predominance of commercial rather than scientific sources of drug information, *even while the physicians themselves were not aware of their own personal sources of their information.* Of course, other sources of influence (patient preference, advice from colleagues, personal experience) could have led to this irrational prescribing as well. Nevertheless, the net result was an irrational choice of drug.

**PRINCIPLE When a physician believes a drug to be effective in the management of a disease despite strong scientific evidence to the contrary, this represents irrational prescribing. Nonscientific factors can and do influence physician prescribing even though the physician may be unaware of their presence and effect.**

### *Prescribing habits can be hard to break*

Physicians continue to have difficulty accepting the fact that some drugs lack demonstrated clinical efficacy, even though the rationale for their use is attractive. Consider the controversy about using an antiseizure medication to control new-onset seizures related to alcohol withdrawal in non-epileptic alcoholics. Patients who have experienced one such seizure related to alcohol withdrawal are at risk of sustaining further seizures during their course of detoxification. Phenytoin is an antiseizure medication with a wide spectrum of activity for a variety of seizure types. The hypothesis that administration of phenytoin to patients experiencing alcohol withdrawal seizures might reduce the chances of their sustaining further seizures is reasonable. Phenytoin has been used in this fashion for more than 20 years. Nevertheless, rigorous clinical studies have failed to demonstrate a significant benefit over placebo in the prevention of subsequent seizures in this specific situation (Alldredge et al. 1989). In addition, the toxicity of intravenous phenytoin (e.g., hypotension, arrhythmias) appears to outweigh the benefits of the drug for these patients.

**PRINCIPLE The temptation to treat for no other reason than "it makes sense" is very hard to resist, even in the face of strong evidence that contradicts the therapeutic strategy. Although the psychology of such behavior may be understandable, all the consequences are borne by the unfortunate patient.**

### *Factors that perpetuate false information about drugs*

The previous two examples demonstrate how irrational use of drugs can begin with a reasonable hypothesis that is not confirmed in subsequent rigorous clinical trials. Once such irrational drug therapy is begun, it can be perpetuated by nonscientific factors affecting the prescribing habits of physicians. Cluff summarized these nonscientific factors, which included the example of a teacher or respected peer, testimonials of colleagues, extrapolation to an incorrect situation from other clinical trials, convenience, persuasiveness of advertising, and availability of liberal samples (Cluff 1967). Thus prescribing habits lacking in scientific justification can be passed on from one generation of physicians to the next for years before such habits are scrutinized under the light of rigorous clinical trials.

---

**WARNING** Irrational prescribing habits can be perpetuated by

- Example of teacher or peer
- Testimonials from a colleague
- Generalizing results from one trial to a different group of patients
- Persuasive advertising
- Availability of free drug samples

---

## 4. Optimizing Selection of Drug and Dose

Once the physician has considered the pathophysiology of the patient's disease and has reviewed the therapeutic options, he or she must choose the *best* therapeutic plan for his or her particular patient. Using the concept of the "value compass" discussed earlier, this choice involves picking the drug and dose regimen designed to maximize the probability of producing clinical efficacy (and minimizing the probability of producing toxicity), to minimize total cost of treatment (including drug cost, monitoring cost, length of hospitalization), to maximize functional outcome, and to maximize patient overall satisfaction. Although this process sounds simple enough, it is probably the area in which the most possibilities exist for the physician to drift away from the path of rational therapeutics. The factors at work here range from several obvious ones to others that are so subtle that most physicians deny they are at work. In this short discussion, we can only mention briefly some of the most important factors involved.

### *The option of no drug treatment*

For many diseases ranging from viral pharyngitis or bronchitis, to occasional insomnia, to some lymphomas and to advanced cancer, there is a real possibility that no drug offers a probability of real benefit with acceptably low risk. In other words, no (drug) treatment may be the best treatment, along with discussion, reassurance, nonpharmacologic treatments (e.g., massage therapy for back pain), and palliation (e.g., treatment of cancer pain with adequate analgesics, even if no chemotherapy is indicated). The physician's prescribing of a medication, however, has taken on roles and connotations far beyond its simplest function of recommending a specific drug to the patient. The prescription itself has come to be viewed as an expected and essential transaction that formally concludes the exchange between the patient and the physician (Manasse 1989). The patient may feel that he or she has not gotten his or her money's worth unless a prescription is given. The physician may feel pressed to provide a prescription to keep the patient happy. In any case, writing a prescription can be quicker and simpler than taking time to explain to the patient why no drug is indicated for his particular problem, or in fact that prescribing a drug may actually decrease the total value of pharmacologic outcome, function, cost, and patient satisfaction.

### *Information about new drugs not provided by the manufacturer*

By the time a drug is approved by the FDA for marketing, a large amount of information about the drug has been provided by the company, reviewed by the FDA, and finally synthesized into the standard package insert familiar to all physicians who have read the *Physicians' Desk Reference.* Even this large amount of reviewed and approved information is incomplete and, in many ways, inadequate to permit the prescriber to make truly informed therapeutic decisions. This deficiency in information provided to prescribers has been briefly but elegantly described (Herxheimer 1987). Herxheimer points out that data comparing a new drug with older drugs of the same class is distinctly missing from the information provided by the manufacturer. The physician must look elsewhere (primary clinical trials, review articles, *The Medical Letter,* etc.) for such comparisons. In addition, although the FDA has already assessed a new drug for its likely therapeutic gain (and this information is publicly available from the FDA), the information is not distributed to the public or to physicians. Also, the data are not sufficient to allow optimal use of the drug for its known and inevitably unknown effects (see Chapter 27).

There are other gaps in the information provided to physicians as well. The physician likely will not know how the maximum dose was arrived at; what the dose–response curve looks like; or how safe the drug is likely to be in pregnant women, children, or the elderly (although this has been slowly changing and improving over the last few years). Warnings and adverse effects tend to be vague, nonquantitative, and difficult to transcribe into practical therapeutic strategies. The physician will likely not know exactly what to communicate to the patient as well. For older, established, commonly used drugs, patient information sheets are available from organizations such as the US Pharmacopeial (USP) Convention, from various software products, and from various disease-related patient support groups. The physician, however, usually acts alone when deciding what to tell the patient about a newer medication.

As a drug is used extensively, further clinical trials likely will be done to increase our knowledge of how to use the drug for new indications, or how to use the drug more wisely, or what adverse responses should be added to the list. For example, the "standard" target concentration of lithium for maintenance treatment of bipolar disorder has been 0.8 to 1.0 mmol/L, while concern about the drug's toxic effects has led some physicians to aim for a lower target concentration of lithium. Only recently has a clinical trial been conducted that clearly shows that the risk of relapse was 2.6 times higher among patients in the low-range group (median level 0.54 mmol/L) than in the standard-range group (median 0.83 mmol/L) (Gelenberg et al. 1989). Although adverse effects were more common in the standard-range group as well, this type of study makes it easier for the thoughtful physician to choose an optimal target dose and plasma concentration.

Finally, experience produces new and more accurate information about other types of therapy as well as drug therapy. For example, early reports about the benefits and risks of carotid endarterectomy described experiences in centers with demonstrated excellence and found 30-day mortality rates of 0.1 to 0.6%. Once this therapeutic procedure began to be performed more routinely, perioperative mortality rates ranged from 1.4% (at trial hospitals) to 2.5% (in non-trial hospitals conducting few procedures of this kind) (Wennberg et al. 1998). Thus, the practicing physician must use caution in translating data about efficacy and safety of various therapies from carefully controlled trials to every-day clinical practice.

### *Increasing knowledge of a drug's adverse effects*

As discussed in Chapter 27, when a new drug is approved by the FDA, it may have been used in only several thousand patients (or even fewer if the drug is on a "fast track.") Therefore, the likelihood of identifying infrequent adverse effects (<1:100 times the drug is given) before approval is low. It is not commonly appreciated, however, that new adverse effects can be noted in "old" drugs that have been in use for years.

For example, phenobarbital has been used in children with new-onset febrile seizures. The patients were at increased risk of sustaining subsequent seizures. Although some reports surfaced concerning possible behavioral and cognitive side effects of the drug, it remained commonly used for this indication. A recent placebo-controlled trial demonstrated that after 2 years, the mean IQ in the group assigned to phenobarbital was 8.4 points lower than in the placebo group. A trend toward lower IQ in the treatment group persisted even 6 months after the drug was discontinued. Finally, the study failed to demonstrate any benefit of reduced risk of subsequent seizures in the treated group (Farwell et al. 1990). For this drug used for this indication, a well-performed study documented significant toxicity that was not balanced by any measurable efficacy.

A case–control study was performed to assess the risk of hip fracture being associated with the use of four classes of psychotropic drugs (Ray et al. 1987). Although patients treated with short-acting hypnotics had no measurable increased risk of hip fracture, those patients who received long-acting hypnotics (odds ratio 1.8), tricyclic antidepressants (odds ratio 1.9), and antipsychotics (odds ratio 2.0) were at increased risk. The additional risk associated with these classes of drugs appeared to be dose-related as well. Although such a case–control study cannot prove a causal relationship, it suggests the possibility that these classes of drugs increase the risk of hip fractures in elderly patients, possibly because of their sedative or hypotensive effects, or perhaps because of more subtle effects on balance.

**PRINCIPLE Even when a drug has been used for years for recognized indications, we should not be surprised when new data surface documenting a new form of drug-induced toxicity. In fact, it is likely that increased experience with a drug will not only lead to new indications for the drug's use, but also provide data that older indications may not be justified.**

### *Does the cost matter?*

For some patients, the cost of a prescription probably is not a factor in determining whether the patient will fill the prescription. The frequent stories of patients angrily calling their physicians to complain about the cost of their most recent prescription, however, suggest that cost actually can be a concern (Babington et al. 1983). Many physicians are surprised when patients call them about cost, since the physician may have no idea what the price of a prescription really is.

There is good evidence that the out-of-pocket cost for prescriptions can make an important difference in patient compliance. One study compared patterns of patient behavior in filling prescriptions for 16 different drugs in two states, New Hampshire and New Jersey (Soumerai et al. 1987). In New Hampshire, the state Medicaid program began a new policy of limiting patients to three paid prescriptions per month. This policy resulted in a drop of 30% in the number of such prescriptions filled, while no change was observed in the comparison state. In the elderly patients taking multiple drugs, the number of prescriptions filled per month fell from an average of 5.2 to 2.8 drugs. Although much of this decrease was accounted for by a drop in "ineffective drugs," decreases in the purchases of "essential" medications such as insulin and diuretics also were observed. The next year, New Hampshire changed its policy by replacing the three-prescription cap with a $1 copayment policy. Prescriptions increased to almost pre-cap levels for most drugs. Savings to Medicaid on drug costs were comparable under both policies.

**PRINCIPLE Cost-reduction strategies can be similar in the amount of money saved, but different in their effect on particular patients. Also, in certain patient populations, the cost of filling a prescription definitely affects patient compliance to having the prescription filled.**

Many, perhaps most, patients will pay directly for prescription costs, although this is changing with increasing patient participation in health-care plans that cover outpatient prescription costs. One study of 54 residents in internal medicine and primary care medicine documented that residents had poor estimates of the actual prices of drugs. Their total mean percent deviation from actual drug price was about 63%. Surprisingly, even when the residents were given a price guide booklet, their exposure to this pricing information did not improve the residents' knowledge of drug costs (Babington et al. 1983). A different study asked medical students, pediatric residents, and pediatricians to evaluate the cost of commonly prescribed medications (Weber et al. 1986). Their estimates were considered adequate in only 40, 52, and 62% of the cases, respectively. In most situations, the adequacy of these estimates did not appear to improve with the length of training of the physician.

These data suggest that when physicians try to pick an optimal drug for a given patient, the price of the medication and the patient's ability to pay for the medication should be important factors to be considered. The impression of some observers that many physicians do not understand the cost of the therapies they are recommending, however, seems to be justified.

### *Anticipation of drug interactions*

Earlier in this Introduction and again in Chapter 30, detailed discussions of the mechanisms and incidence of drug interactions have been included. The physician must consciously think about the possibility of initiating an adverse drug interaction whenever a drug is added or subtracted from a patient's total drug regimen. This deliberate step should form a conscious part of the decision to pick the best drug (and dose) for the individual patient.

For example, consider a patient already receiving warfarin who requires a sedative-hypnotic agent. A benzodiazepine would be preferable to a barbiturate given the former's equal efficacy, decreased toxicity, and decreased probability of altering the clearance (and thereby steady-state concentration) of warfarin.

One study indicated that physicians' prescribing of new drugs frequently leads to potential or real drug interactions (Beers et al. 1990). In a survey of 424 randomly selected adults seeking care at a university-affiliated hospital emergency department, 47% of visits led to the addition of one or more new medications. In 10% of the visits in which one or more medications was added, a new medication produced the potential for an adverse interaction that was of real clinical importance. The best predictor of whether a potential interaction would be introduced was the number of medications used by the patient at the time of presentation to the emergency room. Perhaps most discouraging, a medication history was recorded for every patient at admission to the emergency room (presumably by an admitting nurse) and was available to the treating physician. The treating physician, however, did not routinely screen for potential drug interactions.

**PRINCIPLE Prescribing physicians should not only have a knowledge base that allows them to anticipate probable drug interactions, but should also have an attitude that encourages them to anticipate the possible effects of any change they make in a patient's drug regimen. In an ideal world, each physician would have immediate access to a computer program that could screen for potential drug–drug interactions in real time, as the physician is writing the prescription. Several software products are now available that can accomplish exactly this task on the physician's personal computer, or on a hospital computer information system available to all prescribers.**

### *Irrational physician beliefs*

Although physicians like to believe that scientific data form the basis for their therapeutic decisions, there are several nonscientific sources of information that can affect a physician's prescribing habits, even when he or she is not aware of them (Avorn et al. 1982). Physician "attitudes" can be even more important than physician "beliefs" in determining prescribing habits (Epstein et al.

1984). Beliefs or attitudes are often influenced by nonscientific factors.

In an editorial, Burnham describes fads and fashions in medical science, and many of the examples focus on the influence of fads on prescribing habits (Burnham 1987). For example, the media hype in 1978 promoting the release of the new NSAID Clinoril (sulindac) led to a flurry of patient demands for the new wonder drug; a similar media blitz with the intended patient demand was associated with the release of Oraflex (benoxaprofen); and all of this was before pharmaceutical companies began advertising prescription drugs on national television. What can account for the fact that Atarax is usually prescribed for itching and Vistaril for nausea, even though they both contain the same active ingredient (hydroxyzine)? Burnham points out that therapies and, even diagnoses, come in and out of fashion, often for no clear or rational reason. He concludes that "Medical fashions have a powerful effect on how we treat, whom we treat, and what we treat, on how patients take care of themselves, and even on the directions of medical science. It shames me to admit that I have given fashion a say in my treatment of patients. . . . The lines are drawn. Which shall it be, science or fashion? Let each decide."

There are attempts to unravel the factors accounting for large differences in practice patterns. Rates of hospitalization for children for illnesses such as asthma or for toxic ingestions and rates for surgical procedures such as hysterectomy can vary widely from county to county, or city to city (Perrin et al. 1989; Wennberg and Gittelsohn 1982; Wennberg and Cooperman 1998). Some think that the amount and cost of hospital care for patients in a community can have more to do with factors such as the number of physicians, their specialties, their preferred procedures, and the number of hospital beds available than with the health status or needs of the residents (Wennberg and Gittelsohn 1982). In modern American medicine, the powerful gatekeeper role of the HMO can play an even more dramatic role in deciding "who shall receive."

Similar differences in physician choices for medical therapy also are evident. For example, physicians confronting similar nonrheumatic patients with chronic atrial fibrillation make different decisions concerning whether or not to give their patients anticoagulant. In one study, physicians with different training (family physicians, general internists, and cardiologists) behaved similarly when confronted with patients with either mitral valve disease or a history of chronic alcohol abuse, but behaved differently when confronted with other patients in atrial fibrillation (Chang et al. 1990). It was found that a physician's treatment decision was strongly related to his or her assessment of the relative risk of embolism versus hemorrhage derived for each case. Cardiologists were least likely to initiate chronic anticoagulation (they judged the risk of embolism to be lower), while family practitioners were most likely to institute anticoagulation (they judged the risk of embolism to be higher). Although these groups of physicians differed in their assessment of the risk of hemorrhage, in fact, none of the groups' estimates of the risk of embolization was close to the best estimate published in recent literature.

When "local" prescribing patterns seem out of step with generally accepted and validated prescribing practices, nonmedical (nonscientific) factors may be playing a role. Several such examples were provided in a study of drug prescribing by a Yugoslavian pediatric service (Stanulovic et al. 1984). For example, an unexpected reduction in the appropriate use of penicillin was triggered by two recent patient deaths thought to be caused by procaine penicillin G-induced rhabdomyolysis. Less effective or more toxic drugs were used in place of penicillins.

**PRINCIPLE Although a physician's recent personal experience is important, it can lead to the physician's overestimating the frequency of his or her most recently recognized adverse drug reaction and underestimating what he or she has not seen recently.**

### *Detailing and counter-detailing*

One source of influence leading to irrational or nonscientific prescribing by physicians is unbalanced, inaccurate, or frankly misleading information provided by pharmaceutical companies in written advertisements or in person in the form of the pharmaceutical detail worker, or manufacturer's representative ("drug rep"). Apparently, the pharmaceutical industry spends about $5000 per year per physician on detailing activities designed to acquaint physicians with specific drug products and to encourage their prescription (Silverman and Lee 1974; Wall Street Journal 1984; Soumerai and Avorn 1990). This amount is more than half of the money spent each year on drug promotion, which also includes activities such as journal advertising, direct mail, free samples, conventions, and so on. "Drug detailing" and advertising can cause physicians to change their beliefs and prescribing habits, even when they are not aware of the impact of the advertising or detailing itself, and even when the physician denies the importance of such factors in his or her therapeutic decisions (Avorn et al. 1982).

The visit of the "drug rep" is often accompanied by the leaving of reprints from drug studies, often published as symposium proceedings. Such reprints, however, can be difficult for the physician to interpret. In one recent analysis of drug studies published in symposium proceedings, the investigators found that articles in symposia sponsored by single drug companies were similar in quality and clinical relevance to articles with other types of sponsors and to articles published in the parent journals. Articles with drug company sponsorship, however, were more likely than articles without drug company support to have outcomes favoring the drug of interest (Cho and Bero 1996).

This subtle and effective combination of printed advertisements and personal contact during visits from detail workers can be difficult to counteract or reverse. Several investigators have explored educational strategies that have various degrees of success. In one study of three educational methods designed to improve antibiotic prescribing in office practice, a mailed brochure had no detectable effect; a drug educator had only a modest effect; but personal visits by a physician produced strong attributable changes in prescribing behavior (Schaffner et al. 1983). This beneficial effect was seen with respect to improving the quality of care and to reducing its cost.

A second study also demonstrated improved therapeutic decisions achieved through educational outreach programs termed "academically based detailing" (Avorn and Soumerai 1983). In this study, two separate interventions for physicians (compared with a control group) were used in an effort to reduce the excessive use of three groups of drugs. Physicians who received only mailed printed materials did not reduce their prescribing of the target drugs relative to control physicians. Those who received a series of mailed "unadvertisements" along with personal educational visits by specially trained clinical pharmacists, however, reduced their prescribing of the target drugs by 14% as compared with control physicians. (Given the target drugs chosen, it was assumed that patients benefited from these changes in prescription habits.) In a subsequent report, the same authors enumerated some of the key factors that make such "academic detailing" successful (Soumerai and Avorn 1990). "Counter-detailing" activities, however, will likely never keep pace with industry-sponsored detailing. The industry has much greater experience and larger budgets for these educational purposes!

### *Physician conflicts of interest*

Although well-intentioned physicians can be influenced without their knowledge by nonscientific arguments made by pharmaceutical companies, an even more subtle but effective process also is occurring that may be causing irrational prescribing, again without the physician's awareness. There is increasing evidence that physicians' decisions concerning which drug to prescribe for a given patient may be increasingly affected by unrecognized conflicts of interest on the part of the physician/prescriber. One physician has framed the problem as follows: "The charge against us is that, in many of our dealings with the industry, we have become corrupt: that in return for needlessly (and sometimes recklessly) prescribing their expensive products, we accept (or even demand) rewards on a breathtaking scale" (Rawlins 1984). When challenged with this idea, most physicians believe that *they* are not affected by promotional activities and that they can receive gifts from drug companies without prescribing that company's products. These earnest denials of conflict of interest may be sincere but incorrect. "The degree to which the profession, mainly composed of honourable and decent people, can practise such self-deceit is quite extraordinary" (Rawlins 1984).

It is tempting to view such harsh judgments as extreme, biased, or inaccurate. Nevertheless, serious work has lent credibility to such statements. Doctors accept gifts from pharmaceutical companies in many forms, often without recognizing the general rule that accepting a gift has complex practical and ethical repercussions (Chen et al. 1989). In an interesting analysis of doctors receiving gifts from drug companies, the authors also point out that such gifts cost patients money and are likely to influence the way society perceives our profession. Most physicians do not realize that by accepting a gift, they incur an obligation to reciprocate in some way. In an extreme situation, physicians may substantially alter their prescribing practices in order to obtain additional free gifts such as free airline tickets, money, paid trips or vacations, and so on (Wilkes and Shuchman 1989). In recent years, when the FDA became increasingly concerned about distinguishing industry promotional from educational activities, the pharmaceutical companies have developed more subtle methods for blending the two.

Such potential and real conflicts of interest have led to the interesting situation in which most physicians maintain that they can accept gifts without becoming biased, whereas several organizations have proposed new guidelines for physician–industry relationships. The Royal College of Physicians proposed that "The overriding principle is that any benefit in cash or kind, any gifts, any hospitality or any subsidy received from a pharmaceutical company must leave the doctor's independence of judgment manifestly unimpaired. When it comes to the margin between what is acceptable and what is unacceptable, judgment may sometimes be difficult: a useful criterion of acceptability may be 'Would you be willing to have these arrangements generally known?' " (Royal College of Physicians 1986). The American College of Physicians (ACP) also felt compelled to issue a position paper concerning the relationship of physicians to the pharmaceutical industry. The ACP was concerned that physicians' receiving excessive or inappropriate gifts impairs public confidence in the integrity of the profession and could compromise the physicians' clinical judgment. The College's primary position was similar to that advocated by its English counterpart, namely, that a useful criterion in determining which activities are acceptable is, would the physician be willing to have such arrangements generally known? (Goldfinger 1990).

Another physician activity that can produce an inherent conflict of interest occurs when physicians sell prescription drugs to their patients at a profit. A bill in the US Congress dealt with this issue, and an editorial posed both sides of the argument (Relman 1987). This is yet another activity in which physician conflict of interest can lead to irrational and suboptimal prescribing.

**PRINCIPLE A physician will have difficulty putting the patient's welfare first and practicing rational therapeutics when he or she consciously or unconsciously has a vested and material interest in which drug is prescribed. Such real and potential conflicts of interest can not only undermine the doctor–patient relationship, but can also undermine public confidence in the profession.**

## 5. Selecting and Following Appropriate Endpoints

### *Appropriate endpoints of efficacy*

When the physician prescribes a new drug, what endpoints should he or she pick to see if the drug is working? In some situations, perhaps the patient should help the physician pick the most appropriate endpoints to follow. For example, a study of the use of methotrexate (MTX) in rheumatoid arthritis demonstrated statistically significant but clinically small (5 to 11%) differences in patients treated with MTX versus placebo with respect to standard measures of physical, social, and emotional function (Tugwell et al. 1990). Yet when patients specified in advance a set of measurements that best described the functions they most wanted the treatment to improve, patients receiving MTX fared about 29% better than patients receiving placebo.

This type of study suggests that although endpoints for certain drugs can be easily picked by the physician (e.g., the prothrombin time in the patient receiving warfarin), in some situations, a combination of endpoints of efficacy must be chosen on the basis of discussions between the patient and the physician. Even a "simple" endpoint of efficacy, however, can turn out to be more difficult to use wisely than expected. Consider the monitoring of the prothrombin time mentioned previously. How often is a medical student told to start a patient on warfarin and then simply to follow the PT result as if that were a simple-minded task? Several clinical studies have suggested that the intensity of anticoagulation in the treatment of patients with proximal-vein thrombosis (Hull et al. 1982) or mechanical prosthetic heart valves (Saour et al. 1990) can be lower than originally believed with equal efficacy and less toxicity. In addition, it now appears that different intensities of anticoagulation are required for different underlying thromboembolic conditions (e.g., prophylaxis during hip surgery, treatment of thrombophlebitis, prevention of embolism in patients with cardiac dysfunction, prevention of thrombus formation in patients with prosthetic heart valves). One study demonstrated that very low doses of warfarin (1 mg per day) can help prevent thrombosis in patients with central venous catheters, even though the prothrombin time was not prolonged at all (Bern et al. 1990). In addition, the prothrombin time itself has changed over the years as there has been growing international standardization of the thromboplastin reagents used in the assay itself.

**PRINCIPLE Choosing appropriate endpoints of efficacy may not be straightforward but should be done prospectively as often as possible. Targets and goals can change as our understanding of the disease or the drugs change over time. Patients may stress endpoints related to cost, functional status, or overall satisfaction, even as physicians traditionally select endpoints related to pharmacologic effect and quantitative evidence of reduction in the severity of illness.**

### *Endpoints reflecting toxicity*

Physicians commonly recognize the occurrence of an adverse drug reaction, even if they do not report it (Koch-Weser et al. 1969; Rogers et al. 1988). It is less clear how often physicians fail to see an ADR even when it occurs. Since most drugs can cause a wide variety of adverse effects, it is difficult for the physician to consider them all and look for them all. For example, many physicians prescribing an NSAID will remember to ask the patient about GI symptoms during subsequent visits but not think to check for the development of renal toxicity, which appears to be more common than is generally appreciated (Whelton et al. 1990; Murray and Brater 1990). Even more worrisome, a recent study with standardized patients revealed that while NSAID-related gastropathy was correctly diagnosed in 93% of patient visits, it was acceptably managed in only 77% of visits (Tamblyn et al. 1997).

Physicians prescribing an aminoglycoside may think to follow the patient for the development of nephrotoxicity but fail to ascertain the development of cochlear or vestibular ototoxicity. Physicians must understand the most likely toxic effects of a drug, must develop a plan to follow the patient to see whether those adverse reactions develop, and must recruit the patient's help and cooperation in carrying out the plan. Whether the patient and physician follow a symptom, a physical finding, the result of a special test, or a laboratory value, following a patient for the development of toxic effects can be a thought-provoking and major clinical undertaking.

### *The prescription as an experiment*

Perhaps 75% of all office visits to a physician end with one or more new prescriptions (Soumerai et al. 1990). Although the writing of the prescription may terminate the office visit, it only serves to begin a new experiment for each patient. There is no certainty that the desired pharmacologic effect will occur. Undesired pharmacologic, immunologic, or idiosyncratic reactions—drug toxicity—also can occur. Thus, the prescription represents the beginning of an experiment that can last for hours (e.g., one dose of subcutaneous terbutaline) or years (chronic daily use of penicillamine). The physician must pick appropriate endpoints of drug efficacy and lower limits of acceptable toxicity and must follow those endpoints over the course of the experiment. The appropriate endpoints should take into account patient preferences, common reactions, and less common but potentially severe or threatening reactions.

**PRINCIPLE Only when the physician approaches each drug prescription as the beginning of a therapeutic experiment of uncertain outcome, and not as a concluding act to an office visit, will the chances that the experiment will be as safe, effective, and productive as possible be maximized.**

## 6. The Therapeutic Alliance Between Physician and Patient

### *Do physicians listen to their patients?*

How can the relationship between the prescribing physician and the patient be improved so that it results in a contract or bond that is maximally satisfying for both parties, and also is most likely to produce therapeutic "experiments" in which efficacy strongly outweighs toxicity? This relationship, or therapeutic alliance, is a complicated one because it is dynamic, reciprocal, and constantly evolving (Kaplan et al. 1989). The patient–physician relationship has been extensively examined and discussed by many, and interesting contradictions have been observed. The patient may desire to tell a physician about a particular problem, but the physician feels he or she is too busy to listen carefully to the patient (Baron 1985). The patient comes seeking advice and guidance, but the physician does not ask about or ignores patient preferences in making difficult choices between therapeutic options. The overall failure of physicians to listen attentively to their patients has been blamed on the high technology, science, and language of modern medicine. Others have pointed out that the apparent dichotomy between science and humanism in medicine is a false dichotomy; an inclusive scientific model for medicine must acknowledge the science of the human domain as well (Engel 1987). Other forces can disrupt the patient–physician bond as, for example, the current pattern of physician remuneration tends to reward doing things to patients rather than talking with and thinking about them (Almy 1980).

### *Patient–physician communication can affect choice of therapy and outcome*

It is becoming increasingly clear that there is a relationship between the way patients and physicians behave and communicate during an office visit and a patient's subsequent health status (Greenfield et al. 1985; Kaplan et al. 1989). The failure of physicians to communicate adequately with their patients causes many problems. One of the largest is noncompliance by the patient, which in various studies has ranged from 10 to 95% (Bond 1990). Although there are many reasons for patient noncompliance, some are related to suboptimal communication between the physician and patient. Even if the physician takes time in the office to educate the patient about medications, perhaps 50% of the statements made about the medication are quickly forgotten by the patient (Bond 1990). Results of patient noncompliance can range from minor to severe. For example, one study found that patients who had recently stopped using their beta-blockers had a transient fourfold increase in the relative risk of angina and myocardial infarction (Psaty et al. 1990). Compliance can be very low even when patients have potentially curable malignant disease (Levine et al. 1987).

Patient compliance, and even outcomes of chronic disease, are positively correlated with certain types of physician–patient communication (Kaplan et al. 1989). After analysis of communication patterns during office visits (according to three broad categories of control, communication, and affect), better patient health status was positively related to more patient and less physician control; more affect (positive or negative) expressed by physician and patient; and more information provided by the physician in response to patient questions.

**SUMMARY**
**Health status and compliance are related to**

- **Greater patient control during the office visit**
- **More affect expressed by the physician**
- **More information provided by the physician in response to the patient's questions**

Although both patient and physician share responsibility for the contract between them, physicians sometimes stop listening to patients before a correct diagnosis has been made, or even before the patient has had time to present his or her chief complaint. The physician may fail to learn enough about the patient and his or her medications to know what the best medication (and dose) might be for managing newly presented problems. The physician might fail to elicit patient input in the process of choosing the best treatment, which could be medical, surgical, or no treatment at all. Work analyzing therapeutic options for men with symptomatic prostatism revealed several things. There are wide differences in the way different physicians treat the problem (the frequency of prostate operations varies from city to city by a factor of four), and there is little scientific evidence to show that one treatment is clearly superior to another in terms of life expectancy (Fowler et al. 1988; Wennberg and Gittelsohn 1982). Ultimately, the "right" therapeutic option is the one chosen by the patient after he has been informed of the relative risks and benefits of each approach (watchful waiting, transurethral prostatectomy). Perhaps the physician's most important role in such a situation is to help educate the patient with respect to the risks and benefits of each therapeutic option. The efficacy of innovative patient education adjuncts such as interactive videodisc programs (Faltermayer 1988) has been explored, and more conventional educational videotapes are now available in doctors' offices and pharmacies on a variety of medical topics.

An intact and dynamic patient–physician bond is necessary for the physician to have the greatest chance of making an accurate diagnosis, and for the patient and physician jointly to select an optimal therapeutic plan. When the patient or physician does not uphold his or her end of the relationship, all kinds of mistakes can be made. When a series of small errors escalates into a major adverse outcome, the breakdown in the process has been termed an adverse medical cascade.

## FINAL COMMENTS

### The Adverse Medical Cascade

At first blush, it would appear that small errors in physician communication with patients, or errors in clinical logic, should not result in large, potentially fatal errors. In certain situations triggered by a relatively minor event, however, "both patient and physician may become helpless victims of a frustrating, uncontrollable, runaway situation, leading to a course of progressively riskier and costlier interventions that seem simultaneously unnecessary and unavoidable" (Ober 1987). One case serves to illustrate this phenomenon, which has been termed the medical cascade effect (Ober 1987; Mold and Stein 1986).

**CASE HISTORY** *A 71-year-old woman with chronic hypertension and normal renal function was begun on captopril, which resulted in excellent control of her blood pressure. Weeks later, she developed a mild case of cystitis that was treated successfully with an oral antibiotic. During that episode, her BUN and creatinine were measured and found to be elevated to 72 and 3.6 mg/dL, respectively. Her captopril was stopped because her physician suspected the presence of an ADR; in addition, he ordered an ultrasound to assess renal size. That study revealed kidneys of normal size and a 4.0 × 4.5-cm abdominal aortic aneurysm that had been totally asymptomatic. The patient was transferred to a university hospital for further evaluation. A review of systems obtained by an intern was positive for leg claudication and orthopnea; an admission EKG revealed an old anteroseptal myocardial infarction.*

*Her BUN and creatinine returned to normal over the next few days. A femoral aortogram could not be completed because of severe atherosclerosis involving the femoral artery; an aortogram obtained via a translumbar approach confirmed a 4.5-cm aneurysm beginning just below the renal arteries, with bilateral renal artery stenosis. A nephrologist felt that surgery to correct the renal artery lesions was not indicated, since the patient's BUN and creatinine had returned to normal. If a repair of the aneurysm were to be attempted, however, then the renal arteries could be repaired at the same time. The surgical team decided the patient should undergo an elective repair of the aortic aneurysm. The surgery was complicated by postoperative shock marked by a low cardiac output and extremely high systemic vascular resistance. Ultimately, the patient developed multiple organ system failure and died from infarction of her entire bowel.*

**Discussion** *This case illustrates a pattern of events that characterizes an adverse medical cascade. A series of unfortunate medical decisions escalates into a disastrous situation that seems to proceed because of an apparently unstoppable momentum. More than 30 years ago, this process was recognized and described as follows, "The disseminated or metastatic form of iatrogenic disease is not an uncommon occurrence, although rarely talked or written about" (Seckler and Spritzer 1966).*

*A variety of factors can help to cause or perpetuate such a cascade; many of these factors are visible in this case. The physician may fail to obtain a complete or accurate database, or may make an error in analyzing the data. Faulty reasoning can lead to misuse or overuse of diagnostic tests. One educator observed that clinical reasoning ". . . has become not a systematic exercise in deductive logic, but a rapid reflex arc that begins with a few perfunctory observations at the bedside, and ends with a profound list of entries in the nurse's order book" (Feinstein 1967). Often there is a tendency for the physician to underestimate the risks of diagnostic tests or of treatment. For example, one risk of doing an unnecessary ultrasound of the kidneys is discovering an unsuspected abdominal aortic aneurysm; the risk of surgical repair in this woman with extensive atherosclerotic disease was underestimated. It is also common for the physician to overestimate the risks of not performing diagnostic tests or a surgical procedure, or to order or use a test in a way for which it was not intended. For example, there were minimal risks to stopping the patient's captopril and watching to see if the elevated BUN and creatinine improved.*

*The surgical team was aware of the fact that the mortality of performing elective repairs of such aneurysms has been dropping steadily over the past 30 years (Thompson et al. 1975; Hicks et al. 1975). The team likely overestimated the risk of mortality from rupture of the aneurysm itself, since the mortality rate for aneurysms between 4 and 6 cm in diameter is about 25%; overall prognosis is related to the size of the aneurysm and the severity of coexistent coronary artery and cerebral vascular diseases; and patients who avoid dying from rupture of the aneurysm are likely to succumb to coronary heart disease or stroke (Dzau and Creager 1994). The presence of severe atherosclerotic heart disease both increases the risk of performing the surgery and decreases the probability of 5-year survival significantly. In such patients with extensive atherosclerotic heart disease and small, asymptomatic aneurysms, analysis of risks and benefits of surgery suggests that it may be best to follow the patient with serial ultrasound examinations and to perform surgery only if symptoms occur, or if there is a significant increase in the size of the aneurysm (Dalen 1987). In retrospect, this patient would certainly have done better had the asymptomatic aneurysm never been discovered. Possibly, the patient was not given all of the relevant facts and thus, was unable to make a fully informed decision about whether or not to proceed with an elective repair of her abdominal aortic aneurysm.*

Insecurity on the part of the patient or family, physician, or consultant can lead to the ordering of more tests, each with its own additional burden of cost and toxicity. Threat of a law suit for a "missed" diagnosis can cause similar effects. In a university hospital with multiple attendings, consultants, residents, cross-covering teams, and so on, a situation can develop in which no one really understands the patient and no one is really in charge of developing a rational diagnostic and therapeutic plan. As was observed years ago, ". . . when the patient offers a puzzling problem to his medical attendant, who, in turn, is backed by a galaxy of specialists, certain events are almost unavoidable. Foremost among them is the 'collusion of anonymity.' Vital decisions are taken without anybody feeling fully responsible" (Balint 1957).

**PRINCIPLE The processes that cause or perpetuate an adverse medical cascade are negative reflections of the positive processes that comprise rational therapeutics.**

In a medical cascade, some or all of the six key steps that characterize a thoughtful therapeutic plan are perverted, leading to a situation in which the chances of a beneficial therapeutic outcome are minimized, whereas the probability of toxicity is maximized. Thus, an adverse medical cascade is an extreme example of how well-intended actions on the part of the physician can lead to adverse, even disastrous, therapeutic outcomes.

## Quality in Pharmacotherapeutics

Good physicians continually strive to optimize the quality of the pharmacotherapeutic decisions they make for and with their patients. As was discussed earlier, recent work in the field of continuous quality improvement has stressed that there are four main points on the compass of quality: medical (or clinical) outcome, patient functional status, cost, and patient satisfaction. It is rarely simple for the thoughtful physician to plan a course of pharmacotherapy that optimizes quality, in the eyes of the patient, based on some complex weighting of these four variables.

For the physician to optimize the quality of his or her therapeutic decisions, he or she must master the facts, skills, attitudes, and behaviors that constitute the core of clinical pharmacology. Although our undergraduate and postgraduate medical curricula tend to emphasize the importance of diagnostic skills and knowledge over those related to therapeutics, the risk of such an unbalanced approach is now clear. Students and physicians can develop appropriate therapeutic skills in the increasing number of courses in medical schools, residency programs, and continuing medical education (CME) programs devoted to these issues. A "core curriculum" of these facts, skills, and attitudes has been outlined in this Introduction. This outline is expanded in subsequent chapters. Since diagnostic and therapeutic drugs comprise such an increasingly important part of medicine in the 1990s, the thoughtful physician must deliberately pay increasing attention to their wise and careful use.

**PRINCIPLE Optimal therapeutic choices are not simple, but they can appear to be. Patients often can compensate physiologically for therapeutic misadventures; patients can improve *despite* our treatments. If therapy fails, the failure is often attributed to progression of disease. Perhaps nowhere else in professional life are mistakes so easily hidden, even from ourselves.**

**However, the rewards for optimizing your therapeutic decisions can be some of the largest ones in medicine. Consider your ability to prevent a stroke, relieve pain, address suffering (nausea, anxiety, depression, shortness of breath, etc.) in the terminally ill, cure pneumonia, correct electrolyte imbalances, relieve depression, or cure leukemia in a way that maximizes medical outcome, optimizes functional outcome, minimizes cost, and produces the greatest patient satisfaction. Practicing rational pharmacotherapeutics is part of what "good doctoring" is all about.**

## REFERENCES

Alarcon GS, Kremer JM, Macaluso M, et al. 1997. Risk factors for methotrexate-induced lung injury in patients with rheumatoid arthritis. *Ann Intern Med* **127**:356–64.

Alldredge BK, Lowenstein DH, Simon R. 1989. Placebo-controlled trial of intravenous diphenylhydantoin for short-term treatment of alcohol withdrawal seizures. *Am J Med* **87**:645–8.

Almy TP. 1980. The healing bond: Doctor and patient in an era of scientific medicine. *Am J Gastroenterol* **73**:403–7.

Anglo-American Workshop on Clinical Pharmacology. 1986. *Clin Pharmacol Ther* **39**:435–80.

Assem ESK. 1985. Drug allergy. In: Davies, DM, editor. *Textbook of Adverse Drug Reactions.* 3rd ed. New York: Oxford University Press. p 611–33.

Avorn J. 1997. Putting adverse drug events into perspective. *JAMA* **277**:341–2.

Avorn J, Chen M, Hartley R. 1982. Scientific versus commercial sources of influence on the prescribing behavior of physicians. *Am J Med* **73**:4–8.

Avorn J, Soumerai SB. 1983. Improving drug-therapy decisions through educational outreach. *N Engl J Med* **308**:1457–63.

Babington MA, Robinson LA, Monson RA. 1983. Effect of written information on physicians' knowledge of drug prices. *S Med J* **76**:328–31.

Balint M. 1957. *The Doctor, His Patient and the Illness.* New York: Int Univ Pr.

Baron RJ. 1985. An introduction to medical phenomenology: I can't hear you while I'm listening. *Ann Intern Med* **103**:606–11.

Bates DW, Spell N, Cullen DJ, et al. 1997. The costs of adverse drug events in hospitalized patients. *JAMA* **277**:307–11.

Beers MH, Ouslander JG. 1989. Risk factors in geriatric drug prescribing: A practical guide to avoiding problems. *Drugs* **37**:105–12.

Beers MH, Storrie M, Lee G. 1990. Potential adverse drug interactions in the emergency room: An issue in the quality of care. *Ann Intern Med* **112**:61–4.

Bender BS, Caranasos GJ, editors. 1989. Geriatric medicine: A problem-oriented approach. *Med Clin N Am* **73**(6).

Berkowitz RL, Coustan DR, Mochizuki TK. 1986. *Handbook for Prescribing Medications During Pregnancy.* 2nd ed. Boston: Little, Brown.

Bern MM, Lokich JJ, Wallach SR, et al. 1990. Very low doses of warfarin can prevent thrombosis in central venous catheters. *Ann Intern Med* **112**:423–8.

Blaschke TF, Meffin PJ, Melmon KL, et al. 1975. Influence of acute viral hepatitis on phenytoin kinetics and protein binding. *Clin Pharmacol Ther* **17**:685–91.

Bond WS. 1990. Medication noncompliance. *Drug News* **9**:33–5.

Briggs GG, Freeman RK, Yaffe SJ. 1990. *Drugs in Pregnancy and Lactation.* 3rd ed. Baltimore: Williams & Wilkins. p xix–xx.

Burnham JF. 1987. Medical practice a la mode: How medical fashions determine medical care. *N Engl J Med* **317**:1220–2.

Chang HJ, Bell JR, Deroo DB, et al. 1990. Physician variation in anticoagulating patients with atrial fibrillation. *Arch Intern Med* **150**:81–4.

Chen M, Landefeld CS, Murray TH. 1989. Doctors, drug companies, and gifts. *JAMA* **262**:3448–51.

Cho MK, Bero LA. 1996. The quality of drug studies published in symposium proceedings. *Ann Intern Med* **124**:485–9.

Cluff LE. 1967. The prescribing habits of physicians. *Hosp Practice* **(Sep.)**:101–4.

Cockerill FR, Wilson WR, Carpenter HA, et al. 1985. Open lung biopsy in immunocompromised patients. *Arch Intern Med* **145**:1398–1404.

Condemi JJ. 1986. Allergy to penicillin and other antibiotics. In: Reese, RE, Douglas, RG, editors. *A Practical Approach to Infectious Diseases.* 2nd ed. Boston: Little, Brown. p 680–97.

Cooper JW. 1996. Probable adverse drug reactions in a rural geriatric nursing home population: A four-year study. *J Am Geriatr Soc* **44**:194–7.

Dalen JA. 1987. Diseases of the aorta. In: Braunwald E, Isselbacher KJ, Petersdorf G, et al. *Harrison's Principles of Internal Medicine.* 11th ed. New York: McGraw-Hill. p 1037–40.

deShazo RD, Kemp SF. 1997. Allergic reactions to drugs and biologic agents *JAMA* **278**:1895–1906.

Dzau VJ, Creager MA. 1994. Diseases of the aorta. In: Braunwald E, Isselbacher KJ, Petersdorf G, et al. *Harrison's Principles of Internal Medicine.* 14th ed. New York: McGraw-Hill. p 1131–3.

Engel GL. 1987. Physician-scientists and scientific physicians: Resolving the humanism-science dichotomy. *Am J Med* **82**:107–11.

Epstein AM, Read JL, Winickoff R. 1984. Physician beliefs, attitudes, and prescribing behavior for anti-inflammatory drugs. *Am J Med* **77**:313–8.

Everitt DE, Avorn J. 1986. Drug prescribing for the elderly. *Arch Intern Med* **146**:2393–6.

Faltermayer E. 1988 October 10. Medical care's next revolution. *Fortune* 126–33.

Farwell JR, Lee YJ, Hirtz DG, et al. 1990. Phenobarbital for febrile seizures—effects on intelligence and on seizure recurrence. *N Engl J Med* **322**:364–9.

Feinstein AR. 1967. *Clinical Judgment.* Baltimore: Williams & Wilkins.

Feinstein AR, Horwitz RI. 1997. Problems in the "evidence" of "evidence-based medicine." *Am J Med* **103**:529–35.

Fowler FJ, Wennberg JE, Timothy RP, et al. 1988. Symptom status and quality of life following prostatectomy. *JAMA* **259**:3018–22.

Gelenberg AJ, Kane JM, Keller MB, et al. 1989. Comparison of standard and low serum levels of lithium for maintenance treatment of bipolar disorder. *N Engl J Med* **321**:1489–93.

Goldfinger SE. 1990. Physicians and the pharmaceutical industry. *Ann Intern Med* **112**:624–6.

Gonzales R, Steiner JF, Sande MA. 1997. Antibiotic prescribing for adults with colds, upper respiratory tract infections, and bronchitis by ambulatory care physicians. *JAMA* **278**:901–4.

Greenblatt DJ, Ehrenberg BL, Gunderman JS, et al. 1989. Pharmacokinetic and electroencephalographic study of intravenous diazepam, midazolam, and placebo. *Clin Pharmacol Ther* **45**:356–65.

Greenfield S, Kaplan S, Ware JE. 1985. Expanding patient involvement in care: Effects on patient outcomes. *Ann Intern Med* **102**:520–8.

Greenman RL, Goodall PT, King D. 1975. Lung biopsy in immunocompromised hosts. *Am J Med* **59**:488–96.

Healy B, Campeau L, Gray R, et al. 1989. Conflict of interest guidelines for a multicenter clinical trial of treatment after coronary-artery bypass-graft surgery. *N Engl J Med* **320**:949–51.

Herxheimer A. 1987. Basic information that prescribers are not getting about drugs. *Lancet* **1**:31–2.

Hicks GL, Eastland MW, DeWeese JA, et al. 1975. Survival improvement following aortic aneurysm resection. *Ann Surg* **181**:863–9.

Hull R, Hirsh J, Jay R, et al. 1982. Different intensities of oral anticoagulant therapy in the treatment of proximal-vein thrombosis. *N Engl J Med* **307**:1676–81.

Jellin JM. 1997. Reducing inappropriate use of antibiotics. *Prescribers Lett.* **4**:55.

Kaplan NM. 1997. Perspectives on the new JNC VI guidelines for the treatment of hypertension. *Hosp Formul* **32**:1224–31.

Kaplan SH, Greenfield S, Ware JE. 1989. Assessing the effects of physician-patient interactions on the outcomes of chronic disease. *Med Care (Phila)* **27**:S110–S127.

Karch FE, Lasagna L. 1975. Adverse drug reactions. *JAMA* **234**:1236–41.

Kase CS, O'Neal AM, Fisher M, et al. 1990. Intracranial hemorrhage after use of tissue plasminogen activator for coronary thrombolysis. *Ann Intern Med* **112**:17–21.

Kim JH, Gallis HA. 1989. Observations on spiraling empiricism: Its causes, allure, and perils, with particular reference to antibiotic therapy. *Am J Med* **87**:201–6.

Klotz U, Avant GR, Hoyumpa A, et al. 1975. The effects of age and liver disease on the disposition and elimination of diazepam in adult man. *J Clin Invest* **55**:347–59.

Klotz U, McHorse TW, Wilkenson GR, et al. 1974. The effect of cirrhosis on the disposition and elimination of meperidine (Pethidine) in man. *Clin Pharmacol Ther* **16**:667–75.

Koch-Weser J, Sidel VW, Sweet RH, et al. 1969. Factors determining physician reporting of adverse drug reactions. *N Engl J Med* **280**:20–6.

Kroenke K. 1985. Polypharmacy: Causes, consequences, and cure. *Am J Med* **79**:149–52.

Kusserow RP. 1989. *Medicare Drug Utilization Review.* Document OAI-01-88-00980, Washington, DC: Office of the Inspector General.

Lakshmanan MC, Hershey CO, Breslau D. 1986. Hospital admissions caused by iatrogenic disease. *Arch Intern Med* **146**:1931–4.

Lamy PP. 1986. The elderly and drug interactions. *J Am Geriatr Soc* **34**:586–92.

Lazarov J, Pomeranz BH, Corey PN. 1998. Incidence of adverse drug reactions in hospitalized patients. *JAMA* **279**:1200–5.

Lennard L, Van Loon JA, Weinshilboum RM. 1989. Pharmacogenetics of acute azathioprine toxicity: Relationship to thiopurine methyltransferase genetic polymorphism. *Clin Pharmacol Ther* **46**:149–54.

Lesar TS, Briceland L, Stein DS. 1997. Factors related to errors in medication prescribing. *JAMA* **277**:312–17.

Levine AM, Richardson JL, Marks G, et al. 1987. Compliance with oral drug therapy in patients with hematologic malignancy. *J Clin Oncol* **5**:1469–76.

Lewis LD, Benin A, Szumlanski CL, et al. 1997. Olsalazine and 6-mercaptopurine-related bone marrow suppression: A possible drug-drug interaction. *Clin Pharmacol Ther* **62**:464–75.

Mackowiak PA, LeMaistre CF. 1987. Drug fever: A critical appraisal of conventional concepts. *Ann Intern Med* **106**:728–33.

Manasse HR. 1989. Medication use in an imperfect world: Drug misuse of public policy. *Am J Hosp Pharm* **46**:929–44, 1141–52.

Masur H, Shelhamer J, Parrillo JE. 1985. The management of pneumonias in immunocompromised patients. *JAMA* **253**:1769–73.

McFadden ER, Elsanadi N, Dixon L, et al. 1995. Protocol therapy for acute asthma: Therapeutic benefits and cost savings. *Am J Med* **99**:651–61.

Melmon KL, Morrelli HF. 1969. The need to test the efficacy of the instructional aspects of clinical pharmacology. *Clin Pharmacol Ther* **10**:431–5.

Melmon KL, Nierenberg DW. 1981. Drug interactions and the prepared observer. *N Engl J Med* **304**:723–5.

Meyer BR. 1988. Improving medical education in therapeutics. *Ann Intern Med* **108**:145–7.

Mold JW, Stein HF. 1986. The cascade effect in the clinical care of patients. *N Engl J Med* **314**:512–4.

Mollman JE. 1990. Cisplatin neurotoxicity. *N Engl J Med* **322**:126–7.

Montamat SC, Cusack BJ, Vestal RE. 1989. Management of drug therapy in the elderly. *N Engl J Med* **321**:303–10.

Moss FM, McNicol MW. 1983. Audits of antibiotic prescribing. *Br Med J* **286**:1513.

Mulrow CD, Cook DJ, Davidoff F. 1997. Systematic reviews: Critical links in the great chain of evidence. *Ann Intern Med* **126**:389–91.

Murray MD, Brater DC. 1990. Adverse effects of nonsteroidal anti-inflammatory drugs on renal function. *Ann Intern Med* **112**: 559–60.

Nelson EC, Mohr JJ, Batalden PB, et al. 1996. Improving health care. Part 1. The clinical value compass. *J Qual Improv* **22**:243–58.

Nelson EC, Splaine ME, Batalden PB, et al. 1996. Measuring clinical outcomes at the front line. In: Caldwell C, editor. *The Handbook for Managing Change in Health Care.* Milwaukee: ASQ Quality Press. Chapt 9, p 225–47.

Nierenberg DW. 1986. Clinical pharmacology instruction for all medical students. *Clin Pharmacol Ther* **40**:483–7.

Ober KP. 1987. Uncle Remus and the cascade effect in clinical medicine. *Am J Med* **82**:1009–13.

Office of Technology Assessment. 1987 Oct. *Prescription Drugs and Elderly Americans: Ambulatory Use and Approaches to Coverage for Medicare.* Washington, DC: US Congress. p 3–1.

O'Hanley P, Easaw J, Rugo H, et al. 1989. Infectious disease management of adult leukemic patients undergoing chemotherapy: 1982–1986 experience at Stanford University Hospital. *Am J Med* **87**:605–13.

Ohnishi A, Tsuboi Y, Ishizaki T, et al. 1989. Kinetics and dynamics of enalapril in patients with liver cirrhosis. *Clin Pharmacol Ther* **45**:657–65.

Osborne OT. 1905. The therapeutic art. *Trans Am Ther Soc* 13–6.

Osborne OT. 1916. What therapy means. *Trans Am Ther Soc* 43–6.

Paladino JA, Kapfer JA, DiBona JR. 1986. Bedside estimation of creatinine clearance: Which method is most accurate while least complex? *Hosp Formul* **21**:709–15.

Parker CW. 1975. Drug allergy. *N Engl J Med* **292**:511–4, 732–6, 957–60.

Perrin JM, Homer CJ, Berwick DM, et al. 1989. Variations in rates of hospitalization of children in three urban communities. *N Engl J Med* **320**:1183–7.

Peters NL. 1989. Snipping the thread of life. *Arch Intern Med* **149**: 2414–20.

Psaty BM, Koepsell TD, Wagner EH, et al. 1990. The relative risk of incident coronary heart disease associated with recently stopping the use of beta-blockers. *JAMA* **263**:1653.

Rawlins MD. 1984. Doctors and the drug makers. *Lancet* **2**:276–8.

Ray WA, Griffin MR, Schaffner W, et al. 1987. Psychotropic drug use and the risk of hip fracture. *N Engl J Med* **316**:363–9.

Relman AS. 1987. Doctors and the dispensing of drugs. *N Engl J Med* **317**:311–2.

Rieder MJ, Uetrecht J, Shear NH, et al. 1989. Diagnosis of sulfonamide hypersensitivity reactions by in vitro "rechallenge" with hydroxylamine metabolites. *Ann Intern Med* **110**:286–9.

Roberts RJ. 1984. *Drug Therapy in Infants: Pharmacological Principles and Clinical Experience.* Philadelphia: WB Saunders.

Rogers AS, Israel E, Smith CR, et al. 1988. Physician knowledge, attitudes, and behavior related to reporting adverse drug events. *Arch Intern Med* **148**:1596–1600.

Royal College of Physicians. 1986. The relationship between physicians and the pharmaceutical industry. *J Roy Coll Physicians Lond* **20**:235–42.

Rubin M, Hathorn JW, Pizzo PA. 1988. Controversies in the management of febrile neutropenic cancer patients. *Cancer Invest* **6**: 167–84.

Saour JN, Sieck JO, Mamo LAR, et al. 1990. Trial of different intensities of anticoagulation in patients with prosthetic heart valves. *N Engl J Med* **322**:428–32.

Saxon A, Beall GN, Rohr AS, et al. 1987. Immediate hypersensitivity reactions to beta-lactam antibiotics. *Ann Intern Med* **107**:204–15.

Schaffner W, Ray WA, Federspiel CF, et al. 1983. Improving antibiotic prescribing in office practice. *JAMA* **250**:1728–32.

Schriger DL, Kalafut M, Starkman S, et al. 1998. Cranial computed tomography interpretation in acute stroke. *JAMA* **279**:1293–7.

Seckler SG, Spritzer RC. 1966. Disseminated disease of medical progress. *Arch Intern Med* **117**:447–50.

Siegel D, Lopez J. 1997. Trends in antihypertensive drug use in the United States. *JAMA* **278**:1745–8.

Silverman M, Lee PR. 1974. *Pills, Profits, and Politics.* Berkeley, CA: University of California Press. p 54–7.

Soumerai S, Avorn J. 1990. Principles of educational outreach ("academic detailing") to improve clinical decision making. *JAMA* **263**:549–56.

Soumerai SB, Avorn J, Ross-Degnan D, et al. 1987. Payment restrictions for prescription drugs under Medicaid: Effects on therapy, cost, and equity. *N Engl J Med* **317**:550–6.

Soumerai ST, Ross-Degnan D, Gortmaker S, et al. 1990. Withdrawing payment for nonscientific drug therapy: Intended and unexpected effects of a large-scale natural experiment. *JAMA* **263**:831–9.

Stanulovic M, Jakovljevic V, Roncevic N. 1984. Drug utilization in paediatrics: Non-medical factors affecting decision making by prescribers. *Eur J Clin Pharmacol* **27**:237–41.

Stewart RB, Caranasos GJ. 1989. Medication compliance in the elderly. *Med Clin N Am* **73**:1551–64.

Stover DE, Zaman MB, Hajdu SI, et al. 1984. Bronchoalveolar lavage in the diagnosis of diffuse pulmonary infiltrates in the immunosuppressed host. *Ann Intern Med* **101**:1–7.

Tamblyn R, Berkson L, Dauphinee WD, et al. 1997. Unnecessary prescribing of NSAIDs and the management of NSAID-related gastropathy in medical practice. *Ann Intern Med* **127**:429–38.

Tatro DS. 1990. *Drug Interaction Facts.* St Louis: Lippincott.

Thompson JE, Hollier LH, Patman RD, et al. 1975. Surgical management of abdominal aortic aneurysms: Factors influencing mortality and morbidity—a 20-year experience *Ann Surg* **181**:654–61.

Thomson PD, Melmon KL, Richardson JA, et al. 1973. Lidocaine pharmacokinetics in advanced heart failure, liver disease, and renal failure in humans. *Ann Intern Med* **78**:499–508.

Tugwell P, Bombardier C, Buchanan WW, et al. 1990. Methotrexate in rheumatoid arthritis: Impact on quality of life assessed by traditional standard-item and individualized patient preference health status questionnaires. *Arch Intern Med* **150**:59–62.

VanArsdel PP, Larson EB. 1989. Diagnostic tests for patients with suspected allergic disease: Utility and limitations. *Ann Intern Med* **110**:304–12.

*Wall Street Journal.* 1984 May 25. *Wall Street Journal;* Sect. A:31,49.

Walson PD, Hammel M, Martin R. 1981. Prescription-writing by pediatric house officers. *J Med Educ* **56**:423–8.

Weber ML, Auger C, Cleroux R. 1986. Knowledge of medical students, pediatric residents, and pediatricians about the cost of some medications. *Pediatr Pharmacol* **5**:281–5.

Weiss ME, Nyhan D, Peng Z, et al. 1989. Association of protamine IgE and IgG antibodies with life-threatening reactions to intravenous protamine. *N Engl J Med* **320**:886–92.

Wennberg DE, Lucas FL, Birkmeyer JD, et al. 1998. Variation in carotid endarterectomy mortality in the Medicare population. *JAMA* **279**:1278–81.

Wennberg J, Gittelsohn A. 1982. Variations in medical care among small areas. *Sci Am* **246**(4):120–34.

Wennberg JE, Cooperman X, editors. 1998. *The Dartmouth Atlas of Health Care*. Chicago, IL: American Hospital Publishing.

Whelton A, Stout RL, Spilman PS, et al. 1990. Renal effects of ibuprofen, piroxicam, and sulindac in patients with asymptomatic renal failure. *Ann Intern Med* **112**:568–76.

Wilcox RW. 1903. The teaching of therapeutics. *Trans Am Ther Soc* 25–34.

Wilkes MS, Shuchman M. 1989 Nov 5. Pitching doctors. *New York Times Magazine*:88–9, 126–9.

PART

# 2

# DRUG THERAPY OF COMMON DISEASES: PROBLEM-BASED THERAPEUTIC DECISIONS

CHAPTER

# 1 CARDIOVASCULAR DISORDERS

## Hypertension

**Brian B. Hoffman, S. George Carruthers**

### *Chapter Outline*



The treatment of hypertension has been strongly influenced by the results of powerful controlled clinical trials over the past three decades and the increasing availability of novel antihypertensive drugs. In order to provide optimal therapy to individual patients, practitioners must keep abreast of developments in this broad field, which includes important elements of preventive cardiology. This section provides a foundation for therapy based on sound principles of clinical pharmacology and evidence-based medicine.

### Definition and Epidemiology

Hypertension is important because elevated blood pressure (BP) confers a greater risk of stroke, heart failure, renal disease, peripheral vascular disease, and coronary artery disease including angina, myocardial infarction, and sudden death. There is a continuous, direct relationship between elevations in blood pressure and increases in these risks. The US Joint National Committee on the Prevention, Detection, Evaluation, and Treatment of Hypertension (Joint National Committee 1997) defined hypertension as a blood pressure greater than 140/90 (systolic/diastolic) mm Hg taken under defined conditions and graded the severity of the elevation of blood pressure into the following categories: *stage 1* (systolic BP 140–159 or diastolic BP 90–99 mm Hg), *stage 2* (systolic BP 160–179 or diastolic BP 100–109 mm Hg), or *stage 3* (systolic BP ≥ 180 mg Hg or diastolic BP ≥ 110 mm Hg). The extent to which blood pressure is elevated plays a role in determining the pace at which the problem should be evaluated and treated. In addition, preexisting cardiovascular risk factors or target-organ damage may have a major impact on the stringency of treating hypertension in individual patients. In general, the higher the blood pressure and the greater the number of risk factors, the greater the urgency and stringency used in treating hypertension. Lowering blood pressure is just one way to prevent complications; attention must also be paid to the presence and reversal of other cardiovascular risk factors such as cigarette smoking, lipid disorders, and especially diabetes. Diabetes is observed more frequently in patients with hypertension, and diabetics have a high prevalence of hypertension. The coexistence of these risk factors greatly increases the likelihood of cardiovascular complications associated with hypertension. The presence of these risk factors should be determined during the evaluation of patients with hypertension by careful history-taking and physical examination, coupled with relatively simple laboratory tests.

### Benefits Versus Risks of Therapy

There is now overwhelming clear and convincing evidence from randomized clinical trials, some conducted decades ago, that the treatment of what was then termed moderate (diastolic BP 105–114 mm Hg) or severe hypertension (diastolic BP ≥ 115 mm Hg) is efficacious in the prevention of clinically important endpoints such as stroke and congestive heart failure. Antihypertensive therapy decreases risk of stroke along the lines forecast from epidemiological studies demonstrating increased risk with elevated blood pressure. However, the effects of antihypertensive therapy have been more limited than expected for improvements in risks of the complications from coronary artery disease, particularly myocardial infarction. For what has been called mild hypertension (diastolic BP > 105 mm Hg), results have varied more substantially in different clinical trials. Nonetheless, there is good evidence that treatment of mild hypertension has efficacy, especially in patients over age 50 and those at higher risk owing to coexisting cardiovascular risk factors such as smoking, hyperlipidemia, and diabetes. Indeed, as a general rule, the greater the risk of complications in hypertensives, the greater the absolute benefit as a consequence of treating the elevated blood pressure. Diabetics with hypertension in the SHEP [The Systolic Hypertension in the Elderly Program (SHEP) Cooperative Research Group 1993], SYST–EUR (Staessen et al. 1997), and HOT (Hansson et al. 1998) studies all had improved outcomes when subjected to active or more aggressive blood pressure lowering. The >80 mm Hg target group in the HOT study had a 50% reduction in major cardiovascular events compared with the >90 mm Hg target group, from more than 24 events per 1000 patient years to less than 12 events per 1000 patient years.

The first step in treating mildly hypertensive patients should be to institute potentially effective nonpharmacologic therapies where appropriate (e.g., weight loss, sodium restriction, curtailment of alcohol intake, smoking cessation, and increased exercise) for 3–6 months. If diastolic pressure remains greater than 95 mm Hg, then drug therapy should then be instituted. This conservative approach avoids premature overtreatment of patients with drugs.

**PRINCIPLE Discovering a disease does not always justify pharmacologic treatment even when such treatment has been proved efficacious.**

## Diagnosis

Because the benefits of drug therapy in mild hypertensive patients are limited and the risks and the costs are shared by all those treated, the one should carefully measure blood pressure to avoid overdiagnosis and overtreatment (Joint National Committee 1997).

**PRINCIPLE Proper therapy begins with proper diagnosis. Especially for those with modest elevations in blood pressure and no other cardiovascular risk factors, repeated measurements over a period of months, coupled with nonpharmacologic approaches to lowering blood pressure, are appropriate before considering the use of antihypertensive medications.**

**PRINCIPLE Risk evaluation must consider both the extent of blood pressure elevation and other cardiovascular risk factors. When the number of patients needed to be treated to prevent an undesirable clinical outcome such as stroke or myocardial infarction is very large, the costs of treatment and the potential for adverse drug events may outweigh potential benefits of therapy.**

## Pathophysiology

### *Systemic hemodynamics*

The term *essential hypertension* arose generations ago because physicians thought that high blood pressure was "essential" for adequate tissue perfusion in patients with extensive blood vessel narrowing. Although the foundation for the term is now viewed as ironically incorrect, its use persists. It is preferable to refer to hypertension as either *primary hypertension* (cause unknown) or *secondary hypertension* associated with a known cause, such as pheochromocytoma. Only a small portion of all patients with hypertension have an underlying disease known to raise blood pressure.

Knowledge of simple hemodynamics provides a rationale for understanding hypertension and its therapy. Blood pressure is the product of cardiac output (CO) and systemic vascular resistance (SVR) ($BP = CO \times SVR$). Increases in either cardiac output or peripheral resistance can produce hypertension. Cardiac output can increase as a function of increased myocardial contractility, heart rate, or venous return. Venous return is a function of the total blood volume (regulated by the kidney) and the percentage of blood volume circulating centrally (regulated by venous tone). Arteriolar smooth muscle tone is the major determinant of SVR.

Because early in the course of hypertension there is frequently a high cardiac output and normal peripheral resistance, elevation in cardiac output may be the initial hemodynamic alteration in primary hypertension. When cardiac output increases, autoregulation ensues to maintain constant blood flow to tissues. The increased flow from increased cardiac output is therefore countered by vasoconstriction. This is often called *functional autoregulation.* As well, however, blood vessel walls can hypertrophy slowly in response to increased flow (*structural autoregulation*). The thickened arteriolar walls will cause disproportionate luminal narrowing for any given constrictor stimulus and amplify the tendency toward hypertension (Folkow 1984). This concept has therapeutic implications. As blood pressure is controlled, structural changes may slowly regress. With increasing duration of therapy, lesser degrees of antihypertensive therapy may suffice for maintenance of the reduction in pressure. Theoretically, this concept justifies attempts to decrease or withdraw therapy once pressure has been normalized with drugs for some time (e.g., 6–12 months).

### *The kidney*

The kidney contributes in many ways to the control of blood pressure (see chapter 6, Renal Disorders and the Influence of Renal Function on Drug Disposition). Renin released from renal juxtaglomerular cells activates the renin–angiotensin–aldosterone (RAA) axis. Renal prostaglandins and renomedullary lipids are vasodilators. However, the paramount role of the kidney in relation to control of blood pressure is regulation of blood volume. When blood pressure rises for any reason, the kidney can excrete more sodium, which lowers blood volume. In turn, the lowering of blood volume tends to decrease cardiac output and to restore pressure toward normal. From this point of view, blood pressure can be restored toward normal as long as the kidneys are functioning appropriately. Guyton (1989) hypothesized that for hypertension to exist there has to be a defect in the ability of the kidney to excrete sodium in response to a rise in blood pressure. In other words, for any given rise in blood pressure, the abnormal "hypertensive" kidney will excrete less sodium than will a normal kidney. Transplantation experiments have provided evidence to support this hypothesis; namely, transplanting a kidney from a normotensive to a nephrectomized hypertensive rat normalizes blood pressure, whereas transplantation of a hypertensive rat's kidney into a normotensive control rat can cause hypertension.

### *The sympathetic nervous system*

The sympathetic nervous system plays a major role in regulating both cardiac output and peripheral resistance. Blood pressure is monitored by arterial baroreceptors that transmit signals to brainstem vasomotor centers. This information is processed and coordinated with information from other areas in the brain, leading to the determination of sympathetic efferent tone. Efferent sympathetic fibers descend into the spinal cord and exit the spinal cord as preganglionic neurons. These exiting fibers then lead to sympathetic ganglia, which activate postganglionic neurons by releasing the neurotransmitter acetylcholine. These neurons, which predominantly use norepinephrine as neurotransmitter, modulate target organs throughout the body. For example, noradrenergic postganglionic neurons are found in the heart, where they increase contractility and heart rate; in arterioles, where they may enhance vasoconstriction; and in veins, where they promote smooth muscle contraction. In the kidneys, sympathetic neurons promote the secretion of renin. Secretion of renin leads to formation of angiotensin II, which enhances vasoconstriction as well as sodium retention via aldosterone effects. Elevated sympathetic nervous system activity may result in transient or sustained hypertension. Other preganglionic nerves innervate the adrenal medulla and stimulate secretion of epinephrine. Epinephrine then circulates as a hormone exerting direct sympathetic effects on distant cells. Conceptually, norepinephrine is the sympathetic neurotransmitter, and epinephrine is the circulating sympathomimetic hormone.

The catecholamines norepinephrine and epinephrine regulate cellular physiology by activating adrenergic receptors, which leads to multiple biological effects (Hoffman and Lefkowitz 1996). There are three known types of adrenergic receptors, termed $\alpha_1$-, $\alpha_2$-, and $\beta$-adrenergic receptors. These receptors are part of the large family of cell surface receptors that signal intracellular effectors via activation of guanine nucleotide regulatory proteins (G proteins). Each of the three types of adrenergic receptors is currently known to have three molecularly cloned subtypes: $\alpha_1$A, $\alpha_1$B, and $\alpha_1$D; $\alpha_2$A, $\alpha_2$B, and $\alpha_2$C; and $\beta_1$, $\beta_2$, and $\beta_3$. These subtypes may share overlapping functions or may selectively activate other biologically important functions. This diversity of adrenergic receptors and their subtypes offers promise in the development of clinically significant selective adrenergic agonists and antagonists.

There is evidence that alterations in sympathetic nervous system activity may play an important pathophysiologic role in the maintenance of hypertension in some patients. As described below, there are a variety of valuable antihypertensive drugs that act on various components of the sympathetic nervous system or on adrenergic receptors. In addition, knowledge about the expression of adrenergic receptors on cells in many organs may suggest secondary (desirable or undesirable) effects of these drugs in the treatment of hypertension.

### *The renin–angiotensin–aldosterone axis*

Renin is secreted by the kidney in response to a decrease in renal blood flow or delivery of sodium to the kidney (see chapter 6, Renal Disorders and the Influence of Renal Function on Drug Disposition). Renin secretion is also stimulated by $\beta$-adrenergic receptors in the kidney. Renin then converts angiotensinogen, made by the liver, into angiotensin I, a decapeptide. Angiotensin-converting enzyme (ACE), which is produced mainly in the lung, then cleaves angiotensin I into angiotensin II, an octapeptide and potent vasoconstrictor. Angiotensin II acts on the zona glomerulosa of the adrenal cortex, causing secretion of aldosterone that enhances reabsorption of $Na^+$ from the distal renal tubule in exchange for $H^+$ and $K^+$, which are excreted in the urine. Activation of the renin system raises blood pressure via enhanced vasoconstriction (angiotensin II) and via increased cardiac output secondary to sodium retention (aldosterone). Angiotensin II activates biological responses via stimulation of two receptor subtypes, called *$AT_1$* and *$AT_2$ receptors.* Angiotensin receptors (and local renin–angiotensin systems expressed in cardiovascular tissues) may also have importance in stimulating cardiac hypertrophy and vascular remodeling in patients with hypertension (Dzau 1993).

There are many other known factors and neurotransmitters involved in blood pressure regulation. These include serotonin, nitric oxide, endothelin and other peptides, as well as prostaglandins and ion pumps and channels. Some of these are the targets for available antihypertensive drugs, whereas others are possible sites for the action of experimental drugs.

## ANTIHYPERTENSIVE DRUGS

### Diuretics

#### *General pharmacology and mechanism of action*

The most commonly used diuretics include thiazides and related drugs, loop diuretics, and aldosterone receptor antagonists. *Diuretics* are agents that affect the kidney to increase urine formation. These agents are also called *natriuretics* because they increase the excretion of sodium. Their sites of action in the nephron are discussed in chapter 6, Renal Disorders and the Influence of Renal Function on Drug Disposition. Evidence supports the hypothesis that an inability to excrete appropriate amounts of sodium in the face of hypertension is a factor that contributes to the maintenance of elevated blood pressure (Guyton 1989). The original rationale for using diuretics to treat hypertension stems from their ability to augment urinary excretion of sodium. In the absence of compensatory mechanisms, this action would tend to decrease total body sodium, reduce blood volume, and secondarily reduce cardiac output. However, it is uncertain exactly how diuretics decrease blood pressure in many hypertensives because the long-term effects of these drugs are due at least in part to a decrease in peripheral vascular resistance.

Experimentation with sulfonamide derivatives led to the discovery of thiazide diuretics in the 1950s. These diuretic, natriuretic, and kaliuretic agents act primarily on the early distal convoluted tubule to inhibit $Na^+$ and $Cl^-$ transport by an interaction with the $Na^+$-$Cl^-$ symporter. The so-called loop diuretics (e.g., furosemide, ethacrynic acid) were subsequently developed. These high-capacity diuretics block the $Na^+$-$K^+$-2Cl cotransport system in the ascending limb of Henle's loop. Aldosterone antagonists such as spironolactone block the receptors for aldosterone in the distal tubule. Antagonism of aldosterone's actions enhances sodium excretion and reabsorption of potassium and hydrogen. Other potassium-sparing diuretics (e.g., triamterene, amiloride) use other mechanisms to counteract the distal tubular loss of potassium induced by thiazide and loop diuretics.

#### *Thiazides and related diuretics*

Thiazides and related drugs are the mainstay of antihypertensive diuretic therapy (for examples of thiazides and related diuretics, see Table 1-1). Inhibition of sodium reabsorption decreases plasma volume causing reflex increases in renin and aldosterone secretion. This adaptation tends to oppose sodium excretion by facilitating distal sodium reabsorption in exchange for potassium and hydrogen losses. The decrease in plasma volume increases proximal tubular avidity to reabsorb salt and water, which also limits sodium excretion. A new steady state then develops, generally at a somewhat lower extracellular vol-

Table 1-1 Thiazides and Related Diuretics

| Drug | Duration of diuretic effect (h) |
|---|---|
| Bendroflumethiazide | 6–12 |
| Benzthiazide | 12–18 |
| Chlorothiazide | 6–12 |
| Chlorthalidone[a] | 48–72 |
| Cyclothiazide | 18–24 |
| Hydrochlorothiazide | 6–12 |
| Hydroflumethiazide | 18–24 |
| Indapamide[b] | |
| Methyclothiazide | <24 |
| Metolazone[c] | 12–24[d] |
| Polythiazide | 24–48 |
| Quinethazone | 18–24 |

Data in part modified from US Pharmacopeia.

[a]Chlorthalidone does not have thiazide ring system but has a sulfonamide group.

[b]An indoline; does not have thiazide ring system but has a sulfonamide group. Although indapamide inhibits sodium reabsorption in cortical diluting segment, its antihypertensive efficacy may be more related to unclear effects on peripheral vasculature. Antihypertensive efficacy may be maintained in patients with renal insufficiency.

[c]Metolazone does not have thiazide ring system but has a sulfonamide group. This drug may be a more efficacious diuretic than thiazides in patients with renal insufficiency.

[d]Sustained-release formulation.

ume. The vigor of this adaptation may vary between responders and nonresponders to the drug's antihypertensive effects. In addition, blood pressure may continue to fall because of a decrease in total peripheral resistance. As a consequence, the antihypertensive effects of thiazides are at least partially dissociated from their effects on blood volume. On the other hand, most of these agents have diminished efficacy in patients with renal insufficiency, for example, serum creatinine concentrations greater than 2.5 mg/mL.

**PRINCIPLE Classification of drugs by their dominant mechanism of action or effects may obscure other useful mechanisms of action and limit understanding of their pharmacologic uses.**

When given orally, thiazide diuretics are absorbed in the intestine with variable bioavailability, are bound to proteins, and are excreted in the urine. They act on the luminal side of the tubule after glomerular filtration and/or proximal tubular secretion. Their half-lives ($t_{1/2}$) vary, but their antihypertensive effects persist for at least 24 hours, allowing once daily dosing. It is not clear whether differences in duration of diuretic action have an impact on a patient's quality of life, but this is something that should be considered, for example, in individual patients experiencing nocturia.

The common agents, with equivalent daily doses, are chlorothiazide, 500 mg; hydrochlorothiazide, 25 mg; chlorthalidone, 25 mg; and bendrofluazide, 2.5 mg. Thiazide diuretics typically have steep dose–response curves that plateau at low doses. Near-maximal antihypertensive effects are usually seen at the doses just indicated in patients with stage 1 or stage 2 hypertension. However, some additional, albeit small, benefit can be gained at double these doses. It is very important to note that at higher doses, although there is little additional antihypertensive benefit, increased potassium wasting and uric acid retention will occur. Also, there is evidence from a case-control study suggesting that the risk of sudden death increases dose-dependently for doses of hydrochlorothiazide greater than 25 mg/day. In other words, the dose–response curves for adverse effects of these drugs is shifted to the right of the dose–response curve for efficacy as an antihypertensive.

**PRINCIPLE Inappropriately high doses of certain drugs may increase adverse effects without providing any additional beneficial effects.**

### *Clinical use and adverse effects of thiazides and related diuretics*

Not only are thiazides usually effective when given once daily as monotherapy, but they also have additional benefits when combined with most other antihypertensive drugs. They can induce reductions in blood pressure averaging up to 20/10 mmHg, depending on the patient population. Typically, about 50% of patients will have a good blood pressure response to monotherapy with a low-dose diuretic. There is some evidence that poor responders in terms of lowered blood pressure tend to have a more marked augmentation in aldosterone concentrations in response to the drug. The long-term efficacy of these drugs is similar to many other classes of antihypertensive medications. Dietary restriction of sodium may allow a reduction in the dosage of diuretics. This restriction also reduces distal availability of sodium for exchange with hydrogen and potassium and limits the hypokalemic metabolic alkalosis induced by diuretics. On the other hand, the addition of a nonsteroidal anti-inflammatory drug (NSAID) may impair the antihypertensive effects of diuretics.

The adverse effects of thiazides have been documented in multiple clinical trials over many years in tens of thousands of patients, possibly more so than any other antihypertensive drug class. Ironically, this large fund of information is often used as a reason to curtail their use. However, as described above, the adverse effects are dose-dependent and often can be minimized by using appropriate lower doses without compromising the efficacy of the drug. In addition, recent controlled trials have found that, in terms of adverse effects, thiazides compare favorably with many other classes of antihypertensive drugs (Grimm et al. 1996).

**PRINCIPLE When little doses work, higher doses do not always work better!**

Diuretics have been found, especially in studies 1 year or less in duration, to increase concentrations of plasma triglycerides and low-density lipoprotein (LDL) cholesterol. Although trials have demonstrated the benefit of lowering elevated concentrations of cholesterol on the incidence of coronary heart disease, the clinical significance of these diuretic-induced relatively small increases is not known. It has been claimed that the failure to demonstrate reduction in coronary artery–related mortality in some controlled trials in patients taking diuretics stems from the consequences of these effects. In addition, diuretics may also elevate plasma glucose concentrations and promote peripheral resistance to insulin. However, these claims should be kept in perspective, especially because diuretics have been the mainstay of most trials demonstrating that antihypertensive therapy is efficacious in decreasing risk of clinically significant endpoints. It should also be emphasized that the adverse effects of thiazides on lipids are likely dose-related, with smaller effects at doses currently recommended in the treatment of hypertension (Ames 1996). A Department of Veterans Affairs Cooperative Study that compared placebo and six drugs in 1292 patients found that an initial trend toward an increase in cholesterol values in the hydrochlorothiazide group was not significantly different from placebo and did not persist at the 1-year follow-up (Materson et al. 1993). Indapamide may have no adverse effects on plasma lipids (Ames 1996).

Because thiazide diuretics (and related drugs in Table 1-1) are sulfonamide derivatives, they may cause allergic reactions, particularly skin rashes. Rarely, vasculitis, interstitial nephritis, pancreatitis, and thrombocytopenia have been reported. Male sexual dysfunction is an uncommon but important adverse effect of thiazide diuretics (Medical Research Council Working Party 1985).

Electrolyte complications stem directly from the mechanisms of action of thiazide diuretics. Hypokalemia is the best known complication. At usual doses, plasma potassium concentrations usually remain greater than 3.4 mmol/L. A potassium concentration of less than 3 mmol/L in a patient taking a low dose of a thiazide (or <3.5 mmol/L when not taking diuretics) should stimulate a search for primary hyperaldosteronism. Some studies have suggested that when thiazide diuretics are taken alone, they may be associated with an increased incidence of sudden death (Multiple Risk Factor Intervention Trial 1982). This effect has been postulated to be due to a reduction in the plasma potassium concentration that could directly predispose patients to ventricular arrhythmias, sudden death, or both. This hypothesis has led to the use of potassium supplementation or potassium-sparing diuretics in conjunction with thiazide usage. It is best to avoid potassium depletion by using the low doses of diuretics, possibly associated with a sodium-restricted diet. Patients with ventricular ectopic activity—or those taking cardiac glycosides, $\beta_2$-adrenergic agonists, or pharmacologic doses of corticosteroids—probably should receive agents to prevent an excessive decrease in the plasma concentration of potassium (Ogilvie et al. 1993). ACE inhibitors are particularly useful in this setting because they have additive antihypertensive effect with thiazides and blunt potassium loss.

**PRINCIPLE Seek drug–drug interactions that not only offer additive efficacy but also decrease the toxicity of one or both drugs.**

Hypomagnesemia results from diuretic-induced enhanced excretion of magnesium by the kidneys. Magnesium depletion predisposes patients to arrhythmias and muscle weakness and will in itself enhance potassium loss. Metabolic alkalosis is encountered especially during exaggerated blood volume depletion caused by diuretics. Diuretic-induced hyperuricemia occasionally may be accompanied by gout. Although it may be tempting to attribute an episode of gout to the drug-induced hyperuricemia, in some but not all studies, the incidence of podagra in patients taking thiazides is no higher than would be predicted by the pretreatment plasma uric acid concentrations.

Hyponatremia is a dose-related potential adverse effect of thiazide use. Thiazide-induced hyponatremia is seen most often in the elderly, especially at daily doses of hydrochlorothiazide of 50 mg (or equivalent) or greater. When therapy at higher doses of diuretics is required, potassium-sparing agents can be used to prevent hypokalemia, but correction of hyponatremia or hypomagnesemia may be overlooked. Increased proximal tubular reabsorption of calcium secondary to decreased plasma volume will cause enhanced calcium reabsorption. Thiazides inhibit urinary calcium excretion and may cause hypercalcemia and unmask latent hyperparathyroidism (see chapter 6, Renal Disorders and the Influence of Renal Function on Drug Disposition).

### *Other diuretics*

**THE LOOP DIURETICS** The loop diuretics are more efficacious diuretics than the thiazides, leading to a greater risk of inducing profound hypovolemia. The hypovolemia may be profound enough to result in what will often be considered paradoxical increases in blood pressure. In addition, high doses of furosemide may cause hearing loss in patients with renal failure (see chapter 6, Renal Disorders and the Influence of Renal Function on Drug Disposition).

For the treatment of hypertension, thiazides are preferable and actually more efficacious as antihypertensive drugs compared with loop diuretics. Using them at marginal autohypertensive doses often is unaccompanied by excessive potassium loss. However, when a patient has renal impairment or significant volume overload, the more powerful loop diuretics *might* be very useful for dual effects (see Table 1-2). Furosemide is used at doses of 20 mg and upward. Patients with renal insufficiency often need higher doses. For a complete discussion of this subject, see chapter 6 (Renal Disorders and the Influence of Renal Function on Drug Disposition). It is very important to emphasize that furosemide should be used in divided doses of two or more per day. The reason is that the duration of diuretic action may be quite short and is likely dose-related; if the drug is administered just once daily, the kidneys will retain sodium avidly after the initial burst of diuretic activity and during the rest of the day. With the ingestion of salt in the diet, negative sodium balance may not be adequately achieved.

**POTASSIUM-SPARING DIURETICS** Major interest in potassium-sparing diuretics has been stimulated by concerns about the potential risk of arrhythmias and sudden death associated with potassium depletion/hypokalemia attributed to thiazide diuretics. In view of circumstantial evidence linking higher doses of thiazide diuretics with increased risk of sudden death, and the very modest benefits seen in reduction of risk from cardiac mortality in studies using those doses of thiazides in the treatment of hypertension, this association may be clinically significant.

Spironolactone is a competitive antagonist that binds to aldosterone receptors, inhibiting the action of aldosterone. It increases sodium excretion and inhibits excretion of hydrogen ion and potassium. Spironolactone undergoes rapid and extensive metabolism in humans. The major fraction of an orally administered dose is converted into the active metabolite canrenone. Canrenone contributes greatly to the pharmacologic effects of spironolactone; this metabolite is further metabolized by the liver and is excreted unchanged in the urine. Although the kinetics have not been extensively studied, canrenone has a relatively long half-life and may accumulate over the course of several days or more, with increasing pharmacologic effect. Spironolactone also may activate estrogen receptors, which limits its use, especially in men, who may experience gynecomastia or mastodynia. This risk appears dose-related and may occur in 30% or more in men taking the drug. Women may experience reduced libido or menstrual irregularities while taking spironolactone. As a consequence, the drug is not a first-line antihypertensive but is particularly attractive in treating patients with primary hyperaldosteronism who are not surgical candidates. In that setting, spironolactone may be desirable because it specially opposes the actions of excess aldosterone. Because it is a competitive inhibitor, effective dosages need to be titrated against the effects of aldosterone, for example, by monitoring changes in sodium and potassium excretion. Spironolactone may cause hyperkalemic metabolic acidosis. Care should be taken in patients with renal insufficiency who already have a predisposition to hyperkalemia or those who are taking potassium supplements, ACE inhibitors, or $AT_1$ antagonists.

Amiloride acts on the collecting tubule to inhibit access of sodium to the transport side independent of aldosterone action (see chapter 6, Renal Disorders and the Influence of Renal Function on Drug Disposition). Potassium and hydrogen excretion is decreased, and as with spironolactone, hyperkalemic metabolic acidosis may occur. The drug is not as effective as thiazide in treating hypertension but can be used in conjunction with thiazides to prevent hypokalemia and alkalosis when diuretic doses of thiazides are considered important. The same cautions mentioned with spironolactone with respect to hyperkalemia and acidosis apply to amiloride.

Triamterene spares potassium (but less so than spironolactone and amiloride). It appears not to have antihypertensive effects on its own. Its sole clinical use in this context is to reduce the likelihood and extent of hypokalemia. Triamterene may reduce the bioavailability of thiazides administered concomitantly. It can also cause interstitial nephritis and renal stones.

**Table 1-2** Loop Diuretics

| DRUG | DURATION OF DIURETIC EFFECT (H) |
|---|---|
| Bumetanide | 4–6 |
| Ethacrynic acid | 6–8 |
| Furosemide | 6–8 |
| Torsemide | 6–8 |

### *Recommendations*

Diuretics have been the mainstay of antihypertensive therapy for more than 30 years. They are effective, inexpensive, and easy to take. Diuretics are useful when used in combination with agents that increase salt and water reabsorption. They are still first-line drugs suitable for most hypertensives, especially the elderly and those with isolated systolic hypertension. But if possible, they should be avoided in patients with allergy to sulfa, hypovolemia, hyponatremia, or gout. Diuretic therapy can decrease renal clearance of lithium; the dose of lithium may require downward adjustment if a diuretic is started. Because thiazides are relatively ineffective in azotemic states, loop diuretics are preferred in that setting, especially to normalize blood volume.

**PRINCIPLE The longer drugs are used, the more useful they become; and the more widespread their use, the more likely that a complete profile on their use and toxicity will become available. Of course, that profile could superficially be more menacing than that of a newer drug, but the profile's completeness should be viewed as an asset, not a liability or a reason for preferring drugs that are less well understood.**

## DRUGS THAT INHIBIT ADRENERGIC NERVOUS SYSTEM EFFECTS

Drugs that inhibit the effects of the adrenergic nervous system were among the first used to treat hypertension. This discussion includes those drugs that are clinically useful today. Adrenergic inhibiting drugs act either to decrease the amount of norepinephrine and epinephrine released from adrenergic terminals and the adrenal medulla or to block the effects of norepinephrine and epinephrine at $\alpha$- and $\beta$-adrenergic receptors. Centrally acting drugs such as clonidine may reduce catecholamine release by stimulating areas of the brain that inhibit sympathetic outflow. Peripherally acting drugs such as reserpine and guanethidine work by depleting the peripheral adrenergic neurons of their catecholamine stores.

### Clonidine and Related Drugs

***Pharmacology and mechanism of action***

Clonidine, a partial $\alpha_2$-adrenergic agonist, was developed as a nasal vasoconstricting decongestant. Because of its nasal decongestant action, investigators anticipated that clonidine would increase blood pressure; however, it was found to actually lower blood pressure in humans. Clonidine that enters the brain has a major effect of inhibiting sympathetic outflow by activating receptors in the vasomotor center, leading to decreased systemic blood pressure. Guanabenz and guanfacine are more recently developed derivatives of clonidine. They probably have many similar actions, although their relative potencies differ from that of clonidine.

The hemodynamic effects of clonidine include decreased peripheral vascular resistance, heart rate, and cardiac output. All probably are related to decreased sympathetic (and secondarily to decreased renin) system(s) activity. In addition, when taken orally, clonidine may enhance vagal tone, which further slows resting heart rate. It has a bioavailability of about 65%. A small dose (0.1 mg) decreases blood pressure in 30 minutes, with a maximum effect achieved in 2–4 hours. The total duration of effect is up to 12 hours. Its plasma half-life is 6–12 hours and doubles in patients with renal failure. The duration of action of guanfacine may be sufficiently long to allow once daily administration (usually at night so that adverse consequences of sedation are minimized). Clonidine should be given at least twice daily for satisfactory control of blood pressure throughout the day. Blood pressure can be further decreased at oral doses up to 1.2 mg or greater per day. However, the incidence and severity of adverse effects increase progressively with doses over 0.3 mg. The marked potency of clonidine has been exploited by the development of a transdermal delivery system using skin patches because sufficient quantities of the drug are systemically available by this route. A single patch can deliver 0.1, 0.2, or 0.3 mg/day continuously for up to 7 days. This delivery system may enhance patient compliance with this medication. Unfortunately, the patch also causes annoying local skin reactions in some patients.

***Clinical use and adverse effects of clonidine***

Clonidine is effective as monotherapy in divided doses of 0.2 to 1.0 mg/day. However, because of its adverse-effect profile, clonidine appears to be most useful when it is used as a second-line, low-dose, antiadrenergic agent—especially in patients with increased sympathetic tone caused by diuretics and/or vasodilators. Furthermore, clonidine is efficacious in a variety of other settings, including ameliorating the hot flushes in the female menopausal syndrome and diminishing symptoms in patients undergoing withdrawal from alcohol, opiates, or nicotine. As a consequence, clonidine may have some advantages in selected hypertensive patients who are trying to withdraw from the use of either alcohol or cigarettes. These all represent "two-for-one" uses in which a single drug can positively impact on more than one indication.

**PRINCIPLE Seek settings in which a single drug can positively impact on more than one indication.**

Sedation and dry mouth are common adverse effects. Other adverse effects include bradycardia, orthostatic hypotension, sleep disturbances, and male sexual dysfunction. Clonidine should generally be avoided or used very cautiously in patients with a history of mental depression. Abrupt discontinuation of clonidine following its chronic use can result in a rebound withdrawal syndrome that includes marked increases in blood pressure and heart rate plus anxiety, sweating, and related symptoms due to marked activation of the sympathetic nervous system. Although the incidence of this potentially life-threatening syndrome is unknown, the risk is probably increased in patients taking higher doses of clonidine and in patients with relatively severe and poorly controlled hypertension. Patients are at risk from marked acute rises in blood pressure and from increased myocardial oxygen demands. As a consequence, caution should be used in treating patients who tend to be noncompliant with medications. This group includes some alcoholics. The clonidine withdrawal syndrome can also theoretically occur with the addition of an $\alpha_2$-adrenergic antagonist such as yohimbine.

***Recommendations***

The adrenergic inhibiting action of central $\alpha$-adrenergic agonists given in low doses makes them a rational choice for treating hypertension in conjunction with other antihypertensive agents. They are very useful in treating diseases that tend to enhance autonomic reflexes. However, adverse effects may limit them as first-line therapeutic agents, and they should be avoided in patients whose concordance with therapy is likely to be poor (for a review, see Houston 1981).

## $\alpha$-Methyldopa

***Pharmacology and mechanism of action***

$\alpha$-Methyldopa was introduced in 1960 and was a mainstay of antihypertensive therapy through the 1970s. $\alpha$-Methyldopa must be transformed in the brain by being converted into active $\alpha_2$-adrenergic agonists (methylnorepinephrine and methylepinephrine) before it exerts its antihypertensive actions. The $\alpha$-adrenergic agonist metabolites of $\alpha$-methyldopa stimulate areas in the brainstem (presumably via $\alpha$-adrenergic receptors) that inhibit sympathetic nerve discharge in a manner similar to that of clonidine. Although $\alpha$-methyldopa is an efficacious drug, the preeminent and limiting adverse effects of $\alpha$-methyldopa are related to depression of central nervous system (CNS) function, particularly lassitude and drowsiness. It has some unusual adverse effects including autoimmune abnormalities that increase with the dose and duration of exposure and include positive Coombs test (rarely leading to hemolytic anemia), positive antinuclear antibody (ANA) tests with occasional lupus-like syndrome, and hepatocellular dysfunction. $\alpha$-Methyldopa's interference with production of dopamine can sometimes unmask signs of Parkinsonism. In rare cases, $\alpha$-methyldopa may cause a fever.

***Recommendation***

$\alpha$-Methyldopa remains an effective and reasonably safe antihypertensive drug when used in the lower dose ranges up to 750 mg/day. Its safety during pregnancy-related hypertension is well established. Nonetheless, its general use in North America and Western European countries has declined markedly with the development of better tolerated medications.

## Reserpine

***Pharmacology and mechanism of action***

Reserpine is one of the active extracts of the Indian snake root plant (*Rauwolfia serpentina*). It was first used by the ancient Egyptians to treat snake bite. Reserpine acts primarily by depleting peripheral norepinephrine through an interaction with storage vesicles in sympathetic nerve endings. There are analogous actions on storage vesicles for norepinephrine and serotonin in the CNS that may contribute to the drug's efficacy and adverse effects. Lowered sympathetic activity produces a fall in peripheral vascular resistance with little or no change in cardiac output.

The half-life of the drug can be estimated from the 2–3 weeks required to reach its maximum antihypertensive effect and the similar time span required to return to baseline pressures after discontinuation of the drug (because recovery involves synthesis of new storage vesicles).

***Clinical use and adverse effects of reserpine***

Historically, reserpine has played a major role in the initiation of effective therapies for hypertension; its effectiveness is enhanced with a diuretic or other agents. Reserpine was used in the early clinical trials that demonstrated that antihypertensive drugs could decrease morbidity and mortality caused by hypertension. Low once-daily doses (e.g., 0.05 mg/day) combined with a thiazide are as effective as 0.25 mg/day alone (Veteran Administration Medical Centers 1982).

Reserpine can frequently cause severe depression. Suicide was common with the early use of high doses (>2 mg/day) of the drug. There is evidence that lower doses of reserpine (0.05–0.25 mg/day) are efficacious but also are associated with many fewer CNS effects. Adverse effects, especially fatigue, are similar to those encountered with other centrally acting agents. Nasal stuffiness may be prominent in some patients treated with reserpine.

Reserpine is an effective and very cheap antihypertensive; when used in low doses in combination with low-dose "diuretics" or other agents that do not inhibit the adrenergic nervous system, the drug appears to have only modest adverse effects. Reports of depression and suicide understandably have limited its use but may not be warranted when the drug is used at doses not exceeding 0.25 mg/day.

**PRINCIPLE Once a drug has developed a compromised reputation, even when that reputation was based on use at excessive doses, it may be difficult for it to be resuscitated.**

## Guanethidine

### *Pharmacology and mechanism of action*

Guanethidine inhibits the release of norepinephrine from peripheral sympathetic nerve endings. Guanadrel is a very similar drug with a shorter duration of action. Guanethidine is taken up in sympathetic neurons via the catecholamine transporter and then enters secretory granules from which it displaces norepinephrine, leading to depletion of this neurotransmitter from the nerve endings. Because the drug appears not to enter the CNS, this action seems to explain the peripheral vasodilation and decrease in blood pressure caused by guanethidine. Depletion of norepinephrine from sympathetic fibers in veins frequently occurs with this drug. Serious adverse effects of the drug are likely due to depletion of norepinephrine; these effects include postural hypotension that may be severe, retrograde ejaculation, and fluid retention. Diarrhea can become marked with guanethidine, although the mechanism of action for this effect is not understood. Because the adverse effects of the drug are so severe and almost inevitable, a therapeutic trial with guanethidine should only be considered in exceptional patients who do not respond to other available antihypertensive drugs or cannot tolerate them. This resistance is exceptional with currently available medications.

## $\alpha$-Adrenergic Receptor Antagonists

### *Pharmacology and mechanism of action*

Prazosin was developed as a direct-acting vasodilator (structurally related to theophyllines) but was subsequently found to be an $\alpha$-adrenergic antagonist. With the discovery of $\alpha_1$- and $\alpha_2$-adrenergic receptors, it became clear that prazosin was very much more potent in blocking $\alpha_1$- than $\alpha_2$-adrenergic receptors. Additional $\alpha_1$-adrenergic receptor selective antagonists have subsequently been developed with different pharmacokinetic profiles and possibly different effects on $\alpha_1$-adrenergic receptor subtypes. These drugs are listed in Table 1-3. Doxazosin and

Table 1-3 $\alpha_1$-Adrenergic Receptor Antagonists

| Drug | Duration of action for hypertension (h) |
|---|---|
| Doxazosin mesylate | 24 |
| Prazosin HCl | 7–10 |
| Terazosin HCl | 24 |

terazosin are similar to prazosin, although their duration of action as autohypertensives is longer, allowing once daily dosing in most patients. Tamsulosin is an $\alpha_1$-adrenergic receptor antagonist that was developed to treat benign prostate hyperplasia rather than hypertension; it has some selectivity for the $\alpha_1$-adrenergic receptor subtype in the prostate, which may contribute to its efficacy in that disease.

The $\alpha$-adrenergic blocking agents that are clinically useful to treat hypertension are selective $\alpha_1$-adrenergic receptor blocking agents. They antagonize the vasoconstrictor actions of norepinephrine and epinephrine. This effect causes arteriolar vasodilatation and lowers peripheral vascular resistance. The action may lead to venodilation and a fall in venous return. The combination of decreased peripheral vascular resistance with decreased venous return impairs the body's response to upright posture and can result in orthostatic hypotension that can be symptomatic, particularly with initial dosing (the so-called "first-dose effect"). However, the orthostatic effects attenuate over time. There is little evidence of loss of efficacy (tachyphylaxis) in the long-term antihypertensive effects of prazosin and related drugs; however, this is in contrast to effects in refractory congestive heart failure for which prazosin's effects quickly wane (see the section on Congestive Heart Failure in this chapter).

### *Clinical use and adverse effects of $\alpha$-adrenergic receptor antagonists*

The typical antihypertensive effect of $\alpha_1$-adrenergic receptor antagonists is similar to the average effects of other major, commonly used antihypertensive drugs. Falls in blood pressure are typically in the range of about 10/10 mm Hg. $\alpha$-Adrenergic antagonists are antihypertensive agents that actually lower LDL cholesterol and raise high-density lipoprotein (HDL) cholesterol (in other words, they have potentially favorable effects on plasma lipids) (Carruthers et al. 1993, Rabkin et al. 1994). Unfortunately there are no data yet to determine whether this effect translates into a reduction of atherosclerotic disease in humans. Prazosin can be used in asthmatic patients because it has a mild relaxant effect on bronchial smooth muscle and may improve exercise-induced asthma. Because $\alpha$-adrenergic antagonists decrease symptomatic urinary hesitancy and bladder neck spasm associated with prostatic hyperplasia, these drugs are very attractive for use in hypertensive men with prostatism.

Adverse effects often occur early in therapy using prazosin. Symptomatic orthostatic hypotension is common with initial large doses (10–50% at $\geq$2 mg) and in patients who are fasting, volume-depleted, salt-restricted, or elderly, or who are taking any other antihypertensive drug. Using an initial dose of 0.5–1.0 mg given at bedtime for a few days minimizes this risk. Similarly, it is important to initiate therapy at analogously low doses with other $\alpha_1$-adrenergic receptor antagonists. Drugs in this class may have an increased risk of causing orthostatic hypotension in the elderly. It is also important to check upright blood pressure before increasing the daily dose of any of these drugs. Fatigue, nonspecific dizziness (unrelated to postural hypotension), and headaches can be caused by these drugs.

***Recommendations***

$\alpha$-Adrenergic antagonists are effective and can be safe antihypertensive drugs. Generally considered to be second-line therapeutic agents in the treatment of hypertension, they may be particularly advantageous in hypertensive patients with prostatism or possibly with vasospasm such as Raynaud's phenomenon or with aortic or mitral valvular insufficiency. These drugs may be neutral or possibly advantageous in hypertensive patients with associated asthma or dyslipidemia. Because they are much more difficult to titrate, phenoxybenzamine and phentolamine are not indicated for the treatment of primary hypertension; phenoxybenzamine can be useful in treating pheochromocytoma.

## $\beta$-Adrenergic Receptor Antagonists

***Pharmacology and mechanism of action***

Propranolol, a nonselective $\beta_1$- and $\beta_2$-adrenergic receptor antagonist, became available in the early 1960s and quickly established the safety and efficacy of this new class of drugs. It is interesting to note that propranolol was originally developed and used to prevent angina. The antihypertensive action of $\beta$-adrenergic receptor blocking agents ("beta-blockers") was unexpected and discovered by serendipity after their initial use in humans. Many $\beta$-adrenergic receptor antagonists with subtle or more markedly distinctive pharmacologic properties have subsequently become available.

$\beta$-Adrenergic blocking agents competitively antagonize the effects of catecholamines at $\beta$-adrenergic receptors. In spite of extensive animal and human experimentation, the mechanism(s) responsible for the antihypertensive effects of $\beta$-adrenergic antagonists remains uncertain. These drugs do not generally cause hypotension when administered chronically to normal individuals but rather are antihypertensive agents. Acutely, $\beta$-adrenergic antagonists decrease heart rate and stroke volume and lower cardiac output. There is an initial increase in peripheral resistance that may be related to blockade of $\beta$-adrenergic receptors in blood vessels that promote vasodilation, leaving unopposed $\alpha$-adrenergic vasoconstrictor actions of catecholamines. However, with chronic treatment, peripheral vascular resistance returns to baseline values or lower. How this transition occurs is not clear. Potentially contributing factors may involve $\beta$-adrenergic-antagonist-induced inhibition of renin secretion or inhibition of presynaptic $\beta_2$-adrenergic receptors that ordinarily enhance the release of norepinephrine. $\beta$-Adrenergic antagonists also may act by an as-yet-undetermined mechanism in the CNS.

**PRINCIPLE When a prototype of a class of drugs has multiple mechanisms that contribute to efficacy, it does not necessarily follow that other drugs in the same class will share each of the useful mechanisms and not have other potentially adverse actions.**

Pharmaceutical ingenuity has led to the development of a multiplicity of $\beta$-adrenergic antagonists with divergent pharmacologic features such as selective affinity for $\beta_1$- rather than $\beta_2$-adrenergic receptors, or partial agonist activity (also called *intrinsic sympathomimetic activity*), and markedly different pharmacokinetic properties. As theoretically attractive as more specialized agents might be therapeutically, one must first determine whether a $\beta$-adrenergic receptor antagonist should be used, then determine whether there are clinically important differences between the agents, and only then make a therapeutic choice based on the differences within the class.

**PRINCIPLE Choose the class of drug first; then choose within the class. But do not assume that drugs within a given class are interchangeable.**

Some $\beta$-adrenergic antagonists have a relatively low affinity for $\beta_2$-adrenergic receptors. They are therefore called *$\beta_1$-adrenergic-selective agents*; however, at clinically useful doses, these drugs may substantially block both $\beta_1$- and $\beta_2$-adrenergic receptors. In other words, the relative selectivity is limited and tends to be overcome as the dose is increased. Furthermore, adverse effects may be seen at very low doses in some asthmatics, which limits the advantage of currently available $\beta_1$-adrenergic-selective drugs (Wilcox et al. 1986).

**PRINCIPLE Claims of receptor selectivity should be viewed with caution; their significance may be influenced by variations in drug concentration, receptor populations, and disease states.**

$\beta_1$-Adrenergic receptor blockade seems critical for antihypertensive effects; however, experimental $\beta_2$-adrenergic-selective blocking agents may not have appreciable antihypertensive effect. Table 1-4 shows the presence and functions of $\beta_1$- and $\beta_2$-adrenergic receptors in human tissues. In addition, there has been considerable recent interest in the possibility that $\beta_3$-adrenergic receptors may be important in regulating lipolysis in humans.

Although it would be very helpful if $\beta_1$-adrenergic-selective antagonists could be used safely in asthmatics, unfortunately, clinically available drugs may still block $\beta_2$-adrenergic receptors in airways. These receptors contribute to bronchodilation. As a consequence, antagonism of these receptors may lead to sharply worsened bronchoconstriction. Therefore, physicians should be very cautious when using any selective $\beta$-adrenergic antagonist in patients in whom $\beta_2$-adrenergic receptor blockade could lead to severe adverse effects. An analogous situation also occurs in diabetics who have hypoglycemic reactions. $\beta_2$-adrenergic receptors, likely on liver cells, are important for the recovery from hypoglycemia via activation of glycogen phosphorylase. If these receptors are blocked, some patients may experience delayed recovery from hypoglycemia. In addition, antagonism of other $\beta_2$-adrenergic receptors may mask some of the symptoms of hypoglycemia—a "double whammy" in these patients.

Some $\beta$-adrenergic receptor antagonists bind to the receptor and stimulate them, albeit with less effect than would epinephrine. These entities are said to be partial agonists or to possess intrinsic sympathomimetic activity. Drugs of this type may have smaller effects than complete antagonists under resting conditions when receptor activation is modest. However, partial agonists serve well to block the effects of increasing concentrations of full agonists such as epinephrine or norepinephrine. For example, a partial agonist might have less effect on resting heart rate than a full agonist yet still effectively block the rise in heart rate that ordinarily occurs upon exercise. The clinical significance of partial agonism is not clear. Table 1-5 shows the categorization of the available $\beta$-adrenergic antagonists according to their various pharmacologic properties.

**Table 1-4 Some Adrenergic Receptor Functions in Human Tissues**

| | Location | Function |
|---|---|---|
| $\alpha_1$ | Arterioles | Constriction |
| | Veins | Constriction |
| | Heart | Inotropy |
| | Bladder sphincter | Contraction |
| | Pupil | Mydriasis |
| | Pilomotor | Contraction |
| $\alpha_2$ | Arterioles | Constriction |
| | CNS | Reduction of sympathetic outflow |
| | Heart | Inotropy |
| | Presynaptic noradrenergic terminals | Reduction of norepinephrine release |
| | Platelets | Aggregation |
| | Adipocytes | Reduction of lipolysis |
| | Various cells | Opposition to $K^+$ entry |
| | Kidney | $Na^+$ retention |
| $\beta_1$ | Heart | Inotropy and chronotropy |
| | Kidney | Renin release |
| $\beta_2$ | Arterioles | Dilation |
| | Heart | Inotropy and chronotropy |
| | Islet cells | Insulin release |
| | Bronchi | Dilation |
| | Presynaptic noradrenergic terminals | Enhancement of norepinephrine release |
| | Various cells | $K^+$ entry |
| | Uterus | Relaxation |
| | Leukocytes | Demargination |
| $\beta_3$ | Adipocytes | Lipolysis |

Some drugs categorized as $\beta$-adrenergic antagonists have additional pharmacologic effects that may be important. Labetalol is also a potent reversible $\beta_1$-adrenergic receptor antagonist. The clinically available form of labetalol consists of a mixture of the four isomers that result from labetalol's having two optical centers. Although this mixture has the capacity to block both $\alpha_1$- and $\beta_1$-adrenergic receptors, each of the separated isomers has different potencies for these receptors. Carvedilol is another $\beta_1$-adrenergic receptor antagonist with some capacity to block $\alpha_1$-adrenergic receptors; in addition, this drug may have other properties that lead to peripheral vasodilation. Carvedilol also has an antioxidant moiety that may contribute to its efficacy, especially in patients with congestive heart failure.

**Table 1-5 β-Adrenergic Receptor Antagonists Used in Primary Hypertension**

| DRUG | SELECTIVITY | ISA | HALF-LIFE (H) |
|---|---|---|---|
| Acebutolol HCl* | $\beta_1$ | + | 4[a] |
| Atenolol $\beta_1$ | 7 | | |
| Betaxolol HCl | $\beta_1$ | 14–22 | |
| Bisoprolol fumarate | $\beta_1$ | 9–12 | |
| Carteolol | + | 6 | |
| Carvedilol | | | |
| Labetalol HCl | 6–8 | $\alpha_1$-Adrenergic receptor antagonist | |
| Metoprolol succinate | $\beta_1$ | 3–7 | Sustained release formulation |
| Nadolol | 20–24 | | |
| Oxprenolol | + | Sustained release formulation | |
| Penbutolol sulfate | 5 | | |
| Pindolol | + | 3–4 | |
| Propranolol HCl | 3–4 | | |
| Timolol maleate | 4 | | |

[a]Acebutolol has a major, active metabolite ciacetolol, which is cardioselective (half-life, 8–13 hr).
ABBREVIATIONS: ISA, intrinsic sympathomimetic activity.

> **PRINCIPLE Drugs in the same class can have very important known (and potentially unknown) differences that may be clinically important.**

The dose of propranolol must be titrated over a relatively large range. On the other hand, the variation in effect from person to person is less with atenolol; consequently, a much more limited dosing range is required for this drug. The more water-soluble antagonists (e.g., atenolol, nadolol) may have a lower rate of penetration into the CNS than more lipid-soluble antagonists. It is possible that these drugs have lower rates of CNS-mediated adverse effects, although comparative data are lacking.

### *Clinical use and adverse effects of β-adrenergic receptor antagonists*

As monotherapy, β-adrenergic antagonists, when studied in direct comparison, have similar efficacy in lowering blood pressure as most other agents. Studies comparing the various β-adrenergic antagonists usually reveal no difference in their antihypertensive effects. β-Adrenergic antagonists may have limited effectiveness as monotherapy in African Americans as a group. However, some individuals may respond well, and these drugs are useful when combined with other agents. There is also evidence suggesting that the efficacy of β-adrenergic antagonists may be lessened in smokers and in the elderly. As shown in Table 1-6, β-adrenergic antagonists have a long list of both indications and relative contraindications. A careful search for any of these factors in an individual patient may determine a decision regarding the choice of which agent to use. β-Adrenergic antagonists may be used with other agents (with the emphasis on those that do not affect the adrenergic system). β-Adrenergic antagonists are especially useful in combination therapy for patients taking vasodilators. In such a setting, the β-adrenergic antagonists interfere with the reflex sympathetic effects stimulated by vasodilation.

Adverse effects of propranolol and other β-adrenergic antagonists are well known. They include fatigue, sleep disturbance, and male sexual dysfunction. $\beta_2$-Adrenergic receptor blockade can aggravate bronchospasm, which may be life-threatening. These drugs may potentially worsen symptoms of peripheral vascular disease including Raynaud's phenomenon and intermittent claudication, although this is unpredictable. Decreased cardiac output and inhibition of $\beta_2$-adrenergic-mediated vasodilatation in muscles may lead to a reduction in exercise tolerance that may be further impaired by diminished free fatty acid flux to exercising muscles. Because β-adrenergic antagonists antagonize the effects of catecholamines, the use of epinephrine in countering severe allergic reactions may require larger than typical doses and may result in severe hypertension in patients receiving nonselective β-adren-

Table 1-6 **Influence of Concomitant Disease on Choice of Therapy**

| | Use in | Avoid in[a] |
|---|---|---|
| Diuretics | Volume overload states | Hyperlipidemia |
| | Renal failure | Gout |
| | Heart failure | Diabetes |
| | | Impotence |
| | | Electrolyte imbalances |
| β-Blocker | Angina | Diabetes |
| | Postmyocardial infarct | Asthma/COPD |
| | Migraine | Heart failure |
| | Tachyarrhythmia | Raynaud phenomenon |
| | Mitral valve prolapse | Peripheral vascular disease |
| | Thyrotoxicosis | Bradyarrhythmia/AV block |
| | Aortic dissection | Depression |
| | Essential tremor | Impotence |
| | Glaucoma | |
| | Hypertrophic cardiomyopathy | |
| | Anxiety states | |
| Sympatholytics | Perimenopausal flushing | Impotence |
| | | Depression |
| | | CNS disease |
| | | Orthostatic hypotension |
| Vasodilators (excluding calcium antagonists) | Heart failure | |
| Calcium-channel blockers | Angina | Bradyarrhythmias |
| | Tachyarrhythmia | Heart failure |
| | Hypertrophic cardiomyopathy | Constipation (verapamil) |
| | Raynaud phenomenon | Edema states (nifedipine) |
| | Migraine | |

[a]Note that the "avoid in" column provides a partial list of adverse effects.

ergic blocking agents because of unopposed α-adrenergic receptor–mediated vasoconstriction.

In type I diabetic patients, these agents mask the sympathetic responses to hypoglycemia, delaying recognition of the hypoglycemic state by both the patient and the physician. β-Adrenergic receptor blocking agents may impair counterregulatory responses necessary for warding off or minimizing the hypoglycemia. Because tight control of blood glucose is important in type I diabetics, and this is associated with potentially frequent hypoglycemic reactions, β-adrenergic antagonists should be used only with considerable caution and if specially required in diabetic patients taking insulin. $\beta_1$-Adrenergic-selective compounds contained to the lower doses of effectiveness may be preferable in this context.

β-Adrenergic receptor blockade can decrease HDL cholesterol concentrations and increase triglyceride concentrations, but the clinical significance of this is unknown. This may be less likely to occur when the drugs have intrinsic sympathomimetic activity. $\beta_2$-Adrenergic receptor stimulation causes entry of potassium into cells. Therefore, antagonists of these receptors can increase potassium concentrations in plasma, especially in association with exercise or other potassium-sparing drugs such as spironolactone, triamterene, or ACE inhibitors.

The effects of β-adrenergic antagonists can adversely influence patients who are susceptible to bradyarrhythmias, atrioventricular (AV) node conduction delays, and heart failure. This is a concern when using the drugs in patients who are taking digitalis or nondihydropyridine calcium antagonists such as verapamil and diltiazem. In theory, bradycardia is less likely to occur when drugs have intrinsic sympathomimetic activity.

Abrupt withdrawal from some β-adrenergic blocking agents may result in a withdrawal syndrome, especially in patients with coronary disease (Rangno 1984). Symptoms may manifest as worsening angina, myocardial infarction, or cardiac arrest. Rebound hypertension is unusual following withdrawal of β-adrenergic blocking agents. But potential rebound can be prevented by tapering the drug or by using β-adrenergic blocking agents with long half-lives.

***Recommendations***

β-Adrenergic antagonists remain a first-line therapy for hypertension. The response rate and acceptance of the drugs are excellent, and their value has been repeatedly demonstrated, especially in patients younger than 65 years of age. The presence of other diseases coexisting with hypertension, or the use of additional antihypertensive agents in a patient, is a determinant of whether β-adrenergic antagonists should be used. Once the decision to use a β-adrenergic antagonist has been made, the pharmacologic differences between them should be exploited. β-Adrenergic antagonists are useful in conjunction with other nonsympatholytic agents, especially vasodilators, and have been used effectively during pregnancy (see chapter 19, Drug Therapy in Pregnant and Breast-Feeding Women). Adverse effects can be avoided by considering patient factors, using the lowest effective doses, and titrating doses appropriately.

## Angiotensin-Converting Enzyme Inhibitors

### *Pharmacology and mechanisms of action*

The renin–angiotensin system plays a major role in the regulation of blood pressure and extracellular fluid volume. Angiotensin-converting enzyme (ACE) inhibitors are a major group of drugs available to inhibit this system. Table 1-7 lists some currently available ACE inhibitors. Although pharmacologic differences among these drugs are often emphasized, the clinical relevance of these distinctions is not obvious.

A number of actions of ACE inhibitors potentially contribute to their antihypertensive effects. The enzyme ACE is a kininase responsible for the conversion of angiotensin I to angiotensin II, a potent endogenous octapeptide that causes arterial smooth muscle contraction. As a consequence, inhibition of this conversion may lead to vasodilation. Angiotensin II stimulates the secretion of aldosterone from the adrenal cortex, leading to increased sodium retention and potassium excretion by the kidney. Inhibition of this action may lead to a decrease in plasma volume. Inhibiting aldosterone secretion by an ACE inhibitor may enhance the action and antagonize fluid retention that may occur with other classes of vasodilating drugs. In addition, angiotensin II may facilitate the release of norepinephrine from sympathetic nerve endings; ACE inhibitors may attenuate the contribution of the sympathetic nervous system to increased peripheral resistance.

Angiotensin-converting enzyme is also the enzyme responsible for metabolizing and inactivating the vasodilator bradykinin and related kinins. As a consequence, ACE inhibitors tend to enhance accumulation of vasodilating substances that may contribute to their antihypertensive actions. Different mechanisms of the ACE inhibitors effects may contribute to efficacy at different times over the course of therapy with this class of drugs. For example, the degree of blood pressure reduction may or may not correlate well with the degree of inhibition of plasma ACE. As with the β-adrenergic antagonists, labeling of a drug class by mechanism does not necessarily define all its important pharmacologic actions.

Angiotensin II has the capacity to activate a variety of biochemical pathways that enhance cell growth. This is potentially particularly important for the cardiac hypertrophy and vascular remodeling that occur in many patients with hypertension. ACE inhibitors can prevent or reverse cardiac hypertrophic changes in hypertensive animals and humans, although most other antihypertensive drugs have efficacy in reducing hypertrophy as well.

Captopril, a sulfhydryl-containing compound, was the first ACE inhibitor approved for treating hypertension. Other ACE inhibitors lacking the sulfhydryl group became available several years later. Enalapril is an inactive prodrug that must be converted by the liver to enalaprilat, the active ACE inhibitor. Lisinopril is an active lysine derivative of enalaprilat. Many additional ACE inhibitors have subsequently become available (see Table 1-7).

Angiotensin-converting enzyme inhibitors are typically well absorbed after oral administration. Food decreases the absorption of captopril by 30% but has no effect on absorption of enalapril. Captopril begins its antihypertensive effects within 30 minutes, and the effects of lisinopril begin within 90 minutes of ingestion. The required conversion of enalapril to enalaprilat in the liver results in its slow accumulation and a delayed peak effect. Elimination of ACE inhibitors is prolonged in patients with advanced renal failure. Although many ACE inhibitors are labeled for use once daily, for a substantial number of patients, especially patients receiving relatively low doses, the antihypertensive effects may not last 24 hours. For these patients, the chosen ACE inhibitor should probably be administered twice daily.

**Table 1-7 Angiotensin Converting Enzyme Inhibitors**

| DRUG | TYPICAL DOSING RANGE (MG/DAY) |
|---|---|
| Benazepril HCl | 5–40 |
| Captopril | 25–150 |
| Enalapril maleate | 5–40 |
| Fosinopril sodium | 10–40 |
| Lisinopril | 5–40 |
| Moexipril HCl | 7.5–15 |
| Quinapril HCl | 5–80 |
| Ramipril | 1.25–20 |
| Trandolapril | 1–4 |

NOTE: Captopril has the shortest duration of action of these ACE inhibitors, requiring 2–3 times daily dosing. Although many other ACE inhibitors are approved in the USA for once daily dosing, some patients will require twice daily dosing to achieve adequate 24-hour blood pressure control. Many patients will not have additional antihypertensive responses to these drugs at the higher end of the approved dose range because of an earlier plateau of the dose–response curve.

SOURCE: Modified from Joint National Committee, 1997.

### *Clinical use and adverse effects of ACE inhibitors*

As with most other within-class comparisons, ACE inhibitors (e.g., captopril, enalapril, lisinopril) have similar capacities to decrease elevated blood pressure, on the order of 10–15/5–12 mm Hg. These agents, like a number of antihypertensives—particularly diuretics—have relatively steep dose–response curves at low doses, with plateauing of the dose–response curve at higher doses.

**PRINCIPLE For drugs with easily measured effects (e.g., blood pressure), the physician may adjust dose based on the patient's actual response to the drug, rather than relying solely on the drug's labeling.**

The ACE inhibitors used as monotherapy have efficacy similar to many other classes of antihypertensives used as monotherapy. Addition of a diuretic to an ACE inhibitor appears to have synergistic effects in lowering blood pressure. This attractive interaction may be due in part to the capacity of ACE inhibitors to antagonize the effects of activation of the renin-angiotensin system typically found in patients receiving a diuretic alone. In addition, hypokalemia caused by diuretics is opposed by combination of the diuretic with an ACE inhibitor because of inhibition of aldosterone secretion.

Angiotensin-converting enzyme inhibitors are effective as antihypertensive agents in about 60–70% of patients. The magnitude of the decrease in blood pressure is proportional to the pretreatment values. Clinical trials have shown that the antihypertensive effects are secondary to a decrease in peripheral vascular resistance with little change in cardiac output and no reflex tachycardia. ACE inhibitors reduce overall renal vascular resistance and can increase renal blood flow. Indeed, the capacity of ACE inhibitors to lower glomerular pressure, possibly owing to preferentially dilating glomerular efferent arterioles, has suggested that these drugs may be especially efficacious in preserving renal function in hypertensive patients with nephropathy, especially type I diabetics (see chapter 6, Renal Disorders and the Influence of Renal Function on Drug Disposition, and chapter 9, Endocrine and Metabolic Disorders). Patients with renovascular hypertension may respond very well to ACE inhibitors, but there are caveats in these patients (see below). These agents are useful in treating severe hypertension, for example, as a vasodilator third-drug therapy added to a regimen of $\beta$-adrenergic antagonists and diuretics.

Excessive declines in blood pressure, even leading to severe orthostatic hypotension, can occur, especially when patients are volume-depleted or taking diuretics. In these settings, angiotensin II may be playing a particularly large role in maintaining blood pressure. In patients at risk, ACE inhibition should be initiated cautiously and with particularly low starting doses (e.g., 2.5 mg lisinopril, 6.25 mg captopril). Skin rashes, disturbance of taste, and mucosal lesions are more common with captopril than with other ACE inhibitors; these adverse effects may be related to its sulfhydryl moiety or to the rather large doses used in early trials. Probably the most common adverse effect of ACE inhibitors is dry cough that occurs in about 10% of patients and is severe in 1–3% of patients. The mechanism is unclear but may relate to the accumulation of peptide mediators that can enhance the cough reflex. Cough may be dose-dependent and is fully reversible with discontinuation of the drug. On the other hand, cough is an unusual adverse effect in patients receiving angiotensin II receptor antagonists (see below).

Early reports of neutropenia and proteinuria with captopril appeared when patients were taking very high doses and had other diseases such as renal failure and connective tissue disease (with associated cytotoxic drug treatments) that may have predisposed them to the toxic effects. These adverse effects are rare. Angioneurotic edema, which can occur with all ACE inhibitors, can be life-threatening and is observed in less than 0.1% of patients. The risk of angioneurotic edema probably is higher in patients in whom drug administration is continued despite the development of mouth ulcers or skin rash.

Because ACE inhibitors decrease aldosterone concentrations, hyperkalemia may result, but it is rarely encountered in patients with normal renal function. Caution should be exercised in administrating ACE inhibitors to patients with renal impairment, type 4 renal tubular acidosis (hyporeninemic hypoaldosteronism) as is seen in diabetic patients, and in combination with potassium-sparing diuretics or potassium supplementation. ACE inhibitors should not be used during pregnancy because of the high risk of renal developmental anomalies.

The ACE inhibitors can exacerbate renal insufficiency in patients with renal vascular stenosis. This complication deserves scrutiny. With decreased renal blood flow during renal artery narrowing, preferential vasodilatation of the glomerular afferent arteriole occurs in order to reduce resistance to blood flow, while tending to preserve glomerular pressure. This adaptation is associated with angiotensin II–induced vasoconstriction of the efferent arteriole. Although this increases postglomerular resistance to blood flow, it increases hydrostatic pressure in the glomerulus and favors glomerular filtration at any perfusion pressure. In this setting of decreased renal blood flow, the filtration fraction is increased, tending to preserve glomerular filtration. Interruption of this compensatory mechanism with an ACE inhibitor can lead to a decrease in glomerular filtration rate (GFR) in the underperfused kidney. In fact, this phenomenon has been exploited with the use of captopril during isotopic renography. The drug exaggerates a difference between the normal (non-angiotensin II–dependent) and renal arterial stenotic (angiotensin II–dependent) kidney. The normal kidney in a patient with unilateral renovascular hypertension can compensate for the effects of ACE inhibition by increasing GFR and keeping serum creatinine concentrations constant. However, when both kidneys are underperfused or when there is a solitary kidney with a stenotic artery, loss of this compensating mechanism leads to rapid reversible rises in serum creatinine concentration. Administration of an ACE inhibitor in any clinical setting of decreased renal perfusion has the potential for worsening the insufficiency.

On the other hand, as indicated above, the effect of ACE inhibitors on postglomerular resistance has a potential long-term advantage in patients with diabetic glomerulopathy. Inhibition of postglomerular tone reduces the transglomerular capillary hydraulic pressure gradient that is thought to play a role in development of glomerular basement membrane damage and subsequent diabetic glomerulosclerosis.

**PRINCIPLE Understanding the pharmacology of new drugs may lead to new diagnostic or therapeutic hypotheses and uses. The actual value and place of these new, potential indications must be established in clinical studies.**

### *Recommendations*

ACE inhibitors are valuable as effective and reasonably safe antihypertensive agents. Their adverse effects are generally predictable, avoidable, or reversible. ACE inhibitors may be considered as first-line therapy, especially for patients in whom diuretics and/or $\beta$-adrenergic antagonists are contraindicated. They are especially useful when combined with diuretics. Of course, using ACE inhibitors to treat patients with heart failure and hypertension exploits the two-for-one principle (see Table 1-6) (see the section on Congestive Heart Failure in this chapter). Because of their additive effects with other agents, they are also useful in treating severe hypertension and as third-drug vasodilator in combined regimens.

## Angiotensin II Receptor Antagonists

### *Pharmacology and mechanism of action*

As described above, ACE inhibitors are useful antihypertensive drugs whose major mechanism of action involves inhibiting the synthesis of angiotensin II. In view of this extensive experience, it is not surprising that angiotensin II receptor antagonists are efficacious in lowering blood pressure in patients with hypertension. Losartan, a nonapeptide angiotensin II receptor antagonist, was the first drug in this class available for treating hypertension. Other examples include valsartan, eprosartan, candesartan, and irbesartan (see Table 1-8).

Angiotensin receptors are coupled to G proteins that contribute to the activation of smooth muscle contraction and growth. They share many signal transduction pathways with $\alpha_1$-adrenergic receptors. Two angiotensin receptors are now known, namely, $AT_1$ and $AT_2$ receptors. $AT_1$ receptors are involved in the mechanism by which angiotensin II stimulates smooth muscle contraction in blood vessels and aldosterone secretion from the adrenal cortex. In response to blockade of these receptors, plasma concentrations of renin and angiotensin II rise. The possible clinical significance of these adaptations is not known. The available angiotensin II receptor antagonists are selective for $AT_1$ receptors.

Losartan is well absorbed after oral administration, and it undergoes extensive first-pass metabolism by the cytochrome P450 system. A very potent active metabolite is produced that is responsible for most of losartin's pharmacologic effects. Although the parent compound has a short half-life (about 2 hours), the main active metabolite has a half-life of about 6–9 hours. Unlike losartan, valsartan is not a prodrug and is not dependent on cytochrome P450 metabolism for activation. Valsartan has a longer half-life and duration of action. Candesartan exhibits noncompetitive antagonism at $AT_1$ receptors, and its very high affinity for these receptors appears to contribute to its long duration of action. The therapeutic relevance of these differences is currently uncertain.

### *Clinical use and adverse effects of angiotensin II receptor antagonists*

Losartan is efficacious in the treatment of hypertension. Its capacity to lower blood pressure as monotherapy is similar to that of many other antihypertensive drugs. How closely the efficacy of angiotensin II receptor antagonists compares with ACE inhibitors will be better known with greater clinical experience. The maximal antihypertensive effects may require 4–6 weeks at a given dose, a time

Table 1-8 Angiotensin II Receptor Antagonists

| DRUG | TYPICAL DOSING RANGE (MG/DAY) |
|---|---|
| Losartan potassium | 25–50 |
| Valsartan | 80–160 |
| Irbesartan | |
| Candesartan | |
| Eprosartan | |

NOTE: The last three drugs are new and no typical dosing range is available.

course found for many antihypertensive drugs. Controlled trials have demonstrated that adding a thiazide diuretic to established therapy has added benefit. Indeed, the actions of angiotensin receptor antagonists can be conceptually linked with those of the better known ACE inhibitors.

The adverse effects of ACE inhibitors due to decreased activation of angiotensin receptors should be expected in patients receiving an angiotensin II receptor antagonist. Specifically, this applies to the adverse effects described above in the ACE inhibitor section for renal function and potassium retention. This also includes the advisory that these drugs not be used in pregnant women because of the importance of the renin–angiotensin system in fetal development, especially in the second and third trimesters. Cough induced by ACE inhibitors is not thought to involve changes in angiotensin II's effects; as expected, cough appears rarely with angiotensin II receptor antagonists. The incidence of angioedema likely will also be less than with ACE inhibitors. However, the experience with the receptor antagonists is so far relatively limited. In addition, the possible consequences, if any, of chronic, marked activation of the renin–angiotensin II system with these drugs remains to be determined.

***Recommendations***

The first marketed angiotensin II receptor antagonist became available in the United States as recently as 1995. As a consequence, the long-term effects of these drugs are not yet known, for neither reduction of risk of clinically important endpoints such as stroke nor potential long-term adverse effects.

**PRINCIPLE It is an obvious truism that long-term consequences of new drugs are generally not known when they are introduced; the physician and patient should balance this uncertainty with the apparent potential advantages of using a new drug.**

Angiotensin II receptor antagonists are effective in lowering the blood pressure of hypertensives and are useful in combination with diuretics. The drugs may be useful in those patients who have unacceptable ACE inhibitor-induced cough. However, to what extent they may share the benefits of ACE inhibitors in hypertensive patients with congestive heart failure or type I diabetes is not yet known. The results of a study designed to compare the safety and efficacy of losartan with captopril in older patients with congestive heart failure had an unanticipated beneficial impact on overall mortality in the losartan group (Pitt et al. 1997). A follow-up study (ELITE 2, an adequately powered multicentered clinical trial) is currently under way to determine whether this was a chance finding or a superior benefit of losartan compared with ACE inhibitors in patients with congestive heart failure.

## Calcium Channel Blockers

***Pharmacology and mechanism of action***

Sustained contraction of blood vessels is a major determinant of peripheral vascular resistance. Because the intracellular concentration of calcium is critical in determining the extent of vascular smooth muscle contraction, it is not surprising that drugs that inhibit calcium entry into vascular smooth muscle cells can play an important role in the treatment of hypertension. Although the mechanisms of action are not completely understood, these drugs inhibit the entry of calcium ions into smooth muscle cells by blocking voltage-gated L-type (i.e., late) calcium channels (also simply called *L channels*). In addition, some of these drugs antagonize entry of calcium into cardiac myocytes and cells in the conduction system of the heart; these actions contribute to negative inotropic effects and alterations in cardiac conductance. See Table 1-9 for general properties of many available calcium-entry blockers.

The first clinically available calcium-entry blocker, namely verapamil, is a congener of papaverine. Many other calcium-entry blockers are now available and have a wide range of structures. The largest group, which in-

**Table 1-9 Calcium Channel Entry Blockers**

| DRUG | DAILY DOSE |
|---|---|
| *Nondihydropyridines* | |
| Diltiazem HCl (Cardizem SR) | 120–360 mg bid |
| (Cardizem CD) | 120–360 mg |
| (Dilacor XR, Tiazac) | |
| Verapamil HCl (Isoptin SR, Calan SR) | 90–480 mg bid |
| (Verelan, Covera HS) | 120–480 mg |
| *Dihydropyridines* | |
| Amlodipine besylate | 2.5–10 mg |
| Felodipine | 2.5–20 mg |
| Isradipine (DynaCirc CR) | 5–20 mg |
| Nicardipine HCl | 60–90 mg bid |
| Nifedipine (Procardia XL) | 30–120 mg |
| (Adalat CC) | |
| Nisoldipine | 20–60 mg |

NOTE: As a group, the dihydropyridines tend to have greater effects on the peripheral vasculature than on the heart. On the other hand, the nondihydropyridines have greater effects on cardiac myocytes as well as inhibitory effects on the sinus and AV nodal conducting systems. Trade names are shown for drugs that are preferably used as long-acting formulations; more rapidly absorbed formulations of these drugs are generally not appropriate therapy for primary hypertension

cludes amlodipine, felodipine, isradipine, nicardipine, and nifedipine, is called *dihydropyridines.* Interestingly, these different structures lead to differences in their sites and modes of action on calcium entry for reasons that are not well understood. Intracellular calcium flux is a final common path for a spectrum of cellular responses to a variety of stimuli. Given that the molecular basis of calcium channels is quite heterogeneous, coupled with the chemical heterogeneity of available calcium channel blockers, the pharmacologic similarities of presently available compounds may be more apparent than real (see clinical use and adverse effects below). The latest addition to the calcium channel blocker class acts mainly on so-called T-type (i.e., transient) calcium channels (also simply called *T channels*), which are distinct from the L channels blocked by other agents described below. The index T-channel blocker is mibefradil, a compound that is structurally unrelated to the other three major groupings typified by verapamil, nifedipine, and diltiazem.

Verapamil can have marked negative inotropic (contractility), chronotropic (heart rate), and dromotropic (atrioventricular node conduction) actions compared with many other calcium-entry blockers. Nifedipine is a relatively selective peripheral smooth muscle dilator. On the other hand, diltiazem lies somewhere in between these two drugs in terms of balance of effects on the heart versus peripheral vasculature. These differences can be exploited by choosing the most appropriate calcium channel antagonist for individual patients. Calcium-entry blockers typically dilate renal arteries, increasing renal blood flow, GFR, and filtration fraction. This combination of effects contributes to a mild diuretic and natriuretic effect. Mibefradil acts predominantly as a vasodilator, but the reflex tachycardia observed with dihydropyridines is blunted by the ancillary property of blocking T channels on the adrenal that blunts sympatho-adrenal activation and by T-channel blockade on the atria that prevents reflex tachycardia. There is usually mild bradycardia, slowing heart rate by 2–5 beats per minute. At usual doses, mibefradil has minimal impact on the L channels on ventricular myocardium, and the usual cardiodepressant effect of L-channel blockers is not observed. However, mibefradil has been withdrawn from the market because of liver toxicity.

For some calcium channel blockers such as nifedipine, prompt-release formulations lead to rapid increases in drug concentration that have relatively short durations. The peak in concentration has been associated with prompt reductions in peripheral vascular resistance and blood pressure that may be associated with reflex tachycardia. There is epidemiological evidence suggesting that use of this type of formulation of nifedipine is associated with potentially adverse outcomes, especially in patients with coexisting ischemic heart disease. In any event, short-acting calcium-entry blockers used in rapid-release formulations require multiple doses (three or more) per day to provide relatively stable control of blood pressure. Based on available evidence, there does not appear to be a role for short-acting formulations of calcium-entry blockers in the treatment of hypertension. Rather, either long-acting (extended or sustained release) formulations or drugs with intrinsic long half-lives, such as amlodipine, are more efficacious and probably safer for treating primary hypertension. Interestingly, the bioavailability of some dihydropyridines may be potentiated by the consumption of grapefruit juice. The interaction is most striking when the calcium channel blocker, such as felodipine, undergoes substantial first-pass metabolism in the small intestine by cytochrome P450 metabolism (CYP3A4) that is impaired by as yet unidentified substances in the grapefruit juice (Bailey et al. 1998).

#### *Clinical use and adverse effects of calcium channel antagonists*

In comparison with other classes of drugs used as monotherapy for hypertension, calcium-entry blockers have similar capacities as antihypertensive agents. Calcium channel blockers are effective when combined with $\beta$-adrenergic antagonists and ACE inhibitors. Verapamil combined with a $\beta$-adrenergic antagonist therapy is more effective in lowering blood pressure than either drug alone. However, as might be expected, the two drugs may have additive effects on the PR interval seen on the electrocardiogram. As a consequence, this combination should generally be avoided. Because calcium channel blockers have other clinical uses, they are ideal in certain two-for-one situations (see Table 1-6).

Many of the adverse effects caused by calcium channel blockers can be predicted from the differences in pharmacologic effects of the different chemical entities. Because nifedipine acts rapidly, especially when given as liquid-containing capsules, symptomatic hypotension and/or orthostatic hypotension can occur and can be associated with rapid heart rate. The practice of breaking nifedipine capsules to speed drug delivery may exacerbate these adverse effects. Indeed, there is no evidence that this approach to administering nifedipine has efficacy in preventing clinically significant endpoints but may increase the risks of adverse events and unpredictable reductions in blood pressure, especially in patients with severe hypertension or coronary artery disease. Bradyarrhythmias and conduction disturbances are more common with verapamil and to a lesser degree with diltiazem. The arrhythmias are particularly prominent when verapamil is taken in combination with other negative chronotropic and dromotropic agents such as β-adrenergic antagonists, quinidine, or digitalis.

Some calcium-entry blockers (e.g., verapamil) may worsen heart failure by virtue of their adverse effects on systolic myocardial function. However, other members of this class, such as amlodipine and felodipine, have small or negligible negative inotropic effects (see Table 1-9). Although these drugs seem to preferentially relax vascular smooth muscle, relaxation of smooth muscle in other organs can lead to esophageal reflux or urinary retention. Constipation is especially common with verapamil and is unusually most prominent in patients with an underlying tendency toward constipation. Ankle edema can occur, especially with nifedipine. This may be secondary to hemodynamic alterations across the capillary, changing Starling forces to favor movement of fluid from the capillary into the interstitium. Because the edema is local and not associated with renal salt and water retention, diuretics are of little use. The adverse effect of ankle edema should not be clinically confused with the development of congestive heart failure. These drugs tend to be neutral in their effect on lipid profiles. In fact, an antiatherosclerotic effect has been reported in animal models, although the significance of these findings for human disease is unclear.

#### *Recommendations*

Calcium channel blockers are effective as first-line therapy, especially in patients for whom diuretics and β-adrenergic antagonists are contraindicated. Calcium channel blockers are useful for hypertensives with other associated conditions (e.g., angina pectoris, atrial tachyarrhythmias) in which the two-for-one concept can be exploited. They are very useful as alternatives for β-adrenergic antagonists in patients for whom those agents are contraindicated (e.g., patients with asthma), especially patients with angina.

### Direct Vasodilators: Hydralazine and Minoxidil

#### *Pharmacology and mechanism of action*

These two agents are no more "direct" than any of the other vasodilating drugs, but they differ from the others in that their actual mechanisms of action remain uncertain. For hydralazine, the mechanism by which it relaxes arterial smooth muscle is unknown. On the other hand, it is now known that an active metabolite of minoxidil—minoxidil N-O sulfate—opens ATP-modulated potassium channels in arteries. Enhanced efflux of potassium from smooth muscle cells tends to hyperpolarize the smooth muscle cells, which in turn lowers intracellular calcium concentrations and inhibits smooth muscle contraction. Interestingly, hydralazine and minoxidil are highly selective for arterial rather than venous smooth muscle. This selective action tends to cause reflex sympathetic activation and venoconstriction with attendant increases in venous return. In turn, cardiac output increases and limits the antihypertensive effectiveness of the vasodilators. The reflex sympathetic effects on the heart increase myocardial contractility and rate and add to the mechanisms of increased cardiac output. At the same time, the kidney retains salt and water, further increasing blood volume and secondarily venous return. The renin system is stimulated by the sympathetic activity. For all these reasons, these agents are not useful as monotherapy and should generally be combined with a diuretic and an adrenergic-inhibiting agent such as a β-adrenergic receptor antagonist. Both hydralazine and minoxidil are well absorbed and have antihypertensive effects for 6 to 12 hours or more. Hydralazine is excreted in the urine mainly as metabolites. Twenty percent of minoxidil is metabolized, 60–70% is conjugated and eliminated, and approximately 10% is excreted unchanged.

#### *Clinical use and adverse effects of vasodilators*

Because these drugs are almost always used as third- or fourth-line therapy, this section concentrates on the use of minoxidil and hydralazine in that context. In comparison with α-adrenergic antagonists, hydralazine produces similar antihypertensive effects with comparatively similar incidences of adverse effects. Trials comparing hydralazine to prazosin showed similar antihypertensive efficacy, but only prazosin was associated with regression of left ventricular hypertrophy (Leenen et al. 1987). Nifedipine as the third drug in a regimen may be more effective than hydralazine.

Minoxidil is a very efficacious orally active antihypertensive agent. Its use originally was reserved to treat refractory hypertension. In large-scale trials, as a third drug given to patients with resistant hypertension, minoxidil produced effective control of blood pressure in over 70% of patients. Minoxidil has been more effective than captopril or hydralazine in double-blind, randomized, control studies of treatment-resistant patients. Minoxidil may have particular utility in patients with renal insufficiency and hypertension refractory to other drugs. Most studies using minoxidil as a third drug have combined it with β-adrenergic antagonists. Patients refractory to β-adrenergic antagonists plus diuretics and minoxidil have responded to the addition of an ACE inhibitor as the fourth drug in the regimen.

Excessive reduction of blood pressure results in orthostatic hypotension. This can be minimized by starting at low doses (e.g., 1.25 mg minoxidil, 25 mg hydralazine). Salt and water retention can occur and may manifest as severe peripheral edema, occasionally with ascites, associated with loss of control of blood pressure. Concomitant use of loop diuretics will be needed in almost all patients with functioning kidneys who respond to minoxidil to reverse the effects of plasma volume expansion. Reflex sympathetic effects can occur and include flushing, palpitations, anxiety, tremulousness, and headache. These are controlled by $\beta$-adrenergic antagonists or other antiadrenergic agents. It may be possible to reduce the dose of $\beta$-adrenergic antagonists once blood pressure is stabilized. Hydralazine and minoxidil in the absence of a sympathetic inhibitor drug can be associated with increasing left ventricular wall mass and ECG changes of left ventricular hypertrophy.

These agents are contraindicated in patients with aortic dissection because they increase cardiac inotropy and lead to increased shear force on the aortic wall. Patients taking hydralazine may develop positive ANA, typically occurring only when doses are greater than 200 mg/day. However drug-induced lupus occurs in only 5–10% of those with positive ANA, usually spares the kidney, and is generally reversible on discontinuation of the drug.

**PRINCIPLE Many syndromes produced by drugs look like spontaneously produced syndromes, but the drugs do not reproduce the pathogenesis, morbidity, or mortality of the disease they mimic. Be aware of the differences between simulating the facade of a disease and causing the disease when it comes time to treat the adverse effect or decide on whether the offending drug can be continued.**

Minoxidil may cause pericardial effusion, usually in patients who have renal failure, heart failure, or severe hypertension requiring high doses. Finally, hirsutism is common with minoxidil, is dose-dependent, and is an important limiting factor to using the drug in women. In fact, minoxidil is now used topically to promote hair growth.

**PRINCIPLE Note how adversity can be put to use for unexpected alternative indications.**

***Recommendations***

Hydralazine should be started at a dosage of 25 mg twice a day and increased gradually to a maximum of 200 mg/day in patients who already are taking diuretics and antiadrenergic therapy. The drug is safe, effective, and relatively inexpensive in this setting. Its use has declined because alternative vasodilators such as ACE inhibitors, $\alpha$-adrenergic antagonists, and calcium channel blockers have become available. Hydralazine, in combination with isosorbide dinitrate, is useful in patients with congestive heart failure who cannot tolerate ACE inhibitors (see the section on Congestive Heart Failure in this chapter). Typically, minoxidil has been reserved to treat refractory hypertensive patients. It may be especially useful in patients with stage 3 hypertension and renal insufficiency. Use of this highly efficacious drug may allow reduction in dosage of other drugs and improvement in the quality of life of patients. The initial dosage should be from 1.25 to 2.5 mg/day, with titration in 2.5- to 5-mg increments up to a maximum dosage of 40–80 mg/day. Obviously, this approach should be highly individualized, especially because less is known about the safety of the systemic administration of minoxidil than for many other antihypertensive drugs. Patients who are taking direct vasodilators but have inadequate control of their blood pressure should have their plasma volume status carefully evaluated. If the patient is volume-overloaded, diuretics should be increased and euvolemia restored before increasing dosage of the vasodilator.

## GUIDELINES FOR MANAGING THE HYPERTENSIVE PATIENT

### Clinical Assessment

Obtaining a thorough patient history is important to determine the following:

- the duration and severity of hypertension
- nonpharmacologic and drug therapies that were or are being used with documented responses, including adverse effects
- the presence or absence of target-organ damage
- the presence or absence of other risk factors for atherosclerosis
- whether findings can be used to reveal secondary hypertension (not discussed here)
- whether other factors might be influencing or exacerbating blood pressure

- whether other drug needs or concomitant conditions in the patient might influence the choice of therapy for hypertension.

Patients with primary hypertension are generally asymptomatic unless target-organ damage has occurred. Headache is unusual except when pressure has increased over a short period of time or is very severe (diastolic pressure exceeding 120 mm Hg).

History of drug use should be recorded. Oral contraceptives, NSAIDs, and licorice-containing compounds (including candy and some forms of chewing tobacco) all can cause or worsen treated and untreated hypertension. Inquiries about diet, especially sodium and alcohol intake, weight change, and patterns of exercise help set priorities for eventual treatment. Assessment of cardiovascular risk factors, including the possible coexistence of diabetes mellitus, should have an important impact on decisions involving selection of drug candidates and therapeutic goals. Coexisting risk factors such as hyperlipidemia, age, family history of premature cardiovascular disease, cigarette smoking, and diabetes have a marked capacity to magnify the risks of any given level of hypertension. In many patients, relatively simple laboratory investigations, generally including measurement of plasma electrolytes, particularly the potassium concentration, assessment of renal function, and possibly an ECG are sufficient studies before initiating therapy.

## Treatment

In the ambulatory patient, the main goal of treatment is to reduce the incidence of target-organ complications of hypertension, such as stroke and congestive heart failure. Also, successful treatment of hypertension reduces the risk that the blood pressure will rise to immediately life-threatening heights requiring emergency treatment.

A two-pronged approach to decrease the elevated blood pressure and decrease impact of coexistent cardiovascular risk factors when possible is optimal. The use of aspirin may play a particularly important role decreasing cardiovascular risk in patients with hypertension. The HOT study (Hansson et al. 1998) involved a factorial design in which half the patients in each blood pressure goal group received aspirin (75 mg once daily) or a matching placebo in a randomized, double-blind design. There was a 36% reduction in myocardial infarction rate in the aspirin-treated patients, from 3.6 to 2.3 myocardial infarctions per 1000 patient years. However, rates of both serious (requiring hospitalization) and less serious rates of bleeding were doubled in the aspirin-treated patients. Because of this trade-off between myocardial infarction on the one hand and serious bleeding on the other, aspirin may not be appropriate for every patient with hypertension. The most useful role for aspirin is likely in older hypertensive patients who have other risk factors for myocardial infarction.

**PRINCIPLE Trade-offs in medicine are common, and they involve benefits versus risks and benefits versus costs. Patients must be involved in discussions that include consideration of trade-offs.**

### *Nonpharmacologic therapy*

Keep in mind that these measures are not always benign and that they should be subjected to the same scrutiny as drug therapy for their efficacy and toxicity. For example, about 50% of the hypertensive population responds to salt restriction with reductions in blood pressure. However, it is fruitless to subject a consult-sensitive hypertensive to restrictive maneuvers that ultimately may compromise compliance with more useful measures. The typical Western diet includes 150–300 mEq of sodium per day. Modest salt restriction to 60–90 mEq can be used as a 4-week trial of therapy in hypertensive patients. If there is no effect on blood pressure, rigorous salt restriction should be discontinued. Periodic 24-hour or spot urinary sodium determinations can help monitor the overall intake of salt and encourage compliance.

Obesity confers an increased risk for cardiovascular disease, either directly or via the association of glucose intolerance and insulin resistance, low HDL and high LDL cholesterol, or hypertension. Once blood pressure has been carefully documented in an obese hypertensive patient, weight reduction should be implemented (or at least attempted). Other dietary factors have been studied in hypertensive patients, but their effectiveness is controversial. Diets containing high potassium, magnesium, and calcium intakes have been reported to lower pressure, although their clinical utility is uncertain.

Alcohol and nicotine are commonly used compounds that can raise blood pressure in susceptible people. Hypertensive patients drinking more than two standard drinks per day should be encouraged to undertake a therapeutic trial of stopping or decreasing ethanol intake in order to determine its effect on their individual blood pressure. Of course, every cigarette smoker should be helped to quit (see chapter 17, Substance Abuse: Dependence and Treatment).

Aerobic exercise such as walking, jogging, or swimming for at least 30 minutes at least three times weekly can reduce blood pressure. On the other hand, isometric exercise may markedly increase blood pressure.

**PRINCIPLE Substantial progress toward a therapeutic endpoint may be made when multiple maneuvers (no one of which has dramatic efficacy) are combined to accomplish the same goal.**

### *Drug therapy*

The decision to intervene with drug therapy is influenced mainly by the extent of blood pressure elevation, evidence of target-organ damage or other cardiovascular disease, and the presence of other cardiovascular risk factors. A classification with specific guidelines for initiating drug therapy based on these factors has been proposed (Joint National Committee 1997).

Some general recommendations for initial selection of a drug for untreated hypertensives can be made based on available clinical evidence. An ideal antihypertensive drug formulation should have a number of important properties (Joint National Committee 1997), such as requiring only once daily dosing, preferably with a duration of action of at least 24 hours with at least 50% peak effect at the end of 24 hours (trough-to-peak ratio) with protection against the rapid rise in blood pressure that may occur on arising from sleep in the morning.

**INITIAL DRUG THERAPY IN UNCOMPLICATED PATIENTS WITH HYPERTENSION** The choice of the initial drug to use in a patient with hypertension remains highly variable in the practice of medicine because of a number of factors, including attitudes of the physician about the desirability of a drug (especially the concern about adverse drug effects) and heavy marketing pressure aimed at influencing the physician's choice of drugs and tending to stress favoring newer drugs. However, based on the extensive experience from randomized clinical trials that demonstrate efficacy in preventing major clinical endpoints, use of diuretics or $\beta$-adrenergic receptor antagonists remain the preferred choice for initial therapy in uncomplicated, otherwise healthy hypertensives who are not at high immediate risk (Joint National Committee 1997). A general approach to treatment, with a goal blood pressure less than 140/90 mm Hg in these patients, is to start a diuretic or $\beta$-adrenergic antagonist at the lowest recommended starting dose.

If the therapeutic response is inadequate, the dose should be titrated upward to the full dose. If the therapeutic effect on blood pressure proves to be insufficient, there are a variety of options. If the patient has had significant adverse effects or has not had any therapeutic effect from the drug (and the physician believes the patient is taking the medication), the initial drug should be discontinued and a substitute chosen from another drug class. On the other hand, if the patient has had a partial therapeutic effect, then the second drug (either a $\beta$-adrenergic receptor antagonist or a diuretic) should be added and its dose titrated upward. Issues relating to patients who do not reach the goal blood pressure using this approach are discussed below.

**INITIAL DRUG THERAPY IN PATIENTS WITH HYPERTENSION WHO HAVE COEXISTING DISEASES** Although $\beta$-adrenergic antagonists and diuretics remain the first line of therapy in uncomplicated patients, a wide range of other factors may suggest that another class of drugs would be appropriate for first-line therapy in selected patients. In general, antihypertensive drugs may have either favorable or unfavorable effects on these conditions. For some diseases, the indication may be very compelling for selecting specific drug classes, for example, ACE inhibitors in type I diabetics with proteinuria (see chapter 9, Endocrine and Metabolic Disorders), ACE inhibitors in patients with congestive heart failure (see the section in this chapter), or $\beta$-adrenergic antagonists in patients with myocardial infarction (see the section in this chapter). Appropriate drug choices have been demonstrated in controlled trials to improve the outcome of the coexisting problem. In many settings, choice of a specific antihypertensive drug may have favorable symptomatic benefit in patients with other diseases (see Table 1-6). For example, in patients with angina, either $\beta$-adrenergic receptor antagonists or calcium-entry blockers can decrease episodes of chest pain (see the section on Coronary Artery Disease in this chapter). Patients with essential tremor or with recurrent migraine may benefit from specific, generally nonselective, $\beta$-adrenergic receptor antagonists. Men with benign prostatic hyperplasia may get marked improvement with an $\alpha_1$-adrenergic receptor antagonist used to treat hypertension.

**PRINCIPLE Search out indications other than primary uses for an agent in a patient who has more than one treatable medical problem; that is, try to get "two for the price of one."**

On the other hand, certain antihypertensive drugs may adversely alter the course of other coexisting diseases. For example, reactive airway diseases such as asthma may be fatally exacerbated by concomitant use of a $\beta$-adrenergic antagonist. Heart block may be increased by $\beta$-adrenergic antagonists or some calcium-entry blockers. Mental depression may be worsened or precipitated in susceptible patients taking drugs such as $\beta$-adrenergic antagonists, clonidine-like drugs, or reserpine. In some settings, the risk is so great (e.g., $\beta$-adrenergic antagonists in asthmatics) that the offending drug is generally contraindicated. On the other hand, the potential adverse effect may be readily detected and reversible should it occur, leaving much more scope for clinical judgment (e.g., diuretics in patients with mild dyslipidemias).

**OTHER SPECIAL PATIENT CONSIDERATIONS** Special considerations in selecting the initial drug also may be influenced by factors other than coexisting diseases (Joint National Committee 1997). Although certain drugs have been heavily marketed as better at preserving quality of life in patients with hypertension on average, evidence to support this contention is modest. Indeed, all drugs recommended for initial treatment of hypertension are generally well tolerated. In any case, if any particular drug has an adverse impact on quality of life in an individual patient, the drug can be discontinued or the dose adjusted as appropriate.

**PRINCIPLE Although knowing about average effects of drugs in large populations is potentially important, the capacity to individualize therapy based on the actual responses in your patient may be much more significant in guiding therapeutic decisions.**

There is some evidence that African-American hypertensive patients on average are more likely to respond to diuretics and calcium-entry blockers than to $\beta$-adrenergic antagonists or ACE inhibitors. On the other hand, particularly if either a $\beta$-adrenergic receptor antagonist or an ACE inhibitor is otherwise preferred because of a coexisting disease, such as myocardial infarction or congestive heart failure respectively, it is appropriate to use drugs in these classes in African-American patients. It may be necessary to use higher doses or encourage salt restriction to achieve the desired efficacy in some of these patients.

Cost of therapy should remain a major consideration in the choice of drugs. Many patients are not insured for the cost of drugs and will not even fill prescriptions for expensive agents. The cost of medication for those who are insured is shared by society as a whole in taxes, insurance rates, and so forth. The determination of the price of a drug in any given geographical area or practice plan is complex and not uniform. However, as a general rule, generic formulations and "older" drugs are cheaper.

**PRINCIPLE When the efficacy of therapy can be easily monitored, there is little disadvantage in choosing the cheapest preparation of a given chemical entity or class.**

The physician and patient should consider prior antihypertensive drug therapy and current antihypertensive drug therapy in choosing modifications in drug therapy. If at all possible, two drugs that are synergistic should be used, and two drugs that have additive adverse effects should be avoided. This commonsensical principle is very useful in guiding multiple-drug therapy. An example can be drawn from the *step-care concept,* whereby addition of a vasodilator to a $\beta$-adrenergic antagonist-plus-diuretic regimen is rational, because the diuretic will counter the vasodilator-induced salt retention and the $\beta$-adrenergic blocking agent will inhibit the reflex sympathetic actions on the heart and venous systems. Other potentially favorable drug pairs include diuretic–ACE inhibitor, diuretic–angiotensin II receptor antagonist, and minoxidil–loop diuretic. Indeed, there may be some justification in the use of fixed drug combination tablets in the treatment of hypertension because this may simplify a patient's drug regimen, possibly having a favorable impact on patient compliance with medical treatment in some cases. However, it is generally advisable to define treatment requirements one drug at a time.

There are combinations of antihypertensive drugs that probably should not be used together as pairs. For example, combinations of two drugs from the same family or class generally makes little sense. Drugs that may share common or overlapping targets may exacerbate adverse drug effects. For example, some drugs may potentially have additive effects in terms of slowing resting heart rate: the combination of a $\beta$-adrenergic receptor antagonist that blocks catecholamine-mediated activation of the sinus node (such as atenolol) and a centrally acting $\alpha_2$-adrenergic receptor agonist (such as clonidine) that decreases sympathetic outflow to the heart and may enhance vagally mediated cardiac slowing can occasionally cause marked bradycardia. In terms of risk of postural hypotension, the combination of an $\alpha_1$-adrenergic receptor antagonist (such as prazosin) with a drug like clonidine may impair the capacity of smooth muscle in veins to contract because of blockade of the $\alpha_1$-adrenergic receptors (prazosin) coupled with inhibition of sympathetic activation of these receptors (clonidine).

To summarize the very important issue of choice of initial therapy, it is worth noting that, in practice, there is no way to predict the response of a given individual to a given drug. Therefore, the physician chooses a candidate drug based on many considerations, including personal experience, drug cost, and coexisting disease, and submits it to an empirical trial starting at low doses. The anticipated adverse effects in the individual (both short- and long-term) are a far greater consideration, because all antihypertensive drugs used as monotherapy produce similar degrees of blood pressure reduction when directly compared in large populations.

***General principles of antihypertensive drug therapy***

Choice of a starting drug in the treatment of hypertension has been discussed above. If this single agent is not sufficiently efficacious, consideration should be given to using two drugs at relatively low doses, rather than "pushing" the dose of a single drug and increasing the risk of adverse effects. At the higher dosage range, even large dose increments produce relatively little further hypotensive effect as the top of the dose–response curve is reached. In contrast, the dose-dependent incidence of adverse effects continues to increase in the higher dosage ranges. Using two drugs in low dosage often exploits additive or synergistic efficacy between drugs, allowing maintenance of these low doses and avoidance or a minimization of adverse effects.

In poorly controlled patients with severe hypertension or those who are at high risk, add drugs, rather than substituting one class of agent for another. When blood pressure is controlled with the use of the added drug, attempts can then be made to reduce or discontinue other agents. In patients with severe hypertension, one may be unsure whether the drug is having an effect and whether the pressure would be much higher in its absence. Withdrawing a useful agent and allowing the pressure to rise might exacerbate the disease and be dangerous to the patient. In treating mild hypertension in low-risk patients, sequential use of drugs as monotherapy can help to determine empirically the most effective agent with the least toxicity in the patient, because it is quite acceptable to take months to control hypertension in these patients.

It is important to use the lowest possible doses to maintain pressure below the target blood pressure. In patients whose blood pressure is well controlled for one year or more, it may be appropriate to attempt to minimize the dosage required to keep the patient at this level (step-down therapy). Such efforts may be especially useful in patients who have undertaken nonpharmacologic approaches to lowering blood pressure, such as weight loss. Because of the implications of lifelong therapy of hypertension, maintaining patients on the lowest possible drug dosage for the longest possible time is justified.

## Special Settings Requiring Consideration for Antihypertensive Therapy

***Very severe hypertension***

Management of patients with very high blood pressure depends on the clinical setting rather than the actual levels of blood pressure. One must be able to distinguish the true hypertensive emergency from less pressing situations, because the risks of lowering blood pressure rapidly are considerable and should be avoided unless absolutely necessary.

A hypertensive emergency is a situation in which elevated blood pressure must be lowered immediately to limit and reverse damage to target organs. Hypertensive emergencies include markedly elevated blood pressure that has led to dissecting aortic aneurysm, encephalopathy, or pulmonary edema. Clinical judgment and experience, rather than controlled clinical trials, indicate that these life-threatening settings require prompt judicious lowering of blood pressure to relieve symptoms and to stop or reverse pathological changes. Hypertensive patients with severe elevations in blood pressure typically have altered cerebral blood flow autoregulation that makes them susceptible to cerebral ischemia at much higher mean arterial pressures than for normotensive subjects, as blood pressure is lowered. Accordingly, it is especially important to avoid precipitous drops in blood pressure unless the situation warrants taking such risks. It has been suggested that the initial goal of therapy in these patients should be to lower mean blood pressure by no more than 25% in the first minutes to 2 hours after start of therapy; at that point blood pressure can be lowered toward 160/100 mmHg over 2 to 6 hours (Joint National Committee 1997). This is a consensus view, trying to balance the benefit of lowered blood pressure against the risk of precipitating cerebral, coronary, or renal ischemia from too rapid a fall in blood pressure; it is not currently feasible to test these recommendations in controlled clinical trials.

Drugs useful in the emergency treatment of hypertension are shown in Table 1-10. The ideal drugs are given intravenously, are titratable, have rapid onset and offset of action, are predictable in their effects, and are easily monitored. Therapy should be given in such a manner to maintain blood flow to all vital organs. Sodium nitroprusside is one drug of choice. Other drugs can be considered. The use of sodium nitroprusside requires intra-

**Table 1-10 Parenteral Drugs for Hypertensive Emergencies**

| |
|---|
| *Vasodilators* |
| Sodium nitroprusside |
| Nicardipine HCl |
| Fenoldapam |
| Nitroglycerin |
| Enalaprilat |
| Diazoxide |
| *Adrenergic receptor antagonists* |
| Labetalol HCl |
| Esmolol HCl |

arterial monitoring of blood pressure in an intensive care unit setting. Other potentially useful intravenous agents include labetalol, diazoxide, fenoldopam, or hydralazine, especially when sodium nitroprusside is not available.

Hypertensive urgencies are defined as those situations in which it is desirable to lower blood pressure over the course of hours (Joint National Committee 1997). Some physicians believe this is appropriate for very high absolute values of blood pressure, hypertension in the setting of papilledema (so-called "malignant hypertension") or progressive target-organ damage, and severe perioperative hypertension. In addition, many physicians believe that elevated blood pressure in its own right, in the absence of significant symptoms or new or progressive target-organ damage, should not be treated as an emergency. These types of guidelines are somewhat ambiguous, depend on clinical judgment, and have not been studied in controlled trials. However, in the absence of demonstrated benefit and the known risks of sudden lowering of blood pressure in severe hypertension, a conservative approach to lowering blood pressure cautiously over substantial periods of time seems warranted. In other words, hypertensive urgencies are probably best managed using oral medications with relatively prompt onset of action, such as $\beta$-adrenergic receptor antagonists, ACE inhibitors, calcium-entry blockers, and loop diuretics when appropriate. Broken capsules of nifedipine administered sublingually (actually swallowing the contents works faster) has been very extensively used in the treatment of hypertensive urgencies. However, this approach leads to particularly unpredictable large falls in blood pressure that may have severe adverse consequences in terms of tissue ischemia. These include stroke or acute myocardial infarction.

As a consequence, there is no justification for using this approach to lower blood pressure in any situation.

Finally, even in the context of very high pressures, if the patient is asymptomatic and there is no advanced retinopathy, then it is safe to slowly decrease blood pressure over days and to use oral agents in an outpatient setting provided that frequent (up to daily) monitoring is feasible if indicated.

**PRINCIPLE In the absence of likely benefit, the physician should not expose patients to the risk of unnecessary treatment merely to make the numbers look better as an end in itself.**

## Hypertension in the Elderly, Including Isolated Systolic Hypertension

Hypertension in the elderly is very common. There is now convincing evidence from multiple controlled clinical trials that treatment of hypertension in the elderly has large beneficial effects on the progress of cardiovascular disease, including development of stroke, coronary heart disease, and congestive heart failure. Thiazide diuretics and calcium channel blockers reduce the risk of these adverse cardiovascular endpoints in the elderly [The Systolic Hypertension in the Elderly Program (SHEP) Cooperative Research Group 1993; Joint National Committee 1997; Staessen et al. 1997]. It may be prudent to initiate therapy with particularly low starting doses of these drugs in the elderly. Therapeutic goals (BP < 140/90) should generally be the same as in younger patients. However, for some elderly patients it may be hemodynamically challenging to markedly lower elevated systolic blood pressure (see below for discussion of isolated systolic hypertension). In those patients, more modest goals for reduction of systolic hypertension may be more appropriate, such as decreases of systolic pressure to less than 160 mmHg. The elderly may have impaired buffering capacity to control blood pressure in the upright position. As a consequence, drugs that are more likely to cause postural hypotension, such has high-dose diuretics, $\alpha_1$-adrenergic receptor antagonists, and drugs interfering with sympathetic nervous system function, should be avoided or used particularly cautiously in the elderly.

Systolic blood pressure is a better predictor of cardiovascular complications than is diastolic blood pressure. Systolic blood pressure may rise markedly with age. This is thought to predominantly relate to age-associated reduction in the compliance of the large arteries. Normally, ejection of the stroke volume from the left ventricle into the aorta stretches the aortic wall. During diastole, blood flows down the arterial tree as the large vessels contract. This *windkessel* effect is useful in distributing the cardiac output more evenly between systole and diastole. With loss of the windkessel effect, systolic pressure is raised, and diastolic pressure tends to fall, in part, because of the more rapid return to the aorta of the reflected pressure wave in the less compliant vasculature. In addition, augmented reflection contributes to pressure overload of the left ventricle and left ventricular hypertrophy.

In the absence of other complicating factors, the pulse pressure (systolic minus diastolic pressure) is a reasonable index of large artery compliance; the index widens with decreased compliance. The mean arterial pressure is a reasonable index of BP=CO × SVR irrespective of changes in aortic wall compliance (Safar and Simon 1986). This concept of systemic hemodynamic change during aging accounts for the observed trends in blood pressure. Isolated systolic hypertension (systolic >160 and diastolic <90 mmHg) is largely a disease of the elderly.

There is now strong evidence from randomized controlled clinical trials demonstrating the effectiveness of drug therapy for isolated systolic hypertension. The Systolic Hypertension in the Elderly Program study [The Systolic Hypertension in the Elderly Program (SHEP) Cooperative Research Group 1993] demonstrated that a diuretic combined with atenolol as second-step therapy, compared with placebo, significantly decreases stroke, acute myocardial infarction, heart failure, and death due to coronary artery disease. The therapeutic goal for systolic blood pressure in that study was less than 140 mmHg. Furthermore, a European study of isolated systolic hypertension in the elderly demonstrated that the calcium-entry blocker nitrendipine causes a marked reduction in risk for stroke in the treated patients (Staessen et al. 1997).

Although there was skepticism in the 1980s about the value of treating diastolic or isolated systolic hypertension in the elderly, randomized clinical trials have demonstrated that drug treatment of these problems in the elderly has a major impact on cardiovascular complications. As a consequence, treatment of these patients is strongly encouraged based on available evidence. On the other hand, relatively little is known about the capacity of various antihypertensive drugs, more often used to treat diastolic hypertension, to decrease blood pressure in patients with isolated systolic hypertension. Whether it is beneficial to lower blood pressure with isolated systolic hypertension with initial values of systolic pressure between 140 and 160 mmHg is unknown.

## Secondary Hypertension

There are many causes of secondary hypertension, but curable secondary hypertension is rarely encountered (probably less than 2% of all hypertensive patients). Secondary hypertension should be especially considered in those patients with severe hypertension, hypertension refractory to medical therapy, the young (less than 35 years), and patients with progressive target damage or advanced retinopathy with hemorrhages, exudates, or papilledema. However, to what extent these factors are actually associated with increased risk of secondary hypertension is unknown. A rapid increase of severity of diastolic blood pressure in a patient with extensive atherosclerotic disease or advanced age suggests the possibility of renovascular hypertension.

### *Pheochromocytoma*

Pheochromocytoma, an endocrine tumor of the adrenal medulla or sympathetic chain, secretes potentially enormous quantities of catecholamines such as norepinephrine and epinephrine in an unregulated fashion. This tumor is life-threatening, has many possible presentations, and can be difficult to diagnose. Approaches to treatment of this rare disease vary from center to center and available information of necessity is generally observational rather than stemming from controlled clinical trials. Depending on circumstances, patients with diagnosed pheochromocytoma often are treated with $\alpha$-adrenergic blocking agents, generally using the irreversible antagonist phenoxybenzamine, followed by $\beta$-adrenergic blocking agents if necessary. Phenoxybenzamine is usually dosed empirically, starting at 10 mg/day, with dose increments determined by symptoms and control of blood pressure. Evidence of the adequacy of $\alpha$-adrenergic receptor blockade can include worsening postural hypotension and nasal stuffiness. Some patients may require 60 mg/day or more to control their hypertensive episodes. Phenoxybenzamine has also been used as long-term therapy in surgically incurable patients. The reversible and rapidly acting $\alpha$-adrenergic receptor antagonist phentolamine has been used for controlling hypertensive crises that complicate pheochromocytoma. Although this is theoretically an attractive drug in this setting, very few physicians are experienced in its use. Indeed, case-report data suggests that rapid infusions of phentolamine may cause sudden and severe hypotension in patients with pheochromocytoma. Because of this, it may be preferable for physicians to use more familiar drugs, such as sodium nitroprusside, in the treatment of hypertensive emergencies in patients with pheochromocytoma.

**PRINCIPLE The best drug to use in an emergency might be a familiar one rather than a theoretically preferable agent that is almost never used in medical practice.**

Methyl paratyrosine, a competitive inhibitor of tyrosine hydroxylase, the rate-limiting step in catecholamine synthesis, may be useful in treating patients with incurable pheochromocytoma.

***Renovascular hypertension***
Renovascular hypertension is defined as hypertension caused by a narrowing of the renal artery (or arteries). This disease occurs more commonly in patients with risk factors for atherosclerosis or evidence of atherosclerosis in the abdominal vessels or elsewhere (e.g., the smoker with peripheral vascular disease). There are still not enough data to determine whether medical or surgical (bypass or angioplasty) therapy is superior, but surgical therapy appears to be useful in the setting of renal insufficiency, a small kidney, or bilateral disease, and of course when medical therapy fails. Investigation should not be undertaken unless the decision has been made a priori to repair the renal artery if a lesion is found.

**PRINCIPLE Do not order tests that will not affect diagnosis or management.**

Multiple drug regimens are usually necessary owing to the severity of the hypertension. Even after successful revascularization, drug therapy is often necessary, especially in older patients with atherosclerosis.

***Primary aldosteronism***
Primary hyperaldosteronism is a disease produced by oversecretion of aldosterone, either from a unilateral lesion or from disease in both adrenal glands. It is commonly associated with hypokalemia. Spironolactone, a specific competitive antagonist of aldosterone, is a medical therapy commonly used to treat primary hyperaldosteronism, especially in patients with bilateral disease or in those who are not candidates for surgery. Although spironolactone is theoretically a very attractive drug for treating this disease, male patients may be especially bothered by the gynecomastia and sexual dysfunction that often accompany treatment with spironolactone. Amiloride may be efficacious in ameliorating hypokalemia and hypertension due to hyperaldosteronism. Whether long-term blockage of aldosterone receptors expressed throughout the body has any benefit in these patients is not known.

Drug-induced hypertension is a potentially reversible cause of secondary hypertension. For example, immunosuppressive drugs such as cyclosporine and high-dose glucocorticoids may commonly cause or worsen hypertension. Recombinant erythropoietin frequently increases blood pressure in patients receiving therapy for anemia associated with severe renal failure. Use of oral contraceptives has been associated with an increased risk of hypertension. Drugs such as cocaine and amphetamines should be considered in the emergency setting of severe unexplained hypertension.

### Hypertension During Pregnancy

Hypertension during pregnancy is defined as blood pressure greater than 140/90 mmHg or an increase of 30/15 mmHg over baseline. It is important to differentiate hypertensive disorders encountered in pregnancy. The pregnant hypertensive patient may have chronic hypertension that developed before pregnancy or before the 20th week of gestation. The goal of treatment in these women is to control hypertension without exposing the fetus to undue risk. With the exception of calcium channel blockers, ACE inhibitors, and angiotensin II receptor antagonists (contraindicated in pregnancy), most commonly used antihypertensive medications can be continued when a women becomes pregnant. It is interesting to note that the largest experience with an antihypertensive drug started during early pregnancy has probably been for $\alpha$-methyldopa. Because of this, it remains a preferred drug in this setting. Although $\beta$-adrenergic antagonists are similarly efficacious in pregnancy, there is concern that use in early pregnancy may lead to retardation of fetal growth (Joint National Committee 1997).

A different problem in pregnant women is that of a previously normotensive woman who may develop pregnancy-induced hypertension. When this occurs in the third trimester and is associated with proteinuria and edema, the term *preeclampsia* is used. The prevention and treatment of preeclampsia are considered in chapter 19, Drug Therapy in Pregnant and Breast-Feeding Women).

## CASE SCENARIOS FOR TREATMENT OF HYPERTENSION

### Cases in Hypertension

What would you do if you were asked to manage the following cases:

A 43-year-old Caucasian woman, BP 154/96?
A 56-year-old woman of South Asian origin, BP 144/88?
A 74-year-old Caucasian man, BP 176/84?
A 68-year-old African-American man, BP 184/112?
A 36-year-old Hispanic woman, BP 144/92?

With only this information, you would be hard pressed to make a rational decision. However, the clinical context of each case provided below will help make your management planning more solidly based. The short case histories are presented to test your knowledge of the management of hypertension under different clinical circumstances. We suggest that you answer the following questions:

- If the patient is not taking antihypertensive treatment, then should I begin treatment?
- If I should treat, then how; and should I consider nonpharmacologic therapy or drug treatments or both?
- If the patient is already on treatment, then should I discontinue or choose different treatment?
- Are other cardiovascular risk management strategies warranted?

Each vignette reflects a common clinical scenario. Review each case and select a particular treatment. The rationale and evidence for suggesting a particular approach are described below. It is hoped that this contextual approach will reinforce key learning issues presented in the chapter and reemphasize why we don't merely "treat the numbers."

## Clinical Circumstances

CASE HISTORY 1 *Case 1 is a 43-year-old Caucasian woman with the following scenario: BP 154/96, premenopausal, overweight but otherwise healthy, body mass index (BMI) 28.3, single parent of two teenagers, "very stressed," alimony payments often delayed, and no family history of hypertension or premature cardiovascular disease. Her lipid profile and blood glucose are unremarkable. She is a nonsmoker and consumes one to five standard drinks of alcohol each week.*

CASE MANAGEMENT 1 If this level of BP is confirmed under appropriate office conditions (using a large cuff if necessary), then this woman can be diagnosed as having stage 1 hypertension. Given her sex (i.e., female), premenopausal status, and lack of risk factors, she is at very low risk of a cardiovascular event within the next decade. However, her obesity, economic circumstances, and stressful lifestyle cannot be ignored. She should be counseled about weight reduction and a heart-healthy diet. Pharmacotherapy can be deferred until she has had at least 1 year of nonpharmacologic treatment. Her BP, lipid status, and glucose tolerance should be monitored on an annual basis as long as she remains overweight with BP at this level.

CASE HISTORY 2 *A 56-year-old woman of South Asian origin presents with the following: BP 152/94, BMI 28.6, type II diabetes for 6 years treated with oral hypoglycemic agents, and well-controlled blood sugars and glycosylated hemoglobin. Before antihypertensive therapy began, her BP ranged from 160 to 182 mm Hg systolic and from 104 to 110 mm Hg diastolic. After a combination of ACE inhibitor and calcium channel blocking agent (CCB) therapy, her BP is now in the range of 140–146/86–90.*

CASE MANAGEMENT 2 This patient likely suffers from metabolic syndrome X—a clustering of hypertension, obesity, late-onset diabetes, and hypertriglyceridemia with suboptimal HDL cholesterol level. Obesity in this disorder is generally of the android type (i.e., central or abdominal location rather than on the buttocks or thighs), and visceral adiposity is likely part of the pathophysiology of the disorder. Her cardiovascular risk is greatly enhanced by the combination of diabetes and hypertension. Although the potential to control her BP might be considered "good," she will benefit by setting a goal diastolic BP at less than 80 through the use of a low-dose diuretic (e.g., 12.5 mg/day hydrochlorothiazide or equivalent) or a once-daily $\alpha$-adrenergic receptor blocking agent (alpha-blocker) such as doxazosin or terazosin. Her glucose control and lipid profile should be monitored to ensure that thiazide therapy does not disturb her electrolyte or metabolic status.

CASE HISTORY 3 *This case is a 74-year-old Caucasian man who is in generally good general health apart from some urinary symptoms attributable to benign prostatic hyperplasia. He has the following scenario: BMI 27.1 and gradually increasing BP, which has been 170–176/76–84 during past 3 months. Results of an ECG showed intraatrial conduction delay and repolarization changes, with occasional ventricular ectopic on rhythm strip.*

CASE MANAGEMENT 3 This man has isolated systolic hypertension, which is usually defined as systolic BP of 160 or greater and diastolic BP of less than 90. A low-dose thiazide diuretic (e.g., 12.5 mg/day hydrochlorothiazide or equivalent) or a long-acting, once-daily dihydropyridine CCB is recommended. A $\beta$-adrenergic receptor blocking agent (beta-blocker, BB) may be added but is not recommended as first-line therapy. Some would argue that his ECG changes are a relative contraindication to the use of a diuretic, whereas his prostatic symptoms may suggest the preferential use of an alpha-blocker. A low-dose thiazide/alpha-blocker combination or a low-dose CCB/alpha-blocker combination will likely be effective in controlling systolic BP, reducing cardiovascular risk, and improving urinary track symptoms in this man, perhaps deferring the need for prostatectomy.

CASE HISTORY 4 *A 68-year-old African-American man has the following clinical circumstance: BMI 23, formerly a heavy smoker, an MI at age 62, and a below-the-knee leg amputation at age 66. His BP before leg surgery was 146–152/92–96 while on CCB therapy. He suffers from winter bronchitis with wheezing exacerbations that have required aerosol bronchodilators on visits to the emergency room and brief courses of oral steroids. His BP was 184/112 and 178/110 on the last two consecutive visits. He carefully complies with current CCB and BB therapy. Further examination reveals absent pulses below both femorals and a systolic–diastolic abdominal bruit.*

CASE MANAGEMENT 4 This patient has several manifestations of arteriopathy. With recent deterioration in BP control despite apparent concordance with treatment, progressive renal artery stenosis with secondary renovascular hypertension should be suspected. Appropriate diagnostic evaluation should be undertaken, and renal artery balloon angioplasty or surgical correction should be considered. Furthermore, his episodes of wheezing may be associated with acute viral bronchitis superimposed on his chronic obstructive airways disease, but a beta-blocker may aggravate bronchoconstriction and should be discontinued. Moreover, there are suitable alternatives such as ACE inhibitors or angiotensin II type 1 ($AT_1$) blocking agents that are more likely to control BP in the setting of renovascular disease. Serum potassium values and renal function should be monitored carefully, especially in the setting of bilateral renal artery disease that is not amenable to revascularization.

**CASE HISTORY 5** *This is a 36-year-old Hispanic woman who is 32 weeks pregnant. She presents with BP 110–114/66–72 and BMI 26.5 when first seen between 8 and 12 weeks of pregnancy. There is no family history of hypertension. Her current BP is 144/92, and she has mild ankle swelling but no proteinuria.*

**CASE MANAGEMENT 5** There is clearly documented de novo increase in BP in this woman, in association with her pregnancy. Although her BP would not be noteworthy otherwise, the BP increase, associated with ankle edema, is consistent with the diagnosis of preeclampsia that threatens both the health of the developing child and the mother herself. Rest should be encouraged, with the use of $\alpha$-methyldopa or one of the beta-blockers that has a good record of safety such as atenolol. Delivery is commonly expedited between 36 and 38 weeks if BP control is inadequate or if fetal development is threatened.

## REFERENCES


Ames RP. 1996. A comparison of blood lipid and blood pressure responses during the treatment of systemic hypertension with indapamide and with thiazides. *Am J Cardiol* **77**:612b–16b.

Bailey DG, Malcolm J, Arnold O, et al. 1998. Grapefruit juice–drug interactions. *Br J Clin Pharmacol* **46**:101–10.

Carruthers SG, Dessain P, Fodor G, et al. 1993. The Alpha Beta Canada Trial Group: comparative trial of doxazosin and atenolol on cardiovascular risk reduction in systemic hypertension. *Am J Cardiol* **71**:575–81.

Dzau VJ. 1993. Local expression and pathophysiological role of renin-angiotensin in the blood vessels and heart. *Basic Res Cardiol* **88**(Suppl 1):1–14.

Folkow, B. 1984. Early structural changes: brief historical background and principle nature of process. *Hypertension* **6**(suppl. III):III-1–III-3.

Grimm R H, Jr, Flack JM, Grandits GA, et al. 1996. Treatment of Mild Hypertension Study (TOMHS) Research Group: long-term effects on plasma lipids of diet and drugs to treat hypertension. *JAMA* **275**:1549–56.

Guyton AC. 1989. Dominant role of the kidneys and accessory role of whole body autoregulation in the pathogenesis of hypertension. *Am J Hypertens* **2**:575–585.

Hansson L, Zanchetti A, Carruthers SG, et al. 1998. Effects of intensive blood-pressure lowering and low-dose aspirin in patients with hypertension: principal results of the Hypertension Optimal Treatment (HOT) randomised trial. *Lancet* **351**:1755–62.

Hoffman BB, Lefkowitz RJ. 1996. Catecholamines, sympathomimetic drugs, and adrenergic receptor antagonists. In: Hardman JG, Gilman AG, Limbird LE, et al., editors. *Goodman and Gilman's The Pharmacologic Basis of Therapeutics.* 9th ed. New York: McGraw Hill. p. 199–248.

Houston MC. 1981. Clonidine hydrochloride: review of pharmacological and clinical uses. *Prog Cardiovasc Dis* **23**:337–50.

Joint National Committee. 1997. The sixth report of the Joint National Committee on prevention, detection, evaluation, and treatment of high blood pressure. *Arch Intern Med* **157**:2413–46.

Leenen FHH, Smith DL, Farkas RM, et al. 1987. Vasodilators and regression of left ventricular hypertrophy: hydralazine versus prazosin in hypertensive humans. *Am J Med* **82**:969–78.

Materson BJ, Reda DJ, Cushman WC, et al. 1993. Department of Veterans Affairs Cooperative Study Group on Antihypertensive Agents: single-drug therapy for hypertension in men: a comparison of six antihypertensive agents with placebo. *N Engl J Med* **328**:914–21.

Medical Research Council Working Party. 1985. MRC trial of treatment of mild hypertension: Principal results. *Br Med J* **291**:97–104.

Multiple Risk Factor Intervention Trial. 1982. Risk factor changes and mortality results. *JAMA* **248**:1465–77.

Ogilvie RI, Burgess ED, Cusson JR, et al. 1993. Report of the Canadian Hypertension Society Consensus Conference: 3. Pharmacologic treatment of essential hypertension. *Can Med Assoc J* **149**: 575–84.

Pitt B, Segal R, Martinez FA, et al. 1997. Randomised trial of losartan versus captopril in patients over 65 with heart failure (Evaluation of Losartan in the Elderly Study, ELITE). *Lancet* **349**:747–52.

Rabkin SW, Huff MW, Newman C, et al. 1994. The Alpha Beta Canada Trial Group: lipids and lipoproteins during antihypertensive drug therapy—comparison of doxazosin and atenolol in a randomized, double-blind trial. *Hypertension* **24**:241–8.

Rangno RE. 1984. Beta blocker withdrawal syndrome. In: Kostis JB, DeFelice EA, editors. *Beta Blockers in the Treatment of Cardiovascular Disease.* New York: Raven Press. p. 275–300.

Safar ME, Simon AC. 1986. Hemodynamics in systolic hypertension. In: Tarazi R, Zanchetti A, editors. *Handbook of Hypertension: Vol. 7. Cardiovascular Aspects.* Amsterdam: Elsevier. p. 225–41.

Staessen JA, Fagard R, Thijs L, et al. 1997. The Systolic Hypertension in Europe (SYST–EUR) Trial Investigators: randomised double-blind comparison of placebo and active treatment for older patients with isolated systolic hypertension. *Lancet* **350**:757–64.

The Systolic Hypertension in the Elderly Program (SHEP) Cooperative Research Group. 1993. Implications of the systolic hypertension in the elderly program. *Hypertension* **21**:335–43.

[Veteran Administration Medical Centers]. 1982a. Low doses v standard dose of reserpine: a randomized, double-blind, multiclinic trial in patients taking chlorthalidone. *JAMA* **248**: 2471–7.

Wilcox PG, Ahmad D, Darke AC, et al. 1986. Respiratory and cardiac effects of metoprolol and bevantolol in patients with asthma. *Clin Pharmacol Ther* **39**:29–34.

# Hypotension

David Robertson

*Chapter Outline*



An evidence-based approach is being used in this text. This approach is ideal in disciplines where a critical mass of carefully controlled studies exist. In many of the more uncommon disorders, there is often an inadequate basis for such an approach. In the autonomic disorders, for example, there are probably fewer than five double-blind studies of chronic drug efficacy in homogeneous dysautonomic populations. Reasons for this include limited numbers of clinical investigators with an interest in these diseases, poorly characterized pathophysiological mechanisms of many entities, and a high likelihood that many autonomic disorders are heterogeneous in etiology, which may require individualized therapy. With increasing interest in autonomic disorders, improved therapy based on optimally designed trials can be anticipated.

## PATHOPHYSIOLOGY

### Upright Posture in Health and Disease

Assumption of upright posture is a major challenge to autonomic cardiovascular homeostasis. The fight-or-flight response is emblematic of sympathetic activation in animals, but in contemporary human subjects, more norepinephrine is synthesized and released each day to facilitate upright posture than for any other single purpose. Just as upright posture is a relatively recent evolutionary capability, the autonomic cardiovascular regulatory mechanisms that enable it have also undergone rapid development and may still be evolving. Under these circumstances, it is not surprising that many people have orthostatic dysregulatory problems of various kinds. Almost all symptoms in these individuals stem from inadequate cerebral perfusion during standing. At least 500,000 Americans have a problem of orthostatic regulation, but fortunately, for the majority of them, the degree of impairment is relatively mild. The purpose of this chapter is to highlight the most important of these disorders and their management.

### Terminology

The terminology to describe problems with cerebral perfusion on standing has long been heterogeneous and confusing. The most important reason for this was the fact that the absolute fall in blood pressure on standing was not a very good predictor of symptoms, and there was a reluctance to use the term *orthostatic hypotension* for individuals who were symptom-free. In 1996, the American Autonomic Society Consensus Conference agreed to define orthostatic hypotension in specific hemodynamic terms whether the individual was symptomatic or not (American Autonomic Society and American Academy of Neurology 1996). These guidelines have subsequently been widely accepted.

> **Orthostatic hypotension:** $\Delta$BP $\geq$20/10 mmHg with or without symptoms
>
> **Orthostatic intolerance:** symptoms on standing, $\Delta$BP $<$20/10 mmHg

### Orthostatic Hypotension

*Orthostatic hypotension* is now defined as a fall in blood pressure of 20/10 mmHg or more within 5 minutes of standing, whether or not there are associated symptoms (American Autonomic Society and American Academy of Neurology 1996). At least 5% of most adult populations have orthostatic hypotension. Therefore, orthostatic hypotension must be viewed as a physical finding rather than a disorder. Many individuals with this finding will have no evidence of impaired cerebral perfusion and may need no special evaluation or therapy. Other patients experience symptoms on standing, which are relieved within one minute of lying down; these people may require therapeutic management. The differential diagnosis (Table 1-11) of orthostatic hypotension is extensive (Robertson and Robertson 1994). Acute hypotension can occur in paroxysmal autonomic syncopes (Kaufmann 1997) that may be due to parasympathetic activation and sympathetic withdrawal (Robertson and Robertson 1981; Onrot, Fogo, et al. 1987; Jordan, Shannon, Black, et al. 1997), but between attacks orthostatic hemodynamics may be normal or near normal (Mosqueda-Garcia et al. 1997).

**Table 1-11 Differential Diagnosis of Orthostatic Hypotension**

| |
|---|
| Autonomic disorders |
| Pure autonomic failure |
| Multiple system atrophy |
| Familial dysautonomia |
| Dopamine-$\beta$-hydroxylase deficiency |
| Baroreflex failure |
| Acute pandysautonomia |
| Secondary autonomic neuropathies |
| Hypovolemia disorders |
| Hemorrhage or plasma loss |
| Overdiuresis |
| Overdialysis |
| Idiopathic hypovolemia |
| Endocrinologic disorders |
| Addison disease |
| Hypoaldosteronism |
| Pheochromocytoma |
| Renovascular hypertension |
| Vascular insufficiency |
| Varicose veins |
| Absent venous valves |
| Arteriovenous malformations |
| Vasodilator excess |
| Mastocytosis (histamine, prostaglandin $D_2$) |
| Hyperbradykininism (bradykinin) |
| Carcinoid (bradykinin) |
| Hypermagnesemia |
| Paroxysmal autonomic syncope |
| Glossopharyngeal syncope |
| Micturition syncope |
| Carotid sinus syncope |
| Swallow syncope |
| Cough syncope |
| Bezold-Jarisch reflex activation |
| Miscellaneous |
| Drugs and toxins |
| Stokes-Adams attacks |
| Mitral valve prolapse syndrome |
| Gastrectomy |
| Hypokinesia, weightlessness, bed rest |

There is a disproportionate prevalence of orthostatic hypotension in older age groups but the mechanism for this is not yet certain (Lipsitz 1996). However, there is an age-related reduction in cell bodies in the intermediolateral column of the spinal cord. Chronic orthostatic hypotension is frequently due to an adverse drug effect, for example, due to tricyclic antidepressants, vasodilators, diuretics, clonidine, or marijuana.

## Orthostatic Intolerance

Perhaps an even greater number of individuals experience symptoms upon standing, but do not have a fall in blood pressure of 20/10 mmHg; tachycardia is quite common but not universal in such patients. Patients with orthostatic symptoms in the absence of orthostatic hypotension are said to have *orthostatic intolerance* (Table 1-12). Although large numbers of individuals transiently experience such symptoms, those with symptoms lasting at least 6 months are said to have *chronic orthostatic intolerance.*

In contrast to patients with orthostatic hypotension, which strikes especially the elderly of both genders, patients with orthostatic intolerance tend to be younger and there is a 4:1 or greater female predominance. When the orthostatic intolerance is accompanied by tachycardia on standing, it is sometimes called *postural tachycardia syndrome,* or *POTS*. When the orthostatic intolerance is accompanied by the finding of mitral valve prolapse, it is sometimes called *mitral valve prolapse syndrome.* It is important to recognize that orthostatic intolerance and all the other terms mentioned here are categories of illness rather than specific pathophysiological entities, somewhat

**Table 1-12 Orthostatic Intolerance: Alternative Names**

| |
|---|
| Hyperadrenergic orthostatic hypotension |
| Orthostatic tachycardia syndrome |
| Postural orthostatic tachycardia syndrome |
| Postural tachycardia syndrome |
| Hyperadrenergic postural hypotension |
| Hyperdynamic $\beta$-adrenergic state |
| Idiopathic hypovolemia |
| Orthostatic tachycardia plus |
| Sympathicotonic orthostatic hypotension |
| Mitral valve prolapse syndrome |
| Soldier's heart |
| Vasoregulatory asthenia |
| Neurocirculatory asthenia |
| Irritable heart |
| Orthostatic anemia |

like the term "fever," which is also a category of illness rather than a true diagnosis.

Among the best established pathophysiologies involved in patients presenting with the syndrome of orthostatic intolerance are partial dysautonomia (Jacob and Biaggioni 1999) and a centrally mediated autonomic dysregulation (Furlan et al. 1997; Low et al. 1999). The tilt table, although widely employed in evaluation of patients with orthostatic symptoms (Kapoor 1999), has not yet allowed a matching of pathophysiology to appropriate therapy, an important future goal. Many other designations and entities such as chronic fatigue syndrome (Freeman and Komaroff 1997), orthostatic hypertension, postural orthostatic tachycardia syndrome, mitral valve prolapse syndrome, vasoregulatory asthenia (Streeten 1987), idiopathic hypovolemia (Fouad et al. 1986), and orthostatic anemia appear in the literature and need to be better defined in relation to the extent to which they overlap with these pathophysiologies. A mismatch between cerebral perfusion and central nervous system needs during upright posture clearly occurs in some patients with orthostatic intolerance (Jacob et al. 1996; Novak et al. 1996; Blaber et al. 1997) and in many of the entities listed above.

Challenges to our understanding of orthostatic intolerance include apparent hypersensitivity to $\alpha$-adrenoreceptors in the face of the often high circulating concentrations of norepinephrine, impaired norepinephrine release in response to tyramine, slightly impaired baroreflex function, raised supine muscle sympathetic nerve activity with an inadequate step-up in response to upright posture and altered norepinephrine metabolism in certain vascular beds. No current hypothesis to explain this disorder adequately addresses all these findings, reflecting the heterogeneity of the disorder.

**SUMMARY**
**Orthostatic intolerance**
**Presentation: Symptoms of inadequate cerebral perfusion on upright posture, usually in the absence of a significant fall (sometimes even an increase) in blood pressure. Symptoms include palpitations, fatigue, altered mentation, headache, nausea and presyncope/syncope**
**Diagnosis: Heart rate increase on standing greater than 30 bpm with no known cause; most symptoms relieved immediately on lying down**
**Therapy: Fludrocortisone, midodrine, clonidine, phenobarbital**

## Neurally Mediated Syncope

Some patients have recurrent episodes of what appears to be vasovagal fainting. Most of the time they may feel well, whether lying, seated or standing, but occasionally with orthostatic stress, they may become presyncopal with bradycardia, nausea, diaphoresis, and pallor; these symptoms may rapidly progress to syncope if supine posture is not immediately restored. Since these patients do not experience symptoms every time they stand, they are not generally classified as having "orthostatic intolerance," but it is possible that the pathophysiology may ultimately be found to overlap with this entity.

**SUMMARY**
**Neurally mediated syncope (neurocardiogenic syncope)**
**Presentation: Episodic, unprovoked bradycardia/hypotension leading to syncope in otherwise healthy individuals**
**Diagnosis: Replication of symptoms, and bradycardia/hypotension with tilt (on standing) in a patient in whom all other causes of syncope have been excluded**
**Therapy: No current proven therapy. Beta-blockers, pacing, and yohimbine have been used.**

## Baroreflex Failure

Acute baroreflex failure presents as severe episodic hypertension, headache, tachycardia, and diaphoresis, closely resembling pheochromocytoma (Robertson et al. 1993). Such pressor crises alternate with periods of hypotension. Plasma norepinephrine is raised during the former and suppressed during the latter. Baroreflex failure results from bilateral damage to glossopharyngeal and vagal nerves or their medullary interconnections. The hallmark of baroreflex failure is an inability to alter heart rate in response to pressor and depressor drugs in a patient who can raise and lower heart rate in response to endogenous sympathetic activation and withdrawal. Patients with baroreflex failure have supranormal pressor responses to the handgrip test, the cold pressor test, and especially the mental arithmetic test, all stimuli that activate sympathetic function. A small dose of clonidine (for example, 0.1 to 0.2 mg orally) often will lower blood pressure precipitously in a patient with baroreflex failure during the pressor phase of this disorder, presumably by central suppression of sympathetic outflow. During the chronic phase of the disorder, orthostatic hypotension may sometimes be seen (Table 1-13). Baroreflex failure usually is accompanied by significant collateral damage to vagal parasympathetic efferent fibers. In the absence of such damage (selective baroreflex failure), quiet rest can lead to unrestrained parasympathetic activation, leading to "malignant vagotonia" with hypotension and bradycardia, sometimes with cardiac arrest of 10 seconds or more (Jordan, Shannon, Black, et al. 1997) (Fig. 1-1).

**SUMMARY**
**Baroreflex failure**
**Presentation: Hypertension and tachycardia punctuated by hypotension with or without bradycardia; pressor crises often resemble pheochromocytoma with headache and diaphoresis**
**Diagnosis: Evidence of baroreflex impairment; heart rate fails to decline with pressor boluses of phenylephrine or heart rate fails to increase with depressor boluses of nitroprusside**
**Therapy: Clonidine, methyldopa, benzodiazepines**

## Pure Autonomic Failure

Pure autonomic failure (idiopathic orthostatic hypotension or PAF) is a degenerative disorder of the autonomic nervous system presenting in middle to late life (Bradbury

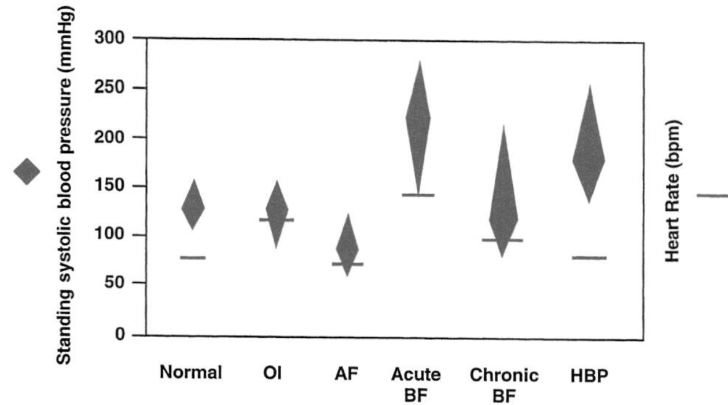


**FIGURE 1-1 Representative standing systolic blood pressures recorded in in-patients and normal subjects. The widest point of each diamond depicts the most common standing systolic pressure seen in typical patients, while the height depicts the range of pressures seen throughout the day. Patients with orthostatic intolerance (OI) have near-normal standing blood pressure, but often a dramatic tachycardia on standing. Patients with autonomic failure (AF) have the lowest standing pressure. In the acute phase (Acute BF), e.g., as in the days to weeks immediately following acute bilateral damage to cranial nerves IX and X, extremely high pressures are seen, in some cases exceeding those seen even in severe hypertension (HBP). After several months (Chronic BF), the standing systolic pressure is usually near normal, but great variability is still seen.**

and Eggleston 1925; Furlan et al. 1995). It remains a diagnosis of exclusion, once secondary dysautonomias such as amyloidosis, diabetes, and other peripheral neuropathies have been excluded. From clinical observations, PAF appears to be confined to the sympathetic and parasympathetic nervous systems (Table 1-14). The adrenal medulla is relatively spared. The initial feature in men can be male erectile dysfunction, but more commonly orthostatic hypotension is the symptom that brings patients to their physician. Hypotension may be so severe that seizures supervene in perhaps 3% of affected patients. Some patients find that leg-crossing helps to maintain upright posture. About 5% of patients with pure autonomic failure have discomfort suggestive of angina pectoris, usually in the absence of significant angiographically demonstrable coronary atherosclerosis. There is often headache or neck discomfort with upright posture in autonomic failure with orthostatic hypotension (Robertson et al. 1994). Patients with pure autonomic failure do not tolerate high altitude well, perhaps because they hyperventilate in this situation.

**Table 1-13 Contrasting Features of Acute versus Chronic Baroreflex Failure**

- Baroreflex failure should be suspected in patients with labile or brittle hypertension in a history of neck injury, neck irradiation, or neck surgery.
- Blood pressure: >30 mmHg pressor response to the cold pressor test; >30 mmHg depressor response to clonidine 0.1 mg
- Loss of bradycardic response to phenylephrine 25–200 $\mu$g intravenously
- Acute baroreflex failure (days)
  - Severe continuous hypertension
  - Incapacitating headache
  - Flushing
  - Tachycardia
  - Marked anxiety
  - Emotional volatility
  - Very elevated plasma and urinary catecholamines
- Chronic baroreflex failure (weeks to years)
  - Blood pressure volatility with hypertension and hypotension
  - Concomitant blood pressure and heart rate excursions
  - Headache and flushing during hypertensive spells
  - Elevated catecholamines during hypertensive episodes
  - Emotional volatility

**PRINCIPLE The forme fruste of a disease can alert the clinician to a less obvious syndrome or disease. If it does not, treatment of a forme fruste alone could be frustrating and counterproductive.**

**Table 1-14 Clinical Features of Autonomic Failure**

| |
|---|
| Orthostatic hypotension |
| Dizziness |
| Dimming of vision |
| Neck or head discomfort |
| Weakness in legs |
| Postprandial angina pectoris |
| Syncope |
| Seizures |
| Male erectile dysfunction |
| Hypohidrosis |
| Nasal stuffiness |
| Constipation or diarrhea |
| Bladder dysfunction |
| Mild anemia |

In this case one should consider the consequence of treating the angina with reducers of preload and afterload. It would likely be unsuccessful and exacerbate other elements of the disease.

Orthostatic hypotension in PAF is usually accompanied by supine hypertension, even when the patient is not taking vasopressor medications (Shannon et al. 1997). However, even when the supine hypertension is quite severe, cardiac function is well preserved and contractility may even be raised (Kronenberg et al. 1990). Usually hypohidrosis or at least an asymmetric distribution of sweating is seen. Nocturia (partly from excessive atrial natriuretic factor release during supine posture) is an invariable accompaniment of dysautonomic orthostatic hypotension and may cause the patient to get up as many as five to eight times per night to pass substantial volumes of urine. Some patients develop signs of neurogenic urinary retention, and these individuals may have repeated urinary tract infections. It is noteworthy that patients with the pure autonomic failure do not usually have fevers as high as healthy subjects; nevertheless, any fever will significantly lower their blood pressure and consequently decrease their functional capacity. A sudden decline in functional mobility in a patient with pure autonomic failure is suggestive of an intercurrent infection, usually of the urinary tract. There is marked hypersensitivity to all pressor and depressor stimuli, especially sympathomimetic amines (Robertson et al. 1984) (Fig. 1-2, Table 1-15).

The pathology of pure autonomic failure has not been completely elucidated, but there is a loss of cells in the intermediolateral column of the spinal cord and secondarily a loss of catecholamine uptake and catecholamine fluorescence in sympathetic postganglionic fibers. Lewy bodies, like those seen in the brain in Parkinson's disease, have been noted at many peripheral sites including the heart. Plasma and urinary concentrations of norepinephrine usually are greatly reduced, sometimes to 10% of normal (Goldstein et al. 1989). In fully developed PAF, the concentration of norepinephrine in plasma is virtually always less than 200 pg/ml and often less than 100 pg/ml (Ziegler et al. 1977). Plasma concentrations of epinephrine in the supine posture are also reduced but usually to a lesser extent than those of norepinephrine. Dopamine (Fig. 1-3) concentrations in urine usually are about 50% of normal values.

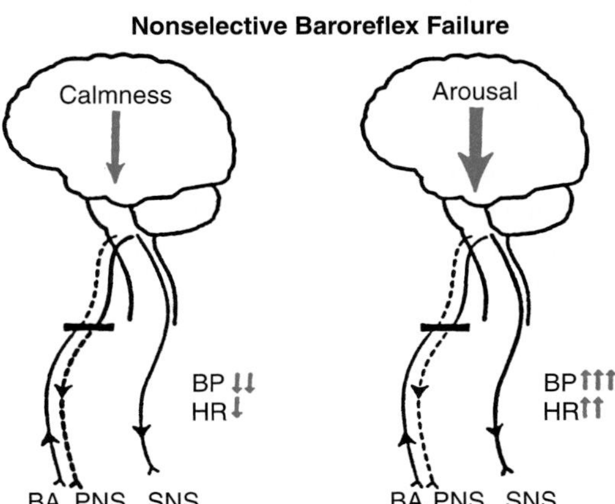


**FIGURE 1-2** Selective baroreflex failure (*top*) contrasted to nonselective baroreflex failure (*bottom*). Efferent sympathetic (SNS) and parasympathetic nerves (PNS) are intact in selective baroreflex failure. In nonselective baroreflex failure, efferent parasympathetic nerves were damaged. Baroreflex afferents (BA) were damaged in selective and nonselective baroreflex failure (Jordan, Shannon, Black, et al. 1997, with permission from *Hypertension*).

Table 1-15 **Comparison of Standing Blood Pressure, Heart Rate, and Catecholamine Values in Patients with Baroreflex Failure, Autonomic Failure, and Essential Hypertension**

| PARAMETER[a] | NORMAL ($n$=12) | BAROREFLEX FAILURE ($n$=11) | AUTONOMIC FAILURE ($n$=12) | ESSENTIAL HYPERTENSION ($n$=8) |
|---|---|---|---|---|
| Mean arterial pressure[b] (mm Hg) | 85±10 | 141±;32* | 69±10*H | 128±16* |
| Plasma norepinephrine (pg/ml) | 524±32 | 1840±320*H | 28±3*H | 570±41 |
| Plasma epinephrine (pg/ml) | 32±5 | 110±21*H | 10±3*H | 38±6 |
| Plasma dopamine (pg/ml) | 28±6 | 64±12* | 11±4H | 32±7 |
| Urinary norepinephrine($\mu$g/day) | 32±5 | 79±9*H | 4±2*H | 39±7 |
| Urinary epinephrine ($\mu$g/day) | 9±3 | 39±9*H | 4±2*H | 10±7 |
| Urinary dopamine($\mu$g/day) | 239±29 | 299±33 | 154±13*H | 277±29 |
| Cold pressor test Δ systolic BP (mm Hg) | +24±7 | +56±14* | −2±6*H | +33±8 |
| Clonidine Δ systolic BP (mm Hg) | −12±5 | −54±14*H | +12±4*H | −26±7 |
| Clonidine Δ plasma norepinephrine | −70±28 | −242±48H | −2±6*H | −106±24 |
| Phenylephrine Δ heart rate | −13±4 | −1±1*H | −1±1*H | −9±4 |

NOTE: Values are means ±SEM. Statistical significance:*$P < 0.05$ (vs. normal subjects); H$P < 0.05$ (vs. patients with essential hypertension). Autonomic failure patients differed significantly from baroreflex failure patients in all variables reported except phenylephrine-induced bradycardia.
[a] To convert norepinephrine picograms/milliliter to nanomoles/liter, multiply by 0.0059. To convert epinephrine picograms/milliliter to nanomoles/liter, multiply by 0.0055. To convert dopamine picograms/milliliter to nanomoles/liter, multiply by 0.0065.
[b] Mean arterial pressure, estimated as 2× diastolic pressure plus systolic pressure, divided by 3.

Patients with pure autonomic failure have a generally good prognosis; many live for 20 years or more after the onset of their disease. A common cause of death in these patients is pulmonary embolus.

SUMMARY

**Pure autonomic failure (idiopathic orthostatic hypotension, Bradbury-Eggleston syndrome)**

**Presentation: Autonomic failure with orthostatic hypotension, male erectile dysfunction, urinary tract problems, loss of sweating, and often supine hypertension and mild anemia**

**Diagnosis: Supine plasma norepinephrine below 100 pg/ml in the absence of another cause of autonomic failure; Lewy bodies in autonomic tissue**

**Therapy: Fludrocortisone, midodrine, erythropoietin, phenylpropanolamine, yohimbine, indomethacin**

## Multiple System Atrophy

In multiple system atrophy (MSA), autonomic failure is widespread and is associated with impairment in other neurologic systems. When autonomic failure dominates the disease presentation, it is sometimes called Shy-Drager syndrome (American Autonomic Society and American Academy of Neurology 1996). The other neurologic systems may be cerebellar, extrapyramidal, pyramidal, neuromuscular, or cortical (Wenning et al. 1997). The autonomic dysfunction in MSA can be viewed as a predominantly central nervous system defect with an inability to engage the postganglionic autonomic system. The result is a constitutive, poorly organized, postganglionic sympathetic release of norepinephrine (Jordan et al. 1997). In these patients, chronic orthostatic hypotension may be a presenting symptom; in other cases, problems with balance due to extrapyramidal or cerebellar involvement may predominate early in the course. In patients with cerebellar involvement, tremor is worsened by nicotine, and MSA patients often spontaneously discontinue smoking at the onset of their disease. A significant minority of patients will also experience a painful neuropathy in the lower extremities. When the chronic orthostatic hypotension antedates other neurologic involvement, it may be very difficult to differentiate the MSA from the more benign pure autonomic failure (Table 1-11). Clinical symptoms of autonomic failure discussed above in terms of pure autonomic failure often apply to patients with MSA.

**PRINCIPLE Habits (e.g., smoking that delivers nicotine) can exacerbate a disease and often may be used as a diagnostic test. Look for the associations and medical opportunities.**

Pathologically, multiple sites within the brain and spinal cord are involved. Sympathetic and parasympathetic postganglionic neurons, however, appear relatively

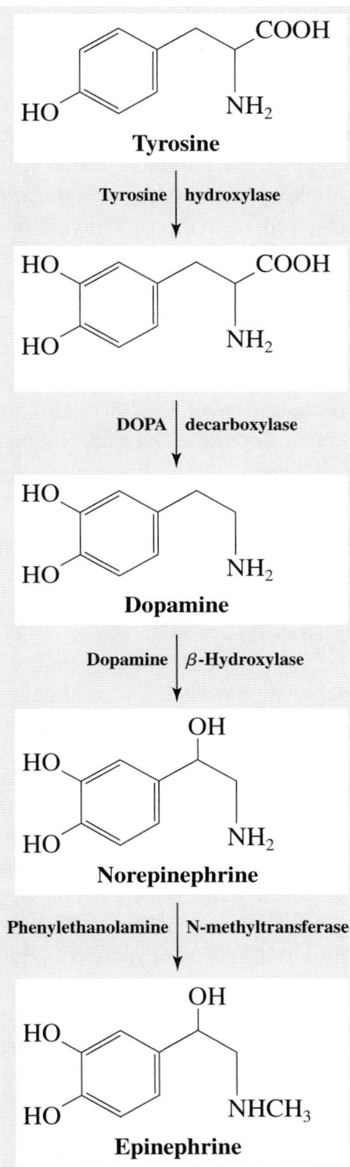


**FIGURE 1-3 The synthesis of norepinephrine and epinephrine. All these enzymatic steps take place in the cytoplasm except for the conversion of dopamine to norepinephrine. Dopamine-β-hydroxylase is confined to the neurotransmitter vesicles.**

spared in most patients. Characteristic cytoplasmic inclusions that are quite distinct from the Lewy bodies encountered in Parkinson disease occur in oligodendroglia and neurons (Papp and Lantos 1992). Very likely, MSA will ultimately be found to represent several distinct clinical entities. Some investigators distinguish between a spinocerebellar degeneration (spontaneous olivospinocerebellar atrophy) and an autonomic dysfunction associated with extrapyramidal involvement (striatonigral degeneration).

Supine blood and urinary concentrations of norepinephrine are often near normal in patients with MSA, but they do not rise appropriately on assumption of the upright posture (Ziegler et al. 1977). Such patients have a constitutive release of peripheral autonomic neurotransmitters in the absence of normal central control. Noteworthy is the biochemical evidence of central abnormalities in the dopamine, acetylcholine, and serotonin systems.

The prognosis is more guarded in MSA than in pure autonomic failure. It is rare for a patient to survive 12 years, although the autonomic abnormalities are rarely the direct cause of death. A significant number of MSA patients develop laryngeal stridor and difficulty in swallowing. This may lead to recurrent episodes of pneumonia, a frequent cause of death. In addition, many patients with MSA experience Cheyne-Stokes or periodic respiration. In some cases this may lead to a critical loss of respiratory drive, so-called Ondine's curse. Pulmonary hypertension may occur during apnea. In spite of the frequency of these two problems, however, one of the most common causes of death in patients with multiple system atrophy is pulmonary embolus.

**SUMMARY**
**Multiple system atrophy (Shy-Drager syndrome)**
**Presentation: Autonomic failure, extrapyramidal symptoms, and cerebellar dysfunction in any combination; cardinal autonomic features are orthostatic hypotension and genitourinary abnormalities**
**Diagnosis: Clinical presentation. The only definitive diagnosis is presence of glial cytoplasmic inclusions at autopsy**
**Therapy: Fludrocortisone, midodrine, antiparkinsonian medications**

## Dopamine-β-Hydroxylase Deficiency

Dopamine-β-hydroxylase deficiency is a genetic disorder in which norepinephrine and epinephrine cannot be normally synthesized due to this enzyme deficit. There is absence of norepinephrine, coupled with a greatly increased dopamine concentration in plasma, cerebrospinal fluid, and urine. DBH deficiency differs from the Riley-Day syndrome (familial dysautonomia) and various other autonomic disorders seen in adults in that the peripheral defect can be localized to the noradrenergic and adrenergic tissues. The clinical presentation of DBH deficiency includes incapacitating orthostatic hypotension, ptosis, retrograde ejaculation, and a difficult perinatal course but otherwise normal development (Robertson et al. 1991). There are no pressor responses to sustained handgrip, the cold pressor test or mental arithmetic. However, sympathetic cholinergic function is intact, as evidenced by normal sweating. Parasympathetic function is also preserved, as evidenced by intact sinus arrhythmia, normal heart rate increase during the Valsalva maneuver, and tachycardia after atropine. The clinical characteristics and the response to autonomic maneuvers of patients with DBH deficiency are shown in Table 1-16.

The most distinguishing feature of these patients is the virtual absence of plasma, urinary, and cerebrospinal norepinephrine and epinephrine together with the greatly increased plasma concentration of dopa and dopamine. These patients have no response to high (8 mg IV) doses of tyramine that would normally increase blood pressure by releasing neuronal norepinephrine. Even the most severely affected patient with pure autonomic failure would be expected to respond to high doses of tyramine with at least some increase in blood pressure. Yet, in DBH-deficient patients, norepinephrine remains undetectable following administration of tyramine, while dopamine concentrations are increased (Fig. 1-3).

In patients with DBH deficiency, central autonomic control as well as mechanisms that release catecholamines are intact, but dopamine, acting as a false neurotransmitter, is released instead of norepinephrine. Dopamine concentrations increase on assumption of the upright posture, during sustained handgrip, and after administration of tyramine. Furthermore, the concentration of plasma dopamine decreases after administration of clonidine. Also, muscle sympathetic nerve traffic, as measured by direct intraneuronal recordings, is present, perhaps even in excess under basal conditions but is otherwise normally modulated by baroreceptor mechanisms in these patients. Therefore, primary autonomic neuronal pathways are intact and responsive to appropriate stimuli, but dopamine instead of norepinephrine is the neurotransmitter in the noradrenergic neuron terminals.

**Table 1-16 Symptoms of Dopamine-β-Hydroxylase Deficiency**

| |
|---|
| Severe orthostatic hypotension |
| Nasal stuffiness |
| Ptosis of the eyelids |
| Retrograde ejaculation in males |
| Complicated perinatal course |
| Hypothermia |
| Hypoglycemia |
| Hypotension |

Patients with DBH deficiency must be identified as early as possible. There are several reasons for this. First, the disease is likely to be fatal in the neonatal period if it is unrecognized. DBH knockout mice have succumbed unless maternally administered dihydroxyphenylserine (DOPS) was provided to bypass pharmacologically the enzyme deficiency. Patients so far encountered as adults have had unusually meticulous care during illnesses in the neonatal period. Second, unlike other dysautonomias, DBH deficiency has a relatively specific and uniquely effective treatment. The administration of DOPS results in the endogenous replacement of dopamine by norepinephrine and a remarkable improvement in blood pressure regulation in these patients (discussed below).

**PRINCIPLE A marvelous reward of understanding the molecular pathogenesis of a disease is devising a disease-specific molecular therapy. In spite of the intellectual attractiveness of such specific intervention, its toxicity relative to nonspecific intervention must be compared before it becomes a "drug of choice."**

The disorder is most easily diagnosed by measuring the ratio of the concentration of norepinephrine to dopamine in plasma. Normally, the norepinephrine/dopamine ratio is approximately 10. In patients with DBH deficiency this ratio has generally been 0.1 or less. The biochemical manifestations of DBH deficiency are so dramatic that they may be said to be pathognomonic.

**SUMMARY**
**Dopamine-β-hydroxylase deficiency (DBH deficiency)**
**Presentation: Lifelong severe orthostatic hypotension**
**Diagnosis: Absent or extremely low levels of norepinephrine and its metabolites in a setting of excessive levels of dopamine and its metabolites**
**Therapy: Dihydroxyphenylserine (DOPS), metyrosine**

## PHARMACOLOGIC AND NONPHARMACOLOGIC THERAPIES

For all disorders associated with chronic orthostatic hypotension (Table 1-17), fludrocortisone is the treatment of choice when nonpharmacologic measures no longer suf-

Table 1-17 **Cardiovascular Manifestations of Autonomic Disorders**

| PARAMETER | AUTONOMIC FAILURE | BAROREFLEX FAILURE | ORTHOSTATIC INTOLERANCE | PAROXYSMAL SYNCOPE |
|---|---|---|---|---|
| Accelerated hypertension | + | ++ | − | − |
| Chronic hypertension | − | ++ | − | − |
| Supine hypertension | ++ | + | − | − |
| Labile hypertension | − | +++ | +/− | − |
| Orthostatic hypotension | +++ | +/− | + | − |
| Supine hypotension | +/− | +/− | +/− | +/− |
| Episodic hypotension | + | +++ | ++ | +++ |
| Postprandial hypotension | +++ | − | − | − |
| Bradycardia | + | +/− | − | − |
| Episodic bradycardia | − | +/− | +/− | +++ |
| Tachycardia | − | +/− | ++ | − |
| Episodic tachycardia | − | +++ | ++ | − |
| Orthostatic tachycardia | +/− | + | +++ | − |
| Supraventricular tachycardia | +/− | +/− | + | − |
| Syncope | +++ | + | ++ | +++ |
| Angina pectoris | + | + | − | |

fice (Fig. 1-4; Table 1-18). The value of fludrocortisone for raising blood pressure in a patient with autonomic failure was first demonstrated by Grant W. Liddle on December 18, 1956, at Vanderbilt University. Fludrocortisone subsequently became the treatment of choice for this purpose (Chobanian et al. 1979; Robertson and Davis 1995). Certain special features of fludrocortisone complicate its successful use. First, most of its blood pressure raising effect is due to sodium retention, which develops over several days; therefore, the full pressor action of fludrocortisone is seen in 1–2 weeks, rather than on the day it is first administered. Doses should be altered no more often than weekly, commencing with a dose of 0.1 mg PO qd. Since patients usually expect a drug to work the first day, it is wise to discuss this delayed action so they are not disappointed by the lack of immediate salutary effect. They should also be aware that they may need to gain 5–8 pounds in order for fludrocortisone to have its maximal favorable effect to raise their blood pressure. Sleeping with 6–8 inches of head upright tilt will prevent excessive nocturnal volume loss, and consequently increase the efficacy of fludrocortisone.

There are occasional complications of fludrocortisone therapy. Almost 50% of patients will develop hypokalemia within 2 weeks and about 5% will also develop hypomagnesemia. The former can be treated with potassium supplementation and the latter with small doses of magnesium sulfate.

Since fluid retention is critical to fludrocortisone's beneficial effect, the drug should not be used in patients who are unable to tolerate an increased fluid load (e.g., congestive heart failure patients). In point of fact, patients with congestive heart failure usually have increased (rather than reduced) orthostatic tolerance and we have seen patients with mild autonomic failure experience a lessening of their orthostatic hypotension when they develop congestive heart failure. We have never encountered a case of pulmonary edema in a patient with autonomic failure that did not respond immediately to assumption of the seated or upright posture. It seems prudent, however, to avoid weight gains greater than 10 pounds.

A common adverse effect of fludrocortisone is headache. This appears to be a greater problem in younger and healthier persons than in elderly or sick persons. Headache has limited the use of fludrocortisone in astronauts, who experience a very high incidence of orthostatic intolerance on return from space. Few patients with severe autonomic failure complain of headache. In patients who need fludrocortisone most of all, the headache is usually not noticed.

Recently, there have been a number of improvements in our understanding of fludrocortisone actions. Whereas it was initially thought that mineralocorticoid receptors acted within the nucleus of the cell to alter gene transcription, it is becoming evident that some actions of mineralocorticoids are due to cell surface receptors that act through second messengers without requiring engagement of the DNA. Such mechanisms might be activated more rapidly than those requiring involvement of cellular transcription machinery. For this reason, a better understanding of the pharmacokinetic profile of fludrocortisone has been important. Fludrocortisone is rapidly and nearly

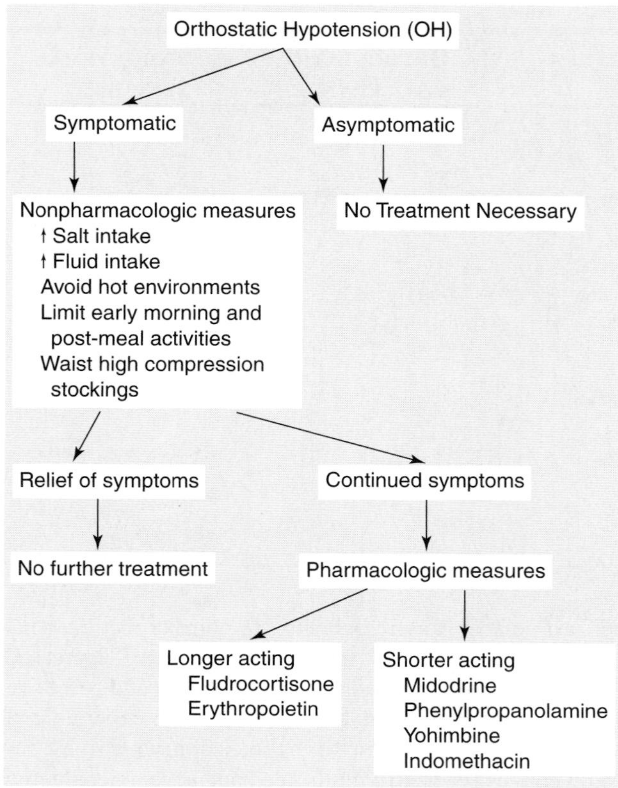


**FIGURE 1-4 Practical management of orthostatic hypotension due to autonomic failure.**

completely absorbed following oral administration and declines with a half-life of 2–3 hours. Because of this relatively short half-life, it may be more efficacious to give the drug in a twice daily regimen rather than the once daily regimen more commonly used. However, many patients have clearly received benefit even with a once daily regimen.

> **PRINCIPLE The efficacy and toxicity of drugs are almost always better understood as data on their mechanism of action appear.**

The recommended dosage in the published literature of fludrocortisone in autonomic failure varies over a wide range (0.05–2.00 mg daily). It is unusual to have any benefit from a dosage smaller than 0.05 mg daily. In practice, 0.1 mg per day is usually the starting dose. That dose can be increased by 0.1 mg oral increments at 1- to 2-week intervals. Few patients will require more than 0.4 mg PO daily. There appears to be little if any glucocorticoid effect at low (0.1–0.2 mg) daily doses of fludrocortisone, but ACTH suppression as manifested by reduced cortisol level can be seen following one oral dose of 2.0 mg fludrocortisone. In using fludrocortisone or any other pressor agent, it is important to be guided by relief of unacceptable symptoms (syncope), rather than any a priori level of upright blood pressure.

**Table 1-18 Drug Treatment of Autonomic Failure and Nonpharmacologic Measures**

| Treatment |
|---|
| Fludrocortisone (9$\alpha$-fluorohydrocortisone) |
| Caffeine |
| Sympathomimetic amines |
| Midodrine HCl |
| Phenylpropanolamine HCl |
| Ephedrine |
| Tyramine + MAO inhibition |
| Cyclooxygenase inhibitors |
| Indomethacin |
| Ibuprofen |
| Ergot alkaloids |
| Ergotamine |
| Dihydroergotamine mesylate |
| Somatostatin analogs |
| Somatostatin |
| Octreotide acetate |
| Dihydroxyphenylserine |
| Antihistamines |
| Diphenhydramine HCl |
| Cimetidine |
| Other drugs |
| Dopamine antagonists |
| Metoclopramide |
| Domperidone |
| $\alpha_2$ Agonists and antagonists |
| Clonidine |
| Methyldopa |
| Yohimbine HCl |
| $\beta$ Antagonists |
| Serotonin antagonists (cyproheptadine) |
| Vasopressin analogs |
| Angiotensin |
| Vasodilators |
| Hydralazine HCl |
| Minoxidil |
| Erythropoietin |
| Nonpharmacologic measures |
| Elevated head of bed |
| Antigravity suit |

ABBREVIATIONS: $\alpha_2$, $\alpha_2$-adrenergic receptor; $\beta$, $\beta$-adrenergic receptor; MAO, monoamine oxidase.

## Midodrine

Midodrine is a prodrug which, following absorption, is metabolized to *desglymidodrine,* an $\alpha_1$-adrenoreceptor agonist that differs from *methoxamine* only in lacking a methyl group on the side chain (McTavish and Goa 1989). There is a long history of successful clinical use of the $\alpha_1$-adrenoreceptor agonist class of drugs. A theoretical advantage of midodrine is that it is absorbed as the prodrug with limited direct effect to constrict the vasculature of the gastrointestinal tract; it is metabolized to desglymidodrine, which has an order of magnitude greater potency to raise blood pressure in the peripheral circulation. It is more than 90% absorbed following oral administration. The peak concentration in plasma occurs in 20–30 minutes and has a half-life of 30 minutes. The plasma concentration of desglymidodrine peaks at 1 hour with a half-life of approximately 3 hours. The metabolites are predominantly excreted through the urinary tract.

Oral midodrine results in all the typical effects of an $\alpha_1$-adrenoreceptor agonist. Such drugs lead to arterial and venous constriction with attendant increased peripheral vascular resistance and central redistribution of blood volume. The trigone and sphincter of the urinary bladder are stimulated. There is contraction of the radial muscle of the iris leading to pupillary dilatation. Pilomotor muscles are stimulated leading to a sensation of hair standing on end (piloerection or horripilation). Noradrenergic sweating may occur transiently.

Midodrine directly raises blood pressure by constriction of arterioles and veins. It is best used to raise blood pressure during the daytime, especially in the morning so that the maximum effect occurs at a time when the patient wants to be up and about. While in the supine posture, for example, during the night, blood pressure is always sufficiently high in autonomic failure and raising it further at that time with this or some other agent is counterproductive. For all these reasons, administration of midodrine early in the day is the means to achieve the greatest benefit.

The initial dose of midodrine typically needs to be increased after a day or so to maintain the same effect as desensitization of the $\alpha_1$-receptor-mediated responses may occur initially. This desensitization does not continue, however, after the first week. Usually midodrine is begun with 2.5 mg at breakfast and lunch, but the dose is escalated at 2.5-mg increments daily until a satisfactory response occurs or a dosage of 30 mg daily is achieved. Many patients will benefit from 5 or 10 mg on arising, a similar dose mid morning and a third dose in the early afternoon. Only by individualization of the use of this drug can its therapeutic benefit be maximized. It is also important that the functional capacity as assessed by *standing time* in severely affected patients and by systolic blood pressure in more mildly affected patients should be the ultimate guide in structuring the regimen. Through personal observation patients may develop considerable facility in the use of agents such as midodrine, and input from knowledgeable and medically sophisticated patients can greatly enhance the efficacy of this agent, particularly in regard to dosage scheduling.

**PRINCIPLE Never underestimate the positive effects of an interested and able patient in attempts at maximizing efficacy and minimizing toxicity.**

The adverse effects of midodrine are entirely predictable from its mechanism of action. Almost all patients receiving effective doses, if carefully questioned, will experience the sensation of gooseflesh (piloerection), paresthesia of the scalp, or pruritus. All three of these symptoms probably relate to effects of smooth muscle contraction on integumentary hairs. In many patients, these symptoms are very mild. In some cases, these symptoms may become a welcome sign that the blood pressure is about to rise. Occasional patients, however, are severely bothered by these sensations. Sometimes it is sufficiently bothersome that they will request discontinuation of the medication. The most serious complication of administration of midodrine is hypertension, particularly in the supine posture, that may be of considerable concern.

**PRINCIPLE When using a drug whose efficacy depends on position, be sure to understand the life habits of the patient. A nighttime worker will clearly have different requirements from those of a daytime worker.**

## Indomethacin

Indomethacin (25–30 mg) will raise blood pressure about 20 mmHg in most but not all severely affected patients with autonomic failure. The response is more dramatic in the postprandial period than at other times of the day. Since patients may have troubling gastrointestinal or central nervous system adverse effects with indomethacin, other nonsteroidal anti-inflammatory drugs (NSAIDs), such as ibuprofen, have also been successfully employed, although their relative efficacies and toxicities have not been compared. The precise mechanism of the pressor action of NSAIDs in autonomic failure is not established.

## Dihydroxyphenylserine

Dihydroxyphenylserine (L-DOPS) is an analog of norepinephrine to which a carboxyl group has been attached. This agent is uniquely beneficial in patients with DBH deficiency (Freeman et al. 1996). The advantage of this agent in this disorder is that L-DOPS is already $\beta$-hydroxylated and can be converted directly into norepinephrine by the enzyme dopa decarboxylase, which lacks substrate specificity (Figs. 1-5 and 1-6).

Although this agent has occasionally been used in other forms of autonomic impairment (Biaggioni, Robertson, Robertson 1994; Kaufmann 1996), it is of greatest benefit in DBH deficiency where it circumvents the enzymatic defect. Dosages of 250–500 mg two or three times daily are dramatically pressor in patients with DBH deficiency. In general, the drug has been well tolerated. Orthostatic tolerance is greatly enhanced during therapy with this agent, and plasma norepinephrine concentrations, previously undetectable, usually rise into the normal range. A concomitant fall in plasma concentrations of dopamine usually occurs, perhaps because the rate-limiting tyrosine hydroxylase activity is decreased by the newly synthesized feedback inhibition actions of norepinephrine now present in the patient's sympathomimetic neurons.

**PRINCIPLE Undeniably, understanding of the molecular mechanisms of disease ultimately leads to development of disease-specific therapeutics. The challenge is to be aware of the opportunity for discovering such agents and to develop a perspective that optimizes their use.**

## Yohimbine

The $\alpha_2$-adrenergic receptor antagonist yohimbine is sometimes useful in patients with autonomic failure (Onrot, Goldberg, Biaggioni, et al. 1987; Seibyl et al. 1989; Freeman et al. 1996). Although it might seem paradoxical that both $\alpha_2$-adrenergic receptor agonists, such as clonidine, and $\alpha_2$-adrenergic receptor antagonists, such as yohimbine, would be employed in treating low blood pressure, they are useful in different subgroups of patients. While clonidine should be restricted to patients who have no sympathetic function remaining (plasma norepinephrine levels ≤25 pg/ml), yohimbine may be useful in proportion to the amount of sympathetic activity the patient still possesses. In a sense, yohimbine may be a particularly physiologic approach in that it enhances the patient's own

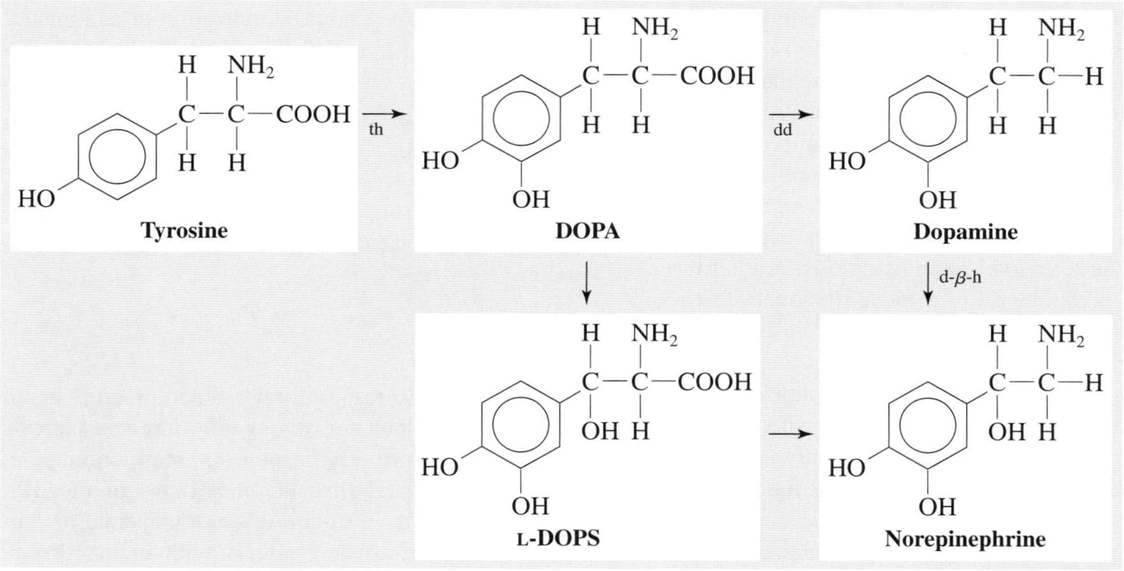

Tyrosine → (th) DOPA → (dd) Dopamine ↓ (d-$\beta$-h) Norepinephrine; DOPA ↓ L-DOPS → Norepinephrine

**FIGURE 1-5 Primary biosynthetic pathway of catecholamines (*solid arrows*) and alternative formation of norepinephrine (*dotted arrow*) from DOPS (Biaggioni and Robertson 1987, with permission from the *Lancet*).**

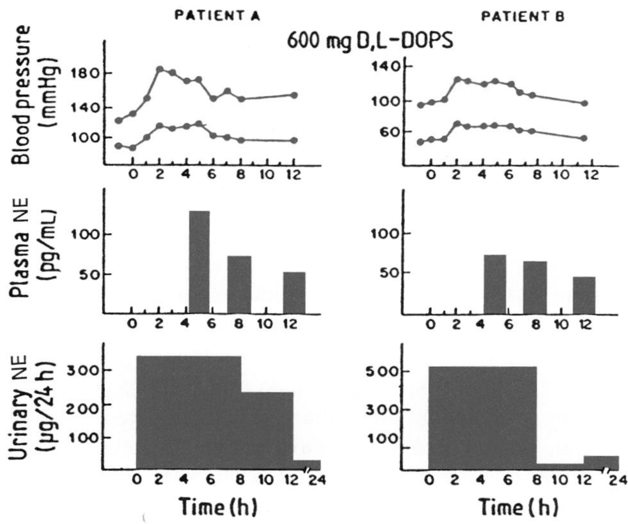


**FIGURE 1-6 Time-course of the changes after 600 mg D,L-DOPS on blood pressure (*upper panels*), plasma norepinephrine (NE) and urinary norepinephrine (Biaggioni and Robertson 1987, with permission from the *Lancet*).**

sympathetic nervous system activation, whereas most other drugs merely supplement or compensate for it. Adverse effects with yohimbine are predominantly anxiety, nervousness, and diarrhea.

**PRINCIPLE When the classification of a disease (e.g., orthostatic hypotension) encompasses pathogenetic and demographic heterogenicity, useful therapies often will remain undiscovered because only a minority subset of the whole will respond well. Remember that most "named diseases" truly are multiple diseases, and judge study results accordingly.**

## Clonidine

The use of $\alpha_2$-adrenergic receptor agonists and antagonists has been extensively studied (Goldberg and Robertson 1983; Onrot, Fogo, et al. 1987, Onrot, Goldberg, Hollister, et al. 1987; Freeman et al. 1996). In the vasomotor center, $\alpha_2$-adrenergic receptor stimulation inhibits sympathetic outflow; on the other hand, centrally active $\alpha_2$-receptor agonists also have direct activity on muscular $\alpha_2$ receptors in the periphery. In the rare patient in whom sympathetic denervation is complete (plasma norepinephrine levels $\leq$25 pg/ml), clonidine does not decrease blood pressure, and the direct effects of clonidine on vascular smooth muscle $\alpha_2$-adrenergic receptors promote smooth muscle contraction. This can result in a dramatic elevation in blood pressure, particularly with oral dosages of 0.4 to 0.8 mg (Robertson et al. 1983). However, the major limitation of clonidine is its depressor effect, observed when this agent is administered to a patient with partial autonomic failure. Sometimes patients with partial autonomic impairment may develop quite severe orthostatic hypotension in response to clonidine. In such patients, although only a low level of sympathetic activity remains, it may be pivotal in the maintenance of blood pressure, and the administration of clonidine, particularly at low doses, may result in incapacitating hypotension. This is especially likely to occur in patients with baroreflex failure. Finally, some patients given clonidine for the management of low blood pressure have marked CNS effects, such as sedation. For all these reasons, clonidine should only rarely be used in the management of orthostatic hypotension.

## Erythropoietin

Recombinant human erythropoietin is available in a preparation with a 165-amino acid sequence "backbone" identical to that of erythropoietin. The recombinant erythropoietin available for clinical use has been given the generic name *epoetin alfa*. It can be given intravenously or subcutaneously. It has the same physiological actions as endogenous erythropoietin. Patients with severe autonomic failure often have mild anemia (hematocrit 32–38), usually in proportion to the degree by which the plasma norepinephrine level is subnormal (Biaggioni, Robertson, Krantz, et al. 1994). This anemia typically elicits an inadequate endogenous erythropoietin response. The anemia is dramatically responsive to epoetin alfa (Hoeldtke and Streeten 1993). For this reason, when simpler measures are insufficient, a trial of epoetin alfa may be undertaken. The greatest disadvantage of this agent is that it must be administered parenterally.

Epoetin alfa usually is administered in doses of 25–75 U/kg three times weekly. An increase in the reticulocyte count usually is detected within 10 days, and an increase in hematocrit is detectable in 2–6 weeks. The goal of using epoetin alfa for patients with autonomic failure is to achieve a hematocrit in the normal gender-based range. This is a somewhat higher target than is usually sought in other diseases for which epoetin alfa has been recommended. It should be recognized that, because epoetin alfa has still been used in only a few hundred patients with autonomic failure, there may be refinements in our use of it in the future.

In addition to the increase in red blood cell count that occurs with epoetin alfa, blood pressure often rises slightly. The mechanism by which this occurs is not entirely clear. It does not appear to be entirely explained by viscosity changes in the blood. The possibility that epoetin alfa might possess an effect on the vasculature heretofore not recognized must remain open.

Occasional patients with autonomic failure experience an acute increase in blood pressure with the first dose, which does not necessarily occur with subsequent doses. The mechanism of this remains unclear. During the period when the hematocrit is increasing, iron deficiency is particularly prone to develop. This should be anticipated in patients with marginal iron levels. Supplementation may be required during the first two months of therapy, and, in some cases, for an indefinite period thereafter.

Many patients are able, once they have reached their target hematocrit to reduce the dosage of epoetin alfa. Some patients are able to be maintained long-term on doses as low as 25 U/kg three times weekly. It is not uncommon for patients to experience a greatly increased sense of well-being and improved appetite on this regimen.

## INDIVIDUALIZATION OF THERAPY

The purpose of therapeutic interventions in patients with chronic orthostatic hypotension is to increase the patient's functional capacity rather than to achieve any particular level of blood pressure (Senard and Montastruc 1996). Factors such as prior ingestion of food and drug as well as the rate of ventilation should be taken into account when assessing the patient's standing time or blood pressure. Hyperventilation lowers (Onrot et al. 1991), and hypoventilation raises blood pressure. Strenuous exercise may markedly lower blood pressure in these patients, but an appropriate exercise program may have long-term benefits.

**PRINCIPLE Be very careful in evaluation of therapy that a surrogate endpoint does not replace more substantial endpoints that are more difficult to measure but more meaningful medically.**

Patient education is the cornerstone of treating individuals with postural hypotension. Many patients discover for themselves that they are less able to carry out vigorous activities following meals. This association may not have been made by other patients, who should be advised to utilize the period before meals for most of their activities and to limit their activities in the hour or so following a large meal.

### Management of Autonomic Failure

Maximizing circulating blood volume is extremely important in treating orthostatic hypotension in severely affected patients with autonomic failure. Even healthy young people pool 350 ml of blood in their legs on standing, and this pooling is, of course, much more marked in patients with autonomic failure. There is a reduction in central blood volume, and most patients have a reduced total blood volume as well. Low-normal values of central venous pressure, right atrial pressure, and pulmonary wedge pressure are frequently seen in severely affected patients with autonomic failure even in the supine position. Liver blood flow is reduced considerably by upright posture, and drug metabolism (e.g., lidocaine) may thus be altered (Feely et al. 1982).

Patients with autonomic failure have inadequately conserved sodium during low salt intake (Bachman and Youmans 1953). This may be due to decreased noradrenergic activity in the kidney, to relatively enhanced dopamine actions, or to other effects. In addition, renin responses to a low-salt diet and upright posture are reduced or absent during autonomic failure (Gordon et al. 1967). Virtually all these patients have elevated supine systemic vascular resistance that does not increase with upright posture. This elevated supine pressure probably also contributes to the failure of the kidney to conserve salt and water. At night, when supine, these patients inappropriately waste sodium in the urine, leading to relative hypovolemia and a degree of orthostatic hypotension that is worse in the morning and improves during the day. It is interesting that angiotensin-converting enzyme (ACE) inhibitors can sometimes reduce blood pressure in spite of the very low plasma renin activity levels present in these patients, raising the possibility of the involvement of a kallikrein mechanism.

**PRINCIPLE Oversimplification of the mechanisms and indications of dominant effects of a drug leads to underutilization of the chemical entity.**

Supine hypertension and its attendant diuresis can be minimized by elevating the head of the bed on blocks to approximately 5–20 degrees (MacLean et al. 1944). In addition to attenuating nocturnal diuresis, this will reduce the notable worsening of symptoms in the morning. Head-up tilt at night also may minimize nocturnal shifts of interstitial fluid from the legs into the circulation. Interstitial fluid in the legs on standing may exert greater support and oppose the tendency of blood to pool. Supine blood pressure usually is highest just after a person goes to bed at night. Most treatment modalities raise supine as well as upright blood pressure. Thus, head-up tilt can minimize the effect of pressor drugs during the night, a time when pressor actions are no longer necessary and may in fact be harmful. Tilt-table conditioning has led to improved functional capacity in some patients with autonomic failure (Hoeldtke et al. 1988).

Salt intake should be liberalized in all patients except those few with coexisting congestive heart failure (Wilcox et al. 1984). Slight pedal edema is well tolerated and implies higher intravascular volume as well as increased interstitial hydrostatic pressure in the legs.

Waist-high, custom-fitted elastic support garments exert graded pressure on the legs and increase interstitial hydrostatic pressure. When the patient stands, this hydrostatic pressure will tend to keep blood from pooling in the legs. However, patients must be cautioned not to wear these stockings at night or when supine, since they will increase central blood volume, contribute to diuresis, and decrease interstitial fluid in the legs. *Note that support stockings are not of much use unless they go at least to the waist.* In fact, an abdominal binder in association with elastic stockings is even more useful. This will serve to augment venous return from the splanchnic bed, a major source of venous pooling. Antigravity suits and shock suits have been used in the past with some success but are quite awkward and bring attention to the patient's problems.

Patients should avoid activities that involve straining, such as lifting heavy objects. Increased abdominal and intrathoracic pressure at these times significantly compromise venous return and can precipitate hypotension. Coughing and straining at stool or with voiding particularly may bring on hypotension. Working with one's arms above shoulder level (e.g., shaving) can lower pressure dramatically, because this maneuver and lifting are often accompanied by an unconscious Valsalva-like increase in thoracic pressure. Ambulation or shifting weight from leg to leg as opposed to standing motionless takes advantage of muscular pumping on the veins. A slightly stooped walking posture may be helpful to the severest patients. Squatting is also a valuable "emergency" mechanism of increasing venous return, particularly when presyncopal symptoms occur. Patients may hang their legs over the side of the bed before standing. This minimizes hemodynamic stress, since assumption of the upright posture is broken down into two movements: (1) assumption of the seated posture and (2) standing from the seated posture.

**PRINCIPLE The appropriate use of measures that are considered adjunctive to drug therapy may be a key determinant of the efficacy of the drug therapy.**

The effect of food on blood pressure in patients with chronic orthostatic hypotension can be important (Sanders 1932; Robertson and Robertson 1981; Jansen and Lipsitz 1995). In normal subjects, there is a slight tachycardia with little or no fall in blood pressure after eating. However, patients with autonomic failure, the elderly, and those taking sympatholytic agents may exhibit large postprandial falls in blood pressure. Digestion shifts blood flow to the hepatic and splanchnic beds, and as already noted, these patients are exquisitely sensitive to changes in circulating blood volume. In addition, several vasoactive substances such as histamine and adenosine, and a variety of vasodilatory gastrointestinal hormones, may be released into the circulation during a meal. These substances, acting either as local vasodilators or systemic hormones, can contribute to the hypotensive response, although their precise role in altering blood pressure is uncertain. Patients should avoid excessive activity in the 2-hour period after meals, since at these times, especially after breakfast, they are most likely to have symptomatic orthostatic hypotension. Patients should also eat smaller meals and limit confections to minimize this effect. In diabetic patients, alterations in insulin levels and the consequences of hypoglycemia may dramatically affect blood pressure and autonomic function (Davis et al. 1997) (Table 1-19). As strange as it may seem, the ingestion of plain water elicits a profound pressor response in most patients with autonomic failure. This effect is evident

**Table 1-19 Stimuli on Blood Pressure in Autonomic Failure**

| *Depressor* | *Pressor* |
|---|---|
| Standing | Lying |
| Food | Water |
| Hyperventilation | Hypoventilation |
| Exercise | Water immersion |
| Straining | Abdominal binding |
| Fever, environmental heat | |

within several minutes, peaks at about 30 minutes, and is sustained for about 1 hour (Jordan, Shannon, Grogan, et al. 1997).

**PRINCIPLE Almost all substances ingested can have pharmacologic/therapeutic importance in the appropriate situation.**

Adenosine may be partially responsible for splanchnic vasodilatation after meals through either local or central mechanisms. Simple measures such as a cup of coffee with meals may lessen this hypotensive response, perhaps because of the ability of caffeine to block adenosine receptors. Pressor agents should be administered in such a way that peak effects occur in the postprandial period when they are needed most. The depressor effect of meals can also be exploited in these patients. Those who have supine hypertension benefit from a small meal or snack at bedtime in order to lower their nocturnal blood pressure. This is especially important in those who have been receiving pressor agents during the day.

**PRINCIPLE Being aware of the effects of routine maneuvers during an average day that can affect the outcome of drug therapy is facilitated by outcome measures that are easy to make and bring about a quick response. Sophisticated therapy uses rather than fights environmental factors.**

Although exhaustive isometric exercise in normal subjects raises blood pressure via sympathetic activation, it can precipitate hypotension in patients with autonomic failure. A graded program of isotonic exercise such as walking may be beneficial (Youmans et al. 1935). More vigorous exercise such as jogging is rarely tolerated because of marked decreases in blood pressure that may occur. Climbing stairs is a common hypotensive stimulus. Exercise, even while a patient is supine, may cause hypotension.

Periods of inactivity and prolonged bed rest should be avoided, since they will worsen tolerance to standing. Prolonged bed rest, even in normal subjects, may cause mild orthostatic hypotension, and even astronauts who are very fit physically experience orthostatic hypotension on return to Earth after the weightlessness of outer space. Even well-trained and healthy young pilots, during the positive G accelerations of aerial maneuvers, may experience quite severe hypotension leading to unconsciousness and seizures. Small wonder that in severely affected patients with autonomic failure, quite mild acceleration, such as that encountered in an ordinary elevator, can bring on symptoms.

The ideal exercise for patients with autonomic failure is swimming. While the patient is submerged in water, his or her tolerance of upright posture is almost unlimited. In this situation, hydrostatic pressure prevents blood pooling in the legs and abdomen, and blood pressure is well maintained. We recommend that our patients undertake a graded program of swimming. Leaving the swimming pool, however, may pose difficulty. Furthermore, patients with the Shy-Drager syndrome may find swimming more of a challenge if the extrapyramidal disease restricts their mobility.

Other stresses can also worsen orthostatic hypotension. Symptoms are more pronounced in hot weather. This is not so much due to volume loss from sweating (which is usually reduced) as to vasodilatation and increased blood flow to the skin. In addition, fever in patients with autonomic failure may contribute markedly to orthostatic hypotension. Patients are also especially at risk in the shower or arising from a hot bath.

Patients should avoid certain nonprescription medications such as diet pills containing phenylpropanolamine or nasal sprays containing phenylephrine or oxymetazoline (a congener of clonidine). Although acutely pressor, these agents, when ingested in excess over time, can lead to significant orthostatic hypotension. All prescription medications should be carefully screened for their potential effects on blood pressure. In particular, antihypertensive medicines prescribed for supine hypertension and drugs such as tricyclic antidepressants can greatly reduce blood pressure. Alcohol tends to lower blood pressure in these patients and can worsen symptoms. On the other hand, alcohol can be exploited in order to treat supine hypertension at night. We often advise our patients to have a glass of wine before retiring, as it elicits a fall of 10–20 mm Hg in blood pressure.

**PRINCIPLE Always be aware that patients have multiple sources of drugs, many of which do not require medical supervision. In addition, it often is hard for doctors to remember that nose drops, for example, do not confine their effects to the nose and that some truly produce hypertension or hypotension.**

Patients with autonomic failure are extremely sensitive to venodilating agents. They have increased sensitivity to the effects of sympathomimetic amines and have an exaggerated sensitivity to $\beta_2$-agonist stimulation compared with $\beta_1$-agonist stimulation (Kronenberg et al. 1990). Consequently, $\beta$ agonists may exert a marked vasodepressor effect in these patients. The dramatic vasoactive effects of many classes of drugs make use of anesthetics especially difficult in these patients (Parris et al. 1984).

Some mechanical aids may allow patients to carry on activities of daily living more easily. For instance, a "derby chair" (a cane when folded, and a small seat when unfolded) can be used by severely affected patients to extend their walking range. Patients may use the cane for support while walking, and when symptoms ensue, they can unfold the chair and sit until they are ready to walk again. Recliner chairs are used so that patients can rest during the day without lying flat. This is especially important when pressor drugs are administered during the day, conferring added risk for supine hypertension.

**PRINCIPLE You cannot be an optimal therapist without being an optimal clinician.**

While atrial tachypacing has been advocated in the management of autonomic failure, our results have been poor. This approach cannot be recommended except in the face of significant persistent bradycardia.

Orthostatic hypotension is a highly variable phenomenon. In many patients, it is completely absent at certain times of the day. In other patients, it may be present in the morning but not later in the day, after a large breakfast but not before breakfast, after climbing a flight of stairs but not before (Robertson et al. 1981). In other individuals, orthostatic hypotension may be present at all times, while its degree remains variable. Other major determinants of the degree of hypotension include hyperventilation (Burnum et al. 1954), fever, and environmental temperature. In the most severely affected patients, admittedly a small subgroup of all patients with orthostatic symptoms, the upright blood pressure can be as low as 60/40 mmHg. At this cuff estimate of blood pressure, the sphygmomanometer is inadequate to assess true intra-arterial blood pressure. For this reason, in severely affected patients, it is useful to monitor the severity of disease and its response to therapy by the standing time.

The standing time is defined as the length of time a patient can stand motionless before the onset of symptoms of orthostatic hypotension. In patients with autonomic impairment, standing motionless is more stressful than walking, because the pumping action of the calf muscles helps venous return during the latter activity. The most common symptoms of orthostatic hypotension are dizziness or lightheadedness, dimming or tunneling of vision, and pain or discomfort in the back of the neck or head. In a small number of patients, slurred speech may be the presenting symptom. As soon as the patient's herald symptoms of orthostatic hypotension appear, he or she is allowed to sit down as the number of elapsed seconds is recorded. If a patient is able to stand for 3 minutes without the onset of symptoms, it is assumed that a reliable blood pressure probably is obtainable, and a sphygmomanometric blood pressure determination is made at that time.

The standing time is primarily of value in monitoring individuals who are unable to stand motionless for as long as 3 minutes. The importance of the standing time is that many individuals who have an increase in standing time from 30 to 120 seconds may have a substantial increase in functional capacity, even though they may have no change in their level of upright blood pressure as assessed by the sphygmomanometer. A patient with a standing time under 30 seconds usually cannot live alone, while a patient with a standing time greater than 60 seconds generally can. Thus, the standing-time determination greatly facilitates the management of the most severely affected patients with orthostatic hypotension.

**PRINCIPLE Understanding the value of a diagnostic test in establishing both the diagnosis and the adequacy of therapy is key to adequate monitoring of the treated and untreated patient.**

## Management of Orthostatic Intolerance

Because orthostatic intolerance is such a heterogeneous disease and because its various pathophysiologies are still incompletely understood, it has been difficult to develop therapeutic regimens genuinely effective for everyone. The most commonly used agents are low-dose propranolol, fludrocortisone plus salt, midodrine, low-dose clonidine or methyldopa, and, where anemia is present, erythropoietin. Results are often disappointing with each of these therapies. The rationale for some of them is to increase blood volume or vascular tone, while for others it is to attenuate the orthostatic tachycardia. Controlled trials conducted over a long period of time are needed to fully evaluate these and other approaches (e.g., phenobarbital, acetazolamide, hydralazine).

## Management of Neurally Mediated Syncope

Because of its resemblance to the vasovagal faint, physicians have sometimes used slightly different approaches in managing neurally mediated syncope, although all the approaches used for orthostatic intolerance have also been employed. Because bradycardia often occurs in association with syncopal attacks, agents that increase heart rate by reducing parasympathetic tone (disopyramide and other muscarinic antagonists) have been employed with varying degrees of success. In a carefully conducted study in a small number of subjects, Mosqueda et al. noted attenuated sympathetic activity on tilt and reasoned that enhancing sympathetic tone with a centrally acting $\alpha_2$-adrenoreceptor antagonist might be beneficial. They showed significant improvement in orthostatic tolerance in patients with neurally mediated syncope in response to oral yohimbine (Mosqueda-Garcia et al. 1996). A larger and more prolonged trial of this agent is needed.

## Management of Baroreflex Failure

The treatment of baroreflex failure is difficult. The initial sustained hypertension phase requires hospitalization in an intensive care unit and control with nitroprusside and sympatholytic agents. In the first two or three days, apneic spells occasionally occur when powerful pain medications are employed, so monitoring is necessary. Once the chronic labile phase is reached, clonidine, either orally or in the form of a clonidine patch is extremely effective, but quite high doses (0.6–2.5 mg daily in divided doses) are sometimes initially required. While commencement with 0.1 mg tid is usual, escalation every other day may be required until blood pressure surges are brought under control. Such agents may make hypotensive episodes worse in some patients. A practical point in the management of patients in the first few weeks after baroreflex failure develops is recognition of the relationship between emotional upset and pressor crises. Patients may over time learn to control the onset of the pressor crises (usually recognized by flushing or headache) by exerting calming self-control. Thus, in some cases, the patients may develop a spontaneous biofeedback treatment of his/her disorder that may result in a reduction in both the number and severity of attacks. Over long periods of time, most patients may be graduated from clonidine to benzodiazepine with continued adequate control.

The patient with selective baroreflex failure may have the additional problem of episodic malignant vagotonia. In such patients, therapy may have to begin with placement of a pacemaker to prevent cardiac arrest, after which long-term management of hypertension by guanethidine or guanedrel, and attenuation of hypotension by fludrocortisone may be the only effective regimen.

## REFERENCES


American Autonomic Society and American Academy of Neurology. 1996. Consensus statement on the definition of orthostatic hypotension, pure autonomic failure, and multiple system atrophy. In: Robertson D, Low PA, Polinsky RJ, editors. *Primer on the Autonomic Nervous System*. San Diego: Academic Press p 334–6.

Bachman DM, Youmans WB. 1953. Effects of posture on renal excretion of sodium and chloride in orthostatic hypotension. *Circulation* **7**:413–21.

Biaggioni I, Robertson D. 1987. Endogenous restoration of norepinephrine by precursor therapy in dopamine $\beta$-hydroxylase deficiency. *Lancet* **2**:1170–2.

Biaggioni I, Robertson D, Krantz S, et al. 1994. The anemia of primary autonomic failure and its reversal with recombinant erythropoietin. *Ann Intern Med* **121**:181–6.

Biaggioni I, Robertson RM, Robertson D. 1994. Manipulation of norepinephrine metabolism with yohimbine in the treatment of autonomic failure. *J Clin Pharmacol* **34**:418–23.

Blaber AP, Bondar RL, Stein F, et al. 1997. Transfer function analysis of cerebral autoregulation dynamics in autonomic failure patients. *Stroke* **28**:1686–92.

Bradbury S, Eggleston C. 1925. Postural hypotension: a report of three cases. *Am Heart J* **1**:73–86.

Burnum JF, Hickam JB, Stead EA. 1954. Hyperventilation in postural hypotension. *Circulation* **10**:362–5.

Chobanian AV, Volicer L, Tifft CP, et al. 1979. Mineralocorticoid-induced hypertension in patients with orthostatic hypotension. *N Engl J Med* **301**:68–73.

Davis SN, Shavers C, Davis B, et al. 1997. Prevention of an increase in plasma cortisol during hypoglycemia preserves subsequent counterregulatory responses. *J Clin Invest* **100**:429–38.

Feely J, Wade D, McAllister CB, et al. 1982. Effect of hypotension on liver blood flow and lidocaine disposition. *N Engl J Med* **307**: 866–9.

Fouad FM, Tadena-Thome L, Bravo E, et al. 1986. Idiopathic hypovolemia. *Ann Intern Med* **104**:298–303.

Freeman R, Komaroff AL. 1997. Does the chronic fatigue syndrome involve the autonomic nervous system? *Am J Med* **102**:357–64.

Freeman R, Young J, Landsberg L, et al. 1996. The treatment of postprandial hypotension in autonomic failure with 3,4-DL-threo-dihydroxyphenylserine. *Neurology* **47**:1414–20.

Furlan R, Jacob G, Piazza S, et al. 1997. Impaired baroreflex modulation of heart rate and muscle sympathetic nerve activity in chronic orthostatic intolerance during gravitational stimulus. *Clin Autonom Res* **7**:240.

Furlan R, Piazza S, Bevilacqua M, et al. 1995. Pure autonomic failure: complex abnormalities in the neural mechanisms regulating the cardiovascular system. *J Autonom Nerv Syst* **51**:223–35.

Goldberg MR, Robertson D. 1983. Yohimbine: a pharmacological probe for study of the $\alpha_2$-adrenoreceptor. *Pharmacol Rev* **35**:143–80.

Goldstein DS, Polinsky RJ, Garty M, et al. 1989. Patterns of plasma levels of catechols in idiopathic orthostatic hypotension. *Ann Neurol* **26**:558–3.

Gordon RD, Kuchel O, Liddle GW, et al. 1967. Role of the sympathetic nervous system in regulating renin and aldosterone production in man. *J Clin Invest* **46**:599–605.

Hoeldtke RD, Cavanaugh ST, Hughes JD. 1988. Treatment of orthostatic hypotension: interaction with pressor drugs and tilt table conditioning. *Arch Phys Med Rehabil* **69**:895–8.

Hoeldtke RD, Streeten DHP. 1993. Treatment of orthostatic hypotension with erythropoietin. *N Engl J Med* **329**:611–5.

Jacob G, Atkinson D, Shannon JR, et al. 1996. Evidence of cerebral blood flow abnormalities in idiopathic hyperadrenergic state. *Circulation* **94** (Suppl 1):1–545.

Jacob G, Biaggioni I. 1999. Orthostatic intolerance and postural tachycardia syndromes. *Am J Med Sci* **317**:88–101.

Jansen RW, Lipsitz LA. 1995. Postprandial hypotension: epidemiology, pathophysiology and clinical management. *Ann Intern Med* **122:**286–95.

Jordan J, Shannon JR, Black B, et al. 1997. Malignant vagotonia due to selective baroreflex failure. *Hypertension* **30**:1072–7.

Jordan J, Shannon JR, Grogan E, et al. 1997. Pressor effects of oral water in primary autonomic failure. *Circulation* **96**:1–740.

Jordan J, Shannon JR, Grogan E, et al. 1999. A potent pressor response elicited by drinking water (letter). *Lancet* **353**:1971–2.

Kapoor W. 1999. Using a tilt table to evaluate snycope. *Am J Med Sci* **317**:110–6.

Kaufmann H. 1996. Could treatment with DOPS do for autonomic failure what DOPA did for Parkinson's disease? *Neurology* **47**: 1370–1.

Kaufmann H. 1997. Syncope: a neurologist's viewpoint. *Cardiol Clin* **15**:177–94.

Kronenberg MW, Forman MB, Onrot J, et al. 1990. Enhanced left ventricular contractility in autonomic failure: assessment using pressure-volume relations. *J Am Coll Cardiol* **15**:1334–42.

Lipsitz LA. 1996. Aging and the autonomic nervous system. In: Robertson D, Low PA, Polinsky RJ, editors. *Primer on the Autonomic Nervous System.* San Diego: Academic Press. p 79–83.

Low PA, Novak V, Spies JM, et al. 1999. Cerebrovascular regulation in the postural tachycardia syndrome (POTS). *Am J Med Sci* **317**:124–33.

MacLean AR, Allen EV, Magath TB. 1944. Orthostatic tachycardia and orthostatic hypotension: defects in the return of venous blood to the heart. *Am Heart J* **24**:145–63.

McTavish D, Goa KL. 1989. Midodrine: a review of its pharmacological properties and therapeutic use in orthostatic hypotension and secondary hypotensive disorders. *Drugs* **38**:757–77.

Mosqueda-Garcia R, Furlan R, Fernandez-Violante R, et al. 1996. Enhancement of central noradrenergic outflow prevents neurally mediated syncope. *Clin Autonom Res* **6**:290.

Mosqueda-Garcia R, Furlan R, Fernandez-Violante R, et al. 1997. Sympathetic and baroreflex function in neurally mediated syncope evoked by tilt. *J Clin Invest* **99**:2736–44.

Novak V, Novak P, Opfer-Gehrking TL, et al. 1996. Postural tachycardia syndrome: time frequency mapping. *J Autonom Nerv Syst* **61**:313–20.

Onrot J, Bernard GR, Biaggioni I, et al. 1991. Direct vasodilator effect of hyperventilation-induced hypocarbia in autonomic failure patients. *Am J Med Sci* **301**:305–9.

Onrot J, Fogo A, Biaggioni I, et al. 1987. Neck tumor with syncope due to paroxysmal sympathetic withdrawal. *J Neurol Neurosurg Psychiatry* **50**:1063–6.

Onrot J, Goldberg MR, Biaggioni I, et al. 1987. Oral yohimbine in human autonomic failure. *Neurology* **37**:215–20.

Onrot J, Goldberg MR, Hollister AS, et al. 1987. Management of chronic orthostatic hypotension. *Am J Med* **80**:454–64.

Papp MI, Lantos PL. 1992. Accumulation of tabular structures in oligodendroglial and neuronal cells as the basic observation in multiple system atrophy. *J Neurol Sci* **107**:172–82.

Parris WC, Goldberg MR, Robertson D. 1984. The anesthetic management of autonomic dysfunction. *Anesthesiol Rev* **11**:17–23.

Robertson D, Davis T. 1995. Recent advances in the treatment of orthostatic hypotension. *Neurology* **45** (Suppl 4):S26–32.

Robertson D, Goldberg MR, Hollister AS, et al. 1983. Clonidine raises blood pressure in idiopathic orthostatic hypotension. *Am J Med* **74**:193–9.

Robertson D, Hollister AS, Biaggioni I, et al. 1993. The diagnosis and treatment of baroreflex failure. *N Engl J Med* **329**:1449–55.

Robertson D, Hollister AS, Carey EL, et al. 1984. Increased vascular beta2-adrenoceptor responsiveness in autonomic dysfunction. *J Am Coll Cardiol* **3**:850–6.

Robertson D, Kincaid DW, Robertson RM. 1994. The head and neck discomfort of autonomic failure: an unrecognized etiology of headache. *Clin Autonom Res* **4**:99–103.

Robertson D, Perry SE, Hollister AS, et al. 1991. Dopamine-$\beta$-hydroxylase deficiency: a genetic disorder of cardiovascular regulation. *Hypertension* **18**:1–8.

Robertson D, Robertson RM. 1981. The Bezold-Jarisch reflex: possible role in limiting myocardial ischemia. *Clin Cardiol* **4**:75–9.

Robertson D, Robertson RM. 1994. Causes of chronic orthostatic hypotension. *Arch Int Med* **154**:1620–4.

Robertson D, Wade D, Robertson RM. 1981. Postprandial alterations in cardiovascular hemodynamics in autonomic dysfunctional states. *Am J Cardiol* **48**:1048–52.

Sanders AO. 1932. Postural hypotension with tachycardia: a case report. *Am Heart J* **7**:808–13.

Seibyl JP, Krystal JH, Price LH, et al. 1989. Use of yohimbine to counteract nortriptyline-induced orthostatic hypotension. *J Clin Psychopharmacol* **9**:67–8.

Senard JM, Montastruc JL. 1996. Which drug for which orthostatic hypotension. *Fundament Clin Pharmacol* **10**: 225–33.

Shannon J, Jordan J, Costa F, et al. 1997. The hypertension of autonomic failure and its treatment. *Hypertension* **30**:1062–7.

Streeten DHP. 1987. *Orthostatic Disorders of the Circulation: Mechanisms, Manifestations, and Treatment.* New York: Plenum. 272 p.

Wenning GK, Tison F, Ben Shlomo Y, et al. 1997. Multiple system atrophy: a review of 203 pathologically proven cases. *Movement Disord* **12**:133–47.

Wilcox CS, Puritz R, Lightman SL, et al. 1984. Plasma volume regulation in patients with progressive autonomic failure during changes in salt intake and posture. *J Lab Clin Med* **104**:331–9.

Youmans JB, Akeroyd JH, Frank H. 1935. Changes in the blood and circulation with changes in posture: the effect of exercise and vasodilatation. *J Clin Invest* **14**:739–53.

Ziegler MG, Lake CR, Kopin IJ. 1977. The sympathetic-nervous-system defect in primary orthostatic hypotension. *N Engl J Med* **296**: 293–7.

# Coronary Artery Disease

Thomas Michel, Mark S. Weinfeld

*Chapter Outline*



Coronary artery disease (CAD) represents an important cause of morbidity and premature death. One-half of all patients with CAD present acutely with myocardial infarction or sudden cardiac death as the first manifestation of their illness. *How can these patients be identified and treated before the onset of a life-threatening event?* Other patients with CAD develop angina pectoris, a chronic or subacute chest pain syndrome caused by transient myocardial ischemia, most commonly due to increased myocardial oxygen demands in the face of flow-limiting coronary artery stenoses from atherosclerosis. *What can ameliorate the symptoms of angina, and how might the underlying disease be most effectively treated?*

Therapies for CAD address interdependent therapeutic goals: to prevent CAD, to treat its acute and potentially life-threatening manifestations, to delay or prevent disease progression, and to ameliorate CAD symptoms (see Fig. 1-7). This chapter focuses on the drugs used for symptomatic treatment of angina pectoris, and addresses the preventive approaches that can be used to minimize the likelihood of developing CAD and/or its complications. The management of patients with acute versus chronic manifestations of CAD clearly involves distinct treatment strategies. The next section of this chapter presents the acute medical and surgical interventions that may be mandated by a patient's presentation with incipient, ongoing, or recent myocardial infarction.

Therapeutic strategies for treatment of coronary artery disease (CAD) may be categorized into three distinct classes:

- Primary or secondary prevention of coronary artery disease. CAD prevention therapies are directed toward reducing a patient's risk for developing coronary atherosclerosis, and/or minimizing the long-term morbidity from the disease once it has become clinically expressed. Drugs in this category include lipid-lowering agents and antihypertensive medications.
- Chronic angina pectoris. Strategies for the treatment of the symptoms of angina principally involve medications that reduce myocardial oxygen demand and include organic nitrate vasodilators, $\beta$-adrenergic receptor blocking drugs, and calcium channel blockers. These drugs are discussed in this chapter.
- Acute coronary syndromes. Therapies using thrombolytic agents, anticoagulants, and antiplatelet drugs complement the use of urgent mechanical interventions for the treatment of acute (or threatened) coronary occlusion, which is most commonly manifest as unstable angina pectoris or acute myocardial infarction. This topic is covered in the section following in this chapter. The sequelae of myocardial infarction include heart failure and sudden cardiac death, topics covered in later sections of this chapter.

## PREVENTION OF CORONARY ARTERY DISEASE

Coronary atherosclerosis is associated with a broad range of risk factors that increase the likelihood of developing the disease (Table 1-20). One important strategy to minimize the morbidity and mortality of coronary artery disease is prevention by modifying the factors that lead to an increased risk for the development of premature atherosclerosis. Modifiable cardiac risk factors include hypertension, diabetes mellitus, cigarette smoking, dyslipidemia, and postmenopausal state (see Table 1-20). Other therapeutic approaches that may attenuate the development of coronary artery disease include regular aspirin ingestion, the treatment of hyperhomocysteinemia with folate and vitamin $B_{12}$, and the use of antioxidant vitamins

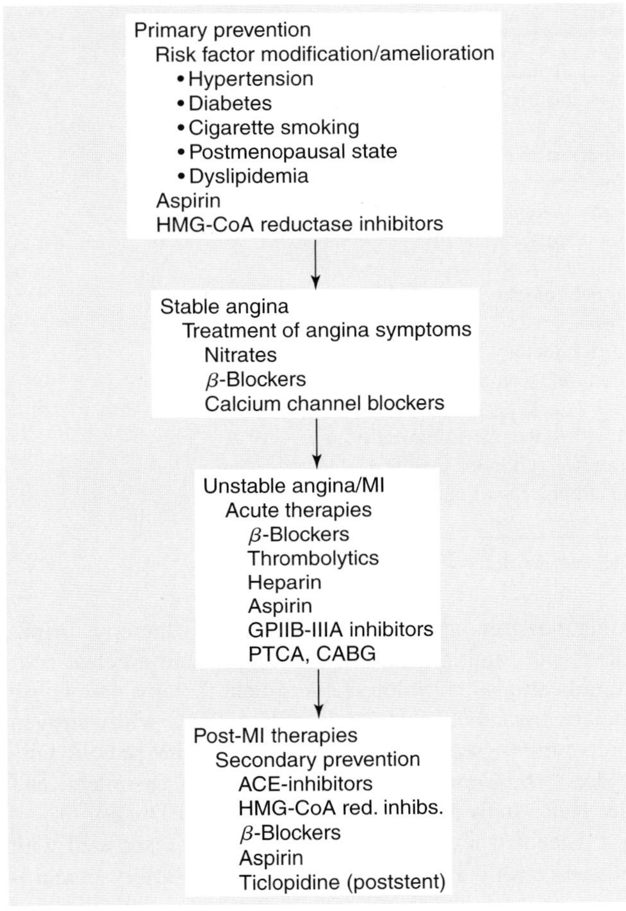


**FIGURE 1-7 Angina and the spectrum of coronary artery disease (CAD). Therapeutic approaches for treatment of symptoms of stable CAD, as well as approaches that prevent the development and/or progression of the disease, are shown. Treatments for the acute manifestations of unstable angina and myocardial infarction (MI) include drugs, as well as invasive therapies such as percutaneous transluminal coronary angioplasty (PTCA) and coronary artery bypass grafting surgery (CABG), and are discussed in chapter 12, Hematologic Disorders. ACE, angiotensin-converting enzyme; GPIIb-IIIa, glycoprotein IIb/IIIa; HMG-CoA, hydroxymethylglutaryl-coenzyme A reductase.**

and/or dietary supplements. Data supporting the use of these therapies varies greatly in quantity and quality, and clinical investigation into prevention of CAD remains an active area of research. Once CAD has become clinically evident following myocardial infarction, various drugs and interventions have been identified that reduce the likelihood of mortality, or of further morbidity, from CAD (secondary prevention).

Hypertension is an important risk factor for the development of coronary artery disease, and control of hypertension lessens morbidity from coronary atherosclerosis. A meta-analysis of nine long-term prospective studies enrolling almost 420,000 subjects showed baseline blood pressure correlates with coronary artery disease death and nonfatal MI (MacMahon et al. 1990). A meta-analysis of 14 large, randomized trials of antihypertensive therapy demonstrated a significantly lower event rate of coronary artery signs and symptoms in treated patients (Collins et al. 1900). Many of the drugs used for the treatment of hypertension also have antianginal effects. For example, patients with CAD and hypertension are commonly treated with β-adrenergic blocking drugs, leading to a combination of salutary effects in blood pressure control, treatment of angina pectoris, and secondary prevention of MI.

**PRINCIPLE Seek settings in which single drug therapy can modulate multiple therapeutic endpoints. The concept of two or more therapeutic targets for one drug leads to compliance and often reduction of cost of care.**

Although a relation between glycemic control and coronary artery disease outcome has been demonstrated for microvascular complications in patients with type I and type II diabetes mellitus, it remains controversial (Gaster and Hirsch 1998). Current recommendations emphasize the importance of glycemic control to decrease retinopathy, nephropathy, and neuropathy, rather than for control of coronary artery disease per se. In addition, strict control of other modifiable risk factors, such as hypertension and smoking cessation, is warranted in diabetic patients.

Perhaps the most important modifiable cardiovascular risk factor is cigarette smoking. The Framingham Heart Study linked increases in cardiovascular mortality of 18% in men and 31% in women for each 10 cigarettes smoked per day (Kannel and Higgins 1990). Discontinuation of tobacco is associated with a rapid decrease in risk of coronary artery disease events, declining to that of nonsmokers within 3 years of smoking cessation (Dobson et al. 1991). Treatment modalities for nicotine addiction have been variably successful, and are discussed in chapter 17, Substance Abuse: Dependence and Treatment.

It has long been known that severe hypercholesterolemia is associated with the development of premature atherosclerosis. More recently, the beneficial effects of

Table 1-20 Risk Factors for Development of Coronary Artery Disease (CAD)

| RISK FACTOR | THERAPY |
|---|---|
| Cigarette smoking | Smoking cessation pharmacotherapies and lifestyle modifications |
| Male sex | Not usually subject to therapeutic intervention |
| Family history | Not usually subject to therapeutic intervention |
| Postmenopausal state | Hormone replacement therapy in many patients |
| Dyslipidemia | Dietary modifications; lipid-lowering agents, especially HMG-CoA reductase inhibitors |
| Hypertension | Antihypertensive medications, often beta-blockers if patient has history of myocardial infarction |
| Diabetes mellitus | Aggressive treatment of other CAD risk factors |
| Hyperhomocyst(e)inemia | Dietary supplements with folate, vitamins $B_6$ and $B_{12}$ |
| *Other risk factors* | |
| Inflammation | { Daily aspirin use is associated with lower CAD mortality, and the use of "antioxidant vitamins" (vitamins C and E) may be beneficial; no role for antimicrobial agents has yet been established. |
| Platelet activation | |
| Oxidative stress | |
| Infection | |

ABBREVIATIONS: HMG-CoA, hydroxymethylglutaryl-coenzyme A; { refers to all "other risk factors".

hydroxymethylglutaryl coenzyme A (HMG-CoA) reductase inhibitors on coronary morbidity and mortality have been established in studies of patients with mild as well as severe hypercholesterolemia (Scandinavian Simvastatin Study Group 1994; Shepherd et al. 1995). Patients with coronary disease or multiple cardiac risk factors should undergo a careful assessment of their dietary intake of fat and cholesterol; dyslipidemias unresponsive to dietary modification should be treated with agents such as hydroxymethylglutaryl-coenzyme A (HMG-CoA) reductase inhibitors, cholesterol-binding resins, or niacin, as discussed in detail in chapter 9, Endocrine and Metabolic Disorders.

Clinical manifestations of coronary disease in premenopausal women are relatively uncommon, but following menopause the incidence of atherosclerosis in women equals that of men. The increased cardiac risk seen after menopause is associated with adverse changes in lipid levels, including changes in lipoproteins: increased LDL and decreased HDL levels (Matthew et al. 1989). In the Nurses' Health Study, hormone replacement therapy was associated with a marked decrease in the relative risk of myocardial infarction and death for subjects using estrogen (Stampfer et al. 1991). Unfortunately, the important cardiovascular benefit of estrogen therapy is partially offset by an increase in the risk of breast cancer in patients taking postmenopausal estrogens. The decision whether to initiate or continue hormone replacement therapy must be highly individualized, taking into account the patient's risks for the development of coronary disease in the context of their risks for breast cancer, thromboembolism, or other possible complications of estrogen therapy. In patients with multiple cardiac risk factors and no clear contraindications to hormone replacement therapy, many physicians treat their postmenopausal patients with estrogen preparations (see chapter 9, Endocrine and Metabolic Disorders; 10, Connective Tissue and Bone Disorders; and 28, Risk Analysis Applied to Prescription Drugs).

Elevated levels of homocysteine are associated with atherosclerotic disease, including coronary artery, cerebrovascular, and peripheral vascular disease (Moghadasian et al. 1997). Potential treatments for some patient subsets include dietary supplementation with vitamin $B_6$, vitamin $B_{12}$, and folate (Welch and Loscalzo 1998). The therapeutic efficacy of these dietary supplements on clinical endpoints remains to be determined, but treatment with these vitamins lowers homocyst(e)ine concentrations and seems warranted at this time.

**PRINCIPLE When the logic of using a drug for an indication is strong but the outcome is unknown, the decision to treat lies in the toxicity of the treatment and availability of a surrogate marker to guide dosage and duration of treatment.**

Antioxidants may influence atherogenesis through multiple mechanisms. Although epidemiological studies have suggested dietary antioxidant vitamins may be protective against coronary artery disease, randomized trials have had inconsistent results. One small randomized trial found that vitamin E supplementation was associated with a 60% reduction in nonfatal myocardial infarction (Stephens et al. 1996). Further studies will be necessary to determine whether any of the multiple antioxidants studied are clinically beneficial.

Large observational trials have found that a patient's aspirin use is associated with a decreased risk of death from CAD, and it has been postulated that mediators of inflammation could play a key role in the pathogenesis of atherosclerosis. In the US Physicians' Health Study, a marker for underlying systemic inflammation (plasma C-reactive protein) was higher at baseline in subjects who subsequently developed myocardial infarction or ischemic stroke. Use of aspirin was associated with a significant decrease in the risk of myocardial infarction in patients with the highest levels of C-reactive protein (Ridker et al. 1997).

**PRINCIPLE One often analyzes the effects of drugs on a disease described by a rubric (e.g., myocardial infarction) that covers a spectrum of pathogenesis and severities. Very often when the disease can be subdivided into subgroups based on severity or the presence of a surrogate marker for severity or predisposition toward disease, it is possible to identify highly effective therapies whose efficacy is diluted if the treatment group is more heterogeneous. The exercise of looking for subgroups that are predictably responsive or not responsive to specific therapy is an important step in individualizing therapy.**

Aspirin, in addition to its anti-inflammatory properties, also is a potent inhibitor of platelet aggregation. Aspirin has been shown to be effective for primary and secondary prevention of cardiovascular events. In the US Physicians' Health Study, an alternate-day dose of 325 mg of aspirin was associated with a 44% decrease in risk of a first myocardial infarction (Steering Committee of the Physicians Health Study Research Group 1989). The 1994 Antiplatelet Trialists' Collaboration found that aspirin therapy decreased the risk of vascular events by approximately one-quarter in patients with a history of a cardiac event, peripheral vascular disease, or atrial fibrillation (Antiplatelet Trialists' Collaboration 1994). The range of the commonly used doses was 75–325 mg per day (Hennekens et al. 1997).

The antiplatelet agent clopidogrel has been studied for secondary prevention. The CAPRIE study suggested that 75 mg per day of clopidogrel may be slightly more effective than aspirin in prevention of vascular events in patients with a history of atherosclerotic disease (CAPRIE Steering Committee 1996). Although further studies will be necessary to validate this finding and to determine its generalizability, the thienopyridines are alternatives to aspirin as antiplatelet agents for primary and secondary prevention of vascular events. Another antiplatelet drug in increasingly common use in selected patients with CAD is ticlopidine, a structural analog of clopidogrel. Ticlopidine, given concomitantly with aspirin, has been shown to reduce the likelihood of abrupt closure of intravascular coronary stents, which are frequently used in percutaneous catheter-based coronary revascularizations (Schomig et al. 1996). These drugs are discussed in chapter 12, Hematologic Disorders.

Seroepidemiological and pathologic evidence has associated atherosclerosis with exposure to infectious agents, including cytomegalovirus and *Chlamydia pneumoniae.* The significance of these associations and potential for intervention are active areas of research (Libby et al. 1997). The role, if any, of antimicrobial agents in the prevention or treatment of CAD remains obscure and intriguing!

## TREATMENT OF STABLE ANGINA PECTORIS

### The Pathophysiology of Angina Pectoris

Angina pectoris is the most common clinical presentation of chronic ischemic heart disease from coronary atherosclerosis. The term was first used by Dr. William Heberden in a report published in 1772: ". . . there is a disorder of the breast marked with strong and peculiar symptoms, considerable for the danger belonging to it, and not extremely rare, which deserves to be mentioned more at length. The seat of it, and sense of strangling, and anxiety with which it is attended, may make it not improperly be called angina pectoris. Those who are afflicted with it are seized while they are walking (more especially if it be up hill, and soon after eating) with a painful and most disagreeable sensation in the breast, which seems as if it would extinguish life, if it were to increase or continue; but the moment they stand still, all this uneasiness vanishes. . . With respect to the treatment of this complaint, I have little or nothing to advance. . ."

But we do!

Heberden believed that angina pectoris arose in the breast, but it has since become clear that angina pectoris reflects the pain of myocardial ischemia. The local metabolic derangements consequent to myocardial ischemia lead to the activation of cardiac afferent nerve fibers, and produce a sensation of discomfort that often is experienced as chest heaviness or pressure, with accompanying feelings of nausea, dyspnea, presyncope and/or diaphoresis. Commonly, patients will deny that they have a sensation of "pain," but rather describe a vague retrosternal chest discomfort that may radiate to the jaw or left arm. A typical angina "attack," provoked commonly by physical exertion or emotional distress, may last a few minutes or as long as half an hour; the provoked ischemia is rarely sufficiently severe so as to cause frank myocardial necrosis.

The presence of myocardial ischemia represents an imbalance between myocardial oxygen supply and demand (Table 1-21) and can reflect a variety of pathophysiologic processes, but most commonly represents a manifestation of atherosclerotic coronary artery disease. Decreases in myocardial blood supply can result from the presence of flow-limiting chronic stenoses in diseased coronary arteries, or can occur acutely due to coronary artery vasospasm or thrombosis. By contrast, increases in myocardial oxygen demand may arise as a result of physical exertion or emotional stress, two common precipitating factors for angina.

Myocardial oxygen demand is principally determined by heart rate, ventricular contractility, and by myocardial wall tension, which in turn is influenced by cardiac preload (ventricular filling pressure), ventricular volume, contractility, and afterload. Mechanical factors that lead to an adaptive increase in wall thickness, such as the hypertrophy consequent to systemic hypertension or aortic stenosis, will lower the ischemic threshold for the development of symptoms of angina. Drugs that ameliorate or prevent angina either decrease myocardial oxygen demand (by slowing the heart rate or decreasing myocardial wall tension), or increase myocardial blood supply (by inducing coronary vasodilatation or preventing coronary vasoconstriction). Three classes of drugs are used in this context: organic nitrate vasodilators, $\beta$-adrenergic antagonists, and calcium channel blockers.

**Table 1-21 Determinants of Myocardial Oxygen Demand and Supply**

*Determinants of myocardial oxygen demand*
- Heart rate
- Ventricular contractility
- Myocardial wall tension
  - Preload
  - Afterload
  - Wall thickness
- Metabolic factors

*Determinants of myocardial oxygen supply*
- Blood flow
  - Pressure
  - Resistance
- Blood $O_2$ content and delivery

## Organic Nitrate Vasodilator Drugs

### *Pathophysiology*

The prototype organic nitrate vasodilator drug is nitroglycerin (properly but not commonly termed glyceryl trinitrate), and has been in clinical use for the treatment of angina pectoris since the late 19th century (Robertson and Robertson 1996). Other clinically important organic nitrate vasodilators include isosorbide dinitrate and isosorbide mononitrate; related compounds such as pentaerythritol tetranitrate share similar properties but are not in widespread clinical use. In vivo, all these organic nitrate vasodilators serve as prodrugs, and become biologically active when they are metabolized to release nitric oxide (NO) by biochemical pathways that remain incompletely understood.

The antianginal effect associated with organic nitrate vasodilator administration is multifactorial. NO released from nitroglycerin induces the relaxation of vascular smooth muscle and results in the dilatation of both arteries and veins. Low concentrations of nitroglycerin produce venodilation, and higher concentrations produce arteriolar dilatation as well. In commonly used doses, nitrates produce dilatation of epicardial coronary arteries. Local factors may differentially influence the metabolism of nitroglycerin to NO. The dilatation of veins results in venous "pooling" of the intravascular volume, and leads to a decrease in both left and right ventricular filling pressures (decreased preload). The dilatation of the large epicardial arteries leads to increases in total coronary flow to the subendocardium, the region most likely to become ischemic. Dilatation of peripheral resistance arteries may also result in a decrease in systemic arterial pressure, an effect that can actually provoke angina if coronary perfusion (which depends on diastolic pressure) is compromised or if reflex tachycardia occurs consequent to systemic hypotension. These undesirable effects, as well as severe headache due to cerebral arterial vasodilatation, are usually seen with the rapid administration of higher doses of nitroglycerin.

The biotransformation of the organic nitrate vasodilators to NO appears to involve the action of extracellular reductants and intracellular reduced thiols (e.g., glutathione), but the precise contributions of enzymatic and nonenzymatic steps to this process is controversial. The production of NO leads to the activation of diverse biochemical pathways, the best characterized of which involves guanylate cyclase activation. Nitric oxide forms a nitroso–heme complex with the soluble isoform of guanylate cyclase, thereby activating the enzyme and increasing the concentration of the second messenger cyclic GMP in target tissues. Cyclic GMP itself has several molecular targets within the cell, including its cognate protein kinase; activation of cGMP-dependent protein kinase leads to the phosphorylation of specific substrates to produce physiological responses characteristic of the target tissue. Vascular smooth muscle cells relax as a consequence of nitroglycerin administration; smooth muscle cells in other tissues are similarly influenced by organic nitrate vasodilators following the metabolism of these drugs to NO. Nitric oxide also inhibits platelet aggregation, and it appears that the antiplatelet effects of nitroglycerin may also have some antianginal role (see Fig. 1-8).

The broad range of physiological responses to nitric oxide in diverse tissues reflects the presence of endogenous enzymatic pathways for the synthesis of nitric oxide as a messenger molecule. In vascular endothelial cells, the enzyme nitric oxide synthase makes NO in response to activation of a variety of cell surface receptors; the enzyme can also be activated by hemodynamic shear stress. The endothelial isoform of nitric oxide synthase (eNOS) is a member of a family of proteins that forms nitric oxide by oxidizing the terminal guanido nitrogen of the amino acid L-arginine. More than a century passed between the common clinical use of organic nitrate vasodilators and the discovery of an enzyme that synthesizes an "endogenous nitrovasodilator." The endothelial nitric oxide synthase belongs to a recently described family of enzymes found in numerous mammalian tissues, and the nitric oxide formed by these different enzyme isoforms appears to play important roles in such disparate processes as blood pressure regulation (endothelial NO synthase), neurotransmission (neural NO synthase) and cytotoxicity (macrophage NO synthase). When eNOS enzyme activity is blocked by the administration of specific enzyme inhibitors, or when the gene encoding eNOS is inactivated (in experimental animals), there is an increase in the resting systemic blood pressure. This suggests that the ongoing synthesis of nitric oxide by endothelial cells is an important determinant of vascular tone.

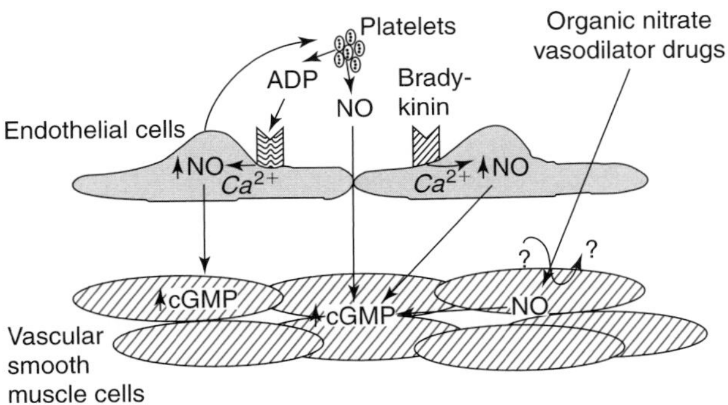


**FIGURE 1-8 Nitric oxide (NO) signaling in the vascular wall. The monolayer of endothelial cells that forms the lining of the vascular wall is surrounded by vascular smooth muscle cells. In response to increases in intracellular calcium induced by stimulation by a variety of cell surface receptors or by hemodynamic shear stress, the endothelial nitric oxide synthase becomes activated and produces NO, which then acts on smooth muscle cells and blood platelets and leads to an increase of intracellular cyclic GMP in these target cells, associated with vasorelaxation and inhibition of platelet aggregation, respectively. Organic nitrate vasodilator drugs undergo reductive metabolism to form NO, in a process thought to involve both enzymatic and nonenzymatic pathways, possibly localized in the particulate fraction of vascular smooth cells.**

**PRINCIPLE When multiple drugs have similar effects on a variety of tissues, first, expect diverse effects of the drug clinically and, second, explore the possibility of a common mechanism working on diverse tissue responses that may create opportunity for one drug having far more value than others in the same class.**

An important pathway for the endogenous activation of endothelial nitric oxide synthase involves the action of the autocoid peptide bradykinin, which binds to its cognate receptor on the endothelial cell surface and stimulates endothelial NO production. Drugs that influence the metabolism of bradykinin, most notably the angiotensin-converting enzyme inhibitors (see section on Hypertension in this chapter), can indirectly activate the endothelial synthesis of NO by inhibiting the catabolism of bradykinin in the vessel wall. This indirect effect of angiotensin-converting enzyme inhibitors on vascular NO production may account in part for the therapeutic effects of this class of drugs. Several other drugs may impinge upon the abundance or biological activity of eNOS. For example, it has been recently shown that some HMG-CoA inhibitors increase the abundance of eNOS in experimental models. Other studies have shown that the oral administration of L-arginine, the substrate for nitric oxide synthases, apparently can have an antiatherogenic effect, possibly by indirect effects that lead to an increase in vascular nitric oxide synthesis. The mechanisms underlying these drug effects remain obscure, and the clinical relevance of these observations remains to be established.

**PRINCIPLE Insist on familiarizing yourself with data on relative efficacy and toxicity when multiple agents are available with a similar mechanism of positive effects.**

**PRINCIPLE When multiple drugs contribute to a common effect expect value in combinations if toxicity is not dependent on the same effects.**

### *Pharmacological properties*

Although the specific metabolic pathways involved in the reduction of organic nitrate vasodilators to NO are incompletely understood, pharmacokinetic profiles of these drugs have been extensively studied (Parker and Parker 1998). Nitroglycerin is effectively absorbed from mucosal surfaces, skin, and the GI tract. Nitroglycerin can be administered by a variety of routes: sublingual, buccal, oral, transdermal, and intravenous. Onset of drug action is most rapid after intravenous or sublingual drug administration. Once absorbed, nitroglycerin has a plasma half-life of only a few minutes, although its bioactive metabolites may persist in the plasma for several tens of minutes. Isosorbide dinitrate is well absorbed from the GI tract, and the drug and its active hepatic metabolites can exert a therapeutic benefit for 3–5 hours following drug administration. Isosorbide mononitrate is similarly well-absorbed but, unlike nitroglycerin and isosorbide dinitrate, the mononitrate does not undergo extensive first-pass hepatic metabolism and therefore has clinical efficacy for a longer period following ingestion.

Tolerance to the effects of organic nitrate vasodilators is a clinically important phenomenon and serves as a major factor limiting the clinical efficacy of this class of drug. Pharmacologic tolerance is defined as the requirement for successively higher doses of a drug to achieve the same pharmacologic effect. The antianginal efficacy of organic nitrate vasodilators can be quantified by measuring a patient's anginal threshold in an exercise test, and this parameter can be determined under varying drug regimens to evaluate approaches that may minimize the development of pharmacologic tolerance to these medications. Tolerance to the therapeutic effects of nitroglycerin does not appear to depend on the route of administration and can be seen with oral, transdermal, and parenteral drug administration. A variety of hypotheses have been put forward to explain the cellular basis for tolerance to organic nitrate vasodilator drugs, but the mechanisms leading to the development of tolerance will likely remain poorly understood so long as the biochemical pathways that lead to NO formation from these drugs remain obscure. Changing the dosing interval or varying the dose can minimize the development of tolerance to oral and transdermal nitrates; for intravenous nitroglycerin, escalating drug doses may be required to maintain a therapeutic effect.

Tolerance can be minimized by adjusting the dosing schedule to permit a daily "nitrate-free interval." Since angina typically is exacerbated during diurnal activities, a dosing schedule can be devised that permits a prolonged nocturnal interval without drug. This is exactly countered by transdermal patches. But, isosorbide dinitrate can be most efficacious when administered on a dosing schedule in which drug is administered in more frequent doses during the day, allowing for a prolonged period without drug overnight to reduce the development of tolerance. For transdermal nitroglycerin, tolerance can be minimized by the simple expedient of removing of the nitroglycerin patch for at least 12 hours each night. Obviously, the withdrawal of an effective drug for a prolonged period could minimize its therapeutic effect. Patients who develop angina during their "nitrate-free interval" often require other antianginal medications (vide infra) to sustain a therapeutic effect. To date, the coadministration of other drugs that might, in theory, attenuate the development of tolerance (including angiotensin-converting enzyme inhibitors and reduced thiol compounds) do not appear to be clinically useful in the prevention of tolerance to the organic nitrate vasodilators.

**PRINCIPLE Pharmacological tolerance is defined as the requirement for increasing drug doses with prolonged therapy in order to reach the same therapeutic effect as was achieved initially. Although drug dosing schedules have been devised that reduce drug tolerance, the development of tolerance to organic nitrate vasodilators represents an important limitation to their efficacy.**

### *Clinical uses of organic nitrate vasodilators*

Nitroglycerin is most commonly used to treat acute episodes of angina in rapid-acting drug formulations, such as sublingual tablets or a metered-dose nitroglycerin oral spray; intravenous nitroglycerin is used in acute coronary syndromes, as discussed in a later section in this chapter.

Sublingual nitroglycerin tablets are easily self-administered, and the drug is rapidly absorbed; nitroglycerin spray has the advantage of having a longer shelf life than the tablets, which lose their efficacy within 3–6 months (Opie 1996). A single 0.4-mg sublingual nitroglycerin tablet (or an equivalent dose of the oral spray) may abrogate an anginal attack within 2 to 5 minutes of its administration, but its therapeutic effect can last for 20 or 30 minutes. Sublingual nitroglycerin also finds an important use in short-term prophylaxis against angina: a patient about to embark on an activity likely to provoke anginal symptoms (e.g., climbing stairs or engaging in sexual relations) may find that the prophylactic use of nitroglycerin may permit these activities to be consummated without angina.

For the treatment of chronic angina, isosorbide dinitrate and isosorbide mononitrate are much more commonly used as oral agents (vide infra) and are rapidly absorbed following ingestion; the enteral administration of nitroglycerin (i.e., pills that are swallowed) is of limited efficacy because of the short duration of its therapeutic effect. Administration of 10 to 30 mg of isosorbide dinitrate two or three times daily (initiating therapy at the lower dose range), with a period of at least 12 hours without drug ingestion, can have a sustained antianginal effect with a low likelihood for the development of tolerance. Similarly, sustained-release isosorbide dinitrate may have greater therapeutic efficacy, with less development of tolerance, when the drug is given in an "eccentric" twice-daily dosing schedule (i.e., two doses during the day, none at night). Isosorbide dinitrate undergoes extensive first-pass hepatic metabolism; by contrast, isosorbide mononitrate does not undergo such extensive first-pass metabolism, and it has a more sustained therapeutic effect than does isosorbide dinitrate. When given in an eccentric dosing schedule (10–20 mg tablets administered 7 hours apart, with a period of >14 hours without drug ingestion), isosorbide mononitrate maintains efficacy in the prevention of angina. A sustained-release preparation of isosorbide mononitrate can be given once daily, and doses of 30–240 mg can be efficacious in long-term therapy.

**PRINCIPLE For initial drug efficacy studies, investigators often have to pick dose and duration of therapy empirically. Optimal therapy may depend on refinement of each. Look for the optimization by extrapolating information from successive studies.**

**PRINCIPLE Bioavailability of the drug is only one determinant of its potential clinical efficacy. Knowledge of the pharmacology of the agent can help to predict whether simple continuous delivery of the drug is appropriate to achieve a desirable clinical effect.**

Transdermal or topical preparations of nitroglycerin are also effective in the prophylaxis of angina pectoris. Nitroglycerin ointment can be applied topically and provides an effective if somewhat messy means for chronic antianginal therapy. For example, in hospitalized patients with chest pain syndromes suggestive of angina, administration of topical nitroglycerin ointment may be titrated to control a patient's anginal symptoms, while doses of the drug that provoke hypotension may be avoided. In the outpatient setting, transdermal nitroglycerin patches may be more convenient. These nitroglycerin patches are available in a wide range of specific formulations and are designed to release between 0.2 and 0.8 mg of drug per hour. Nitroglycerin patches are usually designed to provide 24 hours of drug delivery; however, prolonged use of transdermal nitroglycerin can rapidly lead to a loss of drug efficacy due to the development of tolerance. Transdermal patches should be removed for at least 12 hours daily to yield a nitrate-free interval and to minimize the development of tolerance. In such a setting the value of constant delivery of a drug by transdermal routes is nullified by the tolerance such delivery can create.

There is little evidence to suggest differences in efficacy between different nitrate preparations. Factors to be considered in choosing an appropriate nitrate regimen include cost, compliance, and patient preference. There are data in a variety of settings for improved patient compliance with medication regimens using less frequent dosing. In comparison with regimens of multiple doses per day, once-daily nitrate regimens may be associated with improved compliance and symptomatic benefit (Brun 1994).

#### *Adverse effects of organic nitrate vasodilators*

The therapeutic effect of organic nitrate vasodilators is associated with more venous rather than arterial dilation, but higher doses of rapidly absorbed nitroglycerin preparations can lead to symptoms related to drug-induced decreases in arterial tone. Headache is a major adverse effect reported by many patients taking organic nitrate vasodilators, and this probably reflects the effects of cerebral arterial dilation. After several days or a few weeks of therapy, patients often develop tolerance to headache, but usually without developing clinically significant tolerance to the therapeutic effects of the drug. Acetaminophen (650–1000 mg) taken 30–60 minutes before drug administration (before applying a topical nitroglycerin patch or swallowing isosorbide di- or mononitrate) may minimize the development of headache in some patients. Other common side effects of the organic nitrate vasodilators include prosyncopal symptoms or frank hypotension. Obviously, if a patient already has hypotension from whatever cause, nitroglycerin must be administered with great caution. It is also important to note that the hemodynamic consequences of venodilation alone can have profound effects in patients dependent on an elevated ventricular preload for optimal cardiac function. For example, in patients with significant aortic stenosis or hypertrophic cardiomyopathy, a decrease in ventricular preload induced by nitroglycerin may acutely depress cardiac output and lead to refractory hypotension even in patients with normal resting blood pressure before the administration of the drug. Patients with moderate aortic stenosis and symptoms of angina may receive some palliation of angina through the use of nitrates, but nitroglycerin must be used with caution in patients with more severe aortic stenosis. In patients receiving sildenafil for erectile dysfunction, nitrates are contraindicated because of the risk of hypotension exacerbated by the actions of this phosphodiesterase inhibitor.

For all these reasons, it is important to caution patients that they be seated when self-administering sublingual nitroglycerin for the first few times, and also to inform patients of the possibility that they may experience a flushing sensation from the drug. Preparing the patient for the development of these adverse effects can help in the patient's interpretation of and reaction to these symptoms.

The adverse effects of headache and presyncope are common to organic nitrate vasodilators in all formulations and routes of administration; unique to the use of transdermal preparations is the development of erythema at the site of drug delivery, which can be minimized by rotating the site at which the drug is applied.

## β-Adrenergic Receptor Antagonists

### *Pathophysiology*

β-Adrenergic receptor blocking agents ("beta-blockers") play a fundamental role in the management of chronic coronary artery disease. These agents provide symptomatic benefit for patients with angina. In addition, β-adrenergic receptor antagonists are among the few classes of drugs with demonstrated efficacy in reducing mortality after myocardial infarction (Furberg et al. 1995).

This class of drugs has multiple effects. β-Adrenergic receptor antagonists competitively inhibit the action of neuronally released and circulating catecholamines on the beta receptors of the cardiac conduction system and myocardium (Hoffman and Lefkowitz 1996). This inhibition decreases myocardial oxygen demand primarily by reducing heart rate and, to a lesser extent, by decreasing myocardial contractility. By blunting the increase in heart rate in response to exercise, β-adrenergic receptor antagonists have an even greater effect on myocardial oxygen demand during activity. In addition, by slowing heart rate and increasing the time for diastolic coronary artery perfusion, beta-blockers secondarily increase myocardial oxygen supply. These effects improve the balance of myocardial oxygen supply and demand, and may decrease ischemia in the patient with stable angina.

β-Adrenergic receptor antagonists also have antiarrhythmic properties that are beneficial to the patient with chronic coronary artery disease. The antagonism of the proarrhythmic effects of catecholamines may contribute to the usefulness of beta-blockers in prevention of death after myocardial infarction.

### *Pharmacologic properties*

The multiple β-adrenergic receptor antagonists may be distinguished by a variety of properties: their receptor subtype specificity, their degree of lipophilicity, their metabolism and pharmacodynamics, and the presence of partial receptor agonism (Opie 1996) (Table 1-22). $\beta_1$-Adrenergic receptors are present in the heart, kidney, and adipocytes, where their stimulation leads to, respectively, increases in heart rate, atrioventricular nodal conduction, contractility; release of renin; and lipolysis. $\beta_2$-Adrenergic receptors are present in the bronchi, peripheral vasculature, and liver, where their stimulation leads to, respectively, bronchodilation, vasodilatation, and glycogenolysis. Although β-adrenergic receptor antagonists may be classified as possessing or lacking selectivity for cardiac $\beta_1$ receptors, this cardioselectivity is relative and diminishes at increasing dosages that are commonly used clinically.

**PRINCIPLE Be careful in ascribing clinical value to the basic pharmacologic differences between drugs. These differences may be pharmacologically real but may only produce minor clinical nuances.**

Differences in lipid solubility affect β-adrenergic receptor antagonist metabolism. Lipophilic β-adrenergic receptor antagonists are metabolized predominantly by the liver and have relatively short half-lives. In the past, strongly lipophilic β-adrenergic receptor blocking agents were routinely given as often as four times per day. Newer formulations of some lipophilic beta-blockers allow these drugs to be taken once a day.

Table 1-22 **Pharmacologic Features of Commonly Used β-Adrenergic Receptor Blocking Drugs**

| FEATURE | LIPOPHILICITY | ROUTE OF ELIMINATION | $\beta_1$-RECEPTOR SELECTIVITY | ISA | USUAL MAINTENANCE DOSE | OTHER |
|---|---|---|---|---|---|---|
| Atenolol | Low | Renal | + | − | 50–100 mg/qd or bid | |
| Metoprolol | Moderate | Hepatic | + | − | 50–100 mg tid | |
| Nadolol | Low | Renal | − | − | 40–80 mg/day | |
| Pindolol | Moderate | Renal and hepatic | − | + | 5–20 mg tid | |
| Propranolol | High | Hepatic | − | − | 60 mg qid | |
| Timolol | Low | Renal and hepatic | −<br>− | − | 20 mg bid | |
| Acebutolol | Low | Hepatic | + | + | 200–600 mg bid | |
| Labetalol | Low | Hepatic | − | − | 100–600 mg/day | α-Receptor blocking activity |
| Penbutolol | High | Hepatic | − | + | 20 mg/day | |

ABBREVIATIONS: ISA, intrinsic sympathomimetic activity.
SOURCE: Modified from Frishman et al. 1986.

Although there are few comparisons of the effect on angina of different dose frequencies for the same β-adrenergic receptor antagonist, issues of pharmacodynamics are fundamental to the appropriate dosage of these medications. In general, antagonists with short half-lives require multiple daily administrations of drug.

**PRINCIPLE For therapeutic indications requiring drug efficacy at all times, drug regimens must be selected with an adequate dosage frequency.**

An understanding of β-adrenergic receptor antagonist pharmacodynamics is also necessary for safe discontinuation of these drugs. After chronic administration, abrupt discontinuation may lead to an exaggerated sympathetic response. Upregulation of β-adrenergic receptors may contribute to this withdrawal phenomenon. In the patient with ischemic coronary artery disease, abrupt withdrawal of β-adrenergic receptor blocking agents may precipitate acute coronary syndromes. This concern is especially important with the use of β-adrenergic receptor antagonists with short half-lives. The gradual, slow taper of beta-blockers may avoid precipitation of ischemia on their discontinuation.

Some β-adrenergic receptor antagonists have partial agonist activity, or intrinsic sympathomimetic activity (ISA). β-Adrenergic receptor antagonists with ISA may be less likely to lead to profound bradycardia or negative inotropy in the resting heart. Beta-blockers with ISA are effective in decreasing anginal symptoms and improving exercise test results in patients with angina. Although small studies have found no difference between β-adrenergic receptor antagonists with and without ISA in effects on symptoms, beta-blockers with ISA may not be as effective as beta-blockers without ISA in preventing exercise-associated ischemia. It is noteworthy that the major trials of β-adrenergic receptor antagonists to decrease mortality after myocardial infarction did not study drugs with ISA.

**PRINCIPLE There are very few drugs whose complete pharmacologic profile is known. It is almost inconceivable that drugs in different categories (e.g., β-adrenergic receptor antagonists and calcium channel antagonists) have the same profiles even if they have some overlapping qualities. Therefore, proof of equivalent efficacy among such drugs for the same indication is required and cannot be assumed.**

***Clinical uses of β-adrenergic receptor antagonists***

As mentioned above, β-adrenergic receptor antagonists are used in the symptomatic treatment of chronic ischemic coronary artery disease. As discussed elsewhere in this chapter, β-adrenergic receptor blocking agents are a mainstay of the chronic treatment of hypertension and of the acute treatment of the acute coronary syndromes, unstable angina and acute myocardial infarction. In addition, beta-blockers are used for treatment of arrhythmia and heart failure.

Another major long-term use of beta-blockers is to decrease mortality after acute myocardial infarction. This decrease in mortality is likely due to prevention of another infarction that leads to sudden death. Although randomized trials have not been performed to assess the relative efficacy for secondary prevention of different $\beta$-adrenergic receptor blocking agents and different regimens of these medications, it is worthwhile to note the drugs and doses actually used in the major trials. These regimens include propranolol [160–240 mg total dose per day (Beta-Blocker Heart Attack Trial Study Group 1984)], metoprolol (200 mg total dose per day [Olsson et al. 1985]), and timolol [20 mg total dose per day (Norwegian Study Group 1981)]. Treatment with atenolol during acute myocardial infarction and continued for the first week (5–10 mg intravenous load, followed by 100 mg total dose per day) is associated with decreased mortality (First International Study of Infarct Survival Collaborative Group 1986). Extrapolation from these data makes atenolol an acceptable agent for longer term secondary prevention of myocardial infarction. These $\beta$-adrenergic receptor antagonists include both $\beta_1$-selective and nonselective blockers and drugs with varying degrees of lipophilicity. As noted above, none of the beta-blockers used in these trials had ISA.

**PRINCIPLE The most reliable approach to achieving drug benefits demonstrated in clinical trials is to use the doses of the medications used in those trials.**

***Adverse effects of β-adrenergic receptor antagonists***

By affecting the balance between the sympathetic and parasympathetic nervous systems, beta-blockers can lead to adverse effects in a variety of systems (Table 1-23). Cardiac conduction and contractility can be decreased. In some patients, $\beta$-adrenergic receptor antagonists can precipitate bradycardia or atrioventricular block. Consequently, their administration should be initiated with caution in patients with significant conduction system disease of the sinus or atrioventricular nodes. Initiation of the use of $\beta$-adrenergic receptor antagonists with ISA is associated with a decrease in resting heart rate, which is not so great as that associated with initiation of agents without ISA. In patients with decreased systolic cardiac function, beta-blockers can precipitate heart failure and should be initiated cautiously. Because $\beta$-adrenergic receptor antagonists can decrease blood pressure, therapy with them should be initiated carefully in patients with low blood pressure. For inpatients at risk for compromise of cardiac conduction or hemodynamics, use of the short-acting, intravenous beta-blocker esmolol may be appropriate. The choice of a specific agent may allow use of a $\beta$-adrenergic receptor antagonist in patients with relative contraindications to their use (Tables 1-23 and 1-24).

Table 1-23 Contraindications to the Use of β-Adrenergic Receptor Blocking Drugs

| |
|---|
| Hypotension |
| Symptomatic bradycardia |
| Advanced atrioventricular conduction block |
| Decompensated congestive heart failure |
| Acute exacerbation of bronchospastic disease |

Use of this class of drugs may lead to worsening of Raynaud's phenomenon. Peripheral vasoconstriction may be less likely with $\beta_1$-selective agents.

Beta-blockers can precipitate bronchospasm in patients with underlying pulmonary disease. As discussed above, this side effect is mediated by blockade of $\beta_2$ receptors and may be decreased with $\beta_1$-selective medications, although cardioselectivity is relative and diminishes at high doses. Beta-receptor antagonists are generally contraindicated in patients with underlying asthma.

This class of drugs can have multiple metabolic side effects. Patients with diabetes mellitus may have mild worsening of glycemic control and blunting of the sympathetically mediated symptoms of hypoglycemia, increasing the risk of hypoglycemic complications. This may contraindicate the use of beta-blockers in diabetics with hypoglycemic reactions, especially if they are taking insulin. $\beta$-Adrenergic receptor antagonists may lead to decreased high density lipoprotein levels and increased triglyceride levels. These lipid effects may be attenuated for beta-blockers with ISA. For patients with diabetes or hyperlipidemia, the physician must balance the benefits and risks of these agents. It is important to note that the benefits of $\beta$-adrenergic receptor antagonists and the ability to substitute other medications for these drugs may vary greatly with the clinical setting. In contrast, for the patient with a recent myocardial infarction, the benefit of beta-blockers may be especially strong.

**PRINCIPLE Because of specific characteristics of individual patients, the same drug may have different degrees of benefit, adverse effects, and risk in different patients.**

Central nervous system adverse effects of $\beta$-adrenergic receptor antagonists include symptoms of fatigue, nightmares, and depression. Although it has been suggested that the more lipophilic beta-blockers may be as-

Table 1-24 Use of β-Adrenergic Receptor Antagonists in the Face of Contraindications

| RELATIVE CONTRAINDICATION | STRATEGY TO CONSIDER |
|---|---|
| Bronchospasm | Use a $\beta_1$-selective receptor antagonist |
| Bradycardia | Start with low dose and increase slowly a beta-blocker with ISA |
| Heart failure | Initiate use of a beta-blocker in a stable patient (with no recent changes in medications, including diuretic dosage). Start with a low dose and increase slowly. |
| Diabetes mellitus | Use a $\beta_1$-selective receptor antagonist |
| Raynaud's phenomenon | Use a $\beta_1$-selective receptor antagonist |

ABBREVIATIONS: beta-blocker, $\beta_1$-adrenergic receptor antagonist; ISA, intrinsic sympathomimetic activity.

sociated with increased incidence of depression, there is no reliable clinical evidence to support this supposition.

Because of their interference with the sympathetic nervous system, $\beta$-adrenergic receptor antagonists may be associated with impotence. In some clinical settings, such as after myocardial infarction, it may be difficult to determine whether medications or psychological factors are responsible for depression or impotence.

Although there is concern about potential effects of $\beta$-adrenergic receptor antagonists on limb perfusion in patients with severe peripheral arterial disease, multiple studies of $\beta_1$-selective and nonselective agents have shown no adverse effects in patients with mild or moderate peripheral arterial disease (Radack and Deck 1991).

#### *Choice of β-adrenergic receptor antagonist*

A variety of $\beta$-adrenergic receptor antagonists are available (see Tables 1-22 and 1-24). There is no body of literature with clear, consistent results demonstrating superior clinical outcomes with one beta-blocker as opposed to another. Consequently, the choice of a specific agent is strongly influenced by differences in class properties (e.g., with or without ISA), data supporting the particular use (e.g., for secondary prevention of myocardial infarction), and the likelihood of the patient to encounter adverse effects (e.g., bronchospasm). As listed in the table, the choice of agent, the dose at initiation, and the pace of dose increase may be influenced by patient characteristics. If not limited by side effects, the dose of the $\beta$-adrenergic receptor antagonist is titrated to parameters of heart rate and blood pressure. During treatment with beta-blockers, patients should be asked about symptoms of associated CNS side effects. In addition, physical examination should include measurement of blood pressure and pulse to observe for hypotension and bradycardia, as well as auscultation of the heart and lungs to detect signs of heart failure.

## Calcium Channel Antagonists

#### *Pharmacology*

Since the development of verapamil in the 1960s, over a dozen calcium channel antagonists have been approved for clinical usage in the United States. A knowledge of the pharmacology, pharmacokinetics, and pharmacodynamics of these agents is fundamental to their appropriate clinical use. Calcium channel antagonists interfere with calcium entry through voltage-dependent calcium channels and slow recovery channels (Opie 1996). Calcium channel antagonists are classified by the type of calcium channel inhibited and by binding site. There are two prototypical types of voltage-activated calcium channels: the L (long-acting) type, which is the target of most approved calcium channel antagonists, and the T (transient) type. Calcium channel antagonists that bind to L-type channels are divided into three classes distinguished by their chemical nature and binding sites. Nifedipine binds to the N binding site and is the prototypic dihydropyridine calcium channel blocker. Other dihydropyridines in clinical use include amlodipine, isradipine, and nicardipine, all sharing pharmacologic profiles similar to that of nifedipine. The two other distinctive calcium channel blocking drugs are diltiazem (a benzothiazepine), which binds to the D binding site, and verapamil (a phenylalkylamine), which binds to the V binding site.

**PRINCIPLE Be careful in ascribing clinical value to the basic pharmacological differences between drugs. These differences may be pharmacologically real, but may only produce minor clinical nuances.**

In contrast to the $\beta$-adrenergic blocking drugs, in which the diverse members of the drug class compete for the same binding sites on their cognate receptors, the binding characteristics of the different calcium channel blocking drugs demonstrate important distinctions from one another. For example, nifedipine, diltiazem and verapamil bind to distinct but partially overlapping sites on the L-type channel, and also show differential affinity for the different physiological states of the channel. For example, verapamil and diltiazem (but not nifedipine) exhibit "frequency dependent antagonism" in that the drug binds preferentially to the inactivated state of the channel. This leads to more pronounced blockade of the L-type channel by verapamil and diltiazem in tissues in which the channel undergoes repetitive cycling through its inactivated state, and may explain in part the pronounced effects of these drugs on pacemaker cells.

Calcium channel antagonists have three basic actions on the cardiovascular system (Robertson and Robertson 1996):

- vasodilatation through action on smooth muscle in the coronary and peripheral vasculature
- decreased contractility through action on cardiac myocytes; and
- decreased automaticity and conduction velocity through slowing of calcium channel recovery in sinus and atrioventricular nodal cells.

The relative strength of these effects varies with the class of the particular calcium channel antagonist and, to a lesser extent, with the particular agent in each class. The classic dihydropyridine nifedipine has a greater effect on vascular smooth muscle than on myocytes or cardiac conduction cells. In vivo, nifedipine is much more selective for vasodilatation relative to negative inotropy than the nondihydropyridines diltiazem and verapamil. In contrast, the nondihydropyridines have greater degrees of negative inotropic, chronotropic, and dromotropic effects relative to their vasodilator effect (see Table 1-25).

**PRINCIPLE Verapamil, diltiazem, and nifedipine are all three categorized as calcium channel blockers, yet there are important differences amongst these drugs in their pharmacologic properties and adverse effect profiles.**

### *Pharmacokinetics*

The different preparations of calcium channel antagonists have varying pharmacokinetics that influence their use. The intravenous forms of diltiazem and verapamil allow for bolus administration and continuous infusion. The short-acting form of nifedipine has a rapid onset of action that may lead to excessively rapid lowering of blood pressure (see section on hypotension in this chapter). The short-acting forms of the dihydropyridines may elicit reflex sympathetic activation, resulting in tachycardia and activation of the renin–angiotensin system. Once-daily administered and long-acting forms of the dihydropyridines may be associated with lesser degrees of activation of the sympathetic and renin–angiotensin systems. As discussed below, differences between short- and long-acting preparations in sympathetic activation may lead to differences in clinical outcomes with long-term use of the dihydropyridines.

**PRINCIPLE Standard and sustained-release formulations of the same drug (e.g., nifedipine) can exhibit distinct clinical features beyond the differences in drug dosing interval.**

### *Clinical uses of calcium channel antagonists*

The variety of clinical indications for the calcium channel antagonists reflects their multiple effects on the peripheral and coronary vasculature, cardiac myocytes, and cardiac conduction tissue (Gersh et al. 1997). In addition to their use in coronary artery disease, calcium channel antagonists are frequently used for chronic hypertension, commonly for supraventricular arrhythmias, and rarely for ventricular arrhythmias. In addition, calcium channel antagonists are used as pulmonary vasodilators in patients with primary pulmonary hypertension. Because of their greater selectivity for vasodilatation, some dihydropyridines have been studied for use in heart failure.

Calcium channel antagonists are used for angina of two etiologies, namely, fixed coronary stenoses and vasospasm-induced angina. In the setting of atherosclerotic narrowing of coronary arteries, calcium channel antagonists favorably alter the balance between myocardial oxygen supply and demand. Dilatation of the peripheral vasculature decreases afterload and consequently decreases myocardial oxygen demand. Dilatation of coronary arteries may lead to increased blood flow and improved myocardial oxygen supply. The nondihydropyridine calcium channel antagonists decrease myocardial oxygen demand through their negative inotropic and chronotropic effects. Clinical studies with calcium channel antagonists in patients with angina have demonstrated efficacy on multiple short-term endpoints, including reduction of anginal symptoms, decreased ischemia on ambulatory monitoring, and increased duration of exercise. Data on longer term

**Table 1-25 Features of the Prototypical Calcium Channel Antagonists**

| DRUG DOSAGE | VASODILATATION (CORONARY FLOW) | SUPPRESSION OF CARDIAC CONTRACTILITY | SUPPRESSION OF AUTOMATICITY (SA NODE) | SUPPRESSION OF CONDUCTION (AV NODE) | INITIAL DOSAGE | MAXIMUM |
|---|---|---|---|---|---|---|
| Nifedipine | 5 | 1 | 1 | 0 | 10 mg tid | 60 mg tid |
| Diltiazem | 3 | 2 | 5 | 4 | 30 mg tid | 120 mg tid |
| Verapamil | 4 | 4 | 5 | 5 | 80 mg tid | 160 mg tid |

NOTE: Other nifedipine-like (dihydropyridine) calcium channel antagonist drugs such as nicardipine and amlodipine share similar cardiovascular effects with nifedipine. This table identifies the relative effects of the drugs in this class on vasodilation and cardiac inotropy and chronotropy graded from 0 to 5, in which 0 means no effect and 5 means significant effect.
SOURCE: Adapted from Julian 1987 and Tiara 1987.

endpoints of morbidity and mortality in patients with coronary artery disease, however, are limited, as discussed below.

Rarely, treatment with calcium channel antagonists, especially the dihydropyridines, may exacerbate anginal symptoms. There are two likely pathophysiologic mechanisms of this adverse effect. Tachycardia due to reflex sympathetic activation may increase myocardial oxygen demand. A coronary steal due to dilatation of coronary blood vessels that are not critically stenotic may decrease myocardial oxygen supply. Concomitant therapy with negative chronotropic agents, such as a $\beta$-adrenergic receptor antagonist, or use of an alternative, nondihydropyridine calcium channel antagonist may avoid worsening of angina with such a patient. This risk is especially great with short-acting formulations of dihydropyridine calcium channel antagonists in patients with stable angina.

**PRINCIPLE Analysis of the effects of only one among many competing therapeutic interventions that may be given singly or in combination can produce major distortion of the efficacy of any of the interventions.**

Calcium channel antagonists are particularly effective in the treatment of vasospastic angina, also known as Printzmetal's or variant angina. In contrast to the chronic angina due to fixed atherosclerotic stenoses and associated with ischemia during increased myocardial oxygen demand, vasospastic angina commonly occurs at rest and is associated with ST segment elevation seen on electrocardiography. Nifedipine, diltiazem, and verapamil are considered equally efficacious for treatment of vasospastic angina.

***Adverse effects of calcium channel antagonists***

Adverse effects from the calcium channel antagonists may occur secondary to excessive therapeutic action or from other effects. Excessive vasodilatation may lead to hypotension. In patients with decreased left ventricular systolic function, the negative inotropy of some calcium channel antagonists may lead to exacerbation of heart failure. In patients with underlying conduction system disease, excessive negative chronotropy may lead to bradycardia or heart block. Heart failure and bradyarrhythmia are more frequently associated with use of diltiazem and verapamil, rather than with the dihydropyridines.

Class side effects of the calcium channel antagonists include headache, facial flushing, dizziness, and pedal edema. These adverse effects of vasodilatation and edema occur more commonly with the dihydropyridines. Gastrointestinal adverse effects include nausea, esophageal reflux, vomiting, and, especially with verapamil, constipation. Rarely, gingival hyperplasia may occur during chronic therapy with verapamil.

Because of these potential adverse effects, the calcium channel antagonists should be used with caution in certain groups of patients. Patients with relatively low baseline blood pressure may develop hypotension. Patients with decreased left ventricular systolic function may be vulnerable to worsening of heart failure. Patients with sick sinus syndrome or atrioventricular nodal block may develop worsening bradyarrhythmia.

Calcium channel antagonists are absolutely contraindicated in arrhythmias involving antegrade conduction down a bypass tract, such as in patients with Wolff-Parkinson-White syndrome, and during antidromic reentrant arrhythmias or atrial fibrillation. In addition, calcium channel antagonists are contraindicated during all but rare forms of ventricular tachycardia and should be avoided during almost all wide complex tachycardias. The dihydropyridines are contraindicated in patients with severe aortic stenosis.

Although there is consensus that calcium channel antagonists should be avoided during an acute coronary syndrome, controversy exists concerning their chronic usage in patients with coronary artery disease, especially after an acute coronary syndrome (see the section in this chapter on acute myocardial infarction). Observational studies suggest that use of calcium channel antagonists, especially short-acting nifedipine, may be associated with increased cardiovascular morbidity and mortality in patients with chronic hypertension (Psaty et al. 1995) or after unstable angina and myocardial infarction (Furberg et al. 1995). Prospective, randomized trials are needed to assess whether this association is valid and, if so, to determine for which calcium channel antagonists such an association may exist. Based on the currently available data, it is reasonable to use long-acting calcium channel blockers but not short-acting agents in patients with coronary artery disease. It is expected that on-going, long-term trials of calcium channel antagonists in patients with coronary artery disease will clarify these issues. Given the concerns about calcium channel blockers and the known efficacy of beta-blockers in patients with coronary artery disease, a conservative approach would include use of other agents, especially β-adrenergic receptor antagonists, as first-line agents for the treatment of angina due to atherosclerotic coronary artery disease (Yusuf 1995). Nevertheless, calcium channel antagonists are useful in subsets of patients with angina. Calcium channel antagonists remain the agents of choice for vasospastic angina and they may be useful in addition to beta-blockers, or may be used instead of beta-blockers in intolerant patients, such as those with asthma.

The number of approved calcium channel antagonists has expanded greatly in recent years, largely because of the development of additional dihydropyridines. These "second-generation" dihydropyridines generally have more selectivity for vasodilatation than nifedipine. In addition, some of these agents, such as amlodipine, have a slower onset of action and longer half-life, allowing for once-daily dosing. Clinical data comparing these dihydropyridines with other calcium channel antagonists are scant.

Other agents, less closely related to the traditional classes, include bepridil, a long-acting calcium channel antagonist, and mibefradil, a T-type calcium channel antagonist. Because of concerns about multiple drug interactions, mibefradil was withdrawn by the manufacturer after its approval for treatment of hypertension and angina. As additional calcium channel antagonists are approved and their theoretical advantages promoted, it is important to use clinical endpoints of comparative trials as the standard to judge new and often expensive agents.

### Combinations of Antianginal Drugs

The complex pathophysiology of angina sometimes necessitates the combination of different classes of antianginal drugs to achieve the desired therapeutic effect. Obviously, care must be taken to avoid adding toxic effects, and the greatest benefit may accrue from using complementary forms of therapy. For example, the combined negative inotropic effects of verapamil plus a β-adrenergic antagonist drug can precipitate heart failure in the patient with compromised ventricular systolic function. In similar fashion, the negative chronotropic effect of a beta-blocker can yield a dangerous slowing of the heart rate when used with the calcium channel blocker verapamil, a drug that also has a marked negative chronotropic effect. However, the same dose of a beta-blocker may attenuate the reflex tachycardia often seen with the use of the dihydropyridine calcium channel blocker nifedipine, leading to an enhanced therapeutic effect. It must be noted that combination therapies using all of the three different antianginal drugs (i.e., organic nitrate plus beta-blocker plus calcium channel blocker) has not been clearly shown to have greater antianginal efficacy than treatment regimens using only two different antianginal drugs.

**PRINCIPLE Combinations of antianginal drugs can be used to provide the most effective relief from the symptoms of angina. Combinations of antianginal drugs that have similar adverse effects can lead to toxicity. Conversely, combinations in which the adverse effects of one drug complement the side effects of another can lead to greater drug efficacy.**

## APPROACH TO THE INDIVIDUAL PATIENT WITH CORONARY ARTERY DISEASE

A carefully individualized treatment plan can help to optimize the care of any patient with coronary artery disease (Fig. 1-9). A detailed patient history, with particular attention to the patient's exercise habits and the presence of any exertional chest discomforts, can provide clues to the existence of occult symptoms of CAD, and may provide important insights into the patient's functional status. Questions that identify the presence of remediable CAD

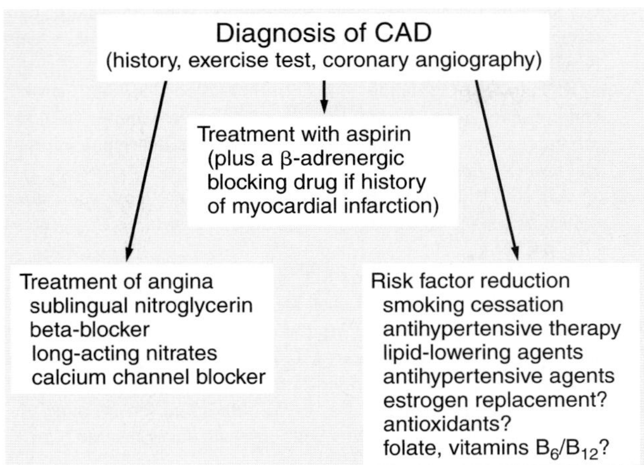


**FIGURE 1-9 An individualized approach to treating the patient with CAD. Patients with an established diagnosis of CAD should take aspirin daily, and therapies may be initiated to attenuate the progression of the disease, and, as necessary, to treat symptoms of angina. These considerations are discussed in detail in the text.**

risk factors, in addition to a careful family history, may serve to guide preventive strategies. A comprehensive physical examination may reveal signs of hypertension, heart failure, or dyslipidemia. Baseline laboratory evaluations include an assessment of renal function, liver-associated enzymes, and determination of the patient's hematocrit, serum lipids, and glucose. These tests serve both to identify the presence of comorbid illnesses and to provide baseline values before the initiation of pharmacotherapy. The choice of other laboratory tests must be individualized for a particular patient.

The baseline electrocardiogram is often normal in the asymptomatic CAD patient at rest, but may show signs of myocardial ischemia during exercise. An exercise tolerance test serves as an effective means of screening for the presence of CAD in the patient with risk factors and/or atypical symptoms suggestive of angina pectoris. In selected patients, the diagnostic yield of standard exercise-electrocardiographic testing can be enhanced by a variety of noninvasive cardiac imaging techniques. Evidence for the presence of significant CAD suggested by these noninvasive tests, and/or the existence of symptoms of angina unresponsive to medical therapies, will often lead to the decision to perform coronary angiography in order to assess coronary anatomy definitively. However, it must be emphasized that the diagnosis of coronary artery disease can often be made on clinical grounds alone, and coronary angiography is not required in order to establish the diagnosis or to initiate therapy. Rather, coronary angiography provides an important diagnostic tool to assess coronary anatomy in selected patients suspected of having such advanced CAD that coronary artery bypass surgery may be indicated, and in those patients in whom disease symptoms remain refractory to medical therapy, therefore leading to consideration of surgical or percutaneous revascularization.

Barring contraindications to its use, there is good reason for all patients with CAD to take aspirin daily. For the patient with symptoms of effort-related angina, short-acting and rapidly absorbed nitroglycerin preparations (sublingual tablets or oral spray) represent an effective initial therapy. Patients should be carefully instructed (vide supra) in the use of nitroglycerin for the treatment of acute attacks of angina, as well as the use of the drug in symptom prophylaxis. A beta-blocker is a good choice as a second antianginal agent; in addition to the utility of this drug class as antihypertensive agents, beta-blockers are efficacious for prevention of secondary infarction in patients with a prior history of myocardial infarction. The presence of effort-related angina, despite the use of these drugs, might lead to the additional administration of either oral or topical nitrates. Contraindications to the use of beta-blockers might lead instead to the use of calcium channel blockers as a second-line antianginal agent; in this context, diltiazem or verapamil may be preferable to the dihydropyridine calcium channel blockers because of the reflex tachycardia elicited by the latter group of agents. Addition of other antianginal drugs has not clearly been shown to be beneficial in clinical trials, but may be of benefit in selected patients.

**PRINCIPLE Combined therapy is particularly attractive when the drugs combined do not share similar mechanisms of either efficacy or toxicity. Then smaller doses of each would be expected to have additive effects on efficacy and insufficient concentrations to produce the toxicity expected of effective monotherapy.**

## INVASIVE THERAPIES FOR CORONARY ARTERY DISEASE

A significant fraction of patients with stable coronary artery disease will remain limited by symptoms of angina despite maximal antianginal drug therapy, or may be intolerant of the adverse effects of these drugs. Maximal medical therapy for angina consists of titration of medications (nitrates, beta-receptor antagonists, and calcium channel blockers) to maximally effective doses that do not lead to adverse cardiovascular effects (including symptomatic bradycardia, hypotension, heart block, or heart failure) or other intolerances. With a realistic goal of reducing symptoms of angina, such patients may undergo percutaneous transluminal coronary angioplasty (often augmented by the use of intravascular stents) or coronary artery bypass grafting. Yet other patients will be discovered upon coronary angiography to have such significant coronary stenoses that surgical revascularization is indicated. There is strong evidence that mortality is lower in selected groups of CAD patients who undergo bypass surgery. For example, coronary artery bypass grafting is almost always indicated for patients with significant stenosis of the left main coronary artery, or in patients with left ventricular dysfunction in whom all three epicardial coronary vessels show significant stenoses. Strategies to modify CAD risk factors should certainly continue following these interventions. Smoking cessation, aggressive lipid-lowering therapies, and continued use of aspirin are clearly indicated in these patients.

In patients who have undergone placement of intracoronary stents, the antiplatelet agent ticlopidine has been shown to reduce the rate of stent thrombosis. Major adverse effects of ticlopidine include rash, granulocytopenia, thrombocytopenia and, rarely, aplastic anemia or agranulocytosis. Typically, ticlopidine is started at or up to 3 days before the time of stent placement at a dose of 250 mg twice daily, and is continued for 2 to 4 weeks following the procedure. A baseline complete blood count is obtained when the drug is initiated, and should be monitored again every week during therapy and at the conclusion of therapy. Other drugs used during acute coronary interventions, including thrombolytic agents, anticoagulants, and inhibitors of platelet glycoprotein IIb/IIIa, and other antiplatelet agents, are discussed in greater detail in the section in this chapter on venous thromboembolic disease and in chapter 12, Hematologic Disorders.

## REFERENCES


Antiplatelet Trialists Collaboration. 1994. Collaborative overview of randomized trials of antiplatelet treatment. I: prevention of vascular death, MI and stroke by prolonged antiplatelet therapy in different categories of patients. *Br Med J* **308**:235.

Beta-Blocker Heart Attack Trial Study Group. 1984. A randomised trial of propranolol in patients with acute myocardial infarction. *Circulation* **69**:761.

Brun J. 1994. Patient compliance with once-daily and twice-daily oral formulations of 5-isosorbide mononitrate: a comparative study. *J Int Med Res* **22**:266.

CAPRIE Steering Committee. 1996. A randomised, blinded trial of clopidogrel versus aspirin in patients at risk of ischaemic events (CAPRIE). *Lancet* **348**:1329.

Collins R, Peto R, MacMahon S, et al. 1900. Blood pressure, stroke, and coronary heart disease. Part 2: short-term reductions in blood pressure: overview of randomised drug trials in their epidemiological context. *Lancet* **335**:827.

Dobson AJ, Alexander HM, Heller RD, et al. 1991. How soon after quitting smoking does risk of heart attack decline? *J Clin Epidemiol* **44**:1247.

First International Study of Infarct Survival Collaborative Group. 1986. Randomised trial of intravenous atenolol among 16 027 cases of suspected acute myocardial infarction: ISIS-1. *Lancet* **2**:57.

Frishman WH, Kafka KR, Meltzer AH. 1986. Antianginal agents. Part 2: Beta-blockers. *Hosp Formul* **21**:62–75.

Furberg CD, Psaty BM, Meyer JV. 1995. Nifedipine: dose related increase in mortality in patients with coronary heart disease. *Circulation* **92**:1326.

Gaster B, Hirsch IB. 1998. The effects of improved glycemic control on complications in type 2 diabetes. *Arch Intern Med* **158**:134.

Gersh BJ, Braunwald E, Rutherford JD. 1997. Chronic coronary artery disease. In: Braunwald E, editor. *Heart Disease: A Textbook of Cardiovascular Medicine.* 5th ed. Philadelphia: WB Saunders. p 1289.

Hennekens CH, Dyken ML, Fuster V. 1997. Aspirin as a therapeutic agent in cardiovascular disease. *Circulation* **96**:2751.

Hoffman BB, Lefkowitz RJ. 1996. Adrenergic receptor antagonists. In: Hardman JG, Gilman AG, Limbird LE, editors. *Goodman and Gilman's the Pharmacologic Basis of Therapeutics.* 9th ed. New York: McGraw-Hill. p 199–248.

Julian DG. 1987. Symposium—concluding remarks. *Am J Cardiol* **59**:37J.

Kannel WB, Higgins M. 1990. Smoking and hypertension as predictors of cardiovascular risk in population studies. *J Hypertens* **8** (Suppl):S3.

Libby P, Egan D, Skarlatos S. 1997. Roles of infectious agents in atherosclerosis and restenosis: an assessment of the evidence and need for future research. *Circulation* **96**:4095.

MacMahon S, Peto R, Cutler J, et al. 1990. Blood pressure, stroke, and coronary heart disease. Part 1: prolonged differences in blood pressure: prospective observational studies corrected for the regression dilution bias. *Lancet* **335**:765.

Matthew KA, Meilahn E, Kuller LH, et al. 1989. Menopause and risk factors for coronary heart disease. *N Engl J Med* **321**:641.

Moghadasian MH, McManus BM, Frolich JJ. 1997. Homocyst(e)ine and coronary artery disease. *Arch Intern Med* **157**:2299.

Norwegian Study Group. 1981. Timolol-induced reduction in mortality and reinfarction in patients surviving acute myocardial infarction. *N Engl J Med* **304**:801.

Olsson G, Rehnqvist N, Sjogren A, et al. 1985. Long-term treatment with metoprolol after myocardial infarction: effect on 3 year mortality and morbidity. *J Am Coll Cardiol* **5**:1428.

Opie LH. 1996. Pharmacologic options for treatment of ischemic disease. In: Smith TE, editor. *Cardiovascular Therapeutics: A Companion to Braunwald's Heart Disease.* Philadelphia: WB Saunders. p 22.

Parker JD, Parker JO. 1998. Nitrate therapy for stable angina pectoris. *N Engl J Med* **338**:520.

Psaty BM, Heckbert SR, Koepsell TD, et al. 1995. The risk of incident myocardial infarction associated with anti-hypertensive drug therapies. *JAMA* **274**:620.

Radack K, Deck C. 1991. Beta-adrenergic blocker therapy does not worsen intermittent claudication in subjects with peripheral arterial disease: a meta-analysis of randomized controlled trials. *Arch Intern Med* **151**:1769.

Ridker PM, Cushman M, Stampfer MJ, et al. 1997. Inflammation, aspirin, and the risk of cardiovascular disease in apparently healthy men. *N Engl J Med* **336**:973.

Robertson RM, Robertson D. 1995. Drugs used for the treatment of myocardial infarction. Hardman JG, Gilman AG, Limbird LE, editors. *Goodman and Gilman's the Pharmacologic Basis of Therapeutics.* 9th ed. New York: McGraw-Hill. p 759–79.

Scandinavian Simvastatin Study Group. 1994. Randomised trial of cholesterol lowering in 4444 patients with coronary heart disease: the Scandinavian Simvastatin Survival Study (4S). *Lancet* **334**: 1383.

Schomig A, Neumann FJ, Kastrati A, et al. 1996. A randomized comparison of antiplatelet and anticoagulant therapy after the placement of coronary-artery stents. *N Engl J Med* **334**:1084.

Shepherd J, Cobbe SM, Ford I, et al. 1995. Prevention of coronary heart disease with pravastatin in men with hypercholesterolemia. West of Scotland Coronary Prevention Study Group. *N Engl J Med* **333**:1301.

Stampfer MJ, Colditz GA, Willett WC, et al. 1991. Postmenopausal estrogen therapy and cardiovascular disease: ten-year follow-up from the Nurses' Health Study. *N Engl J Med* **325**:756–62.

Steering Committee of the Physicians' Health Study Research Group. 1989. Final report on the aspirin component of the ongoing Physicians' Health Study. *N Engl J Med* **321**:129.

Stephens MG, Parsons A, Schofield PM, et al. 1996. Randomized controlled trial of vitamin E in patients with coronary disease: Cambridge Heart Antioxidant Study (CHAOS). *Lancet* **347**:781.

Tiara N. 1987. Differences in cardiovascular profile among calcium antagonists. *Am J Cardiol* **59**:24B–9B.

Welch GN, Loscalzo J. 1998. Homocysteine and atherothrombosis. *N Engl J Med* **338**:1042.

Yusuf S. 1995. Calcium antagonists in coronary artery disease and hypertension. *Circulation* **92**:1079.

# Acute Myocardial Infarction

**Christopher P. Cannon, Peter H. Stone**

*Chapter Outline*



## OVERVIEW OF PATHOPHYSIOLOGIC MECHANISMS

During the past two decades understanding of the pathophysiologic mechanisms considered responsible for the acute coronary syndromes (Q-wave myocardial infarction [MI], non-Q-wave MI, and unstable angina) have dramatically evolved. In the mid-to-late 1970s episodic coronary vasospasm was thought to be responsible for the development of unstable angina and acute MI (Oliva et al. 1973; Maseri et al. 1978). In the mid-to-late 1980s and mid-1990s rupture of plaques and subsequent thrombus formation were considered paramount (Davies and Thomas 1985; Davies 1990), while coronary vasoconstriction was considered inconsequential. The different acute coronary syndromes were perceived simply to represent different points on a continuum of plaque rupture and thrombus formation: the continuum ranging from a ruptured plaque with little or no thrombus (often asymptomatic), to a ruptured plaque with moderate thrombus leading to only partial coronary occlusion (unstable angina and MI associated with ST-segment depression on the electrocardiogram), to a ruptured plaque with extensive thrombus and complete occlusion of the artery (MI associated with ST-segment elevation). In the mid-to-late 1990s, however, evidence has accumulated that makes this two-component pathophysiologic model of the acute coronary syndromes simplistic and inadequate for some patients. Recent evidence from atherectomy samples, for example, indicates that a substantial number of patients with unstable angina, and perhaps those with non-Q-wave MI as well, may have manifest their disease because of a rapid cellular proliferation of the atherosclerotic plaque itself, with little contribution from either major thrombus formation or vasoconstriction (Flugelman et al. 1993; Arbustini et al. 1995). These three mechanisms (ruptured plaque, thrombus formation, and rapid cellular proliferation) may also be closely interrelated in a given patient, with a substantial contribution from each.

Recent experience with thrombolytic therapy has substantially clarified important differences in the pathophysiologic mechanisms underlying different types of acute MI and has dramatically improved mortality in certain subsets of patients. Patients whose acute MI is manifested by ST-segment *elevation* experience a dramatic benefit from thrombolytic therapy: before thrombolytics were available, mortality was approximately 13% at one month [Gruppo Italiano per lo Studio della Streplochinasi nell'Infarto Miocardico (GISSI) 1986; ISIS-2 (Second International Study of Infarct Survival) Collaborative Group 1988b], whereas in the current era of reperfusion therapy, mortality has fallen to approximately 6.3% (The GUSTO Investigators 1980). In contrast, among patients whose MI is not associated with ST-segment elevation, thrombolytic therapy is not of value [The TIMI IIIB Investigators 1994; Fibrinolytic Therapy Trialists' (FTT) Collaborative Group 1994]. Angiographic studies have suggested that this difference is due to the initial status of the infarct-related artery: patients with ST-segment elevation exhibit 100% occlusion of the artery, whereas patients without ST-segment elevation exhibit a severely stenotic, but nevertheless patent, coronary artery (Fig. 1-10) (DeWood et al. 1986; The TIMI IIIA Investigators 1993). Consequently, patients with "acute MI with ST-segment elevation" versus "non-ST-segment elevation MI/unstable angina" can be classified on the basis of the underlying pathophysiology and also on their response to the administration of acute reperfusion therapy (Fig. 1-10).

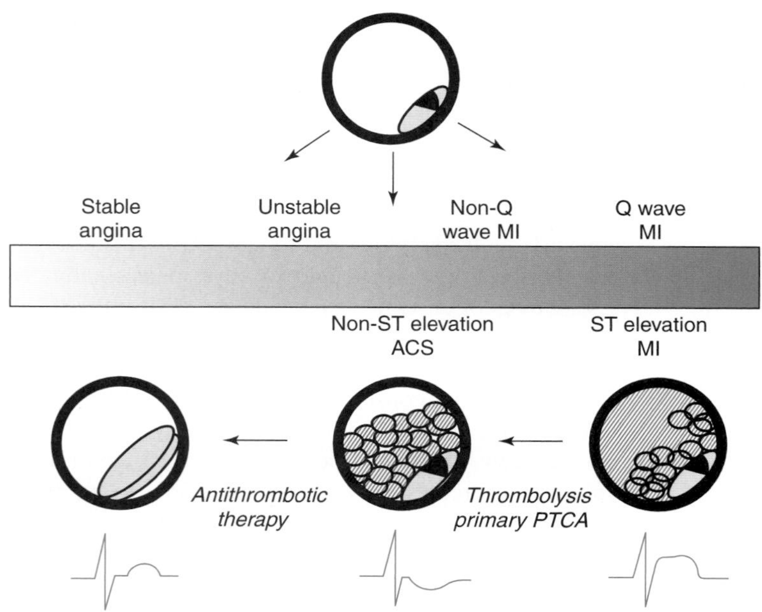


**FIGURE 1-10 The new paradigm of acute coronary syndromes. The various clinical syndromes of coronary artery disease can be viewed as a spectrum, ranging from patients with stable angina to those with acute Q-wave MI. Across the spectrum of the acute coronary syndromes, atherosclerotic plaque rupture leads to coronary artery thrombosis: in acute Q-wave MI, which usually presents with ST-segment elevation on the electrocardiogram, complete coronary occlusion is present. In those with unstable angina or non-Q-wave MI, a flow-limiting thrombus is usually present. In patients with stable angina, thrombus is rarely seen. (Adapted from Cannon 1995.)**

**PRINCIPLE Acute myocardial infarction associated with ST-segment elevation is due to sudden coronary plaque rupture and 100% occlusive thrombus; MI associated with ST-segment depression or unstable angina may be due to plaque rupture and subocclusive thrombus or rapid cellular proliferation.**

The benefit of thrombolytic therapy for acute ST-segment elevation MI is related to *early* achievement of patency of the infarct-related artery. Early, successful coronary reperfusion limits the size of the infarct, decreases LV dysfunction, and improves survival (Braunwald 1989; 1993). The primary goal in the treatment of acute ST-segment elevation MI, therefore, is to maximize early reperfusion; adjunctive antithrombotic and anti-ischemic therapy are important to assure and maintain successful reperfusion. For patients with acute coronary syndromes without ST-segment elevation, on the other hand, antithrombotic and anti-ischemic medications become the *primary therapy* (Fig. 1-10).

The "open artery theory" is the paradigm by which thrombolytic therapy is understood to be beneficial in acute ST-segment elevation MI: Patients who achieve normal antegrade flow (TIMI grade 3 flow) (TIMI Study Group 1985) at 90 minutes have the lowest mortality (i.e., 3.6%), patients with antegrade flow but at a reduced rate (TIMI grade 2 flow) have an intermediate mortality of 6.6%, and patients with total occlusion or only a trickle of flow (TIMI grade 0 or 1 flow) have the highest mortality of 9.5% ( $P < 0.00001$) (Cannon and Braunwald 1994). An "open artery" not only optimizes blood flow to enhance local myocardial function, it also provides an "exoskeleton" to limit left ventricular (LV) dilatation and LV dysfunction, as well as reduces electrical instability post MI.

## Importance of Time to Treatment

Time is a critical determinant in the success of the administration of any thrombolytic regimen (The GUSTO Angiographic Investigators 1993). In GISSI-1, patients who were treated within one hour from the onset of chest pain had a 50% reduction in mortality [Gruppo Italiano per lo Studio della Streptochinasi nell'Infarto Miocardico (GISSI) 1986]. In the TIMI 2 trial, for each hour earlier that a patient was treated, there was a decrease in the absolute mortality by 1% (Timm et al. 1991) that translates into an additional 10 lives saved per 1000 treated (Cannon et al. 1994). Figure 1-11 illustrates the crucial time-dependence of administration of thrombolytic therapy.

**PRINCIPLE The time from onset of MI to restoration of coronary blood flow is a critical determinant of the amount of myocardium preserved and mortality.**

## SPECIFIC THROMBOLYTIC AGENTS

The specific thrombolytic agents currently available for use in the United States are noted in Table 1-26. All of the thrombolytic (fibrinolytic) agents currently available are plasminogen activators. They all work enzymatically, directly or indirectly, to convert the single-chain plasminogen molecule to the double-chain plasmin (which has potent intrinsic fibrinolytic activity) by splitting a single bond at the arginine 560-valine 561 site, exposing the active enzymatic center of plasmin (Ryan et al. 1996). High-

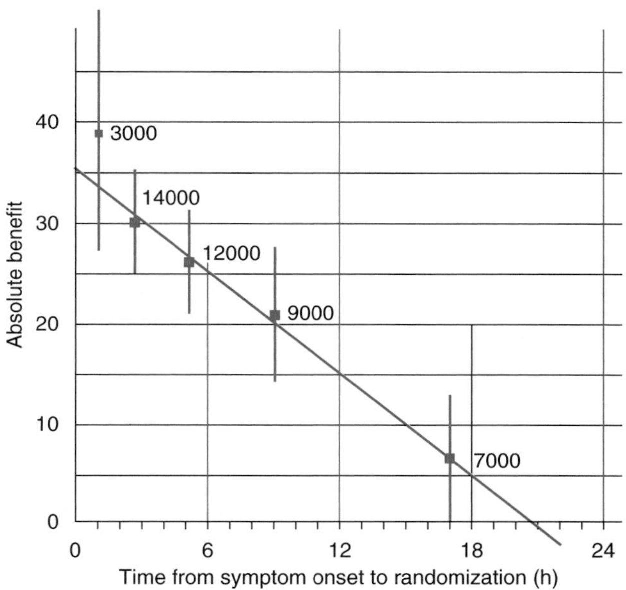


FIGURE 1-11 **Absolute reduction in 35-day mortality versus delay from symptom onset to randomization and treatment among 45,000 patients with ST-segment elevation or bundle branch block BBB. Absolute benefit refers to absolute benefit per 1000 patients with ST elevation or left BBB who are given fibrinolytic therapy (±SD). Loss of benefit per hour of delay to randomization is 1.6 (SD0.6) per 1000 patients. [From Fibrinolytic Therapy Trialists' (FTT) Collaborative Group 1994. Used with permission.]**

Table 1-26 **Comparison of US Food and Drug Administration-Approved Thrombolytic Agents**

| FACTOR | STREPTOKINASE | ASPAC | TPA |
|---|---|---|---|
| Dose | 1.5 million U in 30–60 min | 30 mg in 5 in | 100 mg in 90 min[a] |
| Circulating half-life | 20 | 100 | 6 |
| Antigenic | Yes | Yes | No |
| Allergic reactions | Yes | Yes | No |
| Systemic fibrinogen depletion | Severe | Severe | Moderate |
| Intracerebral hemorrhage | ~0.3% | ~0.6% | ~0.6% |
| Recanalization rate, 90 min[b] | ~40% | ~63% | ~79% |
| Lives saved per 100 treated | ~2.5% | ~2.5% | ~3.5% |
| Cost per dose (approx. US $) | 290 | 1700 | 2200 |

[a]Accelerated tPA given as follows: 15-mg bolus, then 0.75 mg/kg over 30 min (maximum 50 mg), then 0.50 mg/kg over 60 min (maximum 35 mg).
[b]Based on the finding from the GUSTO (Global Utilization of Streptokinase and tPA for Occluded Arteries) Trial that accelerated tPA saves one more life per 100 treated than does SK.
ABBREVIATIONS: Approx., approximate; APSAC, anisoylated plasminogen–streptokinase activator complex; tPA, tissue plasminogen activator.

lights of differences in dosing pharmacokinetics, recanalization rates, complication rates, and cost are shown in Table 1-26. Thrombolytic agents are administered intravenously; intracoronary use of these agents for acute MI is now virtually obsolete. Additional agents are being developed (e.g., prourokinase, staphylokinase, and various mutant plasminogen activators) (Ryan et al. 1996).

Thrombolysis has been shown to reduce mortality in numerous placebo-controlled trials using streptokinase [Gruppo Italiano per lo Studio della Streptochinasi nell'Infarto Miocardico (GISSI) 1986; ISIS-2 (Second International Study of Infarct Survival) Collaborative Group 1988], anistreplase (anisoylated plasminogen streptokinase activator complex [APSAC]) (AIMS Trial Study Group 1988), and the 3-hour regimen of tissue plasminogen activator (tPA) (Asset Study Group 1988). The Fibrinolytic Therapy Trialists' overview of all the large placebo-controlled studies showed a reduction in mortality of an absolute 2.6% for patients with ST-segment elevation MI treated within the first 12 hours after the onset of symptoms [Fibrinolylic Therapy Trialists' (FTT) Collaborative Group 1994]. The benefit from treatment between 6 and 12 hours after the onset of symptoms is greater with tPA (LATE Study Group 1993) than with streptokinase [EMERAS (Estudio Multicentrico Estreptoquinasa Republicas de America del Sur) Collaborative Group 1993]. Patients presenting with left bundle branch block and a strong clinical history of acute MI also derive a large benefit from thrombolysis (The GUSTO Investigators 1980). However, as noted above, those without ST-segment elevation or left bundle branch block do not benefit from thrombolysis and indeed may be harmed (The GUSTO Investigators 1980; The TIMI IIIB Investigators 1994).

**PRINCIPLE A clear challenge to the physician is to subcategorize patients with the disease to segregate those who can benefit from therapy from those who cannot.**

## Selection of Appropriate Thrombolytic Regimen

Given the importance of rapid reperfusion, one would expect that a more aggressive thrombolytic regimen, administered rapidly and as a partial bolus, that achieves a higher rate of early infarct-related vascular patency, would be associated with a lower mortality. Tissue plasminogen activator (tPA) was observed in the TIMI 1 trial to achieve reperfusion of occluded coronary arteries by 90 minutes in nearly twice as many patients as streptokinase, suggesting that it would be a superior agent.

The GUSTO trial (The GUSTO Investigators 1993) was the best direct comparison of four thrombolytic regimens: "accelerated" (15-mg bolus followed by the remainder over a 90-minute infusion) or "front-loaded" tPA and concomitant IV heparin, streptokinase with IV heparin, streptokinase with subcutaneous heparin, and a combination of tPA and streptokinase with IV heparin. The lowest 30-day mortality was observed with tPA (6.3%), compared with streptokinase and subcutaneous heparin (7.2%), streptokinase and IV heparin (7.4%), and combined tPA and streptokinase with IV heparin (7.0%). The tPA and heparin regimen also achieved higher 90-minute infarct-related artery patency, and the significant improvement in mortality was seen after only 24 hours following tPA infusion. The 14% mortality reduction associated with tPA versus streptokinase was highly significant ($P = 0.001$), although there was a significant excess of hemorrhagic stroke associated with tPA ($P = 0.03$) compared with streptokinase (0.7% of patients treated with tPA vs. 0.5% of patients treated with streptokinase). To put their results in full clinical perspective, the GUSTO investigators developed the concept of "net clinical benefit," i.e., the occurrence or absence of either death or a disabling stroke. When comparing the net clinical benefit from using tPA, streptokinase, or the combinations of low-dose streptokinase and low-dose tPA, tPA still produced a clear benefit compared with the other three regimens (9 fewer deaths or disabling strokes per 1000 patients treated with tPA). Other complications of acute MI were generally less frequent when tPA was used as compared with use of streptokinase. The complications included allergic reactions, congestive heart failure, cardiogenic shock, and atrial and ventricular arrhythmias (Ryan et al. 1996).

The majority of recent studies indicate that accelerated tPA with IV heparin is currently the most effective therapy for achieving early reperfusion and enhanced survival in acute MI, but it is also substantially more expensive and is associated with more intracranial hemorrhage (Ryan et al. 1996). The cost–benefit ratio is greatest in patients presenting early after onset of symptoms with a large area of injury (e.g., anterior acute MI) and at low risk of intracranial hemorrhage. In groups with smaller potential for survival benefit and a greater risk for intracranial hemorrhage, streptokinase appears to be the agent of choice, particularly in view of the cost (Ryan et al. 1996).

A number of proposals for selection of thrombolytic regimens after GUSTO have been suggested. Additional considerations include avoiding reuse of streptokinase or anistreplase for at least 2 years (preferably indefinitely) because of a high prevalence of potentially neutralizing antibody titers (Ryan et al. 1996).

## Current Guidelines for Thrombolysis

The guidelines for administration of thrombolytic therapy are described in Table 1-27. Thrombolysis is indicated for patients presenting within 12 hours of onset of symptoms if they have ST-segment elevation (or left bundle branch block) provided they have no contraindications to thrombolytic therapy (Table 1-28). Less clear indications include patients who are older than 75 years of age, those who can be treated only more than 12–24 hours after the onset of acute MI, and those who are hypertensive but present with high-risk MI. Patients should not be treated if the time to treatment is less than 24 hours and their ischemic symptoms have resolved, or if they present only with ST-segment depression.

## Primary Angioplasty as an Alternative to Thrombolysis

An alternate method of achieving coronary reperfusion is use of immediate or "primary" percutaneous transluminal coronary angioplasty (PTCA), without concomitant administration of thrombolytic therapy (see Table 1-29).

**PRINCIPLE Initial randomized trials (Grines et al. 1993; Zijlstra et al. 1993) and a recent meta-analysis (Weaver et al. 1997) have shown that primary percutaneous transluminal coronary angioplasty (PTCA) appears to be more beneficial in reducing death or MI than administration of a thrombolytic agent.**

**Table 1-27 Recommendations for Administration of Thrombolytic Therapy**

| | |
|---|---|
| *Class I* | (Conditions for which there is evidence and/or general agreement that treatment is beneficial, useful, and effective) |
| | 1. ST elevation (>0.1 mV, >2 contiguous leads); time to therapy, <12 hours; age, <75 years. |
| | 2. Bundle branch block (obscuring ST-segment analysis) and history suggesting acute MI. |
| *Class IIa* | (Conditions for which there is conflicting evidence, but the weight of evidence is in favor of usefulness and efficacy) |
| | 1. ST elevation, age 75 years or older. |
| *Class IIb* | (Usefulness and efficacy is less well established by evidence/opinion) |
| | 1. ST elevation, time to therapy 12–24 hours. |
| | 2. BP on presentation >180 mm Hg systolic and/or diastolic >110 mm Hg associated with high-risk MI. |
| *Class III* | (Conditions for which treatment is not useful and may be harmful) |
| | 1. ST elevation, time to therapy >24 hours, ischemic pain resolved. |
| | 2. ST-segment depression only. |

ACC/AHA guidelines: Ryan et al. 1996.
ABBREVIATIONS: BP, blood pressure; MI, myocardial infarction; ST, segment of the electrocardiogram.

Table 1-28 **Contraindications and Cautions for Thrombolytic Use in Myocardial Infarction**

Contraindications

- Previous hemorrhagic stroke at any time; other strokes or cerebrovascular events within 1 year
- Known intracranial neoplasm
- Active internal bleeding (does not include menses)
- Suspected aortic dissection

Cautions/relative contraindications

- Severe uncontrolled hypertension on presentation (blood pressure >180/110 mm Hg)
- History of prior cerebrovascular accident or known intracerebral pathology not covered in contraindications
- Current use of anticoagulants in therapeutic doses (INR ≥2–3); known bleeding diathesis
- Recent trauma (within 2–4 weeks), including head trauma or traumatic or prolonged (>10 min) CPR or major surgery (<3 wk)
- Noncompressible vascular punctures
- Recent (within 2–4 weeks) internal bleeding
- For streptokinase/anistreplase: prior exposure (especially within 5 day–2 yr) or prior allergic reaction
- Pregnancy
- Active peptic ulcer
- History of chronic severe hypertension

SOURCE: From White and Van de Werf 1998.
ABBREVIATIONS: CPR, cardiac-pulmonary resuscitation; INR, international normalized ratio.

However, as with thrombolysis, rapid time to treatment is critical to success (Cannon and Braunwald 1996; Cannon et al. 1996). Patients are most suitable candidates for primary PTCA if they have a contraindication to thrombolytic therapy such as risk of bleeding and if they are in a facility where restoration of antegrade flow can occur within 60–90 minutes of acute MI (Ryan et al. 1996). The logistic problems associated with having a catheterization laboratory available for primary PTCA may be very difficult in many hospitals.

## ANTITHROMBOTIC THERAPY

In addition to achieving reperfusion in patients with acute MI, especially those with MI associated with ST-segment elevation, it is essential to provide adjunctive therapy to maintain patency of the coronary arteries and to decrease myocardial oxygen demands.

Following rapid treatment and early restoration of infarct-related artery patency for ST-segment elevation MI, reocclusion of the artery or its clinical correlate, repeat infarction, could reverse the benefits of early patency. Indeed, reocclusion is associated with a nearly threefold increase in mortality (Ohman et al. 1990). Reinfarction following successful reperfusion therapy has also been found to be associated with a two- to threefold increase in mortality (Mueller et al. 1995; Cannon et al. 1997). As such, prevention of both reocclusion and repeat infarction become important targets for antithrombotic therapy following thrombolytic therapy.

Table 1-29 **Meta-analysis of Primary PTCA versus Thrombolysis**

| | RATE (%) | | | |
|---|---|---|---|---|
| STUDY GROUP | PTCA | LYTIC THERAPY | ODDS RATIO (95% CI) | ABSOLUTE RISK REDUCTION (%) 95% CI) |
| *Mortality* | | | | |
| Streptokinase | 4.0 | 5.9 | 0.66 (0.29–1.50) | 1.9 (−2.7–4.1) |
| 3- to 4-h tPA | 3.5 | 5.7 | 0.60 (0.24–1.41) | 2.2 (−2.2–4.3) |
| Accelerated tPA | 5.0 | 7.2 | 0.68 (0.42–1.08) | 2.2 (−0.5–4.0) |
| Total | 4.4 | 6.5 | 0.66 (0.46–0.94) | 2.1 (0.4–3.4) |
| *Death Plus Nonfatal Reinfarction* | | | | |
| Streptokinase | 5.6 | 13.0 | 0.40 (0.21–0.75) | 7.4 (−2.9–10.0) |
| 3- to 4-h tPA | 5.6 | 10.3 | 0.51 (0.26–0.99) | 4.8 (0.1–7.4) |
| Accelerated tPA | 8.7 | 12.0 | 0.70 (0.48–1.08) | 3.3 (0.0–5.9) |
| Total | 7.2 | 11.9 | 0.58 (0.44–0.76) | 4.6 (2.6–6.3) |
| *Nonfatal Reinfarction* | | | | |
| Total | 2.9 | 5.3 | 0.53 (0.34–0.80) | 2.4 (1.0–3.4) |

SOURCE: Adapted from Weaver et al. 1997.
ABBREVIATIONS: CI, confidence interval; PTCA, percutaneous transluminal coronary angioplasty; tPA, tissue plasminogen activator.

## Aspirin

Aspirin is a critical antithrombotic agent in patients with coronary artery disease particularly in the setting of the administration of thrombolytic therapy (Figs. 1-12 and 1-13).

**PRINCIPLE In the setting of acute ST-segment elevation MI, aspirin decreased reocclusion by more than 50% (Roux et al. 1992) decreased repeat infarction by nearly 50%, and reduced morality by 25% [ISIS-2 (Second International Study of Infarct Survival) Collaborative Group 1988]. In patients with non-ST-segment elevation MI or unstable angina, aspirin reduced the risk of death or MI by more than 50% (Lewis et al. 1983; Cairns et al. 1985; Theroux et al. 1988; The RISC Group 1990).**

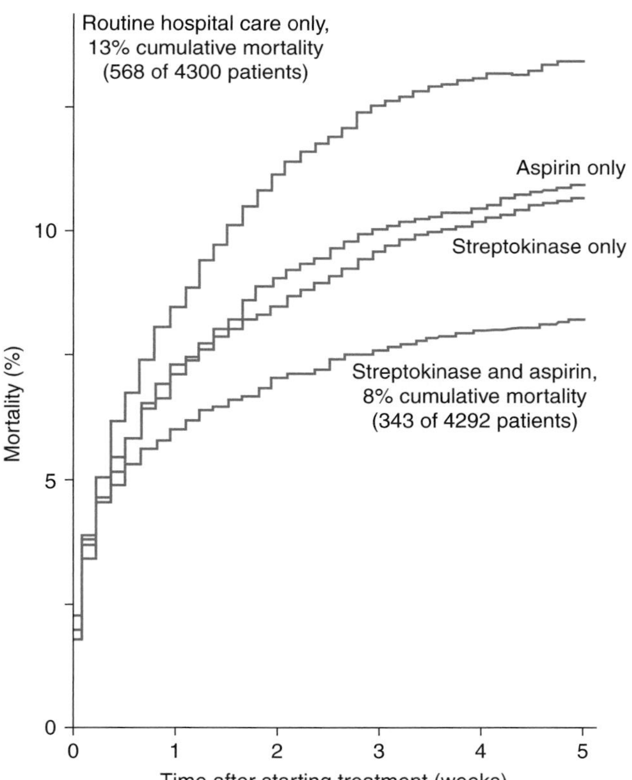


FIGURE 1-12 **Cumulative mortality from vascular causes up to day 35 in the ISIS-2 Trial. [From Receptor Suppression Using Integrilin Therapy (PURSUIT) Trial Investigators 1998. Used with permission.]**

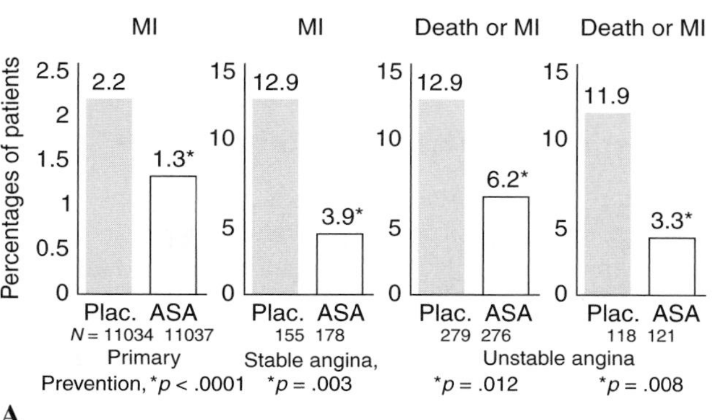


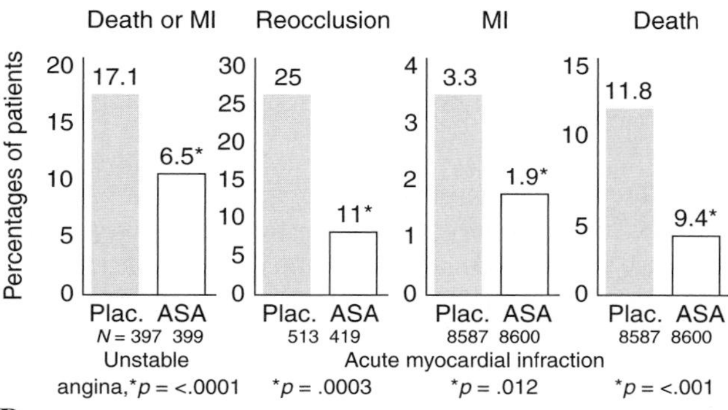


FIGURE 1-13 **(A) and (B) Benefit of aspirin across the spectrum of acute coronary syndromes. The risk of subsequent MI was reduced by aspirin compared with placebo in healthy subjects and thus was effective primary prevention. Similarly, patients with stable angina had a reduced incidence of MI. In unstable angina, the incidence of death or MI was reduced by more than 50% in each of three trials. In acute MI, aspirin reduced reocclusion of the infarct-related artery, repeat infarction, and mortality. (Reproduced from Cannon 1995. Used with permission.)**

Of note, the dosage of aspirin in the ISIS-2 trial was 162 mg daily [ISIS-2 (Second International Study of Infarct Survival) Collaborative Group 1988], and in the four unstable angina trials, dosages were 75, 325, 650, and 1300 mg per day, with equal efficacy, and slightly more bleeding at the higher doses. A dosage of 162–325 mg daily is currently recommended.

Following MI, aspirin also reduces subsequent cardiac events and provides secondary prevention (Klimt et al. 1986; Antiplatelet Trialists' Collaboration 1994). These benefits with chronic antiplatelet therapy have now been observed to persist for up to 4 years of follow-up (Antiplatelet Trialists' Collaboration 1994). Aspirin has had a dramatic effect in reducing adverse clinical events and thus constitutes primary therapy for all acute coronary syndromes.

## Glycoprotein IIb/IIIa Inhibitors

The appreciation that aspirin is a relatively weak antiplatelet drug has led to the development of a class of drugs that inhibit platelet aggregation by binding to the platelet glycoprotein (gp) IIb/IIIa receptor (Lefkovits et al. 1995).

**PRINCIPLE By preventing the final common pathway of platelet aggregation, i.e., fibrinogen-mediated crosslinkage, these agents are more efficacious inhibitors than aspirin, and inhibit platelet aggregation in response to all types of stimuli (e.g., thrombin, adenosine diphosphate, and collagen).**

Three gpIIb/IIIa inhibitors are approved for use in the United States, namely, abciximab for use in coronary angioplasty, and tirofiban and eptifibatide for unstable angina/non-ST-elevation MI with the latter also approved for angioplasty. Several agents are being tested in the setting of thrombolytic therapy. There are three broad categories of gpIIb/IIIa inhibitors: 1) the monoclonal antibody to the gpIIb/IIIa receptor, abciximab (ReoPro), 2) the intravenous peptide and nonpeptide small molecule inhibitors, such as eptifibatide and tirofiban, and 3) the oral gpIIb/IIIa inhibitors, such as xemilofiban, orbofiban, and sibrafiban.

Abciximab, the monoclonal antibody, binds very tightly to the gpIIb/IIIa receptor (Coller et al. 1986). Consequently, antiplatelet effects persist much longer than the infusion period—a potential benefit on improving efficacy. On the other hand, if bleeding occurred, discontinuing the drug infusion will not quickly reverse the antiplatelet effect; transfusion of platelets however, will allow the antibodies to redistribute among all the platelets, thereby decreasing the level of platelet inhibition.

**PRINCIPLE When toxicity can be acute and severe, consider countermeasures in addition to discontinuation of the drug before therapy is initiated.**

The peptide and peptidomimetic inhibitors (e.g., tirofiban and eptifibatide) are competitive antagonists of the gpIIb/IIIa receptor (Tcheng et al. 1995; Kereiakes, Kleiman et al. 1996). The extent of platelet inhibition is directly related to the drug concentration in the blood. Since both inhibitors have short half-lives, antiplatelet activity returns toward normal after a few hours when the drug infusion is stopped (Tcheng et al. 1995; Kereiakes, Kleiman et al. 1996), providing a potential benefit for avoiding bleeding complications. On the other hand, for prolonged antiplatelet effect, the drug needs to be given intravenously for a longer period of time.

The third group of gpIIb/IIIa competitive inhibitors are orally available agents under development. These compounds are generally pro-drugs, which are absorbed and then converted to active compounds in the blood (Kereiakes, Runyon et al. 1996; Cannon et al. 1998). The oral agents all have longer half-lives, such that they can be given twice or three times daily in order to achieve relatively steady levels of gpIIb/IIIa inhibition. With oral dosing, long-term therapy (i.e., >1 year) is possible. However, the long half-life also means that if bleeding occurs, the drug must be removed from the circulation in order to reduce the antiplatelet effect. This can currently be accomplished acutely by hemodialysis or charcoal hemoperfusion in emergency situations.

### *Use of glycoprotein IIb/IIIa inhibition in unstable angina and non-Q-wave myocardial infarction*

Two agents, tirofiban and eptifibatide, are currently approved for the treatment of unstable angina and non-Q-wave MI. The combination of tirofiban, heparin, and aspirin significantly lowered the rate of death, MI, or recurrent refractory ischemia at 7 days compared with heparin plus aspirin alone (12.9% vs. 17.9%, respectively, a 34% risk reduction, $P = 0.004$) [The Platelet Receptor Inhibition for Ischemic Syndrome Management in Patients Limited by Unstable Signs and Symptoms (PRISM-PLUS) Trial Investigators 1998). The 30-day rate of death or MI was also decreased by 31%, from 11.9% to 8.7% ($P = 0.03$). The rate of major hemorrhage was not significantly increased for patients treated with tirofiban/heparin/aspirin versus heparin plus aspirin (4.0% vs. 3.0%; not significant [NS]).

Eptifibatide was studied in the PURSUIT trial, involving 10,948 patients with unstable angina and non-Q-wave MI. Eptifibatide plus heparin and aspirin decreased the rate of death or MI at 30 days from 15.7% to 14.2% compared with heparin and aspirin alone ($P = 0.04$) [Receptor Suppression Using Integrilin Therapy (PURSUIT) Trial Investigators 1998].

Glycoprotein IIb/IIIa inhibition was first shown to be beneficial during high-risk coronary angioplasty, e.g., for patients with acute coronary syndromes, and resulted in 25–50% decrements in ischemic complications (The EPIC Investigators 1994; The EPILOG Investigators 1997; The

CAPTURE Investigators 1997; The IMPACT-II Investigators 1997; The RESTORE Investigators 1997). Significant benefit was found to persist for up to 3 years (Topol et al. 1997). Benefit from administration of gpIIb/IIIa inhibitors has also been observed when placing coronary stents and when performing "primary PTCA" for acute ST-segment elevation MI. Consequently, given this broad experience with gpIIb/IIIa inhibitors in PTCA, especially in high-risk patients with acute coronary syndromes, their use has become a new therapeutic standard for coronary intervention (Fig. 1-14).

***Potential risks***

The major concern with the gpIIb/IIIa inhibitors is bleeding. Some studies suggested that gpIIb/IIIa inhibitors are associated with increased bleeding (The EPIC Investigators 1994), but careful evaluation has suggested that excessive bleeding is more associated with excessive heparinization and prolongation of the aPTT (activated partial thromboplastin time) rather than with use of the gpIIb/IIIa inhibitors per se (The EPILOG Investigators 1997; The IMPACT-II Investigators 1997; The RESTORE Investigators 1997; Cannon et al. 1998). Use of lower doses of heparin and careful monitoring of the level of anticoagulation reduces risk of bleeding complications in patients receiving gpIIb/IIIa inhibitors.

**PRINCIPLE Assigning appropriate risk to simultaneously assessed therapeutic agents is crucial to generating appropriate efficacy.**

Thrombocytopenia is the other major adverse effect of gpIIb/IIIa inhibition. Platelet counts falling below 100,000 occur in approximately 1–2% of patients treated with gpIIb/IIIa inhibitors, and platelet counts falling to <50,000 occur in fewer than 0.5% of patients [The EPILOG Investigators 1997; The IMPACT-II Investigators 1997; The Platelet Receptor Inhibition for Ischemic Syndrome Management in Patients Limited by Unstable Signs and Symptoms (PRISM-PLUS) Trial Investigators 1998]. In the initial trials, thrombocytopenia generally occurred on either the first day after beginning therapy, or after approximately 2 weeks of therapy. The mechanism by which it occurs is not well understood. Fortunately, it is nearly always reversible, with platelet counts returning to normal after a few days.

## Heparin

In acute ST-segment elevation MI, heparin is also an important adjunctive agent to decrease reocclusion following administration of tPA. Although no difference in infarct-related artery patency was seen at 90 minutes (Topol et al. 1989), there is higher patency between 18 hours and 5 days in patients randomized to receive intravenous heparin (Bleich et al. 1990; Hsia et al. 1990; de Bono et al. 1992). The benefit of heparin may be due to decreased risk of reocclusion. Further analyses of these studies demonstrated that improved patency was greatest in patients who had effective anticoagulation, with an aPTT of less than 2 times control or >60 seconds. More recent anal-

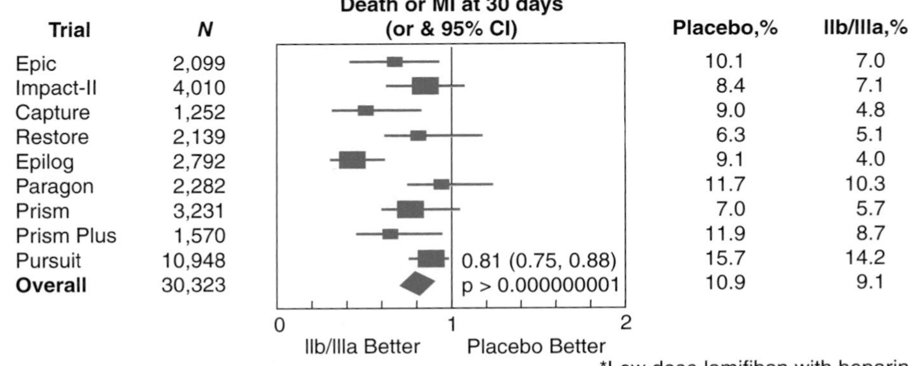


FIGURE 1-14 Overview of large trials with glycoprotein IIb/IIIa inhibition in unstable angina and angioplasty. Death or MI at 30 days, with odds ratio (OR) and 95% confidence interval (CI). (Adapted from Topol 1998. Used with permission.)

yses suggest a target range of 50–70 seconds as optimal (Granger et al. 1996).

Following the use of streptokinase or anistreplase (APSAC), the role of heparin is less clear. Patients treated with streptokinase with intravenous or subcutaneous heparin in the GUSTO-I trial had similar infarct-related artery patency at 90 minutes and 24 hours, but those receiving intravenous heparin had significantly higher patency at 5 to 7 days (84% vs. 72%, $P = 0.04$) (The GUSTO Investigators 1993). Nonetheless, the overall mortality and the rate of clinical repeat infarction were the same between these two groups (The GUSTO Investigators 1993). However, patients randomized to the subcutaneous administration arm of the study received intravenous heparin when recurrent ischemia developed. Therefore intravenous heparin may be considered optional in streptokinase-treated patients. Subcutaneous heparin is not beneficial in preventing repeat infarction or death compared with placebo [Gruppo Italiano per lo Studio della Soprovivenza nell'Infarto Miocardico (GISSI-2) 1990; International Study Group 1990; ISIS-3 (Third International Study of Infarct Survival) Collaborative Group 1992].

**Heparin administered IV to achieve a target aPTT of 50–70 seconds is critical to assure patency following tPA administration, but is optional following administration of streptokinase.**

In unstable angina and non-ST-segment elevation MI, heparin is an important component of primary therapy [The Platelet Receptor Inhibition for Ischemic Syndrome Management in Patients Limited by Unstable Signs and Symptoms (PRISM-PLUS) Trial Investigators 1998; Cannon et al. 1998]. In a recent meta-analysis (Oler et al. 1996) active treatment with aspirin and heparin lowered the risk of death or MI compared with aspirin treatment alone: 33% reduction in death or MI at 2–12 weeks (7.9% vs. 10.4%; RR=0.67, 95% C.I. 0.44–1.02). These data support the use of aspirin plus heparin in acute coronary syndromes.

## Low-Molecular-Weight Heparins

A major advance in the use of heparin has been the development of low-molecular-weight heparins (LMWHs). Inhibition of factor Xa leads to reduced thrombin generation and inhibition of factor IIa (thrombin) leads to reduced thrombin activity. These drugs are obtained by depolymerization of standard, unfractionated heparin and selecting out those portions with lower molecular weight (Hirsh and Levine 1993). As compared with unfractionated heparin, which has nearly equal anti-IIa and anti-Xa activity, LMWHs have modified ratios of anti-IIa to anti-Xa activity of either 1:2 (dalteparin) or 1:3 (enoxaparin or nadroparin).

**Low-molecular-weight heparin selectively inhibits factor Xa compared with thrombin (factor 11a). LMWHs may have advantages over unfractionated heparins (Theroux et al. 1992; Gold et al. 1993; Hirsh and Levine 1993; Hirsh and Fuster 1994a; Granger et al. 1995; Warkentin et al. 1995; FRISC Study Group 1996). See chapter 12, Hematologic Disorders, for additional information.**

The LMWHs have several potential advantages over standard, unfractionated heparin. First, they may be more potent antithrombic agents than either unfractionated heparin or the direct thrombin inhibitors because LMWHs inhibit both thrombin generation and thrombin activity. LMWH also induces a greater release of tissue factor pathway inhibitor than standard heparin and is not neutralized by platelet factor 4. From a safety perspective, LMWH does not increase capillary permeability (which may lead to fewer bleeding complications) (Hirsh and Levine 1993; Hirsh and Fuster 1994a), and LMWH may also produce a lower rate of thrombocytopenia (Warkentin et al. 1995). Finally, the high bioavailability of LMWH allows for subcutaneous administration and the ability to treat for longer periods of time (i.e., at home). This use would both avoid any "rebound" effect after stopping heparin early (Theroux et al. 1992; Gold et al. 1993; Granger et al. 1995) and potentially allow for greater "passivation" of the thrombotic lesion. Another critical advantage is that LMWHs do not require monitoring of aPTT to assure therapeutic effects.

The LMWHs have been found to be efficacious in patients with unstable angina/non-ST-segment elevation MI. Dalteparin plus aspirin reduced death or MI over the first 6 days compared with aspirin alone (1.8% vs. 4.8%, $P = 0.001$) (FRISC Study Group 1996). Moreover, no difference has been observed between dalteparin and intravenous heparin (Klein et al. 1997). The ESSENCE (Evaluation of the Safety and Efficacy of Enoxaparin in Non-ST elevation Coronary Events) trial compared enoxaparin with intravenous heparin in 3000 patients with unstable angina and non-Q-wave MI. Enoxaparin was superior to unfractionated heparin with regard to the occurrence of death, MI, or recurrent ischemia at 14 days (16.6% vs. 19.8%, $P = 0.019$) ) and at 30 days (19.8%

vs. 23.3%, $P = 0.016$) (Fig. 1-15) (Cohen et al. 1997). Consequently, based on available data, LMWH appears to be a significant improvement over standard unfractionated heparin. Studies are also in progress to determine whether LMWH is of value in the setting of ST-segment elevation MI treated with thrombolytic therapy.

## Direct Thrombin Inhibitors

Direct thrombin inhibitors have also undergone extensive evaluation, although with less promising results than shown in the above studies. One such agent is the anticoagulant hirudin, which binds in a 1:1 relationship to thrombin, the last step in the coagulation cascade. Although hirudin reduced the rate of recurrent MI following thrombolytic therapy, there was no difference in the primary endpoint, death, or in MI or severe congestive heart failure and/or shock, at 30 days (Antman 1996). Hirudin was compared with unfractionated heparin in more than 12,000 patients across the full spectrum of acute coronary syndromes in the GUSTO IIb trial. There was a reduction in repeat infarction (5.4% vs. 6.3%, $P = 0.04$), but only a trend toward reduction in death or MI at 30 days (8.9% vs. 9.8%, $P = 0.06$) [The Global Use of Strategies to Open Occluded Coronary Arteries (GUSTO) IIb Investigators 1996]. Other direct thrombin inhibitors have also been tested, and again, only modest improvements or none were observed compared with heparin (Gold et al. 1993; Molhoek et al. 1997). Hirudin does provide the advantage of achieving aPTT in the target range almost twice as frequently as heparin. No episodes of thrombocytopenia were reported for hirudin.

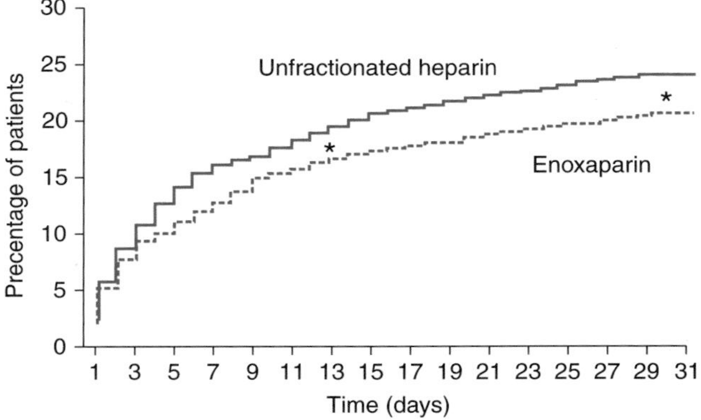


**FIGURE 1-15 Primary result from the ESSENCE trial, which showed a benefit of enoxaparin over intravenous heparin. (From Cohen et al. 1997. Used with permission.)**

## Warfarin and/or Oral Anticoagulation

Anticoagulant therapy with warfarin has been shown to be beneficial following MI. In pooled data from seven randomized trials between 1964 and 1980, oral anticoagulant therapy over a 1- to 6-year period reduced the rate of death or MI by 20% (Hirsh and Fuster 1994b). Subsequently, three large studies evaluating warfarin after MI (both ST-segment elevation and non-ST-elevation MI) demonstrated a 24% reduction in mortality ($P = 0.027$) and a 34–53% reduction in repeat infarction (Anonymous 1994b). Consequently, warfarin monotherapy appears to be at least as effective as aspirin after MI.

There are several circumstances in which benefit or potential benefit with warfarin therapy exceeds that of aspirin. First, warfarin is superior to aspirin in prevention of systemic emboli in patients with atrial fibrillation (The Stroke Prevention in Atrial Fibrillation Investigators 1990; Hirsh and Fuster 1994b). In addition, beneficial effects in reducing systemic emboli have also been observed in patients after MI with documented LV dysfunction (Loh et al. 1997). In selected patients at risk for systemic emboli, warfarin affords a second beneficial effect.

**PRINCIPLE The concept of seeking multiple positive effects from a single agent applies when many drugs can be chosen to affect a primary indication.**

The Coumadin Aspirin Reinfarction Study (CARS) evaluated the combination of aspirin (80 mg) and fixed-dose warfarin (1 or 3 mg, not adjusted to a prothrombin time) compared with aspirin alone (160 mg) for patients early after MI. No benefit was observed with the combinations of fixed-dose warfarin plus aspirin with regard to recurrent MI, cardiac death, or nonfatal ischemic stroke [Coumadin Aspirin Reinfarction Study (CARS) Investigators 1997]. More recently, a trial in men at risk for ischemic heart disease, using a slightly higher 4.1-mg average dose of warfarin, titrated to international normalized ratio of prothrombin time (INR) of 1.5, found a significant reduction in coronary death or MI for those using the combination of warfarin and aspirin at 75 mg daily compared with placebo (8.7% vs. 13.3% for placebo) (The Medical Research Council's General Practice Research Framework 1998), but no significant difference between the combination versus aspirin alone (8.7% vs. 10.2%) or versus warfarin alone (10.3%). In this trial there was an increase in hemorrhagic strokes among patients treated with the combination (0.9%) versus those treated with warfarin alone (0.1%) or with aspirin alone (0.2%), and

0% (no increase) with placebo ($P = 0.009$) (The Medical Research Council's General Practice Research Framework 1998).

**Warfarin is a suitable alternative to aspirin following MI as monotherapy, but there is no evidence to support a combination regimen of warfarin plus aspirin.**

## Novel Antiplatelet Agents

### *Clopidogrel*

Clopidogrel, like its structural analog ticlopidine, is a thienopyridine derivative that inhibits platelet aggregation, increases bleeding time, and reduces blood viscosity. The two agents achieve their antiaggregatory action by inhibiting the binding of adenosine diphosphate (ADP) to its platelet receptors.

Clopidogrel has been tested for secondary prevention in a study of 19,185 patients, with recent MI, stroke, or documented peripheral arterial disease (CAPRIE Steering Committee 1996). Over an average 2-year follow-up, clopidogrel was associated with an 8.7% reduction relative to aspirin in the combined endpoint of ischemic stroke, MI, or vascular death (5.32 vs. 5.83% per year; $P = 0.042$) (Fig. 1-16) (CAPRIE Steering Committee 1996). Clopidogrel produced a significant 19.2% reduction in MI

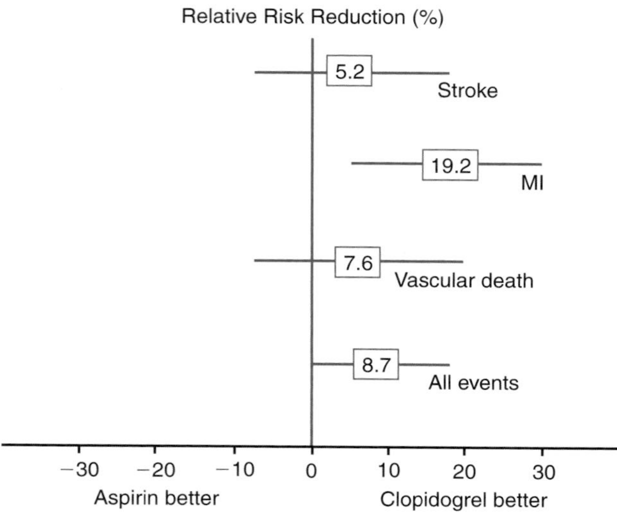


**FIGURE 1-16 Benefit of clopidogrel compared with aspirin in patients with symptomatic atherosclerosis. Relative risk reduction for each component of the primary composite endpoint (*P* 0.008 for MI, and *P* 0.04 for composite endpoint). (Data from Gent 1997, and reproduced with permission from Topol 1998.)**

($P = 0.008$), whereas there were nonsignificant 5.2% and 7.6% reductions in stroke and vascular death, respectively (Fig. 1-16) (Gent 1997). On the basis of these data, the FDA recently approved clopidogrel for secondary prevention of vascular events among patients with symptomatic atherosclerosis.

# $\beta$-ADRENERGIC RECEPTOR ANTAGONISTS

$\beta$-Adrenergic receptor blocking agents ("beta-blockers") function as competitive antagonists at $\beta$-adrenergic receptors expressed in many cells. Selective $\beta_1$-adrenergic receptor blocking agents act at receptor sites found primarily in the myocardium, inhibiting catecholamine-mediated increases in cardiac contractility and nodal conduction rates. $\beta_2$-Adrenergic receptors are found mainly in vascular and bronchial smooth muscle, and inhibition at these receptor sites can lead to vasoconstriction and bronchospasm. $\beta$-Adrenergic receptor blocking agents are thought to exert their beneficial effects in the acute coronary syndromes by inhibiting catecholamine-mediated beta-1 activation, leading to decreased contractility and heart rate, thereby improving the oxygen supply: demand balance. These drugs may also have antiarrhythmic effects, as evidenced by an increase in the threshold for ventricular fibrillation in animals and a reduction in complex ventricular arrhythmias in humans (Rossi et al. 1983; Yusuf et al. 1983; Morganroth et al. 1985). Finally, beta-blockers may prevent plaque rupture by reducing the mechanical stresses imposed on the plaque (Lee et al. 1991).

## Use of Beta-Blockers for Myocardial Infarction with ST-Segment Elevation

Beta-blockers were among the first therapeutic interventions designed to limit the size of acute MI. Recent studies have demonstrated that administering the beta-blocker within an appropriate time window following onset of acute MI has clinical benefit (Fig. 1-17) (Yusuf et al. 1985; Ryan et al. 1996). In the largest trial, the First International Study of Infarct Survival (First International Study of Infarct Survival Collaborative Group 1986), more than 16,000 patients with suspected MI were treated with intravenous atenolol, 5 to 10 mg, within 12 hours of the onset of symptoms followed by oral doses of 100 mg daily. The difference in mortality between those receiving atenolol and the controls was evident by the end of day 1; the 7-day mortality was reduced from 4.3% to 3.7% ($P < 0.02$). Meta-analyses from 27 randomized trials, to-

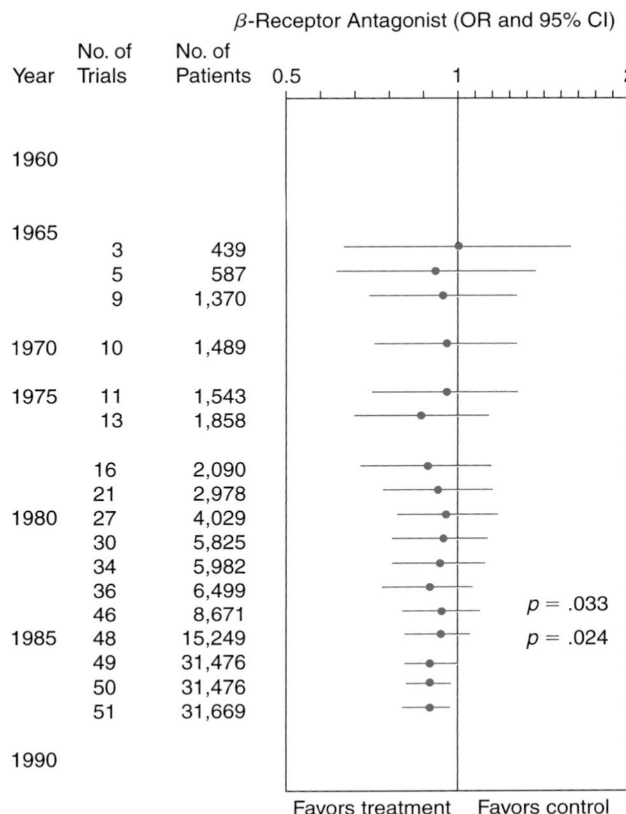


**FIGURE 1-17 Results of 51 randomized clinical trials of the effects of oral or intravenous followed by oral β-adrenergic receptor blockers for the treatment of acute MI. The odds ratio and 95% confidence intervals for an effect of treatment on mortality use are shown. (From Antman et al. 1992. Used with permission.)**

taling about 27,000 patients, indicate that early intravenous, followed by oral treatment with beta-blockers reduced mortality by 13% in the first week (95% confidence interval [CI] −2% to −25%, $P < 0.02$) (Yusuf et al. 1988a; Lee et al. 1991). The reduction in mortality was greatest in the first 2 days (about 25%), supporting the value of early initiation of beta-blockade (Yusuf et al. 1988a). Early treatment also reduced nonfatal repeat infarction by about 19% (95% CI, −5% to −33%, $P < 0.01$) and nonfatal cardiac arrest by about 16% (95% CI, −2% to −30%, $P < 0.02$). Composite endpoints of death, nonfatal repeat infarction, and nonfatal arrest were reduced by 16% ($P < 0.001$) (Cannon and Braunwald 1994). Data from the ISIS-1 trial suggest that the reduction in mortality is largely due to prevention of cardiac rupture and ventricular fibrillation (First International Study of Infarct Survival Collaborative Group 1986). Detailed analyses of the results based on various subgroups (age, sex, site of infarction, initial heart rate, risk category, presence or absence of ventricular arrhythmia, etc.) indicated a benefit in all groups.

When beta-blockers have been used in conjunction with thrombolytic therapy they provide incremental benefit, particularly if they can be administered early after the onset of symptoms of infarction. In the TIMI II trial (The TIMI Study Group 1989) patients with persisting ST-segment elevation who were randomized to receive only oral metoprolol (15 mg IV, followed by oral metoprolol 50 mg bid for one day and then 100 mg bid thereafter) in addition to intravenous alteplase, experienced a 49% lower incidence of subsequent nonfatal repeat infarction ($P = 0.02$) and a 27% lower incidence of recurrent ischemia ($P = 0.005$) compared with those patients randomized to receive only oral metoprolol beginning 6 days after the acute event. Those patients who were treated within 2 hours of the onset of symptoms had the greatest reduction of the composite endpoint of death or repeat infarction compared with those treated late with only oral metoprolol.

**PRINCIPLE Early IV adjunctive treatment with a beta-blocker along with thrombolytic therapy is particularly effective in reducing death and repeat infarction in patients with acute myocardial infarction.**

A number of studies have classified the mechanism of death into "sudden" and "non-sudden," based on the duration of time from the onset of symptoms to actual death. Sudden death is variably defined as "instantaneous" to "within 2 hours of symptoms" and is presumably due to arrhythmias or cardiac rupture; non-sudden deaths are those occurring later after the onset of symptoms and are presumably due to nonarrhythmic causes, such as repeat infarction, and may include a few noncardiac deaths. Tabulation of the results from the available studies indicates a highly significant reduction of approximately 30% in the incidence of sudden death and a nonsignificant reduction of only about 12% in the incidence of non-sudden death (Fig. 1-18) (Yusuf et al. 1985). The fact that beta-blockers are particularly effective in reducing sudden death and in reducing mortality among patients with complex ventricular ectopy (Friedman et al. 1984) suggests that these drugs exert their beneficial effect primarily by reducing the frequency and severity of arrhythmias (Byington and Furberg 1990).

Long-term mortality benefits of beta-blockers following an index MI (i.e., secondary prevention) seem to be

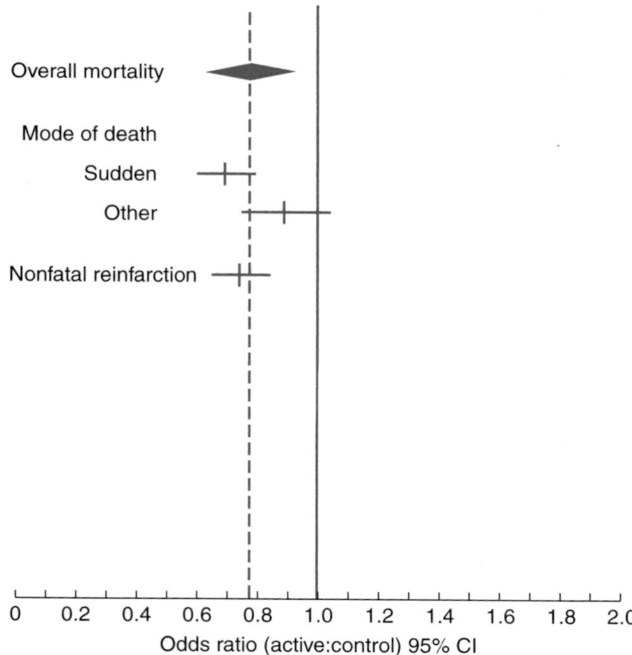


**FIGURE 1-18 Sudden death, other death, and nonfatal repeat infarction in long-term $\beta$-adrenergic receptor blocker trials that reported these endpoints separately: odds ratios (active:control), together with approximate 95% confidence ranges. See original article for citation of specific trials. (From Yusuf et al. 1985. Used with permission.)**

similar for nonselective and $\beta_1$-adrenergic receptor-selective antagonists that have been evaluated (Yusuf et al. 1985) (Fig. 1-19). However, the presence of intrinsic sympathomimetic activity reduced the benefit to nonsignificance (Yusuf et al. 1985). It is noteworthy that there is a significant relationship between the magnitude of heart rate reduction observed on the active agent and the magnitude of reduction in mortality (Fig. 1-20A) (Kjekshus 1986).

Many of the large-scale clinical trials have also reported the effect of long-term use of beta-blockers on nonfatal repeat infarction. Results from pooled analyses indicate that beta-blockers are associated with reduced risk, having an odds ratio of 0.74 (95% CI, 0.66–0.83; $P < 0.001$). As observed for mortality, there is also a significant relationship between the magnitude of reduction in heart rate and the reduction in nonfatal recurrent MI ($r = 0.54$; $P < 0.05$) (Fig. 1-20B) (Kjekshus 1986). This observed benefit of reducing nonfatal repeat infarction is in addition to the benefit on mortality.

The magnitude of benefit from long-term use of beta-blockers is also dependent on the patient's risk of mortality associated with their index MI. Post hoc analyses from the Beta Blocker Heart Attack Trial (BHAT) (Furberg et al. 1984) indicate that those MI patients without electrical or mechanical complications experienced only a 6% relative benefit from the use of propranolol. MI patients with electrical complications experienced a 52% relative benefit, and those with mechanical complications experienced a 38% relative benefit, and those with both mechanical and electrical complications experienced a 25% relative benefit. Considering the low cost of many beta-blockers, and their substantial benefit, such therapy has a relatively favorable cost-effectiveness ratio: an estimated cost of therapy per year of life saved would be \$13,000 in low-risk patients, \$3,600 in medium-risk patients, and \$2,400 in high-risk patients (Goldman et al. 1988).

The benefits from routine use of beta-blockers seem to persist as long as the active agent is continued (Olsson et al. 1988; Yusuf et al. 1993). It is therefore most appro-

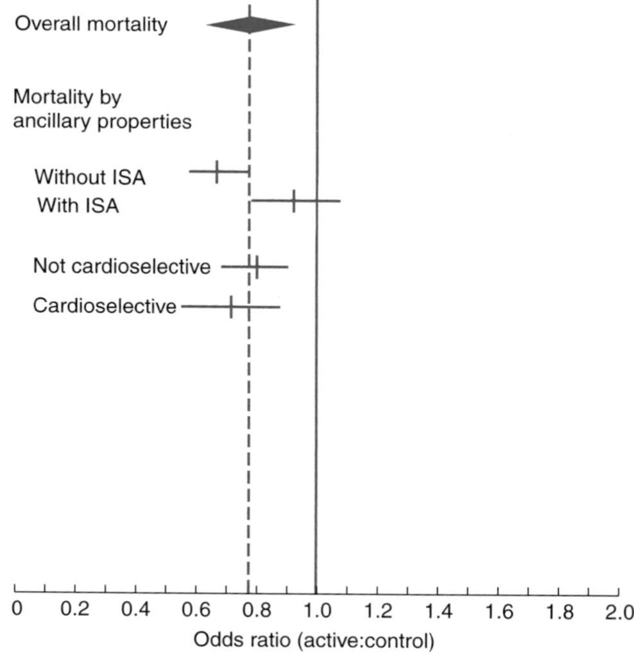


**FIGURE 1-19 Mortality in long-term $\beta$-adrenergic receptor blocker trials, by ancillary properties of agent tested: odds ratios (active:control), together with approximate 95% confidence intervals. See original article for citation of specific trials. (From Yusuf et al. 1985. Used with permission.)**

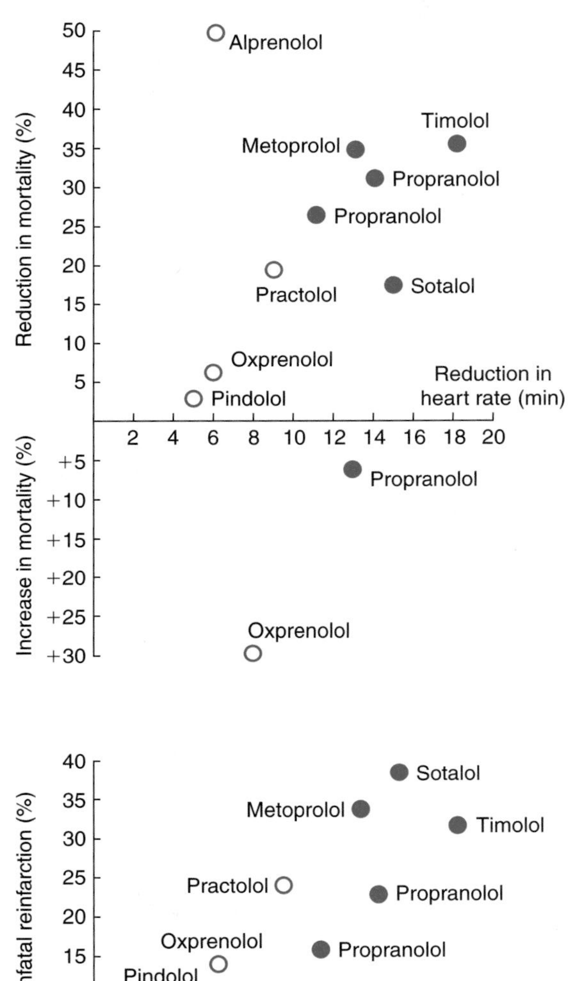


**FIGURE 1-20** **(A) Relation between reduction in heart rate (difference between treatment groups) and percentage of reduction in mortality in large, prospective, double-blind trials with $\beta$-adrenergic receptor blockers. Open circles, beta-blockers with intrinsic sympathomimetic activity: $r$ 0.6: $P < 0.05$. See original article for citation of specific trials. (B) Relation between reduction in heart rate and percentage of reduction in recurrent nonfatal infarctions in large, prospective, double-blind trials with beta-blockers. Open circles, beta-blockers with intrinsic sympathomimetic activity; $r$ 0.59; $P < 0.05$. See original article for citation of specific trials. (From Kjekshus 1986. Used with permission.)**

priate after MI to maintain beta-blocker therapy indefinitely in patients who can tolerate it (Stone and Sacks 1996).

The benefits of beta-blockers in long-term secondary prevention appear to extend to most patient subgroups. The Beta-Blocker Pooling Project (Beta-Blocker Pooling Project Research Group 1988) combined the results of nine large trials and found that, although high-risk patients were most likely to benefit from beta-blocker therapy, lower risk patients also benefited, even though the absolute and relative benefits were small. The experience using beta-blockers in the elderly is limited; however, available data indicate that the benefit may even be greater in patients older than 50 to 60 than in younger patients. Benefit appeared to be similar in both men and women.

The adverse effects from prolonged beta-blockers have generally been relatively modest (The Beta Blocker Heart Attack Trial Research Group 1982). In studies that report it, the incidence of heart failure is slightly but significantly higher in patients receiving beta-blocker (5.9%) than in patients receiving placebo (5.4%) (pooled odds ratio: 1.16, 95% CI, 1.01–1.34) (Yusuf et al. 1985). However, even patients with a history of mild or moderate congestive heart failure actually experienced greater benefit from beta-blockade than did patients without congestive heart failure (Byington and Furberg 1990).

## Use of Beta-Blockers for Unstable Angina and Myocardial Infarction with ST-Segment Depression

Only one placebo-controlled trial [Holland University Nifedipine/Metoprolol Trial (HINT) Research Group 1986] specifically examined the effectiveness of beta-blockers in unstable angina. In this study, patients who had not received beta-blockers were randomized to receive metoprolol, the L-channel calcium antagonist nifedipine, or both. Patients already taking beta-blockers were randomized to either nifedipine or placebo. The use of beta-blockers alone was associated with a 25% reduction in recurrent ischemia or MI at 48 hours, although this difference was not statistically significant. However, the addition of nifedipine to existing beta-blockade was associated with a 20% reduction in short-term cardiac endpoints.

Other trials of beta-blockers' use in unstable angina have been small and uncontrolled. A meta-analysis of these trials (Yusuf et al. 1988) showed a 13% reduction in progression from unstable angina to MI, but no significant reduction in mortality. However, a number of randomized trials have shown a clear benefit in lowering mortality from beta-blockers in other coronary syndromes, including acute MI, stable angina, and postinfarction angina, as discussed above.

**SUMMARY**

***β*-Adrenergic receptor blocking agents remain a cornerstone of the acute treatment of MI. Treatment is generally initiated intravenously, especially if it can be administered within 12 hours of onset of symptoms, followed by continuation using oral formulations. The recent ACC/AHA guidelines for the administration of beta-blockers to patients with acute MI are noted in Table 1-30 (Ryan et al. 1996). Beta-blockers are consistently useful for secondary prevention following MI (Stone and Sacks 1996) and should be maintained indefinitely.**

## NITRATES

The clinical effects of nitrates are mediated through several distinct mechanisms, including the following: 1) dilation of large coronary arteries and arterioles with redistribution of blood flow from epicardial to endocardial regions. Nitroglycerin provides an exogenous source of nitric oxide in vascular endothelium, facilitating coronary vasodilation even when damaged endothelium is unable to generate endogenous nitric oxide because of coronary artery disease. It is important to emphasize that these coronary vasomotor effects may either increase or decrease collateral flow. 2) Peripheral venodilation leads to an increase in venous capacitance and a substantial decrease in preload, thus reducing myocardial oxygen demand. Nitrates are consequently of particular value in treating patients with LV dysfunction and congestive heart failure. 3) Peripheral arterial dilation, typically of a modest degree, may decrease afterload. In addition (4), nitrates relieve dynamic coronary constriction, including that induced by exercise. Nitrates may also have an inhibitory effect on platelet aggregation in patients with unstable angina (Diodati et al. 1990), though the clinical significance of this finding is unclear.

### Use of Nitrates for Myocardial Infarction with ST-Segment Elevation

Early studies demonstrated that nitrates may be of value to reduce infarct size and to improve regional myocardial function when administered early in the course of acute MI (Bussmann et al. 1981; Jugdutt and Warnic 1988; Antman et al. 1992). A meta-analysis of these earlier studies before the acute reperfusion era indicated that nitrates reduced the odds of death after acute MI by 35% (95% CI, 28–49%, $P < 0.001$) (Yusuf et al. 1988). However, it should also be noted that use of nitroprusside was found in early studies to actually exacerbate myocardial infarction by causing a coronary steal phenomenon. Routine use of nitroprusside to limit infarct size has led to conflicting results (Cohn et al. 1982; Durrer et al. 1982; Passamani 1982), and its use cannot be recommended.

Recent studies have reinvestigated the use of nitrate therapy in the setting of concomitant thrombolytic therapy and aspirin administration. The GISSI-3 trial [Gruppo Italiano per lo Studio della Sopravivenza nell'Infarto Miocardico (GISSI-3) 1994] randomly assigned 19,394 patients to a 24-hour infusion of nitroglycerin (beginning within 24 hours of onset of pain), followed by topical nitroglycerin (10 mg daily) for 6 weeks (with patch removed at bedtime, allowing a 10-hour nitrate-free interval to avoid development of tolerance), or control. Approximately 50% of patients in the control group received nitrates on the first day or two at the discretion of their physician. There was an insignificant reduction in mor-

**Table 1-30 Recommendation for Administration of β-Adrenergic Receptor Antagonists**

| | |
|---|---|
| *Class I* | (Conditions for which there is evidence and/or general agreement that treatment is beneficial, useful, and effective)<br>1. Patients without a contraindication to *β*-adrenergic receptor (beta-blocker) therapy who can be treated within ≤ 12 h of onset of MI, irrespective of administration of concomitant thrombolytic therapy.<br>2. Patients with continuing or recurrent ischemic pain.<br>3. Patients with tachyarrhythmias, such as atrial fibrillation with rapid ventricular response.<br>4. As secondary prevention for all patients who can tolerate beta-blocker therapy. |
| *Class II* | (Conditions for which beneficial effects are less well established, but weight of evidence favors their use)<br>Patients with non-Q-wave MI |
| *Class III* | (Conditions for which evidence suggests treatment is not useful and may be harmful)<br>Patients with moderate or severe left ventricular failure or other contraindications to beta-blocker therapy |

SOURCE: From American College of Cardiology/American Heart Association (ACC/AHA) Guidelines: Ryan et al. 1996.
ABBREVIATIONS: MI, myocardial infarction; Q wave, segment of electrocardiogram.

tality at 6 weeks in the group randomly assigned to nitrate therapy alone, compared with the control group (6.5% vs. 6.9%, respectively). GISSI-3 evaluated lisinopril in a similar fashion; 6-week mortality was reduced slightly. At both 6-week and 6-month follow-up, the combined use of lisinopril and nitrates led to a greater reduction in mortality when compared with the group that received no nitrate therapy or lisinopril alone. The other large trial, ISIS-4, compared 28-day treatment of controlled-release oral isosorbide mono-nitrate with placebo control (as well as intravenous magnesium sulfate vs. control and the ACE inhibitor captopril vs. placebo control) in a 2 × 2 × 2 factorial design of 58,050 patients with suspected MI (ISIS-4 1995). Nitrate therapy led to a minor reduction in 35-day mortality compared with the control group (7.34% vs. 7.54%; NS). In both GISSI-3 and ISIS-4, the statistical power to detect potential beneficial effects of routine nitrate therapy was reduced by the extensive early use (greater than 50%) of nonprotocol nitrate in the control patients. When data from all randomized control trials of nitrate use in the management of acute MI are combined, there is a small relative reduction in mortality (5.5%) that is statistically significant ($P = 0.03$).

A review of evidence from all pertinent randomized clinical trials does not support routine use of long-term nitrate therapy in patients with uncomplicated acute MI (Ryan et al. 1996). However, it is reasonable to use intravenous nitroglycerin for the first 24 to 48 hours in more complicated patients, such as those with acute MI and recurrent ischemia, congestive heart failure, or those who require management of hypertension. It should be continued orally or topically in patients with congestive heart failure and large transmural MIs as well.

### Use of Nitrates in Patients with Unstable Angina

Despite a clear benefit when applied in patients with chronic coronary artery disease or ischemic left heart failure, there are no data from randomized placebo-controlled trials that demonstrate an effect of nitrates with respect to relief of symptoms or reduction in morbid events in patients with unstable angina. In patients receiving continuous nitrates, tachyphylaxis may be seen as early as 24–48 hours after initiation of therapy. This problem can be overcome by increasing the dose as needed until symptom relief is achieved. Once a patient has been pain-free for 24 hours, it is advisable to switch to a topical or oral form of nitrate therapy, with a nitrate-free interval of 6–8 hours each day.

## CALCIUM CHANNEL-BLOCKING AGENTS

Calcium channel-blocking agents inhibit the entry of calcium into vascular smooth muscle cells and myocardial cells during the action potential. This $Ca^{++}$ entry blockade leads to direct effects of vasodilatation, negative inotropy, negative chronotropy (decreased heart rate), and negative dromotropy (decreased atrioventricular [AV]-nodal conduction) (Stone et al. 1980). The systemic vasodilatation leads to reflex sympathetic activation which, in turn, promotes an increase in AV-nodal conduction. The net clinical effects of the calcium channel blockers consist of a composite of their direct effects and their reflex-mediated indirect effects. The two major categories of calcium channel blockers, the dihydropyridines (including nifedipine, amlodipine, nicardipine) and the non-dihydropyridines (including diltiazem and verapamil) differ fundamentally: the dihydropyridines have greater vascular selectivity, leading to more peripheral vasodilatation, and the potential for increased reflex sympathetic activation, whereas the non-dihydropyridines have greater myocardial selectivity with a greater negative inotropic, chronotropic, and dromotropic effect. Both types of calcium channel blockers inhibit coronary vasoconstriction and lower blood pressure. Consequently, the principal anti-ischemic effects of the calcium channel blockers are to decrease myocardial oxygen demand by lowering blood pressure (dihydropyridines and non-dihydropyridines) and lowering contractility and heart rate (non-dihydropyridines only), as well as to prevent coronary vasoconstriction if it is present. It should be noted that if reflex sympathetic activation predominates, as may be observed with use of immediate release dihydropyridines, then the increase in contractility and heart rate may lead to an exacerbation of the myocardial oxygen supply: demand imbalance.

The calcium channel blockers may also exert a fundamental cardioprotective effect of limiting $Ca^{++}$ influx during ischemia, thereby limiting the amount of necrosis that ensues from a given ischemic result (Stone et al. 1980).

### Use of Calcium Channel Blockers for Myocardial Infarction

#### *Dihydropyridine calcium channel blockers (nifedipine and nicardipine)*

Early studies investigated the use of calcium channel blockers, particularly the dihydropyridines, for the early treatment of MI, but they were not found to be useful

(Fig. 1-21) (Held et al. 1989). Patients were generally included regardless of the direction of ST-segment deviation on presentation. The dihydropyridines were studied in particular because they could be safely combined with beta-blockers without the concern for excessive reduction in myocardial contractility or bradycardia. The available formulation of dihydropyridines in this early era consisted of short-acting (immediate-release) nifedipine. This formulation of nifedipine actually was found to be detrimental when used without a beta-blocker, which blunts the increased reflex sympathetic activity induced by nifedipine (Muller, Morrison, et al. 1984; Sirnes et al. 1984; Wilcox et al. 1986; The Israeli Sprint Study Group 1988; Goldbourt et al. 1993). When combined with a beta-blocker, nifedipine was found to be significantly beneficial in decreasing symptomatic manifestations of acute MI (Muller, Morrison, et al. 1984). Many of the studies are not methodologically comparable because the doses tested

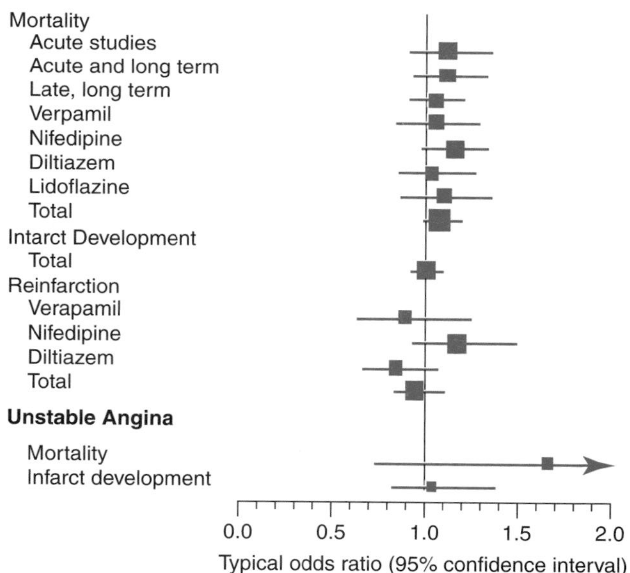


**FIGURE 1-21 Typical odds of death, infarct development, and repeat infarction by disease, type of trials, and drug. Areas of squares are proportional to numbers of patients. *Bars* indicate 95% confidence intervals. *Portions to left* of vertical line (corresponding to odds ratio of <1) indicate risk with treatment; *portions to right* of vertical line indicate increased risk with treatment. Upper 95% confidence limit for effect on mortality in unstable angina 6.2. Note that treatment does not seem to reduce risk of any event. See original article for citation of specific trials. (From Held et al. 1989. Used with permission.)**

varied, and both the underlying disease manifestations and the timing from onset of the acute ischemic manifestation to initiation of the study drug were different.

Nevertheless, nifedipine has been uniformly unsuccessful in reducing either mortality or the rate of repeat infarction (Fig. 1-21). A recent update of a pooled analysis (Yusuf et al. 1991) of stable coronary patients in a coronary regression trial with either nifedipine (Lichtlen et al. 1990) or nicardipine (Waters et al. 1990) showed a trend toward an increase in mortality (7.4% vs. 6.5%; odds ratio: 1.16; 95% CI, 0.99–1.35; $P = 0.07$) and a nonsignificant increase in repeat infarction (3.5% vs. 3.1%; odds ratio:1.19; 95% CI, 0.92–1.53).

Use of the calcium blockers to treat pathophysiologic disturbances associated with acute MI nevertheless remain potentially useful, such as treating hypertension with a dihydropyridine in combination with a beta-blocker. Treatment of supraventricular tachycardias with non-dihydropyridine L-channel blockers (diltiazem and verapamil) may also be useful, especially if treatment with a beta-blocker is contraindicated.

***Verapamil and diltiazem***

Verapamil and diltiazem can be considered together because their net pharmacologic effects include slowing the heart rate and, in some instances, reducing myocardial contractility (Stone et al. 1980), thereby reducing myocardial oxygen demand. These agents have been given to patients as secondary prevention after their index MI was stabilized. A recent pooled analysis (Yusuf et al. 1991) indicated that verapamil and diltiazem had no effect on mortality following acute MI, but that they exerted a significant effect on reducing the rate of repeat infarction (6.0% vs. 7.5%; odds ratio: 0.79; 95% CI, 0.67–0.94; $P < 0.01$). The effect seems similar for both agents.

Although the overall results of trials with verapamil have found no benefits on mortality, subgroup analysis suggests that immediate-release verapamil initiated several days after acute MI in patients who were not candidates for a beta-blocking agent may be useful in reducing the incidence of the composite endpoint of repeat infarction and death, provided LV function is well preserved and there is no clinical evidence of heart failure. In a placebo-controlled trial of almost 1800 patients, verapamil 360 mg/day, started in the second week after acute MI and continued for a mean of 16 months, had no effect on mortality compared with that of the control group, but reduced major event rates (death or repeat infarction) from 21.6% in the control group to 18.0% in the active treatment group ($P = 0.03$) (The Danish Verapamil Infarction

Trial II-DAVITII 1990). In patients who did not have heart failure while in the coronary care unit, verapamil significantly reduced both mortality (from 11.8% in the control group to 7.7% in the active treatment group, $P = 0.02$) and major events (from 19.7% in the control group to 14.6% in the active treatment group, $P = 0.01$); however, there was no effect on either endpoint among patients who experienced congestive heart failure while in the coronary care unit (phs45). Verapamil is detrimental to patients with heart failure or bradyarrhythmias during the first 24 to 48 hours after acute MI (Held and Yusuf 1993; Ryan et al. 1996).

Data from the Multicenter Diltiazem Postinfarction Trial (MDPIT) and the Diltiazem Reinfarction Study (DRS) (Gibson et al. 1986; Anonymous 1988e) suggest that patients with non-Q-wave MI or those with Q-wave infarction, preserved LV function, and no evidence of heart failure may also benefit from treatment with immediate-release diltiazem. In the DRS, patients were treated with either diltiazem (90 mg every 6 hours) or placebo initiated 24 to 72 hours after the onset of MI, and continued for 14 days (Gibson et al. 1986). There was no difference in mortality, but diltiazem decreased both the rate of repeat infarction (from 9.3% in the control group to 5.2% [$P < 0.03$]) and the rate of refractory post-infarction angina (from 6.9% in the control group to 3.5% [$P = 0.03$]). In the MDPIT, patients were treated either with diltiazem (240 mg per day) or placebo 3–15 days after the MI onset and followed for a mean of 25 months. There was no difference in mortality in the two treatment groups (Multicenter Diltiazem Postinfarction Trial Research Group 1988). A significant bidirectional interaction was observed, however, between diltiazem and the presence of pulmonary congestion at the time of the index MI (Fig. 1-22). In the 1,909 patients without pulmonary congestion, diltiazem was associated with a significant reduction in cardiac events at one year from 11% in the control group to 8%, whereas in the 490 patients with pulmonary congestion, diltiazem increased the cardiac event rate from 18% in the control group to 26%. A similar pattern was observed with respect to the ejection fraction, which was dichotomized at 40% (Multicenter Diltiazem Postinfarction Trial Research Group 1988). The results of MDPIT may be confounded by the fact that 53% and 55% of placebo- and diltiazem-treated patients, respectively, received concomitant beta-blocker therapy. Also, both the MDPIT and DRS projects were conducted in an era when the use of aspirin was not as prevalent as it is today, raising further uncertainty about the relevance of their findings for contemporary management of acute MI (Ryan et al. 1996). Of particular clinical importance is the detrimental mortality effect of diltiazem in patients with LV dysfunction.

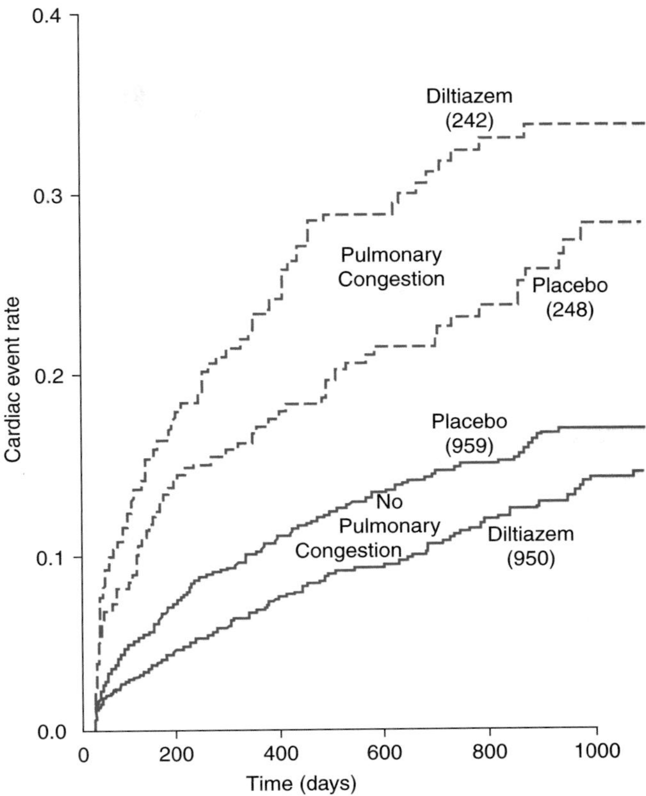


**FIGURE 1-22 Diltiazem-treated patients with pulmonary congestion had a higher rate of cardiac events than patients receiving placebo; diltiazem-treated patients without pulmonary congestion had a lower rate of cardiac events than patients receiving placebo. The values in parentheses are numbers of patients. (From Multicenter Diltiazepam Postinfarction Trial Research Group 1988. Used with permission.)**

It should be emphasized that there have been no studies comparing the efficacy of verapamil or diltiazem with that of a beta-blocker. β-Adrenergic receptor blocking agents more consistently reduce both mortality and repeat infarction and should be recommended for those patients who can tolerate these drugs. Verapamil or diltiazem may be a reasonable alternative for those patients who cannot tolerate a beta-blocker, for example, patients with asthma. It should be noted, however, that many patients who cannot tolerate a beta-blocker because of concern of excessive bradycardia or congestive heart failure may experience similar complications from diltiazem or verapamil.

Table 1-31 **Recommendation for Use of Calcium Channel Blockers**

| | |
|---|---|
| *Class I* | (Conditions for which there is evidence and/or general agreement that treatment is beneficial, useful, and effective) None. |
| *Class IIa* | (Conditions for which there is conflicting evidence, but the weight of evidence is in favor of usefulness and efficacy) |
| | Verapamil or diltiazem may be given to patients in whom beta-blockers are ineffective or contraindicated (i.e., bronchospastic disease) for relief of ongoing ischemia or control of a rapid ventricular response with atrial fibrillation after acute MI in the absence of CHF, LV dysfunction, or AV block. |
| *Class IIb* | (Conditions for which beneficial effects are less well established, but weight of evidence favors their use) |
| | In non-ST-segment-elevation MI, diltiazem may be given to patients without LV dysfunction, pulmonary congestion, or CHF. It may be added to standard therapy after the first 24 hours and continued for 1 year. |
| *Class III* | (Conditions for which evidence suggests treatment is not useful and may be harmful) |
| | Short-acting nifedipine is generally contraindicated in routine treatment. |
| | Diltiazem and verapamil are contraindicated in patients with acute MI and associated LV dysfunction or CHF. |

SOURCE: From ACC/AHA Guidelines, Ryan et al. 1996.
ABBREVIATIONS: AV, atrioventricular; CHF, congestive heart failure; LV, left ventricular; MI, myocardial infarction; ST, segment of the electrocardiogram.

### Use of Calcium Channel Blockers in Patients with Unstable Angina

Several small randomized trials have examined the use of nifedipine and diltiazem in unstable angina. A meta-analysis of these trials (Held et al. 1989) showed no reduction in MI or death rates in patients given these calcium antagonists (Fig. 1-21). The largest trial [Holland University Nifedipine/Metoprolol Trial (HINT) Research Group 1986] was discontinued prematurely because of a trend towards more nonfatal MIs in patients receiving nifedipine alone. When combined with a beta-blocking agent, however, patients receiving nifedipine had a decreased rate of MI and death compared with those taking a placebo. Several studies, have shown symptomatic benefit from calcium antagonists (Gerstenblith et al. 1982; Muller, Turi, et al. 1984; Gibson et al. 1986). Consequently, evidence for use of calcium channel blockers in patients with unstable angina does not suggest any beneficial effect on mortality or progression of myocardial infarction, but does support their use for relief of refractory symptoms. Because of randomized trials showing an increased risk of death in patients treated with calcium channel blockers in the setting of acute MI, particularly in patients with LV dysfunction (Multicenter Diltiazem Postinfarction Trial Research Group 1988), calcium antagonists should be used only in patients with refractory symptoms despite the use of nitrates and beta-blockers.

The most recent ACC/AHA guidelines concerning use of the calcium channel blockers are shown in Table 1-31 (Ryan et al. 1996).

## ANGIOTENSIN-CONVERTING ENZYME INHIBITORS

Angiotensin-converting enzyme (ACE) inhibitors have become a mainstay in the acute treatment of patients with acute MI because they prevent the deleterious left ventricular chamber remodeling that may occur after MI and because they may prevent the progression of vascular pathology. The LV dysfunction associated with acute MI leads to a perceived reduction in circulating blood volume and blood pressure, which is compensated by an increase in the renin–angiotensin–aldosterone system as well as an increase in sympathetic tone. These effects lead to salt and water retention as well as vasoconstriction, which in turn further dilate the left ventricle and cause progressive LV dysfunction. This vicious cycle can be interrupted by ACE inhibitors, which block the increased renin–angiotensin activity and thereby prevent the progressive dilation and dysfunction. The recent overview by the ACE Inhibitor Myocardial Infarction Collaborative Group 1998, which included observations in almost 100,000 patients with acute MI treated within 36 hours of the onset of chest pain, found a 7% reduction in 30-day mortality when ACE inhibitors were given to all patients with acute MI, with most of the benefit observed in the first week. The absolute benefit was particularly large in some high-risk groups, such as those in Killip class II or III (23 lives saved per 1000 patients) and those with an anterior MI (11 lives saved per 1000 patients) (ACE Inhibitor Myocardial Infarction Collaborative Group 1998). ACE inhibitor therapy also reduced the incidence of nonfatal congestive heart failure (14.6% vs. 15.2%, $P = 0.01$), but was associated with an excess of persistent hypotension (17.6% vs. 9.3%, $P = 0.01$) and renal dysfunction (1.3% vs. 0.6%, $P = 0.01$). In the overview >85% of the lives saved attributed to ACE inhibitor therapy occurred in the anterior MI subgroup, a group that represented 37% of the overall population (Pfeffer 1998). Of note, an analysis of survival relative to the time from onset of symptoms to treatment with either control or ACE inhibitor did not show a time-related trend within the first 36 hours.

**PRINCIPLE Unlike aspirin and reperfusion strategies, it is not critical to introduce the ACE inhibitor in the hyperacute phase of acute MI (Pfeffer 1998). There is still benefit from ACE inhibitor therapy when administered at any time following MI, although benefit is lessened if therapy is delayed by days or weeks.**

The time-dependent priority decisions are the use of aspirin, reperfusion, and beta-blockade, followed by reevaluation for ACE inhibitor therapy (Pfeffer 1998). The current recommendations for use of ACE inhibitors for acute MI are shown in Table 1-32.

Of note, ACE inhibitors may also protect against progression of atherosclerosis and the development of MI by their antiproliferative and antimigratory effects on smooth muscle cells, neutrophils, and mononuclear cells, by enhancing endogenous fibrinolysis, and by improving endothelial dysfunction (Lonn et al. 1994). Studies suggest that patients treated with ACE inhibitors experience fewer MIs and episodes of unstable angina, not related to hemodynamic effects and ventricular remodeling, and further studies are in progress to determine the role of such therapy in routine secondary prevention.

**SUMMARY AND CONCLUSIONS**

**Many advances have occurred in the treatment of acute coronary syndromes over recent years. The summary of recommendations is illustrated as a decision tree in Figures 1-23 and 1-24. In ST-segment elevation MI, new aggressive thrombolytic regimens improve early reperfusion and improve survival. The current focus is on bolus administration of thrombolytic agents, with glycoprotein IIb/IIIa inhibition and low-molecular-weight heparin administered as adjuncts. In unstable angina and non-ST-elevation MI, two major advances are gpIIb/IIIa inhibition and low-molecular-weight heparin. Beta-blockers, nitrates, and calcium channel blockers provide an important foundation to reduce myocardial oxygen demand. Following acute coronary syndromes, beta-blockers, antithrombotic agents (such as aspirin, clopidogrel or warfarin), and ACE inhibitors provide important secondary prevention. Risk factor modification is critical after MI, with attention devoted to cessation of smoking, control of hypertension, and lipid lowering with aggressive dietary and pharmacologic means, as necessary.**

With the great number of new medical treatments available and under development, the outcome for patients with acute coronary syndromes will continue to improve as we enter the next millennium.

Table 1-32 **Recommendation for Use of Angiotensin-Converting Enzyme Inhibitors**

| | |
|---|---|
| *Class I* | (Conditions for which there is evidence and/or general agreement that treatment is beneficial, useful, and effective) |
| | Patients with the first 24 hours of MI with ST elevation in ≥2 anterior leads or with CHF |
| | Patients with MI and EF <40% or with CHF and systolic dysfunction during and after convalescence |
| *Class IIa* | (Conditions for which there is conflicting evidence, but the weight of evidence is in favor of usefulness and efficacy) |
| | All other MI patients with first 24 h |
| | Asymptomatic patients with EF40–50% and previous MI |
| *Class IIb* | (Conditions for which beneficial effects are less well established, but weight of evidence favors their use) |
| | Patients recently recovered from MI with normal or midly abnormal LV function |

SOURCE: From ACC/AHA Guidelines: Ryan et al. 1996.
ABBREVIATIONS: CHF, congestive heart failure; EF, ejection fraction; MI, myocardial infarction; ST, segment of the electrocardiogram.

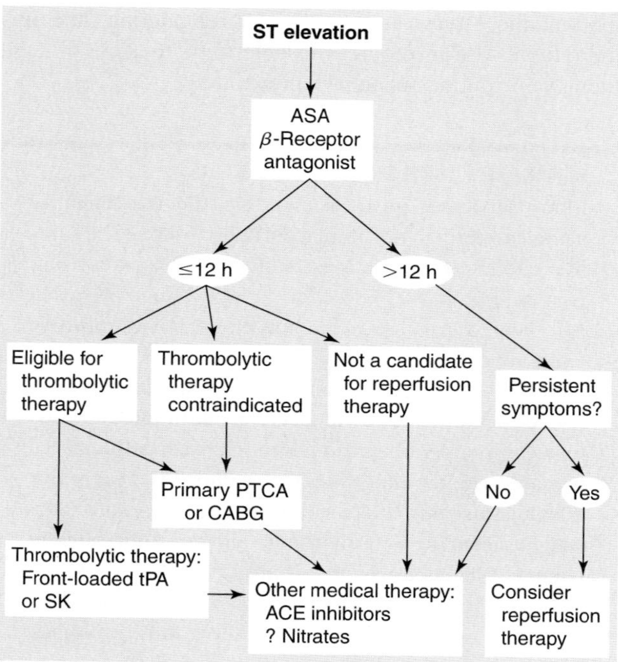


FIGURE 1-23 **Recommendations for management of patients with ST-segment elevation. All patients with ST-segment elevation on the electrocardiogram should receive aspirin (ASA), β-adrenergic receptor blockers (in the absence of contraindications), and an antithrombin (particularly if tissue-type plasminogen activator [t-PA] is used for thrombolytic therapy). The role of glycoprotein IIb/IIIa inhibitors in the setting of thrombolytic therapy is unclear. Whether heparin is required in patients receiving streptokinase (SK) remains a matter of controversy; the small additional risk for intracranial hemorrhage may not be offset by the survival benefit afforded by adding heparin to SK therapy. Patients treated within 12 hours who are eligible for thrombolytics should expeditiously receive either front-loaded TPA or SK or be considered for primary percutaneous transluminal coronary angioplasty (PTCA). Primary PTCA is also to be considered when thrombolytic therapy is absolutely contraindicated. Coronary artery bypass graft (CABG) may be considered if the patient is less than 6 hours from onset of symptoms. Individuals treated after 12 hours should receive the initial medical therapy noted above and, on an individual basis, may be candidates for reperfusion therapy or angiotensin-converting enzyme (ACE) inhibitors (particularly if left ventricular function is impaired). (From ACC/AHA Guidelines, Ryan et al. 1996.)**

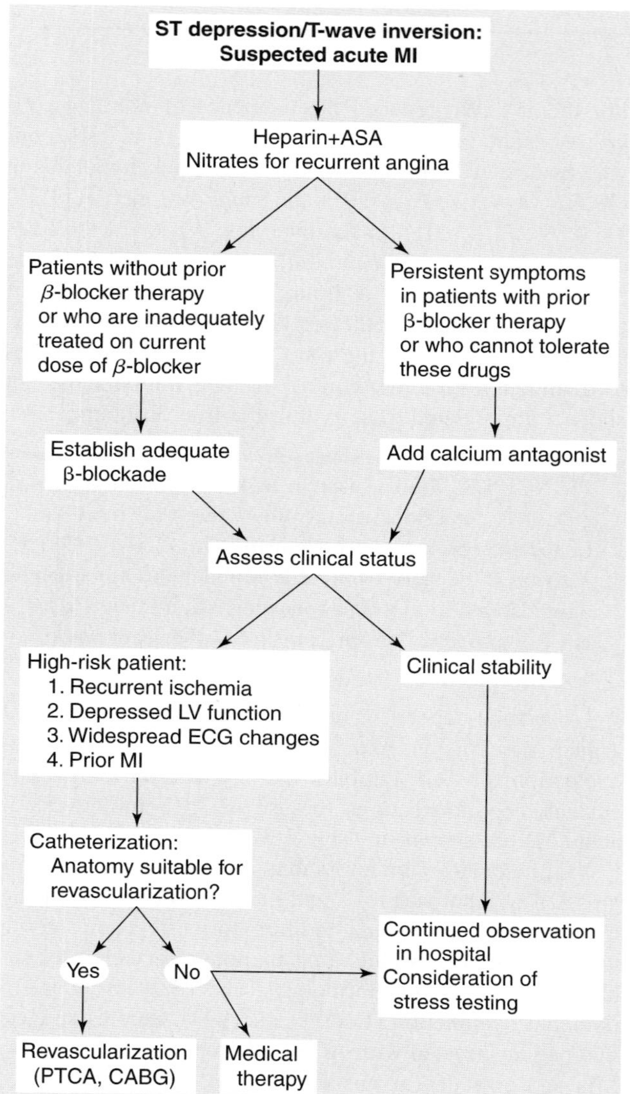


FIGURE 1-24 **Recommendations for management of patients with acute myocardial infarction (AMI) without ST-segment elevation. All patients without ST elevation should be treated with an antithrombin (heparin or low-molecular-weight heparin) and aspirin (ASA). Glycoprotein IIb/IIIa inhibitors may be used instead of ASA. Nitrates should be administered for recurrent episodes of angina. Adequate β-adrenergic receptor blockade (beta-blockade) should then be established; when this is not possible or contraindications exist, a calcium antagonist (verapamil or diltiazem) can be considered. High-risk patients should be sorted by priority (triage) to cardiac catheterization with plans for revascularization if they are clinically suitable; patients who are clinically stable can be treated more conservatively, with continued observation in the hospital and consideration of a stress test to screen for myocardial ischemia that can be provoked. LV indicates left ventricular; ECG, electrocardiographic; PCTA, percutaneous transluminal coronary angioplasty; CABG, coronary artery bypass graft. (From ACC/AHA Guidelines, Ryan et al. 1996.)**

## REFERENCES

ACE Inhibitor Myocardial Infarction Collaborative Group. 1998. Indications for ACE inhibitors in the early treatment of acute myocardial infarction: systematic overview of individual data from 100,000 patients in randomized trials. *Circulation* **97**:2202–12.

AIMS Trial Study Group. 1988. Effect of intravenous APSAC on mortality after acute myocardial infarction: Preliminary report of a placebo-controlled clinical trial. *Lancet* **1**:545–9.

Anticoagulants in the Secondary Prevention of Events in Coronary Thrombosis (ASPECT) Research Group. 1994. Effect of long-term oral anticoagulant treatment on mortality cardiovascular morbidity after myocardial infarction. *Lancet* **343**:499–503.

Antiplatelet Trialists' Collaboration. 1994. Collaborative overview of randomised trials of antiplatelet therapy-I: prevention of death myocardial infarction and stroke by prolonged antiplatelet therapy in various categories of patients. *Br Med J* **308**:81–106.

Antman EM. 1996. Hirudin in acute myocardial infarction: Thrombolysis and Thrombin Inhibition in Myocardial Infarction (TIMI) 9B trial. The TIMI 9B Investigators. *Circulation* **94**:911–21.

Antman EM, Lau J, Kupelnick B, et al. 1992. A comparison of results of meta-analyses of randomized control trials and recommendations of clinical experts. Treatments for myocardial infarction. *JAMA* **268**:240–8.

Arbustini E, DeServi S, Bramucci E, et al. 1995. Comparison of coronary lesions obtained by directional coronary atherectomy in unstable angina, stable angina, and restenosis after either atherectomy or angioplasty. *Am J Cardiol* **75**:675–82.

ASSET Study Group. 1988. Trial of tissue plasminogen activator for mortality reduction in acute myocardial infarction. Anglo-Scandinavian Study of Early Thrombolysis (ASSET). *Lancet* **2**:525–30.

Beta-Blocker Pooling Project Research Group. 1988. The Beta-Blocker Pooling Project (BBPP): Subgroup findings from randomized trials in post-infarction patients. *Eur Heart J* **9**:8–16.

Bleich SD, Nichols T, Schumacher RR, et al. 1990. Effect of heparin on coronary patency after thrombolysis with tissue plasminogen activator in acute myocardial infarction. *Am J Cardiol* **66**:1412–7.

Braunwald E. 1989. Myocardial reperfusion, limitation of infarct size, reduction of left ventricular dysfunction, and improved survival: Should the paradigm be expanded? *Circulation* **79**:441–4.

Braunwald E. 1993. The open-artery theory is alive and well-again. *N Engl J Med* **329**:1650–2.

Bussmann WD, Passek D, Seidel W, et al. 1981. Reduction of CK and CK-MB indexes of infarct size by intravenous nitroglycerin. *Circulation* **63**:615–22.

Byington RP, Furberg CD. 1990. Beta-blockers during and after acute myocardial infarction. In: Francis, Alpert, editors. *Modern Coronary Care*. Boston, MA: Little, Brown. p 511–39.

Cairns JA, Gent M, Singer J, et al. 1985. Aspirin, sulfinpyrazone, or both in unstable angina. *N Engl J Med* **313**:1369–75.

Cannon CP. 1995. Optimizing the treatment of unstable angina. *J Thromb Thrombolysis* **2**:205–18.

Cannon CP, Antman EM, Walls R, et al. 1994. Time as an adjunctive agent to thrombolytic therapy. *J Thromb Thrombolysis* **1**:27–34.

Cannon CP, Braunwald E. 1994. GUSTO, TIMI and the case for rapid reperfusion. *Acta Cardiol* **49**:1–8.

Cannon CP, Braunwald E. 1996. Time to reperfusion: the critical modulator in thrombolysis and primary angioplasty. *J Thromb Thrombolysis* **3**:109–17.

Cannon CP, Lambrew CT, Tiefenbrunn AJ, et al. 1996. Influence of door-to-balloon time on mortality in primary angioplasty results in 3,648 patients in the Second National Registry of Myocardial Infarction (NRMI-2) [abstract]. *J Am Coll Cardiol* **27** (Suppl A): 61A–2A.

Cannon CP, McCabe CH, Borzak S, et al. 1998. A randomized trial of an oral platelet glycoprotein IIb/IIIa antagonist, sibrafiban, in patients after an acute coronary syndrome: Results of the TIMI 12 trial. *Circulation* **97**:340–9.

Cannon CP, Sharis PJ, Schweiger MJ, et al. 1997. Prospective validation of a composite end point in thrombolytic trial of acute myocardial infarction (TIMI 4 and 5). *Am J Cardiol* **80**:696–9.

CAPRIE Steering Committee. 1996. A randomised, blinded, trial of clopidogrel versus aspirin in patients at risk of ischaemic events (CAPRIE). *Lancet* **348**:1329–39.

Cohen M, Demers C, Gurfinkel EP, et al. 1997. A comparison of low-molecular-weight heparin with unfractionated heparin for unstable coronary artery disease. *N Engl J Med* **337**:447–52.

Cohn J, Franciosa JA, Francis GS, et al. 1982. Effect of short-term infusion of sodium nitroprusside on mortality rate in acute myocardial infarction complicated by left ventricular failure. *N Engl J Med* **306**:1129–35.

Coller BS, Folts JD, Scutter LE, et al. 1986. Antithrombotic effect of a monoclonal antibody to the platelet glycoprotein IIb/IIIa receptor in an experimental model. *Blood* **68**:783–6.

Coumadin Aspirin Reinfarction Study (CARS) Investigators. 1997. Randomised double-blind trial of fixed low-dose warfarin with aspirin after myocardial infarction. *Lancet* **350**:389–96.

Davies MJ, Thomas AC. 1985. Plaque fissuring: the cause of acute myocardial infarction, sudden death, and crescendo angina. *Br Heart J* **53**:363–73.

Davies MJ. 1990. A macro and micro view of coronary vascular insult in ischemic heart disease. *Circulation* **82** (Suppl II):II-38–46.

de Bono DP, Simoons MI, Tijssen J, et al. 1992. Effect of early intravenous heparin on coronary patency, infarct size, and bleeding complications after alteplase thrombolysis: results of a randomized double blind European Cooperative Study Group trial. *Br Heart J* **67**:122–8.

DeWood MA, Stifter WF, Simpson CS, et al. 1986. Coronary arteriographic findings soon after non-Q wave myocardial infarction. *N Engl J Med* **315**:417–23.

Diodati J, Theroux P, Latour J-G, et al. 1990. Effects of nitroglycerin in therapeutic doses on platelet aggregation in unstable angina pectoris and acute myocardial infarction. *Am J Cardiol* **66**: 683–8.

Durrer JD, Lie KI, VanCapell JFL, et al. 1982. Effect of sodium nitroprusside on mortality in acute myocardial infarction. *N Engl J Med* **306**:1121–28.

EMERAS (Estudio Multicentrico Estreptoquinasa Republicas de America del Sur) Collaborative Group. 1993. Randomised trial of late thrombolysis in patients with suspected acute myocardial infarction. *Lancet* **342**:767–72.

Fibrinolytic Therapy Trialists' (FTT) Collaborative Group. 1994. Indications for fibrinolytic therapy in suspected acute myocardial infarction: collaborative overview of early mortality and major morbidity results from all randomised trials of more than 1000 patients. *Lancet* **343**:311–22.

First International Study of Infarct Survival Collaborative Group. 1986. Randomised trial of intravenous atenolol among 16,027 cases of suspected acute myocardial infarction: ISIS-1. *Lancet* **2**:57–66.

Flugelman MY, Virmani R, Correa R, et al. 1993. Smooth muscle cell abundance and fibroblast growth factors in coronary lesions of patients with nonfatal unstable angina. *Circulation* **88**:2493–500.

Friedman LM, Byington RP, Capone RJ, et al. 1984. Effect of propranolol in patients with myocardial infarction and ventricular arrhythmia. *J Am Coll Cardiol* **7**:1–8.

FRISC Study Group. 1996. Low molecular weight heparin (Fragmin) during instability in coronary artery disease (FRISC). *Lancet* **347**:561–68.

Furberg CD, Hawkins CM, Lichstein E, et al. 1984. Effect of propranolol in post-infarction patients with mechanical or electrical complications. The Beta Blocker Heart Attack Trial Study Group. *Circulation* **69**:761–5.

Gent M. 1997. Benefit of clopidogrel in patients with coronary disease. *Circulation* **96** (Suppl I):1–467.

Gerstenblith G, Ouyang P, Achuff SC, et al. 1982. Nifedipine in unstable angina: a double-blind randomized trial. *N Engl J Med* **306**: 885–9.

Gibson RD, Boden WE, Theroux P, et al. 1986. Diltiazem and reinfarction in patients with non-Q-wave myocardial infarction. *N Engl J Med* **315**:423–9.

Gold HK, Torres FW, Garabedian HD, et al. 1993. Evidence of a rebound coagulation phenomenon after cessation of a 4-hour infusion of a specific thrombin inhibitor in patients with unstable angina pectoris. *J Am Coll Cardiol* **21**:1039–47.

Goldbourt U, Behar S, Reicher-Reiss H, et al. 1993. Early administration of nifedipine in suspected acute myocardial infarction: the Secondary Prevention Reinfarction Israel Nifedipine Trial 2 Study. *Arch Intern Med* **153**:345–53.

Goldman L, Sia BST, Cook EF, et al. 1988. Cost and effectiveness of routine therapy with long-term beta-adrenergic antagonists after acute myocardial infarction. *N Engl J Med* **319**:152–7.

Granger CB, Hirsh J, Califf RM, et al. 1996. Activated partial thromboplastin time and outcome after thrombolytic therapy for acute myocardial infarction: results from the GUSTO-I Trial. *Circulation* **93**:870–87.

Granger CB, Miller JM, Bovill EG, et al. 1995. Rebound increase in thrombin generation and activity after cessation of intravenous heparin in patients with acute coronary syndromes. *Circulation* **91**:1929–35.

Grines CL, Browne KF, Marco J, et al. 1993. A comparison of immediate angioplasty with thrombolytic therapy for acute myocardial infarction. *N Engl J Med* **328**:673–9.

Gruppo Italiano per lo Studio della Sopravivenza nell'Infarto Miocardico: GISSI-2. 1990. A factorial randomised trial of alteplase versus streptokinase and heparin versus no heparin among 12,490 patients with acute myocardial infarction. *Lancet* **336**:65–71.

Gruppo Italiano per lo Studio della Sopravivenza nell'Infarto Miocardico (GISSI-3). 1994. GISSI-3: effects of lisinopril and transdermal glyceryl trinitrate singly and together on 6–week mortality and ventricular function after acute myocardial infarction: *Lancet* **343**:1115–22.

Gruppo Italiano per lo Studio della Streptochinasi nell'Infarto Miocardico (GISSI). 1986. Effectiveness of intravenous thrombolytic treatment in acute myocardial infarction. *Lancet* **1**:397–401.

Held PH, Yusuf S, Furberg CD. 1989. Calcium channel blockers in acute myocardial infarction and unstable angina: an overview. *Br Med J* **229**:1187–92.

Held PH, Yusuf S. 1993. Effects of beta-blockers and calcium channel blockers in acute myocardial infarction. *Eur Heart J* **14** (Suppl F):18–25.

Hirsh J, Fuster V. 1994a. Guide to anticoagulation therapy. Part 1: Heparin. *Circulation* **89**:1449–68.

Hirsh J, Fuster V. 1994b. Guide to anticoagulation therapy. Part 2: Oral anticoagulants. *Circulation* **89**:1469–80.

Hirsh J, Levine M. 1993. Low molecular weight heparin. *Blood* **79**: 1–17.

Holland University Nifedipine/Metoprolol Trial (HINT) Research Group. 1986. *Br Heart J* **56**:400–4134.

Hsia J, Hamilton WP, Kleiman N, et al. 1990. A comparison between heparin and low-dose aspirin as adjunctive therapy with tissue plasminogen activator for acute myocardial infarction. *N Engl J Med* **323**:1433–37.

International Study Group. 1990. In-hospital mortality and clinical course of 20,891 patients with suspected acute myocardial infarction randomised between alteplase and streptokinase with or without heparin. *Lancet* **336**:71–5.

ISIS-2 (Second International Study of Infarct Survival) Collaborative Group. 1988. Randomised trial of intravenous streptokinase, oral aspirin, both, or neither among 17,187 cases of suspected acute myocardial infarction: ISIS-2. *Lancet* **2**:349–60.

ISIS-3 (Third International Study of Infarct Survival) Collaborative Group. 1992. ISIS-3: a randomised comparison of streptokinase vs tissue plasminogen activator vs anistreplase and of aspirin plus heparin vs aspirin alone among 41,299 cases of suspected acute myocardial infarction. *Lancet* **339**:753–70.

ISIS-4. 1995. A randomized factorial trial assessing early oral captopril, oral mononitrate, and intravenous magnesium sulphate in 58,050 patients with suspected acute myocardial infarction. *Lancet* **345**:669–685.

Jugdutt BI, Warnic JW. 1988. Intravenous nitroglycerin therapy to limit myocardial infarct size, expansion, and complications: effect of timing, dosage, and infarct location. *Circulation* **78**:1088–92.

Kereiakes DJ, Kleiman NS, Ambrose J, et al. 1996. Randomized, double-blind, placebo-controlled dose-ranging study of tirofiban (MK-383) platelet IIb/IIIa blockade in high risk patients undergoing coronary angioplasty. *J Am Coll Cardiol* **27**:536–642.

Kereiakes DJ, Runyon JP, Kleiman NS, et al. 1996. Differential dose-response to oral xemilofiban after antecedent intravenous abciximab. Administration for complex coronary intervention. *Circulation* **94**:906–10.

Kjekshus JK. 1986. Importance of heart rate in determining beta-blocker efficacy in acute and long-term acute myocardial infarction intervention trials. *Am J Cardiol* **57**:43F–9F.

Klein W, Buchwald A, Hillis SE, et al. 1997. Comparison of low-molecular-weight heparin with unfractionated heparin acutely and with placebo for 6 weeks in the management of unstable coronary artery disease. Fragmin in Unstable Coronary Artery Disease Study (FRIC). *Circulation* **96**:61–8.

Klimt CR, Knatterud GL, Stamler J, Meier P. 1986. Persantine-Aspirin Reinfarction Study. Part II. Secondary coronary prevention with persantine and aspirin. The PARIS II Investigator Group. *J Am Coll Cardiol* **7**:251–69.

LATE Study Group. 1993. Late Assessment of Thrombolytic Efficacy (LATE) study with alteplase 6–24 hours after onset of acute myocardial infarction. *Lancet* **342**:759–66.

Lee RT, Grodzinsky AJ, Frank EH, et al. 1991. Structure-dependent dynamic mechanical behavior of fibrous caps from human atherosclerotic plaques. *Circulation* **83**:1764–70.

Lefkovits J, Plow EF, Topol EJ. 1995. Platelet glycoprotein IIb/IIIa receptors in cardiovascular medicine. *N Engl J Med* **332**: 1553–9.

Lewis HD, Davis JW, Archibald DG, et al. 1983. Protective effects of aspirin against acute myocardial infarction and death in men with unstable angina. *N Engl J Med* **309**:396–403.

Lichtlen PR, Hugenholtz PG, Rafflenbenl W, et al. 1990. Retardation of angiographic progression of coronary artery disease by nifedipine: results of the International Nifedipine Trial on Antiatherosclerotic Therapy (INTACT). The INTACT Group. *Lancet* **335**:1109–13.

Loh E, Sutton MS, Wun CC, et al. 1997. Ventricular dysfunction and the risk of stroke after myocardial infarction. *N Engl J Med* **336**:251–7.

Lonn EM, Yusuf S, Jha P, et al. 1994. Emerging role of angiotensin-converting enzyme inhibitors in cardiac and vascular protection. *Circulation* **90**:2056–69.

Maseri A, Severi S, DeNes M, et al. 1978. "Variant" angina: one aspect of a continuous spectrum of vasospastic myocardial ischemia. Pathogenic mechanisms, estimate incidence, clinical and coronarographic findings in 138 patients. *Am J Cardiol* **42**:1019–35.

Molhoek P, Tebbe U, Laarman GJ, et al. 1997. Hirudin for the improvement of thrombolysis with streptokinase in patients with acute myocardial infarction. Results of the HIT-4 Study [abstract]. *Circulation* **96** (Suppl I):1–205.

Morganroth J, Lichstein E, Byington R, et al. 1985. Beta-blocker heart attack trial: impact of propranolol therapy on ventricular arrhythmias. *Prev Med* **14**:346.

Mueller HS, Forman SA, Manegus MA, et al. 1995. Prognostic significance of nonfatal reinfarction during 3-year follow-up: results of the Thrombolysis in Myocardial Infarction (TIMI) phase II clinical trial. *J Am Coll Cardiol* **26**:900–7.

Muller JE, Morrison J, Stone PH, et al. 1984. Nifedipine therapy in patients with threatened and acute myocardial infarction. A randomized double-blind, placebo-controlled comparison. *Circulation* **69**:740–7.

Muller JE, Turi ZG, Pearle DL, et al. 1984. Nifedipine and conventional therapy for unstable angina pectoris: a randomized double-blind comparison. *Circulation* **69**:728–39.

Multicenter Diltiazem Postinfarction Trial Research Group. 1988. The effect of diltiazem on mortality and reinfarction after myocardial infarction. *N Engl J Med* **319**:385–92.

Ohman EM, Califf RM, Topol EJ, et al. 1990. Consequences of reocclusion after successful reperfusion therapy in acute myocardial infarction. *Circulation* **82**:781–91.

Oler A, Whooley MA, Oler J, et al. 1996. Adding heparin to aspirin reduces the incidence of myocardial infarction and death in patients with unstable angina. A meta-analysis. *JAMA* **276**:811–5.

Oliva PB, Potts DE, Pluss RC. 1973. Coronary arterial spasm in Prinzmetal angina. Documentation by coronary arteriography. *N Engl J Med* **232**:745–51.

Olsson G, Oden A, Johansson L, et al. 1988. Prognosis after withdrawal of chronic post-infarction metoprolol treatment: a 2–7 year follow-up. *Eur Heart J* **9**:365–72.

Passamani ER. 1982. Nitroprusside in myocardial infarction [editorial]. *N Engl J Med* **306**:1168–9.

Pfeffer MA. 1998. ACE inhibitors in acute myocardial infarction: patient selection and timing. *Circulation* **97**:2192–4.

Receptor Suppression Using Integrilin Therapy (PURSUIT) Trial Investigators. 1998. Inhibition of platelet glycoprotein IIb/IIIa with eptifibatide in patient with acute coronary syndromes without persistent ST-segment elevation: a randomized, placebo-controlled clinical trial. The Platelet Glycoprotein IIb/IIIa in Unstable Angina. *N Engl J Med* **339**:436–43.

Rossi PRF, Yusuf S, Ramsdale D, et al. 1983. Reduction of ventricular arrhythmias by early intravenous atenolol in suspected acute myocardial infarction. *Br Med J* **286**:506–10.

Roux S, Christeller S, Ludin E. 1992. Effects of aspirin on coronary reocclusion and recurrent ischemia after thrombolysis: a meta-analysis. *J Am Coll Cardiol* **19**:671–7.

Ryan TJ, Anderson JL, Antman EM, et al. 1996. ACC/AHA guidelines for the management of patients with acute myocardial infarction: a report of the American College of Cardiology/American Heart Association Task Force on Practice Guidelines (Committee on Management of Acute Myocardial Infarction). *J Am Coll Cardiol* **28**:1328–1428.

Sirnes PA, Overskeid K, Pedersen TR, et al. 1984. Evolution of infarct size during the early use of nifedipine in patients with acute myocardial infarction: the Norwegian Nifedipine Multicenter Trial. *Circulation* **70**:638–44.

Stone PH, Antman EM, Muller JE, et al. 1980. Calcium channel blocking agents in the treatment of cardiovascular disorders. Part II. Hemodynamic effects and clinical applications. *Ann Intern Med* **93**:886–904.

Stone PH, Sacks FM. 1996. Strategies for secondary prevention. In Manson JE, Ridker PM, Gaziano JM, Hennekens CH, editors. *Prevention of Myocardial Infarction.* New York: Oxford Univ. Press, 463–510.

Tcheng JE, Harrington RA, Kottke-Marchant K, et al. 1995. Multicenter, randomized, double-blind, placebo-controlled trial of the platelet integrin glycoprotein IIb/IIIa blocker Integrelin in elective coronary intervention. *Circulation* **91**:2151–57.

The Beta Blocker Heart Attack Trial Research Group. 1982. A randomized trial of propranolol in patients with acute myocardial infarction. I. Mortality results. *JAMA* **247**:1707–14.

The CAPTURE Investigators. 1997. Randomised placebo-controlled trial of abciximab before and during coronary intervention in refractory unstable angina: the CAPTURE study. *Lancet* **349**:1429–35.

The Danish Verapamil Infarction Trial II-DAVIT II. 1990. Effect of verapamil on mortality and major events after acute myocardial infarction *Am J Cardiol* **66**:779–85.

The EPIC Investigators. 1994. Use of a monoclonal antibody directed against the platelet glycoprotein IIb/IIIa receptor in high risk angioplasty. *N Engl J Med* **330**:956–61.

The EPILOG Investigators. 1997. Platelet glycoprotein IIb/IIIa receptor blockade and low-dose heparin during percutaneous coronary revascularization. *N Engl J Med* **336**:1689–96.

The Global Use of Strategies to Open Occluded Coronary Arteries (GUSTO) IIb Investigators. 1996. A comparison of recombinant hirudin with heparin for the treatment of acute coronary syndromes. *N Engl J Med* **335**:775–82.

The GUSTO Angiographic Investigators. 1993. The comparative effects of tissue plasminogen activator, streptokinase, or both on coronary artery patency, ventricular function and survival after acute myocardial infarction. *N Engl J Med* **329**:1615–22.

The GUSTO Investigators. 1980. An international randomized trial comparing four thrombolytic strategies for acute myocardial infarction. *N Engl J Med* **303**:897–902.

The GUSTO Investigators. 1993. An international randomized trial comparing four thrombolytic strategies for acute myocardial infarction. *N Engl J Med* **329**:673–82.

The IMPACT-II Investigators. 1997. Randomised placebo-controlled trial of effect of eptifibatide on complications of percutaneous coronary intervention: IMPACT-II. *Lancet* **349**:1422–28.

The Israeli Sprint Study Group. 1988. Secondary Prevention Reinfarction Israeli Nifedipine Trial (SPRINT): a randomized intervention trial of nifedipine in patients with acute myocardial infarction. *Eur Heart J* **9**:354–64.

The Medical Research Council's General Practice Research Framework. 1998. Thrombosis prevention trial: randomised trial of low-intensity oral anticoagulation with warfarin and low dose aspirin in the primary prevention of ischaemic heart disease in men at increased risk. *Lancet* **351**:233–41.

The Platelet Receptor Inhibition for Ischemic Syndrome Management in Patients Limited by Unstable Signs and Symptoms (PRISM-PLUS) Trial Investigators. 1998. Inhibition of the platelet glycoprotein IIb/IIIa receptor with tirofiban in unstable angina and non-Q-wave myocardial infarction. *N Engl J Med* **338**:1488–97.

The RESTORE Investigators. 1997. The effects of platelet glycoprotein IIb/IIIa blockade with tirofiban on adverse cardiac events in patients with unstable angina or acute myocardial infarction undergoing coronary angioplasty. *Circulation* **96**:1445–53.

The RISC Group. 1990. Risk of myocardial infarction and death during treatment with low dose aspirin and intravenous heparin in men with unstable coronary artery disease. *Lancet* **336**:827–30.

The Stroke Prevention in Atrial Fibrillation Investigators. 1990. Preliminary report of the Stroke Prevention in Atrial Fibrillation Study. *N Engl J Med* **322**:863–8.

The TIMI Study Group. 1989. Comparison of invasive and conservative strategies after treatment with intravenous tissue plasminogen activator in acute myocardial infarction results of the thrombolysis in myocardial infarction (TIMI) phase II trial. *N Engl J Med* **320**:618–627.

The TIMI IIIA Investigators. 1993. Early effects of tissue-type plasminogen activator added to conventional therapy on the culprit lesion in patients presenting with ischemic cardiac pain at rest. Results of the Thrombolysis in Myocardial Ischemia (TIMI IIIA) Trial. *Circulation* **87**:38–52.

The TIMI IIIB Investigators. 1994. Effects of tissue plasminogen activator and a comparison of early invasive and conservative strategies in unstable angina and non-Q-wave myocardial infarction. Results of the TIMI IIIB Trial. *Circulation* **89**:1545–56.

Theroux P, Ouimet H, McCans J, et al. 1988. Aspirin, heparin or both to treat unstable angina. *N Engl J Med* **319**:1105–11.

Theroux P, Waters D, Lam J, et al. 1992. Reactivation of unstable angina after the discontinuation of heparin. *N Engl J Med* **327**:141–5.

TIMI Study Group. 1985. The Thrombolysis in Myocardial Infarction (TIMI) Trial: phase I findings. *N Engl J Med* **312**:932–6.

Timm TC, Ross R, McKendall GR, et al. 1991. Left ventricular function and early cardiac events as a function of time to treatment with t-PA: a report from TIMI II [abstract]. The TIMI Investigators. *Circulation* **84** (Suppl II):II-230.

Topol EJ. 1998. Toward a new frontier in myocardial reperfusion therapy. Emerging platelet preeminence. *Circulation* **97**:211–18.

Topol EJ, Ferguson JJ, Weisman HF, et al. 1997. Long term protection from myocardial ischemic events after brief integrin $B_3$ blockade with percutaneous coronary intervention. *JAMA* **278**:479–84.

Topol EJ, George BS, Kereiakes DJ, et al. 1989. A randomized controlled trial of intravenous tissue plasminogen activator and early intravenous heparin in acute myocardial infarction. *Circulation* **79**:281–6.

Warkentin TE, Levine MN, Hirsh J, et al. 1995. Heparin-induced thrombocytopenia in patients treated with low-molecular-weight heparin or unfractionated heparin. *N Engl J Med* **332**:1330–5.

Waters D, Lesperance J, Francetich M, et al. 1990. A controlled clinical trial to assess the effect of a calcium channel blocker upon the progression of coronary atherosclerosis. *Circulation* **82**:1940–53.

Weaver WD, Simes J, Betriu A, et al. 1997. Comparison of primary coronary angioplasty and intravenous thrombolytic therapy for acute myocardial infarction: A quantitative review. *JAMA* **278**:2093–8.

White HD, Van de Werf FJ. 1998. Thrombolysis for acute myocardial infarction. *Circulation* **97**:1641.

Wilcox RG, Hampton JR, Banks DC, et al. 1986. Trial of early nifedipine in acute myocardial infarction: the TRENT study. *Br Med J Clin Res* **293**:1204–8.

Yusuf S, Collins R, MacMahon S, et al. 1988. Effect of intravenous nitrates on mortality in acute myocardial infarction: an overview of the randomized trials. *Lancet* **1**:1088–92.

Yusuf S, Held P, Furberg C. 1991. Update of effects of calcium antagonists in myocardial infarction or angina in light of the second Danish Verapamil Infarction Trial (DAVIT-II) and other recent studies. *Am J Cardiol* **67**:1295–7.

Yusuf S, Lessem J, Jha P, et al. 1993. Primary and secondary prevention of myocardial infarction and strokes: an update of randomly allocated, controlled trials. *J Hypertens* **11** (Suppl 4):S61–S73.

Yusuf S, Peto R, Lewis J, et al. 1985. Beta-blockade during and after myocardial infarction: an overview of the randomized trials. *Prog Cardiovasc Dis* **27**:335–71.

Yusuf S, Sleight P, Rossi PRF, et al. 1983. Reduction in infarct size, arrhythmias, chest pain and morbidity by early intravenous betablockade in suspected acute myocardial infarction. *Circulation* **67** (Pt 2):32–41.

Yusuf S, Wittes J, Friedman L. 1988a. Overview of results of randomized clinical trials in heart disease. I. Treatments following myocardial infarction. *JAMA* **260**:2088–93.

Yusuf S, Wittes J, Friedman L. 1988b Effect of propranolol in postinfarction patients with mechanical or electrical complications. Overview of results of randomized clinical trials in heart disease. II. Unstable angina, heart failure, primary prevention with aspirin, and risk factor modification. *JAMA* **260**:2259–63.

Zijlstra F, de Boer MJ, Hoorntje JCA, et al. 1993. A comparison of immediate coronary angioplasty with intravenous streptokinase in acute myocardial infarction. *N Engl J Med* **328**:680–4.

# Heart Failure

J. Malcolm O. Arnold

*Chapter Outline*



## DEFINITIONS

Heart failure is a clinical syndrome of cardiac dysfunction associated with reduced exercise tolerance due to dyspnea or fatigue (Fig. 1-25). It needs to be diagnosed correctly and distinguished from other conditions that can produce similar symptoms or signs such as chronic lung disease, constrictive pericarditis, and renal failure, to name only a few. Since it is the end product of other diseases, comorbid diseases usually exist, not infrequently leading to difficulties in attributing the principal cause of symptoms. This is particularly the case with chronic lung disease, since smoking can cause both lung disease and ischemic heart disease, with myocardial infarction (MI) subsequently causing heart failure. In addition, severe chronic lung disease can cause isolated right heart failure. Most of the large clinical trials, which direct our current therapies, have addressed left ventricular systolic failure, and therefore it will be the main focus of this section.

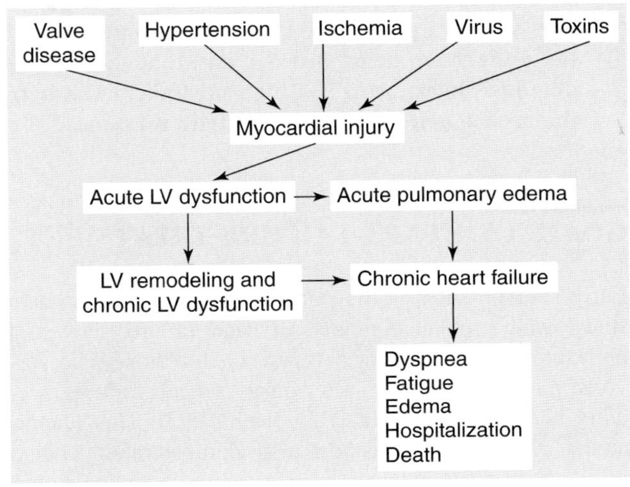


**FIGURE 1-25 Principle causes and manifestations of heart failure.**

Some additional descriptors of heart failure are frequently used. Congestive heart failure certainly describes the situation where there is clear "congestion" of both the pulmonary and systemic circulations with fluid overload and edema peripherally and in the lungs. However, not all patients experience congestion, despite marked cardiac dysfunction, and, while this is poorly understood, it probably reflects different patterns of neurohormonal activation. Similarly, "forward" and "backward" heart failure have been used and have been helpful to explain and describe some of the cardinal features of the clinical syndrome. Nonetheless, they focus predominantly on the heart as a pump, and we are now aware that the signs of congestion attributed to "backward" failure are not merely due to passive congestion but also reflect neurohormonal activation especially of the renin–angiotensin–aldosterone (RAA) system associated with additional fluid retention. The term "decompensated" heart failure describes acute exacerbations, interspersed with periods of stable symptoms perhaps with no evidence of pulmonary or systemic congestion. These periods are sometimes called "compensated" heart failure and, although this implies a stable and perhaps nonprogressive state, frequently the underlying heart dysfunction is silently progressive despite apparent clinical stability.

**Key Point: A proper concept of clinical heart failure needs to take into account the multiple causes of cardiac dysfunction, the fact that symptoms may not be a good reflection of the progression of the underlying heart disease, and that the correct diagnosis bears with it a high mortality even with the recent major advances in drug therapies.**

## GOALS OF HEART FAILURE TREATMENT

Early studies, such as the population-based Framingham study using clinical diagnosis of heart failure, showed a high mortality of 69% at 5 years but, for those who survived more than 90 days after onset of heart failure, mortality was 56% at 5 years (Ho et al. 1993). The Scandinavian CONSENSUS study also demonstrated a high mortality of 52% at 1 year for patients with severe symptoms at rest (The CONSENSUS Trial Study Group 1987). Subsequent large-scale, placebo-controlled clinical trials have documented the high mortality at different stages of clinical symptomatology even when patients are treated in specialized heart failure centers within those clinical trials. As new therapeutic advances are added to previously proven therapies, there have been incremental gains with further reductions in mortality. Yet, progressive lowering in left ventricular ejection fraction (LVEF) and worsening of symptoms are strong predictors of a poor outcome, which remains worse than that of some forms of cancer. Although pump failure is the most common mode of death, sudden unexpected death can occur in up to 40% of patients whose death is attributed to their heart failure (Uretsky and Sheaham 1997). Although sudden death may be caused by an arrhythmia, it is not always a ventricular tachyarrhythmia and may be bradyarrhythmia or electromechanical dissociation in the setting of a large, acute myocardial infarction. Patients with heart failure also die suddenly from cerebral vascular accidents and pulmonary emboli. Improving survival remains the primary long-term therapeutic target in the management of heart failure. Other important therapeutic targets include the prevention of progression of disease, the relief of symptoms, improvement of quality of life, and reduction in hospitalizations.

In the Framingham study, the most prevalent cause of heart failure was considered to be hypertension in more than 70% of cases (Kannel and Belanger 1991) but, in the modern era of clinical trials and as attested to in clinical practice, nearly 70% of heart failure is now attributed to a primary etiology of ischemic heart disease (Gheorgiade and Bonow 1998). Heart failure will therefore become a global health problem, since ischemic heart disease is predicted to be the leading cause of death in the world by the year 2020 (Murray and Lopez 1997). As the "baby boomer" population ages and as our population life expectancy increases, the total burden of cardiovascular disease will increase and will accelerate in other cultures as the lifestyles of the "developed" world are adopted. Already, heart failure is one of the most common causes for hospital admission in the elderly population and is a significant contributor to increased length of stay and to both hospital and community health costs. In recognition of the importance of the problem and the need for appropriate and carefully managed therapy, specialized clinics have been developed to improve the delivery of care. They have been successful in the investigation of new drugs and therapeutic approaches and have demonstrated improvement in patient symptoms with a substantial reduction in hospitalizations, at least in the short term (Rich et al. 1995; Fonarow et al. 1997; Hanumanthu et al. 1997; West et al. 1997). Thus, the provision of cost-effective therapies within a cost-conscious health-care delivery system is another important therapeutic goal of heart failure treatment.

Although this section focuses predominantly on the treatment of heart failure, the above serves to emphasize that the patient presents not just with heart failure but with the comorbid illnesses that have often led to the development of that clinical syndrome. In younger people, idiopathic dilated cardiomyopathy may occur, and this is often thought to be the result of a previous viral myocarditis in an otherwise healthy individual. In the older population, these patients may have concomitant ischemic heart disease, dyslipidemia, hypertension, diabetes, smoking, obesity, peripheral and cerebrovascular disease, renal disease, arthritis, gout and depression. Heart failure patients, therefore, need to be treated as whole persons rather than as a mere conglomerate of diseases.

**PRINCIPLE The management of heart-failure patients requires a broad-based, multidisciplinary approach to treat not just the presenting symptoms and signs of heart failure but also the attendant risk factors, precipitating and aggravating causes, and comorbid illnesses.**

Nonetheless, each disease has a specific treatment and most large-scale clinical trials address only one problem at a time. This has led, quite appropriately, to the use of multiple drugs in the management of patients with heart failure, but a consequence has been the possibility of drug–drug interactions, increased drug adverse effects, complicated drug regimens, and potential confusion for the patient with errors in drug administration. Variously referred to as noncompliance, poor adherence, and lack of concordance, all result in the patient's heart condition not remaining adequately controlled and in acute exacerbations with worsening symptoms necessitating hospital readmissions. This emphasizes the need for specialized treatment clinics where a multidisciplinary approach can be implemented, patient education can be emphasized, and rapid convenient access to care is provided (Abraham and Bristow 1997; Massie and Shah 1997; Arnold et al. 1999). With some therapies, especially diuretic therapy, the patient can be given instructions as to how to adjust their own diuretic dose based on their weight and symptoms. Thus, patient education to improve concordance with complicated treatment regimens is an additional and perhaps underrecognized therapeutic goal in community practice.

**Key Point: The goals of HF treatment are to reduce mortality, morbidity, and hospitalizations, with an improvement in patient symptoms and quantity and quality of life in the setting of cost-effective proven therapies and active patient-centered education.**

## PATHOPHYSIOLOGY AND TREATMENT OF HEART FAILURE

Since the early 1980s, our pathophysiologic construct of heart failure has changed significantly and this is reflected in our current therapies. The principal therapies in the early 1980s were digoxin and diuretics. Important advances in understanding the hemodynamics of heart failure occurred with the development of indwelling catheters to measure cardiac filling pressures and cardiac output in response to treatment. Such studies described the failing heart as a defective pump and at the same time allowed the conceptual development of the influence of preload and afterload on that pump function, the mismatch between loading conditions and pump function, and the introduction of vasodilator therapies, which resulted in the first clinical trial showing that vasodilator therapy (hydrallazine and nitrates) could improve morbidity and mortality in heart failure (Cohn et al. 1986). However, some vasodilators with substantial acute and even chronic hemodynamic effects did not show benefits with respect to mortality. This finding enhanced the view that some of the successful vasodilators, such as angiotensin-converting enzyme (ACE) inhibitors, were showing important benefits by reducing excessive neurohormonal activation. This observation resulted in the development of the neurohormonal hypothesis of heart failure, which has held sway over the last number of years and has greatly influenced our understanding of heart failure and the direction of treatment and has been reviewed in detail elsewhere (Packer 1992).

Multiple interventions have been tested to interfere with hormones that are abnormally elevated in heart failure or abnormally suppressed, but at the time of writing this section, ACE inhibitors, beta blockers, and spironolactone remain the most important neurohormonal modulators, although other intriguing neurohormonal antagonists or modulators are being actively studied in clinical trials (Fig. 1-26). An important focus of current research is the prevention of progressive myocardial damage, and much attention is focused on the role of cytokines and oxidative stress in causing cell suicide or apoptosis. The purpose of this section, however, is to address therapies of proven benefit, although the potential for new therapies offers exciting possibilities.

The current management of heart failure can be likened to the treatment of cancer, for which rational combination drug therapy is applied to tackle the cell cycle at different stages. The modern treatment of heart failure also involves multiple approaches, which need to be combined in a rational manner, and this is clearly to be distinguished from irrational administration of multiple drugs.

## CLINICAL SCENARIOS FOR TREATMENT DECISIONS

Left ventricular dysfunction lies within a spectrum between predominantly systolic and predominantly diastolic dysfunction. Most patients with heart failure have some combination of both, yet it remains clinically possible and helpful to attempt to categorize patients according to their position on that spectrum.

Predominant *diastolic dysfunction* can be an abnormality of either the active or passive filling phase in diastole, resulting in impaired left ventricular filling, elevated left atrial pressures, pulmonary congestion, and symptoms of dyspnea (Grossman 1991; Lenihan et al. 1995; Dauterman et al. 1998). Additional complications can include right ventricular failure, atrial fibrillation, and consequent systemic embolism. The true incidence of di-

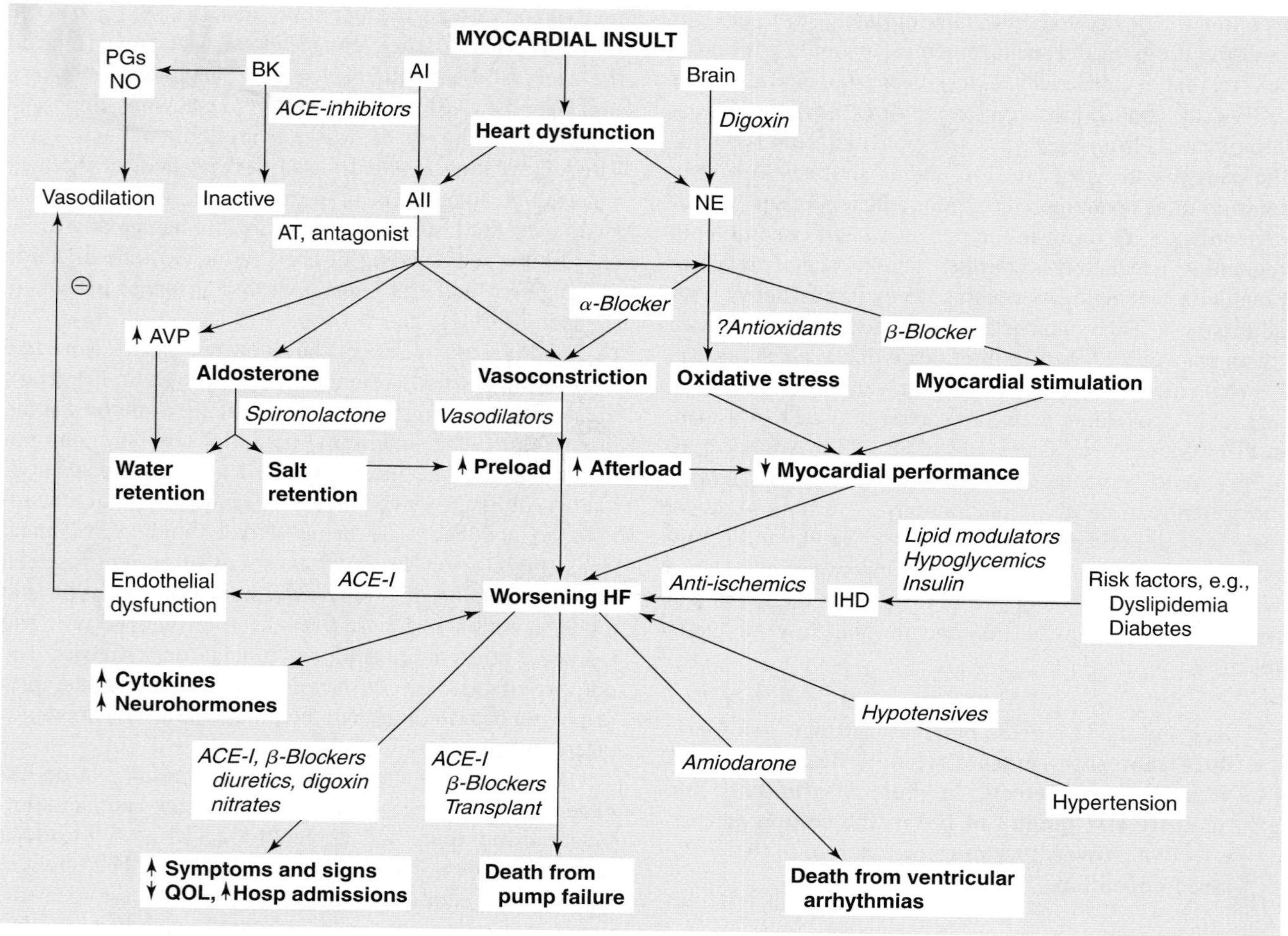


**FIGURE 1-26 Pathophysiologic schema linking mechanisms and drug treatments based on survival benefits of ACE inhibitors and β-adrenergic receptor blockers.**

astolic heart failure differs in different countries and ethnic communities but overall may contribute to 30–40% of clinically symptomatic heart failure. The most common cause of diastolic dysfunction is hypertension with left ventricular hypertrophy, and this can be aggravated as the patient ages or has diabetes. Acute and chronic ischemia (which cause stunned and hibernating myocardium), infiltrative myocardial disease (such as amyloid), and hypertrophic cardiomyopathy will also cause diastolic dysfunction. A patient with diastolic dysfunction can be recognized as having typical symptoms of heart failure, principally being dyspnea on exertion, and acute exacerbations when the diastolic filling period is reduced during tachycardia or in combination with loss of atrial contraction in atrial fibrillation. The patient will be more likely to have a fourth heart sound rather than a third heart sound (assuming the patient remains in sinus rhythm) and will be less likely to have a displaced apex on clinical examination or an enlarged heart on chest X-ray. The ECG may show evidence of left ventricular hypertrophy.

To guide appropriate treatment, it is recommended that an objective test of left ventricular function is made in all patients at the time of initial diagnosis. The choice of tests may depend on local expertise and availability. The diagnosis can be confirmed if the patient has abnormal ventricular filling patterns on echocardiographs or radionuclide ventriculography. The presence of changes in filling patterns can be diagnostic for diastolic dysfunction, but the absence of their detection does not exclude the diagnosis, which may be a presumptive diagnosis based on typical symptoms and the presence of hypertension, amyloidosis, or left ventricular hypertrophy. In this situation it may be referred to as heart failure with preserved systolic function.

The importance of detecting diastolic dysfunction is to be able to treat the underlying cause. There have not been major clinical trials investigating the range of therapies in diastolic heart failure but, in the setting of preserved systolic function, acute relief of symptoms can occur with diuretic therapy, nitrate therapy, prolongation of diastolic filling with rate-limiting drugs such as $\beta$-adrenergic receptor antagonists (beta blockers) and some calcium-channel antagonists, and correction and maintenance of sinus rhythm if the patient is in atrial fibrillation. Regression of left ventricular hypertrophy with treatment will be a slower and more long-term process and occurs with several types of drugs including ACE inhibitors. Long-term clinical trials of hypertension have not always included heart failure as an independent clinical endpoint or may not have followed patients long enough over the natural history of hypertension to detect changes in heart failure, but several trials that have identified heart failure as an endpoint have shown that it is decreased with the appropriate long-term management of hypertension. More clinical trials are needed in this important area since most of the current, large-scale clinical trials in heart failure have included only patients with LVEFs ≤40% and have therefore studied a population of patients with predominant systolic dysfunction.

Chronic *systolic heart failure* has been investigated in large clinical trials in patients with differing severity of symptoms, in patients with chronic left ventricular systolic dysfunction who have minimal symptoms or are asymptomatic, and in patients following acute MI who have left ventricular systolic dysfunction but have not yet developed chronic symptoms. To assess the impact of treatment, symptoms, neurohormones, LVEF, hospitalizations, and mortality have been used as endpoints. Although mortality is the most important endpoint, the absolute extension of life for some patients may be modest, and some patients say that they would prefer to have symptomatic relief even if their life were not prolonged. Thus, whereas symptomatic relief does not always translate into mortality benefit, it should not be ignored as an appropriate therapeutic target, although drugs that have been proven to do both are obviously preferred. ACE inhibitor and, more recently, the addition of some beta blockers and spironolactone have been shown to improve both. Although diuretics and nitrates clearly can improve symptoms acutely, information on their impact on long-term mortality is not known, but is clinically inferred to be beneficial. This seems a reasonable conclusion based on clinical experience and short-term clinical trials. It is unlikely that a placebo-controlled trial will be designed to address mortality and routine diuretic therapy. The same situation existed with digoxin until recently, when the development of ACE inhibitors provided an ethical alternative to digoxin and allowed the design and completion of the DIG (Digoxin Investigators Group) trial. Whether development of new drugs in the future will allow the optimal use of diuretic therapy to be addressed remains to be seen.

A number of national and international guidelines for the diagnosis and management of heart failure have been published over the last few years and provide excellent reviews of current treatment options and approaches (Johnstone et al. 1994; ACC/AHA guidelines, Williams et al. 1995; ESC 1995; Advisory Council 1999).

## NONPHARMACOLOGIC THERAPY

The importance of patient education has been stressed previously and multidisciplinary approaches including patient education have been shown to reduce hospitalizations for heart failure. Also, most clinical trials with study nurses include patient education as part of the close follow-up. These trials usually have found the placebo arm of the trial to have a clinical event rate less than predicted. By inference, therefore, it could be assumed that patient education and close follow-up is helpful. This also underpins much of clinical medicine and has been shown to be helpful in other disease states such as diabetes. However, within heart failure, the independent benefit of patient education has not been dissected apart from the other multiple interventions that are concurrently used. Nonetheless, it makes sense for patients to understand the nature of their illness, the warning signs of worsening in their condition, and what to do when their symptoms change. Depending on the resources available and the education level of the patient, a tailored approach can be developed that allows the patient some control over his or her illness, some control over medications such as diuretics and nitrates, and the knowledge that a rapid response to a change in his (her) condition with prompt access to medical care can prevent progressive deterioration in symptoms and improve quality of life (Uretsky et al. 1998). Reinforcement of this education is necessary. Patients and physicians also need to be educated with regard to which medications, such as NSAIDs, may cause a worsening in fluid retention. If resources are limited, physicians need to identify and target patients with recurrent hospital admissions and aggressively attempt to identify issues of salt and water indiscretion or medication noncompliance. Once the patient can see a direct link between the cause and the consequence, the education process will be enhanced. A diet without added table salt and with avoidance of processed foods and foods rich in salt is appropriate for most patients with symptomatic heart failure. Patients with more severe heart failure may require fluid restriction to 1–1.2 L per day with less than 2 g of sodium in the diet. A multidisciplinary approach allows a dietitian to actively reinforce these concepts and to provide healthy alternatives and at the same time discuss diabetic, low-calorie, low-cholesterol, and low-fat diets for appropriate patients. Involving other health-care professionals can also allow psychological and emotional responses to illness to be addressed (Sullivan and Hawthorne 1996).

The role of exercise in cardiac rehabilitation is well established for patients after post-MI and has been investigated in heart failure. As a surrogate endpoint, many drugs can improve exercise performance, although that does not necessarily translate into improved survival. Exercise tolerance, however, remains an important clinical symptom for patients. Reducing pulmonary congestion, improving the loading conditions of the heart, and improving overall pump function with medications will decrease symptoms and improve exercise capacity. This will allow the patient to be more active and to enjoy a better quality of life.

It has also become recognized that patients with heart failure do less and therefore develop deconditioning of their skeletal muscle. Training will improve muscle energetics with increased strength and endurance, although the best forms of exercise for heart failure patients has not been well defined. If a cardiac rehabilitation program exists with specific protocols and advice for heart failure patients, then this would be currently recommended by clinical consensus. However, cardiac rehabilitation programs are not available in all communities, and many heart failure patients are elderly and may have difficulty getting out to formal programs. In these scenarios, simple clinical common sense can encourage patients whose heart failure is stable to engage in light, regular activity up to but just short of producing symptoms. The type of activity can be dictated by what the patient enjoys doing most, but is usually walking. Patients can be encouraged to walk at their own pace; to make small amounts of effort frequently rather than pushing themselves hard all at once; and to avoid sudden, unexpected, or prolonged exertion. Planning the day's activities in advance and avoiding exertion after a heavy meal or at times of the day when the temperatures are more extreme is appropriate. More strenuous activity can be considered, but should be optimized by a specific exercise prescription following formal functional testing. Lifting heavy objects is best avoided, and a helpful clinical guideline for patients is that they can lift an object if they can do so without holding their breath or grunting or groaning, or while continuing to speak in conversational tones. When to have sexual relations with their partner is probably best decided on an individual patient basis. Although these guidelines are conservative, they provide a basis on which patients can be encouraged to do more, especially if supervised. Formal cardiopulmonary exercise testing is generally not required but can be helpful in patients being evaluated for heart transplantation.

**Key Point: The ability to provide multidisciplinary interventions with frequent patient follow-up, either in the office or by telephone with rapid access to medical care if the patient's condition should change, is an ideal that cannot always be achieved in practice within current health care systems. The importance of the personal and economic burden of heart failure to patients and society, as well as its increase over the next few decades, should spur health-care organizations to consider the economic benefits of interventions that can reduce hospitalizations and improve patients' functional capacity and quality of life in their home environment.**

## INHIBITORS AND ANTAGONISTS OF THE RENIN-ANGIOTENSIN-ALDOSTERONE SYSTEM

### Angiotensin-Converting Enzyme Inhibitors

The principal mechanism of action of ACE inhibitors is to inhibit the formation of angiotensin II, which results in less vasoconstriction and less aldosterone production with consequently less salt and water retention (Fig. 1–26). The myocardial and connective tissue growth effects of angiotensin II are also prevented, as is the effect of angiotensin II on apoptosis (cell suicide) and progressive myocyte loss. Less angiotensin II will also decrease sympathetic stimulation and arginine vasopressin release. Despite long-term ACE inhibitor therapy, angiotensin II concentrations can gradually increase through alternative pathways for production, but the clinical significance is not known. The ACE enzyme is also kininase II, which causes the breakdown of bradykinin to inactive fragments. ACE inhibition therefore results in increased bradykinin with increased vasodilatation, prostaglandin formation, and nitric oxide production. This additional vasodilatation is helpful, but the magnitude of its contribution to clinical outcomes is not known, and debate persists with regard to the significance of aspirin on this mechanism (see below). The accumulation of bradykinin is also believed to cause bronchial irritation and cough.

The use of ACE inhibitors has become the cornerstone in the management of systolic heart failure over the last decade. This is because many small- to moderate-sized trials have shown improvement in hemodynamics, symptoms, and exercise performance of patients and several large landmark clinical trials have demonstrated improved survival (The CONSENSUS Trial Study Group 1987; The SOLVD Investigators 1991; Cohn et al. 1991). ACE inhibitors are, therefore, recommended in all heart failure patients with significant systolic dysfunction (usually defined as LVEF <35–40% or a left ventricular end diastolic dimension by echo of >60 mm) if there are no contraindications such as previous angioedema in response to an ACE inhibitor, shock, significant hyperkalemia, significant unilateral or bilateral renal artery stenosis, or severe aortic stenosis. The last two conditions should be corrected before the use of ACE inhibitors. In both situations less severe disease is not an absolute contraindication but ACE inhibitors should be used with caution and should be monitored closely to avoid significant deterioration in renal function or presyncope/syncope, respectively. ACE inhibitors are also indicated for asymptomatic but significant systolic dysfunction, and they can be used in diastolic dysfunction in which they are effective to control blood pressure and cause regression of left ventricular hypertrophy (see the hypertension section of this chapter). However, in diastolic dysfunction, they are not yet considered mandatory but are considered an appropriate and effective treatment along with other drugs and the choice is often made on the basis of comorbid conditions such as ischemic heart disease, renal dysfunction, diabetes, or arrhythmias. Many ACE inhibitors are available for use (Table 1-33) and questions remain as to which one, which dose, and which dosing interval.

With regard to whether one ACE inhibitor is better than the other, enalapril, captopril, lisinopril, ramipril, and trandolapril have been studied in large mortality trials to treat or prevent heart failure. For these drugs, we know the doses that are effective in improving survival. All of the ACE inhibitors have similar hemodynamic effects and benefits on major surrogate endpoints such as symptoms or exercise capacity. It is, therefore, generally assumed that they are all effective in the management of systolic heart failure. Additional properties that have been demonstrated include a reduction in the risk of MI [this has been seen in several of the large clinical trials (Lonn and Yusuf 1994) and has been independently and prospectively investigated in the HOPE and PEACE studies using ramipril and trandolapril, respectively], improvement in endothelial function (e.g., this has been demonstrated for quinapril in the TREND study [Mancini et al. 1996]), and a reduction in sudden death (e.g., trandolapril in the TRACE study [Kober et al. 1995]). It is likely that these additional benefits, either potential or proven, apply to most ACE inhibitors. Some adverse effects are common to all ACE inhibitors and include angioedema, cough, hypotension and renal dysfunction, though the last two mentioned are often predictable and potentially avoidable in many patients with careful adjustment of diuretic dose.

With regard to which dose is appropriate, this is an issue of considerable clinical importance, since the doses used in clinical practice are generally lower than those used in the major clinical trials. One point of view would be that, if the physician wishes to translate the benefits of a clinical trial to an individual patient, it is necessary to use the doses that were proven to be beneficial in that clinical trial. However, clinical trials by design tend to use relatively large doses in an attempt to ensure a potential benefit and to avoid the possibility of not showing a benefit of an effective drug because the dose chosen was too low. Also, in clinical practice, physicians tend to use lower doses to avoid a perceived risk of adverse effects

**Table 1-33 Angiotensin-Converting Enzyme Inhibitors Commonly Used for Chronic Heart Failure Treatment**

| Drug | Usual starting dose (mg) | Dose range | Time to onset (h) | Peak effect (h) | $T_{1/2}$ (h) | Prodrug | Route of elimination |
|---|---|---|---|---|---|---|---|
| Captopril | 6.25 | 6.25–50 mg tid | 0.3 | 1 | 2 | N | Renal |
| Enalapril maleate | 2.5 | 2.5–20 mg bid | 1 | 4–6 | 11 | Y | Renal |
| Lisinopril | 2.5 | 5–35 mg/day | 1 | 4–6 | 13 | N | Renal |
| Ramipril | 2.5 | 5–10 mg bid | 1–2 | 3–6 | 12 | Y | R+H 70/30 |
| Quinapril | 5 | 10–20 mg bid | 1 | 4 | 3 | Y | Renal |
| Trandolapril | 1 | 1–4 mg/day | 2 | 6–8 | 16–24 | Y | R+H 30/70 |

ABBREVIATIONS: R+ H, renal + hepatic.

and may not adequately adjust the dose of diuretics that could often help to prevent adverse effects such as hypotension or renal dysfunction. If the patient improves symptomatically then the physician may be satisfied. This is not an adequate treatment endpoint since many trials have not shown a good association between short-term improvement in symptoms and long-term improvement in survival. Two trials have addressed the appropriate dose of ACE inhibitors. The NETWORK study, of 1532 patients with clinical heart failure but not limited to predominantly systolic dysfunction, found no differences between enalapril 2.5, 5, and 10 bid in the incidence of the primary endpoint of mortality, heart failure–related hospitalization, or worsening heart failure, but followed patients for only 6 months (The NETWORK Investigators 1998a). The ATLAS study of 3,164 patients has recently been published in which 2.5 to 5 mg of lisinopril was compared with 32.5 to 35 mg daily over 5 years of follow-up (ATLAS investigators 1999). The trial showed no differences in mortality, though there was a small nonsignificant trend in favor of the higher dose lisinopril. The higher dose lisinopril was significantly better at reducing hospitalizations and was as well tolerated as the low dose when the patients were followed carefully within the context of the clinical trial and by experienced physicians and nurses. At this time, therefore, dosages for patients should continue to be titrated toward the clinical trial doses of ACE inhibitor with appropriate reductions in diuretic dosage if required. Although neither the ATLAS nor NETWORK trial were placebo-controlled, even small doses of ACE inhibitors appeared to have an acceptably comparable survival outcome, which provides reassurance that, if a patient cannot tolerate higher doses of an ACE inhibitor, even low doses may provide benefit.

Apart from the previously mentioned clinical situations of lower blood pressure and renal dysfunction, in which lower doses of ACE inhibitors may be required despite optimization of diuretic dosing, lower doses of ACE inhibitors may cause renal dysfunction in small elderly women in whom the serum creatinine may not be an adequate reflection of the glomerular filtration rate because of their small lean body mass. None of the large clinical trials adjusted the dose based on body mass. Higher doses may be required in patients with poorly controlled hypertension (see the hypertension section of this chapter) or significant mitral regurgitation (see below). ACE inhibitors should be introduced in low doses in patients who are considered unstable, have hypotension, have had recent increases in diuretic dose, or are suspected of having renal artery stenosis or aortic valve stenosis (if severe, ACE inhibitors should be avoided). Since it is a goal of treatment to have patients accept an ACE inhibitor and continue treatment indefinitely, it is important to optimize the conditions under which the drug is introduced so that patients develop confidence in it and do not subsequently believe that they are intolerant because of an acute lowering of blood pressure or worsening renal function.

Debate persists as to whether there are advantages or disadvantages in short-acting versus long-acting ACE inhibitors. Both have been shown to have beneficial effects on symptoms and mortality. Theoretical considerations are that short-acting drugs may produce greater acute peak effects, but may not adequately inhibit the renin-angiotensin system over a 24-hour period, and may be less forgiving if a dose is missed. Possible advantages of long-acting medications are that there may be better patient concordance with the treatment regimen especially since they are likely to be taking other drugs. Long-acting drugs may provide better inhibition of angiotensin II formation and may give a more gradual and better tolerated peak effect. From a practical standpoint, a single dose may be given at bed time when peak hemodynamic effects of diuretics will not occur simultaneously and when a subsequent decrease in blood pressure is unlikely to be symptomatic. Currently the choice is made on individual physician and patient preferences that include the familiarity of a physician with the titration of a particular drug to appropriate doses and, at times, patient preferences for a medication that may be available in a generic form and is therefore cheaper. Patients who are still at work, or are frequently out of their home during the middle of the day, may be more likely to miss a midday dose of medication, and this should be taken into account. Some physicians prefer to give a short-acting ACE inhibitor when it is being introduced to patients with a lower blood pressure, so that any hypotensive effect is short-lived, and they can monitor the response over a reasonable period of time in their outpatient clinic.

#### *Chronic symptomatic systolic heart failure*

Angiotensin-converting enzyme inhibitors are recommended in all patients if there are no contraindications. The CONSENSUS, SOLVD (Studies of Left Ventricular Dysfunction), and VHeft trials established the effectiveness of ACE inhibitors over placebo and other effective vasodilators (The CONSENSUS Trial Study Group 1987; The SOLVD Investigators 1991; Cohn et al. 1991). Treatment improves survival, reduces heart failure hospitalizations, and decreases symptoms. Enalapril was studied in all three trials. Treatment should be continued indefinitely unless newer therapies are proven to be better.

**Key Point: All patients with symptomatic LV systolic dysfunction should receive ACE inhibitors as primary therapy to improve survival and to reduce heart failure symptoms and hospitalizations, if no contraindication exists. The dose should be titrated toward that used in clinical trials. If adverse effects occur, patients should remain on an ACE inhibitor where possible, but at a lower dose.**

***Asymptomatic left ventricular systolic dysfunction***

The SOLVD prevention study demonstrated a trend for improved survival and a definite decrease in heart failure hospitalizations when patients were treated with enalapril over 5 years of follow-up (The SOLVD Investigators 1992). This well-designed clinical trial has established the role and indication for ACE inhibitors in people with very mild symptoms or asymptomatic systolic dysfunction with LVEF <35%. It is recommended that all such patients should be treated with an ACE inhibitor if there is no contraindication.

**Key Point: All patients with significant LV systolic dysfunction (e.g., LVEF <35%), even if asymptomatic, should be treated with ace inhibitors if no contraindication exists.**

***Left ventricular dysfunction or heart failure after myocardial infarction***

The goal of the prevention or treatment of heart failure after MI is to minimize the size of the infarct with thrombolysis, to reduce ischemia, to prevent extension of the infarct, to reduce expansion of the infarct, and to prevent remodeling of the ventricular cavity thus maintaining the more elliptical rather than a spherical shape of the ventricle in the long term.

A variety of ACE inhibitor strategies has been addressed in large clinical trials, and most are effective. After myocardial infarction, ACE inhibitors have been shown to be complementary to the benefits of $\beta$-adrenergic receptor antagonists, and they therefore can be used in combination (Vantrimpont et al. 1997). It is recommended that ACE inhibitors be introduced in patients post-MI who have heart failure during their MI or have significant left ventricular systolic dysfunction by echo or radionuclide angiography (LVEF ≤40%). ACE inhibitors should be introduced in low doses early after MI and should be titrated over a course of days to weeks toward clinical trial doses (ACE Inhibitor Myocardial Infarction Collaborative Group 1998b). If significant LV dysfunction persists in the outpatient clinic, then the ACE inhibitor should be continued indefinitely.

This recommendation is based on the following trials. The SAVE (Survival And Ventricular Enlargement) trial introduced captopril at a mean of 10 days after MI in patients with an LVEF less than 40% who were free of heart failure at the time of randomization (Pfeffer et al. 1992). It was the first post-MI ACE inhibitor trial to show benefits on morbidity and mortality. The TRACE (TRandolapril And Cardiac Evaluation trial) used echocardiography to identify patients and found comparable results (Kober et al. 1995). The AIRE (Acute Infarction Ramipril Evaluation) trial enrolled patients with clinical heart failure at the time of their infarct without a prior need to document left ventricular function and showed benefit (The AIRE Study Investigators 1993) that persisted in the AIREX study (Hall et al. 1997). These results are supported by the SMILE (Survival of Myocardial Infarction Long-term Evaluation) study (early introduction of zofenopril to patients with acute anterior infarction and not receiving thrombolysis) (Ambrosiori et al. 1995) and the Chinese cardiac study (early introduction of captopril in patients with suspected acute infarction) (Chinese Cardiac Study Collaborative Group 1995b). The GISSI-3 (Gruppo Italiano per lo Studio della Sopravvivenza nell'Infarto Miocardico 1994; Gruppo Italiano per lo Studio della Sopravvivenza nell'Infarto Miocardico 1996) and ISIS-4 (ISIS-4 Collaborative Group 1995a) trials introduced oral ACE inhibitors to all patients within 24 hours of their MI and showed small but significant decreases in 30-day mortality. The last two studies together showed that the majority of lives saved were saved within the first week of treatment, which supports the early introduction of ACE inhibitors (Latini et al. 1995; Pfeffer et al. 1995; ACE Inhibitor Myocardial Infarction Collaborative Group 1998b). The HEART (Healing and Early Afterload Reducing Therapy) trial compared a strategy of early low doses of ramipril with early titrated high doses of ramipril with delayed (14 days) high doses of ramipril (Pfeffer et al. 1997). Early introduction of titrated high doses of ramipril provided echocardiographic benefit and similar results were obtained in CATS (Captopril And Thrombolysis Study, van Gilst 1996). The early introduction of low doses with titration to higher doses as the patient's clinical condition allows is the preferred option since the CONSENSUS II study showed that intravenous doses of enalaprilat within 24 hours of MI can lower blood pressure significantly with potential adverse events (Swedberg et al. 1992).

> **Key Point: In addition to other proven therapies, ACE inhibitors should be introduced in low doses in the first few days after MI, and titrated to higher doses over several days as clinical condition allows, in patients with heart failure or poor systolic function.**

### *Reduction of myocardial infarction and prevention of heart failure*

When ACE inhibitors were first studied in patients with LV systolic dysfunction, treatment unexpectedly reduced the risk of myocardial infarction by 23%, independent of LVEF, cause of heart disease, use of other medications, diabetes status, and blood pressure (Yusuf et al. 1992, Pfeffer et al. 1992, Lonn et al. 1994). The HOPE (Heart Outcomes Prevention Evaluation 2000) study prospectively tested the ability of an ACE inhibitor, ramipril, to reduce the composite clinical outcome of cardiovascular death, myocardial infarction, or stroke, as well as each outcome separately in 9541 high-risk patients (55 years or older) without evidence of LV systolic dysfunction. The results have recently been published and conclusively demonstrated that ramipril 10 mg OD reduced the composite primary outcome by 22%, cardiovascular death by 25%, myocardial infarction by 20%, and stroke by 31%, all with a very high level of statistical significance (HOPE investigators, 2000). The results could not be fully attributed to the small observed decrease in blood pressure and were consistent amongst the broad range of patients in different subgroups including patients with diabetes.

Prevention of myocardial infarction will prevent LV systolic dysfunction and the HOPE study also demonstrated a significant reduction (22%) in the risk of developing heart failure. These combined observations will broaden the indications for ramipril, a long acting ACE inhibitor, to move patients at high risk of cardiovascular clinical events. Whether the results apply to other ACE inhibitors or patients at lower risk is currently being prospectively evaluated in clinical trials such as PEACE.

> **Key Point: A very large clinical trial has clearly demonstrated that ramipril 10 mg OD can reduce the risk of developing heart failure in a broad spectrum of high-risk patients with cardiovascular disease but without known LV systolic dysfunction.**

## Modifying the Effects of Angiotensin-Converting Enzyme Inhibitors

### *Combination of ACE inhibitor and neutral endopeptidase inhibitor*

Both neutral endopeptidase (NEP) and ACE are cell-surface metalloproteases with structural similarities at interactive sites. NEP inactivates bradykinin and atrial natriuretic peptide (ANP), therefore a NEP inhibitor prevents the breakdown of both these compounds, potentiating their biological actions. In addition to vasodilatation, ANP also has natriuretic and antiproliferative properties. Some new drugs (e.g., omepatrilat) have been developed that inhibit both ACE and NEP and offer a broader modulation of neurohormones than ACE inhibitors alone. Initial small clinical trials are promising, but the true role of these compounds in the future treatment of heart failure awaits longer-term outcomes of clinical trials. At least in theory, they represent a potential advance over ACE inhibitors.

### *Angiotensin receptor blockers (ARB)*

As stated above, angiotensin II concentrations can accumulate in patients receiving chronic treatment with ACE inhibitors. This is believed to be principally because of alternative pathways by which angiotensin II can be produced. Several enzymes are potentially important in this regard, although the one that has received the most attention to date is chymase. It may be particularly important in the heart, though its direct contribution to the production of angiotensin II in a normal heart has been variously estimated depending on the techniques used. It does appear, however, that its activity may be upregulated in heart failure, which might make it of increasing importance. An ARB, which would block the action of angiotensin II on the $AT_1$ receptor, would therefore be effective independent of the route through which angiotensin II is produced, giving more complete blockade of the actions of angiotensin II. Two potential limitations might decrease this benefit. First, ACE inhibitors also increase vasodilatation through bradykinins, prostaglandins, and nitric oxide mechanisms. ARBs would not share this possible benefit but as stated previously, the magnitude of this benefit has remained unclear. Second, the other major angiotensin receptor in humans is the $AT_2$ receptor. Selective ARBs will block negative feedback to the production of angiotensin II, which will therefore circulate in higher concentrations and be free to stimulate the $AT_2$ receptor. The function of the $AT_2$ receptor was unknown until recently, but it appears to have antigrowth effects that counteract the growth and proliferative effects of $AT_1$-receptor stimulation. Therefore, it remains possible that increased $AT_2$-receptor stimulation might actually be beneficial.

Two studies have been published on clinical outcomes in heart failure patients treated with ARBs. The ELITE (Evaluation of Losartan In The Elderly) trial studied more than 700 patients over the age of 65 with symptomatic heart failure who had not previously been treated with an ACE inhibitor (Pitt et al. 1997). Patients were randomized to receive either captopril 50 mg orally t.i.d. or losartan 50 mg orally daily. Although the primary outcome of changes in serum creatinine was not different between the groups, a surprising improvement in survival was seen in the group treated with losartan and this was attributed principally to a reduction in sudden death. Losartan was better tolerated than captopril, and this has been a consistent finding with the ARBs as a class. The total number of events in the trial was small, and therefore, these results were provocative and exciting.

The ELITE-2 trial of 3152 patients was designed to closely duplicate the ELITE trial and confirm losartan as being more effective and better tolerated than captopril. However, in contrast to the original ELITE trial, losartan was not shown to be superior to captopril though it was better tolerated (results presented at AHA annual meeting, Nov. 1999). This calls into question some of the theoretical advantages of ARBs over ACE inhibitors but more trials are required with other ARBs and in a broader range of heart failure patients.

**Key Point: ACE inhibitors remain the therapy of choice in patients with systolic heart failure though ARBs may be considered in patients who are truly intolerant to ACE inhibitors for reasons such as angioedema or cough. Every effort should be made to safely continue patients on ACE inhibitors whenever possible.**

Theoretically, a combination of ACE inhibitors and ARBs may give more complete blockade of the renin–angiotensin system. This was prospectively tested in the RESOLVD (Randomized Evaluation of Strategies for Left Ventricular Dysfunction) pilot study, which investigated dose-response relationships between an ACE inhibitor, enalapril, alone or in combination with an ARB, candesartan (RESOLVD Pilot Study Investigator, 1999). Unlike losartan, which is a competitive antagonist, candesartan has been called an "insurmountable" antagonist, as it decreases the maximum response to angiotensin II and has a prolonged duration of effect at the receptor level. This study was designed as a dose-ranging study for safety and was not powered to detect significant changes in clinical events. Overall, it appeared that the combination of the two drugs together was better than either alone in terms of ventricular dilatation and its surrogate marker, plasma brain natriuretic peptide (BNP). At this point in time, combination therapy cannot be recommended in routine clinical practice until further safety data and long-term trials are performed and some are currently ongoing (e.g., VAL-HEFT, which is a placebo-controlled trial of valsartan plus ACE inhibitors in patients with New York Heart Association class II to IV heart failure, and CHARM which is evaluating candesartan plus ACE inhibitors in a very broad range of patients not just with systolic heart failure but also with diastolic heart failure, and candesartan vs placebo in patients intolerant of ACE inhibitors). Similar trials with ARBs are also being conducted in post-MI patients (e.g., OPTIMAAL with losartan and VALIANT with volsartan).

An additional randomization was performed at the end of the RESOLVD pilot study trial to look at the further safety and benefits of metoprolol. This represents an ongoing direction of heart failure management, blocking neurohormonal activation on several fronts concurrently.

**PRINCIPLE The theoretic or intellectual appeal of a new drug must be balanced against the enormous usefulness of meaningful data that have been acquired during the use of "standard" therapy.**

***Renin inhibitors***

These have been investigated in small trials of heart failure, but currently no compounds have been released with an indication for management of heart failure (Kleinert 1995; Lin and Frishman 1996).

## Aldosterone Antagonists

Aldosterone production is increased in heart failure and promotes salt and water retention and myocardial fibrosis. A large survival trial, RALES (Randomized Aldactone Longevity Evaluation Study), studied the addition of spironolactone 25–50 mg OD to standard therapy with ACE inhibitors and diuretics in 1663 patients with severe heart failure, NYHA class III–IV at enrollment but who had NYHA Class IV symptoms in the previous 6 months, with serum potassium less than 5 mmol/L and creatinine less than 221 mmol/L (Pitt et al. 1999). Total mortality was significantly reduced by 30% and represented a reduction in both sudden death and death from progressive heart failure. Hospitalization for heart failure was reduced 35% and symptoms of heart failure improved. Gynecomastia or breast pain occurred in 10% of men on spironolactone. The incidence of serious hyperkalemia was minimal in both groups. At 2 years of follow up, the mean daily dose of spironolactone was 26 mg. These important results support the more widespread addition of low doses of spironolactone to ACE inhibition in patients with severe systolic heart failure and stable renal function. The benefits were consistent among subgroups and the survival curves began to separate early at 3 months. Other aldosterone antagonists without side-effects of gynecomastia, e.g., eplerenone, are currently being investigated.

**Key Point: Low-dose spironolactone should be considered, in addition to ACE inhibition, in patients with severe chronic systolic heart failure.**

## SYMPATHETIC ANTAGONISTS

The most widely studied sympathetic antagonists are $\beta$-adrenergic receptor antagonists (beta blockers), which have a variety of ancillary properties but are most commonly distinguished by being either $\beta_1$-adrenergic receptor antagonists (cardioselective), or $\beta_1$- and $\beta_2$-adrenergic receptor antagonists (nonselective). Some are also vasodilators, others combine alpha receptor blockade, and most recently an additional antioxidant property has been proposed to be of importance. Clearly, $\beta$-adrenergic receptor antagonists are an important drug where hypertension, ischemia, or arrhythmias are the etiology or precipitating aggravating factors in the development of heart failure. Currently some beta blockers are recommended in treatment of stable mild-to-moderate systolic heart failure (see below) and in acute left ventricular systolic dysfunction associated with MI (see section on acute myocardial infarction of this chapter). However, their introduction and use in heart failure requires closer initial monitoring than with ACE inhibitors with which they should be used in combination rather than as a substitute. Increased awareness of how they should be prescribed should increase their safety profile and wider acceptance.

Several large clinical trials have firmly established the benefits of beta blockers acutely in MI and also to prevent complications after MI (see section on acute myocardial infarction of this chapter). Indeed, those patients with evidence of heart failure at the time of their myocardial infarction or with the worst heart function seem to get at least as much benefit and perhaps more. However, since patients with acute pulmonary edema are dependent on sympathetic activation to increase heart rate and to maintain blood pressure to vital organs, it is widely recognized that acute use of beta blockers in this scenario or in unstable heart failure will cause acute worsening of the heart failure condition. Because of this, it at first appears counterintuitive that they would be helpful in the long-term management of chronic heart failure. Activation of the sympathetic nervous system is prominent in patients with heart failure and when marked, is associated as a strong indicator of worse prognosis. Chronic overactivation of the sympathetic nervous system will cause vasoconstriction and increase afterload on the heart, which, along with increased heart rate, will be an additional burden on the failing pump. In severe cases of catecholamine toxicity, direct myocardial damage has been recognized for some time, but recently the role of the sympathetic nervous system in contributing to the state of oxidative stress in the myocardium and contributing to apoptosis has attracted a lot of research.

The cardioselective $\beta$-adrenergic receptor antagonist, metoprolol, has been the beta blocker studied over the longest period of time in chronic systolic heart failure (Table 1-34). The fact that the medication was studied carefully over many years has substantially contributed to our knowledge of how to safely use it. Beta blockers should be started in low doses and increased gradually under close supervision. Over a period of weeks to months, doses can be substantially increased. During the first months of therapy, depending on the patient's condition and the rapidity with which the dose is increased, there is a likelihood that some patients will notice some worsening in their heart failure symptoms as a result of the pharmacologic effect of the beta-blocker action to depress cardiac function. The patient should be educated that this is not unexpected. The dose of diuretic can be increased, and further increases to $\beta$-adrenergic receptor antagonist should be postponed until the patient's condition is again stable. In the long term, beta blockers have a biological benefit on heart function with an improvement in the left ventricular ejection fraction, reduction in hospitalizations for heart failure, and improved survival. Because of their beta-blocking effects on heart rate, they may not always cause an early improvement in functional capacity. Although the metoprolol in dilated cardiomyopathy (MDC) trial showed reduction in the need for transplantation (Waagstein et al. 1993), it is recommended that they be

Table 1-34 β-Adrenergic Receptor Antagonists Commonly Used for Chronic Heart Failure Treatment

| | Usual starting dose (mg) | Dose range | $T_{1/2}$ (h) | $\beta_1$ Receptor selectivity | $\alpha$ Receptor blockade | PAA | Renal excretion | Liver metabolism |
|---|---|---|---|---|---|---|---|---|
| Metoprolol succinate | 5 bid | 50–75 mg bid | 3–7 | ++ | 0 | 0 | N | Y |
| Carvedilol | 3.125 bid | 25 mg bid | 7–10 | 0 | ++ | 0 | N | Y |
| Bisoprolol | 1.25 daily | 1.25–5 mg od | 10–12 | ++ | 0 | 0 | Y | Y |

ABBREVIATIONS: PAA, partial agonist activity.

introduced mainly in patients with mild to moderate disease and only in patients who are stable. Therefore, the ideal patient would more likely be a stable outpatient rather than a patient acutely admitted to the hospital for severe heart failure. At this time, patients with more than moderate symptoms and a marked reduction in left ventricular ejection fraction may be best evaluated for the appropriateness of beta-blocker therapy by a physician with a special interest in heart failure. The trials that support this approach to decrease mortality are the U.S. carvedilol trials (Packer, Bristow, et al. 1996), the Australian/New Zealand carvedilol trial in patients with ischemic heart disease (Australia/New Zealand Heart Failure Research Collaborative Group 1997b), and the recently completed CIBIS-II study with bisoprolol in 2667 patients (CIBIS-II Investigators, 1999) and the MERIT-HF study with metoprolol CR/XL in 3991 patients (MERIT-HF Study Group, 1999) which were discontinued early because of a beneficial effect on survival. While both trials attempted to include sicker patients with NYHA class 3–4 heart failure, the placebo mortality rates were less than in the recently presented BEST trial with bucindolol in 2708 patients (Eichhorn et al. 1999) which was also stopped early but because of an inability to clearly slow overall benefit in favor of bucindolol. Whether this represents differences between beta blockers or differences between study populations is not known but they are most appropriately used in combination with ACE inhibitors in patients with chronic stable heart failure and, as yet, should not be routinely used in the much sicker population. Other trials are ongoing, e.g., carvedilol versus metoprolol in heart failure (COMET), carvedilol in patients with severe heart failure (COPERNICUS) and carvedilol after MI (CAPRICORN).

**WARNING** β-Adrenergic receptor antagonists should not currently be introduced in patients with severe or unstable heart failure.

Carvedilol is of interest since, in addition to being a nonselective β-adrenergic receptor blocker, it is an alpha blocker and may therefore give more broad-based sympathetic antagonism, but is also a significant antioxidant, which could help to decrease oxidative stress and to reduce apoptosis though the clinical significance of this and its quantification is as yet uncertain. Its alpha-blocking properties may allow a reduction in afterload at the time that the beta-blocker effects depress LV function, and this may be helpful. However, the alpha-blocking properties may also cause hypotension, and the clinician is therefore challenged to determine whether the hypotension is due to the alpha-blocking effects, requiring a reduction in diuretic dose, or the beta-blocking effects to depress LV function, in which case a diuretic dose may need increasing. Hence the current need to use carvedilol and other beta blockers in stable patients, to increase the dose gradually, to maintain close follow-up, and to be familiar with the assessment and treatment of heart failure patients. When ACE inhibitors were first introduced in the treatment of heart failure, caution was advised but appropriate education of physicians and patients has led to their widespread use and recommendation as first-line therapy to be introduced in the primary-care physician's office. Early concerns about adverse effects have lingered and may currently contribute to some underutilization of ACE inhibitors; the same scenario may unfold with the use of sympathetic antagonists.

If a patient develops adverse effects to the sympathetic antagonist, the patient can be instructed to go back to the previous tolerated dose and to be seen in outpatient clinic or office. The physician may then wish to adjust any other therapy and halve the next dose increment. As such, the dosing intervals for these agents can be individualized to the patient's condition and response though, in most instances, target doses are achieved in 6–12 weeks.

Because of the known effects of acute administration of beta blockers to worsen acute heart failure, it has been commonplace to automatically stop beta-blocker therapy if the patient is admitted to the hospital with heart failure. This may not, however, be a logical automatic response. $\beta$-Adrenergic receptor antagonists are known to cause rebound neurohormonal activation if stopped suddenly, but this has not been carefully evaluated in heart failure patients. Second, there is now strong clinical evidence for the benefit of beta blockers in chronic heart failure to improve survival and to reduce hospitalizations. However, no drugs, including ACE inhibitors, will abolish heart failure hospital admissions. Therefore, a hospital admission does not automatically imply the failure of that therapy since the sympathetic antagonist may have already reduced the number of admissions in that patient. Nonetheless, common sense would dictate that if the patient is in acute severe heart failure, the dose of beta blocker could be reduced, then held until their condition restabilizes. Phosphodiesterase inhibitors, such as milrinone or amrinone, should be used as intravenous positive inotropes, if required, instead of catecholamines whose actions could be blocked by the $\beta$-adrenergic receptor antagonist. If the drug is discontinued, this should be viewed as temporary and consideration should be given to reintroducing medication once the acute event has stabilized. In patients with a less severe acute exacerbation of heart failure, the dose of beta blocker may be reduced but not discontinued, and heart failure may be treated with diuretics and nitrates and optimization of other medications. If the exacerbation is mild, then the beta blocker may be continued at its previous dose and the diuretic dose increased. The most common contraindications to $\beta$-adrenergic receptor antagonists in heart failure apart from pulmonary edema or very severe heart failure, are severe reactive airways disease or symptomatic bradycardia or heart block.

**Key Point: $\beta$-Adrenergic receptor antagonists are indicated in stable patients with chronic systolic heart failure and mild to moderate symptoms while following standard heart failure treatment including ACE inhibitors. A low dose should be introduced, then titrated slowly over several weeks with close follow-up.**

Centrally acting alpha agonists will reduce sympathetic outflow, and clonidine has been shown in very small trials to have some hemodynamic benefit, but large clinical trials have not been performed because of its other adverse effects of sedation and depression. Moxonidine is an imidazoline agonist and also reduces central sympathetic outflow. It has been investigated in heart failure (MOXCON study) but the trial was discontinued because of early adverse events probably because of the choice of too high a dose.

## OTHER DRUG TREATMENTS FOR HEART FAILURE

### Other Vasodilator Drugs

Hydralazine and nitrates are of importance because they were the first vasodilators tested that were shown to be better than placebo in improving survival in heart failure (Cohn et al. 1986). However, most other pure vasodilators have not been helpful, and indeed, some such as prostacyclin have been harmful. Subsequent studies have shown ACE inhibitors to be better than a combination of hydralazine and nitrates (Cohn et al. 1991), which remain a second-line choice in patients who cannot tolerate ACE inhibitors (Johnstone et al. 1994; ACC/AHA guidelines, Williams et al. 1995). There is a growing clinical consensus that an ARB may be a preferable second-line choice to hydralazine and nitrates (except in the setting of renal dysfunction), but there are no trials that have compared the two. The doses aimed for in the VHeft I and VHeft II trials were hydralazine 75 qid and isosorbide dinitrate 40 mg orally qid, but the combination of hydralazine and nitrates often was not well tolerated by patients because of frequent adverse effects.

Nitrates alone have not been adequately tested to determine whether they have an additional effect on mortality in chronic heart failure but do provide additional benefits with respect to symptoms and signs of heart failure when used alone or in combination with ACE inhibitors (Elkayam et al. 1999). They have the advantage that they can be used as sublingual tablet or spray for short-term relief of acute exertional dyspnea, as oral long-acting tablet formulations, as transdermal preparations in people who dislike taking tablets, with the advantage that the patch can be wiped off when the effect is achieved or adverse effect occurs, and as intravenous solution for acute pulmonary edema. Furthermore, since at least two-thirds of patients with heart failure have ischemic heart disease, nitrates are clearly useful to improve ischemia and have advantages over some anti-ischemic therapies that have negative inotropic effects. Multiple modes of administration, along with patient flexibility and self-administration, and the anti-ischemic effects of nitrates, make them widely used and recommended as additional vasodilating therapy. The dose can be titrated to therapeutic response, but an 8- to 12-hour nitrate-free interval is recommended to avoid the development of tolerance.

## Diuretics

Loop diuretics such as furosemide and ethacrynic acid primarily inhibit reabsorption of $Na^+$ and $Cl^-$ in the thick ascending limb of the loop of Henle. Bumetanide may have an additional action on the proximal tubule but does not appear to act on the distal tubule and is more chloruretic. Torsemide acts mainly on the ascending limb of the loop of Henle. Thiazide diuretics inhibit reabsorption of $Na^+$ and $Cl^-$ in the distal tubules. Spironolactone blocks aldosterone receptors in the distal nephron and collecting ducts, which are also the site of action of other $K^+$-sparing diuretics that block $Na^+$ exchange with $K^+$ and $H^+$ (see chapter 6, Renal Disorders and the Influence of Renal Function on Drug Disposition).

Diuretics can clearly save lives when used in acute pulmonary edema but there are no long-term mortality trials demonstrating improved survival in chronic heart failure. Nonetheless, they are very effective for treating the signs and symptoms of heart failure and thus are widely used. Since their action is complementary to that of digoxin and other drugs used in the treatment of heart failure, they are used in combination with these drugs and are not used alone for treatment of chronic heart failure. They are effective in controlling the signs and symptoms in both systolic and diastolic heart failure. They are indicated in all patients who have current or previous evidence of systemic or pulmonary congestion. An occasional patient with low cardiac filling pressures, low cardiac output, and no current or past evidence of systemic or pulmonary congestion, can sometimes be treated without concomitant diuretic therapy. The dose of diuretic should be tailored to the individual patient with the endpoint of optimizing other drugs such as ACE inhibitors that have been shown to improve survival but to give additional help in normalizing cardiac filling pressures and controlling edema. The patient should be educated about signs and symptoms of congestion and, in conjunction with a low salt diet and at times reduced fluid intake, the patient may take an additional dose of the diuretic or a single dose of another diuretic in combination if their daily morning weight increases by 3 pounds or more. Most of the guidelines for the use of diuretics are derived from clinician consensus and small clinical trials. However, RALES (see above) has demonstrated a survival benefit for low dose spironolactone (25–50 mg OD) when added to ACE inhibitor therapy in patients with severe heart failure.

Where symptoms and signs of congestion are very mild, some patients may require only a very low dose of a diuretic such as hydrochlorothiazide (25 to 50 mg orally daily), furosemide (20 mg orally daily), or bumetanide (0.5 mg daily) (Table 1-35). To avoid the potassium-lowering effects of diuretics, combination diuretics containing triamterene, amiloride, or spironolactone appear logical, but should be used cautiously, since the patients should also be on an ACE inhibitor, which will help to conserve potassium and may cause hyperkalemia in combination with a potassium-sparing diuretic. An occasional patient can maintain normal fluid balance with a diuretic every second or third day but, for simplicity of drug regimen, in most cases diuretics are given on a daily basis. Convention is to take the diuretic in the morning though, in a stable patient, the timing could be changed to the afternoon or the evening if this is more socially acceptable because of planned activities. A disadvantage of the evening dose of diuretic is that it may have a prolonged effect causing nocturia and disturbed sleep. Some small studies of patient preference have suggested that the shorter-acting diuretic, bumetanide, appears to avoid this problem if taken in the evening when patients are at work during the day.

In most patients with moderate heart failure and chronic symptoms, a loop diuretic such as furosemide will be required, and a thiazide diuretic alone is insufficient. In the setting of renal dysfunction or failure, a loop diuretic would have to be introduced earlier and in higher doses to obtain an effective diuresis. Patients need to be reminded about the synergistic effect between diuretic and a low-salt diet. Physicians vary as to whether they would increase furosemide to 40 mg orally bid or to 80 mg orally daily. With a single morning dose, the diuresis may be more convenient for active patients, but the peak effect may occur concurrently with peak blood pressure lowering of ACE inhibitors, if also taken in the morning, causing postural hypotension. This can be circumvented by taking a long-acting ACE inhibitor at night. Twice-a-day dosing of furosemide may provide a gentler diuresis from the patient's perspective, but the second dose may sometimes be omitted or forgotten, the lower doses will be less effective in the setting of renal dysfunction, and the sec-

Table 1-35 Oral Diuretics Commonly Used for Chronic Heart Failure Treatment

| Drug | Usual Oral Starting Dose (mg) | Dose Range | Time to Onset of Diuresis (min) | Peak Effect (h) | (h) | Diuresis $T_{1/2}$ (min) | Comments |
|---|---|---|---|---|---|---|---|
| Furosemide | 40 | 20–250 | | 1–2 | 4–8 | 4 h | Flexible convenient dosing; ototoxicity at high doses; hypokalemia an adverse effect |
| Bumetanide | 1 | 0.5–4 | 30–60 | 1–2 | 4–6 | 60–90 | Shorter duration of action than other loop diuretics |
| Ethacrynic acid | 50 | 50–150 | <30 | 2 | 6–8 | 60 | Used if "resistance" to furosemide or sulfonamide allergy |
| Torsemide | 5 | 5–40 | <60 | 1–2 | 6–8 | 210 | Recently withdrawn from Canadian market |
| Hydrochlorothiazide | 50 | 25–100 | 120 | 4–6 | 6–12 | 5–15 | Flat dose–response curve; metabolic side effects at higher doses |
| Metolazone | 2.5 | 25–100 | 60 | 2 | 12–24 | NA | Combination with furosemide may give marked diuresis with decreased $K^+$, increased urea |
| Spironolactone | 25 | 25–50 | 24–48 hr | 2–3 days | 2–3 days | 20 h | May produce increased $K^+$ with ACE inhibitors, K supplements, and renal dysfunction; gynecomastia in men |

ond dose later in the day may contribute to nocturia unless taken in the early afternoon.

In severe heart failure, further increases in loop diuretics are frequently required despite optimal dosing with ACE inhibitors and digoxin. Since elevated filling pressures will continue to cause symptoms and increase wall stress with possible further progression of ventricular dilatation, an important goal of heart failure therapy is to normalize filling pressures and relieve congestion where possible (Stevenson et al. 1998). Once the dose of loop diuretic such as furosemide has been increased to ≥80 mg orally b.i.d., it is often appropriate to consider the addition of a second diuretic such as hydrochlorothiazide, metolazone, or spironolactone. This combination therapy may not be required on a chronic basis, but can be used for acute exacerbations, or periodically if the patient's daily home weight increases. Hydrochlorothiazide can be added in doses of 25 to 50 mg daily with good effect. If higher doses are required, it may be reasonable to consider metolazone in doses of 2.5, 5, or 10 mg daily. Since the synergistic effect of metolazone with a loop diuretic can be substantial, it is best to start with a dose of 2.5 mg and to adjust the dose daily, based on the morning weight. It is unusual for metolazone 10 mg orally daily to have to be continued long term. Chronic therapy with metolazone has the increased risk of overdiuresis and metabolic abnormalities, especially a low potassium. In general, it is advised to aim for a serum potassium ≥4.0 mEq/L to avoid the complications of hypokalemia including muscle cramps or fatigue, serious ventricular arrhythmias, and digoxin toxicity. When metolazone is used, additional potassium supplementation is indicated, and electrolytes and renal function should be measured more frequently. The patient who has to take doses on three or more consecutive days should at the physician's office have blood tests done and a full clinical assessment. Metolazone remains an excellent backup for the patient to have at home and is ideal for use as the occasion arises following careful education of the patient. Spironolactone should be strongly considered in all patients whose heart failure is worsening requiring increasing diuretics despite optimization of other drugs (see RALES above). Doses higher than 25–50 mg OD, in combination with ACE inhibitors or potassium supplements, increase the risk of hyperkalemia. Spironolactone may be particularly helpful in patients who tend to have low potassium, but electrolytes and renal function require closer monitoring. In patients with significant right-sided heart failure, spironolactone is helpful because of hyperaldosteronism, though diuresis is not as immediate as that achieved by metolazone.

**Key Point: Most patients with heart failure should be treated with diuretics, initially in low doses, but with appropriate dose increases or combination diuretics if symptoms and signs persist or progress.**

In patients with chronic gastric and hepatic congestion, anorexia is a problem and may be associated with poor absorption of diuretics leading to a vicious cycle of clinical deterioration (see chapter 6, Renal Disorders and the Influence of Renal Function on Drug Disposition). In these circumstances, intravenous diuretics are extremely helpful and necessary. Return of the patient's appetite is an excellent sign of the relieved congestion. A single intravenous dose of diuretic given in the emergency room may temporarily alleviate some symptoms and signs, but a longer course of intravenous therapy may be required to allow successful reinstitution of oral therapy and restabilization of signs and symptoms. Depending on clinical and social circumstances, this may be achieved as an outpatient, but frequently patients need to be admitted briefly. Chronic outpatient intravenous therapy through indwelling lines is rarely needed if other medications have also been optimized. The goal of therapy is to provide chronic stability of symptoms with lowered filling pressures. Removal of the need for recurring intravenous therapy is a sign of success.

In significant pulmonary edema or severe peripheral edema with ascites, large bolus doses of loop diuretics such as furosemide may cause significant fluid shifts and electrolyte abnormalities with clinical instability of blood pressure and potassium. Also, high-bolus plasma concentrations of furosemide carry an increased risk of ototoxicity. Intravenous infusions of furosemide can be used to lessen ototoxicity, to increase clinical stability, and to allow frequent dose adjustments over a short period of time to achieve and maintain an effective diuresis. Once again, electrolyte and renal function should be monitored closely. Potassium supplementation will be required, and if the patient continues to have symptoms or signs of low potassium, serum magnesium and calcium should also be checked and corrected if abnormal. This is often required before intracellular stores of potassium can be repleted.

Apparent "resistance" to diuretic therapy may be due to inadequate dosing or lack of appropriate combination therapy. However, chronic diuretic therapy does result in hypertrophy of the distal convoluted tubule, and therefore the dose of the diuretic may need to be increased. In some small studies, switching from furosemide to ethacrynic acid or bumetanide has been reported to be successful. Since it is the concentration of diuretics in the lumen of the loop of Henle that dictates the extent of diuresis, marked proteinuria, which binds furosemide in the lumen may decrease the diuresis. Other classes of diuretics such as carbonic acid anhydrase inhibitors are rarely used. If the patient continues to appear to be resistant to diuretics, then salt and fluid intake should be carefully reassessed in addition to the use of other drugs such as NSAIDs or licorice, or other causes of edema such as the nephrotic syndrome or peripheral venous disease.

## Digoxin

Digoxin inhibits the ($Na^+/K^+$)-ATPase pump and, in response, the cell exchanges calcium for sodium with the increased intracellular $Ca^{2+}$ enhancing excitation–contraction coupling. Digoxin also decreases sympathetic tone and increases vagal tone, probably by sensitization of baroreceptor function. The increased vagal tone and, to a lesser extent, digoxin's direct depression of AV nodal conduction both lead to a slowed ventricular response in atrial fibrillation.

Initial small clinical trials of digoxin gave conflicting results (Yusef et al. 1992). The use of digoxin varied widely between individual physicians, and practice patterns also varied considerably between different countries. Two larger studies looking at withdrawal of digoxin in patients with symptomatic systolic heart failure either not on ACE inhibitors (PROVED study) or on ACE inhibitors (RADIANCE study) were better designed and showed that stopping digoxin therapy was associated with a worsening of symptoms (Uretsky et al. 1993; Packer et al. 1993). Two other studies comparing digoxin with captopril and enalapril also showed benefits of digoxin therapy, though less than that seen with the ACE inhibitors (The Captopril-Digoxin Multicenter Research Group 1988; Davies et al. 1991).

The recently completed DIG (Digitalis Investigators Group) trial gave an answer to a problem that had not been addressed in two hundred years (The Digitalis Investigation Group 1997c) and supports the use of digoxin as a second-line drug after ACE inhibitors if patients continue to be symptomatic or have been recently hospitalized. Since digoxin had been one of the few drugs available for the treatment of heart failure, no randomized placebo-controlled mortality trials had been conducted until the introduction of ACE inhibitors provided an alternative background therapy in combination with diuretics. There was a concern about increased mortality because all other studies conducted in trials large enough to examine mortality had shown that other positive inotropes increased mortality. The DIG trial demonstrated that digoxin, when used in patients with chronic systolic heart failure, did not increase mortality, but also did not improve survival. However, although total survival was not improved in patients with systolic heart failure, there was a strong trend for a decrease in risk of death attributed to worsening heart failure and a significant decrease in hospitalizations for heart failure. Total hospitalizations showed only a small decrease, since there was an increase in hospitalizations for suspected digoxin toxicity. The benefit of digoxin to reduce hospitalizations for heart failure was seen in the different subgroups studied, though the effect tended to be slightly greater among patients at high risk—low LVEF, enlarged heart, or more severe symptoms. Of additional interest was the observation that digoxin also did not have an adverse effect in a subgroup of almost 1000 patients who had symptoms and signs of heart failure with an LVEF ≥45% and were therefore presumed to have predominant diastolic dysfunction. An adverse effect had been postulated since digoxin's positive inotropic effects would be associated with increased intracellular calcium, which might aggravate diastolic dysfunction and delay diastolic filling. Some have suggested that, because of the demonstrated effects on heart failure hospitalizations in the DIG study, the cheap price of digoxin, and its relatively low incidence of adverse effects when used in the doses employed in the DIG study, digoxin should be used more widely even to prevent the patient's first hospitalization for heart failure. As the data on total mortality were not beneficial, this approach has not been universally adopted, especially in countries with traditionally low use of digoxin.

Since the DIG study excluded patients with atrial fibrillation, the overall results of that trial may have underestimated the benefits of digoxin in the clinical population of heart failure patients. Although digoxin may not be an effective single drug in sustained or paroxysmal atrial fibrillation with normal systolic function, it is beneficial in patients with atrial fibrillation and heart failure. In these circumstances it can improve ventricular rate response at rest with further amelioration of heart failure symptoms. It is therefore generally indicated in most patients with symptomatic heart failure and chronic atrial fibrillation. However, even though the ventricular rate appears controlled at rest, it may not be during exercise and this can be assessed by a 24-hour ambulatory ECG monitor or an exercise stress test. If the ventricular rate is poorly controlled during activity or exercise, then additional therapy with a low-dose beta blocker is indicated because of the recent proven benefits of beta blockers on survival. If this is not effective for rate control or because of side effects, on an individual patient basis, very cautious use of rate limiting calcium channel antagonists may be considered and atrioventricular (AV) nodal ablation with insertion of a permanent pacemaker is helpful in a small subset of patients. If the atrial fibrillation is of recent onset, electrical cardioversion should be considered, and maintenance of sinus rhythm should be attempted with an antiarrhythmic drug. The current most commonly favored is amiodarone in low-maintenance doses of 200 mg orally daily for conversion and maintenance of sinus rhythm. The dose of digoxin should be reduced by half when patients are on amiodarone. In patients with heart failure and chronic atrial fibrillation, warfarin is strongly recommended.

The symptomatic benefit of digoxin can be discussed with patients such that they are aware that the drug will relieve symptoms if they are troublesome, but overall, will not prolong life.

**Key Point: Digoxin has not become a mandatory drug in symptomatic heart failure, but is considered useful by many clinicians for the relief of symptoms.**

Clearly, it would be most helpful to be able to identify those who obtained the beneficial effects of digoxin from those who did not. As stated above, certain clinical characteristics such as severe symptoms and large hearts identify patients who will benefit more. Yet, digoxin can be a toxic drug with life-threatening ventricular arrhythmias. The DIG study did not resolve this issue completely, but has shed light on some aspects. A dose of digoxin was chosen based on sex, weight, and renal function. The dose was between 0.125 and 0.5 mg per day, and a median daily dose was 0.25 mg at randomization; 86% of patients remained on this treatment at 1 year. In a subgroup of 1485 patients, digoxin serum concentrations were measured at one month and one year, and 88% of patients had digoxin concentrations at one month between 0.5 and 2.0 ng/mL (0.6–2.6 mmol/L). Thus, although a direct correlation between improvement in symptoms and digoxin serum concentration was not reported in the publication, and although digoxin concentrations have not been reported to correlate with mortality, it appears that any beneficial effects on heart failure symptoms occurred with trough digoxin serum concentrations in lower therapeutic range and at a mean for the DIG study of 0.9 ng/mL (1.1 nmol/L) at one month. Therefore, to minimize potential adverse effects of digoxin, the consensus viewpoint at the present time is to aim for trough digoxin concentrations (before dosing or at least 8–12 hours after the dose attained in the DIG study) around 1–1.5 nmol/L and to maintain adequate serum potassium >4.0 mmol/L. Routine repeat plasma concentration measurements were not performed in the DIG study and are probably not required in stable outpatients, though, they can be helpful if noncompliance is suspected.

Adverse effects of digoxin have been well characterized and include nausea, vision disturbances, fatigue, gynecomastia in men, and arrhythmias. Cardiac toxicity of digoxin is accentuated in hypokalemia and may occur with "therapeutic" plasma levels. The dose of digoxin should be reduced in renal failure and during concomitant administration of amiodarone, quinidine, or verapamil, although the last-named is generally not recommended in the treatment of systolic dysfunction because of its negative inotropic effects. It may, however, be appropriate to use in predominant diastolic dysfunction. Digoxin should not be taken concurrently with cholestyramine or antacids that combine with digoxin in the gut and reduce absorption. When very sick patients are admitted to the hospital and put on bed rest, the digoxin level may decrease as a result of improved renal blood flow.

**WARNING** The dose of digoxin should be reduced in renal failure and with concurrent use of quinidine, amiodarone, and verapamil to reduce risk of digoxin toxicity.

Digitoxin has a longer duration of action and is extensively metabolized by the liver and can be used in patients with significant renal dysfunction (ESC 1997). It has a half-life of 5–7 days.

## Calcium-Channel Antagonists

Amlodipine and felodipine can be recommended as being safe to use in patients with heart failure based on the PRAISE and VHeft III trials (Packer, O'Connor, et al. 1996; Cohn et al. 1997). They are, therefore, useful additional therapy in patients with hypertension or symptomatic ischemic heart disease. Diltiazem, verapamil, and other dihydropyridines are not recommended as they have been shown to increase morbidity and mortality in patients with significant systolic heart failure. There may be rare circumstances where they can be used if there is a specific precipitating cause of heart failure such as uncontrolled ventricular rate in atrial fibrillation or severe hypertension, that cannot be controlled by other mechanisms, since the control of that aggravating cause may improve heart function and offset negative inotropic effects. This should only, however, be done by physicians specializing in management of heart failure. It is not known at this time whether amlodipine has independent benefits in patients with nonischemic cardiomyopathy. This is being tested in the PRAISE-2 trial since subgroup analysis of the original PRAISE trial showed that nonischemic patients seemed to obtain benefit. Why this should occur is hypothesized, but the actual mechanism is not known and has not been confirmed, though it is known that amlodipine is an antioxidant. Mibefradil has been withdrawn from the market because of significant drug–drug interactions. A large, as yet unpublished, study in heart failure (MACH-1) showed that it did not worsen the heart failure state but neither did it improve it. Mibefradil was of interest since it was a T-channel calcium antagonist and did not have rate-limiting properties.

## Other Neurohormonal Antagonists

Neurohormonal activation has been the focus of much research in heart failure over the past ten years. Many attempts have been made to develop antagonists to neurohormones found to be elevated in heart failure and that also would have a theoretical or proven adverse effect. For example, elevated endothelin levels are associated with worsened survival, and studies have addressed the potential benefit of endothelin antagonists. Unfortunately, some promising molecules such as bosantan have significant hepatic adverse effects. Vasopressin antagonists, antioxidants, antigrowth factors, and other agents may dramatically increase our armamentarium of therapies.

Each new therapy is usually added on top of the previous battery of drugs, which have individually or in combination been shown to be effective. The most effective drugs may become replacements for previous drugs, but for the foreseeable future, patients with heart failure will continue to be treated with multiple drugs. This continues to pose a challenge to physicians since heart failure patients will be treated with other drugs for comorbidities and the risk of drug–drug interactions will increase as occurred in the recent mibefradil trials. Close monitoring of response is crucial.

## Positive Inotropes

Chronic administration of positive inotropes other than digoxin is associated with increased mortality and is not recommended (Arnold 1993). Short-term use of positive inotropes is indicated in patients with acute decompensations of heart failure associated with poor tissue perfusion or resistant pulmonary edema. Low doses may be sufficient to improve renal blood flow and to initiate a diuresis. Higher doses will further increase cardiac contractility, and dopamine, dobutamine, milrinone, and amrinone are widely used in this regard. Milrinone and amrinone have a particular role in a patient who is taking a beta blocker, since they work on the phosphodiesterase enzyme to increase contractility rather than through the beta receptor. Higher doses of positive inotropes may cause an inappropriate tachycardia and, along with isoproterenol and adrenaline, may decrease diastolic filling and may increase myocardial oxygen consumption, which could be detrimental.

For unstable outpatients, short-term intravenous infusions of positive inotropes have been studied but, in some cases, have been associated with increased mortality (Dies et al. 1986) or no benefit (Elis et al. 1998), whereas other studies have shown symptomatic benefit (Miller et al. 1990). They would appear to play a role in patients who are waiting transplantation or as a palliative treatment for patients who wish to stay at home rather than be admitted to the hospital frequently for their severe heart failure. Caution and careful monitoring is required since their effect on mortality is potentially adverse. The OPTIME trial is currently investigating the effect of intravenous milrinone on hospitalizations for patients with heart failure.

Drugs that sensitize myocardial calcium (e.g., pimobendan, levosimendan) are currently under investigation and their role has yet to be defined though early studies with levosimendan appear promising.

## Other, Less Often Used Therapies

In small studies, growth hormone has beneficial effects and several current trials will clarify its role in the management of chronic systolic heart failure. Other supplements such as coenzyme Q10 and thiamine, although apparently innocuous and possibly helpful, cannot currently be recommended until large clinical trials have been reported.

## Warfarin and Aspirin

Warfarin is indicated in patients with atrial fibrillation, documented left ventricular mural thrombus, a past history of systemic embolism, or in patients intolerant to or allergic to aspirin. The dose of coumadin needs to be adjusted to maintain an international normalized ratio of prothrombin time (INR) of between 2 and 3. Standard contraindications and duration of therapy apply. Acetylsalicylic acid (aspirin) is indicated in all patients with a history of ischemic heart disease and can be used in doses of 80 to 325 mg per day, usually in a coated formulation. Higher doses of aspirin are sometimes used in patients with concurrent transient ischemic attacks. Aspirin use is important to reduce the risk of further ventricular damage as it will reduce the risk of MI, especially in the setting of unstable angina. Ticlopidine and clopidogrel are also platelet inhibitors but work on ADP mechanisms and not the cyclooxygenase enzyme and may be slightly more effective than aspirin for vascular disease but are considerably more expensive and have some additional adverse effects (see section on Cerebrovascular Disorders in chapter 7, Treatment of Neurologic Disorders, and other sections of this chapter).

Since it is probable that some of the benefits of ACE inhibitors work through the bradykinin and prostaglandin mechanism, there are theoretical reasons for believing that aspirin might diminish the efficacy of ACE inhibitors. This has been supported in some in vitro work, in some small clinical trials, and retrospectively there seems to be decreased efficacy of ACE inhibitors in the SOLVD trial (The SOLVD Investigators 1992). Larger prospective studies are required in this regard, though, based on the current indirect or retrospective data, some have suggested that 80 mg of aspirin or warfarin should be considered (Cleland et al. 1993; Gheorghiode et al. 1998). Whether the alternatives ticlopidine or clopidogrel should be used is not known. A large clinical trial (WATCH) is currently underway to compare warfarin, aspirin, and clodipogrel in heart failure patients.

## Antiarrhythmic Agents

Because of underlying myocardial disease and elevated filling pressures, ventricular arrhythmias are very common in heart failure. In all cases of ventricular arrhythmias, every effort should be made to optimize heart failure medications to normalize filling pressures and to decrease myocardial wall stress in addition to treating ischemia. ACE inhibitors are important, but it is not clear whether their benefit is an indirect effect through improvement of hemodynamics, wall stress, and the general heart failure condition (Guindo 1996), or whether it is a direct effect through improvement in potassium homeostasis or direct antiarrhythmic effects (Campbell 1996). Electrolyte imbalances must be avoided, and a potassium concentration of at least 4.0 m/Eq/L, with correction of magnesium and calcium, should be maintained. Both beta blockers and spironolactone in combination with ACE inhibitors have been shown to reduce sudden death as well as total mortality (see above). If there has been an episode of resuscitated sudden death, syncope or presyncope associated with rapid ventricular tachycardia, or worsening heart failure associated with arrhythmia, amiodarone would appear to be the drug of choice, although an automatic implantable defibrillator can be considered in some centers for some patients.

In patients with ventricular ectopics, even though frequent, the treatment is less clear. These are certainly associated with increased mortality, but may be a marker as much as a cause. The GESICA trial showed benefit of amiodarone in an open-label design (Doval et al. 1994), but the CHF-STAT double-blind trial of amiodarone did not (Singh et al. 1995). Meta-analysis of the use of amiodarone showed an overall benefit (Amiodarone Trials Meta-Analysis Investigators 1997a) as did the EMIAT trial post-MI (Julian et al. 1997), which enrolled a significant number of patients with heart failure. Other antiarrhythmic drugs have either negative inotropic effects or significant adverse effects or have not been studied in heart failure. For these reasons, if an antiarrhythmic drug needs to be started, then in most cases amiodarone can be chosen. Beta blockers may also be considered in appropriate patients alone or in combination with amiodarone, and there is some evidence to suggest the combination might be better. For the patient taking amiodarone, thyroid-stimulating hormone (TSH), liver function tests, and chest X-ray should be monitored, and the dose of digoxin should be reduced by half. The usual minimum target maintenance dose of amiodarone in heart failure is 200 mg daily.

As noted previously, ventricular arrhythmias are not the only cause of sudden death, and routine monitoring for ventricular arrhythmias is not considered necessary unless they are suspected as a cause of symptoms.

Atrial fibrillation occurs frequently in patients with heart failure but, if of recent onset, attempts should be made to restore and maintain sinus rhythm to control ventricular response and to reestablish coordinated atrial contraction. Amiodarone is again the drug most commonly used, though flecainide and other type 1A agents are occasionally used under close supervision.

## MODIFIABLE RISK FACTORS FOR HEART FAILURE

Since ischemic heart disease is now the most common cause of systolic heart failure, its associated risk factors such as hypertension, dyslipidemia, glucose intolerance, smoking, and obesity, should be appropriately and aggressively managed (see respective sections of this chapter and other chapters). Patient noncompliance remains a major problem in acute exacerbations and requires active patient education, reinforcement, simplification of drug regimens, and reduction of avoidable adverse effects (Miller et al. 1997). Mitral regurgitation is often believed to be an inevitable consequence of systolic heart failure, but should also be treated appropriately. In some cases, surgical repair of the mitral valve or replacement should be considered, but aggressive diuresis and increasing ACE inhibitor doses to as high as can be tolerated will help to reduce preload and afterload with reductions in the regurgitant fraction. It is important to remember that, in the presence of significant mitral regurgitation, the left ventricular ejection fraction may be an overestimate of underlying myocardial function.

## MECHANICAL HEART FAILURE TREATMENTS

Since ischemic heart disease is now one of the most common causes of heart failure, myocardial ischemia should be treated aggressively and, where appropriate, percutaneous coronary angioplasty or bypass surgery is indicated. The risks of bypass surgery in patients with low ejection fraction are gradually becoming less, and minimally invasive cardiac surgery may offer additional hope for suitable patients. The timing of valve surgery is critical to reduce perioperative mortality and to enhance postoperative recovery of myocardial function. Mitral valve repair is now being considered more frequently as a definitive operation or as an adjunct of bypass surgery.

For acute and severe exacerbations of heart failure, intra-aortic balloon pump and mechanical ventilation are being used more widely. Left ventricular assist devices continue to be perfected in selected centers as a bridge to transplantation. Transplantation is still the treatment of choice for younger patients with irreversible end-stage heart failure but is not widely available because of the relative paucity of donors. The total artificial heart is not yet a practical reality. Cardiomyoplasty, to surgically wrap the latissimus dorsi muscle around the heart and synchronously pace it, has had variable results, and its proper role has not yet been defined. Similarly, the role of implantation of myocardial cells and the use of associated growth factors remain in the experimental stages.

Left ventricular aneurysmectomy is appropriate for selected patients. Volume reduction therapy to attempt to restore a spherical heart to an ellipsoid shape, in conjunction with a mitral valve repair procedure, has generated considerable interest but its long-term role as a surgical treatment for heart failure remains unclear and requires further clinical trials. An automatic implantable cardiodefibrillator is effective to internally cardiovert rapid ventricular tachycardia or ventricular fibrillation and has a role for patients who have had such symptomatic arrhythmias or have been resuscitated from sudden death. Since it does not alter the natural pathophysiology of left ventricular dysfunction, is expensive, is not readily available in all countries, and is not always accepted readily by the patient if it fires frequently, its role in the management of heart failure requires clinical trials. Trials are ongoing to investigate different electronic pairing modalities to "resynchronize" the failing heart.

Continuous positive airway pressure is effective in acute pulmonary edema and is currently being tested in clinical trials to determine if it can favorably alter the progression of heart failure in appropriate patients who have sleep disordered breathing and in whom it may effectively reduce transmyocardial pressures and perhaps sympathetic outflow to the heart.

## TREATMENT CONSIDERATIONS

### Special Patient Populations

Renal dysfunction is often the reason for underutilization of ACE inhibitors. A small, but stable, increase in serum creatinine is common and to be expected after the introduction of ACE inhibitors, because of the mechanism of action on the efferent glomerular arteriole. Greater increases in creatinine can occur, from an apparently normal creatinine before introduction of ACE inhibitors, in significant renal artery stenosis or in small elderly women in whom lean body mass results in a lower serum creatinine that is not a true reflection of glomerular filtration rate. With creatinines up to 200 $\mu$mol/L (2.2 mg/dL) ACE inhibitors can still be introduced with careful downward titration of the diuretic dose and close monitoring after each increase in ACE inhibitor dose. With creatinines between 200 and 300 $\mu$mol/L (2.2–3.4 mg/dL), the ACE inhibitors are probably best introduced by specialists in the management of heart failure. With creatinines above 300 $\mu$mol (3.4 mg/dL), ACE inhibitors may be best avoided in the majority of situations, although if the patient is on some form of dialysis, ACE inhibitors can be reintroduced. Available evidence suggests that ARBs are no less likely to cause renal dysfunction than ACE inhibitors. Hydralazine and nitrates can be considered an alternative as can increased dose of diuretics, beta blockers, and nitrates. Spironolactone and other potassium-sparing diuretics generally should be avoided in patients with significant renal dysfunction because of the risk of hyperkalemia.

Hypotension is another common cause for under utilization of ACE inhibitors. Routine clinical follow-up should include supine and standing blood pressures. If there is no symptomatic postural hypotension and renal function is stable, then patients can often tolerate the introduction of ACE inhibitors. Hypotension is less frequent if the JVP is elevated, since this indicates elevated filling pressures. Hyponatremia may be associated with an increased likelihood of hypotension, since it reflects a marked increase in the activation of the renin–angiotensin–aldosterone system but, in this setting, ACE inhibitors are also more effective and will correct hyponatremia when introduced carefully. To avoid systemic hypotension, the dose of diuretics should be decreased and, in appropriate cases, the timing of the peak effect of the diuretic dose and that of the ACE inhibitors or other vasodilators should be separated.

Cough does occur in patients taking an ACE inhibitor, but patients should be reassured that this is not damaging. However, an intractable severe cough may necessitate discontinuation of treatment. Physicians should carefully evaluate the patients to make sure that pulmonary congestion and worsening heart failure are not the cause of the cough before automatically attributing it to the ACE inhibitor. Withdrawal of the drug with reintroduction of a different ACE inhibitor at a lower dose may help to clarify cause and effect and may allow the patient to regain confidence in the medication. It should be noted, however, that the cough is a class effect to all ACE inhibitors if the dose is sufficient to block the breakdown of bradykinin. In the future, if large clinical trials show equivalence or superiority of ARBs, they may become a suitable or preferred alternative to ACE inhibitors. Symptomatic treatment of more minor degrees of the cough can be helpful, and some small studies have suggested that sodium dicromoglycate works in some patients.

Gout occurs frequently in heart failure patients because of diuretics, and standard preventative measurements are appropriate. NSAIDs are widely used for the acute management of gout, but are problematic in patients with heart failure because of their effects on the kidney to cause salt and fluid retention. If they are used, patients should be carefully educated to monitor their home daily weights and to increase their dose of diuretic for weight gain of 3 lbs or more. If a patient already has fluid retention or has unstable heart failure, NSAIDs are best avoided. Colchicine can be started early during the attack of gout, but short courses of prednisone are effective and well tolerated. After the acute attack, long-term prophylaxis with lower doses of diuretics and allopurinol is required.

## Acute Pulmonary Edema

Acute pulmonary edema is a life-threatening emergency requiring admission to the hospital and intravenous treatment for prompt relief. The underlying cause should be addressed and treated (e.g., thrombolysis for acute MI). Patients should sit upright for relief of dyspnea, with $O_2$ therapy (40–100%, 2–4 L/min) by mask or nasal prongs. Intravenous furosemide 40–80 mg usually initiates a diuresis within 30 minutes, but higher doses may be required if there is renal dysfunction. In general, the oral dose taken at home is the initial dose chosen for IV dose. A transient increase in afterload can occur, but is usually not clinically significant. An acute vasodilation is then followed by diuresis. Repeat boluses can be given as required but, if the patient did not previously have chronic heart failure and volume overload, then excessive diuresis will cause hypotension. This is relevant since nitrates are now widely used in the early treatment of pulmonary edema and will also lower blood pressure (BP). Nitrates may be administered as a sublingual tablet or spray, transdermal paste or patch, or intravenous infusion (initial dose, 5–10 μg/min) and are particularly useful in the setting of acute MI or chronic ischemic heart disease. Lower doses will cause venodilation and decrease preload, whereas higher doses (>40–50 μg/min) will also decrease afterload. Sodium nitroprusside is an alternative IV veno- and arteriolar vasodilator (3–300 μg/min) with prompt onset of action and short half-life. Thiocyanate toxicity can occur with prolonged use of nitroprusside in the setting of renal dysfunction. Both drugs require hemodynamic monitoring [noninvasive may suffice for nitroglycerine though intraarterial blood pressure (BP) measurement is usual for nitroprusside] and the doses used are individually titrated to the patient response. Invasive monitoring of right atrial pressure, pulmonary artery pressures, and cardiac output should be considered in sick patients especially if they are slow to respond to initial therapy.

Intravenous morphine (2-mg aliquots) has beneficial direct arteriolar and venous vasodilation, in addition to sympathetic and antilytic effects. Its use is well established in clinical practice, but it produces nausea and vomiting in addition to sedation. Intravenous digoxin (0.125–0.25 mg) is sometimes given for its positive inotropic effects to increase cardiac output. More control over changes in cardiac output may be achieved acutely with intravenous dobutamine (2–20 μg/kg per min) or dopamine (2–20 μg/kg per min), the latter being preferred in patients with severe hypotension and low renal blood flow. Both drugs can be combined with nitroglycerine and nitroprusside. Intravenous amrinone (5–10 μg/kg per min) and milrinone (50 μg/kg bolus over 10 min, 0.375–0.75 μg/kg per min), as phosphodiesterase inhibitors, which combine positive inotropy with peripheral vasodilation, can also be used in combination with other intravenous drugs and are of particular importance for patients previously on beta blockers or not responding to sympathomimetic agents. Combination drug therapy will increase risk of arrhythmias and other adverse effects. Total intravenous fluid load should be minimized.

Endotracheal intubation with mechanical ventilation has been used increasingly and earlier in acute pulmonary edema to reduce the work of breathing. Continuous positive airway pressure may also be helpful in milder cases. Intra-aortic balloon pumps are inserted particularly in patients undergoing revascularization procedures.

## Other Manifestations of Cardiomyopathy

Acute viral myocarditis can be life-threatening, but immunosuppressant therapy has not been shown to be helpful. Aggressive supportive therapy with standard drugs is needed, though in some cases transplantation is required.

Infiltrative cardiomyopathies are difficult to treat and have restrictive, diastolic, and systolic components. An underlying cause should be sought and treated with specific therapy if it is available. Otherwise, standard therapy is appropriate and may require increased doses of diuretics.

Right ventricular failure secondary to lung disease or pulmonary hypertension and pulmonary emboli is difficult to treat, and even high doses of vasodilators are often not effective in lowering pulmonary artery pressures. Prevention of recurrent pulmonary emboli with coumadin is important, and oxygen therapy for chronic obstructive pulmonary disease will help to ameliorate the progressive nature of the illness by reducing pulmonary artery pressures. An atrial septal defect should not be forgotten as a cause of right heart failure, but once right heart failure has become established, closure of the defect would be less effective.

SUMMARY

**Since chronic heart failure is a potentially fatal disease, it must be managed aggressively. Causative factors need correcting and patient education is important. All patients with symptomatic chronic heart failure should be on an ACE inhibitor if there is no**

**contraindication. In stable patients with mild to moderate symptoms, β-adrenergic receptor antagonists such as metoprolol CR/TL, carvedilol, or bisoprolol, started in low doses and titrated carefully, can be considered. Spironolactone in low doses is indicated as additional therapy in patients with severe heart failure. Diuretics, digoxin, and nitrates are helpful to relieve symptoms. As effective new drugs are introducedinto our therapeutic armamentarium for chronic heart failure, important issues to be addressed will include whether the new drug is added in combination or can be considered as a substitution. The cost-effectiveness of different drugs and multidisciplinary management approaches will become increasingly important as the economic burden of heart failure increases as baby boomers get older, as life expectancy is prolonged, and as ischemic heart disease becomes more prevalent globally. Patient preferences should be considered and outpatient therapy should be maximized with careful attention to prophylaxis of precipitating and aggravating causes to reduce hospitalizations. As underlying mechanisms are more fully elucidated, specific targeted treatments will be successful and progressively replace therapies that manage only the symptoms but not the disease process.**

## REFERENCES


Abraham WT, Bristow MR. 1997. Specialized centers for heart failure management. *Circulation* **96**:2755–7.

ACE Inhibitor Myocardial Infarction Collaborative Group. 1998b. Indications for ACE Inhibitors in the early treatment of acute myocardial infarction: systematic overview of individual data from 100,000 patients in randomized trials. *Circulation* **97**:2202–12.

Adams KF Jr, Zannad F. 1998. Clinical definition and epidemiology of advanced heart failure. *Am Heart J* **135**:S204–15.

Advisory Council. 1999. Consensus recommendations for the management of chronic heart failure. Membership of the advisory council to improve outcomes nationwide in heart failure. *Am J Cardiol* **83**(2A):1A–38A.

Ambrosioni E, Borghi C, Magnani B, et al. 1995. The effect of the angiotensin-converting-enzyme inhibitor zofenopril on mortality and morbidity after anterior myocardial infarction. The Survival of Myocardial Infarction Long-term Evaluation (SMILE) Study Investigators. *N Engl J Med* **332**:80–5.

Amiodarone Trials Meta-Analysis Investigators. 1997a. Effect of prophylactic amiodarone on mortality after acute myocardial infarction and in congestive heart failure: meta-analysis of individual data from 6500 patients in randomised trials. *Lancet* **350**:1417–24.

Arnold JMO. 1993. The role of phosphodiesterase inhibitors in heart failure. *J Pharmacol Ther* **57**:161–70.

Arnold JMO, Howlett J, Nigam R, et al. 1999. The Canadian CHF-Clinics Network: Implementation and initial results. *Can J Cardiol* **15**(Suppl D):120D.

[ [NAMES?]. 1998. Assessment of Treatment with Lisinopril and Survival Trial. ATLAS Study Investigators. Results presented at American College of Cardiology Annual Meeting; [DATES?] March 1998; [CITY?]. PLACE OF PUBLICATION: PUBLISHER? PAGES?].

Australia/New Zealand Heart Failure Research Collaborative Group. 1997b. Randomised, placebo-controlled trial of carvedilol in patients with congestive heart failure due to ischaemic heart disease. *Lancet* **349**:375.

Baig MK, Mahon N, McKenna WJ, et al. 1998. The pathophysiology of advanced heart failure. *Am Heart J* **135**:S216–30.

Califf RM, Vidaillet H, Goldman L. 1998. Advanced congestive heart failure: what do patients want? *Am Heart J* **135**:S320–6.

Campbell RWF. 1996. Antiarrhythmic mechanisms of ACE-I. *Heart* **76** (Suppl 3):79–82.

Chinese Cardiac Study Collaborative Group. 1995b. Oral captopril versus placebo among 13,634 patients with suspected acute myocardial infarction: interim report from the Chinese Cardiac Study (CCS-1). *Lancet* **345**:686–7.

CIBIS-II Investigators and Committees. 1999. The Cardiac Insufficiency Bisoprolol Study II-(CIBIS-II): a randomized trial. *Lancet* **353**: 9–13.

Cleland JGF, Bulpitt CJ, Rodney HF, et al. 1995. Is aspirin safe for patients with heart failure? *Br Heart J* **74**:215–19.

Cohn JN, Arichibald DG, Phil M, et al. 1986. Effect of vasodilator therapy on mortality in severe congestive heart failure. Results of a Veterans Administration cooperative study. *N Engl J Med* **314**:1547–52.

Cohn JN, Johnson G, Ziesche S, et al. 1991. A comparison of enalapril with hydralazine-isosorbide dinitrate in the treatment of chronic congestive heart failure. *N Engl J Med* **325**:303–10.

Cohn JN, Ziesche S, Smith R, et al. 1997. Effect of the calcium antagonist felodipine as supplementary vasodilator therapy in patients with chronic heart failure treated with enalapril: V-HeFT III. Vasodilator-Heart Failure Trial (V-HeFT) Study Group. *Circulation* **96** (3):856–63.

Cowie MR, Moster A, Wood DA, et al. 1997. The epidemiology of heart failure. *Eur Heart J* **18**:208–25.

Dauterman KW, Massie BM, Gheorghiade M. 1998. Heart failure associated with preserved systolic function: a common and costly clinical entity. *Am Heart J* **135**:S310–19.

Davies RF, Beanlands DS, Nadeau C, et al. 1991. Enalapril versus digoxin in New York Association Class II-III congestive heart failure: results of a randomized, double-blind multicenter trial. *J Am Coll Cardiol* **18**:1602–9.

Dies F, Krell MJ, Whitlow P, et al. 1986. Intermittent dobutamine in ambulatory outpatients with chronic cardiac failure [abstract]. *Circulation* **74** (Suppl II):38.

Doval HC, Nul DR, Grancelli HO, et al. 1994. Randomized trial of low-dose amiodarone in severe congestive heart failure. Grupo de Estudio de la Sobrevida en la Insuficiencia Cardiaca en Argentina (GESICA). *Lancet* **344**:493–8.

Eichhorn E on behalf of BEST Investigators. Nov. 1999. β Blocker Evaluation of Survival Trial (BEST). Preliminary results presented at American Heart Association 72nd Annual Scientific Meeting.

Elis A, Bental T, Kimchi O, Ravid M, Lishner M. 1998. Intermittent dobutamine treatment in patients with chronic refractory congestive heart failure: a randomized, double-blind, placebo-controlled study. *Clin Pharmacol Ther* **63**:682–85.

Elkayam U, Johnson JV, Shotan A, et al. 1999. Double-blind, placebo-controlled study to evaluate the effect of organic nitrates in patients with chronic heart failure treated with angiotensin-converting enzyme inhibitor. *Circulation* **99**:2652–57.

[ESC] European Society of Cardiology. 1995. The Task Force on Heart Failure of the European Society of Cardiology. Guidelines for the diagnosis of heart failure. *Eur Heart J* **16**:741–51.

[ESC] European Society of Cardiology. 1997. The Task Force of the Working Group on Heart Failure of the European Society of Cardiology. The treatment of heart failure. *Eur Heart J* **18**: 736–53.

Fonarow GC, Stevenson LW, Walden JA, et al. 1997. Impact of a comprehensive heart failure management program on hospital readmission and functional status of patients with advanced heart failure. *J Am Coll Cardiol* **30**:725–32.

Gheorghiade M, Bonow RO. 1998. Chronic heart failure in the United States: a manifestation of coronary heart disease. *Circulation* **97**:282–9.

Gheorghiade M, Cody RJ, Francis GS, et al. 1998. Current medical therapy for advanced heart failure. *Am Heart J* **135**:S231–48.

Grossman W. 1991. Diastolic dysfunction in congestive heart failure. *N Eng J Med* **325**:1557–1564.

Gruppo Italiano per lo Studio della Sopravvivenza nell'Infarto Miocardico (GISSI-3). 1994. GISSI-3: effects of lisinopril and transdermal glyceryl trinitrate singly and together on 6-week mortality and ventricular function after acute myocardial infarction. *Lancet* **343**:1115–22.

Gruppo Italiano per lo Studio della Sopravvivenza nell'Infarto Miocardico (GISSI-3). 1996. Six-month effects of early treatment with lisinopril and transdermal glyceryl trinitrate singly and together withdrawn six weeks after acute myocardial infarction: the GISSI-3 trial. *J Am Coll Cardiol* **27**:337–44.

Guindo J, Bayés Genis AB, Dominguez de Rozas JM, et al. 1996. Sudden death in heart failure. *Heart Failure Reviews* **1**:249–60.

Hall AS, Murray GD, Ball SG, et al. 1997. Follow-up study of patients randomly allocated ramipril or placebo for heart failure after acute myocardial infarction: AIRE Extension (AIREX) Study. AIREX Study Investigators. *Lancet* **349**:1493–7.

Hanumanthu S, Butler J, Chomsky D, et al. 1997. Effect of a heart failure program on hospitalization frequency and exercise tolerance. *Circulation* **96**:2842–8.

The Heart Outcomes Prevention Evaluation Study Investigators 2000. Effects of an angiotension-converting enzyme inhibitor, ramipril, on death from cardiovascular causes, myocardial infarction and stroke in high-risk patients. *N Engl J Med*; Jan 20th issue (currently on NEJM prerelease website www.nejm.org) Nov 10th posting 1999.

Heidenreich PA, Lee TT, Massie BM. 1997. Effect of beta-blockade on mortality in patients with heart failure: a meta-analysis of randomized clinical trials. *J Am Coll Cardiol* **30**:27–34.

Ho KKL, Anderson KM, Kannel WB, et al. 1993. Survival after the onset of congestive heart failure in Framingham Heart Study subjects. *Circulation* **88**:107–15.

ISIS–4 (Fourth International Study of Infarct Survival) Collaborative Group. 1995a. ISIS-4: a randomized factorial trial assessing early oral captopril, oral mononitrate, and intravenous magnesium sulphate in 58050 patients with suspected acute myocardial infarction. *Lancet* **345**:669–85.

Johnstone DE, Abdulla A, Arnold JMO. 1994. Diagnosis and management of heart failure. Canadian Cardiovascular Society's Consensus Conference. *Can J Cardiol* **10**:613–31.

Julian DG, Camm AJ, Frangin G, et al. 1997. Randomised trial of effect of amiodarone on mortality in patients with left ventricular dysfunction after recent myocardial infarction (EMIAT). *Lancet* **349**:667–74.

Kannel WB, Belanger AJ. 1991. Epidemiology of heart failure. *Am Heart J* **121**:951.

Kleinert HD. 1995. Renin inhibition. *Cardiovasc Drugs Ther* **9**:645–55.

Kober L, Torp-Pedersen C, Carlesen JE, et al. 1995. A clinical trial of the angiotensin-converting-enzyme inhibitor trandolapril in patients with left ventricular dysfunction after myocardial infarction. The Trandolapril Cardiac Evaluation (TRACE) Study Group. *N Engl J Med* **333**:1670–76.

Latini R, Maggioni AP, Flather M, et al. 1995. ACE Inhibitor use in patients with myocardial infarction: summary of evidence from clinical trials. *Circulation* **92**:3132–3137.

Lenihan DJ, Gerson MC, Hoit BD, et al. 1995. Mechanisms, diagnosis, and treatment of diastolic heart failure. *Am Heart J* **130**:153–66.

Lin C, Frishman WH. 1996. Renin inhibition: a novel therapy for cardiovascular disease. *Am Heart J* **131**:1024–1034.

Lonn EM, Yusuf S, Jha P, et al. 1994. Emerging role of angiotensin-converting enzyme inhibitors in cardiac and vascular protection. *Circulation* **90** (4):2056–69.

Mancini GBJ, Henry GC, Macaya C, et al. 1996. Angiotensin-converting enzyme inhibition with quinapril improves endothelial vasomotor dysfunction in patients with coronary artery disease: the TREND (Trial on Reversing Endothelial Dysfunction) Study. *Circulation* **94**:258–65.

Massie BM, Shah NB. 1997. Evolving trends in the epidemiologic factors of heart failure: rationale for preventive strategies and comprehensive disease management. *Am Heart J* **133**:703–12.

McDonagh TA, Morrison CE, Lawrence A, et al. 1997. Symptomatic and asymptomatic left-ventricular systolic dysfunction in an urban population. *Lancet* **350**:829–33.

MERIT-HF Study Group. 1999. Effect of metoprolol CR/XL in chronic heart failure: Metoprolol CR/XL Randomized Intervention Trial in Congestive Heart Failure (MERIT-HF). *Lancet* **353**:2001–7.

Miller NH, Hill M, Kottke T, et al. 1997. The multilevel compliance challenge: recommendations for a call to action. A statement for healthcare professionals. *Circulation* **95**:1085–90.

Murray CJ, Lopez AD. 1997. Alternative projections of mortality and disability by cause 1990–2020: Global Burden of Disease Study. *Lancet* **349**:1498–504.

O'Connor CM, Gattis WA, Swedberg K. 1998. Current and novel pharmacologic approaches in advanced heart failure. *Am Heart J* **135**:S249–63.

Packer M. 1992. Treatment of chronic heart failure. *Lancet* **340**:92–5.

Packer M, Bristow M, Cohn J, et al. 1996. The effect of carvedilol on morbidity and mortality in patients with chronic heart failure. *N Engl J Med* **334**:1349–55.

Packer M, Gheorghiade M, Young JB, et al. 1993. Withdrawal of digoxin from patients with chronic heart failure treated with angiotensin-converting-enzyme inhibitors. The RADIANCE Study. *N Engl J Med* **329**:1–7.

Packer M, O'Connor CM, Ghali JK, et al. 1996. Effect of amlodipine on morbidity and mortality in severe chronic heart failure. Prospective Randomized Amlodipine Survival Evaluation Study Group. *N Engl J Med* **335**:1107–14.

Pearson TM, Peters TD. 1997. The treatment gap in coronary artery disease and heart failure: community standards and the post-discharge patient. *Am J Cardiol* **80**:45H–52H.

Pfeffer MA, Braunwald E, Moyé L, et al. 1992. Effect of captopril on mortality and morbidity in patients with left ventricular dysfunction after myocardial infarction. The SAVE Investigators. *N Engl J Med* **327**:669–77.

Pfeffer MA, Greaves SC, Arnold JMO, et al. 1997. Early versus delayed angiotensin-converting enzyme inhibition therapy in acute myocardial infarction. The Healing and Early Afterload Reducing Therapy (HEART) Trial Investigators. *Circulation* **12**:2643–51.

Pfeffer MA, Hennekens CH, et al. 1995. When a question has an answer: rationale for our early termination of the HEART trial. The HEART Study Executive Committee. *Am J Cardiol* **75**:1173–5.

Pitt B, Segal R, Martinez FA, et al. 1997. Randomised trial of losartan versus captopril in patients over 65 with heart failure (Evaluation of Losartan in the Elderly Study, ELITE). *Lancet* **349**:747–52.

Pitt B, Zannad F, Remme WJ, et al. 1999. The effect of spironolactone on morbidity and mortality in patients with severe heart failure. *Lancet* **341**:709–17.

Rich MW, Beckham V, Wittenberg C, et al. 1995. Multidisciplinary intervention to prevent the readmission of elderly patients with congestive heart failure. *N Engl J Med* **333**:1190–5.

Schulman KA, Mark DB, Califf RM. 1998. Outcomes and costs within a disease management program for advanced congestive heart failure. *Am Heart J* **135**:S285–92.

Singh SN, Fletcher RD, Fisher SG, et al. 1995. Amiodarone in patients with congestive heart failure and asymptomatic ventricular arrhythmia. *N Engl J Med* **333**:77–82.

Soriano JB, Hoes AW, Meems L, et al. 1997. Increased survival with $\beta$-blockers: importance and ancillary properties. *Prog Cardiovasc Dis* **39**:445–56.

Stevenson LW, Massie BM, Francis GS. 1998. Optimizing therapy for complex or refractory heart failure: a management algorithm. *Am Heart J* **135**:S293–309.

Sullivan MJ, Hawthorne MH. 1996. Nonpharmacologic interventions in the treatment of heart failure. *J Cardiovasc Nurs* **10**:47–57.

Swedberg K, Held P, Kjekshus J, et al. 1992. Effects of the early administration of enalapril on mortality in patients with acute myocardial infarction. Results of the Cooperative North Scandinavian Enalapril Survival Study II (CONSENSUS II). The CONSENSUS II Study Group. *N Engl J Med* **327**:678–84.

The Acute Infarction Ramipril Efficacy (AIRE) Study Investigators. 1993. Effect of ramipril on mortality and morbidity of survivors of acute myocardial infarction with clinical evidence of heart failure. *Lancet* **343**:821–8.

The Captopril-Digoxin Multicenter Research Group. 1988. Comparative effects of therapy with captopril and digoxin in patients with mild to moderate heart failure. *JAMA* **259**:539–44.

The CONSENSUS Trial Study Group. 1987. Effects of enalapril on mortality in severe congestive heart failure. Results of the Cooperative North Scandinavian Enalapril Survival Study (CONSENSUS). *N Engl J Med* **316**:1429–35.

The Digitalis Investigation Group. 1997c. The effect of digoxin on mortality and morbidity in patients with heart failure. *N Engl J Med* **336**:525–33.

The NETWORK Investigators. 1998a. Clinical outcome with enalapril in symptomatic chronic heart failure; a dose comparison. *Eur Heart J* **19**:481–9.

The RESOLVD Pilot Study Investigators. 1999. Comparison of candesartan, enalapril and their combination in congestive heart failure: Randomized Evaluation of Strategies for Left Ventricular Dysfunction (RESOLVD) Pilot Study. *Circulation* **100**:1056–64.

The SOLVD Investigators. 1991. Effect of enalapril on survival in patients with reduced left ventricular ejection fractions and congestive heart failure. *N Eng J Med* **325**:293–302.

The SOLVD Investigators. 1992. Effect of enalapril on mortality and the development of heart failure in asymptomatic patients with reduced left ventricular ejection fraction. *N Engl J Med* **327**:685–91.

Uretsky BF, Pina I, Quigg RJ, et al. 1998. Beyond drug therapy: nonpharmacologic care of the patient with advanced heart failure. *Am Heart J* **135**:S264–84.

Uretsky BF, Sheahan RG. 1997. Primary prevention of sudden cardiac death in heart failure: will the solution be shocking? *J Am Coll Cardiol* **30**:1589–97.

Uretsky BF, Young JB, Shadhidi FE, et al. 1993. Randomized study assessing the effect of digoxin withdrawal in patients with mild to moderate chronic congestive heart failure: results of the PROVED trial. The PROVED Investigative Group. *J Am Coll Cardiol* **22**:955–62.

Van Gilst WH, Kingma JH, Peels KH, et al. 1996. Which patient benefits from early angiotensin-converting enzyme inhibition after myocardial infarction? Results of one-year serial echocardiographic follow-up from the Captopril and Thrombolysis Study (CATS). The CATS Investigators. *J Am Coll Cardiol* **28**:114–21.

Vantrimpont P, Rouleau JL, Wun CC, et al. 1997. Additive beneficial effects of beta-blockers in the Survival and Ventricular Enlargement (SAVE) Study. *J Am Coll Cardiol* **29** (2):229–36.

Waagstein F, Bristow MR, Swedberg K, et al. 1993. Beneficial effects of metoprolol in idiopathic dilated cardiomyopathy. The Metoprolol in Dilated Cardiomyopathy (MDC) Trial Study Group. *Lancet* **342**:1441–46.

West JA, Miller NH, Parker KM, et al. 1997. A comprehensive management system for heart failure improves clinical outcomes and reduces medical resource utilization. *Am J Cardiol* **79**:58–63.

Williams JF Jr, Bristow MR, Fowler MB, et al. 1995. Guidelines for the evaluation and management of heart failure: Report of the American College of Cardiology/American Heart Association Task Force on Practice Guidelines (Committee on Evaluation and Management of Heart Failure). *Circulation* **92**:2764–84.

Yusuf S, Garg R, Held P, et al. 1992. Need for a large randomized trial to evaluate the effects of digitalis on morbidity and mortality in congestive heart failure. *Am J Cardiol* **68**:64G–70G.

Yusuf S, Pepine CJ, Garces C, et al. 1992. Effect of enalapril on myocardial infarction and unstable angina in patients with low ejection fractions. *Lancet* **340**:1173–8.

# Arrhythmias

**Dan M. Roden**

*Chapter Outline*



## ARRHYTHMIAS: MECHANISMS

### Normal Cardiac Excitation

In the normal heart, the specialized "pacemaker" tissue of the sinus node, located in the high right atrium (at its junction with the superior vena cava), depolarizes rhythmically, usually 60–80 times per minute. Impulses are then propagated rapidly (Fig. 1-27) from the sinus node throughout the atria, causing atrial systole and propelling atrial blood through the mitral and tricuspid valves into the ventricles. Atrial depolarization is inscribed on the surface electrocardiogram as the P wave. The wave of impulses then enters the atrioventricular (AV) node, located in the lower atrial septum. Depolarization in the AV node is considerably slower than elsewhere in the heart, and 150—200 ms elapse before the propagating wave front emerges from the AV node and enters the specialized conducting system of the ventricles. The passage of impulses in the conduction system, whose fibers are located in the subendocardium of both ventricles, is extremely rapid, and activation of the ventricles then proceeds from subendocardial conducting system fibers transmurally to the epicardium, inscribing the QRS complex of the electrocardiogram. Following depolarization, ventricular cells repolarize, inscribing the T wave of the normal electrocardiogram. The time from QRS onset to the end of T wave (QT interval) is frequently used as a measurement of repolarization time (action potential duration) in individual cells in the ventricle.

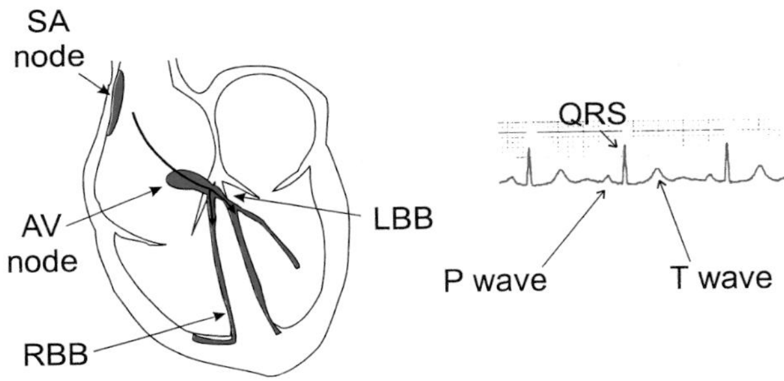


**FIGURE 1-27 Normal impulse propagation in the heart. Impulses arise in the sinus node and propagate through the atria, the atrioventricular (AV) node, and right and left bundle branches of the conducting system (RBB, LBB). The normal ECG is inscribed as a result of this normal propagation, and subsequent ventricular repolarization (T wave).**

Any deviation from the above description of a normal heart beat is an *arrhythmia*. Such deviations can arise because the heart rate is faster or slower than usual although the activation sequence described above is intact (sinus tachycardia and sinus bradycardia, respectively). Impulse propagation described above may fail, most commonly in or just below the AV node, causing heart block or bundle branch block. Single or multiple beats may arise from ectopic sites (i.e., not the sinus node) and propagate to excite the heart prematurely and in an abnormal sequence. If such ectopic activity arises in the atrium, the result is atrial premature contraction(s) (APCs) and in the ventricle, ventricular premature contraction(s) (VPCs). These may occur as isolated beats or consecutively (atrial or ventricular tachycardia).

The fundamental cellular event responsible for normal electrical activity in the heart is the cardiac action potential. The configuration and duration of action potentials in various regions of the heart (atrium, ventricle, AV node, etc.) vary substantially even under physiologic conditions. With disease, action potential durations or configurations vary even further, causing or contributing to arrhythmias. The crucial molecular events that control the changes in transmembrane voltage occurring during a cardiac action potential are ion currents flowing across the membrane of heart cells during excitation and recovery from excitation (Roden and George 1997). Ion currents flow through specific pore-forming protein complexes, termed ion channels, located in the membrane of individual cardiac cells. Ion channels open and close in response to stimuli such as changes in voltage, and it is the coordinated activity of multiple ion channels that results in the cardiac action potential (Fig. 1-28). Most drugs that are now used in the treatment of cardiac arrhythmias have as their major mechanism of action blocking of one or more cardiac ion current(s).

## Cellular Mechanisms in Arrhythmias

Three major cellular mechanisms for arrhythmias have been identified: enhanced automaticity, triggered automaticity, and reentry (Roden 1995).

In *enhanced automaticity*, propagation of the impulse wave originates from cell(s) outside the sinus node that are undergoing spontaneous depolarization, at a rate faster than in the sinus node.

*Triggered automaticity* refers to spontaneous beat(s) whose appearance depends on previous (normal) sinus beats. The cellular correlates of triggered automaticity are afterdepolarizations, depolarizations in the cardiac action potential that occur before or after full repolarization of the cell, early afterdepolarizations (EADs) or delayed afterdepolarizations (DADs), respectively (Fig. 1-29). For example, arrhythmias occurring when the QT interval is prolonged (described further below) frequently arise when the underlying sinus rate is slow; EADs have been implicated in their genesis, and maneuvers to increase heart rate can abolish EADs in vitro and are used to treat these arrhythmias. Arrhythmias due to intracellular calcium overload (e.g., with digitalis intoxication) may arise as a result of DADs and are exacerbated by antecedent rapid sinus rates.

The fundamental principle of *reentrant excitation* is that two sites in the heart are connected by more than a single pathway for propagation. A propagating impulse blocks (through a variety of mechanisms) in one of these pathways, propagates via the other to the distal site, and then returns to the original site via the initial pathway. One good example is the atrioventricular reentrant tachycardia (AVRT) occurring in the Wolff-Parkinson-White (WPW) syndrome (Fig. 1-30). Subjects with WPW are born with accessory pathway(s), or bypass tracts, connecting atrium and ventricle. Atrioventricular conduction with sinus beats occurs via both the AV node and the accessory pathway, resulting in the typical short PR and delta wave characteristic of preexcitation (Fig. 1-30A). If conduction block occurs in the pathway, impulses can propagate from atrium to ventricle via the AV node, and

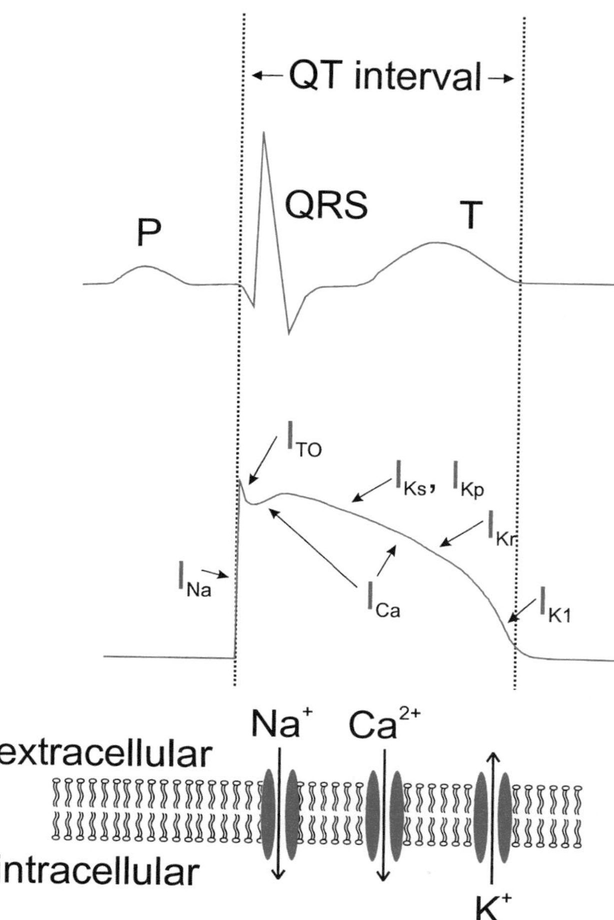


FIGURE 1-28 **Relationship between surface ECG (top) and ventricular action potential (middle). The QRS complex of the ECG corresponds to ventricular depolarization (action potential upstroke), while the QT interval is determined by the duration of the action potential. Ion currents moving through pore-forming membrane proteins, termed ion channels, are diagrammed in the bottom panel. Sodium and calcium currents move into cells (and depolarize them) while potassium currents move out of cells and repolarize them. Multiple potassium currents, including $I_{Kr}$, $I_{Ks}$, $I_{TO}$, $I_{K1}$, and $I_{Kp}$, have been identified, and each appears to play an especially prominent role during specific portions of the action potential, as indicated. Ion current amplitudes vary as a function of factors such as antiarrhythmic drugs, adrenergic tone, heart rate, location of the cell in the heart, and disease. As a result, there is substantial cell-to-cell variability in the shape and duration of individual action potentials, since these are determined by the integrated behavior of all membrane currents.**

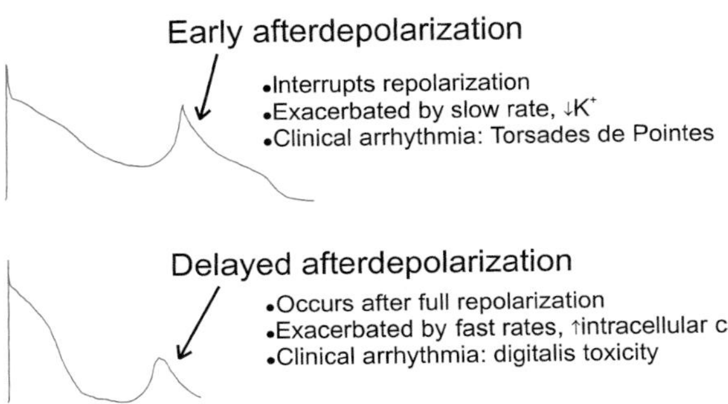


**FIGURE 1-29 Contrasting appearances and basic and clinical features of early and delayed afterdepolarizations. (Adapted from Roden DM. 1992. Treatment of cardiovascular disorders: arrhythmias. In: Melmon KL, Morrelli HF, Hoffman BB, et al., editors. *Clinical Pharmacology: Basic Principles in Therapeutics*. New York: McGraw-Hill. p 151-85. Reproduced with permission of the McGraw-Hill Companies.)**

then reenter the atrium via the accessory pathway (or rarely vice versa) (Fig. 1-30B). Reentrant excitation can also occur in anatomically fixed circuits within and around the AV node (AV nodal reentrant tachycardia, AVNRT), at the rim of a healed myocardial infarction (monomorphic ventricular tachycardia), and within the atrium (atrial flutter). In yet other cases, reentrant excitation can occur not because of anatomically fixed pathways, but because an abnormal milieu (e.g., due to myocardial ischemia) permanently or transiently creates sufficient heterogeneity in the electrophysiologic properties of specific regions of the heart to promote reentry. In such cases a reentrant pathway is not fixed, and multiple reentrant vortices may meander around the atria (atrial fibrillation) or the ventricle (ventricular fibrillation).

## Mechanisms of Antiarrhythmic Drug Action

Some antiarrhythmic drugs have been available for decades, from the time before the recognition of specific cardiac ion currents, so some preconceptions about mechanisms of drug action are being reinterpreted in the context of modern molecular and cellular biology. Four major mechanisms of antiarrhythmic drug action have been recognized: sodium channel block, calcium channel block, action potential prolongation, and antiadrenergic activity (Table 1-36). Blocking of cardiac sodium channels raises the threshold for excitation (makes tissue harder to excite) and slows impulse propagation. Sodium channel blockers can be antiarrhythmic either by slowing conduction so extensively (particularly in diseased tissue) that impulse propagation fails completely, disrupting reentrant arrhythmias, or by preventing propagation from or suppressing activity of automatically firing foci. However, it is now recognized that conduction slowing can also promote arrhythmias (see below). Calcium channels are widely distributed in the heart, in vascular tissues, and elsewhere. Many calcium channel blockers (e.g., see sections in this chapter on hypertension and coronary artery disease) have preferential effects on the vasculature, and are used in antihypertensive or antianginal therapy. Some calcium channel blockers (verapamil, diltiazem) also have activity for cardiac tissues. The major effect of these drugs is to slow or block impulse propagation in the AV node; consequently, their greatest utility is to terminate or prevent reentrant arrhythmias whose circuit includes the AV node (AVNRT, AVRT) and to slow rapid ventricular rates in other supraventricular arrhythmias (atrial fibrillation, atrial flutter, atrial tachycardia). As with calcium channel blockers, $\beta$-adrenergic receptor blockers ($\beta$-blockers) are especially effective in arrhythmias involving the AV node or in controlling ventricular response in supraventricular arrhythmias. $\beta$-Blockers are also effective in some ventricular arrhythmias, as described further below. Prolongation of cardiac action potential duration, particularly if it is accomplished in a uniform fashion (i.e., in a way that reduces heterogeneity of action potential durations), should, in theory, suppress many reentrant arrhythmias. Blocking of cardiac potassium currents is one common mechanism whereby drugs prolong cardiac action potentials, and modern molecular techniques have identified multiple different potassium currents whose blocking can achieve this effect and indeed suppress arrhythmias such as atrial fibrillation. However, a major liability of many available potassium channel blocking agents is the potential to precipitate new arrhythmias (one example of the phenomenon of proarrhythmia described below).

Some drugs suppress arrhythmias through mechanisms not directly related to blocking of ion channels or adrenergic receptors. Digitalis glycosides slow impulse propagation through the AV node by their indirect vagomimetic effects and are useful in control of ventricular rate during supraventricular arrhythmias. Magnesium has been used, with some success, in specific situations such as arrhythmias related to digitalis intoxication or arrhythmias related to excess action potential prolongation. Its mechanism of action is unknown. Some trials have also indicated that intravenous magnesium administered early in the course of a myocardial infarction can improve long-term survival (Woods and Fletcher 1994), but other studies have disputed this outcome [ISIS-4 (Fourth International Study of Infarct Survival) Collaborative Group 1955]. The rapid intravenous administration of a bolus of

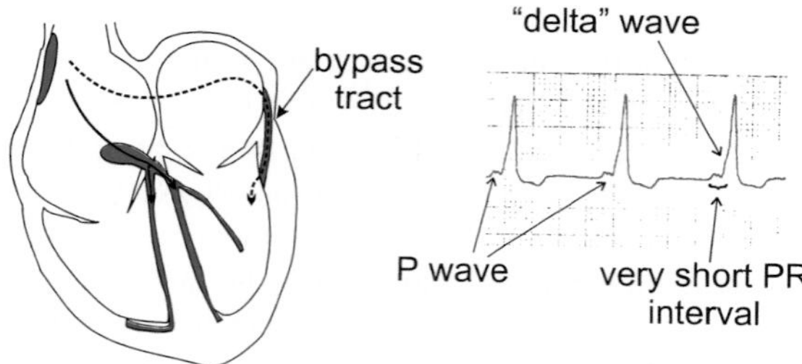


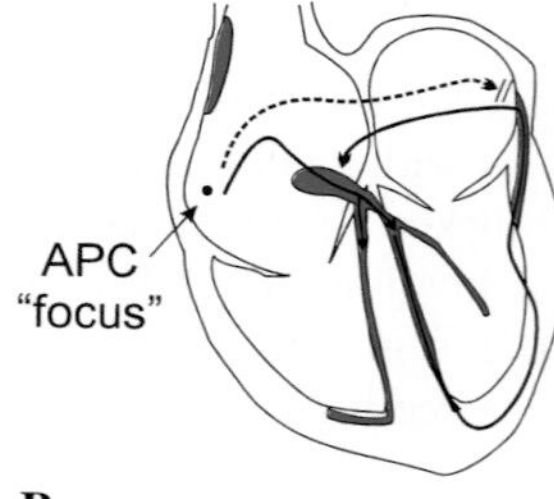


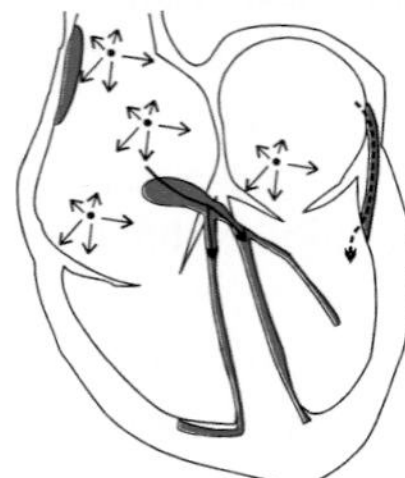


**FIGURE 1-30** Mechanisms in the Wolff-Parkinson-White (WPW) syndrome. *A*: Pathways for cardiac depolarization during sinus rhythm. In addition to the normal pathways (as in Fig. 1-27), there is an accessory pathway capable of bypassing conduction through the AV node. Therefore, during sinus rhythm, a portion of the ventricle is activated prematurely (accounting for a short PR interval), and in an ectopic fashion (accounting for a delta wave). *B*: Initiation of AV reentry in WPW. An impulse fails to propagate in the bypass tract but continues to conduct through the normal pathways, e.g., with an atrial premature complex (APC). Under these conditions, there is a longer PR interval, and no delta wave. However, the propagating wavefront can reenter the atrium via the bypass tract, and thus initiate sustained AV reentry (see text). *C*: Occasionally patients with WPW may develop atrial fibrillation. Atrioventricular conduction can then take place across the bypass tract and result in a bizarre appearance of the QRS complexes and an extraordinarily rapid heart rate (>300/min in this example). While this syndrome is unusual, it is important to recognize since drugs commonly used in atrial fibrillation, e.g., verapamil, digitalis, can be fatal (see text).

**Table 1-36 In Vitro Electrophysiologic Actions of Antiarrhythmic Drugs**

| | ELECTROPHYSIOLOGIC ACTIONS | | | | | | |
|---|---|---|---|---|---|---|---|
| | | ↓K+ CURRENT | | | | | |
| **DRUG** | ↓$I_{Na}$ | $I_{Kr}$ | OTHER[a] | ↓$I_{Ca}$ | | **β-BLOCKADE** | **OTHER ACTIONS** |
| Adenosine | | | | | | | Acute AV nodal block |
| Amiodarone HCl | xx | xx | x | x | | | Sympatholytic; antithyroid |
| Azimilide[b] | | xx | xx | x | | | |
| Bepridil HCl | | | xx | xx | | | |
| Bretylium tesylate | | | xx | | | | Acute norepinephrine release followed by inhibition of presynaptic uptake. |
| Digoxin | | | | | | | Vagotonic |
| Diltiazem HCl | | | | xx | | | |
| Disopyramide | xx | | xx | | | | Anticholinergic |
| Dofetilide[b] | | xx | | | | | |
| Esmolol HCl | | | | | | xx | |
| Flecainide acetate | xx | x | | | | | |
| Ibutilide fumarate | | x | | | ↑$I_{Na}$ | | |
| Lidocaine | xx | | | | | | |
| Magnesium | | | | x (?) | | | |
| Mexiletine HCl | xx | | | | | | |
| Moricizine HCl | xx | | | | | | |
| Procainamide HCl | xx | xx[c] | | | | | Ganglionic blockade |
| Propafenone HCl | xx | x | x | | | xx[d] | |
| Propranolol HCl | | | | | | xx | |
| Quinidine | xx | xx | x | x | | | α-Blockade |
| Sotalol HCl | | xx | x | | | xx | |
| Tedisimil[b] | | x | xx | | | | |
| Tocainide HCl | xx | | | | | | |
| Verapamil HCl | | | x | xx | | | |

SYMBOLS: xx, in vitro action that likely mediates clinical actions; x, other demonstrable action of uncertain clinical significance; (?), possible clinical effect but not yet proven.
[a]Blocker of other $K^+$ currents or known to prolong action potentials through presumed but not yet demonstrated $K^+$ current block.
[b]Investigational drug.
[c]The active metabolite *N*-acetylprocainamide (NAPA) blocks $I_{Kr}$.
[d]The extent of β-blockade by propafenone is highly variable and is inversely related to the activity of CYP 2D6 (see chapter 25, Drug Interactions).
ABBREVIATIONS: AV, arteriovenous; α- and β-blockade, α- and β-adrenergic receptor antagonism; *I*, current.

adenosine produces transient AV nodal block; adenosine is especially useful in terminating reentrant arrhythmias involving the AV node (Camm and Garratt 1991). β-Blockers as well as a number of "nonelectrophysiologic" interventions, e.g., aspirin (Antiplatelet Trialists Collaboration 1988), hydroxymethylglutaryl-coenzyme A (HMG-CoA) reductase inhibitors (Scandinavian Simvastatin Survival Study Group 1994; Shepherd et al. 1995), and angiotensin-converting enzyme (ACE) inhibitors (The SOLVD Investigators 1992; Pfeffer et al. 1992) appear to reduce mortality in patients with advanced heart disease. The mechanism whereby these interventions exert this effect (some of which may be antiarrhythmic) is uncertain, but indirect effects such as stabilization of coronary artery disease, rather than direct modulation of cardiac electrophysiology, seem likely.

Although it has become conventional to subclassify antiarrhythmics according to their major ionic mechanism of action, most available drugs exert multiple potential antiarrhythmic (and proarrhythmic) pharmacologic actions (Table 1-36), "classes" I–IV, respectively. In addition, the specific detailed characteristics of blocking, e.g., how much more extensively a drug blocks channels at fast vs. slow rates or in depolarized vs. normal tissue (Snyders et al. 1991), may vary considerably among drugs of the same class. In addition, drugs whose major ionic mechanisms of action in the heart are similar may have very different profiles of noncardiac adverse effects. Although classification schemes are widely promulgated, their actual utility in selecting a drug for a specific patient is more limited (Task Force of the Working Group on Arrhythmias of the European Society of Cardiology 1991). To the extent that individual ion channel blocking properties can be associated with adverse effects, particularly proarrhythmia, classification schemes may be useful in predicting such events.

## APPROACH TO THE PATIENT WITH ARRHYTHMIAS

### Symptoms Associated with Arrhythmias: Why Treat?

Treatment for arrhythmias is undertaken either to suppress symptoms or to prevent morbidity or mortality due to arrhythmias. The most common symptoms associated with arrhythmias are palpitations (a feeling of the heart beating rapidly or irregularly), light-headedness, and/or transient loss of consciousness (syncope). Palpitations are most frequently due to APCs, VPCs, or atrial fibrillation. The severity of symptoms associated with arrhythmias is strongly dependent on the extent of underlying heart disease. For example, patients with AVNRT or AVRT (who generally have otherwise normal hearts) may have heart rates in excess of 250 bpm and yet may note only light-headedness or palpitations. On the other hand, patients with sustained monomorphic ventricular tachycardia, who usually have advanced underlying heart disease due to remote myocardial infarction(s), may present with slower tachycardia rates but nevertheless more severe symptoms such as recurrent syncope due to severe hypotension, without even premonitory palpitations. The most extreme occurrence is the syndrome of sudden cardiac death, which kills 300,000–500,000 Americans each year and which usually arises from ventricular fibrillation in a patient with advanced myocardial scarring. In ventricular fibrillation, all effective contractile function ceases, and the patient will die within minutes unless effective cardiopulmonary resuscitation is initiated.

In atrial fibrillation, the AV node is bombarded by multiple impulses, and the ventricular rate is often very rapid (150–180 bpm in an untreated patient), with symptoms such as dyspnea, chest pain, and palpitations. In patients with the WPW syndrome, the development of atrial fibrillation can result in much faster rates, because the ventricle may be excited not only via the AV node but also via atrioventricular conduction over the accessory pathway (Fig. 1-30C). Although this arrhythmia ("pre-excited atrial fibrillation") is very rare, it is crucial to recognize, since the use of AV nodal blocking drugs, such as digitalis, has been associated with paradoxical increases in ventricular rate, and the development of ventricular fibrillation; deaths in patients with WPW are probably attributable to this mechanism (Klein et al. 1979).

Some patients with atrial tachycardia (in which an automatic focus fires repetitively at rapid rates, resulting in heart rates of 150–200 bpm) may present with advanced heart failure but no specific arrhythmia symptoms such as palpitations. In such cases of "tachycardia-induced cardiomyopathy," normal contractile function may return several weeks after suppression of the arrhythmia (Shinbane et al. 1997). Similar advanced contractile dysfunction can also be seen in occasional patients with persistent atrial flutter or atrial fibrillation with rapid rates (Zipes 1997).

Patients with severe symptoms due to recurrent or ongoing arrhythmias can and should be treated. On the other hand, in patients with milder symptoms (e.g., palpitations due to APCs or VPCs), many treatments may—as described further below—confer risk; indeed, in these patients the risk of therapy may exceed any potential benefit, and therapy should be deferred. In patients who are asymptomatic, currently available data described below indicate that therapy should not be undertaken except in very specialized instances (e.g., tachycardia-induced cardiomyopathy). Some studies do indicate that certain arrhythmias (e.g., VPCs) that occur in patients with advanced heart disease are a marker for an increased risk for sudden cardiac death due to ventricular fibrillation (Hallstrom et al. 1992). Ongoing trials are currently assessing whether antiarrhythmic therapies can prolong life in such individuals, but currently available data do not, in general, support antiarrhythmic interventions.

### Evaluation of Antiarrhythmic Therapy

As with all other forms of therapy, clinicians using antiarrhythmic therapies should first ensure that the potential benefits of treatments outweigh the potential risks. Benefits can be maximized by establishing the correct arrhythmia diagnosis and subsequent selection of the most appropriate treatment. Risks can be minimized by appropriate dose selection based on sound pharmacokinetic principles, appropriate drug selection to minimize noncardiac adverse effects, and maneuvers to minimize the risk of proarrhythmia.

The best, commonly available tool for appropriate arrhythmia diagnosis is the 12-lead electrocardiogram. This may allow distinction of, for example, supraventricular from ventricular arrhythmias (Wellens 1986). Although the electrocardiograms (ECGs) in these arrhythmias can occasionally resemble each other, the distinction is clinically important because treatments directed at supraventricular tachycardia (e.g., intravenous verapamil) can result in catastrophic hemodynamic collapse if the arrhythmia is actually ventricular tachycardia (Stewart et al. 1986). In addition, diagnostic criteria have been developed for specific forms of ventricular tachycardia and for specific subtypes of supraventricular tachycardia, including AVRT and AVNRT. This information can be useful in selection of drug therapy, as well as in guiding nonpharmacologic approaches described further below. The signal-averaged ECG (SAECG) is a specialized variant designed to detect slow conduction that is the substrate for reentrant ventricular arrhythmias in patients who have had a remote myocardial infarction or other myocardial scar; the extent to which an SAECG adds information to other readily obtained predictors of risk (such as ejection fraction) is controversial and the test has not been widely adopted.

In patients presenting with intermittent symptoms such as palpitations or light-headedness, a diagnosis should be established before therapy is initiated. If symptoms are frequent, a 24- or 48-hour continuous recording of cardiac rhythm (Holter monitor) can frequently help in establishing the diagnosis. When symptoms are more sporadic, patient-activated or automatic "event recorders," which can record cardiac rhythm at specific times over weeks or months, should be considered. Tilt table testing can be used to investigate vasovagal and other forms of bradycardia-related syncope. However, the sensitivity and specificity of the technique are unclear. Clinically occurring sustained tachyarrhythmias can sometimes be reproduced (and their mechanisms and response to therapy can be evaluated) during programmed electrical stimulation of the heart, which includes pacing and recording specific intracardiac sites using electrode catheters. However, "nonclinical" arrhythmias, to which the patient may not be susceptible in ordinary life, may also be elicited by these techniques.

## Noncardiac Adverse Effects of Antiarrhythmic Drugs

Many antiarrhythmic agents commonly cause noncardiac adverse effects, and this can have an important impact on selection of antiarrhythmic therapy. For example, disopyramide exerts prominent anticholinergic effects, which may include not only dry mouth and constipation, but increased intraocular pressure and urinary hesitancy. As a consequence, disopyramide should generally not be used in patients with glaucoma or prostatism. Another problem with noncardiac adverse effects of antiarrhythmic drugs is the potential to introduce diagnostic confusion. For example, a relatively common adverse effect during long-term use of procainamide is the drug-induced lupus syndrome, a major manifestation of which is arthralgias and arthritis. Use of procainamide in a patient with, for example, rheumatoid arthritis would therefore be undesirable, because it would be difficult to establish whether a flare of symptoms was due to the drug or the underlying disease. Similarly, the use of amiodarone is undesirable in patients with lung disease. Common noncardiac adverse effects of antiarrhythmic drugs are listed in Table 1-37.

## The Problem of Proarrhythmia

The recognition that drugs designed to suppress arrhythmias can, in some patients, actually increase arrhythmias or provoke new ones is probably the single most important factor currently guiding selection and use of antiarrhythmic therapy. For example, not only are drugs incompletely effective in preventing ventricular fibrillation, but they may also increase risk of sudden death in some patients. Therefore, many clinicians choose to use nonpharmacological therapy (described below), rather than drugs, as primary therapy in such patients. Proarrhythmia is not attributable to a single mechanism. Rather, multiple proarrhythmia "syndromes" have now been identified, and underlying mechanisms elucidated (Table 1-38). Treatment of all these syndromes includes recognition, withdrawal of offending agents, and specific mechanism-based therapies described below.

***Digitalis intoxication***

The drug that was first associated with the development of abnormal rhythms was probably digitalis (see also the section in this chapter on congestive heart failure). Although it is said that intoxication with digitalis glycosides can produce virtually any arrhythmia, certain arrhythmias should raise a particular suspicion. Typically, arrhythmias related to digitalis glycoside toxicity are manifest as ectopic rhythms such as atrial tachycardia or VPCs, thought to be due to DAD-related triggered automaticity, with sinus slowing or AV nodal block, owing to the drug's indirect vagomimetic effects. In advanced cases, digoxin concentrations are generally >2 ng/ml. For asymptomatic arrhythmias due to digitalis intoxication, discontinuation of the drug and observation are probably sufficient. For more advanced cases, the therapy of choice is anti-digoxin antibodies (Antman et al. 1990). Temporary pacing may be required.

Table 1-37 **Adverse Effects of Antiarrhythmic Drugs**

| Drug | Major adverse effects[a] | Underlying disease in which potential for drug toxicity creates relative contraindication |
|---|---|---|
| Amiodarone HCl | Pulmonary fibrosis | Lung disease |
| | Liver dysfunction | Advanced liver disease (?) |
| | Peripheral neuropathy | Preexisting neuropathy |
| | Thyroid dysfunction, photosensitivity, corneal microdeposits | |
| β-Blockers | Adverse effects secondary to β-blockade, e.g., bronchospasm | Asthma, insulin-dependent diabetes with symptomatic hypoglycemia |
| Calcium channel blockers | Congestive heart failure | LV dysfunction |
| | AV block | Underlying conduction system disease |
| Disopyramide phosphate | Congestive heart failure | LV dysfunction |
| | Torsades de pointes | Baseline QT prolongation; hypokalemia |
| | Urinary retention | Prostatism |
| | Increased intraocular pressure | Glaucoma |
| Flecainide acetate, moricizine HCl | Increased mortality post-MI | Coronary artery disease |
| | bradyarrhythmias | Conduction system disease |
| Ibutilide fumarate | Torsades de pointes | Baseline QT prolongation; hypokalemia |
| Lidocaine, mexiletine HCl, tocainide HCl | Tremors | Parkinson disease |
| | Seizures | Seizure disorder |
| Procainamide HCl | Lupus-like syndrome | Chronic arthritis |
| | Agranulocytosis | Preexisting blood dyscrasia |
| Propafenone HCl | Bronchospasm | Asthma |
| | Congestive heart failure | LV dysfunction |
| | Bradyarrhythmias | Conduction system disease |
| Quinidine | Diarrhea | Chronic GI disease |
| | Torsades de pointes | Baseline QT prolongation; hypokalemia |
| Sotalol HCl | Side effects secondary to β-blockade, e.g., bronchospasm | Asthma, insulin-dependent diabetes with symptomatic hypoglycemia |
| | Torsades de pointes | Baseline QT prolongation; hypokalemia |

[a]Only examples of toxicities that may give rise to patient-specific management situations are listed.
ABBREVIATIONS: AV, atrioventricular; GI, gastrointestinal; LV, left ventricular; MI, myocardial infarction; QT, portion of the electrocardiogram that shows depolarization and repolarization (action potential duration).

***Proarrhythmia due to sodium channel block***

Four distinct forms of proarrhythmia have been associated with treatment with sodium channel blockers. First, in patients with atrial flutter, sodium channel block can slow the flutter rate, e.g., from 300/min to 200/min. When the atrial flutter rate is 300/min, the usual AV nodal response is 2:1 block, i.e., a ventricular rate of 150/min. However, when the flutter rate slows to 180–200/min, 1:1 AV nodal conduction can occur, with a ventricular rate that is therefore faster than that seen before the drug was administered. Because the effects of sodium channel block increase at fast rates, patients with this syndrome often present with wide QRS complexes, making the distinction from ventricular tachycardia difficult (Crijns et al. 1988). Treatment includes drugs such as calcium channel blockers to increase the degree of AV nodal block. Second, slow conduction in the rim of an old myocardial infarction plays a prominent role in the genesis and maintenance of sustained monomorphic ventricular tachycardia. The use of sodium channel blockers can, in some patients, increase the frequency of episodes of this arrhythmia, likely by further slowing conduction (Morganroth et al. 1986; Coromilas et al. 1995). β-Blockade has been effective in some cases (Myerburg et al. 1989), possibly by slowing sinus rate and thereby decreasing the extent of sodium channel block. In addition, some data suggest intravenous sodium (as bicarbonate or chloride) may be useful (Chouty et al. 1987). Third, sodium channel block reduces

**Table 1-38 Proarrhythmia Syndromes**

| SYNDROME | POSTULATED MECHANISM[a] | CLINICAL FEATURES | SPECIFIC THERAPY[a] |
|---|---|---|---|
| *Digitalis toxicity* | DADs due to intracellular calcium overload | VPCs or atrial tachycardia with AV block | Mild cases: observe<br>Severe cases: anti-digoxin antibodies |
| *Sodium channel block-related*: | | | |
| Atrial flutter with 1:1 AV conduction | Slowing of conduction in the atrial flutter circuit →fewer impulses exciting the AV node→↓AV block →faster ventricular rate | Fast regular ventricular rate | AV nodal block |
| Incessant VT | Conduction slowing within a reentrant VT circuit | Frequently recurring, often slow, VT | ?Sodium infusion<br>? $\beta$-Blockers |
| Increased threshold for pacing or defibrillation | Increased threshold for excitability | | |
| Increased mortality during long-term treatment | Increased risk for ischemic VF | | |
| *Action potential prolongation*: | | | |
| Torsades de pointes | EADs, triggered activity, intramural reentry | QT prolongation, dispersion and lability; pause-dependent onset | Magnesium<br>Maintain serum $K^+ > 4.5$ mEq/L maneuvers to increase heart rate: isoproterenol, pacing<br>?inhibition of triggered activity: calcium channel blockers $\beta$-blockers |
| Increased mortality during long-term treatment (*d*-sotalol) | Torsades de pointes degenerating to VF | | |

[a]Treatment always includes recognition and withdrawing offending agent(s).
ABBREVIATIONS: AV, atrioventricular; DAD, delayed afterdepolarization; EAD, early afterdepolarization; QT, portion of the electrocardiogram that shows depolarization and repolarization (action potential duration); VF, ventricular fibrillation; VPC, ventricular premature contraction; VT, ventricular tachycardia.

excitability of the heart. In patients with pacemakers or implantable cardioverter-defibrillators (ICDs) discussed further below, increased output of the devices may be required for effective function. Rarely, ventricular arrhythmias occurring in the presence of sodium channel blockers cannot be effectively terminated by internal or external direct current (DC) cardioversion, and deaths have been reported (Winkle et al. 1981; Oetgen et al. 1983). For this and other reasons, management of patients with ICDs is left to specialized clinical electrophysiologists.

The fourth proarrhythmia syndrome occurring during treatment with sodium channel blockers is an increase in mortality during long-term treatment. This was established by the Cardiac Arrhythmia Suppression Trial (CAST), a landmark study that tested, in a placebo-controlled, randomized, double-blind fashion, the then-prevailing wisdom that suppression of VPCs in patients convalescing from a myocardial infarction would reduce the incidence of sudden death. In CAST, patients with VPCs and a recent myocardial infarction were randomly assigned to one of three sodium channel blocker therapies, which was then titrated to the dose that appeared to suppress VPCs on a 24-hour Holter monitor. Once the effective dose and drug were established, patients were randomly assigned to continue drug or placebo. Remarkably, mortality among patients randomized to drug was 2 to 3 times that among those randomized to placebo [The Cardiac Arrhythmia Suppression Trial (CAST) Investigators 1989; The Cardiac Arrhythmia Suppression Trial II Investigators 1991]. The mechanism underlying this striking, and previously undefined, effect of sodium channel block remains uncertain. However, conduction slowing with an increased risk of sustained ventricular arrhythmias (including ventricular fibrillation) seems likely. It has been argued that other sodium channel blockers might not produce the same effect as the three drugs tested in CAST (encainide [no longer available], flecainide, and moricizine). However, preclinical data suggest this may be a "class action" of sodium channel block (Nattel et al. 1981) and other, less well designed, studies with mexiletine and with disopyramide (IMPACT Research Group 1984; UK Rythmodan Multicentre Study Group 1984) showed a very similar trend to increased mortality. Perhaps the most important implications of CAST were the recognition that "surrogate" endpoints (in this case, VPCs as a surrogate for arrhythmic death) should be used with extreme caution in clinical medicine unless well-validated, and that physicians should recognize that their own biases, which so often drive therapy in areas in which data are not available, may be erroneous.

***Proarrhythmia due to QT prolongation***

In some patients, therapy with action potential prolonging drugs such as sotalol, quinidine, or ibutilide can be associated with marked prolongation of the QT interval and induction of a morphologically distinctive polymorphic ventricular tachycardia, torsades de pointes (Ben-David and Zipes 1993; Roden 1993; Tan et al. 1995). Torsades de pointes can also occur during treatment with "noncardiovascular" drugs; common examples include terfenadine, cisapride, haloperidol, and thioridazine (Tan et al. 1995). Many such cases are attributable to inhibition of drug elimination, and thus accumulation of drug to unusually high plasma concentrations, due to coadministration of an inhibitor of CYP3A4 (see chapter 22, Pharmacogenetics, and chapter 25, Drug Interactions). Occasional cases are also unrelated to drug therapy and can be attributed to the syndrome of congenital QT prolongation, marked bradyarrhythmias, hypokalemia, or acute central nervous system injury. It is interesting that most drugs that have been associated with torsades de pointes appear to target a single, specific cardiac potassium current, termed $I_{Kr}$. Mutations in the gene that encodes the channel responsible for $I_{Kr}$ are now recognized as a cause of congenital long QT syndrome, a disease associated with QT prolongation, torsades de pointes, and sudden death (Sanguinetti et al. 1995). Thus, the molecular genetic data as well as the clinical data both suggest that block of other potassium channels may be a more effective way of achieving the antiarrhythmic effect of prolonging the action potential, possibly without causing torsades de pointes.

Risk factors for torsades de pointes have been identified. These include female gender (Makkar et al. 1993), hypokalemia, bradycardia, and high drug dosages or plasma concentrations of drugs listed above. An exception is quinidine, where the reaction can occur with the first dose and at "subtherapeutic" plasma concentrations. Other data suggest that advanced heart failure, recent conversion from atrial fibrillation (Choy et al. 1996), and very rapid intravenous administration of drug (Carlsson et al. 1993) may also increase risk. Uncontrolled clinical trials suggest that potassium supplementation (to a concentration above 4.5 mEq/L) and intravenous magnesium (Tzivoni et al. 1988) should be the first approaches to therapy, as they are relatively simple and unlikely to do harm. If these are ineffective, maneuvers to increase the heart rate to >90 bpm are usually effective; this can be accomplished by isoproterenol or by temporary pacing.

Most recognized cases of torsades de pointes occur shortly after starting culprit drug(s). However, a specific $I_{Kr}$ blocker, the dextrorotatory isomer of sotalol (*d*-sotalol), was found in SWORD (Survival with Oral *d*-Sotalol), a large study with a CAST-like design, to increase long-term mortality compared to placebo in patients judged to be at risk for sudden death (Waldo et al. 1996). Since the drug is not a sodium channel blocker, a mechanism different from that in CAST seems likely; torsades de pointes occurring during chronic term outpatient treatment is one leading possibility (Fig. 1-31).

***Amiodarone and proarrhythmia***

Amiodarone is a drug that is associated with a relatively low risk of proarrhythmia. The mechanism whereby this drug, which prolongs the QT interval and blocks sodium channels, does not appear to cause a high risk for proarrhythmia is not yet understood (Lazzara 1989). Amiodarone has cumbersome pharmacokinetics: an elimination half-life of months has been measured after withdrawal of the drug during chronic therapy, indicating very slow accumulation in tissues. Because of this slow accumulation, loading regimens extending over several weeks are usu-

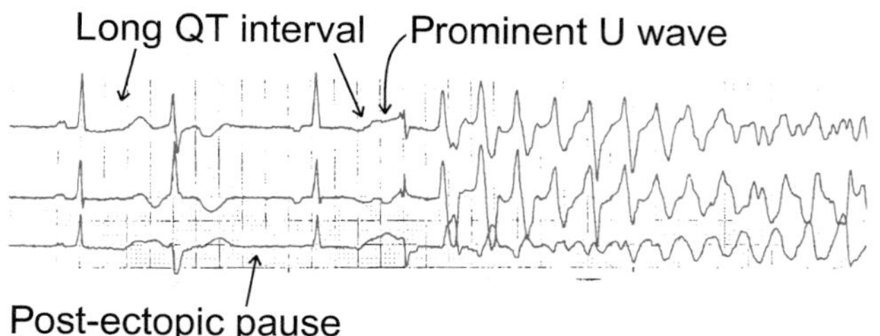


**FIGURE 1-31 Torsades de pointes in a patient receiving sotalol. This 3-lead tracing shows a sinus beat, an ectopic beat followed by a pause, and a post-pause sinus beat with a remarkably long and deformed QT interval and prominent U wave. The tachycardia starts after this U wave. This pattern of pause-dependence and QTU changes is typical of torsades de pointes.**

ally used during initiation of therapy. Bradycardia and multiple noncardiac adverse effects (including potentially fatal pulmonary fibrosis) are well recognized during long-term treatment of amiodarone. Despite its usual pharmacokinetics and adverse effect profile, amiodarone is increasingly assuming a role as a first line antiarrhythmic drug because of its relative lack of proarrhythmia and on account of its demonstrated superior efficacy compared to other drugs in some clinical settings, described below.

## Pharmacokinetic Principles in the Use of Antiarrhythmic Drugs

The necessity for adjustment of loading and/or maintenance dosages when there are alterations in volume of distribution or in drug-eliminating organ(s) is a well-established principle in clinical pharmacology and especially applicable to antiarrhythmic drugs with their narrow margins between drug doses associated with efficacy and those associated with toxicity (see chapter 23, Clinical Pharmacokinetics and Pharmacodynamics). For some drugs, therapeutic ranges of plasma concentrations have been established. For other drugs, metabolism and elimination are so highly variable (often with varying contributions of active metabolites to overall drug efficacy) that therapeutic ranges of plasma concentrations have not been well validated. In these cases, the most appropriate approach to therapy is to initiate therapy with low dosages and to escalate upward only if adverse effects are absent and efficacy is not present. For antiarrhythmic drugs, as with all other forms of therapy, the potential that concomitant therapy can modulate drug disposition and thereby modulate drug effect is widely recognized (see chapter 25, Drug Interactions). Important pharmacokinetic considerations for antiarrhythmic drugs are included in Tables 1-39 and 1-40.

**Table 1-39 Drugs Used for the Acute Therapy of Arrhythmias**

| Drug | Indication | Typical initial dose[a] | Maintenance infusion | Dosage adjustment | Therapeutic plasma concn | Cost of initial dose ($)[b] |
|---|---|---|---|---|---|---|
| Adenosine | PSVT | 6 mg | | | | Adenocard $26 |
| Amiodarone HCl | VT, VF | 150 mg | 0.25–0.5 mg/min | | | Cordarone $69 |
| Bretylium tosylate | VT, VF | 150 mg | 1–4 mg/min | Renal failure | | Generic $6 |
| Diltiazem HCl | AF (rate control) | 15 mg | 5–15 mg/hr | | | Cardizem $13 |
| Esmolol HCl | AF (rate control) | 30 mg | 3–12 mg/min | | | Brevibloc $7 |
| Ibutilide fumarate | AF (conversion) | 1 mg | | | | Corvert $137 |
| Lidocaine | VT, VF | 200 mg (3–4 mg/kg) | 1–4 mg/min | CHF, liver disease, β-Blockers | 2–5 μg/ml | Xylocaine $1 |
| $MgSO_4$ | Torsades de pointes | 1 g | Renal failure | | | Generic $2 |
| Metoprolol succinate | | VT, VF, PSVT | 10 mg | | | Generic $15 |
| Procainamide HCl | VT, VF, AF (conversion) | 1 g | 1–4 mg/min | Renal failure | 4–8 μg/ml | Generic $11 |
| Verapamil HCl | PSVT | 5 mg | | | | Generic $2 |

[a]All initial doses are administered as infusions (over 5–30 minutes, depending on the drug), with the exception of adenosine, which is administered as a rapid bolus dose through a large bore intravenous line. When no maintenance dose is listed, the drug is administered as a single or multiple boluses.

[b]Source of drug prices is *Mosby's GenRx* 1998. Current prices may vary from those quoted, but comparative prices among products are expected to be similar. The reader should check on local prices at the time of prescribing.

ABBREVIATIONS: AF, atrial fibrillation or flutter; CHF, congestive heart failure; concn, concentration; PSVT, paroxysmal supraventricular tachycardia; VF, ventricular fibrillation; VT, ventricular tachycardia.

**Table 1-40 Drugs Used for the Long-Term Therapy of Arrhythmias**

| Drug | Indication | Total daily dose[a] (usually divided) | Dosage adjustment | Therapeutic plasma concn ($/month)[b] | Cost of therapy at low-end of typical daily dose | |
|---|---|---|---|---|---|---|
| Amiodarone HCl | AF, VT, VF | 200–400 mg/day | | —[c] | Cordarone | $91 |
| Digoxin | AF (rate control), PSVT[d] | 0.125–0.25 mg/day | Renal failure(↓) amiodarone HCl, quinidine, cyclosporine, verapamil HCl (↓) | 0.5–2.0 ng/ml | Generic<br>Lanoxin | $2<br>$7 |
| Diltiazem HCl | AF (rate control) | 120–360 mg/day[e] | | | Generic<br>Cardizem | $12<br>$53 |
| Disopyramide phosphate | AF | 300–600 mg/day[5] | Renal failure (↓); phenytoin, rifampin (↑) | 2–5 $\mu$g/ml[3] | Generic<br>Norpace | $14<br>$77 |
| Flecainide acetate | PSVT, AF | 100–300 mg/day | | | Tambocor | $46 |
| Metoprolol succinate[f] | AF (rate control), PSVT, VT, VF | 100–200 mg/day | | | Toprol XL | $20 |
| Mexiletine HCl | VT, VF[d] | 450–750 mg/day | Liver disease (↓); phenytoin, rifampin (↑) | 1–2 $\mu$g/ml | Generic<br>Mexitil | $62<br>$71 |
| Moricizine HCl | VT, VF[4] | 600–900 mg/day | | —[c] | Ethmozine | $87 |
| Procainamide HCl | AF, VT, VF | 2–5 g/day (alternate[e]) | Renal failure (↓) | 4–8 $\mu$g/ml[c] (NAPA: 10–20 $\mu$g/ml) | Generic<br>Pronestyl | $10<br>$97 |
| Propafenone HCL | PSVT, AF | 450–900 mg/day | Renal failure (↓) | —[c] | Rythmol | $76 |
| Propranolol HCl[f] | PSVT, AF (rate control), VF, VT | 80–240 mg/day | | | Generic<br>Inderal | $1<br>$28 |
| Quinidine gluconate | AF, VT, VF | 648–1944 mg/day | Phenytoin, rifampin (↑) | 2–5 $\mu$g/ml[c] | Quinaglute Dura-tabs | $50 |
| Sotalol HCl | AF, VT, VF | 160–320 mg/day | Renal failure (↓) | | Betapace | $97 |
| Tocainide HCl | VT, VF[d] | 1200–1800 mg/day | Renal failure (↓) | | Tonocard | $72 |
| Verapamil HCl | AF (rate control), PSVT | 240–480 mg/day (alternate[e]) | | | Generic<br>Calan | $4<br>$43 |

[a]Oral loading regimens are typically used for 1–3 months before reduction to maintenance doses.
[b]Source of drug prices is *Mosby's GenR$_x$* 1998. Current prices may vary from those quoted, but comparative prices among products are expected to be similar. The reader should check on local prices at the time of prescribing.
[c]Active metabolite(s) may contribute to clinical effects during long-term therapy. The best studied of these is NAPA (*N*-acetylprocainamide). Compared with the parent drug, NAPA exerts different electrophysiologic effects, undergoes no metabolism (is eliminated unchanged by the kidneys), and has a different range of therapeutic concentrations.
[d]Not drug of first or second choice for this indication.
[e]Sustained-release formulation also available.
[f]Many other $\beta$-blockers also available and effective.
ABBREVIATIONS: as in Table 1–39.

## Nonpharmacologic Therapy of Arrhythmias

Chronic or recurrent symptomatic bradyarrhythmias are treated with permanent pacemakers. Transient bradyarrhythmias, such as those occurring with digitalis toxicity or myocardial infarction, may occasionally respond to interventions such as isoproterenol or atropine, but temporary pacemakers may also be required.

In the 1970s, surgical procedures were developed to section accessory atrioventricular connections and thereby to cure patients with the WPW syndrome and frequently recurring and/or life-threatening arrhythmias. In the late 1980s, techniques were developed to allow permanent interruption of such accessory pathways via radiofrequency energy applied through catheters advanced to specific locations in the heart (Manolis et al. 1994). These procedures cause minimal discomfort, do not require general anesthesia, and require minimal (or no) in-patient hospitalization. Radiofrequency catheter ablation is now widely used to cure permanently patients with the WPW syndrome, and with many other forms of reentrant arrhythmias utilizing a fixed pathway (AVNRT, atrial flutter, some forms of ventricular tachycardia). The procedures are highly effective with a minimal risk of adverse effects, and data on their cost-effectiveness are now being reported. For example, modeling studies suggest that catheter ablation for patients with WPW who have had a cardiac arrest is highly cost-effective, but is not in those who are asymptomatic (Hogenhuis et al. 1993); the management decision in an individual patient is guided by model data such as these, as well as by individual patient characteristics (e.g., whether the patient has a job, such as truck driving or piloting airplanes, in which syncope or dizziness might be dangerous). In addition, catheter ablation can also be curative in patients with foci of abnormal automaticity (some forms of atrial tachycardia, some forms of ventricular tachycardia). In patients with atrial fibrillation and poorly controlled ventricular responses, interruption of AV nodal transmission by ablation of the AV node, with placement of a permanent pacemaker, may be an option. Techniques are currently being evaluated for applying radiofrequency lesions to interrupt or to prevent the development of atrial fibrillation.

Another form of nonpharmacologic therapy for arrhythmias is the implantable cardioverter-defibrillator. The ICD device is placed, like a pacemaker, subcutaneously in the pectoral region and is connected by a specialized lead to the right ventricular endocardium. The device senses cardiac rhythm. Should a very fast tachycardia (e.g., ventricular fibrillation) occur, the device can initiate pacing and/or defibrillating therapies to "rescue" the patient. Pacing therapies are preferred because they are painless, while shocks are painful. Currently available devices are quite sophisticated, offering features such as programmability of the characteristics of tachycardia to be treated, antibradycardia pacing, and storage (with retrieval capability by telemetry) of electrical signals corresponding to abnormal rhythms. ICDs have had their greatest impact in the management of patients with rapid ventricular tachycardia or ventricular fibrillation (McAnulty et al. 1997). Trials are completed (but not yet reported in full) to assess whether patients judged to be at very high risk for such arrhythmias, but in whom no event has yet occurred, should receive ICDs or other forms of antiarrhythmic therapy (Buxton et al. 1993). Preliminary data suggest ICDS may be useful in some of these patients.

Like drug therapy for arrhythmias, nonpharmacologic therapies do have recognized risks. The risks of radiofrequency catheter ablation include cardiac perforation, damage to the AV node (with a subsequent need for a permanent pacemaker), and formation of intracardiac thrombi with subsequent embolization. In experienced hands, these risks are very small. First-generation ICDs, implanted in the mid-1980s, included a 2% operative mortality, as placement of those devices required thoracotomy. With current-generation devices, mortality should be near zero. The major complications related to ICD placement and therapy include infection (which usually requires removal of the whole system), lead failures (which usually manifest as ICD shock(s) when the underlying rhythm is normal), and inappropriate shock(s) because of supraventricular arrhythmias such as sinus tachycardia or atrial fibrillation with a rapid ventricular response.

# THERAPY FOR SPECIFIC ARRHYTHMIAS

This section will outline options available for management of specific arrhythmias. Before initiating therapy for any arrhythmia, the clinician should ensure that reversible causes have been sought and corrected and that a specific arrhythmia diagnosis, corresponding to the patient's symptoms when present, has been established. The most common reversible causes of arrhythmias include treatment with digitalis, antiarrhythmic drugs or other arrhythmogenic agents (theophylline, sympathomimetic agents), illicit drug use (cocaine), and severe disturbances of normal physiology, such as acute myocardial ischemia, severe hypoxia, or hypokalemia. When an obvious reversible cause is identified and treated, long-term antiarrhythmic therapy may not be necessary. It should, however, be emphasized that relatively mild degrees of hypokalemia are extremely common in patients who have been resuscitated from ventricular fibrillation. The mechanism appears to be epinephrine-induced sequestration of potassium within skeletal muscle cells via $\beta_2$-receptor-mediated mechanism (Brown et al. 1983). Attributing a cardiac arrest to mild hypokalemia under these circumstances would be a major error.

A major distinction should be made between acute therapy for ongoing cardiac arrhythmias and chronic long-term therapy designed to prevent recurrences. In the acute situation, patients are being continuously monitored, the potential benefits of terminating the arrhythmia are immediately obvious, and the risks are minimized by the use of intravenous therapies and by continuous patient monitoring, allowing prompt identification and treatment of proarrhythmia should it arise. During long-term therapy, the potential benefits continue, but the risks of therapy may be considerably different. Different forms of therapy are generally used for acute and for long-term management of arrhythmias (Tables 1-39 and 1-40).

## Atrial Premature Contractions and Ventricular Premature Contractions

Isolated ectopic beats arising from any location in the heart are common. They can occur in patients without structural heart disease, but are more frequent in patients with advanced heart disease. Ventricular arrhythmias arising de novo (e.g., during surgery) should prompt a search for underlying triggers such as hypoxia or myocardial ischemia. Most patients with ectopic beats are asymptomatic and treatment is therefore not justified. Occasionally patients are highly symptomatic with palpitations. In such instances, reassurance and detailed description of the risks associated with long-term antiarrhythmic therapy are frequently sufficient to convince the patient that treatment is undesirable. $\beta$-Blockers can sometimes be effective. Only very rarely should treatment with antiarrhythmic drugs, such as flecainide, moricizine, or propafenone (in patients with no structural heart disease) or sotalol or amiodarone (in those with heart disease), be undertaken.

## Atrial Fibrillation

Atrial fibrillation is the most common rhythm disturbance requiring intervention. Although a number of clinical situations associated with reversible atrial fibrillation have been identified (e.g., pericarditis, hyperthyroidism, pulmonary embolism), most patients with atrial fibrillation have structural heart disease and no such precipitator. The most common underlying heart disease is probably ventricular hypertrophy secondary to hypertension, although atrial fibrillation can occur in virtually any type of heart disease. In addition, the arrhythmia is well documented to occur in subjects with no underlying heart disease, and a very rare familial form was described recently (Brugada et al. 1997).

One of the most feared consequences of atrial fibrillation is the development of intra-atrial thrombi, with subsequent embolization to the cerebral arteries that causes stroke. Data from multiple well-controlled randomized clinical trials have consistently demonstrated that therapy with warfarin to maintain an international normalized ratio of prothrombin time (INR) of 2–3 reduces the incidence of stroke by approximately two-thirds, from 4–5% per year to 1–2% per year, with an acceptably low incidence of intracerebral hemorrhage (Singer 1996). On the basis of these data, patients with chronic atrial fibrillation with at least one additional risk factor for stroke (age >65, diabetes, hypertension, prior stroke) should receive anticoagulant therapy with warfarin. It is not yet known whether similar considerations apply to patients with paroxysmal atrial fibrillation; many clinicians prescribe anticoagulants to patients with paroxysmal atrial fibrillation if they have these additional risk factors. Although aspirin is widely used as an alternative to warfarin, studies to determine its efficacy in this situation have yielded inconsistent results (Singer 1996).

Patients developing atrial fibrillation in the absence of AV nodal blocking drugs or AV nodal disease will generally have ventricular responses in excess of 150/min. Symptoms such as palpitations, dyspnea, or exacerbation of congestive heart failure or angina are common. Mechanisms that account for the symptoms include the rapid rate, the irregularity of the rate, and loss of atrial "kick" that results in decreased cardiac output. In patients presenting with serious symptoms, such as hypotension, rapidly progressive congestive heart failure, or angina, the treatment of choice is sedation followed by direct current (DC) cardioversion despite the risk of thromboemboli. In patients who are less symptomatic, rate control with digitalis, intravenous calcium channel blockers (diltiazem or verapamil), and/or $\beta$-blockers is most appropriate. The specific choice of AV nodal blocking drug depends in part on underlying heart disease. In patients with advanced heart disease, $\beta$-blockers and calcium channel blockers are relatively contraindicated.

### *Acute therapy of atrial fibrillation*

An important consideration in evaluating the patient who presents with atrial fibrillation is the likely duration of the arrhythmia. If the patient can clearly time the onset of the arrhythmia to <48 hours before presentation, then it is usually considered that the risk of thromboembolism with elective DC cardioversion or pharmacologic cardioversion is small. Oral propafenone and flecainide as well as intravenous ibutilide, procainamide, sotalol, flecainide and propafenone (the latter three formulations are not available in the United States) have been reported effective in acutely converting atrial fibrillation. Flecainide and propafenone should be used with caution in patients with underlying heart disease. The efficacy of ibutilide in conversion of acute atrial fibrillation is not known, since most clinical trials studied patients that had the arrhythmia for at least several weeks, and it is known that a long duration of atrial fibrillation is a powerful predictor of lack of drug efficacy. In trials of patients with atrial fibrillation of >3 weeks duration, ibutilide converted <50% of patients to sinus rhythm, and was associated with a 1–6% incidence of torsades de pointes (Ellenbogen et al. 1996). In one large randomized trial, procainamide was less effective than ibutilide but may have fewer side effects (Stambler et al. 1997).

In patients in whom atrial fibrillation has been present for >48 hours or in patients who cannot time the onset of atrial fibrillation, cardioversion should be deferred. The conventional approach in this situation is to initiate anticoagulation with heparin and warfarin and to maintain rate control with digitalis, calcium channel blockers, and/or $\beta$-blockers. Once the INR rises to 2–3, warfarin and AV nodal block are continued for at least 3 weeks, following which elective DC cardioversion can be undertaken with a minimal risk of thromboembolism. An alternate strategy is to perform transesophageal echocardiography to ascertain whether thrombus is present in the left atrium. If it is, then a conventional strategy such as that outlined above is pursued. If it is not, immediate cardioversion is undertaken. A large randomized trial, ACUTE (Assessment of Cardioversion Using Transesophageal Echocardiography), is under way to assess the outcomes and costs of these two strategies.

***Long-term therapy for atrial fibrillation***

Once atrial fibrillation has been converted to normal rhythm, the next question the clinician faces is whether to initiate long-term therapy to maintain sinus rhythm. Because drugs are incompletely effective and carry the risk of proarrhythmia, many clinicians will manage patients presenting with their first episode of atrial fibrillation by cardioversion, but not long-term suppressive therapy. This approach is justified by the finding that approximately 25% of patients in whom sinus rhythm was restored and treatment with placebo was undertaken were still in sinus rhythm at 6–12 months (Coplen et al. 1990).

In patients presenting with recurrent atrial fibrillation, many clinicians will initiate antiarrhythmic drug therapy to maintain sinus rhythm either before or after elective DC cardioversion. The advantage of initiating therapy before cardioversion is that some patients will "pharmacologically" cardiovert, thus avoiding the need for a DC cardioversion. Because of the risk of proarrhythmia, it is the practice of many physicians to hospitalize patients for initiation of antiarrhythmic therapy. In one series, the risk of serious adverse effects within 24–48 hours of in-patient initiation of antiarrhythmics was 13.4%, with an increased risk in the elderly and in patients with previous myocardial infarction (Maisel et al. 1997). In general, approximately 50% of patients treated with antiarrhythmic drugs (e.g., propafenone, flecainide, amiodarone, quinidine, sotalol) remain in sinus rhythm after 6–12 months (Kerr et al. 1988; Coplen et al. 1990; Juul-Möller et al. 1990). The success of antiarrhythmic therapy is determined not only by the risk of noncardiac adverse effects and proarrhythmia discussed above, but also by chronicity of atrial fibrillation and extent of underlying heart disease. Many clinicians feel that rare recurrences of atrial fibrillation during long-term drug treatment need not prompt a switch in drugs. In addition, because of limited efficacy and the risks of therapy, some clinicians prefer to avoid suppressive therapy altogether, or to merely try one or two drugs, before pursuing a strategy of rate control and anticoagulation only in patients with atrial fibrillation. Whereas with this approach the risk of proarrhythmia is essentially eliminated, symptoms may persist, and some data suggest the insidious deterioration of left ventricular performance with maintained atrial fibrillation. The choice of approaches in an individual subject is determined largely by patient symptoms as convincing evidence is not available. A large randomized trial, AFFIRM, is now under way testing which of the two strategies (rate control vs. rhythm control) is optimal for patients with chronic or recurrent atrial fibrillation.

## Atrial Flutter

The management of this arrhythmia has traditionally been lumped together with atrial fibrillation, and such a combined approach is justified by the fact that, in many cases, patients with atrial flutter will also have episodes of atrial fibrillation (and vice versa). Atrial flutter is a reentrant rhythm that utilizes a fixed circuit that includes much of the right atrial septum and free wall, as well as an "isthmus" between the inferior vena cava and the tricuspid valve annulus. The electrocardiogram shows distinctive regular sawtooth (flutter, "F") waves in the inferior leads. Occasionally, the electrocardiogram of patients with atrial fibrillation may appear to display similar relatively regular atrial depolarizations. However, on close inspection, such "flutter-fibrillation" is generally found to be irregular both in amplitude and periodicity and should be treated as atrial fibrillation.

While conventional clinical wisdom has suggested that thromboembolism may be somewhat less prevalent in patients with atrial flutter than those with atrial fibrillation, more recent data suggest that, as in atrial fibrillation, patients with atrial flutter and advanced heart disease are also susceptible to this complication. Therefore, most experts will use anticoagulation in patients with atrial flutter, just as in atrial fibrillation. Because the atrial rate in atrial flutter is constant, the ventricular response tends to change in increments. Therefore, in patients with atrial flutter, rates may jump abruptly from relatively low values to relatively fast values.

Drugs that are used to maintain sinus rhythm in atrial fibrillation may also be effective in atrial flutter. It is interesting that drugs whose major action is to prolong the action potential (ibutilide, sotalol) may be more effective than drugs whose major effect is to slow conduction (flecainide). In patients with recurrent atrial flutter and no evidence of atrial fibrillation, catheter ablation directed at the isthmus in the circuit can be successful in effecting a permanent cure.

## Paroxysmal Supraventricular Tachycardia

The typical patient with paroxysmal supraventricular tachycardia (PSVT) presents with paroxysms of arrhythmia, often dating to childhood, and no structural heart disease. AVNRT and AVRT account for >90–95% of such cases, so acute treatment is interruption of impulse propagation in the AV node, which is a portion of both circuits and is especially susceptible to drug block (Table 1-41). The drug of choice is adenosine, administered as a rapid intravenous bolus. Calcium channel blockers (verapamil, diltiazem) are also highly effective (DiMarco et al. 1990). Other therapies that have been used include intravenous $\beta$-blockers (propranolol, esmolol, metoprolol), and drugs that directly (edrophonium) or indirectly (phenylephrine) increase vagal tone, and hence interrupt AV nodal transmission. In rare patients, the mechanism underlying PSVT is actually an automatic or reentrant focus within the atrium. In these cases, the use of AV nodal blocking drugs generally does not affect the tachycardia but does cause AV block. This outcome establishes that the AV node is not a crucial part of the arrhythmia mechanism, and therefore suggests these less common underlying causes.

In patients with recurrent episodes of symptomatic PSVT, radiofrequency catheter ablation is becoming the treatment of choice. Basic electrophysiologic and clinical data support the efficacy of verapamil (Tonkin et al. 1980). In addition, well-designed, randomized, controlled clinical trials have shown that chronic oral therapy with propafenone or flecainide can provide highly effective long-term therapy (Henthorn et al. 1991; UK Propafenone PSVT Study Group).

## Ventricular Tachycardia or Fibrillation

The last decade has seen revolutionary changes in the management of ventricular arrhythmias. These changes have occurred because therapy, which was previously essentially empiric and driven by physician bias, is now approached on the basis of the results of randomized clinical trials. Ventricular tachycardia (VT) is said to be sustained when some intervention (cardioversion or administration of a drug) is required for its termination, while the term nonsustained ventricular tachycardia is used to describe VT that terminates by itself (or lasts <30 seconds). In the vast majority of patients, sustained ventricular tachycardia reflects the presence of advanced structural heart disease. The approach to therapy for ventricular fibrillation is the same as that for fast ventricular tachycardia. In patients with coronary artery disease and myocardial scarring due to remote myocardial infarction, sustained ventricular tachycardia is most often due to microreentry in the border zone between normal tissue and scar. In patients with various forms of cardiomyopathy unrelated to coronary artery disease, sustained ventricular tachycardia may be due to reentry because of abnormal myocardial architecture (including scarring) or to automatic mechanisms; however, in practice, the distinction is not readily made. In addition, a number of rarer syndromes of ventricular tachycardia have been delineated, each with its own distinctive mechanism and therapies. These are listed in Table 1-42, and include various forms of monomorphic ventricular tachycardia occurring in the absence of structural heart disease (often—unlike other forms of VT—responsive to verapamil), polymorphic ventricular tachycardia with long QT intervals (the torsades de pointes syndrome described above), polymorphic ventricular tachycardia with short QT intervals (often seen with acute myocardial ischemia), and ventricular tachycardia occurring in patients with arrhythmogenic right ventricular dysplasia (where some data indicate so-

**Table 1-41 A Mechanistic Approach to Supraventricular Tachycardia**

| | | ECG features | | Management | |
|---|---|---|---|---|---|
| Sign or symptom | Underlying heart disease | Baseline | During tachycardia | Acute[a] | Long term[b] |
| AV nodal reentry | Unusual[a] | Normal | Regular narrow complex tachycardia | Adenosine, verapamil HCl, diltiazem, intravenous β-blocker | Verapamil, flecainide acetate, propafenone HCl |
| AV reentry utilizing a bypass tract for retrograde (ventricle → atrium) conduction | Unusual[a] | Normal or delta wave | Regular narrow complex tachycardia | Adenosine, verapamil HCl, diltiazem, intravenous β-blocker | Verapamil, flecainide acetate, propafenone HCl |
| AV reentry utilizing a bypass tract for anterograde (ventricle → atrium) conduction | Unusual[a] | Normal or delta wave | Regular tachycardia with wide QRS complexes | Adenosine, verapamil HCl, diltiazem, intravenous β-blocker (diagnosis may be difficult to establish due to ECG) | (Multiple bypass tracts relatively frequent; electrophysiologic evaluation indicated) |
| Atrial fibrillation | Common | | Irregularly irregular ventricular rate, often 120–180/min in the absence of AV nodal block | *To control rate*: Digitalis, verapamil HCl, diltiazem, intravenous β-blocker *To convert:* Ibutilide (IV), procainamide HCl (IV), propafenone HCl (PO), DC-cardioversion | *To control rate*: Digitalis, verapamil HCl, diltiazem, β-blocker *To maintain sinus rhythm*: Quinidine, amiodarone HCl, sotalol HCl, propafenone HCl, flecainide acetate, disopyramide phosphate |
| "Pre-excited" atrial fibrillation (antegrade atrioventricular conduction via a bypass tract) | Unusual[a] | Delta wave | Irregularly irregular ventricular rate which may exceed 300/min. Beat-to-beat variability in QRS morphology | Procainamide DC-cardioversion- *Avoid digitalis, calcium channel blockers* | (Electrophysiologic evaluation indicated before any attempt at long-term drug therapy; ablation often the treatment of choice) |
| Atrial flutter | Common | | Distinctive saw-tooth-like "flutter" waves (II, III, aVF). Ventricular rate can be regular or irregular, depending on AV nodal transmission | As with atrial fibrillation | As with atrial fibrillation (consider ablation) |

Table 1-41 A Mechanistic Approach to Supraventricular Tachycardia (Continued)

| | | ECG FEATURES | | MANAGEMENT | |
|---|---|---|---|---|---|
| SIGN OR SYMPTOM | UNDERLYING HEART DISEASE | BASELINE | DURING TACHYCARDIA | ACUTE[a] | LONG TERM[b] |
| Atrial tachycardia | Patient can present with tachycardia-induced heart failure if incessant | Regular narrow complex tachycardia; unusual P-wave axis | Digitalis, verapamil HCl, diltiazem, intravenous $\beta$-blocker, occasionally rapid atrial pacing | | As with atrial fibrillation (consider ablation) |

[a]Although these arrhythmias usually present in patients with no major underlying heart disease, they certainly can occur in patients with other types of heart disease. In these cases, the diagnosis may be more difficult (because, for example, the underlying ECG may be abnormal for some other cause).

[b]Radiofrequency catheter ablation is highly effective to "cure" AV nodal reentry, AV reentry, and atrial flutter, and less often atrial tachycardia. In cases of pre-excited atrial fibrillation (Fig. 1-30C), electrophysiologic evaluation with radiofrequency catheter ablation is indicated to prevent dangerously rapid ventricular rates. In patients with atrial fibrillation without a bypass tract (the vast majority) and ventricular rates that remain rapid despite AV nodal blocking drugs, catheter ablation of the AV node to create third heart block (which then requires placement of a permanent pacemaker) has been used.

ABBREVIATIONS: DC, direct current; IV, intravenous; PO, per os (by mouth, orally); QRS is a segment of the electrocardiogram (see Figs. 1-27 and 1-28)

talol may be especially effective). These entities are not further discussed here.

In light of these varying mechanisms and approaches to therapy, the most important determinant of long-term treatment of ventricular arrhythmias is an assessment of the extent and nature of underlying heart disease. Not only may this influence the specific choice of therapies (as described in Table 1-40), but also extensive left ventricular dysfunction can preclude certain drug therapies (Table 1-37).

### *Acute therapy of sustained ventricular arrhythmias*

In patients with cardiovascular collapse due to ventricular fibrillation or rapid ventricular tachycardia, cardiopulmonary resuscitation using standard protocols is required. In patients with severe symptoms (hypotension, angina, heart failure) due to ongoing ventricular tachycardia, the treatment of choice is sedation followed by cardioversion. Following acute management, drug therapy is generally instituted to prevent recurrences of ventricular tachycardia. In patients with less severe symptoms, an initial trial of drug therapy in an attempt to pharmacologically convert the rhythm to normal can be undertaken. Among patients presenting with sustained monomorphic ventricular tachycardia, the initial drug generally attempted is lidocaine. The calculated loading dose of lidocaine is generally 3–4 mg/kg, but administration of this large dose as a single bolus results in transient supratherapeutic plasma concentrations and may produce seizures. Therefore, the loading regimen is generally administered as a series of slow bolus infusions, followed by a maintenance infusion. In patients with congestive heart failure, the magnitude of both the total loading dose and the maintenance infusion rate should be reduced, while in patients with liver disease, only the maintenance dose requires reduction (Thompson et al. 1973). If administration of a loading dose of lidocaine is ineffective in terminating the tachycardia, initiation of a maintenance infusion is pointless. Rather, a second drug, for example, procainamide, should be tried.

In patients with frequent episodes of ventricular fibrillation or hemodynamically destabilizing ventricular tachycardia, suppressive drug therapy should be attempted even if the tachycardia episodes themselves terminate spontaneously. In patients with sustained monomorphic ventricular tachycardia due to coronary artery disease and remote myocardial infarction, at least one trial suggests that intravenous sotalol (which combines $\beta$-blockade with action potential prolonging characteristics, but is not available in the intravenous form in the United States) is more effective than lidocaine (Ho et al. 1994). Bretylium has been found to be roughly equivalent to lidocaine in preventing recurrences of ventricular fibrillation in patients resuscitated from cardiac arrest (Heissenbuttel and Bigger 1979). Amiodarone has been found to be equivalent to or slightly superior to bretylium (Kowey et al. 1995), and some anecdotes suggest it is especially effective if acute myocardial ischemia is present (Wolfe et al. 1991). Other intravenous drugs that have been used include procainamide and, occasionally, $\beta$-blockers (again if acute ischemia is thought to be present), but controlled data to assess their efficacy is lacking. Intravenous procainamide, bretylium, and amiodarone can all cause severe hypotension.

**Table 1-42 A Mechanistic Approach to Sustained Ventricular Tachycardia**

| | | ECG FEATURES | | MANAGEMENT | |
|---|---|---|---|---|---|
| SIGN OR SYMPTOM | UNDERLYING HEART DISEASE | BASELINE | DURING VT | ACUTE[a] | LONG TERM[b] |
| VT in CAD | Remote transmural MI | Q waves | Monomorphic VT; bizarre QRS *or* polymorphic fast VT | Lidocaine, procainamide HCl, amiodarone HCl, bretylium tosylate | ICD, amiodarone HCl (RFA for some with monomorphic VT) |
| | Active ischemia | ST segment changes | Very fast polymorphic VT; 1st beat close-coupled | Amiodarone, β-blocker | Revascularization |
| VT in dilated cardiomyopathy | Severe diffuse ↑contractility | Variable; LBBB common | Multiple morphologies | Lidocaine, procainamide HCl, amiodarone HCl, bretylium tosylate | ICD, amiodarone HCl (RFA in selected patients) |
| RVOT VT | None | Normal | LBBB + tall R inferiorly (II, III, aVF) | Verapamil, β-blocker | Verapamil, β-blocker, RFA |
| Fascicular VT | None | Normal | RBBB + LAD; QRS may be relatively narrow | Verapamil, β-blocker, adenosine | Verapamil, β-blocker, RFA |
| Torsades de pointes | Variable (see text) | ↑QTU; bradycardia | Polymorphic VT (150–230/min); 1st beat late-coupled | Magnesium, potassium, isoproterenol, pacing | Pacing + β-blocker |
| ARVD | RV disease, often localized | T-wave changes V1–V3; positive signal-averaged electrocardiogram | LBBB; often similar to RVOT VT | Lidocaine, procainamide HCl, amiodarone HCl, bretylium tosylate | ICD, sotalol HCl |
| Brugada syndrome | None; may be common in Southeast Asia | Intermittent RBBB + ST-segment elevation V1–V3 | VF | Lidocaine, procainamide HCl, amiodarone HCl, bretylium tosylate | ICD |

[1]All drug therapy intravenous; direct current cardioversion is initial therapy when there is hemodynamic instability (e.g., hypotension, angina).
ABBREVIATIONS: ARVD, arrhythmogenic right ventricular dysplasia; ICD, implantable cardioverter-defibrillator; LAD, left axis deviation; LBBB, left bundle branch block; MI, myocardial infarction; RBBB, right bundle branch block; RFA, radiofrequency catheter ablation; RV, right ventricle; RVOT, right ventricular outflow tract; VF, ventricular fibrillation; VT, ventricular tachycardia.

As treatment for ventricular tachycardia or fibrillation is being started, an immediate search for underlying causes or exacerbating factors should be undertaken. These include hypokalemia, the presence of some antiarrhythmic drugs, or acute myocardial ischemia. In patients in whom a clear precipitator for ventricular tachycardia or fibrillation can be identified, for example, acute myocardial ischemia, treatment directed at the underlying cause is generally all that is required to prevent recurrences. However, in patients in whom an underlying cause cannot be readily identified, long-term antiarrhythmic therapy is generally undertaken. Historical controls suggest that, in this group, annual recurrence rates are approximately 50%.

***Long-term therapy for sustained ventricular arrhythmias***

A number of trials have been conducted (Table 1-43) to compare the efficacy of antiarrhythmic drugs and to determine the best way of predicting whether antiarrhythmic

Table 1-43 Selected Randomized Trials of Antiarrhythmic Therapies

| Trial | Population | Treatments[a] (N) | | Primary endpont | Outcome | Reference | Comment |
|---|---|---|---|---|---|---|---|
| BHAT | Post-MI | Placebo (1912) | Propranolol (1916) | Total mortality | ↓Mortality 27% | Beta-Blocker Heart Attack Trial Research Group 1982<br>Beta-Blocker Heart Attack Trial Research Group 1983 | Dose adjusted by extent of $\beta$-blockade |
| Norwegian multicenter trial | Post-MI | Placebo (939) | Timolol 10 mg bid (945) | | ↓Mortality 45%<br>↓Reinfarction 28% | The Norwegian Multicenter Group 1981 | |
| Metoprolol post-MI | Post-MI | Placebo (697) | Metoprolol (698) | Mortality | ↓Mortality 36% | Hjalmerson et al. (1981) | |
| IMPACT | Post-MI + PVCs | Placebo (313) | Mexiletine (317) | PVC frequency | ↑Mortality 58% (NS);<br>↓PVCs at 1 and 4 months but not 12 months | IMPACT Research Group 1984 | Underpowered for mortality, but large effect presaged CAST result |
| UK Rhymodan Multicentre Study Group | Post-MI | Placebo (995) | Disopyramide (990) | | ↑Mortality 29% (NS) | UK Rythmodan Multicentre Study Group 1984 | Underpowered for mortality, but large effect presaged CAST result |
| CAST | Post-MI + PVCS | Placebo (743) | Flecainide, encainide (755) | Mortality | ↑Mortality 142% in 10 months | The Cardiac Arrythmia Suppression Trial (CAST) Imvestigators 1989<br>Echt at el. 1991 | Flecainide and encainide arms stopped because of death rate |
| CAST-II | Post-MI + PVCs + ↓EF | Placebo (660) | Moricizine HCl (665) | Mortality | ↑Mortality 17% (NS) | The Cardiac Arrythmia Suppression Trial II Investigators 1991 | Significant ↑mortality with drug in 1st 2 weeks of therapy |
| CASCADE | resuscitated from VF | Empiric amiodarone (113) | Antiarrhythmic drugs, guided by EP testing (115) | Mortality + ICD discharges + resuscitation from VF | Fewer events with amiodarone; high overall recurrence rate | Greene and the CASCADE investigators 1993 | |
| ESVEM | VT inducible by PES + >10 VPCs/hr | Drug selection by PES (242) | Drug selection by VPC suppression (244) | Recurrent VT + death | Outcome did not depend on method of drug selection NS | Mason 1993a, 1993b | Outcome appeared better with sotalol than other drugs studied (not a primary outcome variable) |
| CHF-STAT | CHF, EF <40%, >10 PVCs/hr, cardiac enlargement | Placebo (338) | Amiodarone (336) | Mortality | NS | Singh et al. 1995 | EF improved in amiodarone group, but no effect on mortality |

**Table 1-43 Selected Randomized Trials of Antiarrhythmic Therapies (Continued)**

| TRIAL | POPULATION | TREATMENTS[a] (N) | | PRIMARY ENDPONT | OUTCOME | REFERENCE | COMMENT |
|---|---|---|---|---|---|---|---|
| GESICA | CHF | standard treatment | Amiodarone (260) | Mortality | ↓Mortality 28% | Doval et al. 1994 | Fewer patients with coronary artery disease than in CHF-STAT |
| EMIAT | Post-MI + ↓EF | Placebo (743) | Amiodarone (743) | Total mortality | NS | Julian et al. 1997 | 35% ↓ in arrhythmic death |
| CAMIAT | Post-MI + PVCS | Placebo (596) | Amiodarone (606) | Arrhythmic death | Arrhythmic death ↓49% | Cairns et al. 1997 | NS for total mortality |
| AVID | Resuscitation from VF or fast VT | ICD (507) | Amiodarone or sotalol (509) | Total mortality | ↓Mortality by 39% at 1 year with ICD | McAnulty et al. 1997 | More patients in ICD arm received β-blockers |
| MADIT | Post-MI + ↓EF + unsustained VT + VT induced by programmed stimulation and resistant to IV procainamide | ICD (95) | Best antiarrhythmic drug (usually amiodarone) (101) | Total mortality | ↓ Mortality 54% with ICD | Moss et al. 1996 | Very small trial ($n$ = 196 total); unexplained excess of "non-cardiac" deaths in non-ICD arm; more patients in ICD arm received β-blockers |
| CIDS | Resuscitation from VF or fast VT | ICD | Amiodarone | | Recruitment completed; patients being followed | Connolly et al. 1993 | |
| MUSTT | Post-MI + ↓EF + nonsustained VT + VT induced by PES | Best conventional cardiovasculer therapy | Antiarrhythmic drugs to suppress inducible VT, or ICD | | Recruitment completed; patients being followed | Buxton et al. 1993 | Preliminary data show ICD benefit |
| AFFIRM | Atrial fibrillation | Rate control | Rhythm control | Death | Ongoing | Wyse et al. 1997 | |
| ACUTE | Atrial fibrillation | Standard therapy | Therapy guided by transesophageal echocardiography | | Ongoing | Steering and Publications Committee of the ACUTE Study 1998 | |

[a]Numbers of patients randomized are in parentheses. Drug salts are as follows: amiodarone, amiodarone HCl; disopyramide, disopyramide phosphate; encainide, encainide HCl; flecainide, flecainide acetate; metoprolol, metoprolol succinate; mexiletin, mexiletin HCl; moricizine, moricizine HCl; propranolol, propranolol HCl; sotalol, sotalol HCl.

ABBREVIATIONS: ACUTE, Assessment of Cardioversion Using Transesophageal Echocardiography; AFFIRM, Atrial Fibrillation Follow-Up Investigation of Rhythm Management; AVID, Antiarrhythmics versus Implantable Defibrillators; BHAT, B-Blocker Heart Attack Trial Research Group; CAMIAT, Canadian Amiodarone Myocardial Infarction Arrhythmia Trial; CASCADE, Cardiac Arrest in Seattle Conventional versus Amiodarone Drug Evaluation; CAST, Cardiac Arrhythmia Suppression Trial; CHF, congestive heart failure; CHF-STAT, Survival Trial of Antiarrhythmic Therapy in Congestive Heart Failure; CIDS, Canadian Implantable Defibrillator Study ; EF, ejection fraction; EMIAT, European Myocardial Infarct Amiodarone Trial Investigators; ESVEM, Electrophysiologic Study versus Electrocardiographic Monitoring ; GESICA, Grupo de Estudio de la Sobrevida en la Insuficiencia Cardiaca Argentina; ICD, implantable cardioverter-defibrillator; IMPACT, International Mexiletine and Placebo Antiarrhythmic Coronary Trial; MADIT, Multicenter Automatic Defibrillator Implantation Trial; MI, myocardial infarction; MUSTT, Multicentre Unsustained Tachycardia Trial; NS, not significant; PES, programmed electrical stimulation of the heart, a technique that may reproduce VT in susceptible patients; PVCs, premature ventricular complexes; VF, ventricular fibrillation; VT, ventricular tachycardia.

drugs will be effective long term in patients who present with sustained ventricular arrhythmias. In CASCADE, empiric therapy with oral amiodarone was found to be superior to what were termed at the time "conventional" agents such as quinidine or procainamide, whose efficacy was thought to be predicted by serial programmed electrical stimulation of the heart (Greene and The CASCADE Investigators 1993). ESVEM (Electrophysiologic Study versus Electrocardiographic Monitoring) tested seven antiarrhythmic drugs in patients with sustained ventricular tachycardia and found sotalol to be most effective, with the fewest adverse effects, compared with drugs such as quinidine, procainamide, mexiletine, and propafenone (Mason 1993). In both ESVEM and CASCADE, recurrence rates of arrhythmias (including sudden cardiac death) were substantial, 10–20% per year, even with the best of drug therapies. The AVID trial (Antiarrythmics versus Implantable Defibrillators) was therefore undertaken to compare placement of ICDs versus best antiarrhythmic drug (generally amiodarone) in patients with hypotensive ventricular tachycardia or those resuscitated from cardiac arrest without underlying precipitator (McAnulty et al. 1997). ICD therapy was found to be more effective than antiarrhythmic drug therapy in this group. Cost-benefit analyses using modeled data as well as actual cost data indicate that the superiority of ICD therapy is obtained at higher cost. One study suggested a cost-effectiveness compared to amiodarone of $74,400 per quality-adjusted life-year saved (Owens et al. 1997); that is, although patients live somewhat longer with the ICD (4.18 vs. 3.68 years), the costs of ICD (including not only the device, $20,000–30,000, but also implant and follow-up costs and anticipated hospitalizations for complications) were higher than those of treatment with chronic amiodarone (including not only the cost of drug but also the cost of monitoring for anticipated toxicity and of treating such toxicity). Nevertheless, the results of such trials form the basis of the current enthusiasm for ICD therapy (as opposed to drugs) as primary treatment in patients presenting with sustained ventricular arrhythmias. Other trials are ongoing in these patients (Table 1-43), and should help further solidify rational selection of therapies in this once largely empiric area.

## Antiarrhythmic Therapy to Reduce the Incidence of Sudden Cardiac Death

Patients with depressed left ventricular performance with or without episodes of asymptomatic nonsustained ventricular tachycardia are recognized to be at especially high risk for sudden cardiac death due to ventricular fibrillation. However, mortality has not been favorably affected by antiarrhythmic drugs in multiple trials, including CAST and SWORD (Table 1-43).

## REFERENCES


Antiplatelet Trialists Collaboration. 1988. Secondary prevention of vascular disease by prolonged antiplatelet treatments. *Br Med J* **296**:320–31.

Antman EM, Wenger TL, Butler VPJ, et al. 1990. Treatment of 150 cases of life-threatening digitalis intoxication with digoxin-specific F(ab′) antibody fragments: Final report of a multicenter study. *Circulation* **81**:1744–52.

Ben-David J, Zipes DP. 1993. Torsades de pointes and proarrhythmia. *Lancet* **341**:1578–82.

Beta-Blocker Heart Attack Trial Research Group. 1982. A randomized trial of propranolol in patients with acute myocardial infarction. I. Mortality results. *JAMA* **247**:1707–14.

Beta-Blocker Heart Attack Trial Research Group 1983. A randomized trial of propranolol in patients with acute myocardial infarction. II. Morbidity results. *JAMA* **250**:2814–9.

Brown MJ, Brown DC, Murphy MB. 1983. Hypokalemia from beta2-receptor stimulation by circulating epinephrine. *N Engl J Med* **309**:1414–9.

Brugada R, Tapscott T, Czernuszewicz GZ, et al. 1997. Identification of a genetic locus for familial atrial fibrillation. *N Engl J Med* **336**:905–11.

Buxton AE, Fisher JD, Josephson ME, et al. 1993. Prevention of sudden death in patients with coronary artery disease: the Multicenter Unsustained Tachycardia Trial (MUSTT). *Progr Cardiovasc Dis* **36**:215–26.

Cairns JA, Connolly SJ, Roberts R, et al. 1997. Randomised trial of outcome after myocardial infarction in patients with frequent or repetitive ventricular premature depolarisations: CAMIAT. The Canadian Amiodarone Myocardial Infarction Arrhythmia Trial Investigators. *Lancet* **349**:675–82.

Camm AJ, Garratt CJ. 1991. Adenosine and supraventricular tachycardia. *N Engl J Med* 325:1621–9.

Carlsson L, Abrahamsson C, Andersson B, et al. 1993. Proarrhythmic effects of the class III agent almokalant: importance of infusion rate, QT dispersion, and early afterdepolarisations. *Cardiovasc Res* **27**:2186–93.

Chouty F, Funck-Brentano C, Landau JM, et al. 1987. Efficacité de fortes doses de lactate molaire par voie veineuse lors des intoxications au flecainide. *La Press Med* **16**:808–10.

Choy AMJ, Darbar D, Dell'Orto S, et al. 1996. Increased sensitivity to QT prolonging drug therapy immediately after cardioversion to sinus rhythm [abstract]. *Circulation* **94**:I202.

Connolly SJ, Gent M, Roberts RS, et al. 1993. Canadian Implantable Defibrillator Study (CIDS): study design and organization. CIDS Co-Investigators. *Am J Cardiol* **72**:103F–8F.

Coplen SE, Antman EM, Berlin JA, et al. 1990. Efficacy and safety of quinidine therapy for maintenance of sinus rhythm after cardioversion. *Circulation* **82**:1106–16.

Coromilas J, Saltman AE, Waldecker B, et al. 1995. Electrophysiological effects of flecainide on anisotropic conduction and reentry in infarcted canine hearts. *Circulation* **91**:2245–63.

Crijns HJ, van Gelder IS, Lie KI. 1988. Supraventricular tachycardia mimicking ventricular tachycardia during flecainide treatment. *Am J Cardiol* **62**:1303–6.

DiMarco JP, Miles W, Akhtar M, et al. 1990. Adenosine for paroxysmal supraventricular tachycardia: dose ranging and comparison with verapamil: assessment in placebo-controlled, multicenter trials. *Ann Intern Med* **113**:104–10.

Doval HC, Nul DR, Grancelli HO, et al. 1994. Randomised trial of low-dose amiodarone in severe congestive heart failure. Grupo de Estudio de la Sobrevida en la Insuficiencia Cardiaca en Argentina (GESICA). *Lancet* **344**:493–8.

Echt DS, Liebson PR, Mitchell LB, et al. 1991. Mortality and morbidity in patients receiving encainide, flecainide, or placebo. CAST Investigators. The Cardiac Arrhythmia Suppression Trial. *N Engl J Med* **324:**781–8.

Ellenbogen KA, Stambler BS, Wood MA, et al., for the Ibutilide Investigators.1996. Efficacy of intravenous ibutilide for rapid termination of atrial fibrillation and atrial flutter: a dose-response study. *J Am Coll Cardiol* **28**:130–6.

Greene HL, the CASCADE Investigators. 1993. The CASCADE Study: randomized antiarrhythmic drug therapy in survivors of cardiac arrest in Seattle. Cardiac Arrest in Seattle, Conventional versus Amiodarone Drug Evaluation Study. *Am J Cardiol* **72:**70F–4F.

Hallstrom AP, Bigger JT, Jr., Roden D, et al. 1992. Prognostic significance of ventricular premature depolarizations measured 1 year after myocardial infarction in patients with early postinfarction asymptomatic ventricular arrhythmia. *J Am Coll Cardiol* **20**: 259–64.

Heissenbuttel RH, Bigger JT, Jr. 1979. Bretylium tosylate: a newly available antiarrhythmic drug for ventricular arrhythmias. *Ann Intern Med* **91**:229–38.

Henthorn RW, Waldo AL, Anderson JL, et al., and the Flecainide Supraventricular Tachycardia Study Group. 1991. Flecainide acetate prevents recurrence of symptomatic paroxysmal supraventricular tachycardia. *Circulation* **83**:119–25.

Hjalmarson A, Herlitz J, Malek I, et al. 1981. Effect on mortality of metoprolol in acute myocardial infarction: a double-blind randomized trial. The Norwegian Multicenter Study Group. *Lancet* **2**: 823–7.

Ho DS, Zecchin RP, Richards DA, et al. 1994. Double-blind trial of lignocaine versus sotalol for acute termination of spontaneous sustained ventricular tachycardia. *Lancet* **344**:18–23.

Hogenhuis W, Stevens SK, Wang P, et al. 1993. Cost-effectiveness of radiofrequency ablation compared with other strategies in Wolff-Parkinson-White syndrome. *Circulation* **88**:II437–46.

IMPACT Research Group. 1984. International mexiletine and placebo antiarrhythmic coronary trial: I. Report on arrhythmia and other findings. *J Am Coll Cardiol* **4**:1148–63.

ISIS-4 (Fourth International Study of Infarct Survival) Collaborative Group. 1995b. ISIS-4: a randomized factorial trial assessing early oral captopril, oral mononitrate, and intravenous magnesium sulphate in 58,050 patients with suspected acute myocardial infarction. *Lancet* **345**:669–82.

Julian DG, Camm AJ, Frangin G, et al. 1997. Randomised trial of effect of amiodarone on mortality in patients with left-ventricular dysfunction after recent myocardial infarction: EMIAT. The European Myocardial Infarct Amiodarone Trial Investigators. *Lancet* **349**:667–74.

Juul-Möller S, Edvardsson N, Rehnqvist-Ahlberg N. 1990. Sotalol versus quinidine for the maintenance of sinus rhythm after direct current cardioversion of atrial fibrillation. *Circulation* **82**:1932–9.

Kerr CR, Klein GJ, Axelson JE, et al. 1988. Propafenone for prevention of recurrent atrial fibrillation. *Am J Cardiol* **61**:914–6.

Klein GJ, Bashore TM, Sellers TD, et al. 1979. Ventricular fibrillation in the Wolff-Parkinson-White Syndrome. *N Engl J Med* **301**: 1080–5.

Kowey PR, Levine JH, Herre JM, et al., and Intravenous Amiodarone Multicenter Investigators Group. 1995. Randomized, double-blind comparison of intravenous amiodarone and bretylium in the treatment of patients with recurrent, hemodynamically destabilizing ventricular tachycardia or fibrillation. *Circulation* **92**:3255–63.

Lazzara R. 1989. Amiodarone and torsades de pointes. *Ann Intern Med* **111**:549–51.

Maisel WH, Kuntz KM, Reimold SC, et al. 1997. Risk of initiating antiarrhythmic drug therapy for atrial fibrillation in patients admitted to a university hospital. *Ann Intern Med* **127**:281–4.

Makkar RR, Fromm BS, Steinman RT, et al. 1993. Female gender as a risk factor for torsades de pointes associated with cardiovascular drugs. *JAMA* **270**:2590–7.

Manolis AS, Wang PJ, Estes NA. 1994. Radiofrequency catheter ablation for cardiac tachyarrhythmias. *Ann Intern Med* **121**:452–61.

Mason JW. 1993. A comparison of seven antiarrhythmic drugs in patients with ventricular tachyarrhythmias. Electrophysiologic Study versus Electrocardiographic Monitoring Investigators. *N Engl J Med* **329**:452–8.

Mason JW. 1993a. A comparison of electrophysiologic testing with Holter monitoring to predict antiarrhythmic-drug efficacy for ventricular tachyarrhythmias. Electrophysiologic Study versus Electrocardiographic Monitoring Investigators. *N Engl J Med* **329**:445–51.

Mason JW. 1993b. A comparison of seven antiarrhythmic drugs in patients with ventricular tachyarrhythmias. Electrophysiologic Study versus Electrocardiographic Monitoring Investigators. *N Engl J Med* **329**:452–8.

McAnulty J, Halperin B, Kron J, et al. 1997. A comparison of antiarrhythmic-drug therapy with implantable defibrillators in patients resuscitated from near-fatal ventricular arrhythmias. The Antiarrhythmics versus Implantable Defibrillator (AVID) Investigators. *N Engl J Med* **337**:1576–83.

Morganroth J, Anderson JL, Gentzkow GD. 1986. Classification by type of ventricular arrhythmia predicts frequency of adverse cardiac events from flecainide. *J Am Coll Cardiol* **8**:607–15.

*Mosby's GenR$_x$* 1998. *Mosby's GenR$_x$ 1998: The Complete Reference for Generic and Brand Drugs.* 8th ed. St. Louis: Mosby–Year Book.

Moss AJ, Hall WJ, Cannom DS, et al. 1996. Improved survival with an implanted defibrillator in patients with coronary disease at high risk for ventricular arrhythmia. Multicenter Automatic Defibrillator Implantation Trial (MADIT) Investigators. *N Engl J Med* **335**:1933–40.

Myerburg RJ, Kessler KM, Cox MM, et al. 1989. Reversal of proarrhythmic effects of flecainide acetate and encainide hydrochloride by propranolol. *Circulation* **80**:1571–9.

Nattel S, Pedersen DH, Zipes DP. 1981. Alterations in regional myocardial distribution and arrhythmogenic effects of aprindine produced by coronary artery occlusion in the dog. *Cardiovasc Res* **15**:80–5.

Oetgen WJ, Tibbits PA, Abt MEO, et al. 1983. Clinical and electrophysiologic assessment of oral flecainide acetate for recurrent ventricular tachycardia: evidence for exacerbation of electrical instability. *Am J Cardiol* **52**:746–50.

Owens DK, Sanders GD, Harris RA, et al. 1997. Cost-effectiveness of implantable cardioverter defibrillators relative to amiodarone for prevention of sudden cardiac death. *Ann Intern Med* **126**:1–12.

Pfeffer MA, Braunwald E, Moye LA, et al. 1992. Effect of captopril on mortality and morbidity in patients with left ventricular dysfunction after myocardial infarction: results of the survival and ventricular enlargement trial. *N Engl J Med* **327**:669–77.

Roden DM. 1992. Treatment of cardiovascular disorders: arrhythmias. In: Melmon KL, Morrelli HF, Hoffman BB, et al., editors. *Clinical Pharmacology: Basic Principles in Therapeutics*. New York: McGraw-Hill. p 151–85.

Roden DM. 1993. Early afterdepolarizations and Torsades de Pointes: implications for the control of cardiac arrhythmias by controlling repolarization. *Eur Heart J* **14H**:56–61.

Roden DM. 1995. Antiarrhythmic drugs. In: Hardman JL, Limbird LE, Molinoff PB, et al., editors. *Goodman and Gilman's The Pharmacological Basis of Therapeutics*. 9th ed. New York: McGraw-Hill. p 839–74.

Roden DM, George AL. 1997. Structure and function of cardiac sodium and potassium channels. *Am J Physiol* **42**:H511–25.

Sanguinetti MC, Jiang C, Curran ME, et al. 1995. A mechanistic link between an inherited and an acquired cardiac arrhythmia: HERG encodes the IKr potassium channel. *Cell* **81**:299–307.

Scandinavian Simvastatin Survival Study Group. 1994. Randomised trial of cholesterol lowering in 4444 patients with coronary heart disease: the Scandinavian Simvastatin Survival Study (4S). *Lancet* **344**:1383–9.

Shepherd J, Cobbe SM, Ford I, et al. 1995. Prevention of coronary heart disease with pravastatin in men with hypercholesterolemia. West of Scotland Coronary Prevention Study Group. *N Engl J Med* **333**:1301–7.

Shinbane JS, Wood MA, Jensen DN, et al. 1997. Tachycardia-induced cardiomyopathy: a review of animal models and clinical studies. *J Am Coll Cardiol* **29**:709–15.

Singer DE. 1996. Anticoagulation for atrial fibrillation: epidemiology informing a difficult clinical decision. *Proc Assoc Am Phys* **108**:29–36.

Singh SN, Fletcher RD, Fisher SG, et al. 1995. Amiodarone in patients with congestive heart failure and asymptomatic ventricular arrhythmia. Survival Trial of Antiarrhythmic Therapy in Congestive Heart Failure. *N Engl J Med* **333**:77–82.

Snyders DJ, Hondeghem LM, Bennett PB. 1991. Mechanisms of drug-channel interactions. In: Fozzard HA, Haber E, Jennings RB, et al., editors. *The Heart and Cardiovascular System: Scientific Foundations*. 2nd ed. New York: Raven Press. p 2165–93.

Stambler BS, Wood MA, Ellenbogen KA. 1997. Antiarrhythmic actions of intravenous ibutilide compared with procainamide during human atrial flutter and fibrillation: electrophysiological determinants of enhanced conversion efficacy. *Circulation* **96**:4298–306.

Steering and Publications Committees of the ACUTE Study. 1998. Design of a clinical trial for the assessment of cardioversion using transesophageal echocardiography (The ACUTE Multicenter Study). *Am J Cardiol* **81**:877–83.

Stewart RB, Bardy GH, Greene HL. 1986. Wide complex tachycardia: misdiagnosis and outcome after emergent therapy. *Ann Intern Med* **104**:766–71.

Task Force of the Working Group on Arrhythmias of the European Society of Cardiology. 1991. The Sicilian gambit: a new approach to the classification of antiarrhythmic drugs based on their actions on arrhythmogenic mechanisms. *Circulation* **84**:1831–51.

Tan HL, Hou CJ, Lauer MR, et al. 1995. Electrophysiologic mechanisms of the long QT interval syndromes and torsade de pointes. *Ann Intern Med* **122**:701–14.

The Cardiac Arrhythmia Suppression Trial (CAST) Investigators. 1989. Preliminary report: Effect of encainide and flecainide on mortality in a randomized trial of arrhythmia suppression after myocardial infarction. *N Engl J Med* **321**:406–12.

The Cardiac Arrhythmia Suppression Trial II Investigators. 1991. Effect of the antiarrhythmic agent moricizine on survival after myocardial infarction. *N Engl J Med* **327**:227–33.

The Norwegian Multicenter Study Group. 1981. Timolol-induced reduction in mortality and reinfarction in patients surviving acute myocardial infarction. *N Engl J Med* **304**:801–7.

The SOLVD Investigators. 1992. Effect of enalapril on mortality and the development of heart failure in asymptomatic patients with reduced left ventricular ejection fractions. *N Engl J Med* **327**:685–91.

Thompson PD, Melmon KL, Richards JA, et al. 1973. Lidocaine pharmacokinetics in advanced heart failure, liver disease and renal failure in man. *Ann Intern Med* **78**:499–9.

Tonkin AM, Aylward PE, Joel SE, et al. 1980. Verapamil in prophylaxis of paroxysmal atrioventricular nodal reentrant tachycardia. *J Cardiovasc Pharmacol* **2**:473–86.

Tzivoni D, Banai S, Schugar C, et al. 1988. Treatment of torsade de pointes with magnesium sulfate. *Circulation* **77**:392–97.

UK Propafenone PSVT Study Group. 1995. A randomized, placebo-controlled trial of propafenone in the prophylaxis of paroxysmal supraventricular tachycardia and paroxysmal atrial fibrillation. *Circulation* **92**:2550–7.

UK Rythmodan Multicentre Study Group. 1984. Oral disopyramide after admission to hospital with suspected acute myocardial infarction. *Postgraduate Med J* **60**:98–107.

Waldo AL, Camm AJ, DeRuyter H, et al. 1996. Effect of d-sotalol on mortality in patients with left ventricular dysfunction after recent and remote myocardial infarction. *Lancet* **348**:7–12.

Wellens HJJ. 1986. The wide QRS tachycardia. *Ann Intern Med* **104**:879–9.

Winkle RA, Mason JW, Griffin JC, et al. 1981. Malignant ventricular tachy-arrhythmias associated with the use of encainide. *Am Heart J* **102**:857–64.

Wolfe CL, Nibley C, Bhandari A, et al. 1991. Polymorphous ventricular tachycardia associated with acute myocardial infarction. *Circulation* **84**:1543–51.

Woods KL, Fletcher S. 1994. Long-term outcome after intravenous magnesium sulphate in suspected acute myocardial infarction: the second Leicester Intravenous Magnesium Intervention Trial (LIMIT-2). *Lancet* **343**:816–9.

Wyse DG, Anderson JL, Antman EM, et al. 1997. Atrial fibrillation follow-up investigation of rhythm management: The AFFIRM study design. *Am J Cardiol* **79**:1198–1202.

Zipes DP. 1997. Atrial fibrillation: a tachycardia-induced atrial cardiomyopathy. *Circulation* **95**:562–4.

# Peripheral Arterial Occlusive Disease

Thomas L. Whitsett

*Chapter Outline*



Atherosclerotic plaques in the larger conducting arteries are a common cause of disability. Proximal arteries in the lower limbs, such as iliac and femoral arteries are the most frequent location of these atherosclerotic lesions. Diabetic patients tend also to have disease in the smaller distal vessels. Peripheral arterial occlusive disease (PAOD) is more common in men and increases with age (Criqui 1997). Prevalence, as determined by noninvasive testing, is about 2% to 3% for men <60 years, 8% for men 60–69 years, and 19% for men >70 years of age. In one study of 5-year outcomes for patients with PAOD, mortality was 29%, worsening claudication 16% (of which patients showed need for surgery 25% and amputation 4%), and 55% were stable or improved (McDaniel and Cronenwett 1989). Atherosclerosis remains clinically silent until luminal narrowing prevents adequate flow to meet metabolic demands typically associated with exertion. The disease may present suddenly because of thromboembolism induced by plaque rupture. Treatment consists of risk-factor modification, exercise training, possible angioplasty or surgical revascularization, and pharmacotherapy. Drug therapy of this disease is the major focus of this chapter.

## PATHOPHYSIOLOGY

Mild PAOD is usually asymptomatic, and a ratio of ankle/brachial systolic pressure index (ABPI) is usually >0.8 at rest. Patients with moderate PAOD have ABPI values of <0.8 and experience symptoms only with exercise. Exercise-induced calf pain, muscle weakness, numbness, or cramping are classical symptoms. These symptoms usually start in the calf and migrate proximally to the hip. Patients with predominantly aortoiliac involvement may experience hip or gluteal pain as an initial symptom. These symptoms are nonspecific, and a variety of musculoskeletal problems can mimic claudication, e.g., spinal stenosis and degenerative disk, hip, or knee disease, as well as certain foot problems.

**PRINCIPLE When two diseases are common and share nonspecific symptoms, a definitive diagnostic test is necessary as a first step in rational therapy.**

Severe PAOD usually has an ABPI of <0.5 and is associated with ischemic pain at rest (i.e., pain in the affected limb while in the supine or leg-elevated position) that is relieved by dangling the foot over the side of the bed, standing, or slowly walking. These conditions threaten loss of tissue. These patients lack healing potential if ulcerations occur and may develop gangrenous lesions as the disease progresses.

Atherosclerotic plaque is the primary lesion of PAOD. Over several years there is progressive plaque growth typically associated with the presence of one or more risk factors (Table 1-44). Major risk factors promote endothelial oxidative stress with the generation of superoxide anions (Cooke 1997). This reduces endothelial nitric oxide production, which appears to be an early factor in the formation of atherosclerotic lesion, as well as other processes (Candipan et al. 1996).

Table 1-44 **Risk Factors Associated with Peripheral Arterial Occlusive Disease (PAOD)**

| | |
|---|---|
| • Cigarette smoking | • Hyperfibrinogenemia |
| • Hyperlipidemia | • Hyperhomocystinemia |
| • Hypertension | • Lipoprotein (*a*) |
| • Diabetes mellitus | • Asymmetric dimethylarginine |
| • Male gender | |
| • Age | |

**PRINCIPLE Definitive approaches to therapy are those aimed at pathogenesis, not those aimed at the end phenotypic abnormality.**

Atherosclerotic plaque contributes to PAOD by two general mechanisms. First, plaque may gradually produce luminal narrowing to the degree that flow is compromised. Patients are often asymptomatic at rest, but with exercise, when demand exceeds inflow capabilities, muscle ischemia occurs, resulting in symptoms of claudication. Rest usually reverses the symptoms within 5 to 10 minutes, and then activity can be resumed. A narrowing of luminal diameter by <70% generally does not limit flow unless exercise exceeds compensatory mechanisms of increasing flow velocity to maintain flow volume. As increasing demand for oxygenated blood produces greater vasodilation with a fixed inflow, perfusion pressure decreases, and ischemic symptoms (claudication) ensue (usually when perfusion pressure falls below 50 mm Hg) (Birdwell and Whitsett 1996).

Second, plaques may rupture, exposing blood to the thrombogenic core, resulting in platelet aggregation followed by thrombus formation. This may cause sudden occlusion of the vessel or may produce emboli that travel to distal vessels. Either process results in an acutely ischemic limb characterized by the five Ps: pulselessness, pallor, pain, paresthesias, and paralysis, depending on the degree and duration of the ischemia. Also, the limb may be relatively cold. Approximately 50% of sudden ischemic peripheral events are due to thromboembolism from either a cardiac source or a diseased proximal vessel. Remember, a sudden worsening of limb perfusion often reflects acute arterial occlusion from a thrombotic and/or embolic process.

**Key Point: The five "P's" of an acutely ischemic limb are**

- **pulselessness**
- **pallor**
- **pain**
- **paresthesias**
- **paralysis**

## THERAPEUTIC OPTIONS

A major challenge in treating patients with PAOD is to identify the optimal therapy for each specific patient, keying on the patient's risks and comorbidity profile. Individuals with severe disease (ischemic pain at rest or nonhealing ulcers) and threatened tissue loss will likely require surgical revascularization. Patients whose claudication limits their lifestyle are candidates for a variety of medical therapies. Patients who do not respond adequately to medical therapies may need angioplasty or surgical revascularization. Mild-to-moderate disease is best treated conservatively. Clearly, treatment of risk factors is more likely to improve morbidity and mortality to a greater degree than simply treating the symptoms of claudication (Table 1-45).

**PRINCIPLE When treating claudication and peripheral arterial disease, it is important to manage the shared risk factors contributing to cardiac and cerebral morbidity and mortality.**

### Exercise Training

Walking as a form of exercise has proven benefits of prolonging the initial and absolute claudication distances (ICD and ACD, respectively). Consider exercise therapy as the gold standard to which other remedies are compared.

The mechanism by which exercise improves claudication distances is not clear. Benefits seem to accrue from more effective redistribution of blood flow and more favorable muscle metabolism (Hiatt et al. 1996). Individuals are best managed in a supervised training program often involving use of a treadmill; resistive training has no effect on walking distance (Hiatt et al. 1994). Training sessions of greater than 30 minutes each, occurring three times weekly and utilizing walking are best correlated with improved performance (Gardner and Poehlman 1995). When such a program is appropriately implemented, the average ICD increased 179% (from 126 m to 351 m), and the ACD increased 122% (326 m to 723 m).

**Key point: A given patient with claudication can anticipate a doubling and possibly tripling of his or her walking distance with a supervised exercise training program.**

### Cessation of Smoking

Cigarette smoking is the major risk factor contributing to PAOD (Hirsch et al. 1997). Continued smoking continues to add measurably to the process (Howard et al. 1998) (Table 1-46). Successful cessation of smoking is rewarded by a reduced rate of myocardial infarction and stroke and

**Table 1-45 Effects of Selected Medical Interventions on the Outcome of PAOD**

| Intervention | Improve claudication symptoms? | Decrease CHD event rates (fatal and nonfatal)? | Decrease mortality |
|---|---|---|---|
| Tobacco cessation strategies | Minimal improvement | Yes | Yes |
| Antiplatelet therapies | Trend toward benefit (ticlopidine) | Yes[a] | Yes[a] |
| Lipid-lowering therapies | Unknown | Hypothesized | Hypothesized |

[a]Aspirin, ticlopidine, and clopidogrel have each been shown to decrease event rates for the pooled outcome of myocardial infarction, ischemic stroke and vascular death. A beneficial effect of improved all-cause mortality rates has not yet been directly demonstrated for any agent but is surmised from trends from multiple investigations (prior trials have not had sufficient power to detect such an effect).
SOURCE: Adapted from Hirsch et al. 1997.

increased survival (Jonason and Bergstrom 1987). Environmental tobacco smoke (secondary smoke) was recently shown to cause a 20% increase in progression of atherosclerosis, whereas active smoking caused a 50% increase (Howard et al. 1998). Medical personnel should remind smokers regularly of the importance of becoming a nonsmoker, and continuing efforts to quit are encouraged.

To stop smoking, behavioral treatment is important but has a success rate of only 15% to 30% after one year. Use of the nicotine patch has a 23% to 27% success rate. Fortunately, PAOD is not a contraindication to use of the patch, as plasma nicotine concentrations are less than achieved with smoking. Bupropion is effective for smoking cessation at one year compared with placebo (see chapter 26, Writing Prescriptions.

**PRINCIPLE Smoking cessation may be the single most important aspect of medical management of peripheral arterial occlusive disease.**

**Table 1-46 Effects of Tobacco on Progression of PAOD**

| |
|---|
| Progression from asymptomatic PAOD to stable claudication |
| Conversion of stable claudication to rest pain (usually requires revascularization) |
| Increased failure rate of limb bypass grafts and PTA |
| Increased amputation rate |
| Accelerated rates of other cardiovascular ischemic events (e.g., MI and stroke) |
| Decreased survival |

SOURCE: Adapted from Hirsch et al. 1997.

## Antiplatelet Therapy

Complications of atherosclerotic plaque involve platelet aggregation and thrombus formation. Antiplatelet agents that have been tested as management for patients with PAOD include aspirin, ticlopidine, and clopidogrel.

### *Aspirin*

Aspirin as given in the Physicians' Health Study (325 mg every other day, compared with placebo-controlled, tested in 22,071 male physicians) did not change the incidence of claudication in the two groups, but there was a 50% reduction in the need for a peripheral arterial revascularization procedure (Goldhaber et al. 1992). The Antiplatelet Trialists' Collaboration 1994) demonstrated an approximately 25% reduction in vascular events associated with the use of aspirin. The most widely tested aspirin regimen was 75 mg to 325 mg once daily.

**Key Point Aspirin use in patients with peripheral arterial occlusive disease is associated with a lower rate of coronary and cerebral vascular events and is associated with a reduced need for peripheral revascularization.**

### *Ticlopidine*

Ticlopidine interferes with platelet membrane function by inhibiting ADP-induced platelet-fibrinogen binding and subsequent platelet–platelet aggregation. It may reduce plasma fibrinogen concentrations and whole-blood viscosity. Although PAOD/claudication is not a US Food and Drug Administration (FDA)-approved indication, there is evidence to suggest efficacy. The most convincing study in patients with intermittent claudication compared ticlopidine 250 mg bid to placebo in 151 patients (Balsano et al. 1989). Whereas there was an approximate 250% increase in ICD with ticlopidine, subjects receiving placebo had a striking 180% improvement. There was greater improvement in ABPI at the end of exercise testing in the ticlopidine group compared with the placebo group. It is noteworthy that a recent study demonstrated greater long-term patency of infrainguinal saphenous vein bypass grafts for subjects receiving ticlopidine compared with those receiving placebo (Becquemin 1997). Also, long-term use of ticlopidine in patients with PAOD resulted in a lower rate of revascularization (Bergqvist et al. 1995). More studies are needed to define the role of ticlopidine in patients with PAOD.

Neutropenia (neutrophils $<1200/mm^3$) occurs in 2.4% of patients, whereas agranulocytosis occurs in 0.8%. A CBC should be performed every two weeks until the end of the third month of therapy. The effect on neutrophils is reversible. The most common adverse effects involve the GI tract and consist of nausea, vomiting, cramps, diarrhea, and gastralgia.

***Clopidogrel***

Clopidogrel has a mechanism of action similar to that of ticlopidine but does not share the problems of neutropenia. In a study of 19,185 patients, clopidogrel 75 mg daily was compared with aspirin 325 mg daily (CAPRIE 1996). In the 6452 patients who entered the study as a result of having PAOD, there was a 23.8% reduction in relative risk of MI, ischemic stroke or vascular death of any variety in favor of clopidogrel. The overall annual event rate for placebo was 5.32% and for clopidogrel, 5.83%, but it was a statistically significant difference. Effect on claudication and quality of life was not tested.

**PRINCIPLE The physician must make every effort to determine whether statistical differences mean clinical differences that justify the risk of therapeutic intervention.**

## Hemorheologic Therapy

***Pentoxifylline***

Pentoxifylline is the only agent in the United States approved by the FDA for the indication of claudication. It reduces the viscosity of blood by improving impaired red-cell membrane flexibility, moderately decreasing plasma fibrinogen levels, and retarding platelet aggregation. To what extent these changes lead to prolonged walking distance in patients with PAOD is unclear. Beneficial effects of two studies are shown in Table 1-47. There is an improvement of about 20% in ICD (Porter et al. 1982; SSG 1989). A meta-analysis reports results for eleven trials demonstrating an average 29.4-meter increase in ICD and a 48.4-meter increase in ACD compared with distance for those taking a placebo (Hood et al. 1996). Again, while this difference was statistically significant, the quality-of-life assessments were not made to determine whether the significance of these results was clinically important. Pentoxifylline generally is well tolerated at doses of 250 mg tid when taken with meals, but is associated with nausea in some patients. Although patients can anticipate greater improvement with exercise training, some individuals cannot walk adequately to obtain this benefit and may experience improvement with pentoxifylline. Whether pentoxifylline adds an additional benefit in the exercise-trained patient with claudication is unknown.

**PRINCIPLE Sometimes the drug has better value without optimal employment of the nondrug "adjuvant" exercise.**

## Metabolic Agents

***Proprionyl-L-carnitine***

Proprionyl-L-carnitine is currently in phase III trials for the treatment of claudication, and the complexities of its action have been reviewed (Hiatt 1997). Carnitine is important for muscle metabolism during times of stress. Patients with PAOD have higher than normal concentrations of carnitine esters, which increase further during exercise. Proprionyl-L-carnitine is thought to act by increasing the amount of free carnitine in muscle and thus favorably affecting energy production. This compound has demonstrated the ability to increase ACD (Table 1-47). The initial dose of 500 mg bid is titrated at 2-month intervals to 2 g daily. It has been well tolerated with no serious adverse effects and appears to improve walking distance and the quality of life (Coot et al. 1992; Brevetti et al. 1995). There is much more to be learned about this compound before it possibly finds a place in the therapy of PAOD. Cases of thrombotic thrombocytopenic purpura were recently reported and usually occurred during the first month of therapy (Bennett et al. 1998).

## Vasodilators

A major therapeutic objective in patients with claudication is to increase blood flow to ischemic tissue. However, vasodilating drugs have not been efficacious therapeutic agents probably because these agents primarily act on ar-

Table 1-47 Randomized, Placebo-Controlled Trials of Drug Therapy in Patients with Claudication

| Drug | Reference | n | Dose | Duration (months) | ΔACD (%) Placebo | Drug | Difference (P value) | Functional Assessment[a] |
|---|---|---|---|---|---|---|---|---|
| Pentoxifylline | Porter et al. 1982 | 128 | 1.2 g/d | 6 | 38 | 56 | 18 (0.19) | No |
| | SSG 1989 | 150 | 1.2 g/d | 6 | 29 | 50 | 21 (0.09) | No |
| | (subset)[b] | 109 | 1.2 g/d | 6 | 30 | 63 | 33 (<0.05) | No |
| Proprionyl-L-carnitine | Brevetti et al. 1995 | 245 | 1–3 g/d | 6 | 43 | 65 | 22 (<0.05) | No |
| | Coto et al. 1992 | 300 | 2 g/d | 6 | 20 | 53 | 33 (<0.05) | No |
| | Hiatt[c] | 155 | 2 g/d | 6 | 23 | 49 | 26 (<0.01) | Improved walking distance, speed, role physical function and body pain |
| Ticlopidine | Balsano et al. 1989 | 151 | 500 mg/d | 21 | 38 | 71 | 33 (<0.01) | No |
| Beraprost | Lievre et al. 1996 | 83 | 60 μg/d | 3 | 41 | 42 | 50 (NS) | No |
| Cilostazol | Money et al. 1998 | 239 | 100 mg/d | 4 | 14 | 43 | 29 (<0.01) | Improved physical function |
| | Beebe et al. 1997 | 419 | 100 mg/d | 6 | 15 | 50 | (<0.01) | Yes |

[a]Functional status defined by the Walking Impairment Questionnaire and Medical Outcomes Study SF-36 (Regensteiner 1997).
[b]Only the subset of patients at the optimal dose is reported.
[c]Unpublished data from company files.
ABBREVIATION: ACD, absolute claudication distance.
SOURCE: Adapted from Hirsch et al. 1997.

terioles that are maximally dilated during ischemia by autoregulation. In other words, the uninvolved arteries are the ones that dilate with the possibility of redistribution or shunting flow away from the site of need. Further, it is possible to lower systemic arterial pressure to such a degree that perfusion of the affected site is impaired.

> WARNING Vasodilators in patients with claudication may shunt flow away from the ischemic tissue or lower systemic perfusion pressure, thereby worsening symptoms of ischemia.

### *Verapamil*

Verapamil may increase the oxygen-extracting capacity of the ischemic lower limb (Bagger et al. 1985). In patients with claudication, verapamil increased ICD 29% and ACD 49% compared with placebo. However, individual dose titration was necessary and varied fourfold (120 mg to 420 mg daily) (Bagger et al. 1997). Much more work is necessary before this class of compound can be considered efficacious for treating claudication.

## Phosphodiesterase Inhibitors

### *Cilostazol*

Cilostazol is a phosphodiesterase inhibitor that decreases platelet aggregation and promotes vasodilatation (Okuda et al. 1993). A multicenter study comparing two doses of cilostazol to placebo demonstrated a dose-dependent increase in ICD and ACD for cilostazol (Beebe et al. 1997; Money et al. 1998). At 100 mg bid there was a 59% increase in ICD and a 51% increase in ACD, whereas patients given placebo improved approximately 20%. This was associated with benefits in quality-of-life measures.

## Prostaglandins

For years, various prostaglandin derivatives have been studied in patients with PAOD. Patients with severe disease have experienced limited success, whereas there is even less experience in patients with claudication alone.

### *Beraprost*

Beraprost is a stable oral analog of prostacyclin ($PGI_2$) with antiplatelet and vasodilating properties. A dose–response study of beraprost compared three doses (20, 40, and 60 μg orally tid) with placebo (Lievre et al. 1996). There was a dose-dependent, up to 129% increase in ICD at 12 weeks for the 60-μg dose, while ACD increased 142%. Further studies with this and other compounds in this class of agents are necessary before their possible role in the therapy of claudication is defined.

### *AS-013*

AS-013 is a pro-drug metabolized to prostaglandin E-1 ($PGE_1$) which is a potent vasodilator and inhibitor of platelet aggregation. In a recent study, three doses of AS-013 (given IV 5 days/week for 4 weeks) were compared with placebo (Belch et al. 1997). Efficacy was demonstrated for increased ICD and improved quality of life. More definitive studies of this drug are required.

### *Prostaglandin E-1*

Prostaglandin E-1 administration IV (5 days/week for 4 weeks, then 2 days/week) was compared with placebo in patients with severe claudication (Diehm et al. 1997). At the conclusion of the study, patients given $PGE_1$ improved walking distance by 104%, whereas those given placebo improved by 60%. This drug requires further study.

## Chelation Therapy

The use of edetate disodium ($Na_2$ EDTA) to chelate calcium has been touted by some physicians as beneficial in treating patients with atherosclerotic problems. However, efficacy for this compound has not been rigorously demonstrated. A recent double-blind, randomized, placebo-controlled study did not demonstrate benefits compared with placebo (Lyngdorf et al. 1996), and chelation carries potential toxicity (e.g., precipitous hypocalcemia). Chelation therapy cannot be recommended for the treatment of atherosclerotic problems at this time.

# APPROACH TO PATIENT MANAGEMENT

The first step in managing patients with claudication is to determine whether their symptoms are due to arterial insufficiency. If so, patients must understand how atherosclerotic occlusive disease not only affects their legs, but it is quite likely at work on their coronary and cerebral vessels. The next step involves modification of risk factors. Every effort should be made to control blood pressure, to reduce LDL cholesterol to levels near 100 mg/dL, and to cease smoking. It is usually useful to encourage an exercise program and to make certain patients understand that when they experience claudication, they are not damaging their legs. Walking for 30 minutes three times weekly, especially in an organized program, has a chance of improving walking distance greater than any medication.

**Table 1-48 Drugs Used in the Treatment of PAOD and Claudication**

| Drug | Common dose | Average Wholesale price (per month)[a] | Comments |
|---|---|---|---|
| Aspirin | 325 mg qd | Generic $1<br>Bayer brand $2 | Usual first-line antiplatelet agent |
| Ticlopidine HCl | 250 mg bid | Generic NA<br>Ticlide $86 | Useful in aspirin-sensitive patients; watch for neutropenia |
| Clopidogrel | 75 mg qd | Generic NA<br>Plavix $72 | Newest antiplatelet agent, fewer side effects than ticlopidine |
| Pentoxifylline | 400 mg tid with meals | Generic NA<br>Trental $57 | Only agent specifically approved for claudication |
| Verapamil HCl | 80 mig tid | Generic $5<br>Calan $48 | Careful titration necessary to avoid worsening pain |
| Proprionyl-L-carnitine; | 500 mg bid | | Still in phase III testing |
| Cilostazol | 100 mg bid | Generic NA<br>Pletal NA | Still in phase III testing |
| Beraprost | 60 μg tid | Experimental | |
| AS-013 | | Experimental | |

[a]Source of non-OTC drug prices is *Mosby's GenR*$_x$ 1998, except Plavix from author's local pharmacy. Current prices may vary from those quoted, but comparative prices among products are expected to be similar. The reader should check on local prices at the time of prescribing.

Pharmacotherapy is usually initiated with aspirin 325 mg daily as a first-line antiplatelet medication (Table 1-48). If the patient has sensitivity to aspirin, then ticlopidine 250 mg bid is often prescribed. Clopidogrel is new and may have effects similar to those of ticlopidine with less adverse effects. It is of distinct value in patients who do not tolerate ticlopidine.

After the patient has achieved maximum benefit from exercise training, risk factor reduction, and use of an antiplatelet drug, the use of pentoxifylline should be considered if the patient still has lifestyle-limiting claudication. If the patient has not achieved a perceived benefit by 8 weeks, it should be discontinued.

If lifestyle-limiting claudication persists at this point, a revascularization procedure (e.g., angioplasty or bypass grafting) could be considered. Remember that the patient must understand the possible risks and anticipated benefits of these procedures to allow for a truly informed decision.

## REFERENCES

Antiplatelet Trialists' Collaboration. 1994. Collaborative overview of randomized trials of antiplatelet therapy. I. Prevention of death, myocardial infarction, and stroke by prolonged antiplatelet therapy in various categories of patients. *Br Med J* **308**:81–106.

Bagger JP, Helligsoe P, Randsbaek F, et al. 1997. Effect of verapamil in intermittent claudication: a randomized, double-blind, placebo-controlled, cross-over study after individual dose-response assessment. *Circulation* **95**:411–14.

Bagger JP, Mathar R, Paulsen PK, et al. 1985. Verapamil induced increment of oxygen extraction in the arteriosclerotic limb. *Cardiovasc Res* **19**:567–69.

Balsano F, Coccheri S, Libretti A, et al. 1989. Ticlopidine in the treatment of intermittent claudication: a 21-month double-blind trial. *J Lab Clin Med* **114**:84–91.

Becquemin J-P. 1997. Effect of ticlopidine on the long-term patency of saphenous-vein bypass grafts in the legs. *N Engl J Med* **337**:1726–31.

Beebe HG, Dawson DL, Cutler BS, et al. 1997. Cilostazol, a new treatment for intermittent claudication: results of a randomized, multicenter trial [abstract]. 70th Scientific Sessions of the American Heart Association; 1997 Nov 9–12; Orlando (FL). *Circulation* **96**(Suppl.):I-12.

Belch JJ, Bell PR, Creissen D, et al. 1997. Randomized, double-blind, placebo-controlled study evaluating the efficacy and safety of AS-013, a prostaglandin E1 prodrug, in patients with intermittent claudication. *Circulation* **95**:2298–302.

Bennett CL, Weinberg PD, Rozenberg-Ben-Dror K, et al. 1998. Thrombotic thrombocytopenic purpura associated with ticlopidine: a review of 60 cases. *Ann Intern Med* **128**:541–4.

Bergqvist D, Almgren B, Dickinson JP. 1995. Reduction of requirement for leg vascular surgery during long-term treatment of claudicant patients with ticlopidine: results from the Swedish Ticlopidine Multicentre Study (STIMS). *Eur J Vasc Endovasc Surg* **10**:69–76.

Birdwell BG, Whitsett TL. 1996. Peripheral vascular disease. In: Kaufman CE, McKee PA, editors. *Essentials of Pathophysiology.* Boston: Little, Brown. Sect. I, chapter 13.

Brevetti G, Perna S, Sabba C, et al. 1995. Propionyl-L-carnitine in intermittent claudication: double-blind, placebo-controlled, dose titration, multicenter study. *J Am Coll Cardiol* **26**:1411–16.

Candipan RC, Wang BY, Tsao PS, et al. 1996. Regression or progression: dependency upon vascular nitric oxide activity. *Arterioscler Thromb Vasc Biol* **16**:44–50.

CAPRIE Steering Committee. 1996. A randomised, blinded trial of clopidogrel versus aspirin in patients at risk of ischaemic events (CAPRIE). CAPRIE Steering Committee. *Lancet* **348**:1329–39.

Cooke JP. 1997. The pathophysiology of peripheral arterial disease: rational targets for drug intervention. *Vasc Med* **2**:227–30.

Coto V, D'Alessandro L, Grattarola G, et al. 1992. Evaluation of the therapeutic efficacy and tolerability of levocarnitine propionyl in the treatment of chronic obstructive arteriopathies of the lower extremities: a multicentre controlled study vs. placebo. *Drugs Exp Clin Res* **18**:29–36.

Criqui MH, Denenberg JO, Langer RD, et al. 1997. The epidemiology of peripheral arterial disease: importance of identifying the population at risk. *Vasc Med* **2**:221–6.

Diehm C, Balzer K, Bisler H, et al. 1997. Efficacy of a new prostaglandin E1 regimen in outpatients with severe intermittent claudication: results of a multicenter placebo-controlled double-blind trial. *J Vasc Surg* **35**:537–44.

Gardner AW, Poehlman ET. 1995. Exercise rehabilitation programs for the treatment of claudication pain: a meta-analysis. *JAMA* **274**:975–80.

Goldhaber SZ, Manson JE, Stampfer MJ, et al. 1992. Low-dose aspirin and subsequent peripheral arterial surgery in the Physicians' Health Study. *Lancet* **340**:143–45.

Hiatt WR. 1997. Current and future drug therapies for claudication. *Vasc Med* **2**:257–62.

Hiatt WR, Regensteiner JG, Carry M, et al. 1996. Effect of exercise training on skeletal muscle histology and metabolism in peripheral arterial disease. *J Appl Physiol* **81**:780–8.

Hiatt WR, Wolfel EE, Meier RH, et al. 1994. Superiority of treadmill walking exercise vs. strength training for patients with peripheral arterial disease. Implication for the mechanism of the training response. *Circulation* **90**:1866–74.

Hirsch AT, Treat-Jacobson D, Lando HA, et al. 1997. The role of tobacco cessation, antiplatelet and lipid lowering therapies in the treatment of peripheral arterial disease. *Vasc Med* **2**:243–51.

Hood SC, Moher D, Barber GG. 1996. Management of intermittent claudication with pentoxifylline: meta-analysis of randomized controlled trials. *Can Med Assoc J* **155**:1053–59.

Howard G, Wagenknecht LE, Burke GL, et al. 1998. Cigarette smoking and progression of atherosclerosis: the Atherosclerosis Risk in Communities (ARIC) study. *JAMA* **279**:119–24.

Jonason T, Bergstrom R. 1987. Cessation of smoking in patients with intermittent claudication. Effects on the risk of peripheral vascular complications, myocardial infarction and mortality. *Acta Med Scand* **221**:253–60.

Lievre M, Azoulay S, Lion L, et al. 1996. A dose-effect study of beraprost sodium in intermittent claudication. *J Cardiovasc Pharmacol* **27**:788–93.

Lyngdorf P, Guldager B, Holm J, et al. 1996. Chelation therapy for intermittent claudication: a double-blind, randomized, controlled trial [letter; comment]. *Circulation* **93**:395–6.

McDaniel MD, Cronenwett JL. 1989. Basic data related to the natural history of intermittent claudication. *Ann Vasc Surg* **3**:273–7.

Money SR, Herd JA, Isaacsohn JL, et al. 1998. Effects of cilostazol on walking distances in patients with intermittent claudication caused by peripheral vascular disease. *J Vasc Surg* **27**:267–75.

*Mosby's GenR$_x$* 1998. *Mosby's GenR$_x$ 1998: The Complete Reference for Generic and Brand Drugs.* 8th ed. St. Louis: Mosby–Year Book.

Okuda Y, Kimura Y, Yamashita K. 1993. Cilostazol. *Cardiovasc Drug Rev* **11**:451–65.

Porter JM, Cutler BS, Lee BY, et al. 1982. Pentoxifylline efficacy in the treatment of intermittent claudication: multicenter controlled double-blind trial with objective assessment of chronic occlusive arterial disease patients. *Am Heart J* **104**:66–72.

Regensteiner JG. 1997. Exercise in the treatment of claudication: assessment and treatment of functional impairment. *Vasc Med* **2**:238–42.

[SSG] Lindgarde F, Jelnes R, Bjorkman H, et al. of the Scandinavian Study Group. 1989. Conservative drug treatment in patients with moderately severe chronic occlusive peripheral arterial disease. *Circulation* **80**:1549–56.

# Venous Thromboembolic Disease

**Brian G. Birdwell, Thomas L. Whitsett**

*Chapter Outline*



**Key Points:**

- **Deep vein thrombosis (DVT) and pulmonary embolism (PE) are different expressions of the same disorder, venous thromboembolic disease.**
- **PE is a leading cause of or contributing factor to in-hospital mortality.**

A robust estimate of the incidence of deep-vein thrombosis (DVT) and pulmonary embolism (PE) found that in 1986 there were over 250,000 cases in the United States, or 107 cases of DVT/PE per 100,000 population (Anderson et al. 1991). Most investigators agree that PE causes or contributes significantly to 10% to 15% of all in-hospital deaths, and DVT of the deep veins of the lower extremities and pelvis is the source of 80% to 90% of pulmonary emboli (Moser 1990; Hull et al. 1996). Thus, it is important to remember that DVT and PE are different expressions of the same disorder, venous thromboembolic disease.

## PATHOPHYSIOLOGY

Virchow's triad of venous stasis, endothelial damage, and hypercoagulability still anchor our concept of the pathophysiology of DVT. Factors related to this triad are common and compounded in many clinical circumstances (Table 1-49). For instance, the anatomic and physiological features of total knee replacement illustrate the interaction of all elements of Virchow's triad. Endothelial damage is unavoidable; surgery induces a hypercoagulable state (a physiologic response: stopping the bleeding caused by injury); and tourniquet use and inactivity result in venous stasis in the leg. Indeed, without anticoagulant prophylaxis, the incidence of DVT after total knee replacement is 60% to 80% (Hull, Delmore, Hirsh et al. 1979; McKenna et al. 1980; Haas et al. 1990; Leclerc et al. 1992;

Table 1-49 Risk Factors for Venous Thromboembolic Disease[a]

| | Virchow's triad | | |
|---|---|---|---|
| Risk factor | Stasis | Venous endothelial injury | Hypercoagulability |
| Major joint surgery | X | X | X |
| Other major surgery | X | | X |
| Malignancy | | X | X |
| Leg injury (esp. with leg immobilization) | | X | X |
| Extended travel | X | | |
| Oral contraceptive use | | | X |
| Stroke with leg paralysis | X | | ? |
| Pregnancy/post-partum | X | | X |
| Illness requiring bedrest (e.g., congestive heart failure) | X | | ? |

[a]Other hypercoagulability factors (e.g., protein C or S deficiency, antiphospholipid antibody syndrome with history of thrombosis, factor V Leiden, oral contraceptives, indwelling subclavian catheters, advancing age) add to deep vein thrombosis/pulmonary embolic disease (DVT/PE) risk.

Clagett et al. 1995; see Table 1-50). The risk is even higher when an individual has other inherited or acquired risk factors.

**PRINCIPLE Risk factors for deep venous thrombosis are cumulative and are present in a large percentage of hospitalized patients.**

## CLINICAL MANIFESTATIONS OF VENOUS THROMBOEMBOLISM

Venous thromboembolism may manifest clinically with leg symptoms, chest symptoms, or both. DVT-associated symptoms characteristically include swelling, pain and/or tenderness, but 75% to 85% of patients presenting with such symptoms do not have DVT (Birdwell et al. 1998). Patients with PE can manifest life-threatening symptoms (hypotension, syncope, respiratory failure) but more typically present with dyspnea on exertion, mild tachypnea, pleuritic chest pain, cough, and rales. Thus, most patients with DVT and PE have common, nonspecific clinical symptoms. Objective testing is required to manage patients appropriately (see "Approach to Patient Management").

**Key Points:**

- **Leg and chest symptoms caused by DVT and PE are nonspecific, and even "classic" presentations may be mimicked by numerous disorders.**
- **Objective testing is required to make the diagnosis of DVT or PE.**

## ANTICOAGULANT THERAPY FOR VENOUS THROMBOEMBOLISM

Heparin and warfarin are the primary pharmacologic agents used to prevent and treat DVT and PE. Recent work with the chemical composition of heparin has produced an important new class of drugs, the low-molecular-weight heparins (LMWHs). Information about doses and costs of standard or unfractionated heparin (UH), LMWHs, and warfarin is presented in Table 1-51. Thrombolytic agents such as urokinase, streptokinase, and tissue plasminogen activator (tPA) are occasionally used in the setting of venous thromboembolism, but evidence of improved outcomes for patients is sparse. These drugs are not reviewed here.

Table 1-50 **Prophylaxis Against Deep Vein Thrombosis for Total Knee Replacement**

| REGIMEN | REFERENCES | TRIALS (*n*) | PATIENTS (*n*) | PATIENTS WITH DVT (*n*) | INCIDENCE (%) | 95% CI | RELATIVE RISK REDUCTION (%) |
|---|---|---|---|---|---|---|---|
| Placebo | Hull, Delmore, Hirsh et al. 1979; McKenna et al. 1980; Haas et al. 1990; Leclerc et al. 1992 | 4 | 116 | 71 | 61 | 52–70 | – |
| Aspirin | Graor et al. 1992 | 1 | 27 | 21 | 79 | 64–94 | – |
| Low-dose heparin | Spiro et al. 1993 | 1 | 225 | 77 | 34 | 28–40 | 44 |
| LMW heparin | Leclerc et al. 1992; Hull et al. 1993; Spiro et al. 1993; Leclerc et al. 1994; Spiro et al. 1994; Aster 1995; Heit et al. 1995 | 7 | 1354 | 399 | 30 | 28–32 | 51 |
| Low–intensity warfarin | Hull et al. 1993; RD Heparin Arthroplasty Group 1994; Leclerc et al. 1994; Spiro et al. 1994; Heit et al. 1995 | 5 | 1033 | 486 | 47 | 44–50 | 23 |
| IPC | Hull, Delmore, Hirsh et al. 1979; McKenna et al. 1980; Haas et al. 1990; Lynch 1990 | 4 | 366 | 41 | 11 | 9–14 | 82 |

NOTE: Pooled data from trials requiring mandatory postoperative venography. Adapted from Clagett et al. 1995. Used by permission.
ABBREVIATIONS: CI, confidence interval; DVT, deep venous thrombosis; IPC, intermittent pneumatic compression; LMW, low-molecular-weight.

## Heparin Preparations

### *Unfractionated heparin*

Unfractionated heparin (UH) was isolated in 1922 and has been used clinically for many years. It is a glycosaminoglycan comprising alternating residue chains of D-glucosamine and iduronic acid. Clinical preparations are heterogeneous with respect to size, ranging from molecular mass of 5000 to 30,000 Da with an average molecular mass of 12,000 Da. UH is usually extracted from bovine lung or porcine intestinal mucosa, and although these preparations are not identical, their biological activities are similar (Majerus et al. 1990). The potent anticoagulant activity of UH is due to a unique pentasaccharide that binds to the plasma inhibitor protein antithrombin III (ATIII) (Hirsh and Levine 1992). This high affinity binding induces a conformational change ATIII (see Fig. 1-32), effectively enhancing the inhibitory effect of ATIII on IIa (thrombin), factor Xa, and factor IXa (Hirsh and Levine 1992). Of these, thrombin is the most sensitive to heparin-catalyzed ATIII inhibition. UH also inhibits the thrombin-mediated activation of factors V and VIII (Hyers et al. 1995).

Unfractionated heparin is poorly absorbed after oral administration and so must be given parenterally, either intravenously or by subcutaneous injection. Intramuscular injection may result in large hematomas and should be avoided. UH is cleared and degraded primarily by the reticuloendothelial system (Majerus et al. 1990), so neither hepatic nor renal insufficiency appreciably alters clearance at therapeutic concentrations (Majerus et al. 1990; Hirsh and Levine 1992).

**Key Points:**

- **Unfractionated heparin (UH) must be administered parenterally.**
- **Renal or hepatic insufficiency do not significantly affect UH clearance.**

Unfractionated heparin is usually given intravenously. It is effective in the treatment of established DVT and PE (Hyers et al. 1995). Achieving a therapeutic activated partial thromboplastin time (aPTT) within the first 24 hours of treatment is key to effective treatment (Hull, Raskob, Rosenbloom et al. 1992; Levine et al. 1994). Failure to achieve therapeutic aPTT within 24 hours is associated with recurrent DVT/PE in 20% to 25% of patients (Hull, Raskob, Rosenbloom et al. 1990; Hull, Raskob, Pineo et al. 1992a, 1992b; Hull, Raskob, Rosenbloom et al. 1992; Raschke et al. 1993) compared with 4% to

Table 1-51 **Drugs Used for Prevention and Treatment of Venous Thromboembolism**

| DRUG | TYPICAL TREATMENT REGIMEN | COST/ DAY[a] | TYPICAL PROPHYLACTIC REGIMEN | COST/ DAY[a] | COMMENTS |
|---|---|---|---|---|---|
| *Unfractionated heparin* | | | | | |
| Heparin sodium | 20,000–40,000 U/24 hr | $10.00 | 5,000 U q8h–q12h | $4.00 | Considerable variation in dose and response. Must follow with aPTT. |
| *Low-molecular-weight heparin* | | | | | |
| Enoxaparin (Lovenox) | 1 mg/kg bid | $94.00 | 30 mg q12h | $35.00 | Predictable dose response based on weight. |
| Dalteparin (Fragmin) | 200 anti-Xa U/kg | $58.00[b] | 5000 anti-Xa U qd | $18.00[b] | Predictable dose response based on weight. |
| Tinzaparin (Innohep) | 175 anti-Xa U/kg qd | NA | 75 anti-Xa U qd | NA | Predictable dose response based on weight. Not available in USA. |
| Ardeparin (Normiflow) | Not evaluated | | 50 anti-Xa U/kg bid | NA | Predictable dose response based on weight. Not available in USA. |
| Nadroparin (Fraxiparin) | 4100 anti-Xa U bid if <50 kg | NA | 41 to 62 U/kg qd | NA | Predictable dose response based on weight. Not available in USA |
| | 6150 anti-Xa U bid if 50–70 kg | NA | | | |
| | 9200 anti-Xa U bid if >70 kg | NA | | | |
| Reviparin (Clivarin) | 6300 anti-Xa U bid if >60 kg | NA | 4200 anti-Xa U qd | NA | Predictable dose response based on weight. Not available in USA. |
| | 4200 anti-Xa U bid if 46–60 kg | | | | |
| | 3500 anti-Xa U bid if 35–45 kg | | | | |
| Danaparoid[c] (Orgaran) | 150–200 anti-Xa U/hr | $454.00 | 750 anti-Xa U bid | $189.00 | A heparinoid; it has low cross-reactivity to heparin products. |
| *Oral anticoagulants* | | | | | |
| Warfarin sodium (Coumadin) | 2–10 mg qd | $0.47–0.75 | 1–5 mg qd | $0.47–0.50 | Follow PT or INR. Generic saves ~40%. |
| Anisindione (Miradon) | 25–250 mg/day | $0.40–2.00 | | NA | Indandione derivative for patients who cannot tolerate warfarin. |

[a]Cost/day is based on the average wholesale price. Source of drug prices is the author's local pharmacy. Current prices may vary from those quoted, but comparative prices among products are expected to be similar. The reader should check on local prices at the time of prescribing.
[b]Based on 9.5 mL vial (10,000 U/mL).
[c]A heparinoid, not a low-molecular-weight heparin.
ABBREVIATIONS: aPTT, activated partial thromboplastin time; anti-Xa, anti-factor Xa; NA, not available.

6% recurrent DVT/PE for those patients whose aPTT reached the therapeutic threshold within 24 hours. Several clinical trials demonstrate that this goal is reliably met via use of heparin protocols, either weight-based (Raschke et al. 1993) or fixed/adjusted (Hull, Raskob, Rosenbloom et al. 1992; see Table 1-52).

**PRINCIPLE Large studies that demonstrate efficacy of a drug for an indication often cannot assure the clinician of optimal dose. That ultimately will be determined by examining multiple studies with reasonably homogeneous patient bases.**

A

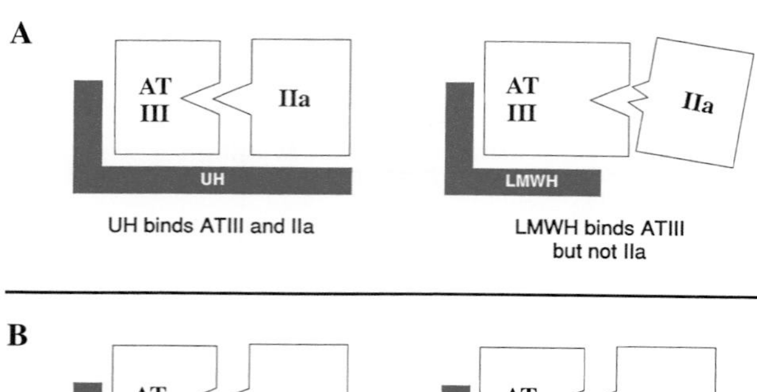


B

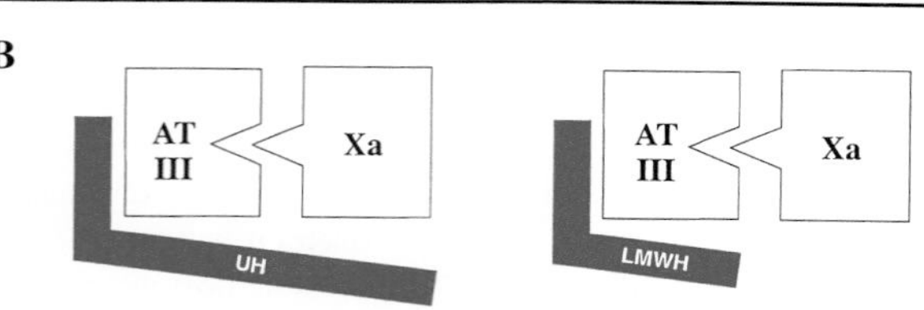


FIGURE 1-32 (A) Inactivation of factor IIa (thrombin). To inactivate factor IIa, both antithrombin III (ATIII) and IIa must be bound to the heparin molecule. Since most low-molecular-weight heparin (LMWH) molecules are too small to bind factor IIa, LMWHs do not inactivate factor IIa. (B) Inactivation of factor Xa. Factor Xa need only bind to the heparin-bound ATIII molecule. Therefore, factor Xa can be inactivated by unfractionated heparin (UH) and LMWHs. (Adapted from Hirsh and Levine 1992. Used by permission.)

**Key Points:**

- **UH treatment of DVT: Failure to achieve therapeutic aPTT within 24 hours is associated with 20–25% rate of recurrence.**
- **Therapeutic aPTT: can be achieved reliably and safely via a standard protocol (Table 1-52).**

### *Low-molecular-weight heparin*

Low-molecular-weight heparins (LMWHs) have been in wide clinical use in Europe and are being introduced in the United States for prevention and treatment of venous thromboembolism, as well as other uses such as for acute coronary syndromes.

Low-molecular-weight heparins are prepared from UH, either by organic chemical methods or heparinase digestion. Properties of LMWHs differ from those of UH in a number of important ways, summarized in Table 1-53 and Fig. 1-32. Each of the LMWH preparations is a unique drug, so different LMWHs should not be regarded as interchangeable. Recommendations for use of each should be based on the strength of evidence for that specific drug.

**PRINCIPLE Prospects of new indications and more sharply focused pharmacologic agents arise when a drug representing new chemistry and efficacy becomes available. The clinician's major responsibility is to understand the basis of claims of differences in indications or effects of similar chemical entities.**

**Key Points:**

- **Low-molecular-weight heparin can be given in once or twice daily subcutaneous injections for either prophylaxis or systemic anticoagulation.**
- **No laboratory monitoring is required with LMWHs.**

### *Safety of heparins*

The most important complication of heparin use is bleeding. Heparin-induced thrombocytopenia (HIT) is less common but potentially catastrophic if associated with arterial and/or venous thromboses. Bleeding and HIT are discussed below.

Clinically significant osteoporosis may complicate heparin administration of greater than 3–6 months' duration (Griffith et al. 1965; Hirsh 1991). Elevation of serum transaminases is not uncommon (Dukes et al. 1984), but the clinical significance of this is uncertain. There are also documented cases of hypoaldosteronism and hyperkalemia (Lechey et al.1981; Edes and Sunderrajan 1985; Levesque et al. 1990), skin necrosis (Levine et al. 1983; Fowlie 1990; Ritchie and Hart 1992; Sallah et al. 1997), dermatitis and skin hypersensitivity (Young 1988; Klein et al. 1989; Korstanje et al. 1989; Valsecchi 1992; Bircher 1994), and priapism (Klein et al. 1972). The incidence of these problems with LMWH is not yet clear but should be considered to be possible complications of LMWHs until greater experience is gained with these drugs.

**BLEEDING CAUSED BY UNFRACTIONATED HEPARIN** The incidence of bleeding with UH therapy for venous thromboembolism is well documented. Several factors have proven to impact bleeding risk with UH. Route of administration—intermittent IV bolus, continuous IV administration, or high-dose subcutaneous—is important: from 1975 to 1981 six studies (Salzman et al. 1975; Glazier and Cornell 1976; Mant et al. 1977; Wilson and Lampman 1979; Fagher and Lundh 1981; Wilson et al. 1981) with a total of 211 patients found a 14% risk of major bleeding, including some fatal bleeding when UH was administered by intermittent IV bolus. The rate

**Table 1-52 Intravenous Unfractionated Heparin (UH) Protocol for Treatment of Venous Thromboembolism**

| | HIGH BLEEDING RISK[a,b] | LOW BLEEDING RISK |
|---|---|---|
| INITIAL UH BOLUS | 5000 U | 5000 U |
| INITIAL UH INFUSION ONLY | 1250 U/hr (24-hr DOSE: 30,000 U) | 1650 U/hr (24-hr DOSE OF 39,600 U) |

All subsequent adjustments are based on the aPTT and are performed identically in high or normal risk patients.

The aPTT is performed as follows (desired range: 55–85 seconds):

- 4 hours after starting heparin. (If therapeutic, do not change dose; repeat aPTT in 4 hours to confirm aPTT stays within range. If still in range, repeat next morning.)
- aPTT and any indicated adjustments in heparin infusion rate are performed per nomogram for the first 24 hours of therapy
- After >24 hours, aPTT is performed daily, unless aPTT <55 seconds, in which case aPTT should be repeated 4 hours after any change in infusion rate.
- If heparin therapy is interrupted for >1 hour:
  - Re-bolus 5,000 U and resume previous IV infusion rate
  - Check aPTT in 4 hours, and proceed per nomogram
- If heparin therapy interrupted for <1 hour:
  - Resume heparin infusion at previous rate, aPTT in 4 hours, and follow nomogram
- Check platelet count daily.

**Nomogram: IV infusion of unfractionated heparin for Treatment of Venous Thromboembolism**

| aPTT (s)[c] | RATE CHANGE (mL/hr)[d] | DOSE CHANGE (U/24 hr) | ADDITIONAL ACTION |
|---|---|---|---|
| ≤45 | +5 | +6000 U | Repeat aPTT in 4 hr. |
| 46–54 | +3 | +3600 U | Repeat aPTT in 4 hr. |
| 55–85 | 0 | 0 | None.[e] |
| 86–110 | –3 | –3600 U | Stop heparin for 1 hr. Repeat aPTT 4 hr after restarting heparin. |
| >110 | –5 | –6000 units | Stop heparin for 1 hr. Repeat aPTT 4 hr after restarting heparin. |

[a]High bleeding risk: 1) Surgery within 2 weeks; 2) recent stroke (e.g., thromboembolic stroke within 2 weeks); 3) history of peptic ulcer disease, gastric ulcer or GI bleeding, or other disorders predisposing to bleeding (e.g., invasive lines, uremia, line failure, etc.); 4) platelet count <150,000.
[b]Data from Hull, Raskob, Rosenbloom et al. 1992.
[c]aPTT measurements using Actin-F5 thromboplastin reagent (Dade, Mississauga, Ontario, CA).
[d]Using heparin 25,000 U in 500 mL (50 U/mL).
[e]During the first 24 hr, repeat aPTT in 4 hr. Thereafter, perform aPTT once daily.
ABBREVIATIONS: aPTT, activated partial thromboplastin time; IV, intravenous; s, seconds; UH, unfractionated heparin.

of major bleeding is 2.6% (20 out of 771 patients) in studies comparing different durations of continuous intravenous UH (Gallus et al. 1986; Hull, Raskob, Rosenbloom et al. 1990), UH alone versus UH and acenocoumarol (Brandjes et al. 1992), and continuous UH versus heparin assay or weight-based nomogram (Raschke et al. 1993; Levine et al. 1994) (see also Table 1-54). Overall, UH used to treat venous thromboembolism is associated with a major bleeding rate of less than 5% (Hyers et al. 1995; Levine, Raskob et al. 1995).

Bleeding with UH in full therapeutic doses is strongly affected by patient-specific factors including surgery or

Table 1-53 **Properties of Unfractionated Heparin and Low-Molecular-Weight Heparin**

| | UNFRACTIONATED HEPARIN | LMW HEPARIN |
|---|---|---|
| Size | 12,000–15,000 Da | 4,000–6,500 Da |
| Anticoagulant effect | Correlates with therapeutic aPTT threshold of ~55 s | Highly correlated with actual body weight |
| Heparin-induced thrombocytopenia (HIT) | 1–3% | <1% |
| Anti-IIa activity | +++ | 0 |
| Anti-Xa activity | ++ | ++++ |
| Route of administration (treatment dose) | Continuous IV infusion | Subcutaneous injection, once or twice daily |

ABBREVIATIONS: anti-IIa, anti-factor IIA (thrombin); anti-Xa, anti-factor Xa; Da, daltons; LMW, low-molecular-weight; s, seconds.

trauma within the previous 14 days, history of GI or genitourinary bleeding, history of peptic ulcer disease, stroke within 14 days, thrombocytopenia (patient count <100,000), and the presence of other clinical disorders predisposing the patient to bleeding. Whether the aPTT is therapeutic or supratherapeutic, bleeding is much more likely in the presence of one or more of these factors (4% versus 1% in a major prospective trial [Hull, Raskob, Rosenbloom et al. 1990, 1992]). Heparin-induced bleeding is primarily a function of patient-specific factors rather than attributable to heparin dosage or supratherapeutic aPTT levels (Hull, Raskob, Rosenbloom et al. 1992).

Unfractionated heparin-associated bleeding can often be managed by simply interrupting the IV infusion, because the anticoagulant effect disappears fairly quickly. The half-life of UH is about 2 to 3 hours. If major hemorrhage occurs, protamine sulfate, a heparin antagonist, may be used. The dose is 1 mg protamine for every 100 units of heparin estimated to remain in the patient. Protamine sulfate can induce anaphylaxis, hypotension, bradycardia, dyspnea, and flushing, particularly if administered at a rate exceeding 50 mg/10 min (Majerus et al. 1990). Resuscitation capacity and appropriate agents to treat anaphylactic shock should be readily available.

**BLEEDING CAUSED BY LOW-MOLECULAR-WEIGHT HEPARINS** In head-to-head trials in the treatment of venous thromboembolism, rates of major bleeding with LMWHs have been at or below those in patients treated with UH for DVT (Hull, Raskob, Pineo et al. 1992a; Prandoni et al. 1992; Simmoneau et al. 1993; Lindmarker et al. 1994; Levine, Raskob et al. 1995; Koopman et al. 1996; Levine et al. 1996) or pulmonary embolism (The Columbus Investigators 1997; Simonneau et al. 1997; Decousus et al. 1998) (Table 1-54). This has held true in the outpatient setting as well (Levine et al. 1996; The Columbus Investigators 1997). Conversely, in randomized DVT prophylaxis trials with LMWHs and warfarin, there has been a trend toward more major bleeding with LMWH (Hull et al. 1993), offset to a degree by greater efficacy in DVT prevention in knee replacement (Hull et al. 1993; RD Heparin Arthroplasty Group 1994; Hamulyak et al. 1994; Leclerc et al. 1996) (see Prophylaxis). Management of bleeding associated with LMWH is not as straightforward as with UH. Protamine sulfate may be used, but the anti-factor Xa activity of LMWH is not fully neutralized by protamine (Woltz et al). The clinical effectiveness of protamine sulfate in this setting remains uncertain (Aster 1995).

**Key Points:**

- **UH treatment of DVT/PE: major bleeding 1–5%**
- **LMWH treatment of DVT/PE: major bleeding 1–3% (consistently lower than UH)**

**HEPARIN-INDUCED THROMBOCYTOPENIA** A modest decrease in platelet count during therapy with UH is common and generally not worrisome. The syndrome of heparin-induced thrombocytopenia (HIT) is caused by heparin-dependent antibodies that bind to a complex of heparin and platelet factor 4 (George 1996). HIT occurs in 1% to 3% of patients treated with heparin for DVT (George 1996). Paradoxically, it is sometimes associated with thrombosis, both arterial ("white clot syndrome") and venous, the very problems heparin is used to prevent (Raskob and George 1997). LMWH appears to induce HIT and HITT (heparin-induced thrombocytopenia with thrombosis) less frequently than UH, but HIT has been

**Table 1-54 Clinical Trials Comparing Unfractionated and LMW Heparins for Initial Treatment of Venous Thromboembolic Disease**

| STUDY | DESIGN | REGIMENS | RECURRENT VTE | MAJOR BLEEDING | DEATH |
|---|---|---|---|---|---|
| Prandoni et al. 1992 | Randomized, open | Nadroparin SC bid (weight-adjusted) | 6/85 (7%) | 1/85 (1%) | 5/85 (6%) |
| | | vs. | | | |
| | | IV heparin aPTT ratio 1.5 to 2.0 | 12/85 (14%) | 3/85 (4%) | 9/85 (11%) |
| Hull, Raskob, Pineo et al. 1992a | Randomized, double-blind | Tinzaparin 175 anti-Xa U/kg SC once daily | 6/213 (3%) | 1/213 (0.5%) | 10/213 (5%) |
| | | vs. | | | |
| | | IV heparin aPTT ratio 1.5 to 2.5 | 15/219 (7%) | 11/219 (5.0%) | 21/219 (10%) |
| Lopaciuk et al. 1992 | Randomized, open | Nadroparin 92 anti-Xa U/kg SC bid | 0/74 (0%) | 0/74 (0%) | 0/74 (0%) |
| | | vs. | | | |
| | | SC heparin aPTT ratio 1.5 to 2.5 | 3/72 (4%) | 1/72 (1%) | 1/72 (1%) |
| Simmoneau et al. 1993 | Randomized, open | Enoxaparin 1 mg/kg SC bid | 0/67 (0%) | 0/67 (0%) | 3/67 (4%) |
| | | vs. | | | |
| | | IV heparin aPTT ratio 1.5 to 2.5 | 3/67 (4%) | 0/67 (0%) | 2/67 (3%) |
| Lindmarker et al. 1994 | Randomized, open | Dalteparin 200 anti-Xa U/kg SC once daily | 5/101 (5%) | 0/101 (0%) | 2/101 (2%) |
| | | vs. | | | |
| | | IV heparin aPTT ratio 1.5 to 3.0 | 3/103 (3%) | 0/103 (0%) | 2/103 (2%) |
| Feissinger et al. 1996 | Randomized, open | Dalteparin 200 anti-Xa U/kg SC once daily | 5/127 (4%) | 0/127 (0%) | 2/127 (2%) |
| | | vs. | | | |
| | | IV heparin aPTT ratio 1.5 to 3.0 | 3/133 (2%) | 2/133 (2%) | 4/133 (3%) |
| Koopman et al. 1996 | Randomized, open, home treatment | Nadroparin SC bid (weight-adjusted) | 14/202 (7%) | 1/202 (0.5%) | 14/202 (7%) |
| | | vs. | | | |
| | | IV heparin aPTT ratio 1.5 to 2.0 | 17/198 ( 9%) | 4/198 (2%) | 16/198 (8%) |
| Levine et al. 1996 | Randomized, open, home treatment | Enoxaparin 1 mg/kg SC bid | 13/247 (5%) | 5/247 (2%) | 11/247 (4%) |
| | | vs. | | | |
| | | IV heparin aPTT 60 to 85 sec | 17/253 (7%) | 3/253 (1%) | 17/253 (7%) |
| COLUMBUS Study[a] Simmoneau et al. 1997 | Randomized, open | Reviparin 3500 to 6300 anti-Xa U SC bid (weight-adjusted) | 27/510 (5%) | 16/510 (3%) | 36/510 (7%) |
| | | vs. | | | |
| | | IV heparin aPTT ratio 1.5 to 2.5 | 25/511 (5%) | 12/511 (2%) | 39/511 (8%) |
| THESEE Study[a] Simmoneau et al. 1997 | Randomized, open | Tinzaparin 175 anti-Xa U/kg SC once daily | 5/304 (2%) | 6/304 (2%) | 12/304 (4%) |
| | | vs. | | | |
| | | IV heparin aPTT ratio 2.0 to 3.0 | 6/308 (2%) | 8/308 (3%) | 14/308 (5%) |

[a]Included patients with pulmonary embolism.
ABBREVIATIONS: aPTT, activated partial thromboplastin time; enoxaparin, enoxaparin sodium; dalteparin, dalteparin sodium; anti-Xa, anti-factor Xa; VTE, venous thromboembolic disease.

reported in patients treated with LMWHs (Warkentin et al. 1995).

A platelet count of ≤100,000/μL appearing on or after the 5th day of heparin treatment is consistent with HIT. It may appear more quickly in susceptible patients who have had recent exposure to heparin (George 1996). A significant drop in platelet count over 2 to 3 days should raise the suspicion of heparin-associated thrombocytopenia (George 1996). There is growing interest in using an assay for IgG antibodies directed against platelet factor 4–heparin complex as further support of the diagnosis of HIT (Aster 1995; Warkentin et al. 1995; George 1996; Raskob and George 1997).

Treatment with UH or LMWH must be stopped if HIT develops. Subsequent use of heparin in any form or amount is contraindicated, even heparin "locks" or heparin flushing of IV lines. Treatment options for patients with HIT include the low-molecular-weight heparinoid danaparoid (Magnani 1993), the defibriniginating agent ancrod (Demers et al. 1991), or a direct thrombin inhibitor, for example, hirudin (Schiele et al. 1995; Schiffmann et al. 1997).

**Key Points:**

- **Treatment with UH or LMWH should be stopped if heparin-induced thrombocytopenia (HIT) occurs.**
- **If the diagnosis of HIT is established, all subsequent use of any heparin is contraindicated.**

***Effectiveness of heparins***

There is a strong association between fatal PE and proximal DVT (i.e., thrombosis of the deep veins of the lower extremities at the level of the popliteal vein and above). Several studies have shown that there is a 10% rate of fatal PE associated with untreated proximal DVT (Coventry et al. 1973; Imperiale and Speroff 1994), and inadequately treated proximal DVT is associated with a 20% to 50% risk of clinically important recurrent venous thromboembolic events. (Hull et al. 1986; Brandjes et al. 1992; Raschke et al. 1993). Effectiveness of treatment of DVT/PE with UH or LMWH will be reflected in improvement in these outcomes. UH treatment saves lives in patients with pulmonary embolism (Barrett and Jordan 1960) and is the treatment standard for both PE and DVT. Treatment of DVT/PE with LMWHs has been tested in a number of clinical trials; outcomes are consistently as good or better than with UH (summarized in Table 1-54).

**Key Points:**

- **UH treatment of DVT/PE saves lives and reduces recurrence.**
- **LMWH is at least as effective as UH in the treatment of DVT and submassive PE.**

## Warfarin

Oral anticoagulants in use today are derivatives of 4-hydroxycoumarin, which include warfarin sodium, phenprocoumon, and acenocoumarol. Warfarin sodium is the preparation widely used in North America, because its absorption is rapid and complete, and its duration of action is predictable (Hirsh et al. 1995). Warfarin and the other oral anticoagulants are vitamin K antagonists. Vitamin K is a cofactor in a carboxylation step that results in biological activation of the clotting factors II, VII, IX, and X and anticoagulant proteins C and S. Warfarin in therapeutic doses (as determined by following the prothrombin time [PT] or the international normalized ratio of prothrombin time [INR]) decreases hepatic production of each vitamin K-dependent coagulation factor by 30% to 50%, but has no effect on the active, carboxylated factors already in the circulation (Majerus et al. 1990).

In appropriate therapeutic doses, warfarin prolongs the PT. Because bleeding is strongly associated with excessive prolongation of PT, warfarin dosage must be monitored carefully by using the INR. The INR is a standardized numerical conversion of the measured PT, using the formula:

$$\text{INR} = [(\text{PT observed})/(\text{PT control})]^{\text{ISI}}$$

The power value ISI, or international sensitivity index, is an intrinsic property of a given thromboplastin. Thromboplastin is the tissue extract used in the measurement of the prothrombin time (Hirsh 1992).

Use of the INR is essential, because there is considerable variation in the ISI of different commercial thromboplastins. Failure to "normalize" the PT measurement via INR calculation may result in under- or overestimate of anticoagulant intensity (Bussen et al. 1992; Hirsh 1992).

**PRINCIPLE When drug therapy is maintained by following a laboratory test, the test itself must be thoroughly understood by the physician if he or she is to apply test results in a rational manner.**

Warfarin interacts with many drugs, and these interactions may enhance or inhibit its effect. Vitamin K consumption also affects warfarin effect. A thorough, evidence-based review of reported drug and food interactions with warfarin was recently published (Wells et al. 1994).

***Warfarin safety***

*Bleeding.* Bleeding is the major complication of warfarin treatment. Rates of major bleeding with high-intensity therapy (INR 2.5–4.5) are 4% to 16% (Levine, Raskob et al. 1995). Bleeding rates are considerably lower in contemporary studies employing the current standard INR range of 2.0–3.0 (see Table 1-55). When the INR is maintained between 2.0 and 3.0, bleeding rates are about 1%; there was only one fatal bleeding episode out of 1,283 patients treated with warfarin. Factors contributing to bleeding risk include intensity of anticoagulant treatment, use of other drugs that interfere with hemostasis (e.g., aspirin), and comorbid conditions [e.g., cerebrovascular disease (Levine, Raskob et al. 1995), peptic ulcers (Stein et al. 1995), and duration of therapy]. It is interesting that

Table 1-55 Bleeding in Trials of Long-Term Warfarin Treatment of Deep Venous Thrombosis/Pulmonary Embolism

| STUDY | PATIENTS (*n*) | BLEEDING (%) TOTAL | MAJOR | FATAL | TARGETED INR |
|---|---|---|---|---|---|
| Hull, Raskob, Pineo et al. (1992b) | 432 | 19 (4.3) | 5 (0.9) | 0 | 2.0–3.0 |
| Brandjes et al (1992) | 120 | 14 (11.7) | 5 (4.2) | 0 | 2.0–3.0 |
| Simmoneau et al. (1993) | 134 | 3 (2.2) | 0 | 0 | 2.0–3.0 |
| Prandoni et al (1992) | 170 | 10 (5.8) | 4 (2.3) | 0 | 2.0–3.0 |
| Hull, Raskob, Rosenbloom et al. (1990) | 199 | 8 (4.0) | 4 (2.0) | 0 | 2.0–3.0 |
| Hull et al. (1986) | 115 | 2 (1.7) | 0 | 0 | 2.0–3.0 |
| Levine, Hirsh et al. (1995) | 113 | 1 (0.9) | 1 (0.9) | 1 (0.9) | 2.0–3.0 |

SOURCE: Adapted from Levine, Raskob et al. 1995. Used by permission.

age has not been shown to be an important risk for warfarin-associated bleeding, with the possible exception of patients 80 years and older (Fihn et al. 1996).

**PRINCIPLE Improved methods for monitoring drug therapy can lead to improved safety and also to new indications as risk/benefit ratios.**

In the absence of clinically significant bleeding, excessive anticoagulation with warfarin is usually managed by interrupting therapy and/or administering vitamin K. There is no fixed formula but INRs less than 5–6 rarely require more than deletion of one or two doses and reassessment of proper dosage. This process should include careful consideration of drug interactions or substantial changes in diet (Wells et al. 1994). At INRs greater than 5 or 6, risk of hemorrhage rises significantly (Levine, Raskob et al. 1995). At INRs of 5–10, either oral vitamin K (2.5 mg) (Weibert et al. 1997) or subcutaneous vitamin K (1–2 mg) may be given. If the INR is above 10, either slow IV vitamin K (0.5 mg) (Shetty et al. 1992) or 3 mg subcutaneous vitamin K are usually effective in bringing the INR to $\leq 5$ within 12 hours, without rendering the patient "warfarin resistant." For serious bleeding or life-threatening hemorrhage associated with warfarin, active clotting factors should be replaced: fresh-frozen plasma or prothrombin complex concentrate, supplemented with vitamin K, is a standard approach.

**Key Points:**

- **Life-threatening bleeding associated with warfarin requires replacement of active clotting factors with fresh-frozen plasma or prothrombin complex concentrate.**
- **Excessive warfarin anticoagulation requires vitamin K**
- **Interruption of warfarin therapy**
- **INR 5–10: may be managed with vitamin K, i.e., oral (2.5 mg) or subcutaneous injection (1–2 mg).**
- **INR 10: subcutaneous vitamin K (2–3 mg) or slow IV vitamin K (0.5 mg)**
- **Reassess warfarin dose, medications, and diet**

WARFARIN-INDUCED SKIN NECROSIS This is a rare complication, usually on the extremities but sometimes the breast, adipose tissue, or penis. It is thought to be related to a short-lived period of protein C deficiency. Because protein C is a vitamin K-dependent protein, patients with inherited protein C deficiency are thought to be particularly susceptible to this malady. The lesion manifests within the first few days of therapy and can be circumvented by being certain that heparin is administered therapeutically to patients before initiation of warfarin therapy (Majerus et al. 1990; Hirsh et al. 1995; Sallah et al. 1997).

If given during pregnancy, warfarin and other oral anticoagulants cause birth defects and abortion (Majerus et al. 1990). They should never be used during the first trimester because of their teratogenic effects.

### *Warfarin effectiveness*

Warfarin therapy for venous thromboembolism is begun on the first or second day of heparin treatment. The duration of treatment may be months to years. The effectiveness of long-term warfarin for preventing recurrence of venous thromboembolism has been demonstrated (Hull, Delmore, Genton et al. 1979). Attention has focused on the intensity and duration of treatment. An INR in the range of 2.0–3.0 is as effective as more intense anticoagulation, but causes less bleeding ([Hull et al. 1982]; see also Table 1-54).

Duration of treatment remains a major issue. Patients remaining on warfarin longer will have more bleeding but fewer recurrent thrombotic episodes (Schulman et al. 1995). Data from randomized trials are needed to determine the optimum duration of treatment. Six months is superior to 6 weeks of treatment for the first episode of DVT (Schulman et al. 1995). Patients whose noninvasive leg test for DVT normalized at 4 weeks were nevertheless found to be better off taking 3 months, rather than only 4 weeks, of warfarin (Levine, Hirsh et al. 1995). Indefinite treatment following a second event has been recommended (Schulman et al. 1997), but definitive data (and recommendations for specific subgroups, e.g., for those with inherited abnormalities) are not yet available. After three or more documented events, indefinite supply of anticoagulation with warfarin is the standard management (Ginsberg 1996).

# APPROACH TO PATIENT MANAGEMENT

## Suspected Venous Thromboembolic Disease

***Suspected deep venous thrombosis***

Patients with symptoms compatible with DVT require objective testing because clinical diagnosis can be inaccurate, notoriously so (Hull et al. 1983; Moser 1990; Birdwell et al. 1998). Treating all patients would subject 75% to 85% of these patients (approximately 400,000 patients in the United States each year) to unnecessary risks of anticoagulant treatment (Anderson et al. 1991; Birdwell et al. 1998). Patients with proximal vein DVT who are not treated face a 10% risk of death from PE and up to 50% likelihood of recurrent thromboembolic events (Coventry et al. 1973; Imperiale and Speroff 1994; Hull et al. 1996). Therefore, to be clinically useful, testing for patients with suspected DVT must separate patients into two groups: those in whom treatment may be safely withheld, and those who require either treatment or further testing.

Contrast venography satisfies this criterion. If venography is normal, treatment may be safely withheld (Hull et al. 1981).*

*Patients with proximal-vein (popliteal vein and above) DVT who are not treated with anticoagulants have clinical complications (fatal PE; recurrent DVT and PE) which can be measured objectively (Hull, Hirsh, Carter et al. 1985a). Therefore, clinical outcome for patients in whom anticoagulants are withheld is the gold standard for negative results of any test for DVT. Venography is the gold standard for the (positive) diagnosis of DVT (Rabinov and Paulin 1972).

An abnormal result (an intraluminal filling defect) is the "gold standard" definition of DVT (Rabinov and Paulin 1972), and anticoagulation is indicated. However, venography is uncomfortable, not always available, and relatively expensive (Birdwell 1996). Noninvasive methods of DVT diagnosis have been developed that identify patients in whom treatment can be withheld. Impedance plethysmography (IPG) must be repeated several times over an 8- to 14-day period, but if the test remains normal, withholding treatment is associated with a vanishingly small risk of fatal pulmonary embolism and very low risk of recurrent venous thrombotic events. In five level I studies of consecutive patients in whom anticoagulants were withheld based on normal serial IPGs, 0 of 1231 patients had a fatal PE (0%, 95% CI 0–0.24%) and 2 of 1231 had recurrent DVT or nonfatal PE (0.2%, 95% CI 0.02–0.59%) (summarized in Raskob 1996). Compression ultrasound (C-US) is the most used test in North America, and recent data support the safety of withholding anticoagulants in symptomatic patients if testing is normal on two tests 5 to 7 days apart (Cogo et al. 1998; Birdwell et al. 1998).

When either IPG or C-US is abnormal, either empiric anticoagulation or confirmation of the presence of DVT with venography is indicated. The positive predictive value (PPV) of abnormal IPG is approximately 90%, and the causes of false-positive results are well documented (Cogo et al. 1998). The PPV of abnormal C-US is less clear, and the causes of false-positives are not well documented. The decision to pursue further testing (e.g., venography) rather than treating on the basis of an abnormal noninvasive test for DVT requires balancing the likelihood of a false-positive test against the estimated risk of serious or fatal bleeding from treatment (see above).

Suspected recurrent DVT is a problematic diagnosis. The best studied and most useful test is IPG (Hull et al. 1983).

***Suspected pulmonary embolism***

Most patients with suspected pulmonary embolism have perfusion/ventilation nuclear lung scanning done initially. If the perfusion lung scan is normal, treatment may be safely withheld (Hull, Raskob, Coates et al. 1990; van Beek et al. 1995). If perfusion/ventilation scan is high probability, this corresponds to an approximate 90% likelihood of PE (i.e., 90% positive predictive value), as compared with the diagnostic gold standard, pulmonary angiography (Hull, Hirsh, Carter et al. 1985b; PIOPED Investigators 1990). Unfortunately, the majority of patients' lung scans are "low," "intermediate," or "indeterminate," none of which effectively separates patients into categories for treating or withholding treatment. As is the case with DVT and venography, all patients with suspected PE could have pulmonary angiography, and management decisions would be unequivocal. However, this is an invasive test with a significant risk of serious complications, including death. Currently, the best supported approach combines the use of specific clinical parameters, lung scanning, and DVT leg testing to identify those who may have anticoagulation safely withheld, versus those who should be treated (or have further testing). (These approaches are summarized in the work of Dalen 1993 and Hull et al. 1994).

### Treatment of Established, Acute Venous Thromboembolic Disease

Patients with PE may present with life-threatening complications, and thrombolytic therapy or even surgical thrombectomy may be considered massive or submassive. PE complicated by hypotension or shock is the best supported indication for thrombolytic therapy (Dalen et al. 1997). However, there is no evidence that lives are saved, and the risk of intracranial hemorrhage is 2% (Dalen et al. 1997). Short-term outcomes (such as better right-heart function, lung perfusion, and pulmonary artery pressures) do appear to improve in some patients (Goldhaber et al. 1993). However, the great majority of patients with PE and/or DVT are best managed initially with heparin. Whether UH or LMWH is used is a function of availability, cost, feasibility of outpatient treatment, comorbidities, etc. Clinical trials are further refining our knowledge of advantages and pitfalls in the use of LMWH. When UH is used, a proven dosing protocol is essential to optimize outcome.

Patients with proximal-vein DVT who have contraindications to immediate anticoagulation often have an inferior vena caval filter placed (Becker et al. 1992; Decousus et al. 1998). For some patients the contraindication to anticoagulation is temporary, as in patients with current bleeding or recent neurosurgery. In most such patients long-term anticoagulation with warfarin should be instituted (or reinstituted) as soon as possible (Becker et al. 1992; Decousus et al. 1998).

Long-term anticoagulation with warfarin is indicated for DVT and PE. Strong evidence suggests an INR of 2.0–3.0 is optimal for long-term treatment (Hyers et al. 1995). "Breakthrough" episodes of DVT or PE do not dictate INRs above 3.0. Instead, the possible causes of failure (e.g., inadequacy of initial heparin treatment, consistency of warfarin administration) should be carefully considered. When failure of warfarin therapy is unequivocally established, placement of an inferior vena caval filter is indicated (Becker et al. 1992).

### Prophylaxis

Warfarin, UH, and LMWH, as well as pneumatic leg compression, have been used to prevent DVT and PE in patients at high risk. Use of LMWH in perioperative prophylaxis, trauma patients, and high-risk medical patients is expanding.

The prophylactic efficacy of no treatment, various drugs, and mechanical devices are compared in Table 1-50 in one of the highest risk settings known: total knee replacement. Evidence-based recommendations for this (Clagett et al. 1995) and many other surgical and medical settings are thoroughly reviewed by the American College of Chest Physicians Consensus Conference on Antithrombotic Therapy, and published every 3 years in a *Chest* supplement (see also references Hirsh et al. 1995; Hyers et al. 1995; Levine, Raskob et al. 1995, Stein et al. 1995).

## CONCLUSION

The primary difficulty in managing venous thromboembolic disease lies in the fact that establishing the diagnosis is not straightforward, symptoms and clinical signs are nonspecific, and both the disease and its treatment carry important risks. Furthermore, treatable DVT may be present in asymptomatic patients. Symptoms compatible with PE or DVT are usually due to other causes. High-risk settings, e.g., orthopedic surgery, challenge our ability to prevent DVT; even with LMWHs and other promising drugs, the incidence of DVT rates remain high, and noninvasive detection of thrombi in that setting is a diagnostic challenge yet to be solved.

Despite these limitations, current treatment of venous thromboembolic disease must be considered an unqualified success. Indeed, it represents medical science at its best, combining molecular biology, clinical epidemiology, and pharmacotherapeutics to improve patient outcomes.

## REFERENCES

Anderson FA, Wheeler HB, Goldberg RJ, et al. 1991. A population-based perspective of the hospital incidence and case-fatality rates of deep vein thrombosis and pulmonary embolism. *Arch Intern Med* **151**:933–8.

Aster R. 1995. Heparin-induced thrombocytopenia and thrombosis. *N Engl J Med* **332**:1374–6.

Barrett MW, Jordan SC. 1960. Anticoagulation drugs in the treatment of pulmonary embolism. *Lancet* **1**:1309–12.

Becker DM, Philbrick JT, Selby JB. 1992. Inferior vena cava filters: indications, safety, effectiveness. *Arch Intern Med* **152**:1985–94.

Bircher A, Itin PH, Stanislaw AB. 1994. Skin lesions, hypereosinophilia, and subcutaneous heparin. *Lancet* **343**:861.

Birdwell B, Raskob G, Whitsett T, et al. 1998. The clinical validity of normal compression ultrasound in patients suspected of having deep venous thrombosis. *Ann Intern Med* **128**:1–7.

Birdwell B. 1996. Contrast venography. In: Hull RD, Raskob GE, Pineo GF, editors. *Venous Thromboembolism: An Evidence-Based Atlas.* Armonk, NY: Futura. p 101–6.

Brandjes DP, Higber H, Buller H, et al. 1992. Acenocoumarol and heparin compared with acenocoumarol alone in the initial treatment of proximal vein thrombosis. *N Engl J Med* **327**:1485–9.

Bussen HI, Force RW, Bianco TM. 1992. Reliance on prothrombin time ratios causes significant errors in anticoagulation therapy. *Arch Intern Med* **152**:258–66.

Clagett GP, Anderson FA, Heit J, et al. 1995. Prevention of venous thromboembolism. *Chest* **108**(Suppl):312S–34S.

Cogo A, Lensing AWA, Koopman MMW, et al. 1998. Compression ultrasonography for diagnostic management of patients with clinically suspected deep vein thrombosis: prospective cohort study. *Br Med J* **316**:17–20.

Coventry MB, Nolan DR, Beckenbaugh RD. 1973. "Delayed" prophylactic anticoagulation: a study of results and complications in 2,012 total hip arthroplasties. *J Bone Joint Surg(Am)* **55**:1487–92.

Dalen JE, Alpert JS, Hirsh J. 1997. Thromboembolic therapy for pulmonary embolism: Is it effective? Is it safe? When is it indicated? *Arch Intern Med* **157**:2550–6.

Dalen JE. 1993. When can treatment be withheld in patients with suspected pulmonary embolism? *Arch Intern Med* **153**:1415–8.

Decousus H, Leizorovicz A, Parent F, et al. 1998. A clinical trial of vena cava filters in the prevention of pulmonary embolism in patients with proximal deep-vein thrombosis. *N Engl J Med* **338**: 409–15.

Demers C, Ginsberg JS, Brill-Edwards P, et al. 1991. Rapid anticoagulation using ancrod for heparin-induced thrombocytopenia. *Blood* **78**:2194–7.

Dukes GE Jr, Sanders SW, Russo J, et al. 1984. Transaminase elevations in patients receiving bovine or porcine heparin. *Ann Intern Med* **100**:646–50.

Edes TE, Sunderrajan EV. 1985. Heparin-induced hyperkalemia. *Arch Intern Med* **145**:1070–2.

Fagher B, Lundh B. 1981. Heparin treatment of deep vein thrombosis. *Acta Med Scand* **210**:357–61.

Feissinger JN, Lopez-Fernandez M, Gatterer E, et al. 1996. One cc daily subcutaneous dalteparin, a low molecular weight heparin, for the initial treatment of acute deep vein thrombosis. *Thromb Haemost* **76**:195–6.

Fihn SD, Callahan CM, Martin DC, et al. 1996.The risk of and severity of bleeding complications in elderly patients treated with warfarin. *Ann Intern Med* **124**:970–9.

Fowlie J, Stanton PD, Anderson JR. 1990. Heparin-associated skin necrosis. *Postgrad Med J* **66**:573–5.

Gallus A, Jackaman J, Tillett J, et al. 1986. Safety and efficacy of warfarin started early after submassive venous thrombosis or pulmonary embolism. *Lancet* **2**:1293–6.

George J. 1996. Heparin-associated thrombocytopenia. In: Hull R, Pineo GF, editors. *Disorders of Thrombosis.* Philadelphia: WB Saunders. p 359–73.

Ginsberg J. 1996. Management of venous thromboembolism. *N Engl J Med* **335**:1816–28.

Glazier RC, Cornell EB. 1976. Randomized progressive trial of continuous versus intermittent heparin therapy. *JAMA* **236**:1365–7.

Goldhaber SZ, Haire WD, Feldstein ML, et al. 1993. Alteplase versus heparin in acute pulmonary embolism: randomized trial assessing right-ventricular function and pulmonary perfusion. *Lancet* **341**:507–11.

Graor RA, Stewart JH, Lotke PA, et al. 1992. RD heparin vs aspirin to prevent deep vein thrombosis after hip or knee replacement surgery [abstract]. 58th Annual Scientific Assembly, American College of Chest Physicians, 118S.

Griffith GC, Nichols G Jr, Asher JD, et al. 1965. Heparin osteoporosis. *JAMA* **193**:91–4.

Haas SB, Insall JN, Scuderi GR, et al. 1990. Pneumatic sequential-compression boots compared with aspirin prophylaxis of deep-vein thrombosis after total knee arthroplasty. *J Bone Joint Surg (Am)* **72**:27–31.

Hamulyak K, Lensing AWA, van der Meer J, et al. 1994. Subcutaneous low-molecular weight heparin or oral anticoagulants for the prevention of deep-vein thrombosis in elective hip and knee replacement? Fraxiparin Oral Anticoagulant Study Group. *Thromb Haemost* **74**:1428–31.

Heit J, Berkowitz S, Bona R, et al. 1995. Efficacy and safety of ardeparin (a LMWH) compared to warfarin for prevention of venous thromboembolism following total knee replacement: a double blind, dose ranging study [abstract]. *Thromb Haemost* **73**:978.

Hirsh J. 1991. Heparin. *N Engl J Med* **324**:1565–74.

Hirsh J. 1992. Substandard monitoring of warfarin in North America: time for change. *Arch Intern Med* **152**:257–8.

Hirsh J, Dalen J, Deylein D, et al. 1995. Oral anticoagulants: mechanism of action, clinical effectiveness, and optimal therapeutic range. *Chest* **108**(Suppl):231S–46S.

Hirsh J, Levine M. 1992. Low molecular weight heparin. *Blood* **79**: 1–17.

Hull R, Delmore T, Genton E, et al. 1979. Warfarin sodium versus low-dose heparin in the long-term treatment of venous thrombosis. *N Engl J Med* **301**:855–8.

Hull R, Hirsh J, Jay R, et al. 1982. Different intensities of oral anticoagulant therapy in the treatment of proximal-vein thrombosis. *N Engl J Med* **307**:1676–81.

Hull R, Hirsh J, Sackett DL, et al. 1981. Clinical validity of a negative venogram in patients with clinically suspected venous thrombosis. *Circulation* **64**:622–5.

Hull RD, Carter CJ, Jay RM, et al. 1983. The diagnosis of acute, recurrent, deep-vein thrombosis: a diagnostic challenge. *Circulation* **67**:901–6.

Hull RD, Delmore TV, Hirsh J, et al. 1979. Effectiveness of intermittent pulsatile elastic stockings for the prevention of calf and thigh vein thrombosis in patients undergoing elective knee surgery. *Thromb Res* **16**:37–45.

Hull RD, et al. 1996. Overview of treatment of venous thromboembolism. In: Hull RD, Raskob GE, Pineo GF, editors. *Venous Thromboembolism: An Evidence-Based Atlas.* Armonk, NY: Futura. p 221–4.

Hull RD, Hirsh J, Carter CJ, et al. 1985a. Diagnostic efficacy of impedance plethysmography for clinically suspected deep-vein thrombosis: a randomized trial. *Ann Intern Med* **102**:21–8.

Hull RD, Hirsh J, Carter CJ, et al. 1985b. Diagnostic value of ventilation-perfusion lung scanning in patients with suspected pulmonary embolism. *Chest* **88**:819–28.

Hull RD, Raskob GE, Coates G, et al. 1990. Clinical validity of a normal perfusion lung scan in patients with suspected pulmonary embolism. *Chest* **97**:23–6.

Hull RD, Raskob GE, Ginsberg JS, et al. 1994. A non-invasive strategy for the treatment of patients with suspected pulmonary embolism. *Arch Intern Med* **154**:289–97.

Hull RD, Raskob GE, Hirsh J, et al. 1986. Continuous intravenous heparin compared with intermittent subcutaneous heparin in the treatment of proximal-vein thrombosis. *N Engl J Med* **315**:1109–14.

Hull RD, Raskob GE, Pineo GF, et al. 1992a. Subcutaneous low molecular weight heparin compared with continuous intravenous heparin in the treatment of proximal-vein thrombosis. *N Engl J Med* **326**:975–83.

Hull RD, Raskob GE, Pineo GF, et al. 1992b. Subcutaneous low molecular weight heparin compared with continuous intravenous heparin in the treatment of proximal vein thrombosis. *N Engl J Med* **326**:975–82.

Hull RD, Raskob GE, Pineo GF, et al. 1993. A comparison of subcutaneous low molecular weight heparin with warfarin for prophylaxis against deep-vein thrombosis after hip or knee implantation. *N Engl J Med* **329**:1370–6.

Hull RD, Raskob GE, Rosenbloom D, et al. 1990. Heparin for 5 days versus for 10 days in the initial treatment of proximal venous thrombosis. *N Engl J Med* **323**:1260–4.

Hull RD, Raskob GE, Rosenbloom D, et al. 1992. Optimal therapeutic level of heparin therapy in patients with venous thrombosis. *Arch Intern Med* **152**:1589–95.

Hyers TM, Hull RD, Weg JG. 1995. Antithrombotic therapy for venous thromboembolic disease. *Chest* **108** (Suppl):335S–51S.

Imperiale TF, Speroff T. 1994. A meta analysis of methods to prevent venous thromboembolism following total hip replacement. *JAMA* **271**:1780–5.

Klein GF, Kofler H, Wolf H, et al. 1989. Eczema-like erythematous, infiltrated plaques: a common side effect of subcutaneous heparin therapy. *J Am Acad Derm* **21**:703–7.

Klein LA, Hall RL, Smith RB. 1972. Surgical treatment of priapism: with a note on heparin-induced priapism. *J Urol* **108**:104–8.

Koopman MW, Prandoni P, Piovella F, et al. 1996. Treatment of venous thrombosis with intravenous unfractionated heparin administered in the hospital as compared with subcutaneous low-molecular-weight heparin administered at home. Tasman Study Group. *N Engl J Med* **334**:682–4.

Korstanje MJ, Bessems MJ, Hardy E, et al. 1989. Delayed-type hypersensitivity reaction to heparin. *Contact Dermatitis* **20**:383–4.

Lechey D, Gantt D, Lim V. 1981. Heparin-induced hypoaldosteronism. *JAMA* **246**:2189–90.

Leclerc JR, Geerts WH, Desjardins L, et al. 1992. Prevention of deep vein thrombosis after major knee surgery: a randomized, double-blind trial comparing a low molecular weight heparin fragment (enoxaparin) to placebo. *Thromb Haemost* **67**:417–23.

Leclerc JR, Geerts WH, Desjardins L, et al. 1996. Prevention of venous thromboembolism after knee arthroscopy: a randomized, double-blind trial comparing enoxaparin with warfarin. *Ann Intern Med* **124**:619–26.

Leclerc JR, Geerts WH, Desjardins L, et al. 1994. Prevention of venous thromboembolism after knee arthroplasty: a randomized, double blind trial, comparing a low molecular weight heparin fragment (enoxaparin) to warfarin [abstract]. *Blood* **84** (Suppl I):246A.

Levesque H, Verdier S, Cailleux N, et al. 1990. Low molecular weight heparin and hypoaldosteronism. *Br Med J* **300**:1437–8.

Levine LE, Bernstein JE, Soltari K, et al. 1983. Heparin-induced cutaneous necrosis unrelated to injection sites. A sign of potentially lethal complications. *Arch Dermatol* **119**:400–3.

Levine MN, Geust M, Hirsh J, et al. 1996. A comparison of low-molecular-weight heparin administered primarily at home with unfractionated heparin administered in the hospital for proximal deep-vein thrombosis. *N Engl J Med* **334**:677–81.

Levine MN, Hirsh J, Gent M, et al. 1994. A randomized trial comparing activated thromboplastin time with heparin assay in patients with acute venous thromboembolism requiring large daily doses of heparin. *Arch Intern Med* **154**:49–56.

Levine MN, Hirsh J, Gent M, et al. 1995. Optimal duration of oral anticoagulant therapy: a randomized trial comparing four weeks with three months of warfarin in patients with proximal deep vein thrombosis. *Thromb Haemost* **74**:606–11.

Levine MN, Raskob GE, Landefeld S, et al. 1995. Hemorrhagic complications of anticoagulant treatment. *Chest* **108**(Suppl):276S–90S.

Lindmarker P, Holmstrom M, Granquist M, et al. 1994. Comparison of once-daily subcutaneous Fragmin with continuous intravenous unfractionated heparin in the treatment of deep-vein thrombosis. *Thromb Haemost* **72**:186–90.

Lopacink S, Meissner AJ, Filipecki S, et al. 1992. Subcutaneous low molecular weight heparin versus subcutaneous unfractionated heparin in the treatment of deep vein thrombosis: a Polish multicenter study. *Thromb Haemost* **68**:14–8.

Lynch JA, Baker PL, Polly RE, et al. 1990. Mechanical measures in the prophylaxis of postoperative thromboembolism in total knee arthroplasty. *Clin Orthop* (Nov): 24–9.

Magnani HN. 1993. Heparin-induced thrombocytopenia (HIT): an overview of 230 patients treated with orgaran (Org 10172). *Thromb Haemost* **70**:554–61.

Majerus PW, Broze GJ, Miletich J, et al. 1990. Anticoagulant, thrombolytic and antiplatelet drugs. In: Gilman AG, Rall TW, Nils AS, et al., editors. *The Pharmacologic Basis of Therapeutics*. New York: Pergamon Press. p. 1311–31.

Mant MJ, O'Brion BD, Thoug KC, et al. 1977. Haemorrhagic complications of heparin therapy. *Lancet* **1**:1133.

McKenna R, Galante J, Rashman F, et al. 1980. Prevention of venous thromboembolism after total knee replacement by high-dose aspirin or intermittent calf and thigh compression. *Br Med J* **280**: 514–7.

*Mosby's GenR$_x$ 1998. Mosby's GenR$_x$1998: The Complete Reference for Generic and Brand Drugs. 8th ed. St. Louis: Mosby–Year Book.*

Moser KM. 1990. Venous thromboembolism. *Annu Rev Respir Dis* **141**:235–49.

PIOPED Investigators. 1990. Value of the ventilation/perfusion scan in acute pulmonary embolism. Results of the prospective investigation of pulmonary embolism diagnosis (PIOPED). *JAMA* **263**: 2753–9.

Prandoni P, Lensing AW, Buller HR, et al. 1992. Comparison of subcutaneous low molecular weight heparin with intravenous standard heparin in proximal deep-vein thrombosis. *Lancet* **339**:441–5.

Rabinov K, Paulin S. 1972. Roentgen diagnosis of venous thrombosis in the leg. *Arch Surg* **104**:134–44.

Raschke RA, Reilly BM, Guidry J, et al. 1993. The weight-based heparin nomogram compared with a 'standard care' nomogram: a randomized controlled trial. *Ann Intern Med* **119**:874–81.

Raskob G. 1996. Impedance plethysmography. In: Hull RD, Raskob GE, Pineo GF, editors. *Venous Thromboembolism: An Evidence-Based Atlas*. Armonk, NY: Futura. p 107–14.

Raskob GE, George J. 1997. Thrombotic complications of antithrombotic therapy: a paradox with implications for clinical practice. *Ann Intern Med* **127**:839–41.

RD Heparin Arthroplasty Group. 1994. RD heparin compared with warfarin for prevention of venous thromboembolic disease following total hip or knee arthroplasty. *J Bone Joint Surg (Am)* **76**: 1174–85.

Ritchie AJ, Hart NB. 1992. Massive tissue necrosis can be induced by heparin (case report). *Acta Haematol* **87**:69–70.

Sallah S, Thomas DP, Roberts HR. 1997. Warfarin and heparin-induced skin necrosis and the purple toe syndrome: infrequent complications of anticoagulant treatment. *Thromb Haemost* **78**:785–90.

Salzman EW, Deykin D, Shapiro RM, et al. 1975. Management of heparin therapy: controlled perspective trial. *N Engl J Med* **292**: 1046–50.

Schiele F, Vuillemenot A, Kramerz J, et al. 1995. Use of recombinant hirudin as antithrombosis treatment in patients with heparin-induced thrombocytopenia. *Am J Hematol* **50**:20–5.

Schiffmann H, Unterhalt M, Harms K, et al. 1997. Successful treatment of heparin-induced thrombocytopenia (HIT) type II in childhood with recombinant hirudin. *Monatsschr Kinderheilkd* **145**:606–12.

Schulman S, Granqvist S, Holmström M, et al. 1997. The duration of oral anticoagulant therapy after a second episode of venous thromboembolism. *N Engl J Med* **336**:393–8.

Schulman S, Rhedin AS, Lindmarker P, et al. 1995. A comparison of six weeks with six months of oral anticoagulant therapy after a first episode of venous thromboembolism. *N Engl J Med* **332**:1661–5.

Shetty HGM, Backhouse G, Bentley DP, et al. 1992. Effective reversal of warfarin-induced excessive anticoagulation with low dose vitamin K. *Thromb Haemost* **67**:13–5.

Simmoneau G, Charbonnier B, Decousus H, et al. 1993. Subcutaneous low-molecular weight heparin compared with continuous intravenous unfractionated heparin in the treatment of proximal deep vein thrombosis. *Arch Intern Med* **153**:1541–6.

Simonneau G, Sors H, Charbonnier B, et al. 1997. A comparison of low molecular weight heparin with unfractionated heparin for acute pulmonary embolism. *N Engl J Med* **337**:663–9.

Spiro TE, Colwell CW, Bona RD, et al. 1993. A Clinical trial comparing the efficacy and safety of enoxaparin, a low molecular weight heparin, and unfractionated heparin for the prevention of deep venous thrombosis after elective knee replacement surgery. *Blood* **82** (Suppl):1642a.

Spiro TE, Fitzgerald RH, Trowbridge AA, et al. 1994. Enoxaparin, a low molecular weight heparin, and warfarin for the prevention of venous thromboembolic disease after elective knee replacement surgery. *Blood* **84** (Suppl I):246 A.

Stein PD, Alpert JS, Copeland JG, et al. 1995. Antithrombotic therapy in patients with mechanical and biological prosthetic heart valves. *Chest* **108**:371–9.

The Columbus Investigators. 1997. Low molecular weight heparin in the treatment of patients with venous thromboembolism. *N Engl J Med* **337**:657–62.

Valsecchi R, Rozzoni M, Cainelli T. 1992. Allergy to subcutaneous heparin. *Contact Dermatitis* **26**:129–30.

van Beek EJ, Kuijer PM, Schenk BE, et al. 1995. A normal perfusion lung scan in patients with clinically suspected pulmonary embolism: frequency and clinical validity. *Chest* **108**:170–3.

Warkentin TE, Levine MN, Hirsh J, et al. 1995. Heparin-induced thrombocytopenia in patients treated with low-molecular-weight heparin or unfractionated heparin. *N Engl J Med* **332**:1330–5.

Weibert RT, The Le D, Kayser SR, et al. 1997. Correction of excessive anticoagulation with low-dose oral vitamin K. *Ann Intern Med* **125**:959–62.

Wells PS, Holbrook AW, Crowther NR, et al. 1994. The interaction of warfarin with drugs and food: a critical review of the literature. *Ann Intern Med* **121**:676–83.

Wilson JR, Bynum LJ, Parker RW. 1981. Heparin therapy in venous thromboembolism. *Am J Med* **70**:808–16.

Wilson JR, Lampman J. 1979. Heparin therapy: a randomized study. *Am Heart J* **97**:155–8.

Woltz M, Welterman A, Nieszpaurl-Los, et al. 1995. Studies on the neutralizing effects of protamine on unfractionated and low molecular weight heparin (Fragmin) at the site of activation of the coagulation system in man. *Thromb Haemost* **73**:439–43.

Young E. 1988. Allergy to subcutaneous heparin. *Contact Dermatitis* **19**:152–3.

# Adverse Effects of Cardiovascular Drugs on the Cardiovascular System

Stanley Nattel

*Chapter Outline*



This chapter will present an overview of adverse effects of cardiovascular drugs on the cardiovascular system. As a paradigm, we will consider drugs used to treat or prevent cardiovascular disease that produce adverse effects that often mimic elements of the disease that they are designed to treat. Sample case histories will be used to illustrate the clinical conundrums that may be presented by such reactions.

**PRINCIPLE Because cardioactive drugs target components of cardiovascular physiology, they are particularly prone to cause adverse cardiovascular effects. In some cases, these manifest as a worsening of the disease being treated, resulting in potential confusion in distinguishing between inadequate therapeutic responses and drug adverse effects.**

## ANTIARRHYTHMIC DRUGS THAT CAUSE CARDIAC ARRHYTHMIAS

CASE HISTORY *A 65-year-old woman experiences palpitations several months after an acute inferior myocardial infarction. Her only treatment is aspirin, 325 mg per day, and hydrochlorothiazide, 50 mg per day. An ECG shows frequent ventricular extrasystoles and her physician treats her with sotalol, 80 mg three times per day. A few days later, she returns to her physician, complaining of dizzy spells. The ECG shows a brief run of 4-beat ventricular tachycardia. Her doctor, concluding that her drug therapy is inadequate to control her arrhythmias, increases the dosage of sotalol to 160 mg twice daily. For the next few days she feels better; however, she suddenly has a fainting spell associated with a seizure. The ambulance brings her to the emergency room, where physical exam is normal apart from some drowsiness. Her ECG shows sinus rhythm at 50/min, an old inferior myocardial infarction (MI) and a QT interval of 0.72 seconds. She is observed and her ECG is monitored. Within an hour, she has a cardiopulmonary arrest associated with a polymorphic ventricular tachyarrhythmia that requires emergency direct current (DC) cardioversion for termination.*

**Discussion** *This history is typical of a patient who develops torsades de pointes arrhythmias in response to a drug that delays ventricular repolarization. When the initial indication for drug therapy is ventricular arrhythmias, this form of adverse effect may be mistaken for inadequate drug action, leading to increases in drug dose and/or the addition of agents with similar actions that worsen the clinical state.*

**PRINCIPLE Always suspect and consider a drug-induced proarrhythmia in a patient on antiarrhythmic drugs who presents with worsening arrhythmias, syncope, or seizures.**

As explained in the section on Arrhythmias in this chapter, torsades de pointes arrhythmias are caused by early afterdepolarizations (EADs). These are a form of abnormal activity that is favored by a variety of factors, most of which delay repolarization, including hypokalemia, bradycardia, hypomagnesemia, and action potential-prolonging drugs (Roden and Hoffman 1985; Nattel and Quantz 1988), along with cellular hypertrophy (Volders et al. 1998). The factors facilitating EADs correspond to and potentially account for a variety of clinical risk factors for torsades de pointes, including hypokalemia, diuretic therapy which can cause hypokalemia, bradyarrhythmias (Kawasaki et al. 1995), heart failure (Lehmann et al. 1996), therapy with class IA or class III antiarrhythmic drugs, and abnormal function of the organ of drug elimination (Roden 1998). In addition, coronary artery disease, female gender, a history of ventricular tachyarrhythmia (Lehmann et al. 1996), and drug dose for all drugs but quinidine (Roden 1998) are risk factors. Multiple risk factors are at least additive in individual patients (Lehmann et al. 1996), suggesting different basic mechanisms and pointing to the great clinical importance of recognizing and avoiding drug therapy that adds risk factors for torsades.

Our patient had multiple risk factors for torsades, some of which (such as female gender and a history of coronary disease) were intrinsic. On the other hand, diuretic therapy, the use of sotalol, and the (possibly indiscriminant) increase in sotalol dose exposed the patient to further increased risk. Syncope, not infrequently with seizures, is a typical presentation of torsades de pointes arrhythmias. A key point is to avoid unnecessary antiarrhythmic drug therapy (isolated ectopic complexes do not require treatment), and when such therapy is needed, to select the drug and dose appropriate to the patient. In addition to therapeutic considerations (i.e., the arrhythmia mechanism targeted), drug and dose selection should consider patient features that increase proarrhythmic risks of specific compounds. The basic mechanistic principles determining antiarrhythmic drug efficacy and proarrhythmia are presented in the section on Arrhythmias in this chapter. A list of special patient groups to consider is given in Table 1-56.

Amiodarone is associated with a generally low risk of proarrhythmia, even among patients with symptomatic coronary disease, congestive heart failure, previous MI, and presenting arrhythmia or ventricular tachycardia and/or ventricular fibrillation (VT/VF). The only subgroup of patients in which amiodarone therapy appears to be contraindicated because of an increased risk of proarrhythmic sudden death is that of patients with congestive heart failure and a history of torsades de pointes (Middlekauff et al. 1995).

Routine hospitalization for the initiation of antiarrhythmic drug therapy has been proposed to limit the risk of proarrhythmia (Maisel et al. 1997). Problems with this approach (Thibault and Nattel 1999) include a relatively low detection rate, low cost-efficacy, and a continuing risk of proarrhythmia after hospital discharge (about half of proarrhythmic events occur after the first three days of therapy for class IA and III drugs, and a much higher percentage are delayed for class IC drugs and amiodarone). Recognizing risk factors and selecting drug and dose carefully for each patient are critical in preventing proarrhythmia. Similar considerations apply for noncardiovascular drugs that can cause proarrhythmia, such as erythromycin, terfenadine, thioridazine, tricyclic antidepressants, and cisapride (that can cause torsades by blocking $I_{Kr}$ [see the section on Arrhythmias, this chapter]) or tricyclic antidepressants (that can cause excess $Na^+$ channel blockade in an overdose setting).

**PRINCIPLE In order to minimize the risk of proarrhythmia, individualize antiarrhythmic drug selection and dose based on risk factors for each patient.**

## ANTIANGINAL DRUGS THAT WORSEN OR MIMIC SYMPTOMS OF CORONARY ARTERY DISEASE

**CASE HISTORY** *A 70-year-old man has stable exertional angina. He is treated with a long-acting nifedipine preparation, 30 mg/day, but his symptoms remain. The nifedipine dose is increased to 60 mg/day, but despite this, his anginal episodes become more frequent, and ankle swelling develops. While shopping in a department store, the patient has a severe anginal attack, for which he takes sublingual nitroglycerin, and he then promptly loses consciousness. He is easily resuscitated and is brought by ambulance to the emergency room with tentative diagnoses of unstable angina with congestive heart failure and suspected ventricular tachyarrhythmias.*

**Discussion** *All of the symptoms presented by this patient may be iatrogenic consequences of his treatment. In a small minority of patients, anginal symptoms can be worsened by dihydropyridine $Ca^{2+}$ antagonists. This worsening of angina may be due to the reflex tachycardia resulting from the strong vasodilating actions of dihydropyridines, or to an unfavorable redistribution of coronary blood flow away from ischemic zones ("coronary steal syndrome"). The clinical manifestations of angina depend on the factors controlling the balance between oxygen supply and demand that determines the occurrence of myocardial ischemia. Metabolic needs of the heart depend on cardiac work, which*

Table 1-56 Special Patient Groups at Increased Risk of Torsades de Pointes or Arrhythmia

| Increased risk of torsades de pointes (avoid class IA and III drugs) | Increased risk of $Na^+$ channel block-related arrhythmias (avoid class IC drugs) |
|---|---|
| Female gender | Coronary artery disease |
| Congestive heart failure | Previous myocardial infarction |
| Index arrhythmia VT/VF | Congestive heart failure |
| Hypokalemia (and diuretics) | Greater drug doses |
| Greater drug doses (except quinidine) | Abnormal ventricular conduction |
| Disease of drug eliminating organ | Index arrhythmia VT/VF |

ABBREVIATIONS: VT/VF, ventricular tachycardia and/or ventricular fibrillation.

*is closely related to the so-called "double product"—the product of heart rate and blood pressure. Ischemia can be favored by drugs that increase heart rate (e.g., dihydropyridines, β-adrenergic agonists including some anti-asthma drugs, theophylline products, anticholinergic agents like tricyclic antidepressants, and drugs used to treat urinary symptoms) or by drugs that increase blood pressure.*

*Peripheral edema is a common consequence of $Ca^{2+}$ antagonist therapy, particularly the dihydropyridines. It can also occur, but is much less frequent, with diltiazem and verapamil. Drug-induced edema is often misdiagnosed as congestive heart failure related to coronary disease. In most cases, the distinction between peripheral edema due to heart failure and that caused by $Ca^{2+}$ antagonists can be made fairly readily on the basis of the presence or absence of chest X-ray findings of significant heart failure and noninvasive indices of cardiac systolic function. Confirmation is obtained by noting the response of peripheral edema to the cessation of the $Ca^{2+}$ antagonist.*

*Vasovagal syncope is often caused by sublingual nitroglycerin therapy, especially in warm environments and when the patient is upright at the time of nitrate ingestion. The clinical picture is usually typical of vasovagal syncope, with gradual onset, often with nausea, sweating, and pallor, then a rapid recovery following a fall and/or minimal cardiopulmonary resuscitation maneuvers. It should be noted that full cardiopulmonary arrest, including convulsions, is uncommon with nitrate syncope but can occur, especially if the patient remains upright after the onset of symptoms. The main risk is overmanagement if the diagnosis of nitrate syncope is not considered and aggressive treatment (such as with pacemakers, antiarrhythmic drugs, or defibrillators) is applied without a clear indication.*

**PRINCIPLE Always consider the possibility of adverse drug reactions when clinical events occur that do not have a clear pathophysiological basis.**

## DRUGS FOR CONGESTIVE HEART FAILURE THAT IMPROVE SYMPTOMS IN THE SHORT TERM BUT WORSEN THE LONG-TERM OUTCOME

CASE HISTORY *A 45-year-old man with heart failure and atypical chest pain is treated with nifedipine. He initially feels better, but 3 months later becomes increasingly short of breath. A chest X-ray shows interstitial pulmonary edema, and he is admitted to the hospital.*

**Discussion** *Historically, the initial focus in the therapy of congestive heart failure (CHF) was on improving the force of cardiac contraction. Subsequently, the important role of afterload in governing function of the failing heart was recognized, and afterload reducers such as nitrates, hydralazine, and angiotensin-converting enzyme inhibitors were found to be effective in reducing symptoms and improving outcome.*

*The dihydropyridine $Ca^{2+}$ channel blockers are potent arterial dilators, and nifedipine has beneficial short-term effects on hemodynamics and symptoms in patients with heart failure (Klugman et al. 1980; Ludbrook et al. 1981). Subsequent controlled studies, however, showed that long-term nifedipine administration is associated with an increased number of episodes of severe heart failure that require hospitalization (Elkayam et al. 1990). Possible explanations of this phenomenon include intrinsic negative inotropic effects of the drug and sympathetic reflex activation. Diltiazem, known to have more direct cardiodepressant effects than nifedipine, clearly worsens the prognosis in patients with heart failure following myocardial infarction (Goldstein et al. 1991). Third-generation dihydropyridine $Ca^{2+}$ antagonists such as amlodipine appear to be safe in patients with heart failure (Packer et al. 1996), perhaps because their slower onset and offset of action elicit a less intense sympathetic reflex. Alternatively, a greater degree of vascular specificity (and consequent absence of cardiodepressant actions) may be involved.*

Another set of compounds that improves symptoms of congestive heart failure in the short term but worsens long-term outcome is the positive inotropic agents (with the exception of digoxin). A variety of such agents, including xamoterol (The Xamoterol in Severe Heart Failure Study Group 1990), ibopamine (Hampton et al. 1997), milrinone (Packer et al. 1991), vesnarinone (Cohn et al. 1998), and pimobendan (Lubsen et al. 1996) have been shown to increase significantly overall mortality in patients with congestive heart failure, despite reproducibly improving hemodynamics and symptoms upon short-term administration. In contrast, $\beta$-adrenoceptor antagonists are known to sometimes worsen symptoms of congestive heart failure acutely, but in patients able to tolerate $\beta$-adrenergic blockers, they consistently improve long-term outcome (Massie 1998). The clear benefits of angiotensin-converting enzyme inhibitors (Massie 1998) also appear to exceed the results expected based on their vasodilating actions alone. The long-term results of congestive heart failure therapy trials lead to the conclusion that outcome in patients with this syndrome does not depend only on the hemodynamic state, rather factors that determine ventricular remodeling (likely by governing the intrinsic "health" of cardiac myocytes) are of utmost importance. In this context, various potentially cardiostimulatory drugs used for noncardiac conditions, such as oral $\beta_2$-adrenergic agonists (Jenne 1998), may also have the potential to worsen outcome in patients with congestive heart failure.

**PRINCIPLE Short-term improvements in the pathophysiology of a cardiac disease may not translate into long-term benefits, and in some cases, quite the opposite is true. Trials of long-term effects on hard endpoints such as mortality are essential for evaluating the potential usefulness of a therapy.**

## ABRUPT WITHDRAWAL OF A VARIETY OF CARDIOACTIVE DRUGS CAN CAUSE A SERIOUS DETERIORATION OF THE CLINICAL STATE

CASE HISTORY *A 65-year-old woman is brought to the emergency room by her family because of confusion and headaches. She had been taking clonidine, 0.2 mg three times per day, and hydrochlorothiazide, 25 mg daily, for hypertension. On examination, she has a blood pressure of 170/120 and a heart rate of 110/minute. Further questioning of the family indicates that she had become depressed after an argument with her children about 36 hours ago and may have stopped taking her medications subsequently.*

**Discussion** *This patient likely presents a case of clonidine withdrawal syndrome. Abrupt withdrawal of long-term clonidine therapy may be followed by rebound sympathetic activation resulting in tachycardia and hypertension (Geyskes et al. 1979). The hypertension may be more severe than that before therapy and occasionally can have features of a hypertensive emergency. Clonidine withdrawal syndromes can be avoided by decreasing the drug gradually over several days before discontinuation. Other drugs whose abrupt withdrawal can cause rebound syndromes include $\beta$-adrenergic receptor antagonists (Nattel et al. 1979) and high-dose nitrates. True withdrawal syndromes occur when intrinsic homeostatic alterations have occurred in response to a drug, and their disappearance outlasts the elimination of the drug from the body. In the case of adrenergic receptors, receptor number is regulated in response to the level of stimulation. An excess of agonist downregulates receptor number, whereas a decrease in stimulation may upregulate receptors. In the case of clonidine, which is an $\alpha$-adrenergic receptor agonist, chronic stimulation of CNS $\alpha$-receptors leads to poorly understood cellular adaptations. When the drug is abruptly discontinued, the unmasking of these adaptations leads to increased sympathetic activation (Augustine et al. 1982). Withdrawal syndromes can be avoided by gradual discontinuation of the drug involved, but need to be differentiated from a simple return to the baseline state following the discontinuation of previously effective therapy. The most straightforward treatment of a withdrawal syndrome is re-introduction of the responsible agent, followed by gradual discontinuation after the clinical situation has stabilized.*

## ANTITHROMBOTIC AGENTS THAT PRODUCE THROMBOTIC COMPLICATIONS

CASE HISTORY *A 42-year-old man is admitted to the hospital with unstable angina. After an initially stormy hospital course with recurrent chest pain, he stabilizes in response to treatment with intravenous heparin and nitroglycerin. Five days after admission, he develops slurred speech and weakness of the right arm. A computed tomography study shows a nonhemorrhagic left hemisphere infarct. A partial thromboplastin time (PTT) measurement demonstrated therapeutic anticoagulation; the platelet count is 50,000/ml.*

**Discussion** *This is a typical case of heparin-induced thrombocytopenia (HIT). With increased therapeutic use of intravenous heparin, the awareness of HIT has increased (Brieger et al. 1998; Walenga and Bick 1998; Warkentin 1998). Moderate thrombocytopenia is a relatively frequent* *complication of heparin therapy (heparin-induced thrombocytopenia or HIT), occurring in about 10–20% of patients and presenting with transient decreases in platelet count to the range of 100–150,000/ml. This relatively benign syndrome has not been associated with thromboembolic complications; these changes have been termed HIT Type I. Much more sinister is Type II HIT which occurs in about 3% of patients receiving intravenous heparin for a week or more. Most cases occur 5–10 days after the initiation of therapy; thrombocytopenia is due to antibodies (generally IgG) that recognize a complex of heparin and platelet factor 4 (PF4). The antigen–antibody complex causes platelet aggregation, thrombosis, and thrombocytopenia. The clinical picture can be confusing, frequently of a patient who develops unexpected thromboembolic events despite therapeutic anticoagulation and then drops their platelet count. A high index of suspicion is essential. The most common types of thromboembolic events are lower limb ischemia, cerebrovascular accidents, and myocardial infarctions, but a host of vascular and graft occlusions can occur. Definitive diagnosis can be made by specific immunological studies (Brieger et al. 1998). A key element of treatment is the discontinuation of all heparin administration, not only therapeutic intravenous infusions but also heparin used to keep lines open. Direct thrombin inhibitors such as hirudin (Greinacher et al. 1999) or argatroban (Matsuo et al. 1992) may be useful in management.*

**CONCLUSIONS**

**Cardioactive medications can cause a host of adverse effects, many of which present like the disease being treated. A high index of suspicion and a knowledge of common adverse effect presentations is essential for the safe use of drugs to treat cardiovascular diseases.**

## REFERENCES


Augustine SJ, Buckley JP, Tachikawa S, et al. 1982. Involvement of central noradrenergic mechanisms in the rebound hypertension following clonidine withdrawal. *J Cardiovasc Pharmacol* **4**:449–55.

Brieger DB, Mak KH, Kottke-Marchant K, et al. 1998. Heparin-induced thrombocytopenia. *J Am Coll Cardiol* **31**:1449–59.

Cohn JN, Goldstein SO, Greenberg BH, et al. 1998. A dose-dependent increase in mortality with vesnarinone among patients with severe heart failure. The Vesnarinone Trial Investigators. *N Engl J Med* **339**:1810–16.

Elkayam U, Amin J, Mehra A, et al. 1990. A prospective, randomized, double-blind, crossover study to compare the efficacy and safety of chronic nifedipine therapy with that of isosorbide dinitrate and their combination in the treatment of chronic congestive heart failure. *Circulation* **82**:1954–61.

Geyskes GG, Boer P, Dorhout Mees EJ. 1979. Clonidine withdrawal. Mechanism and frequency of rebound hypertension. *Br J Clin Pharmacol* **7**:55–62.

Goldstein RE, Boccuzzi SJ, Cruess D, et al. 1991. Diltiazem increases late-onset congestive heart failure in post-infarction patients with early reduction of ejection fraction. *Circulation* **83**:52–60.

Greinacher A, Volpel H, Janssens U, et al. 1999. Recombinant hirudin (lepirudin) provides safe and effective anticoagulation in patients with heparin-induced thrombocytopenia: a prospective study. *Circulation* **99**:73–80.

Hampton JR, van Veldhuisen DJ, Kleber FX, et al. 1997. Randomised study of effect of ibopamine on survival in patients with advanced severe heart failure. Second Prospective Randomised Study of Ibopamine on Mortality and Efficacy (PRIME II) investigators. *Lancet* **349**:971–7.

Jenne JW. 1998. Can oral $\beta_2$ agonists cause heart failure? *Lancet* **352**:1081–82.

Kawasaki R, Machado C, Reinoehl J, et al. 1995. Increased propensity of women to develop torsades de pointes during complete heart block. *J Cardiovasc Electrophysiol* **6**:1032–8.

Klugmann S, Salvi A, Camerini F. 1980. Hemodynamic effects of nifedipine in heart failure. *Br Heart J* **43**:440–6.

Lehmann MN, Hardy S, Archibald D, et al. 1996. Sex difference in risk of torsade de pointes with *d,l*-sotalol. *Circulation* **94**:2535–41.

Lubsen J, Just H, Hjalmarsson AC, et al. 1996. Effect of pimobendan on exercise capacity in patients with heart failure: main results from the Pimobendan in Congestive Heart Failure (PICO) trial. *Heart* **76**:223–31.

Ludbrook PA, Tiefenbrun AJ, Sobel BE. 1981. Influence of nifedipine on left ventricular systolic and diastolic function: relationship to manifestations of ischemia and congestive failure. *Am J Med* **71**:683–92.

Maisel WH, Kuntz KM, Reimold SC, et al. 1997. Risk of initiating antiarrhythmic drug therapy for atrial fibrillation in patients admitted to a university hospital. *Ann Intern Med* **127**:281–4.

Massie M. 1998. 15 years of heart-failure trials: what have we learned? *Lancet* **352**(Suppl I):29–33.

Matsuo T, Kazuomi K, Chikahira Y, et al. 1992. Treatment of heparin-induced thrombocytopenia by use of argatroban, a synthetic thrombin inhibitor. *Br J Haematol* **82**:627–9.

Middlekauff HR, Stevenson WG, Saxon LA, et al. 1995. Amiodarone and torsades de pointes in patients with advanced heart failure. *Am J Cardiol* **76**:499–502.

Nattel S, Quantz MA. 1988. Pharmacological response of quinidine induced early after depolarisations in canine cardiac Purkinje fibres: insights into underlying ionic mechanisms. *Cardiovasc Res* **22**:808–17.

Nattel S, Rangno RE, Van Loon G. 1979. Mechanism of propranolol withdrawal phenomena. *Circulation* **59**:1158–64.

Packer M, Carver JR, Rodeheffer RJ, et al. 1991. Effect of oral milrinone on mortality in severe chronic heart failure. The PROMISE study research group. *N Engl J Med* **325**:1468–75.

Packer M, O'Connor CM, Ghali JK, et al. 1996. Effect of amlodipine on morbidity and mortality in severe chronic heart failure. Prospective randomized amlodipine survival evaluation study group. *N Engl J Med* **335**:1107–14.

Roden DM. 1998. Taking the "idio" out of "idiosyncratic": predicting torsades de pointes. *PACE* **21**:1029–34.

Roden DM, Hoffman BF. 1985. Action potential prolongation and induction of abnormal automaticity by low quinidine concentrations in canine Purkinje fibers. Relationship to potassium and cycle length. *Circ Res* **56**:857–67.

The Xamoterol in Severe Heart Failure Study Group. 1990. Xamoterol in severe heart failure. *Lancet* **336**:1–6.

Thibault B, Nattel S. 1999. Optimal management with class I and class III antiarrhythmic drugs should be done in the outpatient setting-protagonist. *J Cardiovasc Electrophysiol* **10**:472–81.

Volders PG, Sipido KR, Vos MA, et al. 1998. Cellular basis of biventricular hypertrophy and arrhythmogenesis in dogs with chronic complete atrioventricular block and acquired torsade de pointes. *Circulation* **98**:1136–47.

Walenga JM, Bick RL. 1998. Heparin-induced thrombocytopenia, paradoxical thromboembolism, and other side effects of heparin therapy. *Med Clin North Am* **82**:635–58.

Warkentin TE. 1998. Clinical presentation of heparin-induced thrombocytopenia. *Semin Hematol* **35**(Suppl 5):9–16.

CHAPTER

# 2 RESPIRATORY DISORDERS
## Introduction and General Approach to Therapy

John A. Abisheganaden, Homer A. Boushey

*Chapter Outline*



## INTRODUCTION TO RESPIRATORY DISORDERS

The major function served by the respiratory system is the exchange of gas between the atmosphere and the circulation. This purpose dictates the system's structure, which consists of three major elements. One element—the tracheobronchial tree—distributes inhaled air to the interface with the circulation and consists of progressive, dichotomous branches of a single central airway, the trachea, into as many as $2^{16}$ final branches, the terminal bronchioles. The second element—the pulmonary circulation—delivers blood to the interface with air, and also consists of a progressively branching system, this time from a single, central vessel, the pulmonary artery, into many final branches, the pulmonary arterioles. The third element—the alveolar bed—is the interface where gas exchange occurs, and is made up of respiratory bronchioles and alveoli, fed by the terminal bronchioles, and alveolar capillaries, fed by the pulmonary arterioles. Together with a spare stroma of fibrous tissue and lymphatic vessels draining the alveoli, the alveolar capillary bed makes up the lung parenchyma. Diseases of the lung are thus often classified as *airway diseases,* that is, those that affect primarily the trachea and bronchi, like asthma and bronchitis; as *pulmonary vascular diseases,* like multiple pulmonary emboli or primary pulmonary hypertension; and *parenchymal lung disease,* that is, those affecting primarily the alveolar bed and its supporting stroma, like diffuse pulmonary fibrosis.

## ROUTES OF DRUG DELIVERY

From the standpoint of therapeutics, the lung presents at least the theoretical opportunity for delivering drugs directly to the structures affected by adding them to inhaled air. This avoids a limitation of delivering drugs by ingestion or by injection, which ultimately deliver drugs to the circulation and hence to all other tissues of the body. The opportunity for direct treatment has been at least partially exploited through the use of aerosols for treating diseases of the airways, but the effectiveness of the lung's natural defenses against inhaled particles and the difficulties in delivering drugs in particles fine enough to reach the alveoli have presented obstacles to this approach for the treatment of alveolar or "parenchymal" lung disease that have so far proved insurmountable.

Inhalation is the preferred mode of delivery of drugs that act directly on the airways, and aerosolized therapies are the mainstay of treatment for the most common forms of airway disease, indeed the most common forms of lung disease, asthma and chronic obstructive bronchitis (Newhouse and Dolovich 1986). Inhalation is the only way to deliver some drugs, like the "mast cell stabilizers," cromolyn sodium and nedocromil, and the anticholinergic agents, ipratropium bromide and tiotropium bromide, and is the preferred route for delivery of others, like $\beta$-adrenergic agonists and corticosteroids. Antibiotics also may be delivered by the inhaled route for chronic airway infection, as in cystic fibrosis, or for the prevention of lung infection in high-risk patients, like those who require prolonged intubation and are prone to nosocomial pneumonia, and those with advanced AIDS who are prone to *Pneumocystis* pneumonia.

In delivering a drug as an aerosol or dry powder, the size and shape of the particles and the pattern on inhalation by which they are entrained into the lungs critically determine the sites of deposition (Newman et al. 1981). Particles with an effective diameter much larger than 15 $\mu$m penetrate poorly beyond the larynx and trachea. A high proportion of particles with a "mass median diameter" of $<1$ $\mu$m penetrate to the alveoli but may be expelled along with exhaled air. For settling in the airways, the optimum size for particles is between 2 and 5 $\mu$m. It is not enough that the mean size of the particles delivered by a particular device be in this range, for the volume of a sphere (or droplet) is a function of the third power of its radius, so the majority of the total dose of drug delivered as an aerosol could be contained in a relatively small proportion of large particles. Ideally, particles should be monodispersed, that is, the range of sizes of particles around the mean should be narrow.

Of the systems currently available for prescribing inhaled therapies, the ones that most closely match the theoretical ideal are metered-dose inhalers and dry-powder inhalers. Both require coordination of inspiration by the patient, so nebulizers are still used for delivering aerosols to patients too young, too old, or too ill to shape their inspiratory effort to conform with the design of the delivery system. Nebulizers are also useful for delivering drugs, like antibiotics, when relatively high doses are needed.

**PRINCIPLE When a drug such as a glucocorticoid or antibiotic can be administered topically, orally, or parenterally, the optimal route must be determined for each indication and even for each patient. Goals of treatment (e.g., therapy, prophylaxis), severity of illness, and other factors must be weighed, as each route offers a different combination of benefits and risks.**

Metered-dose inhalers (MDIs) deliver drug from a canister with a chlorofluorocarbon (CFC) propellant. The high volatility of the propellant ensures that the particles sprayed from the device will shrink promptly into the respirable range. These devices are convenient, portable, and inexpensive, and have become the most common means for delivering inhaled medication. One problem with their design is their reliance on CFC propellants, for the industrial use of CFCs has been identified as a cause of depletion of ozone from the stratosphere. Under an international agreement, MDIs containing CFCs will be replaced by ozone-friendly non-CFC propellant MDIs. One has already been approved. This MDI is driven by hydrofluoroalkane (HFA-134a), which does not deplete ozone, and the inhaler has proved as effective as the usual CFC-containing albuterol inhalers in producing bronchodilation (Dockhorn et al. 1995).

**PRINCIPLE We do not often concern ourselves with the environmental effects of drugs but the example above, and examples with the environmental effects of clinically useful antibiotics, should remind us to.**

Another problem with MDIs is that the "puff" of aerosol is sprayed at high velocity, so entrainment of the medication into the airstream requires that it be activated during inhalation; this inhalation must be kept slow for particles not to impact on the posterior pharyngeal wall. Even with well-coordinated inspiration, $<10\%$ of the dose delivered from the device is delivered beyond the larynx. The rest is swallowed and delivered to the gut, where any drug absorbed is subjected to first-pass metabolism by the liver.

To reduce the demands for perfect coordination of inhalation, "spacers" or reservoir devices have been developed. These are large-volume devices placed between the MDI and the patient. The "puff" from the device is thus held in a contained space, giving the patient time to coordinate initiation of a slow inspiration and the particles time to evaporate, with large particles settling onto the device's walls. These devices improve airway delivery of medication and greatly reduce oropharyngeal deposition and subsequent delivery to the GI tract.

Delivery of medication from MDI delivery with a spacer is efficient. Delivery of 4–12 puffs of 90 *micrograms* of albuterol by this method is at least as effective as delivery of 2.5–5.0 *milligrams* by conventional nebulizer in the treatment of asthmatic bronchoconstriction.

**PRINCIPLE The mechanism of drug delivery can be the key determinant of the dose-effect relationship.**

Dry powder inhalers scatter a fine powder dispersed by the turbulence of air inhaled directly through the device. Dry powder inhalers are easy to use and when used correctly, appear to deliver a higher proportion of drug to the airways (Borgstrom et al. 1996). Generating the turbulence necessary for scattering the particles requires brisk inhalation, which may present a problem for some patients with severe airflow obstruction, and some patients find the dry powder irritating. Others sense so little irritation that they complain they cannot tell whether any medication was delivered.

However an inhaled medication is delivered, its ultimate fate is poorly understood. Four possible fates seem likely: it is deposited on the oropharyngeal mucosa, swallowed, and delivered to the gut; it is deposited on the tracheobronchial mucosa and is either absorbed into the bronchial circulation or carried up to the mouth on the mucociliary escalator and swallowed; it is delivered to the alveolar bed and is either taken up by phagocytic cells or absorbed into the pulmonary circulation; or it does not settle onto any surface and is expelled with the next exhalation. Understanding the fate of inhaled particles has become more important with the recognition that sufficient quantities of inhaled corticosteroids can be absorbed into the circulation to cause systemic toxicity. The development of an inhaled corticosteroid that was fully metabolized by a single pass through the liver (99% "first-pass metabolism") thus seemed important, for drug deposited in the mouth and pharynx no longer presented any risk for systemic toxicity (Harding 1990). It became apparent, however, that inhaled corticosteroids are well absorbed from the bronchial and alveolar surfaces and delivered to pulmonary or azygous venous systems, bypassing the liver in gaining access to the systemic circulation (Lipworth 1995).

**PRINCIPLE When delivering a drug to a local site of interest the physician must survey effects of the drug beyond the site of application. Corticosteroids delivered to the skin are absorbed and can have systemic effects. Many other drugs that are placed locally have more distant effects, for example, "nonabsorbable antibiotics" delivered to the gut, many drugs "delivered" to the skin, β-adrenergic antagonists "delivered" to the eye, contraceptives "delivered" to the cervix and so forth.**

Drugs to treat pulmonary disease may be given orally. The oral dose usually is much higher than the inhaled dose required to achieve the same effect (by a ratio of >20:1); consequently, systemic adverse effects may be more common and severe. When delivery by either route is possible, the inhaled route is preferable and the oral route should be reserved for the few patients unable to use inhalers or nebulizers. Another consideration that sometimes leads to the selection of a drug formulation for oral therapy is patient preference. Several studies have shown that patients comply poorly with regular use of inhaled therapies (Rand et al. 1992), and are generally believed to adhere more reliably to oral therapy. This may partially account for the initial success of oral leukotriene receptor antagonists as a treatment for mild asthma, even though they appear less predictably efficacious in controlling asthma than do inhaled corticosteroids (Mullen et al. 1998).

**PRINCIPLE Compliance is critical for an efficacy of chronic therapy. The means of drug application may be an important determinant of a patient's willingness to take therapy regularly.**

Administering drugs by subcutaneous, intramuscular, or intravenous injection is generally reserved for patients too severely ill to inhale medication or to absorb drugs from the GI tract. Adverse effects are generally more frequent and severe with this route because of the higher plasma concentrations achieved.

## REFERENCES


Borgstrom L, Derom E, Stahl E, et al. 1996. The inhalation device influences lung deposition and bronchodilating effect of terbutaline. *Am J Respir Crit Care Med* **1996**:1636–40.

Dockhorn R, Vanden Burgt JA, Ekholm BP, et al. 1995. Clinical equivalence of a novel non-chlorofluorocarbon-containing salbutamol sulfate metered-dose inhaler and a conventional chlorofluorocarbon inhaler in patients with asthma. *J Allergy Clin Immunol* **96**: 50–6.

Harding SM. 1990. The human pharmacology of fluticasone propionate. *Respir Med* **84** (Suppl A):S25–9.

Lipworth BJ. 1995. New perspectives on inhaled drug delivery and systemic bioactivity. *Thorax* **50**:105–10.

Mullen B, Driskell JE, Yancey SW. 1998. A statistical comparison of the efficacy of leukotriene modifiers and inhaled corticosteroids. *J Allergy Clin Immunol* **101**:S232.

Newhouse MT, Dolovich MB. 1986. Control of asthma by aerosols. *N Engl J Med* **315**:870–4.

Newman SP, Pavia D, Moren F, et al. 1981. Deposition of pressurized aerosols in the human respiratory tract. *Thorax* **36**:52–5.

Rand CS, Wise RA, Nides M, et al. 1992. Metered-dose inhaler adherence in a clinical trial. *Am Rev Respir Dis* **146**:1559–64.

# Obstructive Lung Diseases: Treatment

John A. Abisheganaden, Homer A. Boushey, Stephen I. Rennard

*Chapter Outline*



## BRONCHODILATORS

The drugs most commonly used for the treatment of pulmonary diseases are bronchodilators, and they are the mainstay for prompt reversal of bronchospasm. Of the three main classes of bronchodilators in current clinical use ($\beta$-adrenergic agonists, methylxanthines, and anticholinergics), the $\beta$-adrenergic agonists are the most effective for acute reversal of airway narrowing in asthma (Chaieb et al. 1989). Short-acting inhaled $\beta_2$-adrenergic agonists remain the treatment of choice for acute exacerbations of asthma and for preventing exercise-induced bronchospasm. Although long-acting $\beta_2$-agonists appear less effective than inhaled corticosteroids as a chronic treatment of asthma (Verberne et al. 1997), they are effective in improving asthma control when added to inhaled corticosteroid therapy. Because corticosteroids improve airway obstruction only gradually, they are generally not considered to be bronchodilators. Methylxanthines, particularly theophylline, have direct inhibitory effects on airway smooth muscle tone and are indeed bronchodilators, but they must be given systemically (by the oral or intravenous route), have important potential toxicities, are less effective in reversing bronchospasm acutely, and appear not to add to the acute bronchodilation produced by inhaled $\beta$-adrenergic agonists (Rossing et al. 1980), so they have fallen from favor as bronchodilators. Anticholinergic agents, once eschewed as bronchodilators because of the ease with which atropine sulfate was absorbed into the systemic circulation and then crossed the blood–brain barrier, have reclaimed an accepted place as bronchodilators with the availability of ipratropium bromide and oxytropium bromide, quaternary ammonium salts of atropine that are poorly absorbed and that do not enter the CNS (Gross and Schloo 1975). Although less effective than $\beta$-adrenergic agents in relieving asthmatic bronchoconstriction, anticholinergic agents appear equally or even more effective in improving airway caliber in chronic obstructive bronchitis and emphysema ("COPD") (Gross and Skorodin 1984b).

### $\beta$-Adrenergic Receptor Agonists

***Background and pharmacology***

Ephedrine has been used to treat asthma for millennia in China; epinephrine was the mainstay of therapy for acute attacks for most of this century; and isoproterenol may still remain the most potent $\beta$-adrenergic receptor agonist known. These have fallen from favor, however, because of their production of unwanted cardiovascular effects and their short duration of action. Ephedrine and epinephrine stimulate both $\alpha$- and $\beta$-adrenergic receptors, and thus cause hypertension as well as bronchodilation. This stimulated the development of isoproterenol in the 1940s, a $\beta$-adrenergic agonist with weak $\alpha$-adrenergic potency. Isoproterenol stimulates both $\beta_1$- and $\beta_2$-receptors, however, and causes tachycardia even when taken only by inhalation. It was suspected also of promoting cardiac arrhythmias, and the release of a high-dose formulation was blamed for an epidemic of asthma deaths in the United Kingdom in the mid-1960s (Stolley and Schinnar 1978). This stimulated the development of second-generation $\beta$-adrenergic agonists that selectively stimulate $\beta_2$-receptors. These agents, including metaproterenol, terbutaline, albuterol, bitolterol, and pirbuterol indeed produce significant bronchodilation with less cardiovascular effects, and additionally have a longer duration of action and are effective when taken orally. These $\beta_2$-selective agonists have supplanted all other $\beta$-adrenergic agents in prescribed therapy for asthma, but even these agents still show substantial $\beta_1$-type activity when given in high doses. Furthermore, up to 50% of the beta receptors in some areas of the heart are of the $\beta_2$-type (Robberecht et al. 1983). Thus, the $\beta_2$-selective agonists have reduced but have not eliminated all risk of cardiac toxicity.

The development of these selective $\beta_2$-agonists resulted from substitutions in the catechol ring of the catecholamine structure (Fig. 2-1) (McFadden 1981). Norepinephrine differs from epinephrine (adrenaline) only in the substitution of the terminal amino group. Modification at this site confers $\beta$-receptor selectivity. Further substitution of the terminal amino group resulted in the development of $\beta_2$-receptor selectivity, as seen with albuterol and terbutaline. Modification of the groups in the catechol ring conferred resistance to degradation by catechol-*O*-methyltransferase, prolonging the duration of action from 60–90 minutes to 3–4 hours, and further conferred resistance against degradation in the gut, enabling oral administration.

***Mechanism of action***

The $\beta_2$-adrenergic receptor consists of a protein that traverses the cell membrane seven times, with three extracellular and three intracellular loops. Direct stimulation of this receptor leads to relaxation of bronchial smooth muscle. This effect has been demonstrated in vitro by the relaxant effect of isoproterenol on human bronchi and lung strips (Zaagsma et al. 1983), and in vivo by a rapid decrease in airway resistance. The molecular mechanisms by which $\beta$-adrenergic agonists relax airway smooth muscle

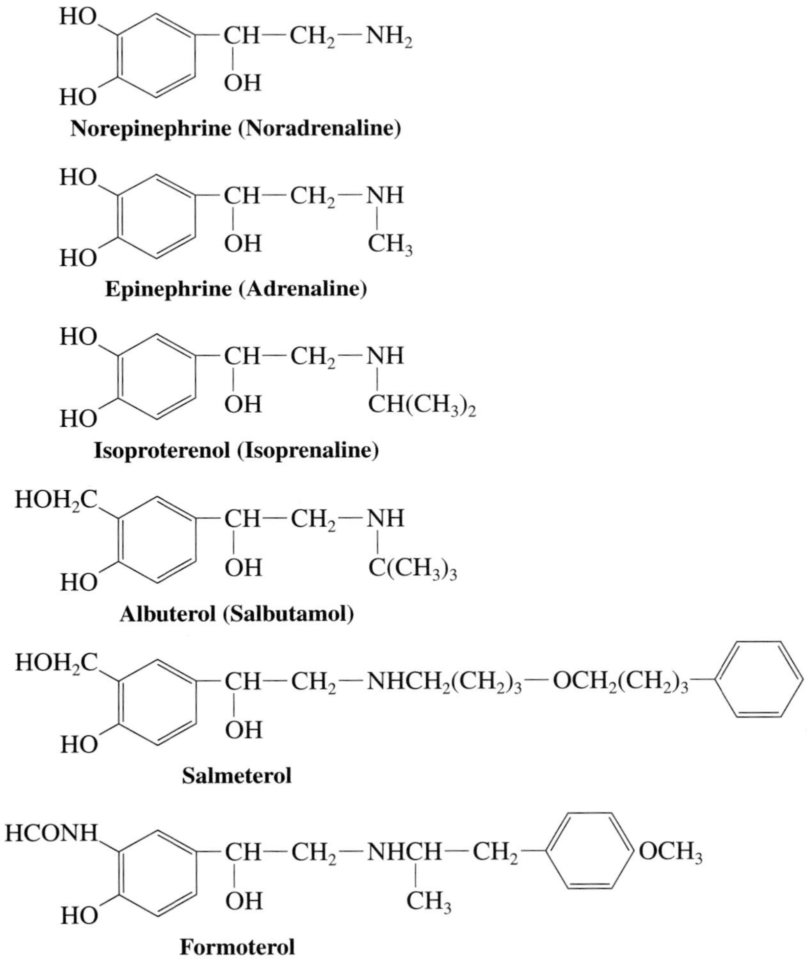

**Norepinephrine (Noradrenaline)**

**Epinephrine (Adrenaline)**

**Isoproterenol (Isoprenaline)**

**Albuterol (Salbutamol)**

**Salmeterol**

**Formoterol**

FIGURE 2-1 **Chemical structure of some adrenergic agonists, showing their evolution from catecholamines.**

include activation of stimulatory guanine-nucleotide-binding protein (G proteins), followed by activation of the cyclic AMP second messenger system. Cyclic adenosine 3′,5′-monophosphate (cAMP) activates a specific kinase (protein kinase A) that phosphorylates several target enzymes and ion channels within the cell, leading to relaxation (Barnes 1995b).

$\beta$-Adrenergic receptors have been found on a wide variety of cells, as on vascular smooth muscle, cardiac conducting cells, skeletal smooth muscle cells, and others. Hence, $\beta$-adrenergic agonists have effects besides promoting bronchodilation; they have been shown, for example, to inhibit mediator release from mast cells, both in vitro (Church and Hiroi 1987) and in vivo (Howarth et al. 1985). $\beta$-Adrenergic agonists also reduce microvascular leakage and thus the development of bronchial mucosal edema caused by exposure to mediators such as histamine (Erjefalt and Persson 1986), and they enhance mucociliary clearance (Pavia et al. 1980). Although these effects may be relevant to the prophylactic use of these drugs, there is no evidence that $\beta_2$-adrenergic agonists have any substantial effect on the chronic inflammation characteristic of bronchial asthma, and their primary and rapid bronchodilator action is still their main indication for treating the bronchoconstriction of a wide range of airway diseases. A summary of the effects of $\beta$-adrenergic agonists in airway cells is presented in Table 2-1.

**PRINCIPLE Drugs can produce their net beneficial effects on an additive basis of multiple and different mechanisms.**

### *Long-acting $\beta_2$-adrenergic agonists*

The novel $\beta_2$-adrenergic agonists salmeterol and formoterol are as potent as albuterol or terbutaline but have a much longer duration of action (Nelson 1995). Both display a higher lipophilicity and have a higher affinity and selectivity than most of the short-acting agonists. The mechanisms responsible for their long duration of action differ. Salmeterol was devised by introducing a long side-chain to a hydrophobic site. The side chain binds to a specific site within the $\beta_2$-adrenergic receptor (an "exo-receptor" near the $\beta_2$-receptor site (Fig. 2-1) that allows prolonged activation of the receptor (Johnson et al. 1993). Formoterol may exert its long duration of action by being retained in the plasmalemma lipid bilayer of airway smooth muscle from which it can leech out and reach the receptor (Anderson 1993). When given by the inhaled route, both salmeterol and formoterol cause bronchodilation that lasts 12 hours or longer. They attenuate exercise-induced bronchospasm for longer than do short-acting $\beta_2$-agonists (Green and Price 1992), and improve nocturnal asthma symptoms (Fitzpatrick et al. 1990). Their onset of action is slow, however, and neither is indicated for the treatment of acute exacerbations of asthma (National Institutes of Health/NHLBI 1995). Some representative inhaled $\beta$-adrenergic agonists in common use today are listed in Table 2-2.

**Table 2-1 Effects of $\beta$-Adrenergic Agonists in Airway Cells**

|  |
|---|
| Relaxation of airway smooth muscle |
| Increased mucociliary clearance |
| Inhibition of plasma exudation and airway edema |
| Increased mucus secretion |
| Inhibition of mast cell mediator release |

### *Tolerance*

A characteristic of many membrane-associated receptors is the phenomenon of tolerance after high-dose or repeated use of the drug. Both in vitro (Hauck et al. 1990) and in vivo (Lipworth et al. 1989) studies show loss of responsiveness to $\beta$-agonist stimulation after repeated agonist exposure, which is likely mediated by receptor uncoupling (destabilization of the high-affinity state of the receptor) and receptor downregulation (Nijkamp et al. 1992). When both short- and long-acting $\beta$-agonists are used on a regular basis, their bronchodilating action is preserved, but they lose effectiveness in inhibiting the bronchospasm caused by allergen, methacholine, and exercise challenge (Cockcroft et al. 1993; Ramage et al. 1994; Bhagat et al. 1995; Kalra et al. 1996). The clinical significance of this is currently unclear. The more readily demonstrable tolerance of extrapulmonary effects is advantageous, because adverse effects tend to decrease with continued use of the drug.

**PRINCIPLE When the mechanisms that are responsible for diminishing both the toxic and the efficacious effects of a drug are the same (e.g., downregulation of $\beta$-adrenergic receptors leading to tolerance to the effects of the drug), special effort must be made to measure efficacy as toxicity wanes.**

### *Genetic polymorphisms of the $\beta_2$-adrenergic receptor*

Recent studies of polymorphism of human $\beta_2$-receptors suggest that some forms of the receptor may be more likely downregulated (Green et al. 1994). Among adult asthmatics taking formoterol, those homozygous for the

Table 2-2 Some Inhaled β-Adrenergic Bronchodilators in Current Clinical Use

| Generic name | Proprietary name | Dose (μg/puff) |
|---|---|---|
| *Short-to-medium acting (3–6 h)* | | |
| Metaproterenol sulfate | Alupent | 650 μg |
| Albuterol | Proventil, Ventolin | 90 μg |
| Bitolterol mesylate | Tornalate | 370 μg |
| Pirbuterol acetate | Maxair | 200 μg |
| Terbutaline sulfate | Breathaire, Bricanyl | 200 μg |
| Fenoterol[a] | Berotec | 200 μg |
| *Long-acting (>12 h)* | | |
| Salmeterol xinafoate | Serevent | 21 μg |
| Formoterol[a] | Fioradil | 12 μg |

[a]Not available in the United States.

"Gly16" polymorphism developed significantly greater loss in bronchodilator responsiveness than did those who were homozygous for Arg16 (Tan et al. 1997). The Gly 16 phenotype also appears to be associated with more frequent nocturnal asthma (Turki et al. 1995). In contrast, the "Gln/Glu27" form of the receptor resists downregulation in vitro and is associated with lower airway hyperreactivity (Hall et al. 1995).

### *Indications and clinical use*

Inhalation of short-acting $\beta_2$-agonists results in rapid bronchodilation (Lemanske and Joad 1990). It is the treatment of choice for exacerbations of asthma and is an essential element of treatment of acute exacerbations of chronic obstructive bronchitis. Although all $\beta_2$-agonists are similarly effective and have similar toxicities in studies of patient groups, there is individual variability in the development of adverse effects, like skeletal muscle tremor, so some patients tolerate some agents better than others.

For relief of mild bronchoconstriction, $\beta_2$-agonists are typically taken as two puffs from a metered-dose inhaler every 4 to 6 hours as needed, but patients should be instructed to take higher doses at more frequent intervals for persistent or severe symptoms while also starting additional treatment (e.g., with an oral or inhaled corticosteroid) or seeking a higher level of care. Dose-response studies show that as many as 12 puffs from an MDI may be necessary to achieve maximal bronchodilation in severe bronchoconstriction, and for severe attacks of asthma requiring emergency care, continuous nebulized therapy may be necessary. Oral administration of β-adrenergic agonists provides no advantage and is more likely to cause systemic adverse effects. Sustained-release oral preparations may be useful in treating nocturnal asthma. Subcutaneous injection of a β-adrenergic agonist has proved useful in some asthmatic patients with "brittle" asthma characterized by sudden and unpredictable episodes of bronchoconstriction (O'Driscoll et al. 1988).

In the past, $\beta_2$-agonists were often prescribed for regularly scheduled use in the belief that this regimen would improve asthma control. A recent multicenter clinical trial showed, however, that regular use of albuterol was neither more beneficial nor more harmful than taking it only as needed (Drazen et al. 1996). The current consensus is that intermittent use of inhaled short-acting $\beta_2$-agonists can control episodic airway narrowing and are a safe, effective, and necessary therapy for asthma (National Asthma Education and Prevention Program Expert Panel, 1997a and 1997b). The frequency of $\beta_2$-agonist usage is useful as a marker of disease activity, because use of more than one canister of a $\beta_2$-agonist per month has been associated with increased risk for death or near death from asthma (Spitzer et al. 1992).

**PRINCIPLE Diseases, like drugs, have characteristic dynamics. Because dose-related response to a drug depends on the severity of the lesion it is to reverse, assessing the dynamics of the disease and matching the kinetics and dynamics of the drug to the severity is crucial in preventing worsening of the disease. Proper matching of drugs to disease simplifies overall management, avoiding overreliance on a drug that provides only transient symptomatic relief.**

$\beta_2$-Adrenergic agonists are also used in chronic obstructive pulmonary disease. These patients' response to anticholinergic drugs may or may not be greater than their response to $\beta_2$-adrenergic agonists (Braun et al. 1989; Karpel 1991). $\beta_2$-Adrenergic agonists improve airflow, functional exercise capacity, and the quality of life for patients with COPD when these drugs are administered on a regular schedule (Guyatt et al. 1987).

Long-acting $\beta_2$-agonists such as salmeterol and formoterol are currently recommended as adjuncts to anti-inflammatory medications for the control of persistent asthma (National Asthma Education and Prevention Program Expert Panel 1997a and 1997b). They are effective for asthmatics with symptomatic or physiologic impairment despite regular use of an inhaled corticosteroid [American Academy of Allergy, Asthma and Immunology (AAAAI) Committee on Drugs 1996; National Asthma Education and Prevention Program Expert Panel 1997a and 1997b].

The final position of long-acting inhaled $\beta_2$-agonists in clinical practice has yet to be fully established (Abisheganaden and Boushey 1998), but several recent studies show that for asthma inadequately controlled by regular treatment with an inhaled corticosteroid, the addition of a long-acting $\beta$-agonist confers greater benefit than does increasing the dose of the inhaled corticosteroid (Greening et al. 1994; Woolcock et al. 1996). Another study has shown greater improvement in symptom control from adding formoterol than from increasing the dose of budesonide, and a greater reduction in the frequency of exacerbations from increasing budesonide. The best effects were achieved with the combination of the high-dose of the inhaled steroid and the long-acting $\beta$-agonist (Pauwels et al. 1997).

**Key Points:** Short-acting $\beta_2$-agonists are the most effective medication for relieving acute bronchospasm. Regularly scheduled, daily use of short-acting $\beta_2$-agonists is no more effective than taking them as needed for relief of symptoms. Increasing usage (>1 canister/month) indicates inadequate control and the need for initiating or intensifying anti-inflammatory therapy. The long-acting $\beta_2$-adrenergic agonists may be used concomitantly with anti-inflammatory medications for long-term control of symptoms, especially of nocturnal symptoms.

### *Adverse effects*

Adverse effects are less common with inhaled therapy than with oral or parenteral administration. At conventional doses, inhalation of drugs by means of an MDI produces fewer adverse effects than inhalation by nebulization. The common adverse effects of $\beta$-adrenergic agonists are listed in Table 2-3.

**Table 2-3 Adverse Effects of $\beta$-Adrenergic Agonist Use**

| |
|---|
| Muscle tremor, jitteriness |
| Nausea and vomiting |
| Tachycardia, arrhythmias (more common in elderly, patients with coronary ischemia), or anginal-type pain |
| Rise in blood pressure |
| Hypokalemia |
| Restlessness, nervousness |
| Hypoxemia (increased *V/Q* mismatch due to pulmonary vasodilation) |
| Rarely—headache, flushing of the skin, dizziness, weakness, sweating |
| Tolerance (tachyphylaxis) |

ABBREVIATIONS: *V/Q*, ratio of ventilation to perfusion.

**PRINCIPLE The inhaled route of administration is preferable to the oral route of administration because it causes fewer adverse effects and is more effective.**

## Anticholinergics

### *Background and pharmacology*

Atropine, a naturally occurring compound, has long been used for treating asthma but has significant toxicity from its ready absorption into the blood stream and its ready passage across the blood–brain barrier. Less soluble quaternary compounds such as atropine methylnitrate and ipratropium bromide were therefore developed. Currently, ipratropium and oxitropium bromide are used widely for treating chronic obstructive pulmonary disease, and they are also useful as additional bronchodilators for acute severe asthma. Both are nonselective anticholinergic agents. Blockade of muscarinic receptors $M_1$ and $M_3$ leads to bronchodilation by relieving intrinsic cholinergic tone and by inhibiting cholinergic reflex bronchoconstriction. Blockade of the prejunctional $M_2$ receptors (autoreceptors), however, leads to an increase in acetylcholine release from nerve endings, an effect that counters the postjunctional blockade of $M_3$ receptors. This suggests that selective $M_3$-blockers would be more effective in blocking cholinergic nerve-induced effects in airways (Barnes 1989) and at least one such drug, tiotropium bromide, is currently in clinical trials.

Ipratropium bromide, the *N*-propyl derivative of atropine, is the most widely used anticholinergic inhaler and is available as an MDI, a solution for nebulization, and a nasal spray (Gross 1988). It is a nonselective anticholinergic, competitively blocking all muscarinic receptor subtypes. Bronchodilation is relatively slow in onset, reaching its maximum 30 to 60 minutes after inhalation but persists for up to 8 hours. The drug usually is given by MDI four times daily on a regular basis, rather than intermittently to control symptoms. When given by inhalation, ipratropium bromide attains negligible serum levels. Although more than 90% of the drug is swallowed, it is minimally absorbed from the gastrointestinal tract. Unlike atropine sulfate, it has little effect on baseline mucus production, mucus transport, or ciliary function. Oxitropium bromide, a novel quaternary nonselective anticholinergic bronchodilator similar to ipratropium bromide, is available in higher doses for inhalation and may lead to more prolonged effects (Frith et al. 1986). Thus, it may be useful in some patients with nocturnal asthma (Coe and Barnes 1986). The recent recognition that at least four subtypes of muscarinic receptors are expressed in the airways has led to a search for receptor-subtype-selective antagonists (Barnes 1993). In this respect, the most promising drug appears to be tiotropium bromide which has the unique property of kinetic selectivity, with rapid dissociation from $M_2$ receptors and slow dissociation from $M_1$ and $M_3$ receptors (Barnes 1998).

### *Mode of action*

Nerve fibers from both the afferent and efferent limbs of the parasympathetic nervous system enter the lung. The parasympathetic preganglionic fibers travel through the vagus nerve and end in ganglia located in the walls of the large and intermediate airways. Postganglionic fibers innervate receptors on smooth muscle and submucosal glands. Anticholinergics are specific antagonists of muscarinic receptors, which are one of the end-receptors of the parasympathetic innervation in the airways. Parasympathetic innervation of the airways is mainly limited to the proximal, conducting airways of the lung. Because anticholinergics can only reverse parasympathetically mediated stimulation of airway smooth muscle contraction, they have little or no effect in normal individuals but have significant bronchodilator effects in patients with chronic obstructive lung disease. The therapeutic benefits of anticholinergic drugs in asthma are derived from this bronchodilator activity and, in some patients, from inhibition of cholinergically stimulated mucous gland secretion.

### *Indications and clinical use*

Both ipratropium bromide and oxitropium bromide are useful bronchodilators in COPD but are less effective in chronic asthma (Gross 1988). Compared with short-acting $\beta_2$-agonists, they have a slower onset but a longer duration of action. These drugs may be more effective in older asthmatics, in whom there may be an element of fixed airway obstruction (Ullah et al. 1981). Nebulized therapy is effective in acute severe asthma, although it is less effective than are $\beta$-agonists (Ward et al. 1981). In clinical trials of asthma, there has been little evidence to support their use in long-term management (Gross and Skorodin 1984a). Although they play an important role in the long-term control of symptoms in COPD, they do not alter the progression of disease (Anthonisen et al. 1994).

Ipratropium bromide has been studied in combination with other therapeutic agents for asthma, including $\beta$-adrenergic agonists, theophylline, and cromolyn sodium. These studies indicate that they may be most effective when they are combined with a $\beta$-agonist (COMBIVENT Inhalation Aerosol Study Group 1994). The addition of ipratropium bromide to nebulized albuterol for acute severe asthma improves bronchodilation and reduces the proportion of patients requiring hospitalization (Schuh et al. 1995). Other situations where anticholinergics may be beneficial include the bronchospasm seen with beta-blockade, anxiety-induced asthmatic episodes, cough-variant asthma syndrome, and cough associated with asthma.

**PRINCIPLE Even when a type of drug is less effective than another first-line type, it may contribute significantly to overall clinical efficacy and lowered toxicity when utilized to produce a deliberate and rational drug interaction.**

**Key Point:** Ipratropium bromide may provide some additive benefit to inhaled $\beta_2$-agonists in severe asthma exacerbations. Their role in the treatment of chronic severe asthma appears to be limited.

Ipratropium nasal spray acts directly on secretory glands to decrease the production of nasal secretions, and it also has a mild decongestant effect. It will probably be used widely in the treatment of vasomotor rhinitis (Grossman et al. 1995).

### *Adverse effects*

Inhaled anticholinergics are generally well tolerated and there is no evidence for tolerance with continued use. When discontinued, a small rebound increase in bronchial responsiveness has been described, the clinical relevance of which is uncertain (Newcomb et al. 1985). Compared with atropine, which causes dryness of the mouth, blurred vision, and urinary retention, systemic adverse effects with inhaled ipratropium bromide are very uncommon because there is virtually no systemic absorption.

## Theophylline

### *Pharmacology and actions*

Theophylline, a methylxanthine, is related in structure to other xanthines such as caffeine and theobromine. Although it has been used for more than 50 years and is known to be a nonselective phosphodiesterase inhibitor, the mechanisms of action responsible for its bronchodilating action are still uncertain (Weinberger and Hendeles 1996). The longest held theory is that it inhibits phosphodiesterase (PDE), increasing intracellular cAMP, so that it results in airway smooth muscle relaxation. Several studies suggest that the drug also has anti-inflammatory effects (Sullivan et al. 1994; Kidney et al. 1995), including inhibition of inflammatory-cell mediator release. These studies indicate that it may have anti-inflammatory or immunomodulatory effects at doses lower than those required for bronchodilation, and this has led to its reevaluation for use in asthma (Barnes and Pauwels 1994). The drug also increases mucociliary clearance, diaphragmatic contractility, and central nervous system respiratory drive. In addition, it may also act as a pulmonary vasodilator. Other beneficial effects of theophylline include attenuation of the late-phase response to allergen (Pauwels et al. 1985), steroid-sparing effects, and improved exercise tolerance (Weinberger and Hendeles 1993).

Theophylline is an effective bronchodilator at serum concentrations of 10 to 20 mg/L. Below 10 mg/L, the improvements in airway function are small, and above 25 mg/L, adverse effects are common and potentially severe; the therapeutic range is therefore estimated as between 10 and 20 mg/L (Weinberger 1984). Consequently, it has a narrow therapeutic range which requires periodic monitoring of plasma concentrations in all patients taking the drug.

Theophylline is available in liquid, beaded capsules, and tablets, including sustained-release formulations that may be given at 8- to 24-hour intervals. Aminophylline, the amino-salt of theophylline, can be administered intravenously. The long-acting formulations make theophylline particularly useful for nocturnal manifestations of airway diseases. Theophylline is rapidly and completely absorbed, but there are large interindividual variations in clearance. Serum levels of theophylline are markedly affected by variations in hepatic metabolism among healthy individuals and also are affected by age, diet, disease states, smoking and drug interactions, all of which contribute to the complexity of using this medication. Many drugs, including cimetidine, oral contraceptives, macrolide antibiotics, and disulfiram can slow its metabolism. Phenytoin, carbamazepine, rifampin, and phenobarbital can increase the rate of its metabolism. The factors affecting theophylline clearance are summarized in Table 2-4.

### *Indications and clinical use*

Theophylline is less effective than inhaled or parenteral $\beta_2$-selective agonists in treating acute severe asthma. A meta-analysis of 13 controlled trials of aminophylline in severe acute asthma found insufficient evidence of benefit to recommend its use (Littenberg 1988).

Regular use of theophylline decreases the frequency and severity of asthmatic symptoms in patients with chronic asthma. It reduces the "as needed" use of inhaled $\beta$-adrenergic agonists (Weinberger and Bronsky 1974; Nassif et al. 1981) and of short courses of corticosteroids (Nassif et al. 1981; Brenner, et al. 1988; Duskieker et al. 1982), and prevents exercise-induced bronchoconstriction (Pollock et al. 1977; Magnussen et al. 1988). Sustained-release theophylline's main use is as adjunctive therapy, and it is particularly effective for controlling nocturnal symptoms of asthma (Barnes et al. 1982; Heins et al. 1988). Although theophylline is less effective than $\beta_2$-agonists and corticosteroids, a minority of asthmatic patients appear to derive clinically important benefit, and even patients on oral steroids may show deterioration in lung function when theophylline is withdrawn (Brenner, et al. 1988). A recent study also indicates additional benefit from adding low-dose theophylline for patients already taking 400 $\mu$g of inhaled budesonide twice daily (Evans et al. 1997). This benefit was evident in improvement in lung function and in a reduction in $\beta$-adrenergic agonist inhaler use.

**Table 2-4 Factors That Affect Theophylline Clearance.**

| |
|---|
| *Increased clearance* |
| Enzyme induction (by rifampicin, phenobarbital, ethanol, etc.) |
| Smoking tobacco, marijuana |
| High-protein, low-carbohydrate diet |
| Barbecued meat |
| Youth |
| *Decreased clearance* |
| Enzyme inhibition (by cimetidine, erythromycin, ciprofloxacin, etc.) |
| Congestive heart failure |
| Liver disease |
| Pneumonia |
| Viral infection and vaccination |
| High-carbohydrate diet |
| Old age |

### *Adverse effects*

Theophylline produces a number of dose-related adverse effects, such as nausea and vomiting, irritability, and insomnia. The gastrointestinal symptoms may be intolerable to some patients, even well within the therapeutic range. The frequency and severity of these adverse effects can be minimized by initiating therapy with a low-dose theophylline, and gradually increasing the dose to achieve therapeutic serum levels. Although the suggestion that theophylline might adversely affect school performance in children taking the drug raised widespread concern (Furukawa et al. 1984; Rachelefsky et al. 1986), subsequent studies have not substantiated this association (Bender et al. 1991; Bender and Milgrom 1992; Lindgren et al. 1992). Avoidance of the drug in children with previous behavior or school difficulties nonetheless seems reasonable. The adverse effects of theophylline are listed in Table 2-5.

Table 2-5 Adverse Effects of Theophylline

| |
|---|
| Nausea and vomiting |
| Gastrointestinal disturbance |
| Headache |
| Restlessness |
| Gastroesophageal reflux |
| Diuresis |
| Cardiac arrhythmias |
| Epileptic seizures |

## ANTI-INFLAMMATORY DRUGS

### Glucocorticoids

These potent anti-inflammatory agents are available in inhaled, oral, and intravenous forms. Neither oral nor intravenous administration causes immediate bronchodilation, and tests of airway caliber show significant improvement only after 6–12 hours (Ellul-Micallef and French 1975; Fanta et al. 1983). Inhaled corticosteroids (ICS) are currently the most potent and effective therapy available for long-term treatment of asthma, and they may also enhance the effects of inhaled $\beta$-agonists (Shenfield et al. 1975; Hui et al. 1982). When used at the recommended dosages and with a spacing device, they are predictably effective, safe, well tolerated, and have few systemic effects. Topical preparations can be used in the treatment of allergic rhinitis. Oral steroids are indicated in several other pulmonary diseases, such as sarcoidosis, interstitial lung diseases, and pulmonary eosinophilic syndromes.

#### *Background and pharmacology*

Corticosteroids were introduced to treat asthma shortly after they were discovered in the 1950s. However, the legitimate fear of adverse effects correctly limited the use of oral or parenteral preparations to the treatment of acute severe attacks of bronchoconstriction and of the rare patient with chronic, extremely severe asthma. Another reason for their slow acceptance was the prevailing belief that asthma primarily reflected disturbances in the function of the adrenergic and cholinergic nervous systems. Inhaled corticosteroids were first given to patients with severe asthma requiring treatment with an oral corticosteroid (Cameron et al. 1973; Gaddie, Petrie, et al. 1973; Gaddie, Reid, et al. 1973; Davies et al. 1977). They were subsequently used in patients in whom sympathomimetics and methylxanthines were ineffective (Siegel et al. 1985; Johnson 1987).

The results of clinical and pathologic studies of asthma in the 1980s gave impetus to their use in less severe asthma. Clinical studies showed that regular use of an inhaled corticosteroid, in contrast to regular use of an inhaled $\beta$-agonist, reduced bronchial reactivity—an effect that was both dose- and time-dependent (Kraan et al. 1985; Kerrebijn et al. 1987). Pathologic studies provided firm evidence that the bronchial mucosa from patients with mild asthma showed the same, highly characteristic pattern of infiltration with lymphocytes, eosinophils, and mast cells that had previously been reported in post mortem studies of asthma fatalities (Dunnill 1960; Laitinen et al. 1985; Djukanovic et al. 1990). Ongoing airway inflammation was demonstrated in allergic (Bradley et al. 1991), nonallergic (Bentley et al. 1992), aspirin-sensitive (Nasser et al. 1996), and occupational asthma (Saetta et al. 1992). These findings suggested that all forms of asthma are associated with airway mucosal inflammation and invited the speculation that prolonged application of an anti-inflammatory agent with the broad potency of a corticosteroid might act on a level fundamental to asthma's pathogenesis, and would thus constitute a "disease-modifying" treatment effect, as opposed to regular use of inhaled $\beta$-agonists, regarded as offering only symptom relief from transient bronchodilation. Indeed, inhaled corticosteroids are currently considered first-line therapy for all but the mildest cases.

#### *Chemistry*

Cortisone, or the active form hydrocortisone (cortisol), was the first glucocorticoid found effective for the treatment of asthma. Modification of the structure of hydrocortisone resulted in derivatives such as prednisolone and dexamethasone, which are highly effective when given systemically for asthma. All anti-inflammatory steroids have a common 2-carbon chain at the 17 position and methyl groups at carbons 18 and 19 (Fig. 2-2). Further substitution at the 17$\alpha$ ester position resulted in a new group of extremely potent steroids (e.g., beclomethasone dipropionate, betamethasone, and budesonide; see Fig. 2-2), which are effective when given topically for skin diseases, and effective when given by inhalation for treating asthma. Substitution of acetyl groups at carbons 16 and 17 led to the formation of triamcinolone acetonide and flunisolide. A relatively new and highly potent glucocorticoid for inhalation use is fluticasone propionate, which has a 17 carbon propionate substitution and a 21 carbon thiofluoromethyl ester. Fluticasone also has two fluorine substitutions at carbons 6 and 9 (Phillips 1990). Although numerous in vitro and ex vivo models have been used to compare the potencies of these various inhaled glucocorticoids, comparative clinical efficacy and safety data are still limited. Drawing on the data that has been published, recent asthma treatment guidelines suggest that the order of potency of current agents is fluticasone > budesonide = beclomethasone > flunisolide = triamcinolone (National Asthma Education and Prevention Program Expert Panel 1997a and 1997b; The British Guidelines on Asthma Management, 1995 and 1997).

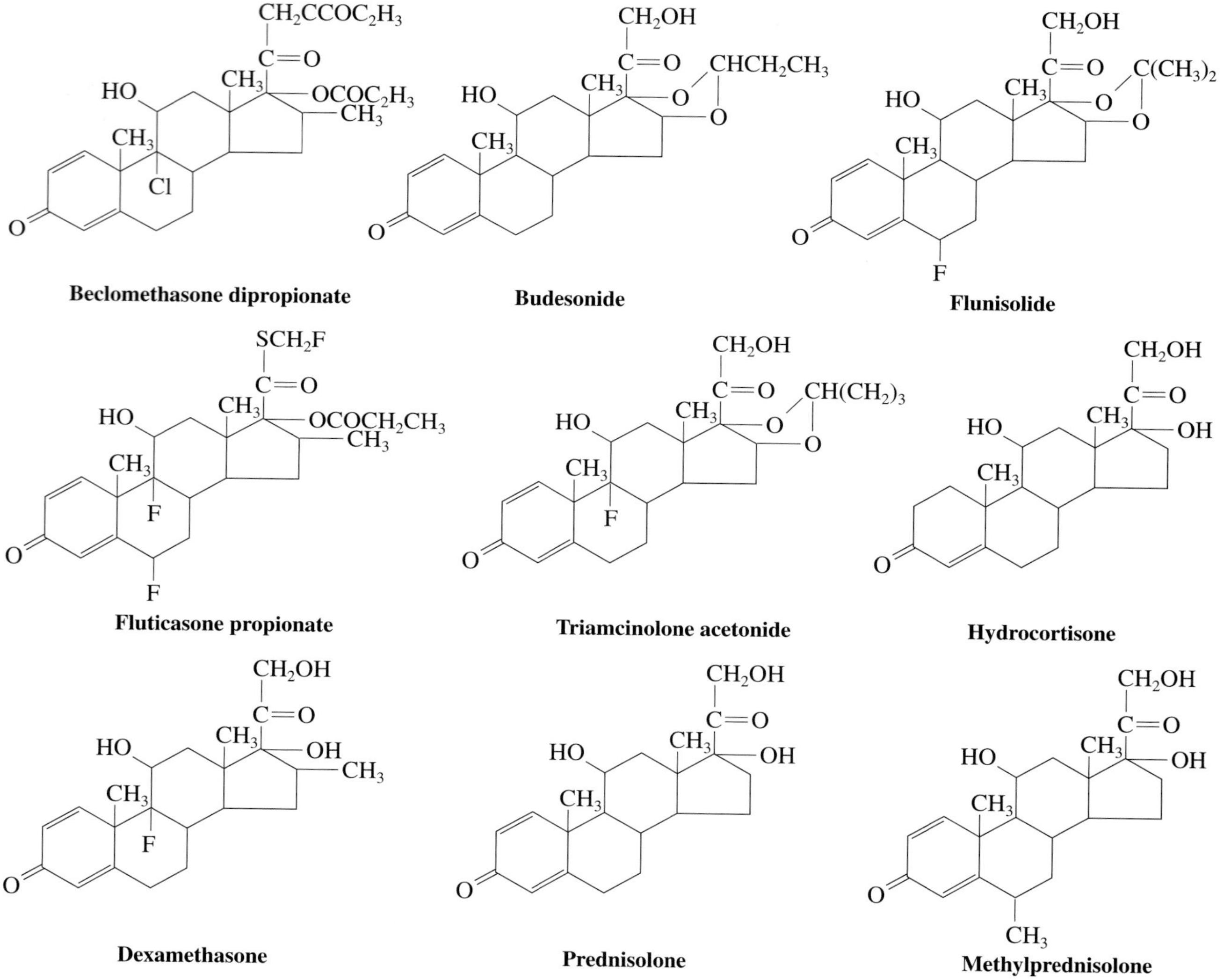

**Beclomethasone dipropionate** **Budesonide** **Flunisolide**

**Fluticasone propionate** **Triamcinolone acetonide** **Hydrocortisone**

**Dexamethasone** **Prednisolone** **Methylprednisolone**

FIGURE 2-2 **The structures of newer inhaled corticosteroids are compared with that of hydrocortisone.**

The critical question is not the relative potencies of the different agents, however. It is rather their relative therapeutic ratios, that is, the ratios of local anti-inflammatory action in the airway mucosa to systemic absorption and toxicity. An early hope in the development of fluticasone, for example, was that its risks of systemic toxicity would be lower because of the complete first-pass metabolism in the liver of any drug absorbed from the GI tract (Thorsson et al. 1997). Reevaluation of this hopeful expectation has been made necessary by the realization of the importance of absorption into the circulation from the bronchial and alveolar surfaces. Whether the increases in therapeutic potency are offset by similar increases in systemic toxicity is actively debated, but resolution of the question will have to await careful trials comparing the therapeutic efficacy and the systemic toxicity of different inhaled corticosteroids.

### *Mechanisms of action*

The efficacy of glucocorticoids is related to many factors, including diminution of inflammatory cell numbers and activity, stabilization of vascular leakage, reduction in mucus production, and an increase in $\beta$-adrenergic responsiveness. Despite the seemingly diverse effects on different physiologic systems, corticosteroids mediate their effects by their influence on the cellular production of proteins, either by directly or indirectly regulating the transcription of certain target genes (Truss and Beato 1993). The steroid molecule first enters cells, then binds to specific glucocorticoid receptors in the cytoplasm to form an active glucocorticoid–receptor complex; this complex then translocates into the nucleus. Here the active complex associates with DNA and alters nuclear gene expression, leading to the synthesis of messenger RNA (mRNA) and the translation of certain proteins (Fig. 2-3). One such protein is lipocortin which inhibits phospholipase $A_2$, leading to inhibition of production of such arachidonic acid metabolites such as prostaglandins, leukotrienes, and platelet-activating factor. Stimulation of protein production may account for corticosteroid enhancement of the expression of neutral endopeptidase, an enzyme that degrades bronchoconstrictor and inflammatory peptides such as bradykinin, and tachykinins.

Corticosteroids also act to inhibit the production of some proinflammatory proteins, like various cytokines (summarized below), lipid mediators (Mitchell et al. 1994), nitric oxide (Robbins et al. 1994), and adhesion molecules (Van De Stolpe et al. 1993). The cellular mechanism appears to involve inhibition of the expression of inducible genes in airway epithelial cells by blocking key transcription factors, such as nuclear factor-6κB and activator protein-1 (Barnes and Adcock 1993). The cells in

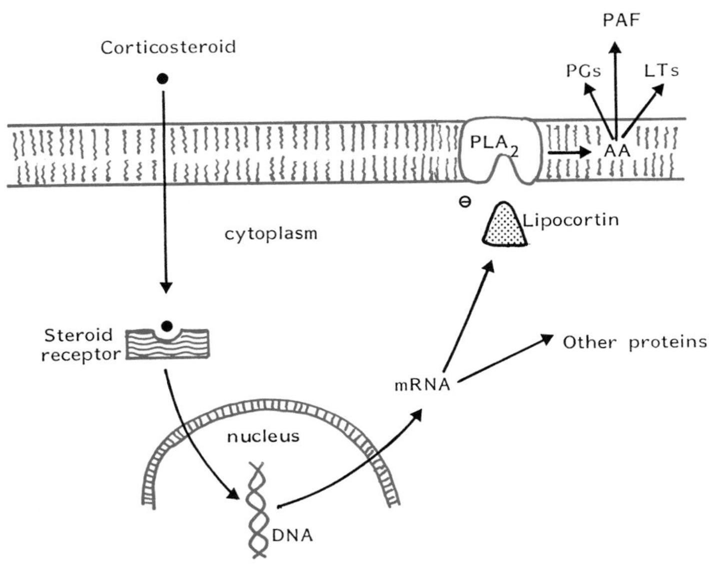


FIGURE 2-3 **Molecular mechanisms of steroid action. Corticosteroids bind to a cytoplasmic glucocorticoid receptor that interacts with steroid-responsive elements of DNA. This leads to the transcription of mRNA, and translation of certain proteins. One such protein is lipocortin, which inhibits phospholipase $A_2$ ($PLA_2$), thus leading to inhibition of formation of prostaglandins (PGs), leukotrienes (LTs), and platelet-activating factor (PAF). Several other proteins, which have not yet been well characterized, are also induced.**

which these effects are most important are probably epithelial cells, mast cells, macrophages, T lymphocytes, dendritic cells, and eosinophils (Schleimer 1990).

***Effects on cytokines***

Inhaled corticosteroids decrease the number of mast cells, eosinophils, and submucosal T lymphocytes in bronchial biopsy specimens from patients with mild or moderate asthma. Study of bronchoalveolar lavage fluid indicates that oral corticosteroid therapy reduces mRNA expression of interleukins IL-4 and IL-5 and granulocyte-macrophage colony-stimulating factor (GM-CSF) and increases the number of cells expressing mRNA for interferon-$\gamma$ (Adelroth et al. 1990; Duddridge et al. 1993; Wilson et al. 1994; Schwiebert et al. 1996). The number of activated T cells in bronchoalveolar lavage fluid is also reduced. These effects on cytokines and inflammatory cells may be responsible for the potent anti-inflammatory action.

***Effect on β-adrenergic receptors***

Corticosteroids potentiate the effects of $\beta$-adrenergic agonists on bronchial smooth muscle, and they appear also to prevent $\beta$-adrenergic-receptor downregulation and therefore tachyphylaxis to $\beta$-adrenergic agonists in airways in vivo (Mak et al. 1995). Systemic corticosteroid treatment, for example, prevents the reduction in the bronchodilator response to albuterol otherwise caused by chronic treatment with formoterol (Tan et al. 1997, 1998). Corticosteroids have also been shown to upregulate $\beta$-adrenergic receptors in human lung (Mak et al. 1996), but whether this effect contributes to their efficacy in asthma is still uncertain.

**PRINCIPLE Drugs can produce their beneficial effects on the basis of multiple and different mechanisms, including unexpected but beneficial drug interactions.**

***Routes of administration***

**INHALED** Several inhaled preparations are available, including beclomethasone dipropionate (BDP), triamcinolone, flunisolide, budesonide, and fluticasone. Inhalation permits control of symptoms without causing significant systemic effects. The recommended doses vary with different preparations because of differences in the amount of medication dispensed per actuation (Table 2-6). At current recommended doses, effects on the hypothalamic–pituitary–adrenal (HPO) axis are minimal, but use of higher doses causes a dose-dependent effect on the HPO axis (Prahl et al. 1987). In most patients, it is hard to show additional clinical benefit from giving doses higher than 400–800 $\mu$g/day of BDP, but some patients may benefit from higher doses (up to 2000 $\mu$g/day of fluticasone (Noonan et al. 1995). Twice-daily administration usually is effective and enhances compliance (Meltzer et al. 1985).

**ORAL** Oral prednisolone and prednisone are the most commonly used oral corticosteroids. They are indicated for use as short-term (7–10 days) burst therapy for exacerbations of asthma and of chronic obstructive bronchitis, and to prevent exacerbations in patients experiencing falls in peak flow or worsening of symptoms requiring frequent $\beta$-agonist inhalation (Harris et al. 1987). They are also used for long-term prevention of symptoms in severe persistent asthma and COPD and for severe, progressive diffuse pulmonary fibrosis. In all instances, the lowest effective dose should be used. Consideration must also be given to coexisting conditions that could be worsened by systemic corticosteroids, such as infection with herpes, varicella, or tuberculosis; hypertension; peptic ulcer disease; and osteoporosis. In asthma, if daily doses are required, efficacy may be improved without an increase in adrenal suppression by delivering the drug at 3 P.M. rather than in the morning (Beam et al. 1992).

**PRINCIPLE The schedule of drug administration may significantly alter both the efficacy and the toxicity of the drug.**

**INTRAVENOUS** Severe acute asthma ("status asthmaticus") and acute exacerbations of chronic obstructive bronchitis are treated with high-dose systemic glucocorticoids combined with frequent nebulization with $\beta$-adrenergic bronchodilator agents. In these circumstances methylprednisolone sodium succinate (1 mg/kg every 6–12 hours) or hydrocortisone sodium succinate (3–4 mg/kg every 6–12 hours) may be administered intravenously (Haskell et al. 1983), but because prednisone and methylprednisolone are well absorbed, oral therapy is equally effective for patients able to take therapy by mouth. Following resolution of severe obstruction, the steroid dose is reduced over 10 to 14 days.

***Indications and clinical use***

Corticosteroids have had a great impact on the management of asthma and are highly effective in altering many of the known clinical consequences of asthma (Barnes 1995a) (see Table 2-7). Intravenous or oral treatment is essential for acute, severe exacerbations; regular oral therapy is sometimes necessary for control of chronic severe asthma, and inhaled therapy is established as the most

**Table 2-6 Estimated Comparative Daily Dosages for Inhaled Corticosteroids**

| Drug | Low Dose | Medium Dose | High Dose |
|---|---|---|---|
| *Adults* | | | |
| Beclomethasone dipropionate | 168–504 μg | 504–840 μg | >840 μg |
| 42 μg/puff | (4–12 puffs — 42 μg) | (12–20 puffs — 42 μg) | (>20 puffs — 42 μg) |
| 84 μg/puff | (2–6 puffs — 84 μg) | (6–10 puffs — 84 μg) | (>10 puffs — 84 μg) |
| Budesonide | 200–400 μg | 400–600μg | >600 μg |
| DPI: 200 μg/dose | (1–2 inhalations) | (2–3 inhalations) | (>3 inhalations) |
| Flunisolide | 500–1,000 μg | 1,000–2,000 μg | >2,000 μg |
| 250 μg/puff | (2–4 puffs) | (4–8 puffs) | (>8 puffs) |
| Fluticasone propionate | 86–264 μg | 264–660 μg | >660 μg |
| MDI: 44, 110, 220 μg/puff | (2–6 puffs — 44 μg) OR | (2–6 puffs — 110 μg) | (>6 puffs — 110 μg) OR |
| | (2 puffs — 100 μg) | | (>3 puffs — 220 μg) |
| DPI: 50, 100, 250 μg/dose | (2–6 inhalations — 50 μg) | (3–6 inhalations — 100 μg) | (>6 inhalations — 100 μg) OR |
| | | (>2 inhalations — 250 μg) | |
| Triamcinolone acetonide | 400–1,000 μg | 1,000–2,000 μg | >2,000 μg |
| 100 μg/puff | (4–10 puffs) | (10–20 puffs) | (>20 puffs) |
| *Children* | | | |
| Beclomethasone dipropionate | 84–336 μg | 336–672 μg | >672 μg |
| 42 μg/puff | (2–8 puffs — 42 μg) | (8–16 puffs — 42 μg) | (>16 puffs — 42 μg) |
| 84 μg/puff | (1–4 puffs — 84 μg) | (4–8 puffs — 84 μg) | (>8 puffs — 84 μg) |
| Budesonide | 100–200 μg | 200–400 μg | >400 μg |
| DPI: 200 μg/dose | | (1–2 inhalations — 200 μg) | (>2 inhalations — 200 μg) |
| Flunisolide | 500–750 μg | >1,000–1,250 μg | 1,250 μg |
| 250 μg/puff | (2–3 puffs) | (4–5 puffs) | (>5 puffs) |
| Fluticasone propionate | 88–176 μg | 176–440 μg | >440 μg |
| MDI: 44, 110, 220 μg/puff | (2–4 puffs — 44 μg) | (4–10 puffs — 44 μg) OR | (>4 puffs — 110 μg) OR |
| | | (2–4 puffs — 110 μg) | (>2 puffs — 220 μg) |
| DPI: 50, 100, 250 μg/dose | (2–4 inhalations — 50 μg) | (2–4 inhalations — 100 μg) | (>4 inhalations — 100 μg) OR |
| | | | (>2 inhalations — 250 μg) |
| Triamcinolone acetonide | 400–800 μg | 800–1,200 μg | >1,200 μg |
| 100 μg/puff | (4–8 puffs) | (8–12 puffs) | (>12 puffs) |

ABBREVIATIONS: DPI, dry powder inhaler; MDI, metered-dose inhaler.

**The most important determinant of appropriate dosing is the clinician's judgment of the patient's response to therapy.** The clinician must monitor the patient's response on several clinical parameters and must adjust the dose accordingly. The stepwise approach to therapy emphasizes that, once control of asthma is achieved, the dose of medication should be carefully titrated to the minimum dose required to maintain control, thus reducing the potential for adverse effect.

The reference point for the range in the dosages for children is based on data on the safety of inhaled corticosteroids in children, which, in general, suggest that the dose ranges are equivalent to beclomethasone dipropionate 200–400 μg/day (low dose), 400–800 μg/day (medium dose), and >800 μg/day (high dose).

Some dosages may be outside package labeling.

Metered-dose inhaler (MDI) dosages are expressed as the actuator dose (the amount of drug leaving the actuator and delivered to the patient), which is the labeling required in the United States. This is different from the dosage expressed as the valve dose (the amount of the drug leaving the valve, all of which is not available to the patient), which is used in many European countries and in some of the scientific literature. Dry powder inhaler (DPI) doses are expressed as the amount of drug in the inhaler following activation.

effective known maintenance or "long-term controller" therapy for the disease. Corticosteroids also are effective in some patients with chronic obstructive bronchitis, and determining the "steroid-responsiveness" of airflow obstruction is important for developing a therapeutic plan. Oral corticosteroids are important in the treatment of infiltrative diseases of the lung parenchyma, like sarcoidosis and diffuse interstitial fibrosis.

### *Adverse effects*

The local adverse effects of inhaled corticosteroids include oropharyngeal candidiasis that occurs in <10% of patients (Rinehart et al. 1975). Use of a spacer/holding chamber and rinsing the mouth after inhalation reduces the incidence of colonization and of clinical infection. Hoarseness and weakness of voice (dysphonia) also may occur, possibly due to atrophy of the vocal cords. The

**Table 2-7 Effects of Inhaled Corticosteroids on the Clinical Consequences of Asthma**

| |
|---|
| *Established effects* |
| Reduction or elimination of need for systemic corticosteroids |
| Reduction of asthmatic symptoms and exacerbations |
| Improvement of lung function (spirometry, peak flow readings) |
| Reduction in diurnal variation in lung function |
| Decrease in need for rescue bronchodilators |
| Reduction in nocturnal awakenings from asthma |
| Improvement of quality of life indices |
| *Other (probable/possible) effects* |
| Reduction in hospitalization and death |
| Reduction in rate of decline in lung function |
| Increase in likelihood of sustained remission of asthma |

incidence of these adverse effects may be related to the local concentrations of steroid and may be reduced by the use of various spacing devices (Toogood et al. 1984).

The systemic adverse effects associated with long-term corticosteroid therapy are well described and include fluid retention, increased appetite and weight gain, osteoporosis, capillary fragility, hypertension, peptic ulceration, hyperglycemia, and psychosis. Two toxicities once thought not to occur from the use of inhaled corticosteroids alone but that have been associated with use of high doses by elderly patients are glaucoma and cataracts (Cumming et al. 1997; Garbe et al. 1997). Very occasionally adverse reactions (such as anaphylaxis) to IV hydrocortisone have been described, particularly in aspirin-sensitive asthmatics (Dajani et al. 1981).

**PRINCIPLE The pattern, frequency, and severity of adverse effects caused by a drug often may relate to the characteristics of the patient taking the drug.**

### *Adrenal suppression*

Steroids inhibit adrenocorticotrophic hormone (ACTH) and cortisol secretion by a negative feedback effect on the pituitary gland (hypothalamic pituitary axis function), and this suppression is dose-dependent, typically occurring at doses of prednisone greater than 7.5 mg/day. Significant suppression after short courses of steroid therapy is not usually a problem, but prolonged suppression may occur after longer periods of time and doses must therefore be reduced slowly.

### *Linear growth*

Because growth in children with asthma may be influenced by many factors (steroid therapy, severity of the asthma, atopy, and gender), evaluating the effects of systemic or inhaled corticosteroids on growth in children with asthma has been challenging and has led to sometimes contradictory findings. A recent meta-analysis of the influence of inhaled beclomethasone in the attainment of expected adult height did not find any significant adverse effects (Allen et al. 1994). Other studies have identified some growth delay in those treated with inhaled corticosteroids, suggesting that some caution may be prudent until this important issue is studied further.

**PRINCIPLE Careful meta-analysis should provoke thinking about the examined subject but does not provide definitive information.**

The local and systemic adverse effects of inhaled steroids are summarized in Table 2-8.

## Cromolyn Sodium and Nedocromil

These drugs have proven efficacy as maintenance therapy for mild asthma and have very little toxicity, but their principal mechanism of action is poorly understood. Cromolyn sodium (sodium cromoglycate) is a derivative of khellin, an Egyptian herbal remedy which was found to protect against allergen challenge but to have no direct bronchodilator action. It is classified as a chromone. Nedocromil sodium is a newer prophylactic drug that has a profile of activity similar to that of cromolyn sodium.

**Table 2-8 Adverse Effects of Inhaled Corticosteroids**

| |
|---|
| *Local adverse effects* |
| Hoarseness (dysphonia) |
| Oropharyngeal candidiasis |
| Throat irritation and cough (due to additives) |
| *Systemic adverse effects* |
| Adrenal suppression |
| Effects on growth in children |
| Weight gain, truncal obesity |
| Dermal thinning, easy skin bruising |
| Cataracts, glaucoma |
| Increased bone turnover, osteoporosis |
| Hypertension, hyperglycemia |
| Peptic ulceration |
| Mood changes, psychosis |
| Disseminated *Varicella* infection |

*Mode of action*

Cromolyn was initially thought to act by stabilizing mast cells, inhibiting mediator release. This action has indeed been demonstrated in murine mast cells, but has been difficult to establish as its in vivo mechanism in humans. Nedocromil is structurally dissimilar to cromolyn but has similar effects in inhibiting the airway responses to challenge with exercise, sulfur dioxide, etc., and the early and late airway responses to antigen (Gonzales and Brogden 1987; Thompson 1989; Novembre et al. 1994; Alton and Norris 1996). Recent evidence suggests that these drugs may block swelling-dependent chloride channels (Heinke et al. 1995), and thus modulate mast cell mediator release and eosinophil recruitment (Eady 1986) or the function of sensory nerves in the airway mucosa. Whatever their precise mechanism of action, their effect is prophylactic, preventing the development of bronchospasm; they do not reverse bronchospasm once it has developed.

*Indications and clinical use*

These drugs are best used as maintenance, preventive therapies for asthma, and they have been shown to improve symptoms, frequency of $\beta$-agonist use, and peak flow in groups of patients (Lal et al. 1993; Schwartz et al. 1996). Their clinical efficacy in individual subjects is variable. They appear to work most consistently in young allergic asthmatics, but many adults with mild asthma also respond (Petty et al. 1989). Dosing recommendations for both drugs are for administration four times a day, although nedocromil has been shown to be clinically effective with twice daily dosing (Creticos et al. 1995). Both are also effective when used 20 minutes before exercise or to an unavoidable allergen exposure (e.g., in animal handlers). Some pediatricians believe that sodium cromoglycate is often the anti-inflammatory drug of first choice in children because it has almost no short-term or long-term adverse effects. It must be delivered by inhalation, as a dry powder, by MDI, or by nebulization.

## OTHER ANTIALLERGY DRUGS

### Ketotifen

Ketotifen is also used in the prophylactic treatment of asthma (Martin and Bagglionlini 1981). One of its prominent effects is antagonism of the histamine receptor $H_1$, an effect which may account for its sedative properties in some patients. It may also act as a membrane stabilizer inhibiting cellular degranulation and histamine release. Controlled studies show both effectiveness and ineffectiveness of ketotifen in asthma. A long-term, placebo-controlled trial of oral ketotifen in children with mild asthma showed no clinical benefit (Loftus and Price 1987). In another study, asthmatic children were able to decrease their oral dose of theophylline with less worsening of symptoms and to have less bronchial hyperreactivity with ketotifen therapy (Sole et al. 1992). The largest, double-blind, placebo-controlled study evaluating ketotifen in atopic asthmatics was conducted in 445 patients. At a dose of 1 mg twice a day, ketotifen enabled reduction of concomitant medication use without increasing symptoms or decreasing pulmonary function (Burns 1985). Overall, ketotifen appears to be an effective adjunctive treatment for asthma in patients above 6 years of age.

### Antihistamines

Some of the early clinical trials that examined the effects of oral $H_1$ antihistamines in asthma found little benefit (Levy and Seabury 1947; Schuller 1983). These earlier trials used first-generation sedating antihistamines that have anticholinergic and antiserotonergic adverse effects. Because the anticholinergic adverse effects were thought to impair mucus secretion, antihistamines were once thought even to be relatively contraindicated in patients with asthma. More recent studies utilizing newer second-generation, nonsedating antihistamines, however, suggest that they actually benefit asthmatic patients. Some act as mild bronchodilators. For example, 20 mg of cetirizine has a bronchodilator action additive to that of albuterol in subjects who had a forced expired volume in one second ($FEV_1$) of 50–80% of the predicted value (Spector et al. 1995). At the very least, it is clear that the new, nonsedating antihistamines do not adversely affect asthma, and they may be useful adjuncts to asthma therapy. Antihistamine treatment of upper respiratory symptoms in patients with concomitant allergic rhinitis and asthma may facilitate the treatment of lower airway symptoms.

> **PRINCIPLE The class name of a drug often does not describe the complete effects of its members. Global decisions about use of a class of drugs for an indication are rarely valid.**

### Mast Cell Stabilizers

Almost 40 drugs were developed as mast cell stabilizers in the past (Church 1978). In vitro, these drugs inhibit the release of mediators from mast cells triggered by allergens. All of them have been disappointing in tests of their efficacy for treatment of clinical asthma. None has become available for clinical use.

### Leukotriene Modifiers

Leukotrienes are biologically active fatty acids derived from the oxidative metabolism of arachidonic acid, an integral part of the cell membrane. These potent mediators are released from mast cells, eosinophils, and basophils, and their actions include contraction of airway smooth muscle, increase in vascular permeability, increase in mucus secretions, and attraction and activation of inflammatory cells. The cellular sources and actions of leukotrienes made them candidates for participation in the pathogenesis of asthma and led to the development of leukotriene modifiers—inhibitors of leukotriene production (5-lipoxygenase inhibitors), and antagonists of leukotriene binding to cell surface receptors (LT-receptor antagonists) (Henderson 1994).

Zafirlukast and montelukast, LT-receptor antagonists, and zileuton, a 5-lipoxygenase (5-LO) inhibitor, have been recently approved by the US Food and Drug Administration (FDA) for the treatment of asthma. All are prepared as oral formulations, and all are classified as alternative controller medications for the treatment of mild persistent asthma (National Asthma Education and Prevention Program Expert Panel 1997a and 1997b). The LT-receptor antagonists attenuate the acute airway response to allergen (Taylor et al. 1991) and exercise challenge (Finnerty et al. 1992), and improve control of asthma when taken chronically (Reiss et al. 1996, 1998). A study comparing zafirlukast with placebo in patients who had mild-to-moderate asthma demonstrated that patients treated with the drug experienced modest improvement in $FEV_1$ (mean improvement of 11% above placebo), improved symptom scores, and reduced albuterol use (average decline of one puff/day) (Spector et al. 1994). LT-receptor antagonists have also been shown to enable reduction of inhaled corticosteroids in moderately severe asthma (Leff et al. 1997). Zileuton, the 5-LO inhibitor, also inhibits exercise-induced bronchospasm, produces prompt and sustained improvements in $FEV_1$ (mean increase of 15%), and reduces the frequency of exacerbations requiring oral corticosteroids (Israel et al. 1993, 1996). A theme of clinical studies of leukotriene modifiers is that a wide range of responses is seen among individuals, with no obvious clinical feature enabling prediction of benefit, with the exception of the small subgroup of asthmatics who have anaphylaxis-like reactions to nonsteroidal anti-inflammatory drugs (NSAIDs), like aspirin. In these patients, leukotriene modifiers effectively blunt the response to aspirin challenge (Christie et al. 1991; Dahlen et al. 1993).

Because zileuton may produce liver toxicity, hepatic enzymes (e.g., ALT) should be monitored in patients taking the medication. Zafirlukast is less likely to cause hepatic inflammation and does not require such monitoring. Both drugs are metabolized in the liver, and interfere with the cytochrome P450 isoenzymes. Hence, zafirlukast can interfere with warfarin metabolism, and zileuton interferes with warfarin, theophylline, and terfenadine metabolism. Cases of pulmonary eosinophilic vasculitis (Churg-Strauss syndrome) have been reported in patients with severe asthma soon after initiating therapy with zafirlukast. It appears that this might not be related to the drug itself, but rather to the reduction in systemic corticosteroids that it permitted, "unmasking" the syndrome in patients in whom it had previously been suppressed (Wechsler et al. 1998).

**PRINCIPLE Drug interactions come in many forms. Sometimes sparing a potentially toxic drug can unmask unsuspected disease.**

The leukotriene modifiers present the advantages of oral efficacy and of little apparent toxicity. They do not appear to be as potent, or as predictably effective as inhaled corticosteroids in chronic, maintenance treatment of asthma. Their final place in asthma management awaits more extensive clinical experience with their efficacy and toxicity as long-term controller therapy for chronic asthma.

## OTHER THERAPIES

### Immunosuppressants

Immunosuppressive therapy is most used for treating diseases of the lung interstitium in which immunologic pathogenetic mechanisms are implicated, like sarcoidosis, diffuse interstitial fibrosis, and the pulmonary vasculitides. The details of these drugs are covered in chapter 10, Connective Tissue and Bone Disorders, and chapter 12, Hematologic Disorders. Some immunosuppressant drugs, like methotrexate, gold, and cyclosporine have been examined as treatments for severe, prednisone-dependent asthma, with varying degrees of success, probably depending on the care with which conditions known to exacerbate asthma were diagnosed and treated (e.g., chronic sinusitis, gastro-esophageal reflux, vocal cord dysfunction) and with which patient understanding of, and adherence to, regular use of standard therapies was ensured (Muranaka et al. 1978; Klaustermeyer et al. 1987; Mullarkey et al. 1988; Shiner et al. 1990; Alexander et al. 1992; Trigg and Davies 1993; Coffey et al. 1994; Nizankowska et al. 1995; Lock et al. 1996).

## Drugs That Act on Mucus

Agents that affect mucus have been in use since antiquity (Ziment 1989c). Clinical trials evaluating the utility of these agents, however, have been difficult for several reasons (Task Group on Mucoactive Drugs 1994). First, there are no clearly accepted valid means to quantify cough or sputum production. Second, it is likely that patients may cough and produce sputum for a variety of reasons, and there are no current guidelines for matching patients to the various classes of agents available.

Secretogogues that stimulate the secretion of ions and fluid can result in thinning of airway secretions. Although this may increase the volume of secretions, expectoration may be made easier. It is likely that iodides work in this manner (Ziment 1989d). Two clinical trials with iodinated glycerol suggested a small but significant improvement in symptoms in patients with COPD (Petty 1990; Repsher 1993). A third trial was unable to confirm this result (Rubin et al. 1996). A similar action has been suggested for ambroxol (Zavattini et al. 1989) and bromhexine (Zuliani et al. 1989), and a similar effect may also be achieved through reflex vagal stimulation induced by a number of expectorants (Ziment 1989b). The diuretic amiloride has also been demonstrated to increase the secretions of ions and fluid, thus thinning airway secretions (Knowles et al. 1990).

*N*-Acetylcysteine and related compounds that have active thiol groups have been suggested to function as mucolytics by virtue of their ability to break disulfide bonds (Colombo et al. 1989; Guffanti et al. 1989; Ventresca et al. 1989; Ziment 1989a). These agents can also function directly as antioxidants and some, such as *N*-acetylcysteine, can enter cells and restore depleted glutathione levels. Although clinical trials with these agents have demonstrated some benefits (Multicenter Study Group 1980), these have usually examined outcomes that are difficult to quantify.

Large quantities of DNA released from necrotic inflammatory cells in the airways can contribute to sputum viscosity, and recombinant human DNase is administered via inhalation to degrade DNA and to improve airway clearance (Shak et al. 1990). Small, but significant, benefits have been observed in patients with cystic fibrosis (Hubbard et al. 1992). Early reports of benefits in patients with chronic bronchitis have not been repeated (Fick et al. 1994), perhaps because DNA content of sputum is lower in chronic bronchitis. DNase is not currently approved for use in chronic bronchitis. One report has suggested that administration of surfactant improves lung function in patients with chronic bronchitis (Anzueto et al. 1997).

Mucoactive agents are not widely used by physicians in the United States (American Thoracic Society 1995). Although some are popular in certain European countries, they are not strongly recommended in the European Respiratory Society guidelines (Siafakas et al. 1995). Nevertheless, it is likely that patients will continue to use such agents, often from nonprescription sources.

**PRINCIPLE Over-the-counter remedies and alternative approaches are likely to be popular with patients when conventional medicine offers little effective therapy.**

### Expectorants

A variety of agents, most often part of traditional pharmacopoeias, have been used as expectorants (Ziment 1989c, 1989e). Many may act as local irritants in the airways or the GI tract, stimulating cough by vagal reflex. Similar mechanisms may lead to thinning of sputum through increased secretion of ions and water. Guaifenesin, ipecac, and benzoin, among others, may have such actions. No general guidelines are available for their use.

### Antitussives

Cough is a complex reflex that can originate from peripheral or central stimuli. Unlike other pulmonary reflexes like sneezing and yawning, cough may be initiated at will. Recurrent or persistent cough may reflect recurrent or persistent disease of the lungs and airways, but also occurs in other conditions, like gastroesophageal reflux and chronic sinusitis. Careful diagnosis is essential before empirical use of long-term treatments.

Peripheral cough receptors are sensitive to local anesthetics, and topical application of agents such as lidocaine or cocaine are routinely used to inhibit cough during bronchoscopy (Pneumology Task Group on BAL 1992). Benzonatate, administered orally, has been suggested to suppress cough by a similar action (Mongan and Culling 1992). Central cough receptors are suppressed by opiates and antitussives such as dextromethorphan (Kamei 1996).

Although suppression of cough may relieve symptoms acutely, cough is an important defense mechanism, and chronic use of antitussives is not recommended in the routine management chronic lung disease (American Thoracic Society 1995; Siafakas et al. 1995).

## Opioids

Opioids are effective inhibitors of cough and may provide relief from sensation of dyspnea and the associated anxiety (Light et al. 1989). Promethazine (Woodcock et al. 1981) and possibly buspirone (Argyropoulou et al. 1993; Singh et al. 1993) may have a similar effect. Benzodiazepines are not effective (Woodcock et al. 1981). Reduced perception of dyspnea may be associated with improved exercise performance (Light et al. 1996), but this has not been uniformly observed. Opioids likely affect perception of dyspnea centrally; no benefit was observed from their administration by the inhaled route (Beauford et al. 1993; Maswood et al. 1995; Leung and Burdon 1996). Since opioids may be associated with respiratory depression, their use as palliatives must be balanced against the risk of causing respiratory failure. Combinations of morphine with promethazine or prochlorperazine may potentiate the dyspnea relieving effect while minimizing respiratory suppression (Light et al. 1996).

## Respiratory Stimulants

Doxapram is a respiratory stimulant approved for use in the United States for reversal of hypoventilation induced by drugs, including general anesthetics, and also for hypercapnia secondary to COPD. Almitrine is a similar agent used in Europe (Connaughton et al. 1985; Winkelmann et al. 1994). Both are believed to increase alveolar ventilation by stimulating peripheral chemoreceptors. A direct action of almitrine on the pulmonary circulation has also been suggested (Saadjiian et al. 1993). Although increasing ventilation may slightly improve blood gases, the increased work of breathing is associated with increased dyspnea (Connaughton et al. 1985; Winkelmann et al. 1994). For this reason, and because of unwanted side effects, neither agent is recommended for routine use in chronic management of COPD (American Thoracic Society 1995; Siafakas et al. 1995). Its proposed uses are limited, as for reversal of acute hypoventilation when prompt intubation is not possible (Kerr 1997). The proposed use of doxapram as an aid to weaning in neonates was not supported by the results of a clinical trial (Barrington and Muttitt 1998), but it may have some use in treating the idiopathic apnea associated with prematurity (Bairam et al. 1992).

## Oxygen

Administration of supplemental oxygen can be lifesaving both in acute respiratory failure and in the management of chronic lung disease. There are several sources of oxygen. In general, oxygen concentrators that require only electricity are the most convenient for home use, but liquid oxygen systems and compressed gas cylinders have advantages in some settings. Oxygen may be given through nasal prongs, masks, transtracheal catheters and endotracheal tubes, with the selection of delivery system determined by the clinical condition of the patient.

Two large controlled prospective studies have demonstrated that chronic use of supplemental oxygen improves survival in patients with COPD and an arterial $P_{O_2}$ <55 Torr (Nocturnal Oxygen Therapy Trial Group 1980; Medical Research Council [MRC]: Medical Research Council Working Party 1981). The target $P_{O_2}$ of 70 Torr is generally achieved with 2 L of nasal oxygen per minute. Improved survival is also suggested in other forms of chronic hypoxic lung disease, and use of oxygen is routine for similar degrees of hypoxemia in these settings (Chailleux et al. 1996). With milder degrees of hypoxemia, the benefits of supplemental oxygen are less clear, so the treatment is recommended only if clinical complications related to hypoxemia are present, such as pulmonary hypertension and polycythemia. Intermittent use of supplemental oxygen is rarely prescribed, except in patients known to develop significant hypoxemia with certain activities, like exercise or sleep. Guidelines for the use of long-term oxygen therapy have been developed (Tiep 1991; American Thoracic Society 1995; Siafakas et al. 1995).

## REFERENCES

Abisheganaden J, Boushey HA. 1998. Long-acting inhaled beta 2-agonists and the loss of "bronchoprotective" efficacy. *Am J Med* **104**:494–7.

Adelroth E, Rosenhall L, Johansson S-A, et al. 1990. Inflammatory cells and eosinophilic activity in asthmatics investigated by bronchoalveolar lavage. *Am Rev Respir Dis* **142**:91–9.

Alexander AG, Barnes NC, Kay AB. 1992. Trial of cyclosporin A in corticosteroid-dependent chronic severe asthma. *Lancet* **339**:324–8.

Allen DB, Mullen M, Mullen B. 1994. A meta-analysis of the effect of oral and inhaled corticosteroids on growth. *J Allergy Clin Immunol* **93**:967–76.

Alton E, Norris AA. 1996. Chloride transport and the actions of nedocromil sodium and cromolyn sodium in asthma. *J Allergy Clin Immunol* **98**:S102–6.

American Academy of Allergy, Asthma and Immunology (AAAAI) Committee on Drugs. 1996. Safety and appropriate use of salmeterol in the treatment of asthma. *J Allergy Clin Immunol* **98**: 475–9.

American Thoracic Society. 1995. Standards for the diagnosis and care of patients with chronic obstructive pulmonary disease. *Am J Respir Crit Care Med* **152**:S78–121.

Anderson GP. 1993. Formoterol: pharmacology, molecular basis of agonism, and mechanism of long duration of a highly potent and selective beta2-adrenoceptor agonist bronchodilator. *Life Sci* **52**:2145–60.

Anthonisen NR, Connett JE, Kiley JP, et al. 1994. Effects of smoking intervention and the use of an inhaled anticholinergic bronchodilator on the rate of decline of FEV1: the Lung Health Study. *JAMA* **272**:1497–1505.

Anzueto A, Jubran A, Ohar JA, et al. 1997. Effects of aerosolized surfactant in patients with stable chronic bronchitis. *JAMA* **278**: 1426–31.

Argyropoulou P, Patakas D, Koukou A, et al. 1993. Buspirone effect on breathlessness and exercise performance in patients with chronic obstructive pulmonary disease. *Respiration* **60**:216–20.

Bairam A, Faulon M, Monin P, et al. 1992. Doxapram for the initial treatment of idiopathic apnea of prematurity. *Biol Neonate* **61**: 209–13.

Barnes PJ. 1989. Muscarinic receptor subtypes: implications for lung disease. *Thorax* **44**:161–7.

Barnes PJ. 1993. Muscarinic receptor subtypes in airways. *Life Sci* **52**:521–7.

Barnes PJ. 1995a. Inhaled glucocorticoids for asthma. *N Engl J Med* **332**:868–75.

Barnes PJ. 1995b. State of the art: beta-adrenergic receptors and their regulation. *Am J Respir Crit Care Med* **152**:838–60.

Barnes PJ. 1998. New therapies for chronic obstructive pulmonary disease. *Thorax* **53**:137–47.

Barnes PJ, Adcock IM. 1993. Anti-inflammatory actions of steroids: molecular mechanisms. *Trends Pharmacol Sci* **14**:436–41.

Barnes PJ, Greening AP, Neville L, et al. 1982. Single-dose slow-release aminophylline at night prevents nocturnal asthma. *Lancet* **1**:299–301.

Barnes PJ, Pauwels RA. 1994. Theophylline in the management of asthma: time for reappraisal? *Eur Respir J* **7**:579–91.

Barrington KJ, Muttitt SC. 1998. Randomized, controlled, blinded trial of doxapram for extubation of the very low birthweight infant. *Acta Pediatr* **87**:191–4.

Beam WR, Weiner DE, Martin RJ. 1992. Timing of prednisone and alteration of airways inflammation in nocturnal asthma. *Am Rev Respir Dis* **146**:1524–30.

Beauford W, Saylor TT, Stansbury DW, et al. 1993. Effects of nebulized morphine sulfate on the exercise tolerance of the ventilatory limited COPD patient. *Chest* **104**:175–8.

Bender BG, Lerner JA, Ikle D, et al. 1991. Psychological change associated with theophylline treatment of asthmatic children: a 6-month study. *Pediatr Pulmonol* **11**:233–44.

Bender BG, Milgrom H. 1992. Theophylline-induced behavior change in children: an objective measure of parent's perceptions. *JAMA* **267**:2621–4.

Bentley AM, Menz G, Storz C, et al. 1992. Identification of T lymphocytes, macrophages, and activated eosinophils in the bronchial mucosa in intrinsic asthma: relationship to symptoms and bronchial responsiveness. *Am Rev Respir Dis* **146**:500–4.

Bhagat R, Kalra S, Swystun VA, et al. 1995. Rapid onset of tolerance to the bronchoprotective effect of salmeterol. *Chest* **108**:1235–9.

Bradley BL, Azzawi M, Jacobson M, et al. 1991. Eosinophils, T-lymphocytes, mast cells, neutrophils, and macrophages in bronchial biopsy specimens from atopic subjects with asthma: comparison with biopsy specimens from atopic subjects without asthma and normal control subjects and relationship to bronchial hyperresponsiveness. *J Allergy Clin Immunol* **88**:661–74.

Braun SR, McKenzie WN, Copeland C, et al. 1989. A comparison of the effect of ipratropium and albuterol in the treatment of chronic obstructive airway disease. [published erratum appears in *Arch Intern Med* 1990 **150**:1242]. *Arch Intern Med.* **149**:544–7.

Brenner M, Berkowitz R, Marshall N, et al. 1988. Need for theophylline in severe steroid-requiring asthmatics. *Clin Allergy* **18**:143–50.

Burns RB. 1985. A multicenter study with ketotifen (Zaditen). *New Engl Regional Allergy Proc* **6**:78–83.

Cameron SJ, Cooper EJ, Crompton GK, et al. 1973. Substitution of beclomethasone aerosol for oral prednisolone in the treatment of chronic asthma. *Br Med J* **4**:205–7.

Chaieb J, Belcher N, Rees PJ. 1989. Maximum achievable bronchodilation in asthma. *Respir Med* **83**:497–502.

Chailleux E, Bauroux B, Binet F, et al. 1996. Predictors of survival in patients receiving domiciliary oxygen therapy or mechanical ventilation. *Chest* **109**:741–9.

Christie PE, Smith CM, Lee TH. 1991. The potent and selective sulfidopeptide leukotriene antagonist: SK&F 104353, inhibits aspirin-induced asthma. *Am Rev Respir Dis* **144**:957–8.

Church MK. 1978. Cromoglycate-like anti-allergic drugs. *Drugs Today* **14**:281–341.

Church MK, Hiroi J. 1987. Inhibition of IgE-dependent histamine release from human dispersed lung mast cells by anti-allergic drugs and salbutamol. *Br J Pharmacol* **90**:421–9.

Cockcroft DW, McParland CP, Britto SA, et al. 1993. Regular inhaled salbutamol and airway responsiveness to allergen. *Lancet* **342**:833–7.

Coe CI, Barnes PJ. 1986. Reduction of nocturnal asthma by an inhaled anticholinergic drug. *Chest* **90**:485–8.

Coffey MJ, Sanders G, Eschenbacher WL, et al. 1994. The role of methotrexate in the management of steroid-dependent asthma. *Chest* **105**:649–50.

Colombo F, Borella F, Rampoldi C, et al. 1989. Thiopronine. In: Braga PC, Allegra L, editors. *Drugs in Bronchial Mucology*. New York: Raven Press. p 103–18.

COMBIVENT Inhalation Aerosol Study Group. 1994. In chronic obstructive pulmonary disease, a combination of ipratropium and albuterol is more effective than either agent alone. An 85-day multicenter trial. *Chest* **105**:1411–9.

Connaughton JJ, Douglas NJ, Morgan AD, et al. 1985. Almitrine improves oxygenation when both awake and asleep in patients with hypoxia and carbon dioxide retention caused by chronic bronchitis and emphysema. *Am Rev Respir Dis* **132**:206–10.

Creticos P, Burk J, Smith L, et al. 1995. The use of twice daily nedocromil sodium in the treatment of asthma. *J Allergy Clin Immunol* **95**:829–36.

Cumming RG, Mitchell P, Leeder SR. 1997. Use of inhaled corticosteroids and the risk of cataracts. *N Engl J Med* **337**:8–14.

Dahlen B, Kumlin M, Margolskee DJ, et al. 1993. The leukotriene receptor antagonist MK–0679 blocks airway obstruction induced by inhaled lysine aspirin in aspirin-sensitive asthmatics. *Eur Respir J* **6**:1018–26.

Dajani BM, Sliman NA, Shubair KS, et al. 1981. Bronchospasm caused by intravenous hydrocortisone sodium succinate (Solu-Cortef) in aspirin-sensitive asthmatics. *J Allergy Clin Immunol* **68**:201–6.

Davies G, Thomas P, Broder I, et al. 1977. Steroid-dependent asthma treated with inhaled beclomethasone dipropionate—a long-term study. *Ann Intern Med* **86**:549–53.

Djukanovic R, Roche WR, Wilson JW, et al. 1990. Mucosal inflammation in asthma. State of the art. *Am Rev Respir Dis* **142**:434–57.

Drazen JM, Israel E, Boushey HA, et al. 1996. Comparison of regularly scheduled with as-needed use of albuterol in mild asthma. *N Engl J Med* **335**:841–7.

Duddridge M, Ward C, Hendrick DJ, et al. 1993. Changes in bronchoalveolar lavage inflammatory cells in asthmatic patients treated with high dose inhaled beclomethasone dipropionate. *Eur Respir J* **6**:489–97.

Dunnill MS. 1960. The pathology of asthma with special reference to changes in the bronchial mucosa. *J Clin Pathol* **13**:27–33.

Duskieker L, Green M, Smith GD, et al. 1982. Comparison of orally administered metaproterenol and theophylline in the control of chronic asthma. *J Pediatr* **101**:281–7.

Eady RP. 1986. The pharmacology of nedocromil sodium. *Eur J Respir Dis* **69**:S112–9.

Ellul-Micallef R, French FF. 1975. Intravenous prednisolone in chronic bronchial asthma. *Thorax* **30**:312–5.

Erjefalt I, Persson CGA. 1986. Anti-asthma drugs attenuate inflammatory leakage into airway lumen. *Acta Physiol Scand* **128**:653–5.

Evans DJ, Taylor DA, Zetterstrom O, et al. 1997. A comparison of low-dose inhaled budesonide plus theophylline and high-dose inhaled budesonide for moderate asthma. *N Engl J Med* **337**:1412–8.

Fanta CH, Rossing TH, McFadden ER. 1983. Glucocorticoids in acute asthma. A controlled clinical trial. *Am J Med* **74**:845–51.

Fick RB, Ansueto A, Mahutte K. 1994. Recombinant DNase mortality reduction in acute exacerbations of chronic bronchitis. *Clin Res* **42**:294A.

Finnerty JP, Wood-Baker R, Thomson H, et al. 1992. Role of leukotrienes in exercise-induced asthma: inhibitory effect of ICI 204219, a potent leukotriene D4 receptor antagonist. *Am Rev Respir Dis* **145**:746–9.

Fitzpatrick MF, Mackay T, Driver H, et al. 1990. Salmeterol in nocturnal asthma: a double-blind, placebo-controlled trial of a long acting inhaled beta2-agonist. *BMJ* **301**:1365–8.

Frith PA, Jenner B, Dangerfield R, et al. 1986. Oxitropium bromide. Dose response and time response study of a new anticholinergic bronchodilator drug. *Chest* **89**:249–53.

Furukawa CT, Shapiro GG, Bierman CW, et al. 1984. A double-blind study comparing the effectiveness of cromolyn sodium and sustained-release theophylline in childhood asthma. *Pediatrics* **76**:453–9.

Gaddie J, Petrie GR, Reid IW, et al. 1973. Aerosol beclomethasone dipropionate: a dose-response study in chronic bronchial asthma. *Lancet* **2**:280–1.

Gaddie J, Reid IW, Skinner C, et al. 1973. Aerosol beclomethasone dipropionate in chronic bronchial asthma. *Lancet* **1**:691–3.

Garbe E, LeLorier J, Boivin J-F, et al. 1997. Inhaled and nasal glucocorticoids and the risks of ocular hypertension or open-angle glaucoma. *JAMA* **277**:722–7.

Gonzales JP, Brogden RN. 1987. A preliminary review of its pharmacodynamic and pharmacokinetic properties, and therapeutic efficacy in the treatment of reversible obstructive airways disease. *Drugs* **34**:560–77.

Green CP, Price JF. 1992. Prevention of exercise induced asthma by inhaled salmeterol xinafoate. *Arch Dis Child* **67**:1014–17.

Green SA, Turki J, Innis M, et al. 1994. Amino-terminal polymorphisms of the human beta2-adrenergic receptor impart distinct agonist-promoted regulatory properties. *Biochemistry* **33**:9414–9.

Greening AP, Ing PW, Northfield M, et al. 1994. Treatment of adult asthmatic patients symptomatic on low dose inhaled corticosteroids: a comparison of the addition of salmeterol to existing inhaled corticosteroid therapy, with increasing the dose of inhaled corticosteroids. *Lancet* **344**:219–24.

Gross NJ. 1988. Ipratropium bromide. *N Engl J Med* **319**:486–94.

Gross NJ, Schloo O. 1975. A new anticholinergic bronchodilator. *Am Rev Respir Dis* **112**:823.

Gross NJ, Skorodin MS. 1984a. Anti-cholinergic, anti-muscarinic bronchodilators. *Am Rev Respir Dis* **129**:856–70.

Gross NJ, Skorodin MS. 1984b. Role of the parasympathetic system in airway obstruction due to emphysema. *N Engl J Med* **311**:421–5.

Grossman J, Banov C, Boggs P, et al. 1995. Use of ipratropium bromide nasal spray in chronic treatment of nonallergic perennial rhinitis, alone and in combination with other perennial rhinitis medications. *J Allergy Clin Immunol* **95**:1123–7.

Guffanti EE, Rossetti S, Scaccabarozzi S. 1989. Carbocysteine. In: Braga PC, Allegra L, editors. *Drugs in Bronchial Mucology*. New York: Raven Press. p 147–70.

Guyatt GH, Townsend M, Pugsley SO, et al. 1987. Bronchodilators in chronic airflow limitation: effects on airway function, exercise capacity, and quality of life. *Am Rev Respir Dis* **135**:1069–74.

Hall IP, Wheatley A, Wilding P, et al. 1995. Association of Glu 27 beta2-adrenoceptor polymorphism with lower airway reactivity in asthmatic subjects. *Lancet* **345**:1213–4.

Harris JB, Weinberger MM, Nassif E, et al. 1987. Early intervention with short courses of prednisone to prevent progression of asthma in ambulatory patients incompletely responsive to bronchodilators. *J Pediatr* **110**:627–33.

Haskell RJ, Wong BM, Hansen JE. 1983. A double-blind, randomized clinical trial of methylprednisolone in status asthmaticus. *Arch Intern Med* **143**:1324–7.

Hauck RW, Bohm M, Gengenbach S, et al. 1990. Beta2-adrenoceptors in human lung and peripheral mononuclear leukocytes of untreated and terbutaline-treated patients. *Chest* **98**:376–81.

Heinke S, Szues G, Norris A, et al. 1995. Inhibition of volume-activated chloride currents in endothelial cells by cromones. *Br J Pharmacol* **115**:1392–8.

Heins M, Kurtin L, Oellerich M, et al. 1988. Nocturnal asthma: slow-release terbutaline versus slow release theophylline therapy. *Eur Respir J* **1**:306–10.

Henderson WR. 1994. The role of leukotrienes in inflammation. *Ann Intern Med* **121**:684–97.

Howarth PH, Durham SR, Lee TH, et al. 1985. Influence of albuterol, cromolyn sodium and ipratropium bromide on the airway and circulating mediator responses to allergen bronchial provocation in asthma. *Am Rev Respir Dis* **132**:986–22.

Hubbard RC, McElvaney NG, Birrer P, et al. 1992. A preliminary study of aerosolized recombinant human deoxyribonuclease I in the treatment of cystic fibrosis. *N Engl J Med* **326**:812–5.

Hui KKP, Conolly ME, Tashkin DP. 1982. Reversal of human lymphocyte beta-adrenoceptor desensitization by glucocorticoids. *Clin Pharmacol Ther* **32**:566–71.

Israel E, Cohn J, Dube L, et al. 1996. Effect of treatment with zileuton, a 5-lipoxygenase inhibitor, in patients with asthma. The Zileuton Clinical Trial Group. *JAMA* **275**:931–6.

Israel E, Rubin P, Kemp JP, et al. 1993. The effect of inhibition of 5-lipoxygenase by zileuton in mild-to-moderate asthma. *Ann Intern Med* **119**:1059–66.

Johnson CE. 1987. Aerosol corticosteroids for the treatment of asthma. *Drug Intell Clin Pharm* **21**:784–90.

Johnson M, Butchers PR, Coleman RA, et al. 1993. The pharmacology of salmeterol. *Life Sci* **52**:2131–43.

Kalra S, Swystun VA, Bhagat R, et al. 1996. Inhaled corticosteroids do not prevent the development of tolerance to the bronchoprotective effect of salmeterol. *Chest* **109**:953–6.

Kamei J. 1996. Role of opioidergic and serotonergic mechanisms in cough and antitussives. *Pulm Pharmacol* **9**:349–56.

Karpel JP. 1991. Bronchodilator responses to anticholinergic and beta-adrenergic agents in acute and stable COPD. *Chest* **99**: 871–6.

Kerr HD. 1997. Doxapram in hypercapnic chronic obstructive pulmonary disease with respiratory failure. *J Emerg Med* **15**:513–5.

Kerrebijn KF, Van Essen-Zandvliet EEM, Neijens HJ. 1987. Effect of long-term treatment with inhaled corticosteroids and beta-agonists on the bronchial responsiveness in children with asthma. *J Allergy Clin Immunol* **79**:653–60.

Kidney J, Dominguez M, Taylor PM, et al. 1995. Immunomodulation by theophylline in asthma. *Am J Respir Crit Care Med* **151**: 1907–14.

Klaustermeyer WB, Noritake DT, Kwong KF. 1987. Chrysotherapy in the treatment of corticosteroid-dependent asthma. *J Allergy Clin Immunol* **79**:720–5.

Knowles MR, Church NL, Waltner WE, et al. 1990. A pilot study of aerosolized amiloride for the treatment of lung disease in cystic fibrosis. *N Engl J Med* **322**:1189–94.

Kraan J, Koeter GH, Van Der Mar TW, et al. 1985. Changes in bronchial hyperreactivity induced by 4 weeks of treatment with antiasthmatic drugs in patients with allergic asthma: a comparison between budesonide and terbutaline. *J Allergy Clin Immunol* **76**: 628–36.

Laitinen LA, et al. 1985. Damage to the airway epithelium and bronchial reactivity in patients with asthma. *Am Rev Respir Dis* **131**:599–606.

Lal S, Dorow PD, Venho KK, et al. 1993. Nedocromil sodium is more effective than cromolyn sodium for the treatment of chronic reversible obstructive airway disease. *Chest* **104**:438–47.

Leff JA, Israel E, Noonan MJ, et al. 1997. Montelukast (MK–0476) allows tapering on inhaled corticosteroids in asthmatic patients while maintaining clinical stability (abstract). *Am J Respir Crit Care Med* **155**:A976.

Lemanske RF, Joad J. 1990. $\beta_2$ receptor agonists in asthma: a comparison. *J Asthma* **27**:101–9.

Leung RPH, Burdon J. 1996. Effect of inhaled morphine on the development of breathlessness during exercise in patients with chronic lung disease. *Thorax* **51**:596–600.

Levy LI, Seabury JH. 1947. Spirometric evaluation of Benadryl in asthma. *J Allergy* **18**:244–50.

Light RW, Muro JR, Sato R. 1989. Effects of oral morphine on breathlessness and exercise tolerance in patients with chronic obstructive pulmonary disease. *Am Rev Respir Dis* **139**:126–33.

Light RW, Stansbury DW, Webster JS. 1996. Effect of 30 mg of morphine alone or with promethazine or prochlorperazine on the exercise capacity of patients with COPD. *Chest* **109**:975–81.

Lindgren S, Lokshin B, Stromquist A, et al. 1992. Does asthma or treatment with theophylline limit children's academic performance? *N Engl J Med* **327**:926–30.

Lipworth BJ, Struthers AD, McDevitt DG. 1989. Tachyphylaxis to systemic but not to airway responses during prolonged therapy with high dose inhaled salbutamol in asthmatics. *Am Rev Respir Dis* **140**:586–92.

Littenberg B. 1988. Aminophylline treatment in severe, acute asthma: a meta-analysis. *JAMA* **259**:1678–84.

Lock SH, Barnes NC, Kay AB. 1996. Double-blind placebo-controlled study of cyclosporin A (CsA) as a corticosteroid sparing agent in corticosteroid-dependent asthma. *Am J Respir Crit Care Med* **153**:509–14.

Loftus BG, Price JF. 1987. Long-term, placebo-controlled trial of ketotifen in the management of preschool children with asthma. *J Allergy Clin Immunol* **79**:350–5.

Magnussen H, Reuss G, Jorres R. 1988. Methylxanthines inhibit exercise-induced bronchoconstriction at low serum theophylline concentration and in a dose-dependent fashion. *J Allergy Clin Immunol* **81**:531–7.

Mak JC, Nishikawa M, Barnes PJ.1996. Glucocorticoids increase beta2-adrenergic receptor transcription in human lung. *Am J Physiol* **268**:L41–6.

Mak JC, Nishikawa S, Shirasiki H, et al. 1995. Protective effects of a glucocorticoid on down-regulation on pulmonary beta2-adrenergic receptors in vivo. *J Clin Invest* **96**:99–106.

Martin U, Bagglionlini M. 1981. Dissociation between the anti-anaphylactic and antihistamine action of ketotifen. *Arch Pharmacol* **316**:186–9.

Maswood AR, Reed JW, Thomas SHL. 1995. Lack of effect of inhaled morphine on exercise-induced breathlessness in chronic obstructive pulmonary disease. *Thorax* **50**:629–34.

McFadden ER. 1981. Beta2-receptor agonists—metabolism and pharmacology. *J Allergy Clin Immunol* **68**:91–6.

Medical Research Council Working Party. 1981. Long term domiciliary oxygen therapy in chronic hypoxic cor pulmonale complicating chronic bronchitis and emphysema. Medical Research Council Working Party. *Lancet* **1**:681–6.

Meltzer EO, Kemp JP, Welch MJ, et al. 1985. Effect of dosing schedule on efficacy of beclomethasone dipropionate aerosol in chronic asthma. *Am Rev Respir Dis* **131**:732–6.

Mitchell JA, Belvisi MG, Akarasereenont P, et al. 1994. Induction of cyclooxygenase-2 by cytokines in human pulmonary epithelial cells: regulation by dexamethasone. *Br J Pharmacol* **113**:1008–14.

Mongan PD, Culling RD. 1992. Rapid oral anesthesia for awake intubation. *J Clin Anesth* **4**:101–5.

Mullarkey MF, Blumenstein BA, Andrade WP, et al. 1988. Methotrexate in the treatment of corticosteroid-dependent asthma. A double-blind crossover study. *N Engl J Med* **318**:603–7.

Multicenter Study Group. 1980. Long-term oral acetylcysteine in chronic bronchitis, a double-blind controlled study. *Eur J Respir Dis* **61**:93–108.

Muranaka M, Miyamoto T, Shida T, et al. 1978. Gold salt in the treatment of bronchial asthma—a double-blind study. *Ann Allergy* **40**:132–7.

Nasser SM, Pfister R, Christie PE, et al. 1996. Inflammatory cell populations in bronchial biopsies from aspirin-sensitive asthmatic subjects. *Am J Respir Crit Care Med* **153**:90–6.

Nassif EG, Weinberger M, Thompson R, et al. 1981. The value of maintenance theophylline in steroid-dependent asthma. *N Engl J Med* **304**:71–5.

National Asthma Education and Prevention Program Expert Panel. 1997a. Clinical practice guidelines. Expert Panel Report 2: Guidelines for the diagnosis and management of asthma. Bethesda, MD: NIH/National Heart, Lung, and Blood Institute.

National Asthma Education and Prevention Program Expert Panel. 1997b. Highlights of the Expert Panel Report 2: Guidelines for the diagnosis and management of asthma. Bethesda, MD: NIH/National Heart, Lung, and Blood Institute.

National Institutes of Health/NHLBI. 1995. Global strategy for asthma management and prevention NHLBI/WHO workshop report March 1993. NIH Publication No. 95–3659. Bethesda, MD: US Dept of Health and National Heart, Lung, and Blood Institute.

Nelson HS. 1995. Drug therapy: beta-adrenergic bronchodilators. *N Engl J Med* **333**:499–506.

Newcomb R, Tashkin DP, Hui KK, et al. 1985. Rebound hyperresponsiveness to muscarinic stimulation after chronic therapy with an inhaled muscarinic antagonist. *Am Rev Respir Dis* **132**:12–5.

Nijkamp FP, Engels F, Hendricks PAJ, et al. 1992. Mechanisms of beta-adrenergic receptor regulation in lungs and its implications for physiological responses. *Physiol Rev* **72**:323–67.

Nizankowska E, Soja J, Pinis G, et al. 1995. Treatment of steroid-dependent bronchial asthma with cyclosporin. *Eur Respir J* **8**:1091–9.

Nocturnal Oxygen Therapy Trial Group.. 1980. Continuous or nocturnal oxygen therapy in hypoxemic chronic obstructive lung disease. *Ann Intern Med* **93**:391–8.

Noonan M, Chervinsky P, Busse WW, et al. 1995. Fluticasone propionate reduces oral prednisone use while it improves asthma control and quality of life. *Am J Respir Crit Care Med* **152**:1467–73.

Novembre G, Frongia GF, Veneruso G, et al. 1994. Inhibition of exercise-induced asthma (EIA) by nedocromil sodium and sodium cromoglycate in children. *Pediatr Allergy Immunol* **5**:107–10.

O'Driscoll BRC, Ruffles SP, Ayres JG, et al. 1988. Long term treatment of severe asthma with subcutaneous terbutaline. *Br J Dis Chest* **82**:360–7.

Pauwels R, Van Renterghem D, Van Der Straeten M, et al. 1985. The effect of theophylline and enprophylline on allergen-induced bronchoconstriction. *J Allergy Clin Immunol* **76**:583–90.

Pauwels RA, Lofdahl C-G, Postma DS, et al. 1997. Effect of inhaled formoterol and budesonide on exacerbations of asthma. *N Engl J Med* **337**:1405–11.

Pavia D, Bateman JRM, Clarke SW. 1980. Deposition and clearance of inhaled particles. *Bull Eur Physiopathol Respir* **16**:335–66.

Petty TL. 1990. The national mucolytic study. Results of a randomized, double-blind, placebo-controlled study of iodinated glycerol in chronic obstructive bronchitis. *Chest* **97**:75–83.

Petty TL, Rollins DR, Christopher K, et al. 1989. Cromolyn sodium is effective in adult chronic asthmatics. *Am Rev Respir Dis* **139**:694–701.

Phillips GH. 1990. Structure-activity relationship of topically active steroids: the selection of fluticasone propionate. *Respir Med* **84**: 19–23.

Pneumology Task Group on BAL. 1992. Clinical guidelines and indications for bronchoalveolar lavage (BAL). Pneumology Task Group on BAL. In: Klech H, Hutter C, Costabel U, eds. European Respiratory Review. Vol. 2, 8–127.

Pollock J, Kiechel F, Cooper D, et al. 1977. Relationship of serum theophylline concentration to inhibition of exercise-induced bronchospasm and comparison with cromolyn. *Pediatrics* **60**:840–4.

Prahl P, Jensen T, Bjerregaard-Andersen H. 1987. Adrenocortical function in children on high-dose steroid aerosol therapy. Results of serum cortisol, ACTH stimulation test and 24 hour urinary free cortisol excretion. *Allergy* **42**:541–4.

Rachelefsky GS, Wo J, Adelson J, et al. 1986. Behavior abnormalities and poor school performance due to oral theophylline use. *Pediatrics* **78**:1133–8.

Ramage L, Lipworth BJ, Ingram CG, et al. 1994. Reduced protection against exercise-induced bronchoconstriction after chronic dosing with salmeterol. *Respir Med* **88**:363–8.

Reiss TF, Altman LC, Chervinsky P, et al. 1996. Effects of montelukast (MK–0476), a new potent cysteinyl leukotriene (LTD4) receptor antagonist, in patients with chronic asthma. *J Allergy Clin Immunol* **98**:528–34.

Reiss TF, Chervinsky P, Dockhorn RJ, et al. 1998. Montelukast, a once-daily leukotriene receptor antagonist, in the treatment of chronic asthma: a multicenter, randomized, double-blind trial. *Arch Intern Med* **158**:1213–20.

Repsher LH. 1993. Treatment of stable chronic bronchitis with iodinated glycerol: a double-blind, placebo-controlled trial. *J Clin Pharmacol* **33**:856–60.

Rinehart JJ, Sagone AL, Balcerzak SP, et al. 1975. Effects of corticosteroid therapy on human monocyte function. *N Engl J Med* **292**:236–41.

Robberecht P, Delhaye M, Taton G, et al. 1983. The human heart beta-adrenergic receptors. *Mol Pharmacol* **24**:169–73.

Robbins RA, Barnes PJ, Springall DR, et al. 1994. Expression of inducible nitric oxide synthase in human bronchial epithelial cells. *Biochem Biophys Res Commun* **203**:209–18.

Rossing TH, Fanta CH, Goldstein DH, et al. 1980. Emergency therapy of asthma: comparison of the acute effects of parenteral and inhaled sympathomimetics and infused aminophylline. *Am Rev Respir Dis* **122**:365–71.

Rubin BK, Ramirez O, Ohar JA. 1996. Iodinated glycerol has no effect on pulmonary function, symptom score, or sputum properties in patients with stable chronic bronchitis. *Chest* **109**:348–52.

Saadjiian A, Philip-Joet F, Barret A, et al. 1993. Nifedipine inhibits the effects of almitrine in patients suffering from pulmonary artery hypertension secondary to chronic obstructive pulmonary disease. *J Cardiovasc Pharmacol* **21**:797–803.

Saetta M, Di-Stefano A, Maestrelli P, et al. 1992. Airway mucosal inflammation in occupational asthma induced by toluene diisocyanate. *Am Rev Respir Dis* **145**:160–8.

Schleimer RP. 1990. Effects of glucocorticoids on inflammatory cells relevant to their therapeutic applications in asthma. *Am Rev Respir Dis* **141**:S59–69.

Schuh S, Johnson DW, Callahan S, et al. 1995. Efficacy of frequent nebulized ipratropium bromide added to frequent high-dose albuterol therapy in severe childhood asthma. *J Pediatr* **126**:639–45.

Schuller D. 1983. The spectrum of antihistamines adversely affecting pulmonary function in asthmatic children. *J Allergy Clin Immunol* **71**:147.

Schwartz HJ, Blumenthal M, Brady R, et al. 1996. A comparative study of the clinical efficacy of nedocromil sodium and placebo: how does cromolyn sodium compare as an active control treatment? *Chest* **109**:945–52.

Schwiebert LA, Beck LA, Stellato C, et al. 1996. Glucocorticosteroid inhibition of cytokine production: relevance to antiallergic actions. *J Allergy Clin Immunol* **97**:143–52.

Shak S, Capon DJ, Hellmiss R, et al. 1990. Recombinant human DNase I reduces the viscosity of cystic fibrosis sputum. *Proc Natl Acad Sci USA* **87**:9188–92.

Shenfield GM, Hodson ME, Clarke SW, et al. 1975. Interaction of corticosteroids and catecholamines in the treatment of asthma. *Thorax* **30**:430–5.

Shiner RJ, Nunn AJ, Chung KF, et al. 1990. Randomized, double-blind placebo-controlled trial of methotrexate in steroid-dependent asthma. *Lancet* **336**:137–40.

Siafakas NM, Vermeire P, Pride NB, et al. 1995. Optimal assessment and management of chronic obstructive pulmonary disease (COPD). The European Respiratory Society Task Force. *Eur Respir J* **8**:1398–1420.

Siegel D, Sheppard D, Gelb A, et al. 1985. Aminophylline increases the toxicity but not the efficacy of an inhaled beta-adrenergic agonist in the treatment of acute exacerbation of asthma. *Am Rev Respir Dis* **132**:283–6.

Singh NP, Despars JA, Stansbury DW, et al. 1993. Effects of buspirone on anxiety levels and exercise tolerance in patients with chronic airflow obstruction and mild anxiety. *Chest* **103**:800–4.

Sole D, Mallozi MC, Toledo EC, et al. 1992. Reduction in the oral doses of theophylline in asthmatic children during concomitant treatment with ketotifen. *Allergol Immunopathol* **20**:57–60.

Spector SL, Nicodemus CF, Corren J, et al. 1995. Comparison of the bronchodilatory effects of cetirizine, albuterol, and both together versus placebo in patients with mild-to-moderate asthma. *J Allergy Clin Immunol* **96**:174–81.

Spector SL, Smith LJ, Glass M, et al. 1994. Effects of 6 weeks of therapy with oral doses of ICI 204,219, a leukotriene D4 receptor antagonist, in subjects with bronchial asthma. Group AAT. *Am J Respir Crit Care Med* **150**:618–23.

Spitzer WO, Suissa S, Ernst P, et al. 1992. The use of beta-agonists and the risk of death and near death from asthma. *N Engl J Med* **326**:501–6.

Stolley PD, Schinnar R. 1978. Association between asthma mortality and isoproterenol aerosols: a review. *Prev Med* **7**:319–38.

Sullivan P, Bekir S, Jaffar Z, et al. 1994. Anti-inflammatory effects of low-dose oral theophylline in atopic asthma. *Lancet* **343**:1006–8.

Tan S, Hall IP, Dewar J, et al. 1997. Association between beta2-adrenoceptor polymorphism and susceptibility to bronchodilator desensitization in moderately severe stable asthmatics. *Lancet* **350**: 995–9.

Tan SK, Grove A, McLean A, et al. 1997. Systemic corticosteroid rapidly reverses bronchodilator subsensitivity induced by formoterol in asthmatic patients. *Am J Respir Crit Med* **156**:28–35.

Tan SK, McFarlane LC, Lipworth BJ. 1998. Concomitant administration of low-dose prednisolone protects against in vivo beta2-adrenoceptor subsensitivity induced by regular formoterol. *Chest* **113**: 34–41.

Task Group on Mucoactive Drugs. 1994b. Recommendations for guidelines on clinical trials of mucoactive drugs in chronic bronchitis and chronic obstructive pulmonary disease. *Chest* **106**:1532–7.

Taylor IK, O'Shaughnessy KM, Fuller RW, et al. 1991. Effect of cysteinyleukotriene receptor antagonist ICI 204.219 on allergen-induced bronchoconstriction and airway hyperreactivity in atopic subjects. *Lancet* **337**:690–4.

The British Guidelines on Asthma Management, 1995. 1997. Review and position statement. *Thorax* **52**:S1–21.

Thompson NC. 1989. Nedocromil sodium: an overview. *Respir Med* **83**:269–76.

Thorsson L, Dahlstrom K, Edsbacker S, et al. 1997. Pharmacokinetics and systemic effects of inhaled fluticasone propionate in healthy subjects. *Br J Clin Pharmacol* **43**:155–61.

Tiep BL. 1991. *Medicare Regulations for Oxygen Reimbursement*. Armonk, NY: Futura Publishing Co.

Toogood JH, Baskerville J, Jennings B, et al. 1984. Use of spacers to facilitate inhaled corticosteroid treatment of asthma. *Am Rev Respir Dis* **129**:723–9.

Trigg CJ, Davies RJ. 1993. Comparison of methotrexate 30 mg per week with placebo in chronic steroid-dependent asthma: a 12-week double blind, cross-over study. *Respir Med* **87**:211–6.

Truss M, Beato M. 1993. Steroid hormone receptors: interaction with deoxyribonucleic acid and transcription factors. *Endocr Rev* **14**:459–79.

Turki J, Pak J, Green SA, et al. 1995. Genetic polymorphisms of the beta2-adrenergic receptor in nocturnal and non-nocturnal asthma: evidence that Gly 16 correlates with the nocturnal phenotype. *J Clin Invest* **95**:1635–41.

Ullah MI, Newman GB, Saunders KB. 1981. Influence of age on response to ipratropium and salbutamol in asthma. *Thorax* **36**: 523–9.

Van De Stolpe A, Caldenhoven E, Raaijmakers JAM, et al. 1993. Glucocorticoid-mediated repression of intercellular adhesion molecule-1 expression in human monocytic and bronchial epithelial cell lines. *Am J Respir Cell Mol Biol* **8**:340–7.

Ventresca GP, Cicchetti V, Ferrari V. 1989. Acetylcysteine. In: Braga PC, Allegra L, editors. *Drugs in Bronchial Mucology*. New York: Raven Press. p 77–102.

Verberne AAPH, Frost C, Roorda RJ, et al. 1997. One year treatment with salmeterol compared with beclomethasone in children with asthma. The Dutch Paediatric Asthma Study Group. *Am J Respir Crit Care Med* **156**:688–95.

Ward MJ, Fentem PH, Smith WHR, et al. 1981. Ipratropium bromide in acute asthma. *Br Med J* **282**:598–600.

Wechsler ME, Garpestad E, Flier SR, et al. 1998. Pulmonary infiltrates, eosinophilia, and cardiomyopathy following corticosteroid withdrawal in patients with asthma receiving zafirlukast. *JAMA* **279**:455–7.

Weinberger M, Hendeles L. 1993. Theophylline. In: Middleton E, Reed CE, Ellis EF, et al., editors. *Allergy: Principles and Practice.* Vol. 120. St. Louis, MO: Mosby–Year Book. p 816–55.

Weinberger M, Hendeles L. 1996. Theophylline in asthma. *N Engl J Med* **334**:1380–8.

Weinberger M. 1984. The pharmacology and therapeutic use of theophylline. *J Allergy Clin Immunol* **73**:525–40.

Weinberger MM, Bronsky EA. 1974. Evaluation of oral bronchodilator therapy in asthmatic children. *J Pediatr* **84**:421–7.

Wilson JW, Djukanovic R, Howarth PH, et al. 1994. Inhaled beclomethasone dipropionate downregulates airway lymphocyte activation in atopic asthma. *Am J Respir Crit Care Med* **149**:86–90.

Winkelmann BR, Kullmer TH, Kneissl DG, et al. 1994. Low-dose almitrine bismesylate in the treatment of hypoxemia due to chronic obstructive pulmonary disease. *Chest* **105**:1383–91.

Woodcock AA, Gross FR, Geedes DM. 1981. Drug treatment of breathlessness: contrasting effects of diazepam and promethazine in pink puffer syndrome. *Br Med J* **283**:343–6.

Woolcock A, Lundback B, Ringdal N, et al. 1996. Comparison of addition of salmeterol to inhaled steroids with doubling of the dose of inhaled steroids. *Am J Respir Crit Care Med* **153**:1481–8.

Zaagsma J, Van Der Heijden PJCM, Van Der Schaar MWG, et al. 1983. Comparison of functional beta-adrenoceptor heterogeneity in central and peripheral airway smooth muscle of guinea pig and man. *J Recept Res* **3**:89–106.

Zavattini G, Leproux GB, Daniotti S. 1989. Ambroxol. In: Braga PC, Allegra L, editors. *Drugs in Bronchial Mucology*. New York: Raven Press. p 263–91.

Ziment I. 1989a. Cysteine and its derivatives. In: Braga PC, Allegra L, editors. *Drugs in Bronchial Mucology*. New York: Raven Press. p 71–5.

Ziment I. 1989b. Drugs modifying the sol-layer and the hydration of mucus. In: Braga PC, Allegra L, editors. *Drugs in Bronchial Mucology*. New York: Raven Press. p 293–322.

Ziment I. 1989c. Historic overview of mucoactive drugs. In: Braga PC, Allegra L, editors. *Drugs in Bronchial Mucology*. New York: Raven Press. p 1–33.

Ziment I. 1989d. Inorganic and organic iodides. In: Braga PC, Allegra L, editors. *Drugs in Bronchial Mucology*. New York: Raven Press. p 251–60.

Ziment I. 1989e. Volatile inhalants and balsams. In: Braga PC, Allegra L, editors. *Drugs in Bronchial Mucology*. New York: Raven Press. p 323–34.

Zuliani G, Marenco G, Daniotti S. 1989. Bromhexine. In: Braga PC, Allegra L, editors. *Drugs in Bronchial Mucology*. New York: Raven Press. p 221–38.

# Asthma

**John A. Abisheganaden, Homer A. Boushey**

### *Chapter Outline*



The philosophy of the treatment of asthma has undergone a sea change in the last 15–20 years. What was once regarded as an intermittent disease of episodic bronchoconstriction possibly mediated by a disturbance in sympathetic or parasympathetic neural function is now regarded as a chronic inflammatory disease of the airways associated with intermittent bouts of symptomatic bronchoconstriction. This shift in the conception of the pathogenesis of the disease revolutionized the approach to its treatment. Recognition that lymphocytic, eosinophilic infiltration of the airway mucosa is chronically present called attention both to the need for chronic, regular therapy (as opposed to episodic use of bronchodilators alone) and to the possibility that irreversible scarring or "remodeling" of the airways might occur over the long term. Coincident with this shift in the conception of asthma's pathophysiology was the recognition that the prevalence, morbidity, and mortality of asthma have increased throughout the developed world, especially in populations shifting from an agrarian, Third World pattern of living to an urban, Western one. The reasons for this increase in asthma are unknown and are beyond the scope of this chapter, but recognition that the increase has occurred—and continues—accounts for the profusion of guidelines for the diagnosis and treatment of asthma, developed by panels of experts in Europe and North America (National Institutes of Health/NHLBI 1995; National Asthma Education and Prevention Program Expert Panel 1997a and 1997b; British Guidelines on Asthma Management, 1995).

A theme of guidelines for the pharmacotherapy of asthma is the broad classification of drugs as "short-term relievers" and "long-term controllers." In the first category are the bronchodilators, with inhaled $\beta_2$-adrenergic agonists occupying the first place. For patients with mild intermittent asthma that causes symptoms on no more than 2 days per week, rarely interferes with function, that causes wakening from sleep less than twice a month, and that is not associated with more than mild reductions in $FEV_1$ or peak flow, as needed use of a $\beta_2$-agonist from an MDI suffices.

**PRINCIPLE As information about pathogenesis is acquired, treatment changes often follow.**

## CHRONIC ASTHMA

For patients with persistent asthma, even if the symptoms are mild, use of a long-term controller mediation is recommended. Because it is predictably effective in improving control of asthma and has been shown to reduce airway mucosal inflammation, the treatment most strongly recommended is regular use of an inhaled corticosteroid, but cromolyn and nedocromil, the leukotriene modifiers, and theophylline are all regarded as acceptable alternatives even though comparisons of relative efficacy are not available. The dose of an inhaled corticosteroid considered appropriate for mild persistent asthma varies depending on the specific product and delivery device. For more severe asthma, higher doses are recommended, as is the combination of treatment with an inhaled corticosteroid and a long-acting $\beta$-adrenergic agonist or theophylline. Table 2-6 summarizes the estimated comparative daily dosage for inhaled corticosteroids. Table 2-9 summarizes the stepwise approach for managing patients with asthma, in which the intensity of therapy is matched to the severity of the disease, as reflected by symptoms, frequency of $\beta$-agonist use, and tests of airway caliber.

The evidence of efficacy of inhaled corticosteroids as a treatment for asthma seems incontrovertible. Inhaled corticosteroids reduce asthmatic symptoms and improve airway caliber and bronchial reactivity. These effects were initially demonstrated with beclomethasone (Gaddie, Petrie, et al. 1973, Gaddie, Reid, et al. 1973; Godfrey and Konig 1974; Klein et al. 1977), and subsequently with triamcinolone, flunisolide, budesonide, and fluticasone (Shapiro et al. 1981; Bernstein et al. 1982; Falliers and Petraco 1982; Meltzer et al. 1982; De Baets et al. 1990; Hoekstra et al. 1996; Sheffer et al. 1996). A meta-analysis of the published literature for inhaled corticosteroids in children confirmed the efficacy of glucocorticoids in improving these clinical outcome measures (Calpin et al. 1997).

A long-term consequence of asthma favorably affected by inhaled glucocorticoids is the accelerated decline in lung function. This decline is believed to reflect airway wall remodeling from the deposition of collagen and growth of vessels, smooth muscle, and secretory cells and glands mediated by the products of inflammatory cells activated in the airways. This process is thought to account for the high proportion of elderly asthmatics who have severe, irreversible airflow obstruction in the absence of any history of cigarette smoking or exposure to fumes or dusts (Brown et al. 1984; Braman et al. 1991). Recent evidence suggests that some remodeling occurs early in the course of asthma, for a delay in initiating corticosteroid therapy lessens the maximal improvement in airway caliber that can be achieved (Dompeling et al. 1992; Haahtela et al. 1994), even in children (Agertoft and Pedersen 1994). The rationale for early institution of anti-inflammatory therapy has been bolstered by studies of bronchial biopsies, sputum, or bronchial lavage, showing that significant inflammation is present in early asthma, even in patients who have had mild symptoms of recent onset (Beasley et al. 1989; Laitinen et al. 1993; Vignola et al. 1998).

Specific instruments assessing the quality of life have shown that regular use of fluticasone by patients with moderately severe asthma improved their assessments of their physical function, vitality, mental health, and general health (Mahajan et al. 1997). Fluticasone has also been shown to reduce oral prednisone requirements while improving asthma control and quality of life variables (Noonan et al. 1995).

That inhaled corticosteroids reduce the risk of hospitalization has been reported by a retrospective epidemiologic study of nearly 17,000 asthmatics enrolled in a prepaid health-care plan (Donahue et al. 1997). The investigators found that the filling of $>8$ prescriptions for $\beta$-agonists in a year was associated with a fourfold excess risk of hospitalization. Filling of prescriptions for an inhaled corticosteroid reduced the risk of hospitalization by 50% overall, and by 70% in those dispensed $>8$ $\beta$-agonists per year. Cromolyn, which was mostly prescribed to children, reduced the relative risk by 20%. Evidence from another recent multicenter study of 852 mild-moderate asthmatics similarly showed an association between use of an inhaled corticosteroid and reduction in the risk of hospitalization (Pauwels et al. 1997).

The other long-term controller therapies have all been shown to improve outcome measures reflecting asthma control, such as symptoms, $\beta$-adrenergic-agonist use, frequency of exacerbations, and peak flow or $FEV_1$ in well-designed, prospective, controlled, double-blind trials, but none is supported by the weight of data showing efficacy of inhaled corticosteroids for virtually all known consequences of the disease. With that said, the limitations of inhaled corticosteroid therapy must also be acknowledged. First, and perhaps most important, it is not curative. Even in patients with mild asthma that is well controlled over 2 years of use of a moderate-to-high dose of an inhaled corticosteroid, 50% or more develop recurrence of symptoms within 6 weeks of stopping the therapy (Chervinsky et al. 1994; Haahtela et al. 1994). Another limitation is that it is not universally effective. Among patients who have survived a near fatal attack of asthma, aggressive

**Table 2-9 Stepwise Approach for Managing Asthma in Adults and Children Over 5 Years Old: Treatment**

| | ***Long-Term Control*** |
|---|---|
| **Step 4**<br>**Severe**<br>**Persistent** | Daily medication:<br>• **Anti-inflammatory: inhaled steroid (high dose)*** AND<br>• Long-acting bronchodilator: either **long-acting inhaled $\beta_2$-agonist** (adult; 2 puffs q 12 hours; child: 1–2 puffs q 12 hours), sustained-release theophylline, or long-acting $\beta_2$-agonist tablets AND<br>• Steroid tablets or syrup long term; make repeated attempts to reduce systemic steroid and maintain control with high-dose inhaled steroid. |
| **Step 3**<br>**Moderate**<br>**Persistent** | Daily medication:<br>• Either<br>– **Anti inflammatory: inhaled steroid (medium dose)***<br>OR<br>– **Inhaled steroid (low-to-medium dose)*** and add a long-acting bronchodilator, especially for nighttime symptoms: either **long-acting inhaled $\beta_2$-agonist** (adult: 2 puffs q 12 hours; child: 1–2 puffs q 12 hours), sustained-release theophylline, or long-acting $\beta_2$-agonist tablets.<br>• If needed<br>– **Anti-inflammatory: inhaled steroids (medium-to-high dose)***<br>AND<br>– Long-acting bronchodilator, especially for nighttime symptoms; either **long-acting inhaled $\beta_2$-agonist**, sustained-release theophylline, or long-acting $\beta_2$-agonist tablets. |
| **Step 2**<br>**Mild**<br>**Persistent** | Daily medication:<br>• **Anti inflammatory**: either **inhaled steroid (low dose)*** or **cromolyn** (adult 2–4 puffs tid-id; child: 1–2 puffs tid-qid) or **nedocromil** (adult: 2–4 puffs bid-qid; child: 1–2 puffs bid-id) (children usually begin with a trial of cromolyn or nedocromil).<br>• Sustained-release theophylline to serum concentration of 5–15 $\mu$g/mL is an alternative, but not preferred, therapy. Zafirlukast or zileuton may also be considered for those $\geq$12 years old, although their position in therapy is not fully established. |
| **Step 1**<br>**Mild**<br>**Intermittent** | No daily medication needed. |
| | ***Quick Relief*** |
| **All Patients** | Short-acting bronchodilator, **inhaled $\beta_2$-agonist** (2–4 puffs) as needed for symptoms.<br>Intensity of treatment will depend on severity of exacerbation. |

SOURCE: NIH guidelines, 1995.

**Preferred treatments are in bold print.**

*See Table 2–6. Estimated Comparative Daily Dosages for Inhaled Steroids.

*The stepwise approach presents general guidelines to assist clinical decision-making. Asthma is highly variable, clinicians should tailor medication plans to the needs of individual patients.*

**Gain control** as quickly as possible. Either start with aggressive therapy (e.g., add a course of oral steroids or a higher dose of inhaled steroids to the therapy that corresponds to the patient's initial step of severity); or start at the step that corresponds to the patient's initial severity and step up treatment, if necessary.

**Step down:** Review treatment every 1 to 6 months. Gradually decrease treatment to the least medication necessary to maintain control.

**Step up:** If control is not maintained, consider step up. Inadequate control is indicated by increased use of short-acting $\beta_2$-agonists and in: step 1 when patient uses a short-acting $\beta_2$-agonist more than two times a week; steps 2 and 3 when patient uses short-acting $\beta_2$-agonist on a daily basis or more than three to four times in 1 day. But before stepping up: Review patient inhaler technique, compliance, and environmental control (avoidance of allergens or other precipitant factors).

A course of oral steroids may be needed at any time and at any step.

Patients with exercise-induced bronchospasm should take two to four puffs or an inhaled $\beta_2$-agonist 5 to 60 minutes before exercise.

Referral to an asthma specialist for consultation or comanagement is *recommended* if there is difficulty maintaining control or if the patient requires step 4 care. Referral may be *considered* for step 3 care.

use of inhaled corticosteroids normalizes bronchial reactivity in some, but has little effect in others (Ruffin et al. 1991). Inhaled corticosteroid treatment is sometimes limited by local toxicity. Some patients, for example, develop disabling hoarseness however they inhale the medication. A serious problem is patient anxiety over potential toxicity, possibly fed by articles in popular literature emphasizing the dangers of osteoporosis and the hazards of systemic glucocorticoid treatment, combined with confusion over the distinctions between oral and systemic corticosteroid treatment and between anabolic steroids and glucocorticoids. These anxieties, possibly combined with aversion to the "stigma" of using an inhaler regularly, may account for the discouragingly low rates of adherence to regular use of an inhaled corticosteroid (Milgrom et al. 1996; Boulet 1998).

## ACUTE ASTHMA

For acute severe asthma, oxygen should be started to maintain the percentage of saturation of hemoglobin with $O_2$ above 90 (>95% in children and pregnant women) and an inhaled $\beta$-agonist should be given by nebulizer (e.g., albuterol at 2.5–5.0 mg dissolved in saline every 20 minutes for three doses or 10–15 mg/hour continuously) or by MDI (four puffs every 20 minutes). For severe attacks, the addition of ipratropium to the nebulizer solution increases bronchodilation and reduces the need for hospitalization (Schuh et al. 1995). For severe attacks, systemic glucocorticoids (e.g., methylprednisolone at 1 mg/kg every 6 hours for 48 hours or prednisone 120 mg/day in divided doses) should be administered promptly and continued until the peak flow or $FEV_1$ has improved to 70% of predicted. Corticosteroids are clearly indicated if peak flow or the $FEV_1$ is <30% of predicted on presentation or is <70% predicted after repeated administration of an inhaled bronchodilator. Giving a short course of corticosteroids to all patients who present for urgent care with more than mild, promptly reversible bronchoconstriction reduces the rate of relapse and return for care (Fanta et al. 1983; Chapman et al. 1991; Rowe et al. 1992; Scarfone et al. 1993; Connett et al. 1994). That inhaled corticosteroids may be equally effective has been suggested by some studies (Levy et al. 1996), but is not yet accepted as a standard practice.

For severe attacks of asthma that fail to respond to treatment with oxygen, aerosolized bronchodilator, and systemic corticosteroid treatment, other treatments are sometimes initiated, such as intravenous administration of a $\beta$-agonist (Salmeron et al. 1994) or of magnesium sulfate (Skorodin et al. 1995) and substituting a mixture of helium and oxygen ("heliox") for oxygen-enriched air (Gluck et al. 1990; Manthous et al. 1995). Although these therapies may be effective in some subgroups, none has so far been proven consistently effective.

## REFERENCES


Agertoft L, Pedersen S. 1994. Effects of long-term treatment with an inhaled corticosteroid on growth and pulmonary function in asthmatic children. *Respir Med* **88**:373–81.

Beasley R, Roche WR, Roberts JA, et al. 1989. Cellular events in the bronchi in mild asthma and after bronchial provocation. *Am Rev Respir Dis* **139**:806–17.

Bernstein IL, Chervinsky P, Falliers CJ. 1982. Efficacy and safety of triamcinolone acetonide aerosol in chronic asthma: results of a multicenter, short-term controlled and long-term open study. *Chest* **81**:20–6.

Boulet LP. 1998. Perception of the role and potential side effects of inhaled corticosteroids among asthmatic patients. *Chest* **113**: 587–92.

Braman SS, Kaemmerlen JT, Davis SM. 1991. Asthma in the elderly: a comparison between patients with recently acquired and long-standing disease. *Am Rev Respir Dis* **143**:336–40.

British Guidelines on Asthma Management, 1995. Review and position statement. *Thorax* **52**:S1–21.

Brown PJ, Greville HW, Finucane KE. 1984. Asthma and irreversible airflow obstruction. *Thorax* **39**:131–6.

Calpin C, Macarthur C, Stephens D, et al. 1997. Effectiveness of prophylactic inhaled steroids in childhood asthma: a systemic review of the literature. *J Allergy Clin Immunol* **100**:452–7.

Chapman KR, Verbeek PR, White JG, et al. 1991. Effect of a short course of prednisone in the prevention of early relapse after the emergency room treatment of acute asthma. *N Engl J Med* **324**:788–94.

Chervinsky P, Van As A, Bronsky EA, et al. 1994. Fluticasone propionate aerosol for the treatment of adults with mild to moderate asthma. *J Allergy Clin Immunol* **94**:676–83.

Connett GJ, Warde C, Wooler E, et al. 1994. Prednisolone and salbutamol in the hospital treatment of acute asthma. *Arch Dis Child* **70**:170–3.

De Baets FM, Goeteyn M, Kerrebijn KF. 1990. The effect of two months of treatment with inhaled budesonide on bronchial responsiveness to histamine and house-dust mite antigen in asthmatic children. *Am Rev Respir Dis* **142**:581–6.

Dompeling E, Van Schayck CP, Molema J, et al. 1992. Inhaled beclomethasone improves the course of asthma and COPD. *Eur Respir J* **5**:945–52.

Donahue JG, Weiss ST, Livingston JM, et al. 1997. Inhaled corticosteroids and the risk of hospitalization for asthma. *JAMA* **277**: 887–91.

Falliers CJ, Petraco AJ. 1982. Control of asthma with triamcinolone acetonide aerosol inhalations at 12-hour intervals. *J Asthma* **19**:241–7.

Gaddie J, Petrie GR, Reid IW, et al. 1973. Aerosol beclomethasone dipropionate: a dose-response study in chronic bronchial asthma. *Lancet* **2**:280–1.

Gaddie J, Reid IW, Skinner C, et al. 1973. Aerosol beclomethasone dipropionate in chronic bronchial asthma. *Lancet* **1**:691–3.

Gluck EH, Onorato DJ, Castriotta R. 1990. Helium-oxygen mixtures in intubated patients with status asthmaticus and respiratory acidosis. *Chest* **98**:693–8.

Godfrey S, Konig P. 1974. Treatment of childhood asthma for 13 months and longer with beclomethasone dipropionate aerosol. *Arch Dis Child* **49**:591–6.

Haahtela T, Jarvinen M, Kava T, et al. 1994. Effects of reducing or discontinuing inhaled budesonide in patients with mild asthma. *N Engl J Med* **331**:700–5.

Hoekstra MO, Grol MH, Bouman K, et al. 1996. Fluticasone propionate in children with moderate asthma. *Am J Respir Crit Care Med* **154**:1039–44.

Klein R, Waldman D, Kershnar H, et al. 1977. Treatment of chronic childhood asthma with beclomethasone dipropionate aerosol: I. A double-blind crossover trial in non-steroid-dependent patients. *Pediatrics* **60**:7–13.

Laitinen LA, Laitinen A, Haahtela T. 1993. Airway mucosal inflammation even in patients with newly diagnosed asthma. *Am Rev Respir Dis* **147**:697–704.

Levy ML, Stevenson C, Maslen T. 1996. Comparison of short courses of oral prednisolone and fluticasone propionate in the treatment of adults with acute exacerbations of asthma in primary care. *Thorax* **51**:1087–92.

Mahajan P, Okamoto LJ, Schaberg A, et al. 1997. Impact of fluticasone propionate powder on health-related quality of life in patients with moderate asthma. *J Asthma* **34**:227–34.

Manthous CA, Hall JB, Caputo MA, et al. 1995. Heliox improves pulsus paradoxus and peak expiratory flow in nonintubated patients with severe asthma. *Am J Respir Crit Care Med* **151**:310–4.

Meltzer E, Kemp J, Orgel A, et al. 1982. Flunisolide aerosol for treatment of severe chronic asthma in steroid-independent children. *Pediatrics* **69**:340–5.

Milgrom H, Bender B, Ackerson L, et al. 1996. Noncompliance and treatment failure in children with asthma. *J Allergy Clin Immunol* **98**:1051–7.

National Asthma Education and Prevention Program Expert Panel. 1997a. Clinical practice guidelines. Expert Panel Report 2: Guidelines for the diagnosis and management of asthma. Bethesda, MD: NIH/National Heart, Lung, and Blood Institute.

National Asthma Education and Prevention Program Expert Panel. 1997b. Highlights of the Expert Panel Report 2: Guidelines for the diagnosis and management of asthma. Bethesda, MD: NIH/National Heart, Lung, and Blood Institute.

National Institutes of Health/NHLBI. 1995. Global strategy for asthma management and prevention NHLBI/WHO workshop report March 1993. NIH Publication No. 95–3659. Bethesda, MD: US Dept of Health and National Heart, Lung, and Blood Institute.

Noonan M, Chervinsky P, Busse WW, et al. 1995. Fluticasone propionate reduces oral prednisone use while it improves asthma control and quality of life. *Am J Respir Crit Care Med* **152**:1467–73.

Pauwels RA, Lofdahl C-G, Postma DS, et al. 1997. Effect of inhaled formoterol and budesonide on exacerbations of asthma. *N Engl J Med* **337**:1405–11.

Rowe BH, Keller JL, Oxman AD. 1992. Effectiveness of steroid therapy in acute exacerbations of asthma: a meta-analysis. *Am J Emerg Med* **10**:301–10.

Ruffin RE, Latimer KM, Schembri DA. 1991. Longitudinal study of near fatal asthma. *Chest* **99**:77–83.

Salmeron S, Brochard L, Mal H, et al. 1994. Nebulized versus intravenous albuterol in hypercapnic acute asthma: a multicenter, double-blind, randomized study. *Am J Respir Crit Care Med* **149**:1466–70.

Scarfone RJ, Fuchs SM, Nager AL, et al. 1993. Controlled trial of oral prednisone in the emergency department treatment of children with acute asthma. *Pediatrics* **2**:513–8.

Schuh S, Johnson DW, Callahan S, et al. 1995. Efficacy of frequent nebulized ipratropium bromide added to frequent high-dose albuterol therapy in severe childhood asthma. *J Pediatr* **126**:639–45.

Shapiro G, Izu A, Furukawa C, et al. 1981. Short-term double-blind evaluation of flunisolide aerosol for steroid-dependent asthmatic children and adolescents. *Chest* **80**:671–5.

Sheffer AL, LaForce C, Chervinsky P, et al. 1996. Fluticasone propionate aerosol: efficacy in patients with mild to moderate asthma. The Fluticasone Propionate Asthma Study Group. *J Fam Pract* **42**:369–75.

Skorodin MS, Tenholder MF, Yetter B, et al. 1995. Magnesium sulfate in exacerbations of chronic obstructive pulmonary disease. *Arch Intern Med* **155**:496–500.

Vignola AM, Chanez P, Campbell AM, et al. 1998. Airway inflammation in mild intermittent and in persistent asthma. *Am J Respir Crit Care Med* **157**:403–9.

# Chronic Obstructive Pulmonary Disease

Stephen I. Rennard

*Chapter Outline*



## PATHOPHYSIOLOGY OF CHRONIC OBSTRUCTIVE PULMONARY DISEASE

Chronic obstructive pulmonary disease is a "grab-bag" term that encompasses the common causes of incompletely reversible intrapulmonary limitation of expiratory flow, including principally emphysema and chronic obstructive bronchitis (Snider et al. 1994; American Thoracic Society. 1995; Siafakas et al. 1995). In emphysema, destruction of alveolar wall results in enlargement of the alveolar airspaces with a resulting loss of lung elastic recoil. In chronic obstructive bronchitis, the combined factors of glandular hypertrophy, goblet cell metaplasia, and inflammation and fibrosis of the airway wall narrow the airway lumen and obstruct airflow, especially in small airways. Although associated with chronic airflow obstruction, cystic fibrosis and bronchiectasis are generally excluded from the rubric of COPD. Cigarette smoking is the major etiologic factor in 80–90% of cases of COPD. Other exposures, $\alpha_1$-protease inhibitor deficiency, and possibly lifelong asthma also play etiologic roles in some cases.

Cigarette smoking can cause several distinct pathologies that contribute to expiratory airflow limitation through different mechanisms. Considering their relationship to a common etiologic exposure, it is not surprising that these conditions are often present concurrently. Thus, although lacking semantic rigor, the term *COPD* has been useful to the clinician to refer to a spectrum of related conditions present in smokers. Historically, much of the therapeutic approach to "COPD" was generic, but recent advances in understanding the underlying etiology and the specific pathophysiologic mechanisms activated have led to more selective and more effective therapies.

**PRINCIPLE Broad clinical classifications permit broadly applicable therapeutic strategies. More specific clinical classifications permit implementation of therapies which may be effective in smaller subsets of patients.**

## TREATMENT OF CHRONIC OBSTRUCTIVE PULMONARY DISEASE

The therapeutic approach to COPD should be viewed in context of the natural history of the disease (Fig. 2-4). On average, smokers lose expiratory airflow, as measured by spirometry, at twice the 20 mL/year rate of nonsmokers (Fletcher et al. 1976). This accelerated loss in lung function is gradual, and while it causes no symptoms in most smokers, it is an independent risk factor for mortality (Sorlie et al. 1989). About 15% of smokers lose enough lung function to develop symptoms. Dyspnea on exertion may be noted when expiratory flow decreases to about 50% predicted. Symptoms then worsen rapidly with further declines in function. Consequently, COPD generally begins when an individual starts to smoke, but remains preclinical until relatively late in the course.

Early diagnosis is now easy and convenient for both patient and physician, for relatively inexpensive and reliable electronic spirometers permitting measurement of expiratory airflow and vital capacity are available.

**PRINCIPLE Improved diagnostic methods can bring quantitative methods to guide diagnosis and treatment into more general use.**

During the early, asymptomatic phase of COPD, the therapeutic goal is to slow the accelerated loss of lung function. The most important step is cessation of cigarette

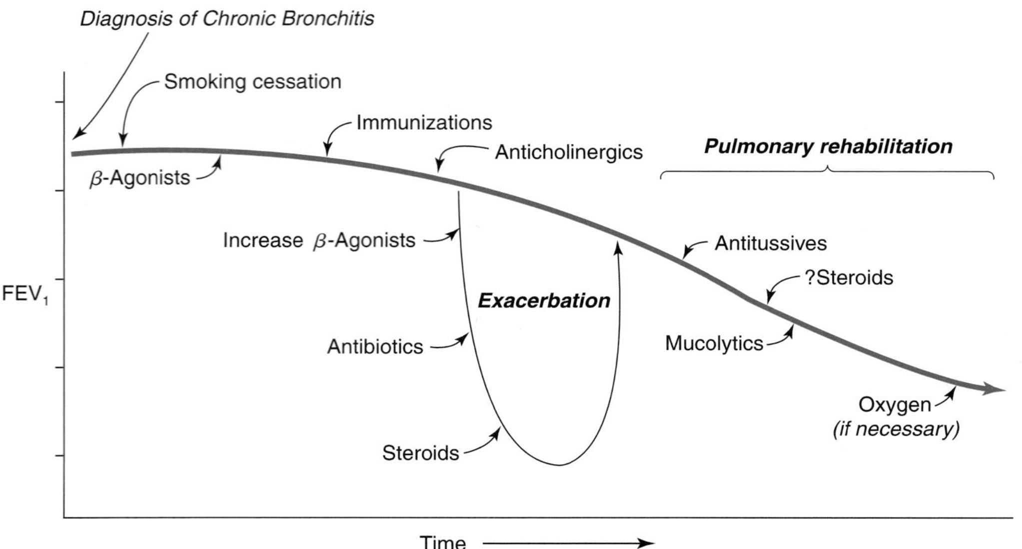


FIGURE 2-4 **Therapy of chronic bronchitis.**

smoking. The Lung Health Study has demonstrated the benefits of quitting (Anthonisen et al. 1994). These results are also supported by cross-sectional studies (Fletcher et al. 1976; Higgins et al. 1984). Smoking cessation also decreases symptoms of cough and sputum production (Buist et al. 1976).

In clinical trials, behavioral approaches are reported to help up to 20% of well-motivated smokers to quit (U.S. Department of Health and Human Services DHHS 1996). Lower rates of smoking cessation are generally observed in clinical practice (Mausner et al. 1968; Russell et al. 1979; Daughton et al. 1998). Nevertheless, even brief interventions may facilitate quitting. Nicotine replacement therapy can approximately double the rate of quitting achieved with behavioral modification alone (Fiore et al. 1994; Silagy et al. 1994; U.S. Department of Health and Human Services DHHS 1996). Transdermal systems may be more effective in the primary practice setting than nicotine gum (Russell et al. 1993; Daughton et al. 1998). The nicotine inhaler and nicotine nasal spray have recently been approved and may be more acceptable to some patients (Schneider et al. 1995, 1996). Bupropion, previously used as an antidepressant, is also effective in facilitating cessation (Hurt et al. 1997).

Severe genetic deficiency of $A_1$-protease inhibitor predisposes to emphysema even in the absence of cigarette smoking (Snider et al. 1994). For individuals with documented inhibitor deficiency and evidence of emphysema, replacement therapy with $A_1$-protease inhibitor purified from pooled blood donors is available. This treatment has been approved in the United States under the orphan drug act, which does not require demonstration of clinical efficacy. Although no randomized controlled trials are available, data from two registries suggest slowing of the progression of disease (Seersholm et al. 1994; The Alpha-1-Antitrypsin Deficiency Registry Study Group 1998). Replacement therapy should not be given to smokers, for cigarette smoke can oxidize and inactivate the inhibitor.

Unless contraindicated, patients with COPD should be vaccinated with the multivalent pneumococcal vaccine [Advisory Committee on Immunization Practice (ACIP) 1989]. In addition, vaccination with the appropriate strain of influenza vaccine should be given annually (Centers for Disease Control and Prevention). Oral vaccination with bacterial extracts to boost mucosal immunity has been in use for some years in Europe. Although recent studies provide some support for benefits of this form of therapy (Anthonisen 1997; Collet et al. 1997), it is not currently recommended in the United States.

## Bronchodilators

The bronchodilators used in asthma are also used in COPD. Anticholinergics, β-agonists, and methylxanthines can all improve airflow and relieve symptoms in COPD. One large trial of regular use of ipratropium showed no effect on the rate of loss of lung function (Anthonisen et al. 1994). Neither β-agonists nor theophylline have been evaluated in this regard.

Early in the symptomatic phase of the disease, some patients may benefit from episodic use of bronchodilators as needed. Short acting $\beta$-agonists are appropriate for this indication. Most patients with COPD, however, always have limitation of expiratory airflow, and regular use of bronchodilators to optimize airflow is the usual therapeutic strategy. For these individuals, regularly scheduled, long-acting $\beta$-agonists or anticholinergics are generally used. The loss of benefit associated with regular use of short acting $\beta$-agonists has not been observed with anticholinergics (Rennard et al. 1996). Bronchodilators of different classes can be combined effectively in COPD patients (Gupta et al. 1993).

Bronchodilators may improve symptoms even while spirometric measures of expiratory airflow are unaffected (Mahler 1985; Taylor et al. 1985). In this regard, dyspnea is related to the work of breathing and to inspiratory effort, and bronchodilators may improve these parameters by reducing hyperinflation, without altering the $FEV_1$ and forced vital capacity measured by spirometry (Sassi-Dambron et al. 1995; Belman et al. 1996; Gorini et al. 1996). In addition, theophylline may have salutary effects—as on diaphragmatic contractility—in addition to bronchodilation. Although objective assessment of airflow obstruction is still necessary for optimal management, the use of bronchodilators in COPD is also guided empirically based on symptoms.

**PRINCIPLE In COPD patients, the "clinical trial of one" can be used to assess the utility of bronchodilators, both alone and in combination.**

As disease progresses, the relative benefits that can be obtained, even with modest bronchodilator responses, increase (Anthonisen and Wright 1986). It is therefore essential to reassess the clinical management program periodically.

Since the only established benefit of bronchodilator therapy is the relief of symptoms, treatment should logically be limited to symptomatic patients. This sensible conclusion can prove problematic in actual clinical practice. Many COPD patients, especially the elderly, do not report symptoms because they have habitually restricted their level of activity to match their pulmonary impairment or attribute their progressive loss of function to aging. This fact of the clinical presentation of COPD emphasizes the importance of objective measurement of lung function in initial assessment. Even patients with large reductions in lung function often report little or no dyspnea. In such patients, a trial of bronchodilator treatment may lead to dramatic improvement. Such patients may recognize only in retrospect that they had been restricted by pulmonary symptoms.

Again because the only established action of bronchodilators is to relieve symptoms, the clinical response reported by the patient is the most important measure of therapeutic success. And again, this sensible principal can prove problematic in practice, for some patients have so restricted their activity through fear of dyspnea that they have become severely deconditioned and are unable to function at the new, higher level now permitted by improved airway function. Both fear and deconditioning can be important, and management often requires a global approach combining optimal physiological treatment, psychological support, and an aggressive program of physical rehabilitation (Ries et al. 1995; Lacasse et al. 1996).

## Glucocorticoids

Glucocorticoids, which have such a central place in the management of asthma, have a smaller place in management of chronic COPD. A minority of patients with COPD respond to short-term administration of a glucocorticoid with an improvement in lung function and a reduction in symptoms. This has been observed in several well-designed clinical trials and is supported by meta-analysis (Callahan et al. 1991). The response may be dramatic, so determining whether an individual patient has "steroid responsive" disease is important. Some clues of likely responsiveness are a history of asthma, blood or sputum eosinophilia, and a good response to a $\beta$-agonist bronchodilator, but the only way to determine responsiveness is with a therapeutic trial. The recommended trial is with 20–30 mg of oral prednisone for 2–3 weeks (American Thoracic Society 1995; Siafakas et al. 1995). If a beneficial response is observed, the patient can be weaned to inhaled glucocorticoids. An initial trial of inhaled corticosteroids is also reasonable (Paggiaro et al. 1998), but a negative response will raise questions of proper inhaler use.

Two cautions must be kept in mind in assessing the response to a therapeutic trial of glucocorticoid therapy. One is that the recommended dose of prednisone can have mood-elevating effects, so a patient's report of an improved sense of well-being should be regarded skeptically unless it is associated with some objective evidence of improvement in airflow. The other caution is that the failure to respond to a course of glucocorticoid treatment in the baseline state does not mean that airflow obstruction will be similarly unresponsive during an exacerbation.

Even in patients with COPD responsive to glucocorticoids, it is not known whether inhaled glucocorticoids slow progression of the disease. Results from four large randomized trials will be available in the near future. The issue is important, for the systemic adverse effects of inhaled corticosteroid therapy that have been reported in adults, cataracts and glaucoma, were reported to occur in elderly patients, the age group most affected by COPD.

**PRINCIPLE Preventive treatments must have a higher margin of safety than treatments that have acute benefits.**

## Other Treatments for Chronic Obstructive Pulmonary Disease

### *Oxygen*

As COPD progresses, oxygen therapy may be necessary for relief of hypoxemia and its consequences. The severity of hypoxemia depends on the degree of ventilation-perfusion mismatching and, in some cases, on hypoventilation. These abnormalities are variably present in individual patients with COPD depending on the underlying pathology. When emphysema predominates, hypoxemia becomes severe only late in the course of disease, and hypoventilation occurs only in its final stages. When chronic obstructive bronchitis predominates, both hypoxemia and hypoventilation occur earlier and are more responsive to treatment. Because treatment of hypoxemia can improve mortality and morbidity, oxygenation should be assessed regularly in patients with an $FEV_1 < 50\%$ of the predicted value (Nocturnal Oxygen Therapy Trial Group 1980; Medical Research Council Working Party 1981). For this purpose, transcutaneous measurement of oxygen saturation is sufficient.

Two large randomized studies have demonstrated supplemental oxygen improved survival in patients with arterial $PO_2 < 55$ Torr ($SaO_2 < 90\%$). The Medical Research Council (MRC) trial (1981) compared no oxygen with oxygen given 15 hours/day, and the NOTT trial (Nocturnal Oxygen Therapy Trial Group 1980) compared oxygen given 12 hours/day with oxygen given "continuously." Survival increased with increasing duration of oxygen treatment. Routine use of oxygen for patients with less severe hypoxemia ($PO_2$ 55–60 Torr) is not supported unless there is evidence of end-organ dysfunction from hypoxemia, for example, mental status changes, polycythemia, cor pulmonale, etc., oxygen is generally recommended if the $PO_2$ is less than 60 Torr. Situational oxygen therapy is also recommended for individuals with transient hypoxemia documented during exercise or sleep.

### *Treatments used in selected patients*

Despite their use for many centuries, no clear evidence-based guidelines are available for mucoactive agents in COPD. As these agents are generally used for symptomatic management, however, cautious empirical trials in appropriate patients represent reasonable clinical practice.

Other medications are sometimes used in special situations. Narcotics and other psychoactive agents has been reported to improve dyspnea in COPD patients. Although respiratory depression may result from such agents, the risk of this complication may be acceptable for relief of suffering, and indeed severe dyspnea can be regarded as a pain equivalent (Light et al. 1989, 1996). Respiratory stimulants have been reported to improve ventilation and, therefore, gas exchange in COPD patients. Clinical benefits have not been demonstrated, and their use is not routinely recommended (American Thoracic Society 1995; Siafakas et al. 1995). Anabolic agents and dietary supplements have been evaluated in COPD patients. To date, clinical benefits have not been demonstrated. It may simply be the case that patients capable of gaining weight are in a better prognostic group (Schols et al. 1998).

### *Surgery*

Surgery may improve lung function in COPD patients. This was first demonstrated in patients with large lung bullae. Removal of these enlarged, nonfunctional, "space-occupying" lesions was shown to allow greater expansion of the remaining, healthier lung and to restore the hyperinflated chest to a more normal volume, thus improving chest mechanics. Pneumoreductive surgery, often referred to as "volume reduction surgery" may achieve much the same result through the removal of emphysematous tissue (Fein et al. 1996; Brenner, McKenna, et al. 1998). Whether such a drastic approach actually leads to a sustained reduction in symptoms and improvement in functional capacity is currently undergoing a large prospective clinical trial sponsored by the National Heart, Lung, and Blood Institute of the National Institutes of Health. Finally, an even more drastic therapeutic option of lung transplantation is an option in carefully selected patients with severe COPD and without significant morbidity from the cardiovascular complications that commonly occur from heavy tobacco use over many years.

## Acute Exacerbations of Chronic Ostructive Pulmonary Disease

Chronic obstructive pulmonary disease is a chronic, progressive illness whose course is frequently punctuated by acute exacerbations. These are characterized by acute increases in cough, sputum production, and dyspnea. They are probably caused most often by viral infections of the respiratory tract, as are most acute exacerbations of asthma, but viral and bacterial causes of tracheobronchitis are difficult to distinguish on clinical grounds. Systemic manifestations, for example, fever, chills, and pleuritic chest pain, should be regarded as signs of more severe infection, for example, pneumonia.

The treatment of acute exacerbations of COPD resembles in many, but not all, ways the treatment of acute exacerbations of asthma. Bronchodilators, given by MDI or nebulizer, supplemental oxygen, and systemic corticosteroid administration are the cornerstones of treatment of both conditions (Albert et al. 1980; Hudson and Monti 1990). Recent studies also support the use of oral prednisone for less severe exacerbations, demonstrating improved resolution (Thompson et al. 1996). As most exacerbations remit spontaneously, however, the necessity for use of glucocorticoids in mild exacerbations remains uncertain.

## Differences in Treatment for Asthma and Chronic Obstruction Pulmonary Disease

One of the differences in the treatment of the two conditions arise from the difference in respiratory drive. In an asthmatic attack, respiratory drive may be presumed to be increased unless the patient is exhausted, so oxygen can be given freely to correct hypoxemia. In COPD, respiratory drive may be diminished and may fall further if the hypoxemic drive to breathing is removed. Oxygen must thus be given judiciously, usually starting at a flow of 2–4 L/min by face mask or nasal prongs, and the patient's clinical status and arterial $P\text{CO}_2$ followed closely for signs of worsening hypoventilation. Also because the drive to breathing may be low in COPD, respiratory failure does not necessarily imply the same extraordinary increase in the work of breathing associated with respiratory failure in asthma, and a trial of noninvasive ventilation may be appropriate (Ambrosino et al. 1995; Confalonieri et al. 1996). In both conditions, intubation and mechanical ventilation are required if respiratory failure has developed or is imminent despite other therapy. Because survival following episodes of respiratory failure may be good, even in patients with advanced COPD, aggressive therapy, including intubation and mechanical ventilation, should not be arbitrarily withheld (Menzies et al. 1989; Rieves et al. 1993; Seneff et al. 1995).

Another difference from the treatment of asthma exacerbations is the earlier use of antibiotics for acute exacerbations of COPD. This practice arose from recognition of chronic bacterial colonization of the lower respiratory tract in many patients with COPD and from the presumption that bacterial overgrowth can lead to exacerbations. Although the benefits of antibiotic treatment demonstrated by well controlled clinical trials are small, they were statistically significant (Orr et al. 1993; Saint et al. 1995). The weight of evidence, including meta-analysis, indicates clinical benefit, and current practice standards endorse empiric treatment with an antibiotic (American Thoracic Society 1995; Siafakas et al. 1995). In general, the data indicate that the more purulent the sputum, the more likely are antibiotics to be effective (Anthonisen et al. 1987).

Several recent trials have suggested that COPD exacerbations may be prevented by chronic treatment. Inhaled glucocorticoids (Paggiaro et al. 1998), ipratropium (Friedman et al. 1996), and early initiation of a course of antibiotics have been suggested. Although such preventive measures are promising, they are not yet recommended by evidence-based guidelines.

## REFERENCES

Advisory Committee on Immunization Practices (ACIP). 1989. Pneumococcal polysaccharide vaccine: recommendations of the immunization practices advisory committee. *Morbid Mortal Wkly Rep* **38**:64–76.

Albert R, Martin T, Lewis S. 1980. Controlled clinical trial of methylprednisolone in patients with chronic bronchitis and acute respiratory insufficiency. *Ann Intern Med* **92**:753–8.

Ambrosino N, Foglio K, Rubini F, et al. 1995. Non invasive mechanical ventilation in acute respiratory failure due to chronic obstructive pulmonary disease: correlates for success. *Thorax* **50**:755–7.

American Thoracic Society. 1995. Standards for the diagnosis and care of patients with chronic obstructive pulmonary disease. *Am J Respir Crit Care Med* **152**:S78–121.

Anthonisen NR. 1997. OM–8BV for COPD. *Am J Respir Crit Care Med* **156**:1713–4.

Anthonisen NR, Connett JE, Kiley JP, et al. 1994. Effects of smoking intervention and the use of an inhaled anticholinergic bronchodilator on the rate of decline of $\text{FEV}_1$: the Lung Health Study. *JAMA* **272**:1497–1505.

Anthonisen NR, Manfreda J, Warren CPW, et al. 1987. Antibiotic therapy in exacerbations of chronic obstructive pulmonary disease. *Ann Intern Med* **106**:196–204.

Anthonisen NR, Wright E. 1986. Bronchodilator response in chronic obstructive pulmonary disease. *Am Rev Respir Dis* **133**:814–9.

Belman MJ, Botnick WC, Shin JW. 1996. Inhaled bronchodilators reduce dynamic hyperinflation during exercise in patients with chronic obstructive pulmonary disease. *Am J Respir Crit Care Med* **153**:967–75.

Brenner M, McKenna RJ, Gelb AF, et al. 1998. Rate of FEV change following lung volume reduction surgery. *Chest* **113**:652–9.

Buist AS, Sexton GJ, Nagy JM, et al. 1976. The effect of smoking cessation and modification on lung function. *Am Rev Respir Dis* **114**:115–22.

Callahan CM, Dittus RS, Katz BP. 1991. Oral corticosteroid therapy for patients with stable chronic obstructive pulmonary disease. *Ann Intern Med* **114**:216–23.

Centers for Disease Control and Prevention. 1998. Prevention and control of influenza: recommendations of the Advisory Committee on Immunization Practices (ACIP). *Morbid Mortal Wkly Rep* **47**(RR–6):1–26.

Collet JP, Shapiro P, Ernst P, et al. 1997. Effects of an immunostimulating agent on acute exacerbations and hospitalizations in patients with chronic obstructive pulmonary disease. The Prevention of Acute Respiratory Infection by an Immunostimulant (PARI-IS) Study Steering Committee and Research Group. *Am J Respir Crit Care Med* **156**:1719–24.

Confalonieri M, Parigi P, Scartabellati A, et al. 1996. Noninvasive mechanical ventilation improves the immediate and long-term outcome of COPD patients with acute respiratory failure. *Eur Respir J* **9**:422–30.

Daughton DM, Susman J, Sitorius M, et al. 1998. Transdermal nicotine therapy and primary care: importance of counseling, demographic and patient selection factors on one-year quit rates. *Arch Fam Med.*

Fein AM, Branman SS, Casaburi R, et al. 1996. Lung volume reduction surgery—This official statement of the Am. Thoracic Society was adopted by the ATS board of directors, May 1996. *Am J Respir Crit Care Med* **154**:1151–2.

Fiore MC, Smith SS, Jorenby DE, et al. 1994. The effectiveness of the nicotine patch for smoking cessation. *JAMA* **271**:1940–7.

Fletcher C, Peto R, Tinker C, et al. 1976. *The Natural History of Chronic Bronchitis and Emphysema.* New York: Oxford Univ. Press. p 1–272.

Friedman M, Witek TJ, Serby CW, et al. 1996. Combination bronchodilator therapy is associated with a reduction in exacerbations. *Am J Respir Crit Care Med* **153**:A126.

Gorini M, Misuri G, Corrado A, et al. 1996. Breathing pattern and carbon dioxide retention in severe chronic obstructive pulmonary disease. *Thorax* **51**:677–83.

Gupta SK, Okerholm RA, Coen P, et al. 1993. Single- and multiple-dose pharmacokinetics of Nicoderm (nicotine transdermal system). *J Clin Pharmacol* **33**:169–74.

Higgins MW, Keller JB, Landis JR, et al. 1984. Risk of chronic obstructive pulmonary disease. *Am Rev Respir Dis* **130**:380–5.

Hudson LD, Monti CM. 1990. Rationale and use of corticosteroids in chronic obstructive pulmonary disease. *Med Clin North Am* **74**:661–90.

Hurt RD, Sachs DP, Glover ED, et al. 1997. A comparison of sustained-release bupropion and placebo for smoking cessation. *N Engl J Med* **337**:1195–1202.

Lacasse Y, Wong E, Guyatt GH, et al. 1996. Meta analysis of respiratory rehabilitation in chronic obstructive pulmonary disease. *Lancet* **348**:1115–9.

Light RW, Muro JR, Sato R. 1989. Effects of oral morphine on breathlessness and exercise tolerance in patients with chronic obstructive pulmonary disease. *Am Rev Respir Dis* **139**:126–33.

Light RW, Stansbury DW, Webster JS. 1996. Effect of 30 mg of morphine alone or with promethazine or prochlorperazine on the exercise capacity of patients with COPD. *Chest* **109**:975–81.

Mahler DA. 1985. Sustained-released theophylline reduces dyspnea in nonreversible obstructive airway disease. *Am Rev Respir Dis* **131**:22–5.

Mausner JS, Mausner B, Rial WY. 1968. The influence of a physician on the smoking of his patients. *Am J Publ Health* **58**:46–53.

Medical Research Council Working Party. 1981. Long term domiciliary oxygen therapy in chronic hypoxic cor pulmonale complicating chronic bronchitis and emphysema. *Lancet* **1**:681–6.

Menzies R, Gibbons W, Goldberg P. 1989. Determinants of weaning and survival among patients with COPD who require mechanical ventilation for acute respiratory failure. *Chest* **95**:398–405.

Nocturnal Oxygen Therapy Trial Group. 1980. Continuous or nocturnal oxygen therapy in hypoxemic chronic obstructive lung disease. *Ann Intern Med* **93**:391–8.

Orr PH, Scherer K, MacDonald A, et al. 1993. Randomized placebo-controlled trials of antibiotics for acute bronchitis: a critical review of the literature. *J Fam Pract* **36**:507–12.

Paggiaro PL, Dahle R, Bakran I, et al. 1998. Multicentre randomised placebo-controlled trial of inhaled fluticasone propionate in patients with chronic obstructive pulmonary disease. *Lancet* **351**:773–80.

Rennard SI, Serby CW, Ghafouri M, et al. 1996. Extended therapy with ipratropium is associated with improved lung function in patients with COPD: a retrospective analysis of data from seven clinical trials. *Chest* **110**:62–70.

Ries AL, Kaplan RM, Limberg TM, et al. 1995. Effects of pulmonary rehabilitation of physiologic and psychosocial outcomes in patients with chronic obstructive pulmonary disease. *Ann Intern Med* **122**:823–32.

Rieves RD, Bass D, Carter RR, et al. 1993. Severe COPD and acute respiratory failure. Correlates for survival at the time of tracheal intubation. *Chest* **104**:854–60.

Russell MAH, Stapleton JA, Feyerabend C, et al. 1993. Targeting heavy smokers in general practice: randomised controlled trial of transdermal nicotine patches. *Br Med J* **306**:1308–12.

Russell MAH, Wilson C, Taylor C, et al. 1979. Effect of general practitioners' advice against smoking. *Br Med J* **2**:231–5.

Saint S, Bent S, Vittinghoff E, et al. 1995. Antibiotics in chronic obstructive pulmonary disease exacerbations: a meta-analysis. *JAMA* **273**:957–60.

Sassi-Dambron DE, Eakin EG, Ries AL, et al. 1995. Treatment of dyspnea in COPD. *Chest* **107**:724–9.

Schneider NG, Olmstead R, Mody FV, et al. 1995. Efficacy of a nicotine nasal spray in smoking cessation: a placebo-controlled, double-blind trial. *Addiction* **90**:1671–82.

Schneider NG, Olmstead R, Nilsson F, et al. 1996. Efficacy of a nicotine inhaler in smoking cessation: a double-blind, placebo-controlled trial. *Addiction* **91**:1293–1306.

Schols AMWJ, Clangen J, Vovovic L, et al. 1998. Weight loss is a reversible factor in the prognosis of chronic obstructive pulmonary disease. *Am J Respir Crit Care Med* **157**:1–7.

Seersholm N, Dirksen A, Kok-Jensen A. 1994. Airways obstruction and two year survival in patients with severe alpha 1-antitrypsin deficiency. *Eur Respir J* **7**:1985–7.

Seneff MG, Wagner DP, Wagner RP, et al. 1995. Hospital and 1-year survival of patients admitted to intensive care units with acute exacerbation of chronic obstructive pulmonary disease. *JAMA* **274**:1852–7.

Siafakas NM, Vermeire P, Pride NB, et al. 1995. Optimal assessment and management of chronic obstructive pulmonary disease (COPD). The European Respiratory Society Task Force. *Eur Respir J* **8**:1398–1420.

Silagy C, Mant D, Fowler G, et al. 1994. Meta-analysis on efficacy of nicotine replacement therapies in smoking cessation. *Lancet* **343**:139–142.

Snider GL, Faling LJ, Rennard SI. 1994. Chronic bronchitis and emphysema. In: Murray JF, Nadel JA, editors. *Textbook of Respiratory Medicine*. San Francisco: W. B. Saunders Company. p 1331–97.

Sorlie PD, Kannel WB, O'Connor G. 1989. Mortality associated with respiratory function and symptoms in advanced age. The Framingham Study. *Am Rev Respir Dis* **140**:379–84.

Taylor DR, Buick B, Kinney C, et al. 1985. The efficacy of orally administered theophylline, inhaled salbutamol, and a combination of the two as chronic therapy in the management of chronic bronchitis with reversible air-flow obstruction. *Am Rev Respir Dis* **131**:747–51.

The Alpha-1-Antitrypsin Deficiency Registry Study Group. 1998. Survival and $FEV_1$ decline in individuals with severe deficiency of $\alpha 1$ antitrypsin. *Am J Respir Crit Care Med* **158**:49–59.

Thompson WH, Nielson CP, Carvalho P, et al. 1996. Controlled trial of oral prednisone in outpatients with acute COPD exacerbation. *Am J Respir Crit Care Med* **154**:407–12.

U.S. Department of Health and Human Services [DHHS]. 1996. Smoking Cessation. Clinical Practice Guideline: U.S. Department of Health and Human Services.

# Cystic Fibrosis

**Moira L. Aitken, Mark Tonelli**

*Chapter Outline*



## PATHOPHYSIOLOGY OF CYSTIC FIBROSIS

Cystic fibrosis (CF) is an autosomal recessive disorder affecting 1:3300 Caucasians, 1:17,000 African-Americans, and 1:90,000 Asians. The gene product is expressed in cells of epithelial origin, with disease manifestations in the lungs, sinuses, pancreas, gastrointestinal tract, hepatobiliary system, sweat glands, and reproductive tract. The term *cystic fibrosis* refers to the original description of the pathologic appearance of disease in the pancreas.

Diagnosis is based on a positive "sweat test" (chloride concentration >60 mEq/L) or genetic testing demonstrating two CF alleles and symptoms compatible with CF. The sweat test is highly sensitive (96%) and specific for CF.

The CF gene is located on the long arm of the 7th chromosome. The deletion of three base pairs (ΔF508) accounts for approximately 70% of all the CF alleles. The CF gene encodes for the cystic fibrosis transmembrane conductance regulator (CFTR), a membrane glycoprotein that influences chloride and sodium ion channels (Al-Awqati 1995). How these ion channel defects lead to organ disease is unknown. One suggestion is that high NaCl concentrations in airway fluid impair bacterial killing by natural antibacterial proteins, or "defensins," in the airways (Smith et al. 1996). Another possibility is that increased sodium absorption and decreased chloride secretion by airway epithelial cells reduce the water content of fluid overlying the epithelium, thus increasing mucus viscosity and slowing ciliary beat frequency, impairing the clearance of bacterial pathogens (Johnson et al. 1991).

## PHARMACOKINETICS IN PATIENTS WITH CYSTIC FIBROSIS

Pharmacokinetics are altered in patients with cystic fibrosis. Renal and hepatic cell function may be directly altered by the effects of disturbances in ion channel function on intracellular pH (Barasch et al. 1991). Loss of bile salts increases hepatic cytochrome P450 activity. The drugs affected range from those that are extensively metabolized, such as sulfamethoxazole and theophylline, to those that are excreted unchanged in the urine, such as the penicillins. Increases in the volume of distribution and clearance, and aminoglycoside binding to DNA in purulent airway secretions, increase dose requirements of aminoglycoside antibiotics given for treatment of airway infections (Spino 1991).

**PRINCIPLE Disease-based alterations in pharmacokinetics can be solely responsible for altered responses to "standard" doses. See also the effects of congestive heart failure on dose requirements of lidocaine, etc.**

## PULMONARY DISEASE IN PATIENTS WITH CYSTIC FIBROSIS

Over the past 50 years, the median life expectancy of CF patients has increased progressively to 31 years (FitzSimmons 1997). The course of the disease is characterized by chronic airflow obstruction and recurrent exacerbations of chronic airway infection. Hemoptysis, pneumothorax, clubbing, and respiratory failure with cor pulmonale may occur. Over 95% of patients die from respiratory failure.

Pathologically, the lungs are normal at birth. The earliest detectable change is plugging of submucosal gland ducts in large airways. Once infection occurs, a self-perpetuating, destructive inflammatory reaction is initiated in the tracheobronchial tree. The neutrophils attracted to the airways themselves release chemoattractants and produce proteases that damage tissues, impair phagocytosis, and interfere with complement and immunoglobulin function, preventing effective clearance of bacteria.

Once infection is established, airway disease progresses rapidly, with bronchiolitis, bronchitis, and some degree of bronchiectasis demonstrable by age 6–24 months. The course thereafter is typically punctuated by recurrent exacerbations, with subjective symptoms of increased cough, sputum production and shortness of breath and, often, anorexia and weight loss. Fever or leukocytosis may be present, spirometric values may be reduced, and the chest radiograph may show subtle changes but rarely shows a frank infiltrate (Greene et al. 1994). The infectious agents most common in exacerbations are *Staphylococcus aureus*, *Haemophilus influenzae,* and *Pseudomonas aeruginosa*. Common respiratory viruses are associated with some pulmonary exacerbations. Eventually, *P. aeruginosa* becomes the dominant organism in 90% of patients.

Impairment in pulmonary function is not apparent in the newborn with CF until peripheral airways are obstructed by mucus. As lung disease progresses, air trapping occurs first (increased residual volume), and airflow obstruction predominates soon thereafter (decreased $FEV_1$ and peak flow). Arterial blood gases show progressive widening of the alveolar–arterial difference with disease progression, and the presence of carbon dioxide retention is an ominous sign (Kerem et al. 1992).

Overinflation, peribronchial cuffing, small infiltrates (mucous plugging) are early findings on chest roentgenogram. Computerized tomography (CT) scanning also reveals bronchiectasis at an early stage. As the disease progresses, routine chest radiographs show bronchiectasis and diffuse fibrosis, most marked in the upper lobes, with scarring and upward retraction of the hila. Hilar and mediastinal adenopathy secondary to chronic infection and enlargement of the pulmonary arteries appear later in the course of the disease.

## PULMONARY TREATMENTS FOR CYSTIC FIBROSIS

### Antibiotics

A key to successful management of cystic fibrosis is antibiotic treatment of airway infection. In general, mild exacerbations can be treated with oral or inhaled antibiotics (Ramsey 1996). Severe exacerbations require intravenous antibiotics. Because bacteria can rarely be eradicated from the airways, the duration of therapy is determined by improvement in clinical parameters, that is, symptoms, physical examination, decreased leukocyte count, and improvement in spirometric measurements. Improvement in pulmonary function usually occurs within 5 days of initiation of treatment and continues for 10–21 days (Redding et al. 1982). Home intravenous therapy has become the mainstay of treatment in many CF centers, with only severely ill patients requiring hospitalization.

The question as to whether maintenance antibiotic therapy should be prescribed is unclear. The most compelling study suggesting that chronic therapy should not be given was a 5-year placebo-controlled, double-blind study of cephalexin treatment in 119 CF patients less than 2 years old. Growth, number of acute exacerbations, hospitalizations and/or hospital days, radiographic abnormalities, and pulmonary function tests did not differ with treatment (Cystic Fibrosis Foundation 1996). Patients treated with cephalexin had less infection with *S. aureus*, but had more with *P. aeruginosa*.

**PRINCIPLE When disease seems to demand chronic treatment with drugs ordinarily used for short courses, the therapist must be very alert to new signs of toxicity.**

Another approach to controlling chronic bronchial infection is to deliver antibiotics, especially aminoglycosides, by inhalation. A recent study of inhaled tobramycin showed improvement in lung function and little increased antibiotic resistance (Ramsey et al. 1999).

## Bronchodilators

Bronchodilators benefit patients with cystic fibrosis who are clinically wheezy or who demonstrate a significant improvement in a test of airflow after a trial of therapy (Cropp 1996; Hordvik et al. 1996). The bronchodilators most often used are $\beta$-agonists given by inhalation. The symptomatic improvements seen in some patients treated with theophylline preparations may reflect improving diaphragmatic contractility. Cromolyn is not effective, even though atopy and bronchial hyperreactivity are common in cystic fibrosis (Sivan et al. 1990). In contrast, anticholinergic bronchodilators seem roughly equivalent to $\beta$-agonists as bronchodilators (Weintraub and Eschenbacher 1989), despite theoretical concerns over further alterations in mucus secretion.

## Anti-inflammatory drugs

Anti-inflammatory agents, including corticosteroids, ibuprofen, and antiproteases, have been examined in CF. A modest benefit of oral corticosteroid treatment on pulmonary function was offset by growth retardation and by the possibility of increased susceptibility to osteoporosis (Eigen et al. 1995). Inhaled steroids seem a reasonable choice in patients with hyperreactive airways and chronic inflammation (but of a nature quite different from that of asthma) and indeed appear to cause modest improvements in spirometry (Wojtczak et al. 1996; Bisgaard et al. 1997). The even more modest benefit from chronic treatment with ibuprofen (Konstan et al. 1995) is offset by concern over renal toxicity in patients who require frequent treatment with nephrotoxic antibiotics, such as the aminoglycosides.

**PRINCIPLE Although it is tempting to use drugs that appropriately affect surrogate endpoints, a number of examples have shown that drugs that alter surrogate endpoints may increase mortality (antiarrhythmics to decrease ventricular premature beats, MER 29 to reduce cholesterol levels, antitumor drugs used to manage nodular lymphomas). The therapist should try to obtain data on mortality before embracing a drug's use because of its effects on surrogate endpoints.**

## Airway clearance

A variety of techniques and devices are used to enhance clearance of mucopurulent secretions. These include physical maneuvers, such as postural drainage, percussion and vibration, autogenic drainage, and use of the Flutter device. Mucolytics are also used to enhance the clearance of airway secretions. The mucolytics tested in chronic bronchitis, such as *N*-acetylcysteine, iodinated products, and guaifenesin have not been studied in patients with CF, so their use can be justified only by extrapolation from studies of their effectiveness in a different disease. A mucolytic specifically developed for treating cystic fibrosis is dornase alpha, or rhDNase. This is a recombinant product of the gene for the enzyme, DNase, that randomly cuts DNA into smaller pieces. Its development was stimulated first by the observation that DNA is highly viscous and, second, by the observation that the purulent sputum of cystic fibrosis has an extraordinarily high DNA content because of DNA release from dead neutrophils. Aerosol administration of this enzyme improves spirometric values and decreases the number of days antibiotic therapy is required (Fuchs et al. 1994; McCoy et al. 1996). It has been associated with voice change, but has not been demonstrated to have serious adverse effects. Unanswered questions regarding the utility of rhDNase are the appropriate time in the course of the disease to initiate therapy, the appropriate dose and duration, and the long-term benefits of treatment (Kanga 1996).

# OTHER DISEASE MANIFESTATIONS

The pulmonary consequences of cystic fibrosis usually dominate this genetic disorder's clinical presentation, but the defect in ion transport affects epithelial and secretory cells of many organs. Many nonpulmonary complications can occur and, in some patients, dominate the course of disease and the required treatment. Pharmacologic treatment of these other manifestations of cystic fibrosis are beyond the scope of this chapter, but can be listed briefly: disorders in sweating with an attendant risk of hyperthermia, chronic sinusitis, impairment of gastrointestinal motility, hepatobiliary disease, pancreatic insufficiency, and azoospermia in men.

"Evidence-based" clinical practice guidelines for cystic fibrosis have been written for the treatment of both the chronic disease and acute exacerbations (Cystic Fibrosis Foundation 1997). The multiorgan nature of the disease, the variability of the underlying genetic mutation, and the variability of phenotypic expression of common genotypes clearly mean, however, that management must be individualized.

## REFERENCES


Al-Awqati Q. 1995. Regulation of ion channels by ABC transporters that secrete ATP. *Science* **269**:805–6.

Barasch J, Kiss B, Prince A, et al. 1991. Defective acidification of intracellular organelles in cystic fibrosis. Nature **325**:70–3.

Bisgaard H, Pedersen S, Nielsen K, et al. 1997. Controlled trial of inhaled budesonide patients with cystic fibrosis and chronic bronchopulmonary *Pseudomonas aeruginosa* infection. *Am J Respir Crit Care Med* **156**:1190–6.

Cropp G. 1996. Effectiveness of bronchodilators in cystic fibrosis. *Am J Med* **100**(Suppl 1A):S19–29.

Cystic Fibrosis Foundation. Clinical Practice Guidelines for Cystic Fibrosis. Bethesda, MD: Cystic Fibrosis Foundation, 1997.

Cystic Fibrosis Foundation. Highlights: Selected proceedings from the 10th annual North American Cystic Fibrosis Conference, Orlando, FL. Orlando, FL: Cystic Fibrosis Foundation, 1996.

Eigen H, Rosenstein B, FitzSimmons S, et al. 1995. A multicenter study of alternate-day prednisone therapy in patients with cystic fibrosis. The CF Foundation Prednisone Trial Group. *J Pediatr* **126**: 515–23.

FitzSimmons S. 1997. Patient Registry 1996 Annual Data Report. Bethesda, MD: Cystic Fibrosis Foundation.

Fuchs H, Borowitz D, Christiansen D, et al. 1994. Effect of aerosolized recombinant DNase on exacerbations of respiratory symptoms and on pulmonary function in patients with cystic fibrosis. *N Engl J Med* **331**:637–42.

Greene K, Takasugi J, Godwin J, et al. 1994. Radiographic changes seen in acute exacerbations of cystic fibrosis in adults: a pilot study. *Am J Radiol* **163**:557–62.

Hordvik N, Sammut P, Judy C, et al. 1996. The effects of albuterol on the lung function of hospitalized patients with cystic fibrosis. *Am J Respir Crit Care Med* **154**:156–60.

Johnson N, Royce F, Villalon M, et al. 1991. Autoregulation of beat frequency in respiratory cells: demonstration by viscous load. *Am J Respir Dis* **144**:1091–4.

Kanga J. 1996. Dornase alfa therapy in cystic fibrosis: who should get it? *Chest* **110**:871–2.

Kerem E, Reisman J, Corey M, et al. 1992. Prediction of mortality in patients with cystic fibrosis. *N Engl J Med* **326**:1187–91.

Konstan M, Byard P, Hoppel C, et al. 1995. Effect of high-dose ibuprofen in patients with cystic fibrosis. *N Engl J Med* **332**:848–54.

McCoy K, Hamilton S, Johnson C, et al. 1996. Effects of 12-week administration of dornase alfa in patients with advanced cystic fibrosis lung disease. The Pulmozyme Study Group. *Chest* **110**:889–95.

Ramsey BW. 1996. Drug therapy: management of pulmonary disease in patients with cystic fibrosis. *N Engl J Med* **335**:179–88.

Ramsey BW, Pepe MS, Otto KL, et al. 1999. Intermittent administration of inhaled tobramycin in patients with cystic fibrosis. Cystic Fibrosis inhaled tobramycin study group. *N Engl J Med* **340**:23–30.

Redding G, Restuccia R, Cotton E, et al. 1982. Serial changes in pulmonary functions in children hospitalized with cystic fibrosis. *Am Rev Respir Dis* **126**:31–6.

Sivan Y, Arce P, Eigen H, et al. 1990. A double-blind, randomized study of sodium cromoglycate versus placebo in patients with cystic fibrosis and bronchial hyperreactivity. *J Allergy Clin Immunol* **85**:649–54.

Smith J, Travis S, Greenberg E, et al. 1996. Cystic fibrosis airway epithelia fail to kill bacteria because of abnormal surface fluid. *Cell* **85**:229–36.

Spino M. 1991. Pharmacokinetics of drugs in cystic fibrosis. *Clin Rev Allergy* **9**:169–209.

Weintraub S, Eschenbacher W. 1989. The inhaled bronchodilators ipratropium bromide and metaproterenol in adults with CF. *Chest* **95**:861–4.

Wojtczak H, Wagener J, Kerby G, et al. 1996. Effect of inhaled beclomethasone dipropionate on airway inflammation in children with cystic fibrosis. *Pediatr Pulmon Suppl* **13**:414A.

# Pneumonia

Michael S. Niederman

### Chapter Outline



Pneumonia can be acquired from sources in the community or in the altered microbial environment of the hospital. It is the sixth most common cause of death in the United States, but the number one cause of death from infectious diseases (Niederman et al. 1993). Recent studies have demonstrated that effective therapy of this illness, often provided empirically by necessity, can reduce mortality for patients with both community-acquired pneumonia (CAP) and hospital-acquired pneumonia (HAP) (Leroy et al. 1995; Gordon et al. 1996; Luna et al. 1997; Meehan et al. 1997; Rello et al. 1997). To achieve this end, it is necessary to provide therapy in a timely fashion, often without knowing the results of diagnostic testing, and to select a regimen that is likely to cover the most common etiologic agents. The complexities of pneumonia bacteriology and the ever-increasing problem of antimicrobial resistance among commonly recovered pathogens have made this increasingly difficult. At the same time that new options for therapy are becoming available, along with new strategies for their application, greater emphasis is being placed on the cost-effectiveness of care, with the resultant emphasis on providing care in the outpatient setting whenever possible. Several national societies have incorporated these issues into the development of guidelines for the therapy of both CAP and HAP (Niederman et al. 1993; Campbell et al. 1996; Bartlett et al. 1998). With a thorough understanding of the clinical issues and current therapeutic options for pneumonia, outcomes are likely to be good, even as the microbiologic complexities of this infection increase.

In this section, the antibiotic principles relevant to the therapy of pneumonia are examined, followed by a review of the clinical issues related to therapy, and a summary of current guidelines for empiric therapy.

## ANTIBIOTIC PRINCIPLES IN TREATMENT OF PNEUMONIA

### Mechanisms of Bacterial Killing

Antibiotics interfere with bacterial growth by preventing the formation of an intact cell wall, by interfering with protein synthesis or by inhibiting common metabolic pathways (Mandell 1994; Niederman 1997). Agents that interfere with cell wall synthesis or with other key metabolic functions of the organism can kill bacteria and are termed "bactericidal." These agents include penicillins, cephalosporins, aminoglycosides, fluoroquinolones, vancomycin, rifampin, and metronidazole. Agents that inhibit the growth of bacteria and rely on host defenses to eliminate the organisms are termed "bacteriostatic" and these agents include the macrolides, tetracyclines, sulfa drugs, chloramphenicol, and clindamycin. In clinical practice, the choice between these two types of agents should be dictated by bacterial susceptibility patterns, since little clinical difference exists between bacteriostatic and bactericidal agents unless the patient is neutropenic or has a deep-seated infection such as endocarditis, meningitis, or osteomyelitis. In these cases, a bactericidal agent is required.

The activity of an antimicrobial agent can be defined by the MIC (minimum inhibitory concentration) of that drug. This is the minimum concentration of that drug that inhibits the growth of one isolate of a pathogen for 24 h under specific in vitro conditions. The $MIC_{90}$ represents the minimum concentrations of that drug that inhibits growth of 90% of the isolates of that pathogen for 24 hours. The lower the MIC number, the more active an agent is against its target pathogen. However, the use of MIC values to predict antimicrobial effect only takes into account whether an agent can achieve adequate concentrations in blood. When an infection is in the tissues, as is the case with pneumonia, then the MIC value may not adequately predict killing at the tissue level. Thus if an agent penetrates well into respiratory secretions (such as a quinolone) and its concentrations exceed those in serum, the MIC values may underestimate the antibacterial effect (Niederman 1998). Conversely a poorly penetrating agent (such as an aminoglycoside) may be less effective clinically at certain sites of respiratory infection than expected on the basis of in vitro MIC values.

Not all bactericidal agents, even if they penetrate to the site of infection, kill bacteria in the same way, and the dosing regimens that are used should reflect the mechanisms of bactericidal activity of the specific drugs (Craig 1998). Thus some agents kill in a concentration-dependent fashion and the higher the serum level relative to the MIC and the higher the area under the concentration-time curve (AUC) relative to the MIC, the more effective the agent. In theory the optimal way to administer these agents would be to take a 24-hour dose and to infuse it once a day to achieve high peak concentrations. On the other hand, there are agents that do not achieve a greater effect with higher concentrations, but rather kill in relation to how long they exceed the MIC of the target organism, and the activity of these agents can be enhanced by maximizing time above the MIC of the target organism. For these drugs, optimal effect could be achieved by continuous infusion to maintain serum concentrations above the MIC.

Craig has recently reviewed and clarified some of these concepts related to bactericidal killing mechanisms (Craig 1998). Agents that kill in a concentration-dependent fashion include the aminoglycosides, the fluoroquinolones, and metronidazole (Table 2-10). With these drugs, the efficacy of an agent can be predicted by the peak/MIC ratio or the AUC/MIC ratio. Studies with quinolones illustrate these concepts well. In a clinical trial with levofloxacin, both clinical and microbiologic success were more likely if the peak/MIC ratio exceeded 12 (Preston et al. 1998). In addition, peak/MIC ratio of at least 8–10 must be maintained to prevent the emergence of bacterial resistance during therapy (Craig 1998). In studies of critically ill patients given ciprofloxacin, the best predictor of clinical and microbiologic efficacy was the AUC/MIC ratio, and if the 24-hour value exceeded 125, outcomes were better than if lower ratios were achieved (Forest et al. 1993). The efficacy of aminoglycosides has also been related to both the AUC/MIC and peak/MIC ratios (Hatala et al. 1996; Craig 1998). Agents that kill in a time-dependent fashion have a saturation of killing effect once the concentrations exceed 4–5 times the MIC, and time of exposure above MIC is the key to their effect. In this group of antimicrobials are β-lactam antibiotics, vancomycin, clindamycin, and the macrolides. Although continuous infusion strategies have been used for some of these agents, it may not be necessary to keep the concentration of antibiotics above the MIC for an entire dosing interval. Using animal models, Craig has shown that with penicillins and cephalosporins, bacteriologic cure will occur 85–100% of the time if the concentration of these agents exceeds the MIC for at least 40% of the dosing interval (Craig 1998). Maximal killing occurs once concentrations exceed the MIC for 60–70% of the dosing interval.

**Table 2-10 Pharmacokinetics of Common Antibiotics**

| |
|---|
| Bactericidal in a concentration-dependent fashion |
| Aminoglycosides [a] |
| Fluoroquinolones [a] |
| Metronidazole |
| Bactericidal in a time-dependent fashion |
| β-Lactams [b] |
| Vancomycin HCl |
| Clindamycin HCl |
| Macrolides |

[a]Prolonged post antibiotic effect against gram-negative bacteria.
[b]Little or no post antibiotic effect against gram-negative bacteria.

One other killing mechanism to consider is the post-antibiotic effect (PAE), which refers to the continued suppression of bacterial growth after the concentration of the antibiotic falls below the MIC of the target organism (Craig 1994, 1998). Although most antibiotics have a PAE against gram-positive organisms, prolonged PAEs against gram-negative organisms occur with the aminoglycosides, quinolones, tetracyclines, macrolides, chloramphenicol, and rifampin. Little or no PAE against gram-negative organisms occurs with β-lactam agents with the exception of the carbapenems (imipenem and meropenem). Fortunately, the agents with a prolonged PAE tend to be the same agents that kill in a concentration-dependent fashion, and this is why once-daily dosing of agents such as the aminoglycosides has been successful (Hatala et al. 1996). With once-daily dosing, high peaks are achieved, thus maximizing concentration-dependent killing, low troughs result, thus minimizing nephrotoxicity, and the prolonged PAE is relied upon to keep killing bacteria at the times that low trough concentrations occur. A recent meta-analysis has shown the efficacy and safety of once-daily aminoglycoside dosing, although this type of regimen is not substantially safer or more effective than traditional dosing schemes (Hatala et al. 1996).

**PRINCIPLE The appropriate use of pharmacokinetics information can do far more than estimate bioavailability, half-lives, and compliance. Selective use can be the difference between optimal and useless therapy.**

## Penetration to Sites of Infection

As discussed, the serum concentration of an antibiotic may not reflect tissue concentrations, with some agents penetrating well and exceeding serum concentrations in lung secretions and tissues, and with other agents penetrating poorly despite substantial concentration in blood. Concentrations of antibiotic can be measured in sputum, in epithelial lining fluid (collected by bronchoalveolar lavage), in the bronchial mucosa (sampled with biopsy), in the lung parenchyma, and in phagocytic cells (recovered by bronchoscopy). It remains uncertain which site-related concentration is most clinically relevant, but probably concentrations in epithelial lining fluid, phagocytes, and lung parenchyma are most relevant for patients with pneumonia.

Concentrations of an antibiotic depend on the permeability of the capillary bed at the site of infection (the bronchial circulation for lung tissue, the pulmonary circulation for the epithelial lining fluid), the degree of protein binding of the drug, and the presence of active transport into the lung (Honeybourne 1994). In the bronchial circulation, the capillary bed is fenestrated, and only small molecules that are not highly protein bound can readily enter the lung parenchyma unless inflammation is present and enhances entry. In the pulmonary circulation, the epithelium is not fenestrated, and lipophilic agents pass easily and enter the epithelial lining fluid. In general, lipophilic agents enter all sites well and are not inflammation-dependent and these include the following: quinolones, the new macrolides (azithromycin, clarithromycin), tetracyclines, clindamycin, and trimethoprim/sulfamethoxazole. On the other hand, the agents that are relatively lipid insoluble, and thus penetrate poorly, and are inflammation-dependent include the following: the aminoglycosides, the penicillins, the cephalosporins, the carbapenems, and the monobactams (Table 2-11). Drugs that enter phagocytes by active transport include the macrolides, quinolones, and clindamycin. Agents that are not actively transported into phagocytes remain in the extracellular space that constitutes 40% of the weight of bronchial tissue, and thus these agents (such as the penicillins) achieve only 40% of their serum concentrations in lung tissue.

Although penetration factors will determine the concentration of an antibiotic at the site of infection, this may not always reflect the activity of the agent. Certain antibiotics, such as the aminoglycosides, are not active at the acidic pH value that are common in the lung at sites of pneumonia (Bodem et al. 1983). In addition, bacteria can become resistant to an antibiotic by binding the antibiotic poorly to its site of action or by extruding the antibiotic from the cell or by having reduced permeability of the porin channels that allow antibiotics to have access to gram-negative organisms (Gold and Moellering 1996).

**Table 2-11 Penetration of Common Antibiotics into Respiratory Secretions**

| |
|---|
| Good penetration (generally lipid-soluble and inflammation-independent) |
| Fluoroquinolones |
| Macrolides: including azithromycin dihydrate and clarithromycin |
| Tetracyclines |
| Clindamycin HCl |
| Trimethoprim/sulfamethoxazole |
| Poor penetration (generally lipid-insoluble and inflammation-dependent) |
| Aminoglycosides |
| β-Lactams: penicillins, cephalosporins, carbapenems, monobactams |

## Clinical Microbiologic Aspects of Key Agents

### *Macrolides/tetracyclines*

Macrolides are bacteriostatic agents that bind to the 50S ribosomal subunit of the target bacteria and inhibit RNA-dependent protein synthesis. The macrolides have had good activity against pneumococci, as well as atypical pathogens (*Chlamydia pneumoniae*, *Mycoplasma pneumoniae*, *Legionella*), but the older erythromycin-type drugs are not active against *Haemophilus influenzae*, and have poor intestinal tolerance, so that prolonged therapy, as well as use in patients with COPD, is difficult. The new macrolide agents include azithromycin (also referred to as an azalide) and clarithromycin. These agents have enhanced activity against *H. influenzae* (including β-lactamase-producing strains), although on an MIC basis, azithromycin is more active (Mandell 1994; Niederman 1997). Erythromycin is active against *Moraxella catarrhalis*, although the new agents have enhanced activity against this pathogen. Among the new macrolides azithromycin is more active against not only *H. influenzae* and *M. catarrhalis*, but also *M. pneumoniae*. On the other hand, clarithromycin is more active against *Streptococcus pneumoniae*, *Legionella,* and *C. pneumoniae* (Mandell 1994; Niederman 1997).

Both of these newer agents are tolerated better by the GI tract than erythromycin, and they penetrate well into sputum, lung tissue, and phagocytes. Clarithromycin, which has an active 14-hydroxy metabolite that is antibacterial, is administered twice a day orally at a 500-mg dose for 10 days in the treatment of CAP. Azithromycin has a longer half-life than clarithromycin, and concentrates in tissues, achieving very low serum levels when administered orally. The dose for oral therapy of CAP is 500 mg on day 1, followed by 250 mg daily on days 2–5. Recently an intravenous preparation of azithromycin has been developed that produces efficacy as monotherapy for CAP not caused by anaerobic or gram-negative organisms. Concentrations of this agent in serum are adequate when the drug is given intravenously. The drug has been effective for patients with bacteremic pneumococcal pneumonia. The dose of the intravenous preparation is 500 mg for 2–5 days, followed by 500 mg of oral therapy for a total of 7–10 days of treatment. The use of most macrolides with the exception of azithromycin can lead to an elevation in theophylline concentrations.

Macrolides remain an important therapeutic option for CAP, and studies in both outpatients and inpatients have shown that these agents lead to favorable outcomes for patients with CAP, when used alone or in combination with a β-lactam agent (Gordon et al. 1996). One concern however, is that pneumococci are becoming increasingly resistant to macrolides, particularly in conjunction with penicillin resistance. In one study, 30–40% of all the pneumococci that were intermediate or high-level penicillin-resistant were also resistant to erythromycin (Clavo-Sanchez et al. 1997). The clinical relevance of these in vitro findings remains to be defined.

The tetracyclines are also bacteriostatic agents that act by binding the 30S ribosomal subunit and interfering with protein synthesis. These agents can be used in CAP because they are active against *H. influenzae* and atypical pathogens, but there are reports of increasing resistance among pneumococci (Mandell 1994; Niederman 1997). Photosensitivity is the major adverse effect, limiting the use of these agents in sun-exposed patients.

### *β-Lactam antibiotics*

These bactericidal antibiotics have in common a β-lactam ring, which is bound to a five-membroid thiazolidine ring in the case of the penicillins and to a six-membroid dihydrothiazine ring in the case of the cephalosporins. Modifications in the thiazolidine ring can lead to agents such as the carbapenems (imipenem and meropenem), whereas absence of the second ring structure characterizes the monobactams (aztreonam). These agents can also be combined with β-lactamase inhibitors such as sulbactam, tazobactam, or clavulanic acid, to create the β-lactam/β-lactamase inhibitor drugs. These agents extend the antimicrobial spectrum of the β-lactams by providing a substrate for the bacterial β-lactamases (sulbactam, clavulanic acid, tazobactam), thereby preserving the antibacterial activity of the parent compound. β-Lactam antibiotics work by interfering with the synthesis of bacterial cell wall peptidoglycans by binding to bacterial penicillin binding proteins.

The penicillins used for respiratory tract infections include the natural penicillins (penicillins G and V), the aminopenicillins (ampicillin, amoxicillin), the antistaphylococcal agents, the antipseudomonal agents, and the β-lactam/β-lactamase inhibitor combinations. The antipseudomonal penicillins include the older carboxypenicillins (ticarcillin) and the ureidopenicillins (piperacillin, azlocillin, mezlocillin), with piperacillin and azlocillin being the most active agents against *Pseudomonas aeruginosa*. The β-lactamase inhibitor combinations include clavulanic acid with either amoxicillin or ticarcillin; sulbactam with ampicillin; and tazobactam with piperacillin.

The cephalosporins span the first to fourth generations. The earlier agents were generally active against gram-positive bacteria, but did not have extended activity to the more complex gram-negative bacteria, or anaerobic bacteria, and were susceptible to destruction by bacterial β-lactamases. The newer generation agents are generally more specialized agents, with broad-spectrum activity, and with more mechanisms to resist breakdown by bacteria. The second-generation and newer agents are resistant to bacterial β-lactamases. The third-generation agents active against penicillin-resistant pneumococci include ceftriaxone and cefotaxime, whereas ceftazidime is active against *P. aeruginosa* (Pallares et al. 1995). The third-generation agents, as mentioned above, may induce β-lactamases among certain gram-negative organisms, and thus promote the emergence of resistance during monotherapy (Chow et al. 1991). The fourth-generation agent, cefepime, is active against pneumococci and *P. aeruginosa*, but is also less likely to induce resistance among the Enterobacteriaceae than the third-generation agents (Niederman 1997).

Imipenem and meropenem are the broadest spectrum agents in this class, being active against gram-positive organisms, anaerobes, and gram-negative organisms including *P. aeruginosa*. They have shown efficacy for patients with severe pneumonia, both community-acquired and nosocomial, and may be effective as monotherapy (Fink et al. 1994; Sieger et al. 1997). Aztreonam is a monobactam that is so antigenically different from the rest of the β-lactams, that it can be used in patients who are allergic to penicillin. It is only active against gram-negative organisms, having a spectrum very similar to the aminoglycosides.

### *Fluoroquinolones*

These bactericidal agents act by interfering with bacterial DNA gyrase, leading to impairment of DNA synthesis for repair, transcription, and other cellular processes, resulting in bacterial cell lysis (Niederman 1998). DNA gyrase is one form of bacterial topoisomerase enzyme that is inhibited by the quinolones, but activity against other similar enzymes is part of the effect of a variety of quinolones. As mentioned above, quinolones kill in a concentration-dependent fashion, related to the $C_{max}$/MIC ratio and to the AUC/MIC ratio of drug concentration relative to organism susceptibility.

There are two features of quinolones that make them well-suited to respiratory infections. First, they penetrate well into secretions and inflammatory cells within the lung, achieving concentrations that in many instances exceed those in serum. Thus, these agents may be clinically more effective than predicted by MIC values. Second, these agents are highly bioavailable after oral administration and thus similar concentrations can be reached whether administered orally or intravenously. This allows for some "borderline" patients (such as nursing home patients) with pneumonia to be managed with outpatient oral therapy and not be admitted solely for the purpose of intravenous therapy to achieve high serum levels of antibiotics (Gentry et al. 1992). In addition, the high bioavailability of these agents permits an easy transition from intravenous to oral therapy of inpatients with pneumonia, facilitating early discharge when the patient is doing well, and permitting ongoing oral therapy with maintenance of high serum concentrations of antibiotics.

Currently, the quinolones fall into several "generations" as defined by Gootz and Brighty (1998). The first-generation agents had gram-negative activity only and were used for urinary tract infections, epitomized by the agent nalidixic acid. The second-generation agents had added gram-positive activity and could be used for systemic infections and included ciprofloxacin, ofloxacin, pefloxacin, fleroxacin, and lomefloxacin. These agents had limited value for respiratory infections because of relatively high MIC values among pneumococci, making it necessary to use high doses to achieve efficacy against this pathogen. The third-generation agents are characterized by better gram-positive activity, particularly against pneumococcus. Approved agents include grepafloxacin, levofloxacin, sparfloxacin, gatifloxacin, and trovafloxacin, Clinafloxacin and moxifloxacin, which are still in development. Among the third-generation agents, the most active against pneumococcus is trovafloxacin, followed by grepafloxacin and sparfloxacin, and then levofloxacin (Table 2-12) (Niederman 1998). These new agents also have long half-lives, allowing once-daily dosing with most of the third-generation agents. In addition, quinolones that are active against pneumococcus are likely to be effective regardless of penicillin susceptibility patterns since penicillin and quinolone resistance do not generally occur together in the same organisms, and pneumococcal resistance rates to new quinolones are low (Niederman 1998). Trovafloxacin is unique among the new quinolones, as it is the only one active against anaerobes (clinafloxacin is active but not available for clinical use), and it is also approved for use against *P. aeruginosa*, making it the second antipseudomonal quinolone available, although it is not quite as active on an MIC basis against this organism as ciprofloxacin. New observations about drug-related hepatotoxicity have limited the widespread use of trovafloxacin.

**Table 2-12 Activity of Fluoroquinolones against Pneumococcus**

| AGENT | $MIC_{90}$ (MG/L)[a] |
|---|---|
| Clinafloxacin | 0.125 |
| Grepafloxacin | 0.25–0.5 |
| Levofloxacin | 1.0 |
| Sparfloxacin | 0.25–0.5 |
| Trovafloxacin | 0.125–0.25 |
| Gatifloxacin | 0.5 |
| Moxifloxacin | 0.25 |

[a]Minimum inhibitory concentration for 90% of strains of that pathogen.

Quinolones can be used for acute exacerbations of chronic bronchitis, CAP, and HAP because of their broad spectrum of activity. They are active against $\beta$-lactamase-producing *H. influenzae* and *M. catarrhalis* making them very useful for patients with COPD. Quinolones are also active against atypical pathogens, with the newer agents being more active against *C. pneumoniae* and *M. pneumoniae* than the older agents (Niederman 1998). The new agents are also highly effective against *L. pneumophila*.

### *Aminoglycosides*

These bactericidal agents act by binding to the 30S ribosomal subunit of bacteria, thus interfering with protein synthesis. Aminoglycosides have primarily a gram-negative spectrum of activity and are usually used in combination with other agents, targeting difficult organisms such as *P. aeruginosa* or other resistant gram-negative bacteria. When combined with certain $\beta$-lactam agents they can achieve antibacterial synergy against *P. aeruginosa*. Amikacin is the least susceptible to enzymatic inactivation by bacteria, whereas tobramycin is more active than gentamicin against *P. aeruginosa*. Aminoglycosides penetrate poorly into lung tissue, and can be inactivated at the acid pH values common in pneumonic lung tissue. Thus in one clinical trial of nosocomial pneumonia therapy, the use of an aminoglycoside with a $\beta$-lactam was no more effective than a $\beta$-lactam alone, and the combination regimen was not more effective in preventing the emergence of pseudomonal resistance during therapy than was the monotherapy regimen with a $\beta$-lactam (Cometta et al. 1994). In the treatment of bacteremic pseudomonal pneumonia, aminoglycoside combination therapy may be more effective than monotherapy (Hilf et al. 1989).

As discussed above, aminoglycosides kill in a concentration-dependent fashion, and can be dosed once-daily to optimize killing while minimizing toxicity. In clinical practice, once-daily dosing is comparable in efficacy and nephrotoxicity to multiple-dose regimens (Hatala et al. 1996). When aminoglycosides are used, it is necessary to monitor serum levels to minimize the occurrence of acute renal failure. Peak concentrations correlate with efficacy, but only have meaning with multiple daily doses, and their utility in once-daily regimens has not been established. Trough concentrations are monitored to minimize toxicity and probably should be followed regardless of the dosing regimen.

Because of poor penetration into tissues, some investigators have used nebulized aminoglycosides for the therapy and/or prevention of gram-negative pneumonia. This approach has been effective in the treatment of infectious exacerbations of cystic fibrosis, but has not been effective as adjunctive therapy to systemic antibiotics in patients with serious respiratory tract infections (Ilowite and Niederman 1990).

## THERAPEUTIC ISSUES IN COMMUNITY-ACQUIRED PNEUMONIA

### The Need and Rationale for Empiric Therapy

Although the identification of a specific etiologic pathogen in a patient with CAP can lead to highly focused therapy, even extensive diagnostic testing does not establish a specific diagnosis in up to half of all pneumonia patients (Bates et al. 1992; Niederman et al. 1993; Mundy et al. 1995). In addition, many diagnostic studies provide an answer too late to assist timely therapy. Sputum cultures often take 24 hours or longer to identify a pathogen, and the results may be nonspecific, yielding respiratory tract colonizers and not true pathogens. Serologic testing may require weeks to detect the fourfold rise in titer needed to definitively identify infection by organisms such as *L. pneumophila*, *C. pneumoniae* and *M. pneumoniae*. More recently, the problem of specific diagnosis in CAP has been complicated by data showing that as many as 40% of patients have mixed infection involving both bacterial pathogens and atypical organisms (Lieberman et al. 1996; Marston et al. 1997). If these findings are correct, then even if a specific agent (such as pneumococcus) is isolated from a definitive culture site (such as blood), it may still be necessary to provide coverage for simultaneous infection with another organism such as *C. pneumoniae* (Kauppinen et al. 1996).

One of the reasons empiric therapy for CAP is possible is that the organisms responsible are relatively predictable. Assessment of the severity of illness, age, the presence of comorbid illness, the presence of risk factors for resistant pathogens, and the site of therapy (outpatient, hospital ward, or intensive care unit) permits the division of patients into different groups, each with a list of likely pathogens. The specific algorithms and suggested therapies are discussed below, but several general microbiologic principles apply. The most common pathogen for any patient with CAP, regardless of risk factors, is pneumococcus. *H. influenzae* is a concern in cigarette smokers, and in those with chronic obstructive pulmonary disease. The role of enteric gram-negative organisms is often debated, but these organisms account for 20–40% of all the pathogens in patients with advanced age, serious cardiopulmonary disease, residence in a nursing home, or with a severe illness requiring ICU care (Niederman et al. 1993; Dahmash and Chowdhury 1994; Leroy et al. 1995). As mentioned, atypical pathogens are probably more common than have been appreciated, and recent studies have shown that they are not confined to young and otherwise healthy patients. They can be found in the elderly as well, and may even spread in epidemic form in nursing homes (Lieberman et al. 1996; Marston et al. 1997; Troy et al. 1997). In severe CAP, the organisms that have been most commonly identified are pneumococcus, *Legionella* species, enteric gram-negative organisms (including *P. aeruginosa* in some series), and *H. influenzae*. Patients who are known to be immune-suppressed or HIV-infected may have different pathogens, and the value of diagnostic testing in these patients may be greater than for other populations. The approach to therapy in this population is beyond the scope of this discussion.

### Antimicrobial Resistance among Common Respiratory Pathogens

Many common bacterial pathogens are becoming increasingly resistant to commonly used antimicrobials, with varying impact on the regimens for and outcomes from empiric therapy. As many as 20–40% of all *H. influenzae* organisms and over 90% of *M. catarrhalis* isolates produce β-lactamase enzymes that can inactivate penicillins and first-generation cephalosporins. This has great impact on the selection of empiric therapy for patients with acute exacerbations of chronic bronchitis, but its impact on CAP therapy is less well-studied. More recently, penicillin-resistant *Streptococcus pneumoniae* (PRSP) has emerged as a common cause of CAP, with as many as 25–40% of all respiratory isolates being penicillin-resistant (Doern et al. 1996). Much of this resistance is of intermediate (MIC of 0.1–1.0 mg/L) rather than high level (MIC ≥ 2.0 mg/L) and thus there has been no demonstrated impact of resistance on mortality in patients with CAP due to PRSP, in the absence of meningitis (Pallares et al. 1995; Plouffe et al. 1996; Clavo-Sanchez et al. 1997). With current levels of resistance, treatment with high-dose penicillin or with selected cephalosporins (cefotaxime, ceftriaxone) or new fluoroquinolones (grepafloxacin, levofloxacin, sparfloxacin, or trovafloxacin) is adequate, and the use of alternative agents such as vancomycin is rarely necessary. However, this situation still needs to be followed closely, since an increasing percentage of isolates in some communities are now highly penicillin-resistant, and many isolates of PRSP are multidrug-resistant, with cross-resistance to both macrolides (up to 40% of penicillin-resistant strains) and trimethoprim/sulfamethoxazole (up to 90% of penicillin-resistant strains) (Plouffe et al. 1996; Clavo-Sanchez et al. 1997). In the future, the new fluoroquinolones may be particularly useful in this setting because penicillin resistance has not been commonly associated with quinolone resistance.

**PRINCIPLE There is perhaps no better illustration of the consequences of misuse of pharmacotherapy than the resistance developing to antibiotics undoubtedly contributed to by widespread unjustified use of antibiotics.**

## The Value of Timely and Effective Empiric Therapy

Since definitive diagnostic information is often not available at the time of acute illness, the initial therapy of CAP is usually empiric, based on an epidemiologic assessment of the patient's risk factors for specific pathogens. In some patients, information can be obtained by examining an expectorated sputum sample by Gram's stain for potential pathogens, but the value of this test for predicting the presence of organisms at the alveolar level is uncertain and controversial (Niederman et al. 1993). Similarly, the value of sputum culture for patients with CAP is uncertain, and may only be useful if unusual or drug-resistant organisms are suspected. If patients receive antibiotic therapy before cultures are obtained, then the diagnostic yield of these studies will be reduced. However, recent data have shown that delays in administration of antibiotics can lead to an increased mortality rate for patients with CAP, and thus it may be unwise to put off therapy for the sole purpose of obtaining diagnostic testing, particularly since such testing has only a 50% likelihood of yielding a specific diagnosis (Niederman et al. 1993; Meehan et al. 1997). In one study of more than 14,000 Medicare patients with CAP, many patients had delays in the administration of the first dose of therapy, taking up to 8 hours after admission for 80% of patients to be treated. Delays of longer than 8 hours were associated with increased 30-day mortality, and there was an incremental increase in mortality for each hour of delay in the initiation of therapy (Meehan et al. 1997). With the advent of highly active fluoroquinolones with high bioavailability after oral administration, it may be useful to give patients a dose of observed therapy in the office setting before sending them to the hospital for admission. The benefits of such prompt therapy still must to be weighed against the potential loss of diagnostic data from the administration of antibiotics before obtaining diagnostic cultures.

**PRINCIPLE When a definitive diagnosis is not likely, and the efficacy of empiric therapy is time limited, the physician may have to choose empiric therapy and a careful monitoring strategy to determine if the choice was correct at the earliest possible time.**

The correct selection of effective initial empiric therapy improves outcome (mortality). This situation has been most clearly demonstrated in patients with severe forms of CAP, in whom effective empiric therapy improved outcome, whereas establishing a specific etiologic diagnosis did not (Moine et al. 1994; Leroy et al. 1995). For example, in one study of 132 patients with CAP, overall mortality rate was 24%. In those in whom an etiologic diagnosis was made, the mortality rate was 31%, whereas in those in whom no specific diagnosis was made, the mortality rate was 8% (Moine et al. 1994). In another study of 286 patients admitted to the ICU with severe CAP, the initial empiric therapy regimen was effective in 194 patients, as judged by clinical response at 72 hours, and ineffective in 92 patients (Leroy et al. 1995). In the latter group, an etiologic pathogen was found to be resistant to initial therapy in 25% of the patients, allowing for a change to a specific and potentially more effective treatment regimen. However, the mortality rate for those who received ineffective initial therapy was 60%, even though specific diagnostic information became available. This high rate of death, in spite of the availability of diagnostic information, points to the limited value of obtaining this information at the time that it becomes available. On the other hand, the patients who received effective empiric therapy had a mortality rate of only 11%, emphasizing the value of accurate therapy, even in the absence of specific diagnostic information.

**PRINCIPLE The burden of the right therapeutic decision must be borne in settings of known diagnostic inadequacy.**

Several recent studies of CAP have shown that atypical pathogens are more common than previously suspected, and that these organisms can occur in patients of all ages, and can be present as copathogens with bacterial agents. This is particularly true for *C. pneumoniae*, and one study has shown that when it was present with pneumococcus, but untreated, the hospital course was more complicated than in pure pneumococcal infection or pure *C. pneumoniae* infection (Kauppinen et al. 1996). These data suggest that certain atypical pathogens can potentiate the severity of infection caused by bacterial organisms. This implies the relatively routine need for atypical pathogen coverage for patients with CAP, and several outcome studies support this possibility. In one study of outpatients with CAP, patients of all ages, with or without comorbid illness had a better outcome if they received macrolide therapy compared with other regimens that did not have atypical pathogen coverage (mostly $\beta$-lactams or trimethoprim-sulfamethoxazole) (Gleason et al. 1997). In another study of nearly 4500 patients with CAP, those who received a $\beta$-lactam combined with a macrolide had a lower mortality than patients who received either $\beta$-lactam monotherapy or therapy with other regimens (Gordon et al. 1996).

## Using Antibiotic Approaches to Shift Care to the Outpatient Setting

A number of studies have shown that some patients with CAP who are being admitted to the hospital have a low risk of mortality and may be able to be treated safely in the outpatient setting (Fine et al. 1997). In one study of 38,039 admitted patients with CAP, evaluated retrospectively with a prognostic scoring system, the authors concluded that 15,500 patients had a low risk of mortality and that many of them could possibly have been managed at home (Fine et al. 1997). This is a particularly important approach to consider, especially because many low-risk patients would prefer outpatient therapy if possible, although few are asked about this decision by their doctors (Coley et al. 1996).

In order to allow home therapy of CAP, several interventions are needed. The first is an accurate way to define which patients need hospitalization and which can be safely managed at home, and the advent of prognostic scoring systems that stratify patients into risk groups will make this easier. However, no scoring system has yet been prospectively validated to define the need for hospital admission, and even if this is done, the decision to hospitalize a patient will still need an "art of medicine" approach. Assuming that a proper scheme for stratification can be developed, there will always be "borderline" patients who could be managed in either setting. To assure safe outpatient care of these patients, home nursing care and possibly home intravenous therapy may be necessary. However, there are two developments in antibiotic therapy that may facilitate home care of these patients. First, a number of new antibiotics can be administered once-daily, making home intravenous therapy with these agents much less cumbersome than with antibiotics administered multiple times per day. Agents that can be used once-daily intravenously for CAP include ceftriaxone, levofloxacin, gatifloxacin, and trovafloxacin. The other development in antibiotic therapy that can facilitate home treatment is the availability of a new group of fluoroquinolones that have excellent gram-positive, gram-negative, and atypical pathogen coverage, can be given once-daily and are highly bioavailable so that they achieve high serum levels even when given orally. These drugs include grepafloxacin and sparfloxacin, which are only available orally, and levofloxacin, gatifloxacin, and trovafloxacin, which are available for both oral and intravenous administration.

The other area in which antibiotic strategies can minimize the need for hospitalization is in the switch from intravenous to oral therapy during the treatment of admitted patients with CAP. Switch therapy can typically be done by the third hospital day, and, once accomplished, the patient can be discharged (Ramirez et al. 1995). It may not even be necessary to observe patients in the hospital on oral therapy, since little seems to happen during this observation period, and thus the switch to oral therapy can coincide with discharge to the outpatient setting (Rhew et al. 1998). Ramirez has applied an aggressive switch therapy program at the Veterans Administration (VA) hospital in Louisville (KY), and has demonstrated a reduction in mortality rate from CAP, with up to half of all patients being switched by the third hospital day (Ramirez 1995). Criteria for switch therapy include subjective improvement in cough, sputum production and dyspnea; absence of fever on at least two occasions 8 hours apart; a falling white blood cell count; and a functioning gastrointestinal tract (Ramirez et al. 1995). The use of aggressive early switch therapy can reduce hospital costs and will likely add to patient satisfaction. Even the presence of bacteremia does not mandate a prolonged course of intravenous therapy, provided that the patient has shown the above signs of clinical improvement. In fact, in one study with 23% of the patients having positive blood cultures, intravenous therapy for 2 days followed by 8 days of oral therapy was as effective as intravenous therapy for 5 days or 10 days (Siegel et al. 1996).

**PRINCIPLE Evidence-based decisions clearly can displace historical conservatism in therapeutic decision.**

## THERAPEUTIC ISSUES IN HOSPITAL-ACQUIRED PNEUMONIA

### Epidemiologic Importance and Attributable Mortality

Hospital-acquired pneumonia is the second or third most common nosocomial infection, but the one that is most likely to lead to a fatal outcome (Campbell et al. 1996). In one study of patients with nosocomial infections, pneumonia was present in 60% of patients in whom the nosocomial infection contributed to death, making HAP the most important hospital-acquired infection from the perspective of mortality (Gross and Van Antwerpen 1983). HAP is a particular problem among patients requiring mechanical ventilation, with up to 20% of a mixed medical-surgical ICU population developing ventilator-associated pneumonia (VAP). The incidence of infection increases with the duration of mechanical ventilation, at a rate of about 1% per day, but since most patients are ventilated for short periods, up to half of all episodes of VAP are of early onset, beginning within the first four days of mechanical ventilation (Fagon et al. 1989; Prod'hom et al. 1994).

Although the crude mortality rate of VAP has been reported as high as 40–70%, not all patients who die with this illness do so because of infection. Rather, many are already seriously ill and would have died even in the absence of pneumonia, and thus they do not have an "attributable mortality" from VAP. Only about half of all deaths in patients with VAP are estimated to be the direct result of infection (Fagon et al. 1993, 1996). Mortality is more likely to be accurately attributable to VAP when certain high-risk organisms such as *P. aeruginosa*, *S. maltophilia*, and *Acinetobacter* spp. are involved (Kollef et al. 1995). In addition, mortality is more likely in medical patients than in surgical or trauma patients (Baker et al. 1996), reflecting the different types of comorbid illness in the two populations.

Attributable mortality is best measured by comparing the outcome of patients who have pneumonia with equally ill patients without pneumonia. However, with this approach, all patients with pneumonia are receiving antibiotic therapy, and thus the presence of excess mortality is a reflection of the ineffectiveness of antibiotic therapy. As with CAP, patients with VAP who receive effective empiric therapy (defined by using agents that are active against the recovered etiologic pathogens), have a lower mortality than patients who receive ineffective initial therapy (Luna et al. 1997). Thus, mortality will be attributable to VAP only as long as we have diagnostic and therapeutic strategies that are not fully effective. One goal of therapy for VAP is to choose antimicrobials that are likely to be effective and thereby to reduce the mortality of this infection.

**PRINCIPLE The speed and accuracy of therapy may often become the key determinant of efficacy.**

### Diagnostic Problems in Hospital-Acquired Pneumonia

Most physicians use a clinical definition of nosocomial pneumonia, which is quite sensitive to the presence of infection, but not highly specific, and many patients who satisfy this definition have noninfectious illness. This definition requires the presence of a new or progressive infiltrate by chest X-ray, plus some evidence of infection such as a positive blood culture, radiographic cavitation, histologic confirmation, or a constellation of clinical features including fever, purulent sputum, and leukocytosis (Campbell et al. 1996). In early studies, as many as two-thirds of all patients who satisfied this clinical definition did not have the diagnosis confirmed by quantitative cultures of bronchoscopic specimens, and many were found to have alternate diagnoses (Chastre et al. 1984). These observations led to efforts to use quantitative cultures (usually obtained by bronchoscopic protected specimen brush or bronchoalveolar lavage) to define the presence or absence of pneumonia. This approach remains controversial, and it does not appear that patients who have pneumonia defined by clinical criteria have a prognosis different from patients who satisfy quantitative culture definitions for pneumonia (Niederman et al. 1994; Timsit et al. 1996). In addition, the outcome of patients managed by clinical judgment is no different from the outcome of those managed by bronchoscopic data, although the latter group is usually subjected to more frequent changes in antibiotic therapy (Sanchez-Nieto et al. 1998).

At the present time, the role of invasive diagnostic methods to guide initial antibiotic therapy of suspected VAP is controversial, and in most patients, the decision is made on the basis of clinical, not bronchoscopic, criteria. The problems associated with withholding therapy until the diagnosis is confirmed by bronchoscopy include not only the delay in therapy but also the possibility of inaccurate interpretation of data resulting from the technical difficulties associated with bronchoscopic collection of culture samples. There is no established benefit for using bronchoscopic criteria in place of clinical criteria (Niederman et al. 1994). It does appear that cultures of tracheal aspirates from intubated patients demonstrate the same organisms that are found by bronchoscopy. Once a clinical diagnosis of pneumonia is made, a reasonable strategy is thus to initiate empiric antibiotic therapy according to standard guidelines (Rumbak and Bass 1994; Campbellet al. 1996), immediately after obtaining a tracheal aspirate. Once culture results become available, the empiric therapy can be broadened or streamlined.

**PRINCIPLE A true clinician accepts the challenge of an empiric decision with thought and logical weighing of the data. The results of a reflexive and thoughtless decision are not likely to have the same outcomes.**

## Issues in Therapy of Hospital-Acquired Pneumonia

Many patients with HAP are routinely treated with a combination of antimicrobial agents, although this may not always be necessary. There are three well-established rationales for the use of combination therapy in nosocomial pneumonia: One is to provide antibacterial synergy against pathogens such as *P. aeruginosa*. This may only be important for neutropenic patients and for those with bacteremia and has been documented to lead to better outcomes in patients with positive blood cultures (Hilf et al. 1989). If synergy is desired, then a β-lactam must be combined with an aminoglycoside, although some synergy between β-lactams and quinolones has been seen in vitro (Miltavic and Wallrauch 1996). The second rationale is the provision of a broader spectrum of antimicrobial activity against a wide range of possible organisms than can be provided by a single agent alone. This is rarely necessary given the broad spectrum agents that are currently approved for use for HAP. The third rationale is the prevention of the emergence of resistance during therapy, a real problem for certain pathogens that are treated with a single agent. It is this last rationale that is most relevant for patients with severe HAP, particularly those with VAP who may be infected with *P. aeruginosa, Acinetobacter* spp. or *S. maltophilia*, all organisms that have been associated with a high attributable mortality and that can develop resistance to commonly used monotherapy regimens (Fink et al. 1994; Kollef et al. 1995).

In the treatment of VAP, a number of monotherapy regimens have been shown to be effective including ceftazidime, meropenem, imipenem, piperacillin/tazobactam, cefepime, ciprofloxacin, and trovafloxacin (Gouin et al. 1993; Fink et al. 1994; Rubinstein et al. 1995; Graham et al. 1997; Sieger et al. 1997). However, with all of these agents there is concern that resistance among *P. aeruginosa* pathogens can emerge, an event observed in 33% of patients treated with ciprofloxacin monotherapy and in over 50% treated with imipenem monotherapy in one clinical trial (Fink et al. 1994). To address this issue, a reasonable approach would be to start all patients with severe VAP, who are at risk for resistant organisms, on a combination antipseudomonal regimen, and to then change to monotherapy if this, or another highly resistant, pathogen is not found in tracheal aspirate cultures.

When using combination therapy, it is best to choose agents from different classes, using either an aminoglycoside/β-lactam regimen or a quinolone/β-lactam regimen. Use of dual β-lactam therapy is not a good approach because the two agents can compete with one another for antibacterial effect and if either induces a bacterial β-lactamase, both agents may be inactivated simultaneously. The currently available antipseudomonal agents include (Table 2-13 ): the aminoglycosides such as gentamicin, tobramycin, and amikacin; the β-lactams such as the extended-spectrum penicillins (piperacillin, ticarcillin), the cephalosporins (ceftazidime, cefepime), the carbapenems (imipenem, meropenem), and the monobactams (aztreonam); the β-lactam/β-lactamase inhibitor combinations (piperacillin-tazobactam or ticarcillin-clavulanate); and the quinolones ciprofloxacin and trovafloxacin.

One class of antibiotics that should be used carefully as monotherapy is the third-generation cephalosporins. With widespread use, these agents promote the emergence of chromosomally mediated β-lactamase-producing Enterobacteriaceae, which can appear sensitive to cephalo-

**Table 2-13 Antipseudomonal Antibiotics**

Aminoglycosides: gentamicin sulfate, tobramycin sulfate, amikacin sulfate
*β-Lactams*
Cephalosporins: ceftazidime, cefepime
Carbapenems: imipenem, meropenem
Monobactams: aztreonam
Penicillins: piperacillin sodium, azlocillin, mezlocillin sodium monohydrate, ticarcillin disodium
β-Lactam/β-lactamase inhibitor combinations: piperacillin/tazobactam, ticarcillin/clavulanic acid
Fluoroquinolones: ciprofloxacin, trovafloxacin

sporins on initial testing, but express resistance once therapy is started (Chow et al. 1991). The emergence of this form of resistance may require the use of combination therapy any time a third-generation cephalosporin is used and can be minimized if these agents are avoided. Other β-lactam agents such as the carbapenems, and the fourth-generation cephalosporin cefepime, may be acceptable alternatives to the third-generation cephalosporins (Kollef et al. 1997, Niederman 1997).

In selecting empiric therapy for VAP, it may be necessary to treat some patients empirically for methicillin-resistant *S. aureus* (MRSA), necessitating the addition of vancomycin to another agent, and thereby using combination therapy. MRSA is likely in patients who have late-onset VAP (after at least 5 days of hospitalization), are treated with corticosteroids, and who have received antibiotics before the onset of VAP (Campbell et al. 1996). The decision about whether to routinely add vancomycin to such at risk patients can be made by looking at a tracheal aspirate Gram's stain for the presence of gram-positive cocci.

## SPECIFIC EMPIRIC THERAPY REGIMENS FOR PNEUMONIA

### Community-Acquired Pneumonia

In the therapy of CAP, patients can be assigned to empiric therapy regimens on the basis of several clinical assessments including place of therapy (inpatient vs. outpatient), presence of advanced age (> age 65) or comorbid illness (serious cardiopulmonary disease), severity of illness (mild, moderate, or severe), and the presence of risk factors for specific pathogens such as penicillin-resistant pneumococcus and *P. aeruginosa* (Niederman et al. 1993).

Among outpatients who are nonsmokers and have no cardiopulmonary disease, regardless of age, the likely organisms are pneumococcus and atypical pathogens, and treatment can be given with an oral macrolide such as azithromycin or clarithromycin, or possibly erythromycin, with doxycycline as an alternative (Niederman et al. 1993). If a patient has mild-to-moderate illness and can be treated out of the hospital but has a smoking history or underlying cardiopulmonary disease, then *H. influenzae* and, in some patients, enteric gram-negative organisms, are also of concern, and therapy must include coverage for these bacteria, along with pneumococcal and atypical pathogens. If an outpatient with cardiopulmonary disease is not from a nursing home and has no specific risk factors for penicillin-resistant *Streptococcus pneumoniae* (PRSP), then gram-negative organisms are not a concern and therapy can be started with a new macrolide or tetracycline to cover all likely pathogens including *H. influenzae*. If, however, an outpatient has cardiopulmonary disease and also has risks for PRSP (such as age >65, alcoholism, immune suppression, β-lactam therapy within 3 months) and/or is from a nursing home, then therapy should be done differently, with the aim of covering PRSP and enteric gram-negative organisms, as well as the other pathogens listed above. This type of patient should be treated with a β-lactam (outpatient intravenous ceftriaxone, or oral cefpodoxime, cefuroxime, high-dose amoxicillin or amoxicillin/clavulanate) plus a macrolide (a new agent, unless the β-lactam agent is resistant to bacterial β-lactamase production, in which case erythromycin can be used). Another alternative for this type of patient would be one of the new oral fluoroquinolones (grepafloxacin, gatifloxacin, levofloxacin, sparfloxacin, or trovafloxacin) (Table 2-14) (Niederman et al. 1993; Bartlett et al. 1998; Niederman 1998).

For patients who have moderate-to-severe illness and who require inpatient therapy, but not ICU admission, two groups should be defined: one with no risks for PRSP and not from a nursing home, and one with either or both of these risk factors (Table 2-15). For the patient without risks for PRSP and not from a nursing home, intravenous azithromycin can be used if no cardiopulmonary disease is present, whereas those with cardiopulmonary disease require a β-lactam/macrolide combination or the use of a new quinolone. Doxycycline could be used in place of a macrolide. If an admitted, non-ICU patient does have risks for PRSP or is from a nursing home, the above approach can be used, but the β-lactams that are acceptable are only ceftriaxone, cefotaxime, piperacillin/tazobactam, cefepime, imipenem, neropenem, or high-dose ampicillin,

Table 2-14 **Therapy of Outpatients with Community-Acquired Pneumonia**

Nonsmoker, all ages, no cardiopulmonary disease
- Macrolide

OR
- Doxycycline

Smoker, + cardiopulmonary disease, all ages, no risks for PRSP, not in nursing home
- New macrolide

OR
- Doxycycline

Smoker, + cardiopulmonary disease, all ages, with risks for PRSP or from nursing home
- β-Lactam (IV ceftriaxone, cefpodoxime sodium, cefuroxime sodium, high dose amoxicillin, amoxicillin-clavulanic acid) PLUS a new macrolide

OR
- New fluoroquinolone

ABBREVIATIONS: PRSP, penicillin-resistant *S. pneumoniae.*

with an intravenous or oral new macrolide. Monotherapy with an intravenous quinolone is another acceptable choice for this population.

In patients with severe CAP requiring admission to an ICU, therapy must be broad spectrum and must involve multiple agents. There are two types of ICU patients, defined by their risk for *P. aeruginosa* infection. Risk factors for this organism include recent antibiotic therapy, corticosteroid therapy, bronchiectasis, and immune suppression. For the ICU patient without these risk factors, therapy should be with a β-lactam (cefotaxime, ceftriaxone, piperacillin/tazobactam, cefepime, imipenem, or meropenem) plus either an intravenous macrolide (erythromycin, azithromycin) or an intravenous quinolone (levofloxacin, trovafloxacin or high-dose ciprofloxacin). In this group, if high-level penicillin resistance is also suspected, the β-lactam should be imipenem or meropenem, or vancomycin should be added. For ICU patients with pseudomonal risk factors, therapy should be with two antipseudomonal agents plus a macrolide, or one antipseudomonal β-lactam plus an antipseudomonal quinolone (ciprofloxacin or trovafloxacin). If PRSP is also likely, the β-lactam agents should be selected with this pathogen in mind.

Table 2-15 **Therapy for Patient with Community-Acquired Pneumonia, Requiring Hospitalization but not ICU**

*No risks for PRSP, not from nursing home*

No cardiopulmonary disease
- Intravenous azithromycin

Cardiopulmonary disease
- Intravenous β-lactam a PLUS oral or IV macrolide or doxycycline

OR
- Intravenous or oral new fluoroquinolone

*Risks for PRSP, or from a nursing home*
- Intravenous β-lactam (only ceftriaxone, cefotaxime, cefepime, imipemem, meropenem, piperacillin/tazobactam, or high dose ampicillin)
- PLUS oral or IV > new macrolide or doxycycline

OR
- Intravenous new fluoroquinolone

ABBREVIATIONS: PRSP, penicillin-resistant *S. pneumoniae.*

## Hospital-Acquired Pneumonia

Guidelines for empiric therapy of nosocomial pneumonia have also been published and involve dividing patients into three groups on the basis of severity of illness, time of onset of infection (early or late), and the presence of risk factors for specific pathogens (Campbell et al. 1996). All patients are at risk for a "core" group of organisms that include nonpseudomonal gram-negative organisms, *S. pneumoniae, H. influenzae*, and methicillin-sensitive *S. aureus*. Patients who are at risk for only these core organisms are those with mild-to-moderate pneumonia, beginning any time, but with no specific organism risk factors as well as patients with severe pneumonia, early onset, and no specific organism risk factors. Therapy for these patients can be with any of a core group of antibiotics which include second-, third-, or fourth-generation cephalosporins, β-lactam/β-lactamase inhibitor combination drugs, quinolones or the combination of clindamycin and aztreonam.

The next group of patients are those with mild-to-moderate illness, onset any time, but risk factors for specific organisms. These patients are at risk for the core bacteria plus other organisms, as dictated by risk factors. Thus, if a patient has had recent abdominal surgery or witnessed aspiration, anaerobes are also a concern, and clindamycin can be added to a core antibiotic, or a β-lactam/β-lactamase inhibitor combination can be used alone. In patients with coma, head trauma, renal failure, or diabetes, *S. aureus* is a concern, and the core agent selected should be effective against this pathogen. In a patient who has been given high-dose steroids or recent antibiotics, or has had a prolonged ICU stay before the onset of pneumonia, then resistant organisms should be treated empirically, even if the patient is not severely ill with HAP. Thus these patients should receive the same regimen as the patient with severe HAP of late onset or severe HAP of early onset, with risk factors. The regimen is a combination antipseudomonal regimen, with vancomycin added if a tracheal aspirate Gram stain shows gram-positive cocci. In all of these patients, particularly the intubated patient in the ICU, the empiric regimen is continued until the results of tracheal aspirate or sputum cultures are known, and then therapy is streamlined. If *P. aeruginosa* or another resistant gram-negative organism is not found, then therapy can be completed with a single agent to which the isolated organism is sensitive.

## REFERENCES


Baker AM, Meredith J, Haponik EF. 1996. Pneumonia in intubated trauma patients: microbiology and outcome. *Am J Respir Crit Care Med* **153**:343–9.

Bartlett JG, Breiman RF, Mandell LA, et al. 1998. Community-acquired pneumonia in adults: guidelines for management. The Infectious Disease Society of America. *Clin Infect Dis* **26**:811–38.

Bates JH, Campbell GD, Barron AL, et al. 1992. Microbial etiology of acute pneumonia in hospitalized patients. *Chest* **101**:1005–12.

Bodem CR, Lampton LM, Miller DP, et al. 1983. Endobronchial pH: relevance to aminoglycoside activity in gram-negative pneumonia. *Am Rev Respir Dis* **127**:39–41.

Campbell GD, Niederman MS, Broughton WA, et al. 1996. Hospital-acquired pneumonia in adults: diagnosis, et al. *Am J Respir Crit Care Med* **153**:1711–25.

Chastre J, Viau F, Brun P, et al. 1984. Prospective evaluation of the protected specimen brush for the diagnosis of pulmonary infections in ventilated patients. *Am Rev Respir Dis* **130**:924.

Chow JW, Fine MJ, Shlaes DM, et al. 1991. *Enterobacter* bacteremia: clinical features and emergence of antibiotic resistance during therapy. *Ann Intern Med* **115**:585–90.

Clavo-Sanchez AJ, Giron-Gonzalez JA, Lopez-Prieto D, et al. 1997. Multivariate analysis of risk factors for infection due to penicillin-resistant and multidrug-resistant Streptococcus pneumoniae: a multicenter study. *Clin Infect Dis* **24**:1052–9.

Coley CM, Yi-Hwei L, Medsger AR, et al. 1996. Preference for home vs. hospital care among low-risk patients with community-acquired pneumonia. *Arch Intern Med* **156**:1565–71.

Cometta A, Baumgartner JD, Lew D, et al. 1994. Prospective randomized comparison of imipenem monotherapy with imipenem plus netilmicin for treatment of severe infections in nonneutropenic patients. *Antimicrob Agents Chemother* **38**:1309–13.

Craig W. 1994. Pharmacodynamics of antimicrobial agents as a basis for determining dosage regimens. *Eur J Clin Microb Infect Dis* **38**:1309–13.

Craig WA. 1998. Pharmacokinetic/pharmacodynamic parameters: rationale for antimicrobial dosing of mice and men. *Clin Infect Dis* **26**:1–12.

Dahmash NS, Chowdhury MNH. 1994. Re-evaluation of pneumonia requiring admission to an intensive care unit: a prospective study. *Thorax* **49**:71–6.

Doern GV, Brueggemann A, Holly HP, et al. 1996. Antimicrobial resistance of *Streptococcus pneumoniae* recovered from patients in the United States during the winter months of 1994 to 1995: results of a 30 center national surveillance study. *Antimicrob Agents Chemother* **40**:1208–13.

Fagon JY, Chastre J, Domart Y, et al. 1989. Nosocomial pneumonia in patients receiving continuous mechanical ventilation: prospective analysis of 52 episodes with use of a protected specimen brush and quantitative culture techniques. *Am Rev Respir Dis* **139**:877.

Fagon JY, Chastre J, Hance A, et al. 1993. Nosocomial pneumonia in ventilated patients: a cohort study evaluating attributable mortality and hospital stay. *Am J Med* **94**:281–8.

Fagon JY, Chastre J, Vaugnat A, et al. 1996. Nosocomial pneumonia and mortality among patients in intensive care units. *JAMA* **275**:866–9.

Fine MJ, Auble TE, Yearly DM, et al. 1997. A prediction rule to identify low-risk patients with community-acquired pneumonia. *N Engl J Med* **366**:243–50.

Fink MP, Snydman DR, Niederman MS, et al. 1994. Treatment of severe pneumonia in hospitalized patients: results of a multicenter, randomized, double-blind trial comparing intravenous ciprofloxacin with imipenem-cilastatin. *Antimicrob Agents Chemother* **38**:547–57.

Forest A, Nix DE, Ballow CH, et al. 1993. Pharmacodynamics of intravenous ciprofloxacin in seriously ill patients. *Antimicrob Agents Chemother* **37**:1073–81.

Gentry LO, Rodriguez-Gomez G, Kohler RB, et al. 1992. Parenteral followed by oral ofloxacin for nosocomial and community-acquired pneumonia requiring hospitalization. *Am Rev Respir Dis* **145**:31–5.

Gleason PP, Kapoor WN, Stone RA, et al. 1997. Medical outcomes and antimicrobial costs with the use of the American Thoracic Society Guidelines for outpatients with community-acquired pneumonia. *JAMA* **278**:32–9.

Gold HS, Moellering RC. 1996. Antimicrobial-drug resistance. *N Engl J Med* **335**:1445–53.

Gootz TD, Brighty KE. 1998. Chemistry and mechanism of action of the quinolone antibacterials. In: Andriole V, editor. *The Quinolones* . San Diego: McGraw-Hill. p 29–80.

Gordon GS, Throop D, Berberian L, et al. 1996. Validation of the therapeutic recommendations of the American Thoracic Society (ATS) guidelines for community acquired pneumonia in hospitalized patients. *Chest* **110**:55S.

Gouin F, Papazian L, Martin C, et al. 1993. A non-comparative study of the efficacy and tolerance of cefepime in combination with amikacin in the treatment of severe infections in patients in intensive care. *J Antimicrob Chemother* **32**:205–14.

Graham D, Klein T, Marti A, et al. 1997. A double-blind, randomized, multicenter study in nosocomial pneumonia (NOS) comparing trovafloxacin with ciprofloxacin + clindamycin/metronidazole [abstract LM–74]. The Trovan Nosocomial Pneumonia Study Group. 37th Interscience Conference on Antimicrobial Agents and Chemotherapy, September 28–October 1, 1997, Toronto.

Gross PA, Van Antwerpen C. 1983. Nosocomial infections and hospital deaths: a case-control study. *Am J Med* **75**:658.

Hatala R, Dinh T, Cook DJ. 1996. Once-daily aminoglycoside dosing in immunocompetent adults: a meta analysis. *Ann Intern Med* **124**:717–25.

Hilf M, Yu VL, Sharp J, et al. 1989. Antibiotic therapy for *Pseudomonas aeruginosa* bacteremia: outcome correlations in a prospective study of 200 patients. *Am J Med* **87**:540–6.

Honeybourne D. 1994. Antibiotic penetration into lung tissues. *Thorax* **49**:104–6.

Ilowite JS, Niederman MS. 1990. Problems and opportunities in the topical treatment of infectious diseases of the respiratory tract. *Adv Drug Delivery Rev* **5**:93–105.

Kauppinen MT, Saikku P, Kujala P, et al. 1996. Clinical picture of *Chlamydia pneumoniae* requiring hospital treatment: a comparison between chlamydial and pneumococcal pneumonia. *Thorax* **51**:185–9.

Kollef MH, Silver P, Murphy DM, et al. 1995. The effect of late-onset ventilator-associated pneumonia in determining patient mortality. *Chest* **108**:1655–62.

Leroy O, Santré C, Beuscart C, et al. 1995. A five-year study of severe community-acquired pneumonia with emphasis on prognosis in patients admitted to an intensive care unit. *Intensive Care Med* **21**:24–31.

Lieberman D, Schlaeffer F, Boldur I, et al. 1996. Multiple pathogens in adult patients admitted with community-acquired pneumonia: a one year prospective study of 346 consecutive patients. *Thorax* **51**:179–84.

Luna CM, Vujacich P, Niederman MS, et al. 1997. Impact of BAL data on the therapy and outcome of ventilator associated pneumonia. *Chest* **111**:676–85.

Mandell LA. 1994. Antibiotics for pneumonia therapy. *Med Clin North Am* **78**:997–14.

Marston BJ, Plouffe JF, File TM, et al. 1997. Incidence of community-acquired pneumonia requiring hospitalization. *Arch Intern Med* **157**:1709–18.

Meehan TP, Fine MJ, Krumholz HM, et al. 1997. Quality of care, process and outcomes in elderly patients with pneumonia. *JAMA* **278**:2080–4.

Miltavic D, Wallrauch C. 1996. In vitro activity of trovafloxacin in combination with ceftazidime, meropenem, and amikacin. *Eur J Clin Microb Infect Dis* **15**:688–93.

Moine P, Vercken JP, Chevret S, et al. 1994. Severe community-acquired pneumonia: etiology, epidemiology, and prognosis factors. *Chest* **105**:1487–95.

Mundy LM, Auwaerter PG, Oldach D, et al. 1995. Community-acquired pneumonia: impact of immune status. *Am J Respir Crit Care Med* **152**:1309–15.

Niederman MS. 1997. The principles of antibiotic use and the selection of empiric therapy for pneumonia. In: Fishman A, editor. *Pulmonary Diseases and Disorders*. New York: McGraw-Hill. p 1939–49.

Niederman MS. 1997. Is crop rotation of antibiotics the solution to a resistant problem in in the ICU? *Am J Respir Crit Care Med* **156**:1029–1031.

Niederman MS. 1998. Treatment of respiratory infections with quinolones. In: Andriole V, editor. *The Quinolones*. San Diego: McGraw-Hill. p 229–50.

Niederman MS, Bass JB, Campbell GD, et al. 1993. Guidelines for the initial management of adults with community-acquired pneumonia: diagnosis, assessment of severity, and initial antimicrobial therapy. *Am Rev Respir Dis* **148**:1418–26.

Niederman MS, Torres A, Summer W. 1994. Invasive diagnostic testing is not needed routinely to manage suspected ventilator-associated pneumonia. *Am J Respir Crit Care Med* **150**:565–9.

Pallares R, Linares J, Vadillo M, et al. 1995. Resistance to penicillin and cephalosporin and mortality from severe pneumococcal pneumonia in Barcelona, Spain. *N Engl J Med* **333**:474–80.

Plouffe JF, Breiman RF, Facklam RR, et al. 1996. Bacteremia with *Streptococcus pneumoniae*: implications for therapy and prevention. *JAMA* **275**:194–8.

Preston SL, Drusano GL, Berman AL, et al. 1998. Pharmacodynamics of levofloxacin: a new paradigm for early clinical trials. *JAMA* **279**:125–9.

Prod'hom G, Leuenberger P, Koerfer J, et al. 1994. Nosocomial pneumonia in mechanically ventilated patients receiving antiacid, ranitidine, or sucralfate as prophylaxis for stress ulcer: a randomized controlled trial. *Ann Intern Med* **120**:653–62.

Ramirez JA. 1995. Switch therapy in adult patients with pneumonia. *Clin Pulm Med* **2**:327–33.

Ramirez JA, Srinath L, Ahkee S, et al. 1995. Early switch from intravenous to oral cephalosporins in the treatment of hospitalized patients with community-acquired pneumonia. *Arch Intern Med* **155**:1273–6.

Rello J, Gallego M, Mariscal D, et al. 1997. The value of routine microbial investigation in ventilator-associated pneumonia. *Am J Respir Crit Care Med* **156**:196–200.

Rello J, Quintana E, Ausina V, et al. 1990. Risk factors for *Staphylococcus aureus* nosocomial pneumonia in critically ill patients. *Am Rev Respir Dis* **142**:1320–4.

Rhew DC, Hackner D, Henderson L, et al. 1998. The clinical benefit of in-hospital observation in "low risk" pneumonia patients after conversion from parenteral to oral antimicrobial therapy. *Chest* **113**:142–6.

Rubinstein E, Lode H, Grassi C, and an. 1995. Ceftazidime monotherapy vs. ceftriaxone/tobramycin for serious hospital-acquired gram-negative infections. Antibiotic Study Group. *Clin Infect Dis* **20**:1217–28.

Rumbak MJ, Bass RL. 1994. Tracheal aspirate correlates with protected specimen brush in long-term ventilated patients who have clinical pneumonia. *Chest* **106**:531–4.

Sanchez-Nieto JM, Torre A, Garcia-Cordoba F, et al. 1998. Impact of invasive and noninvasive quantitative culture sampling on outcome of ventilator-associated pneumonia: a pilot study. *Am J Respir Crit Care Med* **157**:371–6.

Siegel RE, Halpern NA, Almenoff PL, et al. 1996. A prospective randomized study of inpatient IV antibiotics for community-acquired pneumonia. *Chest* **110**:965–71.

Sieger B, Berman SJ, Geckler RW, et al. 1997. Empiric treatment of hospital-acquired lower respiratory tract infections with meropenem or ceftazidime with tobramycin: a randomized study. The Meropenem Lower Respiratory Tract Infection Group. *Crit Care Med* **25**:1663–70.

Timsit JF, Chevret S, Valcke J, et al. 1996. Mortality of nosocomial pneumonia in ventilated patients: influence of diagnostic tests. *Am J Respir Crit Care Med* **154**:116–23.

Troy CJ, Peeling RW, Ellis AG, et al. 1997. *Chlamydia pneumoniae* as a new source of infectious outbreaks in nursing homes. *JAMA* **277**:1214–8.

# Pulmonary Vascular Disease

Sean P. Gaine

*Chapter Outline*



## PATHOGENESIS AND PATHOPHYSIOLOGY OF PULMONARY VASCULAR DISEASE

The normal pulmonary circulation is a high-flow, low-pressure circuit. The right ventricle poorly tolerates acute increases in pulmonary artery pressure. Progressive increases in pulmonary vascular resistance initially result in right ventricular hypertrophy but eventually in right ventricle decompensation, right heart failure and, ultimately, death. The first step in management is to identify the underlying cause of the pulmonary hypertension and to determine its reversibility. Attention is then focused on reducing pulmonary vascular tone, optimizing right ventricular function and preventing thrombosis.

The classification of pulmonary hypertension based on the underlying cause is outlined in Table 2-16. Primary pulmonary hypertension (PPH) is defined by an increased pulmonary arterial pressure in the absence of an identifiable cause (Rubin 1993). All other causes of pulmonary artery hypertension are termed secondary pulmonary hypertension (SPH).

Alveolar hypoxia is a potent stimulus for pulmonary arterial vasoconstriction, and chronic hypoxia may produce polycythemia which, by increasing plasma viscosity, may exacerbate the hypertension. These mechanisms are important in the pulmonary hypertension of chronic obstructive bronchitis and of disorders of ventilation (e.g., sleep apnea syndrome). Acute massive or recurrent pulmonary emboli cause pulmonary hypertension by direct obliteration of the pulmonary vascular bed, as well as reflex and hypoxemically induced vasoconstriction. The SPH seen in association with emphysema, advanced bullous lung disease, and parenchymal lung disease results from both obliteration of the vascular bed and vasoconstriction from hypoxemia.

**Table 2-16 Classification of Pulmonary Hypertension**

1. Parenchymal lung disease
   - Chronic obstructive lung disease
   - Idiopathic pulmonary fibrosis
   - Sarcoidosis
2. Disorders of ventilation
   - Sleep apnea syndrome
   - Kyphoscoliosis
3. Left heart obstruction or dysfunction
4. Vascular obstruction
   - Chronic thromboembolic disease
   - Mediastinal fibrosis
   - Schistosomiasis
5. Intrinsic pulmonary vascular disease
   - Primary pulmonary hypertension
   - Collagen vascular disease
   - Sickle cell disease
   - Congenital heart disease
   - Portal hypertension
   - High altitude

Disease of the left heart, like left ventricular failure and mitral valve disease, produce secondary, postcapillary pulmonary hypertension by increasing pulmonary venous pressure. Although mitral valve replacement or treatment of left ventricular failure may produce a fall in the pulmonary artery pressure, the vascular remodeling that occurs with severe or long-standing pulmonary hypertension from any cause can lead to irreversible increases in pulmonary vascular resistance.

Vascular obstruction by parasites in schistosomiasis, clot in chronic thromboembolic disease, or extrinsic compression in mediastinal fibrosis or tumor can all lead to pulmonary hypertension. Intrinsic pulmonary vascular disease can be caused by a number of different stimuli and conditions (Fig. 2-5). Despite heterogeneous etiologies, three distinct pathologic features are consistent: medial hypertrophy, an indicator of vasoconstriction; intimal proliferation, a marker of vascular remodeling; and in situ thrombosis, suggesting endothelial dysfunction and local activation of thrombosis. Therapy in intrinsic pulmonary

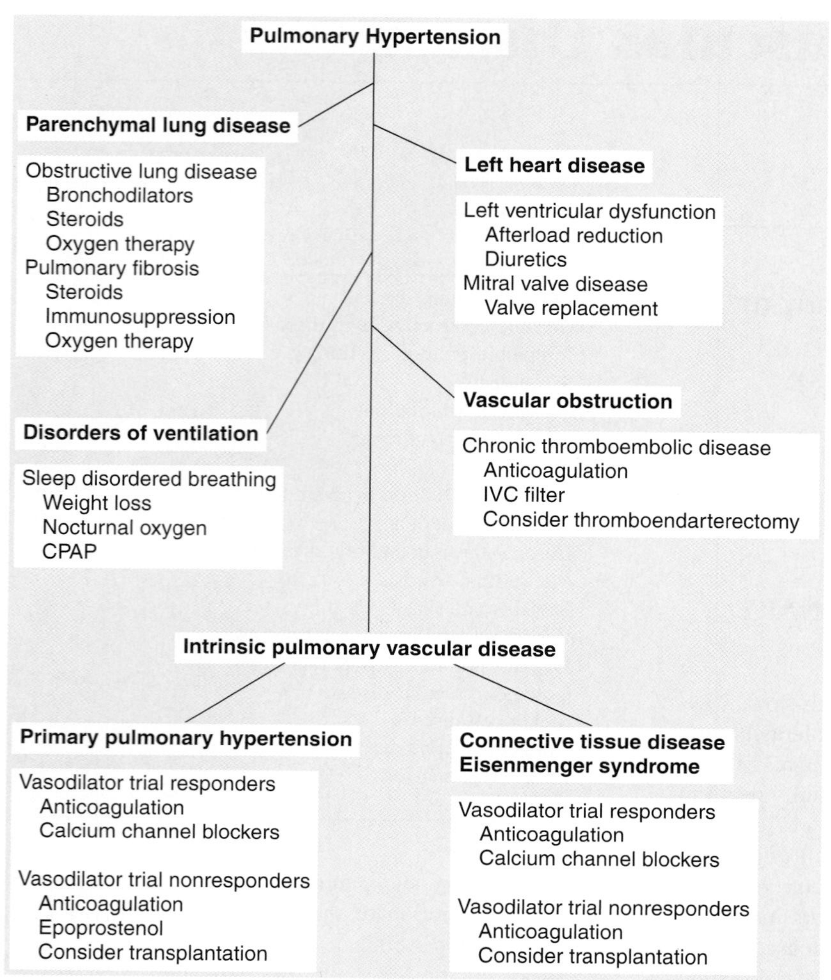


FIGURE 2-5 **Pulmonary hypertension.**

vascular disease focuses on each of these characteristic pathologic findings.

## TREATMENT OF PULMONARY VASCULAR DISEASE

### Main Actions of Therapies and General Approach

The first step in treatment is to identify and treat the underlying cause of disease. Therefore, in pulmonary hypertension secondary to COPD or to parenchymal lung disease, improving gas exchange with bronchodilators and administering supplemental oxygen may significantly reduce PA pressure. Likewise, in patients with interstitial pulmonary fibrosis (IPF), pulmonary hypertension may improve significantly in response to oxygen, steroids, and immunosuppression. Individuals with obstructive sleep apnea or disorders of ventilation may benefit from nocturnal CPAP (chronic positive airway pressure) (Weitzenblum et al. 1988). Surgical intervention with a pulmonary thromboendarterectomy may be warranted in selected patients with chronic thromboembolic disease (Moser et al. 1987).

### Approach to Vasodilator Therapy

Vasoconstriction is commonly present in both primary and secondary pulmonary hypertension. Vasodilators may thus be beneficial in many types of intrinsic pulmonary vascular disease, but they do not currently have a role in pulmonary hypertension secondary to parenchymal lung disease or left-sided heart disease. Treatment with vasodilators in pulmonary hypertension can be unpredictably hazardous, and great care is essential to reduce the risk of serious adverse events, such as profound systemic hypotension and sudden death.

**PRINCIPLE Drugs with poorly documented efficacy and well-documented toxicity should be used cautiously if at all. Caution in this regard means setting the lower limits of acceptable toxicity before starting therapy and assessing the effects of the drugs frequently.**

Patients diagnosed with intrinsic pulmonary vascular disease should be considered for a right heart catheterization and vasodilator trial before empirical vasodilator therapy is initiated (Galie et al. 1995). This procedure enables assessment of the severity of pulmonary hypertension and of left-sided cardiac function and also allows prediction of survival (Rich et al. 1987; D'Alonzo et al. 1991). Assessing the response to short-acting agents such as inhaled nitric oxide (Pepke et al. 1991), epoprostenol (Rubin et al. 1982) or adenosine (Morgan et al. 1991), at the time of catheterization also provides a guide to therapy. A decrease in mean pulmonary artery pressure and an increase in cardiac output roughly predict sustained hemodynamic improvement and prolonged survival with oral vasodilators (Rich and Brundage 1987; Rich et al. 1992). Approximately 20–30% of patients with PPH demonstrate an acute response to vasodilators (Rich and Brundage 1987), but the response rate is lower in secondary forms of intrinsic pulmonary vascular disease, such as scleroderma. Oral vasodilators are contraindicated in patients whose systemic arterial pressure, cardiac output, or oxygen saturation significantly decrease during the vasodilator trial.

## Calcium Channel Blockers

Although there are no prospective randomized trials of oral vasodilators in the treatment of primary or secondary pulmonary hypertension, evidence suggests a beneficial role for calcium channel blockers in PPH. Patients who show a favorable acute response to a calcium channel blocker during right heart catheterization demonstrate improved survival, and regression of right ventricular hypertrophy with sustained therapy (Rich and Brundage 1987; Rich et al. 1992). Calcium channel blockers must be used with extreme caution, for they may result in worsening gas exchange, right heart failure, hypotension, and death (Paker et al. 1984; Weir et al. 1989). Whereas calcium channel blockers are initiated cautiously at a low dose, the final dose attained in order to achieve benefit is generally higher than that used to treat systemic hypertension (Rubin et al. 1983; Rich and Brundage 1987; Rich and Kaufmann 1991). The most commonly used agents are amlodipine (2.5–20 mg/day), nifedipine (30–240 mg/day) and diltiazem (120–900 mg/day). Relatively minor adverse effects include salt retention and edema. Abrupt discontinuation can lead to fatal rebound pulmonary hypertension (Rich and Brundage 1987).

## Epoprostenol

Epoprostenol (prostacyclin, prostaglandin $I_2$, Flolan®), an arachidonic acid metabolite, was recently approved for treatment of PPH (Epoprostenol 1996). Epoprostenol is a potent vasodilator with a short half-life (3–5 min) that is delivered through a permanent indwelling catheter by a continuous infusion pump. In a randomized trial in PPH, epoprostenol improved hemodynamics and exercise tolerance, and prolonged survival in severe PPH (NYHA III–IV) (Rubin et al. 1990; Barst et al. 1994, 1996). A trial evaluating the efficacy of epoprostenol in the treatment of SPH in scleroderma is under way.

Minor adverse effects of epoprostenol include jaw pain, headache, rash, diarrhea, and joint pain. More serious adverse effects are related predominantly to the cumbersome drug delivery system and include life-threatening line sepsis or discontinuation of drug delivery. Epoprostenol should be avoided in postcapillary pulmonary hypertension because of the risk of acute pulmonary edema (Rubin et al. 1990). Dose increments are required frequently during the first year of therapy to preempt the recurrence of symptoms. The reason for this increased dose requirement is unknown but is speculated to be due to either enhanced drug degradation or the increase of vasoconstrictive mediators such as thromboxane.

Epoprostenol may help control PPH in patients awaiting lung transplantation and may even enable deferment or avoidance of lung transplantation (Gaine and Rubin 1998). The absence of an acute vasodilator response to epoprostenol does not rule out long-term improvement in hemodynamics with therapy, suggesting alternative modes of action, such as antiplatelet or antiproliferative properties (Barst et al. 1996).

## Other Therapies for Pulmonary Vascular Disease

### *Chronic oxygen therapy*

Chronic oxygen therapy is indicated in patients with pulmonary hypertension who have documented hypoxemia, either at rest or with exercise. Patients with intrinsic vascular disease are not usually hypoxemic in the absence of right to left intracardiac shunting or reduced cardiac output. However, hypoxemia is frequently observed in parenchymal lung disease such as COPD and IPF. In these patients chronic oxygen therapy improves survival (Nocturnal Oxygen Therapy Trial Group 1980; Report of the Medical Research Council Working Party 1981; Owens et al. 1991). The benefits of oxygen are probably multifactorial, for its effects on pulmonary hemodynamics are variable and improvements are slow to develop (Timms et al. 1985).

### *Anticoagulation*

Several factors seem logically to predispose to thrombus formation in pulmonary hypertension: pulmonary vascular endothelial dysfunction, venous stasis from right heart failure, and impaired mobility. Two nonrandomized studies have indeed suggested that anticoagulation prolongs life in PPH (Fuster et al. 1984; Rich et al. 1992). Anticoagulation has thus been recommended for patients with SPH. Heparin may be an alternative in those with contraindications to warfarin.

**PRINCIPLE Unless the effect of a drug is immediate, unequivocal, and definitive, the value of an open study must be questioned. Even when a drug has dramatic effects controlled studies are necessary to develop convincing information about the appropriate indications for its use. There is little excuse except provisionally, for accepting an open study as definitive for establishing an indication for drug use.**

### *Diuretics, inotropes, and glycosides*

Diuretic therapy is frequently required to control edema and to reduce right ventricular end-diastolic volume in advancing right heart failure. In patients with severe right heart failure, low-dose dopamine may improve right ventricular contractility and enhance diuresis. In parenchymal lung disease ankle edema may occur as a result of salt retention secondary to hypoxia or steroid use and may not indicate worsening right heart function.

Digoxin has been shown to benefit patients with hypoxemic pulmonary hypertension and left heart dysfunction (Mathur et al. 1981), but its value in other forms of pulmonary hypertension is controversial. Digoxin may also have a role in counteracting the negative inotropic effect of calcium channel blockers (Rich and Brundage 1987) and in antagonizing the neurohumoral activation of PPH and right heart failure (Nootens et al. 1995).

### *Nonpharmacologic therapy*

Lung transplantation (double or single) is effective for severe pulmonary hypertension unresponsive to maximum medical therapy (Rubin 1997; Gaine and Rubin 1998). Atrial septostomy, the controlled opening of a right to left shunt at the atrial level, is reserved for patients with severe right-sided heart failure or recurrent syncope. This procedure, by decompressing the right ventricle and improving cardiac output may provide palliation and improved survival (Rich and Lam 1983; Kerstein et al. 1995).

## REFERENCES


Barst RJ, Rubin LJ, Long WA, et al. 1996. A comparison of continuous intravenous epoprostenol (prostacyclin) with conventional therapy for primary pulmonary hypertension. The Primary Pulmonary Hypertension Study Group. *N Engl J Med* **334**:296–302.

Barst RJ, Rubin LJ, McGoon MD, Caldwell EJ, et al. 1994. Survival in primary pulmonary hypertension with long-term continuous intravenous prostacyclin. *Ann Intern Med* **121**:409–15.

D'Alonzo G, Barst RJ, Ayres SM, et al. 1991. Survival in patients with primary pulmonary hypertension. Results from a national prospective registry. *Ann Intern Med* **115**:343–9.

Epoprostenol. 1996. Epoprostenol for primary pulmonary hypertension. *Med Lett Drugs Ther* **38**(968):14–5.

Fuster V, Steele PM, Edwards WD, et al. 1984. Primary pulmonary hypertension: natural history and the importance of thrombosis. *Circulation* **70**:580–7.

Gaine SP, Rubin LJ. 1998. Medical and surgical treatment options for pulmonary hypertension. *Am J Med Sci* **315**:179–84.

Galie N, Ussia G, Passarelli P, et al. 1995. Role of pharmacologic tests in the treatment of primary pulmonary hypertension. *Am J Cardiol* **75**:55A–62A.

Kerstein D, Levy PS, Hsu DT, et al. 1995. Blade balloon atrial septostomy improves survival in patients with severe primary pulmonary hypertension. *Circulation* **91**:2028–35.

Mathur P, Powles R, Pugsley S, et al. 1981. Effect of digoxin on right ventricular function in severe chronic airflow obstruction. *Ann Intern Med* **95**:283–8.

Morgan J, McCormack D, Griffiths M, et al. 1991. Adenosine as a vasodilator in primary pulmonary hypertension. *Circulation* **84**:1145–9.

Moser KM, Daily PO, Peterson K, et al. 1987. Thromboendarterectomy for chronic, major vessel thromboembolic pulmonary hypertension: immediate and long term results in 42 patients. *Ann Intern Med* **107**:560–5.

Nocturnal Oxygen Therapy Trial Group. 1980. Continuous or nocturnal oxygen therapy in hypoxemic chronic obstructive lung disease. *Ann Intern Med* **93**:391–8.

Nootens M, Kaufmann E, Rector T, et al. 1995. Neurohumoral activation in patients with right ventricular failure from pulmonary hypertension: relation to hemodynamics and endothelin levels. *J Am Coll Cardiol* **26**:1581–5.

Owens MW, Anderson WM, George RB. 1991. Indications for spirometry in outpatients with respiratory disease. *Chest* **99**:730–4.

Paker M, Medina N, Yushak M. 1984. Adverse hemodynamic and clinical effects of calcium channel blockade in pulmonary hypertension secondary to obliterative pulmonary vascular disease. *J Am Coll Cardiol* **4**:890–901.

Pepke Z, Higenbottam T, Dinh-Xuan A, et al. 1991. Inhaled nitric oxide as a cause of selective pulmonary vasodilatation in pulmonary hypertension. *Lancet* **338**:1173–4.

Report of the Medical Research Council Working Party. 1981. Long term domiciliary oxygen therapy in chronic hypoxic cor pulmonale complicating chronic bronchitis and emphysema. Report of the Medical Research Council Working Party. *Lancet* **1**:681–6.

Rich S, Brundage BH. 1987. High dose calcium channel blocking therapy for primary pulmonary hypertension: evidence for long term reduction in pulmonary artery pressure and regression of right ventricular hypertrophy. *Circulation* **76**:135–41.

Rich S, Dantzker DR, Ayres SM, et al. 1987. Primary pulmonary hypertension. A national prospective study. *Ann Intern Med* **107**:216–23.

Rich S, Kaufmann E, Levy PS. 1992. The effect of high doses of calcium-channel blockers on survival in primary pulmonary hypertension. *N Engl J Med* **327**:76–81.

Rich S, Kaufmann E. 1991. High dose titration of calcium channel blocking agents for primary pulmonary hypertension: guidelines for short-term drug testing. *J Am Coll Cardiol* **18**:1323–7.

Rich S, Lam W. 1983. Atrial septostomy as palliative therapy for refractory primary pulmonary hypertension. *Am J Cardiol* **51**:1560–1.

Rubin LJ. 1993. ACCP Consensus Statement. Primary pulmonary hypertension [review]. *Chest* **104**:236–50.

Rubin LJ, Groves BM, Reeves JT, et al. 1982. Prostacyclin-induced acute pulmonary vasodilation in primary pulmonary hypertension. *Circulation* **66**:334–8.

Rubin LJ, Mendoza J, Hood M, et al. 1990. Treatment of primary pulmonary hypertension with continuous intravenous prostacyclin (epoprostenol). Results of randomized trial. *Ann Intern Med* **112**:485–91.

Rubin LJ, Nicod P, Hillis LD, et al. 1983. Treatment of primary pulmonary hypertension with nifedipine. *Ann Intern Med* **99**:433–8.

Timms R, Khaja F, Williams G. 1985. Hemodynamic response to oxygen therapy in chronic obstructive pulmonary disease. *Ann Intern Med* **102**:29–36.

Weir E, Rubin L, Ayres S, et al. 1989. The acute administration of vasodilators in primary pulmonary hypertension: experience from the National Institutes of Health Registry on Primary Pulmonary Hypertension. *Am Rev Respir Dis* **140**:1623–30.

Weitzenblum E, Krieger J, April M, et al. 1988. Daytime pulmonary hypertension in patients with obstructive sleep apnea syndrome. *Am Rev Respir Dis* **138**:345–9.

# Idiopathic Pulmonary Fibrosis

**Naseema B. Merchant, Paul W. Noble**

### *Chapter Outline*



The interstitial lung diseases are a heterogenous group of diseases characterized by inflammation and fibrosis in the lung parenchyma or small airways (e.g., bronchioles). Diffuse pulmonary fibrosis is an interstitial lung disease characterized by chronic inflammation and progressive fibrosis. It sometimes results from repeated or chronic exposure to environmental antigens (e.g., "pigeon breeder's lung") or as the end-stage of repeated or chronic hypersensitivity pneumonitis, and it also occurs in association with systemic collagen-vascular diseases, such as scleroderma and lupus erythematosus. It most commonly presents, however, without any predisposing condition, and is then described as "idiopathic." This form is the most common severe form of interstitial lung disease. An understanding of its presentation, and treatment of *idiopathic pulmonary fibrosis* (IPF), will enable a general approach to this heterogenous group of diseases.

Interstitial pulmonary fibrosis accounts for more than 30,000 hospitalizations and more than 5,000 deaths in the US annually (Lynch and Standiford 1993). It most often presents with progressive dyspnea; hypoxemia; diffuse, often predominantly basilar, bilateral interstitial infiltrates on the chest radiograph; and a restrictive pattern on pulmonary function testing (Crystal et al. 1984; Panos and King 1991; Lynch and Chavis 1992). Lung biopsies reveal a mixture of fibrosis and inflammatory cell infiltration in the pulmonary interstitium and alveolar walls. With progression of inflammation and fibrosis, the lung architecture is destroyed and distorted, terminating eventually in pulmonary hypertension and respiratory failure.

## PATHOPHYSIOLOGY OF IDIOPATHIC PULMONARY FIBROSIS

The etiology of IPF is unknown. One hypothesis is that this disorder occurs in a susceptible individual following an insult, such as an infection with a respiratory virus that shares antigen recognition sites with some protein endogenous in the pulmonary interstitium, so that the disease is autoimmune in nature, but efforts to identify a viral cause have so far been unsuccessful. Whatever the initial stimulus, chronic inflammation is thought to play the key role in promoting injury and a fibrotic response. This ongoing process involves inflammatory and immune effector cells. Increased number of neutrophils and macrophages are typically found in the air spaces (Crystal et al. 1976; 1981). Products of these or other cells stimulate fibroblast proliferation and activity, and the resulting fibrosis distorts normal lung architecture, obliterating alveolar capillaries and reducing lung distensibility. The precise factors responsible for attracting and activating neutrophils and macrophages are unknown, but once alveolar macrophages are activated, they themselves recruit more cells by releasing cytokines, chemotactic factors, and growth factors, which amplify the inflammatory response. As inflammation proceeds, collagen deposition by fibroblasts under the effect of several fibroblast growth factors ultimately leads to fibrosis (King et al. 1994).

## GENERAL APPROACH TO THERAPY FOR IDIOPATHIC PULMONARY FIBROSIS

The median survival of patients with IPF after diagnosis is less than 5 years (Hay and Turner-Warwick 1988), and because no treatment is known to reverse interstitial fibrosis, therapy is directed at modulating the inflammatory and immune processes that appear to incite the fibrotic process (Turner-Warwick 1984; Raghu 1987; Hay and Turner-Warwick 1988; King 1993). This is why it is thought to be important to diagnose the condition and to initiate treatment early, in order to prevent progression of the disease (King et al. 1994). The therapeutic goals are to prevent further fibrosis and to maintain lung function. But except for identifying early pulmonary fibrosis in patients sensitive to an airborne antigen they can avoid, the treatments now available even for these modest, limited goals of therapy are only partially effective and have substantial toxicities. Few patients respond favorably to treatment, and even after an initially favorable response, the disease may progress despite continued therapy.

Few randomized controlled clinical trials of different treatments for IPF have been performed, so much of the standard approach to treatment is based on the knowledge that the disease involves inflammation and unregulated fibrosis and that it may involve a disorder in immune function. The treatments most used are thus systemic corticosteroids for their anti-inflammatory action and immunosuppressants, for example, cyclophosphamide or azathioprine. Interstitial pulmonary fibrosis does not respond quickly, so whatever agents are used, they need to be continued for at least 3–6 months before their effectiveness can be assessed (King et al. 1994).

At present, the best available data suggest that early treatment, when symptoms, radiographic and pulmonary function changes are mild, offers the best chance of improvement. Although it is by no means clear that every patient needs to be treated, there is general agreement that a trial of therapy is advisable for all patients with evidence of progression of disease or with moderate to severe impairment on presentation. Logically, aggressive anti-inflammatory therapy should be given to patients with evidence of ongoing active inflammation, but some experts initiate treatment with corticosteroids even when lung biopsy specimens show mainly fibrosis with little or no inflammation. The logic underlying this approach is that histopathological changes in IPF tend to be heterogenous, with areas of fibrosis mixed with regions of inflammation and with regions that appear unaffected. The approach to patients with mild disease and those with physiologic impairment but with some contraindication to therapy is to follow them carefully at 3- to 6-month intervals for signs of deterioration and need for therapy. Elderly patients with chronic progressive disease and severe abnormalities on pulmonary function tests tend to have a shorter duration of symptoms before clinical presentation and a more rapid subsequent deterioration than do younger patients. They are also at greater risk for drug-induced adverse effects. Although few elderly patients have a significant objective response to therapy, those with severe or progressive disease should still be given a 3- to 6-month treatment trial in the hope that the disease may be reversible or progression slowed (Lynch and Standiford 1993; King et al. 1994). If improvement is seen after this initial course of intensive treatment, the best results seem to be obtained with a very slow taper of medications to achieve the optimal balance between efficacy and toxicity.

## DRUG THERAPY FOR IDIOPATHIC PULMONARY FIBROSIS

### Corticosteroids

Corticosteroids have potent anti-inflammatory effects and have been the mainstay of treatment for IPF for more than three decades. The rationale for their use is that they are expected to reverse or suppress active, ongoing alveolitis. A favorable response to a 3- to 6-month trial of therapy occurs in approximately 10–30% of cases and even complete reversal of evidence of disease may rarely occur (Rudd et al. 1981; Crystal et al. 1984; Panos and King 1991; Lynch and Chavis 1992). Difference in responsiveness to corticosteroid treatment may be related to the differences in the balance of active inflammation (thought to be responsive) and of pulmonary fibrosis (thought to be unresponsive) accounting for pulmonary impairment.

Therapy is initiated with prednisone 1.0–2.0 mg/kg per day, not to exceed a total dose of 100 mg/day as a single daily oral dose. This initial treatment is continued for approximately 2 to 3 months, when the response to treatment is assessed by analyzing changes in symptoms, in the infiltrates on the chest radiograph, and in pulmonary function tests. If the response is considered to be favorable, the dose is tapered by 1–2 mg/week, until a dose of 0.5 mg/kg per day is reached. This dose is continued for about an additional 3 to 6 months, and is further reduced to 0.25 mg/kg daily and maintained for at least 6 months (total one year), if no clinical deterioration is noted. If clinical deterioration occurs during this taper, the dose of prednisone should be raised to the level that maintains stability. No clear guidelines exist regarding optimal duration of treatment. Most clinicians recommend treatment for up to 1 year with or without other immunosuppressive therapy and then gradual taper treatment with follow-up assessments at 3- to 6-month intervals. If there is no objective evidence of a response to corticosteroids, therapy should be tapered and discontinued.

Short courses of high-dose corticosteroid therapy have been recommended to arrest clinical deterioration in patients with rapidly progressive disease. Pulse therapy in the form of methylprednisolone given intravenously (1–2 g once per week) has been used in these patients. The adverse effects of pulse methylprednisolone therapy include all of those associated with high-dose treatment with any corticosteroid given systemically (mood changes, acute psychosis, hypertension, glucose intolerance, etc.) and include also a metallic taste, flushing, and headache. The net incidence of severe adverse effects with pulse therapy may be lower than with chronic low-dose corticosteroid therapy, but this point has not been analyzed critically (Lynch and Standiford 1993). The potential complications of corticosteroid therapy are numerous (alteration in appetite, weight gain, altered visual acuity, irritability, hyperglycemia, osteoporosis, vertebral compression fractures, aseptic necrosis of femoral head, opportunistic infections, poor wound healing, hypertension, cataracts, adrenal insufficiency, myopathy, peptic ulcer disease, etc.) and patients should be monitored frequently for early detection and treatment of complications as they occur.

### Cyclophosphamide

Cyclophosphamide is a potent alkylating agent of the nitrogen mustard group and is sometimes used as a second-line agent in patients who either did not respond to or could not tolerate corticosteroids or in patients who responded to an initial course of high-dose corticosteroid treatment, but in whom chronic use of an alternate therapy seems preferable (Weese et al. 1975; Johnson et al. 1989). Its mode of action involves the depletion of lymphocytes and suppression of lymphocyte function. The rate of favorable responses has been reported to be as high as 50% by some authors (Rudd et al. 1981). The recommended dose is 2 mg/kg given daily as a single dose, usually given in combination with oral prednisone at 0.25 mg/kg per day. Most patients tolerate doses in the range of 100–150 mg/day. Because the response to cyclophosphamide, like the response to a high-dose of a corticosteroid, is delayed, a minimum of 4–6 months of therapy is necessary to assess the response. Although no data exist as to the optimal duration of treatment, it is recommended that cyclophosphamide be given for not less than 3 months and probably for as long as 9–12 months in patients whose clinical status stabilizes or improves, as documented by follow-up studies (King et al. 1994). Cyclophosphamide's most worrying adverse effects are leukopenia and thrombocytopenia, so patients treated with this drug should be periodically monitored with complete blood and platelet counts. Other potential toxicities include hemorrhagic cystitis (one-third of patients), bladder cancer, hematologic malignancies, bone marrow toxicity, stomatitis, alopecia, oligospermia, opportunistic infections, and, ironically, interstitial pneumonitis that may be indistinguishable from IPF.

### Azathioprine

Azathioprine (AZA) is a purine analogue that is converted to mercaptopurine in body tissues (King et al. 1994). It appears to act by the substitution of purines in DNA synthesis and by inhibiting adenosine deaminase, the deficiency of which inhibits the lymphocyte function. Some recent studies have shown encouraging results with the combination of AZA and low-dose prednisone in patients with IPF (Weese et al. 1975). The recommended dose is 2 mg/kg (max. 200 mg/day), though an optimal dose has not yet been determined. As with the other therapies discussed, a therapeutic trial of at least 3 to 6 months is necessary before the response to therapy can be assessed. Although azathioprine appears to be slightly less effective than cyclophosphamide, its use is associated with fewer serious adverse effects (Lynch and Standiford 1993). It is this lower risk of toxicity that principally accounts for azathioprine's place as an alternative to cyclophosphamide in patients with progressive IPF refractory to steroids. Some experts even prefer it for corticosteroid-responsive patients suffering from corticosteroid adverse effects. Complete blood counts should be monitored because of potential bone marrow toxicity.

Potential toxicities include leukopenia, anemia, pure red cell aplasia, thrombocytopenia, pancytopenia, nausea, vomiting, diarrhea, peptic ulcer disease, mild LFT abnormality, severe hepatitis (rarely), progressive cirrhosis, cholestasis and, again ironically, diffuse alveolar damage and pneumonitis (seen most often in renal transplant recipients).

### Antifibrotic Therapy

An alternate approach to treating IPF that has begun to attract attention is the direct targeting of fibrosis itself, rather than the targeting of altered immune function and inflammation as precursors of fibrosis. An example of this approach is the use of colchicine, a potent alkaloid historically used for the treatment of gout but that has also been found to have antifibrotic and anti-inflammatory properties. Published data affirming its efficacy are pending at this time, and whereas colchicine presents the advantages of familiarity, low cost, and low toxicity, its role in the treatment of IPF is controversial.

Another agent that has been used for its putative antifibrotic actions is D-penicillamine, a chelating agent that interferes with collagen cross-linking in vitro. It may also suppress humoral and cellular immunity. Reports of D-penicillamine's use are so far limited to isolated case reports or small series, so the usefulness of this drug in the management of IPF is not known.

### Novel Drug Therapies

The National Heart, Lung, and Blood Institute reviewed some new therapies under investigation in August 1994 and published the workshop summary in March 1995 (Hunninghake and Kalica 1995). These therapies appear promising for the future and could potentially be breakthroughs. These novel therapies include cytokine inhibitors, growth factor inhibitors, antifibrotic agents, antiproteases, novel anti-inflammatory agents, antioxidants, and gene therapy.

## SUPPORTIVE THERAPY

Most patients with IPF do not respond to treatment, and even in the fortunate minority who do respond, complete reversal is rare. All patients should be assessed for hypoxemia during rest as well as during exertion. In such patients, supplemental oxygen therapy can relieve dyspnea and extend the period of independent activity. Physical therapy and pulmonary rehabilitation may help patients learn energy-saving techniques, again enabling them to perform more of their activities of daily living.

## LUNG TRANSPLANTATION

When trials of anti-inflammatory and immunosuppressive treatment have proved ineffective, lung transplantation should be considered. Transplantation is usually reserved for relatively young patients without other significant illnesses and with progressively severe disease, especially when complicated by pulmonary hypertension. This intervention is definitive as a treatment, but of course carries all of the risks of surgery and immunosuppression common to organ transplantation and the additional risk of bronchiolitis obliterans in the transplanted lungs.

## CONCLUSION

The long-term prognosis of IPF is variable, but it is most often a relentlessly progressive disease. The severity of impairment at the time of diagnosis and its progression over the 3 to 6 months thereafter are important determinants of the decision as to whether to initiate therapy. If treatment is initiated, the relative contributions of alveolar inflammation and of fibrosis to pulmonary impairment are likely determinants of the response. Although the mainstays of therapy are currently systemic corticosteroids and immunosuppressants, the identification of cellular mediators in the affected lung tissue and improved concepts of how these interact to injure tissue and promote fibrosis will lead to different forms of specific therapies in the future.

## REFERENCES


Crystal RG, Bitterman PB, Rennard SI, et al. 1984. Interstitial lung diseases of unknown cause. Disorders characterized by chronic inflammation of the lower respiratory tract [review, two parts]. *N Engl J Med* **310**:154–66, 235–44.

Crystal RG, Fulmer JD, Roberts WC, et al. 1976. Idiopathic pulmonary fibrosis: clinical histologic, radiographic, physiologic, scintigraphic, cytologic and biochemical aspects. *Ann Intern Med* **85**:769–88.

Crystal RG, Gadek JE, Ferrans VJ, et al. 1981. Interstitial lung disease: current concepts of pathogenesis, staging and therapy. *Am J Med* **70**:542–68.

Hay J, Turner-Warwick M. 1988. Interstitial pulmonary fibrosis. In: Murray J, Nadel J, editors. *Textbook of Respiratory Medicine*. Philadelphia: W B Saunders. p 1445–61.

Hunninghake GW, Kalica AR. 1995. Approaches to the treatment of pulmonary fibrosis. *Am J Respir Crit Care Med* **151**:915–8.

Johnson MA, Kwan S, Snell NJ, et al. 1989. Randomized controlled trial comparing prednisolone alone with cyclophosphamide and low dose prednisolone in combination in cryptogenic fibrosing alveolitis. *Thorax* **44**:280–8.

King T, Cherniack R, Schwartz M. 1994. Idiopathic pulmonary fibrosis and other interstitial lung diseases of unknown etiology. In: Murray J, Nadel J, editors. *Textbook of Respiratory Medicine*. Vol. 2. Philadelphia: W B Saunders. p 1827–49.

King T. 1993. Idiopathic pulmonary fibrosis. In: Schwartz M, King TJ, eds. *Interstitial Lung Diseases*. St. Louis: Mosby–Year Book. p 367–403.

Lynch J, Standiford T. 1993. What are your best tools for diagnosing and managing IPF? *Intern Med* **14**:19–38.

Lynch JI, Chavis A. 1992. Chronic interstitial lung disorders. In: Victor L, ed. *Clinical Pulmonary Medicine*. Boston: Little Brown. p 193–264.

Panos R, King T. 1991. Idiopathic pulmonary fibrosis. In: Lynch JI, DeRemee R, eds. *Immunologically Mediated Pulmonary Diseases*. Philadelphia: Lippincott. p 1–39.

Raghu G. 1987. Idiopathic pulmonary fibrosis: a rational clinical approach. *Chest* **92**:148–54.

Rudd R, Haslam P, Turner-Warwick M. 1981. Cryptogenic fibrosing alveolitis: Relationships of pulmonary physiology and bronchoalveolar lavage to response to treatment and prognosis. *Am Rev Respir Dis* **124**(1):1–8.

Turner-Warwick M. 1984. Interstitial lung disease: approaches to therapy. *Semin Respir Med* **6**:92–102.

Weese W, Levine B, Kazemi H. 1975. Interstitial lung disease resistant to corticosteroid therapy: Report of three cases treated with azathioprine and cyclophosphamide. *Chest* **67**:57–60.


# Drug-Induced Lung Disease

Naseema B. Merchant, Paul W. Noble

### *Chapter Outline*



Drug toxicity is a major challenge faced by clinicians today. It is currently estimated that 2–5% of hospital admissions are related to adverse drug reactions, with about 0.3% of hospital deaths being drug-related (Classen et al. 1991). The list of drugs implicated in lung injury has grown rapidly over the last two decades. To date, more than 150 agents have been reported to have adverse effects on the lungs (Rosenow 1994), affecting the airways, lung parenchyma, vasculature, pleura, respiratory muscles including the diaphragm and even the respiratory centers in the brain. Drug adverse effects are generally due to the pharmacologic effects of the drug or idiosyncratic reactions. The mechanisms of drug-induced lung injury are classified in four general categories (Table 2-17) (Rosenow 1994), but a wide variety of clinical syndromes have been described.

## DRUGS THAT AFFECT THE AIRWAYS

Cough, bronchospasm, and constrictive bronchiolitis can all result from drug toxicity.

### Angiotensin-Converting Enzyme Inhibitors

Angiotensin-converting enzyme (ACE) inhibitors produce an irritating cough in about 10% of treated patients, beginning a few days to several months after initiation of the drug (Gibson 1989; Sebastian et al. 1991; Israili and Hall 1992; Simons et al. 1992). The clinical presentation is characterized by a dry cough and occurs with all of the ACE inhibitors (Israel-Biet et al. 1991). Aggravation of preexisting asthma as well as recurrence of asthma are known to occur (Popa 1987; Bucknall et al. 1988). The mechanism appears to be related to the accumulation of bronchomotor mediators such as bradykinin and other kinins (Usberti et al. 1985; Morice et al. 1987). Discontinuation of the drug leads to cessation of symptoms in a few days, with recurrence of symptoms upon readministration of the drug. Nebulized cromolyn sodium and oral NSAIDs, for example, indomethacin and sulindac, may also relieve the cough (Nicholls and Gilchrist 1987). A life-threatening complication of ACE inhibitors is angioneurotic edema (Israili and Hall 1992).

### Aerosols

Aerosolized mucolytics like *N*-acetylcysteine and deoxyribonuclease, given to liquefy secretions responsible for bronchial obstruction, can also cause bronchial edema. Concomitant use of bronchodilators is recommended to prevent aggravation of bronchospasm (Kory et al. 1968; Lourenso and Cotromanes 1982). Aerosol therapy with sodium cromoglycate is associated with remarkably few adverse effects, apart from cough, caused by transient irritation of the upper airways (Cox 1969; Sheffer et al. 1975). Metaproterenol and albuterol MDIs have also been reported to cause cough and even bronchospasm (Yarbrough et al. 1985). If the preservative in solutions of bronchodilators such as isoproterenol, isoetharine, and racemic epinephrine contains sulfites, then nebulized treatment may paradoxically produce cough and bronchospasm because of sulfite sensitivity (Koepke et al. 1983, 1984). Cough and bronchospasm have also been reported with the use of aerosolized pentamidine in HIV patients with *Pneumocystic carinii* pneumonia (PCP) (Montgomery et al. 1987). The mechanisms proposed include nonspecific irritation from inhaled particles, histamine release (Israel-Biet et al. 1991), and inhibition of cholinesterases by pentamidine. Pretreatment with either an anticholinergic agent or a $\beta$-adrenergic agonist prevents symptoms in most cases (Smith et al. 1988). Cough is also a common adverse effect of inhalation of beclomethasone dipropionate from an MDI, occurring in approximately 40% of cases (Israel-Biet et al. 1991). The causative agent may be oleic acid, a dispersant used in beclomethasone MDIs (Shim and Williams 1987a, 1987b). Prior treatment with $\beta$-adrenergic agonists may reduce the cough.

**Table 2-17 Mechanisms of Drug-Related Pulmonary Toxicity**

| |
|---|
| Direct cytotoxicity |
| Injury due to intracellular accumulation of lipoid substances |
| Oxidant injury |
| Immune-mediated injury |

### Aspirin and Other Nonsteroidal Anti-Inflammatory Agents

Approximately 2–5% of patients with asthma are sensitive to aspirin (ASA), with abrupt, severe worsening of their asthma sometimes with symptoms of an anaphylactic-like reaction, being the most serious outcome. In one study, up to 8% of attacks requiring admission to an ICU were probably precipitated by the use of ASA (Picado 1989). The bronchospasm may be related to inhibition of production of bronchodilatory prostaglandins or increased production of leukotrienes. Interestingly, continued administration of aspirin on the days following an ASA-induced attack may not cause further bronchospasm. The return of ASA-sensitivity may require that the patient stop taking aspirin (or other NSAIDs) for several days. Almost all of the NSAIDs can produce the same adverse effects as aspirin. Drugs such as indomethacin, mefenamic acid, flufenamic acid, meclofenamic acid, ibuprofen, fenoprofen, ketoprofen, naproxen, diclofenac, and phenylbutazone are absolutely contraindicated in patients with ASA-induced asthma as they can cause life-threatening bronchospasm. ASA intolerance should be considered in all asthmatics, but it is especially common in patients with adult-onset asthma and nasal polyps. Use of $\beta$-agonists reverses bronchospasm caused by ASA and related drugs but large doses may be required (Israel-Biet et al. 1991). Prevention of ASA-induced adverse effects requires avoidance of all NSAIDs and all NSAID-containing products. Consistent with the idea that the mechanism of ASA-induced asthma involves an alteration in prostaglandin metabolism is the remarkable efficacy of leukotriene synthesis inhibitor or receptor antagonists to prevent attacks (Christie et al. 1991). In fact, regular use of a leukotriene receptor antagonist improves overall asthma control in ASA-sensitive asthmatics (Dahlen et al. 1993).

## $\beta$-Adrenergic Antagonists

$\beta$-Adrenergic antagonists are known to induce clinical bronchospasm. Even $\beta$-adrenergic antagonists given as eye drops (e.g., timolol) can cause severe worsening of asthma in mild asthmatic subjects (Everitt and Avorn 1990). Propranolol has been shown to cause an increase in airway resistance even in normal individuals (Chester et al. 1981). These effects appear to be mediated by blockade of $\beta_2$-receptors. Although the nonselective $\beta$-adrenergic antagonists are well recognized as dangerous in asthmatics, even the $\beta_1$-selective $\beta$-adrenergic antagonists are also potentially dangerous, because their "selectivity" is modest. Inhaled agonists and anticholinergic medications are the treatment of choice for beta-blocker-induced bronchoconstriction (Ind et al. 1989). If topical or systemic $\beta$-adrenergic antagonists have to be used, in an individual with obstructive lung disease, they should be used in conjunction with aerosolized $\beta_2$-selective agonists (Rosenow 1994) for prevention of potential bronchospasm. Propafenone, an antiarrhythmic agent structurally similar to propranolol, has been reported to cause bronchoconstriction in some asthmatic patients.

## Miscellaneous Agents

Drug-induced constrictive bronchiolitis has been described with D-penicillamine, and rarely with gold salts and sulfasalazine prescribed for collagen-vascular diseases. The mechanism of injury is still unknown, and corticosteroids may not be an effective treatment (Israel-Biet et al. 1991).

# DRUGS THAT AFFECT THE PULMONARY PARENCHYMA

Several patterns of parenchymal lung disease from drug toxicity are recognized.

## Pulmonary Infiltrates with Eosinophilia

More than 30 drugs have been reported to cause pulmonary infiltrates with eosinophilia (Table 2-18). The clinical presentation may be fairly sudden with the rapid onset of fever, cough, shortness of breath and widespread pulmonary infiltrates. This syndrome generally starts to resolve within a few days of stopping the drug, but severe cases may require corticosteroid therapy (Cole 1977).

## Interstitial Pneumonitis and Fibrosis

### *Amiodarone*

Pulmonary toxicity from amiodarone develops in about 6% of treated patients, with up to 10–20% of these reactions being fatal (Martin and Rosenow 1988; Kennedy 1990). Typically, pulmonary toxicity presents with cough and dyspnea and a chest radiograph showing peripheral upper lobe infiltrates. The risk of pulmonary toxicity is low with a daily dose of less than 400 mg or an amiodarone serum concentration of less than 2.5 mg/L (Rotmensch et al. 1984). Most patients respond to discontinuation of amiodarone and the addition of corticosteroids (Zaher et al. 1983; Martin and Rosenow 1988), but fatalities are known to occur. Continuation of amiodarone when patients manifest features of toxicity may lead to an irreversible fibrosis.

### *Bleomycin*

Bleomycin causes pulmonary toxicity in approximately 10% of treated patients; as many as 10% of this group will have a fatal outcome (Rosenow 1994). The risk for pulmonary complications increases with the use of more than 450 U of drug, with age over 70 years, with concomitant or prior radiation, and with the supplemental administration of oxygen. The interaction with oxygen therapy is persistent, so supplemental oxygen should be used with caution in patients treated with bleomycin within the past year (Goldiner et al. 1978; Gibson 1989). The treatment of oxygen-potentiated bleomycin toxicity requires keeping the inspired oxygen concentration ($FIo_2$) as low as possible, and adding high-dose corticosteroid therapy (Rosenow 1994). If responsive, bleomycin pulmonary

**Table 2-18 Drugs That Cause Pulmonary Infiltrates with Eosinophilia**

| | |
|---|---|
| Acetylsalicylic acid | Naproxen |
| *p*-Aminosalicylic acid | Nitrofurantoin |
| Carbamazepine | Penicillin |
| Gold | Sulfasalazine |
| Imipramine HCL | Sulfonamides |
| Methotrexate sodium | |

toxicity reverses slowly; the chest radiographic normalizes over 6–12 months, whereas pulmonary function returns to normal over about two years (Van Barneveld et al. 1987).

***Miscellaneous agents***
Several other drugs may cause interstitial alveolar infiltrates, which are thought to reflect immunologically mediated injury to alveolar cells, causing desquamation and initiating fibrosis. This occurs with some cytotoxic and immunosuppressive drugs, especially busulphan, carmustine and methotrexate. Nitrofurantoin and gold salts may also produce this pattern of toxicity.

### Pulmonary Edema

Several drugs are known to cause noncardiogenic or cardiogenic pulmonary edema. Acetylsalicylic acid can cause a noncardiogenic pulmonary edema when serum salicylate concentration exceeds 40 mg/dL (Heffner and Sann 1981; Rosenow 1994). The mechanism is probably related to a direct effect on the alveolar capillary membrane and a resultant increase in vascular permeability. Treatment of severe salicylate-induced pulmonary edema requires, in addition to discontinuing the drug, mechanical ventilation, forced alkaline diuresis, or even hemodialysis. Heroin, and rarely other opiates, are also known to cause noncardiogenic pulmonary edema which usually develops within a few hours of narcotic use, although the onset may be delayed for as long as 24 hours and may first appear after hospitalization. Heroin-induced pulmonary edema is believed to be a consequence of overdose. Treatment is mainly supportive and includes naloxone therapy to reverse respiratory depression, administration of supplemental oxygen, and, if necessary mechanical ventilation with PEEP. Early recovery is generally the rule unless the course is prolonged by aspiration pneumonia, which is a frequent complication (Stern et al. 1968). Noncardiogenic pulmonary edema may also be caused by propoxyphene, cocaine, hydrochlorothiazide, tocolytics, tricyclic antidepressants, and high-dose oxygen therapy itself (Frank and Massaro 1980; Pisani and Rosenow 1989; Roy et al. 1989; Kavaru et al. 1990).

## DRUGS THAT AFFECT THE PULMONARY VASCULATURE

Aminorex and dexfenfluramine, appetite suppressants, have been implicated in causing pulmonary hypertension.

Talc, used as a filler in many different medications intended for oral use, is injected IV by addicts who crush, dissolve, and inject oral medications like meperidine or methadone. Toxic effects include granulomatous inflammation in the pulmonary arterial bed. With vascular occlusion, pulmonary hypertension may result. Another pattern of response, perhaps related to the size of the particles injected, is granulomatous interstitial pneumonitis (Waller et al. 1980; Crouch and Churg 1983). For both patterns of toxicity, the response to corticosteroid treatment is variable, but is usually poor.

## OTHER DRUG EFFECTS

### Drugs that Affect the Pleura and the Mediastinum

Drugs may adversely affect the pleura and the mediastinum (Table 2-19) (Sostman et al. 1977; Sasame and Boyd 1979; Michael and Rudin 1981; Rinne 1981).

### Miscellaneous Drug Effects

Certain drugs can induce a syndrome that closely resembles systemic lupus erythematosus and that may involve the lungs with pleurisy and pleural effusions. Drugs commonly implicated in this category include hydralazine, procainamide, isoniazid, and sulfonamides. The syndrome usually regresses when the drug is withdrawn (Ginsberg 1980). Several drugs are capable of affecting the respiratory neuromuscular apparatus, acting on the respiratory center (sedatives, hypnotics), on the peripheral nerves supplying respiratory muscles, on the neuromuscular junction (paralytic agents, aminoglycosides) and on respiratory muscles (corticosteroids) (Aldrich and Prezant 1990).

SUMMARY
**Drugs are not yet perfectly safe and likely never will be. Because early recognition of an unwanted reaction and withdrawal of the responsible agent is fundamental to treatment, awareness of the possibility of a potential drug reaction and of the danger of potential toxicity is of utmost importance.**

Table 2-19 **Drugs That Affect the Pleura and the Mediastinum**

| | |
|---|---|
| Pleural effusion | Bromocriptine mesylate, busulfan, methysergide maleate |
| Mediastinal lipomatosus | Corticosteroids |
| Mediastinal adenopathy | Methotrexate sodium, mitomycin, hydantoin, phenylbutazone |

## REFERENCES


Aldrich T, Prezant D. 1990. Adverse effects of drugs on the respiratory muscles. *Clin Chest Med* **11**:177–89.

Bucknall CE, Neilly JB, Carter R, et al. 1988. Bronchial hyperreactivity in patients who cough after receiving angiotensin converting enzyme inhibitors. *Br Med J* **296**:86–8.

Chester E, Schwartz H, Flemming G. 1981. Adverse effect of propranolol on airway function in nonasthmatic chronic obstructive lung disease. *Chest* **79**:540–4.

Christie PE, Smith CM, Lee TH. 1991. The potent and selective sulfidopeptide leukotriene antagonist: SK&F 104353, inhibits aspirin-induced asthma. *Am Rev Respir Dis* **144**:957–8.

Classen C, Pestotnik SL, Evans RS, et al. 1991. Computerized surveillances of adverse drug events in hospitalized patients. *J Am Med Assoc* **266**:2847–51.

Cole P. 1977. Drug-induced lung disease. *Drugs* **13**:422–44.

Cox J. 1969. Review of chemistry: pharmacology, toxicity, metabolism, specific side-effect, anti-allergic properties in vitro and in vivo of disodium cromoglycate. In: Pepys J, Frankland A, editors. *Disodium Cromoglycate in Allergic Airway Disease*. London: Butterworth. p 13–25.

Crouch E, Churg A. 1983. Progressive massive fibrosis of the lung secondary to intravenous injection of talc. *Am J Clin Pathol* **80**:520–6.

Dahlen B, Kumlin M, Margolskee DJ, et al. 1993. The leukotriene receptor antagonist MK–0679 blocks airway obstruction induced by inhaled lysine aspirin in aspirin-sensitive asthmatics. *Eur Respir J* **6**:1018–26.

Everitt D, Avorn J. 1990. Systemic effects of medications used to treat glaucoma. *Ann Intern Med* **112**:120–5.

Frank L, Massaro F. 1980. Oxygen toxicity. *Am J Med* **69**:117–26.

Gibson GR. 1989. Enalapril-induced cough. *Arch Intern Med* **149**:2701–3.

Ginsberg W. 1980. Drug-induced systemic lupus erythematosus. *Semin Respir Med* **2**:51–8.

Goldiner P, et al. 1978. Factors influencing postoperative morbidity and mortality in patients treated with bleomycin. *Br Med J* **1**:1664–7.

Heffner J, Sann S. 1981. Salicylate-induced pulmonary edema: clinical features and prognosis. *Ann Intern Med* **95**:405–9.

Ind P, et al. 1989. Anticholinergic blockage of beta-blocker-induced bronchoconstriction. *Am Rev Respir Dis* **139**:1390–4.

Israel-Biet D, Labrune S, Huchon G. 1991. Drug-induced lung disease. *Eur Respir J* **4**:465–78.

Israili ZH, Hall WD. 1992. Cough and angioneurotic edema associated with angiotensin-converting enzyme inhibitor therapy. A review of the literature and pathophysiology. *Ann Intern Med* **117**:234–242.

Kavaru M, Ahmad M, Amirthalingam K. 1990. Hydrochlorothiazide-induced pulmonary edema. *Cleveland Clin J Med* **57**:181–4.

Kennedy JJ. 1990. Clinical aspects of amiodarone pulmonary toxicity. *Clin Chest Med* **11**:119–29.

Koepke J, Christopher KL, Chai H, et al. 1984. Dose dependent bronchospasm from sulfites in isoetharine. *JAMA* **251**:2982–3.

Koepke J, Selner J, Dunhill A. 1983. Presence of sulphur dioxide in commonly used bronchodilator solutions. *J Allergy Clin Immunol* **72**:504–8.

Kory R, Hirsch S, Giraldo J. 1968. Nebulization of *N*-acetyl cysteine combined with a bronchodilator in patients with chronic bronchitis: a controlled study. *Chest* **54**:504–9.

Lourenso R, Cotromanes E. 1982. Clinical aerosols: therapeutic aerosols. *Arch Intern Med* **142**:2299–308.

Martin W, Rosenow EC. 1988. Amiodarone pulmonary toxicity. *Chest* **93**:1067–75.

Michael JR, Rudin ML. 1981. Acute pulmonary disease caused by phenytoin. *Ann Intern Med* **95**:452–4.

Montgomery A, Debs R, Luce J. 1987. Aerosolized pentamidine as sole therapy for *Pneumocystis carinii* pneumonia in patients with acquired immune deficiency syndrome. *Lancet* **2**:480–3.

Morice AH, Lowry R, Brown MJ, et al. 1987. Angiotensin-converting enzyme and the cough reflex. *Lancet* **2**:1116–8.

Nicholls MG, Gilchrist NL. 1987. Sulindac and cough induced by converting enzyme inhibitors [letter]. *Lancet* **1**:872.

Picado C, Castillo JA, Montserat JM, et al. 1989. Aspirin intolerance as a precipitating factor of life-threatening attacks of asthma requiring mechanical ventilation. *Eur Respir J* **2**:127–9.

Pisani R, Rosenow EC. 1989. Pulmonary edema associated with tocolytic therapy. *Ann Intern Med* **110**:714–8.

Popa V. 1987. Captopril-related (and induced?) asthma. *Am Rev Respir Dis* **136**:999–1000.

Rinne U. 1981. Pleuropulmonary changes during long term bromocriptine treatment for Parkinson's disease. *Lancet* **1**:44.

Rosenow EC. 1994. Drug-induced pulmonary disease. *Disease-a-month* **60**(5):255–310.

Rotmensch H, Belhassen D, Swanson B. 1984. Steady-state serum amiodarone concentration: relationships with antiarrhythmic efficacy and toxicity. *Ann Intern Med* **101**:462–9.

Roy T, et al. 1989. Pulmonary complication after tricyclic antidepressant overdose. *Chest* **96**:852–6.

Sasame M, Boyd M. 1979. Superoxide and hydrogen peroxide production and NADPH oxidation stimulated by nitrofurantoin in lung microsomes: possible implications for toxicity. *Life Sci* **24**:1091–6.

Sebastian J, et al. 1991. Angiotensin-converting enzyme inhibitors and cough. *Chest* **99**:36–9.

Sheffer A, Rocklin R, Goetzl E. 1975. Immunologic compounds of hypersensitivity reactions to cromoglycate sodium. *N Engl J Med* **293**:1220–4.

Shim C, Williams MH Jr. 1987a. Cough and wheezing from beclomethasone dipropionate aerosol. *Chest* **91**:207–9.

Shim CS, Williams MH Jr. 1987b. Cough and wheezing from beclomethasone dipropionate aerosol are absent after triamcinolone acetronide. *Ann Intern Med* **106**:700–3.

Simons S, et al. 1992. Cough and ACE inhibitors. *Arch Intern Med* **152**:1698–700.

Smith D, Herd D, Gazzard B. 1988. Reversible bronchoconstriction with nebulised pentamidine [letter]. *Lancet* **2**:905.

Sostman H, Matthay R, Putman C. 1977. Cytotoxic drug induced lung disease. *Am J Med* **62**:608–15.

Stern WZ, Spear PW, Jacobson HG. 1968. The roentgenographic findings in acute heroin intoxication. *Am J Roentgenol Radium Ther Nucl Med* **103**:522–32.

Usberti M, Federico J, DiMinno G. 1985. Effects of angiotensin II on plasma ADH, prostaglandin synthesis and water secretion in normal human. *Am J Pathol* **248**:254–9.

Van Barneveld R, et al. 1987. Natural course of bleomycin-induced pneumonitis: a follow-up study. *Am Rev Respir Dis* **135**:48–51.

Waller B, Brownlee W, Roberts W. 1980. Self-induced pulmonary granulomatosis. A consequence of intravenous injection of drugs intended for oral use. *Chest* **78**:90–4.

Yarbrough J, Mansfield L, Ting S. 1985. Metered dose inhaler-induced bronchospasm in asthmatic patients. *Ann Allergy* **55**:25–7.

Zaher C, et al. 1983. Low dose steroid therapy for prophylaxis of amiodarone-induced pulmonary infiltrates [letter]. *N Engl J Med* **308**:779.

CHAPTER

# 3 GASTROINTESTINAL DISORDERS

Gabriel Garcia

*Chapter Outline*



Many common symptoms relate to dysfunction or disease of the gastrointestinal (GI) tract. Digestive diseases afflict 12% of all American adults and account for 16% of all absences from work. In a study of 25,000 illnesses in a group of Cleveland families, acute diarrheal illness was one of the most common illnesses reported, second only to the common cold (Dingle et al. 1964). Therefore, some of the most commonly used drugs are those directed at symptoms and diseases of the alimentary tract.

## SPECIAL FEATURES OF THE CLINICAL PHARMACOLOGY OF THE DIGESTIVE TRACT

The therapy of diseases of the alimentary system presents a number of special challenges that arise from the several special characteristics of the digestive tract. The digestive tract is the usual route of administration for most drugs; they may have a direct action within the GI tract or on its mucosal lining at relatively high concentrations. For example, salicylates and other nonsteroidal anti-inflammatory drugs (NSAIDs) may produce bleeding or erosive gastritis by a direct toxic effect on gastric mucosa.

A therapeutic benefit from certain drugs can be achieved without the drug's entering the circulatory system. Some drugs exert their action solely within the lumen of the GI tract. For example, the poorly absorbed antacids function only within the lumen of the stomach and duodenum to neutralize gastric acid. Some antibiotics (e.g., neomycin) or disaccharides (e.g., lactulose), useful for their action on the GI flora, are poorly absorbed and exert their effects locally.

The presence of an enterohepatic cycle dependent on intestinal absorption, hepatic uptake, and biliary excretion may be exploited in the design of therapeutic regimens. Poisoning or overdoses with drugs that have an extensive enterohepatic circulation, such as theophylline, may be successfully treated with oral activated charcoal even after the initial dose has been completely absorbed (Park et al. 1986).

The GI tract harbors a rich microbial flora, and some drugs require metabolism by bacteria to attain their full therapeutic activity. The action of sulfasalazine in the treatment of ulcerative colitis depends on the cleavage of its azo bond by bacteria of the colon (Goldman and Peppercorn 1975). Bacteria may lead to the production of toxic metabolites from otherwise safe drugs. If cyclamates represent a carcinogenic hazard (the magnitude of this risk is uncertain in humans), they may do so because of bacterial conversion to a known carcinogen. Bacterial enzymes are further complemented by metabolizing enzymes of the intestinal mucosa that may modify drug pharmacokinetics, as in the case of cyclosporine A (Yee et al. 1995).

Because the alimentary tract is the route of administration of most drugs, there are potentially many drug–drug and drug–food interactions that could influence the absorption and effectiveness of various therapeutic agents (see chapter 5, Nutrition; chapter 24, Adverse Drug Reactions; and chapter 25, Drug Interactions). Examples of these include the adsorption of tetracycline by aluminum, calcium, or magnesium antacids; and the binding and inactivation of digitalis glycosides by the bile acid sequestrant cholestyramine (see chapters 24 and 25). Because food may have a marked effect on the rate of absorption of drugs and vitamins and on their unwanted effects, it is very important to consider the impact of meals on the rate of absorption and effectiveness of orally administered drugs (Pantuck et al. 1975).

The gut is one of the richest endocrine organs of the body, and endogenous control or exogenous manipulation of GI hormones may be critical in control of symptoms.

Finally, it is worth noting that disease and dysfunction of the GI tract may influence the effectiveness of any therapeutic regimen that uses orally administered drugs. For example, patients with AIDS and *Candida*-related esophagitis frequently fail to respond to oral ketoconazole. The bioavailability of ketoconazole is reduced as a result of gastric achlorhydria, commonly seen in patients with AIDS. This effect can be reversed by concurrent administration of dilute hydrochloric acid (Lake-Bakaar et al. 1988). Similarly, it is unsound to extrapolate expected drug effects from one population to another when the rates of coexisting diseases (e.g., parasitic infestations, diarrheal illnesses) are different in the population tested from those in the target population.

**PRINCIPLE The effects of disease of one organ on the diagnosis and treatment of disease in another organ should make the "specialist" aware that focus on the disorders of a single organ system cannot be allowed to result in underappreciation of the complex relationships between organ systems.**

A general principle, shared with other organ systems, is that an understanding of the pathophysiology of a symptom or symptom complex in an individual patient usually will result in more selective and more effective therapy. For example, diarrhea as a symptom of enteric infection is more effectively and more definitively treated by specific therapy directed at the enteric pathogen than by nonspecific antidiarrheal agents. Sometimes therapy must be empirically directed at symptoms without a full understanding of their genesis; usually this practice is reserved for temporary control of symptoms during diagnostic evaluation or for those instances in which diagnostic analysis has failed to yield a full understanding of the cause of symptoms.

**PRINCIPLE Continued use of drugs to control symptoms, without a comprehensive effort to understand the disease process that underlies these symptoms, is incomplete and dangerous medicine, delaying correct diagnosis and specific therapy.**

Some GI symptoms may be controlled or eliminated by withdrawal of an offending agent. Many drugs produce GI symptoms; when such drugs are withdrawn or decreased in dose, symptoms usually abate or disappear. Orally administered drugs often exert a direct toxic effect on the GI mucosa. Salicylates are believed to interfere with the integrity of the gastric epithelial membrane, allowing back diffusion of hydrogen ions. Neomycin causes malabsorption partly because of its direct toxicity on the small intestinal epithelium.

Drug dependency is not as frequent in patients with GI disease as it is in patients with disease of other organ systems. However, the individual who abuses laxatives may so interrupt normal reflex function as to become functionally dependent on laxatives. Once again, the withdrawal of laxatives and appropriate changes in diet, with reeducation of and dependence on GI reflex function, will result in a successful return to normal physiology.

**PRINCIPLE In most societies, addiction is not considered important unless the drug predominantly affects the central nervous system (CNS). Such an attitude is unrealistic. Furthermore, education of the patient during withdrawal may be the critical determinant of success of such withdrawal.**

Patients commonly attribute GI symptoms to specific foods. Although many of these cause-and-effect relationships fade under controlled scrutiny (Koch and Donaldson 1964), others, such as diarrhea and distension after ingestion of milk by individuals with deficiency of intestinal lactase, have a firm basis in the pathophysiology of the GI system. In such patients the undigested lactose is fermented by colonic bacteria, with generation of hydrogen gas and organic acids. Much more rarely, however, foods are the cause of intestinal disease rather than of intestinal symptoms; in these instances, there usually is a genetic predisposition (see chapter 22, Pharmacogenetics). An example is celiac sprue, in which the injury to the intestinal mucosa is caused by a genetically determined sensitivity to dietary gluten (wheat protein). Both the mucosal injury and the malabsorption syndrome are reversed by fastidious withdrawal of gluten from the diet. Far less common than celiac disease, but greatly overdiagnosed, is the problem of food allergy. Milk-protein allergy is the best studied and most clearly documented (Host 1997). Withdrawal of the offending protein, such as cow's milk, may result in dramatic improvement in diarrhea or extraintestinal signs, and reversal of the morphologic abnormality of the intestinal mucosa (Gryboski 1985).

When GI disease impairs digestive or absorptive function, resulting nutritional deficiencies are managed by replacement of missing factors or supplemental administration of deficient nutrients, or both (see chapter 5, Nutrition). Intuitively one might think that loss by disease or surgical resection of the acid- and pepsin-producing cells of the stomach might adversely affect digestion and could, therefore, call for replacement therapy. In practice, the peptic activity of the stomach is unnecessary for the individual eating a diet of cooked proteins. Such is not the case with disease or resection of the exocrine pancreas. Although the reserve is very great (90% of the pancreas must be destroyed before maldigestion occurs), such dysfunction can have very serious effects on intestinal digestion and nutrition. Under these circumstances, oral administration of pancreatic enzymes may improve the digestion and absorption of food (Graham 1977).

Replacement therapy may also be required for restoration of nutrients lost because of malabsorption associated with GI disease. The patient with pernicious anemia, who lacks gastric intrinsic factor, requires vitamin $B_{12}$ by injection. The patient with steatorrhea due to pancreatic or intestinal disease may well require supplemental replacement of vitamins by oral or parenteral routes (see chapter 5, Nutrition).

Gastrointestinal therapeutics may require interruption of normal or abnormal physiological processes. Often a process that is qualitatively normal but quantitatively excessive can result in GI disease. Thus, peptic ulcer of the duodenum is associated with normal or excessive gastric acid secretion and may be treated by pharmacological inhibition or neutralization of acid secretion.

**PRINCIPLE Understanding the pathogenesis of a disease and the pharmacology of a drug clearly allows the imaginative and effective design of new uses for old drugs. For most informed physicians, the main challenge in therapy is in construction of a new and logical hypothesis, in testing it with sound design, and in drawing valid conclusions related to the cause-and-effect relationship of drug–patient response.**

Therapy is often directed at decreasing the functional stimulus to actively inflamed or diseased organs. An example of this principle is the effort to decrease the secretory responses of the pancreas in the presence of acute pancreatitis. By decreasing the flow of acid and food into the duodenum, one may decrease neural and hormonal stimuli to pancreatic secretion. In severe pancreatitis, this may require nasogastric suction; under milder conditions, small-volume feedings might minimize the pancreatic and gastric secretory response. Similarly, the inflamed small intestine or colon in Crohn's disease or ulcerative colitis is "put at rest" to diminish diarrhea, abdominal pain, and cramping by decreasing dietary intake or, more drastically, by changing to an elemental diet resulting in a decreased residue and decreased stimulus to bowel function (see chapter 5, Nutrition). In the most symptomatic individuals, bowel rest is not achieved without placing the patient on a nothing-by-mouth regimen and substituting intravenous (IV) administration of fluids and medications. Total parenteral nutrition is used to prevent the worsening catabolic state associated with inadequate intake of calories and nitrogen when standard IV therapy is prolonged (see chapter 5, Nutrition).

In the absence of defined etiology or specific therapy, empirical therapy of proven utility should be used, even if the mechanism of its benefit is not understood. This empirical approach to therapy is of particular importance in inflammatory diseases such as regional enteritis and ulcerative colitis; controlled clinical trials have shown the benefit of anti-inflammatory drugs such as corticosteroids and sulfasalazine, although the pathophysiological basis of this therapeutic benefit is not completely known.

**PRINCIPLE When a drug whose pharmacology is reasonably well understood is empirically found to have efficacy in a disease whose pathogenesis is poorly understood, the finding of efficacy ultimately may shed light on the mechanism of disease.**

## DRUG-INDUCED GI DISORDERS

The GI tract is at risk of damage by direct contact with orally administered drugs as well as by their systemic effects. Drug-related erosive gastritis, ulcers, and diarrhea are common adverse effects of medications. The consequences can lead to serious complications or death. Because the offending agents are readily available and frequently used, it is important to discuss these adverse effects in detail.

### Erosive Gastritis and Ulcers

Many medications cause erosions and ulcerations of the GI tract (e.g., alcohol, potassium chloride, corticosteroids, aspirin). Aspirin and NSAIDs are used by millions of people on a daily basis for long periods of time; they can cause both acute and chronic injury to the mucosa of the

GI tract. These drugs bind to the active site of cyclooxygenase (COX) and prevent the conversion of arachidonate to prostaglandin H (Miyamoto et al. 1976). There are two forms of COX: COX-1 appears responsible for normal cellular functions in all cells, and COX-2 is expressed by cells only as a result of inflammation or injury (Meade et al. 1993). NSAIDs with COX-2 selectivity should preserve normal housekeeping functions of cells, and these drugs may lead to less inherent gastrointestinal toxicity. However, currently available NSAIDs are not selective; the availability of COX-2-selective NSAIDs may likely change the toxicity profile of these drugs, although not all of the toxicity due to NSAIDs is related to a prostaglandin-dependent mechanism.

Endoscopic studies of acute drug injury, best characterized for aspirin, typically show the development of submucosal hemorrhage or active bleeding within 2 hours of ingestion of the drug. Acute drug-induced injury to the gastroduodenum can be diminished by enteric coating of the drug or by measures that decrease stomach content of acid (Lanza et al. 1980). Approximately 25–50% of patients who use NSAIDs on a regular basis will complain of dyspepsia; however, only rarely are GI symptoms severe enough to result in the inability to continue using the medications. Endoscopic studies have shown erosive gastritis in about 40–50% and ulcers of the stomach or duodenum in about 10–25% of chronic NSAID users. Unfortunately, the presence or absence of symptoms does not necessarily predict the findings at endoscopy (Graham and Smith 1988). In addition, the drugs that cause the greatest degree of acute hemorrhagic gastritis are not the ones that necessarily lead to a higher rate of ulceration during chronic use. As a consequence, endoscopic measurements of acute drug injury do not accurately predict the differences in rates of ulcer formation from chronic use of different NSAIDs (Carson, Strom, Soper, et al. 1987). Studies have demonstrated that the risk for a complicated gastrointestinal disease requiring hospitalization in NSAID users is two to five times that for nonusers (Carson, Strom, Morse, et al. 1987; Gabriel et al. 1991). This risk is constant, dose-related, and occurs without significant warning in patients with no prior history of gastrointestinal disease. This results in more than 100,000 hospitalizations and 16,000 deaths annually (Singh et al. 1996).

The impact of *Helicobacter pylori* infection on the incidence of peptic ulcers in patients on NSAIDs is yet to be determined. Both NSAIDs and *H. pylori* are known causes of peptic ulcer disease (Kurata and Nogawa 1997). A reduction in the incidence of peptic ulcers following *H. pylori* eradication in patients taking NSAIDs suggests that some ulcers in NSAID users may be related to *H. pylori* infection (Chan et al. 1997). The results of this study support the notion that patients taking NSAIDs should be screened for *H. pylori* infection and treated with anti-*Helicobacter* therapy before NSAID therapy is initiated.

**PRINCIPLE Many symptoms that appear to be adverse effects of drugs could be caused by disease. A major therapeutic error would be to attribute all adverse events to a drug that could cause them when the relative risks of such cause and effect are low and when the drug is vitally important to the patient's well being.**

Prophylactic therapy with misoprostol, a synthetic prostaglandin E analog with antisecretory and cytoprotective properties, decreased the incidence of gastric ulcers in patients with osteoarthritis who were taking NSAIDs continually and had abdominal pain (Silverstein et al. 1986; Dajani 1987). Ulcers were visualized in 21.7% of placebo recipients, and in 4.2% and 0.7% of misoprostol-treated patients (100 or 200 $\mu$g four times daily, respectively) in three upper endoscopies over a 3-month period of surveillance. The effect on abdominal pain was not as clear-cut because 30% of misoprostil-treated patients and 43% of placebo recipients still had abdominal pain during follow-up, despite healing of the ulcer. Diarrhea occurred in 39% of patients receiving the higher dose of misoprostol but in only 13% of placebo-treated patients (Graham et al. 1988). If the serious GI complications of long-term use of NSAIDs are attributable only to their propensity to cause ulcers, then misoprostil should be widely used. However, the toxicity of long-term use of misoprostil and its ability to prevent ulcers over a long period of therapy with NSAIDs are yet to be determined (Herting and Nissen 1986).

**PRINCIPLE Surrogate endpoints must be evaluated as carefully as any other drug effect. However, the physician must be careful to distinguish one type of endpoint from another when reading studies or treating patients.**

## Diarrhea

Diarrhea can be defined as an abnormal increase in stool frequency, weight, or liquidity. The former two are relatively straightforward to measure; the wet weight of stools is cumbersome to quantify but likely to be the factor that most easily correlates with the patient's complaint. The average person eating three meals each day is likely to have 9000 mL of fluid traversing the duodenum, 1000 mL traversing the ileocecal valve, and 100 mL exiting as stool. Because the fluid balance of the gut must be exceedingly well controlled in order to have a normal water content in stools, minor changes in absorptive capacity of the bowel can likely play a major role in determining stool water content despite the ability of the bowel to adjust to changes in the delivery of abnormal quantities of fluid (Fine et al. 1989).

Diarrhea has many diverse causes but can be classified mechanistically into malabsorptive, maldigestive, or secretory processes; inflammatory states; and deranged intestinal motility (Fordtran 1967). The differential diagnosis of diarrhea is lengthy and has been previously reviewed (Fine et al. 1989). As with other GI symptoms, it is important to judge its severity and prognosis so that the need for treatment can be established, and to identify and specifically treat the underlying condition if possible and necessary.

Drug-induced diarrhea may be caused by any of the mechanisms mentioned above. Most commonly, diarrhea is caused by the use of laxatives or stool softeners. These may be poorly absorbed sugars such as lactulose and sorbitol that are fermented by intestinal bacteria in the colon or poorly absorbed salts of magnesium (sulfate, oxide, or hydroxide) or sodium (sulfate or citrate) ions. The diarrhea that ensues is characterized by a stool osmolality higher than that of plasma. Other commonly used laxatives (ricinoleic acid, phenolphthalein, dioctyl sodium sulfosuccinate, and senna) cause diarrhea characterized by its continuance even during fasting and a stool osmolality gap of less than 50 mOsm/kg (Binder 1977).

The most common nosocomial diarrhea, and the most serious drug-induced diarrhea, is pseudomembranous colitis due to *Clostridium difficile,* a condition facilitated by antibiotic therapy. Most patients with antibiotic-related diarrhea have a benign illness that begins during administration of the drug and lasts less than 1 week following discontinuation of the offending agent. A small percentage of patients will develop severe diarrhea with evidence of invasive colitis (fever, tenesmus, mucus, or bloody stools) that persists after the antibiotic is discontinued. Patients in this group are usually elderly and in the hospital or a skilled nursing facility. The antibiotics most frequently implicated are ampicillin or amoxicillin, clindamycin, and cephalosporins (Bartlett 1981). In patients with pseudomembranous colitis, laboratory studies generally reveal hypoalbuminemia and fecal leukocytes, flexible sigmoidoscopy generally demonstrates the characteristic 3- to 20-mm pseudomembranes bordered by normal or hyperemic colonic mucosa, and analysis generally reveals the presence of *C. difficile* toxin in the stool.

Therapy consists of discontinuing the implicated antibiotic, maintaining an adequate state of hydration and nutrition, and instituting enteric isolation procedures to limit person-to-person spread. Specific antibiotic therapy directed against *C. difficile* should be given to patients with signs and symptoms of moderate to severe colitis, or to those who fail to improve following nonspecific measures and discontinuation of antibiotics. Oral vancomycin and metronidazole appear to be equally efficacious; bacitracin may have equal activity, although it has not been as extensively studied. Parenteral metronidazole should be administered only to patients who cannot take oral medications. Therapy is generally accompanied by rapid defervescence and loss of diarrhea within 7 days; toxin generally is still present in the stool at the end of successful therapy. Relapses occur in 20–25% of patients treated with any of the three antibiotics and are heralded by recurrent symptoms within 7 days of the end of therapy. Relapses may be treated with another course of antibiotics if the seriousness of the colitis warrants specific treatment (Fekety 1997). Prevention of *C. difficile* colitis can be attempted by limiting the use of unnecessary broad-spectrum antibiotics and tailoring antibiotic therapy to culture results with drugs that have a narrow spectrum.

An alternative treatment for antibiotic-related pseudomembranous colitis involves administration of cholestyramine, which binds the toxin, leading to symptomatic improvement. However, this approach is not as efficacious as specific antibiotic therapy, should not be used in seriously ill patients, and may also bind oral vancomycin, rendering it inactive (Taylor and Bartlett 1980).

**PRINCIPLE Understanding the details of the pharmacology of a drug and the pathogenesis of a disease occasionally leads to otherwise nonobvious use of the drug in the disease with gratifying rewards for having considered the hypothesis.**

## TREATMENT OF GI DISORDERS

### Nausea and Vomiting

Vomiting is a complex clinical behavior that results in the evacuation of stomach contents and involves coordinated activity of the GI tract and the nervous system. It is frequently preceded by nausea (an unpleasant sensation that has been felt by most people but is difficult to describe) and retching, or contractions of the diaphragm and chest wall against a closed glottis.

The neurophysiology of vomiting has been studied in detail in cats since the 1950s (Borison and Wang 1953). Findings in studies of cats have generally been very relevant to humans. In brief, a vomiting center (VC), which is located in the dorsal portion of the lateral reticular formation of the medulla, does not itself carry out the act of vomiting but coordinates the many organs involved in the intricate act of vomiting. The VC can be stimulated by a chemoreceptor trigger zone (CTZ) located in the area postrema of the medulla on the floor of the fourth ventricle. The CTZ, in turn, is sensitive to chemical stimulation, including direct application of drugs such as apomorphine or toxins such as uremic plasma. Dopamine receptors in the CTZ likely play a role in the act of vomiting; dopamine agonists such as apomorphine or levodopa initiate vomiting, and dopamine antagonists such as metoclopramide or domperidone diminish vomiting (Jenner and Marsden 1979). The VC can also be stimulated by afferent nerve stimuli originating in the gut, the pharynx, the vestibular system, and probably other sites in the body; these stimuli travel via vagal fibers stimulated by mechanoreceptors (sensitive to distension or abnormal gut motility) or chemoreceptors (enterochromaffin cells). Serotonin, acting on 5-$HT_3$ and to a lesser extent 5-$HT_4$ receptors, mediate the vomiting induced by chemotherapeutic drugs but not that caused by pregnancy or motion sickness (Stott et al. 1989). The latter appears to be modulated by drugs that affect the histamine $H_1$ receptor and the muscarinic cholinergic receptor. Vomiting induced by stimulation of abdominal visceral afferent nerves by ingested toxins or CTZ stimulation by apomorphine is blocked by selective 5-$HT_3$ receptor antagonists (Andrews et al. 1990). Higher CNS influences may also affect the VC.

The vomiting act is preceded by a prodrome consisting of nausea, cold sweats, pupillary dilatation, tachycardia, and salivation. Vagal efferent nerve fibers relax the proximal stomach, contract the esophagus longitudinally and pull the proximal stomach into the thorax, evacuate the upper small intestine into the stomach via a retrograde giant contraction, and empty the lower intestine into the colon (Lang et al. 1993). The vomiting of gastric contents is caused by the compression of the stomach through a strong simultaneous contraction of the diaphragm and abdominal muscles.

Numerous conditions can cause nausea and vomiting, and most can be explained from these neurophysiological relationships. Structural abnormalities of the GI tract may lead to nausea and vomiting by either of two general mechanisms: mechanical obstruction of a hollow viscus (such as congenital pyloric stenosis, achalasia, or Crohn's disease of the small intestine) or by a nonobstructing lesion affecting any or all components of the wall of GI organs (such as an antral peptic ulcer, erosive gastritis, acute cholecystitis). Systemic conditions may have local or distant effects on the gut or on any neuromuscular component of the vomiting reflex; examples are drugs, diabetes mellitus (either through ketoacidosis or local effects on the innervation of the stomach leading to gastroparesis), uremia, pregnancy, adrenal insufficiency, or infiltration by mass lesions (tumors, amyloid) in critical areas of the nervous system or the intrinsic musculature of the stomach wall. Finally, psychiatric illness may manifest itself as predominantly a vomiting disorder, most vividly seen in bulemia. These conditions and others that can lead to nausea and vomiting have been discussed in detail (Malagelada and Camilleri 1984; Hanson and McCallum 1985).

The therapy of nausea and vomiting must first be directed at identifying the underlying condition that has precipitated the problem. Healing a pyloric channel ulcer with antisecretory therapy or the surgical removal of an acutely inflamed, calculous gallbladder is the appropriate therapy to manage the vomiting that frequently accompanies these disorders. However, there are many conditions accompanied by vomiting that have no specific treatment (e.g., viral gastroenteritis or hepatitis) or have vomiting as a predictable effect of therapy (e.g., cisplatin chemotherapy, total nodal radiation). In these cases, the vomiting must be managed without being able to address its cause directly.

Drugs for nausea and vomiting have typically been tested in patients given highly emetogenic chemotherapy. Lessons from these experiments may not apply to nausea and vomiting caused by vestibular disorders or other CNS causes. Management of vomiting in situations for which therapy is indicated must take into account the neurophysiological correlates of vomiting as well as learned responses resulting from prior associations. This has been best studied in situations for which vomiting is predictable and severe, such as that caused by the IV infusion of high doses of cisplatin during the therapy of various solid tumors. Even if there has been no prior experience with emetogenic chemotherapy, one must expect the patient to develop purely anticipatory nausea and vomiting. Such nausea and vomiting can be triggered by sights, odors, or any other memory associated with prior episodes of vomiting. These symptoms have been successfully treated with behavioral modification techniques or anxiolytic–amnesic agents such as lorazepam, or both (Laszlo et al. 1985).

Gastric distension can be avoided by beginning therapy following an overnight fast or, if there is an impediment to emptying the stomach, by evacuating its contents using a nasogastric tube. Maintaining adequate hydration is an important goal during potentially dehydrating therapy, and a large-bore IV line with adequate fluid replacement must be used. Prevention of nausea and vomiting, rather than rescue therapy, should be the goal of treatment (see chapter 23, Pharmacokinetics and Pharmacodynamics).

Drug therapy of vomiting is aimed at the interruption of the vomiting reflex at any and all levels. Phenothiazines such as prochlorperazine were first used for this purpose in the 1950s, and since that time, agents with similar, substantial antidopaminergic effects have been used. These include the butyrophenones such as droperidol and substituted benzamides such as metoclopramide (Wampler 1983) (see chapter 8, Psychiatric Disorders). Corticosteroids such as dexamethasone or methylprednisolone have been found to be useful, although the nature of their antiemetic action is unclear (Markman et al. 1984). Similarly, natural or synthetic cannabinoids have been used in antiemetic therapy following the empirical observation of an antiemetic effect in habitual users who were undergoing chemotherapy. However, their mechanism of action is unknown, and their efficacy has not yet been adequately demonstrated in well designed studies (Carey et al. 1983). Ondansetron, a selective inhibitor of 5-$HT_3$ receptors, was observed to prevent the vomiting induced by cisplatin in laboratory animals and patients (Cubeddu et al. 1990; Marty et al. 1990). Studies also suggested that cisplatin treatment increased the release of serotonin from enterochromaffin cells, as measured by urinary excretion of 5-hydroxyindolacetic acid and plasma chromogranin A levels (Cubeddu et al. 1990, 1995), thus providing a possible mechanism for cisplatin-induced emesis and the beneficial effect of the drug. In addition, 5-$HT_3$ receptors are concentrated in the area postrema—the location of the CTZ and the entry site for most vagal afferents (Tyers and Freeman 1992). Thus, there is evidence for both a peripheral and central action of serotonin in the pathophysiology of vomiting.

Because single agents lack universal effectiveness in the prevention of vomiting, regimens using combinations of drugs are sensible and useful. The goal of combining drugs for this indication is the same as for any indication for which combinations are used. The combination should result in a nausea-free patient and should minimize or abolish the potential adverse effects of the high doses of agents that would be necessary if they were used alone. One should choose combination therapy using agents whose efficacy is proved, whose modes of action are different, and whose potential toxicities are nonoverlapping.

**PRINCIPLE Drug combinations can be useful when single agents fail to provide the desired efficacy or freedom from toxicity. Knowledge of the mode of action, pharmacology, and toxicity of drugs as single agents is useful in the rational planning of combination therapy. Drugs may have additive or even unique toxicities when used together, and the therapist must be alert to make observations that may not be predicted by studies on single agents.**

The information learned from drug studies of patients receiving highly emetogenic drugs is applicable to other clinical situations and should be used to plan therapy of patients who vomit for other reasons. For example, the routine care of patients with severe vomiting from an exacerbation of chronic pancreatitis should include nasogastric suction to empty the stomach, fluid and caloric support by the parenteral route, and prevention or treatment of nausea and vomiting as necessary to maintain patient comfort. This does not exclude therapy that may be specific to the underlying disease, such as surgery to drain pseudocysts or endoscopic sphincterotomy to remove a common bile duct stone. Therapy that is specific to the underlying disease should always be a part of the patient's management.

## Peptic Ulcer Disease

Peptic ulcer disease is a heterogeneous group of illnesses whose hallmark is a mucosal defect in the stomach or duodenum that extends through the muscularis mucosa. It is a common disorder, with lifetime prevalences approaching 10% and point prevalences of 1–2% in American males (Grossman 1980). Peptic ulcers are caused by ulcerogenic factors (acid and pepsin), the breakdown of normal mucosal defenses usually by NSAID use, or infection with *H. pylori* (Graham 1989). Because acute mucosal breaks, such as those caused by endoscopic biopsies, heal rapidly in patients despite constant bathing by acid and pepsin, the interplay of aggressive and protective factors cannot be understated. Even in patients with gastrinomas, whose mucosal surfaces are constantly bathed with large amounts of pepsin and acid, peptic ulceration is an intermittent, albeit severe, condition with spontaneous exacerbations and remissions and multiple recurrences over the lifetime of affected individuals. Because there are now effective and safe methods to heal an acute peptic ulcer, the most important problem facing the therapist is not how to heal an ulcer, but how to prevent its recurrence and its complications.

Because 80 to 95% of patients with gastric or duodenal ulcers are infected with *H. pylori* (Peterson 1991), and because duodenal ulcers develop far more frequently in patients infected with *H. pylori* than in uninfected persons (Sipponen et al. 1989), the role of *H. pylori* in the pathogenesis of peptic ulcers has been established. However, only 15 to 20% of *H. pylori*-infected patients are estimated to develop a peptic ulcer during their lifetime, so factors other than *H. pylori* infection must be important. Factors that are important in maintaining an intact mucosal barrier include the production of mucus and bicarbonate by surface epithelial cells with maintenance of a surface barrier to injury, and the ability to maintain adequate mucosal blood flow during and after a break in the surface defense mechanisms. Studies of rabbits administered antibodies against prostaglandins, and of NSAID-induced gastric erosions and ulcerations, suggest that endogenous prostaglandins may play a critical role in protecting the integrity of the surface epithelium, although the ability of exogenous prostaglandins to reproduce these beneficial effects is at best partial. Endogenous sulfhydryl compounds, through their capacity to be free-radical scavengers, and epidermal growth factor may also contribute to mucosal resistance to injury (Soll 1990).

Traditional therapy against peptic ulceration has been directed against the acid- or ulcer-promoting factors. Therapies include the buffering of stomach acid with antacids and use of agents that block parietal cell acid secretion. Antacids were the first drugs to be used in promoting the healing of peptic ulcers. With time, the development of insoluble and nonabsorbable antacids such as aluminum hydroxide and magnesium trilisate allowed therapy without the systemic absorption of alkali seen with sodium bicarbonate and milk that had led to systemic alkalosis, hypercalcemia, and renal insufficiency (Weberg et al. 1988). Their relative ease of administration and low cost made them very popular among patients with ulcers, but their high incidence of adverse effects (diarrhea, binding of coadministered drugs) and cumbersome regimens with up to seven daily doses made the search for alternate modes of therapy necessary (Lam 1988).

Basic physiological observations of the nature of the stimuli that cause parietal cells to secrete acid led to therapies with anticholinergic agents and histamine $H_2$ receptor antagonists. Therapy with anticholinergic agents such as probanthine and atropine was attempted but essentially abandoned when it became clear that doses necessary to achieve enough acid reduction to heal ulcers also led to predictable adverse effects such as dry mouth, blurred vision, and urinary retention. Pirenzepine, a relatively $M_1$-selective antimuscarinic agent, may lead to enough reduction of acid secretion to promote ulcer healing without the high incidence of anticholinergic effects from inhibition of myocardial and smooth muscle function and salivary secretion (Feldman 1984; Carmine and Brogden 1985).

Histamine $H_2$ receptor antagonists were developed specifically for the treatment of duodenal ulcer disease. All are competitive inhibitors of the action of histamine at $H_2$ receptors; their structure is based on modifications of a molecule with the histamine imidazole ring structure (cimetidine), furan ring (ranitidine), and thiazole ring (famotidine and nizatidine). $H_2$ receptor antagonists became the drugs of choice in the healing of peptic ulcers because they are safe and are easy to administer once or twice daily in regimens that result in healing of 80 to 90% of peptic ulcers after 4 to 8 weeks of therapy. Drug-related adverse effects have been unusual. Antiandrogenic effects leading to gynecomastia and drug interactions secondary to cytochrome P450 enzyme inhibition have been attributed to cimetidine but not the others; presumably these are related to the imidazole ring structure and not to its $H_2$ receptor antagonism (McCarthy 1983; Powell and Donn 1983). Because lymphocytes and cardiac muscle have $H_2$ receptors, immune modulation and bradycardia seen with $H_2$ receptor blocking agents ("$H_2$ blockers") is likely to be a generic adverse effect of this class of drugs, or perhaps in the future an alternate indication for using $H_2$ blockers (Siegel et al. 1982).

Prostaglandins such as misoprostil can lead to suppression of acid secretion and can lead to rates of ulcer healing comparable to those produced with the $H_2$ blockers. However, the need to administer these drugs two to four times daily and their diarrheogenic and uterotonic effects make them unlikely first-line drugs for the therapy of peptic ulcer disease (Sontag 1986).

Omeprazole, a substituted benzimidazole that inhibits $(H^+ + K^+)$-ATPase, the proton pump of the parietal cell, can lead to sustained achlorhydria in humans by abolishing gastric acid secretion (McArthur et al. 1986). The result is an accelerated rate of ulcer healing in patients with peptic ulcer disease or severe erosive or ulcerative esophagitis (Archambult et al. 1988). Although this agent appears to offer distinct advantages over other antisecretory drugs because of its efficacy, the sustained achlorhydria it induces may have as-yet-undetected adverse effects. Laboratory animals that are treated with relatively large doses of this agent have developed chronic elevations in serum gastrin concentrations and enterochromaffin cell hyperplasia, which is sometimes accompanied by malignant carcinoid tumors (Havu 1986). However, these concerns have not been borne out in observations in patients following decades of proton pump inhibitor use (Maton et al. 1989; McCloy et al.1995).

Attempts to heal ulcers by methods that do not reduce gastric acid is a desirable goal in the rare patient intolerant to acid-reduction therapy or as adjunctive therapy. Cessation of smoking and ingestion of alcohol or NSAIDs is important. The capacity of prostaglandins to induce healing is not as great as that of antisecretory therapy (Brand et al. 1985). Prostaglandins appear to be useful in the prevention of NSAID-induced gastric ulcers; however, their superiority to antisecretory drugs in achieving this goal has not yet been tested.

Sucralfate (a sulfated disaccharide complex with aluminum hydroxide) acts by mechanisms other than the reduction of gastric acid production to promote ulcer healing. Sucralfate binds to the ulcer base, forms complexes with pepsin, and stimulates local production of bicarbonate and mucus. One or more of these mechanisms may be responsible for its mode of action. It is as effective as $H_2$ blockers in the promotion of ulcer healing and maintains the gastric acid barrier to microorganisms during the healing process (Marks 1987). This may be important in hospitalized patients who are at risk for extensive colonization of the stomach with bacteria, because such colonization may predispose patients to develop aspiration pneumonia. Adverse effects include constipation and nausea. The absorption of sucralfate from the GI tract has not been well studied; 0.5 to 2.2% of $^{14}$C-labeled sucrose sulfate administered as sucralfate is excreted unchanged in the urine by normal subjects (Giesing et al. 1982). If a significant amount of aluminum is absorbed and deposited in tissues, resulting in chronic aluminum toxicity and the potential for encephalopathy, then the usefulness of sucralfate may be limited to short-term therapy. To date, however, no cases of aluminum toxicity have been assessed in patients only on sucralfate therapy.

The initial approach to the treatment of a gastric or duodenal ulcer involves testing for *H. pylori* infection. Eradication of *H. pylori* infections prevents ulcer recurrence; the 12-month rate of recurrence falls from 90–100% to 0–15% (Graham et al. 1992; Van der Hulst et al. 1997). Diagnosis of *H. pylori* can be performed with excellent accuracy by gastric mucosal biopsy, serological tests, or urease breath tests (Thijs et al. 1996). *H. pylori* is difficult to eradicate and requires either the coadministration of a proton pump inhibitor or $H_2$ blocker, a bismuth preparation, and two antimicrobial agents, or the combined use of three antimicrobial agents. A standard 2-week regimen of 400 mg metronidazole three times daily, 500 mg amoxicillin three times daily, and 40 mg omeprazole daily would be expected to eradicate *H. pylori* in more than 90% of patients (Bell et al. 1995). An NIH Consensus Development Conference recommended that all patients who have documented duodenal or gastric ulcers and who are infected with *H. pylori* receive antimicrobial therapy to eradicate the infection (NIH Consensus Development Panel 1994). Confirmation of eradication is possible either by a repeat endoscopic biopsy or by urease breath test. When eradication has been documented, subsequent reinfection has been unusual, particularly in highly industrialized nations (Borody et al. 1989).

Treatment of peptic ulcers not associated with *H. pylori* infection must be guided by host factors, the location of the ulcer, and whether complications (e.g., perforation, penetration, gastric outlet obstruction, bleeding, intractable pain) have occurred. Several simple, safe, and effective regimens are available to the therapist. Uncomplicated duodenal ulcers can heal with agents that effectively decrease nocturnal acid production without affecting daytime acid production; increasing the degree of acid suppression accelerates the healing process (Jones et al. 1987). A typical regimen of 800 mg cimetidine once nightly has been shown to heal duodenal ulcers in 80% of patients after 4 weeks of treatment and in 95% of patients after 8 weeks. Similar results would be expected with 300 mg ranitidine or 40 mg famotidine nightly, and more rapid healing occurs with more profound acid suppression from using proton pump inhibitors.

The healing of gastric ulcers not associated with *H. pylori* infection by different drugs and regimens correlates best with total duration of treatment but correlates poorly with the ability to suppress acid production over 24 hours (Howden et al. 1988). To achieve the healing rates of 90% or more that are typically seen with 8 weeks of antisecretory therapy in patients with duodenal ulcer, patients with gastric ulcer should be treated for 10 to 12 weeks. This may indicate that the pathogenesis of gastric ulcer may depend less on acid–peptic aggressive factors and more on local mucosal defenses. A typical regimen would be 400 mg cimetidine twice daily or 150 ng ranitidine twice daily. Patients with gastric ulcers should have documentation of complete healing of their ulcer in 10 to 12 weeks by gastroscopy and biopsy to exclude the small chance of a malignant ulcer. If an unhealed gastric ulcer is present, then operative resection should be considered even when biopsies do not reveal malignant tissue because of the possibility of gastric cancer.

Complications of peptic ulcers such as perforation, penetration, GI bleeding, gastric outlet obstruction, and intractable pain have in the past led to operative therapy of peptic ulcer disease. Because of the relatively morbid nature of surgery for peptic ulcer disease and its potential mortality even in otherwise healthy subjects, the advent of new drug therapies for peptic ulcer disease have led to attempts to manage nonemergent complications of ulcers without surgery. Whether this more conservative approach will ultimately benefit patients is yet to be proved.

Patients in whom symptomatic ulcers recur frequently despite the eradication or absence of *H. pylori* infection, or in whom a complication not requiring emergent surgery has occurred, should be considered candidates for prophylactic acid-suppressive therapy with an $H_2$ blocker, at half the usual dose required for healing, or 1 g sucralfate twice daily. This maintenance therapy can be expected to result in ulcer recurrence rates of less than 30% yearly (Bodemar and Walan 1978). The appropriate length of prophylactic therapy is controversial. Elderly patients with serious coexisting illnesses should probably receive lifelong prophylactic therapy because the potential for ulcer-related morbidity and mortality is greater in this group (Piper et al. 1975). Whether young patients without comorbid illnesses benefit from maintenance therapy is also unclear. A model proposed to evaluate the outcome of patients treated with intermittent versus maintenance therapy predicted that the point prevalence of ulcers at any time would be 16.5% in the intermittently treated group and 3% in the maintenance-therapy group and thus may result in patients intermittently treated being at greater risk for complications (Pounder 1981). Failure of prophylactic therapy should signal the need for more aggressive acid-reduction therapy and possibly surgery.

## Reflux Esophagitis

Failure of the gastroesophageal junction to provide a barrier to gastric and duodenal contents can result in reflux esophagitis. Although heartburn is an extremely common complaint, and is both recurrent and generally not progressive, up to 20% of patients referred to a specialist with symptomatic reflux esophagitis may develop complications such as esophageal stricture or Barrett's esophagus, a premalignant condition. Although antacids and lifestyle changes (low-fat diet, elevation of the head of the bed, no recumbent position after meals, no smoking) can improve the symptoms of patients with reflux esophagitis, nificant minority of patients have chronic and disabling symptoms that require more aggressive management.

The success of therapy for reflux esophagitis, whether measured by symptomatic relief or by improvement in endoscopic and histological evidence of inflammation of the esophagus, is directly related to two factors: the degree of acid suppression and the improvement in emptying of esophageal contents. Therapy with proton pump inhibitors, either used singly or in combination with prokinetic agents such as cisapride, is superior to therapy with $H_2$ blockers in both healing reflux esophagitis and in preventing recurrence (Vigneri et al. 1995). However, therapy is not curative because the underlying motor disorder that results in an incompetent gastroesophageal barrier is not fixed by treatment. Also, not all patients respond to therapy: reflux of alkaline stomach contents or bile salts may perpetuate the esophageal injury, and eradication of *H. pylori* infection may heal the gastric mucosa and increase stomach acid production. This results in a minority of patients requiring a surgical antireflux procedure because of complications (stricture, nonhealing ulcers, bleeding), or persistent symptoms, particularly in young patients (Spechler 1992).

## Constipation

Constipation is generally perceived by people as an inability to have stools frequently; some complain of a sensation of incomplete evacuation of their rectum, or stools that are too firm, or too difficult to pass. Associated symptoms may include flatulence, bloating, or abdominal pain. These are common problems for which patients spend hundreds of millions of dollars for drugs in the United States every year. Most drugs are used to increase the frequency and water content of the stool. The frequency of bowel movements depends greatly on the diet, the use of drugs that may change (particularly decrease) GI motility or the water content of stools, the level of physical activity, and water intake. One study found that 99% of healthy adults in Britain have stools more than twice a week and no more than three times daily (Connell et al. 1965). However, people commonly perceive the absence of a daily bowel movement as a sign of illness because of concerns about "the accumulation of toxins." Constipation may affect up to 20% of the population at any given time, and more than 60% of elderly outpatients use a laxative (Talley et al. 1993).

The physician who cares for a patient complaining of chronic constipation must first address whether the patient truly has a problem. If complaints suggest an underlying organic illness of the digestive tract (a sudden decrease in stool frequency or caliber, the presence of blood in the stool, or associated systemic complaints), then evaluation aimed at ruling out serious organic disease must be undertaken. Colonoscopy or a barium enema may be considered. If the patient complains of an inability to initiate a bowel movement, or if he or she has a sense of incomplete evacuation of the rectum, then anorectal manometry and defecography may be useful diagnostic tests (Mahieu et al. 1984). If the patient complains of infrequent bowel movements, then measurement of colonic transit time using radioopaque markers and anorectal manometry may be useful in determining the presence and segmental location causing the delayed transit (Wald 1986).

The majority of patients who have chronic constipation do not have serious organic disease. Reeducation regarding "normal stool habits" and the benefits from increasing their physical activity and amount of fiber in their diet may suffice (Badiali et al. 1995). Patients should be encouraged to respond promptly to their urge to defecate. If necessary, a postprandial routine following breakfast or dinner should be established, to take advantage of the gastrocolic reflex. A careful search of the history of medications for those that may cause constipation should be performed. Nonessential drugs should be discontinued, and essential medications that can possibly alter GI mobility should be changed, if possible. The use of laxatives other than increased fiber intake to treat patients with chronic constipation is generally reserved for those who fail to respond to simple nonpharmacological measures.

Laxatives are generally classified into five categories: bulk-forming, emollients, lubricants, stimulants, and osmotic laxatives (Tedesco and DiPiro 1985). Preparations have been assigned to these categories on the basis of their presumed mechanism of action. For many drugs, the mechanism of action is poorly understood or the current concepts of drug action differ from those presumed at the time the classification was constructed (Binder and Donowitz 1975; Donowitz 1979).

***Bulk-forming agents***

Bulk-forming agents are generally complex plant polysaccharides or cellulose derivatives that swell on contact with water. The most commonly used products contain powdered psyllium seed, methylcellulose, or raw bran. The dose of the product needs to be adjusted so that the patient is ingesting a total of 15 g or more of dietary fiber daily; little else may be required if the patients can increase the daily intake of fiber from foods. Softer, bulkier stools should be achieved within 24 to 48 hours. No systemic absorption of the agent is predicted, but systemic effects of high fiber intake occur. These can include lowering of serum lipid concentrations by agent binding of cholesterol excreted in the bile (Anderson and Gustafson 1988). An adequate amount of water (8 to 16 oz of water per typical 4- to 6-g dose) should be simultaneously ingested; this will prevent the rare but predictable GI obstruction that can follow the use of these agents. If strictures of the GI tract are already present at the time it is started, a bulk-forming agent may precipitate obstruction.

***Emollient laxatives***

Emollient laxatives increase water secretion in the intestine and colon and act as surfactants to improve fecal mixing. Commonly used products include docusate sodium or docusate calcium. All of these preparations are used in doses of 50 to 360 mg/day. Traditionally, these agents have been used in hospitalized patients following myocardial infarction or surgery, when straining at defecation should be avoided but activity and fluid intake may be restricted. They have little role in the management of chronic constipation, except when the patient is fluid-restricted or incapable of increasing his or her dietary fiber or activity.

***Lubricants***

Lubricants are mineral oil products. They coat the bowel and decrease colonic absorption of water, allowing easier passage of stools. Doses of 15 to 30 mL/day result in soft stools within hours. Because of the potential of aspiration pneumonia, the malabsorption of fat-soluble vitamins with chronic use, or the irritation of the perianal area and development of pruritus ani, these agents should not be used when potentially less toxic products are available and have not been tried.

***Stimulant laxatives***

Stimulant laxatives are derivatives of anthraquinones (cascara sagrada, or "holy peel," senna) and dimethylethane (bisacodyl) that are felt to stimulate intestinal motility. More likely they work by increasing fluid secretion in the small intestine and colon. A bowel movement can be expected 6–8 hours after an oral dose or 15 to 60 minutes after the preparation is taken rectally. The drugs may damage the myenteric plexus and have a potential for causing serious acute (severe abdominal cramps, electrolyte and acid-base disorders, erythema multiforme) and chronic (melanosis coli, atonic colon) adverse effects (Smith 1968). These agents are not recommended for chronic use, and even their short-term use can cause toxicity that exceeds that of the osmotic laxatives.

***Osmotic laxatives***

Osmotic laxatives are poorly absorbed by the intestine and colon and result in net water movement into the GI tract along an osmotic gradient. They include lactulose, sorbitol, and ions of magnesium, sulfate, phosphate, and citrate. The onset of action generally is within 30 minutes to 3 hours after oral administration. These drugs have the capability of causing abdominal cramps, electrolyte and acid-base disorders, and volume depletion. Their use is generally limited to clinical settings when prompt evacuation of bowel contents is needed (e.g., following the use of activated charcoal or potassium-binding resins used in poisonings and hyperkalemia, or in preparation for GI endoscopy or surgery). These agents rarely may be required for patients with acute exacerbations of chronic constipation or acute constipation associated with a self-limited process (Koletzko et al. 1989). A balanced salt solution containing polyethylene glycol (Golytely, Colyte) works in a similar manner but causes little net water movement across the intestinal wall.

## Diarrhea

Diarrhea is generally defined as the passing of watery stools or an increased frequency of relatively loose stools. Acute diarrhea is a common condition. It affects adults in developed countries once a year on the average. This illness is not likely to lead to consultation with a health-care worker unless the patient is an infant or small child, or unless the illness is particularly severe. Chronic diarrhea, lasting longer than 3 weeks, is an uncommon condition. It requires a diagnostic workup that can be extensive and often requires a specialist. After illnesses that are managed with specific therapy have been identified and treated, the management of either acute or chronic diarrhea may be similar.

Acute diarrhea is generally regarded as an attempt by the GI tract to get rid of disease-causing microorganisms and toxins. This is believed to be adaptive, and therapy meant merely to decrease the number and volume of stools is generally not recommended. More likely, however, diarrhea provides an efficient way to disseminate and to propagate the organisms that cause it and is an adaptive mechanism of the parasite and not the host.

The mechanisms by which diarrhea occurs fall under four general categories: increased osmolality of intestinal contents, decreased fluid absorption, increased intestinal secretion, and abnormal intestinal motility. Any of these mechanisms may be responsible for diarrhea from any given cause. For example, loss of mature intestinal cells in villus tips due to an acute rotavirus infection is likely to lead to decreased mucosal absorptive surface, decreased fluid absorption, and a self-limited lactose intolerance and osmotic diarrhea with ingestion of milk (Starkey et al. 1986). *Escherichia coli* or *Vibrio cholera* infections cause diarrhea through an enterotoxin that causes net excretion of chloride by the enterocyte (Moss and Vaughan 1989).

The ability of acute diarrhea to cause severe dehydration in children, which often leads to death in areas of the world where poverty and malnutrition are common, makes it an important worldwide health-care problem. In industrialized countries, acute diarrhea is likely to be due to a viral agent (rotavirus, Norwalk virus, or similar viruses) and requires no specific treatment. Travelers to less developed nations are exposed to diarrheal illnesses not common in their native countries (cholera, enterotoxigenic *E. coli* infections, *Entamoeba histolytica*) and must be aware of the symptoms and correct management of these illnesses (see chapter 24, Adverse Drug Reactions). When diarrhea occurs in a traveler, is accompanied by signs of dysentery (temperature greater than 103°F, systemic symptoms, bloody stools, or severe abdominal or rectal pain), or lasts longer than 14 days, one must consider a bacterial or protozoan cause. Further evaluation is necessary to determine whether specific antimicrobial therapy will be necessary.

For the vast majority of people with diarrhea who do not have an invasive infection and will have a self-limited condition, the goal of therapy is to maintain an adequate state of hydration. Simple measures such as avoiding substances that may increase intestinal secretion and motility (caffeinated beverages, alcoholic beverages, spicy foods, milk products) and adequate intake (2–3 L or more per day) of fruit juices and noncarbonated beverages generally are sufficient.

Oral solutions of rehydration represent a major advance in the therapy of severe diarrhea. They take advantage of glucose-coupled sodium uptake and solvent drag in the small intestine. Both are processes that result in absorption of sodium and free water even in the face of bacterial toxin-induced secretory diarrhea (Field et al. 1989). When moderate or severe dehydration is already present and the potential for further dehydration is high (such as during cholera), a solution high in sodium is necessary in order to prevent hyponatremia. The World Health Organization has recommended an oral rehydration solution containing 90 mEq/L of sodium, 20 mEq/L of potassium, 80 mEq/L of chloride, 30 mEq/L of bicarbonate, and 20 g/L of glucose. For a less serious degree of dehydration or to prevent it from occurring, solutions containing 45 to 50 mEq/L of sodium are commercially available (e.g., Infalyte powder, Pedialyte liquid). If dehydration is very severe (>10% of body weight loss) or if the diarrheal illness is accompanied by vomiting or inability to comply with oral fluid therapy, then IV fluids will be necessary.

If diarrhea is not accompanied by signs suggestive of an invasive infection, then symptomatic therapy with antidiarrheals should be considered. Two different classes of agents have been proved to be useful: opiates and NSAIDs. Adsorptive compounds such as kaolin or pectin have been used to treat diarrhea for centuries. They alter stool composition, turning loose stool into lumpy stool. They do not decrease stool volume or frequency and are not recommended (Ludan 1988).

Opiates (e.g., diphenoxylate with atropine, loperamide, deodorized tincture of opium) decrease intestinal motility, increase mucosal absorption, and decrease fluid and electrolyte secretion. Presumably they act on intestinal mu opioid receptors. Their net effect is to reduce stool volume and to alleviate tenesmus and abdominal cramps. Loperamide (4 mg at the onset of diarrhea, and 2 mg after each bowel movement not to exceed 16 mg in 24 hours) is useful for treating "traveler's diarrhea" from multiple causes (DuPont et al. 1990). A theoretical advantage of this drug is that it crosses the blood–brain barrier poorly and is likely to have few CNS effects. Opiates are not recommended for children under 2 years of age because they can blunt alertness and interfere with oral rehydration therapy.

Although the NSAIDs such as aspirin or indomethacin can decrease stool volume in the setting of acute infectious diarrhea, the effect is not to the degree that would make them clinically useful. Bismuth subsalicylate in large doses (30 to 60 mL every 30 minutes for eight doses following the onset of diarrhea) can decrease stool frequency and abdominal pain in mild-to-moderate acute, self-limited diarrhea. However, this amount of salicylate may lead to toxic salicylate concentrations in the blood. It is not recommended for patients with renal failure or with concomitant use of other salicylates (see chapter 11, Dermatologic Disorders). Loperamide is more effective for treating severe diarrhea (DuPont et al. 1990).

Specific antimicrobial treatment is currently recommended for symptomatic cases of diarrhea caused by *Shigella* spp., *C. difficile, Salmonella typhi* with typhoid fever, *Giardia lamblia, Entamoeba histolytica,* and *Vibrio cholerae*. Certain patients with *E. coli* (enterohemorrhagic or enterotoxigenic *E. coli,* infants with enteropathogenic or enteroadherent *E. coli*), *Salmonella* infections without typhoid fever, or prolonged *Campylobacter jejuni* diarrhea may also benefit from specific antimicrobial treatment. Details of specific antimicrobial therapy change frequently and are best obtained from a frequently revised guide (Gilbert 1999) (see chapter 14, Infectious Diseases). However, most bacterial causes of diarrhea can be treated effectively with 500 mg ciprofloxacin twice daily for 5 days. This empirical therapy may be used while awaiting the results of specific cultures (Goodman et al. 1990).

Therapy for chronic diarrhea is generally directed at the underlying disease. If the underlying disease cannot be identified or cured, then the general principles of management of acute diarrheal states are implemented. Other drugs may be considered to manage difficult cases of chronic diarrhea. Clonidine and lithium carbonate increase sodium chloride absorption in the gut; they have been used in chronic secretory diarrheas due to tumors elaborating vasoactive intestinal peptide (VIPomas) with limited success (O'Dorisio et al. 1989). Somatostatin or its analog octreotide decreases fluid and electrolyte secretion, decreases intestinal motility, and may decrease the release of a secretagogue from tumors such as VIPomas or nonmalignant tissue (Maton 1989). Because of its reduction of release of growth hormone, somatostatin should not be used in children.

## REFERENCES

Anderson JW, Gustafson NJ. 1988. Hypocholesterolemic effects of oat and bean products. *Am J Clin Nutr* **48**(3, Suppl):749–53.

Andrews PL, Davis CJ, Bingham S, et al. 1990. The abdominal visceral innervation and the emetic reflex: pathways: pharmacology, and plasticity. *Can J Physiol Pharmacol* **68**:325–45.

Archambult AP, Pare P, Bailey RJ, et al. 1988. Omeprazole (20 mg daily) versus cimetidine (1200 mg daily) in duodenal ulcer healing and pain relief. *Gastroenterology* **94**(5, pt. 1):1130–4.

Badiali D, Corazziari E, Habib FL, et al. 1995. Effect of wheat bran in treatment of chronic nonorganic constipation: a double-blind controlled trial. *Dig Dis Sci* **40**:349–56.

Bartlett JG. 1981. Antibiotic-associated pseudomembranous colitis. *Hosp Pract (Off)* **16**(12):85–8.

Bell GD, Powell KU, Burridge SM, et al. 1995. Rapid eradication of *Helicobacter pylori* infection. *Aliment Pharmacol Ther* **9**:41–6.

Binder HJ. 1977. Pharmacology of laxatives. *Annu Rev Pharmacol Toxicol* **17**:355–67.

Binder HJ, Donowitz M. 1975. A new look at laxative action. *Gastroenterology* **69**:1001–5.

Bodemar G, Walan A. 1978. Maintenance treatment of recurrent peptic ulcer by cimetidine. *Lancet* **1**:403–7.

Borison H, Wang S. 1953. Physiology and pharmacology of vomiting. *Pharmacol Rev* **5**:193–230.

Borody TJ, Cole P, Noonan S, et al. 1989. Recurrence of duodenal ulcer and *Campylobacter pylori* infection after eradication. *Med J* **151**:431–5.

Brand DL, Roufail WM, Thomson AB, et al. 1985. Misoprostol, a synthetic PGE1 analog, in the treatment of duodenal ulcers: a multicenter double-blind study. *Dig Dis Sci* **30**(11, Suppl):147s-158s.

Carey MP, Burish TG, Brenner DE. 1983. Delta-9-tetrahydrocannabinol in cancer chemotherapy: research problems and issues. *Ann Intern Med* **99**:106–14.

Carmine AA, Brogden RN. 1985. Pirenzepine: a review of its pharmacodynamic and pharmacokinetic properties and therapeutic efficacy in peptic ulcer disease and other allied diseases. *Drugs* **30**:85–126.

Carson JL, Strom BL, Morse ML, et al. 1987. The relative gastrointestinal toxicity of the nonsteroidal anti-inflammatory drugs. *Arch Intern Med* **147**:1054–9.

Carson JL, Strom BL, Soper KA, et al. 1987. The association of nonsteroidal anti-inflammatory drugs with upper gastrointestinal tract bleeding. *Arch Intern Med* **147**:85–8.

Chan FKL, Sung JJY, Chung SCS, et al. 1997. Randomized trial of eradication of *Helicobacter pylori* before non-steroidal anti-inflammatory drug therapy to prevent peptic ulcers. *Lancet* **350**:975–9.

Connell AM, Hilton C, Irvine G, et al. 1965. Variation of bowel habit in two population samples. *Br Med J* **5470**:1095–9.

Cubeddu LX, Hoffmann IS, Fuenmayor NT, et al. 1990. Efficacy of ondansetron (GR 38032F) and the role of serotonin in cisplatin-induced nausea and vomiting. *N Engl J Med* **322**:810–6.

Cubeddu LX, O'Connor DT, Parmer RJ. 1995. Plasma chromogranin A: a marker of serotonin release and emesis associated with cisplatin chemotherapy. *J Clin Oncol* **13**:681–7.

Dajani EZ. 1987. Perspective on the gastric antisecretory effects of misoprostol in man. *Prostaglandins* **33**(Suppl):68–77.

Dingle J, Badger G, Jordan W. 1964. *Illness in the Home: A Study of 25,000 Illnesses in a Group of Cleveland Families*. Cleveland, OH: Case Western Reserve University Press, pp 19–32.

Donowitz M. 1979. Current concepts of laxative action: mechanisms by which laxatives increase stool water. *J Clin Gastroenterol* **1**:77–84.

DuPont HL, Flores SJ, Ericsson CD, et al. 1990. Comparative efficacy of loperamide hydrochloride and bismuth subsalicylate in the management of acute diarrhea. *Am J Med* **88**:15s-19s.

Fekety R. 1997. Guidelines for the diagnosis and management of *Clostridium difficile*-associated diarrhea and colitis. American College of Gastroenterology, Practice Parameters Committee. *Am J Gastroenterol* **92**:739–50.

Feldman M. 1984. Inhibition of gastric acid secretion by selective and nonselective anticholinergics. *Gastroenterology* **86**:361–6.

Field M, Rao MC, Chang EB. 1989. Intestinal electrolyte transport and diarrheal disease. *N Engl J Med* **321**:800–6, 879–83.

Fine K, Krejs G, Fordtran J. 1989. Diarrhea. In: Sleisenger MH, Fordtran JS, editors. *Gastrointestinal Disease*. Philadelphia: WB Saunders, pp 1043–72.

Fordtran JS. 1967. Speculations on the pathogenesis of diarrhea. *Fed Proc* **26**:1405–14.

Gabriel SE, Jaakkimainen L, Bombardier C. 1991. Risk for serious gastrointestinal complications related to use of non-steroidal anti-inflammatory drugs: a meta-analysis. *Ann Intern Med* **115**:787–96.

Giesing D, Lanman R, Runser D. 1982. Absorption of sucralfate in man. *Gastroenterology* **82**:1066.

Gilbert DN, Moellering RC, Sande MA. 1999. *The Sanford Guide to Antimicrobial Therapy*. 29th ed. Hyde Park, VT, Antimicrobial Therapy, Inc.

Goldman P, Peppercorn MA. 1975. Drug therapy: sulfasalazine. *N Engl J Med* **293**:20–3.

Goodman LJ, Trenholme GM, Kaplan RL, et al. 1990. Empiric antimicrobial therapy of domestically acquired acute diarrhea in urban adults. *Arch Intern Med* **150**:541–6.

Graham DY. 1977. Enzyme replacement therapy of exocrine pancreatic insufficiency in man: relation between in vitro enzyme activities and in vivo potency in commercial pancreatic extracts. *N Engl J Med* **296**:1314–7.

Graham DY. 1989. *Campylobacter pylori* and peptic ulcer disease. *Gastroenterology* **96**(2, pt. 2, Suppl):615–25.

Graham DY, Agrawal NM, Roth SH. 1988. Prevention of NSAID-induced gastric ulcer with misoprostol: multicenter, double-blind, placebo-controlled trial. *Lancet* **2**:1277–80.

Graham DY, Lew GM, Klein PD, et al. 1992. Effect of treatment of *Helicobacter pylori* infection on the long-term recurrence of gastric or duodenal ulcer: a randomized, controlled study. *Ann Intern Med* **116**:705–8.

Graham DY, Smith JL. 1988. Gastroduodenal complications of chronic NSAID therapy. *Am J Gastroenterol* **83**:1081–4.

Gryboski JD. 1985. The role of allergy in diarrhea: Cow's milk protein allergy. *Pediatr Ann* **14**:31–2.

Hanson JS, McCallum RW. 1985. The diagnosis and management of nausea and vomiting: a review. *Am J Gastroenterol* **80**:210–8.

Havu N. 1986. Enterochromaffin-like cell carcinoids of gastric mucosa in rats after life-long inhibition of gastric secretion. *Digestion* **35**(Suppl 1):42–55.

Herting RL, Nissen CH. 1986. Overview of misoprostol-clinical experience. *Dig Dis Sci* **31**(2, suppl.):47s-54s.

Host A. 1997. Cow's milk allergy. *J Roy Soc Med* **90**:34–9.

Howden CW, Jones DB, Peace KE, et al. 1988. The treatment of gastric ulcer with antisecretory drugs: relationship of pharmacological effect to healing rates. *Dig Dis Sci* **33**:619–24.

Jenner P, Marsden CD. 1979. The substituted benzamides—A novel class of dopamine antagonists. *Life Sci* **25**:479–85.

Jones DB, Howden CW, Burget DW, et al. 1987. Acid suppression in duodenal ulcer: a meta-analysis to define optimal dosing with antisecretory drugs. *Gut* **28**:1120–7.

Koch J, Donaldson R. 1964. A survey of food intolerances in hospitalized patients. *N Engl J Med* **271**:657–60.

Koletzko S, Stringer DA, Cleghorn GJ, et al. 1989. Lavage treatment of distal intestinal obstruction syndrome in children with cystic fibrosis. *Pediatrics* **83**:727–33.

Kurata JH, Nogawa AN. 1997. Meta-analysis of risk factors for peptic ulcer. *J Clin Gastroenterol* **24**:2–17.

Lake-Bakaar G, Tom W, Lake BD, et al. 1988. Gastropathy and ketoconazole malabsorption in the acquired immunodeficiency syndrome (AIDS). *Ann Intern Med* **109**:471–3.

Lam SK. 1988. Antacids: the past, the present, and the future. *Baillieres Clin Gastroenterol* **2**:641–54.

Lang IM, Sarna SK, Dodds WJ. 1993. Pharyngeal, esophageal, and proximal gastric responses associated with vomiting. *Am J Physiol* **265**:G963–72.

Lanza FL, Royer GJ, Nelson RS. 1980. Endoscopic evaluation of the effects of aspirin, buffered aspirin, and enteric-coated aspirin on gastric and duodenal mucosa. *N Engl J Med* **303**:136–8.

Laszlo J, Clark RA, Hanson DC, et al. 1985. Lorazepam in cancer patients treated with cisplatin: a drug having antiemetic, amnesic, and anxiolytic effects. *J Clin Oncol* **3**:864–9.

Ludan AC. 1988. Current management of acute diarrheas: use and abuse of drug therapy. *Drugs* **3**(Suppl 4):18–25.

Mahieu P, Pringot J, Bodart P. 1984. Defecography: I. Description of a new procedure and results in normal patients. *Gastrointest Radiol* **9**:247–51.

Malagelada JR, Camilleri M. 1984. Unexplained vomiting: a diagnostic challenge. *Ann Intern Med* **101**:211–8.

Markman M, Sheidler V, Ettinger DS, et al. 1984. Antiemetic efficacy of dexamethasone: randomized, double-blind, crossover study with prochlorperazine in patients receiving cancer chemotherapy. *N Engl J Med* **311**:549–52.

Marks IN. 1987. The efficacy, safety and dosage of sucralfate in ulcer therapy. *Scand J Gastroenterol* **140**(Suppl):33–8.

Marty M, Pouillart P, Scholl S, et al. 1990. Comparison of the 5-hydroxytryptamine3 (serotonin) antagonist ondansetron (GR 38032F) with high-dose metoclopramide in the control of cisplatin-induced emesis. *N Engl J Med* **322**:816–21.

Maton PN. 1989. The use of the long-acting somatostatin analogue, octreotide acetate, in patients with islet cell tumors. *Gastroenterol Clin North Am* **18**:897–922.

Maton PN, Vinayek R, Frucht H, et al. 1989. Long-term efficacy and safety of omeprazole in patients with Zollinger-Ellison syndrome: a prospective study. *Gastroenterology* **97**:827–36.

McArthur KE, Jensen RT, Gardner JD. 1986. Treatment of acid-peptic diseases by inhibition of gastric $H^+,K^+$-ATPase. *Annu Rev Med* **37**:97–105.

McCarthy DM. 1983. Ranitidine or cimetidine. *Ann Intern Med* **99**: 551–3.

McCloy RF, Arnold R, Bardhan KD, et al. 1995. Pathophysiological effects of long-term acid suppression in man. *Dig Dis Sci* **40**(2 Suppl):96S-120S.

McFarland RJ, Bateson MC, Green JR, et al. 1990. Omeprazole provides quicker symptom relief and duodenal ulcer healing than ranitidine. *Gastroenterology* **98**:278–83.

Meade EA, Smith WL, DeWitt DL. 1993. Differential inhibition of prostaglandin endoperoxide synthase (cyclooxygenase) isozymes by aspirin and other non-steroidal anti-inflammatory drugs. *J Biol Chem* **268**:6610–4.

Miyamoto T, Ogino N, Yamamoto S, et al. 1976. Purification of prostaglandin endoperoxide synthetase from bovine vesicular gland microsomes. *J Biol Chem* **251**:2629–36.

Moss J, Vaughan M. 1989. Guanine nucleotide-binding proteins (G proteins) in activation of adenylyl cyclase: lessons learned from cholera and "travelers' diarrhea." *J Lab Clin Med* **113**:258–68.

NIH Consensus Development Panel. 1994. *Helicobacter pylori* in peptic ulcer disease. *JAMA* **272**:65–9.

O'Dorisio TM, Mekhjian HS, Gaginella TS. 1989. Medical therapy of VIPomas. *Endocrinol Metab Clin North Am* **18**:545–56.

Pantuck EJ, Hsiao KC, Kuntzman R, et al. 1975. Intestinal metabolism of phenacetin in the rat: effect of charcoal-broiled beef and rat chow. *Science* **187**:744–6.

Park GD, Spector R, Goldberg MJ, et al. 1986. Expanded role of charcoal therapy in the poisoned and overdosed patient. *Arch Intern Med* **146**:969–73.

Peterson WL. 1991. *Helicobacter pylori* and peptic ulcer disease. *N Engl J Med* **324**:1043–8.

Piper DW, Greig M, Coupland GA, et al. 1975. Factors relevant to the prognosis of chronic gastric ulcer. *Gut* **16**:714–8.

Pounder RE. 1981. Model of medical treatment for duodenal ulcer. *Lancet* **1**:29–30.

Powell JR, Donn KH. 1983. The pharmacokinetic basis for $H_2$-antagonist drug interactions: concepts and implications. *J Clin Gastroenterol* **5**(Suppl 1):95–113.

Rotter JI, Shehat T, Petersen GM. 1992. Peptic ulcer disease. In: King RA, Rotter JI, Motulsky AG, editors. *The Genetic Basis of Common Diseases*. New York: Oxford University Press, pp 240–78.

Siegel JN, Schwartz A, Askenase PW, et al. 1982. T-cell suppression and contrasuppression induced by histamine $H_2$ and $H_1$ receptor agonists, respectively. *Proc Natl Acad Sci USA* **79**: 5052–6.

Silverstein FE, Kimmey MB, Saunders DR, et al. 1986. Gastric protection by misoprostol against 1300 mg of aspirin: an endoscopic study. *Dig Dis Sci* **31**(2, Suppl):137s-141s.

Singh G, Ramey DR, Morfeld D, et al. 1996. Gastrointestinal tract complication of non-steroidal anti-inflammatory drug treatment in rheumatoid arthritis—a prospective observational cohort study. *Arch Intern Med* **156**:1530–6.

Sipponen P, Seppala K, Aarynen M, et al. 1989. Chronic gastritis and gastroduodenal ulcer: a case-control study on risk of coexisting duodenal or gastric ulcer in patients with gastritis. *Gut* **30**:922–9.

Smith B. 1968. Effect of irritant purgatives on the myenteric plexus in man and the mouse. *Gut* **9**:139–43.

Soll AH. 1990. Pathogenesis of peptic ulcer and implications for therapy. *N Engl J Med* **322**:909–16.

Sontag SJ. 1986. Prostaglandins and acid peptic disease. *Am J Gastroenterol* **81**:1021–8.

Spechler SJ. 1992. Comparison of medical and surgical therapy for complicated gastroesophageal reflux disease in veterans. The Department of Veterans' Affairs Gastroesophageal Reflux Disease Study Group. *N Engl J Med* **326**:786–92.

Starkey WG, Collins J, Wallis TS, et al. 1986. Kinetics, tissue specificity and pathological changes in murine rotavirus infection of mice. *J Gen Virol* **67**:2625–34.

Stott JRR, Barnes GR, Wright RJ, et al. 1989. The effect on motion sickness and occulomotor function of GR38032F: a 5-$HT_3$-receptor antagonist with anti-emetic properties. *Br J Clin Pharmacol* **27**:147–57.

Talley NJ, Weaver AL, Zinsmeister AR, et al. 1993. Functional constipation and outlet delay: a population-based study. *Gastroenterology* **105**:781–90.

Taylor ND, Bartlett JG. 1980. Binding of *Clostridium difficile* cytotoxin and vancomycin by anion exchange resins. *J Infect Dis* **141**:92–7.

Tedesco FJ, DiPiro JT. 1985. Laxative use in constipation. American College of Gastroenterology's Committee on FDA-Related Matters. *Am J Gastroenterol* **80**:303–9.

Thijs JC, Vanzwet AA, Thijs WJ, et al. 1996. Diagnostic test for *H. pylori*. *Am J Gastroenterol* **91**:2125–9.

Tyers MB, Freeman AJ. 1992. Mechanism of the anti-emetic activity of 5-HT3 receptor antagonists. *Oncology* **49**:263–8.

Van der Hulst RWM, Rauws EAJ, Koycu B, et al. 1997. Prevention of ulcer recurrence after eradication of *Helicobacter pylori:* a prospective long-term follow-up study. *Gastroenterology* **176**: 1082–6.

Vigneri S, Termini R, Leandro G, et al. 1995. A comparison of five maintenance therapies for reflux esophagitis. *N Engl J Med* **333**:1106–10.

Wald A. 1986. Colonic transit and anorectal manometry in chronic idiopathic constipation. *Arch Intern Med* **146**:1713–6.

Wampler G. 1983. The pharmacology and clinical effectiveness of phenothiazines and related drugs for managing chemotherapy-induced emesis. *Drugs* **25**(Suppl 1):35–51.

Weberg R, Aubert E, Dahlberg O, et al. 1988. Low-dose antacids or cimetidine for duodenal ulcer? *Gastroenterology* **95**:1465–9.

Yee GC, Stanley DL, Pessa LJ, et al. 1995. Effect of grapefruit juice on blood cyclosporine concentration. *Lancet* **345**:955–6.

CHAPTER

4

# HEPATIC DISORDERS AND THE INFLUENCE OF LIVER FUNCTION ON DRUG DISPOSITION

Gabriel Garcia

*Chapter Outline*



A drug or a toxin will be the cause of disease in 50% or more of patients hospitalized for the management of liver disease, whether this be fulminant hepatic failure or complications of cirrhosis. This chapter discusses injury to the liver by drugs and environmental toxins and outlines principles of management of patients with drug-induced liver disease. Those few liver diseases that have specific drug therapy are also discussed; the rest of the chapter focuses on the management of the complications of endstage liver disease.

## WITHDRAWAL OF POTENTIALLY HEPATOTOXIC SUBSTANCES

Because many acute and chronic forms of liver injury may be caused by exposure of the patient to toxic substances, the physician must obtain a detailed history of drug use (both prescription and OTC pharmaceuticals), use of vitamins and hormones, and exposure to environmental or industrial toxins.

### Drug-Induced Liver Disease

The liver's pivotal role in the processing of foreign substances also makes it susceptible to injury by those xenobiotics. Some chemical agents are predictable or intrinsic hepatotoxins: The injury they induce is generally dose-related, is observed above a threshold dose in all hosts, and can be reproduced in experimental animals. These agents often produce tissue injury that results in metabolic defects and in cell death or dysfunction. Examples of such direct hepatotoxins include the chlorinated hydrocarbons (e.g., carbon tetrachloride) and acetaminophen. Other agents may act indirectly by interfering with a metabolic activity essential to cell function and survival.

Another group of chemical agents depend on idiosyncrasy of the host for their toxicity: Their injury is generally not dose-related, is observed in only a few patients exposed to the drug (generally within 1–4 weeks after the onset of drug use), and may not be reproducible in other species. In certain cases, such as dapsone-induced hepatic injury, features of systemic hypersensitivity as allergy (fever, rash, eosinophilia, lymphocytosis, and lymphadenopathy) are present. In some cases, involvement of the immune system can be documented, confirming the presence of a true drug allergy. Liver biopsy obtained during the illness also may be typical of an allergic reaction, with eosinophilic and/or granulomatous infiltration and cellular necrosis (Mohle-Boetani et al. 1992).

With some drugs, liver injury depends on a metabolic idiosyncrasy that leads to accumulation of a metabolite that is capable either of inciting intrinsic liver damage or an allergic reaction. These reactions can occur over a much longer period of time than would be expected in a typical hypersensitivity reaction and can result from genetic or acquired qualitative or quantitative differences in the handling of drugs. For example, patients with phenytoin-induced liver damage are unable to detoxify a potentially toxic metabolite, the arene oxide; this inability is related to decreased liver epoxide hydrolase activity in affected individuals (Spielberg et al. 1981).

Liver biopsy in drug-induced liver disease generally shows cytotoxic or cholestatic injury. Cytotoxic injury may be accompanied by necrosis or steatosis; cholestatic lesions may be exudative or bland. Less common types of injury include vascular (large or small hepatic vein occlusion, peliosis hepatis, or other sinusoidal lesions), granulomatous, or neoplastic (benign and malignant) lesions. The purpose of a liver biopsy in patients with possible drug-induced liver injury is to establish the diagnosis, to suggest or establish another cause for the liver injury, and occasionally to stage the degree of liver injury.

Although the histologic pattern of the injury to the liver may be useful in determining the presence of drug-induced liver disease, one must remember that the liver has a limited repertoire of responses to injury. The findings in the liver biopsy in patients with drug injuries may mimic other metabolic or infectious diseases and may suggest a common pathway of injury. For example, microvesicular fatty change is a characteristic histologic finding in patients with valproic acid-induced hepatic failure, Reye's syndrome, and Jamaican vomiting disease, all conditions that are most commonly seen in children. Because a similar histologic picture has been seen in animals treated with 4-pentenoic acid, the hypothesis was put forth that a metabolite of the omega-oxidation pathway might be responsible for hepatoxicity caused by these seemingly disparate drug and metabolic insults. Such a metabolite of valproic acid has been isolated, and administration of this metabolite to rats has led to microvesicular fatty change (Lewis et al. 1982).

**PRINCIPLE The full spectrum of a drug's toxicity is not known when it is first used. Considerable experience with the drug in patients and careful observation are required to link an infrequent adverse response to a drug. Establishing a mechanism for an adverse response is even more difficult. However, once a mechanism is defined, it can often be retrospectively used to detect undiscovered reactions of an analogous nature.**

Reproduction of the clinical and biochemical signs of liver injury on rechallenge with the drug can be useful in allowing the therapist the certainty of the connection between the drug and the idiosyncratic drug reaction. This is most important clinically when no alternate therapy exists for a serious disorder. The therapist must weigh the potential benefit of greater diagnostic certainty by observing the response to rechallenge with the rare possibility that it may lead to a life-threatening injury.

The toxins or drugs that most commonly cause liver injury have changed over time as toxic or less effective agents have been removed from the workplace, the environment, and the pharmacy shelf. Predictably, new drugs and environmental agents have led to liver injury not suspected during the studies that determined their efficacy. Every time a drug is used, the therapist must be alert to the possibility of drug toxicity mimicking another disease and be aware of the relationships between drugs that can be used to predict similar toxicities. The reader is referred to a standard text of hepatotoxicity for an extensive list of drugs and chemicals that result in liver injury and for discussion of their clinical manifestations (Zimmerman 1978).

## Removal of Offending Dietary Constituents

Ordinary dietary constituents may occasionally produce liver injury or adverse effects in a genetically susceptible individual. Treatment must then be directed at the removal of such substances from the diet. For example, removal of galactose-containing carbohydrates reverses jaundice, ascites, and hepatosplenomegaly in infants with galactosemia (Hsia and Walker 1961). Removal of protein may reverse coma in a child with a urea cycle enzyme deficiency or in a cirrhotic patient with portal–systemic encephalopathy. Reduction of carbohydrate ingestion improves fatty infiltration of the liver and hepatomegaly in patients who have a genetic susceptibility to carbohydrate-induced type IV hyperlipidemia, or in patients receiving total parenteral nutrition containing high concentrations of glucose.

## Avoidance of Certain Toxic Food Substances

Naturally occurring organic compounds have also been associated with liver injury in man. The alkaloid senecio, which is found in certain herbal teas, produces hepatic vein occlusion. Aflatoxin is produced by a fungus, *Aspergillus flavus,* that grows on grains and nuts. In animals, prolonged consumption of aflatoxin may lead to cirrhosis or hepatoma. In humans, the level of aflatoxin in the diet has been found to be a cocarcinogen with hepatitis B infection in an epidemiologic study of hepatocellular carcinoma in rural China (Yeh et al. 1989). Mushrooms of the *Amanita* genus contain several toxins, of which α-amanitin and phalloidin can produce extensive hepatocellular necrosis that is frequently fatal (Welper and Opitz 1972).

### Removal of "Toxic" Endogenous Substances

Several endogenous substances (e.g., iron, copper, ammonia, bile acids, porphyrins) may accumulate as a result of disorders in intermediary metabolism or acquired liver injury. They may contribute further to liver injury and lead to other systemic effects. Therapy directed at removal of these substances often is beneficial, particularly if instituted during the precirrhotic phase of some of these illnesses. For example, D-penicillamine is used to remove copper in patients with Wilson disease (Scheinberg and Sternlieb 1960; Sternlieb 1980), and phlebotomy is used to reduce the body burden of iron in patients with idiopathic hemochromatosis (Bassett et al. 1980).

## PRINCIPLES OF TREATMENT OF LIVER DISEASE

### Replacement of Depleted Constituents: Role of Dietary Therapy

Although removal of hepatotoxic substances is critical in the therapy of some hepatic disorders, attention must also be directed to replenishing substances that are likely to become deficient in patients with hepatic disease. Three categories of deficiencies should be considered:

- Vitamins and minerals that are depleted because of dietary deficiencies
- Vitamins and nutrients that are diminished as a result of impairment of the enterohepatic circulation
- Endogenous substances that become depleted as a result of impairment of hepatic function

Patients with cholestatic liver disease are unable to excrete bile at a normal rate, and an intestinal luminal deficiency of bile salts results. As a consequence, the absorption of fat-soluble vitamins as well as other lipid substances is impaired and deficiencies may develop. Malabsorption of vitamin K will lead to an impairment of the hepatic synthesis of vitamin K–dependent clotting factors. Similarly, vitamin A and D malabsorption may lead to the clinical syndromes typical of their deficiencies (see chapter 5, Nutrition). In early stages of cholestasis, these deficiencies may be very difficult to detect.

Severe liver damage is almost always associated with impairment in the production of serum proteins that are synthesized in the liver. Intravenous administration of salt-poor albumin, plasma, or plasma fractions may be necessary to lessen these acquired deficiencies, especially in patients with clinically important bleeding who are deficient in hepatically generated clotting factors II, VII, IX, and X.

### Temporizing

One of the most dramatic and imperfectly understood properties of the liver is its capacity to regenerate. After surgical removal of two-thirds of the rat liver, the liver mass is restored within 7–10 days. A similar percentage of the human liver can be surgically removed, and sufficient regeneration can occur to support hepatic function at "normal" levels. The therapist must take advantage of this remarkable regenerative capability. There are many occasions when temporizing (i.e., making the deliberate decision not to treat with drugs) is the best therapeutic decision, allowing normal physiologic processes to reestablish homeostasis.

**PRINCIPLE The use of time as a therapeutic approach is subject to the same principles as the use of drugs, devises, or procedures. The decision not to give a drug has its own inherent potential efficacy and toxicity; like any other therapeutic maneuver, consideration of relative risks and benefits is necessary.**

The physician who waits and watches a patient with liver injury has an opportunity to observe the pattern of the disease and judge whether the liver injury will spontaneously resolve or whether it will become fulminant. This may require days or weeks of observation following acute viral or drug-induced hepatitis. Attention to the state of nutrition and hydration, and prompt identification and treatment of complications such as infection or electrolyte and acid–base disturbances, are key to the proper management of the patient. If fulminant hepatic failure develops (i.e., the presence of encephalopathy within 8 weeks of an acute liver injury in a patient without evidence of prior liver disease), then the patient should be observed in an intensive care unit, and determination of whether the patient is a candidate for liver transplantation should be quickly made.

As a result of improved surgical and anesthetic techniques, better immunosuppressive regimens, and improved preservation of removed organs, liver transplantation is now a well-established therapeutic option for many patients whose liver disease has been complicated by liver failure. Five-year survival rates of greater than 60% have been achieved in patients undergoing treatment for end-stage cirrhosis or fulminant hepatic failure. Absolute contraindications for liver transplantation include sepsis, malignancy outside the hepatobiliary tree, and active substance abuse (Starzl et al. 1989).

**PRINCIPLE The use of devices and procedures as alternatives to drugs for the same indications is becoming a major responsibility of the therapist. However, it should be recognized that the requirements to put devices on the market and to use procedures are considerably less stringent than those that control the marketing of a drug.**

Patients presenting with jaundice may have conditions causing either extrahepatic biliary obstruction or intrahepatic cholestasis. The therapist must choose between mechanical decompression of the biliary tract and careful observation based on bedside evaluation and biliary-imaging studies. Patients in whom there is a high clinical suspicion of obstruction of the common bile duct and secondary cholangitis require prompt decompression (surgical or endoscopic) of the infected biliary tree and antibiotic therapy to treat and contain the bacterial infection. In the patient without clinical evidence of cholangitis, the choice to observe the patient during withdrawal of potentially hepatotoxic agents or identification of viral hepatitis will not expose patients with intrahepatic disease to unnecessary operative morbidity and mortality. Delay of an operative procedure until its need is established will not expose the patient to undue injury because the development of secondary biliary cirrhosis takes weeks and may be surgically reversed after its onset (Bunton and Cameron 1963).

### Prophylactic Therapy

Viral hepatitis A and B can often be prevented or attenuated by vaccination or postexposure prophylaxis with immune serum globulin. Other examples of prophylactic therapy in patients with liver disease include the phlebotomy of asymptomatic patients who have hemochromatosis, or chelation therapy of asymptomatic patients who have Wilson disease. However, most prophylactic measures are not as specific as the measures that can be taken to prevent the severe complications of these latter diseases. For example, such measures include the use of lactulose, cleansing enemas, and poorly absorbed antibiotics to prevent hepatic encephalopathy in a cirrhotic patient with gastrointestinal (GI) bleeding and may include the avoidance of surgery in the decompensated cirrhotic patient in whom the stress of anesthesia may precipitate irreversible hepatic failure. Prevention of GI hemorrhage with $H_2$-receptor antagonists in patients with fulminant hepatic failure is another example (MacDougall et al. 1977).

## MANAGEMENT OF COMPLICATIONS OF ADVANCED LIVER DISEASES

### Portal Hypertension

Portal hypertension is defined as an abnormal rise in the portal venous pressure gradient (portal vein pressure–central venous pressure). It is generally a consequence of the disruption of lobular and sinusoidal architecture that accompanies cirrhosis from any cause. Portal hypertension also may result from hypertension or obstruction at any level of the hepatic venous circulation, from thrombosis of the portal vein (presinusoidal causes) to obliteration or thrombosis of major or terminal hepatic veins (postsinusoidal causes). Although the initiating event leading to portal hypertension is not known, it results in increased intrahepatic and portal–systemic collateral resistance and in increased mesenteric venous capacitance and portal blood flow. The major consequences of portal hypertension include:

- The development of a collateral circulation through the submucosa of the GI tract, the peritoneal surfaces, and the anterior abdominal wall
- An increase in lymphatic flow exiting through the thoracic duct
- An increase in plasma volume and cardiac output with a loss of effective arterial tone

As one would predict by Poiseuille's law, changes in portal pressure are generally caused by changes in vascular resistance or blood flow because changes in the length of blood vessels or blood viscosity are not hemodynamically significant events in most clinical situations. A hyperdynamic state with high blood flow and low peripheral vascular resistance is the rule in patients with cirrhosis and portal hypertension. This is accompanied by increases in plasma volume and by both increased resistance and increased blood flow through the portal circulation as a result of expansion of collateral channels (Groszmann et al. 1988). Serious clinical manifestations that accompany these changes include hemorrhage from GI varices (predominantly esophageal, less commonly gastric or hemorrhoidal), hepatic encephalopathy, and ascites (Grace 1993).

Patients with chronic liver disease who develop symptoms and signs of portal hypertension must be considered candidates for liver transplantation if their underlying liver disease is amenable to this treatment modality. Because the 1-year mortality following the development of variceal hemorrhage, ascites, or hepatic encephalopathy can be as high as 80% in patients with chronic liver disease, the physician has the opportunity to improve both the length and the quality of life by a procedure whose overall 5-year survival is 70% (Starzl et al. 1989).

## Esophageal Variceal Hemorrhage

### *Medical management*

Esophageal varices are large esophageal veins with an extensive capillary network that are formed when portal pressures are elevated. Esophageal varices are at risk for bleeding when the portal pressure, as estimated by the hepatic venous pressure gradient, exceeds 12 mmHg (Garcia-Tsao et al. 1985). Esophageal variceal hemorrhage is a dramatic, unpredictable clinical event in the natural history of cirrhosis that has a high mortality (30–50% per episode of bleeding), and a 70% chance of recurrence, most of which occur within 6 months (Baker et al. 1959; Graham and Smith 1981). Patients at highest risk for bleeding generally have large varices, high portal pressures, and a variety of endoscopically described local signs (red wales, cherry-red spots, and varices-on-varices—collectively named red color signs) (Beppu et al. 1981). Massive GI bleeding in patients with advanced liver disease usually stems from variceal bleeding, but other causes include portal hypertensive gastropathy, peptic ulcer disease, and Mallory-Weiss tears. Emergency upper endoscopy can differentiate among these causes, and an experienced therapeutic endoscopist can achieve local control of the hemorrhage through variceal banding or sclerotherapy, chemical coagulation, or thermal coagulation. Although the ultimate prognosis for patients following variceal hemorrhage is dictated by the seriousness of the underlying liver disease, attempts at medical management of variceal bleeding can reduce the need for massive blood transfusion and high-risk of surgery done under emergency conditions.

Medical management of patients with acute variceal bleeding should take place in an intensive care unit where the patient can be monitored closely. Attention to the hemodynamic status of the patient requires monitoring of urine output, central venous and arterial pressures, hematocrit, electrolytes, and acid–base status. The goal of transfusion therapy should be to reverse hypovolemia and to provide adequate oxygen-carrying capacity. Because overexpansion of the blood volume may raise portal pressures and raise the likelihood of continued bleeding, patients should not be transfused to a normal hematocrit—usually a hematocrit of 30% is adequate.

The diagnosis of the cause of upper GI bleeding in patients with cirrhosis is established by endoscopy. If esophageal varices are the cause, then initial control of bleeding should be performed by variceal sclerotherapy or banding. Success rates for the control of acute bleeding with either procedure vary from 80% to 100%; randomized controlled clinical trials have failed to demonstrate major differences in success rates, although ligation in expert hands appears to be accompanied by fewer complications (Infante et al. 1989; Stiegmann et al. 1992; Laine et al. 1993; Lo et al. 1995).

Medical therapy of variceal bleeding, with vasopressin and somatostatin or their analogues, is aimed at reduction of portal pressure. Both vasopressin and somatostatin decrease splanchnic blood flow, portal pressure, and collateral flow as measured by azygos vein flow. The potential benefits of these agents are the ability to institute therapy at the time of first suspicion of the diagnosis of acute variceal bleeding and the relative ease of administration. If acute GI hemorrhage is due to gastric varices or portal hypertensive gastropathy, lowering of portal pressure with use of these agents is of theoretical but as-yet unproven use.

Vasopressin, or antidiuretic hormone, was isolated and chemically synthesized in the 1950s (duVigneaud et al. 1954). Secretion of this hormone by the hypothalamus is induced by hyperosmolarity, volume depletion, emotional or physiological stress, pharmacologic agents, and painful stimuli (Schrier 1979). Its half-life in the circulation after secretion or intravenous (IV) administration is approximately 10 minutes; it is inactivated by peptidases in many tissues, but principally in the kidney (Rabkin et al. 1979). In addition to its renal antidiuretic effect, vasopressin causes constriction of vascular smooth muscle, as well as contraction of smooth muscle in the uterus and GI tract, leading to increased propulsive forces of both organs. Therapy with a continuous IV infusion of vasopressin has been shown by some (Merigan et al. 1962; Conn et al. 1975; Chojkier et al. 1979; Mallory et al. 1980) but not by others (Fogel et al. 1982) to be effective in stopping variceal bleeding; it has not been shown to improve survival. The intense vasospasm that can accompany the use of vasopressin can compromise blood flow in the coronary, cerebral, and mesenteric circulations, leading to ischemia and infarction. Because of the high rate of serious complications, attempts to reduce the systemic effects of vasopressin have included the simultaneous use of systemic vasodilators (nitroglycerin, nitroprusside) or the use of glypressin (the triglycyl hormonogen of vasopressin) that causes fewer systemic effects (Gelman and Ernst 1979; Freeman et al. 1982; Groszmann et al. 1982). Controlled trials of vasopressin plus nitroglycerin versus vasopressin alone have generally favored the combination therapy (Gimson et al. 1986; Tsai et al. 1986; Bosch et al. 1989); however, no study has shown the combination to be more effective than traditional therapy with balloon tamponade (Teres et al. 1990). Although nitroglycerin could be administered by sublingual or transdermal routes, continuous intravenous administration has been preferred because of the ease to make timely adjustment to systemic blood pressure.

Somatostatin was first isolated as a polypeptide that inhibited the secretion of growth hormone by the pituitary gland (Brazeau et al. 1973). It is found in many tissues throughout the body but is most concentrated in the GI tract and pancreas (Arimura et al. 1975). The physiologic functions of somatostatin in the GI tract are yet to be defined; in general, it inhibits the secretion of GI hormones and pancreatic juice, and inhibits motility of the GI tract. Infusion of somatostatin to normal volunteers and patients with cirrhosis leads to a reduction in mesenteric blood flow and portal pressures without significant hemodynamic effects on the systemic circulation (Bosch et al. 1981). The half-life of somatostatin is measured in minutes, and it must be administered intravenously. Octreotide, a cyclic octapeptide with similar biological activity, can be administered subcutaneously and has a half-life of 1–2 hours. It is therefore easier to administer than the native molecule (O'Donnell and Heaton 1988). Randomized controlled clinical trials have demonstrated that somatostatin is comparable to vasopressin or sclerotherapy in controlling acute variceal bleeding (Kravetz et al. 1984; Jenkins et al. 1985; Bagarani et al. 1987; Burroughs et al. 1990; Hsia et al. 1990; Saari et al. 1990). Only one randomized trial has evaluated the comparative efficacy of octreotide and vasopressin and found them to be similar (Hwang et al. 1992). The combination of octreotide with sclerotherapy, when compared with sclerotherapy alone, has had conflicting results in the two published randomized clinical trials (Besson et al. 1995; Primignani et al. 1995).

***Surgery and other treatments***

When all medical treatments fail to control variceal bleeding, surgery to decompress the portal circulation or devascularize the distal esophagus will control bleeding. Shunt surgery has a high mortality and is often complicated by hepatic encephalopathy in patients with poor hepatic reserve (Reynolds et al. 1981). However, surgery leads to less recurrent bleeding than does sclerotherapy and may be favored in patients with relatively good liver function (Cello et al. 1987). Esophageal transection, in experienced hands, is a simpler procedure that can be as effective as variceal sclerotherapy in the control of active bleeding (Huizinga 1985: Teres et al. 1987; Inokuchi et al. 1990) and has been used to control bleeding in patients failing conventional therapy (McCormick et al. 1992).

Transjugular intrahepatic portosystemic stent shunts (TIPSS) placed by a radiologic procedure between branches of the hepatic and portal veins have been proposed as alternates to surgical shunts. No randomized controlled trials have been reported to date, but success as a salvage procedure in consecutive series of patients with variceal bleeding refractory to endoscopic or medical therapy have led to widespread use of this technique (Rossle et al. 1994).

Because the seriousness of the underlying liver disease affects both short- and long-term survival following variceal bleeding, the physician can use well-established prognostic indicators to guide the management of patients with active variceal bleeding. Patients with acute variceal bleeding should be treated with variceal sclerotherapy until obliteration of distal esophageal varices is achieved. If rebleeding occurs, then patients with adequate hepatic reserve should have surgery or TIPSS to control bleeding. The choice of operation should take into account the experience of the surgeon. The success of these surgical and endoscopic techniques is related to the expertise of the operator. Liver transplantation remains an option for acceptable candidates with refractory bleeding.

**PRINCIPLE Therapeutic options that involve invasive techniques introduce a new variable in determining both efficacy and toxicity: the experience and technical skill of the individual physician.**

***Prevention***

Prophylactic therapy aimed at the prevention of the first variceal bleed has been attempted with agents that reduce portal pressure ($\beta$-adrenergic receptor blocking agents; i.e., "beta-blockers"), sclerotherapy, and surgical shunts. Patients with varices at high risk for bleeding should be considered for prophylactic therapy. Five randomized controlled clinical trials using propranolol and two similar trials using nadolol showed a treatment benefit for either therapy in the prevention of the first variceal hemorrhage (Pascal et al. 1987; Ideo et al. 1988; Lebrec et al. 1988; The Italian Multicenter Project for Propranolol in Prevention of Bleeding 1989; Andreani et al. 1990; The Prova Study Group 1991; Conn et al. 1991). It is difficult to predict which patients are most likely to experience a fall in portal pressure and which dose of beta-blockers would be optimal without invasive studies to measure the portal pressure gradient directly. In addition, the acute hemodynamic response to drug therapy may not predict the long-term efficacy of treatment. When patients have had serial estimates of portal pressure, the group that had a sustained fall in portal pressure below 12 mmHg had no recurrent bleeding (Lebrec et al. 1984). However, serial invasive hemodynamic studies are not feasible in this patient population, and dosing of beta-blockers based on patient tolerance is used. Neither prophylactic shunt surgery nor endoscopic sclerotherapy has been shown conclusively to lead to fewer episodes of bleeding or greater survival, despite initial enthusiasm for both procedures (The Veterans Affairs Cooperative Variceal Sclerotherapy Group 1991a).

About 70% of patients with an initial variceal bleed will suffer at least one episode of rebleeding, usually within the first 6 months of the initial bleed (Graham and Smith 1981). The clinician must choose from pharmacological, endoscopic, and surgical techniques for the prevention of recurrent variceal bleeding. Nonselective $\beta$-adrenergic receptor antagonists have been shown to decrease the number of rebleeding episodes by one-third (66% to 44%), although the small reduction in mortality in the treated groups did not achieve statistical significance (D'Amico et al. 1995). This small reduction of mortality may be more of a reflection on the severity of the inherent liver disease than the inefficacy of beta-blockers used to reduce the number of bleeding episodes. Endoscopic therapy with sclerotherapy has been shown to be as effective as therapy with nonselective $\beta$-adrenergic receptor antagonists in the prevention of rebleeding, but at a higher cost (D'Amico et al. 1995; Grace 1993). Endoscopic variceal ligation has been shown to decrease recurrent variceal bleeding and improve survival compared with sclerotherapy (Laine and Cook 1995). Combination therapy with sclerotherapy and nonselective $\beta$-adrenergic receptor antagonists (with or without long-acting nitrates) has been studied in randomized controlled trials and may offer an advantage over nonselective $\beta$-adrenergic receptor antagonists used alone (O'Connor et al. 1989). Finally, patients who rebleed after medical or endoscopic therapy may be managed by a procedure not yet subjected to rigorous study (TIPSS) or by portosystemic shunt surgery. Randomized controlled trials of shunt surgery have yielded inconsistent results (Jackson et al. 1971; Resnick et al. 1974; Rueff et al. 1976; Reynolds et al. 1981; Grace et al. 1988).

## Ascites

The development of ascites—a collection of free fluid in the peritoneal cavity—is a common clinical feature of end-stage liver disease. A combination of avid renal sodium reabsorption and a decreased "effective" arterial volume leads to an increased extracellular fluid volume. The formation of ascites in cirrhotic patients and the current hypotheses concerning the interplay among hormonal, hemodynamic, and neural mechanisms have been reviewed (Epstein 1988; Arroyo 1996).

Ascites can be associated with untoward clinical events. It is a source of significant discomfort, frequently leads to anorexia and vomiting in an already-malnourished patient, and may predispose the patient to serious bacterial infections. For these reasons, massive ascites should always be treated. Therapy for lesser degrees of ascites should be individualized because survival of the patient will depend on the seriousness of the underlying liver disease and not the presence or absence of ascites. The physician should obtain a sample of the ascitic fluid for total granulocyte count and bacterial culture at the bedside because spontaneous bacterial peritonitis can present without the usual signs and symptoms of inflammation and peritoneal irritation (Runyon et al. 1987, 1988). Granulocytic ascites should be treated presumptively for spontaneous bacterial peritonitis.

### *Medical management*

Important general measures for the management of ascites include withdrawal of potentially toxic agents (alcohol because of its direct toxic effects on the liver; nonsteroidal anti-inflammatory drugs because of their tendency to reduce the glomerular filtration rate) and adherence to a nourishing, sodium-restricted diet. Mobilization of ascites can be achieved with a negative sodium balance. Spontaneous diuresis generally ensues in most patients with new-onset ascites that spontaneously excrete relatively large amounts of sodium in the urine when they are on a sodium-restricted diet. However, these are the minority of patients with cirrhotic ascites (Bernardi et al. 1993). Very severe sodium restriction (500 mg/day or less), although in theory desirable, can make meals so unappetizing that caloric intake becomes compromised.

If the response to sodium restriction is inadequate, then the therapist may proceed to other potential therapeutic modalities with greater efficacy, but also greater risk. Therapy with diuretics is discussed elsewhere (see chapter 6, Renal Disorders and the Influence of Renal Function on Drug Disposition). Spironolactone and loop diuretics are most commonly used to treat cirrhotic ascites. Regimens that lead to a modest natriuresis (100–400 mg/day of spironolactone and/or 20–240 mg/day of furosemide or 5–20 mg/day of torsemide) are best suited for treatment of cirrhotic ascites. The goal of therapy is to produce a rate of diuresis that does not exceed the capacity for reabsorption of ascitic fluid by the systemic circulation: approximately 700–900 mL/day (Shear et al. 1970). Therapy should start with the lowest doses necessary and increase until weight loss of 0.5–1.0 kg/day is achieved. Because mobilization of fluid from peripheral edema is more efficient than from the peritoneal cavity, the 0.5–1.0 kg/day guidelines may be exceeded as long as the patient has peripheral edema.

The most significant adverse events of diuretic therapy are hepatic encephalopathy and renal failure. Encephalopathy occurs in 25% of patients hospitalized for therapy of tense ascites and has been attributed to increased renal ammonia production in the face of hypovolemia-induced alkalosis and hypokalemia (Sherlock et al. 1966). Overt renal failure occurs in 20% of cirrhotic patients hospitalized for the treatment of ascites, particularly in those with no peripheral edema (Sherlock et al. 1966; Shear et al. 1970). Hyponatremia and hypokalemia are common adverse events but are usually clinically silent. The therapist should not underestimate the toxicity of diuretic therapy; the physician should follow endpoints of efficacy (daily weight, physical exam) and toxicity (physical exam, electrolytes, renal function tests) to guide therapy. About 10% of patients with cirrhotic ascites will be resistant to diuretic therapy and will require other treatment modalities.

**PRINCIPLE The rate of improvement may determine the likelihood of toxicity. Rapid success for the physician may lead to serious trouble for the patient.**

#### *Other treatment modalities*

Large-volume paracentesis is a technique by which 4–6 L of fluid a day are removed from the peritoneal cavity in patients with massive ascites. Intravenous administration of albumin is generally used to replace protein losses gram for gram (Ginés et al. 1988). One might have predicted that the length of hospitalization and the incidence of serious acid–base or electrolyte abnormalities might be reduced in patients treated by paracentesis compared with diuretic therapy. However, a surprising finding—counter to traditional teaching—is that patients are less likely to develop azotemia and hypovolemia when therapeutic paracentesis is used (Ginés et al. 1987). Therapeutic paracentesis, either as repeated large-volume paracentesis or as total paracentesis, with concomitant plasma volume expansion with albumin, has been shown to be more effective than diuretic therapy in patients hospitalized for tense ascites (Ginés et al. 1987; Salerno et al. 1987; Titó et al. 1990). Although therapeutic paracentesis may lead to a higher rate of spontaneous bacterial peritonitis, presumably because of dilution of opsonins through direct removal and replacement with albumin (Runyon 1988), it remains the standard of therapy in the patient with diuretic-resistant ascites (Arroyo et al. 1996).

Return of ascites to the central venous circulation by reinfusion devices (extracorporeal or internal) has been proposed as treatment for massive ascites that would not result in protein losses. The best studied technique is peritoneovenous shunting achieved using Le Veen or Denver shunts, in which a tube containing a one-way valve is tunneled under the skin to connect the peritoneal cavity with a vein of the central circulation. Studies of peritoneovenous shunts compared with therapeutic paracentesis show comparable patient survival. Both techniques induce more rapid diuresis than is generally achieved with diuretics alone; however, surgical mortality and serious morbidity (e.g., massive hemorrhage, infection, premature shunt closure) in patients with serious, end-stage liver disease is appreciable in the shunted groups (Stanley et al. 1989). A peritoneovenous shunt can be considered for patients who are not liver transplant candidates and who are having serious adverse events or lack of efficacy with therapeutic paracentesis. Similarly, because TIPSS results in a lowering of portal pressures, it can be considered for a patient refractory to large-volume paracentesis. However, the only randomized clinical trial published to date reported higher mortality in the TIPSS group than in a medically treated group.

**PRINCIPLE The theoretical and intellectual appeal of a new treatment must be balanced against the well-established data concerning efficacy and toxicity of customary therapy. The eventual role of newer therapeutic modalities can become clear only as data accumulate concerning their true efficacy and toxicity.**

## Spontaneous Bacterial Peritonitis

Ascitic fluid infection is common in patients with cirrhotic ascites and advanced liver disease, and is termed spontaneous bacterial peritonitis (SBP). The prevalence of infected ascites in cirrhotic patients hospitalized with ascites has been estimated at 10 to 27% (Ginés et al. 1987). Approximately 85% of patients with infected ascites have suggestive signs or symptoms. Any deterioration in a previously stable cirrhotic patient with ascites should prompt sampling of ascitic fluid. Recurrence rates are 20 to 25% after 1 year (Singh et al. 1995).

Paracentesis can be performed safely in any cirrhotic patient without spontaneous skin or mucosal bleeding, with a complication rate of less than 1% due to bleeding, perforated viscus, or an ascitic leak. Fluid should always be sent for cell count and differential, and 10 mL each inoculated into anaerobic and aerobic culture bottles at the bedside. Ascites should be presumed to be infected, and empirical antibiotic therapy started, if the white cell count in ascitic fluid exceeds 250 cells/mm$^3$, or if the patient has signs or symptoms suggestive of infection. The Gram stain is negative in most patients with SBP; if the Gram stain is positive and many organisms are seen, GI tract perforation and secondary peritonitis must be ruled out.

Most ascitic fluid infections are caused by *Escherichia coli,* streptococci, or *Klebsiella* organisms; 1% of infections are anaerobic. Third-generation cephalosporins (cefotaxime 2 g IV q8h for 5 days) have been shown to be superior to ampicillin plus tobramycin, are predictably well distributed in ascitic fluid, and are not nephrotoxic (Felisart et al. 1985). Oral ofloxacin has shown efficacy in the uncomplicated inpatient with neutrocytic ascites (Navasa et al. 1996). Prevention of recurrent SBP, or of first episodes of SBP in patients with low-protein ascites, can be achieved by numerous regimens: daily TMP-SMZ (Singh et al. 1995), daily norfloxacin (Ginés et al. 1990), or weekly ciprofloxacin (Rolachon et al. 1995).

## Hepatic Encephalopathy

Hepatic encephalopathy (HE) is a syndrome that accompanies severe hepatic insufficiency, disorders of ammonia metabolism from inherited urea cycle enzyme deficiencies, and portosystemic shunting. It is characterized by an altered mental status. Abnormal concentrations or production of ammonia, amino acids, short-chain fatty acids, endogenous GABA receptor ligands, and false neurotransmitters, and abnormalities of the ($Na^+ + K^+$)-ATPase have been implicated in the pathogenesis of this syndrome, but no specific abnormality appears to explain all the clinical manifestations. The diagnosis of HE rests on finding symptoms and signs of a metabolic encephalopathy (impaired cognitive or motor function, asterixis, incontinence, or frank coma) in a patient with signs of serious liver disease or portal hypertension. Abnormal electroencephalograms and elevated serum ammonia and cerebrospinal glutamine concentrations are generally seen in patients with overt hepatic encephalopathy, and their presence helps support the diagnosis (Fraser and Arieff 1985). However, more subtle degrees of HE may be present in the majority of patients with cirrhosis and may only be detected by serial psychometric testing (Gitlin et al. 1986).

### *Medical management*

General therapeutic measures are important in the management of patients with HE. Endogenous or exogenous factors potentially precipitating encephalopathy must be sought and reversed. These can include nitrogen loads from azotemia or GI hemorrhage, hypokalemia, hyponatremia, alkalosis, dehydration, psychoactive drugs, dietary protein overload, constipation, and severe infections. Most patients dramatically improve after withdrawal of drugs or alcohol, treatment of infection, removal of blood from the GI tract and institution of simple support measures.

Preventive measures must be exercised in all patients with advanced liver disease. These include avoiding the use of psychoactive drugs, maintaining soft stools, and limiting protein intake if there is a history of protein intolerance.

Efficacy of treatment can best be monitored by careful staging of hepatic encephalopathy and coma. This must be performed frequently and regularly. For patients with lesser degrees of encephalopathy, standard tests of cognition and fine motor skills—as simple as asking the patient to sign his or her name or draw the face of a clock, or perform a trail test or a number connection test—can show dramatic differences over time as the severity of encephalopathy changes.

Most proven specific drug therapy is aimed at reduction of ammonia production or increased ammonia metabolism. Drugs used for this purpose may be delivered orally or by enema. Reduction of ammonia production can be achieved by dietary protein restriction, particularly with a vegetarian diet (Bianchi et al. 1993), antibiotic therapy, or poorly absorbed carbohydrates. Neomycin, an antibiotic poorly absorbed from the GI tract, may work by decreasing colonic urease activity through quantitative reduction in bowel flora (Conn et al. 1977). A recommended dosage is 2–4 g daily in divided doses. Because of its low oral bioavailability, treatment with oral neomycin is rarely complicated by ototoxicity or nephrotoxicity. However, other antibiotics such as metronidazole that inhibit bacterial urease activity may be indicated in patients with renal insufficiency (Morgan et al. 1982).

Lactulose (or other sugars that are not readily absorbed by the small bowel) can reach the colon, where it is metabolized by bacteria to small organic acids. These result in acidification of the stool, which favors conversion of ammonia to ammonium ion and traps the latter in the colonic lumen. The organic acids also stimulate an osmotic catharsis that expels the trapped ammonium. The oral dose of lactulose is titrated to cause two or three soft stools a day. Patients must be observed for severe diarrhea during treatment with lactulose. The diarrhea itself may cause dehydration or hypernatremia and aggravate the encephalopathy (Conn et al. 1977). The efficacy of lactulose is not merely due to its cathartic effect, because tap water enemas are ineffective despite a similar cleansing effect (Uribe et al. 1987). Oral lactitol or lactose (in lactase deficient patients) achieve a similar degree of efficacy, are more palatable, and may cause less flatulence (Uribe et al. 1980; Blanc et al. 1992). Similarly, substances that enhance ammonia metabolism such as sodium benzoate (10 g/day) or ornithine aspartate (27 g/day) have efficacy similar to lactulose (Herlong et al. 1980; Sushma et al. 1992).

Although substances such as flumazenil that antagonize endogenous benzodiazepines would be expected to improve patients with HE, the effects seen are transient and small in magnitude (Groeneweg et al. 1996).

#### *Nutritional support*

The finding of abnormal plasma and cerebrospinal amino acid profiles in patients with hepatic encephalopathy, and interest in the false-neurotransmitter hypothesis, has led to the use of amino acid solutions enriched with branched-chain amino acids (BCAA). The purpose of such therapy is to alter the plasma amino acid profile to one with fewer aromatic amino acids, the potential precursors of false neurotransmitters. Merely removing protein or amino acids from the diet would not cause this change because plasma amino acid concentrations depend primarily on endogenous production and metabolism. In a controlled study of BCAA solution versus neomycin in the therapy of patients with spontaneous encephalopathy, treatment with BCAA led to fewer deaths and better recovery from encephalopathy within a 14-day period of treatment (Cerra et al. 1985).

Nutritional support for the hospitalized patient with serious liver disease needs to be adjusted for the presence of encephalopathy. Patients without encephalopathy who require parenteral nutrition should be given relatively low concentrations of standard amino acid solutions, and the concentration should be increased as tolerated to deliver a total of 1–1.5 g of protein per kilogram of body weight daily. The presence of encephalopathy should lead to therapy with a BCAA-enriched formula until the patient recovers. Attempts to convert to standard amino acid formulas once the patient recovers are desirable. There is no evidence to show that prolonged therapy with BCAA is necessary as long as precipitating factors are identified and corrected (Blackburn and O'Keefe 1989).

## SPECIFIC DRUG THERAPY AIMED AT AN UNDERLYING DISEASE

### Gallstones

#### *Pathophysiology*

Gallstone disease afflicts approximately 10% of the adult population of the United States (Ingelfinger 1968). There are two distinct classes of gallstones: cholesterol stones and pigment stones. In western countries, 90% of the stones removed are either pure or mixed cholesterol stones. Cholesterol gallstones form in the gallbladder following a nucleation event that results in a nidus capable of supporting deposition and growth of cholesterol crystal. Several factors predispose patients to develop cholesterol gallstones. Bile may become supersaturated because of biliary hypersecretion of cholesterol, or hyposecretion of bile salt or lecithin. An imbalance may develop between nucleation factors (such as gallbladder mucin) and antinucleating factors yet to be characterized. Finally, impaired gallbladder function may lead to stasis and the development of biliary sludge (Holzbach 1986). The prevalence of cholesterol gallstones increases with age and is heterogeneously distributed among racial and ethnic groups. Other risk factors include female sex, massive obesity, rapid weight loss (particularly in patients using some lipid-lowering drugs [see below]), parity, ileal dysfunction, and cystic fibrosis.

Pigment stones may be brown or black (Soloway et al. 1977). Black pigment stones generally occur in patients with hereditary hemolytic disorders or other conditions that lead to decreased red blood cell survival. Brown pigment stones generally are seen in Asian women who are malnourished and have evidence of recurrent biliary tract infection.

The advent of real-time ultrasonography as a rapid and reliable screening test for the evaluation of abdominal pain and jaundice, coupled with progress in surgical and perioperative management of patients, has led to the frequent removal of diseased gallbladders containing gallstones. Approximately 500,000 cholecystectomies are performed each year in the United States. Patients with asymptomatic gallstones will not have biliary complications frequently enough to risk the potential hazard of prophylactic surgery (Gracie and Ransohoff 1982; Ransohoff et al. 1983). The same caution also applies to patients with diabetes mellitus or renal insufficiency who have asymptomatic gallstones, despite the fact that they may be at increased risk for serious morbidity or mortality should they require emergency surgery (Friedman et al. 1988).

The development of biliary colic or biliary complications occurs in about 2 to 2.6% of patients with asymptomatic gallstones yearly (Ransohoff and Gracie 1993). Once symptomatic gallbladder disease develops, the potential for serious complications (e.g., acute gangrenous cholecystitis, ascending cholangitis, common bile duct obstruction, pancreatitis) is frequent enough that specific therapy needs to be considered. Because of the safety and efficacy of cholecystectomy, it remains the treatment of choice for the vast majority of patients with symptomatic gallstones. In an otherwise healthy adult younger than 50 years old, an elective cholecystectomy can be performed with less than 0.1% mortality (Jarvinen and Hasrbacka 1980).

### *Medical treatment*

Interest in nonsurgical therapy for gallstone disease has been fueled by the small but finite number of deaths that occur each year from gallbladder surgery, by the fact that gallstone disease tends to occur with advancing age in patients with comorbid illnesses that make surgery more hazardous, and by the fact that physicians seem to understand its pathogenesis and a medical way to intercede. The recognition of the importance of bile supersaturation in the formation and growth of cholesterol gallstones has led to medical therapy specifically designed to change the physicochemical properties of bile. Both chenodeoxycholic acid (CDCA) and its $\beta$-epimer ursodeoxycholic acid (UDCA), major bile acids of humans and bears, respectively, are effective in dissolving gallstones in selected patients (Schoenfield et al. 1981; Roda et al. 1982).

Both CDCA and UDCA act by expanding the total bile acid pool and decreasing the secretion of biliary cholesterol, thereby decreasing the amount of time supersaturated bile is present in the gallbladder (Ward et al. 1984). Other bile acids such as cholic acid that fail to decrease the secretion of cholesterol into bile do not have a beneficial effect on bile lithogenicity or gallstone dissolution. CDCA also inhibits 3-hydroxy-3-methylglutaryl coenzyme A (HMG-CoA) reductase, the rate-limiting step in cholesterol biosynthesis; the same mechanism has been suggested but not proved for UDCA. CDCA inhibits the synthesis of other bile acids, whereas UDCA does not. UDCA forms a liquid-crystalline phase in the bile rather than a micellar phase.

The largest study of gallstone dissolution in the United States—the National Cooperative Gallstone Study—enrolled 916 adults who had radiolucent, noncalcified gallstones discernible on an oral cholecystogram (OCG) (Schoenfield et al. 1981). Patients were randomly allocated to receive 750 mg/day of CDCA, 375 mg/day of CDCA, or placebo for 2 years. Patients in the highest-dose group had 13.5% complete dissolution and 27% partial dissolution, using the presence of stones by OCG as the endpoint. When therapy was extended to 3 years, a total of 20% of patients treated with 750 mg/day of CDCA achieved total dissolution. Adverse effects of therapy included dose-related diarrhea that occurred in 40% of patients treated with 750 mg/day and was likely due to bile acid-induced colonic secretion of water and electrolytes. CDCA also increased the serum cholesterol concentration by 20 mg/dL, most of which was low-density lipoprotein (LDL) cholesterol. The high-density lipoprotein (HDL) cholesterol concentration was unchanged, and the triglyceride concentrations were mildly decreased. Minor elevations of aminotransferase concentrations were seen in 30% of patients receiving 750 mg/day, and clinically significant but reversible liver disease was seen in 3% of the group. Lithocholic acid, a product of intestinal bacterial $\alpha$-hydroxylation of CDCA, has been implicated in this adverse effect. Analysis of the effect of treatment on bile lithogenicity has suggested that an optimum effect is not achieved until 15 mg/kg CDCA daily is administered; at this dose one would expect more of the dose-related adverse effects than were seen at 750 mg/day.

When UDCA therapy is compared with CDCA therapy, the two drugs are equally efficacious at doses with equivalent effects on bile lithogenicity (Enrico et al. 1982; Erlinger et al. 1984; Fisher et al. 1985; Podda et al. 1989). UDCA is better tolerated by patients because it produces essentially no diarrhea, hypercholesterolemia, or abnormal liver tests. Because of its relative lack of serious adverse effects, it can be used at its optimum dose of 10 mg/kg daily and may ultimately lead to more rapid and frequent dissolution of the stones. In study populations not optimally selected, the total gallstone dissolution rate is approximately 20% at 2 years. However, the range of gallstone dissolution seen in studies of UDCA has been wide and seems to be dependent on the characteristics of the study subjects. The best results (>50% total dissolution after 12–24 months of therapy) have been seen in women with small (<15 mm) floating stones in functioning gallbladders. Stones with a small calcified nidus or an incomplete rim of calcification also may be dissolved, albeit with less success. Patients on drugs or diets that promote cholesterol saturation of bile (estrogens, cholestyramine, or clofibrate, but not lovastatin) are less likely to respond. The addition of specific inhibitors of HMG-CoA reductase may enhance the efficacy of oral bile salts, given their ability to further reduce biliary cholesterol saturation (Logan and Duane 1990).

Because medical dissolution of gallstones does not lead to removal of the diseased gallbladder, the issue of recurrence of the stones is important. About 50% of patients who have had successful dissolution of their gallstones with oral bile salt therapy have had recurrent gallstones within 5 years of discontinuation of oral bile salt therapy. Low doses of oral bile acids may not prevent recurrent gallstones. In 53 patients whose gallstones were dissolved during therapy with CDCA, subsequent therapy with either 375 mg/day of CDCA or placebo resulted in a recurrence rate of 27% during a 2- to 4.5-year follow-up period (Marks et al. 1984). Not all recurrent gallstones are symptomatic; thus whether patients whose gallstones are successfully dissolved will require lifelong therapy to prevent recurrent stones is an issue yet to be resolved. Attempts to modify other factors that contribute to stone formation such as modifying nucleating or antinucleating factors or improving gallbladder motility may play a future role in prevention of recurrence of stones.

**PRINCIPLE The efficacy and toxicity seen during short-term drug therapy should not be extrapolated to chronic drug treatment without proof. Only drug trials designed to assess efficacy and toxicity during chronic administration will give an accurate answer.**

Other nonsurgical approaches to gallstone dissolution being evaluated at this time include extracorporeal shock wave lithotripsy (ESWL) and contact dissolution with the potent cholesterol-dissolving agent methyl tert-butyl ether (MTBE) delivered by needle puncture into the gallbladder. Because ESWL can fragment large stones into smaller (and potentially more easily dissolved) fragments, it may find its role in extending the usefulness of UDCA dissolution therapy in patients with large stones or stones that have calcified rims. However, ESWL may produce fragments that are small enough to exit the gallbladder and cause bile duct or pancreatic duct obstruction; 2% of patients in the largest published series had pancreatitis. ESWL can cause damage to other organs as well; 4% of patients had gross hematuria, presumably due to contusion of the right kidney (Sackmann et al. 1988).

Dissolution with MTBE is an attractive option because of the rapidity with which gallstone dissolution may be achieved following catheterization of the gallbladder. Potential adverse effects of MTBE are those related to small-bowel delivery and absorption of the drug (duodenitis, hemolysis, general anesthesia) or to the transhepatic gallbladder puncture (bleeding, bile peritonitis) (Allen et al. 1985; Thistle 1987).

Current clinical studies suggest that patients with symptoms from gallstone that are neither severe nor life-threatening should be considered for gallstone dissolution therapy if they are older than 50 years, have a high operative risk because of associated illnesses, and have clinical and radiological features that predict a high rate of dissolution (one to three floating, radiolucent stones less than 1.5 cm in diameter in a functioning gallbladder). Therapy should be continued beyond the point of gallstone dissolution, and possibly indefinitely, in order to avoid the high rate of recurrence. It seems prudent to consider for further clinical investigation only those bile acids that increase cholesterol secretion into bile and that are not biotransformed into potentially toxic secondary bile acids.

**PRINCIPLE Studies that prove the efficacy of a drug cannot encompass all the clinical indications nor the eventual regimen that will prove to be most useful. The therapist must use all the available basic and clinical data to decide the best use of the drug in individual patients and must be able to modify use of the drug based on experience and on further postmarketing testing of the drug.**

### *Surgical intervention*

Once gallstone disease is complicated by acute cholecystitis, common bile duct obstruction, pancreatitis, or ascending cholangitis, surgical measures are often necessary to provide adequate drainage of the biliary tree. This is generally performed by removal of the gallbladder and endoscopic cholangiography, papillotomy, and extraction of stones from the common bile duct. Systemic antibiotics should be administered to patients with cholangitis in order to prevent or treat septicemia and to help sterilize the biliary tree. Antibiotics are selected to provide coverage for the organisms that generally infect the biliary tract (gram-negative bacilli and anaerobes), taking into consideration the ability of the drug to be excreted into bile. Extended-spectrum penicillins and cephalosporins have been found to be clinically useful as single-agent therapy (see also chapter 14, Infectious Diseases).

## Viral Hepatitis

General measures important in the care of patients with acute viral hepatitis include maintenance of adequate oral fluid intake and nutrition, and observation for the signs of fulminant viral hepatitis. These signs include altered mental status, the presence of ascites, and evidence of other signs of portal hypertension. If a patient is unable to keep himself or herself adequately nourished and hydrated, or if there are signs of hepatic failure, then hospitalization is necessary for adequate patient management. Antiemetics may be useful in the management of nausea and vomiting and should be administered when adequate hydration does not relieve this complaint. Strict isolation is not necessary, even in cases of viral hepatitis A and E (which are transmitted by the oral–fecal route), unless the patient is incontinent and unable to properly dispose of his or her own urine and stool. However, frequent hand washing and the use of care and gloves when handling potentially infectious material (blood, stool, other body secretions) is mandatory.

### *Hepatitis A*

The agent that causes outbreaks of water-borne or food-related fecally and orally transmitted viral hepatitis worldwide has been identified as the hepatitis A virus (HAV), a small RNA virus classified as enterovirus 72. This infection is not associated with a chronic carrier state; although the disease can be severe, it is only rarely fulminant. Reduced contamination of the water supply and improved handling of sewage have resulted in fewer children being exposed to HAV and a larger pool of adults not being immune. This loss of "herd immunity" leads to occasional outbreaks following the ingestion of contaminated food or water.

Clinically recognizable hepatitis A can be prevented in 80–90% of acutely exposed patients treated intramuscularly with 0.02 mL/kg of standard immune serum globulin (Stokes and Neefe 1945). Controlled clinical trials have supported the use of immune serum globulin having an anti-HAV titer of at least 1:2000 within 2 weeks of a household exposure. This finding should be extended to situations in which the likelihood of acute exposure to HAV is high. This includes exposures to infected children in day care centers or other group care settings, and infectious food handlers. Similarly, prophylaxis is warranted for travelers to areas with an active hepatitis A epidemic. A safe and effective vaccine made from formalin-inactivated, attenuated virus is now commercially available. It was proven to be safe and effective in the prevention of hepatitis A in children at high risk of infection in the United States. It confers immunity against infection as early as 2 weeks after the first dose of vaccine (Werzberger et al. 1992).

### *Hepatitis E*

A disease similar to hepatitis A occurring in developing countries in Asia, Africa, and Central and South America is now known to be due to the hepatitis E virus (HEV). This disease is similar in its epidemiology to hepatitis A; however, it is absent from the United States except in imported cases, and it may cause fulminant hepatitis in pregnant, malnourished women. No specific treatment is available. Although serological tests for this disease are still in the developmental stage, the prevalence of anti-HEV antibodies in blood samples from anicteric individuals living in areas where active HEV outbreaks are occurring is low. This suggests that there are relatively few anicteric cases and that immune globulin prepared from these sources may not be efficacious in preventing this disease (Ramalingaswami and Purcell 1988).

### *Hepatitis B*

Hepatitis B virus (HBV) is endemic in Asia, equatorial Africa, and the Americas. HBV infection leads to a chronic carrier rate of 5 to 10% of these populations and to serious chronic morbidity and mortality from end-stage liver disease and hepatocellular carcinoma (Weissberg et al. 1984; McMahon et al. 1990). It is transmitted from mother to child by blood contamination at the time of birth, between people of any age through intimate contact, and by percutaneous exposure to infectious blood or blood products (Alter et al. 1990). Prevention of transmission following exposure in children of HBV-carrier mothers (Stevens et al., 1987), or in settings of high risk for transmission in sexually active homosexual men (Hadler et al. 1986), has been achieved with the use of hepatitis B immune globulin (HBIG; anti-HBs titer >1:100,000) and/or the hepatitis B vaccine. The currently recommended regimen for postexposure prophylaxis is 0.06 mL/kg HBIG intramuscularly (1 mL in neonates) followed by hepatitis B vaccine at 0, 1, and 6 months.

**VACCINES** Currently available hepatitis B vaccines are made from the small hepatitis B surface antigen (HBsAg) particles extracted from the plasma of chronic carriers of the virus, or are manufactured in yeast by recombinant DNA techniques. Both vaccines stimulate antibody formation against a single determinant. About 5–10% of patients vaccinated do not develop significant titers of anti-HBs, in particular the elderly, the immunosuppressed, and patients with significant comorbid disorders. In otherwise healthy young adults, nonresponsiveness appears to be a recessive trait (Alper et al. 1989) linked to the major histocompatibility complex (MHC). This nonresponsiveness may be circumvented by the inclusion in the vaccine of highly immunogenic epitopes from the pre-S gene product large HBsAg molecule, present in very small numbers in HBV-carrier plasma, but able to be produced in large numbers in yeast by recombinant DNA techniques.

**PRINCIPLE When a fundamental mechanism of drug resistance is revealed (e.g., MHC restriction) and the molecular means to circumvent it are discovered, look for the same concept to be explored for other drugs with other indications (vaccines).**

The efficacy of both the plasma and recombinant vaccines is 90–95% in the prevention of HBV infection (Szmuness et al. 1980; Francis et al. 1982; Hadler et al. 1986). Protection against infection is correlated with antibodies to HBsAg (anti-HBs) titers above 10 IU/L (Szmuness et al. 1980; Francis et al. 1982; Hadler et al. 1986). The length of time that anti-HBs are still detectable in vaccinees is related to the peak titer of anti-HBs achieved by the vaccine. A large number of vaccinees who achieved anti-HBs titers > 10 IU/L after their initial vaccination may lose anti-HBs over the following decade; however, loss of anti-HBs is associated with continued protection against clinical hepatitis B in adults (Hadler et al. 1986) and in infants (West et al. 1994; Whittle et al. 1995). This suggests that immunity persists even after loss of anti-HBs and that protection against clinical disease, but only to a lesser degree against infection, may be prolonged or lifelong in otherwise healthy adults who achieve an initial response to the vaccine. The excellent immunogenicity and long-term clinical effectiveness of the hepatitis B vaccine argues against routine monitoring of quantitative anti-HBs titers and the use of booster injections. However, it would seem reasonable to give postexposure prophylaxis to prior recipients of the vaccine whose postvaccine anti-HBs titers were never determined and who present following a significant exposure with undetectable anti-HBs titers [Recommendations of the Immunization Practices Advisory Committee (ACIP) 1991b].

**ANTIVIRAL THERAPY** Antiviral therapy in patients with chronic hepatitis B is used to eradicate the infection and to prevent further spread of the infection and progression of the liver disease. Resolution of the infection traditionally has been defined as loss of serum HBsAg and development of anti-HBs. This definition describes a person who is felt to be no longer infectious, not likely to have abnormal aminotransferases, and not prone to further progression of their liver disease. A partial response, which results in loss of viremia but persistence of HBsAg, is also associated with improvement in symptoms, lower aminotransferases and less inflammation on the liver biopsy (Hoofnagle and DiBisceglie 1997).

Alpha interferon results in loss of serum HBV DNA in one-third of treated viremic patients, and about two-thirds of these patients will lose HBsAg over the following 5 years (Wong et al. 1993). Patients most likely to respond to interferon are those with HBV DNA levels (<100 pg/mL), high ALT levels (>200 IU/L), short duration of hepatitis, and no coinfection with HIV or HDV (Perrillo et al. 1990). Most studies show that only a small minority of patients who lose HBeAg and HBV DNA with interferon alpha-2b treatment reactivate their infection over time. For those whose disease failed to respond to interferon, retreatment with interferon or increasing the dose or length of treatment has not been shown to improve the overall response to treatment significantly.

Treatment with interferon may result in a flare, which includes a transient twofold or greater increase in aminotransferase levels, usually during the second or third month of therapy. This flare is felt to represent an interferon-induced activation of the immune system and a rapid lysis of hepatocytes infected with hepatitis B virus. This flare is seen twice as commonly in patients who respond to interferon treatment as in nonresponders. During the flare, patients may experience symptoms or signs of liver disease. Patients with advanced stages of liver disease may experience decompensation (hepatic encephalopathy, sterile or infected ascites, variceal bleeding, or death) (Nevens et al. 1993). Treatment should in general be limited to patients with well-compensated liver disease, as the decompensated patient will experience potentially life-threatening complications. During a flare, interferon therapy should be continued as tolerated, and the patient should be monitored more frequently. Treatment with interferon should cease if significant adverse effects or any evidence of decompensation occurs during a flare (Perrillo et al. 1995).

Adverse effects of interferon are common. They include fevers, chills, myalgias, headache, and anorexia, which occur soon after the first injection. They occur in nearly all patients treated with regimens that have been proven effective. Bone marrow suppression, hair loss, depression, irritability, and confusion can occur after days to weeks of therapy, as can immune adverse effects such as thyroiditis, arthritis, and hepatitis. Despite the many adverse effects, interferon is relatively well tolerated, and more than 90% of patients do not need dose adjustments or discontinuation of standard-dose therapy (Perrillo et al. 1990).

There are no other treatments that have been proven to be of long-term benefit to patients with chronic hepatitis B. However, there are many agents for which pilot studies suggest activity against hepatitis B virus that may become important management options or the basis for combination therapy in the future. These agents under investigation for the patient who does not respond to interferon include nucleoside analogs (Trepo et al. 1997; Dienstag et al. 1995), immunomodulators, and DNA or protein immunization techniques.

The best studied is lamivudine, a 2′,3′-dideoxy cytosine analog. Short-term therapy (25, 100, or 300 mg daily for 12 weeks) has been associated with a profound suppression of HBV replication of rapid onset, which was sustained for the length of the study and associated with loss of HBeAg in 12% of study subjects (Dienstag et al. 1995). Cessation of therapy was generally accompanied by return of serum HBV DNA to pretreatment levels, although a small number of patients had a sustained loss of HBV DNA (19%) or HBeAg (12%), and normalization of ALT. Subsequent pilot studies have confirmed these observations. A randomized controlled trial with 6 or 12 months of therapy with either 25 or 100 mg of lamivudine daily documented improvement in histology in 66% and 58% of treated patients versus 30% of placebo recipients (Lai et al. 1997). Drug-resistant mutants were isolated from 15% of treated patients, their appearance usually accompanied by a rise in serum HBV DNA levels. Patients with HIV infection being treated with combination nucleoside analog and protease inhibitor therapy, as well as immunosuppressed organ transplant recipients, can respond to lamivudine with loss or marked fall of detectable serum HBV DNA. The drug is well-tolerated and rapidly absorbed after oral administration; serious side effects are rare and may include anemia, neutropenia, elevated aminotransferases, and peripheral neuropathy.

**LIVER TRANSPLANTATION** Liver transplantation had been previously avoided in patients with chronic hepatitis B. Studies from the University of Pittsburgh showed nearly universal HBV recurrence and an accelerated postoperative injury frequently resulting in liver failure and death. A 20% excess mortality attributable to HBV recurrence was seen, and a frequently fatal fibrosing cholestatic syndrome was described. However, data from a multicenter study in France suggested that postoperative HBIG infusion can prevent recurrence of infection and disease in >80% of patients, independent of the presence or level of serum HBV DNA (Samuel et al. 1993). Our current policy is the use of 45 mL (10,000 IU) of HBIG IV daily for the first seven postoperative days, then every 6 to 8 weeks as required to maintain an anti-HBs titer greater than 1:150. This policy has resulted in no recurrent HBV in the last 12 patients with liver transplants. Patients with infections with precore mutants (HBeAg negative, HBV DNA positive) may have a worse prognosis because of a higher rate of recurrent disease. Recurrent HBV infection should probably be treated with lamivudine or famciclovir; up to 30% of patients may respond to interferon alfa (Bartholomew et al. 1997).

### *Hepatitis D*

Hepatitis B can be complicated by simultaneous infection with the hepatitis D virus (HDV), a small RNA virus most closely related to viroids of plants. This virus is defective and requires simultaneous hepatitis B infection for infection and multiplication in most hosts. Hepatitis D infection is frequently associated with a rapidly progressive chronic active hepatitis or cirrhosis, or with a fulminant acute presentation. There are no known preventive measures, other than avoiding sexual contact with people with HDV infection or their blood products. Treatment with $\alpha$-interferon is not effective in the HDV–HBV coinfected patient (Di Marco et al. 1996).

### *Hepatitis C*

The hepatitis C virus (HCV), an RNA virus similar to flaviviruses, was isolated and characterized from the plasma of a chimpanzee infected with a plasma concentrate known to have transmitted non-A non-B hepatitis to humans (Kuo et al. 1989). HCV infection is a major public health problem. The overall prevalence of chronic hepatitis C infection is 1.8%, with estimates of about 4 million Americans infected with HCV. Death from chronic hepatitis C occurs in over 8000 patients in the United States each year, generally from hepatocellular carcinoma or from complications of cirrhosis (Alter and Mast 1994). Hepatitis C generally follows a parenteral exposure to infected blood or blood products; it is transmitted less effectively by nonparenteral routes. Greater than 85% of patients with acute hepatitis C will develop a persistent infection and chronic hepatitis on liver biopsy. Most patients have abnormal aminotransferases (ALT) and have detectable serum HCV RNA and chronic hepatitis on liver biopsy. About one-third of patients with persistent HCV infection have a persistently normal ALT; they can be distinguished from the 15% of infected patients that clear HCV spontaneously by the presence of serum HCV RNA. Cross-sectional studies of patients with chronic HCV infection suggest that about 20–25% of patients will eventually develop cirrhosis, usually after an average of 20–30 years from the time of infection (Tong et al. 1995). The established risk factors for the development of increased rates of fibrosis include alcohol use of more than 50 g/day, male gender, long-term infection, and age of onset of infection of 40 years or older (Poynard et al. 1997). Once cirrhosis is present, the probability of decompensation (variceal bleeding, ascites, or encephalopathy) is about 4% per year, and the probability of developing hepatocellular carcinoma is about 1.5% per year (Fattovich et al. 1997).

**DRUG THERAPY** Therapy with $\alpha$-interferon has limited success in chronic hepatitis C (Hoofnagle and Di-

Bisceglie 1997). Interpretation of the literature is hampered by different measures of success used in the treatment trials. To compare efficacy across different studies and populations, it is important to agree on the measures of success. The most rigorous is the loss of serum HCV RNA that lasts at least 6 months following the cessation of therapy, which has been termed a virological sustained response. Patients who fulfill this definition of success 6 months after the end of interferon therapy have a 96% likelihood of having no detectable serum HCV RNA at 1–8 years after therapy and will demonstrate an improved hepatic activity index on follow-up liver biopsies. Treatment is recommended for patients with persistently elevated aminotransferases for more than 6 months, a positive serum HCV RNA assay, and a liver biopsy specimen demonstrating either portal or bridging fibrosis and at least moderate degrees of inflammation (NIH Consensus Development Conference Panel Statement 1997).

Approximately 22% of all patients treated with $\alpha$-interferon 3 MU TIW for 12–18 months or consensus interferon 9–15 $\mu$g TIW for 12–18 months will have sustained loss of serum HCV RNA and normalization of ALT (Poynard et al. 1995). More than 95% of patients treated with interferon who will achieve sustained loss of virus will lose serum HCV RNA by the end of the third month of therapy; this has led to a policy of stopping therapy after 3 months if this goal cannot be reached. Factors associated with a greater rate of response to interferon include absence of cirrhosis, genotype 2 or 3, and a low viral titer. Whether therapy delays the onset of primary liver cancer or affects the natural history of chronic hepatitis C is still debated.

Ribavirin is a synthetic nucleoside analogue that has activity against many DNA and RNA viruses. Combination therapy with interferon 3 MU TIW and 1000–1200 mg/day of ribavirin increased the sustained response rate from 6% to 43% in the initial therapy of Taiwanese noncirrhotic patients with chronic hepatitis C (Lai et al. 1996). Other studies have shown an improved response with combination therapy, albeit less dramatic; a Swedish multicenter study showed an increase in response rate from 18% to 36% that was genotype specific (range 19–52%) (Reichard et al. 1998). In this study, patients treated with ribavirin had more GI adverse effects and had a unique adverse effect of reversible hemolytic anemia. Cough, rash, and pruritus have also been associated with ribavirin use.

## Alcoholic Liver Disease

Alcohol consumption greater than 80 g/day for 15 years or more has been associated with the development of clinically significant liver disease. The major pathological manifestations of alcohol-induced liver injury are fatty liver, alcoholic hepatitis, cirrhosis, and hepatocellular carcinoma. The death rate from alcoholic liver disease in a given country is proportional to the consumption of alcohol. In individuals with alcoholic liver disease, prognosis deteriorates once severe clinical manifestations of the disease occur. Patients with alcoholic liver disease have at least a 35% death rate during the year following their first episode of jaundice, ascites, or hematemesis (Graham and Smith 1981). Longer survival is seen in those who abstain from alcohol. Therefore, the most important treatment modality for patients with alcoholic liver disease is lifelong abstinence, and all other potential treatments must be considered adjunctive therapy.

Because alcohol metabolism mediated by alcohol dehydrogenase leads to production of acetaldehyde, the pathogenesis of alcohol-related liver injury has generally been attributed to direct or indirect effects of acetaldehyde, a toxic metabolite that readily forms protein adducts that interfere with enzymes and repair mechanisms, and promote collagen deposition (Lieber 1998). The enhanced bioavailability of alcohol in women and certain individuals can be related to gender and ethnic differences in gastric alcohol dehydrogenase (Lieber 1998). However, because the actual mechanism of hepatocellular injury is unknown, recent trials have embarked on empirical therapy based on theoretical mechanisms of injury that may never be proved correct.

One must distinguish between attempts at reducing mortality in patients with acute exacerbations of alcoholic liver disease and attempts to halt progression of chronic alcoholic liver disease. The former requires general measures of care for critically ill patients and the possibility of prednisolone therapy in selected patients with serious acute alcoholic hepatitis. The latter includes attempts to reduce injury and resultant fibrosis. Corticosteroids, colchicine, and propylthiouracil (PTU) have been studied in randomized clinical trials as potential therapies for alcoholic liver disease.

**ACUTE ALCOHOLIC HEPATITIS** In patients with acute alcoholic hepatitis, corticosteroids have been repeatedly studied because of their potential effects on mediators of inflammation and fibrogenesis. Data supporting their use have been mixed; a randomized, placebo-controlled multicenter study of 263 patients showed no efficacy of prednisolone (Mendenhall et al. 1984). The same study suggested a long-term but no short-term benefit associated with use of oxandrolone (80 mg/day for 1 month). Because of the possibility that failure to demonstrate efficacy was due to the presence of an overwhelming number of patients with a favorable clinical outcome in the studies to date, another multicenter, randomized, placebo-controlled study was designed. The purpose was to enroll only those patients predicted to have a high 30-day mortality because of the presence of high concentrations of serum bilirubin, markedly prolonged prothrombin time and/or the presence of spontaneous hepatic encephalopathy (Carithers et al. 1989). The 30-day mortality was 2/35 in the treatment group versus 11/31 in the control group, and the improved survival was seen in the group with encephalopathy. A study treating only the sickest patients with acute alcoholic hepatitis found a more striking treatment advantage (Ramond et al. 1992). However, few patients seen in a standard practice with acute severe alcoholic hepatitis would fit the study criteria under which these patients were enrolled because it excluded patients with systemic infections, diabetes, pancreatitis, and GI bleeding. These are frequent precipitants or comorbid conditions in acute alcoholic hepatitis.

The use of PTU in patients with alcoholic hepatitis arises from the suggestion that a hypermetabolic state making the centrilobular area of the liver relatively susceptible to ischemic or toxic damage is fundamental to the pathogenesis of alcoholic liver disease and its characteristic early lesion of perivenular fibrosis. In hospitalized patients with mild-to-moderate alcoholic hepatitis, administration of 300 mg/day of PTU did not result in decreased mortality (7/31 in the treatment group versus 7/36 in placebo recipients) or improved tests of liver function (Halle et al. 1982). However, in a randomized, placebo-controlled study of 310 outpatients with various degrees of alcoholic liver injury, a significant survival advantage was seen in the PTU treatment group over the placebo group, despite continued alcohol ingestion (Orrego et al. 1987). The high dropout rate in this study led to insufficient data for analysis of the effect on tests of liver function.

**ALCOHOLIC CIRRHOSIS** Colchicine is a relatively safe drug when used over years of continual treatment. It is relatively inexpensive and has been shown to inhibit in vitro fibrogenesis. It was studied in Mexico City in a randomized, placebo-controlled trial of 100 patients with predominantly alcoholic cirrhosis (Kershenobich et al. 1988). Patients who received 1 mg/day of colchicine had a median survival of 11 years; those randomized to placebo had a median survival of 3.5 years. Enhanced survival was accompanied by histological improvement as determined by follow-up needle biopsies of the liver. Interpretation of the data from this study is made difficult by high rates of noncompliance and dropout and by persistent use of alcohol in both groups. Also, a lower serum albumin concentration in the control group at baseline may indicate failure of randomization to balance treatment and placebo groups with respect to this important marker of the severity of liver disease.

Until more definitive studies are conducted in patients with similar conditions, the therapist must make a decision for his or her patients based on inconclusive and conflicting data. One may consider the relatively safe and inexpensive therapy with colchicine in patients with chronic stable alcoholic cirrhosis as an adjunct to abstinence and await further data on steroids and antithyroid drugs. One may also identify a subgroup of patients who are likely to have a poor prognosis (such as those with acute severe alcoholic hepatitis with spontaneous hepatic encephalopathy) and choose to treat them with prednisolone because it is the drug with most promise in this setting.

Because the effects of these three drugs on tests of liver function or other predictors of success is still unclear, one is faced with the use of potentially harmful drugs without the ability to individualize drug dosage, minimize adverse effects, or monitor efficacy.

**PRINCIPLE Physicians almost never have information adequate to optimize therapy. The clinician can gain some solace in knowing that more information is coming and that a number of answers will involve new indications for old drugs (e.g., colchicine, PTU, corticosteroids for cirrhosis; aspirin for myocardial infarction). When experimental results are conflicting and final conclusions are unclear, choose the least toxic drug and monitor the patient carefully. Be prepared to change the therapeutic plan as new or confirmed data are published.**

## Acknowledgment

I am indebted to Drs. James L. Boyer and L. Frederick Fenster, whose section on hepatic disorders in a prior edition of this textbook inspired and formed the framework for the current chapter.

## REFERENCES

Allen MJ, Borody TJ, Bugliosi TF, et al. 1985. Rapid dissolution of gallstones by methyl tert-butyl ether: preliminary observations. *N Engl J Med* **312**:217–20.

Alper C, Kruskall M, Marcus-Bagley D, et al. 1989. Genetic prediction of nonresponse to hepatitis B vaccine. *N Engl J Med* **321**:707–12.

Alter MJ, Hadler SC, Margolis HS, et al. 1990. The changing epidemiology of hepatitis B in the United States: need for alternative vaccination strategies. *JAMA* **263**:1218–22.

Alter MJ, Mast EE. 1994. The epidemiology of viral hepatitis in the United States. *Gastroenterol Clin North Am* **23**:437–55.

Andreani T, Poupon RE, Balkau B, et al. 1990. Preventive therapy of first gastrointestinal bleeding in patients with cirrhosis: results of a controlled trial comparing propranolol, endoscopic sclerotherapy and placebo. *Hepatology* **12**:1412–9.

Arimura A, Sato H, Dupont A, et al. 1975. Somatostatin: abundance of immunoreactive hormone in rat stomach and pancreas. *Science* **189**:1007–9.

Arroyo V, Ginés P, Gerbes AL, et al. 1996. Definition and diagnostic criteria of refractory ascites and hepatorenal syndrome in cirrhosis. *Hepatology* **23**:164–76.

Bagarani M, Albertini V, Anza M, et al. 1987. Effect of somatostatin in controlling bleeding from esophageal varices. *Ital J Surg Sci* **17**:21–6.

Baker L, Smith C, Lieberman G. 1959. The natural history of esophageal varices. *Am J Med* **26**:228–37.

Bartholomew MM, Jansen RW, Jeffers LJ, et al. 1997. Hepatitis B virus resistance to lamivudine given for recurrent infection after orthotopic liver transplantation. *Lancet* **349**:20–22.

Bassett ML, Halliday JW, Powell LW. 1980. Hemochromatosis—Newer concepts: diagnosis and management. *Dis Mon* 26:1–44.

Beppu K, Inokuchi K, Koyanagi N, et al. 1981. Prediction of variceal hemorrhage by esophageal endoscopy. *Gastrointest Endosc* **27**:213–8.

Bernardi M, Di Marco C, Trevisani F, et al. 1993. Renal sodium retention during upright posture in preascitic cirrhosis. *Gastroenterology* **105**:188–93.

Besson I, Ingrand P, Person B, et al. 1995. Sclerotherapy with or without octreotide for acute variceal bleeding. *N Engl J Med* **333**:555–60.

Bianchi GP, Marchesini G, Fabbri A, et al. 1993. Vegetable versus animal protein diet in cirrhotic patients with chronic encephalopathy: a randomized cross-over comparison. *J Intern Med* **233**:385–92.

Blackburn G, O'Keefe S. 1989. Nutrition in liver failure. *Gastroenterology* **97**:1049–51.

Blanc P, Daures JP, Rouillon JM, et al. 1992. Lactitol or lactulose in the treatment of chronic hepatic encephalopathy: results of a meta-analysis. *Hepatology* **15**:222–8.

Bosch J, Groszmann RJ, Garcia-Pagan JC, et al. 1989. Association of transdermal nitroglycerin to vasopressin infusion in the treatment of variceal hemorrhage: a placebo-controlled clinical trial. *Hepatology* **10**:962–8.

Bosch J, Kravetz D, Rodes J. 1981. Effects of somatostatin on hepatic and systemic hemodynamics in patients with cirrhosis of the liver: comparison with vasopressin. *Gastroenterology* **80**:518–25.

Brazeau P, Vale W, Burgus R, et al. 1973. Hypothalamic polypeptide that inhibits the secretion of immunoreactive pituitary growth hormone. *Science* **179**:77–9.

Bunton G, Cameron R. 1963. Regeneration of liver after biliary cirrhosis. *Ann NY Acad Sci* **111**:412–21.

Burroughs AK, McCormick PA, Hughes MD, et al. 1990. Randomized double-blind placebo-controlled trial of somatostatin for variceal bleeding: emergency control and prevention of early variceal bleeding. *Gastroenterology* **99**:1388–95.

Carithers RL, Herlong HR, Diehl AM, et al. 1989. Methylprednisolone therapy in patients with severe alcoholic hepatitis: a randomized multicenter trial. *Ann Intern Med* **110**:685–92.

Cello J, Grendell J, Crass R, et al. 1987. Endoscopic sclerotherapy versus portacaval shunt in patients with severe cirrhosis and acute variceal hemorrhage. *N Engl J Med* **316**:11–5.

Cerra FB, Cheung NK, Fischer JE, et al. 1985. Disease-specific amino acid infusion (F080) in hepatic encephalopathy: a prospective, randomized, double-blind, controlled trial. *J Parenter Enter Nutr* **9**:288–95.

Chojkier M, Groszmann RJ, Atterburg CE. 1979. A controlled comparison of continuous intra-arterial and intravenous infusions of vasopressin in hemorrhage from esophageal varices. *Gastroenterology* **77**:540–6.

Conn HO, Grace ND, Bosch J, et al. 1991. Propranolol in the prevention of the first hemorrhage from esophageal varices: Results of a randomized double blind cooperative clinical trial. *Hepatology* **13**:902–12.

Conn HO, Leevy CM, Vlahcevic ZR, et al. 1977. Comparison of lactulose and neomycin in the treatment of chronic portal–systemic encephalopathy: a double-blind controlled trial. *Gastroenterology* **72**:573–83.

Conn HO, Ramsby GR, Starer EM. 1975. Intra-arterial vasopressin in the treatment of upper gastrointestinal hemorrhage: a prospective, controlled trial. *Gastroenterology* **68**:211–21.

D'Amico G, Pagliaro L, Bosch J. 1995. The treatment of portal hypertension: a meta-analytic review. *Hepatology* **22**:332–54.

Dienstag JL, Perrillo RP, Schiff ER, et al. 1995. A preliminary trial of lamivudine for chronic hepatitis B infection. *N Engl J Med* **333**:1657–61.

Di Marco V, Giacchino R, Timitilli A. 1996. Long-term interferon-alpha treatment of children with chronic hepatitis delta: A multicentre study. *J Viral Hepat* **3**:123–8.

du Vigneaud V, Gish D, Katsoyannis P. 1954. A synthetic preparation possessing biological properties associated with arginine vasopressin. *J Am Chem Soc* **76**:4751–2.

Enrico R, Bazzoli F, Labate A, et al. 1982. Ursodeoxycholic acid vs. chenodeoxycholic acid as cholesterol gallstone-dissolving agents: a comparative randomized study. *Hepatology* **2**:804–9.

Epstein, M. 1992. *The Kidney in Liver Disease*. Philadelphia: Hanley & Belfus. pp 75–108.

Erlinger S, Le Go A, Husson J, et al. 1984. Franco-Belgian Cooperative Study of ursodeoxycholic acid in the medical dissolution of gallstones: a double-blind, randomized, dose-response study, and comparison with chenodeoxycholic acid. *Hepatology* **4**:308–14.

Fattovich G, Giustina G, Degos F, et al. 1997. Morbidity and mortality in compensated cirrhosis type C: a retrospective follow-up study of 384 patients. *Gastroenterology* **112**:463–72.

Felisart J, Rimola A, Arroyo V, et al. 1985. Randomized comparative study of efficacy and nephrotoxicity of ampicillin plus tobramycin versus cefotaxime in cirrhotics with severe infections. *Hepatology* **5**:457–62.

Fisher MM, Roberts EA, Rosen IE, et al. 1985. The Sunnybrook Gallstone Study: A double-blind controlled trial of chenodeoxycholic acid for gallstone dissolution. *Hepatology* **5**:102–7.

Fogel MR, Knauer CM, Andres LL, et al. 1982. Continuous intravenous vasopressin in active upper gastrointestinal bleeding. *Ann Intern Med* **96**:565–9.

Francis DP, Hadler SC, Thompson SE, et al. 1982. The prevention of hepatitis B with vaccine: report of the centers for disease control multi-center efficacy trial among homosexual men. *Ann Intern Med* **97**:362–6.

Fraser CL, Arieff AI. 1985. Hepatic encephalopathy. *N Engl J Med* **313**:865–73.

Freeman JG, Cobden I, Lishman AH, et al. 1982. Controlled trial of terlipressin (Glypressin) versus vasopressin in the early treatment of oesophageal varices. *Lancet* **2**:66–8.

Friedman LS, Roberts MS, Brett AS, et al. 1988. Management of asymptomatic gallstones in the diabetic patient: a decision analysis. *Ann Intern Med* **109**:913–9.

Garcia-Tsao G, Groszmann RJ, Fisher RI, et al. 1985. Portal pressure predicts presence of gastroesophageal varices and variceal bleeding. *Hepatology* **5**:419–24.

Gelman S, Ernst E. 1979. Nitroprusside prevents adverse hemodynamic effects of vasopressin. *Arch Surg* **113**:1465–71.

Gimson AE, Westaby D, Hegarty J, et al. 1986. A randomized trial of vasopressin and vasopressin plus nitroglycerin in the control of acute variceal hemorrhage. *Hepatology* **6**:410–3.

Ginés P, Arroyo V, Quintero E, et al. 1987. Comparison of paracentesis and diuretics in the treatment of cirrhotics with tense ascites: results of a randomized study. *Gastroenterology* **92**:234–41.

Ginés P, Rimola A, Planas R, et al. 1990. Norfloxacin prevents spontaneous bacterial peritonitis recurrence in cirrhosis: results of a double-blind, placebo-controlled trial. *Hepatology* **12**:716–24.

Ginés P, Titó L, Arroyo V, et al. 1988. Randomized comparative study of therapeutic paracentesis with and without intravenous albumin in cirrhosis. *Gastroenterology* **94**:1493–1502.

Gitlin N, Lewis DC, Hinkley L. 1986. The diagnosis and prevalence of subclinical hepatic encephalopathy in apparently healthy, ambulant, nonshunted patients with cirrhosis. *J Hepatol* **3**:75–82.

Grace ND. 1993. Management of portal hypertension. *Gastroenterologist* **1**:39–58.

Grace ND, Conn HO, Resnick RH, et al. 1988. Distal splenorenal versus portal–systemic shunts after hemorrhage from varices: a randomized controlled trial. *Hepatology* **8**:1475–81.

Gracie W, Ransohoff D. 1982. The natural history of silent gallstones: the innocent gallstone is not a myth. *N Engl J Med* **307**:798–816.

Graham DY, Smith JL. 1981. The course of patients after variceal hemorrhage. *Gastroenterology* **80**:800–9.

Groeneweg M, Gyr K, Amrein R, et al. 1996. Effect of flumazenil on the electroencephalogram of patients with portosystemic encephalopathy: results of a double blind, randomized, placebo-controlled multicentre trial. *Electroencephalogr Clin Neurophysiol* **98**:29–34.

Groszmann RJ, Kravetz D, Bosch J, et al. 1982. Nitroglycerin improves the hemodynamic response to vasopressin in portal hypertension. *Hepatology* **2**:757–62.

Hadler SC, Francis DP, Maynard JE, et al. 1986. Long-term immunogenicity and efficacy of hepatitis B vaccine in homosexual men. *N Engl J Med* **315**:209–14.

Halle P, Pare P, Kaptein E, et al. 1982. Double-blind, controlled trial of propylthiouracil in patients with severe acute alcoholic hepatitis. *Gastroenterology* **82**(5, pt. 1):925–31.

Herlong HF, Maddrey WC, Walser M. 1980. The use of ornithine salts of branched-chain ketoacids in portal–systemic encephalopathy. *Ann Intern Med* **93**:545–50.

Holzbach R. 1986. Recent progress in understanding cholesterol crystal nucleation as a precursor to human gallstone formation. *Hepatology* **6**:1403–46.

Hoofnagle JH, DiBisceglie AM. 1997. The treatment of chronic viral hepatitis. *N Engl J Med* **336**:347–56.

Hsia D, Walker F. 1961. Variability in the clinical manifestations of galactosemia. *J Pediatr* **59**:872–83.

Hsia HC, Lee FY, Tsai YT, et al. 1990. Comparison of somatostatin and vasopressin in the control of acute esophageal variceal hemorrhage: a randomized controlled study. *Chin J Gastroenterol* **7**:71–8.

Huizinga W. 1985. Esophageal transection versus injection sclerotherapy in the management of bleeding esophageal varices in patients at high risk. *Surg Gynecol Obstet* **160**:539–46.

Hwang SJ, Lin HC, Chang CF, et al. 1992. A randomized controlled trial comparing octreotide and vasopressin in the control of acute esophageal variceal bleeding. *J Hepatol* **16**:320–5.

Ideo G, Bellati G, Fesce E, et al. 1988. Nadolol can prevent the first gastrointestinal bleeding in cirrhosis: a prospective, randomized study. *Hepatology* **8**:6–9.

Infante R, Esnaola S, Villeneuve J. 1989. Role of endoscopic variceal sclerotherapy in the long-term management of variceal bleeding: a meta-analysis. *Gastroenterology* **96**:1087–92.

Ingelfinger FJ. 1968. Digestive disease as a national problem: V. Gallstones. *Gastroenterology* **55**:102–4.

Inokuchi K, et al. 1990. Improved survival after prophylactic portal nondecompression surgery for esophageal varices: a randomized clinical trial. Cooperative Study Group of Portal Hypertension of Japan. *Hepatology* **12**:1–6.

Jackson FC, Perrin EB, Smith AG, et al. 1971. A clinical investigation of the portacaval shunt: II. Survival analysis of the therapeutic operation. *Ann Surg* **174**:672–701.

Jarvinen H, Hasrbacka J. 1980. Early cholecystectomy for acute cholecystitis: a prospective randomized study. *Ann Surg* **191**:501–5.

Jenkins SA, Baxter JN, Corbett W, et al. 1985. A prospective randomized controlled clinical trial comparing somatostatin and vasopressin in controlling acute variceal hemorrhage. *Br Med J* **290**:275–8.

Kershenobich D, Vargas F, Garcia-Tsao G. 1988. Colchicine in the treatment of cirrhosis of the liver. *N Engl J Med* **318**:1709–13.

Kravetz D, Bosch J, Teres J, et al. 1984. Comparison of intravenous somatostatin and vasopressin infusions in treatment of acute variceal hemorrhage. *Hepatology* **4**:442–6.

Kuo G, Choo QL, Alter HJ, et al. 1989. An assay for circulating antibodies to a major etiologic virus of human non-A, non-B hepatitis. *Science* **244**:362–4.

Lai CL, Liaw YF, Leung NWY, et al. 1997. 12 months of lamivudine (100 mg od) therapy improves liver histology: results of a placebo controlled multicenter study in Asia. *J Hepatol* **26**:79.

Lai MY, Kao JH, Yang PM, et al. 1996. Long-term efficacy of ribavirin plus interferon alfa in the treatment of chronic hepatitis C. *Gastroenterology* **111**:1307–12.

Laine L, Cook D. 1995. Endoscopic ligation compared with sclerotherapy for treatment of esophageal variceal bleeding: a meta-analysis. *Ann Intern Med* **123**:280–7.

Laine L, El-Newihi LM, Migikovsky B. 1993. Endoscopic ligation compared with sclerotherapy for the treatment of bleeding esophageal varices. *Ann Int Med* **119**:1–7.

Lebrec D, Poynard T, Bernuau J, et al. 1984. A randomized controlled study of propranolol for prevention of recurrent gastrointestinal bleeding in patients with cirrhosis: a final report. *Hepatology* **4**:355–8.

Lebrec D, Poynard T, Capron JP, et al. 1988. Nadolol for prophylaxis of gastrointestinal bleeding in patients with cirrhosis: a randomized trial. *J Hepatol* **7**:118–25.

Lewis JH, Zimmerman HJ, Garrett CT, et al. 1982. Valproate-induced hepatic steatogenesis in rats. *Hepatology* **2**:870–3.

Lieber C. 1998. Hepatic and other medical disorders of alcoholism. *J Stud Alcohol* **59**:9–25.

Lo GH, Lai KH, Cheng JS, et al. 1995. A prospective, randomized trial of sclerotherapy versus ligation in the management of bleeding esophageal varices. *Hepatology* **22**:466–71.

Logan GM, Duane WC. 1990. Lovastatin added to ursodeoxycholic acid further reduces biliary cholesterol saturation. *Gastroenterology* **98**:1572–8.

MacDougall B, Bailey R, Williams R. 1977. $H_2$ receptor antagonists and antacids in the prevention of acute gastrointestinal hemorrhage in fulminant hepatic failure, two controlled trials. *Lancet* **1**:617–9.

Mallory A, Schaeffer JU, Cohen JR. 1980. Selective intra-arterial vasopressin infusion for upper gastrointestinal hemorrhage: a controlled trial. *Arch Surg* **115**:30–2.

Marks J, Lan S, National Cooperative Gallstone Study Committee. 1984. Low dose chenodiol for the prevention of gallstone recurrence following dissolution therapy: The National Cooperative Gallstone Study. *Ann Intern Med* **100**:376–81.

McCormick PA, Kaye GL, Greenslade L, et al. 1992. Esophageal staple transection as a salvage procedure after failure of acute injection sclerotherapy. *Hepatology* **15**:403–6.

McMahon BJ, Alberts R, Wainwright RB, et al. 1990. Hepatitis B-related sequelae. Prospective study in 1400 hepatitis B surface antigen-related sequelae. *Arch Intern Med* **150**:1051–4.

Mendenhall C, Anderson S, Garcia-Pont P. 1984. Short-term and long-term survival in patients with alcoholic hepatitis treated with oxandrolone and prednisolone. *N Engl J Med* **311**:1464–9.

Merigan TC Jr, Plotkin GR, Davidson CS. 1962. Effect of intravenously administered posterior pituitary extract on hemorrhage from bleeding esophageal varices. *N Engl J Med* **266**:134–5.

Mohle-Boetani J, Akula SK, Holodnyi M, et al. 1992. The sulfone syndrome in a patient receiving dapsone prophylaxis for *Pneumocystis carinii* pneumonia. *West J Med* **156**:303–6.

Morgan MH, Read AE, Speller DCE. 1982. Treatment of hepatic encephalopathy with metronidazole. *Gut* **23**:1–7.

Navasa M, Follo A, Llovet JM, et al. 1996. Randomized, comparative study of oral ofloxacin versus intravenous cefotaxime in spontaneous bacterial peritonitis. *Gastroenterology* **111**:1011–7.

Nevens F, Goubau P, Van Eyken P, et al. 1993. Treatment of decompensated viral hepatitis B-induced cirrhosis with low doses of interferon alpha. *Liver* **13**:15–9.

NIH Consensus Development Conference Panel Statement. 1997. Management of hepatitis C. *Hepatology* **26**:2S–11S.

O'Connor KW, Lehman G, Yune H, et al. 1989. Comparison of three nonsurgical treatments for bleeding esophageal varices. *Gastroenterology* **96**:899–906.

O'Donnell L, Heaton K. 1988. Recurrence and re-recurrence of gall stones after medical dissolution: a long-term follow-up. *Gut* **29**:655–8.

Orrego H, Blake J, Blendis L, et al. 1987. Long-term treatment of alcoholic liver disease with propylthiouracil. *N Engl J Med* **317**:1421–7.

Pascal JP, Cales P, Multicenter Study Group. 1987. Propranolol in the prevention of first upper gastrointestinal tract hemorrhage in patients with cirrhosis of the liver and esophageal varices. *N Engl J Med* **317**:856–61.

Perrillo R, Tamburro C, Regenstein F, et al. 1995. Low-dose, titratable interferon alfa in decompensated liver disease caused by chronic infection with hepatitis B virus. *Gastroenterology* **109**:908–16.

Perrillo RP, Schiff ER, Davis GL, et al. 1990 . A randomized, controlled trial of interferon alfa-2b alone and after prednisone withdrawal for the treatment of chronic hepatitis B. The Hepatitis Interventional Therapy Group. *N Engl J Med* Aug **323**:295–301.

Podda M, Zuin M, Battezzati PM, et al. 1989. Efficacy and safety of a combination of chenodeoxycholic acid and ursodeoxycholic acid for gallstone dissolution: a comparison with ursodeoxycholic acid alone. *Gastroenterology* **96**:222–9.

Poynard T, Bedossa P, Chevallier M, et al. 1995. A comparison of three interferon alfa-1b regimens for the long-term treatment of chronic non-A, non-B hepatitis. *N Engl J Med* **332**:1457–62.

Poynard T, Bedossa P, Opolon P. 1997. Natural history of liver fibrosis progression in patients with chronic hepatitis C. *Lancet* **349**:825–32.

Primignani M, Andreoni B, Carpinelli L, et al. 1995. Sclerotherapy plus octreotide versus sclerotherapy alone in the prevention of early rebleeding from esophageal varices: a randomized double-blind placebo-controlled multicenter trial. *Hepatology* **21**:1322–7.

Rabkin R, Share L, Payne P, et al. 1979. The handling of immunoreactive vasopressin by the isolated perfused rat kidney. *J Clin Invest* **63**:6–13.

Ramalingaswami V, Purcell R. 1988. Waterborne non-A, non-B hepatitis. *Lancet* **1**:571–3.

Ramond MJ, Poynard T, Rueff B, et al. 1992. A randomized trial of prednisolone in patients with severe alcoholic hepatitis. *N Engl J Med* **326**:507–12.

Ransohoff D, Gracie WA. 1993. Treatment of gallstones. *Ann Intern Med* **11**:606–19.

Ransohoff D, Gracie W, Wolfenson L, et al. 1983. Prophylactic cholecystectomy or expectant management for silent gallstones. *Ann Intern Med* **99**:199–204.

Recommendations of the Immunization Practices Advisory Committee (ACIP). 1991b. Hepatitis B virus: a comprehensive strategy for eliminating transmission in the United States through universal childhood vaccination. *Morb Mortal Wkly Rep* Nov 22;**40**(RR-13):1–25.

Reichard O, Norkrans G, Fryden A, et al. 1998. Randomised, double-blind, placebo-controlled trial of interferon alpha-2b with and without ribavirin for chronic hepatitis C. The Swedish Study Group. *Lancet* **351**:83–7.

Resnick R, Iber FL, Ishihara A, et al. 1974. A controlled study of the therapeutic portacaval shunt. *Gastroenterology* **67**:843–57.

Reynolds RB, Donavan AJ, Mikkelsen WP, et al. 1981. Results of a 12-year randomized trial of portacaval shunt in patients with alcoholic liver disease and bleeding varices. *Gastroenterology* **80**:1005–11.

Roda E, Bazzoli F, Labate A, et al. 1982. Ursodeoxycholic acid vs. chenodeoxycholic acid as cholesterol gallstone-dissolving agents: a comparative randomized study. *Hepatology* **2**:804–10.

Rolachon A, Cordier L, Bacq Y, et al. 1995. Ciprofloxacin and long-term prevention of spontaneous bacterial peritonitis: results of a prospective controlled trial. *Hepatology* **22**:1171–4.

Rossle M, Haag K, Ochs A, et al. 1994. The transjugular intrahepatic portosystemic stent-shunt procedure for variceal bleeding. *N Engl J Med* **330**:165–71.

Rueff B, Degos F, Degos JD, et al. 1976. A controlled study of therapeutic portacaval shunt in alcoholic cirrhosis. *Lancet* **1**:655–9.

Runyon B. 1988. Patients with deficient ascitic fluid opsonic activity are predisposed to spontaneous bacterial peritonitis. *Hepatology* **8**:632–5.

Runyon B, Umland E, Merlin T. 1987. Inoculation of blood culture bottles with ascitic fluid; improved detection of spontaneous bacterial peritonitis. *Arch Intern Med* **147**:73–5.

Runyon BA, Canawati HN, Akriviadis EA. 1988. Optimization of ascitic fluid culture technique. *Gastroenterology* **95**:1351–5.

Saari A, Klvilaakso E, Inberg M, et al. 1990. Comparison of somatostatin and vasopressin in bleeding esophageal varices. *Am J Gastroenterol* **85**:804–7.

Sackmann M, Delius M, Sauerbruch T, et al. 1988. Shock-wave lithotripsy of gallbladder stones: the first 175 patients. *N Engl J Med* **318**:393–7.

Salerno F, Badalamenti S, Tempini S, et al. 1987. Repeated paracentesis and i.v. albumin infusion to treat tense ascites in cirrhotic patients. *J Hepatol* **5**:102–8.

Samuel D, Muller R, Alexander G, et al. 1993. Liver transplantation in European patients with the hepatitis B surface antigen. *N Engl J Med* **329**:1842–47.

Scheinberg IH, Sternlieb I. 1960. The long-term management of hepatolenticular degeneration. *Am J Med* **29**:316–33.

Schoenfield L, Lachin J, Steering Committee of the National Cooperative Gallstone Study. 1981. A controlled trial of the efficacy and safety of chenodeoxycholic acid as cholesterol gallstone-dissolving agents: a comparative randomized study. *Ann Intern Med* **95**:257–82.

Schrier R. 1979. Osmotic and nonosmotic control of vasopressin release. *Am J Physiol* **236**:F321–F332.

Shah V, Garcia-Cardena G, Sessa WC, et al. 1998. The hepatic circulation in health and disease: report of a single topic symposium. *Hepatology* **27**:279–88.

Shear L, Ching S, Gabuzda GJ. 1970. Compartmentalization of ascites and edema in patients with hepatic cirrhosis. *N Engl J Med* **282**:1391–6.

Sherlock S, Senewiratne B, Scott A, et al. 1966. Complications of diuretic therapy in hepatic cirrhosis. *Lancet* **1**:1049–53.

Singh N, Gayowski T, Yu VL, et al. 1995. Trimethoprim-sulfamethoxazole for the prevention of spontaneous bacterial peritonitis in cirrhosis: a randomized trial. *Ann Intern Med* **122**:595–8.

Soloway R, Trotman B, Ostrow J. 1977. Pigment gallstones. *Gastroenterology* **72**:167–82.

Spielberg SP, Gordon GB, Blake DA, et al. 1981. Predisposition to phenytoin hepatotoxicity assessed in vitro. *N Engl J Med* **305**:722–7.

Stanley MM, Ochi S, Lee KK, 1989. Peritoneovenous shunting as compared with medical treatment in patients with alcoholic cirrhosis and massive ascites. Veterans Administration Cooperative Study on Treatment of Alcoholic Cirrhosis With Ascites. *N Engl J Med* **321**:1632–8.

Starzl T, Demetris A, Van Thiel D. 1989. Liver transplantation (first of two parts). *N Engl J Med* **321**:1013–22.

Sternlieb I. 1980. Copper and the liver. *Gastroenterology* **78**:1615–28.

Stevens CE, Taylor PE, Tong MJ, et al. 1987. Yeast-recombinant hepatitis B vaccine: efficacy with hepatitis B immune globulin in prevention of perinatal hepatitis B virus transmission. *JAMA* **257**:2612–6.

Stiegmann GV, Goff JS, Michaletz-Odony P. 1992. Endoscopic sclerotherapy as compared with endoscopic ligation for bleeding esophageal varices. *N Engl J Med* **326**: 1527–32.

Stokes J Jr, Neefe J. 1945. The prevention and attenuation of infectious hepatitis by gamma globulin. *JAMA* **127**:44–5.

Sushma S, Dasarathy S, Tandon RK, et al. 1992. Sodium benzoate in the treatment of acute hepatic encephalopathy: a double-blind randomized trial. *Hepatology* **16**:138–44.

Szmuness W, Stevens CE, Harley EJ, et al. 1980. Hepatitis B vaccine: demonstration of efficacy in a controlled clinical trial in a high-risk population in the United States. *N Engl J Med* **303**: 833–41.

Teres J, Baroni R, Bordas JM, et al. 1987. Randomized trial of portacaval shunt stapling transection and endoscopic sclerotherapy in uncontrolled variceal bleeding. *J Hepatol* **4**:159–67.

Teres J, Planas R, Panes J, et al. 1990. Vasopressin/nitroglycerin infusion vs. esophageal tamponade in the treatment of acute variceal bleeding: a randomized controlled trial. *Hepatology* **11**:964–8.

The Italian Multicenter Project for Propranolol in Prevention of Bleeding. 1989. Propranolol prevents first gastrointestinal bleeding in nonascitic cirrhotic patients: final report of a multicenter randomized trial. *J Hepatol* **9**:75–83.

The Prova Study Group. 1991. Prophylaxis of first hemorrhage from esophageal varices by sclerotherapy, propranolol or both in cirrhotic patients: a randomized multicenter trial. *Hepatology* **14**:1016–24.

The Veterans Affairs Cooperative Variceal Sclerotherapy Group. 1991a. Prophylactic sclerotherapy for esophageal varices in alcoholic liver disease: a randomized, single-blind, multicenter clinical trial. *N Engl J Med* **324**:1779–84.

Thistle J. 1987. Direct contact dissolution of gallstones. *Semin Liver Dis* **7**:311–6.

Titó LI, Ginés P, Arroyo V, et al. 1990. Total paracentesis associated with intravenous albumin in the management of cirrhosis and ascites. *Gastroenterology* **98**:146–152.

Tong MJ, Neveen SEF, Reikes AR, et al. 1995. Clinical outcomes after transfusion-associated hepatitis C. *N Engl J Med* **332**:1463–6.

Trepo C, Jezek P, Atkinson GF, et al. 1997. Long-term effects of famciclovir in chronic hepatitis B. Results of a phase IIB study. *J Hepatol* **26**:74.

Tsai YT, Lay CS, Lai KH, et al. 1986. Controlled trial of vasopressin plus nitroglycerin versus vasopressin alone in the treatment of bleeding esophageal varices. *Hepatology* **6**:410–3.

Uribe M, Campollo O, Vargas F, et al. 1987. Acidifying enemas (lactitol and lactose) vs. nonacidifying enemas (tap water) to treat acute portal–systemic encephalopathy: a double-blind, randomized clinical trial. *Hepatology* **7**:639–43.

Uribe M, Marquez MA, Garcia-Ramos G, et al. 1980. Treatment of chronic portal–systemic encephalopathy with lactose in lactase-deficient patients. *Dig Dis Sci* **25**:924–8.

Ward A, Brogden R, Heel R, et al. 1984. Ursodeoxycholic acid: a review of its pharmacological properties and therapeutic efficacy. *Drugs* **27**:95–131.

Weissberg J, Andres L, Smith C, et al. 1984. Survival in chronic hepatitis B: analysis of 379 patients. *Ann Int Med* **101**:613–6.

Welper W, Opitz K. 1972. Histological changes in the liver biopsy in *Amanita phalloides* intoxication. *Hum Pathol* **3**:249–54.

Werzberger A, Mensch B, Kuter B, et al. 1992. A controlled trial of a formalin-inactivated hepatitis A vaccine in healthy children. *N Engl J Med* **327**:453–7.

West DJ, Watson B, Lichtman J, et al. 1994. Persistence of immunologic memory for twelve years in children given hepatitis B vaccine in infancy. *Pediatr Infect Dis J* **13**:745–7.

Whittle HC, Maine N, Pilkington J, et al. 1995. Long-term efficacy of continuing hepatitis B vaccination in infancy in two Gambian villages. *Lancet* **345**:1089–92.

Wong DK, Cheung AM, O'Rourke K, et al. 1993. Effect of alpha interferon treatment in patients with hepatitis B e antigen-positive chronic hepatitis B. A meta-analysis. *Ann Intern Med* **119**:312–23.

Yeh F, Yu M, Mo C, et al. 1989. Hepatitis B virus, aflatoxins, and hepatocellular carcinoma in southern Guangxi, China. *Cancer Res* **49**:2506–9.

Zimmerman H. 1978. *Hepatotoxicity: The Adverse Effects of Drugs and Other Chemicals on the Liver.* New York: Appleton-Century-Crofts.

CHAPTER

# 5 NUTRITION

Elizabeth M. Ross, Irwin H. Rosenberg

*Chapter Outline*

**MACRONUTRIENTS AND ENTERAL AND PARENTERAL NUTRITION**

**OBESITY**

**VITAMINS AND MINERALS**

There are many therapeutic modalities available to the practicing physician. Some patients require medication, some require the application of a device, and others may benefit from physiotherapy—but all require adequate nutrition. The chapter stresses the fact that decisions about nutrition are therapeutic decisions! Nutritional problems are highly prevalent. On the hospital ward, one-third to one-half of hospitalized patients show some signs of undernutrition (Weinsier et al. 1979; Coats et al. 1993; Naber et al. 1997). In the outpatient setting, few Americans are eating according to dietary guidelines (Bowman et al. 1998), and more than one-half of adult Americans are overweight (Flegal et al. 1998). Many nutritional interventions have been shown to be highly effective when formally studied. Supplemental nutrition has been shown to decrease postoperative complications when given preoperatively to malnourished patients (Klein et al. 1997), and to improve rates of recovery of functional status in elderly malnourished women after hip fracture (Delmi et al. 1990). Targeted vitamin and mineral supplementation affects many positive outcomes including reduction of fracture rates in elderly men and women (vitamin D and calcium) (Chapuy et al. 1992; Dawson-Hughes et al. 1997) and preventing neural tube defects (folate) (MRC Vitamin Study Research Group 1991). Over the past two decades, the management of the severely ill patient has been altered radically by the introduction and refinement of total parenteral nutrition (TPN). Correct nutritional management therefore deserves high priority in both inpatient and ambulatory settings. Yet, despite this, insufficient attention frequently is given to the nutritional aspects of patient management.

**PRINCIPLE It would be limiting for a physician to have no tools to interdict disease, worse would be to misuse or neglect those that could work, and most inappropriate would be to use a tool so that harm were the only noticeable effect. Nutrition therapy should not be any more neglected than drug therapy.**

Good medical practice requires that every patient—whether in the hospital or in the clinic—be given a nutritional plan. Such a plan will take into account the nutritional status of the patient, the nature of his or her disease, and the social circumstances concerning food availability and cooking. In almost every way, formulating a nutritional plan is like prescribing a drug; it requires attention to detail and knowledge of metabolism and pathophysiology, as well as the life style of the patient. It also requires setting clear-cut objectives that can be followed to assess the adequacy of the "prescription," and monitoring for both efficacy and unacceptable complications.

**PRINCIPLE Nutritional interventions should be thought of as drugs. Diagnosis directs the need to use them and the strategy for their use. Evaluation of efficacy and toxicity is needed in precisely the same way as for prescribing drugs.**

In this chapter we consider the pathophysiologic concepts underlying nutritional status in health and disease, and the basis for a qualitative and quantitative approach to the nutritional management of the patient.

## MACRONUTRIENTS AND ENTERAL AND PARENTERAL NUTRITION

### Macronutrient Assessment

As for other areas of medical evaluation, assessment of nutritional status consists of taking the patient's history, physical examination, laboratory assays, and other diagnostic tests. The three goals of nutrition assessment, as listed in Box 1 are to identify patients who are malnourished, to identify patients at risk for malnutrition, and to monitor the efficacy of nutritional interventions. These goals must not be overlooked or delegated to nonmedical personnel. Malnourished patients have longer mean hospital stays than well-nourished patients, and higher rates of morbidity and mortality (Sullivan et al. 1990; Coats et al. 1993; Naber et al. 1997; Gariballa et al. 1998). In addition, most serious acute illnesses and injuries are associated with hormone- and cytokine-mediated hypermetabolism and hypercatabolism, and they place even well-nourished patients at an increased risk for loss of weight and, most important, loss of lean body mass. Losses of greater than 10% of premorbid body weight place patients at increased risk of morbidity and mortality (Heimburger and Weinsier 1997).

1. Goals of Nutrition Assessment

- To identify malnourished patients
- To identify patients at risk for malnutrition
- To monitor nutritional therapy

#### *Patient history*

As in medicine in general, the history is the most important aspect of the nutritional evaluation. All patients should be questioned about the magnitude and duration of recent weight loss. Keep in mind, however, that patient reports of weight loss are insensitive, therefore, compare historical findings against medical records when possible. If weight loss is present, the etiology should be pursued. When structuring the interview, keep the five general categories of etiology of malnutrition listed in Box 2 in mind. In addition to identifying patients with established malnutrition, it is also important to identify patients with acute or chronic conditions that may potentially affect their nutritional status. In all cases, functional, economic, social, and psychologic concerns that may influence nutritional status should not be overlooked.

2. Etiologies of Malnutrition

- Inadequate intake
- Impaired absorption
- Decreased utilization
- Increased losses
- Increased requirements

#### *Physical examination*

The physical examination in patients likely to be malnourished based on the general impression and history, should include the data listed in Figure 5-1. In acutely ill patients at risk for nutrition-related complications, pertinent positives and negatives should be recorded as a baseline. Height and weight should be measured and recorded. Weight should be compared with tables of ideal weights. In general, patients with weights below 80% of ideal weight are considered to be underweight and may be malnourished. Height and weight should be used to calculate the body mass index, a measure of weight corrected for height (Box 3); patients with BMIs of less than 18.5 are considered to be underweight and possibly malnourished. It is important to consider hydration status, premorbid weight, and loss of height in mind when interpreting these measures. Easily pluckable hair, edema, and poor wound healing are the most commonly seen of the signs listed. Hair pluckability is measured by firmly tugging at hair at the top of the head. Removal of more than three hairs is indicative of protein malnutrition (Heimburger and Weinsier 1997).

3. Body Mass Index (BMI)

$$\text{BMI} = \text{weight/height}^2$$
measured in kilograms/meters$^2$
or in pounds/inches$^2 \times 704.5$

Anthropometric measures such as the triceps skin fold, which reflects fat stores, and the midarm muscle circumference, which reflects muscle mass, are useful indices of malnutrition in research and as clinical tools in experienced hands. Highly abnormal values have been shown to be associated with poor clinical outcome (Klein et al. 1997). These measures, however, have limited utility for the generalist clinician. They are subject to a great deal of measurement-associated variability and can be confounded by age, hydration status, and/or level of physical activity. Their specificity has been estimated to be in the range of 70 to 80% (Klein et al. 1997).

### *Laboratory tests*

Laboratory assessments of malnutrition are most helpful in the context of the overall clinical impression for several reasons. First, no laboratory gold standard for malnutrition exists. Second, all of the currently used assays have many potential confounders, and their specificity is therefore quite limited. In particular, factors that place patients at risk for malnutrition and malnutrition itself often cause similar changes in various commonly used assays. Finally, well-designed investigation of these various measures has been limited. Because of these concerns, it is important not to consider the results of laboratory tests in isolation. Selected nutritional measures are discussed below.

**CREATININE HEIGHT INDEX** The creatinine height index (CHI) provides a measure of the severity of muscle wasting. The rate of production of creatinine from skeletal muscle creatine phosphate is constant, and urinary creatinine, therefore, reflects skeletal muscle mass assuming negligible consumption of creatine and a constant serum creatinine. Measurements of 24-hour urinary creatinine, collected while the patient consumes a meat-free diet, are compared with tables of standard values (see Table 5-1). Values of less than 60% of predicted suggest a severe deficit of muscle mass, values of 60 to 80% suggest a moderate deficit, and values of 80% are considered normal (Gibson 1990; Heimburger and Weinsier 1997). Collections of >24 hours can cause false-negative results on this test; collections of <24 hours and muscle wasting due to causes other than malnutrition can cause false-positive results.

**URINE UREA NITROGEN** The urine urea nitrogen (UUN) can be used to determine the severity of hypercatabolic states and risk for protein malnutrition. As long as protein intakes are relatively low (i.e., under 20 g), carbohydrate intakes are adequate (i.e., over 100 g), and the BUN is stable, urine urea nitrogen can be used as an index of the degree of catabolism: 5 to 10 g/day indicates mild catabolism, 10 to 15 g/day indicates moderate catabolism, and <15 g/day indicates severe catabolism (Heimburger and Weinsier 1997). Fluid overload and incomplete urine collections can cause false-negative results; high protein intakes, gastrointestinal bleeding, glucocorticoids, diuresis, and >24-hour urine collections can cause false-negative results. The UUN can also be used in a calculation of nitrogen balance as a measure of the adequacy of nutritional therapy, as discussed in the section on monitoring, below.

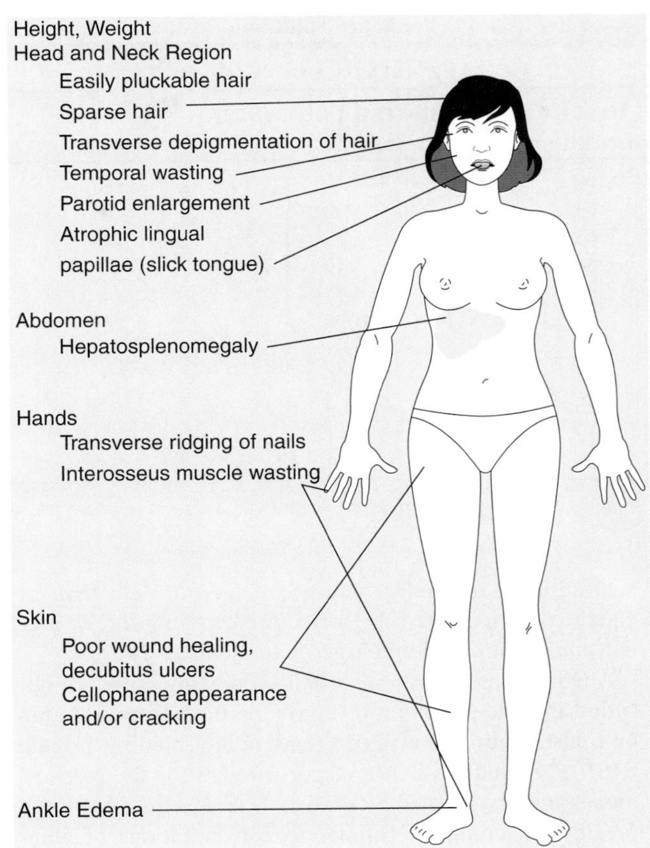


FIGURE 5-1 **Physical examination for protein-calorie malnutrition.**

**SERUM ALBUMIN AND OTHER PLASMA PROTEINS** Reduced albumin concentrations in plasma are associated with an increased risk for medical complications (Klein et al. 1997). Many factors affect serum concentration of albumin including changes in rates of synthesis, redistribution between the extravascular and intravascular spaces, gastrointestinal, skin, and urinary losses, and the state of hydration. In pure energy malnutrition, or marasmus, rates of albumin degradation are reduced and there is redistribution of albumin from the extravascular to the intravascular space. Consequently, serum albumin concentrations either remain normal or are only mildly reduced. With increased metabolic stress, e.g., during infection, inflammation, or injury (including surgery), however, rates of degradation are increased, rates of synthesis decreased, and albumin is redistributed from the intravascular to the extravascular space (Gibson 1990). Serum albumin con-

Table 5-1 Predicted Values for 24-Hour Urinary Creatinine[a]

| Female | | Male | |
|---|---|---|---|
| Height (inches) | Predicted creatinine (mg/24 h) | Height (inches) | Predicted creatinine (mg/24 h) |
| 60 | 875 | 64 | 1359 |
| 61 | 900 | 65 | 1368 |
| 62 | 925 | 66 | 1426 |
| 63 | 949 | 67 | 1467 |
| 64 | 977 | 68 | 1513 |
| 65 | 1006 | 69 | 1555 |
| 66 | 1044 | 70 | 1569 |
| 67 | 1076 | 71 | 1642 |
| 68 | 1109 | 72 | 1691 |
| 69 | 1141 | 73 | 1739 |
| 70 | 1174 | 74 | 1785 |

[a]Tables covering a wider range of heights can be found in many standard nutrition texts.

centration is markedly reduced; values of less than or equal to 2.8 indicate a high risk for kwashiorkor, or protein malnutrition (Heimburger and Weinsier 1997).

Other plasma proteins often used as measures of nutrition include prealbumin (thyroxine-binding prealbumin or transthyretin), transferrin, and retinol-binding protein (RBP). Prealbumin is a transport protein for thyroid hormones and exists in the circulation as a retinol-binding–prealbumin complex. Similar to concentrations of albumin, all three of these proteins are reduced in both protein–energy malnutrition and infection, as well as inflammation and injury. Prealbumin and RBP concentrations are increased during renal failure, transferrin concentrations are increased during iron deficiency, and RBP concentrations are decreased during vitamin A deficiency (Gibson 1990). The chief clinical utility of monitoring prealbumin and RBP is in assessing the effectiveness of nutritional interventions. These are discussed below.

**IMMUNE FUNCTION MEASURES** The total lymphocyte count and delayed hypersensitivity often are used as markers of nutritional status; however, their clinical usefulness is limited by their lack of specificity (Klein et al. 1997).

### *Patterns of protein–calorie malnutrition*

Two general types of protein–calorie malnutrition exist. Patients without an acute illness or injury, a history of weight loss over months to years, a wasted appearance, body weight $<80\%$ of the standard for height or BMI less than 18.5, a low creatine-height index, and a 24-hour urine urea nitrogen $\leq 5$ g and a mildly low or normal albumin are likely to be suffering from marasmus. Patients with an acute illness or injury, easy pluckability of their hair, edema, poor wound healing, and an albumin less than 2.8 are likely to be suffering from kwashiorkor (Heimburger and Weinsier 1997). Patients with marasmus may develop kwashiorkor with superimposed acute illness or injury. These patients are at an exceptionally high degree of nutritional risk and must be distinguished from patients with the two forms of protein-calorie malnutrition, because their nutritional needs markedly differ.

## Nutritional Therapy: Enteral and Parenteral Nutrition

### *Selection of appropriate patients*

Many hospitalized patients and outpatients are candidates for nutrition support enterally or parenterally. The broad categories of patients likely to benefit from this treatment are presented in Box 4. Nutrition support is given to patients to prevent loss of lean body mass and to optimize recovery from illness and injury.

4. Which Patients Need Nutrition Support?

- Nothing by mouth (NPO) > 5 days
- High risk for malnutrition due to illness or injury
- Malnourished and requiring elective surgery

### *Energy requirements*

The first step in designing a prescription for nutrition for an individual patient is to calculate the patient's daily energy requirement. As shown in Box 5, the total daily energy requirement (TDR) consists of three components: the

**Table 5-2 Harris-Benedict Equations for Estimating Basal Metabolic Rate**

| | |
|---|---|
| Men: | BMR = 66 + (13.8 × W) + (5 × H) − (6.8 × A) |
| Women: | BMR = 655 + (9.6 × W) + (1.8 × H) − (4.7 × A) |

NOTE: Where W = weight in kilograms, H = height in centimeters, A = age in years.

basal metabolic rate (BMR), plus the energy expenditure of activity (EAA), and the thermic effect of food (TEF).

> 5. Total Daily Energy Requirement
>
> TDR = BMR + EAA + TEF

There are many methods for measuring the BMR. In the laboratory, BMR is measured by direct calorimetry using chambers designed to measure heat loss, or by indirect calorimetry in which oxygen consumption and carbon dioxide production are measured and used to estimate heat production. Indirect calorimetry is unavailable in many clinical settings, and is currently too cumbersome and expensive for routine use; however, predictive equations based on indirect calorimetry were developed by Harris and Benedict in 1919; are shown in Table 5-2, and provide a clinically useful estimate that is accurate to ±14% (Heimburger and Weinsier 1997).

**INDIVIDUALIZING ENERGY REQUIREMENTS** Energy requirements should be individualized for obese patients, those with marasmus, and those either at risk for or with kwashiorkor. A patient's activity should also be taken into account in the calculation. The thermic effect of food is small, and for practical purposes can be omitted.

**OBESE PATIENTS** In individualizing energy requirements for the obese patient (defined for this purpose as ≥130% of ideal body weight) the use of ideal rather than actual body weight forms the basis for estimation of energy needs, has no deleterious nutritional effects, and is associated with reduced insulin requirements (Choban et al. 1997).

**PATIENTS WITH MARASMUS** In chronically malnourished or starved patients without illness or injury, the BMR falls to between 70% and 90% of normal. If these patients are overfed with carbohydrates, they are subject to life-threatening hypophosphatemia as glucose is oxidized and phosphorus is required for ATP production at faster rates than it can be removed from bone. These patients are also subject to heart failure as metabolic rate and consequently cardiac output increases. Energy delivery to patients who are felt to be hypometabolic should therefore be limited to 0.8 times the BMR (estimated) on days 1 and 2 and then may slowly be increased to 2 times the BMR over the following week if weight gain is desired (Heimburger and Weinsier 1997).

**PATIENTS WITH OR AT RISK FOR KWASHIORKOR**
Acutely ill or injured patients have increased energy requirements. In these patients, the degree of stress should be estimated clinically and the calculated BMR (estimated) should be multiplied by stress factors, as listed in Table 5-3, to calculate total energy needs.

**ESTIMATING NEEDS SECONDARY TO ACTIVITY** Activity is generally not a significant contributor to energy needs in acutely ill or injured hospitalized patients, but in outpatients able to tolerate more normal levels of activity, total daily energy requirements may be estimated by multiplying the estimated BMR by a representative activity factor per unit of time of activity as shown in Table 5-4. Interestingly enough, given their lack of energy expenditure due to activity, the daily energy requirement of ill persons is usually only slightly greater than the requirement of the healthy individual.

> **PRINCIPLE While clinical clichés can be attractive and seem by their age and nature to ring true, be certain that they are based on evidence before using them. How efficacious is it to "feed a fever?"**

### *Protein requirements*

The next step is to calculate the individual patient's requirements for protein. The normal healthy adult requires approximately 0.8 g of protein per kilogram of body weight per day (Food and Nutrition Board 1989); healthy

**Table 5-3 Adjustments to the Basal Metabolic Rate (Estimated) for Acute Illness or Injury**

| CONDITION | STRESS FACTOR |
|---|---|
| Elective surgery | 1.1 |
| Bone fractures | 1.2–1.3 |
| Severe infection | 1.3–1.5 |
| Major burns | 2 |

Table 5-4 **Estimation of Energy Needs of Active Patients**

| ACTIVITY | REPRESENTATIVE VALUE FOR ACTIVITY FACTOR PER UNIT OF TIME OF ACTIVITY |
|---|---|
| $\phi$: Sleeping, reclining | BMR × 1.0 |
| *Very Light:* sitting, standing, driving, typing, sewing, ironing | BMR × 1.5 |
| *Light:* walking 2–3 mph, shopping, washing clothes, carpentry, electrical work, golf | BMR × 2.5 |
| *Moderate:* walking 3–4 mph, gardening, scrubbing floors, biking, tennis | BMR × 5.0 |
| *Heavy:* running, climbing, working with pick or axe, swimming, football | BMR × 7.0 |

ABBREVIATIONS: BMR, basal metabolic rate (estimated).

elders probably require slightly more (Campbell et al. 1994). In the unstressed individual, adaptation to starvation involves a shift from glucose to ketone bodies as a source of energy for most tissues. This minimizes the breakdown of endogenous proteins for gluconeogenic substrates. In stressed individuals, this adaptive response to starvation does not occur. Gluconeogenesis increases markedly in response to increased circulating concentrations of catecholamines, glucagon, and other mediators, perhaps to supply the needs of neutrophils and young fibroblasts that can only utilize glucose and hypoxic tissues that utilize large amounts of glucose per ATP produced. Glucose infusions do not counteract this process. Hypercatabolic patients, therefore, should be supplied with increased amounts of protein to minimize loss of endogenous protein and its attendant complications (Blackburn 1977). The degree of hypercatabolism can be estimated using the urine urea nitrogen as described above. General guidelines shown in Table 5-5 can also be used to individualize protein requirements for the patients' estimated degree of hypercatabolism.

### *Determining the optimal route for nutrition support*

Nutrition support can be delivered via the gastrointestinal tract (enteral nutrition) or by vein (parenteral nutrition). The enteral route is more physiologic and less costly and should be used whenever possible. Use of the enteral route is generally felt to preserve the integrity of the gut and to reduce rates of bacterial translocation and sepsis, although the evidence for modulation of infection in humans may not be convincing (Reynolds et al. 1997).

### *Enteral nutrition*

**ROUTES OF ADMINISTRATION** Enteral formulas may be administered orally or via nasogastric, nasoduodenal, percutaneous gastrostomy, and jejunostomy tubes. Oral feeding requires an intact swallowing mechanism, and a high degree of patient compliance (as well as a mental status that permits this). Nasally placed tubes are suitable for short term but not long-term use. The use of large-bore nasogastric tubes may be uncomfortable, but allows for monitoring of gastric residual volumes. Nasogastric placement allows intermittent bolus feeding; placement in the small intestine limits the risk of aspiration, but may cause some abdominal discomfort.

Percutaneously placed gastric tubes for enteral feeding or jejunal tubes are appropriate for long-term use. Placement in the stomach and small intestine have the same advantages and disadvantages as those described for nasally placed tubes. Feedings to the small intestine may be administered via intraoperatively placed jejunostomy tubes earlier than gastric feedings would be tolerated (Klein et al. 1997).

**CHOICE OF FORMULA** When choosing a particular formula, primary considerations include energy density, protein content, route of administration, and cost (Heimburger and Weinsier 1997). Energy densities of commercially available formulas range from 1 to 2 kcal/mL. The more concentrated formulas are useful for patients who require restriction of fluid volume. Formulas varying in protein complexity, fiber content, and lactose content also are available. Disease-specific formulas designed for patients with renal disease, liver disease, pulmonary disease, or critical illness also are available. The composition of these formulas is generally based on plausible rationale; however, their clinical efficacy has often not been rigorously studied. Descriptions of specialized enteral feeding formulas, as well as their advantages and disadvantages, are presented in Table 5-6.

Table 5-5 Protein Requirements in Normal and Hypercatabolic States

| Degree of hypercatabolism | Estimated protein requirement (g protein/kg body weight/day) |
|---|---|
| None | 0.8 |
| Elderly, none | 1.0–1.1 |
| Mild (elective surgery, mild infection) | 1.3–1.5 |
| Moderate (infection, major surgery, trauma) | 1.5–1.7 |
| Severe (sepsis, burns up to 30% BSA) | 1.7–2.0 |
| Markedly severe (burns over 30% BSA) | |
| Increased protein losses due to wounds or fistulas | 2.0–2.5 |

### *Parenteral nutrition*

Parenteral nutrition should be used in patients who cannot or are not likely to tolerate the enteral route because of a nonfunctional gastrointestinal tract or the likelihood of complications of enteral therapy such as aspiration.

**ROUTE OF ADMINISTRATION** Parenteral nutrition can be administered via peripheral intravenous lines and central lines. The ability to administer total parenteral nutrition (TPN) via a peripheral line is limited by the tonicity of TPN. Concentrations above 10% dextrose are very hypertonic (>500 mosm/L) and too corrosive to use in smaller peripheral veins. Lipid emulsions in concentrations of 10 to 20% by volume have the advantage of delivering a highly concentrated source of calories in an isotonic solution. With the use of such emulsions, it is possible to administer close to 2000 kcal/day by peripheral vein, employing 2.5 L of 10% dextrose with appropriate amino acids and 1000 mL of a 10% lipid emulsion. When more calories are provided as lipids, intakes above 2500 kcal/day can be accomplished. Nutritional support via peripheral veins is most attractive for younger patients whose peripheral veins offer a continuing reliable conduit, when caloric requirements may be met relatively easily,

Table 5-6 Special Enteral Formulas

| Formula type | Description | Potential advantages | Disadvantages (caveats) |
|---|---|---|---|
| Elemental | Proteins supplied as amino acids and oligopeptides | May be better tolerated in patients with malabsorption | Unpalatable, expensive unproven benefit |
| High fiber | Increased fiber content | May prevent constipation and diarrhea | Must maintain good hydration |
| Lactose-free | Low lactose content | Useful in patients with lactose intolerance | |
| Renal failure | Low protein, proportionately high in essential amino acids, low potassium | May allow for adequate protein synthesis with minimal urea production, minimizing solute load | |
| Chronic hepatic insufficiency | Low protein, proportionately high in BCAAs | BCAAs do not require processing by the liver; high BCAA formula may help to establish positive nitrogen balance without causing encephalopathy | Expensive, conflicting evidence of efficacy |
| Pulmonary disease | Low carbohydrate High fat | Calorie for calorie, carbohydrate metabolism produces more $CO_2$ than fat; therefore, high-fat, low-carbohydrate formula may help to optimize the $P_{CO_2}$ | Benefit in terms of $CO_2$ production may be too small to be clinically significant |
| Fat malabsorption | MCT formulas | Bile salts, high levels of pancreatic enzymes, and reesterification to triglycerides in enterocytes not required for absorption | Intakes above 400 kcal/day may cause diarrhea |
| Critical illness | High glutamine formulas | Glutamine is an important fuel for the gut; may preserve gut integrity | Evidence for efficacy limited to animal models |

ABBREVIATIONS: BCAA, branched-chain amino acids; MCT, medium-chain triglyceride.

and when nutrition support is likely to be necessary for only a short term.

Parenteral nutrition by central vein is normally provided through a catheter passed via the subclavian vein into the superior vena cava. Aseptic placement by an experienced physician and careful catheter care by a trained nurse are essential to minimize the considerable risk of infectious complications.

**FORMULA COMPOSITION** Two sources of nonprotein calories for intravenous administration are commercially available: dextrose solutions and lipid emulsions. Both can provide energy through their oxidation, and both are capable of sparing body protein by providing calories that inhibit breakdown of protein for gluconeogenesis. Although dextrose alone and the combination of dextrose and lipid result in weight gain, repletion of protein is optimal with a combined regimen (MacFie et al. 1981). TPN can be administered as 2–in–1 dextrose and amino acid mixtures with lipid given separately or as 3–in–1 admixtures of dextrose, amino acid, and lipid.

***Dextrose*** Carbohydrate solutions for intravenous administration are composed of a monohydric form of dextrose containing 3.4 calories (kcal)/g and can be used in concentrations up to 70%. Maximal suppression of gluconeogenesis occurs when infusions of glucose approach 400 g, or about 1600 kcal/day. There appears to be a limit to the capacity to derive energy from infused glucose. The limits of the nitrogen-sparing effects of glucose infusion are observed at about 35 kcal/kg per day, or 5–7 mg/kg per minute. Above these amounts, one can expect increased synthesis of fat from glucose and deposition of fat in the liver with consequent hepatomegaly, right upper quadrant pain, and abnormalities in liver function tests.

***Lipid*** Lipid emulsions for IV use are derived from soybean or safflower oils, or combinations of both. They supply 9 kcal/g, or 1.1 kcal/mL of a 10% fat emulsion and 2 kcal/mL of a 20% fat emulsion. Lipid emulsions contain essential fatty acids (EFA); they supply nearly 50% of fatty acids as linoleic (omega–6) and 4 to 8% as linolenic (omega–3) acids (in which the double bond is 6 or 3 carbons, respectively, from the omega-carbon). The requirement for EFAs can be met by weekly provision of 500 mL of a 10% lipid emulsion or 250 mL of a 20% emulsion; however, it is normally recommended that more than 20% of total daily nonprotein calories be provided as lipid. As noted above, lipids lower the tonicity of TPN solutions and high proportions are often used when administering TPN by peripheral vein; however, lipid should not supply more than 60 to 70% of the daily nonprotein calories. Lipid emulsions should be delivered at slow rates to prevent immunosuppression. Two alternative forms of lipids, medium-chain triglycerides (MCTs) and emulsions containing increased amounts of omega–3 fatty acids are currently under investigation. MCT is almost completely oxidized and is not stored or accumulated in the liver and, theoretically, may be associated with less immunosuppression than standard formulas. Clinical trials thus far have not established clear benefits of MCT emulsions (Ulrich et al. 1996). The omega–3 fatty acids are metabolized into eicosanoids with less inflammatory profiles than those produced from arachidonic acid. Human studies have thus far showed potentially favorable modifications of eicosanoid profiles, but have not demonstrated clinically significant endpoints of altered inflammation or immune responses (McCowen et al. 1998).

***Amino Acids*** Commercial mixtures of amino acids for intravenous administration contain essential and nonessential amino acids in a ratio of about 1:4, and supply 4 kcal/g. They are available in concentrations from 3.5 (3.5 g/mL) to 15% (15 g/mL). The optimal calorie/nitrogen ratio appears to be about 160:1 cal/g. At a ratio of 100:1, weight loss and negative nitrogen balance have been observed. Glutamine-enriched and branched-chain amino acid (BCAA)-enriched amino acid formulas are also available. Glutamine is an amino acid important for the synthesis of purines and pyrimidines, and an important fuel for lymphoid tissue and gastrointestinal tissue. It becomes depleted in hypercatabolic states, when it may become conditionally essential. Glutamine-enriched formulas may decrease long-term but not short-term mortality after bone marrow transplantation. Also, they have been shown to improve protein synthetic rates and small bowel mucosal height in a rat model of peritonitis. These findings have not been confirmed in human studies. BCAA-enriched formulae may reduce encephalopathy in patients with hepatic failure and may be utilized more efficiently in patients with uremia than standard formulas, but they have not been shown beneficial in septic patients (McCowen et al. 1998).

***Water*** The 70-kg adult normally requires about 30 mL of water per kilogram of body weight per day, or about 1 mL of fluid per kilocalorie per day. The increased fluid and electrolyte requirements of patients with fever, diarrhea, short-bowel syndrome, or extensive drainage from fistula must be provided. In patients with limitations of fluid intake imposed by cardiac failure or cirrhosis, total fluid volume will be an important factor in selecting solutions and their rates of infusion.

***Vitamins, Minerals, and Trace Elements*** Vitamins and minerals should be added to parenteral alimentation solutions within the ranges shown in Table 5-7. Deficiency syndromes of biotin, selenium, zinc, or copper have been reported when these materials have been excluded from parenteral solutions. This experience reinforces the need to include all essential nutrients in parenteral solutions, particularly when prolonged IV therapy is needed. About 150 to 200 mEq of chloride and 90 to 120 mEq of sodium are required per day. Patients with fistulas of the GI tract or those with gastroduodenal drainage may require up to twice these amounts. Patients receiving TPN who are malnourished at baseline often require large amounts of phosphate, potassium, and magnesium, especially during the initiation of TPN. Calcium intake is designed to meet or exceed calcium excretion in urine and stool as predicted from studies of calcium balance. Adequate zinc is required for nutritional restitution, for positive nitrogen balance, and for wound healing. The requirements of zinc may be two or three times normal (or 12–17 mg for each liter of fluid lost) in patients with diarrhea and GI fistulas (Alpers et al. 1995).

### *Considerations in selected clinical settings*

**SHORT BOWEL SYNDROME** The degree of malabsorption in short bowel syndrome depends on the length of bowel resected, the site of resection, and the expected or measured function of the remaining gut. Patients with extensive small bowel resection often require nutritional support, and lifelong TPN is generally required in patients with less than 100 cm of remaining jejunum or with a jejunostomy in those with less than 50 cm of remaining jejunum or ileum and a functioning colon. In other cases, temporary TPN is generally required while awaiting gut adaptation or the return of the ability to eat or receive tube feedings. Nighttime tube feedings and oral rehydration formulas may reduce the needs for TPN (Klein et al. 1997).

**INFLAMMATORY BOWEL DISEASE** Patients with exacerbations of inflammatory bowel disease (IBD) are often placed on "bowel rest" and given TPN. Randomized, controlled trials (RCTs) do not support this practice. In RCTs, patients with exacerbations of both ulcerative colitis and Crohn's disease treated with bowel rest and TPN did not achieve remission more frequently than those eating or receiving tube feeding. Elemental formulas provide little benefit over standard formulas in improving remission rates. TPN and bowel rest, however, may improve rates of fistula closure (Klein et al. 1997).

**ACUTE PANCREATITIS** In patients with mild to moderate pancreatitis (by Ransom criteria or CT scan), bowel rest and TPN do not provide any benefit compared with

**Table 5-7 Typical Daily Total Parenteral Nutrition Prescription for Adult Patients**

| | | | |
|---|---|---|---|
| Calories: 30–40 kcal/kg of IBW | Lipid: 1/3 nonprotein calories | | |
| Protein: 1.0–1.5 g/kg of IBW | Dextrose: 2/3 nonprotein calories | | |
| *Electrolytes and Minerals* (mEq) | | *Vitamins* | |
| Sodium | 90–120 | A (IU) | 3300 |
| Potassium | 90–150 | C (mg) | 100 |
| Calcium | 12–16 | D (IU) | 200 |
| Magnesium | 15–200 | E (IU) | 10 |
| Chloride | 12–16 | K (mg)[a] | — |
| Acetate | 20–30 | | |
| | | Thiamine, $B_1$ (mg) | 3 |
| Phosphorus (mmol) | 20–40 | Riboflavin, $B_2$ (mg) | 3.6 |
| Sulfate | 12–16 | Pyridoxine, $B_6$ (mg) | 4 |
| | | Niacinamide (mg) | 40 |
| *Trace Elements* | | $B_{12}$ ($\mu$g) | 5 |
| Zinc (mg) | 3–9 | Pantothenate (mg) | 15 |
| Copper (mg) | 1–1.6 | Biotin ($\mu$g) | 60 |
| Manganese (mg) | 0.5 | Folic acid ($\mu$g) | 60 |
| Chromium ($\mu$g) | 10–15 | | |
| Selenium ($\mu$g) | 40 | | |
| Molybdenum ($\mu$g) | 20 | | |
| Iron (mg) | 2–3[b] | | |

[a]Vitamin K is added to the TPN or administered IM 5 mg/week.
[b]Doses >5 mg/day have been associated with anaphylactoid or other types of adverse reactions.
ABBREVIATIONS: IBW, ideal body weight; microgram, often abbreviated mcg, is "$\mu$g" here.

oral feeding. This issue has not been investigated in the setting of severe pancreatitis. Jejunal feedings and intravenous lipid emulsions do not stimulate pancreatic secretions significantly and are generally well tolerated in patients with pancreatitis (Klein et al. 1997).

**CIRRHOSIS AND ACUTE HEPATIC ENCEPHALOPATHY** Enteral nutrition has been shown to improve liver function, encephalopathy, and Child's score in patients hospitalized for complications of cirrhosis in one trial, BCAA-enriched TPN formulas have not been shown to improve rates of recovery from acute encephalopathy compared with standard formulas. Other trials comparing BCAA-enriched TPN to dextrose-only solutions showed significant improvements in recovery with the BCAA-enriched formulas, but this scenario is less clinically relevant (Klein et al. 1997).

**PERIOPERATIVE** Preoperative TPN given to malnourished patients has been shown to decrease the risk of postoperative complications by approximately 10% (Klein et al. 1997), whereas postoperative TPN given to similarly malnourished patients who did not receive preoperative TPN increased rates of postoperative complications (Klein et al. 1997). Postoperative enteral feeding of underweight women after surgery for hip fracture increased speed of rehabilitation, decreased postoperative complications, and reduced the length of stay (Delmi et al. 1990).

### *Monitoring and potential complications*

Monitoring is essential both to assess the adequacy of nutritional support and to identify potential complications. Assays useful for monitoring nutritional therapy include those reflecting protein balance, concentration of proteins, glucose, electrolytes, and triglycerides in serum.

**PROTEIN BALANCE** The 24-hour UUN, along with an estimate of protein intake, can be used to determine the adequacy of protein delivery in patients receiving both enteral and parenteral nutrition. Protein balance is calculated as shown in Box 6. In the equation for protein catabolic rate, the value of 4 g nitrogen is added to the UUN to estimate nonurine nitrogen losses (via feces, sweat, lost skin, and hair), and the factor 6.25 converts nitrogen grams to protein grams (since nitrogen accounts for one-sixth of dietary protein) (Heimburger and Weinsier 1997). Protein balance in patients with large nonurinary losses or uremia cannot be calculated by this means. Methods of calculating balance in patients with uremia can be found in handbooks of nutrition (Heimburger and Weinsier 1997; Alpers et al. 1995).

> 6. Protein Balance
>
> Protein balance (g/day) = Protein intake − Protein catabolic rate
>
> Protein catabolic rate = [24-hour urinary urea nitrogen (UUN) (g) + 4] × 6.25

**SERUM PROTEINS** Increases in prealbumin (half-life, 48 hours) and retinol binding protein (half-life, 12 hours) concentrations can be useful to monitor the response to nutritional therapy (Gibson 1990). Prealbumin is more easily performed, more widely available, and less costly. Unfortunately, as discussed above, these measures are confounded by multiple factors beyond the nutritional status and must be used and interpreted with this in mind.

**ELECTROLYTES AND REFEEDING SYNDROME** As discussed above, both in the settings of enteral and parenteral nutrition, overfeeding with carbohydrates may cause hypophosphatemia, hypomagnesemia, and hypokalemia, as well as heart failure. Starting feeding with energy delivery low and increasing gradually as described above and supplying electrolytes as needed should prevent these complications.

**SERUM GLUCOSE** Hyperglycemia is a common complication of both enteral and parenteral nutrition. Both overfeeding and/or endogenous gluconeogenesis can play a role in the development of hyperglycemia. Hyperglycemia can interfere with white blood cell function. Temporarily discontinuing feeding or slowing delivery rates, depending on the magnitude of the hyperglycemia, along with the addition of insulin to TPN and/or using a "sliding-scale" formula for insulin replacement can prevent and treat this complication.

**SERUM TRIGLYCERIDES** When administered intravenously, lipid particles are metabolized in a way, similar to chylomicrons. Before administering lipids, serum triglycerides should be obtained as a baseline measurement and monitored periodically. Serum triglyceride levels above the 500 to 1000 range may be complicated by pancreatitis.

**COMPLICATIONS OF ENTERAL AND PARENTERAL FEEDING** Other than those discussed above, complications of enteral feeding include aspiration, diarrhea, and dehydration. When patients on enteral feeding develop diarrhea, it is important to rule out etiologies other than the hyperosmolality of the formula. Causes including medications (sorbitol-containing elixirs, magnesium-containing antacids, oral and possibly intravenous antibiotics, lactulose, etc.), infection, and gastrointestinal pathology should be investigated. Psyllium or pectin may offer some benefit under most conditions. Dilution of feeding formulas at the onset of feeding generally is unnecessary. Intestinal ileus and altered mental status are the most common causes of aspiration. Aspiration may be minimized by placement of the feeding tube in the duodenum or jejunum and by elevation of the head. Dehydration can be seen with diarrhea, or the use of concentrated formulas. The concentrated formula should only be used when truly necessary.

An important complication of TPN is line infection. Aseptic placement, careful care of the site, and periodic surveillance of the line insertion site including cultures are instrumental in preventing this complication.

## OBESITY

Overnutrition is a much more prevalent problem than undernutrition in many developed countries. Data from the most recent National Health and Examination Survey, NHANES III, indicates that one-half of all men and women and almost two-thirds of African Americans are overweight (BMI ≥ 25). Over the last ten years the prevalence of obesity (BMI ≥ 30) has increased from 12 to 20% in men and from 16 to 25% in women (Flegal et al. 1998). Multiple epidemiologic studies have shown overweight and obesity to be associated with increased morbidity and mortality. In well-designed randomized, controlled trials among overweight and obese individuals, weight loss has resulted in decreases in incidence of and risk factors for obesity-related disease and obesity-associated morbidities. All patients should therefore be assessed for overweight and obesity periodically, and patients should receive treatment as appropriate. Available treatment modalities consist of diet, exercise, behavior modification, pharmacotherapy, and weight loss surgery.

### Obesity Assessment

Periodic evaluation for obesity should consist of measurement of the body mass index (BMI), measurement of waist circumference, assessment of risk status, and assessment of motivation for weight loss [National Heart, Lung, and Blood Institute (NHLBI) 1998].

***Body mass index***
The BMI is a measure of weight corrected for height and reflects total body fat (Taylor et al. 1998). In observational studies, higher BMIs have been associated with increased risk of morbidity and mortality relative to normal BMIs (Manson et al. 1995). The BMI can therefore be used to stratify patients into risk groups for complications of obesity (see Table 5-8). The BMI may overestimate body fat in patients with large muscle mass, in those with edema, and in those who have experienced loss of height, and underestimate body fat in patients who have lost muscle mass.

Table 5-8 **Classification of Weight by Body Mass Index**

| BMI | Classification |
|---|---|
| <18.5 | Underweight |
| 18.5–24.9 | Normal |
| 25.0–29.9 | Overweight |
| 30.0–34.9 | Obesity (class I) |
| 35.0–39.9 | Obesity (class II) |
| >40 | Extreme obesity (class III) |

***Waist circumference***
Waist circumference reflects abdominal adiposity (Taylor et al. 1998). Observational studies suggest abdominal fat is an independent predictor of risk factors and morbidity when the BMI is not markedly increased (NHLBI 1998). Thresholds for risk based on waist circumference are shown in Table 5-9.

Table 5-9 **Waist Circumference and Thresholds for High Health Risk**

| Gender | High risk |
|---|---|
| Male | >120 cm (40 in) |
| Female | >88 cm (35 in) |

***Patient history***
Patients should be questioned regarding history of obesity-associated diseases, risk factors for obesity-associated diseases, and obesity-associated complications (see Table 5-10). The presence or absence of these "risk factors" will help to determine the appropriate intensity of therapy. Finally, the patient's level of motivation to pursue weight-loss therapy should be assessed. When assessing the level of motivation, the considerations highlighted in Table 5-11 should be taken into account (NHLBI 1998).

### Treatment for Obesity

Weight loss has been shown in randomized, controlled trials to decrease blood pressure in overweight and obese hypertensive and normotensive individuals, to improve glucose control in overweight and obese patients with type

Table 5-10 **Obesity-Associated Diseases and Risk Factors**

| *Obesity-Associated Diseases* | *Risk Factors for Obesity-Associated Disease* |
|---|---|
| Coronary heart disease | Cigarette smoking |
| Other atherosclerotic disease | Hypertension |
| Type 2 diabetes mellitus | High LDL |
| Sleep apnea | Low HDL |
| | Impaired fasting glucose (fasting glucose 110–125 mg/dL) |
| | Family history of premature CHD |
| | Age: male >45, female >55 (or postmenopausal) |
| *Obesity-Associated Complications* | *Other Risk Factors* |
| Gynecologic abnormalities | High triglycerides (>400 mg/dL) |
| Osteoarthritis | Physical inactivity |
| Gallstones and their complications | |
| Stress incontinence | |

2 diabetes, and to decrease total and LDL cholesterol and triglycerides and decrease HDL cholesterol in patients with dyslipidemia (NHLBI 1998). Patients who are obese, or who are either overweight or have a high waist circumference and two or more risk factors (as defined above) or a high degree of motivation for weight loss should be treated (NHLBI 1998) (see Table 5-12). Treatment consists of modification of the diet, increased exercise, behavioral therapy, and, in certain circumstances, pharmacotherapy and weight-loss surgery. Dietary therapy and pharmacotherapy will be discussed below.

### *Dietary therapy*

Traditionally, two types of diets, the low calorie diet (LCD) and the very low calorie diet (VLCD) have generally been used for medically guided weight loss (see Table 5-13). The LCD consists of reducing energy intake to 500 to 1000 kcal below usual intake, or approximately 1000 to 1200 kcal/day for a woman and 1200 to 1500 kcal/day for a man. Theoretically, a deficit of 500 to 1000 kcal/day will produce a weight loss of 70 to 140 g/day or 1 to 2 pounds/week. In clinical trials, LCDs have resulted in weight loss of 8% of baseline body weight over 6 months and long-term weight loss of 4% of baseline body weight after more than one year (NHLBI 1998). The VLCD restricts energy intake to below 800 kcal/day (generally 400 to 500 kcal). The VLCD can consist of 1.5 g of protein per kilogram of ideal body weight per day in the form of lean meat, fish, and poultry with small amounts of carbohydrates or commercially formulated liquid diets added to prevent de novo carbohydrate synthesis and muscle wasting. VLCDs are generally administered for 12 to 15 weeks, and weight loss over 6 months averages approximately 13%. Although early problems stemming from formulas lacking complete proteins and adequate electrolytes, vitamins, and minerals have been corrected, VLCDs do not allow gradual introduction of life style changes that can be maintained, and they sometimes are complicated by gallstones. VLCDs have not resulted in long-term weight loss superior to that seen with LCDs (NHLBI 1998). Goals of weight loss therapy are listed in Table 5-14.

### *Pharmacotherapy*

Long-term weight loss achieved via conventional means is often poor, and adjuvant use of medications has been studied as a possible means of improving maintenance of the lowered weight. In 1992, Weintraub published a controlled trial of fenfluramine, a serotonin releaser, and phentermine, in the maintenance of weight loss achieved by conventional means. Both of these medications function as anorexiants or appetite suppressants. At follow-up after 210 weeks,

Table 5-11 **Factors to Evaluate When Assessing Level of Motivation**

| |
|---|
| Reason and readiness for weight loss |
| Previous history of weight loss attempts |
| Social support |
| Patient's understanding of obesity-associated morbidities |
| Attitude toward physical activity |
| Time availability |
| Barriers to change |
| Financial considerations |

Table 5-12 **Patients Who Should Be Treated for Obesity**

| |
|---|
| Obese |
| Overweight + more than 2 risk factors |
| Waist circumference over threshold + more than 2 risk factors |
| Overweight or waist circumference over threshold with more than 2 risk factors + motivation |

Table 5-13 Weight Loss Diets

| | LOW-CALORIE DIET (LCD) | VERY LOW CALORIE DIET (VLCD) |
|---|---|---|
| Kilocalories/day | 1000–1200 | 400–500 |
| Short-term weight loss (6 months to one year) | 8% | 13% |
| Long-term weight loss (over one year) | 4% | 4% |

Table 5-14 Goals of Weight Loss Therapy

Initial goal: 10% weight reduction of body weight over six months
Target energy intake: 500–1000 kcal/day reduction from usual intake
Target diet composition:
- 30% calories as fat (<10% as saturated fat)
- 15% calories as protein
- 55% calories as carbohydrate

Vitamin and mineral needs should be met
Diet should be individualized to patient's food preferences
Patient education should include
- Energy value and macronutrient composition of foods
- Reading nutrition labels
- Low-calorie food shopping
- Low-calorie food preparation

Patient should be advised to
- Limit portion sizes
- Avoid alcohol
- Maintain adequate intake of water

SOURCE: National Heart, Lung, and Blood Institute 1998.

maintenance of weight loss was significantly higher in the medication group compared with the placebo group (Weintraub et al. 1992). Subsequently, weight-loss medications, which had formerly been used as short-term therapy, began to be used long term. Current recommendations (NHLBI 1998) for patients suitable for use of weight loss medications are summarized in Table 5-15.

Four medications, fenfluramine; dexfenfluramine, a serotonin reuptake inhibitor; sibutramine, a norepinephrine, dopamine, and serotonin reuptake inhibitor; and orlistat, a pancreatic lipase inhibitor will result in decreased fat absorption, have been approved for long-term use by the Food and Drug Administration. FDA approval, however, was subsequently withdrawn for fenfluramine and dexfenfluramine, and these drugs were voluntarily taken off the market by their manufacturers because of reports of increased risk of valvular heart disease (Jick et al. 1998; Khan et al. 1998). Data regarding efficacy and adverse effects of the last two medications are shown in Table 5-16.

**PRINCIPLE The risks and benefits of any new therapy, particularly when they are not anticipated by known pharmacologic profiles, take considerable time to reveal themselves. The therapist must maintain a systematic update on any therapy he or she uses and understand how and where to look for follow-up studies.**

## VITAMINS AND MINERALS

In developed countries such as the United States, classical micronutrient deficiency diseases are very rarely seen. Increased risk for chronic disease due to inadequate micronutrient status, however, is quite common. Numerous epidemiologic studies have suggested that poor micronutrient nutrition increases the risk of chronic disease, cancer, and infection. Poor vitamin C status has been associated with cataract formation and macular degeneration (Jacques et al. 1994); poor folate, vitamin $B_6$, and vitamin $B_{12}$ status cause hyperhomocystinemia (Selbub et al. 1993), which has been associated with the development

Table 5-15 Guidelines for Pharmacotherapy for Obesity Treatment

BMI > 30 or BMI > 27 with hypertension, congestive heart failure, type 2 diabetes, or sleep apnea
<1 lb weight loss/week after 6 months of LCD, exercise, behavior therapy
If <4.4 lb weight loss in first month, discontinue
Continue as long as efficacy maintained and adverse effects are mild and manageable
Use as part of a comprehensive program of diet, exercise, and behavior therapy

SOURCE: BMI, body mass index; LCD, low-calorie diet.

Table 5-16 Weight Loss Medications

| MEDICATION | FDA APPROVAL STATUS | EFFICACY—WEIGHT LOSS (LBS) AT INDICATED FOLLOW-UP[a] | ADVERSE EFFECTS | PRECAUTIONS |
|---|---|---|---|---|
| Sibutramine | approved | 6.2 (at one year) 12.1 (at 24 weeks) | Increase in heart rate and blood pressure | Should not be used in patients with a history of hypertension, congestive heart failure, coronary artery disease, arrhythmias, or stroke |
| Orlistat | approved | 4.9 (at 16 weeks) | Decrease in fat-soluble vitamin absorption, soft stools, anal leakage; possible increased incidence of breast cancer | Patients may require replacement of fat-soluble vitamins |

[a]Compared with placebo.

of atherosclerotic vascular disease (Beresford and Boushey 1997), and poor intakes of folate, vitamin A, and antioxidant nutrients have been associated with various cancers. Micronutrient supplementation has been shown to reduce the risk of osteoporotic fracture (Chapuy et al. 1992; Dawson-Hughes et al. 1997) and neural tube defects (MRC Vitamin Study Research Group 1991). Trials are under way to study the use of folate in colon cancer prevention.

A potent example of the changing concepts of the relation between micronutrient status and chronic disease is the relation among B vitamins (especially folate), circulating homocysteine levels, and cardiovascular disease risk. In this case, homocysteine is not only a functional marker of the integrity of enzymatic and metabolic systems, which are dependent on folate, vitamin $B_{12}$, and vitamin $B_6$, but also in a way, homocysteine is analogous to cholesterol, as it represents a risk factor associated with cardiovascular disease and stroke. Homocysteine may therefore be used as an indication of B vitamin status or as a predictor of risk of cardiovascular disease or possibly both.

**PRINCIPLE Cardiovascular disease, osteoporosis, and neural tube defects have replaced xerophthalmia, beri-beri, and scurvy as the results of inadequate vitamin and mineral nutrition. Adequate vitamin and mineral nutrition is an essential part of the diet-disease relationship and has to be considered in any patient with these "chronic degenerative diseases."**

## Micronutrient Assessment

Every patient should receive some assessment of micronutrient status as part of their primary health care. During health maintenance visits, the physician should attempt to identify those whose usual diets might place them at increased risk of chronic disease. In patients with medical and surgical conditions, the physician also should consider the impact of the disease processes and their treatments on micronutrient status. The physician should be aware of the potential effects of using tobacco and alcohol on the micronutrient status, and of genetic syndromes associated with dependency on megadose micronutrient supplementation.

Nutritional deficiencies tend to evolve slowly until they become clinically recognizable, as is typical for other medical conditions.

**PRINCIPLE When an event occurs slowly and is subtle until grossly evident, the therapist may have difficulty recognizing the problem. Anticipation and prevention become more important.**

Although there are exceptions, the first step in depletion usually is a fall in circulating concentrations of the vitamin. This is followed by decreased urinary excretion, and finally by diminished concentration of the vitamin in tissue. In the case of certain nutrients, this last stage can be demonstrated by a fall in vitamin content of circulating blood cells. Tissue depletion is accompanied by diminished coenzyme function or fat-soluble synthetic function, and these disturbances lead to functional abnormalities in vitamin-dependent metabolic pathways. At this stage of functional disturbance, symptoms of deficiency are most likely to be noted, although their manifestations may be very subtle. At more advanced stages of deficiency, visible signs appear, including changes in the skin and mucous membranes that represent pathologic manifestations of functional abnormalities. Since deficiencies can be more effectively treated early in their course, it is important to target patients at risk for further evaluation and treatment before they develop overt deficiencies.

SUMMARY
**Timeliness is important in the detection of nutritional deficiencies as it is in the diagnosis and treatment of other diseases. The earlier the abnormality is corrected, the more readily and effectively therapy will work to reverse it.**

Historical assessment involves two components: the regular dietary intake (a modified diet history) and the level of nutrition, the latter of which reflects the interaction of diet and disease. There are two levels of dietary assessment, qualitative and quantitative. Qualitative assessment involves a history of what the patient usually eats and what he or she avoids, any recent weight changes, whether the patient is following a special diet, and if supplements or vitamins are taken. If this qualitative assessment suggests that there may be problems in nutrition, a detailed quantitation may be needed. This is usually done by a qualified dietitian, who utilizes methods such as 24-hour recalls and questionnaires regarding the frequency of food intake. Standard food composition tables are currently widely available as the database for computer programs that can be used to estimate intakes of various nutrients.

## Nutritional Health Maintenance

Nutrient requirements for healthy individuals are set periodically by the Food and Nutrition Board of the National Academy of Sciences. The last complete set of recommendations was published in 1989 (Food and Nutrition Board 1989), and at the time of this writing these recommendations are under revision. Updated recommendations for several nutrients have been released in draft form (Food and Nutrition Board 1997; Food and Nutrition Board 1998). Recommended dietary allowances are shown in Table 5-17, with recently revised values in italics. Requirements may be increased during pregnancy and lactation and may differ at different ages.

For the great majority of healthy individuals, maintenance of normal vitamin and mineral status can be accomplished by eating a variety of foods in proportions outlined in the USDA food guide pyramid, as recommended in the Dietary Guidelines for Americans (USDA 1995) and shown in Figure 5-2 and Table 5-18. Unfortunately, recent data suggest that only 12% of Americans are currently following these recommendations (Bowman et al. 1998). A few questions regarding usual dietary intakes should help the physician to ascertain whether the patient is eating a well-balanced diet.

## The Patient with Active Medical Problems or Significant Surgical History

The Recommended Dietary Allowances (RDA) describe nutrient requirements in healthy people. Requirements of individual patients may differ from the RDA due to medical illnesses or their treatments, surgical alterations in gastrointestinal anatomy, habits such as drinking and smoking, and genetic conditions. The physician must therefore individualize nutritional assessment and treatment for each particular patient as would be done for any other therapeutic decision.

SUMMARY
**The recommended allowances of nutrients can only be used as guidelines for the average healthy person and in no way can substitute for careful individualization to the needs of the patient.**

### *Patients with abnormalities that affect micronutrient processing*

**ABNORMALITIES OF DIGESTION AND ABSORPTION** Abnormalities in digestion and absorption can cause single abnormality or multiple micronutrient deficiencies. Vitamin $B_{12}$, which is in its coenzyme form in foods, must be cleaved from its enzyme before absorption can take place. Acid is required for this process, and patients with achlorhydria for any reason, including atrophic gastritis, use of proton pump inhibitors, etc., may develop vitamin $B_{12}$ deficiency on this basis. Pancreatic enzymes are also necessary for the absorption of $B_{12}$, and pancreatic enzymes and bile salts are necessary for the digestion and absorption of the fat-soluble vitamins, vitamins A, D, E, and K. Patients with pancreatic exocrine dysfunction or cholestasis of any etiology are at risk for deficiency of

Table 5-17 **Recommended Dietary Allowances (1989, 1998[a])**

| Nutrient | Young Adult M | Young Adult F | Adult M | Adult F | Older Adult M | Older Adult F | Elder M | Elder F | Lactation Pregnancy | 1st–6th Month | 6th–12th Month |
|---|---|---|---|---|---|---|---|---|---|---|---|
| Vitamin A (μg RE) | 1000 | 800 | 1000 | 800 | 1000 | 800 | n/a | n/a | 800 | 1300 | 1200 |
| Vitamin D (IU) | *200* | *200* | *200* | *200* | *400* | *400* | *600* | *600* | *200* | *200* | *200* |
| Vitamin E (IU α-TE) | 10 | 18 | 10 | 18 | 10 | 18 | n/a | n/a | 10 | 12 | 11 |
| Vitamin K (μg) | 70 | 60 | 80 | 65 | 80 | 65 | n/a | n/a | 70 | 95 | 90 |
| Vitamin C (mg) | 60 | 60 | 60 | 60 | 60 | 60 | n/a | n/a | 70 | 95 | 90 |
| Thiamin (mg) | *1.2* | *1.1* | *1.2* | *1.1* | *1.2* | *1.1* | *1.2* | *1.1* | *1.4* | *1.5* | *1.5* |
| Riboflavin etc. (mg) | *1.3* | *1.1* | *1.3* | *1.1* | *1.3* | *1.1* | *1.3* | *1.1* | *1.4* | *1.6* | *1.6* |
| Niacin (mg NE) | *16* | *14* | *16* | *14* | *16* | *14* | *16* | *14* | *18* | *17* | *17* |
| Vitamin B6 (mg) | *1.3* | *1.3* | *1.3* | *1.3* | *1.7* | *1.5* | *1.7* | *1.5* | *1.9* | *2.0* | *2.0* |
| Folate (μg) | *400* | *400* | *400* | *400* | *400* | *400* | *400* | *400* | *600* | *500* | *500* |
| Vitamin $B_{12}$ (μg) | *2.4* | *2.4* | *2.4* | *2.4* | *2.4* | *2.4* | *2.4* | *2.4* | *2.6* | *2.8* | *2.8* |
| Calcium (mg) | *1000* | *1000* | *1000* | *1000* | *1200* | *1200* | *1200* | *1200* | *1000* | *1000* | *1000* |
| Phosphorus (mg) | *700* | *700* | *700* | *700* | *700* | *700* | *700* | *700* | *700* | *700* | *700* |
| Magnesium (mg) | *400* | *310* | *420* | *320* | *420* | *320* | *420* | *320* | *350,360* | *310,320* | *310,320* |
| Iron (mg) | 10 | 15 | 10 | 15 | 10 | 10 | n/a | n/a | 30 | 15 | 15 |
| Zinc (mg) | 15 | 12 | 15 | 12 | 15 | 12 | n/a | n/a | 15 | 19 | 16 |
| Iodine (μg) | 150 | 150 | 150 | 150 | 150 | 150 | n/a | n/a | 175 | 200 | 200 |
| Selenium (μg) | 70 | 55 | 70 | 55 | 70 | 55 | n/a | n/a | 65 | 75 | 75 |

[a]The RDAs listed in italics are released only in draft form at the time of this writing.
ABBREVIATIONS: RE, retinoic acid, α-TE, α-tocopherol.

multiple fat-soluble vitamins. Additionally, in fat malabsorption, unabsorbed fatty acids can bind cations such as calcium, magnesium, and zinc, creating unabsorbable complexes and leading to deficiency. Vitamins and minerals are absorbed at various sites along the small intestine; small intestinal disease affecting absorptive ability, therefore, has the potential to cause deficiencies of multiple micronutrients. Distal ileal resection or disease or a lack of intrinsic factor due to pernicious anemia or gastric resection, can cause selective deficiency of vitamin. Additionally, parasitic microorganisms residing in the gastrointestinal tract, and bacterial overgrowth in the small intestine may cause micronutrient deficiencies by consuming micronutrients before they can be absorbed.

**ABNORMALITIES OF STORAGE, PROCESSING, AND ACTIVATION** Patients with cirrhosis may develop deficiencies in vitamins that require processing and activation in the liver, such as vitamin D which the liver hydroxylates to 25-hydroxycholecalciferol (vitamin $D_3$), and vitamin $B_6$, which the liver coverts from pyridoxine to pyridoxal and pyridoxal phosphate. Hepatic stellate cells store vitamin A, and hepatic parenchymal cells synthesize retinol-binding protein that is required for release of vitamin A from the liver and transport to the tissues. In cirrhosis, patients generally have low levels of retinol, RBP, and transthyretin, and abnormal dark adaptation is common. Because of loss of stellate cells, however, supplementation in these patients may result in toxicity. The kidney is responsible for removing RBP from the circulation and hydroxylating vitamin D to 1α,25-hydroxycholecalciferol (vitamin $D_2$). Patients with chronic renal insufficiency are therefore at risk for both vitamin A toxicity and vitamin A deficiency.

**ABNORMALITIES OF TRANSPORT** Many vitamins and minerals require proteins for transport. The fat-soluble vitamins are transported from the gut to the liver on chylomicrons. Rare disorders of chylomicrons, such as abetalipoproteinemia, are therefore associated with vitamin E deficiency. Transcobalamin II transports vitamin to the

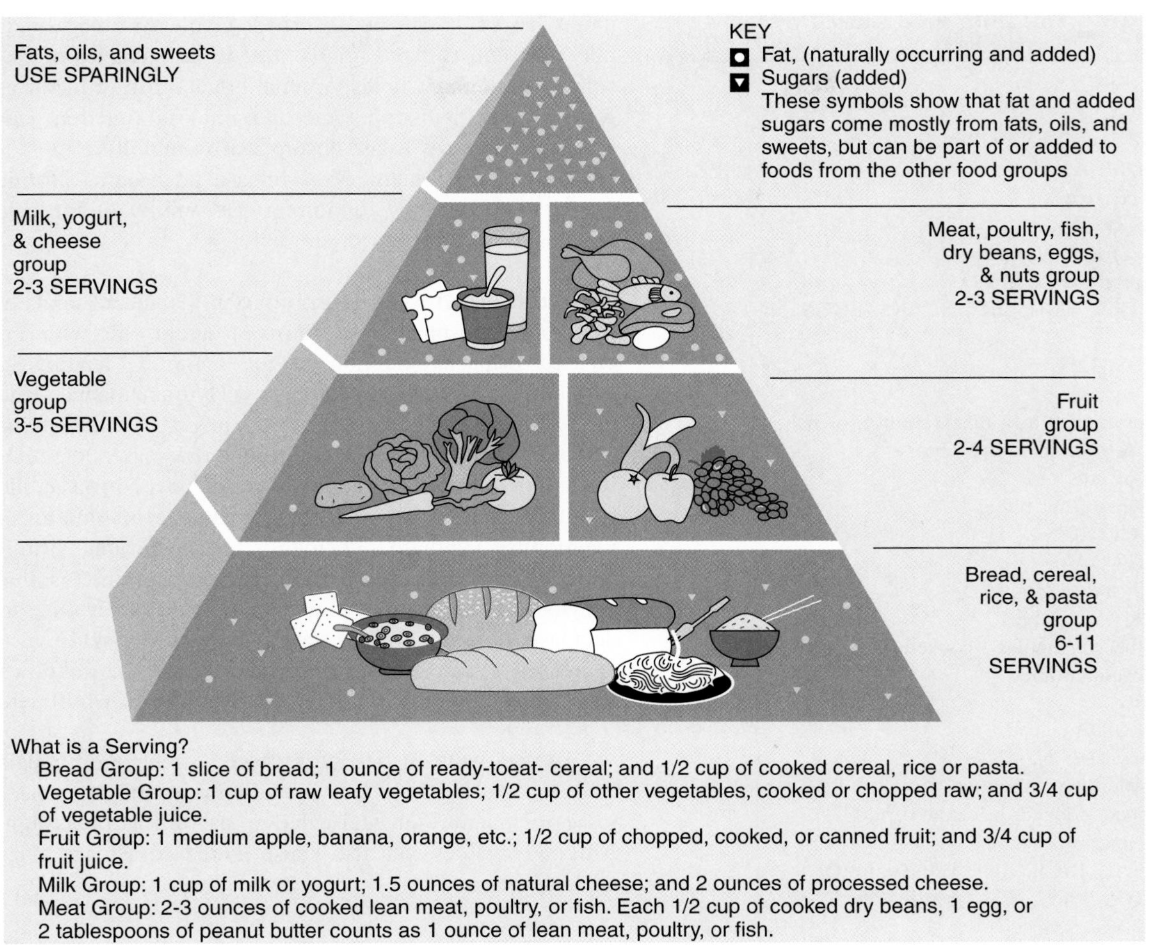


FIGURE 5-2 **The USDA food guide pyramid.**

tissues. Hereditary transcobalamin II deficiency can cause vitamin deficiency.

**ABNORMALITIES OF EXCRETION** The kidney filters and resorbs many water-soluble vitamins and excretes magnesium. In chronic renal insufficiency, patients are at risk for deficiencies of water-soluble vitamins, particularly vitamin $B_6$ and folate, and magnesium toxicity.

### *Patients with increased requirements*

Various groups of patients may be at increased risk for micronutrient deficiencies on the basis of increased requirements. Women who are pregnant or lactating have increased requirements for many micronutrients secondary to needs of the growing fetus and synthesis of breast milk. Elders, whose skin synthesis of vitamin D may be impaired and individuals living at higher latitudes, where wavelengths of light necessary for skin synthesis are not present during winter months, have increased needs for vitamin D from dietary sources. Cigarette smokers require increased amounts of antioxidant vitamins, in particular vitamins C and E, because of increased free radical production. Alcoholics may have increased requirements for vitamin C, the B vitamins, magnesium, and zinc due to multiple etiologies including decreased intake, decreased absorption, decreased stores, increased renal excretion, and decreased bioavailability. Patients with conditions leading to increased hematopoiesis, such as leukemia and

**Table 5-18 The USDA Food Guide Pyramid—Serving Sizes**

FATS, OILS, SWEETS
USE SPARINGLY
MILK, YOGURT, CHEESE GROUP
2–3 SERVINGS/DAY
*One serving consists of:*
1 cup of milk or yogurt
1 1/2 ounces of natural cheese
2 ounces of processed cheese
MEAT, POULTRY, FISH, DRY BEANS, EGGS, NUTS GROUP
2–3 SERVINGS/DAY
*One serving consists of:*
2–3 ounces of cooked lean meat, poultry, or fish
1 to 1 1/2 cups of cooked dry beans
2/3 to 1 cup of nuts
4–6 tablespoons of nut butter
VEGETABLE GROUP
3–5 SERVINGS/DAY
*One serving consists of:*
1 cup raw leafy vegetables
1/2 cup of other vegetables—cooked or chopped raw
3/4 cup of vegetable juice
FRUIT GROUP
2–4 SERVINGS/DAY
*One serving consists of:*
1 medium apple, banana, orange
1/2 cup chopped, cooked, or canned fruit
3/4 cup fruit juice
BREAD, CEREAL, RICE, AND PASTA GROUP
6–11 SERVINGS/DAY
*One serving consists of:*
1 slice of bread
1 ounce ready-to-eat cereal
1/2 cup cooked cereal, rice, or pasta

SOURCE: *Nutrition and Your Health: Dietary Guidelines for Americans* (USDA 1995).

hemolytic anemia, have increased needs for folate due to its role in nucleic acid synthesis.

### *Drug-nutrient interactions*

Patients may have increased or decreased needs for various micronutrients on the basis of food-nutrient interactions.

**DRUGS CAUSING INTERFERENCE WITH NUTRIENT DIGESTION AND ABSORPTION** Medications leading to achlorhydria such as histamine-2 ($H_2$) blockers and proton pump inhibitors may cause vitamin absorption by reducing its digestion from food proteins or by allowing overgrowth of small intestinal bacteria that consume the vitamin before it can be absorbed. Cholestyramine binds bile salts and can potentially lead to deficiencies of fat-soluble vitamins. Cholestyramine binds intrinsic factor as well. Colchicine disrupts intestinal mucosal function. Sulfasalazine reduces folate absorption by inhibiting its mucosal transport system. Slow-release potassium chloride may reduce ileal pH, inhibiting the activity of intrinsic factor and leading to vitamin deficiency.

**DRUGS THAT ALTER METABOLISM** Isoniazid binds to pyridoxal phosphate and forms a hydrazone with increased urinary excretion of the complex, leading to symptoms of vitamin $B_6$ deficiency. Hydralazine may lead to $B_6$ deficiency by a similar mechanism. Pyrimethamine and methotrexate block dihydrofolate reductase, potentially leading to symptoms of folate deficiency. Nitrous oxide converts vitamin $B_{12}$ to a form incapable of binding to methionine synthase. Phenytoin, phenobarbital, primidone, and carbamazepine may induce hepatic microsomal enzymes or inhibit intestinal calcium transport leading to decreased vitamin $D_3$ and serum calcium. Phenytoin also decreases serum folate concentrations by an unknown mechanism. Barbiturates induce catabolism of riboflavin.

**DRUGS THAT ALTER EXCRETION** Amphotericin B is toxic to renal distal tubular epithelium, leading to urinary losses of magnesium and calcium, as well as potassium. Aminoglycosides can also cause increased urinary magnesium losses.

**MICRONUTRIENT EFFECTS ON DRUG REQUIREMENTS** Varying intakes of dietary or supplemental vitamin K may interfere with optimal warfarin anticoagulation. Large doses of vitamin C may interfere with warfarin, as well as heparin therapy. Supplemental folate may counter the effects of phenobarbital, primidone, phenytoin, and supplemental vitamin $B_6$ may counter the effects of levodopa but not carbidopa.

**OTHER DRUG AND NUTRIENT ISSUES** Many medications may cause anorexia or nausea. If a patient complains of these symptoms, the medication list should be examined and substitution should be made if necessary. Other medications, such as calcium channel blockers, and cholestyramine may cause constipation by various mechanisms, and patients may limit their food intake because of fear of this symptom. Selective serotonin reuptake inhibitors may reduce or increase food intake, while other psychotropic medications such as phenothiazines, tricyclic antidepressants, and benzodiazepines promote appetite when administered chronically. If tranquilizers are given to geriatric patients in whom there may be decreased drug metabolism, then excessive somnolence may occur, leading to the opposite effect—disinterest and a decreased food intake.

**PRINCIPLE There are so many ways for diet to influence the outcome of disease or therapy that it must always be considered as part of a therapeutic regimen. Reconsider food-drug interaction when drugs are not performing as expected (either too well or unexpectedly poorly).**

#### *Physical examination and laboratory evaluation*

Physical findings associated with vitamin deficiencies are shown in Table 5-19. As noted, these findings may not be present until deficiency is present in an advanced state.

Laboratory assessment for micronutrient status, taken alone, is seldom diagnostic. Although for some nutrients, such as iron and folate, there are excellent diagnostic tests for deficiency, for other nutrients, such as calcium and selenium, there are no good laboratory indicators of status. A few highly clinically useful assays, such as the vitamin $D_3$ assay for vitamin D status (Beresford and Boushey 1997) and the serum cobalamin assay for vitamin $B_{12}$ status (Food and Nutrition Board 1997), have normal values defined on the basis of population distributions, and may be insensitive when prevalence is high. A full discussion of laboratory assays for micronutrient status is beyond the scope of this text, and the reader is referred to specialized texts for a complete discussion (Gibson 1990).

## Nutritional Prevention

Patients at increased risk for chronic disease due to inadequate or imbalanced dietary intakes should receive appropriate counseling. This counseling should include education regarding the potential long-term negative health effects of the patient's current diet and specific dietary advice. This may be done by the physician, or in referral with a registered dietitian. Implementation will involve

Table 5-19 Findings in Micronutrient Deficiency

| NUTRIENT | FINDINGS IN DEFICIENCY |
|---|---|
| Vitamin A | Xerophthalmia<br>Rapidly growing tissues may revert to undifferentiated state |
| Vitamin D | Bone pain, proximal muscle weakness, rickets (children), osteomalacia (adults), osteoporosis |
| Vitamin E | Myopathy, weakness, ataxia, impaired reflexes, ophthalmoplegia, retinopathy, bronchopulmonary dysplasia, hemolytic anemia |
| Vitamin K | Easily bruised, bleeding |
| Vitamin C | Scurvy |
| Thiamine ($B_1$) | *Dry beriberi:*<br>Chronic progressive polyneuropathy, extreme muscle weakness<br>*Wet beriberi:*<br>Edema, high output cardiac failure<br>*Wernicke–Korsakoff syndrome:*<br>Horizontal nystagmus, ophthalmoplegia, wide-based gait, global confusional state, short-term memory defect (Korsakoff psychosis) |
| Riboflavin ($B_2$) | Burning and itching of the eyes, corneal vascularization, nasolabial and scrotal seborrheic dermatitis, cheilosis, angular stomatitis, glossitis, hypoplastic anemia |
| Niacin ($B_3$) | *early:*<br>Anorexia, lassitude<br>*late: Pellagra:*<br>Diarrhea (sometimes vomiting), dermatitis (exposed areas), dementia (more correctly: mental status changes including irritability, sleeplessness, confusion, delirium, delusions), death |
| Vitamin $B_6$ | Neuritis, weakness, irritability, nervousness, insomnia, hyperirritability and seizures in infants, eczema and seborrheic dermatitis, hypochromic microcytic anemia, hyperoxaluria and renal stones, hyperhomocystinemia and increased risk of atherosclerosis |
| Folate | Megaloblastic anemia, glossitis, malabsorption (megaloblastic changes in gut), atherosclerosis |
| Vitamin $B_{12}$ | Macrocytic anemia, affective and thought disorders, subacute combined degeneration, megaloblastic GI tract, tobacco amblyopia |

changes in habits and behavior, and compliance should be carefully monitored by regular follow-up. Selected instances in which supplementation may be helpful are discussed below.

## Vitamin and Mineral Supplementation

Adequate vitamin and mineral nutrition is best achieved by proper diet; supplementation should be employed by indication only. The major indications for the use of supplements in medical management are 1) the treatment of specific or multiple deficiencies and 2) the prevention of diseases or degenerative conditions related to inadequate vitamin and mineral nutrition. Rarely, vitamins are used in high doses in the treatment of uncommon genetic disorders that impair the absorption or utilization of a specific vitamin.

**PRINCIPLE Not all vitamin and mineral preparations are the same. Select the dose and nutrient content that are appropriate for the specific indication for use.**

For the great majority of healthy individuals, maintenance of normal vitamin and mineral status or prevention of deficiency is accomplished by attention to a diet that uses a variety of food sources and meets usual caloric requirements, as discussed above. There are, however, circumstances under which vitamin and/or mineral supplementation should be recommended even for healthy individuals. Up to 30% of elders are unable to digest vitamin $B_{12}$ in food due to achlorhydria resulting from atrophic gastritis. In such patients, vitamin $B_{12}$ supplements may be required. Vitamin D is important for the prevention of osteoporosis, and skin production of vitamin D can be reduced in the elderly. Vitamin D is present only in a few foods including fortified milk, liver, eggs, fatty fish, and butter, and those unable to consume amounts of these foods necessary to meet recommended vitamin intakes should use supplements. Iron supplements are needed to meet the needs of some menstruating women. Those who are on special restricted diets for weight loss or other reasons (for example, strict vegetarians avoiding all animal products), or persons with multiple food allergies, benefit from vitamin and mineral supplements. In spite of the hype encouraging megadoses of vitamins, there is rarely a need for doses of vitamins or minerals beyond 100% of the RDA.

Higher doses of vitamins are needed to prevent deficiency in patients at increased risk owing to some conditions described above or in order to reverse an established deficiency. Multivitamin-and-mineral preparations for pregnancy ordinarily contain higher doses of certain vitamins and minerals such as folate and iron because of the special increased requirements. Patients who drink alcohol excessively and those with malabsorption may require therapeutic doses of vitamins (5 to 10 times preventive doses) to overcome excessive losses. In clinical settings where vitamin deficiency is manifest, recommended vitamin doses are commonly five to ten times the RDA of the daily requirement so that repletion and restitution of normal metabolic pathways will be achieved as quickly (Food and Nutrition Board 1998).

Usually vitamins and minerals are administered by mouth, but for those who cannot take oral medication, parenteral routes of medication may be used. The patient with pernicious anemia or who has had extensive gastric or distal ileal surgery presents a special instance in the treatment and prevention of vitamin $B_{12}$ deficiency, and under such clinical circumstances, parenteral vitamin $B_{12}$ therapy is generally used; however, because large amounts of crystalline vitamin $B_{12}$ can be absorbed by simple diffusion, large oral doses may also be effective in these patients.

As noted above, some individuals may express a genetic defect in the absorption, transport, or metabolism of a given vitamin and thus present with a nutritional deficiency disease despite the usual dietary intakes of the vitamin. These rare genetic syndromes usually are discovered in early infancy and are called vitamin dependency syndromes to distinguish them from vitamin deficiency syndromes. Substantial improvement of vitamin-dependent metabolic pathways in some of these patients can be achieved with very high doses of the relevant vitamin. To achieve normal function, doses as high as 1000 times the usual requirement may be needed (Food and Nutrition Board 1998).

There are claims for so-called megadoses of vitamins that are neither based on sound therapeutic principles nor safe. Vitamins, like all other therapeutic substances, have their proper dose range for appropriate indications, as noted above and in Table 5-19. This is true of both water-soluble and fat-soluble vitamins. Some doses are safe and adequate but others are potentially toxic. The difference between a preventive or therapeutic dose and a toxic dose is highly variable among nutrients: toxic/therapeutic dose ratios for vitamins may vary from 10- to 300-fold. One of the physician's responsibilities with respect to using vitamins is to see that self-administered vitamins are taken in safe dosages as supplements, not in so-called megadoses that provide no added benefit and risk toxic accumulations. Toxicity syndromes for vitamin A, vitamin D, niacin, and iron have been associated with chronic disease or death (Ross et al. 1997).

Some examples of the use of vitamins may be instructive.

**CASE HISTORY 1** *A 95-lb woman, aged 75, who is not very active, has a caloric requirement of only 1000 calories. The small amount of food required to meet this caloric need may not contain adequate amounts of vitamins and minerals to meet the usual, or the extra, needs of the elderly. A vitamin-mineral preparation that contains 100% of the RDA for all vitamins along with some zinc, chromium, and magnesium would be a prudent recommendation for the prevention of vitamin and mineral deficiency.*

**CASE HISTORY 2** *A middle-aged male presents to a physician with early findings of liver disease. The patient has been obtaining in excess of 50% of his calories from alcohol for some years and presents with folate deficiency anemia and some peripheral neuropathy suggestive of multiple B-vitamin deficiencies. This patient should be treated with vitamin therapy containing 5 to 10 times the requirement of the B vitamins with a dose of folic acid of at least 1 mg/day. Vitamin-mineral preparations containing higher doses of iron are not indicated under these circumstances because of the tendency of alcoholics to have increased total body iron. Also, high doses of vitamin A may exacerbate the hepatotoxic effects of alcohol.*

In addition to dose and route of supplementation, another important consideration when planning a supplementation regimen is the supplement's chemical composition. Magnesium oxide, a form of magnesium commonly used for fortification of foods and supplementation, is highly insoluble and causes diarrhea and is therefore not an effective supplement. Magnesium gluconate is a better choice for oral magnesium supplementation (Manson et al. 1995).

**PRINCIPLE The form of a chemical entity and the excipients used in the product are important determinants of the effects of nutritional supplement.**

## REFERENCES


Alpers DH, Stenson WF, Bier DM. 1995. *Manual of Nutritional Therapeutics*, 3rd edition. Boston: Little Brown and Company.

Beresford SAA, Boushey CJ. 1997. Homocysteine, folic acid, and cardiovascular disease risk. In: Bendich A, Deckelbaum RJ, editors. *Preventive Nutrition: The Comprehensive Guide for Health Professionals*. Totowa, NJ: Humana Press.

Blackburn GL. 1977. Nutritional assessment and support during infection. *Am J Clin Nutr* **30**:1493–7.

Bowman SA, Lino M, Gerrior SA, et al. 1998. *The Healthy Eating Index: 1994–1996*. USDA, Center for Nutrition Policy and Promotion. CNPP-5.

Campbell WW, Crim MC, Dallal GE, et al. 1994. Increased protein requirements in elderly people: new data and retrospective reassessments. *Am J Clin Nutr* **60**:501–9.

Chapuy MC, Arlot ME, Duboeuf F, et al. 1992. Vitamin $D_3$ and calcium to prevent hip fractures in elderly women. *N Engl J Med* **327**:637–42.

Choban PS, Burge JC, Scales D, et al. 1997. Hypoenergetic nutrition support in hospitalized obese patients: a simplified method for clinical application. *Am J Clin Nutr* **66**:546–50.

Coats KG, Morgan SL, Bartolucci AA, et al. 1993. Hospital-associated malnutrition: a reevaluation 12 years later. *J Am Diet Assoc* **93**: 27–33.

Dawson-Hughes B, Harris SS, Krall EA, et al. 1997. Effect of calcium and vitamin D supplementation on bone density in men and women 65 years of age or older. *N Engl J Med* **337**:670–6.

Delmi M, Rapin CH, Bengoa JM, et al. 1990. Dietary supplementation in elderly patients with fractured neck of the femur. *Lancet* **335**:1013–6.

Flegal KM, Carroll MD, Kuczmarski RJ, et al. 1998. Overweight and obesity in the United States: prevalence and trends, 1960–1994. *Int J Obes* **22**:39–47.

Food and Nutrition Board, Commission on Life Sciences, National Research Council. 1989. *Recommended Dietary Allowances*, 10th edition. Subcommittee on the 10th edition of the RDAs. Washington, DC: National Academy Press.

Food and Nutrition Board, Institute of Medicine. 1997. *Dietary Reference Intakes for Calcium, Phosphorus, Magnesium, Vitamin D, and Fluoride*. Standing Committee on the Scientific Evaluation of Dietary Reference Intakes. Washington, DC: National Academy Press.

Food and Nutrition Board, Institute of Medicine. 1998. *Dietary Reference Intakes for Thiamin, Riboflavin, Niacin, Vitamin $B_6$, Folate, Vitamin $B_{12}$, Pantothenic Acid, Biotin, and Choline*. Standing Committee on the Scientific Evaluation of Dietary Reference Intakes. Washington, DC: National Academy Press.

Gariballa SE, Parker SG, Taub N, et al. 1998. Influence of nutritional status on clinical outcome after acute stroke. *Am J Clin Nutr* **68**:275–81.

Gibson RS. 1990. *Principles of Nutritional Assessment*. New York: Oxford University Press.

Heimburger DC, Weinsier RL. 1997. *Handbook of Clinical Nutrition*, 3rd Edition. St Louis: Mosby-Year Book, Inc.

Jacques PF, Chylack LT Jr, Taylor A. 1994. Relationships between natural antioxidants and cataract formation. In: Frei B, editor. *Natural Antioxidants in Human Health and Disease*. Orlando (FL): Academic Press. p 513–33.

Jick H, Vasilakis C, Weinrauch LA, et al. 1998. A population-based study of appetite-suppressant drugs and the risk of cardiac-valve regurgitation. *N Engl J Med* **339**:719–24.

Khan MA, Herzog CA, St. Peter JV, et al. 1998. The prevalence of cardiac valvular insufficiency assessed by transthoracic echocardiography in obese patients treated with appetite-suppressant drugs. *N Engl J Med* **339**:713–8.

Klein S, Kinney K, JeeJeebhoy K, et al. 1997. Nutrition support in clinical practice: review of published data and recommendations for future research directions. *J Parenter Enteral Nutr* **21**:133–156.

Lindenbaum J, Rosenberg IH, Wilson PW, et al. 1994. Prevalence of cobalamin deficiency in the Framingham elderly population. *Am J Clin Nutr* **60**:2–11.

MacFie J, Smith RC, Hill GL. 1981. Glucose or fat as a non-protein energy source? A controlled clinical trial in gastrointestinal patients requiring intravenous nutrition, *Gastroenterology* **80**: 103–7.

Manson JE, Willett WC, Stampfer MJ, et al. 1995. Body weight and mortality among women. *N Engl J Med* **333**:677–85.

McCowen KC, Chan MD, Bistrian BR. 1998. Total parenteral nutrition. *Curr Opin Gastroenterol* **14**:157–163.

MRC Vitamin Study Research Group. 1991. Prevention of neural tube defects: results of the Medical Research Council Vitamin Study. *Lancet* **338**:131–7.

Naber TH, Schermer T, de Bree A, et al. 1997. Prevalence of malnutrition in nonsurgical hospitalized patients and its association with disease complications. *Am J Clin Nutr* **66**:1232–9.

National Heart, Lung, and Blood Institute (NHLBI). 1998. Clinical Guidelines on the Identification, Evaluation, and Treatment of Overweight and Obesity in Adults: The Evidence Report. Expert Panel on the Identification, Evaluation, and Treatment of Overweight and Obesity in Adults. Bethesda, MD: National Heart, Lung, and Blood Institute.

Reynolds JV, Kanwar S, Welsh FKS, et al. 1997. Does the route of feeding modify gut barrier function and clinical outcome in patients after major upper gastrointestinal surgery? *J Parenter Enteral Nutr* **21**:196–201.

Roe DA. 1989. *Diet and Drug Interactions*, New York: Van Nostrand Reinhold.

Ross EM, Rosenberg IH, Dawson-Hughes B, et al. 1997. Should the "normal" 25-hydroxy vitamin D level be increased? [abstract]. *Am J Clin Nutr* **66**:206.

Selbub J, Jacques PF, Wilson PWF, et al. 1993. Vitamin status and intake as primary determinants of homocysteinemia in an elderly population. *JAMA* **270**:2693–8.

Sullivan DH, Patch GA, Walls RC, et al. 1990. Impact of nutrition status on morbidity and mortality in a select population of geriatric rehabilitation patients. *Am J Clin Nutr* **51**:749–58.

Taylor RW, Keil D, Gold EJ, et al. 1998. Body mass index, waist girth, and waist-to-hip ratio as indexes of total and regional adiposity in women: evaluation using receiver operating characteristic curves. *Am J Clin Nutr* **67**:44–9.

Ulrich H, Pastores SM, Katz DP, et al. 1996. Parenteral use of medium chain triglycerides: a reappraisal [review]. *Nutrition* **12**:231–238.

USDA. 1995. *Nutrition and Your Health: Dietary Guidelines for Americans.* 4th edition. Home and garden bull. no. 232. 43p.

Weinsier RL, Hunker EM, Krumdieck CL, et al. 1979. Hospital malnutrition. A prospective evaluation of general medical patients during the course of hospitalization. *Am J Clin Nutr* **32**:418–26.

Weintraub M, Sundaresan PR, Schuster B, et al. 1992. Long-term weight control study. *Clin Pharmacol Ther* **51**:615–8.

CHAPTER

# 6 RENAL DISORDERS AND THE INFLUENCE OF RENAL FUNCTION ON DRUG DISPOSITION

D. Craig Brater

### *Chapter Outline*



The treatment of renal disorders, as well as the influences of renal disease on drugs, constitutes a broad area in the field of medicine. Entire books have been written on these topics. This chapter is, therefore, limited in its scope and focuses on understanding the pathophysiology of renal disorders and experimentally validated therapeutics. The first part of this chapter describes frequently encountered renal disorders. The next part discusses ways in which drugs affect the kidney. The third and final section of this chapter examines the implications of decreased renal function on pharmacokinetics and pharmacodynamics; dosing regimens are also examined in this section. Although this chapter does not discuss all diseases of the kidney, the principles of therapeutics that are reviewed here can be extrapolated to them.

## PHARMACOTHERAPY OF COMMON RENAL DISORDERS

### Acute Renal Failure

#### *Pathophysiology*

Acute renal failure (ARF) is a syndrome in which a rapid decline in renal function occurs that manifests as increases in concentrations of blood urea nitrogen (BUN) and especially creatinine in serum. Decreased urinary output (oliguria or rarely anuria) may also occur. ARF can occur in patients with normal renal function, or it may be superimposed on chronic renal insufficiency (CRI). In addition, factitious increases in BUN and/or creatinine concentrations can occur. For example, excess tissue catabolism or antianabolic agents like the tetracyclines can cause increases in BUN concentrations. Drugs such as cimetidine, which blocks the secretory component of creatinine elimination, can increase serum concentrations of creatinine without altering glomerular filtration rate (GFR) (Zaltman et al. 1996). In these settings, no actual decline in renal function has occurred.

When a patient is seen for the first time, determining whether the patient has ARF or CRI is sometimes difficult. Anemia, osteodystrophy, neuropathy, and shrunken kidneys are more consistent with CRI. Hyperphosphatemia and hypocalcemia can develop quickly during ARF and are less helpful clues. Differentiating ARF superimposed on CRI also can be difficult because renal function in most patients with CRI declines progressively over time. As a consequence, it is sometimes enigmatic whether a patient manifests the natural progression of his or her intrinsic renal disease or, alternatively, whether an acute and possible remedial insult has occurred. A graph of creatinine clearance (or less accurately the reciprocal of serum creatinine concentrations) against time usually reveals a linear deterioration in renal function when intrinsic renal disease progresses naturally (Mitch et al. 1976). Negative deviation from such a plot indicates a new insult and serves as presumptive evidence of ARF until proved otherwise.

Once a diagnosis of ARF is established, its pathogenesis must be determined so that a rational therapeutic strategy can be developed. To facilitate diagnosis, ARF can be attributed to three broad etiologies, as shown in Fig. 6-1 (Thadhani et al. 1996; Nolan and Anderson 1998). Both noninvasive and invasive tests (none of which are specific) can be used to formulate a diagnosis. For example, assessment of the urinary sediment can be helpful: red blood cell casts and proteinuria focus the physician's attention on glomerulonephritis or vasculitis, calcium oxalate or uric acid crystals raise the possibility of urinary tract calculi causing obstruction, granular casts implicate a nephrotoxic insult, and eosinophiluria raises the specter of interstitial nephritis.

The differential diagnosis is often between prerenal azotemia and acute tubular necrosis (ATN). In the former, the kidney behaves as if volume depletion were present. This fact has been used to develop indices that help discriminate between these two entities (Table 6-1) (Klahr and Miller 1998). These indices are not absolute, and they do not apply to patients who have received diuretics, contrast agents, or osmotic agents, including endogenous glucose. In addition to these indices, the BUN concentration rises disproportionally to the creatinine concentration in prerenal azotemia.

If noninvasive assessment and other clinical clues (e.g., exposure to drugs, vascular surgical procedures, presence of decompensated cardiac or hepatic disease) do not allow a firm diagnosis, invasive studies such as arteriography, renal biopsy, or retrograde pyelography may be indicated. Fortunately, such procedures often can be avoided.

**Table 6-1 Indices to Differentiate Prerenal Azotemia from Acute Tubular Necrosis**

| PRERENAL AZOTEMIA | INDEX | ATN |
|---|---|---|
| >1.020 | Specific gravity | ~1.010 |
| >1.5 | U/P osmolality | <1.1 |
| >40 | U/P creatinine | <20 |
| <20 | [Sodium] in urine (mEq/L) | >40 |
| <1 | $FE_{Na}$ (%) | >1 |
| <7 | $FE_{uric\ Acid}$ (%) | >15 |

ABBREVIATIONS: ATN, acute tubular necrosis; FE, fractional excretion ([clearance of marker/creatinine clearance] × 100); P, plasma concentration; U, urinary concentration.

### *Clinical pharmacology of drugs used in acute renal failure*

**OBSTRUCTION OF THE RENAL ARTERIES** Obstruction of the renal arteries is not amenable to drug therapy. However, it often is associated with elevated blood pressure that can further damage the kidney. Hypertension should be controlled as discussed in chapter 1, Cardiovascular Disorders. In this setting, however, use of angiotensin-converting enzyme (ACE) inhibitors can further impair renal function. When both renal arteries are tightly obstructed or when renal perfusion is severely diminished (as may occur in end-stage heart failure), residual glomerular filtration becomes dependent on efferent arteriolar constriction from intrarenal production of angiotensin II. Inhibition of ACE can thereby result in a precipitous fall in renal function.

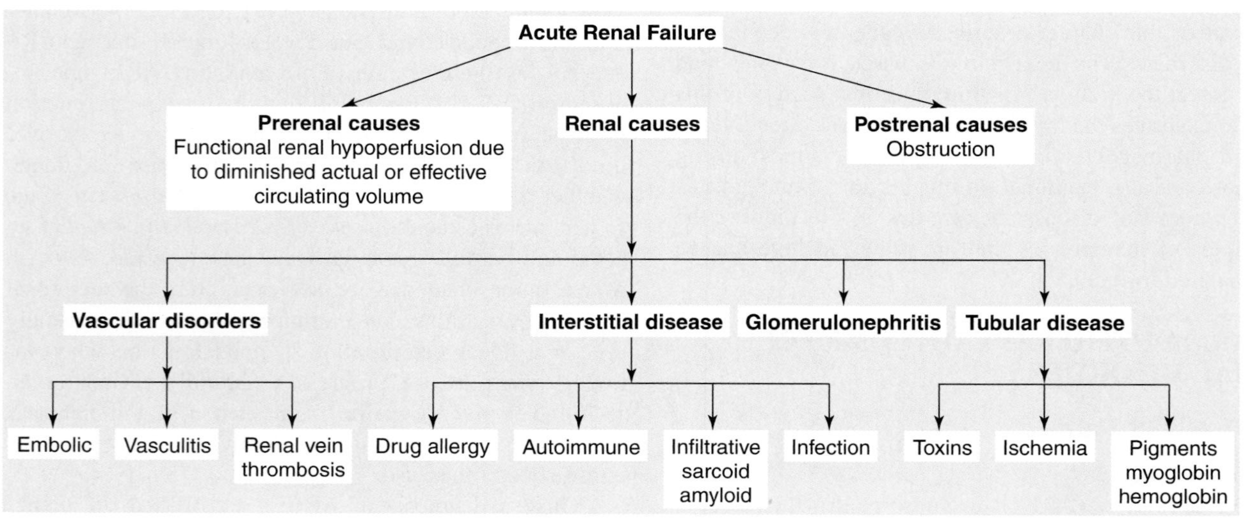


FIGURE 6-1 **Classification of types of acute renal failure.**

**PRERENAL AZOTEMIA** Treatment of prerenal azotemia depends on the underlying disorder. Volume repletion quickly restores renal function in depleted patients. In contrast, treatment of conditions such as severe heart failure or hepatorenal syndrome may not fully restore renal perfusion to normal, and patients may remain with some degree of prerenal azotemia. In fact, the degree of prerenal azotemia can sometimes be used as a helpful guide to therapy. For example, a patient with severe decompensated heart failure might present with a markedly elevated BUN-creatinine ratio. With therapy and diuresis, this ratio should diminish, although it may not return to normal. With further diuresis, the ratio might begin to escalate again, indicating overly vigorous diuresis and the onset of iatrogenic relative volume depletion, not worsening heart failure. In some patients, this may even occur despite the persistence of peripheral edema. A proper response to this scenario would be a decrease in the dose of diuretic and/or liberalized sodium intake.

**GLOMERULONEPHRITIDES AND VASCULITIDES** Glomerulonephritides and vasculitides are treated with immunosuppressive agents that are discussed elsewhere (see chapter 10, Connective Tissue and Bone Disorders). Because the precise etiology of these syndromes is unknown, such therapy is empiric and should be guided by well-controlled clinical trials that are relevant to the patient being treated.

> **PRINCIPLE It may be necessary to treat a patient with a disease of unclear etiology or pathophysiology. In such situations, it is even more important to base therapeutic decisions on evidence from quality clinical trials.**

**ACUTE TUBULAR NECROSIS** ATN represents a syndrome wherein an insult to the kidney (often ischemic) has progressed to a stage of cell death. Before this stage occurs, renal dysfunction may be reversible by ameliorating the original insult. For example, if renal ischemia has occurred because of hypotension during a surgical procedure or due to vasoconstriction induced by the use of a nonsteroidal anti-inflammatory drug (NSAID) (see the section on adverse effects of drugs on renal function), then prompt restoration of blood pressure or stopping the offending NSAID can restore renal perfusion before an ischemic insult to tubular cells occurs.

Once ATN is manifest, it is generally characterized by poor reabsorption of sodium and inability to concentrate or dilute the urine. This feature accounts for the indices listed in Table 6-1. Treatment of ATN has focused on either conversion of oliguric to nonoliguric renal failure or treatment of established ATN. Patients with ATN usually are subdivided into those with oliguria (urine output <20 mL/h) and those who are nonoliguric. Nonoliguric renal failure appears to be less severe than does oliguric in that patients have fewer complications, require less dialysis, and have lower mortality rates (Anderson et al. 1977; McMurray et al. 1978; Minuth et al. 1976). These observations have provoked controversy as to whether patients with oliguric ARF should be treated with the objective of converting them to a nonoliguric state. It appears that nonoliguric patients have a less severe renal insult accounting for their better prognosis. Converting oliguric to nonoliguric renal failure is helpful only insofar as fluid management becomes a bit less complex. This benefit is often small.

Mannitol or loop diuretics appear beneficial in treating pigment-induced ARF but their efficacy after other insults is vigorously debated (Thadhani et al. 1996). Mannitol depends on the kidney for excretion. Its pharmacokinetics are markedly altered in patients with renal disease so that its half-life increases from about 1 to 36 hours (Cloyd et al. 1986). As a consequence, if mannitol does not improve renal function in a patient with ARF, then it persists in plasma, where its osmotic effect can cause intravascular volume expansion sufficient to precipitate heart failure (Warren and Blantz 1981; Borges et al. 1982). In this setting, its pharmacodynamics as an osmotic agent in the systemic circulation are deleterious. In contrast, in patients with cerebral edema, the systemic osmotic effect is beneficial. Therefore, the benefit-risk assessment for the drug is dependent on the clinical indication and the patient's renal status. A tenuous potential beneficial effect in ARF seems outweighed by substantial risks.

The utility of loop diuretics in patients with ARF is also debatable. Some investigators have argued that they may help improve prognosis by converting the patient from the oliguric to the nonoliguric state (Cantarovich et al. 1973). On the other hand, other studies have demonstrated no benefit, or at best, a need for a diminished number of dialysis sessions (Minuth et al. 1976; Epstein et al. 1975; Alkhunaizi and Schrier 1996). In the absence of convincing data, it seems illogical to use diuretics for most patients with ARF. If they are to be tried, it is recommended that a single 200 mg intravenous (IV) bolus dose of furosemide (or the equivalent of another loop diuretic) be administered. If there is no response, then no more doses should be given.

**PRINCIPLE As often as possible, therapeutic decisions should be based on clear and compelling evidence from clinical trials, not untested hypotheses that are merely biologically plausible.**

"Renal dose dopamine" (≤3 μg/kg per minute) theoretically increases renal blood flow without systemic effects. It has been embraced for prophylaxis against development of ARF in patients at risk (e.g., patients in the intensive care unit) and for treatment of established ARF. More recent data argue against efficacy of dopamine in either setting and also point out its risks, including cardiac arrhythmias. Overall, there are no data to support efficacy of renal dose dopamine in patients at risk of or who have developed ARF (Conger 1988; Alkhunaizi and Schrier 1996; Thadhani et al. 1996; Nolan and Anderson 1998).

Other treatments for ARF have been similarly disappointing. Recently evaluated and theoretically beneficial modalities include calcium antagonists, atrial natriuretic factor, and various growth factors (Conger 1988; Simon 1995; Alkhunaizi and Schrier 1996; Thadhani et al. 1996; Nolan and Anderson 1998). Unfortunately, none have been efficacious. Overall, with the exception of induced diuresis for pigment-induced ARF, no therapies have been proven to be beneficial.

What recourse, then, does the clinician have in such patients? First, one must be alert to preventive measures. For example, patients at high risk of ARF from contrast agents (such as diabetics with moderate renal insufficiency) need hydration and may benefit from nonionic contrast agents (Simon 1995). Second, most hospital-acquired ARF is associated with sepsis and multiorgan failure (Minuth et al. 1976; Anderson et al. 1977; McMurray et al. 1978; Klahr and Miller 1998; Nolan and Anderson 1998). Strategies to minimize the risk of infection and good supportive care should be helpful. Last, if renal replacement therapy is needed, then biocompatible dialysis membranes result in better outcomes (Simon 1995). It is to be hoped that drugs useful in treating established ARF will be developed in the future. Until such time, the clinician should not be lured into using theoretical but unproven (not to mention disproven) therapies. To do so may actually harm these already seriously ill patients.

## Chronic Renal Insufficiency

### *Pathophysiology*

Chronic renal insufficiency can result from many disorders such as hypertension, diabetes mellitus, polycystic kidney disease, collagen–vascular diseases, and so forth. Once a decline in renal function occurs by way of any insult, inexorable progression of renal dysfunction usually occurs (Mitch et al. 1976). No matter what the etiology, end-stage kidneys all show interstitial fibrosis and glomerulosclerosis, raising the hypothesis that a single mechanism accounts for the progressive deterioration of renal function. A possible unifying mechanism of continuing renal injury has led to the hypothesis that the final common pathway of the process occurs by glomerular hyperfiltration, as illustrated in Fig. 6-2 (Brenner 1983; Klahr et al. 1988). Simplistically, once a renal insult has occurred, remnant nephrons must work harder. They suffer increased glomerular pressures and glomerular hyperfiltration. Hyperfiltration is associated with a loss in glomerular permselectivity that results in protein filtration and possibly in direct tissue injury. Both these effects cause glomerular mesangial injury and stimulation, the culmination of which is glomerulosclerosis.

The hyperfiltration hypothesis has led to a number of potential therapeutic interventions to arrest the progression of renal disease over and above vigorous treatment of the primary disease (Maki et al. 1995; Peterson et al. 1995). The observation that dietary protein in experimental animals caused glomerular hyperfiltration has led to studies indicating that diminished protein intake (usually 0.6 g of protein per kilogram body weight per day) slows

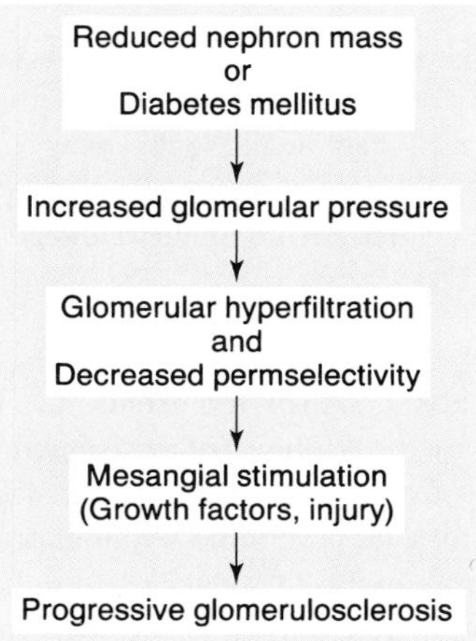


**FIGURE 6-2 Schematic representation of the glomerular hyperfiltration hypothesis of progressive renal dysfunction. [From Brater DC. 1992. Treatment of renal disorders and the influence of renal function on drug disposition. In: Melmon KL, Morrelli HF, Hoffman BB, et al., editors. *Clinical Pharmacology: Basic Principles in Therapeutics*. 3rd ed. New York: McGraw-Hill. pp 270–308. Reproduced with permission of the McGraw-Hill Companies.]**

the rate of progression of renal disease (Zeller 1987; Klahr et al. 1994; Pedrini et al. 1996). In some patients this benefit is outweighed by protein-calorie malnutrition; the degree of protein restriction must be tailored to individual patients.

Studies also have shown that ACE inhibitors diminish glomerular hyperfiltration by ameliorating the intrarenal effects of angiotensin II (Brenner 1983; Ihle et al. 1996; Maschio et al. 1996). These drugs reverse or arrest microalbuminuria in normotensive diabetic patients, and they slow the progression of renal disease (Ihle et al. 1996; Maschio et al. 1996). They are primary agents for prevention of renal disease in both diabetic patients and in patients with other causes of renal insufficiency. This efficacious effect is independent of their blood pressure–lowering effect and may be unique to ACE inhibitors. For calcium-channel antagonists, data are conflicting (Maki et al. 1995; Peterson et al. 1995).

The diminished renal function in patients with CRI results in a number of conditions often requiring pharmacologic therapy. Loss of nephron mass affects solute homeostasis. Even though patients with CRI have an obligate sodium loss of 20–30 mEq/day, compromised ability to excrete larger amounts of sodium commonly ingested usually results in a need for diuretics to enhance sodium excretion.

Diminished ability to excrete phosphate causes its elevation in plasma with a reciprocal lowering of calcium concentrations, which in turn stimulates release of parathyroid hormone (Hruska and Teitelbaum 1995). Ordinarily, parathyroid hormone, among other effects, stimulates 1-hydroxylation of 25-hydroxycholecalciferol (25[OH]$D_3$ or 25-hydroxyvitamin $D_3$) by the kidney, which restores concentrations of calcium toward normal. However, the diminished nephron mass results in decreased capacity to synthesize 1,25-dihydroxyvitamin $D_3$ (1,25[OH]$_2D_3$) such that pharmacologic replacement is needed. Correction of the serum calcium concentration without lowering the phosphate concentration may cause precipitation of calcium phosphate in soft tissue. Therefore, concomitant treatment of hyperphosphatemia is important.

Historically, aluminum-containing antacids were used to irreversibly bind dietary phosphate in the gut precluding its absorption. Aluminum is no longer preferred because it has been found to accumulate in patients with CRI, possibly causing dementia and contributing to renal osteodystrophy. Instead, calcium salts should be taken with meals to bind dietary phosphate. The dose of calcium products and the dose of vitamin D analogs are adjusted to normalize serum phosphate concentrations and keep calcium concentrations at the upper limit of normal to maximally suppress parathormone secretion (Hruska and Teitelbaum 1995).

Diminished renal function is also associated with a decrease in the kidney's ability to synthesize erythropoietin, accounting for the anemia of patients with CRI (Fried 1973; Erslev 1975). Pharmacologic doses of human erythropoietin normalize red cell mass in patients with CRI, reverse the iron overload that occurs in many transfusion-dependent patients, and improve their quality of life (Eschbach et al. 1989). Because many patients treated with erythropoietin become hypertensive, their blood pressure should be followed closely. In addition, they can become iron-deficient.

All patients with CRI become hyperuricemic, but few develop gout. An extensive literature documents that the risks of asymptomatic hyperuricemia—de novo, secondary to diuretics, or due to CRI—are negligible (Berger and Yu 1975; Fessel 1979; Foley and Weinman 1984; Langford et al. 1987). Rare patients develop gout: only 15 episodes occurred over 5 years in 3,693 patients with thiazide-induced hyperuricemia (Langford et al. 1987). The risk of urolithiasis is negligible: 1 stone in about 300 patients with hyperuricemia compared with 1 stone in about 850 normouricemic patients (Fessel 1979); and uric acid nephropathy is so unusual that some experts question its existence as a distinct clinical entity (Foley and Weinman 1984). Hyperuricemia in patients with CRI should only be treated if patients are symptomatic, with attacks of gout or with uric acid nephrolithiasis.

### *Clinical pharmacology of drugs used in chronic renal insufficiency*

Pharmacotherapy in patients with CRI is aimed at preserving renal function and at treating disorders that arise from the loss of nephron mass itself. Preservation of renal function first entails treatment of primary diseases such as hypertension or diabetes mellitus that can cause further decrements in renal function if they are not controlled (Maki et al. 1995; Peterson et al. 1995). The pharmacology and clinical pharmacokinetics of drugs used in these disorders are discussed in chapters 1 and 9, Cardiovascular Disorders and Endocrine and Metabolic Disorders, respectively. Other primary causes of CRI such as polycystic kidney disease are untreatable, although complications such as infection, which hastens renal deterioration, can be treated. Another therapeutic goal is to arrest or slow the progress of renal deterioration, as discussed above.

Strategies for maintaining calcium and phosphate homeostasis have changed. The heretofore universal use of aluminum-containing antacids to bind phosphate in the gut has for the most part been abandoned in order to avoid aluminum toxicity. Similarly, calcium citrate is no longer favored as a phosphate binder and calcium replacement because citrate increases aluminum absorption. Instead, calcium carbonate or calcium acetate should be used to bind phosphate and simultaneously supplement calcium (Sheikh et al. 1989). If hyperphosphatemia is not controlled, judicious use of aluminum-containing antacids can be used if ingested with meals. If plasma phosphate is normal but calcium remains depressed, $1,25[OH]_2D_3$ is used to restore calcium homeostasis and thereby reverse secondary hyperparathyroidism (Hruska and Teitelbaum 1995).

Reversal of erythropoietin deficiency is now possible through use of the genetically engineered human hormone. In virtually all patients, including those treated with chronic dialysis, red cell mass can be restored to normal within 12 weeks. Lack of response implies another disorder such as blood loss, myelofibrosis, iron deficiency, or some other etiology. The increased iron needs for new red blood cell propagation results in iron deficiency in more than 40% of patients; many, if not most, patients require iron supplements. Hypertension, or worsened hypertension, develops in about one-third of patients, although the mechanism is uncertain.

Treatment of symptomatic hyperuricemia entails either decreasing the rate of synthesis of uric acid or increasing its excretion. The latter is not a therapeutic option in patients with CRI since uricosuric agents are ineffective because of the decreased renal function. Allopurinol is used, but at decreased doses to avoid accumulation of its potentially toxic active metabolite, oxypurinol. Allopurinol and oxypurinol decrease production of uric acid by inhibiting xanthine oxidase. Allopurinol itself has a bioavailability of about 65%. It is eliminated quickly with a half-life of about 1.5 hours. With chronic dosing, oxypurinol accumulates because its half-life is 15–30 hours, accounting for the satisfactory response to once-daily dosing. In contrast to allopurinol, which is metabolized in the liver, oxypurinol is excreted in the urine. Patients with CRI accumulate oxypurinol, which has a half-life in patients with severe CRI of about 1 week. If the dose of allopurinol is not decreased to about one-third of normal or less in such patients, severe oxypurinol toxicity, which manifests as a systemic vasculitis, can occur (Young et al. 1974).

Most patients with CRI require treatment with diuretics at some point during the course of their disease, either as antihypertensive agents or to reverse sodium accumulation. The pharmacology of diuretic agents will be subsequently discussed in the section on fluid and electrolytes. Because diuretics used in patients with CRI are for the most part restricted to loop diuretics, their use is discussed here.

The diminished filtered sodium in patients with CRI often makes diuretic therapy vexing because even highly efficacious loop diuretics are limited in their effects. As a consequence, patients can easily ingest sufficient sodium to overcome any drug-induced diuresis and natriuresis, making dietary restriction of sodium a mainstay of therapy in patients with CRI. The loop diuretics bumetanide, ethacrynic acid, furosemide, and torsemide all must reach the lumen of the nephron to exert an effect (Odlind and Beermann 1980). Renal clearance of these diuretics decreases in parallel with the diminished renal perfusion of CRI, so that less drug reaches the site of action. For example, in patients with severe renal insufficiency, only one-fifth as much furosemide reaches the urine compared with administration of the same dose to a patient with normal renal function (Brater et al. 1986; Voelker et al. 1987). This means that larger doses must be given to attain effective amounts of diuretic in the urine.

Residual nephrons in patients with CRI respond normally to amounts of loop diuretic reaching them, with a maximal fractional excretion of sodium of about 20% (Brater et al. 1986; Voelker et al. 1987). In a patient with normal GFR, this level of response amounts to a maximal sodium excretion rate of about 3 mEq/min, a substantial natriuresis even if sustained over only a short period of time. In contrast, a patient with a GFR of 10–15 mL/min has a maximal sodium excretion rate of only about 0.3 mEq/min. Even if sustained over several hours, this magnitude of response may be inadequate in many patients, mandating ancillary measures for removing sodium, such as dialysis. If a therapeutic trial is possible, then occasional patients with CRI respond to a combination of loop and thiazide diuretics. The rationale for such therapy is discussed in the section on fluid and electrolytes.

Maximal doses of loop diuretics in patients with severe CRI (GFR $< 15$ ml/min) are 8–10 mg of oral or IV bumetanide, 200 mg of IV or 400 mg of oral furosemide, and 50–100 mg of oral or IV torsemide. Higher doses add no incremental efficacy and simply risk toxicity. Although the therapeutic margin of loop diuretics is large, ototoxicity that usually is reversible can occur. Ototoxicity usually has been reported with large doses infused rapidly in patients with renal insufficiency particularly if concomitantly treated with other ototoxic drugs such as aminoglycoside antibiotics.

Studies with both bumetanide and furosemide (but not torsemide) in patients with heart failure have shown a delay in absorption, although the total quantity of diuretic absorbed (i.e., bioavailability) is unaltered (Brater et al. 1982; Vasko et al. 1985). Moreover, patients in the decompensated state show a greater delay of absorption than when they have been treated to a stable clinical condition (Vasko et al. 1985). The clinical importance of these observations is that patients with decompensated heart failure absorb some loop diuretics so slowly that they may require treatment by IV dosing.

## Urinary Tract Infections

### *Pathophysiology*

Urinary tract infections (UTIs) encompass infections from the urethra to the kidney itself. In addition, vaginitis often presents with symptoms consistent with a UTI, although it can usually be distinguished from a true UTI by superficial burning that occurs after urination as opposed to true dysuria.

Therapeutic strategies in patients with a UTI are dictated by the type of infection (Table 6-2) (Stamm and Hooton 1993). Recurrent infection of the male urinary tract suggests the likelihood of an underlying pathologic condition, either anatomic or a set of host factors increasing susceptibility to infection. In contrast, uncomplicated UTI is frequent in women, with 10–20% of all women suffering a UTI during their lifetime (Stamm and Hooton 1993; Johnson and Stamm 1989). A search for an underlying pathologic condition in women with UTI is indicated only when infections recur; three or more infections in a woman during a 1-year period warrant further investigation.

Asymptomatic bacteriuria is frequent, particularly in elderly patients, affecting up to 20% of women and 10% of men over 65 years of age. The percentage is even higher in nursing home residents. There is no evidence that asymptomatic bacteriuria leads to progressive renal insufficiency or other complications; thus, it need not be treated (Abrutyn et al. 1994). If symptoms occur, treatment is, however, indicated. The exception to this general rule is pregnancy, wherein even asymptomatic bacteriuria (which occurs frequently) should be treated, accounting for the rationale for screening urinalyses throughout pregnancy (Stamm and Hooton 1993).

When a patient presents with a UTI, it is important to distinguish upper (pyelonephritis) from lower (cystitis) tract infection. Table 6-3 offers clinical signs and symptoms that can help differentiate upper from lower UTI (Johnson and Stamm 1989). However, up to one-third of patients with the characteristic presentation of cystitis have concomitant upper tract infection. If a patient is treated for cystitis and treatment failure occurs or relapse with the same organism occurs within 2 weeks of the completion of therapy, then upper tract infection should be assumed.

### *Clinical pharmacologic considerations in treating urinary tract infections*

Tradition has dictated that treatment of any UTI requires antecedent cultures and sensitivity testing. However, patients with signs and symptoms suggesting lower tract disease and pyuria (two to five white blood cells per high-power field) or a positive leukocyte esterase dipstick can be treated cost-effectively without the guidance of a urine culture (Johnson and Stamm 1989; Stamm and Hooton 1993). Moreover, microscopic hematuria and particularly bacteriuria in the presence of typical symptoms of cystitis are highly specific, although not as sensitive as pyuria (Johnson and Stamm 1989).

If cultures of urine are obtained in a patient with signs and symptoms of a UTI, then the usual cutoff value of $10^4$ bacterial colonies per milliliter is too rigid, and $10^2$ colonies per milliliter should be considered confirmatory of infection (Johnson and Stamm 1989).

Adequate treatment of uncomplicated cystitis can be accomplished with a variety of drugs and a variety of regimens (Table 6-4). Therapeutic regimens for 1-day, 3-day, and for longer 7- to 10-day courses of antibiotics have been assessed. One day of therapy is effective and inexpensive and entails fewer adverse effects than longer courses of treatment, although relapse occurs more frequently. If a 1-day regimen is used, then trimethoprim alone is as effective as trimethoprim plus sulfamethoxazole and has fewer adverse effects. In addition, fewer relapses occur with these two drugs compared with ampicillin, amoxicillin, nitrofurantoin, or an oral cephalosporin (Johnson and Stamm 1989). Three days of therapy with trimethoprim, trimethoprim plus sulfamethoxazole, amoxicillin, or doxycycline has the same efficacy as a 10-day course of treatment but has as low an incidence of adverse effects as a 1-day course and is intermediate in expense. It represents the best regimen for most patients (Johnson and Stamm 1989; Hooton et al. 1995). Fluoroquinolones are also effective for UTIs but should be kept in reserve to avoid development of resistant organisms.

**PRINCIPLE Selection of an antibiotic to treat uncomplicated cystitis and selection of duration of treatment represent a complex balancing of related issues of broadness and coverage, duration of drug therapy, failure rate and treatment, cost of antibiotic, and associated costs (e.g., cultures, repeat visits, time). "Optimal" strategies may, to some extent, be related to patient preferences and patient populations.**

Upper tract infections and those with a greater likelihood of resistant pathogens (Table 6-5) require more ag-

**Table 6-2 Categories of Urinary Tract Infections**

1. Young female with acute uncomplicated cystitis
   - Differentiate from urethritis due to *Chlamydia* trachoma, gonorrhea, or herpes simplex
   - Differentiate from vaginitis due to *Candida* or *Trichomonas*
   - If consistent symptoms and pyuria are present (by microscopic exam or positive leukocyte esterase dipstick)
     - No culture pre- or posttreatment
     - Therapy with a 3-day course of trimethoprim/sulfamethoxazole (fluoroquinolones reserved for allergic or complicated patients)
2. Young female with recurrent cystitis
   - Occurs in 20%
   - Usually exogenous reinfection
   - No need for urologic examination
   - Treatment options
     - Continuous prophylaxis
     - Postcoital prophylaxis
     - Patient-initiated therapy when symptoms develop
3. Young female with acute uncomplicated pyelonephritis
   - Infectious organisms: 80% are *E. coli*; 20–30% are resistant to amoxicillin and first-generation cephalosporins
   - Urine and blood cultures if sick enough for hospitalization
   - If hospitalized, use parenteral antibiotics for 48 to 72 h
   - If fever and pain for more than 72 h, work up for obstruction or perinephric or intrarenal abscess
   - Treat for 2 weeks
   - Urine culture 2 weeks after completion of therapy
4. Adults of either sex with complicated UTIs (see Table 6–5)
   - Many causative organisms; therefore definitive treatment is guided by cultures
   - Initial treatment empiric
     - If mild disease, use fluoroquinolones
     - If severe disease, use imipenem or ampicillin plus gentamicin
   - Treat 10 to 14 days
   - Urine culture 1 to 2 weeks after completion of treatment
5. Asymptomatic bacteriuria
   - Screen all pregnant women during the first trimester and treat; after completion of treatment obtain monthly urine cultures
   - Occurs in up to 40% of elderly adults, particularly if in nursing homes
     - Rarely becomes symptomatic
     - No benefit from treating
6. Young male with acute UTI
   - Pretreatment culture
   - Treat for 7 days (same drugs as those for young women)
   - No need for urologic examination unless recurrent
7. Catheter-associated UTI
   - Most common cause of gram-negative sepsis in a hospitalized patient
   - No treatment if asymptomatic
   - If symptomatic, treat as complicated UTI

**Table 6-3 Signs and Symptoms to Differentiate Upper from Lower Urinary Tract Infection**

*Upper Tract Infection*
- Localized flank, low back, or abdominal pain
- Systemic signs and symptoms
  - Fever
  - Rigors
  - Sweats
  - Headache
  - Nausea
  - Vomiting
  - Malaise
  - Prostration

*Lower Tract Infection*
- Dysuria
- Frequency
- Nocturia
- Urgency
- Frequent small voidings
- Incontinence
- Suprapubic tenderness—occurs in only about 10% of patients but is specific for cystitis

SOURCE: From Brater DC. 1992. Treatment of renal disorders and the influence of renal function on drug disposition. In: Melmon KL, Morrelli HF, Hoffman BB, et al., editors. *Clinical Pharmacology: Basic Principles in Therapeutics*. 3rd ed. New York: McGraw-Hill. pp 270–308. Reproduced with permission of the McGraw-Hill Companies.

gressive therapy and guidance by culture and sensitivity testing (Stamm and Hooton 1993). Intravenous antibiotic therapy is sometimes necessary, with the choice of antibiotics dependent on local sensitivity patterns, aspects of patient history that might indicate the infecting organism, and severity of illness. Once culture results identify the infecting organism, oral drug dosing can commence, as long as the patient can tolerate oral medications, and an effective oral antibiotic with high bioavailability is available. Treatment for 14 days is usually indicated. If relapse occurs, then a 6-week course of therapy should be used.

**Table 6-5 Patient Factors Indicating the Likelihood of Complicated Urinary Tract Infection**

- Hospital-acquired
- Pregnancy
- Indwelling bladder catheter
- Recent urinary tract instrumentation
- Urinary tract anatomic abnormality
- Urinary tract stone
- Recent antibiotic use
- Diabetes mellitus
- Immune compromise

SOURCE: From Brater DC. 1992. Treatment of renal disorders and the influence of renal function on drug disposition. In: Melmon KL, Morrelli HF, Hoffman BB, et al., editors. *Clinical Pharmacology: Basic Principles in Therapeutics*. 3rd ed. New York: McGraw-Hill. pp 270–308. Reproduced with permission of the McGraw-Hill Companies.

If the patient has not improved within 3 days of therapy, then a complication such as nephrolithiasis, obstruction, or abscess must be considered (Johnson and Stamm 1989; Stamm and Hooton 1993).

Some patients have recurrent UTIs. If infections occur three or more times per year, then prophylactic therapy is cost-effective (Stamm and Hooton 1993). Therapy is guided by results of urine cultures. Treatment should last for 6 months; if symptomatic recurrences continue, then prophylactic therapy may need to be indefinite.

Chlamydial infection is worthy of specific comment. This common pathogen should be particularly suspected in women with a stuttering and prolonged onset of dysuria and other lower urinary tract symptoms. Both the patient and his or her sexual partner should be treated with a 7-day course of either erythromycin or tetracycline (Komaroff 1984).

**Table 6-4 Drugs Commonly Used in the Treatment of Uncomplicated Cystitis (3-Day Course)**

| Regimen | Usual dose | Cost for 3 days of therapy (AWP[a]) | | Comment |
|---|---|---|---|---|
| Trimethoprim/sulfamethoxazole | 160/800 mg bid | Generic | $2 | First choice due to better efficacy, comparable toxicity, and lower cost |
| | | Bactrim | $8 | |
| Cefadroxil | 100 mg qid | Duricef | $22 | |
| Amoxicillin | 500 mg tid | Generic | $2 | |
| | | Amoxil | $4 | |
| Macrocrystalline nitrofurantoin | 100 mg qid | Macrodantin | $17 | |
| | | Macrobid | $17 | |
| Ciprofloxacin HCl | 250 mg bid | Generic | NA | Cost and concerns about resistance relegate fluoroquinolones to reserve status. |
| | | Cipro | $17 | |

[a]Average wholesale price (AWP). Source of drug prices is *Mosby's GenR$_x$* 1998. Current prices may vary from those quoted, but comparative prices among products are expected to be similar. The reader should check on local prices at the time of prescribing.
ABBREVIATIONS: NA, not available.

## Urinary Tract Stones

### *Pathophysiology*

Urinary tract stones can be formed from many constituents in urine including calcium, uric acid, cystine, oxalate, and even some drugs and metabolites of drugs excreted in the urine (e.g., triamterene, oxypurinol). Formation of a stone requires a nidus and supersaturated urine, both of which combine to produce precipitation, followed by crystal growth and aggregation or agglomeration. Growth of the crystal and aggregation may be the most important elements because a simple precipitate still can be excreted in the urine.

A predilection to formation of a stone can occur by several general mechanisms (Table 6-6). Increased excretion of the precipitant can occur from a variety of disorders. For example, hypercalciuria can occur from hyperparathyroidism or other primary disorders or can be idiopathic, which in turn has been classified as either absorptive or renal (Pak 1979; Coe et al. 1992; Bushinsky 1998). Similar examples can be enumerated for causes of hyperuricosuria, hyperoxaluria, and cystinuria (Coe et al. 1992; Bushinsky 1998).

**PRINCIPLE Making a specific diagnosis (the basis of the hyperexcretion) is required to target therapy specifically toward the pathogenesis of the underlying disorder.**

An increase in the likelihood of precipitation from supersaturated urine can occur through simple physical factors such as urinary pH and volume. A low urine volume can increase saturation beyond the point of solubility. A corollary of this principle is that increased fluid intake is a reasonable prescription for any patient with nephrolithiasis, no matter what the cause. The solubility of many stone constituents is influenced by pH. An alkaline urine greatly increases the solubility of uric acid and cystine and is a therapeutic goal in patients suffering from these types of stones (Coe et al. 1992; Bushinsky 1998). On the other hand, the persistently alkaline urine seen in renal tubular acidosis diminishes the solubility of calcium salts and can cause not only nephrolithiasis, but also nephrocalcinosis.

The urine contains inhibitors of crystallization. Pyrophosphate and citrate serve this function, as do urine proteins like nephrocalcin, uropontin, and Tamm-Horsfall mucoprotein (Coe et al. 1992; Bushinsky 1998). Some stone disorders are characterized by hypocitraturia that can be corrected by administration of alkali (e.g., sodium or potassium bicarbonate) or citrate-containing salts (Coe et al. 1992; Bushinsky 1998).

**Table 6-6 Factors That Predispose to Formation of Urinary Tract Stones**

| |
|---|
| *Enhanced Precipitation from Urine* |
| Increased excretion of the precipitant (e.g., hypercalciuria, hyperuricosuria, hyperoxaluria, cystinuria) |
| Decreased saturability of the urine |
| Urine pH decreasing solubility |
| Low urine volume |
| *Decrease in Inhibitors of Crystallization* |
| Hypocitraturia |
| Decreased urinary pyrophosphate |
| Deficits in other inhibitors |

SOURCE: From Brater DC. 1992. Treatment of renal disorders and the influence of renal function on drug disposition. In: Melmon KL, Morrelli HF, Hoffman BB, et al., editors. *Clinical Pharmacology: Basic Principles in Therapeutics*. 3rd ed. New York: McGraw-Hill. pp 270–308. Reproduced with permission of the McGraw-Hill Companies.

### *Clinical pharmacology of drugs to treat urinary tract stones*

The treatment used requires a diagnosis of the cause of the formation of the stone (Coe et al. 1992; Bushinsky 1998). The first step is to analyze the stone itself. Seventy-five percent will be calcium oxalate, and from 40 to 75% of these will prove to be due to hypercalciuria. Another 5 to 25% will be accounted for by hyperuricosuria (Coe and Favus 1986). Other causes of stone formation are uncommon. If hyperexcretion of a substance that causes a stone is found, then further workup entails identification of pathogenesis. For example, if hypercalciuria is found, then assessment for hyperparathyroidism or for the different forms of idiopathic hypercalciuria should ensue. Relatively simple methods for such assessment have been described. They are feasible for most patients in an outpatient setting and do not require complex or expensive analytic techniques (Pak et al. 1980; Coe et al. 1992). Three consecutive 24-hour urine collections during which patients eat their normal diet plus a fasting blood sample each day usually suffices. Blood and urine are measured for calcium, magnesium, phosphate, uric acid, and creatinine. Urine is additionally measured for oxalate, citrate, cystine, pH, and volume.

Once the cause of the stone formation is established, the clinician must decide whether to treat. Because the median time to recurrence of untreated calcium-containing stones is about 7 years and because drug treatment entails potential adverse effects, it is reasonable to defer drug treatment until more than one episode has occurred (Uribarri et al. 1989). Some experts disagree and believe treatment should commence after the first stone (Coe et al. 1992). Conservative measures such as increasing fluid intake and decreasing calcium and uric acid intake should be recommended. Therapy is based on the pathogenesis of the stone as summarized in Table 6-7.

Hyperparathyroidism is usually remedied surgically. Most hypercalciuria is idiopathic, making this diagnosis the most common in patients with nephrolithiasis. Thiazide diuretics are effective for both absorptive and renal hypercalciurias. Some experts recommend these diuretics for both forms of this disorder (Coe et al. 1992; Bushinsky 1998). Others argue that more specifically directed therapy is appropriate. Sodium cellulose phosphate may be used to retard absorption of calcium in patients with the absorptive form of this disorder. Thiazides are then reserved for patients with renal hypercalciuria. If sodium cellulose phosphate is used, then substantial negative calcium balance that may adversely affect bone metabolism can occur; patients should be monitored for such an adverse effect.

Chronic use of thiazide diuretics causes mild volume depletion that, in turn, stimulates proximal and distal tubular reabsorption of solute, including calcium (Breslau et al. 1976). The net result is decreased excretion of calcium in urine with amelioration of stone formation. Interestingly, it appears that this therapy results in a net positive calcium balance and increased bone density that appear protective against hip fracture in elderly patients.

Although uric acid stones are less common than are calcium-containing stones, calcium stones in the setting of hyperuricosuria responds to measures that decrease urinary excretion of uric acid, such as dietary restriction of purines or the use of allopurinol (Coe et al. 1992; Bushinsky 1998). The mechanism by which decreases in uric acid excretion diminish formation of calcium stones depends on the fact that the precipitated uric acid serves as a nidus for stone formation. Because even normal excretion of calcium results in a supersaturated urine, a nidus of uric acid allows epitaxial crystal growth with calcium salts (usually oxalate).

Treatment of hyperuricosuria with allopurinol depends mainly on the activity of its active metabolite, oxypurinol. Both compounds decrease uric acid formation by inhibiting xanthine oxidase, the enzyme that converts hypoxanthine to xanthine, and also xanthine to uric acid. With chronic therapy, oxypurinol (with a half-life of 15–30 hours) accumulates in excess of allopurinol (half-life of 1.5 hours) and accounts for the majority of inhibition of xanthine oxidase. Oxypurinol depends on renal function for elimination (e.g., in patients with end-stage renal disease, its half-life is about 1 week). It can accumulate

**Table 6-7 Treatment of Urinary Tract Stones**

| CAUSE | TREATMENT |
|---|---|
| *Hypercalciuria* | |
| Hyperparathyroidism | Parathyroidectomy |
| Idiopathic | |
| Absorptive | Sodium cellulose phosphate or thiazide diuretics |
| Renal | Thiazide diuretics |
| *Hyperuricosuria* | Allopurinol |
| | Alkali |
| *Distal renal tubular acidosis* | Alkali |
| | Potassium citrate |
| *Hyperoxaluria* | |
| Metabolic | Pyridoxine HCl |
| Enteric | Cholestyramine and/or oral calcium |
| *Cystinuria* | D-Penicillamine |
| | Tiopronin |
| *Normocalciuric idiopathic* | Alkali |
| | Thiazides |

SOURCE: From Brater DC. 1992. Treatment of renal disorders and the influence of renal function on drug disposition. In: Melmon KL, Morrelli HF, Hoffman BB, et al., editors. *Clinical Pharmacology: Basic Principles in Therapeutics*. 3rd ed. New York: McGraw-Hill. pp 270–308. Reproduced with permission of the McGraw-Hill Companies.

to toxic concentrations in patients with renal insufficiency unless doses are diminished in relationship to the level of renal function. Oxypurinol toxicity resembles a hypersensitivity reaction with skin rash, fever, hepatitis, nephritis, and eosinophilia (Young et al. 1974).

Stones in patients with distal renal tubular acidosis usually are calcium phosphate, and their formation is a result of not only increased calcium and phosphate excretion but also the additional pathogenetic factors of alkaline pH and hypocitraturia (Coe et al. 1992). Because the urine is already alkaline, treatment with alkali seems paradoxical; however, so doing increases urinary citrate that acts as an inhibitor of stone formation.

Hyperoxaluria can generally be classified as metabolic or enteric, each of which has a variety of causes. The former is rare, and the latter is usually associated with inflammatory bowel disease, intestinal bypass surgery, or malabsorption syndromes. Metabolic hyperoxaluria is treated with pyridoxine. Enteric hyperoxaluria is treated with restriction of dietary fat or replacement of pancreatic enzymes if there is associated steatorrhea, restriction of dietary oxalate, or use of oral calcium carbonate supplements and/or cholestyramine. Calcium supplements bind with enteric oxalate to prevent its absorption. The binding of bile acids by cholestyramine diminishes saponification of dietary fats that bind calcium in the proximal intestine. Thus, more calcium becomes available for binding with oxalate.

Cystinuria is a rare metabolic disorder that is occasionally associated with stone formation. Therapy consists of increasing fluid intake to dilute the urine and ingesting large doses of alkali to alkalinize the urine. The latter is only marginally beneficial because cystine's solubility does not appreciably increase until the urine pH exceeds 7.5, a value close to the maximum physiologic pH of about 8.0. If these conservative maneuvers fail, then either D-penicillamine or tiopronin can be used (Coe et al. 1992; Bushinsky 1998). D-Penicillamine is used as a last resort in patients with cystinuria because of its adverse effects, particularly nephrotoxicity, which usually first manifests as proteinuria from membranous glomerulonephritis. Other common adverse effects include rash, loss of taste, stomatitis, thrombocytopenia, and leukopenia (Stein et al. 1980). Up to 50% of patients will have an adverse effect, and up to one-third will have to discontinue the drug.

Some patients with nephrolithiasis have no identifiable metabolic abnormality. They are classified as normocalciuric idiopathic stone formers. These patients are best treated with alkali to increase urinary citrate, which seems the logical first approach to therapy in these patients.

## Urinary Incontinence

### *Pathophysiology and assessment*

Urinary incontinence affects 15 to 30% of community dwelling elderly patients and more than 50% of nursing home residents. The incidence increases with age, and women are affected twice as frequently as men (NIH Consensus Statement 1988; Fantl et al. 1994; Genadry 1995; AHCPR 1996). This condition is underreported by patients, underdiagnosed by physicians, and undertreated by health care providers. From a public health perspective, there is a substantial need to educate both the public and the health care community (NIH Consensus Statement 1988).

Incontinence results from instability of bladder contractions and/or diminished bladder neck contraction. There is either an increased stimulus to void and/or a decreased ability to prevent voiding. There are four different patterns of urinary incontinence (see Table 6-8). It is important to distinguish among these types of incontinence because treatment varies.

Investigation of the problem entails a detailed history and examination. History should focus on the pattern of incontinence and its precipitants. Examination includes a careful neurologic assessment of the pelvis. Routine studies that should be obtained include a urinalysis, serum creatinine concentration, and determination of postvoid residual volume. Other simple studies such as urine culture, blood glucose, and urinary cytology should be obtained as indicated. If diagnosis is still in question, then other specialized tests can be considered, including a cystometrogram, electrophysiologic sphincter testing, cystourethroscopy, and uroflowmeter (in men only). Other tests are limited to specialized patients or their utility is debated (NIH Consensus Statement 1988; AHCPR 1996).

**Table 6-8 Types of Urinary Incontinence**

*Stress incontinence due to dysfunction of the bladder outlet*
Causes include dysfunction of the urethral sphincter as occurs in postmenopausal women with estrogen deprivation and decreased bladder neck support as occurs in multiparity.

*Urge incontinence due to uninhibited bladder contractions*
Causes include CNS lesions that impair inhibition of bladder contractions, infection, tumors, and idiopathic causes.

*Overflow incontinence due to an overdistended bladder*
Causes include impaired detrusor contraction due to neurologic abnormalities and outflow obstruction due to medications, tumors, strictures, and prostatic hypertrophy.

*Mixed incontinence due to a combination of factors*

### *Clinical pharmacology of drugs for urinary incontinence*

As much as possible, treatment is aimed at the underlying pathophysiology. When pharmacologic therapy is inadequate, a variety of surgical procedures can be considered. Unfortunately, much information about efficacy and comparative trials are either lacking or weakly designed so that guidance is of limited value. (Black and Downs 1996).

Concomitant with drug therapy, a variety of behavioral therapies should be implemented. These include pelvic muscle exercises, biofeedback, bladder training, and scheduled toileting (NIH Consensus Statement 1988; AHCPR 1996). Pharmacologic therapy in postmenopausal women includes estrogen (NIH Consensus Statement 1988; Wein 1995; AHCPR 1996). A meta-analysis of estrogen's efficacy showed improvement in symptoms no matter what the type of incontinence; objective measures of efficacy were equivocal (Fantl et al. 1994). Therapies aimed at decreasing bladder contractility in urge incontinence entail either anticholinergic agents or direct-acting smooth muscle relaxants (Table 6-9). Therapy to enhance bladder outlet function includes the use of $\alpha$-adrenergic receptor agonists. Other drugs have shown efficacy likely due to mixed and nonspecific effects (Fantl et al. 1994; NIH Consensus Statement 1988; Genadry 1995; AHCPR 1996, Wein 1995).

## Erectile Dysfunction

### *Pathophysiology*

The prevalence and demographics of erectile dysfunction are poorly characterized. The physiology of attaining an erection is complex (NIH Consensus Conference: Impotence 1993; Utiger 1998). Stimulation from the CNS and/or a penile/spinal cord reflex parasympathetic arc results in penile parasympathetic activation. Postsynaptic parasympathetic neurons plus endothelium release nitric oxide, which stimulates guanylate cyclase, forming cyclic GMP (cGMP). cGMP relaxes trabecular smooth muscle and helicine arteries of the penis causing expansion of lacunar spaces, which trap blood by compressing venules of the corpus cavernosum against the tunica albuginea, resulting in penile tumescence.

Erectile dysfunction can occur from psychological, neurological, vascular, or a combination of factors. Evaluation of patients should include a detailed medical history, including sexual history, and a psychosocial evaluation. Physical examination should include a focused neurological examination of the pelvis. Laboratory tests include morning serum testosterone and prolactin concentrations (NIH Consensus Conference: Impotence 1993). Results of these tests may dictate additional studies, but it is important to emphasize that many of the additional studies that have been suggested in the literature either have no normative data or stem from poorly designed trials.

The epidemiology of erectile dysfunction is poorly defined (NIH Consensus Conference: Impotence 1993; Benet and Melman 1995). Twenty-five percent of cases are due to adverse drug reactions, and a careful drug history is essential (NIH Consensus Conference: Impotence 1993; Benet and Melman 1995). Other causes are chronic diseases (particularly those affecting the vasculature), prior surgery, and trauma. The prevalence increases with age.

### *Therapy of erectile dysfunction*

Psychosocial interventions are beyond the scope of this discussion but are vitally important components of a comprehensive therapeutic regimen (NIH Consensus Conference: Impotence 1993; Utiger 1998). If patients are hypogonadal, then testosterone should be given either intramuscularly or via a transdermal patch. Importantly, if men have normal serum testosterone concentrations, then testosterone has no benefit and should not be administered (NIH Consensus Conference: Impotence 1993; Mulligan and Schmitt 1993; Utiger 1998). If the patient is hyper-

Table 6-9 Drugs Used to Treat Urinary Incontinence

| MECHANISM | DRUG | USUAL DOSE |
|---|---|---|
| Decrease bladder contraction | Prophantheline bromide | 7.5–30 mg at least tid |
| | Oxybutynin chloride | 2.5–5 mg tid or qid |
| | Dicyclomine HCl | 10–20 mg tid |
| | Flavoxate HCl | 100–200 mg tid or qid |
| Increase bladder outlet contraction | Phenylpropanolamine | 25–100 mg bid |
| | Pseudoephedrine | 15–30 mg tid |
| Nonspecific | Estrogens | |
| | Tricyclic antidepressants | |

prolactinemic, then bromocriptine or similar agents should be used (NIH Consensus Conference: Impotence 1993). Yohimbine has been advocated in the past; more recent rigorous studies indicate no benefit (NIH Consensus Conference: Impotence 1993; Montague et al. 1996).

Current therapeutic approaches can be divided into mechanical (including surgery) and pharmacologic. Surgical procedures include penile implants and vascular surgery (NIH Consensus Conference: Impotence 1993; Montague et al. 1996; Utiger 1998). The former is effective but may preclude use of other therapies. A recent clinical guidelines panel of the American Urological Association concluded that "chances of success do not appear high enough to justify routine use" of vascular surgery and that such procedures should be viewed as experimental (Montague et al. 1996). A nonsurgical mechanical option is a vacuum constriction device (NIH Consensus Conference: Impotence 1993). The mainstays of therapy are pharmacologic.

Drug therapy of erectile dysfunction can be given by either intracavernosal injection, as a urethral suppository, or as an oral agent (NIH Consensus Conference: Impotence 1993; Montague et al. 1996; Goldstein et al. 1998; Utiger 1998). Papaverine, phentolamine, or alprostadil ($PGE_1$) can be injected into the corpus cavernosum. All act by directly causing vasodilation and smooth muscle relaxation. Their effects do not require a stimulus either locally or from the CNS. All can result in prolonged erections and may cause fibrosis over time. Patients should be counseled to call their physician if erections persist longer than 4 hours. In turn, their physician must know how to treat priapism (NIH Consensus Conference: Impotence 1993; Montague et al. 1996). Alprostadil has recently been formulated as an intraurethral suppository. It has similar efficacy to injection.

An oral agent, sildenafil, has recently become available (Goldstein et al. 1998; Utiger 1998). Sildenafil inhibits cGMP phosphodiesterase type 5. This is the isozyme of phosphodiesterase predominantly expressed in the corpus cavernosum. By inhibiting this enzyme, sildenafil increases cGMP locally, which then causes vasodilation and smooth muscle relaxation (Utiger 1998). It is important to stress that sildenafil's efficacy requires that cGMP be formed in the first place, meaning that CNS and/or local stimulation are required so that penile parasympathetic nerves are activated (Utiger 1998). In contrast to the other modalities discussed, sildenafil requires an intact libido.

Adverse effects of sildenafil are predictable based on its pharmacology and the distribution of type 5 phosphodiesterase (Utiger 1998). Headache, flushing, dyspepsia, and visual disturbances (change in perception of color hue or brightness) can occur. Sildenafil can be dangerous in patients taking nitrates or antihypertensive preparations because the hypotensive effects of nitrates may be potentiated.

## Fluid and Electrolyte Disorders

### *Pathophysiology*

A number of diseases and drugs themselves cause abnormalities in fluid and electrolyte status. Understanding the physiology of renal regulation of electrolyte and volume homeostasis is necessary to correct abnormalities thereof.

**VOLUME AND OSMOLARITY** Serum sodium concentration is not a reflection of total-body sodium. In turn, whether a patient has fluid volume excess or deficits is a function of total-body sodium surfeit or deficiency. Thus, a patient can be volume-expanded yet be hyponatremic, as often occurs in patients with congestive heart failure (CHF). The serum sodium concentration is an index of osmolarity. A patient with hyponatremia is hyposmolar unless solutes other than sodium are circulating in plasma (e.g., elevated blood glucose concentration). Osmolarity, in turn, is determined by free-water homeostasis. A patient with severe CHF and hyponatremia thereby has a diminished concentration of sodium in serum because of free-water retention that is independent of overall sodium and volume homeostasis.

Figure 6-3 schematically depicts a renal tubule that highlights the major components of regulation of sodium and water, and thus the control of volume and osmolarity. Various autocoids can affect tubular function. For example, volume depletion increases circulating catecholamine concentration and activates the systemic and intrarenal renin-angiotensin systems. Stimulation of proximal tubular receptors for norepinephrine and angiotensin II stimulate sodium reabsorption (DiBona 1985). Conversely, volume expansion activates atrial stretch receptors that release atrial natriuretic peptide, causing an increase in GFR and filtered sodium with resulting increased sodium excretion (de Bold 1985).

Iso-osmotic reabsorption of 60 to 70% of ions and water occurs in the proximal tubule. Sodium and water reabsorption passively follow the active reabsorption of organic solutes such as glucose and amino acids. In addition, sodium is actively reabsorbed (Rector 1983). Normally, more than 85% of filtered bicarbonate is reabsorbed as sodium bicarbonate. High permeability to water

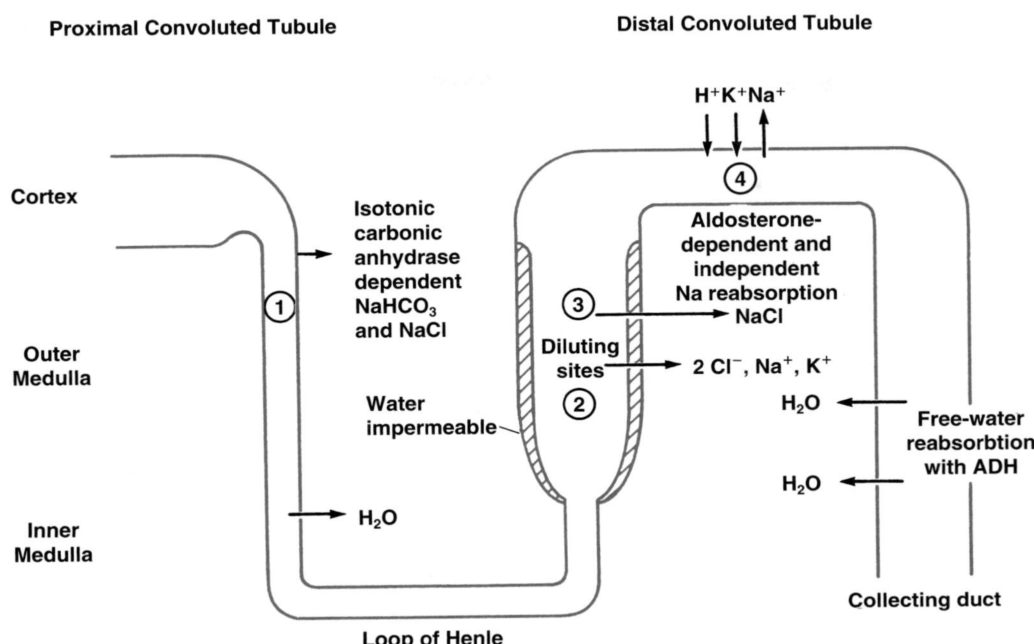


F I G U R E 6 - 3 **Diagram of a nephron indicating functional areas involved in regulation of salt and water homeostasis. Circled numbers represent sites of action of diuretics (see Table 6-10). (From Brater DC. 1992. Treatment of renal disorders and the influence of renal function on drug disposition. In: Melmon KL, Morrelli HF, Hoffman BB, et al., editors. *Clinical Pharmacology: Basic Principles in Therapeutics*. 3rd ed. New York: McGraw-Hill. pp 270–308. Reproduced with permission of the McGraw-Hill Companies.)**

in the proximal tubule allows the passive reabsorption of water in parallel with active reabsorption of sodium.

In the thick loop of Henle, reabsorption of 20 to 30% of the filtered sodium as sodium chloride occurs via active transport of two $Cl^-$ ions coupled to one $Na^+$ and one $K^+$ ion (Greger 1985). Saturation of this transport system cannot be demonstrated under physiologic conditions. This means that increased rejection of solute from the proximal nephron can be reclaimed at the loop of Henle and that the contribution of the loop to overall sodium reabsorption can increase dramatically.

The thick ascending limb of the loop of Henle is impermeable to water. Solute reabsorption from a segment of the nephron that is impermeable to water ultimately renders the tubule fluid hypotonic to plasma. This hypotonic fluid consists of two hypothetical volumes, one isoosmotic with plasma and the other free of osmotic activity (solute-free water or *free water*). Therefore, production of free water occurs in the ascending limb of the loop of Henle and beyond. In the cortical segment of the limb, fluid actually becomes hypotonic. As a consequence, this segment is also referred to as the diluting segment. Production of dilute urine depends on the delivery of sodium chloride to that site (i.e., if less sodium is delivered to the diluting site, then less dilution can occur), active transport of solute, and the tubule's impermeability to water. The tubular fluid in the early distal region remains hypotonic, and if there is no stimulus for conservation of water, then this dilute fluid will be excreted in the urine, thereby providing a mechanism for excretion of free water. Considered in another way, this capacity to excrete a dilute urine (i.e., free water) provides the body's defense against hypo-osmolarity. For example, ingestion of distilled water would cause hyponatremia and hypo-osmolarity unless the kidney could excrete the water load. Conversely, impaired ability to excrete a water load caused by drugs (see the section on adverse effects of drugs on renal function) or disease states can result in a hypo-osmolar state and hyponatremia.

The thick ascending limb of the loop of Henle also contributes to the ability to concentrate the urine. The active reabsorption of solute coupled with passive transport of urea at this segment allows the development of a hypertonic medullary interstitium. This hypertonic interstitium provides the osmotic driving force for water reabsorption when the kidney needs to conserve water. Any interruption of this capacity, then, impairs a patient's ability to conserve water and subjects him or her to the risk of a hyperosmolar state and hypernatremia.

In the distal tubule (including the collecting duct) reabsorption of the remaining 5% of filtrate occurs. In this segment, reabsorption of sodium enhances secretion of potassium and hydrogen ions partly dependent on aldosterone. In this segment of the nephron, sodium and potassium move in opposite directions, whereas in all more proximal nephron sites, sodium and potassium movement is parallel. Therefore, anything that decreases sodium reabsorption at more proximal sites also decreases potassium reabsorption and can lead to potassium depletion. In contrast, a decrease in reabsorption of sodium at the distal tubule results in retention of potassium.

The tubule's permeability to water in the collecting duct is increased by antidiuretic hormone (ADH) that is secreted by the pituitary in response to both osmotic and nonosmotic stimuli (Schrier and Berl 1975). An increase in serum osmolarity causes increased ADH release with retention of free water by the kidney in order to correct the hyperosmolar state. In addition, activation of the sympathetic nervous system also stimulates ADH release even during hypo-osmolar states. This pathophysiology accounts for the free-water retention and hyponatremia that occurs in patients with heart failure, liver disease, and other disorders including hypovolemic states.

As noted above, release of ADH must be coupled with an osmotic driving force for free-water reabsorption to occur. In other words, a hypertonic medullary interstitium is necessary to achieve maximal concentration of urine in response to ADH.

Overall, then, two interdependent regulatory systems are responsible for the normalization of volume and osmolarity: 1) extracellular fluid volume is primarily regulated by the retention or excretion of sodium, and 2) total solute concentration (i.e., osmolarity) is regulated by variation in water intake and by the renal excretion of water modulated by ADH.

**POTASSIUM HOMEOSTASIS** More than 90% of the potassium filtered at the glomerulus is reabsorbed in the proximal tubule. In the distal tubule, both reabsorption and secretion of potassium occur. In the presence of mineralocorticoids such as aldosterone that stimulate distal sodium reabsorption, potassium is actively secreted. In addition, reabsorption of sodium leaves behind nonabsorbable anions that make the lumen electronegative, facilitating excretion of potassium. Impaired secretion of potassium and its retention may occur if delivery of sodium to the distal tubule is reduced by any of a number of mechanisms. Reduction in mineralocorticoid concentration also enhances retention of potassium. Decreased production of aldosterone most often occurs in patients with mild renal disease due to diabetes mellitus (Schambelan et al. 1972). This syndrome can also be caused by drugs that decrease aldosterone secretion such as NSAIDs and ACE inhibitors.

Hyperkalemia may occur in patients who have an impaired ability to excrete potassium, such as those with renal insufficiency, or who have systemic acidemia, which causes potassium to shift extracellularly. In addition, hemolysis and any type of tissue necrosis result in release of potassium to the extracellular space. Commercially available premixed electrolyte solutions, salt substitutes, and low-sodium pharmaceutical products prepared with potassium (e.g., potassium penicillin G) are sources of excess potassium that should be avoided in patients with impaired ability to excrete potassium.

Depletion of potassium occurs in primary or secondary adrenocortical overactivity, with use of diuretics that inhibit sodium reabsorption proximal to sites at which sodium and potassium exchange, and during both acidosis and alkalosis of any cause.

**CALCIUM HOMEOSTASIS** Control of concentrations of calcium in plasma depends on the interaction between parathyroid hormone and vitamin D. These hormones exert their effects on bone, the intestinal epithelium, and the kidney to maintain calcium homeostasis (Reichel et al. 1989). Vitamin $D_3$ is either ingested in the diet or synthesized by the skin on exposure to sunlight. The liver then converts vitamin $D_3$ to $25[OH]D_3$, which in turn is further hydroxylated by the kidney to form $1{,}25[OH]_2D_3$. This final product modulates the effects of parathyroid hormone on bone, increases intestinal absorption of calcium, and increases renal reabsorption of calcium. Parathyroid hormone is released when serum calcium concentrations decrease. The hormone induces release of calcium from bone, stimulates 1-hydroxylation of $25[OH]D_3$ by the kidney, and promotes renal reabsorption of calcium. Thus, the effects of parathyroid hormone and vitamin $D_3$ in concert preserve calcium homeostasis by their effects on multiple organs.

In the kidney, handling of calcium generally parallels that of sodium (Agus et al. 1982). Calcium that is not bound to albumin is freely filtered at the glomerulus, after which it undergoes reabsorption throughout the length of the nephron. Inhibition of reabsorption of sodium at a particular nephron site also results in less reabsorption of calcium; the converse also is true.

When the calcium homeostasis of a patient is evaluated, the usual value reported from the laboratory is the total concentration of calcium in serum. That concentration includes the unbound calcium plus the majority of calcium in serum that is bound to albumin. Changes in the concentration of albumin can affect total concentrations of calcium in serum without affecting the physiologically relevant unbound (also referred to as ionized or free) concentration. In settings of abnormal concentrations of albumin in serum the measured total concentration of calcium in serum can be "normalized" by adding 0.8 mg/dL to the calcium concentration for every 1 g/dL that the serum albumin is below a "normal" value of 4 g/dL.

**ACID–BASE BALANCE** The body's extracellular fluid environment is maintained relatively constant at approximately pH 7.4; intracellular fluid generally is more acidic. Blood pH is determined by the $P\text{CO}_2$ and bicarbonate concentration, such that $\text{pH} = 7.1 + \log [\text{HCO}_3^-]/(0.03 \times P\text{CO}_2)$.

Cell metabolism releases large quantities of $CO_2$ and hydrogen ion. The hydrogen ion is fixed (buffered) by combination with bases and subsequently eliminated (by renal secretion or excretion), so that release, fixation (buffering), and excretion are constantly at steady state. If blood bicarbonate concentration is too low (e.g., from excessive loss in urine or diarrhea), then acidemia results. Conversely, administration or endogenous generation of bicarbonate reduces the concentration of hydrogen ion and results in alkalemia.

Most acid is excreted as $CO_2$ by the lungs. However, the kidney must eliminate 1–2 mEq of hydrogen ion ($H^+$) per kilogram per day to maintain acid–base balance. Removal of this excess hydrogen ion is accomplished by the secretion of hydrogen ion into the urine. To acidify the urine, three processes must operate effectively: 1) reabsorption of bicarbonate, 2) formation of titratable acid, and 3) production of ammonia. The buffering of acid excretion by phosphate and ammonia allows a greater capacity for elimination of hydrogen ion. Without these buffers, urinary pH would rapidly fall so low as to preclude further secretion of $H^+$ by tubular cells.

The tubular secretion of hydrogen ion results in removal of luminal bicarbonate so that bicarbonate is reabsorbed; further hydrogen ion secretion acidifies the urine. Most hydrogen is secreted in the proximal nephron in exchange for sodium, and the process serves to reclaim most of the filtered bicarbonate. Reabsorption of bicarbonate is facilitated by carbonic anhydrase. Acidemia and alkalemia occur when exogenous administration or production of endogenous acid or alkali exceeds removal by metabolism and/or excretion. The metabolic acidosis of uncontrolled diabetes mellitus provides a good example. In this condition, breakdown of fat occurs so rapidly that acetoacetic acid and $\beta$-hydroxybutyric acid accumulate. The accumulation of ketoacids exceeds the normal buffering and excretory mechanisms responsible for acid–base regulation, and diabetic acidemia ensues. If insulin is administered, then ketoacid production decreases, and acid–base balance is restored.

Metabolic acidosis may result from either production or administration of acid ($H^+$) at a rate faster than can be excreted by the normal kidney, from selective loss of base ($HCO_3^-$), or from the inability of a diseased kidney to excrete normal amounts of acid. Loss of base usually occurs via gastrointestinal losses such as during diarrhea, or it is due to failure of the kidney to reabsorb bicarbonate, in which case the acidosis is accompanied by an inappropriately alkaline urine. This defect may be the result of a primary abnormality in reabsorption of bicarbonate in the proximal tubule or of a defect in the ability to maintain a hydrogen ion gradient in the distal tubule (Morris et al. 1972). In addition, drugs such as carbonic anhydrase inhibitors can cause excessive loss of bicarbonate. Last, hyporeninemic-hypoaldosteronism or similar pathophysiologic syndromes caused by NSAIDs or ACE inhibitors diminish the hydrogen secretory ability of the distal tubule causing renal wasting of $HCO_3^-$ and a metabolic acidosis.

Generation of a metabolic alkalosis occurs when acid is lost or bicarbonate is gained in excess of endogenous production of acid. Acid loss can occur due to vomiting, nasogastric suctioning, or by the kidney during potassium depletion or states of mineralocorticoid excess. With each millimole of acid lost, a millimole of bicarbonate is generated systemically. Bicarbonate also can be gained by exogenous administration.

Maintenance of a metabolic alkalosis occurs during depletion of volume, potassium, or chloride, as compensation for a respiratory acidosis (elevated $P\text{CO}_2$), or with hypersecretion of aldosterone (Coe 1977). Persistence of any of these conditions maintains a metabolic alkalosis, and successful therapy requires reversal of all the contributing factors in a given patient.

There is an expected degree of respiratory compensation for each metabolic disturbance in acid–base status. For example, in a simple primary metabolic acidosis, each decrement in the serum bicarbonate concentration is accompanied by a predictable, compensatory reduction in the arterial $P\text{CO}_2$. When the response to metabolic acidosis results in a greater-than-predicted or lesser-than-predicted change in $P\text{CO}_2$, the presence of a separate, independent respiratory acid–base disorder should be suspected. The physician can recognize the presence of mixed acid–base disturbances because of the deviation from the predictable compensatory response. By defining the separate components of the mixed disturbance, the physician can design a more comprehensive therapeutic program.

### *Clinical pharmacology of drugs used to treat fluid and electrolyte disorders*

**RATIONAL USE OF DIURETICS FOR DISORDERS OF VOLUME** Hypovolemia is readily treated by administering fluids appropriate to the patient's condition: whole blood, packed red blood cells, isotonic saline, lactated Ringers solution, or more dilute saline solutions may be indicated. Increased total body sodium (usually with an increase in total body water) is treated with diuretics.

The rational use of diuretics requires an understanding of the pathogenesis of the entity being treated, the mechanisms by which the kidney handles sodium and water (Fig. 6-3), and the pharmacology of the diuretics. Such knowledge is the basis for establishing rational endpoints for efficacy and toxicity during diuretic therapy. The diuretics are one of the most important groups of pharmacologic agents acting directly on the kidney. Although they are given to produce negative sodium balance, they also affect tonicity, acid–base regulation, potassium balance, and calcium homeostasis. Understanding their diverse nondiuretic effects allows their rational use in nonedematous disorders (see below).

Edema is tantamount to an increase in total body exchangeable sodium. Decreased renal excretion of sodium may be primarily due to reduced GFR and thereby be due to renal dysfunction per se. More commonly, the kidney is not diseased but is responding to signals (many or most of which are unknown) stimulated by diseases of other organ systems. These signals affect the regulation of tubular function causing enhanced reabsorption of sodium (Frazier and Yager 1973).

When a diuretic produces a natriuresis, the sodium is initially lost from the intravascular space; therefore, rational therapy entails clinical assessment of the patient's vascular volume. For example, a patient in CHF with an increased intravascular volume predictably tolerates a rapid diuresis more readily than does a patient with a normal or decreased intravascular volume, as occurs in cirrhosis. The maximum rate to mobilize ascitic or pleural fluid safely is approximately 0.5 L/day (Shear et al. 1970). As a consequence, when reduction of intravascular volume would be potentially harmful, diuretic-induced weight loss should be limited to 0.5 kg/day. Patients with peripheral edema and those with expanded intravascular volumes can withstand more rapid mobilization of fluid.

Just as sodium and water are handled differently along the length of the tubule (Fig. 6-3), diuretics act by different mechanisms and at different sites along the nephron (Table 6-10). In addition, as indicated in this table, routes of access of diuretics to their site(s) of action differ.

**Table 6-10** Routes of Access to Sites of Action, Sites of Action of, and Efficacy of Diuretics

| DIURETIC | ROUTE OF ACCESS TO SITE OF ACTION | SITE OF ACTION[a] | RELATIVE EFFICACY |
|---|---|---|---|
| Carbonic anhydrase inhibitors | Organic acid secretion | Proximal tubule (1) | 2 |
| Osmotic diuretics | Glomerular filtration | Proximal tubule and thick ascending limb of loop of Henle (1, 2, 3) | 6 |
| Loop diuretics | Organic acid secretion | Thick ascending limb of loop of Henle (2) | 10–15 |
| Thiazide diuretics | Organic acid secretion | Proximal tubule (clinically negligible) and distal tubule (3) | 4 |
| Potassium-retaining diuretics | | | 1 |
| Amiloride HCl | Organic base secretion | Distal tubule and collecting duct (4) | 1 |
| Spironolactone | Peritubular circulation | Distal tubule and collecting duct (4) | 1 |
| Triamterene | Organic base secretion | Distal tubule and collecting duct (4) | 1 |

[a]Numbers in parentheses refer to the site of action shown schematically in Fig. 6-3.
SOURCE: From Brater DC. 1992. Treatment of renal disorders and the influence of renal function on drug disposition. In: Melmon KL, Morrelli HF, Hoffman BB, et al., editors. *Clinical Pharmacology: Basic Principles in Therapeutics*. 3rd ed. New York: McGraw-Hill. pp 270–308. Reproduced with permission of the McGraw-Hill Companies.

All diuretics except spironolactone must reach the lumen of the nephron to inhibit sodium reabsorption. Osmotic diuretics are filtered at the glomerulus and reach this site by that mechanism. The remaining diuretics depend on secretion to reach the urine. The carbonic anhydrase inhibitors, loop diuretics, and thiazides are acidic drugs and are secreted through the organic acid secretory system of the proximal tubule (Odlind and Beermann 1980). In contrast, amiloride and triamterene are secreted by the organic base secretory system (Besseghir and Roch-Ramel 1987; Kau 1978). Because the majority of diuretics must reach the tubular lumen to cause their effects, it follows that any impairment of delivery of diuretic to this site will result in diminished response.

Understanding the overall response to a diuretic is facilitated by a few simple principles. First, when a diuretic interferes with the reabsorption of sodium at any site in the tubule, it results in inhibition of other renal functions related to reabsorption of sodium at that site (e.g., calcium reabsorption) and to an enhanced effect of reabsorption of sodium at all more distal tubular sites (e.g., increased exchange with potassium). In other words, interference with reabsorption of sodium in the proximal tubule leads to increased delivery of sodium chloride to the ascending limb of the loop of Henle and the distal tubule. This facilitates the creation of free water and increases potassium loss, respectively. Similarly, interference with reabsorption of sodium in the ascending limb of the loop of Henle interferes with the ability to reabsorb free water but continues to potentiate excretion of potassium. Finally, interference with sodium reabsorption at the distal nephron and the collecting duct reduces excretion of potassium.

A second consideration is that diuretics act only if sodium reaches their site of action. Thus, more distally acting diuretics lose their effectiveness if proximal sodium reabsorption is increased, as occurs in a number of edema-forming states. Finally, diuretics acting at different sites or at the same site by different mechanisms may be additive or synergistic in their effects, and the effect of combining drugs can be used to great clinical advantage.

**PRINCIPLE Understanding the details of mechanism of action of drugs may lead the physician to use drug combinations in more rational and productive ways.**

***Carbonic Anhydrase Inhibitors*** The first orally effective diuretic was acetazolamide. Its synthesis was stimulated by the observation that sulfanilamide, a sulfonamide antibiotic, increased urinary excretion of sodium bicarbonate, leading to a metabolic acidosis. Studies showed that the mechanism of this effect is inhibition of carbonic anhydrase. Acetazolamide was then developed by synthesizing derivatives of sulfanilamide.

Currently, acetazolamide is used more for its beneficial effects in glaucoma than as a diuretic. It might seem surprising that acetazolamide is only a weak diuretic, because 60% or more of filtered sodium is reabsorbed in the proximal tubule where it acts. However, this is the case because only a fraction of proximal tubular reabsorption of sodium is as $NaHCO_3$ and thereby linked to carbonic anhydrase. In addition, much of the sodium rejected from the proximal tubule under the influence of acetazolamide is reabsorbed at more distal nephron sites, particularly the thick ascending limb of the loop of Henle.

Acetazolamide occasionally is used as a diuretic in patients who are poorly responsive or refractory to large doses of potent loop diuretics (Table 6-11). Some of these patients, particularly those with heart failure, have increased proximal tubular reabsorption of sodium. In that setting, the loop diuretic is limited in its efficacy because less sodium is being delivered to the loop of Henle. Coadministration of acetazolamide in this setting can cause a clinically important diuresis. This additive effect is predictable based on known renal physiology and the separate tubular sites of action of diuretics.

**PRINCIPLE In general, drugs that produce similar effects by different mechanisms are good candidates to maximize effects that are insufficient when only one is used.**

Most diuretics also are used for a variety of other indications unrelated to sodium reabsorption (Martinez-Maldonado et al. 1973) (Table 6–11). Because carbonic anhydrase is important for intraocular fluid formation, inhibitors of this enzyme decrease intraocular pressure and are therefore used to treat glaucoma. Acetazolamide is also effective by unknown mechanisms as prophylaxis and for treatment of altitude sickness.

***Osmotic Diuretics*** The most common setting of osmotic diuresis is a disease rather than therapy, namely, that caused by renal excretion of glucose that occurs in uncontrolled diabetes mellitus. Osmotic agents (e.g., mannitol) have been used as diuretics in patients with ARF, but as has been discussed above in this chapter, it seems that the risks of this therapy outweigh any potential benefit.

Table 6-11 **Therapeutic Uses of Diuretic Agents**

| TYPE OF DIURETIC | DIURETIC USES | OTHER USES |
|---|---|---|
| Carbonic anhydrase inhibitors | With loop diuretics in patients with resistance to diuretics | Glaucoma, metabolic alkalosis, altitude sickness |
| Osmotic agents | Acute renal failure | Cerebral edema |
| Loop diuretics | Edematous disorders, acute renal failure, hypertension in patients with $CL_{Cr}$ below 40 mL/min or in those with extensive fluid retention | Hypercalcemia, hyponatremia, renal tubular acidosis |
| Thiazide diuretics | Edematous disorders | Hypertension, hypercalciuria, diabetes insipidus |
| Potassium-retaining diuretics | Edematous disorders (particularly primary or secondary hyperaldosteronism; e.g., cirrhosis) | Potassium and/or magnesium loss |

SOURCE: From Brater DC. 1992. Treatment of renal disorders and the influence of renal function on drug disposition. In: Melmon KL, Morrelli HF, Hoffman BB, et al., editors. *Clinical Pharmacology: Basic Principles in Therapeutics*. 3rd ed. New York: McGraw-Hill. pp 270–308. Reproduced with permission of the McGraw-Hill Companies.
ABBREVIATIONS: $CL_{Cr}$, creatinine clearance

On the other hand, the osmotic effect of mannitol is highly effective in short-term treatment of cerebral edema (Table 6-11). This use may be associated with a pronounced diuresis and even unwanted hypotension. Scrupulous attention must be paid to the patient's vital signs to make certain that excessive volume depletion is avoided.

***Loop Diuretics*** Loop diuretics are the most effective diuretics available (Table 6-10). For this reason and because they are often effective when other diuretics are not, they also are called *high-ceiling* diuretics. Their site of action is the thick ascending limb of the loop of Henle, where they block the $2Cl^-$, $Na^+$,$K^+$ reabsorption pump (Fig. 6-3). This segment normally reabsorbs 20 to 30% of filtered sodium. Because the loop diuretics are able to block virtually all reabsorption of the ion at this site, and because only small amounts of sodium can be reclaimed at more distal sites in the nephron, these agents cause excretion of up to 20% of the sodium that is filtered at the glomerulus. If response to a loop diuretic is assessed relative to the amount of diuretic reaching the site of action within the tubular lumen (reflected by amounts in the urine), then a classic pharmacologic concentration–response curve results. The upper plateau of the response curve represents the reabsorptive capacity of the thick ascending limb of the loop of Henle (Fig. 6-4). The figure schematically illustrates this relationship and contrasts the efficacy of a loop diuretic with the lesser response that occurs to a thiazide diuretic.

Many patients require loop diuretics to control edema, particularly those patients with severe heart failure, severe cirrhosis, nephrotic syndrome, or renal insufficiency. If creatinine clearance is less than about 40 mL/min, then other diuretics are unlikely to be effective and loop diuretics usually are needed. Patients may require large doses of these drugs, but the magnitude of their effect demands that small doses be tried first, followed by upward titration adjusting to the clinical response. Thus, 40 mg of furosemide, or the equivalent dose of other loop

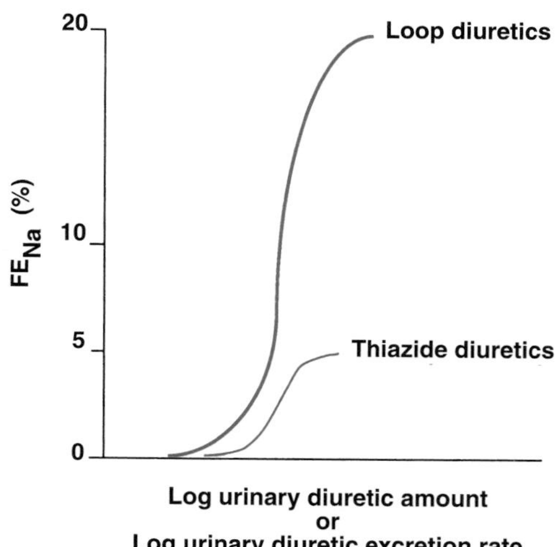


FIGURE 6-4 **Schematized "dose"-response relationship for loop and thiazide diuretics: fractional excretion of sodium ($FE_{Na}$) in relation to diuretic amount and rate. (From Brater DC. 1992. Treatment of renal disorders and the influence of renal function on drug disposition. In: Melmon KL, Morrelli HF, Hoffman BB, et al., editors. *Clinical Pharmacology: Basic Principles in Therapeutics*. 3rd ed. New York: McGraw-Hill. pp 270–308. Reproduced with permission of the McGraw-Hill Companies.)**

diuretics, is given first. If inadequate, the dose can be doubled sequentially until a response ensues or until a maximum tolerated dose is reached. The maximum single dose that should be tried differs for different clinical conditions (Table 6-12). Nothing is gained by administering larger doses than those listed, and toxicity, which is usually auditory, may occur.

The loop diuretics are intense but relatively short-acting in their effects, with duration of action ranging from 2 to 3 hours for bumetanide to about 6 hours with torsemide. Once an effective dose is found, it may need to be administered several times a day, particularly for the short-acting agents. The frequency of administration is also determined for each individual and depends on the amount of cumulative excretion of sodium that is needed and the amount of sodium restriction that the patient will tolerate. For example, if the goal is to cause a net loss of 150 mEq of sodium and each dose of diuretic causes 75 mEq to be excreted, twice-daily dosing would be sufficient if the patient ingested no sodium. If the patient ingests 250 mEq of sodium, then dosing at least three times a day is necessary.

Other renal effects of loop diuretics are useful for treating hypercalcemia, hyponatremia, and occasionally renal tubular acidosis (Table 6-11). The major site of reabsorption of calcium is the thick ascending limb of the loop of Henle (Agus et al. 1982). Thus, by inhibiting solute reabsorption at this segment of the nephron, loop diuretics increase excretion of calcium and are effective adjunctive therapy of hypercalcemia. Most patients with hypercalcemia are volume-depleted, so the first step of therapy is replacement of volume with saline. The saline diuresis in and of itself will increase excretion of calcium and is sufficient for many patients. If additional therapy is needed, loop diuretics plus replacement of fluid losses sufficient to prevent volume depletion can be helpful.

**PRINCIPLE The physician can make use of valuable interactions between drugs, water, and electrolytes.**

By increasing delivery of $Na^+$, $Cl^-$, and water to the diluting segment (where $Na^+$ and $Cl^-$ are reabsorbed) loop diuretics increase free-water formation; in other words, they cause excretion of water in excess of sodium (Schrier et al. 1973). If patients who are hyponatremic have loop diuretic-induced volume losses replaced with isotonic or hypertonic saline, then there will be a net gain of sodium relative to water. This sequence causes the concentration of sodium in serum to increase. This strategy is only rarely used, particularly because overly rapid correction of chronic hyponatremia can be deleterious (Lauriat and Berl 1997).

In some patients with distal renal tubular acidosis who are unable to maintain an adequate systemic pH with conventional therapy, loop diuretics allow excretion of an acid urine and facilitate correction of the metabolic acidosis.

Both the effects on urinary acidification and formation of free water are not primary uses of loop diuretics, but they illustrate that knowledge of a drug's pharmacology can be coupled with known pathophysiology to allow its logical use for otherwise not obvious indications (Table 6-11).

***Thiazide Diuretics*** After discovery of the carbonic anhydrase inhibitors, it was deemed desirable to find a diuretic that would increase urinary excretion of sodium

**Table 6-12 Maximum Single Doses of Loop Diuretics**

| | Dose (mg) | | | | |
|---|---|---|---|---|---|
| | Furosemide | | Bumetanide | Ethacrynic acid | Torsemide |
| Clinical condition | IV | PO | IV & PO | IV & PO | IV & PO |
| Renal insufficiency | | | | | |
| $20 < CL_{Cr} < 50$ | 80 | 160 | 2 | 100 | 50 |
| $CL_{Cr} < 20$ | 200 | 400 | 8–10 | 250 | 100 |
| Nephrotic syndrome | 120 | 240 | 3 | 150 | 50 |
| Cirrhosis | 40 | 80 | 1 | 50 | 20 |
| Congestive heart failure | 80–120 | 240 | 2–3 | 150 | 50 |

SOURCE: Adapted from Brater DC. 1992. Treatment of renal disorders and the influence of renal function on drug disposition. In: Melmon KL, Morrelli HF, Hoffman BB, et al., editors. *Clinical Pharmacology: Basic Principles in Therapeutics*. 3rd ed. New York: McGraw-Hill. pp 270–308. Reproduced with permission of the McGraw-Hill Companies.

ABBREVIATIONS: $CL_{Cr}$, creatinine clearance

chloride. Systematic study of the diuretic effects of chemical modifications of compounds having carbonic anhydrase inhibitory activity resulted in the discovery of chlorothiazide. Additional derivatives have resulted in the large group of thiazide diuretics.

Thiazide diuretics block electroneutral reabsorption of sodium chloride at the distal convoluted tubule, connecting tubule, and early collecting duct, causing diuresis, natriuresis, and chloruresis (Stokes 1989). These segments are collectively referred to as the distal tubule. At suprapharmacologic concentrations, all thiazides inhibit carbonic anhydrase. However, in clinically used doses, any such effect at the proximal tubule is negligible. The enhanced distal delivery of $Na^+$ caused by thiazides predictably facilitates secretion of potassium; these drugs deplete potassium. Because the distal tubule reabsorbs only about 5% of filtered sodium, the maximal effect of thiazides is much less than is that of loop diuretics (Table 6-10) (Fig. 6-4). However, these drugs are still adequate for many patients with mild edematous disorders unless patients have concomitant renal dysfunction. In such cases, limited filtration of sodium and decreased delivery of thiazides into the tubular lumen compromise their efficacy. In such patients, loop diuretics may be required.

The dose-response curve for a thiazide diuretic is illustrated in Fig. 6-4. At maximal doses, all have the same ceiling efficacy; that is, the maximal response to each is the same. These drugs differ from each other only in terms of cost and their duration of action (Table 6-13).

**Table 6-13 Duration of Action of Thiazide Diuretics**

| DIURETIC | DURATION OF ACTION (h) |
|---|---|
| *Short-Acting* | Up to 12 |
| Chlorothiazide | |
| Hydrochlorothiazide | |
| *Intermediate-Acting* | 12–24 |
| Bendroflumethiazide | |
| Benzthiazide | |
| Cyclothiazide | |
| Hydroflumethiazide | |
| Metolazone | |
| Quinethazone | |
| Trichlormethiazide | |
| *Long-Acting* | >24 |
| Chlorthalidone | |
| Indapamide | |
| Methyclothiazide | |
| Polythiazide | |

SOURCE: From Brater DC. 1992. Treatment of renal disorders and the influence of renal function on drug disposition. In: Melmon KL, Morrelli HF, Hoffman BB, et al., editors. *Clinical Pharmacology: Basic Principles in Therapeutics*. New York: McGraw-Hill. pp 270–308. Reproduced with permission of the McGraw-Hill Companies.

**PRINCIPLE The relative potencies of drugs that produce equivalent efficacy and toxicity should have little importance to the wise therapist.**

Historically, the greatest use of thiazide diuretics has been as antihypertensive agents (see chapter 1, Cardiovascular Disorders). Their chronic use triggers homeostatic reflexes that restore blood volume. This effect makes them useful in treating hypercalciuria and diabetes insipidus (Table 6-11). As discussed above, some patients with nephrolithiasis have idiopathically increased urinary excretion of calcium (Pak 1979). When chronic use of thiazide leads to increased reabsorption of solute (including calcium) at proximal nephron sites, the diminished excretion of calcium can help reduce formation of renal stones (Breslau et al. 1976). This effect also will cause slight increases in concentration of calcium in serum. Thus, although loop diuretics can be used to lower the serum calcium concentration, thiazide diuretics can increase it. These effects are predictable based on the pharmacology of the drugs and the physiology of calcium homeostasis.

**PRINCIPLE Fully defining the mechanisms of action of drugs often leads to new understanding of the pathogenesis of disease and new indications for the drugs.**

The increased proximal tubular reabsorption of solute that occurs with chronic administration of thiazide can affect the concentrations of other cations. Because the major component of lithium reabsorption occurs at the proximal tubule, use of thiazides predictably increases reabsorption of lithium such that it can accumulate to potentially toxic concentrations. As a consequence, patients concomitantly treated with thiazides and lithium should be given lower-than-usual doses of lithium and doses should be guided by measuring the concentration of lithium in serum.

The increased proximal reabsorption of solute with chronic use of thiazide also is accompanied by increased reabsorption of water. In addition, the distal site at which thiazides act is responsible for generating a dilute urine.

As a consequence, thiazide diuretics impair the ability to maximally dilute the urine. On the one hand, this effect predisposes to hyponatremia if patients treated with thiazides ingest large amounts of hypotonic fluids. On the other hand, thiazides can be useful therapy in diabetes insipidus (Table 6-11). Patients with central diabetes insipidus are plagued by a maximally dilute urine that can result in urine volumes of up to 20 L/day. Thiazides in such patients often can diminish urinary output to about 10 L/day, a nontrivial decrease that improves the quality of these patients' lives. Thus, a diuretic agent actually can be used to diminish the volume of urine. This paradoxical effect makes sense once understanding of the site of action and pharmacology of the drug is coupled with understanding of the pathophysiology of central diabetes insipidus.

**PRINCIPLE The rewards of thinking about mechanisms of drug and disease can yield very satisfying results that would not occur if one classified drugs simply by their rubric mechanisms of action.**

The mechanisms of other effects of thiazides are poorly understood. Disruption of glucose homeostasis is a good example. In patients with borderline control of blood glucose concentrations, institution of thiazides may cause significant hyperglycemia. Some have attributed this adverse effect to depletion of potassium or to reduced secretion of insulin; there is little support for these hypotheses.

***Potassium-Retaining Diuretics*** In the distal nephron and collecting duct, sodium exchanges with $K^+$ and $H^+$. By blocking luminal sodium channels, amiloride and triamterene interfere with this process. (Frelin et al. 1987). Sodium reabsorption at these nephron segments also is stimulated by aldosterone. Cells responsive to aldosterone contain cytoplasmic receptors that bind mineralocorticoids. Receptor binding results in translocation of the hormone-receptor complex to the nucleus, where synthesis of mRNA coding for $Na^+$ pumps is stimulated. This entire sequence of events can be inhibited by spironolactone, which blocks the receptor for aldosterone.

Thus, there are two different mechanisms by which this class of drugs blocks $Na^+$ reabsorption. Amiloride and triamterene block sodium absorption independent of aldosterone, whereas spironolactone directly antagonizes the effects of aldosterone. This latter mechanism of action provides the rationale for specifically using spironolactone in patients with primary or secondary hyperaldosteronism. The dose of spironolactone needed will be dependent on the endogenous level of mineralocorticoid in each individual patient. Each patient must undergo titration until an effective dose is reached. The appropriate dose can be gauged by monitoring urinary electrolyte concentrations. A pharmacologic effect has been reached when a urine characterized by low amounts of $Na^+$ and high amounts of $K^+$ reverses to one in which $Na^+$ is in excess of $K^+$. Because the mechanism of action of spironolactone (antagonism of aldosterone receptors) leads to a decrease of protein synthesis, the duration of effect of spironolactone is one or more days, and the plateau of effect is not reached until 3 or 4 days of therapy. Therefore, in titrating the drug, doses should not be increased more frequently than every 3 or 4 days. This delay is also due to the fact that steady-state concentrations of an active metabolite of spironolactone may not be achieved for 3 to 7 days.

The actions of amiloride and triamterene contrast with those of spironolactone. They are shorter-acting, making dosage adjustments possible on a daily basis if necessary. These agents are preferable to spironolactone if a potassium-retaining diuretic is needed in a patient without excess mineralocorticoid.

Because only a small amount of sodium is reabsorbed at the site of action of these agents, they produce only weak natriuresis and diuresis in most patients (Table 6-10). Their primary use, then, is to correct or prevent potassium and/or magnesium deficiency (Table 6-11). Potassium-retaining diuretics are most frequently used in combination with thiazide diuretics. Preparations often contain fixed doses of each drug. The rationale for these preparations is that the combination is presumed to have a neutral effect on potassium and magnesium excretion while maintaining the efficacious diuretic or antihypertensive effects. The rationale for using these combination products, however, has some flaws. First, because only about 5% of patients receiving thiazide diuretics become potassium-depleted, the remaining 95% of patients do not require additional therapy with potassium-retaining diuretics. Second, potassium-retaining diuretics may produce hyperkalemia in about 5% of patients, an effect that may be more dangerous than depletion of potassium. Third, patients with a true need for potassium-retaining diuretics often require amounts that are not available in fixed-combination preparations. As a consequence, when used, each of these drugs should be individually titrated to the desired effect. The most rational use of potassium-sparing diuretics is in patients who have actually become hypokalemic or hypomagnesemic rather than as prophylaxis for such imbalance.

**PRINCIPLE There is nothing inherently advantageous or disadvantageous about fixed-dose combination products. They may be tested in the usual clinical settings where their components are or can be given separately for relative rates of efficacy and toxicity. Then the decision about their general utility can follow. In comparisons of fixed-dose products with their separate entities, relative price for a given effect should also be considered.**

Blockade of $H^+$ exchange for $Na^+$ by these drugs causes renal tubular acidosis, type IV. Patients with mild renal insufficiency or with diabetes mellitus may be particularly susceptible. Other adverse effects of potassium-retaining diuretics are not extensions of their pharmacologic effects. Rarely, the metabolite of triamterene can precipitate in concentrated urine. High doses of spironolactone have antiandrogenic effects that can cause gynecomastia and male sexual dysfunction (Ochs et al. 1978).

More recently, spironolactone has been shown to decrease mortality and morbidity in patients with congestive heart failure. This benefit likely represents a direct cardiac effect (Pitt et al. 1999).

***Combinations of Diuretics*** The rationale for combining potassium-retaining and other diuretics has been discussed. Other combinations of diuretics are used to obtain additive or even synergistic natriuretic effects in patients who respond poorly to single agents. Such patients invariably have severe disease, such as end-stage heart failure, severe renal insufficiency, severe cirrhosis with persistent ascites, and so forth. In spite of receiving maximal doses of loop diuretics, the sodium excretion in these patients is inadequate. By blocking additional sites of sodium reabsorption in the nephron, a greater response often can be achieved. The most useful combination of agents for this purpose is that of a loop plus a thiazide diuretic. Response to a loop diuretic alone can be considerably blunted by increased reabsorption of sodium at sites distal to the thick ascending limb. In fact, chronic dosing of loop diuretics appears to cause hypertrophy of distal tubule cells with an enhanced capacity to reabsorb sodium (Ellison 1991). Blocking reclamation of sodium at these distal sites with thiazide diuretics can often increase response and can occasionally result in a pronounced diuresis in patients with minimal or no response to a loop diuretic alone. This effect is schematically shown in Fig. 6-5. Patients should be carefully monitored for volume and potassium status when such combinations are used.

Some patients, particularly those with severe heart failure, have increased proximal tubular reabsorption of sodium that blunts response to more distally acting agents. Addition of an agent with proximal effects such as acetazolamide can be a helpful adjunct to therapy in some of these patients. It is best to try combinations of thiazides

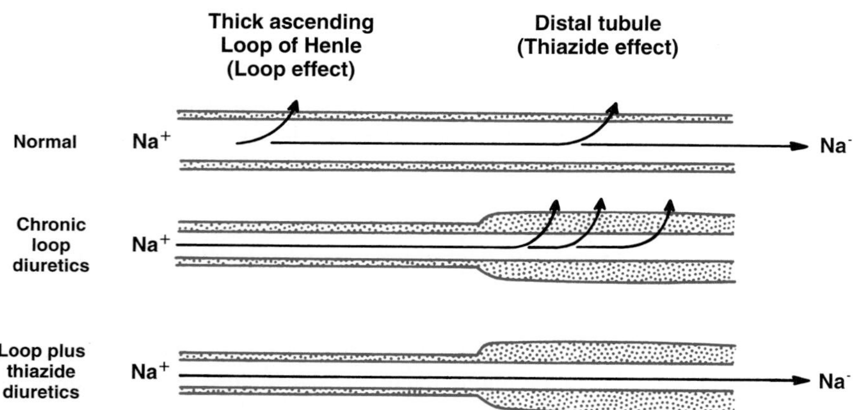


FIGURE 6-5 **Schematic illustration of the synergy between loop and thiazide diuretics. Chronic therapy with loop diuretics causes hypertrophy at the distal tubule with enhanced reabsorption of sodium. Inhibition of this site by thiazide diuretics amplifies the effects of the loop diuretic. (From Brater DC. 1992. Treatment of renal disorders and the influence of renal function on drug disposition. In: Melmon KL, Morrelli HF, Hoffman BB, et al., editors. *Clinical Pharmacology: Basic Principles in Therapeutics*. 3rd ed. New York: McGraw-Hill. pp 270–308. Reproduced with permission of the McGraw-Hill Companies.)**

and loop diuretics first and reserve addition of acetazolamide for those still unresponsive. Fortunately, such patients are rarely encountered.

**TREATMENT OF DISORDERS OF OSMOLARITY (HYPER- AND HYPONATREMIA)** Treatment of hyper- or hyponatremia is dictated by its pathogenesis. The first step in therapy is to decipher the pathophysiology of the disorder (Narins et al. 1982).

Hypernatremia may be caused by loss of free water, as in diabetes insipidus of central or nephrogenic origin. The former can be treated with the vasopressin analog 1-deamino-$\delta$-D-arginine vasopressin (DDAVP); thiazide diuretics also may be helpful. Hypernatremia may also occur from sodium excess including such iatrogenic causes as parenteral administration of hypertonic sodium, mistaken feeding of high-sodium-containing formulas to infants, and so forth. In addition, a number of drugs can cause hypernatremia.

Hyponatremia has many causes that dictate disparate treatments (Narins et al. 1982). Some patients present with acute, symptomatic hyponatremia that often is iatrogenic, for example, caused by receipt of large volumes of hypotonic parenteral fluids postoperatively. Whether and how fast hyponatremia should be corrected is a vigorously debated issue (Lauriat and Berl 1997). Rapid correction of the concentration of sodium in serum (within hours) by administration of hypertonic saline with or without loop diuretics seems appropriate for most causes of severe, acute hyponatremia. In contrast, patients with insidious onset of hyponatremia should be slowly corrected. Rapid reversal in such patients can cause osmotic disequilibrium of the CNS causing myelinolysis with considerable morbidity and mortality. In this circumstance, the serum concentration of sodium should be corrected no more rapidly than 2.5 mEq/L per hour. Total correction should not exceed 20 mEq/L per day (Lauriat and Berl 1997).

Patients with chronic hyponatremia may not need treatment with other than fluid restriction to 500 mL/day. If chronic therapy is needed, then demeclocycline or lithium can be used, taking advantage of the nephrogenic diabetes insipidus that both these drugs can cause (Forrest et al. 1978). Of these drugs, demeclocycline usually is preferable because of its relatively safe profile.

**TREATMENT OF POTASSIUM ABNORMALITIES** Hyperkalemia can be treated acutely by maneuvers that shift the ion into cells. Administration of bicarbonate or $\beta_2$-adrenergic receptor agonists drives potassium intracellularly. Infusion of glucose plus insulin also causes potassium to enter cells. Treatment of chronic hyperkalemia entails use of sodium polystyrene sulfonate, an ion-exchange resin that prevents absorption of potassium by binding it in the gut.

Treatment of hypokalemia is confounded by the fact that concentrations of potassium in serum poorly reflect the state of intracellular potassium stores. For example, at normal systemic pH, reduction of the serum potassium concentration to less than 3 mEq/L reflects a deficit of 400 mEq or more of total body potassium. As the serum potassium concentration falls further, total body potassium deficits rise exponentially. A correlation between the concentration of potassium in serum with pH indicates that about a 0.5–1.0 mEq/L rise in potassium concentration will occur for each fall of 0.1 pH unit in arterial blood. Such estimates of potassium requirements represent averages and are applicable only as guidelines to individual cases. Less potassium should be replaced than the estimated deficit and at the same time that the causative abnormalities in pH are being corrected. Careful monitoring of the effects of therapy is required.

Because the physiological effect of potassium is reflected in the electrocardiogram, it can be monitored to assess the efficacy and safety of rapid replacement of KCl. The intracellular potassium concentration measured by the ECG may be more useful than its serum concentration.

**TREATMENT OF CALCIUM ABNORMALITIES** Most hypercalcemic patients are volume-depleted. The mainstay of their therapy is restoration of normal intravascular volume. Initial therapy of hypercalcemia relies on the parallel reabsorption of sodium and calcium by the nephron. Thus, decreased reabsorption of sodium results in increased excretion of calcium. Parenteral administration of saline often is sufficient to cause calciuresis. If not, then loop diuretics can be used, but scrupulous attention must be paid to preventing contraction of volume.

Chronic treatment of hypercalcemia depends on the cause. For example, hyperparathyroidism is usually treated surgically, that associated with sarcoidosis responds to steroids, and so forth. The most vexing form of hypercalcemia to treat is that caused by malignancy. In such a case, the hypercalcemia may be due to destruction of bone, synthesis of bone-resorbing prostaglandins, or synthesis of other bone-resorbing factors such as parathyroid hormone-like peptide by the tumor (Mundy and Guise 1997). Other than using indomethacin in patients with the rare tumors that produce prostaglandin-mediated hypercalcemia, only nonspecific therapy is available. Oral phosphate, mithramycin, glucocorticoids, and bisphosphonates can be used (Mundy and Guise 1997). Bisphosphonates have become the mainstay of therapy.

Hypocalcemia, if not factitious due to hypoalbuminemia, can be treated with calcium supplements given orally with or without vitamin D analogs. Of the latter, $1,25[OH]_2D_3$ has the shortest duration of action; this feature can be advantageous if patients become hypercalcemic.

**TREATMENT OF ACID–BASE ABNORMALITIES** Treatment of acidemia due to metabolic acidosis requires defining and treating the underlying disease (i.e., treatment of diabetic acidosis, correction of poor tissue perfusion, removal of acidifying drugs, etc.). If one needs to treat the acidemia, then the bicarbonate deficit must be calculated. The clinician must then remember that usually approximately one-half the acid load is buffered intracellularly and one-half extracellularly. In severe acidemia, bicarbonate replacement to restore intra- and extracellular pH is greater than would be calculated on the assumption that only one-half the acid load is buffered in the cell. The objective of therapy with bicarbonate is to restore buffering capacity. Replacement should be slow and cautious because improvement in the patient's clinical condition will recruit endogenous mechanisms for correcting the abnormality. Therefore, a calculated replacement dose of bicarbonate may prove excessive, resulting in alkalemia.

Alkalemia, hypokalemia, or changes in ionized calcium may occur with bicarbonate therapy and complicate the disease state. As acidemia develops, potassium leaves cells and is excreted by the kidney. Depletion of total exchangeable potassium may be masked by an apparently normal or even mildly elevated concentration of potassium in serum caused by the acidemia. Abrupt correction of the acidemia may move potassium back into cells, resulting in hypokalemia with its attendant effects on muscular, neuromuscular, and cardiac functions.

Metabolic alkalosis can be subdivided into that which is saline-responsive (where urinary chloride excretion is <10 mEq/day) and that which is saline-unresponsive (where urinary chloride excretion is >10 mEq/day) (Narins et al. 1982). There are multiple causes of each of these entities, but the former responds to treatment with saline alone; the latter requires therapy of the primary abnormality, replacement of chloride deficits, and concomitant replacement of potassium losses.

## ADVERSE EFFECTS OF DRUGS ON RENAL FUNCTION

Drugs can adversely affect renal function in a variety of ways. Drug-induced nephrotoxic effects can mimic almost any renal disease. Thus, whenever a patient presents with a renal disorder, adverse drug reactions should be considered in the differential diagnosis. If a renal syndrome is not appropriately attributed to an offending drug, then therapy with that drug will continue while additional misdirected treatment is aimed at some other cause. The patient is likely to worsen and potentially incur irreversible renal damage.

**Table 6-14 Types of Adverse Effects of Drugs on Renal Function and Their Prototypes**

| MECHANISM | EXAMPLES OF DRUGS OR EFFECTS |
|---|---|
| Factitious toxicity | Glucocorticoids, tetracyclines, cimetidine |
| Altered renal hemodynamics | ACE inhibitors, NSAIDs, cyclosporine |
| Glomerular damage | |
| "Toxic" | NSAIDs, gold, penicillamine |
| Immunologic | Sulfonamide vasculitis, drug-induced lupus, organic solvents |
| Interstitial damage | |
| "Toxic" | Cyclosporine, analgesics, heavy metals |
| Immunologic | Penicillins, sulfonamide derivatives |
| Renal tubular damage | Aminoglycosides |
| Precipitation in collecting system | Sulfonamides, oxypurinol, triamterene, increased uric acid excretion |

SOURCE: Adapted from Brater DC. 1992. Treatment of renal disorders and the influence of renal function on drug disposition. In: Melmon KL, Morrelli HF, Hoffman BB, et al., editors. *Clinical Pharmacology: Basic Principles in Therapeutics*. 3rd ed. New York: McGraw-Hill. pp 270–308. Reproduced with permission of the McGraw-Hill Companies.

ABBREVIATIONS: ACE, angiotensin-converting enzyme; NSAID, nonsteroidal anti-inflammatory drug.

The manner in which drugs adversely affect renal function can be categorized (Table 6-14). Examples of each type of effect are briefly discussed. An exhaustive listing of drugs and their effects on the kidney is beyond the scope of this chapter.

## Factitious Increases in Creatinine

As indicated in the section on ARF, factitious increases in BUN and creatinine concentrations can occur that could lead to an erroneous diagnosis of renal insufficiency. For example, the catabolic effect of glucocorticoids and the antianabolic effect of tetracyclines can elevate the BUN concentration. Drugs such as cimetidine can block the secretory component of creatinine elimination, causing its concentration in plasma to increase in patients who already have renal dysfunction (Zaltman et al. 1996). The secretory component of creatinine's elimination entails only about 15% of its overall excretion in subjects with normal renal function. Thus, in a healthy person competition for secretion is quantitatively unimportant, and an effect of cimetidine on this component of excretion would not be noticeable. In contrast, as renal function declines, the secretory component becomes noticeable and interference with that secretion can cause a readily detectable increase in creatinine concentrations, without any alteration in GFR being present.

## Decreased Renal Perfusion

Renal perfusion can be impaired by a number of drugs. Any adverse reaction sufficient to cause systemic hypotension or reduce cardiac output can diminish renal perfusion. Such an effect may result in prerenal azotemia or, if extreme, can result in ARF. Common drugs that can cause adverse hemodynamic effects are ACE inhibitors and NSAIDs.

During states of already severely compromised renal blood flow, maintenance of glomerular filtration depends on intrarenal generation of angiotensin II (AII), which constricts the glomerular efferent arteriole, and intrarenal generation of prostacyclin, which dilates the afferent arteriole. Inhibition of AII formation with any ACE inhibitor in this setting will result in prompt decrements in GFR, which may progress to acute oliguric renal failure. This syndrome occurs most often in patients with severe bilateral renal artery stenosis, in those with severe stenosis of a solitary functioning kidney, or in patients with profoundly low cardiac output. In fact, in the absence of severe cardiac disease, ARF from an ACE inhibitor should prompt an evaluation of the patient for renal artery stenosis.

In clinical conditions of diminished actual or effective circulating volume, renal perfusion becomes dependent on local synthesis of vasodilating prostaglandins (PGs). Prostacyclin is synthesized by the renal vascular endothelium. In such settings, inhibition of renal PGs by NSAIDs allows unopposed vasoconstriction by assorted autocoids, causing acute and sometimes profound decreases in renal perfusion. Patients susceptible to this effect include those who are volume-depleted, whether by disease or diuretics, and those with CHF, cirrhosis, or renal insufficiency (including nephrotic syndrome) (Dunn and Zambraski 1980). When such patients are to receive a NSAID, their renal function should be assessed within several days of commencing therapy in order to detect an adverse effect while it is reversible.

Cyclosporine has multiple effects on the kidney, one of which is to cause renal vasoconstriction. The mechanism of this effect is unknown, but it may cause the hypertension that is frequently associated with cyclosporine's use. Whether this vasoconstrictive effect of cyclosporine is the mechanism of the progressive decline in renal function that occurs with chronic use of this agent is unclear.

## Glomerular Injury

Drugs can affect the glomerulus either by a "toxic" effect (meaning the mechanism is not known) or by causing glomerulonephritis. A toxic effect includes not only hemodynamically mediated decrements in GFR discussed above but also drug-induced nephrotic syndrome that does not appear to have an immunological basis. Chronic use (e.g., months or years of therapy) of NSAIDs can rarely result in nephrotic syndrome that is unusual histologically in that glomeruli appear benign in the setting of a marked interstitial nephritis (Clive and Stoff 1984). Thus, this syndrome represents the paradox of a primarily interstitial disease that becomes clinically manifest because of what appears to be a secondary glomerulopathy.

Gold salts and penicillamine commonly cause proteinuria, the mechanism of which is unknown (Hall et al. 1987). Patients receiving these drugs need regular monitoring for urinary protein in order to detect this adverse effect early when it is still reversible.

Other drugs cause glomerulonephritis. The vasculitides that rarely occur with sulfonamide antibiotics can include a glomerular component. Several drugs including procainamide, hydralazine, isoniazid, and phenytoin can cause a systemic lupus erythematosus syndrome (Hess

1988). Presumably, the development of antibodies to these drugs is causal. In contrast to spontaneously occurring lupus, the drug-induced syndrome usually does not manifest glomerulonephritis. The reasons for this difference are unknown.

Organic solvents, including gasoline, cause renal tubular injury (see below). They have also been implicated in antiglomerular basement membrane antibody-mediated glomerulonephritis, including an association with pulmonary involvement (i.e., Goodpasture syndrome).

## Interstitial Injury

Interstitial nephritis can be caused by a number of drugs. The NSAIDs can produce an interstitial inflammatory infiltrate. Cyclosporine also causes an interstitial reaction that may be the mechanism by which its use over time results in declines in renal function in many patients (Myers et al. 1984).

The entity of analgesic nephropathy is likely different from the interstitial nephritis caused by NSAIDs noted above. Analgesic nephropathy has an interstitial component, but this may be secondary rather than primary scarring. The hallmark of analgesic nephropathy is papillary necrosis. The mechanism of the progression from this lesion to end-stage renal disease is unknown. Development of analgesic nephropathy requires years of persistent ingestion of the analgesic. The reasons for distinct geographic distribution (e.g., Scandinavia, Switzerland, Australia, the southeastern United States) are unknown. Likewise, the offending agent(s) is unclear (DeBroe and Elseviers 1998).

Originally phenacetin was presumed to be a major cause of analgesic nephropathy. However, removal of phenacetin from the market in countries with a high prevalence of this syndrome has not decreased its frequency. Many investigators now feel that causality is related to combination products somehow having an additive or synergistic toxic effect on the kidney. Whether currently marketed nonsalicylate NSAIDs will cause this syndrome is unknown. Case reports of NSAID-induced papillary necrosis have appeared (Clive and Stoff 1984) but analgesic nephropathy per se has not been noticed despite widespread use of these agents.

**PRINCIPLE If a drug is banned for the wrong reason, its therapeutic value is unjustly lost and possibly lost forever.**

Heavy metals, particularly lead, cause interstitial nephropathy. Exposure usually occurs through occupational exposure and has been implicated in causing "saturnine" gout and hypertension. Immunologically mediated interstitial nephritis has been described with penicillins and other drugs (Neilson 1989). In some cases, drug-induced development of antibodies to renal tubular basement membranes has been documented. Histologically, this lesion reveals an inflammatory infiltrate with many eosinophils; in fact, systemic eosinophilia and eosinophiluria may aid the diagnosis.

Finding eosinophils in the urine is highly specific for this disorder but is not sensitive because many false negatives occur. Patients usually manifest this syndrome after days, weeks, or even longer duration of therapy. Renal function declines in the absence of other causes. Stopping the medication usually results in prompt resolution. Administration of a structurally dissimilar drug usually is safe. For example, patients suffering interstitial nephritis from furosemide can be successfully managed with ethacrynic acid. In contrast, substituting bumetanide for the structurally similar furosemide would not be wise.

## Damage to the Collecting System

Just as minerals can precipitate in the urinary collecting system, some drugs also can crystallize and serve as the nidus for stone formation. The risk of this effect is greatest if urine flow is low and drugs attain high concentrations in the urine. Sulfonamide diuretics are classic examples of this phenomenon. In fact, this property precluded use of some of them. This risk also historically led to the use of preparations containing several different sulfonamide antibiotics because they had additive antibacterial effects but did not entail an additive risk of precipitation in urine. Thus, with a combination of sulfonamides, the efficacy of a large dose of a single agent could be attained but each component would not reach sufficient concentrations in urine to precipitate. This simple strategy improved the benefit-to-risk ratio.

Oxypurinol (the active metabolite of allopurinol) and triamterene have rarely been found as renal stones in patients. If a patient with no history of nephrolithiasis develops renal colic while taking one of these drugs, one should suspect stones generated from the drug.

Drugs can increase excretion of uric acid by several mechanisms sufficient to cause precipitation and uropathy from uric acids. Rapid necrosis of large malignancies (particularly lymphomas) can cause a sudden increase in the production and excretion of uric acid resulting in ARF (tumor lysis syndrome). Pretreatment of such patients with allopurinol inhibits formation of uric acid, and pretreatment with intravenous fluids helps to increase urine volume. Both of these actions, along with alkalinizing the urine, help reduce the risk of developing uric acid nephropathy.

### Effects on Renal Tubules

Effects of drugs on renal tubular function can result in alterations in fluid and electrolyte homeostasis. As shown in Table 6-15, virtually any fluid and electrolyte disorder can be caused by drugs. Space does not permit discussion of the mechanisms for the effects listed. Nevertheless clinicians should consider a drug-induced cause for any electrolyte disorder encountered in a patient.

## EFFECTS OF RENAL IMPAIRMENT ON DRUG DISPOSITION

Well over 100 commonly prescribed drugs are eliminated by the kidney. Many others are metabolized or conjugated, usually in the liver, and the polar metabolites are excreted by the kidney. Therefore, renal impairment can result in the accumulation of exogenously administered drugs or their polar metabolites. To compensate for such accumulation, doses of affected drugs must be adjusted to attain concentrations similar to those obtained in patients with normal renal function.

The pharmacologic and biochemical characteristics of a drug sometimes allow prediction of whether renal dysfunction is likely to affect their disposition (Table 6-16). If a drug has a wide therapeutic margin, accumulation has little if any consequence and dose adjustment is less critical (unless the drug needs to be given at the very highest end of its therapeutic range). Penicillin derivatives and many cephalosporins are examples of this type of drug, unless very high doses of penicillin G are being given (e.g., for pneumococcal meningitis).

Drugs can bind to plasma proteins, the most important of which are albumin, which binds acidic compounds and $\alpha_1$ acid glycoprotein that binds basic compounds. Patients with renal insufficiency accumulate endogenous organic acids that normally are excreted by the kidney. These compounds are able to displace acidic drugs from albumin's binding sites (Reidenberg and Drayer 1984). The clinical importance of this effect depends on the degree of binding of the drug. For drugs bound less than 90%, the magnitude of effect is so small as to be irrelevant. In contrast, drugs bound more than 90% may be importantly affected by changes in protein binding.

The extent of protein binding also predicts the potential for removal of the drug by dialysis. Substantial binding means that only small amounts of drug are free in plasma. Since only the free fraction can be removed by dialysis, only negligible amounts of drugs that are more than 90% bound to plasma proteins are removed by dialytic procedures (excepting hemoperfusion). The drug's volume of distribution also can help predict its removal by hemodialysis. Drugs with volumes of distribution on the order of total body water or less (i.e., 0.7 L/kg) are likely restricted to the extracellular space and are accessible to dialysis. A large volume of distribution implies that the majority of drug is not dialyzable. Thus, a drug with a small volume of distribution and low protein binding (e.g., aminoglycoside antibiotics) would be predicted to be substantially removed by dialytic procedures and likely require supplemental dosing after dialysis. In contrast, even though a drug with a large volume of distribution may pass through a dialysis membrane, so little of it is in the plasma relative to overall body stores that the total amount removed is negligible.

Knowing the amount of a drug or active metabolite that is excreted in the urine allows one to predict the potential for clinically important accumulation of drug or metabolite in patients with renal insufficiency. Unless the drug has a wide therapeutic margin, if 30% or more is excreted unchanged in urine, then adjustment of the dose will likely be needed in patients with renal insufficiency.

Data describing the amount of drug removed by a dialytic procedure can be used to help predict likely need for adjustment of dose. If no drug is removed by dialysis, then the only dose adjustment needed is that for the patient's endogenous level of renal function (presumably end stage). In contrast, if more than 30% of a dose of a drug is removed by a dialytic procedure, then supplemental dosing to replace the amount removed may be necessary. In addition, dialysis, particularly hemodialysis or hemoperfusion, occasionally is considered for therapeutic intervention in settings of overdose. For such adjuncts to be helpful, the dialytic procedure should increase endogenous clearance of the poison by 30% or more. For increments less than this value, the risks of the procedure likely outweigh any benefits.

The foregoing discussion implies that one can make reasonable predictions as to the need for adjusting therapy even for drugs that have not been explicitly studied in patients with renal insufficiency. Although lack of quantitative guidelines makes dose adjustments tentative, a worse problem is ignoring the need to do so. When no information about a particular drug is available, consider using a drug of the same class but with no dependence on the kidney for elimination. For example, rather than using a modified dose of atenolol as a selective $\beta$-adrenergic receptor antagonist in a patient with renal insufficiency, one could administer metoprolol, which is eliminated by the liver and needs no dose adjustment in

**Table 6-15 Examples of Fluid and Electrolyte Disorders Caused by Drugs**

| DISORDER | DRUG | MECHANISM |
|---|---|---|
| Hypernatremia | Osmotic cathartics (e.g., lactulose) | Intestinal water loss |
| | Povidone-iodine | Cutaneous water loss |
| | Lithium | Decreased renal response to ADH |
| | Demeclocycline HCl | Decreased renal response to ADH |
| | Vinblastine sulfate | Decreased renal response to ADH |
| Hyponatremia | Thiazide diuretics | Decreased function of "diluting segment" |
| | Amiloride HCl | Decreased function of "diluting segment" |
| | Chlorpropamide | Increased response to ADH |
| | Cyclophosphamide | Increased response to ADH |
| | Cisplatin | Unknown |
| | Carboplatin | Unknown |
| | Antidepressants | Unknown |
| Hyperkalemia | Cardiac glycosides | Shift from intracellular stores |
| | Succinylcholine chloride | Shift from intracellular stores |
| | Arginine HCl | Shift from intracellular stores |
| | Potassium salts | Increased intake |
| | $\beta$-Adrenergic antagonists | Hyporenin and/or hypoaldosterone |
| | NSAIDs | Hyporenin and/or hypoaldosterone |
| | ACE inhibitors | Hyporenin and/or hypoaldosterone |
| | Heparin sodium | Hyporenin and/or hypoaldosterone |
| | Cyclosporine | Hyporenin and/or hypoaldosterone |
| | Potassium-retaining diuretics | Decreased potassium secretion |
| | Trimethoprim | Decreased potassium secretion |
| Hypokalemia | Glucose | Distribution into cells |
| | Insulin | Distribution into cells |
| | $\beta_2$-Adrenergic agonists | Distribution into cells |
| | Theophylline | Distribution into cells |
| | Laxatives | Increased elimination (GI losses) |
| | Carbonic anhydrase inhibitors | Decreased tubular reabsorption |
| | Osmotic diuretics | Decreased tubular reabsorption |
| | Loop diuretics | Decreased tubular reabsorption |
| | Thiazide diuretics | Decreased tubular reabsorption |
| | Carbenoxolone | Increased mineralocorticoid effect |
| | True licorice | Increased mineralocorticoid effect |
| | Penicillins | Increased secretion due to non-reabsorbable anion |
| Metabolic acidosis | | |
| Increased anion gap | Biguanides | Lactic acidosis |
| | Papaverine HCl | Unmeasured anions |
| | Nalidixic acid | Unmeasured anions |
| | Nitroprusside | Unmeasured anions |
| | Iron | Unmeasured anions |
| | Salicylates | Unmeasured anions |
| | Paraldehyde | Unmeasured anions |
| | Methanol | Unmeasured anions (metabolites) |
| | Ethylene glycol | Unmeasured anions (metabolites) |
| | Toluene | Unmeasured anions |
| Normal anion gap | Laxatives | Gastrointestinal $HCO_3^-$ loss |
| | Cholestyramine | Gastrointestinal $HCO_3^-$ loss |
| | Carbonic anhydrase inhibitors | Renal $HCO_3$ loss |
| | Toluene | Decreased $H^+$ secretion |
| | Amphotericin B | Decreased $H^+$ secretion |
| | Lithium | Decreased $H^+$ secretion |
| | NSAIDs | Decreased $H^+$ secretion |

**Table 6-15 Examples of Fluid and Electrolyte Disorders Caused by Drugs (Continued)**

| DISORDER | DRUG | MECHANISM |
|---|---|---|
| | Potassium-retaining diuretics | Decreased $H^+$ secretion |
| | $NH_4Cl$ | Exogenous acid |
| | Arginine HCl | Exogenous acid |
| | Lysine | Exogenous acid |
| | Histidine | Exogenous acid |
| Metabolic alkalosis | Potassium-losing diuretics | Renal $K^+$ loss |
| | Tolazoline HCl | Gastrointestinal $H^+$ loss |
| | Drug-induced vomiting | Gastrointestinal $H^+$ loss |
| Hypercalcemia | Milk plus soluble alkali | Increased gastrointestinal $Ca^{2+}$ absorption |
| | Vitamin D | Increased gastrointestinal $Ca^{2+}$ absorption |
| | Vitamin D | Increased mobilization from bone |
| | Vitamin A | Increased mobilization from bone |
| | Tamoxifen citrate | Increased mobilization from bone |
| | Thiazide diuretics | Decreased renal excretion |
| Hypocalcemia | Anticonvulsants | Increased degradation of endogenous vitamin D |
| | Glutethimide | Increased degradation of endogenous vitamin D |
| | Plicamycin | Decreased mobilization from bone |
| | Calcitonin | Decreased mobilization from bone |
| | EDTA | Chelation of calcium |
| | Phosphate | Physicochemical complexing |
| Hypermagnesemia | $Mg^{2+}$ salts | Increased intake |
| Hypomagnesemia | Laxatives | Decreased GI absorption |
| | Potassium-losing diuretics | Increased renal loss |
| | Aminoglycoside antibiotics | Increased renal loss |
| | Cisplatin | Increased renal loss |
| | Amphotericin | Increased renal loss |
| Hyperphosphatemia | Drug-induced rhabdomyolysis | Tissue release |
| Hypophosphatemia | Glucose | Distribution into cells |
| | Insulin | Distribution into cells |
| | Aluminum- and magnesium-containing antacids | Decreased GI absorption |

SOURCE: Adapted from Brater DC. 1992. Treatment of renal disorders and the influence of renal function on drug disposition. In: Melmon KL, Morrelli HF, Hoffman BB, et al., editors. *Clinical Pharmacology: Basic Principles in Therapeutics*. 3rd ed. New York: McGraw-Hill. pp 270–308. Reproduced with permission of the McGraw-Hill Companies.

patients with renal insufficiency. The converse would apply to patients with liver disease.

## Effects of Renal Function on Pharmacokinetic Variables

### *Absorption*

No primary influences of variation in renal function on drug absorption have been identified. The potential exists for a number of secondary influences. For example, dehydration from salt wasting might affect perfusion to and absorption from intramuscular or intestinal sites. Potassium depletion might significantly affect gastrointestinal motility and thereby change the degree and/or rate of absorption of a drug. The clinician should be aware of the potential for a variety of changes in absorption kinetics and prospectively derive therapeutic and toxic endpoints to follow in each patient.

### *Distribution*

The kidney may affect distribution of a drug by several mechanisms. Changes in acid-base balance may affect the amount of ionized drug relative to nonionized drug. A pH favoring the nonionized form of a weak acid or base can facilitate its distribution out of plasma and into tissues. For example, with salicylate, a more acidic systemic pH increases the relative amount of nonionized salicylate and increases the amount reaching the CNS. The larger the amount in the CNS, the greater the chances of CNS toxicity (Hill 1993). Presumably, the acidemia of uremia would enhance distribution of salicylate into the CNS.

Protein binding is another major determinant of a drug's distribution. Diminished binding to albumin of acidic drugs frequently occurs in patients with renal insufficiency, because accumulated endogenous organic acids displace exogenously administered xenobiotics (Rei-

**Table 6-16 Drug Characteristics Having Implications for Patients with Renal Compromise or Receiving Hemodialysis**

| CHARACTERISTIC | IMPLICATIONS |
|---|---|
| Therapeutic margin | If the drug has a wide therapeutic margin, its accumulation poses less risk. |
| Protein binding | A high degree of binding (>90%) to albumin makes displacement likely; a high degree of binding to either albumin or $\alpha_1$-acid glycoprotein means little drug is available for removal by dialysis. |
| Amount of drug excreted in the urine unchanged | If 30% or more of a drug is excreted in the urine unchanged, it is highly likely to accumulate in patients with severe renal insufficiency. |
| Active metabolites are excreted in the urine | The metabolites can accumulate with attendant effects. |
| Volume of distribution | A small volume of distribution (that of total body water or less; i.e., ≤0.7 L/kg) means the drug may be accessible for removal by dialysis if it is not highly protein-bound; a large volume of distribution means little if any removal by dialysis. |
| Dialyzability | Removal of more than 30% of the body burden of drug during a typical 4- to 6-h dialysis procedure means supplemental dosing may be necessary; in overdose settings, an increment in endogenous clearance of more than 30% indicates that dialysis may be useful therapeutically. |

SOURCE: From Brater DC. 1992. Treatment of renal disorders and the influence of renal function on drug disposition. In: Melmon KL, Morrelli HF, Hoffman BB, et al., editors. *Clinical Pharmacology: Basic Principles in Therapeutics*. 3rd ed. New York: McGraw-Hill. pp 270–308. Reproduced with permission of the McGraw-Hill Companies.

denberg and Drayer 1984). This decreased binding increases the percentage of free (unbound) drug in plasma. A popular misconception is that such an effect results in increased concentrations of unbound, pharmacologically active drug, causing an enhanced effect, including toxicity. In the majority of instances, however, there is no increase in concentration of unbound drug and therefore no change in response unless it is caused by pharmacodynamic factors (Greenblatt et al. 1982).

Consider an example of phenytoin. Reductions in protein binding of phenytoin during uremia or in a patient with hypoalbuminemia can lead to misinterpretation of its concentrations in serum. In both clinical conditions, protein binding of phenytoin is decreased; unbound concentrations are unchanged, although total concentrations are diminished. When concentrations of phenytoin in plasma are obtained, the clinical laboratory measures only its total concentration. This could be misinterpreted as being too low even though unbound concentrations are usual and "therapeutic." If the clinician is misled and increases the dose of phenytoin in an attempt to attain a total concentration in the usual therapeutic range, an increase in the unbound concentration of phenytoin could result in toxicity.

This problem could be avoided by measuring unbound concentrations of phenytoin. Alternatively, one must redefine the therapeutic range of the drug in uremic and hypoalbuminemic patients. The therapeutic range for this drug in terms of its total concentration in plasma is about one-half to two-thirds of the value obtained in healthy individuals.

Displacement of drug from albumin binding sites in patients with renal insufficiency has been misinterpreted (Greenblatt et al. 1982). It is mistakenly cited as a mechanism for altered response to drugs in patients with renal disease. However, because unbound concentrations of drug may not change, this mechanism cannot explain altered response to drugs in many, if not most, uremic patients. It also follows that protein binding usually does not influence drug dosing. Clinicians should avoid false conclusions regarding drug disposition from what may be incomplete data in the medical literature, namely, studies of highly bound drugs that quantify only total and not unbound concentrations.

### *Metabolism*

The kidney metabolizes numerous drugs, but its quantitative contribution to overall clearance of drugs is for the most part unknown (Anders 1980). The proximal tubule has high levels of glucuronyl transferase and sulfotransferase (Besseghir and Roch-Ramel 1987). Renal glucuronidation may be substantial; for example, approximately 20% of an IV dose of furosemide and 50% of a dose of morphine may be glucuronidated by the kidney itself. The proximal tubule also contains mixed-function cytochrome P450 oxidases, but in lower amounts than in the liver. There are no data that allow conclusions about the quantitative importance of this potential pathway for drug metabolism (Besseghir and Roch-Ramel 1987; Anders 1980).

The kidney metabolizes proteins. In patients with normal renal function, up to 30% of insulin's elimination occurs via metabolism by the kidney. This component of overall elimination diminishes in patients with renal insufficiency and partially accounts for the decreased insulin requirement as a patient's renal function deteriorates. Many therapeutic peptides and proteins are small enough to be filtered by the glomerulus. They are then metabolized by peptidases of the brush border of the proximal tubule so that no or only negligible amounts of unchanged peptide appear in the final urine. However, decreased function results in retention of such agents with a need to modify the dose. In addition to actual metabolism by the kidney, the kidney excretes many drug metabolites that are formed in the liver. Renal insufficiency does not necessarily mean that metabolites of drugs will accumulate because other excretory pathways such as biliary excretion exist. Many drug metabolites have no pharmacologic effects, but some do (Verbeeck et al. 1981).

Sometimes the active metabolites exert pharmacologic effects similar to those of the parent compound (e.g., primidone). Others account for all the pharmacologic activity of the parent (e.g., enalapril). In additional examples, the metabolite has a different pharmacologic profile from that of the parent drug. For example, normeperidine excites the CNS and can cause seizures, in contrast to the sedating and analgesic effects of meperidine (Szeto et al. 1977). In order to safely use drugs in patients with renal insufficiency, one must not only know the pharmacologic profile of the parent drug, but also its active or toxic metabolite(s). In patients with renal disease, one should avoid using drugs that form active metabolites.

### *Excretion*

**FILTRATION** The integrity of the glomerulus, the size and charge of the molecule to be filtered, and the extent of protein binding determine the amount of a drug that is filtered. Highly protein-bound drugs are not appreciably filtered because only the unbound (free) drug is able to pass through the glomerulus. Protein binding, however, does not preclude substantial elimination by the kidney, because postglomerular secretory sites can efficiently excrete many drugs (see below). The glomerulus offers no barrier to filtration of most drugs that are free in plasma. Exceptions include larger proteins and dextran.

The status of the glomerulus is reflected by its rate of filtration and its integrity as a sieve. In the nephrotic syndrome this integrity is compromised, with loss of protein in the urine. One might predict that highly protein-bound drugs could be carried out with the protein into the urine, significantly increasing their excretion rate. This phenomenon has been investigated for phenytoin and clofibrate, both of which are highly bound to albumin. Their excretion is increased in patients with the nephrotic syndrome. However, there also is a concomitant decrease in protein binding of the two drugs with no change in the clinically important amount of free drug in the serum (Gugler et al. 1975).

The clinical significance of decrements in glomerular filtration rate on drug kinetics is widely known. The scope of agents is so broad that the clinician should consult the literature whenever drugs are prescribed to uremic patients.

**SECRETION** At the pars recta, or straight segment of the proximal tubule, active secretion of organic acids and bases into the tubular lumen occurs (Table 6-17). By competing for anionic secretion, probenecid significantly prolongs the half-life of the penicillins, an effect that was used historically to deliberately increase their efficacy. In contrast, inadvertent administration of probenecid, salicylates, or other NSAIDs with methotrexate has resulted in unexpected severe methotrexate toxicity, including death (Aherne et al. 1978). Each of these drugs inhibits tubular secretion of methotrexate, prolonging its duration of action and increasing its toxicity. Similarly, histamine $H_2$ antagonists can compete with procainamide and *N*-acetylprocainamide for secretion, potentially causing accumulation to toxic concentrations (Somogyi et al. 1983). When patients need concomitant administration of the drugs listed in Table 6-17, one should be alert to possible drug interactions.

For drugs with narrow therapeutic indices, alternative drugs may be sought, or careful plans for dose adjustment should be made. Digoxin is not only filtered at the glomerulus, but a clinically important component also is secreted in the distal nephron via P-glycoprotein (Okamura et al. 1993). Quinidine, verapamil, diltiazem, flecainide,

**Table 6-17 Examples of Drugs That are Secreted either as Organic Acids or Bases by the Kidney**

*Acids* (anionic transport system)
- Cephalosporins (most)
- Loop diuretics
- Methotrexate sodium
- NSAIDs (including salicylate)
- *p*-Aminohippurate sodium (PAH)
- Penicillins (most)
- Probenecid
- Sulfonamides (most)
- Thiazide diuretics

*Bases* (cationic transport system)
- Amiloride HCl
- Choline
- Ephedrine and pseudoephedrine
- Histamine $H_2$ antagonists (cimetidine, famotidine, nizatidine, ranitidine)
- Mepiperphenidol
- Morphine
- *N*-Methylnicotinamide (NMN)
- Quinine sulfate

SOURCE: Adapted from Brater DC. 1992. Treatment of renal disorders and the influence of renal function on drug disposition. In: Melmon KL, Morrelli HF, Hoffman BB, et al., editors. *Clinical Pharmacology: Basic Principles in Therapeutics*. 3rd ed. New York: McGraw-Hill. pp 270–308. Reproduced with permission of the McGraw-Hill Companies.

amiodarone, cyclosporine, and spironolactone can block digoxin's secretion and thereby cause increases in its concentration in serum. This interaction is greatest with quinidine, which causes the serum digoxin concentration to double in at least 90% of patients (Bigger and Leahy 1982). The magnitude and clinical implications of the interaction are much more variable with the other drugs noted above. Individual patients need close monitoring when these possible inhibitors of digoxin secretion are coadministered.

**REABSORPTION** Reabsorption from the tubular lumen back into the systemic circulation occurs with a number of drugs (Table 6-18). Clinically important factors affecting this transport process are urine flow rate and pH. High rates of urine formation decrease the concentration of a drug in the distal tubule and decrease the time for the agent to diffuse from the lumen. Increased renal clearance results. This process occurs to a significant extent with phenobarbital, but the effect has not been investigated for clinical importance during the use of other drugs.

A number of drugs demonstrate urine pH-dependent kinetics that follows the principle of passive nonionic diffusion. For both weak acids and weak bases, the nonionized form of the drug is more readily reabsorbed across the lipid cell membrane than is the ionized form. The $pK_a$ of the drug and the pH of the urine determine the relative amounts of ionized versus nonionized component, as illustrated in Fig. 6-6.

This effect is clinically important for a number of agents. Salicylate is a weak acid, and alkalinization of the urine increases its rate of excretion. This fact is clinically used to advantage in cases of salicylate overdose. Administration of sodium bicarbonate IV raises serum bicarbonate, then excretion of bicarbonate in urine, thereby raising urine pH and rate of excretion of salicylate. Although phenobarbital is a weak acid, its excretion is less pH- and more flow-dependent. Even though a number of sulfa antibiotics are weak acids with pH-dependent kinetics, the increment in their renal clearance caused by changes in urine pH is not significant when compared with overall clearance.

Weak bases similarly follow pH-dependent kinetics. Excretion of amphetamine is highly dependent on urine pH. At alkaline pH, only 2.7% of the drug is excreted in 16 hours, whereas 57% is eliminated during the same period at acidic urine pH. Ephedrine and pseudoephedrine also have significantly decreased renal clearance at alkaline urine pH. Children with renal tubular acidosis and persistently alkaline urine have developed severe pseudoephedrine toxicity due to accumulation of the drug when they are given "normal" doses (Brater et al. 1980).

It should be apparent that clinicians need to be aware of the influence of pH on drug disposition. They should

**Table 6-18 Drug Elimination Dependent on Urinary pH**

*Weak Acids* (increased excretion in alkaline urine)
- Chlorpropamide
- Methotrexate sodium
- Phenobarbital
- Salicylates
- Sulfonamide derivatives

*Weak Bases* (increased excretion in acidic urine)
- Amphetamine
- Ephedrine
- Mexiletine HCl
- Pseudoephedrine
- Quinine sulfate
- Tocainide HCl

SOURCE: From Brater DC. 1992. Treatment of renal disorders and the influence of renal function on drug disposition. In: Melmon KL, Morrelli HF, Hoffman BB, et al., editors. *Clinical Pharmacology: Basic Principles in Therapeutics*. 3rd ed. New York: McGraw-Hill. pp 270–308. Reproduced with permission of the McGraw-Hill Companies.

**Weak Acids**

$$HA \rightarrow H^+ + A^-$$

$$K_a = \frac{(H^+)(A^-)}{(HA)}$$

$$-\log K_a = pK_a = -\log(H^+) - \log\frac{(A^-)}{(HA)}$$

or

$$pK_a = pH - \log\frac{(A^-)}{(HA)}$$

or

$$pH - pK_a = \log\frac{(A^-)}{(HA)} = \log\frac{(\text{ionized drug})}{(\text{nonionized drug})}$$

Therefore, for a weak acid, as pH increases, the concentration of ionized drug increases.

**Weak Bases**

$$BH^+ \rightarrow B + H^+$$

$$K_a = \frac{(B)(H^+)}{(BH^+)}$$

$$-\log K_a = pK_a = -\log(H^+) - \log\frac{(B)}{(BH^+)}$$

or

$$pK_a = pH - \log\frac{(B)}{(BH^+)}$$

or

$$ph - pK_a = \log\frac{(B)}{(BH^+)} = \log\frac{(\text{nonionized drug})}{(\text{ionized drug})}$$

Therefore, for a weak base, as pH increases, the concentration of nonionized drug increases.

**FIGURE 6-6 Relationship between pH and the ionization of weak acids and bases. (From Brater DC. 1992. Treatment of renal disorders and the influence of renal function on drug disposition. In: Melmon KL, Morrelli HF, Hoffman BB, et al., editors. *Clinical Pharmacology: Basic Principles in Therapeutics*. 3rd ed. New York: McGraw-Hill. pp 270–308. Reproduced with permission of the McGraw-Hill Companies.)**

be alert to a patient's urinary pH, a clinical measurement that is often obtained but too little heeded.

**DIALYSIS** Just as dialytic procedures are used to remove accumulated endogenous end products of metabolism, they also can remove drugs. The amount removed can be sufficient to require supplemental dosing. In poisoning, dialysis may speed the elimination of the toxin (e.g., ethylene glycol) or a toxic metabolite (e.g., oxalate). As noted above, several characteristics of drug disposition can help predict removal of a drug by dialysis. Intuitively, a high degree of protein binding restricts the concentration of unbound (free) and therefore dialyzable drug. Similarly, a large volume of distribution means that only a small portion of the total body burden of drug is in plasma and accessible to dialytic removal. These considerations apply not only to conventional hemodialysis, but also to the newer techniques of continuous AV hemofiltration (CAVH) and continuous venovenous hemofiltration (CVVH). For these latter two techniques, ultrafiltration through the dialysis membrane is the sole mode of elimination and dialytic removal is equal to the unbound fraction times the ultrafiltration rate. This value can be used to estimate whether supplementary drug dosing needs to be given and, if so, the amount. For conventional hemodialysis, updated reference sources should be kept accessible so that the need for supplemental dosing can be determined in individual patients.

Hemoperfusion techniques may allow removal of substantially greater amounts of some drugs than can be accomplished with dialysis or ultrafiltration methods. In fact, these methods are so efficient that for some drugs and toxins, nearly all drug entering the hemoperfusion cartridge is removed. However efficient this removal of drug from blood may be, it still may not remove a clinically important amount of drug from the body. For example, if only a minor percentage of the total amount of drug in the body is circulating in plasma, even if hemoperfusion removes all the circulating drug, most of it is still left in body reservoirs inaccessible to the cartridge yet still in equilibrium with the plasma. As soon as hemiperfusion is stopped, these reservoirs serve to refill the circulating compartment such that decrements in circulating concentrations of drug caused by hemoperfusion are only transient. This phenomenon accounts for the lack of efficacy of hemoperfusion in treating poisoning with highly lipid-soluble sedative-hypnotics having large volumes of distribution (e.g., glutethimide, methaqualone).

It is noteworthy that most drugs are negligibly removed by peritoneal dialysis. This finding is in contrast to the substantial absorption of many drugs from the peritoneal space. The mechanism for this unidirectional peritoneal transport is unknown.

## Dosing Regimens

In patients with renal disorders, the clinician often needs to decrease the maintenance dose of drug administered to prevent its accumulation and toxicity. Perturbations of any of the pathways of renal handling of drugs may necessitate alterations in dosage regimens. With a number of drugs, such as the aminoglycoside antibiotics and digoxin, various experimentally validated guidelines to therapy exist. These suffice only as first approximations, and the clinician cannot assume that the predicted concentration of drug in serum derived from a nomogram or formula will be attained in a specific patient. When possible, patients should be monitored for serum concentrations of drugs that have a narrow therapeutic margin. In addition, disease states may alter not only the relation between dose and serum concentration attained, but also between concentration and effect. Determination of the concentration of drugs in serum is useful and beneficial, but is not a substitute for and must be supplemented with clinical endpoints of efficacy and toxicity for each drug administered.

There are two general approaches to decreasing the total amount of administered drug: 1) maintaining the same dose as in patients with normal renal function and giving it at wider intervals (variable interval regimen); and, 2) administering smaller doses at the same dosing interval (variable dosage regimen). Most reports emphasize the approach using variable intervals. This may not be ideal for all drugs. If the goal is a regimen that provides constant concentrations in plasma within a certain range, then the most effective method of maintaining that level is with an IV infusion. This approach often is not practical in clinical settings, and in its stead, intermittent dosing of the drug is recommended. Obviously, small amounts of a drug given at closely spaced intervals more nearly approximates a continuous infusion than does administration of large amounts of the drug at widely spaced time intervals (the total amount of drug administered being the same).

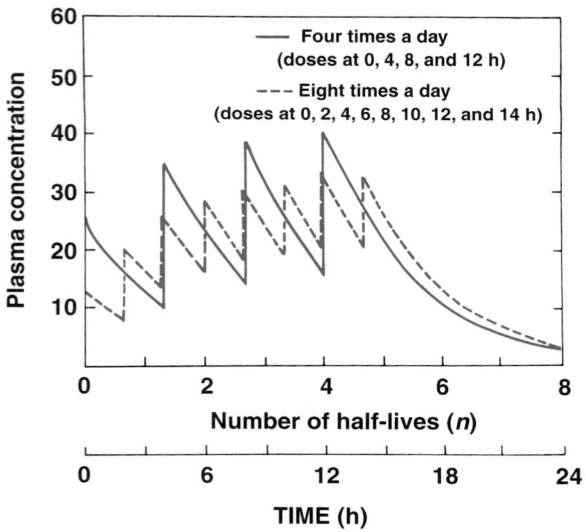


**FIGURE 6-7 Serum concentrations of a drug related to dosing interval. The same total amount of drug is administered in both examples. Half as much drug is administered twice as frequently in the regimen depicted by the broken line compared with that depicted by the solid line. (From Brater DC. 1992. Treatment of renal disorders and the influence of renal function on drug disposition. In: Melmon KL, Morrelli HF, Hoffman BB, et al., editors. *Clinical Pharmacology: Basic Principles in Therapeutics*. 3rd ed. New York: McGraw-Hill. pp 270–308. Reproduced with permission of the McGraw-Hill Companies.)**

Figure 6-7 illustrates this concept. Frequent dosing provides less variation in peak and nadir concentrations of drug. If the range of effective concentrations of the drug is wide, then the efficacy of the two methods may not differ. However, if the therapeutic range is narrow, then wide swings from peak to trough may result in periods during which concentrations of drug are subtherapeutic and other periods when they are toxic. Monitoring concentrations and clinical signs of pharmacologic effect in serum 1 hour after administration of a drug, and just before administration of the next dose, should enable the clinician to ascertain the appropriateness of the dosing regimen.

**PRINCIPLE The kidney is often a major determinant of drug kinetics, efficacy, and toxicity. Renal function must be considered in the development of most therapeutic strategies.**

## REFERENCES

Abrutyn E, Mossey J, Berlin JA, et al. 1994. Does asymptomatic bacteriuria predict mortality and does antimicrobial treatment reduce mortality in elderly ambulatory women? *Ann Intern Med* **120**:827–33, 1994.

[AHCPR] Agency for Health Care Policy and Research. 1996. Managing acute and chronic urinary incontinence. AHCPR Urinary Incontinence in Adults Guideline Panel. *Am Fam Phys* **54**:1661–72.

Agus ZS, Wasserstein A, Goldfarb S. 1982. Disorders of calcium and magnesium homeostasis. *Am J Med* **72**:473–88.

Aherne GW, Piall E, Marks V, et al. 1978. Prolongation and enhancement of serum methotrexate concentrations by probenecid. *Br Med J* **1**:1097–9.

Alkhunaizi AM, Schrier RW. 1996. Management of acute renal failure: new perspectives. *Am J Kidney Dis* **28**:315–28.

Anders MW. 1980. Metabolism of drugs by the kidney. *Kidney Int* **18**:636–47.

Anderson RJ, Linas SL, Berns AS, et al. 1977. Nonoliguric acute renal failure. *N Engl J Med* **296**:1134–8.

Benet AE, Melman A. 1995. The epidemiology of erectile dysfunction. *Urol Clin North Am* **22**:699–707.

Berger L, Yu TF. 1975. Renal function in gout: IV. An analysis of 524 gouty subjects including long-term follow-up studies. *Am J Med* **59**:605–13.

Besseghir K, Roch-Ramel F. Renal excretion of drugs and other xenobiotics. *Renal Physiol* **10**:221–41.

Bigger JT, Leahey EB. 1982. Quinidine and digoxin. An important interaction. *Drugs* **24**:229–39.

Black NA, Downs SH. 1996. The effectiveness of surgery for stress incontinence in women: a systematic review. *Br J Urol* **78**:497–510.

Borges HF, Hocks J, Kjellstrand CM. 1982. Mannitol intoxication in patients with renal failure. *Arch Intern Med* **142**:63–6.

Brater DC, Anderson SA, Brown-Cartwright D. 1986. Response to furosemide in chronic renal insufficiency: Rationale for limited doses. *Clin Pharmacol Ther* **40**:134–9.

Brater DC, Kaojarern S, Benet LZ, et al. 1980. Renal excretion of pseudoephedrine. *Clin Pharmacol Ther* **28**:690–4.

Brater DC, Seiwell R, Anderson S, et al. 1982. Absorption and disposition of furosemide in congestive heart failure. *Kidney Int* **22**: 171–6.

Brenner BM. 1983. Hemodynamically mediated glomerular injury and the progressive nature of kidney disease. *Kidney Int* **23**:647–55.

Breslau N, Moses AM, Wiener IM. 1976. The role of volume contraction in the hypocalciuric action of chlorothiazide. *Kidney Int* **10**:164–70.

Bushinsky DA. 1988. Nephrolithiasis. *J Am Soc Nephrol* **9**:917–24.

Cantarovich F, Galli C, Benedetti L, et al. 1973. High dose furosemide in established acute renal failure. *Br Med J* **4**:449–50.

Clive DM, Stoff JS. 1984. Renal syndromes associated with nonsteroidal antiinflammatory drugs. *N Engl J Med* **310**:563–72.

Cloyd JC, Snyder BD, Cleeremans B, et al. 1986. Mannitol pharmacokinetics and serum osmolality in dogs and humans. *J Pharmacol Exp Ther* **236**:301–6.

Coe FL. 1977. Metabolic alkalosis. *JAMA* **238**:2288–90.

Coe FL, Parks JH, Asplin JR. 1992. The pathogenesis and treatment of kidney stones. *N Engl J Med* **327**:1141–52.

Conger J. 1998. Prophylaxis and treatment of acute renal failure by vasoactive agents: The fact and the myths. *Kidney Int Suppl* **53**: S-23–6.

de Bold AJ. 1985. Atrial natriuretic factor: a hormone produced by the heart. *Science* **230**:767–70.

DeBroe ME, Elseviers MM. 1998. Analgesic nephropathy. *N Engl J Med* **338**:446–52.

DiBona GF. 1985. Neural regulation of renal tubular sodium reabsorption and renin secretion. *Fed Proc* **44**:2816–22.

Dunn MJ, Zambraski EJ. 1980. Renal effects of drugs that inhibit prostaglandin synthesis. *Kidney Int* **18**:609–22.

Ellison DH. 1991. The physiologic basis of diuretic synergism: its role in treating diuretic resistance. *Ann Intern Med* **114**:886–94.

Epstein M, Schneider NS, Befeler B. 1975. Effect of intrarenal furosemide on renal function and intrarenal hemodynamics in acute renal failure. *Am J Med* **58**:510–5.

Erslev AJ. 1975. Biogenesis of erythropoietin. *Am J Med* **58**:25–30.

Eschbach JW, Kelly MR, Haley NR, et al. 1989. Treatment of the anemia of progressive renal failure with recombinant human erythropoietin. *N Engl J Med* **321**:158–63.

Fantl JA, Cardozo L, McClish DK. 1994. Estrogen therapy in the management of urinary incontinence in postmenopausal women: a meta-analysis. First report of the Hormones and Urogenital Therapy Committee. *Obstet Gynecol* **83**:12–8.

Fessel WJ. 1979. Renal outcomes of gout and hyperuricemia. *Am J Med* **67**:74–82.

Foley RJ, Weinman EJ. 1984. Urate nephropathy [review]. *Am J Med Sci* **288**:208–11.

Forrest JN, Cox M, Hong C, et al. 1978. Superiority of demeclocycline over lithium in the treatment of chronic syndrome of inappropriate secretion of antidiuretic hormone. *N Engl J Med* **298**:173–7.

Frazier HS, Yager, H. 1973. The clinical use of diuretics. *N Engl J Med* **288**:246–249, 455–9.

Frelin C, Vigne P, Barbry P, et al. 1987. Molecular properties of amiloride action and of its $Na^+$ transporting targets. *Kidney Int* **32**:785–93.

Fried, W. 1973. Erythropoietin. *Arch Intern Med* **131**:929–38.

Genadry RR. 1995. Evaluation and conservative management of women with stress urinary incontinence. *Maryland Med J* **44**:31–35.

Goldstein I, Lue TF, Padma-Nathan H, et al. 1998. Oral sildenafil in the treatment of erectile dysfunction. *N Engl J Med* **338**:1397–1404.

Greenblatt DJ, Sellers EM, Koch-Wester J. 1982. Importance of protein binding for the interpretation of serum or plasma drug concentrations. *J Clin Pharmacol* **22**:259–63.

Greger R. 1985. Ion transport mechanisms in thick ascending limb of Henle's loop of mammalian nephron. *Physiol Rev* **65**:760–97.

Gugler R, Shoeman DW, Huffman DH, et al. 1975. Pharmacokinetics of drugs in patients with the nephrotic syndrome. *J Clin Invest* **55**:1182–4.

Hall CL, Fothergill NJ, Blackwell MM, et al. 1987. The natural course of gold nephropathy: long term study of 21 patients. *Br Med J* **295**:745–8.

Hess E. 1988. Drug-related lupus. *N Engl J Med* **318**:1460–2.

Hill JB. 1973. Salicylate intoxication. *N Engl J Med* **288**:1110–3.

Hooton TM, Winter C, Tiu F, et al. 1995. Randomized comparative trial and cost analysis of 3-day antimicrobial regimens for treatment of acute cystitis in women. *JAMA* **273**:41–5.

Hruska KA, Teitelbaum SL. 1995. Renal osteodystrophy. *N Engl J Med* **333**:166–74.

Ihle BU, Whitworth JA, Shahinfar S, et al. 1996. Angiotensin-converting enzyme inhibition in nondiabetic progressive renal insufficiency: a controlled double-blind trial. *Am J Kidney Dis* **27**:489–95.

Johnson JR, Stamm WE. 1989. Urinary tract infections in women: Diagnosis and treatment. *Ann Intern Med* **111**:906–17.

Kau ST. 1978. Handling of triamterene by the isolated perfused rat kidney. *J Pharmacol Exp Ther* **206**:701–9.

Klahr S, Levey AS, Beck GJ, et al. 1994. The effects of dietary protein restriction and blood pressure control on the progression of chronic renal disease. *N Engl J Med* **330**:877–84.

Klahr S, Miller SB. 1998. Acute oliguria. *N Engl J Med* **338**:671–5.

Klahr S, Schriener G, Ichikawa I. 1988. The progression of renal disease. *N Engl J Med* **318**:1657–66.

Komaroff AL. 1984. Acute dysuria in women. *N Engl J Med* **310**: 368–75.

Langford HG, Blaufox MD, Borhani NO, et al. 1987. Is thiazide-produced uric acid elevation harmful? Analysis of data from the hypertension detection and follow-up program. *Arch Intern Med* **147**:645–9.

Lauriat SM, Berl T. 1997. The hyponatremic patient: practical focus on therapy. *J Am Soc Nephrol* **8**:1599–1604.

Maki DD, Ma JZ, Louis TA, et al. 1995. Long-term effects of antihypertensive agents on proteinuria and renal function. *Arch Intern Med* **155**:1073–80.

Martinez-Maldonado M, Eknoyan G, Suki WN. 1973. Diuretics in nonedematous states. Physiological basis for the clinical use. *Arch Intern Med* **131**:797–808.

Maschio G, Alberti D, Janin G, et al. 1996. Effect of the angiotensin-converting-enzyme inhibitor benazepril on the progression of chronic renal insufficiency. *N Engl J Med* **334**:939–45.

McMurray SD, Luft FC, Maxwell DR, et al. 1978. Prevailing patterns and predictor variables in patients with acute tubular necrosis. *Arch Intern Med* **138**:950–5.

Minuth AN, Terrell JB, Suki WN. 1976. Acute renal failure: a study of the course and prognosis of 104 patients and of the role of furosemide. *Am J Med Sci* **271**:317–24.

Mitch WE, Walser M, Buffington GA, et al. 1976. A simple method of estimating progression of chronic renal failure. *Lancet* **2**:1326–8.

Montague DK, Barada JH, Belker AM, et al. 1996. Clinical guidelines panel on erectile dysfunction: summary report on the treatment of organic erectile dysfunction. The American Urological Association. *J Urol* **156**:2007–11.

Morris RC, Sebastian A, McSherry E. 1972. Renal acidosis. *Kidney Int* **1**:322–40.

*Mosby's GenR$_x$* 1998. *Mosby's GenR$_x$ 1998: The Complete Reference for Generic and Brand Drugs*. 8th ed. St. Louis: Mosby–Year Book.

Mulligan T, Schmitt B. 1993. Testosterone for erectile failure. *J Gen Intern Med* **8**:517–21.

Mundy GR, Guise TA. 1997. Hypercalcemia of malignancy. *Am J Med* **103**:134–45.

Myers BD, Ross J, Newton L, et al. 1984. Cyclosporine-associated chronic nephropathy. *N Engl J Med* **311**:699–705.

Narins RG, Jones ER, Stom MC, et al. 1982. Diagnostic strategies in disorders of fluid, electrolyte and acid-base homeostasis. *Am J Med* **72**:496–520.

Neilson EG. 1989. Pathogenesis and therapy of interstitial nephritis. *Kidney Int* **35**:1257–70.

NIH Consensus Conference: Impotence. 1993. *JAMA* **270**:83–90.

NIH Consensus Statement. 1988. Urinary incontinence in adults. *NIH Consens Statement* Oct 3–5(5):1–32.

Nolan CR, Anderson RJ. 1998. Hospital-acquired acute renal failure. *J Am Soc Nephrol* **9**:710–8.

Ochs HR, Greenblatt DJ, Bodem G, et al. 1978. Spironolactone. *Am Heart J* **96**:389–400.

Odlind B, Beermann B. 1980. Renal tubular secretion and effects of furosemide. *Clin Pharmacol Ther* **27**:784–90.

Okamura NO, Hirai M, Tanigawara Y, et al. 1993. Digoxin-cyclosporin A interaction: modulation of the multidrug transporter P-glycoprotein in the kidney. *J Pharmacol Exp Ther* **266**:1614–9.

Pak CYC. 1979. Physiological basis for absorptive and renal hypercalciurias. *Am J Physiol* **237**:F415–23.

Pak CYC, Britton F, Peterson R, et al. 1980. Ambulatory evaluation of nephrolithiasis: Classification, clinical presentation, and diagnostic criteria. *Am J Med* **69**:19–30.

Pedrini MT, Levey AS, Lau J, et al. 1996. The effect of dietary protein restriction on the progression of diabetic and nondiabetic renal diseases: a meta-analysis. *Ann Intern Med* **124**:6273–2.

Peterson JC, Adler S, Burkart JM, et al. 1995. Blood pressure control, proteinuria, and the progression of renal disease. *Ann Intern Med* **123**:754–62.

Pitt B, Zannard F, Remme WJ, et al. 1999. The effect of spironolactone on morbidity and mortality in patients with severe heart failure. *N Engl J Med* **341**:709–17.

Rector FC. 1983. Sodium, bicarbonate, and chloride absorption by the proximal tubule. *Am J Physiol* **244**:F461–71.

Reichel H, Koeffler HP, Norman AW. 1989. The role of the vitamin D endocrine system in health and disease. *N Engl J Med* **320**: 980–91.

Reidenberg MM, Drayer DE. 1984. Alteration of drug-protein binding in renal disease. *Clin Pharmacokinet* **9**(Suppl 1):18–26.

Schambelan M, Stockigt JR, Biglieri EG. 1972. Isolated hypoaldosteronism in adults. A renin-deficiency syndrome. *N Engl J Med* **287**:573–8.

Schrier RW, Berl T. 1975. Nonosmolar factors affecting renal water excretion. *N Engl J Med* **292**:81–8, 141–5.

Schrier RW, Lehman D, Zacherle B, et al. 1973. Effect of furosemide on free water excretion in edematous patients with hyponatremia. *Kidney Int* **3**:30–4.

Shear L, Ching S, Gabuzda GJ. 1970. Compartmentalization of ascites and edema in patients with hepatic cirrhosis. *N Engl J Med* **282**:1391–6.

Sheikh MS, Maguire JA, Emmett M, et al. 1989. Reduction of dietary phosphorus absorption by phosphorus binders. A theoretical, in vitro, and in vivo study. *J Clin Invest* **83**:66–73.

Simon EE. 1995. New aspects of acute renal failure [review]. *Am J Med Sci* **310**:217–21.

Somogyi A, McLean A, Heinzow B. 1983. Cimetidine-procainamide pharmacokinetic interaction in man: Evidence of competition for tubular secretion of basic drugs. *Eur J Clin Pharmacol* **25**: 339–45.

Stamm WE, Hooton TM. 1993. Management of urinary tract infections in adults. *N Engl J Med* **329**:1328–34.

Stein HB, Patterson AC, Offer RC, et al. 1980. Adverse effects of D-penicillamine in rheumatoid arthritis. *Ann Intern Med* **92**:24–9.

Stokes JB. 1989. Electroneutral NaCl transport in the distal tubule. *Kidney Int* **36**:427–33.

Szeto HH, Inturrisi CE, Houde R, et al. 1977. Accumulation of normeperidine, an active metabolite of meperidine, in patients with renal failure or cancer. *Ann Intern Med* **86**:738–41.

Thadhani R, Pascual M, Bonventre JV. 1996. Acute renal failure. *N Engl J Med* **334**:1448–60.

Uribarri J, Oh MS, Carroll HJ. 1989. The first kidney stone. *Ann Intern Med* **111**:1006–9.

Utiger RD. 1998. A pill for impotence. *N Engl J Med* **338**:1458–9.

Vasko MR, Brown-Cartwright D, Knochel, JP, et al. 1985. Furosemide absorption altered in decompensated congestive heart failure. *Ann Intern Med* **102**:314–18.

Verbeeck RK, Branch RA, Wilkinson GR. 1981. Drug metabolites in renal failure: pharmacokinetic and clinical implications. *Clin Pharmacokinet* **6**:329–45.

Voelker JR, Cartwright-Brown D, Anderson, S, et al. 1987. Comparison of loop diuretics in patients with chronic renal insufficiency. *Kidney Int* **32**:572–8.

Warren SE, Blantz RC. 1981. Mannitol. *Arch Intern Med* **141**:493–7.

Wein AJ. 1995. Pharmacology of incontinence. *Urol Clin North Am* **22**:557–77.

Young JL, Boswell RB, Nies AS. 1974. Severe allopurinol hypersensitivity. Association with thiazides and prior renal compromise. *Arch Intern Med* **134**:553–8.

Zaltman JS, Whiteside C, Cattran DC, et al. 1996. Accurate measurement of impaired glomerular filtration using single-dose oral cimetidine. *Am J Kidney Dis* **27**:504–11.

Zeller KR. 1987. Effects of dietary protein and phosphorus restriction on the progression of chronic renal failure [review]. *Am J Med Sci* **294**:328–40.

CHAPTER

# 7 TREATMENT OF NEUROLOGIC DISORDERS

## Headache

Thomas N. Ward

### *Chapter Outline*



The complaint of headache has been recorded since the earliest surviving writings. It is the most common medical reason for a patient to consult a neurologist (Kurtzke et al. 1986). Head pain is nearly universal; more than 90% of the population has had an episode of headache within the preceding year (Linet et al. 1989). Approximately 10% of the population has migraine, with the remainder having mostly tension-type headache (TTH).

## PATHOPHYSIOLOGY OF HEADACHE

There are numerous types and etiologies of headache. The most important distinction is between secondary headache (e.g., due to an underlying condition such as a brain tumor) and primary headache (such as migraine, TTH, etc.). Most headaches are primary and a discussion of secondary headaches is beyond the scope of this chapter.

In 1988, the International Headache Society (IHS) published a diagnostic classification for headaches (Headache Classification Committee of the IHS 1988). Although most useful for research purposes, this classification scheme does have heuristic value. However, not all patients fit into these categories, and some headaches are unclassifiable. The major primary (benign) headache types include migraine without aura (formerly called common migraine), migraine with aura (formerly classic migraine), tension-type headache (many previous names including tension headache, muscle contraction headache, psychogenic headache, etc.). There are other primary headache types such as cluster headache, which is uncommon but severe.

Migraine typically has several phases: a prodrome (possibly related to hypothalamic and/or brainstem mechanisms), sometimes an aura, the head pain itself, and finally a postdrome (Blau 1980). The aura, experienced by only a minority of migraine sufferers, is a reversible neurologic phenomenon, most often visual (e.g., an enlarging blind spot with a shimmering edge, flashing lights, zigzag lines), but sometimes sensory (migrating paresthesias), motor (hemiparesis and/or hemiplegia), or aphasic. The aura may precede the headache, occur during it, or not be followed by headache (aura without migraine).

Migraine pain may be hemicranial or bilateral, pounding or sharp, and often is moderate or severe in intensity. Frequently there is associated light and sound sensitivity, and nausea and/or vomiting. Physical exertion tends to worsen the pain, whereas rest seems to help. Migraine attacks generally last 4–72 hours. Longer bouts are termed "status migrainosus."

Tension-type headache is more common than migraine, although the two conditions may coexist, and some experts suggest that these entities may be at opposite ends of a continuum (Raskin 1988). TTH tends to be less severe than migraine, although individual attacks may last longer. The pain is usually bilateral, nonpulsatile, and not worsened by routine physical activity. The associated symptoms of migraine (nausea, vomiting, light and sound sensitivity) are not part of the IHS criteria for TTH; nonetheless, some patients have headaches with features of both.

Analgesic-rebound headache (ARH), one type of chronic daily headache, may affect several million people in the United States. ARH is a condition provoked by the overuse of certain analgesics by migraineurs. Briefly, increasing intake of such remedies beyond a certain threshold (probably more than 2 days per week) leads to an escalation in headache frequency ("transformed migraine") (Kudrow 1982; Mathew et al. 1990). An analogous situation may occur with frequent use of ergotamine drugs (ergotamine-dependency headaches).

Although TTH is the most common headache type, its pathophysiology is not well understood. However, in recent years there has been an explosion of knowledge about migraine. Both vascular and neural, and/or chemical changes appear to be involved.

Formerly, it was believed that vasoconstriction of cerebral vessels was responsible for the aura, whereas vasodilatation produced the head pain. Drugs specific for migraine, such as ergotamine tartrate, diminished the amplitude of vascular pulsation as well as the headache (Graham and Wolff 1938). Subsequently, evidence emerged that showed that while vascular changes certainly occur during migraine, neither the aura nor the head pain is specifically related to their occurrence (Olesen et al. 1990). It also was demonstrated that depletion of serotonin (5-hydroxytryptamine, 5-HT) by reserpine caused depression and worsened migraine, and that intravenous 5-HT relieved acute migraine, albeit with transient significant side effects (essentially an iatrogenic carcinoid attack) (Kimball et al. 1960). It has become apparent that migraine is much more than blood vessels constricting and dilating inappropriately.

The trigeminovascular system may also be involved (Moskowitz 1984). It has been shown that inflammatory neuropeptides such as substance P and calcitonin gene-related peptide (CGRP) are released antidromically from unmyelinated trigeminal nerve endings near blood vessels. Their release results in neurogenic inflammation, and many of the drugs used to treat acute migraine target this system (Moskowitz 1992).

Serotonin (5-HT) receptors have been classified (Silberstein 1994). There are currently seven families of 5-HT receptors, with various subgroups within families (Table 7-1). The 5-$HT_1$ and 5-$HT_2$ families are of particular interest in the pathogenesis and treatment of migraine. Newer specific agents such as sumatriptan (Imitrex) and other "triptans" are 5-$HT_{1D/1B}$ agonists, which diminish neurogenic inflammation by acting on these receptors located on trigeminal nerve terminals. They also act on blood vessels, where they exhibit modest vasoconstrictor effects.

Additional abnormalities occur in migraineurs. The highest concentration of serotonin in the central nervous system is found in the dorsal raphe nucleus in the upper brainstem, and this area (perhaps also including the periaqueductal gray and adjacent region) has been shown by positron emission tomography to be active during migraine attacks (Weiller et al. 1995). Whether this region represents the "migraine generator" or is merely an active area during migraine attacks requires further study. Of note, certain migraine drugs that cross the blood–brain barrier (e.g., dihydroergotamine, zolmitriptan) bind to sites in the dorsal raphe (Goadsby and Gundlach 1991).

The identification of a chromosomal locus for familial hemiplegic migraine, a rare form of migraine, within the $CACNL_{1A4}$ gene, near the site for episodic ataxia type 2, has led to speculation that migraine may be a calcium channelopathy (Ophoff et al. 1996). Especially low levels of magnesium in the occipital cortices of migraineurs and abnormalities of high-energy phosphate metabolism have been reported (Ramadan et al. 1989). Alterations of dopaminergic systems have been described, accounting for some prodromal symptoms (e.g., yawning, lethargy) and associated symptoms during attacks (e.g., nausea, vomiting) (Peroutka 1997).

Comorbid conditions (illnesses that coexist with another condition at a greater frequency than in the general population) have been identified for migraine (Rapoport and Lipton 1996). Knowledge of these conditions may offer insights into pathogenesis but also suggests both therapeutic opportunities and pitfalls (Table 7-2).

**PRINCIPLE Awareness of the presence of comorbid illnesses may allow for greater insight into disease pathophysiology, and even pharmacotherapy.**

## THERAPEUTIC OPTIONS

Headache treatment may be divided into nonpharmacologic and pharmacologic categories. The pharmacologic category may be further divided into acute/abortive therapy (to alleviate or terminate a headache episode), and

**Table 7-1 Serotonin Receptor (5-HT) Subtypes**

| | | | | | | |
|---|---|---|---|---|---|---|
| 5-$HT_{1A}$ | 5-$HT_{2A}$ | 5-$HT_3$ | 5-$HT_4$ | 5-$HT_{5A}$ | 5-$HT_6$ | 5-$HT_7$ |
| 5-$HT_{1B}$ | 5-$HT_{2B}$ | | | 5-$HT_{5B}$ | | |
| 5-$HT_{1D}$ | 5-$HT_{2C}$ | | | | | |
| 5-$HT_{1E}$ | | | | | | |
| 5-$HT_{1F}$ | | | | | | |

After Silberstein 1994.

**Table 7-2 Conditions Comorbid with Migraine**

| |
|---|
| Mitral valve prolapse/palpitations |
| Raynaud's phenomenon |
| Anxiety |
| Depression |
| Phobias |
| Bipolar disorder |
| Epilepsy |

prophylactic/preventative therapy (to reduce the frequency, severity, and/or duration of headache episodes).

## Nonpharmacologic Approaches

Nonpharmacologic approaches to headache therapy consist of maintenance of a healthy lifestyle, regular habits (adequate sleep, meals), and avoidance of factors that trigger headaches to the extent possible for the individual. Behavioral medicine measures such as biofeedback, cognitive therapy, stress management, and relaxation measures may be helpful in selected cases. Physical measures such as exercise, massage, and other maneuvers may be beneficial, especially for TTH. Withdrawal of overused medications under appropriate medical supervision in cases of analgesic-rebound headache or ergotamine-dependency headaches may lead to significant improvement in certain patients with chronic daily headache.

## Acute/Abortive Therapies

The main thrust of the discussion of pharmacologic management will be directed toward migraine headache. The acute/abortive therapies may be divided into analgesics (to lessen pain) and more specific migraine therapies (to terminate the attack). The route of administration chosen is critical; many migraineurs experience significant gastrointestinal dysfunction during an attack even in the absence of vomiting. Oral medications may not be adequately absorbed, and therefore, measures to correct the dysmotility (e.g., administering metoclopramide or cisapride), or alternative routes of administration, should be considered (Volans 1975).

***Nonspecific analgesics***
There are both simple and combination analgesics used for headache relief. Simple analgesics that are utilized for migraine may also be helpful in TTH. If given orally, the general principle is to give an adequate dose either early in the attack or with administration of metoclopramide or cisapride. The most common of these nonspecific analgesics are listed in Table 7-3. Many of the simple analgesics are available "over-the-counter/off-the-shelf"

**Table 7-3 Nonspecific Acute Headache Medications**

| Drug or Combination | Typical Adult Dosing (tablets or capsules PO) | Average Wholesale Price (per 100 tab/cap)[a] | Comments |
|---|---|---|---|
| Aspirin 325 mg | 2–3 tablets at onset | Generic \$1<br>Bayer Aspirin \$6 | Aspirin may cause dyspepsia, bleeding |
| Acetaminophen 325 mg | 2–3 tablets at onset<br>650 mg prn | Generic \$2<br>Tylenol \$7 | Acetaminophen useful in children at lower doses and during pregnancy. |
| Acetaminophen 250 mg<br>Aspirin 250 mg<br>Caffeine 65 mg | 1–2 tablets at onset | Generic \$4<br>Excedrin \$10 | Caffeine may enhance absorption and efficacy |
| Aspirin 325 mg<br>Butalbital 50 mg<br>Caffeine 40 mg | 1–2 tablets at onset, then one q4h | Generic \$4<br>Fiorinal \$54 | Butalbital is sedating, and potentially addictive (C III) |
| Acetaminophen 325 mg<br>Isometheptene mucate 65 mg<br>Dichloralphenazone 100 mg | 1–2 capsules at onset, repeat up to 5/day | Generic \$16<br>Midrin \$39 | Contains isometheptene (a mild vasoconstrictor) dichloralphenazone (a sedative); useful in tension-type headache and mild to moderate migraine; useful in adolescents |
| Ibuprofen 200 mg | 2–3 tablets at onset, repeat q4h as needed | Generic \$2<br>Motrin \$12 | May cause dyspepsia, GI bleeding |

Many of the above are combined with narcotics such as codeine, oxycodone, or propoxyphene. Use of these drugs more than 2 days per week may cause analgesic-rebound headache.

[a]Source of non-OTC drug prices is *Mosby's GenR$_x$* 1998. Current prices may vary from those quoted, but comparative prices among products are expected to be similar. The reader should check on local prices at the time of prescribing.

(OTC), without a prescription (and without medical supervision). Products that contain combinations of ingredients (e.g., Excedrin) are also available OTC. Prescription medications in combination may include acetaminophen or aspirin, caffeine, and/or butalbital. Codeine and other oral narcotics are sometimes used, but side effects such as nausea, as well as lack of efficacy, are common. One combination that may be particularly helpful for mild-moderate attacks (either migraine or TTH) is Midrin (Diamond 1976). Many of the prophylactic agents may also diminish the frequency and/or severity of TTH.

***Ergot derivatives***

Ergotamine tartrate has been a standard migraine treatment for decades (Table 7-4). Available in oral preparations with caffeine, and also as suppositories, it has a broad range of receptor activity and suppresses neurogenic inflammation, as well as causes vasoconstriction (McCarthy and Peroutka 1989). This agent is rather poorly tolerated, with many patients experiencing nausea; overuse may cause ergotism, so limits must be placed on its use with frequent clinical monitoring.

Dihydroergotamine mesylate (DHE-45), available for decades for intravenous or intramuscular use, recently was approved and marketed as a nasal spray (Migranal, Table 7-4). Like ergotamine, it has a broad range of receptor activity and suppresses neurogenic inflammation. It seems to be more of a venoconstrictor than an arterial constrictor. Used intravenously, it has a rapid onset of action in both migraine and cluster headaches, but causes significant nausea and/or vomiting, usually necessitating premedication with an antiemetic, and/or dosage adjustment. Given intramuscularly, or subcutaneously, it has a much slower onset of action than sumatriptan, but after 3 hours achieves similar efficacy with a much lower 24-hour headache recurrence rate (Winner et al. 1996). Dihydroergotamine crosses the blood–brain barrier and binds to brainstem structures, including the dorsal raphe nucleus, which might explain the low recurrence rate associated with its use (Goadsby and Gundlach 1991).

***Triptans***

The observations that abnormalities of 5-HT were associated with migraine and that administration of 5-HT relieved migraine (albeit with significant side effects) led to the development of sumatriptan (Imitrex). A similar group of drugs, the "triptans," is being developed (Table 7-5). As sumatriptan has been the most extensively studied and has been in widespread clinical use, it will be discussed in some detail.

Unlike ergotamine tartrate and dihydroergotamine, sumatriptan is a relatively specific 5-$HT_1$ agonist (Table 7-6). It is available in the United States as a 6-mg pre-

**Table 7-4 Ergot Derivatives for Acute Headache**

| Drug or Combination | Typical Adult Dose | Average Wholesale Price (units as noted)[a] | Comments |
|---|---|---|---|
| Caffeine 100 mg<br>Ergotamine tartrate 1 mg tablets | 1–2 tabs at onset, may repeat every 30 min as needed; limit 6/attack, 10/week | Generic $52<br>Cafergot $91 (per 90 tablets)<br>Wigraine $61 (per 100 tablets) | May cause nausea or vomiting. Arterial vasoconstrictor. Overuse may cause ergotism, ergotamine-dependency headaches. Avoid in patients with vascular disease. |
| Caffeine 100 mg<br>Ergotamine tartrate 2 mg suppositories | 1/4 to 1 suppository at onset; limit 2/attack, 5/week | Generic $21<br>Cafergot $49<br>Wigraine $23 (per 12 suppositories) | As above. Need to find effective subnauseating dose. |
| Dihyroergotamine mesylate 1 mg/ml for injection | 1 mg IM at onset; may repeat at one hour; limit 3 mg/day, 6 mg/week<br>May also be used 0.25–1.0 mg IV q8h, with antiemetic | DHE 45 $107 (per 10 ampules) | May take up to 3 hours to achieve full effect; lower recurrence rate than triptans.<br>IV route much more rapid onset. |
| Dihydroergotamine nasal spray | One spray (0.5 mg) in each nostril, may repeat in 15 minutes | Migranal<br>Not available | Consider use of antiemetic as well. Similar concerns as with other ergotamine preparations listed above. |

[a]Source of non-OTC drug prices is *Mosby's GenR$_x$* 1998. Current prices may vary from those quoted, but comparative prices among products are expected to be similar. The reader should check on local prices at the time of prescribing.

Table 7-5 Triptans

| DRUG | TYPICAL ADULT DOSE/ROUTE | AVERAGE WHOLESALE PRICE (UNITS AS NOTED)[a] | COMMENTS |
|---|---|---|---|
| Sumatriptan<br>25-mg tablet | 25–100 mg PO, up to 300 mg per day | Imitrex \$108 per 9 tablets | Arterial vasoconstrictor. Typical triptan sensations (paresthesia, throat or chest tightness) may occur. Avoid in patients with vascular disease. |
| syringe 6 mg/0.5 ml | 6 mg SC bid, prn | Imitrex \$71 per 2 syringes | |
| Zolmitriptan<br>2.5-, 5-mg tablets | 2.5–5 mg at onset; may repeat up to 10 mg/day; limited to 3 attacks per month | Zomig tablets, NA | As above (with central action) |
| Naratriptan[b]<br>2.5-mg tablets | 2.5 mg | Amerg tablets, NA | As above (with central action) |
| Rizatriptan[b]<br>5-, 10-mg tablets | 5–10 mg | Maxalt tablets, NA | As above (with central action) |
| Eletriptan[c]<br>40-, 80-mg tablets | 40–80 mg | NA | As above (no central action) |
| VML 251[c] | ? | NA | As above |
| Almotriptan[c]<br>? 150-mg tablets<br>? 6-mg injection | ? 150 mg PO<br>? 6 mg SC | NA | Not yet tested in the USA |

[a]Source of non-OTC drug prices is *Mosby's GenR*$_x$ 1998. Current prices may vary from those quoted, but comparative prices among products are expected to be similar. The reader should check on local prices at the time of prescribing. NA, not available.
[b]FDA approval likely in 1998.
[c]Not yet approved by FDA.
ABBREVIATIONS: bid, twice a day; PO, by mouth orally; prn, as required; SC, subcutaneous.

loaded syringe, 6-mg vials, 25- and 50-mg tablets, and 5- and 20-mg nasal spray. Following subcutaneous injection, $t_{max}$ is approximately 15 minutes, with a $t_{1/2}$ of 2 hours (Fowler et al. 1991). Typical "triptan sensations" may include paresthesias, flushing, and throat and/or chest tightness. Relief of head pain is less rapid with the nasal spray, and slower still with tablets. Approximately 80% a of patients given sumatriptan injection experience headache relief, but up to 40% will have recurrence of headache within 24 hours. Sumatriptan does not appreciably

Table 7-6 Dihydroergotamine vs. Sumatriptan Binding to Various Receptor Subtypes

| RECEPTORS | $K_i$ VALUES (NM) | |
|---|---|---|
| | DIHYDROERGOTAMINE | SUMATRIPTAN |
| *Serotonin* | | |
| $5\text{-HT}_{1D}$ | 19 | 17 |
| $5\text{-HT}_{1A}$ | 1.2 | 100 |
| $5\text{-HT}_{1B}$ | 18 | 61 |
| $5\text{-HT}_2$ | 78 | >10,000 |
| $5\text{-HT}_3$ | 10,000 | >10,000 |
| *Adrenergic* | | |
| $\alpha_1$ | 6.6 | >10,000 |
| $\alpha_2$ | 3.4 | >10,000 |
| $\beta$ | 960 | >10,000 |
| *Dopaminergic* | | |
| $D_1$ | 700 | >10,000 |
| $D_2$ | 98 | >10,000 |

From McCarthy and Peroutka 1989.

cross the blood–brain barrier. It is interesting that if patients use the injection during their aura phase, the headache may occur anyway, despite significant levels of drug in the blood. This drug is also effective in terminating attacks of cluster headache. Rarely, serious cardiac toxicity, including myocardial infarction, may occur.

There have been reports that some sumatriptan nonresponders may respond to other triptans. Zolmitriptan (Zomig) is known to cross the blood–brain barrier (as does rizatriptan and to a lesser extent naratriptan) and binds to receptors in the dorsal raphe nucleus. Whether this "central action" will result in additional clinical benefit is unclear.

***Antiemetic drugs***

Nausea and vomiting are often prominent features of the migraine attack, and dopaminergic abnormalities have been reported in migraineurs. Antidopaminergic drugs may also have efficacy against migraine pain. Metoclopramide 10 mg may be used to reverse the gastrointestinal dysmotility that occurs, and thereby enhance the efficacy of drugs taken orally. It may also be given intravenously before administration of dihydroergotamine to diminish nausea and vomiting. As with other dopamine-blocking agents, metoclopramide may provoke dystonic reactions, such as akathisia, and repeated use raises concerns about causing tardive movement disorders. Promethazine (Phenergan), especially when used as a suppository, is efficacious, does not cross the blood–brain barrier significantly, and may be less likely to cause dystonic reactions. Prochlorperazine (Compazine) may also be used as a suppository, but 10 mg intravenously has significant efficacy for acute migraine attacks (Jones et al. 1989). Other neuroleptics, such as chlorpromazine (Thorazine) given per rectum or intravenously, have been utilized.

***Opioids***

The role of narcotics in the treatment of headache is controversial. Certainly, while meperidine (Demerol) remains one of the most commonly prescribed emergency room approaches, giving a medication with a brief duration of action (under 4 hours) for a condition lasting 4–72 hours makes little sense. Narcotics may not only relieve pain but also induce sleep (known to be beneficial in migraine), but studies have shown superior results for other nonnarcotic remedies (Belgrade et al. 1989). Overuse and misuse of narcotics by headache sufferers is a significant problem. Overuse may lead to both addiction and analgesic-rebound headaches. This author prescribes narcotics in very limited circumstances. For appropriate patients, narcotics may be used as "rescue therapy," to try to prevent a trip to the emergency room, after other treatment measures have failed. Transnasal butorphanol (Stadol NS) may be used. One puff in one nostril is equipotent to $\geq$5 mg of morphine. Its advantages are rapid onset of action, and absorption with efficacy even in the presence of vomiting. However, butorphanol is very sedating and may produce dysphoria. The patient self-administers the drug, usually with an antiemetic, and goes to bed. This is a very potent agent and its use should be monitored and limited. Sometimes having the pharmacist dilute the bottle in half with an equal volume of normal saline allows better tolerability (Butorphanol nasal spray for pain 1993; PDR 1996).

## Prophylactic/Preventative Agents

Prophylactic/preventative agents are often employed when patients suffer more than four attacks per month, have prolonged severe attacks with neurologic deficits, or have headaches unresponsive to acute/abortive therapies. Currently, the best approach to selecting a prophylactic agent is to base the choice on the patient's comorbid medical condition(s). The principle is to start at the lowest possibly effective dose, observe the headache pattern over several weeks, then adjust the dose based on efficacy and side effects. The use of a headache calendar is essential to monitoring progress.

**PRINCIPLE Selecting appropriate endpoints to follow (e.g., headache frequency, adverse effects) and following them closely with the aid of a log or calendar are crucial to the success of this clinical drug trial.**

The major categories of prophylactic medications for migraine are beta-blockers, heterocyclic antidepressants, and calcium channel drugs (Table 7-7) (Capobianco et al. 1996). Special drugs not in these categories are methysergide (Sansert), cyproheptadine (Periactin), and divalproex sodium (Depakote). Many other agents have been advocated for prophylaxis of headache, often based solely on anecdotal reports. Monoamine oxidase inhibitors (phenelzine, others) have been utilized, but the side-effect profile (tyramine reactions leading to hypertensive crisis) makes this category dangerous. Vitamin $B_2$ (riboflavin) 400 mg/day has recently been reported as reducing migraine attacks (Schoenen et al. 1998), and magnesium replacement in migraine prophylaxis remains unproven.

Prophylactic agents appear to work by several different mechanisms. Beta-blockers may act on 5-$HT_2$ receptors to prevent the genesis of nitric oxide, and if migraine really is a calcium channelopathy, the potential actions of

**Table 7-7 Selected Drugs Useful In Migraine Prophylaxis**

| Drug | Typical Adult Dose | Average Wholesale Price (per 100 tablets)[a] | Comments |
|---|---|---|---|
| **β-Adrenergic blockers** | | | Useful for coexisting hypertension, tremor, palpitations. May cause hypotension, worsen asthma, CHF, depression, Raynaud's. β-Adrenergic blockers with intrinsic sympathomimetic activity (e.g. pindolol) are ineffective in migraine. |
| Propranolol 40 mg | 40–320 mg/day, divided bid or tid | Generic $2<br>Inderal $60 | |
| Atenolol 25 mg | 25–100 mg per day, divided bid | Generic $9<br>Tenormin $88 | |
| **Antidepressants** | | | Useful for coexisting depression, "fibromyalgia." May worsen palpitations. Sedating. May cause weight gain. |
| Amitriptyline 25 mg | 10–150 mg at bedtime | Generic $2<br>Elavil $37 | Dry mouth may respond to pilocarpine 5–10mg PO tid (contraindicated in asthma). |
| Nortriptyline 25 mg | 10–150 mg at bedtime | Generic $16<br>Pamelor $95 | |
| Doxepin 25 mg | 10–150 mg at bedtime | Generic $4<br>Sinequan $44 | Has fewer anticholinergic side effects, also is available as liquid 10 mg/ml. |
| **Calcium channel blockers** | | | Useful for coexisting hypertension, Raynaud's, esophageal spasm. May cause hypotension. |
| Verapamil 40 mg | 120–480 mg per day divided tid | Generic $21<br>Calan $33 | Available also in sustained-release formulation. |
| Amlodipine 2.5 mg | 2.5–10 mg per day | Generic NA<br>Norvase $103 | |
| **Miscellaneous** | | | |
| Cyproheptadine 4 mg | 2–16 mg per day | Generic $2<br>Periactin $41 | Useful in children, but sedating and promotes weight gain. |
| Methysergide maleate 2 mg | 2–8 mg per day | Generic NA<br>Sansert $171 | Idiosyncratic reaction of retroperitoneal, endocardiac, pulmonary fibrosis. May work rapidly to relieve headache. Drug holiday after 6 months' therapy suggested. Vasoconstrictor. |
| Phenelzine sulfate 15 mg | 15–45 mg per day in divided doses | Generic NA<br>Nardil $40 | May work quickly, but risk of tyramine reaction limits its use. May cause orthostatic hypotension. |
| Divalproex sodium 250 mg | 250–750 mg bid | Generic NA<br>Depakote $61 | Useful in epilepsy, bipolar disorder. Side effects include weight gain, tremor, hair loss. May cause spina bifida if taken during pregnancy. |

[a]Source of non-OTC drug prices is *Mosby's GenR*$_x$ 1998. Current prices may vary from those quoted, but comparative prices among products are expected to be similar. The reader should check on local prices at the time of prescribing. NA, not available.

calcium channel agents and magnesium are apparent (Olesen et al. 1995). Many of the prophylactic agents interact with serotonin receptors, and some act on GABA receptors (Cutrer and Moskowitz 1996).

## APPROACH TO PHARMACOTHERAPY

Children with primary headaches may respond to many of the same measures used for adults, with appropriate adjustment for age and size, although migraine therapies have not been as extensively studied in children (Wikinson 1993). Cyproheptadine (Periactin) has been advocated for use in children with migraine.

Nonpharmacologic approaches represent the treatment of choice for the pregnant migraineuse. When necessary, judicious use of acetaminophen (orally or per rectum), certain narcotics (e.g., meperidine), and antiemetics (e.g., prochlorperazine) that are considered relatively safe during pregnancy is reasonable. Admission to the hospital for intravenous hydration is an appropriate option when necessary. Fortunately, most pregnant migraine sufferers improve during the second and third trimesters (Silberstein 1993).

Optimal headache therapy allows the patient to have an acceptably low rate of attacks, with effective measures available to control those attacks. Triggers should be identified and avoided when possible. Prophylactic agents are utilized to lower the frequency, severity, and/or duration of episodes, chosen based on comorbidity. For example, beta-blockers might be chosen for prophylaxis in the migrain patient with mitral valve prolapse or palpitations but avoided in the migraineuse with depression or Raynaud's phenomenon. Heterocyclic antidepressants might help sleep disturbances, but might worsen palpitations. Calcium channel agents might be preferred for the patient with cold extremities. Divalproex sodium would be appropriate if a seizure disorder or bipolar disease was present. Methysergide (Sansert) is useful when rapid response is desired, but long-term use is associated with the rare occurrence of retroperitoneal, pulmonary, or cardiac valvular fibrosis. Many of these agents may also improve tension-type headache (especially the heterocyclic antidepressants). Occasionally, combinations of prophylactic agents may be necessary to achieve sufficient benefit.

**PRINCIPLE The approach to treating any particular patient must be individualized.**

After a good therapeutic response has been achieved for an arbitrary period of time (36 months), attempts at gradual reduction of the preventive drugs may be considered, depending on the status of the patient's comorbid medical illnesses. Reinstitution of the medications may be necessary in case of relapse.

The selection of acute headache therapy may be based on either a "step-care" approach (starting with simple, and/or inexpensive drugs) and moving to more expensive care as needed or a "stratified care" approach (based on the characteristics of the headache attacks). The latter approach seems more efficient. Several review articles have proposed rational approaches to management of patients with headache (Rapoport and Sheftell 1993; Capobianco et al. 1996).

Migraine attacks evolving slowly, with little nausea, may respond to oral medications. An adequate dose of an OTC product, prescription nonsteroidal anti-inflammatory drug (NSAID), or combination product may be sufficient, especially if taken early during the attack or during migraine aura. If unsuccessful, addition of metoclopramide or cisapride may help. An oral triptan (sumatriptan, zolmitriptan, others) in adequate doses is another option. Oral ergotamine (Wigraine, others) may be effective, but has a significant adverse event profile and may necessitate the use of an antiemetic.

Suppositories are an effective alternative route of administration for patients with migraine, especially when nausea and vomiting are prominent. Acetaminophen suppositories may be particularly helpful during pregnancy.

Indomethacin suppositories 50 mg are useful in selected patients, as are ergotamine suppositories, but the 2-mg dose is often poorly tolerated. It is prudent to recommend one-fourth to one-third of a suppository initially and to adjust the amount used to a subnauseating dose that relieves headache.

Several products are currently available as nasal sprays (Table 7-8). Lidocaine (1 mL of 4% dripped into the nostril) may provide rapid relief but has a high recurrence rate (Maizels et al. 1996). Sumatriptan nasal spray, like injectable sumatriptan, has a rapid onset of action, but dihydroergotamine has a lower recurrence rate (Ziegler et al. 1994; Fowler et al. 1995; Touchon 1997). Transnasal butorphanol is effective, but it should be prescribed only as rescue therapy to avoid causing rebound headaches and abuse.

Injectable medications for headache relief can be administered by patients after appropriate education (Table 7-9). This route is appropriate when simpler measures have failed, especially if vomiting is present. The intravenous (IV) route of administration for medications given in the emergency room or clinic remains the most reliable. Metoclopramide followed by a subnauseating dose of dihydroergotamine is effective in approximately 90% of patients (Callaham and Raskin 1986). Intravenous neuroleptics such as prochlorperazine may also be effective. Side effects of sedation and orthostatic hypotension may necessitate hospitalization; acute dystonic reactions are managed with diphenhydramine or benztropine mesylate.

Intractable headache may respond to steroids, albeit slowly, and repetitive use may result in serious side effects including GI hemorrhage and aseptic necrosis of joints (Rapoport and Sheftell 1993). Narcotics may be employed but ideally in limited amounts, when other options have failed or are inappropriate.

Utilizing a comprehensive approach of both nonpharmacologic and pharmacologic treatments, with a plan tailored to the particular patient's clinical situation, the vast majority of headache patients can be helped.

**Table 7-8 Nasal Sprays**

| |
|---|
| Lidocaine 4% |
| Transnasal butorphanol (Stadol NS) |
| Dihydroergotamine mesylate (Migranal) |
| Sumatriptan (Imitrex) |

Table 7-9 **Common Injectable Medications for Headache**

| DRUG | TYPICAL ADULT DOSE | AVERAGE WHOLESALE PRICE (PER 100 TABLETS)[a] | COMMENTS |
|---|---|---|---|
| Hydroxyzine HCl injection 25 mg/mL | 25–50 mg IM | Generic $2 per 10 mL<br>Vistaril $10 per 10 mL | Antiemetic; sedating. |
| Metoclopramide HCl injection 10 mg/2-mL vial | 10 mg IM or IV | Generic $19 for 25 vials (2 mL)<br>Reglan $53 for 25 vials (2 mL) | If given IV, must be diluted and given slowly. Antiemetic, may provoke akathisia, dystonia. May relieve migraine pain. |
| Prochlorperazine injection 5 mg/mL | 10 mg IM or IV | Generic $55 for 25 vials (2 mL)<br>Compazine $179 for 25 vials (2 mL) | Antiemetic. May provoke akathisia, dystonia. May relieve migraine pain. |
| Chlorpromazine HCl injection 25 mg/mL | 10 mg IV, repeat every 15 minutes as needed | Generic $26 for 25 vials (1 mL)<br>Thorazine $73 for 10 vials (1 mL) | Antiemetic. See above. May cause marked orthostatic hypotension from alpha-receptor blocking effects. |
| Ketoralac tromethamine injection 30 mg/mL | 30–60 mg IM, or 30 mg IV | Generic NA<br>Toradol $72 for 10 vials (1 mL) | May cause dyspepsia, bleeding, other side effects of NSAID class. |
| Dihydroergotamine mesylate injection 1 mg/mL | 0.25–1.0 mg IM or IV | Generic NA<br>DHE 45 $107 for 10 vials (1 mL) | Should be proceeded by antiemetic. Initial DHE dose, then 0.5 mg IV. May repeat 0.5 mg IV if no increase in nausea and no headache relief after 15–20 min. Need to titrate to effective subnauseating dose. |
| Sumatriptan succinate 6 mg/0.5 mL syringe | 6 mg SC, may repeat | Generic NA<br>Imitrex $67 for 2 syringes | Rapidly effective in approximately 80% of migraine patients. High rate of recurrence (up to 40% within 24 hours). |
| Meperidine HCl injection 100 mg/mL | 50–150 mg IM | Generic $7 for 10 vials (1 mL)<br>Demerol $7 for 10 vials (1 mL) | Sedating. Short duration of action. Consider use of antiemetic as well. Addictive. Used only when standard, nonopioid therapies are ineffective. |

[a]Source of non-OTC drug prices is *Mosby's GenR*$_x$ 1998. Current prices may vary from those quoted, but comparative prices among products are expected to be similar. The reader should check on local prices at the time of prescribing. NA, not available.

## REFERENCES


Belgrade MJ, Ling LJ, Sahleevogt MB, et al. 1989. Comparison of single-dose meperidine, butorphanol, and dihydroergotamine in the treatment of vascular headache. *Neurology* **39**:590–2.

Blau JN. 1980. Migraine prodromes separated from the aura: complete migraine. *Br Med J* **281**:658–60.

Butorphanol nasal spray for pain. 1993. *Med Lett* **35**:105.

Callaham M, Raskin N. 1986. A controlled study of dihydroergotamine in the treatment of acute migraine headache. *Headache* **26**:168–71.

Capobianco DJ, Cheshire WP, Campbell JK. 1996. An overview of the diagnosis and pharmacologic treatment of migraine. *Mayo Clin Proc* **71**:1055–66.

Cutrer FM, Moskowitz MA. 1996. The actions of valproate and neurosteroids in a model of trigeminal pain [Wolff Award 1996]. *Headache* **36**:579–85.

Diamond S. 1976. Treatment of migraine with isometheptene, acetaminophen, and dichloralphenazone combination: a double-blind, crossover trial. *Headache* **15**:282–7.

Fowler P, Fuseau E, Chilton J, et al. 1995. The clinical pharmacology of sumatriptan nasal spray. *Cephalalgia* **15**(Suppl 14):238.

Fowler PA, Lacey LP, Thomas M, et al. 1991. The clinical pharmacology, pharmacokinetics, and metabolism of sumatriptan. *Eur Neurol* **31**:291–4.

Goadsby PJ, Gundlach AL. 1991. Localization of $^3$H-dihydroergotamine-binding sites in the cat central nervous system: relevance to migraine. *Ann Neurol* **29**:91–4.

Graham JR, Wolff HG. 1938. Mechanism of migraine headache and action of ergotamine tartrate. *Arch Neurol Psychiatry* **39**:737.

[Headache Classification Committee of the IHS]. 1988. Classification and diagnostic criteria for headache disorders, cranial neuralgias and facial pain. Headache Classification Committee of the International Headache Society. *Cephalalgia* **8**(Suppl 7):1–96.

Jones J, Sklar D, Dougherty J. 1989. Randomized double-blind trial of intravenous prochlorperazine for the treatment of acute headache. *JAMA* **261**:1174–6.

Kimball RW, Friedman AP, Vallejo E. 1960. Effect of serotonin in migraine patients. *Neurology* **10**:107.

Kudrow L. 1982. Paradoxical effects of frequent analgesic use. *Adv Neurol* **33**:335–41.

Kurtzke JF, Bennett DR, Berg BO, et al. 1986. On national needs for neurologists in the United States. *Neurology* **36**:383–8.

Linet MS, Stewart WF, Celentano DD, et al. 1989. An epidemiologic study of headache among adolescents and young adults. *JAMA* **261**: 2211–6.

Maizels M, Scott B, Cohen W, et al. 1996. Intranasal lidocaine for treatment of migraine: a randomized, double-blind, controlled trial. *JAMA* **276**:319–21.

Mathew NT, Kurman R, Perez F. 1990. Drug induced refractory headache—clinical features and management. *Headache* **30**:634–8.

McCarthy BG, Peroutka SJ. 1989. Comparative neuropharmacology of dihydroergotamine and sumatriptan (GR 43175). *Headache* **29**:420–2.

Moskowitz MA. 1984. The neurobiology of vascular head pain. *Ann Neurol* **16**:157–68.

Moskowitz MA. 1992. Neurogenic versus vascular mechanisms of action of sumatriptan and ergot alkaloids in migraine [review]. *Trends Pharmacol Sci* **13**:307–11.

Olesen J, Friberg I, Olsen TS. 1990. Timing and topography of cerebral flow, aura and headache during migraine attacks. *Ann Neurol* **28**:791–8.

Olesen J, Thomsen LL, Lassen LH, et al. 1995. The nitric oxide hypothesis of migraine and other vascular headaches. *Cephalalgia* **15**:94–100.

Ophoff RA, Terwindt GM, Vergouwe MN, et al. 1996. Familial hemiplegia migraine and episodic ataxia type-2 are caused by mutations in the $Ca^{2+}$ channel gene CACNL1A4. *Cell* **87**:543–52.

[PDR] 1996. *Physicians' Desk Reference.* 50th ed. Oradell, NJ: Medical Economics. p 775.

Peroutka SJ. 1997. Dopamine and migraine [review]. *Neurology* **49**:650–6.

Ramadan NM, Halvorson H, Vande-Linde A, et al. 1989. Low brain magnesium in migraine. *Headache* **29**:590–3.

Rapoport A, Lipton R. 1996. Pharmacologic treatment of migraine. In: Samuels M, Feske S, editors. *Office Practice of Neurology.* New York: Churchill Livingstone. p 1115.

Rapoport AM, Sheftell FD. 1993. Comprehensive approach to headache treatment. In: Rapoport AM, Sheftell FD, editors. *Headache: A Clinician's Guide to Diagnosis, Pathophysiology, and Treatment Strategies.* Costa Mesa, California: PMA Publishing Corp. p 247.

Raskin NH. 1988. *Headache.* 2nd ed. New York: Churchill Livingstone. p 224.

Schoenen J, Jacquy J, Lenaerts M. 1998. Effectiveness of high-dose riboflavin in migraine prophylaxis: a randomized, controlled trial. *Neurology* **50**:466–70.

Silberstein SD. 1993. Headaches and women: treatment of the pregnant and lactating migraineur. *Headache* **33**:533–40.

Silberstein SD. 1994. Serotonin (5-HT) and migraine [review]. *Headache* **34**:408–17.

Touchon JA. 1997. A comparison of intranasal dihydroergotamine (DHE) and subcutaneous sumatriptan 6 mg in the acute treatment of migraine. In: Olesen J, Zfelt-Hausen P, editors. *Headache Treatment: Trial Methodology and New Drugs*, Philadelphia: Lippincott-Raven. p 213.

Volans GN. 1975. The effect of metoclopramide on the absorption of effervescent aspirin in migraine. *Br J Clin Pharmacol* **2**:57–63.

Weiller C, May A, Limmroth V, et al. 1995. Brain stem activation in spontaneous human migraine attacks. *Nat Med* **1**:658–60.

Wikinson M. 1993. Headaches in children. In: Rapoport AM, Sheftell FD, editors. *Headache: A Clinician's Guide to Diagnosis, Pathophysiology and Treatment Strategies.* Costa Mesa, California: PMA Publishing Corp. p 185.

Winner P, Ricalde O, Le Force B, et al. 1996. A double-blind study of subcutaneous dihydroergotamine vs. subcutaneous sumatriptan in the treatment of acute migraine. *Arch Neurol* **53**:180–4.

Ziegler D, Ford R, Kriegler J, et al. 1994. Dihydroergotamine nasal spray for the acute treatment of migraine. *Neurology* **44**:447–53.

# Seizures

Richard S. McLachlan

*Chapter Outline*



## DEFINITION OF SEIZURES

A seizure is the outward manifestation of a sudden excessive electrical discharge of neurons in the brain. The successful management of seizure disorders depends on the ability of the treatment to either abolish these "nervous discharges" or prevent their spread through the nervous system. As many as 10% of people will have a seizure sometime during their life but most of these people do not have epilepsy. Epilepsy, which has a prevalence of 0.7% or 1 in 150 people, is a condition characterized by recurrent spontaneous seizures (Engel 1989). Thus, a child with febrile convulsions, an alcoholic with alcohol withdrawal seizures, or a person with hepatic encephalopathy and seizures, is not considered to have epilepsy. Nonetheless, the treatment of each of these conditions is governed by the same pharmacologic, physiologic, and clinical principles as the treatment of epilepsy.

**Key Points**

- **A seizure is the clinical expression of a sudden, excessive discharge of neurons.**
- **Epilepsy is characterized by recurrent spontaneous seizures.**

### Classification of Seizures and Epileptic Syndromes

Although at the cellular level all seizures have the same underlying basis of excessive neuronal activity, they can be expressed in many different ways. Based on clinical observations and an understanding of basic mechanisms of seizures, various classifications have been proposed, the simplest being to consider seizures as two types: focal and generalized. Focal seizures are those in which the neuronal discharge onset is in a localized area of the cerebral cortex; in generalized seizures, the neuronal discharge is widespread at onset or has a rapid, diffuse propagation from a deep (formerly termed "centrencephalic") source. A corollary to this rather simplistic view is that an apparent generalized seizure may actually be focal in onset in the cortex with secondary generalization.

**Key Point**

- **Seizures can be classified into two fundamental categories: focal and generalized.**

The International Classification of Seizures (Commission on Classification and Terminology of the International League Against Epilepsy 1981) expands on this simple scheme (Table 7-10). Such a classification allows for more accurate communication between physicians and

**Table 7-10 International Classification of Seizures**

I Partial Seizures
  Simple partial (consciousness not impaired)
  Complex partial (consciousness impaired)
  With secondary generalization
II Generalized Seizures
  Absence
  Myoclonic
  Clonic
  Tonic
  Tonic-clonic
  Atonic
III Unclassified

serves as a basis for management decisions when treating someone with seizures.

**PRINCIPLE Investigation and treatment of seizures are facilitated by first classifying the seizure type.**

The International Classification is based on the clinical description of the seizure as well as the electroencephalogram (EEG) findings. The most common seizure types are the generalized tonic-clonic (previously grand mal) and complex partial (previously psychomotor) with or without secondary generalization. Absence (previously petit mal) seizures of childhood and the other seizure types are less common. The generalized seizures are all more common in childhood, whereas the partial (focal) seizures predominate in adults. The latter imply a lesion that can be either recent or old, requiring investigation with neuroimaging; generalized seizures in epilepsy are idiopathic or inherited. Acute symptomatic (nonepileptic) focal seizures occur as a result of irritation of the cortex by blood, infection, or inflammation, whereas nonepileptic generalized seizures often occur on the basis of metabolic derangement. The International Classification of the Epilepsies (Commission on Classification and Terminology of the International League Against Epilepsy 1989), which attempts to classify the many different epilepsy syndromes, is less useful to the practicing clinician than the International Classification of Seizures.

**PRINCIPLE Epilepsy and seizures have many causes. Symptomatic management of seizures while ignoring treatment of the underlying disease does not represent optimal therapeutics.**

# THERAPEUTIC OPTIONS

## Mechanism of Action of Antiepileptic Drugs

The firing rate of neurons during a seizure is 200–900 hertz, some 10–50 times the activity of normal neurons. This increased neuronal activity and the associated change in cell membrane potentials (called a paroxysmal depolarization shift) are reflected in the EEG as interictal spikes or ictal activity. The factors that induce a transition from an interictal state to a seizure are not clear, but a requirement is the attainment of a critical mass of bursting neurons by recruitment of more and more neurons into the abnormal activity, ultimately resulting in clinical manifestations. The most common mechanism by which antiepileptic drugs appear to control seizures is through an effect on voltage-regulated sodium channels that stops the high-frequency burst activity of neurons (Table 7-11). Drugs such as carbamazepine, phenytoin, valproic acid, lamotrigine, and topiramate, modulate sodium channels and are effective for controlling generalized tonic-clonic and complex partial seizures. A smaller number of drugs act at voltage-dependent calcium channels that are particularly localized to neurons in the thalamus. Ethosuximide, for example, modulates calcium-channel activity in the thalamus consistent with its effectiveness in controlling generalized absence seizures. Other drugs, such as barbiturates and the benzodiazepines, enhance gamma-aminobutyric acid (GABA) receptor chloride current, augmenting neuronal inhibition. Similarly, vigabatrin and tiagabine increase inhibition through specific actions that increase extracellular GABA concentrations. Finally, some of the newer drugs such as topiramate have been developed to decrease the activity of excitatory glutamate receptors.

**PRINCIPLE All of the antiepileptic drugs have complex and often multiple effects on neuronal activity, and to attribute the antiseizure effect of a drug to any one of these mechanisms would be misleading.**

## When to Start Antiepileptic Drugs?

Treatment of the first seizure is controversial (Beghi et al. 1993). A meta-analysis of 16 studies of individuals presenting with a first seizure found that the average recurrence risk was 51% (Berg and Shinnar 1991). Consequently, drug treatment may be unnecessary in up to half of these patients. However, the seizure recurrence rate ranges from 20 to 80%, depending on various risk factors that must be considered before initiating treatment with an antiepileptic drug (Table 7-12). Focal seizures, neurologic deficit, cognitive impairment, abnormal EEG, and family history of seizures have all been suggested to increase the risk of recurrence (Chadwick 1991). Under

**Table 7-11 Principle Mechanism of Action of Antiepileptic Drugs**

1. Decrease activity of voltage-dependent $Na^{+}$ channels.
2. Decrease activity of voltage-dependent $Ca^{++}$ channels (especially in the thalamus).
3. Augment GABA activity.
4. Decrease glutamate receptor activity.

ABBREVIATIONS: GABA, $\gamma$-aminobutyric acid.

**Table 7-12 Factors Influencing Treatment of First Seizures**

| |
|---|
| Seizure type |
| Seizure syndrome |
| Age and/or sex of patient |
| Neurologic examination |
| EEG & MRI/CT results |
| Family history of seizures |
| Potential drug side effects |
| Driving |
| Psychological reaction of patient |
| Cost of medication |

ABBREVIATIONS: CT, computerized tomography; EEG, electroencephalograph; MRI, magnetic resonance imaging.

some circumstances, such as a febrile convulsion or other provoked seizure, it is unnecessary to treat with an antiepileptic drug; on the other hand, a single prolonged seizure or status epilepticus as a first seizure should probably be treated. Psychosocial issues such as the psychological reaction of the patient to the seizure and the potential impact of a second seizure on ability to drive and work must also be considered.

In contrast to treatment in children (Camfield et al. 1989), treatment of the first seizure with an antiepileptic drug in adults may not result in a substantial reduction in seizure recurrence because compliance is less than satisfactory. Noncompliance with taking daily medications is common after only one seizure (but improves considerably after a second seizure), particularly in the one-third of patients who have some type of adverse drug effects. The decision to start an antiepileptic drug after one seizure should be made in collaboration with the patient after a clear explanation of the potential benefits and risks of treatment.

**PRINCIPLE The risk of seizure recurrence after an initial seizure varies considerably depending on a number of factors which should be considered before initiating antiepileptic drug treatment.**

## When to Stop Antiepileptic Drugs?

There is no consensus on the remission rate of epilepsy over time. The largest study of outcome in 1091 patients found that 86% achieved a remission of 3 years' duration after 9 years' follow-up (Cockerell et al. 1995). Successful withdrawal from antiepileptic drug is most likely to occur after a seizure-free interval of 2–5 years, with a single type of partial or generalized seizure, a normal EEG, and a normal neurologic examination (American Academy of Neurology 1996; Schmidt and Gram 1996). This is based on evidence that risk of seizure recurrence is 30–40% without medication in such patients (MRC 1991; Shinnar et al. 1994). Factors that influence recurrence after a first seizure will also affect the recurrence risk in individual patients when antiepileptic drugs are withdrawn. Partial seizures are more likely to recur than generalized seizures. In addition, the epilepsy syndrome must be considered. Children with benign rolandic epilepsy rarely have seizures after age 14 years, whereas drug withdrawal in a patient with juvenile myoclonic epilepsy usually results in relapse of seizures no matter how long the patient has been seizure-free. Adults and particularly adolescents are more likely to relapse than are children. Drug withdrawal should be done slowly over a period of 3–6 months, although more rapid withdrawal over 6–8 weeks may also be effective (Tennison et al. 1994).

**Key Point**

- **Risk of seizure recurrence after withdrawal of antiepileptic drug medication is 30 to 40%.**

## ANTIEPILEPTIC DRUGS

The most commonly used drugs for treatment of seizures in North America are carbamazepine, phenytoin, valproic acid, and phenobarbital, but a number of others are used regularly (Table 7-13). After a lull in drug development for epilepsy, recent years have seen the introduction of a number of new, highly effective, and relatively safe compounds (Table 7-14). Most of these new drugs are currently indicated as adjunctive therapy for the management of patients with epilepsy who are not satisfactorily controlled by conventional therapy. However, there is mounting evidence that these drugs are also effective in monotherapy. Other less frequently used drugs are listed in Tables 7-15 and 7-16. Some of the last-mentioned drugs

**Table 7-13 Traditional Antiepileptic Drugs**

| |
|---|
| Carbamazepine |
| Clobazam |
| Clonazepam |
| Ethosuximide |
| Phenobarbital |
| Phenytoin |
| Primidone |
| Valproate sodium |
| Valproic acid |

Table 7-14 "New" Antiepileptic Drugs

| |
|---|
| Felbamate |
| Gabapentin |
| Lamotrigine |
| Oxcarbamazepine |
| Pregabalin |
| Remacemide |
| Tiagabine |
| Topiramate |
| Vigabatrin |
| Zonisamide |

are of questionable efficacy or are associated with excessive toxicity. Very general dosing guidelines are found in Table 7-17.

**PRINCIPLE Drug treatment is only part of the management of epilepsy. Patient education and attention to psychosocial issues are equally important.**

## Carbamazepine

Carbamazepine, a tricyclic compound, is the drug of choice for both partial and generalized tonic-clonic seizures in female and most male patients, because it avoids the cosmetic effects of phenytoin and generally is associated with low toxicity. Absorption depends on whether it is given as tablets, suspension, chewable tablets, or controlled release tablets. Carbamazepine is 75% protein bound and primarily metabolized in the liver to the active compound carbamazepine-10,11-epoxide. Dose-related adverse effects include lethargy, diplopia, ataxia, and headache. Carbamazepine can also have an antidiuretic effect resulting in hyponatremia and fluid retention. Myoclonus can be induced by carbamazepine. Rash and other hypersensitivity reactions can occur. Some patients will experience adverse effects with the initiation of therapy, but this usually can be overcome by starting with a low dose of 100–200 mg daily and working up to a full therapeutic dose over 2 or 3 weeks. Because carbamazepine produces autoinduction of its own metabolism, a paradoxic fall in blood concentrations often occurs as the drug dose is increased with an associated reduction in the potential for adverse effects.

Table 7-15 Seldom Used Antiepileptic Drugs

| |
|---|
| Clorazepate |
| Ethotoin |
| Mephenytoin |
| Mephobarbital |
| Methsuximide |
| Nitrazepam |
| Paramethadione |
| Phenacemide |
| Phensuximide |

Table 7-16 Drugs of Limited Usefulness or Whose Use Is Not Established

| | |
|---|---|
| Acetazolamide | Medroxyprogesterone acetate |
| Allopurinol | Nimodipine |
| Amantadine | Potassium bromide |
| Corticotropin (ACTH) | Sulthiame |
| Corticosteroids | Vitamin $B_6$ (pyridoxine) |
| Gamma globulin | Vitamin D |
| Flunarizine | Vitamin E |

**Key Point**

- **Carbamazepine and most other antiepileptic drugs require gradual titration to full dose over days to weeks. The exception is phenytoin.**

Induction of the cytochrome P450 enzyme systems in the liver also results in a potential for interaction with a number of other drugs. There is a risk of aplastic anemia and hepatitis, both of which are rare and probably no more common than with several other anticonvulsants. Small elevations of liver enzymes or lowered white blood cell count may occur, but these conditions are not usually clinically significant. A disadvantage to carbamazepine therapy is lack of a parenteral preparation for use in patients with a tendency for sequential seizures or status epilepticus. Oxcarbamazepine, a new drug similar to carbamazepine, is now available in some countries.

## Phenytoin

Phenytoin is highly effective in controlling partial seizures and all types of generalized seizures except absence. It is a reliable drug for severe, intractable, generalized tonic-clonic (grand mal) seizures that occur in association with mental retardation. The cosmetic adverse effects, which include coarsening of facial features, gum hypertrophy, hirsutism, and acne, can be troublesome, particularly in young women. Chronic therapy can occasionally result in osteomalacia, mild peripheral neuropathy, or cerebellar degeneration with irreversible gait ataxia. The last-mentioned tends to occur in patients who are difficult to control and may in part be related to frequent seizures. Vestibulocerebellar and cognitive dysfunction occur with high

Table 7-17 Daily Dose of Commonly Prescribed Antiepileptic Drugs

| | Dose (mg)[a] | Adult Range (mg) | Child Dose (mg/kg) | Protein Binding (%) | Half-life (hr) |
|---|---|---|---|---|---|
| Carbamazepine | 600 | 400–1200 | 10–30 | 75 | 8–24 |
| Phenytoin | 300 | 200–400 | 5–10 | 90 | 7–42[b] |
| Valproic acid | 1250 | 750–3000 | 15–60 | 90 | 6–16 |
| Phenobarbital | 90 | 30–240 | 3–7 | 50 | 80–120 |
| Ethosuximide | 750 | 500–1500 | 15–30 | 0 | 20–60 |
| Clobazam | 30 | 10–80 | 0.5–1 | 85 | 10–30 |
| Gabapentin | 1200 | 900–3600 | — | 0 | 5–7 |
| Lamotrigine | 200 | 100–600 | — | 55 | 15–70 |
| Vigabatrin | 1500 | 1000–4000 | — | 0 | 5–13 |
| Topiramate | 200 | 100–800 | — | 15 | 20–30 |
| Tiagabine | 32 | 32–80 | — | 96 | 5–8 |

[a]This is a low initial target dose.
[b]"Half-life" is not really an appropriate term for phenytoin as it may have zero-order kinetics at clinically relevant doses.

serum concentrations. Rare adverse events include acute hypersensitivity reactions, hematological changes, hepatitis, pseudolymphoma, lupus erythematosus, and dyskinesias. In the elderly, when used at low daily doses of 100–200 mg (which is often all that is required to control a mild seizure tendency), phenytoin can produce less cognitive dysfunction than does carbamazepine. Phenytoin potentially interacts with many other drugs. The availability of phenytoin in capsules, tablets, suspension, and an injectable solution provides flexibility in drug utilization. Intramuscular administration is not recommended because it results in crystallization of the drug at the injection site with subsequent slow and erratic absorption. Serum concentration monitoring is particularly important with phenytoin to avoid the problems related to its nonlinear kinetics. Fosphenytoin is a new, less toxic, water-soluble phenytoin prodrug for parenteral administration (see below).

## Valproic Acid

The serendipitous discovery in 1963 that valproic acid, a carboxylic acid and organic solvent, had antiepileptic properties has led to its current wide acceptance as one of the major antiepileptic drugs. Initially proposed as a facilitator of inhibitory GABA activity, it more likely acts directly on neuronal membranes to reduce excitability. Although approved primarily for the treatment of absence seizures, it has a broad spectrum of antiepileptic activity against most seizure types and therefore is extensively used for partial, tonic-clonic, myoclonic, and atonic seizures as well. It is useful in patients with more than one seizure type such as the combination of absence and generalized tonic-clonic convulsions for which two anticonvulsants are otherwise usually required. Valproic acid is also effective for the treatment of partial seizures, particularly if these progress to secondary generalization, but efficacy superior to that of other anticonvulsants such as carbamazepine or phenytoin has not been demonstrated.

Toxicity is low, reversible, and generally mild in nature. Gastrointestinal complaints, which are common, can largely be abolished by using the enteric-coated preparation (sodium valproate) to prevent gastric irritation.

**Key Point**

- **Enteric-coated valproate sodium is preferable to valproic acid.**

Weight gain, particularly in females, can be a problem, and some patients develop postural tremor, hair loss, and, less frequently, lethargy. The weight gain in women can be associated with hyperinsulinism, menstrual irregularities, hyperandrogenism, and polycystic ovaries (Isojarvi et al. 1996). Hyperammonemia, which occurs in at least 50% of patients, is almost always asymptomatic but rarely can be associated with stupor or coma. This is a separate condition from the well-publicized but rare fatal hepatotoxicity, which has occurred primarily with polytherapy in children younger than 2 years who have evidence of other neurologic dysfunction in addition to seizures (Dreifuss et al. 1987). Pancreatitis, pseudodementia, and a Parkinsonian syndrome are other rare adverse effects.

A disadvantage of valproic acid therapy is the relatively poor correlation of serum concentration with clinical effectiveness and toxicity compared with other drugs. Therapeutic monitoring does not predict clinical efficacy as accurately as with other antiepileptic drugs. Its pharmacologic activity can also persist for days to weeks after the drug is cleared from serum. Drug interactions with resulting toxicity or increase in seizures are not uncommon with valproic acid, particularly when it is combined with a barbiturate, phenytoin, or lamotrigine, but the lack of interference with oral contraceptives is an advantage.

### Barbiturates

Although seldom prescribed as a drug of first choice in adults, phenobarbital is still widely used, more than 75 years after its introduction, as the initial treatment for many seizure disorders in children, particularly infants. It has broad effectiveness but is primarily used for generalized tonic-clonic seizures in children, as an alternative choice for partial epilepsy which is uncontrolled with other drugs in adults and in status epilepticus. The low cost of phenobarbital is a distinct advantage for many patients. Studies indicate that cognitive and behavioral alterations in the form of sedation, hyperactivity, and impaired school performance occur in up to 50% of children, but general experience suggests that most children tolerate the drug well. There is no consensus on the impact of such adverse effects on children in comparison to other antiepileptic drugs (Pal et al. 1998). Clobazam, valproate, and some of the newer drugs are being used with increasing frequency in young patients who previously would have been treated with phenobarbital.

Primidone, a less commonly used barbiturate, is metabolized rapidly to phenobarbital and phenylethylmalonamide. Because all three of these components have independent antiepileptic activity, a failure of phenobarbital to control seizures should not exclude a trial of primidone, which is best used as an alternative choice for uncontrolled generalized tonic-clonic or partial seizures in adults. Although occasional patients appear to achieve better seizure control with the rarely used barbiturate, mephobarbital (methylphenobarbital), overall it is equal in clinical effect to phenobarbital. Sedation is the most common adverse effect of the barbiturates in adults, but another distressing, often unreported concern, is sexual dysfunction in men particularly with the use of primidone. Development of tolerance is not usually a problem but stopping these drugs after long-term use can be difficult; patients may develop withdrawal symptoms of transient irritability and sleeplessness.

### Ethosuximide

Ethosuximide is used almost exclusively as the drug of choice for the treatment of absence seizures in childhood. It has been suggested but never convincingly demonstrated that ethosuximide may precipitate grand mal seizures. Gastrointestinal symptoms, lethargy, and headache are the main dose-related adverse effects; on rare occasions, an acute psychosis may occur. Drug interactions are not usually a problem.

### Benzodiazepines

The drugs in this class of antiepileptic compounds are used largely as alternative therapy (clobazam, clonazepam, clorazepate, nitrazepam) for seizures uncontrolled by other drugs or as initial treatment (diazepam, lorazepam) for status epilepticus. They are particularly useful for treating myoclonic seizures. In patients with epilepsy compounded by anxiety, the mood-altering properties of these medications can be utilized in an attempt to provide a dual approach to the control of seizures. All seizure types will potentially respond to benzodiazepines, but their use is limited by the common sedative and cognitive adverse effects, as well as the frequent development of tolerance with breakthrough of seizures usually after several months of therapy. This is least likely with clobazam. Drug holidays or alternating treatment with different benzodiazepines may delay the onset of the last-mentioned problem. Drooling is a frequent minor but annoying complication in children, particularly with nitrazepam. Although lorazepam has a relatively short half-life, it may occasionally be used as maintenance therapy or to prevent clusters of repetitive seizures that occur in some patients.

## OTHER ANTIEPILEPTIC DRUGS

About 30% of patients are refractory to the standard antiepileptic medications described above. In up to 50% of these refractory patients, the newer antiepileptic drugs are of benefit in controlling seizures and/or reducing drug toxicity when used as adjunctive therapy. However, a systematic review of randomized controlled trials revealed no conclusive evidence of differences in efficacy or tolerability among these newer antiepileptic drugs (Marson et al. 1996). Although these data showed that the drug with the highest efficacy was topiramate and the most tolerated drug was lamotrigine, statistically, there were few differences between any of the drugs (Chadwick

1997). Despite these results, when treating individual patients, there are usually individual factors which favor the selection of one drug over another (Dichter and Brodie 1996). Most of the new antiepileptic drugs are approved for adjunctive therapy in patients with uncontrolled seizures, but there is no reason to believe they will not also be effective when used as monotherapy. Randomized controlled comparisons with the traditional drugs are under way. Overall efficacy of the new antiepileptic drugs may be comparable to the traditional drugs, but clinical experience suggests they are associated with fewer adverse effects. No teratogenicity has yet been demonstrated. A disadvantage of the new antiepileptic drugs for some patients is their high cost, which often runs into hundreds of dollars a month.

## Gabapentin

Despite its name and structural similarity to GABA, gabapentin does not exert its antiseizure activity through any effect on GABA mechanisms. Its mechanism of action is unknown. It has demonstrated efficacy for the treatment of partial and secondarily generalized seizures, and there is increasing evidence that it may be useful in the management of pain. Toxicity is low in comparison with other antiepileptic drugs, but this may in part relate to a suggested dosage that is somewhat lower than necessary for achieving seizure control. Fatigue, dizziness, and diplopia can occur, particularly at dosages greater than 1200 mg daily. No serious idiosyncratic reactions have been reported with gabapentin. Drug interactions are not a problem since the drug is not metabolized or protein bound and does not induce hepatic enzymes. The short half-life is about 6 hours; a three time daily dosing schedule is necessary. Initially, it was thought that a rapid dose titration over 3 days could be used, but this often results in adverse effects. Increments at weekly intervals provide a better strategy. The efficacy and tolerability of gabapentin in children remains to be determined. Pregabalin, a related compound is currently undergoing clinical trials.

## Lamotrigine

Lamotrigine is a phenyltriazine compound chemically unrelated to other antiepileptic drugs. Its broad spectrum of activity and effectiveness in all seizure types are advantages in patients who have, for example, both generalized tonic-clonic and absence seizures. Lamotrigine is a weak folate antagonist, but its antiseizure effect relates to its action on voltage-sensitive sodium channels possibly with resulting presynaptic decrease in release of excitatory amino acid transmitters. As with other new antiepileptic drugs, it was initially approved as adjunctive therapy for partial seizures.

The main dose-related adverse effects of lamotrigine are dizziness, diplopia, blurred vision, headache, somnolence, and ataxia particularly when used with other drugs. Emotional and behavioral changes are less common. Lamotrigine is not a hepatic enzyme inducer. Lamotrigine's half-life may be increased when it is given with valproate and decreased when used with carbamazepine. The dosing schedule may require modification depending on what additional drugs are being taken. Normally, in adults, lamotrigine can be started at 25 or 50 mg daily with dose increments every 2 weeks aiming for 100 mg twice daily. If lamotrigine is being added to valproate, the initial dose is typically 25 mg every second day with increments every 2 weeks.

The incidence of acute hypersensitivity reaction seems to be somewhat greater with lamotrigine than with other antiepileptic drugs. Rash appears in about 5% of patients and appears to be more common in children. A number of cases of Stevens–Johnson syndrome and toxic epidermal necrolysis have been reported. The incidence of these allergic reactions may be related to the rapidity of dose escalation, particularly when lamotrigine is used with valproate. Pseudolymphoma, similar to that caused by phenytoin, has also been described.

## Vigabatrin

Vigabatrin is an irreversible inhibitor of GABA transaminase, the enzyme responsible for the catabolism of GABA. Increased brain GABA concentrations have been documented. Vigabatrin is particularly effective for complex partial seizures, but it is also useful for generalized tonic-clonic and other seizure types as well. Evidence suggests that vigabatrin may be the drug of choice for treatment of infantile spasms (Chiron et al. 1997). Myoclonus, similar to that occasionally seen with carbamazepine, can be induced by vigabatrin. Although it has a half-life of only 5–13 hours, the vigabatrin-induced enzyme changes in the nervous system can persist for 5 days. Consequently, blood concentration monitoring can be misleading.

Vigabatrin is generally well tolerated, with the most frequent adverse effects being somnolence, fatigue, and weight gain. Acute behavioral disturbances can occur in 3 to 5% of patients, the most severe of which is psychosis. White matter vacuolization, which occurs in rodents and dogs, has not been documented to occur in humans. However, a retinopathy with peripheral visual field constriction has been reported in up to one-third of patients (Eke et al. 1997). It is now suggested that formal visual field assessments be performed prior to starting the drug and at 6- to 12-month intervals thereafter. Rebound seizures and psychiatric symptoms have been reported after abrupt discontinuation of vigabatrin. Vigabatrin may reduce phenytoin concentration by about 20%.

### Topiramate

Topiramate is a sulfamate-substituted monosaccharide that superficially would be closest in action to the carbonic anhydrase inhibitor acetazolamide. It is effective for multiple seizure types including partial and various generalized seizures, reflecting several apparent mechanisms of action including potentiation of GABA-responses, impairment of glutamate receptor activity, and blockade of voltage-dependent sodium channels. It may be particularly effective in Lennox–Gastaut syndrome. A starting dose of 25–50 mg daily can be titrated at weekly intervals to 100 mg twice daily, with further escalation as necessary. In addition to the usual antiepileptic drug adverse effects of somnolence and ataxia, topiramate can induce cognitive changes in the form of confusion and abnormal thinking, particularly with rapid dose escalation. This effect may disappear after a few weeks. Weight loss can occur, particularly in overweight individuals. Kidney stones have occurred in 1.5% of patients. Unusual but not uncommon adverse effects of topiramate are limb paresthesias and speech disturbance.

### Felbamate

Felbamate is a dicarbamate compound related to meprobamate that was approved in the United States in 1993 and withdrawn from the market shortly thereafter, following the infrequent occurrence of aplastic anemia and hepatic failure. The mechanism of action is unknown. Half-life is 14–22 hours. Drug interactions are common and often clinically significant. Felbamate has been used for both partial and generalized seizures but appears to be most effective in Lennox–Gastaut syndrome.

### Tiagabine

Tiagabine is nipecotic acid with an attached lipophilic anchor to allow passage across the blood–brain barrier. It blocks GABA uptake by presynaptic neurons and glial cells, leading to increased GABA concentrations. Suggested starting doses are 4–8 mg daily increasing weekly to 30–80 mg/day. Adverse effects are generally mild as dizziness, asthenia, nervousness, or tremor. No serious idiosyncratic reactions have been reported in early use. Tiagabine is more rapidly metabolized in the presence of cytochrome P450 enzyme inducers. Considering the short half-life, a three times daily dosing schedule is generally required.

## APPROACH TO PHARMACOTHERAPY

Since the majority of patients with epilepsy require only one drug to control seizures, the initial management should be with monotherapy. By using this approach, the adverse effects are minimized, compliance is better, and the cost is less than with polypharmacy (Reynolds and Shorvon 1981). Furthermore, adding rather than substituting a second antiepileptic drug may provide only marginal benefit to seizure control (Schmidt 1982). Adverse effects increase when more than one drug is used, occurring in 20 to 30% of patients on monotherapy, 30 to 40% on two antiepileptic drugs, and 40 to 50% on three or more. However, recent evidence suggests that toxicity may relate more to total drug load rather than number of drugs administered (Deckers et al. 1997). In other words, it is the total dose of the drug(s) that is important. For example, high-dose monotherapy is as likely to cause toxicity as polytherapy with low or medium doses of two or more drugs, a strategy that can be effective for some patients. With polytherapy, there is the potential for clinically relevant drug–drug interactions.

**PRINCIPLE Monotherapy is preferable to polytherapy.**

### Seizure Type

The type of seizure and, in some cases, the epilepsy syndrome must be the first consideration when selecting an antiepileptic drug. Table 7-18 illustrates a protocol of drug of first choice for different seizure types and epilepsy syndromes. Two randomized, double-blind trials in adults demonstrated that carbamazepine and phenytoin are drugs of first choice for complex partial seizures (Mattson et al. 1985, 1992). In addition, these two drugs, along with valproate sodium, were equally effective for the treatment of secondarily generalized tonic-clonic seizures. Although phenobarbital and primidone were comparable to the other drugs in their ability to control seizures, they were not

**Table 7-18 Antiepileptic Drug of Choice Based on Seizure Type and in Some Epilepsy Syndromes**

| | |
|---|---|
| *Generalized Seizures* | |
| Tonic-clonic | CBZ = PHT = VPA |
| Absence | ESM = VPA |
| Myoclonic, tonic, atonic | VPA |
| Multiple types | VPA |
| *Partial Seizures* | |
| Simple or complex | CBZ = PHT |
| Secondarily generalized | CBZ = PHT = VPA |
| *Syndromes* | |
| Febrile convulsions | PB = VPA |
| Infantile spasms | VGB |
| Lennox–Gastaut syndrome | VPA |
| Juvenile myoclonic epilepsy | VPA |
| Benign rolandic epilepsy | CBZ = PHT |

ABBREVIATIONS: CBZ, carbamazepine; ESM, ethosuximide; PB, phenobarbital; PHT, phenytoin; VGB, vigabatrin; VPA, valproic acid.

recommended as drugs of first choice because of more adverse effects. Other randomized trials have supported the equivalence of antiepileptic drugs in controlling seizures in adults (Heller et al. 1995) and children (de Silva et al. 1996) but with a variation in degree of toxicity. However, even differences in toxicity have been challenged in a recent randomized comparison of phenobarbital and phenytoin in children that showed no difference in efficacy or toxicity between the two drugs (Pal et al. 1998).

## Age and Sex

There can be considerable variation in the pharmacokinetics of antiepileptic drugs with age, particularly in the very young and the elderly. In the first weeks of life, the (long) half-life of many antiepileptic drugs may require lower doses than usual; however, in young children ages 1–10 years, higher doses are often necessary because of their high metabolic rate which shortens drug half-life. Children younger than 2 years of age have five times the risk of fatal hepatotoxicity from valproate. Patients over age 60 years may develop toxicity as drug metabolism slows, often requiring a lower dose of drugs such as phenytoin. The elderly are particularly susceptible to the cognitive and sedative effects of carbamazepine.

In addition to the potential problems during pregnancy, a number of other considerations must be made when prescribing antiepileptic drugs to females. These include hirsutism, acne, and gum hypertrophy, all of which can occur with phenytoin and occasionally barbiturates. Women appear to be more susceptible to weight gain from valproate and the associated endocrine disturbances (Isojarvi et al. 1996). Antiepileptic drugs such as phenytoin, carbamazepine, and topiramate, all of which are hepatic enzyme inducers, may reduce the effectiveness of birth control pills, but any such interaction is usually clinically insignificant and should not be a reason to deny use of this form of contraception.

## Pharmacologic Properties

Many aspects of antiepileptic drug pharmacokinetics, such as dosing frequency, drug interactions, and need for drug serum concentration monitoring, influence ease of use of a drug. For example, phenytoin can be a difficult drug to use because of its nonlinear, zero-order kinetics. If blood concentrations are on the steep part of the curve relating concentration to dosage, then very small dose increments of 25–50 mg/day may be necessary to avoid toxic effects. An advantage of phenytoin and some other drugs with a long half-life is the ability to use them as a single daily dose in some patients. Phenytoin is the only drug which does not require some type of upward titration of dose at the start of treatment.

Slight differences in the pharmacologic properties of generic preparations, particularly involving bioavailability related to more rapid absorption, may be reflected in poor seizure control or increased adverse effects. Selected patients may experience fewer problems with proprietary or trade name preparations, assuming they can afford the greater cost of such drugs.

**PRINCIPLE Understanding of drug pharmacokinetics will help guide rational therapy.**

## Serum Antiepileptic Drug Concentrations

The introduction of antiepileptic drug blood concentration monitoring added a new dimension to the assessment of response to treatment. Measures of total and, in some cases, free nonprotein-bound blood concentrations provide an objective guide to altering antiepileptic drug management in patients who continue to have seizures or are experiencing adverse effects (Larkin et al. 1991). Antiepileptic drug concentrations are also useful for assessing compliance.

Many physicians fall into a trap of relying excessively on antiepileptic drug serum concentrations by attempting dosage adjustments purely on the basis of the blood result, while ignoring what is happening to the patient. If a patient is seizure-free and has no adverse effects, it often does not matter whether the serum antiepileptic drug concentration is below or above the "therapeutic range." For example, treating low serum concentrations in well-stabilized, asymptomatic patients does not result in any change in seizures but does cause an increase in adverse effects (Woo et al. 1988).

**PRINCIPLE The therapeutic range of an antiepileptic drug is only a guide to proper drug dosage and is helpful only when placed in context to what is happening to the patient.**

### Blood Monitoring for Potential Toxicity

Antiepileptic drugs commonly alter blood counts as well as liver or renal function but rarely cause serious toxicity. Elevations in liver enzymes, mild leukopenia, or thrombocytopenia generally do not require stopping therapy, unless the patient is symptomatic or the test results are worsening over time. Routine blood monitoring, in an attempt to predict severe adverse reactions such as aplastic anemia, liver failure, or pancreatitis is ineffective and expensive (Camfield et al. 1986). Recommendations regarding routine monitoring (Pellock and Willmore 1991) are presented in Table 7-19.

Although no evidence exists to support the utility of baseline assessments of complete blood count, platelets, liver enzymes, and other tests before initiation of antiepileptic drug treatment, these tests may be performed to screen for any preexisting blood abnormality. Patients taking antiepileptic drugs who were previously healthy and who have no new symptoms suggesting illness do not require routine blood monitoring. If a patient develops unexplained symptoms, then blood tests can be carried out. Patients who have difficulty communicating new symptoms such as the mentally impaired should be watched closely for changes in behavior and have their blood work monitored once or twice a year. Such monitoring can also be carried out in high-risk patients such as those with a family history of diseases such as aplastic anemia, liver failure, or mitochondrial disease, if the physician keeps in mind that there is no evidence that the results will predict a drug reaction (Willmore et al. 1991).

**Table 7-19 Recommendations for Routine Blood Monitoring of Patients Taking Antiepileptic Drugs**

1. Before antiepileptic drug treatment, do baseline assessment.
2. Asymptomatic patients require no further monitoring.
3. Consider monitoring in high-risk patients or those with multiple handicaps.

## STATUS EPILEPTICUS

Recurrent generalized tonic-clonic seizures without recovery of consciousness is a medical emergency. Other forms of status epilepticus such as nonconvulsive status or focal motor status are only slightly less worrisome, since any of these can result in potential brain damage from excitotoxic and other forms of injury.

Although rapid treatment of status epilepticus is critical, taking time to observe the seizure activity and to examine the patient for evidence of raised intracranial pressure or focal signs before instituting pharmacologic treatment is equally important (Recommendations of the Epilepsy Foundation of America's Working Group on Status Epilepticus 1993). Table 7-20 outlines the drug treatment of convulsive status epilepticus. There is presently no clear evidence favoring a preferential choice of drugs. If a benzodiazepine is used, a long-acting antiepileptic drug such as phenytoin should be given at the same time to prevent breakthrough seizures when the benzodiazepine wears off. Potential problems encountered with parenteral phenytoin are phlebitis, hypotension, and arrhythmias, especially if the drug is administered too rapidly. Fosphenytoin, although rapidly hydrolyzed to phenytoin, has the advantage of not causing phlebitis and being usable as an intramuscular injection (Fierro et al. 1996). The disadvantage is the cost which is about 10 times that of phenytoin. The loading dose of 30 mg/kg is roughly $1\frac{1}{2}$ times that of phenytoin.

If seizures do not stop with these measures, then the patient should be treated in the intensive care unit (ICU) where respiratory and other monitoring facilities are available. Once again, there is a choice of several options, none of which have systematically been studied in relation to the others as far as efficacy. These drugs all cause general anesthesia with the attendant risk of respiratory depression requiring monitoring of vital signs and the EEG. The anaesthetic barbiturates should be drugs of last resort in view of their tendency to accumulate and cause protracted coma.

## ANTIEPILEPTIC DRUGS AND PREGNANCY

The incidence of malformations in infants of mothers with epilepsy who are treated with antiepileptic drugs is 2–3 times the incidence in the general population. Exposure of the fetus to phenytoin, carbamazepine, valproate, or phenobarbital is associated with a 6 to 8% risk of mal-

**Table 7-20 Drug Treatment of Convulsive Status Epilepticus**

| | ADULT DOSE | PROBLEMS |
|---|---|---|
| A. *First or second choice* | | |
| Lorazepam IV 2 mg/min | 2–8 mg | Tolerance<br>Respiratory depression |
| OR | | |
| Diazepam IV 5 mg/min | 5–20 mg | |
| B. *First or second choice* | | |
| Phenytoin IV 50 mg/min (saline) | 1000 mg (to load) | Phlebitis<br>Hypotension<br>Arrhythmia<br>Precipitates in $D_5W$ |
| OR | | |
| Fosphenytoin sodium IV or IM | 1500 mg | Cost |
| C. *Continuing seizures, transfer to ICU* | | EEG monitor<br>Respiratory depression |
| Phenobarbital IV 100 mg/min | 1000 mg (to load) | |
| OR | | |
| Pentobarbital sodium IV 50–100 mg/hr | 250 mg bolus then continuous infusion | |
| OR | | |
| Thiopental sodium IV 200 mg/hr | 250 mg bolus then continuous infusion | |
| OR | | |
| Midazolam HCL IM or IV 20–30 mg/hr | 10 mg bolus then continuous infusion | |
| D. *Other options* | | |
| Isoflurane | Anesthesia | Anesthesia machine |
| Propofol IV 0.3–3 mg/kg per hr | Anesthesia | Hypotension |
| Paraldehyde | | |
| • Rectal | 5–10 mg in mineral oil | Pulmonary edema |
| • IV 10% solution | 25 ml/hr | Pulmonary edema |

formation (Delgado-Escueta and Janz 1992). The risk is increased with high-dose polytherapy. The newer antiepileptic drugs may be associated with less teratogenicity, but further study is required before this is known. Women of child-bearing age who take antiepileptic drugs should be on a folic acid supplement, since this reduces the risk of teratogenicity considerably, particularly with respect to neural tube defects. Since the drug effect occurs in the first trimester, folate must be taken before conception.

**Key Point**

- **Folic acid supplements are recommended for women of child-bearing age on antiepileptic drugs.**

Ultrasound examination should be done during the 18th to 22nd weeks and amniocentesis for alpha-fetoprotein levels done when necessary. A theoretical basis exists for using vitamin K supplementation in the newborn and possibly in the mother before delivery to reduce the risk of a bleeding tendency induced by an antiepileptic drug.

Unless the patient has been seizure-free for two years, antiepileptic drugs should be continued during pregnancy since, in many women, the risk of convulsions increases during this time. Postpartum breast feeding is not contraindicated since only small amounts of antiepileptic drugs are found in breast milk. Rarely, infant sedation occurs with some drugs.

The treatment of convulsions related to eclampsia was controversial until two trials in 1995 demonstrated that magnesium sulfate was more effective than phenytoin or diazepam in controlling seizures and also improved both maternal and neonatal outcome (The Eclampsia Trial Collaborative Group 1995; Lucas et al. 1995).

## SEIZURE PROPHYLAXIS FOLLOWING NEUROSURGERY

The incidence of epilepsy following supratentorial craniotomy for nontraumatic lesions (tumor, aneurysm, arteriovenous malformation, abscess) is about 20%. However, routine prophylaxis postoperatively with antiepileptic drugs to prevent seizures has been shown to be ineffective (Foy et al. 1992; Kuijlen et al. 1996). The prophylactic use of antiepileptic drugs following head trauma with or without craniotomy remains controversial and is a more difficult question to address, since the risk of posttraumatic seizures ranges from 5 to 50% depending on the nature and degree of trauma. A recent systematic review of 10 randomized controlled trials found that seizures were reduced with prophylactic antiepileptic drug treatment in the first week after head injury, but that there was no effect on later occurrence of seizures (Schierhout and Roberts 1998).

## REFERENCES


American Academy of Neurology. 1996. Practice Parameter: A guideline for discontinuing antiepileptic drugs in seizure-free patients—Summary Statement. Quality Standards Subcommittee. *Neurology* **47**:600–2.

Beghi E, Ciccone A, the First Seizure Trial Group. 1993. Recurrence after a first unprovoked seizure. Is it still a controversial issue? First Seizure Trial Group. *Seizure* **2**:5–10.

Berg AT, Shinnar S. 1991. The risk of seizure recurrence following a first unprovoked seizure: A quantitative review. *Neurology* **41**:965–72.

Camfield C, Camfield P, Smith E, et al. 1986. Asymptomatic children with epilepsy: little benefit from screening for anticonvulsant-induced liver, blood or renal damage. *Neurology* **36**:838–41.

Camfield P, Camfield C, Dooley J, et al. 1989. A randomized study of carbamazepine versus no medication after a first unprovoked seizure in childhood. *Neurology* **39**:851–2.

Chadwick D. 1991. Epilepsy after first seizures: risks and implications [editorial]. *J Neurol Neurosurg Psychiatry* **54**:387–9.

Chadwick DW. 1997. An overview of the efficacy and tolerability of new antiepileptic drugs. *Epilepsia* **38**:S59–S62.

Chiron C, Dumas C, Jambaque I, et al. 1997. Randomized trial comparing vigabatrin and hydrocortisone in infantile spasms due to tuberous sclerosis. *Epilepsy Res* **26**:389–95.

Cockerell OC, Johnson AL, Sander JWAS, et al. 1995. Remission of epilepsy: results from the National General Practice Study of Epilepsy. *Lancet* **346**:140–4.

Commission on Classification and Terminology of the International League Against Epilepsy. 1981. Proposal for revised clinical and electroencephalographic classification of epileptic seizures. *Epilepsia* **22**:489–501.

Commission on Classification and Terminology of the International League Against Epilepsy. 1989. Proposal for revised classification of epilepsies and epileptic syndromes. *Epilepsia* **30**:389–99.

de Silva M, MacArdle B, McGowan M, et al. 1996. Randomised comparative monotherapy trial of phenobarbitone, phenytoin, carbamazepine, or sodium valproate for newly diagnosed childhood epilepsy. *Lancet* **347**:709–13.

Deckers CLP, Hekster YA, Keyser A, et al. 1997. Reappraisal of polytherapy in epilepsy: a critical review of drug load and adverse effects. *Epilepsia* **38**:570–5.

Delgado-Escueta AV, Janz D. 1992. Consensus guidelines: preconception counseling, management, and care of the pregnant woman with epilepsy. *Neurology* **42**:149–60.

Dichter MA, Brodie MJ. 1996. New antiepileptic drugs. *N Engl J Med* **334**:1583–90.

Dreifuss FE, Santilli N, Sweeney KP, et al. 1987. Valproic acid hepatic fatalities: a retrospective review. *Neurology* **37**:379–85.

Eke T, Talbot JF, Lawden MC. 1997. Severe persistent visual field constriction associated with vigabatrin. *Br Med J* **314**:180–1.

Engel JJ. 1989. *Seizures and Epilepsy*. Philadelphia: FA Davis.

Fierro LS, Savulich DH, Benezra DA. 1996. Clinical review: safety of fosphenytoin sodium. *Am J Health-Syst Pharm* **53**:2707–12.

Foy PM, Chadwick DW, Rajgopalan N, et al. 1992. Do prophylactic anticonvulsant drugs alter the pattern of seizures after craniotomy? *J Neurol Neurosurg Psychiatry* **55**:753–7.

Heller AJ, Chesterman P, Elwes RDC, et al. 1995. Phenobarbitone, phenytoin, carbamazepine, or sodium valproate for newly diagnosed adult epilepsy: a randomised comparative monotherapy trial. *J Neurol Neurosurg Psychiatry* **58**:44–50.

Isojarvi JIT, Laatikainen TJ, Knip M, et al. 1996. Obesity and endocrine disorders in women taking valproate for epilepsy. *Ann Neurol* **39**:579–84.

Kuijlen JMA, Teernstra OPM, Kessels AGH, et al. 1996. Effectiveness of antiepileptic prophylaxis used with supratentorial craniotomies: a meta-analysis. *Seizure* **5**:291–8.

Larkin JG, Herrick AL, McGuire GM, et al. 1991. Antiepileptic drug monitoring at the epilepsy clinic: a prospective evaluation. *Epilepsia* **32**:89–95.

Lucas MJ, Leveno KJ, Cunningham FG. 1995. A comparison of magnesium sulfate with phenytoin for the prevention of eclampsia. *N Engl J Med* **333**:201–5.

Marson AG, Kadir ZA, Chadwick DW. 1996. New antiepileptic drugs: a systematic review of their efficacy and tolerability. *Br Med J* **313**:1169–74.

Mattson RH, Cramer JA, Collins JF, et al. 1985. Comparison of carbamazepine, phenobarbital, phenytoin and primidone in partial and secondarily generalized tonic-clonic seizures. *N Engl J Med* **313**:145–51.

Mattson RH, Cramer JA, Collins JF. 1992. A comparison of valproate with carbamazepine for the treatment of complex partial seizures and secondarily generalized tonic-clonic seizures in adults. The Department of Veterans Affairs Epilepsy Cooperative Study No. 264 Group. *N Engl J Med* **327**:765–71.

[MRC] Medical Research Council. 1991. Randomized study of antiepileptic drug withdrawal in patients in remission. Antiepileptic Drug Withdrawal Group. *Lancet* **337**:1175–80.

Pal DK, Das T, Chaudhury G, et al. 1998. Randomised controlled trial to assess acceptability of phenobarbital for childhood epilepsy in rural India. *Lancet* **351**:19–23.

Pellock JM, Willmore LJ. 1991. A rational guide to routine blood monitoring in patients receiving antiepileptic drugs. *Neurology* **41**:961–4.

Recommendations of the Epilepsy Foundation of America's Working Group on Status Epilepticus. 1993. Treatment of convulsive status epilepticus. *JAMA* **270**:854–9.

Reynolds EH, Shorvon SD. 1981. Monotherapy or polytherapy for epilepsy. *Epilepsia* **22**:1–10.

Schierhout G, Roberts I. 1998. Prophylactic antiepileptic agents after head injury: a systematic review. *J Neurol Neurosurg Psychiatry* **64**:108–2.

Schmidt D, Gram L. 1996. A practical guide to when (and how) to withdraw antiepileptic drugs in seizure-free patients. *Drugs* **52**:870–4.

Schmidt D. 1982. Two antiepileptic drugs for intractable epilepsy with complex partial seizures. *J Neurol Neurosurg Psychiatry* **45**: 1119–24.

Shinnar S, Berg AT, Moshe SL, et al. 1994. Discontinuing antiepileptic drugs in children with epilepsy: a prospective study. *Ann Neurol* **35**:534–45.

Tennison M, Greenwood R, Lewis D, et al. 1994. Discontinuing antiepileptic drugs in children with epilepsy: comparison of a six-week and a nine-month taper period. *N Engl J Med* **330**:1407–10.

The Eclampsia Trial Collaborative Group. 1995. Which anticonvulsant for women with eclampsia? Evidence from the collaborative eclampsia trial. *Lancet* **345**:1455–63.

Willmore LJ, Triggs WJ, Pellock JM. 1991. Valproate toxicity: risk-screening strategies. *Child Neurol* **6**:3–6.

Woo E, Chan YM, Yu YL, et al. 1988. If a well stabilized epileptic patient has a subtherapeutic antiepileptic drug level, should the dose be increased? A randomized prospective study. *Epilepsia* **29**:129–39.

# Cerebrovascular Diseases

**Arturo Tamayo, Vladimir Hachinski**

*Chapter Outline*



## ISCHEMIC STROKE

Stroke is a medical emergency and refers to the neurologic damage resulting from an acute impairment of cerebral blood flow caused by vascular occlusion (ischemic stroke) or hemorrhage (hemorrhagic stroke). Acute ischemic stroke is usually caused by occlusion of an intracranial artery (Fieschi et al. 1989). In 1991, about 500,000 Americans had a stroke (400,000 ischemic stroke), and more than 143,000 died (Adams et al. 1994). Despite recent advances in stroke care, successful management through dedicated stroke units is the most effective means of managing stroke (Kaste 1995).

### Cerebrovascular Terminology

The term *transient ischemic attack* (TIA) is arbitrarily defined as a sudden, brief, and reversible episode manifested with a neurologic or retinal deficit lasting usually no longer than 24 hours. In 50% of cases, TIAs last less than 1 hour with the remaining 50% lasting only minutes (Ad Hoc Committee on Cerebrovascular Disease 1975). TIAs are an important warning diagnosis, indicating a high risk for subsequent stroke (2 to 8%/year), the highest risk occurring within the first year (Oxfordshire Community Stroke Project 1983). In a practical sense, patients with symptoms remaining for more than 2 hours are considered to have suffered a "stroke" and are treated as such.

A *lacunar infarct* is a term based on neuropathologic findings and refers to a small (0.2–5 $mm^3$), deep infarct attributable to primary arterial disease that involves a penetrating branch (100–400 $\mu$m) of a large cerebral artery (Fisher 1969).

### Risk Factors

The identification of risk factors is of the utmost importance in the primary prevention of stroke. Both diastolic and systolic pressures are independent risk factors for hypertension (Colandrea et al. 1970). In the Framingham study (Kannel et al. 1981), the relative risk for stroke in hypertensive men was 3.1 and in hypertensive women 2.9. Controlling blood pressure decreases stroke risk up to 42% (Table 7-21) (SHEP Cooperative Research Group 1991). Cardiac ailments, usually involve emboli (thromboemboli, atheromatous emboli, etc.) from the left side of

Table 7-21 Cerebrovascular Risk Factors

| Diseases | |
|---|---|
| Established Risk Factors | Possible Risk Factors |
| 1. Hypertension | 1. Hyperuricemia |
| 2. Cardiac disease (see Table 7-22) | 2. Hypothyroidism |
| 3. Diabetes mellitus | 3. Migraine |
| 4. Polycythemia | |
| 5. Hyperfibrinogenemia | |
| 6. Dyslipoproteinemia | |
| 7. Homocysteinemia | |
| **Personal Habits and Characteristics** | |
| Established Risk Factors | Possible Risk Factors |
| 1. Age | 1. Oral contraceptives |
| 2. Gender | 2. Sedentary lifestyle |
| 3. Race | 3. Obesity |
| 4. Cigarette smoking | |
| 5. Alcohol | |
| 6. Drugs | |

the heart, aorta, or carotid artery, or from the right side through a patent foramen ovale, predisposing to stroke as mentioned in Table 7-22. Diabetes mellitus is a well-known atherogenic factor and often coexists with hypertension, dyslipidemia, and obesity (Barrett-Connor et al. 1988). Polycythemia, via mechanisms of increased blood viscosity and reduced blood flow, is a risk factor for men between 35 and 64 years of age (Kannel et al. 1972).

Hyperfibrinogenemia has been shown to be associated with stroke in men (Wolf et al. 1985) but little information concerning its treatment and risk reduction is available. Migraine as a risk factor is still a controversial issue, but increasingly the relationship seems coincidental (Bogousslavsky et al. 1988).

Homocyst(e)inemia accelerates atherosclerosis (Berwanger et al. 1995). Hypercholesterolemia is also considered a risk factor on the basis of the relationship with the atherogenesis processes and cerebrovascular diseases (Hachinski et al. 1996). In the United States, 16,000 strokes were attributed to smoking (Bengtsson et al. 1988) owing to chronic hypoxia, polycythemia, endothelial injury, and atherosclerosis (Wolf et al. 1988). The presence of cardiac arrhythmias seen during alcohol binges, "holiday heart," can result in cardiac embolism, and during abstinence, thrombocytosis has been seen (Camargo 1989). Drugs such as amphetamines or cocaine can lead to arterial vasospasm, cerebral infarction, and hemorrhage (Norris and Hachinski 1991). Birth control pills with estrogen doses up to 50 $\mu$g are quite safe, unlike early high-estrogen compounds (Petit et al. 1996). Obesity and a sedentary lifestyle are associated with atherosclerosis because of increased levels of lipoproteins and hypertension (Wolf et al. 1992).

There are other factors not completely understood, but which probably also play a role in stroke, such as sex, age, and ethnic background (Bengtsson et al. 1988).

Table 7-22 Causes of Embolic Stroke

| |
|---|
| High-risk Factors[a] |
| Atrial fibrillation |
| Mitral stenosis |
| Prosthetic heart valve |
| Acute myocardial infarct (up to 6 weeks) |
| Intraventricular thrombus |
| Myxoma |
| Bacterial and marasmic endocarditis |
| Dilated cardiomyopathy (ischemic or not) |
| Intermediate-risk Factors |
| Mitral regurgitation |
| Thyrotoxicosis with atrial fibrillation |
| Sick sinus syndrome |
| Minor Risk Factors[b] |
| Mitral prolapse |
| Mitral calcification |
| Patent foramen ovale |
| Aneurysm within the auricular septum |
| Calcified aortic stenosis |
| Left ventricular wall dysfunction |
| Aortic arch atheromatous plaque |

Modified from Hart 1992.
[a]The absolute risk is high: >6% per year.
[b]The absolute risk and recurrence is <1% per year. The embolic mechanism is not well known.

## Protective Factors

A diet rich in fruits, vegetables, and potassium resulted in a reduction of stroke and death by up to 40% (Whelton et al. 1997). Estrogens have a protective effect in premenopausal women, increasing serum high density lipoproteins (Stamler et al. 1963). Exercise reduces blood pressure and boosts high density lipoproteins (Paffenbarger et al. 1970). Alcohol in small quantities increases high density lipoproteins and could protect against atherosclerosis (Stampfer et al. 1988).

**PRINCIPLE Control of risk factors and enhancement of protective factors are the keystones to stroke prevention.**

## Clinical Presentation

Stroke should be suspected whenever a patient has the characteristic sudden onset of focal neurologic signs, such as hemiparesis, aphasia, hemianopia, or altered consciousness (Caplan 1993). Symptoms of stroke can develop in isolation but they usually occur in combination. The most important differential diagnosis of ischemic stroke is intracranial hemorrhage. In the event the patient is comatose and no history is available, other diagnoses to be considered, include; hypoglycemia, drug overdose, seizures, or craniocerebral trauma (Bogousslavsky et al. 1988) (Table 7-23).

**Table 7-23 Common Patterns of Neurologic Abnormalities in Patients with Acute Ischemic Stroke**

| |
|---|
| Left (Dominant) Hemisphere |
| Aphasia; right hemiparesis; right-sided sensory loss; right visual field defect; poor right conjugate gaze; dysarthria; difficulty in reading, writing, or calculating |
| Right (Nondominant) Hemisphere |
| Neglect of the left visual space, left visual field defect, left hemiparesis, left-sided sensory loss, poor left conjugate gaze, extinction of left-sided stimuli, dysarthria, spatial disorientation |
| Brain Stem/Cerebellum/Posterior Hemisphere |
| Motor or sensory loss in all four limbs, crossed signs, limb or gait ataxia, dysarthria, disconjugate gaze, nystagmus, amnesia, bilateral visual field defects |
| Small Subcortical Hemisphere or Brainstem |
| Pure Motor Stroke |
| Weakness of face and limbs on one side of the body without abnormalities of higher brain function, sensation, or vision |
| Pure Sensory Stroke |
| Decreases sensation of face and limbs on one side of the body without abnormalities of higher brain function, motor function, or vision |

Adapted from Caplan 1993.

## General Initial Approach

Although the clinical features of intracranial hemorrhage and ischemic stroke overlap, management is markedly different. Therefore, differentiation between the two is paramount. Computed tomography (CT) of the brain helps make this distinction (Bamford 1992). Absence of blood on CT supports a diagnosis of ischemic stroke. Early detection of edema, hydrocephalus, or hypodensity (possible in approximately 50 to 60% of cases) may indicate a more serious ischemic injury and may predict hemorrhagic transformation, thereby dictating a change in acute treatment (Horowitz et al. 1991). Magnetic resonance imaging (MRI) is more sensitive than CT, but MRI features of acute hemorrhage can be nonspecific.

MRI is particularly helpful in cases with suspected brain stem or cerebellar infarction difficult to detect with CT (Shuaib et al. 1992). Once a diagnosis is made, treatment is given with consideration to potential etiology such as a cardiac source of embolism (Table 7-22) versus artery–artery embolism from carotid arteries or aortic arch. A carotid ultrasound, a transthoracic or transesophageal echocardiogram, and a Holter monitoring should be ordered. In arterial dissection, angiography is the diagnostic test of choice. In prothrombotic states, a coagulation screen must be performed to determine whether a deficiency in antithrombin III, protein C, or protein S exists, or whether anticardiolipin antibodies are present. In case of vasculitis, angiography and immunologic screening must be undertaken (Adams et al. 1994).

## Pathophysiology

Arterial occlusion and the consequent lowering of cerebral blood flow (CBF) result in a complex series of events (ischemic cascade) that transform ischemic tissue into infarction (Ginsberg and Pulsinelli 1994)(Figure 7-1). The most significant event is that of homeostatic ionic and sodium pump failure. This leads to the extracellular accumulation of potassium ($K^+$) and intracellular sodium ($Na^+$), resulting in a decrease in the energy reserve and phospholipid metabolism (Siesjo 1984). The neuronal damage seems to be related to intracellular calcium ($Ca^{2+}$) flux, which participates in the initiation of the production of free radicals.

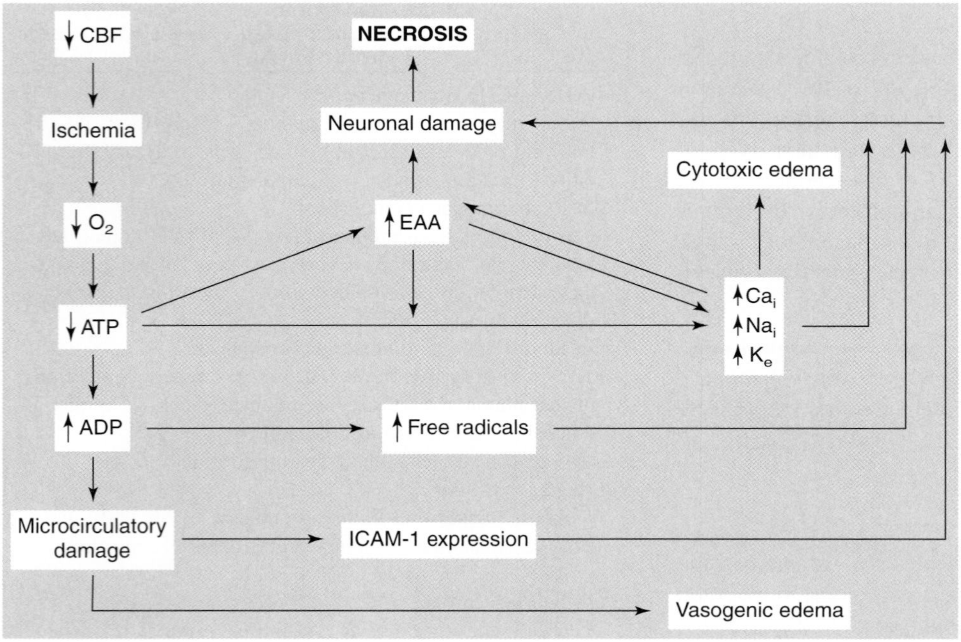

**FIGURE 7-1 Main steps of the ischemic cascade. EAA, excitatory amino acids; $Ca_i$, intracellular calcium; $Na_i$, intracellular sodium, $K_e$, extracellular potassium, ICAM-1, intercellular adhesion molecules.**

In the ischemic neuron, the threshold for electric silence and edema occurs when CBF is below 0.16–0.18 mL/g per minute, for at least 2 hours. The threshold for ($Na^+ + K^+$)-ATPase pump failure occurs when CBF falls to <0.05 mL/g per minute, with structural damage showing up early owing to energetic failure. The reversibility of the ischemic process relies upon the energy capacity of the neurons during ischemia, satisfactory CBF levels, and ischemic time (Raucgke 1983). In the peri-infarct penumbra tissue, while electrical neuronal function is diminished, the neurons themselves are viable until the amount of ATP produced falls below 50% of normal values (Garcia and Anderson 1989). The breakdown of energy-producing metabolites causes lactic acidosis, ion pump failure, and eventually, irreversible membrane damage (Garcia and Anderson 1989; Sacchetti et al. 1997).

## ACUTE INTERVENTION FOR ISCHEMIC STROKE

The "targets of opportunity" for pharmacotherapeutic approaches that may be useful in preventing the cascade of events that occur in acute ischemic stroke are illustrated in Figure 7-2.

### Pharmacology of Reperfusion in Acute Ischemic Stroke

Since the 1950s, many attempts have been made to modify coagulation and fibrinolytic mechanisms pharmacologically to induce the earliest possible recanalization of a cerebral artery in stroke, avoiding extension of necrosis to the penumbra area. Several of the pharmacologic approaches with the most solid clinical research are described below.

#### Tissue plasminogen activator

The European Cooperative Acute Stroke Study (ECASS) (Hacke et al. 1995) was a randomized, prospective, multicenter, double-blind, placebo-controlled study of 620 patients who had sustained acute ischemic hemispheric stroke. Patients received tissue plasminogen activator (tPA) 1.1 mg/kg or placebo within 6 hours of the onset of stroke. No significant benefit with respect to the primary endpoint (Barthel index) was seen. However, 109 patients (17.4%) included in the analysis had protocol violations and should have been barred from enrollment because they fulfilled at least one exclusion criterion (Kasner and Grotta 1997). Another study of tPA was con-

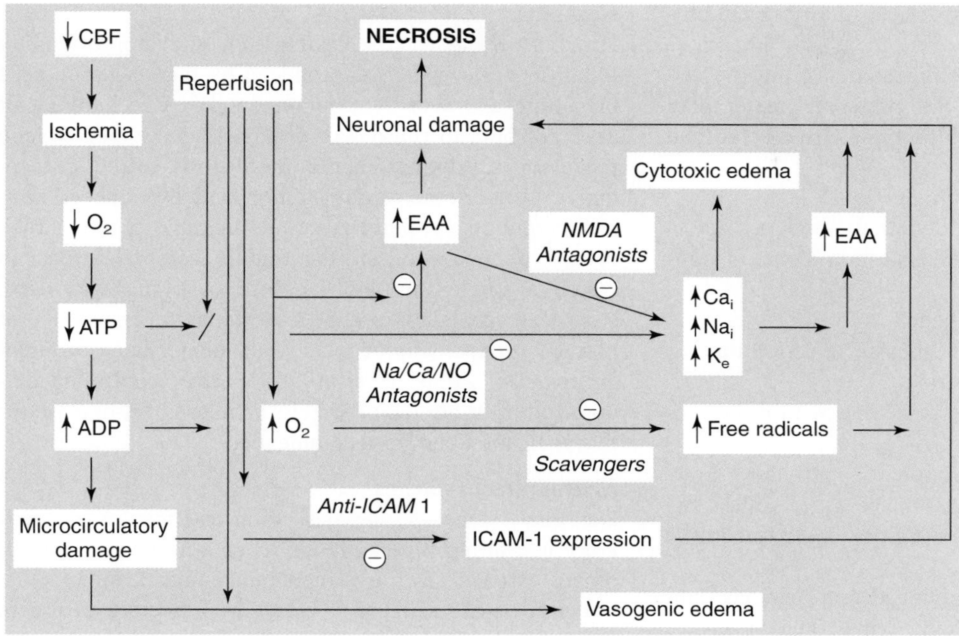


**FIGURE 7-2 How treatments for acute ischemic stroke are supposed to interrupt the ischemic cascade. Bold arrows indicate the possible negative effects of reperfusion. EAA, excitatory amino acids; $Ca_i$, intracellular calcium; $Na_i$, intracellular sodium, $K_e$, extracellular potassium, ICAM-1, intercellular adhesion molecules. (Adapted with permission from Sacchetti et al. 1997.)**

ducted by the National Institute of Neurological Disorders and Stroke (NINDS 1995). It was a prospective, multicenter, double-blind, placebo-controlled study of 624 patients using 0.9 mg/kg or placebo within 3 hours of the onset of symptoms. The study was divided into two parts, each with a specific primary endpoint. In the first part, the effect of tPA within 24 hours of stroke was measured on the basis of complete resolution of deficit or improvement. The second part measured improvement at 3 months. The group receiving tPA showed a 12% greater chance of total recovery or near total recovery, and a 6% chance of bleeding into the brain. In both the ECASS and NINDS studies of intravenous tPA for stroke, the major complication of treatment was intracranial hemorrhage, even though intravenous heparin was prohibited for the first 24 hours. Analysis of these trials is under way to identify risk factors for thrombolysis related hemorrhage. Based on these results, the following recommendations of the Stroke Council from the American Heart Association (Adams et al. 1994, 1996) appear to be reasonable and appropriate at this time:

1. Intravenous tPA (0.9 mg/kg, maximum 90 mg) with 10% of the dose given as a bolus followed by an infusion lasting 60 minutes within 3 hours of the onset of the stroke. Delayed administration (more than 3 hours after onset or when time of onset of stroke cannot be ascertained reliably) is not recommended because of the high risk of thrombolytic complications.
2. Streptokinase is not indicated for management of ischemic stroke.
3. The diagnosis of stroke must be made by a stroke expert, and assessed by imaging studies. If CT demonstrates early changes of a recent major infarction such as sulcal effacement, mass effect, edema, or possible hemorrhage, thrombolytic therapy should be avoided.
4. Patient exclusion criteria:
   a. Current use of oral anticoagulants, a prothrombin time >15 seconds, or an INR (international normalized ratio of prothrombin time) <1.7.
   b. Use of heparin in the previous 48 hours.
   c. Platelet count less than $100{,}000/mm^3$.

d. Another stroke or a serious head injury in the previous 3 months.
e. Major surgery within the preceding 14 days.
f. Pretreatment systolic blood pressure greater than 185 mm Hg or diastolic blood pressure greater than 110 mm Hg.
g. Rapidly improving neurologic signs.
h. Isolated, mild neurologic deficits such as ataxia alone, sensory loss alone, dysarthria alone, or minimal weakness.
i. Prior intracranial hemorrhage.
j. Blood glucose less than 50 mg/dL or >400 mg/dL.
k. Seizure at the onset of stroke.
l. Gastrointestinal or urinary bleeding within the preceding 21 days.
m. Recent myocardial infarction.

5. Thrombolytic therapy should not be given unless the patient is in an intensive care unit or dedicated stroke service.
6. Caution is advised before giving tPA to persons with severe stroke (total hemiplegia with coma or severe obtundation and/or fixed eye deviation).
7. The risks and potential benefits of tPA should be discussed with the patient and his or her family before treatment is initiated.

The use of tPA in patients with acute, ischemic stroke remains controversial. Reference to consensus guidelines is useful, but we should not be surprised when results of new clinical trials lead to revisions in such guidelines.

**Key Point**

- **Tissue plasminogen activator has burst open the door to acute stroke therapy.**

***Streptokinase***

Streptokinase is a protein derived from $\beta$-hemolytic streptococci, activates plasminogen indirectly, and has been found effective in acute myocardial infarction (GISSI-2) (Gruppo Italiano 1990). Three large, randomized trials using streptokinase in subjects with acute, ischemic strokes [Donnan et al. 1995; Multicentre Acute Stroke Trial-Italy (MAST-I) Group 1995; Hommel et al. 1996] were stopped because the interim analysis found a significantly higher rate of symptomatic intracerebral hemorrhages and deaths.

***Urokinase***

Urokinase is a native plasminogen activator originally found in urine, which is produced by human tissue cells in culture and also by recombinant DNA technology. It does not bind to fibrin. Pro-urokinase is the single-chain precursor of urokinase and is more fibrin-selective. It requires intra-arterial administration and experienced neurointervention. Preliminary results in subjects with stroke caused by occlusion of the middle cerebral artery, in which a single intra-arterial dose of 6 mg was used, showed recanalization in 58% of patients versus 14% of placebo group, without increase in hemorrhage in either groups (Del Zoppo et al. 1996). Further controlled randomized trials are required before the use of urokinase for this indication can be recommended.

***Neuroprotective drugs***

Neuronal membrane depolarization and release of excitatory neurotransmitters are key events in the pathophysiologic cascade leading to cell injury and death in acute ischemic stroke (Figure 7-1). Neuroprotective treatment promotes survival of brain cells by interfering with different steps in this cascade (see Figure 7-2). Since no neuroprotective drug has been proven safe and effective for acute stroke, none has been approved by the U.S. Food and Drug Administration.

***Lubeluzole***

Lubeluzole is a benzothiazole compound that prevents increase in extracellular glutamate concentrations and inhibits glutamate-induced nitric-oxide-related neurotoxicity thus reducing the infarct volume. Phase III trials showed that low doses (7.5 mg over 1 hour as a loading dose, followed by a continuous infusion of 10 mg/day for 5 days) were safe, but they did not affect mortality or clinical outcome (Diener 1998). Final analyses are being conducted, with reports to be published in late 1999.

***Nimodipine***

Although nimodipine is commonly used in patients with subarachnoid hemorrhage, a meta-analysis of studies of its use in patients with acute ischemic stroke (Mohr et al. 1994) found no significant difference between nimodipine- and placebo-treated patients.

***Chlormethiazole***

GABA ($\gamma$-aminobutyric acid) is released from presynaptic terminals following the onset of cerebral ischemia, suggesting that the GABAergic inhibitory mechanism is impaired and that stimulation of the GABA (A) receptor might balance the excitotoxic cascade. Chlormethiazole is an anticonvulsant and a sedative, and it has been found to protect in global and focal ischemic injury in stroke models (Cross et al. 1991). A phase III clinical trial is ongoing with doses of 75 mg/kg per day. Further information may become available at the end of 1999.

***N-Methyl-D-aspartate antagonists***

Four drugs of the NMDA antagonist class have been tested: selfotel, eliprodil, cerestat, and magnesium. Both selfotel and eliprodil (Fisher 1995) were found to have severe adverse effects without showing any benefit. Cerestat (Turrini 1996) is currently in phase III study. Magnesium causes a voltage-dependent block of the ion channel of the NMDA receptor, thus acting as a noncompetitive NMDA antagonist (Harrison and Simmonds 1985). A large proportion of patients treated with magnesium improved neurologically, and the need for institutional care after stroke was reduced by 6 months (Wahlgren 1997). Nevertheless, further studies are required to learn more about its use for this indication.

***Free-radical scavengers***

Oxygen free radicals damage brain cells during reperfusion into the ischemic area following spontaneous or induced recanalization. Formation of superoxide, hydrogen peroxide, and hydroxyl radicals may result in peroxidation injury of lipid membranes, protein oxidation, and damage of DNA (Chan 1994). Tirilazad is currently in a phase III trial, although results of phase II trials suggest it is unlikely to be beneficial (Haley et al. 1995).

***Immunologic modulation of intracellular adhesion molecule-1***

Local expression of the intracellular adhesion molecule (ICAM-1) promotes leukocyte adhesion and infiltration, resulting in increased tissue damage. Anti-ICAM-I antibody has been shown to reduce infarct size in animals, particularly in models of reperfusion, but a phase III trial involving 625 subjects randomized within 6 hours of onset demonstrated that the use of enlimomab (ICAM-1) was detrimental compared with placebo (The Enlimomab Acute Stroke Trial Investigators 1997).

Citicoline is a membrane component precursor of CDP-choline and is believed to have a double neuroprotective effect late in the ischemic cascade by stabilizing the neuronal membrane and inhibiting the formation of free radicals (D'Orlando and Sandage 1995). Although the phase III trial is not complete, preliminary studies demonstrate significant improvement in recovery at an oral dose of 500 mg/day for 6 weeks with no important adverse effects. Citicoline trials include patients recruited within 24 hours of symptom onset. This suggests that if citicoline does prove effective in the treatment of stroke, its mechanism of action may be directed toward the later aspects of the ischemic cascade, or toward neuronal recovery.

**Neuroprotective drugs: many have been culled, but none have yet been proven for acute ischemic stroke.**

## The Concept of Combination Therapy in Acute Ischemic Stroke

Studies with tPA have demonstrated that pharmacologic reperfusion can be effective, but it also can result in further tissue damage. We do not know exactly which subgroup of patients is at risk for reperfusion injury. The ideal anti-ischemic treatment should help to restore CBF. It should also counteract the cascade of biochemical events leading from ischemia to neuronal death and the damaging events that occur after reperfusion. We therefore need to enlarge the therapeutic window by using drugs that are able to antagonize the events induced by ischemia, to recanalize the occluded vessel (with thrombolytics), and to protect tissue (the penumbra) from reperfusion injury. A trial of combination therapy with tPA and a neuroprotective agent represents the next step forward from single-agent studies in acute ischemic stroke (Sacchetti et al. 1997).

## Antithrombotic or Antiplatelet-aggregating Drugs

The rationale for anticoagulation in acute stroke is to prevent extension of a thrombus with a subsequent progressive neurologic deficit, in addition to preventing recurrence of cerebrovascular episodes. Heparin, when it combines with antithrombin III, inactivates factor X, and inhibits conversion of prothrombin to thrombin. Since 1983, the value of heparin in acute ischemic stroke has been challenged by controversial results. In 1995, the Chinese study of low-molecular-weight heparin used within 48 hours of the onset of symptoms showed that it was effective in improving outcomes at 6 months (Kay et al. 1995). These results are completely different from those of the International Stroke Trial (IST), which demonstrated that no heparin regimen offered any clinical advantage among 19,435 patients when evaluated at 6 months (IST 1997), and to those of the TOAST study (Trial of Org 10172 in Acute Stroke Treatment) (The Publications Committee for the Toast 1998), which evaluated 1281 patients at 3 months. Therefore, utilization of any type of heparin or heparinoid at any dose in acute ischemic stroke is not routinely recommended at this time.

## Hemodilution

Isovolemic or hypervolemic hemodilution (lowering of the hematocrit by 15% or more) results in reduction in blood viscosity and improvements in CBF. In April 1998, the Multicentre Austrian Hemodilution Stroke Trial (MAHST) found hemodilution to be safe, but failed to demonstrate a significant beneficial effect over the pure rehydration regimen in patients with acute ischemic stroke, and is therefore not recommended (Aichner et al. 1998).

# CHRONIC INTERVENTION (PRIMARY AND SECONDARY STROKE PREVENTION)

Cerebral infarction can be the consequence of an arterial obstruction because of an atherosclerotic plaque of the carotid system or aortic arch that can embolize to medium or small vessels. It is well known that the first step in the formation of an arterial thrombus is platelet adhesion to injured endothelium (Ohlstein et al. 1990).

## Antiplatelet Therapy

Current knowledge in the pathophysiology of platelet performance has led to focusing on platelet inhibition (aggregation and adhesion). Multiple studies have determined eight different sites where platelet inhibition is possible. Five sites are currently under experimentation with three used pharmacologically in clinic: cyclooxygenase inhibitors, ADP inhibitors, and cAMP and cGMP stimulants (Harker and Fuster 1986).

### *Aspirin*

Aspirin inhibits platelet cyclooxygenase and is the drug of choice in prevention of stroke. There remains an important controversy regarding optimal dosage. Several important trials have been undertaken with high doses or low doses of aspirin. Meta-analyses have also been reported.

Several studies have examined the efficacy of aspirin doses greater than 325 mg per day. The first controlled trial comparing aspirin 1300 mg/day with placebo showed that the aspirin group experienced a 31% reduction in recurrent events and mortality (Canadian Cooperative Study Group 1978). A French study showed a reduction in recurrent events and mortality up to 40% in the group receiving aspirin 1000 mg per day (Bousser et al. 1983). Five years later, in a European study (ESPS), the use of aspirin 975 mg/day plus dipyridamole 225 mg/day was demonstrated to be superior to placebo [European Stroke Prevention Study (ESPS) Group 1987].

Other studies have examined the efficacy of "low-dose" aspirin (dose ≤325 mg/day). In 1991, a Swedish trial of 1360 patients (SALT) used 50 mg of aspirin in comparison with placebo. The aspirin group showed an 18% reduction in stroke recurrence and death (The SALT Collaborative Group 1991). The same year, a Dutch trial did not find any difference between two low doses (80 mg vs. 283 mg/ day) in reduction of stroke recurrence and death, but unfortunately no control group was included (The Dutch TIA Trial Study Group 1991). In another study, patients with potential cardiac- embolic sources were included; nevertheless, there was an overall reduction of stroke by 15% (UK-TIA Study Group 1991). In 1996, the European group compared aspirin (50 mg/day) with dipyridamole or placebo and found a nonsignificant trend showing reduction of stroke recurrence rate in the aspirin group (17.7% less) and the dipyridamole group (15.8% less) compared with the placebo group [European Stroke Prevention Study (ESPS-2) Working Group 1996].

Several meta-analyses of trials in which aspirin was used to prevent stroke have been done. The Antiplatelet Trialists' Collaboration (ATC) reported that 29,000 patients receiving aspirin at low doses (≤325 mg/day) experienced 22% fewer new events. A second report (Antiplatelet Trialists' Collaboration 1994) included 100,000 patients receiving low- dose aspirin and found a reduction in mortality and stroke recurrence of 25% (Antiplatelet Trialists' Collaboration 1988). The authors recommend using low doses of aspirin; however, the results are biased by the inclusion of patients with cerebrovascular and coronary diseases.

There is no appropriate comparative trial that establishes an optimal aspirin dose. Furthermore, meta-analysis of all therapeutic trials comparing aspirin with placebo found the global reduction from high doses (>325 mg/ day) versus low doses (≤325 mg/day) of aspirin was not significant (Barnett et al. 1995). The aspirin dosage of 1300 mg/day often recommended to stroke patients for secondary prevention is based upon the following arguments:

1. Follow-up prospective studies of patients under chronic treatment with aspirin showed that the aspirin effect is not maintained, with some patients developing "aspirin resistance" on low doses. An increase in dosage renews the biological effect. Eight percent of patients will develop dose-independent resistance (Grotemeyer et al. 1993).

2. Although inhibition of thromboxane $A_2$ production occurs with low doses of aspirin, the platelet also produces 12-hydroxy-eicosatetraenoic acid, a by-product of the creation of the intraplatelet arachidonic acid (lipid-oxygenase). The rate of synthesis of this compound is not modified with lower doses of aspirin, which is probably explained by the resistance mentioned above (Buchanan and Brister 1995).
3. Experimental studies on endothelial injury have reported a clear association between high doses of aspirin and diminished thrombus formation, embolus number, and recurrence rate (Vesvres et al. 1993).
4. The North American Symptomatic Carotid Endarterectomy Trial (NASCET) revealed that the postsurgery stroke recurrence rate was 5 times as frequent in patients with lower doses of aspirin (Dyken et al. 1992). Currently, a prospective, double-blind, randomized trial (Aspirin in Carotid Endarterectomy [ACE]) is comparing the final outcomes in all patients submitted to surgery when given different aspirin doses (low or high). The study ended in July 1998.
5. The main complications of aspirin are gastric intolerance (gastritis and duodenitis) and bleeding. It appears that these complications are not proportional to the dosage given and can be diminished by the use of enteric-coated preparations (Hawthorne et al. 1991).

#### *Dipyridamole and other antiplatelet agents*

Dipyridamole diminishes platelet aggregation apparently by raising platelet levels of cyclic adenosine monophosphate (cAMP) and of cyclic guanosine monophosphate (cGMP) (Alheid et al. 1989). No study to date has shown dipyridamole's superiority over aspirin (at either low or high dose). In 1996, the European group showed dipyridamole's superiority to placebo [European Stroke Prevention Study (ESPS-2) Working Group 1996). In addition, combining dipyridamole 400 mg/day and aspirin 50 mg/day led to a reduction of 37% in the risk of subsequent strokes. However, these beneficial effects of dipyridamole plus aspirin do not supersede those of high-dose aspirin (1300 mg) as monotherapy.

**PRINCIPLE Aspirin remains the initial drug of choice for stroke prevention.**

#### *Ticlopidine and clopidogrel*

Those patients who demonstrate "aspirin failure" (having a stroke while taking aspirin), and/or adverse effects of aspirin, are candidates for the use of ticlopidine or clopidogrel (McTavish et al. 1990). Both ticlopidine and clopidogrel help to prevent platelet activation, aggregation, and release of platelet granules, interfering with platelet membrane function by inhibiting ADP-induced platelet–fibrinogen binding and platelet–platelet interactions (Di Minno et al. 1985).

Two multicenter studies evaluated ticlopidine. The first did not include patients with cerebral infarcts and was found to reduce the risk of recurrent stroke up to 23.3% (Gent et al. 1989). The second study included patients with transient ischemic attack and minor infarcts who were compared with patients receiving aspirin 1300 mg/day. The study found that the 3-year event rate for nonfatal stroke or death from any cause was 17% for subjects receiving ticlopidine and 19% for subjects receiving aspirin: a 12% reduction in relative risk with ticlopidine. The rates of fatal and nonfatal stroke at 3 years were 10% for the ticlopidine group and 13% for the aspirin group—a 21% reduction in relative risk with ticlopidine (Hass et al. 1989).

Ticlopidine's adverse effects include diarrhea (12.5%) and neutropenia (2.4%), which was severe in 0.8% of cases and reversible in all patients when the drug was withdrawn. For this reason, monitoring the white blood cell count (WBC) every 15 days for 3 months must be done. Infrequent but more serious complications are thrombotic thrombocytopenic purpura and aplastic anemia (some cases are fatal) (McTavish et al. 1990).

Through a multicenter trial (CAPRIE), clopidogrel (75 mg/day) was shown to be safe and had fewer adverse effects or secondary reactions than ticlopidine (CAPRIE Steering Committee 1996). It proved marginally more effective than aspirin at 325 mg/day. How it would compare with aspirin at 1300 mg/day is unknown.

## Anticoagulants

No study showed benefit of anticoagulants in secondary prevention of ischemic stroke in patients with atherosclerotic pathology. For patients with certain cardiac disorders that carry an embolism risk of 5% per year or greater (Table 7-22), anticoagulation therapy has been shown to reduce risk of stroke.

#### *Cardiac patients in sinus rhythm*

A systematic review of anticoagulant trials for survivors of myocardial infarction suggests that long-term use reduces the risk of stroke and vascular death (Antman et al. 1992). A large, randomized controlled trial is now under way: the Warfarin Aspirin Recurrent Stroke Study (WARSS) comparing warfarin with aspirin in a double-blind, placebo-controlled trial. The results will not be available to the end in 1999. Another study, the Stroke Prevention in Recurrent Ischaemia Trial (SPIRIT), comparing warfarin plus aspirin with placebo in a single-blind trial, showed high hemorrhage incidence in preliminary data (Hart 1997). Thus there are insufficient data for the initiation of oral anticoagulation in patients with sinus rhythm.

***Patients with atrial fibrillation***

A systematic review of five trials on the value of anticoagulants in the primary prevention of stroke in patients with atrial fibrillation showed a 68% overall reduction in the annual risk of stroke. The absolute rate of stroke was 4.5% in the control group versus 1.4% in the treated group (Atrial Fibrillation Investigators 1994). However, the results of this trial cannot be extrapolated directly to patients in atrial fibrillation who have survived a TIA or an acute ischemic stroke, because their absolute risk of recurrent stroke is much higher. The average annual risk of stroke among control patients in the five primary prevention trials was just over 4%, compared with 12% among control patients in the European Atrial Fibrillation Trial (EAFT) (European Atrial Fibrillation Trial Study Group 1995). In the EAFT, anticoagulants reduced the risk of stroke by two-thirds, from 12 to 4% per year, and of the primary outcome event (stroke, myocardial infarction, systemic embolism, or vascular death) by about 50%, reducing the annual rate of events from 17% in control to 8% in anticoagulant- allocated patients.

Anticoagulants rather than antiplatelet agents are used in patients with atrial fibrillation for long-term secondary prevention after a TIA or an ischemic stroke has occurred. An INR between 2.0 and 4.0 is the goal (European Atrial Fibrillation Trial Study Group 1995). Ischemic stroke survivors and TIA patients are a fairly heterogeneous group, and certain factors may make clinicians reluctant to prescribe long-term warfarin: a history of uncontrolled hypertension, recent gastrointestinal bleeding, alcoholic liver disease, confusion or dementia, tendency to fall, and difficulties with access to an anticoagulant clinic. These factors increase the likelihood of overdoing anticoagulation and the risk of intracranial bleeding (Hart et al. 1995). Recently (April 1998), investigators published the results of a prospective cohort study (SPAFIII) among 892 patients with *nonvalvular* atrial fibrillation. These were categorized as being at low risk for stroke recurrence based on the absence of recent congestive heart failure or left ventricular fractional shortening of 25% or less, previous thromboembolism, systolic blood pressure greater than 160 mm Hg, or female sex at age older than 75 years. These patients did not benefit substantially from treatment with warfarin, since their rate of stroke during aspirin therapy was sufficiently low that warfarin could only minimally reduce the absolute rate of stroke (1% per year). In contrast, patients in atrial fibrillation with one or more of the four thromboembolic risk factors have much higher rates of stroke (averaging 8% per year) (The SPAFIII Writing Committee for the Stroke Prevention in Atrial Fibrillation Investigators 1998).

Answers regarding the optimal duration of anticoagulation in these patients in atrial fibrillation (particularly in patients over the age of 70 years), as well as how to balance efficacy and risk of bleeding, have yet to be determined.

**PRINCIPLE Cardiac embolism is the only proven indication for anticoagulation in stroke.**

## DRUG TREATMENT OF OTHER TYPES OF STROKE

### Hemorrhagic Stroke

Hemorrhages can be distinguished by their location; epidural or subdural, subarachnoid or intraparenchymal. This distinction is fundamental because the management and treatment are different. Subarachnoid hemorrhage and epidural or subdural hematomas need prompt neurosurgical assessment (Blecic and Bogousslavsky 1995).

### Medical Management of Intracerebral Hemorrhage

The treatment must be specific to the patient's underlying condition with nonhypertensive intracerebral hemorrhage (ICH) (Table 7-24). Intraparenchymal bleeding can occur as a complication of anticoagulation. Vitamin K and fresh frozen plasma should be used for patients on warfarin therapy. Protamine and ε-aminocaproic acid are useful in cases of heparin-induced hemorrhage (1000 IU of protamine inactivates 5000 IU of heparin) (Babikian et al. 1989). The risk of parenchymal bleeding increases to 6–20% (Adams et al. 1994, 1996; NINDS 1995) when intravenous thrombolytic agents are used to treat cerebral ischemia. Fresh frozen plasma, aprotinin at 4 mg/kg intravenously, or tranexamic acid at 25 mg/kg intravenously followed by oral tranexamic acid at 1000 mg qid have

Table 7-24 **Treatment of Intracerebral Hemorrhage**

| | |
|---|---|
| Treat increased intracranial pressure if present. | |
| For secondary ICH following anticoagulation and thrombolysis: | |
| Heparin sodium: | Stop heparin sodium infusion. |
| | Check aPTT and platelet count. |
| | Heparin sodium inactivation with IV protamine sulfate. |
| | (1000 IU inactivates 5000 IU of heparin sodium.) |
| Warfarin sodium: | Stop warfarin sodium. |
| | Concentrate of coagulation factors I, II, VII, and IX with dose correlation to INR, or administer fresh-frozen plasma. |
| | Vitamin K in subacute treatment (30 mg/kg). |
| Thrombolysis: | Stop lytic agent. |
| | Fresh-frozen plasma, aprotinin 4 mg/kg intravenously. |
| | Or tranexamic acid 25 mg/kg intravenously, followed by oral tranexamic acid 1000 mg qid. |
| For subarachnoid hemorrhage: | |
| Aneurysmal: | Requires immediate surgical approach. |
| | Calcium channel blockers to prevent vasospasm. |
| | Antifibrinolytic agents (see text). |
| | Free-radical scavengers (tirilazad mesylate). |
| Nonaneurysmal: | Calcium channel blockers. |

Modified from Brandt et al. 1996.
ABBREVIATIONS: aPTT, activated prothrombin time; ICH, intracerebral hemorrhage; INR, international normalized ratio of prothrombin time.

been recommended as an emergency treatment (Brandt et al. 1996).

Intracerebral hemorrhage in the young is often attributed to the abuse of illicit or prescription drugs, including methamphetamine, phenylpropanolamine, cocaine, phencyclidine, pentazocine-pyribenzamine, or methylphenidate. If the patient is taking aspirin, treatment should be discontinued (Minematsu and Yamaguchi 1995).

**PRINCIPLE The medical management of intracerebral hemorrhage must be specific to the patient's underlying condition.**

## Medical Management of Subarachnoid Hemorrhage

Medical management of subarachnoid hemorrhage (SAH) is focused on prevention of possible complications, and surgery is elected in those cases secondary to an aneurysmal rupture.

**PRINCIPLE Neurosurgical assessment in subarachnoid hemorrhage, and subdural or epidural hematomas, is of the utmost importance.**

### *Antifibrinolytic therapy*

The rationale for antifibrinolytic therapy is that the perianeurysmal clot formed by the initial hemorrhage can support the aneurysmal wall and prevent rerupture. Fibrinolytic activity of the cerebrospinal fluid is stimulated after SAH, and enhanced lysis could lead to dissolution of this supportive clot (Fodstad and Nilsson 1981). Both ε-aminocaproic acid and tranexamic acid inhibit plasminogen activation of plasmin, thus stabilizing the fibrin clot. An intravenous loading dose of ε-aminocaproic acid (5 g) followed by a constant infusion (1 to 1.5 g/h) may permit rapid achievement of therapeutic levels. However, there is controversy regarding its efficacy, and severe adverse effects (e.g., fulminant myopathy with rhabdomyolysis, myoglobinuria, and pulmonary thromboembolism) make its use debatable (Adams and Love 1992).

### *Agents to prevent vasospasm and ischemic stroke*

Nizofenone (OKY-1581) is an agent that protects against ischemia and the development of edema after SAH. It is a selective antagonist of thromboxane $A_2$ synthetase. In a double-blind, multicenter clinical trial in Japan, the improvement was modest, and its use is declining (Ohta et al. 1986). It is not available in the United States.

Nimodipine and nicardipine are both calcium-entry blockers that have been evaluated for this indication. The influx of extracellular calcium is an important factor in sustaining contraction of smooth muscle and is a critical element in the process of cellular ischemia (Weir 1984). Both drugs have shown efficacy during the acute treatment of SAH as prophylactic agents to help prevent vasospasm. Nicardipine has the advantage over nimodipine of being water soluble, allowing parenteral administration. Preliminary results of one large randomized placebo-controlled double-blind trial reported a 30% decline in the incidence of symptomatic vasospasm (Haley et al. 1990).

SUMMARY

**Stroke is a medical emergency. Current knowledge regarding its treatment is not only based on its management during the acute phase, but also, pertinent measures to avoid risk factors (primary prevention) are of utmost importance.**

**Diagnosis and management of acute stroke are best accomplished when trained personnel are the care givers, ideally carried out in a stroke unit. Differentiation between an ischemic and hemorrhagic stroke (CT scan) is the first question to answer. In those with an acute ischemic stroke, with time elapsed from the onset of less than 3 hours (therapeutic window) and severity of less than or equal to 33% of the middle cerebral artery territory, reperfusion with intravenous tPA (if there is no other contraindication) has shown benefit. In patients with an acute stroke who do not qualify for thrombolysis, a neuroprotectant (within the first five hours of onset) to prevent further ischemic damage in the penumbra area, is the option. Shortly, upon trials results, combination therapy will be the next step forward from single-agent management. Not all patients are candidates for the same treatment. The decision requires a balance between risks and benefits.**

**The therapeutic options for secondary prevention (chronic treatment) are based upon the etiology of ischemic stroke. Patients with arterial obstruction because of an atherosclerotic plaque of the carotid system, aortic arch, or even small vessel disease (penetrating arteries) will benefit from life-long antiplatelet therapy. Aspirin is the first choice followed by ticlopidine or clopidogrel. Warfarin is used for those stroke patients with a known cause of cardioembolism or prothrombotic states.**

**The acute management of a hemorrhagic stroke (intracerebral hemorrhage) must be specific to the patient's condition (treat intracranial hypertension if present) and etiology (e.g., hypertension, as a complication of anticoagulation or thrombolysis). For SAH, calcium-channel blockers and immediate surgical approach are mandatory.**

**It is essential to know that stroke is an active, multivariate complex process, allowing multiple therapeutic approaches. This is changing the passive attitudes of the past and improving the prognosis of our patients with stroke.**

## REFERENCES

[Ad Hoc Committee on Cerebrovascular Disease.] 1975. A classification and outline of cerebrovascular diseases. Part II. *Stroke* **6**:565–616.

Adams HJ, Jr, Brott TG, Crowell RM, et al. 1994. Guidelines for the management of patients with acute ischemic stroke. A statement for healthcare professionals from a Special Writing Group of the Stroke Council, American Heart Association. *Circulation* **90**:1588–1601.

Adams HJ Jr, Brott TG, Furlan RM, et al. 1996. Guidelines for Thrombolytic Therapy for Acute Stroke: a supplement to the guidelines for the management of patients with acute ischemic stroke. A statement for healthcare professionals from a Special Writing Group of the Stroke Council, American Heart Association. *Stroke* **27**: 1711–8.

Adams HP, Love BB. 1992. Medical management of aneurysmal subarachnoid hemorrhage. In: Barnett HJM, Mohr JP, Stein BM & Yatsu FM, editors. *Stroke, Pathophysiology, Diagnosis and Management*. 2nd ed. New York: Churchill-Livingstone. p 1029–54.

Aichner FT, Fazekas F, Brainin M, et al. 1998. Hypervolemic hemodilution in acute ischemic stroke. The Multicenter Austrian Hemodilution Stroke Trial (MAHST). *Stroke* **29**:743–9.

Alheid U, Reichwehr I, Foerstermann U. 1989. Human endothelial cells inhibit platelet aggregation by separately stimulating platelet cyclic AMP and cyclic GMP. *Eur J Pharmacol* **164**:103–10.

American Heart Association (AHA). 1993. Heart and Stroke Facts: 1994 Statistical Supplement. Dallas, Tx: American Heart Association.

Antiplatelet Trialists' Collaboration. 1988. Secondary prevention of vascular disease by prolonged antiplatelet treatment. *Br Med J* **296**:320–31.

Antiplatelet Trialists' Collaboration. 1994. Collaborative overview of randomised trials of antiplatelet therapy. I. Prevention of death, myocardial infarction, and stroke by prolonged antiplatelet therapy in various categories of patients. *Br Med J* **308**:81– 106.

Antman EM, Lau J, Kupelnick B, et al. 1992. A comparison of results of meta-analyses of randomized control trials and recommendations of clinical experts. Treatments for myocardial infarction. *JAMA* **268**:240–8.

[Atrial Fibrillation Investigators]. 1994. Risk factors for stroke and efficacy of antithrombotic therapy in atrial fibrillation. Analysis of pooled data from five randomized controlled trials. [Published erratum *Arch Intern Med* 1994. **154**:2254]. *Arch Intern Med* **154**:1449–57.

Babikian V, Kase C, Pessin M, et al. 1989. Intracerebral hemorrhage in stroke patients anticoagulated with heparin. *Stroke* **20**:1500–3.

Bamford J. 1992. Clinical examination in diagnosis and subclassification of stroke. *Lancet* **339**:400–2.

Barnett HJM, Eliasziw M, Meldrum HE. 1995. Drugs and surgery in the prevention of ischemic stroke [review]. *N Engl J Med.* **333**:238–48.

Barrett-Connor E, Khaw KT. 1988. Diabetes mellitus: an independent risk factor for stroke? *Am J Epidemiol* **128**:116–23.

Bengtsson C, Lapidus L, Stendahl C, et al. 1988. Hyperuricaemia and risk of cardiovascular disease and overall death: a 12-year follow-up of population study of women in Gothenburg, Sweden. *Acta Med Scan* **224**:549–55.

Berwanger CS, Jeremy JY, Stansby G. 1995. Homocysteine and vascular disease. *Br J Surg* **82**:726–31.

Blecic S and Bogousslavsky J. 1995. Current management of acute stroke. In: Fisher M, editor. *Stroke Therapy*. Boston, MA: Butterworth- Heinemann. p 247–66.

Bogousslavsky J, Regli MD, Van Melle G, et al. 1988. Migraine stroke. *Neurology* **38**:223–7.

Bogousslavsky J, Van Melle G, Regli F. 1988. The Lausanne Stroke Registry. Analysis of 1000 consecutive patients with first stroke. *Stroke* **19**:1083–93.

Bousser MG, Eschwege E, Haguenau M, et al. 1983. "AICLA" controlled trial of aspirin and dypyridamole in the secondary prevention of athero-thrombotic cerebral ischemia. *Stroke* **14**:5–14.

Brandt T, Grau AJ, Hacke W. 1996. Severe stroke. *Baillieres Clin Neurol* **5**:515–41.

Buchanan MR, Brister SJ. 1995. Individual variations in the effects of ASA on platelet function implications for the use of ASA clinically. *Can J Cardiol* **11**:221–7.

Camargo CA. 1989. Moderate alcohol consumption and stroke. The epidemiologic evidence. *Stroke* **20**:1611–26.

Canadian Cooperative Study Group. 1978. A randomized trial of aspirin and sulfinpyrazone in threatened stroke. *N Engl J Med* **299**:53–9.

Caplan LR. 1993. *Stroke: A Clinical Approach*, 2nd ed. Boston, MA: Butterworth-Heinemann.

CAPRIE Steering Committee. 1996a. A randomised, blinded, trial of clopidogrel versus aspirin in patients at risk of ischaemic events (CAPRIE). *Lancet* **348**:1329–39.

Chan P. 1994. Oxygen radicals in focal cerebral ischemia. *Brain Pathol* **4**:59–65.

Colandrea MA, Friedman GD, Nichaman MZ, et al. 1970. Systolic hypertension in the elderly: an epidemiologic assessment. *Circulation* **41**:239–45.

Cross AJ, Jones JA, Baldwin HA, et al. 1991. Neuroprotective activity of chlormethiazole following transient forebrain ischemia in the gerbil. *Br J Pharmacol* **104**:406–11.

D'Orlando KJ, Sandage BW. 1995. Citicoline (CDP-Choline): Mechanisms of action and effects in ischemic brain injury. *Neurol Res* **17**:281–4.

Del Zoppo GJ, Higashida RT, Furlan AJ, et al. 1996. The Prolyse in Acute Cerebral Thromboembolism Trial (PROACT): Results of 6 mgs dose tier. The PROACT Investigators. *Stroke* **27**:164–8.

Di Minno G, Cerbone AM, Mattioli PL, et al. 1985. Functionally thrombasthenic state in normal platelets following the administration of ticlopidine. *J Clin Invest* **75**:328–38.

Diener HC. 1998. Multinational randomized controlled trial of lubeluzole in acute ischemic stroke. The European and Australian Lubeluzole Ischemic Stroke Study Group. *Cerebrovasc Dis* **8**: 172– 81.

Donnan GA, Davis SA, Chambers BR, et al. 1995. Trials of streptokinase in severe acute ischaemic stroke. *Lancet* **345**:578–9.

Dyken ML, Barnett HJM, Easton D, et al. 1992. Low-dose aspirin and stroke. "It ain't necessarily so" [editorial]. *Stroke* **23**:1395–9.

European Atrial Fibrillation Trial Study Group. 1995. Optimal oral anticoagulant therapy in patients with nonrheumatic atrial fibrillation and recent cerebral ischemia. *N Engl J Med* **333**:5–10.

European Stroke Prevention Study (ESPS) Group. 1987. Principal end points. *Lancet* **2**:1351–4.

European Stroke Prevention Study (ESPS-2) Working Group. 1996. Secondary stroke prevention: aspirin/dipyridamole combination is superior to either agent alone and to placebo [abstract]. *Stroke* **27**:195.

Fieschi C, Argentino GL, Lenzi ML, et al. 1989. Clinical and instrumental evaluation of patients with ischemic stroke within the first six hours. *J Neurol Sci* **91**:311–22.

Fisher CM. 1969. The arterial lesions underlying lacunes. *Acta Neuropathol (Berl)* **12**:1–20.

Fisher M. 1995. Potentially effective therapies for acute ischemic stroke. *Eur Neurol.* **35**:3–7.

Fodstad H, Nilsson IM. 1981. Coagulation and fibrinolysis in blood and cerebrospinal fluid after aneurysmal subarachnoid haemorrhage: effect of tranexaminic acid. *Acta Neurochir* **56**:25.

Garcia JH, Anderson ML. 1989. Physiopathology of cerebral ischemia. *CRC Crit Rev Neurobiol* **4**:303–23.

Gent M, Blakely JA, Easton JD, et al. 1989. The Canadian-American Ticlopidine Study (CATS) in thromboembolic stroke. *Lancet* **1**:1215–20.

Ginsberg MD, Pulsinelli WA. 1994. The ischemic penumbra, injury thresholds, and the therapeutic window for acute stroke. *Ann Neurol* **36**:553–4.

Grotemeyer KH, Scharafinski H, Husstedt IW. 1993. Two year follow-up of aspirin responders and non-responders: a pilot study including 180 post-stroke patients. *Thromb Res* **71**:397–403.

Gruppo Italiano. 1990. GISSI-2: A factorial randomised trial of alteplase versus streptokinase and heparin versus no heparin among 12,490 patients with acute myocardial infarction. Gruppo Italiano per Studio della Sopravivenza nell'Infarto Miocardico. *Lancet* **336**:65–71.

Hachinski V, Graffagnino C, Beaudry M, et al. 1996. Lipids and stroke. A paradox resolved. *Arch Neurol* **53**:303–8.

Hacke W, Kaste M, Fieschi C, et al. for the ECASS Study Group. 1995. Intravenous thrombolysis with recombinant tissue plasminogen activator for acute hemispheric stroke: The European Acute Stroke Study (ECASS) *JAMA* **274**:1017–25.

Haley EC Jr, Kassell NF, Alves WM, et al. 1995. Phase II trial of tirilazad in aneurysmal subarachnoid hemorrhage. A report of the cooperative aneurysm study. *J Neurosurg* **82**:786–90.

Haley EC, Torner JC, Kassell NF, et al. 1990. Cooperative randomized study of nicardipine in subarachnoid haemorrhage. Preliminary report. In: Sano K, Takakara K, Kassell NF, et al., editors. *Cerebral Vasospasm. Proceedings of the Fourth International Conference on Cerebral Vasospasm.* Tokyo: University of Tokyo Press.

Harker LA, Fuster V. 1986. Pharmacology of platelet inhibitors. *J Am Coll Cardiol* **8**:21b.

Harrison NL, Simmonds MA. 1985. Quantitative studies on some antagonists of *N*-methyl-D-aspartate in slices of rat cerebral cortex. *Br J Pharmacol* **84**:381–91.

Hart RG, Boop BS, Anderson DC. 1995. Oral anticoagulants and intracranial hemorrhage. Facts and hypotheses. *Stroke* **26**:1471–7.

Hart RG. 1992. Cardiogenic embolism to the brain. *Lancet* **339**: 589–94.

Hart RG. 1997. Oral anticoagulants for secondary prevention of stroke. *Cerebrovasc Dis* **7**(Suppl 6):24–9.

Hass WK, Easton JD, Adams HP Jr, et al. 1989. A randomized trial comparing ticlopidine hydrochloride with aspirin for the prevention of stroke in high-risk patients. *N Engl J Med* **321**:501–7.

Hawthorne AB, Maluda YR, Cole AT, et al. 1991. Aspirin-induced gastric mucosal damage: prevention by enteric- coating and relation to prostaglandin synthesis. *Br J Clin Pharmacol* **32**:77–83.

Hommel M, Cornu C, Boutitie F, et al. 1996. Thrombolytic therapy with streptokinase in acute ischemic stroke. The Multicentre Acute Stroke Trial-Europe Study Group. *N Engl J Med* **335**:145–50.

Horowitz SH, Zito JL, Donnarumma R, et al. 1991. Computed tomographic-angiographic findings within the first five hours of cerebral infarction. *Stroke* **22**:1245–53.

IST. 1997. The International Stroke Trial (IST): a randomised trial of aspirin, subcutaneous heparin, both, or neither among 19,435 patients with acute ischaemic stroke. *Lancet* **349**:1569–81.

Kannel WB, Gordon T, Wolf PA. 1972. Hemoglobin and the risk of cerebral infarction. The Framingham Study. *Stroke* **128**:409–19.

Kannel WB, Wolf PA, McGee DL, et al. 1981. Systolic blood pressure, arterial rigidity, and risk of stroke: the Framingham Study. *JAMA* **245**:1225–28.

Kasner SE, Grotta JC. 1997. Emergency identification and treatment of acute ischemic stroke. *Ann Emerg Med* **30**: 642–53.

Kaste M, Palomaki H, Sarna S. 1995. Where and how should elderly stroke patients be treated? *Stroke* **26**:249–53.

Kay R, Wong SA, Yu L, et al. 1995. Low-molecular-weight heparin for the treatment of acute ischemic stroke. *N Engl J Med* **333**: 1588–93.

McTavish D, Faulds D, Goa KL. 1990. Ticlopidine. An updated review of its pharmacology and therapeutic use in platelet-dependent disorders. *Drugs* **40**:238–59.

Minematsu K, Yamaguchi T. 1995. Management of intracerebral hemorrhage. In: Fisher M, editor. *Stroke Therapy*. Boston, MA: Butterworth-Heinemann. p 351–72.

Mohr JP, Orgogozo JM, Harrison MJG, et al. 1994. Meta-analysis of oral nimodipine trials in acute ischemic stroke. *Cerebrovasc Dis* **4**:197–203.

Multicentre Acute Stroke Trial-Italy (MAST-I) Group. 1995. Randomised controlled trial of streptokinase, aspirin, and combination of both in treatment of acute ischaemic stroke. *Lancet* **346**:1509–14.

NINDS. 1995. The National Institute of Neurological Disorders and Stroke rt-PA Stroke Study Group. Tissue plasminogen activator for acute ischemic stroke. International Stroke Trial Collaborative Group. *N Engl J Med* **333**:1581–7.

Norris JW, Hachinski VC. 1991. Stroke prevention: past, present, and future. In: Norris JW, Hachinski VC, editors. *Prevention of Stroke*. New York: Springer-Verlag. p 1–18.

Ohlstein EH, Storer B, Nambi P, et al. 1990. Endothelin and platelet function. *Thromb Res* **57**:967.

Ohta T, Kikuchi H, Hashi K, et al. 1986. Nizofenone administration in the acute stage following subarachnoid haemorrhagia: results of a multi-center controlled double- blind clinical study. *J Neurosurg* **64**:420.

Oxfordshire Community Stroke Project. 1983. Incidence of stroke in Oxfordshire: first year's experience of a community stroke register. *Br Med J* **287**:713–7.

Paffenbarger RA Jr, Laughlin ME, Gima AS, et al. 1970. Work activity of longshoremen as related to death from coronary heart disease and stroke. *N Engl J Med* **282**:1109– 14.

Petit DB, Sidney S, Bernstein A, et al. 1996. Stroke in users of low-dose oral contraceptives. *N Engl J Med* **335**:8–15.

Ramirez-Lessepas M, Quinanes MR, Nino HH. 1986. Treatment of acute ischemic stroke. Open trial with continuous intravenous heparinization. *Arch Neurol* **43**:386–90.

Raucgke NE. 1983. Pathophysiology of brain ischemia. *Ann Neurol* **13**:2–10.

Sacchetti ML, Toni D, Fiorelli M, et al. 1997. The concept of combination therapy in acute ischemic stroke. *Neurology* **49**(Suppl 4):S70–4.

SHEP Cooperative Research Group. 1991. Prevention of stroke by antihypertensive drug treatment in older persons with isolated systolic hypertension: final results of the Systolic Hypertension in the Elderly Program (SHEP). *JAMA* **265**:3255–64.

Shuaib A, Lee D, Pelz D, et al. 1992. The impact of magnetic resonance imaging on the management of acute ischemic stroke. *Neurology* **42**:816–8.

Siesjo BK. 1984. Cerebral circulation and metabolism. *J Neurosurg* **60**:883–908.

Stamler J, Pick R, Katz LN, et al. 1963. Effectiveness of estrogens for therapy of myocardial infarction in middle-aged men. *JAMA* **183**:632–8.

Stampfer MJ, Colditz GA, Willett WC, et al. 1988. A prospective study of moderate alcohol consumption and the risk of coronary disease and stroke in women. *N Engl J Med* **319**:267–72.

The Dutch TIA Trial Study Group. 1991. A comparison of two doses of aspirin (30 mg vs 283 mg a day) in patients after transient ischemic attack or minor ischemic stroke. *N Engl J Med* **325**: 1261–6.

The Enlimomab Acute Stroke Trial Investigators. 1997. The Enlimomab Acute Stroke Trial: final results [abstract]. *Neurology* **48**(Suppl 2):A270.

The Publication Committee for the TOAST 1998. The Publications Committee for the Trial of ORG 10172 in Acute Stroke Treatment (TOAST) investigators. Low molecular weight heparinoid, ORG 10172 (danaparoid), and outcome after acute ischemic stroke. *JAMA* **279**:1265–72.

The SALT Collaborative Group. 1991. Swedish aspirin low-dose trial (SALT) of 75 mg aspirin as secondary prophylaxis after cerebrovascular ischaemic events. *Lancet* **338**:1345–9.

The SPAF III writing committee for the Stroke Prevention in Atrial Fibrillation Investigators. 1998. Patients with nonvalvular atrial fibrillation at low risk of stroke during treatment with aspirin. *JAMA* **279**:1273–7.

Turrini R. 1996. A pivotal safety and efficacy of cerestat (aptiganel HCL/CNS 1102) in acute ischemic stroke patients. *Stroke* **27**: 173–5.

UK-TIA Study Group. 1991. The United Kingdom Transient Ischaemic Attack (UK-TIA) aspirin trial: final results. *J Neurol Neurosurg Psychiatry* **54**:1044–54.

Vesvres MH, Doutremepuich F, Lalanne MCI, et al. 1993. Effects of aspirin on embolization in an arterial model of laser-induced thrombus formation. *Haemostasis* **23**:8–12.

Wahlgren NG. 1997. Pharmacological treatment of acute stroke. *Cerebrovasc Dis* **7**(Suppl 3):24–30.

Weir B. 1984. Calcium antagonist, cerebral ischemia and vasospasm. *Can J Neurol Sci* **11**:239–41.

Whelton PK, He J, Cuttler JA, et al. 1997. Effects of oral potassium on blood pressure. *JAMA* **277**:1624–32.

Wolf PA, Belanger AJ, D'Agostino RB. 1992. Management of risk factors. *Neurol Clin* **10**:177–92.

Wolf PA, D'Agostino RB, Kannel WB, et al. 1988. Cigarette smoking as a risk factor for stroke: the Framingham Study. *JAMA* **259**:1025–9.

Wolf PA, Kannel WB, Meeks SL, et al. 1985. Fibrinogen as a risk factor for stroke, the Framingham study. *Stroke* **16**: 139–43.

# Parkinson's Disease

David J. Coffey

*Chapter Outline*



## UNDERLYING PATHOPHYSIOLOGY

Parkinson's disease, first described by James Parkinson in 1817 in his *Essay on the Shaking Palsy*, is a chronic, progressive neurologic disease with its diagnosis based on the clinical triad of akinesia/bradykinesia, rigidity, and tremor (Parkinson 1817). All of the other clinical features including postural instability, shuffling gait, reduced eye-blink rate, paucity of facial expression, flexion posture, drooling, micrographia, and so forth, may be useful in suspecting the condition, but are probably related to the basic clinical triad.

The pathophysiologic basis of Parkinson's disease relates to dysfunction of the pathways connecting the substantia nigra with the corpus striatum. Symptoms begin after the loss of 80% or more of the cells of the substantia nigra (pars compacta) and the tonic inhibition they normally provide to the striatum. In idiopathic Parkinson's disease, this loss of cells possibly occurs as a result of oxidative stress due to environmental toxins (as yet unidentified) in persons who are somehow susceptible. Susceptibility may have some relation to inheritance (possibly mitochondrial) but does not follow typical mendelian patterns in most cases.

There are a number of conditions that mimic Parkinson's disease and are loosely grouped in the category of "parkinsonian syndromes." These include several naturally occurring diseases of uncertain etiology that have parkinsonian features in addition to other symptoms and signs not usually found in Parkinson's disease (hence, "Parkinson-plus syndromes"). A number of toxins can cause parkinsonian syndrome, most notably conventional antipsychotic agents and antiemetics, especially those of the phenothiazine and butyrophenone classes (e.g., metoclopramide, prochlorperazine, haloperidol) (Table 7-25).

WARNING The neuroleptic-induced symptoms of a slight "masked" facies, stiffness of the trunk and limbs, lack of arm swing, tremor of the hands, and mumbling speech are often mistaken for Parkinson's disease, rather than being recognized as a common adverse drug reaction.

## PHARMACOTHERAPY OPTIONS

In general, Parkinson's disease is improved by agents that oppose acetylcholine action or promote dopamine action at CNS receptors. As long ago as the latter part of the nineteenth century, Orderstein and Charcot described remedies for Parkinson's disease that were herbal extracts containing scopolamine and hyoscine, now recognized to be anticholinergic in nature (Orderstein 1867; Charcot 1872–3). Since the middle of the twentieth century, synthetic anticholinergic agents have been available and have been beneficial in management of the rigidity and tremor of Parkinson's disease. Akinesia/bradykinesia are most often the most disabling symptoms of the disease, however, and it was not until the introduction of treatment with levodopa (a precursor of dopamine capable of crossing the blood–brain barrier) that these symptoms could be largely controlled.

The doses of levodopa (L-dopa) required to reverse bradykinesia also caused significant peripheral side effects such as hypotension and nausea. In the early 1970s, it was demonstrated that peripheral conversion of L-dopa to dopamine could be inhibited by carbidopa, allowing smaller doses of L-dopa to achieve effective treatment of symptoms (Cotzias et al. 1967; Papavasiliou et al. 1972).

**PRINCIPLE The primary treatment strategy for Parkinson's disease has focused on restoring the normal balance between dopaminergic and cholinergic neurotransmission within the CNS.**

**Table 7-25 Classification of Parkinsonism**

| PRIMARY (IDIOPATHIC) PARKINSONISM, OR PARKINSON'S DISEASE | SECONDARY (ACQUIRED, SYMPTOMATIC) PARKINSONISM |
|---|---|
| Multiple-system degeneration | |
| ("parkinsonism plus") | Infectious |
| Progressive supranuclear palsy (PSP) | Postencephalitic |
| Multiple-system atrophy (MSA) | AIDS related |
| Striatonigral degeneration | Subacute sclerosing panencephalitis related |
| Olivopontocerebellar atrophy | Creutzfeldt–Jacob disease related |
| Shy–Drager syndrome | Prion diseases related |
| Lytico–Bodig syndrome | Drug-induced |
| (parkinsonism-dementia-ALS complex) | Dopamine receptor blockers |
| Corticobasal ganglionic degeneration | (e.g., antipsychotics, antiemetics) |
| Progressive pallidal atrophy | Reserpine |
| Parkinsonism-dementia complex | Tetrabenazine |
| Autosomal-dominant Lewy body disease | $\alpha$-Methyldopa |
| Diffuse (cortical) Lewy body disease | Lithium |
| Pick's disease | Flunarizine |
| | Cinnarizine |
| | Toxin-induced (agent) |
| | MPTP |
| | Carbon monoxide |
| | Manganese |
| | Mercury |
| | Carbon disulfide |
| | Cyanide |
| | Methanol |
| | Ethanol |
| | Vascular |
| | Multi-infarct |
| | Trauma |
| | Pugilistic encephalopathy |
| | Other |
| | Parathyroid abnormalities |
| | Hypothyroidism |
| | Hepatocerebral degeneration |
| | Brain tumor |
| | Normal-pressure hydrocephalus |
| | Noncommunicating hydrocephalus |
| | Syringomesencephalia |

Adapted from Jankovic 1997.
ABBREVIATIONS: ALS, amyotrophic lateral sclerosis; MPTP, 1-methyl-4-phenyl-1,2,3,6-tetrahydropyridine.

The combined use of carbidopa-levodopa (CD-LD) remains the central treatment for Parkinson's disease, though other adjunctive treatments have been developed. A useful way to categorize pharmacologic therapies is to divide them into "symptomatic" versus "neuroprotective" treatments. At present, most if not all strategies are symptomatic, but hope for neuroprotective agents is high. The basis of this hope began with the tragic discovery that self-administered MPTP (*N*-methyl-4-phenyl-1,2,3,6-tetrahydropyridine), a synthetic congener of meperidine used by drug abusers, caused a number of young people to develop all the symptoms of advanced Parkinson's disease. Once injected, MPTP is converted by a person's own monoamine oxidase, type B (MAO-B) into $MPP^+$, a positively charged and highly reactive ion that is specifically toxic to dopamine-producing cells in the pars compacta of the substantia nigra. Subsequent research has shown that pretreatment with the MAO inhibitors selegiline (deprenyl or Eldepryl) can prevent this toxicity. It became clear that environmental toxins can cause Parkinson's disease, and therefore, preventative strategies of neuroprotection might be clinically useful (Heikkila et al. 1983; Langston et al. 1983).

**PRINCIPLE By causing disease, drugs or xenobiotics may tell us much about pathophysiology or may allow new models of disease to be developed with which to evaluate new therapeutic agents. The discovery of unexpected toxicity of drugs or chemicals may prove useful to the prepared observer.**

## Dopaminergic Agonists

Study of the pharmacology of dopamine has led to a much more detailed appreciation of the complex receptors involved. No fewer than five classes of dopamine receptor are now recognized, and they have been cloned. All five classes comprise only two types, $D_1$ and $D_2$, depending on which population of striatal cells they stimulate and whether they increase or decrease (respectively) cAMP. $D_1$-type receptors are concentrated in striatal cells, whereas $D_2$-type receptors are concentrated in matrix. The $D_1$-type receptors constitute the direct output pathway, while $D_2$-type receptors constitute the indirect output pathway.

The five subtypes of dopamine receptors are designated by subscript numerals. $D_1$ (also called $D_{1a}$) and $D_5$ are of the $D_1$-type, while $D_2$, $D_3$, and $D_4$ are of the $D_2$-type. Dopamine normally stimulates the $D_2$ neurons of the indirect pathway and inhibits the $D_1$ neurons of the direct pathway. If striatal dopamine is depleted, as in Parkinson's disease, both pathways are affected. The direct pathway is underactive, and the indirect pathway is overactive. It is hoped that further study will lead to development of agents that specifically affect those receptor subtypes that yield beneficial effects and not those that lead to adverse effects (Seeman and Van Tol 1994; Uitti and Ahlskog 1996).

### L-*Dopa*

The mainstay therapy for Parkinson's disease is dopamine replacement via levodopa. Levodopa given orally is absorbed into the bloodstream and enters the brain via the large, ventral amino-acid transport systems. These transport systems can theoretically transport less levodopa if competitively inhibited by dietary protein, and fluctuations in dietary protein intake may be the cause of otherwise unpredictable changes in motor ability in patients receiving L-dopa (Carter et al. 1989).

**PRINCIPLE Interactions between dietary components and drugs are frequent and can alter a drug's efficacy or toxicity. Such drug–nutrient interactions are becoming recognized more frequently.**

Once absorbed, levodopa can be metabolized either in blood or brain by two different enzymatic pathways. L-Dopa is either converted by decarboxylase (AAAD, aromatic L-amino acid decarboxylase) to dopamine, or by catechol-*O*-methyltransferase (COMT) to 3-*O*-methyldopa. Dopamine, in turn, is degraded either by COMT to 3-*O*-methyltyramine, which is then metabolized to homovanillic acid by monoamine oxidase, or dopamine may be directly converted by monoamine oxidase to 3,4-dihydroxyphenylacetic acid (Figure 7-3). Each of these metabolic pathways has been manipulated in the effort to manage Parkinson's disease.

**PRINCIPLE A drug's selectivity of action, and even its therapeutic index, may be modulated by using knowledge of the drug's metabolic pathways to design specific inhibitors of biotransformation reactions. Such exploitation of a drug's biotransformation is yet another way in which knowledge of a drug's pharmacokinetic properties is essential to the practice of rational therapeutics.**

### *Carbidopa*

As mentioned earlier, carbidopa (CD) administered in combination with levodopa (LD) in varying proportions can make more dopamine available to the brain by inhibiting peripheral activity of AAAD. CD-LD combination products (Sinemet) are available as 10/100 mg, 25/100 mg, or 25/250 mg formulations. To achieve optimal inhibition of AAAD, a daily minimum of 60–75 mg of CD is recommended in any combination regime with LD.

### *Long-acting levodopa preparations*

For several years, CD-LD has been available in a slowly dissolving matrix that allows rate-controlled dissolution and absorption. The original effect was to prolong the duration of effective plasma concentrations. Consequently, some patients have fewer "peak effect" dyskinesias and may also benefit from less "wearing off" effect. The main drawback of these formulations is longer latency to "on" effect and somewhat lower overall plasma concentration. Sometimes a combination of regular and long-acting preparations will achieve a more desirable ef-

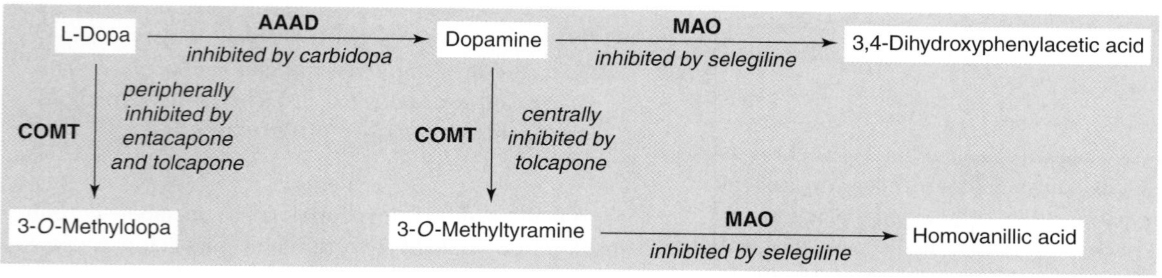


**FIGURE 7-3 Metabolism of levodopa either in blood or brain by two different enzymatic pathways. L-Dopa is either converted by decarboxylase in the form of aromatic L-amino acid decarboxylase (AAAD) to dopamine, or by catechol-*O*-methyltransferase (COMT) to 3-*O*-methyldopa. Dopamine in turn is metabolized to by COMT to 3-*O*-methyltyramine and then to homovanillic acid by monoamine oxidase, or dopamine may be directly converted by monoamine oxidase to 3,4-dihydroxyphenylacetic acid. Effects of pharmaceuticals are shown.**

fect. For reasons that are not clearly established, not all patients experience a smoothing out of motor fluctuations, regardless of approach.

***Direct-acting dopamine agonists***

Through the years, a number of pharmacologic agents have been developed that have the ability to penetrate the CNS and to stimulate the dopamine receptors directly. The original indication for their use was as adjunctive therapy to levodopa, but current practice sometimes calls for their use as monotherapy. Potential theoretical advantages of the direct-acting agents include the following: that they do not require enzymatic conversion, that they are stored and released by the degenerating neurons of the nigrostriatal system, and the possibility that direct-acting agents may be developed with the capability of stimulating receptor subtypes in a highly specific and effective way. By decreasing the overall amount of endogenous and exogenous dopamine turnover, there should be less autooxidation of dopamine into free radical byproducts that are potentially toxic.

However, for reasons not yet clear, currently available dopamine agonists simply have not worked as well as levodopa in monotherapy. Is this because they are only recently being recommended as initial treatment? This question may be answered in time, since the newer agents have been approved in monotherapy of newly diagnosed patients.

Currently available direct-acting agents are listed in Table 7-26 and include bromocriptine (Parlodel™), pergolide (Permax™), pramipexole (Mirapex™), and ropinirole (Requip™). Each of these compounds has unique specificities for interaction with different receptor subtypes. The ergot derivatives bromocriptine and pergolide have agonist activity at $D_2$ receptors, 5-$HT_1$ and 5-$HT_2$ receptors, and $\alpha_1$-adrenergic and $\alpha_2$-adrenergic receptors. Bromocriptine and pergolide also interact with $D_1$ receptors. Whereas bromocriptine is a $D_1$ antagonist, pergolide is a $D_1$ agonist. The newer non-ergoline agents ropinirole and pramipexole are more specific. Both bind with high affinity to $D_2$-like receptors (especially $D_3$ receptors) and have no affinity for $D_1$ receptors. Ropinirole has no appreciable affinity for serotonergic or adrenergic receptors. Pramipexole is very similar in that its primary effect is $D_2$-like (with strong affinity for $D_3$) and not $D_1$-like, but it has low-affinity binding to $\alpha_1$-adrenergic receptors, and has some affinity for the serotonin receptor 5-$HT_{1A}$ and histamine 2 ($H_2$) receptors. The receptor affinity profiles may translate into effects that are clinically important (Jankovic 1997; Watts 1997). For example, the agents

**Table 7-26 In Vitro Receptor Affinity of Direct-Acting Dopamine Agonists**

| | Receptor | | | | | |
|---|---|---|---|---|---|---|
| Dopamine Agonist | $D_2$ | $D_3$ | $D_1$ | 5-$HT_1$ | 5-$HT_2$ | $\alpha_1$-Adr |
| Ropinirole (Requip) | +++ | ++++ | 0 | 0 | 0 | 0 |
| Bromocriptine mesylate (Parlodel) | ++ | + | − | + | + | + |
| Pergolide mesylate (Permax) | +++ | ++++ | + | + | + | + |
| Pramipexole (Mirapex) | +++ | ++++ | + | 0 | 0 | 0 |

ABBREVIATIONS: $\alpha_1$-Adr, $\alpha_1$-adrenergic; $D_{1-3}$, dopamine; 5-HT, serotonin.

without $D_1$ agonist properties may have lower incidence of adverse side effects including hallucinations and dyskinesias. To date, however, studies directly comparing the different dopamine agonists have not been done. Nevertheless, the newer non-ergoline agents do not have the ergot-related potential side effects of erythromelalgia, burning dysesthesias, livedo reticularis, and pulmonary/retroperitoneal fibrosis (Tulloch 1997).

## Nondopaminergic Agents

A compilation of Parkinson's disease therapies, both dopaminergic agonists and nondopaminergic agents, is shown in Table 7-27.

***Amantadine***

Amantadine is a unique agent, which was developed initially as an antiviral agent in the 1960s, then coincidentally was shown to have antiparkinsonian effects later. To this date, the exact mechanism by which it works is uncertain; dopaminergic, anticholinergic, and even glutamate antagonistic properties have all been proposed. It has moderate efficacy and is given in doses per os (PO) of 100 mg bid to 100 mg tid. It may be used alone or in combination with other agents, particularly CD-LD. Amantadine is excreted renally and can accumulate in patients with azotemia. Ankle edema and livedo reticularis are common side effects.

***Anticholinergic agents***

A number of these agents are available. They were the first synthetically prepared drugs for treating Parkinson's disease and are more effective in treating tremor and rigidity than akinesia/bradykinesia. They are generally not as effective as dopaminergic agonists and often produce significant side effects, including dizziness, nausea, dry mouth, constipation, urinary retention, and pupillary dilation. When cognitive impairment is present, they also tend to worsen confusion, delirium, or hallucinations.

***Neuroprotective agents***

As previously mentioned, the first agent thought to be neuroprotective was selegiline (formerly deprenyl). While being used in eastern Europe as a marginally effective antidepressant, selegiline was found to slow or prevent progression in Parkinson's patients. This was rationalized to occur for several possible reasons.

1. It may contribute to general well-being because of its antidepressant properties.
2. It is metabolized to methamphetamine, which is stimulatory. (Amphetamines historically had been given to Parkinson's patients in the pre-levodopa era, with marginal success.)
3. It has histaminic effects.
4. It primarily acts as an inhibitor of MAO-B.

It is the last-mentioned possible mechanism of action that has drawn the most attention. Because selegiline has MAO-B specificity, it does not carry the risks of "tyramine effect" associated with general MAO-inhibiting drugs. More importantly, it has been shown to block MPTP toxicity to the substantia nigra, by preventing conversion of MPTP to the toxic oxidative metabolite $MPP^+$. This property of possible "neuroprotection" from highly oxidative toxic compounds led to several clinical trials in which selegiline, alone or in combination with levodopa, was associated with prolongation of time to disability (Parkinson Study Group 1989; Tetrud and Langston 1989). Questions still remain as to whether this delay of progression to disability is because of actual neuroprotective effects or is due to symptomatic improvement. Nonetheless, the idea that oxidative stress is of pivotal importance in the mechanism of nigral cell death has become central. It is possible that dopamine turnover itself is a source of oxidative stress, and that strategies to minimize dopamine turnover may slow progression. Such strategies may include the following:

- Use of selegiline PO 5 mg once or twice daily (higher doses may lead to loss of MAO-B specificity).
- Reduction of CD-LD total dose to the minimal effective dose.
- Possible early use of long-acting (slow-release) formulations of CD-LD if peak-dose effects can be minimized. Studies are currently under way to test this hypothesis.
- Early or concurrent use of direct-acting agonists to allow lower overall levodopa dosages.
- Possible use of COMT-inhibiting agents for the same purpose. It should be noted that COMT inhibitors may not actually be levodopa-sparing, since they increase the area under the time–plasma concentration curve (see below).
- Use of conventional antioxidants such as $\alpha$-tocopherol and ascorbic acid. While the efficacy of these agents in Parkinson's disease is unproven, they are safe and are often recommended for other indications as well.

***COMT inhibitors***

Inhibitors of catechol-*O*-methyl transferase are novel medications, intended specifically to block that enzyme's ability to metabolize levodopa and dopamine, both pe-

**Table 7-27 Drugs Used to Treat Parkinson's Disease**

| Class/Drug | Formulations | Typical Starting Dose or Maintenance Dose (md) | Average Wholesale Price[a] ($/Month of Therapy) | Comments |
|---|---|---|---|---|
| *Dopamine replacement* | | | | |
| Carbidopa-levodopa (CD-LD) | 10/100 mg<br>25/100 mg<br>25/250 mg | 25/100 mg tid | Generic $28<br>Sinemet $96<br>$129 | A minimum of 60–75 mg of CD is required each day to inhibit peripheral decarboxylase. |
| Long-acting CD-LD | 25/100<br>50/200 | 50/200 bid | Sinemet $73 | |
| *Direct-acting dopamine agonists* | | | | Slow, careful titration of these agents allows best balance of effect and side effects. |
| Ergot derivatives | | | | |
| Bromocriptine mesylate | 2.5, 5 mg | 1.25 mg bid | Generic $32<br>Parlodel $47 | |
| Pergolide mesylate | 0.05, 0.25, 1 mg | 1 mg tid (md) | Permax $318 | |
| Nonergoline drugs | | | | |
| Pramipexole | 0.125, 0.25, 1, 1.5 mg | NA | Mirapex $222 | |
| Ropinirole mesylate | 0.25, 0.5, 1,2,5 mg | NA | Requip $105 | |
| *Anticholinergic agents* | | | | More effective for tremor than for bradykinesia and rigidity; useful in young people to delay use of L-dopa. Elderly do not tolerate as well. |
| Benztropine mesylate | 0.5, 1, 2 mg | 1 mg qd | Generic $1 | |
| Biperiden HCl | 2 mg | 2 mg tid | Cogentin $6 | |
| Trihexyphenidyl HCl (benzhexol) | 2, 5 mg | 2 mg tid (md) | Akineton $23<br>Generic $5 | |
| Procyclidine HCl | 5 mg | 2.5 mg tid | Artane $14<br>Kemadrin $21 | |
| *Antiviral agent* | | | | |
| Amantadine | 100 mg | 100 mg bid | Generic $10<br>Symmetrel $51 | |
| *MAO-B inhibitor* | | | | |
| Selegiline HCl (deprenyl) | 5 mg | 5 mg bid | Eldepryl $188 | Doses >10 mg per day may cause loss of MAO-B selectivity. |
| *COMT inhibitors* | | | | |
| Entacapone | NA | NA | NA | Acts peripherally; still experimental. |
| Tolcapone | 100/200 mg | 100 mg PO tid | Tasmar $220 | Acts peripherally and centrally. |

[a]Source of drug prices is *Mosby's GenR*$_x$ 1998. Current prices may vary from those quoted, but comparative prices among products are expected to be similar. The reader should check on local prices at the time of prescribing.
ABBREVIATIONS: COMT, catechol-*O*-methyltransferase; MAO-B, monoamine oxidase, type B; md, maintenance dose; NA, not available.

ripherally and centrally. The net result should be to produce an increase in peripheral and central levodopa bioavailability, as well as a higher central dopamine concentration. The net effect of dopamine should be prolonged, with greater area under the curve after each due to L-dopa. It should be noted that, unlike direct-acting agonists, COMT inhibitors are not levodopa-sparing. In fact, they increase levodopa availability by increasing the plasma concentration-over-time curve of levodopa, without increasing the maximum concentration. In this way, they probably have an advantage over simply increasing the oral dose of levodopa (Mannisto 1994; Nutt et al. 1994). There are two COMT inhibitors that will likely soon be available, with slightly different properties.

Entacapone inhibits COMT peripherally in circulating erythrocytes, thereby allowing less levodopa to be converted to 3-*O*-methyldopamine in the plasma. Since it does not affect COMT in gut or liver, the first-pass effect on levodopa is not inhibited. Unlike carbidopa, entacapone does not increase maximum levodopa concentration, but slows its elimination peripherally. Entacapone's short half-life of 1.5–3.5 hours requires administering it with each levodopa dose. Entacapone has no central effect. It has been shown to improve motor fluctuations in patients treated with levodopa (Parkinson Study Group 1997).

Tolcapone, on the other hand, acts both centrally and peripherally. Tolcapone is given on a t.i.d. dosing schedule and inhibits not only the 3-*O*-methylation of levodopa in plasma, but also 3-*O*-methylation of dopamine in the brain. Theoretically, this combined action may be of further benefit than peripheral COMT inhibition alone, but this remains to be proven. Tolcapone has been shown to improve motor function in patients who exhibit a "wearing-off" phenomenon with levodopa treatment (Rajput et al. 1997).

In November 1998, after postmarketing surveillance revealed cases of acute fulminant liver failure (potentially fatal) in patients receiving tolcapone, the manufacturer of the drug issued a warning that appears in a black box on the official package insert. The warning (approved by the FDA) states that tolcapone should not be used by patients until there has been a complete discussion of the potential risks of using the drug, and the patient has provided written informed consent. The warning is accompanied by the suggestion that the medicine be discontinued in patients who show no apparent benefit, or who have clinical or laboratory evidence of liver disease. If the prescriber elects to use tolcapone in selected patients, a prescribed program of intensive monitoring of liver function is also recommended.

**PRINCIPLE This recent development with tolcapone reminds us that drugs are approved by the FDA with incomplete knowledge of the nature, severity, and incidence of rare adverse reactions. Physicians must be prepared to contribute to postmarketing adverse reaction surveillance systems (e.g., the MedWatch program organized by the FDA), and they must also be prepared to react appropriately when such new information becomes available.**

## GENERAL APPROACHES TO TREATMENT OF PARKINSON'S DISEASE

For many diseases, monotherapy results in optimal drug treatment, but in treating Parkinson's disease, combination therapy is usually more valuable. The typical patient who presents over the age of 60 has usually been aware of symptoms for several years and has sufficient signs to warrant a trial of treatment with CD-LD. Some practitioners advocate beginning treatment with long-acting CD-LD right away, either alone or in combination with prompt-release CD-LD. The dosing intervals and strengths should reflect the respective half-lives, initially, with adjustments based on the patient's subjective and objective responses.

Early on, diet may play a minimal role. Some patients find that taking food with the medicine minimizes the side effect of nausea, without an apparent detrimental effect on drug absorption. At later stages, dietary protein intake may be associated with reduced absorption of CD-LD as previously noted.

In special circumstances, such as when treating young patients who present with Parkinson's disease, levodopa replacement might be postponed in favor of a trial of treatment with either amantadine, a direct-acting dopamine agonist, or an anticholinergic agent. This last choice may be especially useful in tremor-predominant cases, since patients with tremor are more likely to benefit from anticholinergic agents than those with bradykinesia or rigidity. Some practitioners who accept the idea that selegiline can be neuroprotective might treat "early" Parkinson's disease with that agent in lieu of others, at least in the early phases of treatment. As noted above, the newer nonergoline, direct-acting dopamine agonists are approved for use as monotherapy in early disease.

Whether as monotherapy or in combination with relatively lowered doses of levodopa, the direct-acting dopamine agonists in general tend to allow lower dopamine turnover, of theoretical advantage in reducing end-organ injury by toxic dopamine metabolites. Selegiline also reduces the effective levodopa dose by 15–20% by decreasing dopamine's rate of turnover. It may be reasonable therefore, for some untreated patients to begin treatment with a combination of carbidopa-levodopa, another direct-acting dopamine agonist, and selegiline. One can rationalize that such a "cocktail" may afford synergistic activity, levodopa sparing, and neuroprotection.

The role for treatment with a COMT inhibitor in early Parkinson's disease has yet to be established. As noted above, these are not "levodopa-sparing" in the usual sense, but could conceivably allow a lower total daily dose of levodopa to be used.

While all of the same parameters for treatment must be considered in later stages, some special problems may develop. Five to 10 years into treatment, many patients develop a higher incidence of treatment-related adverse events, including peak-dose dyskinesias, "end-of-dose" phenomena, and unpredictable "on-off" fluctuations in motor performance. These effects are frustrating to patient and doctor alike, in part because it is often quite challenging to correct them. For one thing, it is sometimes hard to tell whether abrupt motor fluctuations are the result of the medication (thereby signaling a need to decrease doses), or a sign that medication dose needs to be increased. Empiric strategies include adding long-acting levodopa preparations, concomitant use of (or switching to) direct-acting agents, selegiline, and dietary manipulation.

At this stage, COMT inhibitors play an unknown role in treatment of late stages of Parkinson's disease, but could contribute to a smoothing of motor performance by prolonging effective plasma concentrations of levodopa and brain concentrations of dopamine.

## REFERENCES


Carter JH, Nutt JG, Woodward WR, et al. 1989. Amount and distribution of dietary protein affects clinical response to levodopa in Parkinson's disease. *Neurology* **39**:552–6.

Charcot JM. 1872–3. Leçons sur les maladies du système nerveux. Paris: Delahaye.

Cotzias GC, Van Woert MH, Shiffer L. 1967. Aromatic amino acids and modification of parkinsonism. *N Engl J Med* **276**:374–9.

Heikkila RE, Manzino L, Cabbat FS, et al. 1983. Protection against the dopaminergic neurotoxicity of 1-methyl-4-phenyl-1,2,3,6-tetrahydropyridine by monoamine oxidase inhibitors. *Nature* **311**:467–9.

Jankovic J. 1997. *Parkinson's Disease and Related Neurodegenerative Disorders*. Kalamazoo, MI: Pharmacia & Upjohn. p 36.

Langston JW, Ballard J, Tetrud J, et al. 1983. Chronic parkinsonism in humans due to a product of meperidine-analog synthesis. *Science* **219**:979–80.

Mannisto PK. 1994. Clinical potential of catechol-*O*-methyltransferase (COMT) inhibitors as adjuvants in Parkinson's disease. *CNS Drugs* **1**:172–9.

Nutt JG, Woodward WR, Beckner RM, et al. 1994. Effect of peripheral catechol-*O*-methyltransferase inhibition on the pharmacokinetics and pharmacodynamics of levodopa in parkinsonian patients. *Neurology* **44**:913–9.

Orderstein L. 1867. Sur la paralysie agitante et la sclérose en plaque généralisé. Doctoral thesis, Martinet, Paris.

Papavasiliou PS, Cotzias GC, Duby S, et al. 1972. Levodopa in parkinsonism: potentiation of central effects with a peripheral inhibitor. *N Engl J Med* **285**:8–14.

Parkinson J. 1817. *An Essay on the Shaking Palsy*. London: Whittingham and Rowland.

Parkinson Study Group. 1989. Effect of deprenyl on the progression of disability in early Parkinson's disease. *N Engl J Med* **321**: 1364–71.

Parkinson Study Group. 1997. Entacapone improves motor fluctuations in levodopa-treated Parkinson's disease patients. *Ann. Neurol* **42**:747–55.

Rajput AH, Martin W, Saint-Hilaire M, et al. 1997. Tolcapone improves motor function in parkinsonian patients with the "wearing off" phenomenon: a double-blind, placebo-controlled, multicenter trial. *Neurology* **49**:1066–71.

Seeman P, Van Tol HH. 1994. Dopamine receptor pharmacology. *Trends Pharmacol Sci* **15**:264–70.

Tetrud JW, Langston JW. 1989. The effect of deprenyl (selegiline) on the natural history of Parkinson's disease. *Science* **245**:519–22.

Tulloch IF. 1997. Pharmacologic profile of ropinirole: a non-ergoline dopamine agonist. *Neurology* **49**(Suppl.):S58–S62.

Uitti RJ, Ahlskog JE. 1996. Comparative review of dopamine receptor agonists in Parkinson's disease. *CNS Drugs* **5**:369–87.

Watts RL. 1997. The role of dopamine agonists in early Parkinson's disease. *Neurology* **49**(Suppl. 1):S34–S48.

# Dementia

Lawrence R. Jenkyn

### *Chapter Outline*



Until the penultimate decade of the twentieth century, no treatment existed for the cognitive symptoms of chronic degenerative brain failure (dementia). In the mid-1980s, pursuant to the previously identified cholinergic deficit in patients with dementia of the Alzheimer type (DAT), reports began to emerge about enhancement of central cholinergic neurotransmitter tone and associated improvement in cognitive function (short-term memory, judgment, insight, problem-solving, praxis, calculations, and language functions). Despite initial optimism, the hope that replacement therapy with a single neurotransmitter would significantly ameliorate cognitive decline in patients with DAT was met with unimpressive broad-spectrum clinical response. Nonetheless, the modest improvements in cognitive abilities in patients with DAT treated with a single agent (tacrine, see below) led to Federal Drug Administration (FDA) approval of this agent for routine clinical use.

Perhaps, the relative lack of efficacy of tacrine spurred more energetic investigation of neuropharmacologic intervention in DAT. The result has been a variety of different therapeutic approaches using polyneurotransmitter stimulants, antiamyloidogenic compounds, antioxidants, nerve growth factors, anti-inflammatory agents, and estrogen replacement therapy.

This era has also witnessed the development of an animal model for amyloid deposition in the brain and the recognition that DAT and other forms of chronic brain failure (CBF) have their origins decades in advance of clinical symptomatology. Noncognitive symptoms accompanying CBF are at least as problematic as the cognitive failure itself; these symptoms require their own forms of intervention.

Complicating the treatment of chronic brain failure is the recognition that clinical diagnosis is not perfectly accurate. Autopsy-proven accuracy rates for clinical diagnoses now approach 90%, up from 50% two decades ago (Rasmusson et al. 1996; Klatka et al. 1997). Physicians now understand that more than one form of chronic brain failure can exist in the same individual (i.e., DAT and vascular dementia) (Korczyn 1991); we lack clear-cut clinical diagnostic criteria for reliably diagnosing other forms of chronic brain failure [Pick's disease (Gearing et al. 1995), Lewy-body disease (Lippa et al. 1994), Parkinson–dementia complex (Geldmacher and Whitehouse 1997), frontal lobe dementia (Neary et al. 1988), etc.]; and even within a particular form of CBF, there are likely to be both clinical and biological heterogeneity resulting in varied presentations.

With these caveats in mind, this chapter will review the currently approved treatments for cognitive symptoms related to DAT, summarize known neuropharmacologic data regarding treatment of noncognitive symptoms from CBF in general, review the extant data concerning primary prevention therapy, and briefly indicate current lines of investigation and the status of unapproved treatments.

## APPROVED TREATMENT FOR COGNITIVE FAILURE IN DEMENTIA OF THE ALZHEIMER TYPE

### The Cholinergic Hypothesis

With the recognition that atherosclerosis of the cerebral vasculature is not the primary cause of cognitive decline in late life (Tomlinson and Blessed 1970), and with the dramatic improvement in motor deficits in patients with Parkinson's disease given single neurotransmitter replacement therapy, neuroscientists of the last quarter of the twentieth century began looking for a similar neurotransmitter deficit in DAT (Perry and Tomlinson 1978). Decreased cholineacetyltransferase (ChAT) activity in the cortex of patients with dementia of the Alzheimer type, cholinergic cell loss in the nucleus basalis of Meynert, the correlation of nucleus basalis cholinergic cell loss with ChAT decline and with neuritic plaque counts, the presence of ChAT and acetylcholinesterase (AChE) in neuritic plaques and neurofibrillar tangles (the acknowledged microscopic correlates of DAT), and the correlation of the severity of dementia with ChAT levels in temporal and parietal cortex and hippocampus in patients with DAT were all observations that supported the hypothesis that replacement of acetylcholine in the cortex of these patients might be useful ("the cholinergic hypothesis") (Mayeux 1990).

Further evidence in favor of the cholinergic hypothesis included the observation that a postsynaptic cholinergic muscarinic blocker (scopolamine) induced memory impairment for new learning in normal human volunteers (Petersen 1977), and that this "scopolamine effect" was antagonized by physostigmine, a centrally active inhibitor of acetylcholinesterase (Drachman and Leavitt 1974). Acetylcholine precursor loading with oral choline (Cohen and Wurtman 1976), lecithin (Bartus et al. 1982), or acetyl-L-carnitine (Passeri et al. 1988) resulted in some observed positive effects in 10 of 43 studies, although these were mostly in areas of noncognitive function (Gershon et al. 1990). Potentially as useful were acetylcholine releasers (4-aminopyridine, 4,5-diaminopyridine, linopirdine), which were poorly studied because of dose-limiting adverse effects (Gibson and Manger 1988); cholinergic agonists (intravenous arecoline [Christie et al. 1981], intraventricular bethanechol [Harbaugh et al. 1984]); with intraventricular therapy undergoing rigorous trial and found to be of no benefit (Penn et al. 1988); and inhibition of acetylcholinesterase within the central nervous system (intravenous or oral physostigmine, intravenous or oral tacrine), with 20 of 33 studies reporting modest positive effects on cognition (Holttum and Gershon 1992).

Poor gastrointestinal absorption and rapid metabolism of physostigmine precluded its use (although current formulations under study have partially surmounted these difficulties); tacrine was the first drug approved by the FDA for this indication.

## Tacrine

This medication was investigated in a number of pilot studies beginning in 1981; an open label trial of 12 patients receiving tacrine found that patients with mild-to-moderate cognitive deficits improved on orientation tasks, but those with severe deficits did not respond at all (Summers et al. 1981). In a single-blind, placebo-controlled trial of tacrine plus lecithin, 5 of 10 subjects improved on the Serial Learning Test, but no such improvement was noted when tacrine was used alone (Kaye et al. 1982). No improvement in free-recall or prompted-recall tasks was observed, however.

In another small prospective trial, 15 subjects receiving tacrine and lecithin showed significant response rates to measures of cognitive function, with decline to baseline levels of cognitive dysfunction in each case when treatment was discontinued (Summers et al. 1986). Subsequent criticism of this clinical trial included the exclusion of 6 of the 23 subjects entered from data analysis because of lack of dementia, the use of scales of cognitive function that were not in common practice or well-validated, the lack of definition of possibly confounding concurrent medications, and lack of a placebo effect (Chatellier et al. 1991). An inspection of the raw data by the FDA indicated that there was no documentation of randomization of the subjects, there was no consistent record of treatment as received by the subject, blinding was not maintained throughout the study, and global ratings of cognitive dysfunction were not recorded while the study was being conducted. The FDA inspection concluded, "at best, we consider the evidence to be the equivalent of uncontrolled, anecdotal clinical information" (FDA 1991). Nonetheless, considerable pressure was exerted to confirm the results, and seven clinical trials were reported in the early 1990s, one of which was deemed pivotal in achieving FDA approval for marketing of tacrine for patients with DAT (*Valley News* 1993).

Chatellier et al. in 1990 found no effect of tacrine on the Mini-Mental State Examination (MMSE) or the Mattis Dementia Rating Scale (DRS) scores in 67 subjects. In this study, 33% experienced nausea and/or vomiting, and 9 of 67 subjects developed significantly elevated liver function tests (LFTs) (Chatellier and Lacomblez 1990). Soon after, in 1991, Molloy et al. entered 34 subjects into a double-blind, placebo-controlled trial of tacrine at 50–100 mg/day, and observed no improvement in measures of cognition. Fourteen of 34 subjects experienced significant hepatotoxicity.

The Canadian Tacrine Study tested tacrine doses less than or equal to 100 mg/day (after titration to the maximum tolerated dose) versus placebo (Gauthier et al. 1990). Fifty-two were enrolled, and 39 with moderate cognitive dysfunction (stages 4–5 on the Global Deterioration Scale of Reisburg et al. [1982]) completed the study. Subjects were maintained on lecithin (4.7 g/day) throughout and were followed for 8 weeks each on either tacrine or placebo, serving as their own controls in a crossover trial with 4-week washout intervals preceding each 8-week treatment interval. Outcome measures included the MMSE, the Modified Mini-Mental State Examination (MMMSE), the Rapid Disability Rating Scale II, Behavioral Scale of Alzheimer's Disease, and the Hierarchic Dementia Scale. Those subjects completing the crossover trial had improvement on their MMSE score of 1.2 points (4%, $P = 0.03$) when they took tacrine compared with placebo. All other cognitive, functional, and behavioral scales showed no significant changes. Thirty-six percent of subjects suffered autonomic dysfunction (abdominal cramps, nausea, vomiting, diarrhea), with 17% experiencing LFT elevations. The investigators concluded that there was no clinically significant beneficial effect from tacrine for these DAT patients overall. This study was criticized for not having an untreated control group, for the possible obscuration of a tacrine effect by lecithin, and for the fact that even a minimally positive result should have been viewed more favorably given the insensitive screening instruments and cognitive scales utilized (Schneider 1990).

One year later, Eagger et al. (1991) reported on 65 subjects who completed a protocol employing titration to a maximum tolerated dose of less than or equal to 150 mg/day. Subjects were then subsequently offered two 13-week double-blind treatment intervals, each after a 4-week washout. In the first treatment period, the subjects were randomized to receive tacrine and lecithin (10.8 g/day) together or placebo. In the second, subjects were randomized to receive tacrine and placebo or lecithin and placebo. Outcome measures included the MMSE, the Abbreviated Mental Test score, and the Activities of Daily Living Scale. The expected decline in the MMSE score is 3 points/year in patients with DAT. In this study, 45% of patients receiving tacrine increased their MMSE score by 3 or more points, whereas only 11% of patients receiving placebo had the same 3-point or more increase ($P < 0.0001$). No effect of lecithin was observed. Improvement was noted on abilities to perform simple tasks and on perceptual, attentional, and executive functions. Memory functions were unimproved. Seventy-two percent of subjects experienced nausea, diarrhea, or vomiting, and 46% registered elevations of their LFTs. This study was criticized for a lack of parallel forms for repeated MMSEs and for several problems with the MMSE: that it was not designed as a measure of change, that it unduly weights measures of speech and praxis, and that it contains only two questions that assess memory function (Eagger et al. 1991).

In 1992, Farlow et al. reported for the Tacrine Study Group (TSG) on 273 subjects who completed a 12-week, double-blind study, which utilized the Alzheimer's Disease Assessment Scale-Cognitive subscale (ADAS-Cog) score, and the Clinical Global Impression of Change (CGIC). The ADAS is a multi-item test battery administered by a psychometrician that examines the areas of memory, attention, praxis, reason, and language (Rosen et al. 1984). It is based on a 115-point scale, 70 of which are cognitive and 45 of which are behavioral points. The CGIC has a 7-point scale, where a score of 3 means no change, a score of 1 means maximum improvement, and a score of 7 means maximum deterioration. The ADAS is expected to decline 7–8 points/year in patients with DAT. In this trial, the primary outcome measure (ADAS-Cog) showed a 2.8-point improvement during the treatment period compared with placebo ($P = 0.015$), with a slight improvement (3.4) in the CGIC ($P = 0.015$). These two statistically significant outcomes favoring tacrine were noted only at the high dosage (80 mg/day). Three secondary outcome measures were also analyzed. The total ADAS score (cognitive plus behavioral) achieved 3.7-point improvement for the tacrine-treated subjects ($P = 0.029$) and the Caregiver-CGIC (CG-CGIC) score improved to 3.5 ($P = 0.028$), again for the 80-mg dose only. The MMSE score was designated a secondary outcome measure and was not significantly different for treated and control subjects. Only 8% of subjects experienced nausea, vomiting, diarrhea, or abdominal pain. Fifty-one percent had elevation of LFTs (25% had alanine transaminase [ALT] or aspartate transaminase [AST] greater than or equal to three times normal). The conclusion of the TSG was that an 80-mg dose of tacrine produced a 6-month gain in cognitive performance, and that weekly testing of LFTs was necessary for those using this medication.

Davis et al. reported in the same year (1992) for the Tacrine Collaborative Study Group (TCSG), a different set of investigators from the TSG, a study of 215 subjects entered into a double-blind, placebo-controlled trial. Study subjects admitted with MMSE scores between 10 and 23 were titrated to best maximum dose of 10 or 20 mg qid over 6 weeks. This was followed by a 2-week washout interval, a 6-week double-blind interval, and a 6-week open-label phase. The TCSG utilized the ADAS as its primary outcome measure. For the duration of this study, a 3-point decline in the ADAS would have been expected for untreated study subjects. Only a 0.7-point decline was noted and was equated to a 5-month gain in performance for those receiving tacrine compared with placebo (equated to nearly three more words recalled from a list of ten, and nearly three more simple commands followed properly). Forty-two percent of patients experienced elevated LFTs (21% had alanine transaminase [ALT] or aspartate transaminase [AST] greater than or equal to three times normal). The TCSG concluded that tacrine may slow the progression of DAT as measured by the ADAS, but that this was not paralleled by improvement recorded by clinicians or caregivers.

Finally, the Tacrine Study Group-II (TSG-II) reported a study of 263 subjects completing a 30-week trial (Knapp et al. 1994). There were three treatment groups and one placebo-control group. The treatment groups were titrated upward from 40 mg/day to 80 mg, 120 mg, and 160 mg per day, respectively. Outcome measures included the ADAS-Cog, the Clinician Information-Based Impression (CIBI), and the Final Comprehension Consensus Assessment (FCCA). A 4-point or better improvement in the ADAS-Cog score was noted in 40% of subjects receiving 160 mg/day compared with 25% receiving placebo ($P = 0.2$), while the CIBI and FCCA scores both improved 42% in patients receiving the same dose ($P = 0.001$). Secondary outcome measures showed improvement as well including the total ADAS score ($P = 0.001$) and the CG-CGIC score ($P = 0.011$) for groups given 80 mg or more per day, whereas improvement in the MMSE score was observed as a secondary outcome measure for the group given 160 mg/day dose only ($P < 0.001$). Conclusions of the TSG-II were that tacrine had demonstrable efficacy for doses up to 160 mg/day, that as many as 40% of subjects may be "responders," and that this response appeared dose-dependent. Adverse effects paralleled the results of the 12-week TSG trial.

Reasons for discrepancies among these clinical trials of tacrine in patients with DAT may include lack of randomized control groups, lack of washout intervals sufficient to prevent carryover effects from best-dose-finding treatment intervals, differing outcome measures, diagnostic inaccuracy regarding the state of enrolled subjects, the heterogeneity of DAT, variable drug dosing, the effects of concomitant medications, variable use of measuring plasma concentrations of tacrine, and the presence or absence of dose titration to optimal dose.

Tacrine is a rapidly absorbed acridine derivative primarily cleared by hepatic transformation with an oral bioavailability of 2 to 3%, a 3.6-hour half-life, and a brain/plasma concentration ratio of 10:1. Depending on the study, 32 to 80% of patients experience cholinergic-mediated adverse effects, and 40% experience sufficient elevations of the liver enzymes AST and ALT (up to 3–5 times normal) to require discontinuation of the medication. Of interest is the lack of recurrent hepatotoxicity on re-exposure in most subjects. Biochemical evidence or hepatitis injury is generally reversible. Nonetheless, ALT and AST levels should be measured biweekly for 16 weeks beginning 4 weeks after treatment is initiated, then monthly for 2 months, then every 3 months thereafter (Tariot 1997). Overall, when nonresponders and those who must drop the medication because of adverse events are included, the clinical response rate in DAT approaches 30%.

In summary, tacrine represents an interesting "first generation" drug limited by a narrow therapeutic spectrum of efficacy given its cost, adverse events (especially cholinergic excess and hepatotoxicity), and short half-life (which must affect compliance with four times per day dosing). With newer, less toxic cholinesterase inhibitors available, it has become a second-line drug for use in those cases in which other medications are ineffective or poorly tolerated, but in patients for whom a cholinergic inhibitor has proved helpful.

## Donepezil

Donepezil, a highly selective centrally active cholinesterase inhibitor with minimal peripheral effects, is potentially useful in subjects with DAT (Rogers and Friedhoff 1996). In a multicenter, double-blind, placebo-controlled, parallel-group design, the investigators subsequently randomized subjects to one of three treatment groups (1, 3, or 5 mg) or placebo, dosed once daily for 12 weeks (Rogers et al. 1996). The primary outcome measures were the ADAS-Cog and the CGIC. Improved ADAS-Cog scores in the 5 mg/day treatment group were observed, as opposed to declining scores in the placebo group. The trial also confirmed a statistically significant 50% relative reduction in clinical deterioration on 5 mg/day (11%) relative to placebo (20%). Adverse events were similar in treatment and control groups, but no adverse events were observed in hematologic tests or clinical biochemistry (Rogers and Friedhoff 1996). Subsequent 15-week and 30-week randomized trials utilizing the same outcome measures showed similar benefits and adverse effects at doses of 5 or 10 mg/day, with a trend toward a greater treatment effect with the 10-mg dose (Rogers et al 1996).

Donepezil is a piperidine-derivative compound cleared by both hepatic and renal mechanisms with selective activity for central nervous system AChE. Its long duration of action (half-life: 70 hours) allows once-daily dosing, and the absence of hepatotoxicity at dosages of 5 or 10 mg/day, have made it the cholinesterase inhibitor of choice for DAT at present.

Abrupt discontinuation of the drug, however, may be accompanied by a rapid decline in cognitive function. Donepezil is currently indicated for mild to moderate degrees of cognitive impairment in patients with DAT but can be offered in selected more severe cases. Its cost, lack of established efficacy in severe cognitive decline, and possibility of prolonging a hopeless circumstance makes its routine use in severely impaired patients unwarranted.

### On The Horizon

Although unapproved for clinical use at the time of this writing, three other centrally active cholinesterase inhibitors (metrifonate, rivastigmine, galanthamine) have shown preliminary efficacy similar to tacrine and donepezil in patients with DAT. The essential features of the two approved and three experimental cholinesterase inhibitors are described in Table 7-28.

## OTHER DRUGS USED TO SLOW PROGRESSION OF DEMENTIA OF THE ALZHEIMER TYPE

The results of a 2-year, placebo-controlled, prospective clinical trial of the effect have been reported of vitamin E and selegiline (a selective monamine oxidase inhibitor) in patients with DAT (Sano et al. 1997). Primary outcome measures included nursing home placement, progression to stage 3 of the Clinical Dementia Rating Scale (CDR), decline in self-care ability, and death. Results showed that either selegiline or vitamin E delayed functional decline by approximately 8 months but, curiously, the combination of the two agents together did not. In this study, the dosage of vitamin E used was 2000 mg/day, quite a bit greater than the typical oral supplement of 400 mg/day.

In addition to its modest effects on cognition, high-dose tacrine (160 mg/day) has been shown to delay nursing home placement when compared with low-dose sustained therapy (Knopman et al. 1996).

## TREATMENT OF NONCOGNITIVE SYMPTOMS IN CHRONIC BRAIN FAILURE

Perhaps more distressing to caregivers of individuals with CBF are the noncognitive symptoms that patients develop. They rob them of their individuality and often cause considerable emotional upset in those around them. Behavior impairment; alterations of mood, perception, and beliefs; and disintegration of the activities of daily living very often are the triggers for family discord, nursing home placement, and subsequent financial impoverishment (Folstein and Bylsma 1994).

Depression is noted in 15 to 20% of patients with DAT in the early stages, and reactive dysphoria (so called grief reaction) may be observed in about 90% of patients when they first become impaired and are still able to be cognizant of their deficit. Anxiety, irritability, and phobias for behaviors such as bathing or changing clothes, as well as apathy are commonly observed. In the middle stages of the dementing disorder, patients may experience delusions, paranoia (someone is stealing a wallet or purse they misplaced, or a "phantom boarder" is living in their place of abode), or the Capgrass syndrome (which is a misidentification of, or failure to recognize familiar faces).

**Table 7-28 Cholinesterase Inhibitors for Dementia of the Alzheimer Type**

| DRUG | DOSE | NAME | AWP ($/MONTH) | ADVANTAGES | CAUTIONS |
|---|---|---|---|---|---|
| Tacrine HCl | 10 mg qid | Cognex | $120 | | Careful monitoring of ALT, AST required |
| | 20 mg qid | | $120 | | |
| | 30 mg qid | | $120 | | |
| | 40 mg qid | | $120 | | |
| Donepezil HCl | 5 mg qd | Aricept | $122 | Once/day dosing, lack of hepatotoxicity | |
| | 10 mg qd | | $122 | Selective for CNS cholinesterase | |
| Rivastigmine | N/A | Excelon | N/A | Selective for CNS cholinesterase | Still under development |
| Metrifonate | N/A | Promem | N/A | Selective for CNS cholinesterase | Still under development |
| Galantamine | N/A | Reminyl | N/A | Selective for CNS cholinesterase | Still under development |

ABBREVIATIONS: ALT, alanine transaminase; AST, aspartate transaminase; AWP, average wholesale price; N/A, not applicable.
Source of drug prices is *Mosby's GenR$_x$* 1998. Current prices may vary from those quoted, but comparative prices among products are expected to be similar. The reader should check on local prices at the time of prescribing.

Hallucinations, usually visual and nonthreatening, are noted in the later stages in 15–30% of cases. Auditory hallucinations are uncommon.

Other unwanted behaviors including overactivity, disruptiveness, perseveration of motor acts, verbal aggression, sleep disorder, wandering, physical aggression, and urinary incontinence, may be secondary to the primary dementing condition or some underlying medical disorder (Folstein and Bylsma 1994). Depression in the early stages, and acute confusional state (delirium) from medication, hypoxemia, infection (pneumonia, urinary tract infection), or anemia need to be identified and treated when present. Once target symptoms are identified and caregivers are educated to observe for an associated pattern that leads to aberrant behavioral expression, neuropharmacologic intervention may be necessary. In general, optimal treatment includes selection of an appropriate drug, using the lowest dose possible, and being vigilant for the development of adverse effects (Rabins 1994).

**PRINCIPLE Different drugs in the same class may have different profiles of adverse effects. These differences can, and should be, consciously exploited by the careful physician.**

Neuroleptic drugs are commonly used to treat patients with behavioral problems (see Table 7-29). In a meta-analysis of 20 double-blind, placebo-controlled studies between 1954 and 1986, it was reported that 60% of subjects evidenced some improvement when treated with neuroleptic medications (Sunderland and Silver 1988). Expected adverse effects of sedation, extrapyramidal movement disorders, orthostatic hypotension, and anticholinergic adverse effects complicated therapy. Placebo effects in such trials approach 40%, and in view of that, only 18% of subjects in 34 double-blind, placebo-controlled trials between 1954 and 1989 improved when compared with patients given placebo (Schneider et al. 1990). Given the toxicity of neuroleptic drugs when used in this patient group (including greater risk of hip fracture), extreme attention to potential benefits and risks is necessary in individual patients.

Treatment of noncognitive symptoms with other classes of drugs has been poorly studied (Schneider and Sobin 1992). Lithium, propranolol, trazodone, carbamazepine, buspirone, and selegiline have all had some evidence of efficacy in small prospective studies. The selective serotonin reuptake inhibitors (fluoxetine, sertraline, paroxetine) have been reported to improve depression and to reduce anxiety and agitation in DAT. Tricyclic antidepressants including nortriptyline and imipramine and the novel antipsychotic agents had variable efficacy reported (Schneider 1993). Hallucinations in parkinsonian patients have responded to use of ondansetron, clozapine, and risperidone, but so far have not been reported to improve in patients with DAT or other forms of CBF. Their empiric use in these patients is expected given that they are approved for other indications. Their relative doses and costs are noted in Table 7-29.

## OTHER NEUROPHARMACOLOGIC INTERVENTIONS FOR CHRONIC BRAIN FAILURE

A review of the rationale for other forms of investigation in the area of neuropharmacologic intervention in CBF is beyond the scope of this chapter. Several recent reviews are available (Aisen and Davis 1997; Doody 1997; Knopman and Morris 1997). Therapeutic approaches include symptomatic treatment of cognitive and behavioral disturbances as described above, with enhanced medical management of systemic ailments and psychosocial intervention for caregivers. Other therapeutic avenues include slowing of symptom progression, prolonging time to symptom onset, and the prevention of disease expression altogether.

Interrupting deposition of amyloid $\beta$-protein or formation of neurofibrillatory tangles may serve these ends. There is growing evidence that estrogen replacement therapy may prove useful for some postmenopausal women in terms of improved cognitive function in general, and a possible prevention or delay of the expression of DAT in selected circumstances. Recognition that an inflammatory response accompanies the neuropathology of DAT has given rise to attempts to modify this process through the use of nonsteroidal anti-inflammatory medications and adrenocorticosteroids.

Antiexcitotoxins (including the benzodiazepines) and anti-apoptosis agents have been proposed. Outcomes of clinical trial with large numbers of subjects observed over long intervals are not yet available.

## FUTURE OUTLOOK

The notion that single or multiple neurotransmitter replacement therapy would reverse the clinical symptoms and signs of DAT and other dementias is waning in the face of limited efficacy as demonstrated in the trials re-

**Table 7-29 Common Neuroleptic Medications Used for Treating Noncognitive Symptoms in Patients with Dementia**

| CLASS | DRUG | USUAL DOSE | | AWP ($/MONTH) | ADVANTAGES | CAUTIONS |
|---|---|---|---|---|---|---|
| Traditional antipsychotics | Haloperidol | 0.5 mg bid | generic | $1 | Less sedating | Greater chance for EPS |
| | | 1 mg bid | Haldol | $24–$48 | | Tardive dyskinesia emerges with chronic use |
| | | 2 mg bid | | | | |
| | Thioridazine HCl | 10 mg tid | generic | $1–$3 | More sedating (for some) | Less chance for EPS |
| | | 25 mg tid | Mellaril | $10–$37 | | Greater chance for anticholinergic adverse effects |
| | | | | | | Tardive dyskinesia emerges with chronic use |
| Novel antipsychotics | Risperidone | 1 mg bid | Risperdal | $114 | Less risk of EPS | Expensive |
| | | 2 mg bid | | $189 | | |
| | | 3 mg bid | | $237 | | |
| | Olanzapine | 2.5 mg bid | Zyprexa | $95 | Less risk of EPS | Expensive |
| | | 5 mg bid | | $189 | | Little experience for this indication |
| | | 10 mg bid | | $464 | | |

ABBREVIATIONS: AWP, Average wholesale price; EPS, extrapyramidal symptoms.
Source of drug prices is *Mosby's GenR*$_x$ 1998. Current prices may vary from those quoted, but comparative prices among products are expected to be similar. The reader should check on local prices at the time of prescribing.

viewed in this chapter. With many new theoretical approaches to explore, the hope remains that improved cognition can be realized in the afflicted. Nonetheless, it will likely be primary prevention of neuronal cell loss through the understanding of the molecular biology of dementing diseases that will ultimately prove most meaningful to these potential patients and their caregivers.

## REFERENCES


Aisen PS, Davis KL. 1997. The search for disease-modifying treatment for Alzheimer's disease [review]. *Neurology* **48** (Suppl. 6):S35–S41.

Bartus RT, Dean RL, Beer B, et al. 1982. The cholinergic hypothesis of geriatric memory dysfunction. *Science* **217**:408–14.

Chatellier G, Lacomblez L, Derouesne C. 1991. Tetrahydroaminoacridine in Alzheimer's disease: a review of its safety and its effectiveness. *Dementia* **2**:200–6.

Chatellier G, Lacomblez L. 1990. Tacrine (tetrahydroaminoacridine; THA) and lecithin in senile dementia of the Alzheimer type: a multicentre trial. Groupe Française d'Etude de la Tetrahydroaminoacridine. *Br Med J* **300**:495–9.

Christie JE, Shering A, Ferguson J, et al. 1981. Physostigmine and arecoline: effects of intravenous infusions in Alzheimer presenile dementia. *Br J Psychiatry* **138**:46–50.

Cohen EL, Wurtman RJ. 1976. Brain acetylcholine: control by dietary choline. *Science* **191**:561–2.

Davis KL, Thal LJ, Gamzu ER. 1992. A double-blind, placebo-controlled multicenter study of tacrine for Alzheimer's disease. The Tacrine Collaborative Study Group. *N Engl J Med* **327**:1253–9.

Doody RS. 1997. Treatment of Alzheimer's disease. *Neurologist* **3**: 333–43.

Drachman DA, Leavitt J. 1974. Human memory and the cholinergic system: a relationship to aging? *Arch Neurol* **30**:113–21.

Eagger SA, Levy R, Sahakian BJ. 1991. Tacrine in Alzheimer's disease. *Lancet* **337**:989–92.

Farlow M, Gracon SI, Hershey LA. 1992. A controlled trial of tacrine in Alzheimer's disease. The Tacrine Study Group. *JAMA* **268**:2523–9.

Folstein MF, Bylsma FW. 1994. Noncognitive symptoms of Alzheimer's disease. In: Terry RD, Katman R, Bick KL, editors. *Alzheimer's Disease*. New York: Raven Press. p 27–40.

Food and Drug Administration [FDA]. 1991. Tacrine as a treatment for Alzheimer's dementia. An interim report from FDA. *N Engl J Med* **324**:349–52.

Gauthier S, Bouchard R, Lamontagne A. 1990. Tetrahydroaminoacridine-lecithin combination treatment in patients with intermediate-stage Alzheimer's disease. The Canadian Tacrine Study. *N Engl J Med* **322**:1272–6.

Gearing M, Schneider JA, Rebeck GW, et al. 1995. Alzheimer's disease with and without coexisting Parkinson's disease changes: apolipoprotein E genotype and neuropathologic correlates. *Neurology* **45**:1985–90.

Geldmacher DS, Whitehouse PJ. 1997. Differential diagnosis of Alzheimer's disease [review]. *Neurology* **48** (5 Suppl. 6):S2–9.

Gershon S, Wright B, Rosenberg DR. 1990. Potential treatment modalities for senile dementia of the Alzheimer's type. *Neurol Forum* **1**:2–4.

Gibson GE, Manger T. 1988. Changes in cytosolic free calcium with 1,2,3,4-tetrahydro-5-aminoacridine, 4-aminopyridine and 3,4-diaminopyridine. *Biochem Pharmacol* **37**:4191–6.

Harbaugh RE, Roberts DW, Coombs DW, et al. 1984. Preliminary report: intracranial cholinergic drug infusion in patients with Alzheimer's disease. *Neurosurgery* **15**:514–8.

Holttum JR, Gershon S. 1992. The cholinergic model of dementia, Alzheimer type: progression from the unitary transmitter concept. *Dementia* **3**:174–85.

Kaye WH, Sitaram N, Weingartner H, et al. 1982. Modest facilitation of memory in dementia with combined lecithin and anticholinesterase treatment. *Biol Psychiatry* **17**:275–80.

Klatka LA, Schiffer RB, Powers JM, et al. 1997. Incorrect diagnosis of Alzheimer's disease: a clinicopathologic study [review] *Arch Neurol* **53**:35–42.

Knapp MJ, Knopman DS, Solomon PR, et al. 1994. A 30-week randomized controlled trial of high-dose tacrine in patients with Alzheimer's disease. The Tacrine Study Group. *JAMA* **271**:985–91.

Knopman DS, Morris JC. 1997. An update on primary drug therapies for Alzheimer's disease. *Arch Neurol* **54**:1406–9.

Knopman DS, Schneider L, Davis KL, et al. 1996. Long-term tacrine (Cognex) treatment: effects on nursing home placement and mortality. *Neurology* **47**:166–77.

Korczyn AD. 1991. The clinical differential diagnosis of dementia: concepts and methodology [review]. *Psychiatr Clin North Am* **14**: 237–49.

Lippa CF, Smith TW, Sweare JM. 1994. Alzheimer's disease and Lewy bodies disease: a comparative clinicopathological study. *Neurology* **35**:81–8.

Mayeux R. 1990. Therapeutic strategies in Alzheimer's disease [review]. *Neurology* **40**:175–80.

Molloy DW, Guyatt GH, Wilson DB, et al. 1991. Effect of tetrahydroaminoacridine on cognition, function and behaviour in Alzheimer's disease. *Can Med Assoc J* **144**:29–34.

*Mosby's GenR$_x$* 1998. *Mosby's GenR$_x$ 1998: The Complete Reference for Generic and Brand Drugs.* 8th ed. St. Louis: Mosby–Year Book.

Neary D, Snowden JS, Northen B, et al. 1988. Dementia of the frontal lobe type. *J Neurol Neurosurg Psychiatry* **51**:353–61.

Passeri M, Iannuccelli M, Ciotti G, et al. 1988. Mental impairment in aging: selection of patients, methods of evaluation and therapeutic possibilities of acetyl-L-carnitine. *Int J Clin Pharmacol Res* **8**: 367–76.

Penn RD, Martin EM, Wilson RS, et al. 1988. Intraventricular bethanechol infusion for Alzheimer's disease: results of double-blind and escalating-dose trials. *Neurology* **38**:219–22.

Perry EK, Tomlinson BE, Blessed G, et al. 1978. Correlation of cholinergic abnormalities with senile plaques and mental test scores in senile dementia. *Br Med J* **2**:1457–9.

Petersen RC. 1977. Scopolamine induced learning failures in man. *Psychopharmacology (Berl.)* **52**:283–9.

Rabins PV. 1994. Noncognitive symptoms of Alzheimer's disease: definitions, treatments, and possible etiologies. In: Terry RD, Katman R, Bick KL, editors. *Alzheimer's Disease*. New York: Raven Press. p 419–29.

Rasmusson DX, Brandt J, Steele C, et al. 1996. Accuracy of clinical diagnosis of Alzheimer's disease and clinical features of patients with non-Alzheimer disease neuropathology. *Alzheimer Dis Assoc Disord* **10**:180–8.

Reisberg B, Ferris SH, de Leon MJ. 1982. The Global Deterioration Scale for assessment of primary degenerative dementia. *Am J Psychiatry* **139**:1136–9.

Rogers SL, Doody R, Mohs R, et al. 1996. E2020 produces both clinical global and cognitive test improvement in patients with mild to moderately severe Alzheimer's disease: results of a 30-week phase III trial. *Neurology* **46** (Suppl.):A217–22.

Rogers SL, Friedhoff LT. 1996. The efficacy and safety of donepezil in patients with mild to moderate Alzheimer's disease: results of a US multicentre, randomized, double-blind, placebo-controlled trial. The Donepezil Study Group. *Dementia* **7**:293–303.

Rosen WG, Mohs RC, Davis KL. 1984. A new rating scale for Alzheimer's disease. *Am J Psychiatry* **141**:1356–64.

Sano M, Ernesto C, Thomas RG, et al. 1997. A controlled trial of selegiline, alpha-tocopherol, or both as treatment for Alzheimer's disease. The Alzheimer's Disease Cooperative Study. *N Engl J Med* **336**:1216–22.

Schneider L. 1990. Tetrahydroaminoacridine and lecithin for Alzheimer's disease [letter, comment on Gauthier et al. 1990]. *N Engl J Med* **323**:919–20.

Schneider LS. 1993. Efficacy of treatment for geropsychiatric patients with severe mental illness [review]. *Psychopharmacol Bull* **29**:501–24.

Schneider LS, Pollock VE, Lyness SA. 1990. A meta-analysis of controlled trials of neuroleptic treatment in dementia. *J Am Geriatr Soc* **38**:553–63.

Schneider LS, Sobin PB. 1992. Non-neuroleptic treatment of behavioral symptoms and agitation in Alzheimer's disease and other dementia. *Psychopharmacol Bull* **28**:71–9.

Summers WK, Majovski LV, Marsh GM, et al. 1986. Oral tetrahydroaminoacridine in long-term treatment of senile dementia, Alzheimer type. *N Engl J Med* **315**:1241–5.

Summers WK, Viesselman JO, Marsh GM, et al. 1981. Use of THA in treatment of Alzheimer-type dementia: pilot study in twelve patients. *Biol Psychiatry* **16**:145–53.

Sunderland T, Silver MA. 1988. Neuroleptics in the treatment of dementia. *Int J Geriatr Psychiatry* **3**:79–84.

Tariot PN. 1997. Treatment strategies in Alzheimer's disease. In: DeKosky ST, Small GW, editors. *Mediguide to Geriatric Neurology*. New York: DalleCorte Publications. p 1–8.

Tomlinson G, Blessed BE, Roth M. 1970. Observations on the brains of demented old people. *J Neurol Sci* **11**:205–42.

*Valley News*. 10 Sep 1993. FDA allows drug: Alzheimer's treatment. p 8.

# Multiple Sclerosis: Current Treatment

George P.A. Rice, George C. Ebers

## *Chapter Outline*



Multiple sclerosis (MS) affects approximately 1 in 500 persons in North America and is the most common seriously disabling disease of young adults. The disease appears to result from immunological attacks on the brain, optic nerves, and spinal cord, commonly starting in young adulthood. Most individuals accrue substantial disability over time. The disease is of vast economic consequence, with annual societal costs in Canada in the billions of dollars.

The cardinal feature is an abnormal immune response probably to unidentified self-antigens in the central nervous system. This process appears to occur in those with a genetic predisposition and might be triggered by something in the environment.

## PATHOGENESIS

### The Immunological Basis

The study of *in vitro* immunological abnormalities in patients with MS has provided relatively little insight into the pathogenesis of the disease. There has been a tendency to describe the immunopathology of the disease in terms of minor deviations from normal in an immunological assay, be it for a new lymphokine, adhesion molecule, or T-cell subset. These association studies have not greatly illuminated the mystery. A few observations appear to be reproducible:

- Lymphocytes are present in the nervous system. Attempts to identify something unique about autoreactive lymphocytes in MS have failed. Preliminary studies suggesting that certain classes of T-cell receptor genes are utilized in patients with MS have not been confirmed (Hashimoto et al. 1992). This is not surprising, given that no diseases have yet been described in which there is faulty expression of T-cell receptor genes. Although lymphocytes from MS patients have been ascribed unusual reactivity to *brain* antigens such as myelin basic protein and proteolipid, this reactivity is also seen in control patients (Olsson et al. 1990).
- Some features of immune activation are present. Activated lymphocytes leave a variety of cytokines in their wake, and this possibly contributes to inflammation and to the process of demyelination. Most treatments applied to MS have been targeted at lymphocytes and their activation. Activation of the immune system, as can happen following viral infection, surgery, or the administration of $\gamma$-interferon, can trigger disease flares (Panitch et al. 1987). Markers of "immune activation" have not yet become established as benchmarks of the disease and are certainly not sufficiently reliable to be used as indicators of disease activity or treatment effects.
- Immunoglobulin synthesis in the central nervous system is increased; the antibodies have a characteristic banding pattern when they are separated by electrophoresis. The antigenic specificity of the immunoglobulin is unknown, as is the relationship of this-B-cell abnormality to the disease (Ebers 1984).

**PRINCIPLE Immune activation in multiple sclerosis:**

- **Lymphocytic pleocytosis in CSF**
- **Increased inflammatory cytokine profiles (serum, CSF, or tissue)**
- **$\gamma$-interferon, tumor necrosis factor, interleukin 2**
- **Reduced immunosuppressive cytokines (serum, CSF, or tissue)**
- **Transforming growth factor-$\beta$, interleukin 10**
- **Possible reduction in "suppressor cell" function**

### A Genetic Predisposition

Genetic factors have been implicated by several compelling observations (reviewed in Ebers 1994a). The hardest evidence is the 30% concordance of the disease between identical twins. The concordance in dizygotic twins is 4%, which approximates that found in nontwin siblings of patients with MS (Ebers et al. 1986). MS-affected family members are found in first-degree relatives of 20% of MS patients. The rarity or absence of MS in certain populations also suggests a genetic role. A major effort is being made to map the genetic determinants of this susceptibility. Several genes might have a role, although no single gene has been yet identified. Populations of MS patients have been recognized to have an overrepresentation of certain HLA types, but the contribution of HLA to MS is likely small. Bearing a certain HLA type is neither sufficient nor essential for the development of MS (Ebers et al. 1982).

### An Environmental Factor

Environmental factors are suggested by the different prevalence rates in genetically similar populations in different parts of the globe (reviewed in Ebers and Sadovnick 1993). The nature of the environmental agent remains a mystery; it seems to act at a population level rather than as an infectious, transmitted agent. Migration studies suggest that it acts early in life.

More than a dozen infectious agents have been linked to MS. All contentions to date have failed the test of reproducibility (chapter 10 of Paty and Ebers 1997).

**PRINCIPLE The etiology of MS appears to be an autoimmune response directed to an undetermined brain antigen, occurring in individuals with a genetic predisposition to this kind of self-reactivity, perhaps influenced by something in the environment acting early in life.**

## CLINICAL FEATURES

Multiple sclerosis commonly begins with episodic sensory, visual, or motor dysfunction secondary to inflammation or loss of myelin. The optic nerve, cerebellum, and brainstem can be involved, resulting in visual failure, incoordination, diplopia, and disequilibrium. Identification of at least two historical attacks, supported by evidence of dysfunction in two different parts of the nervous system, offers a reasonable mandate for making a clinical diagnosis. When the evidence from the history and the clinical examination is less compelling (e.g., one clinical attack with only one abnormality on the neurological examination), magnetic resonance imaging is a useful diagnostic adjunct. Typical white matter lesions are seen in

90% of patients. The diagnosis can also be supported by identification of oligoclonal bands in spinal fluid (present in 80 to 90%) and by electrophysiological identification of slowed conduction times in white matter pathways, such as the visual or auditory projections.

The clinical course pursues a relapsing-remitting pattern in the majority of patients at the outset. About 20% of these patients will pursue an extremely benign course. A progressive deterioration, commonly unrelated to acute attacks, develops in the majority of these patients over time for reasons that are unclear. In approximately 20%, the clinical course is progressive from the beginning.

**PRINCIPLE Clinical forms of multiple sclerosis**

- **Relapsing-remitting, 80%. Of these, 80% will develop a progressive deterioration over time (secondary progression), and 20% will accrue little or no disability over time (benign MS).**
- **Primary progressive (no relapses), 20%.**

Survival is only moderately shortened by MS, but disability, to the point of requiring walking assistance (cane, walker, or wheelchair), develops in about 50% of patients by 15 years and in the majority by 25 years (Weinshenker et al. 1989a). The disease course can be extremely variable. The factors that identify a poor outcome are only partially understood. Early disability accrual and the occurrence of frequent attacks in the first 2 years suggest a more aggressive subsequent course (Weinshenker et al. 1989b). A high burden of disease on the magnetic resonance scan bodes for a more ominous disease course (Filippi et al. 1994).

## TREATMENT OF THE DISEASE

The disease is not curable but is treatable (Ebers 1994b). Although treatment is focused on the suppression of lymphocytes, the essence of MS management is the management of complications of the disease.

### The Difficulty of MS Clinical Trials

Encouraging pilot studies are usually unsupported by confirmatory data evolving from phase III trials. Several reasons account for this. Disease progression is generally slow and can be difficult to measure. The clinical outcome measures commonly used in clinical trials are still relatively crude. Most of them are based upon the Kurtzke disability scale, an ordinal scale that ranges from 0 = normal; 6 = dependence on one cane; 6.5 = dependence upon bilateral assistance; to 10 = death due to MS. Measurement is prone to inter- and intrarater variability, and the score largely reflects one domain of function, namely, ambulation. New approaches to measurement of global disability are being evaluated (Rudick et al. 1997).

Patients are commonly selected for trials on the basis of selected disease activity (attacks or progression). Such patients tend to regress to the mean rate of relapse or progression, or even improve, in the short term. This emphasizes the importance of the placebo group. Recently, magnetic scanning has achieved wide usage as a surrogate marker for treatment trials. The burden of disease visualized on these scans does correlate with disability, although only weakly. It is expected that validation of the MRI as an outcome measure will come. The identification of drugs that affect MRI outcomes, but not clinical outcomes, poses a challenging ethical conundrum for regulatory authorities.

A variety of targets has been selected for immune intervention. Students should be cautioned that clinical experimentation in MS is entirely empiric because the cause of the disease is a total mystery. A modest claim for treatment effect with a new agent is weak evidence for novel immunological insight into a disease process.

**PRINCIPLE A disease whose etiology is poorly understood, whose progress is unpredictable, and whose incidence is relatively low usually awaits an unexpected therapeutic observation to become eventually its therapy of choice.**

### Intervention for the Acute Attack

Attacks on the nervous system can result in serious disability. The average duration of an attack is about 6 weeks. Although spontaneous recovery can occur, persistent deficits become common as years pass by. For patients with acute attacks, corticosteroids (intravenous methylprednisolone or oral prednisone) remain the mainstay of treatment (Beck et al. 1992; Beck et al. 1993). Preliminary studies in which steroid equivalent doses have been compared have failed to show a difference between the oral and the intravenous route (Alam et al. 1993). The drug effect is likely at the blood–brain barrier, based upon suppression of gadolinium enhancement (Miller et al. 1992).

Methylprednisolone is commonly administered as an infusion of 1 g daily for 3 to 5 days, followed by a tapering course of prednisone (generally 1 mg/kg for 7 to

10 days and a brief taper thereafter [Beck et al. 1992]). Physicians are cautioned against long-term use of steroids; the side effects can be major problems, and, most important, this class of drugs has not been shown convincingly to alter long-term disability.

**PRINCIPLE Therapies that ameliorate suffering in a disease with characteristic remissions and exacerbations but that do not alter long-term progress must be titrated to a useful endpoint but not given without a strategy for discontinuation.**

## Prevention of the Acute Attack

In the first few years following the development of MS, the average patient can expect approximately one attack per year (Weinshenker and Sibley 1992). Until 1993, there were few options for the prevention of acute attacks in patients with relapsing-remitting disease. Azathioprine has been shown to have a modest effect in reducing attack frequency (about one-third) with marginal effects on disability. The effect is not seen until the second year of treatment. The drug is given at a daily dosage of 2 to 3 mg/kg (Goodkin et al. 1991).

Some interferons have been shown recently to reduce the frequency of attacks. Recombinant $\beta$-interferons reduce the frequency of clinical attacks by a modest degree (about one-third), but they have a more compelling effect on MRI measures of disease activity (The IFN$\beta$ Multiple Sclerosis Study Group 1993; Jacobs et al. 1996). The accrual of disability is less convincingly reduced (Rice and Ebers 1998), but further studies are under way. The following are interferons currently available for attack prevention:

Interferon $\beta$1b (Betaseron) 8 mU SC q2d
Interferon $\beta$1a (Avonex) 6 mU IM weekly
Interferon $\beta$1a (Rebif) 6 mU SC tiw

Differences among $\beta$-interferons in the various studies probably represent dose effects. The mechanism of action is unclear. Interferons probably affect the expression of hundreds of genes, several of which relate to the immune system. Mild lymphopenia is one clear effect (The IFN$\beta$ Multiple Sclerosis Study Group 1993). Favorable effects of interferon on lymphocyte activation have not been correlated with clinical outcome in individual patients. Interferons are reasonably well tolerated; injection site reactions and flulike symptoms are the major side effects. Neutralizing antibodies to interferons may negate their effectiveness but appear to be self-limited (Rice et al. 1999).

Several other agents are being tested for their ability to prevent attacks. These agents have been selected for a variety of reasons. Intravenous immunoglobulins appear to have a beneficial effect. Long-term efficacy and practicality are uncertain.

Other agents have been chosen for their ability to modulate the outcome of an animal model of MS (experimental allergic encephalomyelitis, EAE). Included in this list are agents like myelin basic protein (MBP) and vaccination with either T-cell receptor peptides (Bourdette et al. 1994) or attenuated MBP-specific T-cell clones (Zhang and Raus 1994). These treatments are reasonably sound for EAE, in which the relevant antigens are better understood. It should be remembered that EAE has not been a very effective crucible for testing drugs for MS. It is also haunting that the alleged quirks in the immune response to myelin and related CNS proteins in EAE have not been shown to be primary events in MS. Much of this work is being tendered without the firm reproducibility of the basic observation that MS patients have an abnormal immune response to myelin components. It was not surprising that treatment of MS patients with myelin basic protein failed to alter the course of the disease (Panitch et al. 1997). Copaxone, a congener of MBP, has been shown to reduce attack frequency by about one-third in patients, although the mechanism is uncertain. It has been approved for use in MS and appears to be well tolerated (Johnson et al. 1995). The costs of these various treatments are summarized in Table 7-30.

## Intervention for Disease Progression

We have only weak medicine for this outcome. Methylprednisolone has a modest effect but only in the short term; patients almost invariably resume their continued progression within a few months of this treatment (Milligan et al. 1987). It is uncertain and unlikely that this drug will have a major impact in the long term, even when given in monthly pulses.

## Prevention of Disease Progression

A variety of lymphocyte poisons has been tried in patients with progressive disease. Azathioprine appears to have a modest effect, but this was deduced only from the meta-analysis of several studies (Yudkin et al. 1991). Not all investigators have been persuaded by the benefit/risk ratio. Considerable interest was lavished upon cyclophos-

Table 7-30 Costs of Commonly Used Treatments for Multiple Sclerosis

| INTERVENTION | DOSAGE | PRICE[a] |
|---|---|---|
| *Attack intervention* (cost per intervention) | | |
| Methylprednisolone | 1 g for 3 days | \$84.11 |
| Prednisone | 60 mg for 1 week, tapering by 10 mg every 3 days thereafter (510 tabs) | \$10.03 |
| *Attack prevention* (monthly cost) | | |
| Interferon $\beta$1b (Betaseron) | 8 mU SC q2d | \$1102.71 |
| Interferon $\beta$1a (Avonex) | 6 mU IM/wk | \$1068.08 |
| Interferon $\beta$1a (Rebif) | 12 mU SC 3×/wk | \$1194.67 |
| *Prevention of disease progression* (monthly cost) | | |
| Azathioprine (Imuran) | 200 mg daily (120 × 50 mg = 1 month's supply) | \$82.35 |
| *Symptomatic treatment* (monthly cost) | | |
| Oxybutinin chloride | 5 mg bid (60 tabs) | \$18.33 |
| Terazosin HCl | 1 mg tid (90 tabs) | \$43.23 |
| Amitriptyline HCl | 50 mg qhs (30 tabs) | \$7.04 |
| Baclofen | 10 mg tid (90 tabs) | \$26.20 |
| Carbamazepine | 200 mg tid (90 tabs) | \$11.92 |

[a]Price in US\$, source is section author. Current prices may vary from those quoted, but comparative prices among products are expected to be similar. The reader should check on local prices at the time of prescribing.

phamide as an immunosuppressive agent following an encouraging report from a Harvard-based study in 1983 (Hauser et al. 1983). This observation could not be corroborated in subsequent trials (The Canadian Cooperative Multiple Sclerosis Study Group 1991; Likosky et al. 1991), and the treatment has been abandoned except by those unmoved by randomized, double-blind, placebo-controlled trials.

**PRINCIPLE In desperate situations, the straws grasped often will not have a rational basis for use even when their toxicity may be severe.**

Several other agents have been tried in progressive disease. Cyclosporine (The Multiple Sclerosis Study Group 1990), methotrexate (Currier et al. 1993), total lymphoid irradiation (Cook et al. 1986), and cladribine (Rice GPA and the Cladribine Study Group 1997) have not made a significant impact on the treatment of progressive MS. It seems likely that MS is unlikely to yield to this kind of treatment, given the number of poisons tried and the extent to which the immune system has been poisoned. Of the cytotoxic drugs, mitoxantrone appears to be the most promising agent for halting disease progression (Edan 1997). Copolymer 1 has not been shown to be effective in progressive MS (Bornstein et al. 1991). The effect of the interferons is under study.

## Interpretation of Future Clinical Trials

Caregivers of MS patients should be optimistic because of the gains made in research in the last few years but are advised to remain skeptical of published results of MS clinical trials. A few questions can be quickly asked to identify the studies destined for replication difficulties.

- Were the outcome measures clearly stated at the outset?
- Were the outcome measures realistic and clinically important?
- Did the behavior of the placebo group bear some resemblance to the natural history of the disease?

If the answer to any of these questions is no, the trial result, historically, has been fragile (Ebers 1994b). Although we have a few promising agents for prevention of attacks, we don't know when is the optimal time to begin treatment and how long to continue.

## TREATMENT OF THE COMPLICATIONS OF MS

### General Management of the Patient in an MS Clinic Setting

Because of the tremendous impact that MS can have on the lives of patients, management is expedited by referral to a regional MS clinic. Once identified, many problems are amenable to management by community-based service agencies (home care, attendant care, MS support groups). Pharmacological intervention, derived from controlled clinical trials and from experience (Paty and Ebers 1997), remains only a small part of patient management.

### Urological Problems

The most common urological abnormality is failure to store urine (vesicourethral dyssynergia), manifest clinically by urgency incontinence. This is best managed by selective alpha blockade at the bladder neck (prazosin, doxazosin, terazosin) to facilitate bladder neck opening. This can be used alone or be supplemented with an anticholinergic (oxybutinin, propantheline) or other relaxant medication (flavoxate). Failure of complete bladder emptying can be helped by drugs that open the bladder neck but is usually best managed with intermittent self-catheterization. Although there is usually some reluctance to pursue intermittent self-catheterization, it is safe, effective, and well tolerated. It carries a remarkably low risk of infection. In-dwelling catheters are to be avoided.

### Spasticity

Although spasticity can serve as an ambulatory aid to MS patients, severe spasticity with pain, adductor spasm, and impaired activities of daily living can pose major challenges. Much can be done before pharmacological treatment is considered. Avoidance of nociceptive stimuli in the abdomen and extremities, management of bowel and bladder, and physiotherapy can make a major impact. Once it has been established that treatment is indicated, it is wise to choose one agent and to titrate the dose (Rice 1987).

For mild spasticity, diazepam (5 to 10 mg at bedtime) and baclofen (10 to 30 mg/day) are effective. For severe spasticity, baclofen can be pushed to dosages in the range of 100 mg/day. Weakness is the principal side effect, and this limits the effectiveness of this agent in individuals who walk with assistance. Baclofen can be given by intrathecal administration. The effect can be quite dramatic, although the clinical benefit is offset by the price of the infusion pump and the not infrequent problems with catheter placement. Tizanidine and vigabatrin are available for those who are intolerant of baclofen.

### Pain and Depression

Pain can affect over 50% of patients with MS. A variety of pain syndromes has been described (Moulin et al. 1988). The most common is a dysesthetic pain in the legs and the lower back. Amitriptyline is the most effective agent. Judicious use of opiate analgesia is reasonable. TENS, acupuncture, and dorsal column stimulation are treatments of last resort.

Paroxysmal pain in the trigeminal field can affect 5 to 10% of MS patients. It can mimic tic douloureux, but MS tic is commonly experienced in the upper and lower face, is more commonly bilateral, and is less trigger sensitive. It usually responds to carbamazepine or baclofen; occasional patients require a surgical procedure.

### Emotional Lability and Depression

Emotional lability is a relatively common problem, resulting from failure of cortical inhibition of limbic circuits, and usually responds to low doses of tricyclic antidepressants.

A heightened awareness for depression is obligatory for all physicians who treat MS patients. The depression responds to the usual agents (tricyclic antidepressants, selective serotonin reuptake inhibitors [SSRIs]).

### Paroxysmal Disorders

Paroxysmal disorders are not infrequent in MS patients, and a variety of syndromes is recognized. The most common is the painful tonic spasm in a lower extremity. These are commonly confused with seizures but are much shorter (15 to 30 seconds) and more frequent. They appear to result from subcortical spontaneous discharges. These symptoms disappear with low-dose carbamazepine, in the order of 200 to 600 mg daily.

### Sexual Dysfunction

Sexual dysfunction is relatively common in MS patients. Genital anesthesia, anorgasmia, incontinence, and fatigue are the principal problems. The management is difficult; counseling can help. Erectile failure may respond to cavernosal alpha blockade, alprostadil administration SC, intrameatal administration, or sildenafil by mouth.

## Fatigue and Heat Sensitivity

Fatigue is a major symptom in patients with MS. The etiology is obscure. Some treatments have been established. Amantadine (100 mg twice daily) has a modest effect. Pemoline (18.75 to 37.5 mg every morning) has a more robust effect, at the expense of some insomnia and occasional drug-induced hepatitis.

4-Aminopyridine looks promising in pilot trials. This potassium channel blocker prevents current leakage from demyelinated axons by prolonging action potentials. It can restore transmission along demyelinated cables.

## Tremor

Tremor is common in MS and can be extremely disabling. It responds poorly to treatment; some patients are helped partially by clonazepam (0.5 to 4.0 mg/day) and ondansteron (8 to 16 mg daily).

## REFERENCES


Alam SM, Kyriakides T, Lawden M, et al. 1993. Methylprednisolone in multiple sclerosis: A comparison of oral with intravenous therapy at equivalent high dose. *J Neurol Neurosurg Psychiatry* **56**: 1219–20.

Beck RW, Cleary PA, Anderson MM, et al. 1992. A randomized, controlled trial of corticosteroids in the treatment of acute optic neuritis. The Optic Neuritis Study Group. *N Engl J Med* **326**:581–8.

Beck RW, Cleary PA, Trobe JD, et al. 1993. The effect of corticosteroids for acute optic neuritis on the subsequent development of multiple sclerosis. The Optic Neuritis Study Group. *N Engl J Med* **329**:1764–9.

Bornstein MB, Miler A, Slagle S. 1991. A placebo-controlled, double blind randomized, two center pilot trial of Cop 1 in chronic progressive multiple sclerosis. *Neurology* **41**:533–9.

Bourdette DN, Whitham RH, Chou YK, et al. 1994. Immunity to TCR peptides in multiple sclerosis. I. Successful immunization of patients with synthetic V beta 5.2 and V beta 6.1 CDR2 peptides. *J Immunol* **152**:2510–19.

Cook SD, Devereux C, Troiano R, et al. 1986. Effect of total lymphoid irradiation in chronic progressive MS. *Lancet* **1**:1405–9.

Currier RD, Haerer AF, Meydrech EF. 1993. Low-dose oral methotrexate treatment of multiple sclerosis: A pilot study. *J Neurol Neurosurg Psychiatry* **56**:1217–8.

Ebers GC. 1984. Oligoclonal banding in MS. *Ann N Y Acad Sci* **36**: 206–12.

Ebers GC. 1984a. Genetics and multiple sclerosis: An overview. *Ann Neurol* **36**(Suppl):S12–4.

Ebers GC. 1984b. Treatment of multiple sclerosis. *Lancet* **343**:275–9.

Ebers GC, Bulman DE, Sadovnick AD, et al. 1986. A population-based study of multiple sclerosis in twins. *N Engl J Med* **315**:1638–42.

Ebers GC, Paty DW, Stiller CR, et al. 1982. HLA-typing in multiple sclerosis sibling pairs. *Lancet* **2**:88–90.

Ebers GC, Sadovnick AD. 1993. The geographic distribution of multiple sclerosis: A review. *Neuroepidemiology*. **12**:1–5.

Edan G, Miller D, Clanet M, et al. 1997. Therapeutic effect of mitoxantrone combined with methylprednisdene in multiple sclerosis: a randomized multicentre study of active disease using MRI and clinical criteria. *J Neurol Neurosurg Psychiatry* **62**:112–8.

Filippi M, Horsfield MA, Morrissey S, et al. 1994. Quantitative brain MRI lesion load predicts the course of clinically isolated syndromes suggestive of multiple sclerosis. *Neurology* **44**:635–41.

Goodkin DE, Bailly RC, Teetzen MI, et al. 1991. The efficacy of azathioprine in relapsing-remitting multiple sclerosis. *Neurology* **41**:20–5.

Hashimoto LL, Mak TW, Ebers GC. 1992. T cell receptor alpha chain polymorphisms in multiple sclerosis. *J Neuroimmunol* **40**:41–8.

Hauser SL, Dawson DM, Lehrich JR, et al. 1983. Intensive immunosuppression in progressive multiple sclerosis: A randomized, three-arm study of high dose intravenous cyclophosphamide, plasma exchange and ACTH. *N Engl J Med* **308**:173–80.

Jacobs LD, Cookfair DL, Rudick RA, et al. 1996. Intramuscular interferon beta 1 a for disease progression in relapsing multiple sclerosis. *Ann Neurol* **39**:285–94.

Johnson KP, Brooks BR, Cohen JA, et al. 1995. Copolymer 1 reduces relapse rate and improves disability in relapsing-remitting multiple sclerosis: Results of a phase III multicenter, double-blind, placebo-controlled trial. *Neurology* **45**:1268–76.

Likosky WH, Fireman B, Elmore R, et al. 1991. Intense immunosuppression in chronic progressive multiple sclerosis: The Kaiser study. *J Neurol Neurosurg Psychiatry* **54**:1055–60.

Linet OI, Ogring FG and the Alprostadil Study Group. 1996. Efficacy and safety of intracavernosal alprostadil in men with erectile dysfunction. *N Engl J Med* **334**:873–7.

Miller DH, Thompson AJ, Morrissey SP, et al. 1992. High dose steroids in acute relapses of multiple sclerosis: MRI evidence for a possible mechanism of therapeutic effect. *J Neurol Neurosurg Psychiatry* **55**:450–3.

Milligan NM, Newcombe R, Compston DA. 1987. A double-blind controlled trial of high dose methylprednisolone in patients with multiple sclerosis. 1. Clinical effects. *J Neurol Neurosurg Psychiatry* **50**:511–6.

Moulin DE, Foley KM, Ebers GC. 1988. Pain syndromes in multiple sclerosis. *Neurology* **38**:1830–4.

Noseworthy JH, Hopkins MB, Vandervoort MK, et al. 1993. An open-trial evaluation of mitoxantrone in the treatment of progressive MS. *Neurology* **43**:1401–6.

Olsson T, Zhi WW, Hojeberg B, et al. 1990. Autoreactive T lymphocytes in multiple sclerosis determined by antigen-induced secretion of interferon-gamma. *J Clin Invest* **86**:981–5.

Panitch H, Francis G and the Oral Myelin Study Group. 1997. Clinical results of a phase three study of oral myelin in relapsing-remitting MS. The Oral Myelin Study Group. *Ann Neurol* **42**:459.

Panitch HS, Hirsch RL, Haley AS. 1987. Exacerbations of multiple sclerosis in patients treated with gamma interferon. *Lancet* **1**:893–5.

Rice GPA. 1987. Pharmacotherapy of spasticity—some theoretical and practical considerations. *Can J Neurol Sci* **14**:510–2.

Rice GPA. 1994. Management of paroxysmal symptoms in multiple sclerosis. Proceedings of the MS forum Modern Management Workshop, Paris, April.

Rice GPA and the Cladribine Study Group. 1997. Cladribine and chronic progressive multiple sclerosis: The results of a multicenter trial [abstract]. *Neurology.*

Rice GPA, Ebers GC. 1998. Interferons and disease progression. *Arch Neurol* **55**: 1578–87.

Rice GPA, Paszner B, Ojer J, et al. 1999. The evolution of neutralizing antibodies in multiple sclerosis patients treated with interferon beta 1b. *Neurology* **52**:1277–9.

Rudick R, Antel J, Confraveux S, et al. 1997. Recommendations from the National Multiple Sclerosis Society Clinical Outcomes Assessment Task Force. *Ann Neurol* **42**:379–82.

The Canadian Burden of Illness Study Group. In press. Burden of illness of multiple sclerosis. 1. Cost of illness. *Can J Neurol Sci.*

The Canadian Cooperative Multiple Sclerosis Study Group. 1991. The Canadian cooperative trial of cyclophosphamide and plasma exchange in progressive multiple sclerosis. *Lancet* **337**:441–6.

The IFN$\beta$ Multiple Sclerosis Study Group. 1993. Interferon beta-1b is effective in relapsing-remitting multiple sclerosis. I. Clinical results of a multicenter, randomized, double-blind, placebo-controlled trial. *Neurology* **43**:655–61.

The IFN$\beta$ Multiple Sclerosis Study Group. 1996. Neutralizing antibodies during treatment of multiple sclerosis with interferon beta 1b: Experience during the first three years. *Neurology* **47**:1277–85.

The Multiple Sclerosis Study Group. 1990. Efficacy and toxicity of cyclosporine in chronic progressive multiple sclerosis: A randomised double-blinded, placebo-controlled clinical trial. *Ann Neurol* **27**:591–605.

Weinshenker BG, Bass B, Rice GP, et al. 1989. The natural history of multiple sclerosis: A geographically based study. I. Clinical course and disability. *Brain* **112**:113–46.

Weinshenker BG, Bass B, Rice GP, et al. 1989. The natural history of multiple sclerosis: A geographically based study. 2. Predictive value of the early clinical course. *Brain* **112**:1419–28.

Weinshenker BG, Sibley WA. 1992. Natural history and treatment of multiple sclerosis. *Curr Opin Neurol Neurosurg* **5**:203–11.

Yudkin PL, Ellison GW, Ghezzi A, et al. 1991. Overview of azathioprine treatment in multiple sclerosis. *Lancet* **338**:1051–5.

Zhang J, Raus J. 1994. T cell vaccination in multiple sclerosis: hopes and facts. *Acta Neurol Belg* **94**:112–5.

# Myasthenia Gravis

Michael W. Nicolle

### *Chapter Outline*



The fatigable weakness characteristic of myasthenia gravis (MG) is a result of impaired neuromuscular transmission at skeletal muscles, mediated by autoantibodies against acetylcholine receptors (AChRs). Over the last two decades, increasingly effective therapies have been developed for MG. These involve either enhancing neuromuscular transmission or suppressing the aberrant autoimmune response. The choice of specific agents is dictated by the timing of benefit, convenience, expense, and the frequency of adverse effects. Although modern therapy has considerably reduced the morbidity and mortality of MG (Genkins et al. 1987; Oosterhuis 1989; Mantegazza et al. 1990; Verma and Oger 1992; Beekman et al. 1997), there is surprisingly little evidence from randomized, controlled trials (RCTs) to endorse individual therapies.

## CLINICAL PRESENTATION OF MYASTHENIA GRAVIS

Although highly variable in its presentation, the clinical hallmark of MG is that of fatigable weakness of skeletal muscles. The initial presentation is often with diplopia and ptosis, reflecting extraocular muscle (EOM) involvement. In 15 to 20% of MG patients, the course is relatively benign with no progression beyond EOM involvement (Genkins et al. 1987; Oosterhuis 1989; Sanders and Scoppetta 1994; Weinberg et al. 1994; Beekman et al. 1997). However the remainder eventually progress to more generalized weakness. Bulbar muscle involvement produces difficulty chewing, facial weakness, dysphagia and dysphonia, and neck weakness may produce a head drop. Involvement of extremity muscles produces mainly proximal and symmetric weakness of arms and legs, which characteristically worsens toward the end of the day or after sustained muscular effort, and which may fluctuate in severity from one day to the next (Genkins et al. 1987; Oosterhuis 1989; Weinberg et al. 1994; Beekman et al. 1997). Because of this fluctuation, a delay of several years before the diagnosis is made is not uncommon (Beekman et al. 1997).

Myasthenia gravis is an uncommon disorder, with an estimated prevalence of 1 in 15–20,000 and an incidence of 3–4 per million (Oosterhuis 1989). However, much is known about its pathogenesis and the lessons learned in the treatment of MG should be instructive in the treatment of less well delineated autoimmune disorders. As with other autoimmune diseases, females are affected more often. Although myasthenia can present at any age, there are two peaks of onset, used to define the two major clinical subgroups. In "early-onset" MG, onset is between 18 and 50 years. "Late-onset" MG, with onset after 50, is more common in males (Oosterhuis 1989; Mantegazza et al. 1990; Sanders et al. 1997). Other groups include juvenile MG, with onset before age 18 (Andrews et al. 1994), and neonatal MG, produced by the transplacental passage of anti-AChR antibodies from a mother with MG to her offspring (Genkins et al. 1987; Oosterhuis 1989; Plauché 1991; Sanders and Scoppetta 1994). In "seronegative" MG, anti-AChR antibodies are not detectable, although the clinical and electrophysiologic features are similar to those of seropositive patients, and there is considerable evidence suggesting a similar humoral mediation (Sanders et al. 1997).

Two other disorders of neuromuscular transmission deserve brief mention. First, the Lambert-Eaton myasthenic syndrome (LEMS) is immunologically and clinically distinct from MG. In LEMS, antibodies against voltage-gated calcium channels on the presynaptic nerve terminal interfere with ACh release and impair neuromuscular transmission. The clinical manifestations of LEMS consist of fatigable muscle weakness, often manifesting as a gait abnormality, autonomic dysfunction, and depression or absence of the deep tendon reflexes. LEMS frequently occurs as a paraneoplastic process in the setting of an underlying small cell carcinoma of the lung. The treatment of LEMS is similar in many respects to that of MG and will not be discussed in this chapter (McEvoy 1994). Second, the congenital myasthenic syndromes (CMSs) have clinical features similar to those of autoimmune myasthenia gravis, although they generally present earlier in life and are often inherited, although they can appear sporadically (Shillito et al. 1993). However, in the CMSs, neuromuscular transmission is impaired by structural abnormalities of proteins, including the AChRs, at the neuromuscular junction, and not by an autoimmune response to the AChRs. Although some symptomatic therapies are effective for both MG and the CMSs, there is no role for immunosuppression in the treatment of CMSs.

Before effective modern medical treatment, the mortality from MG was as high as 25 to 30% and was especially high in late-onset MG or when a thymoma was present (Drachman 1987; Oosterhuis 1989; Beekman et al. 1997; Massey 1997). Individuals succumbed to aspiration pneumonia as a result of dysphagia, or to respiratory failure because of weakness of the respiratory muscles. Without effective treatment, 15 to 22% of patients achieved long-lasting remission, and another 34 to 39% improved (Drachman 1987; Oosterhuis 1989; Verma and Oger 1992; Massey 1997). Although the mortality from MG is now <5%, involvement of the bulbar or respiratory muscles continues to be a major source of morbidity (Donaldson et al. 1990; Mantegazza et al. 1990; Thomas et al. 1997).

## NEUROMUSCULAR TRANSMISSION AND THE PATHOPHYSIOLOGY OF MYASTHENIA GRAVIS

Depolarization of the peripheral motor nerve terminal opens voltage-gated calcium channels in the presynaptic nerve terminal membrane (Fig. 7-4). The ensuing calcium influx promotes the fusion of vesicles containing acetylcholine (ACh) with the nerve terminal membrane, as well as exocytosis of their contents. ACh then diffuses across the synaptic cleft and binds reversibly with AChRs on the postsynaptic skeletal muscle surface (Fig. 7-4). The AChR consists of five subunits arranged around a central ion channel, with ACh-binding sites on each of the two $\alpha$-subunits (Fig. 7-4). Normally there is a steady-state relationship between degradation and synthesis of muscle surface AChRs, with a half-life of 6–13 days (Weinberg et al. 1994). The binding of ACh induces AChR opening, permitting an influx of cations, predominantly $Na^+$, into the muscle fiber, and resulting in an excitatory end-plate potential (EPP). If the EPP is of sufficient amplitude, muscle-surface voltage-gated sodium channels are opened, generating an action potential that ultimately results in muscle contraction. Normally there is a "safety margin" for neuromuscular transmission, in which an excess of released ACh interacts with more AChRs than are

A

Nerve terminal
Vesicles
VGCC
$Ca^{2+}$
ACh
AChE
AChR
Muscle

B

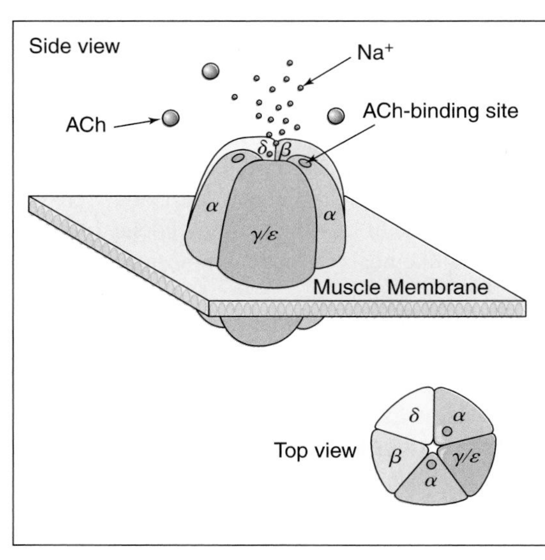


FIGURE 7-4 **(A)** The neuromuscular junction showing acetylcholine-containing vesicles within the presynaptic nerve terminal, the postsynaptic muscle endplate, and other components involved in neuromuscular transmission. **(B)** The acetylcholine receptor (side and top views) in the muscle membrane showing the five subunits arranged around a central cationic channel. ACh, acetylcholine; AChE, acetylcholinesterase; AChR, acetylcholine receptor; $Ca^{2+}$, calcium; $Na^+$, sodium; VGCC, voltage-gated calcium channel.

needed. After binding to the AChRs, ACh dissociates and is hydrolyzed by acetylcholinesterase (AChE) in the synaptic cleft (Fig. 7-4), or simply diffuses away from the neuromuscular junction.

In MG, antibodies against the AChRs interfere with neuromuscular transmission, reducing the EPP amplitude. If this falls below the threshold for generation of action potentials, the clinical result is weakness (Drachman et al. 1987; Keesey 1989). Anti-AChR antibodies interfere with neuromuscular transmission through one of three mechanisms (Drachman et al. 1987). Some bind to the cholinergic binding site on the AChR $\alpha$-subunit, blocking access to ACh. Others crosslink adjacent AChRs, increasing their internalization into muscle and resulting in fewer available muscle surface AChRs. Finally, the most important pathophysiologic mechanism is likely damage to the muscle endplate by complement-fixing anti-AChR antibodies. Continuing AChR resynthesis by muscle cells allows some recovery from these processes (Weinberg et al. 1994). Differences between patients in the proportion of antibodies with these functions may explain the variable responses to treatments such as acetylcholinesterase inhibitors (AChEIs) and plasma exchange.

Anti-AChR antibodies are usually of the immunoglobulin class IgG, and there is considerable variation both within and between individuals in mechanism and precise specificity for the AChRs (Willcox and Vincent 1988). Across a population of myasthenia patients, antibody titers correlate poorly with clinical severity (Oosterhuis et al. 1983), although in a single patient a change in the antibody levels sometimes correlates with clinical changes for better and for worsening (Komiya and Sato 1987).

The thymus is abnormal in 80 to 90% of MG patients and likely plays a central role in exposing autoreactive B and T lymphocytes to the AChR or AChR-like structures, present in thymic myoid cells and cortical thymic epithelial cells (Hohlfeld and Wekerle 1994). Most patients (65%) with early-onset generalized disease have a hyperplastic thymus, enriched for AChR-reactive B and T lymphocytes, and the site of considerable AChR antibody production (Willcox and Vincent 1988). A thymoma is present in 10 to 20% of all MG patients, and 24 to 38% of patients with late-onset disease. These epithelial thymic tumors can be discovered before or after the onset of MG (Mantegazza et al. 1990). Thymomas are rarely, if ever, found in seronegative MG (Sanders and Scoppetta 1994; Beekman et al. 1997), and are less common in ocular MG (Weinberg et al. 1994). The prognosis of MG in the setting of a thymoma is worse, with more severe disease and a higher mortality (Genkins et al. 1987; Mantegazza et al. 1990). In 10 to 20% of MG patients, the thymus is atrophic, in keeping with the normal age-related involution seen in control subjects (Genkins et al. 1987; Mantegazza et al. 1990). When analyzed closely, however, small islands of hyperplastic thymus may be found.

## DIAGNOSIS

The diagnosis of myasthenia gravis relies on recognition of the characteristic clinical features. The weakness in MG can be temporarily reversed by an intravenous injection of the short-acting acetylcholinesterase inhibitor edrophonium, the "tensilon test." Although sensitive, it is not specific for the diagnosis of MG (Weinberg et al. 1994; Beekman et al. 1997), and a positive result does not predict a response to oral AChEIs (Evoli et al. 1988). Although routine electrophysiologic studies in patients with myasthenia gravis may be normal, repetitive nerve stimulation at 3 Hz results in a progressive decrement in the motor nerve amplitude. This is the electrophysiologic correlate to muscle fatigue (Keesey 1989). The sensitivity of this test is low in ocular MG (Keesey 1989), and there are false-positives in other disorders with impaired neuromuscular transmission (Weinberg et al. 1994). Single-fiber electromyogram (SFEMG), which looks for differences (jitter or blocking) in the arrival of action potentials from muscle fibers belonging to the same motor unit, is highly sensitive for detecting impaired neuromuscular transmission, but is also nonspecific (Keesey 1989). Antibodies against the acetylcholine receptor (AChR antibody) are present in 75 to 94% of patients with generalized disease, in 29 to 79% with ocular MG, and nearly always in the presence of a thymoma (Vincent and Newsom-Davis 1985; Evoli et al. 1988; Somnier 1993; Weinberg et al. 1994; Beekman et al. 1997; Sanders et al. 1997). In about 10% of individuals with initially negative AChR antibody levels, subsequent levels will be positive (Weinberg et al. 1994; Sanders et al. 1997). Although useful for the diagnosis, there is a poor correlation between AChR antibody titers and clinical severity, likely reflecting the diverse mechanisms of anti-AChR antibodies (Oosterhuis et al. 1983). Low levels of anti-AChR antibodies can be found but only extremely rarely in other conditions (Somnier 1993).

## THERAPY OF MYASTHENIA GRAVIS

### Principles of Therapy

The ultimate goal in treating immune-mediated MG is to induce a sustained or permanent remission. This involves the symptomatic correction of impaired neuromuscular transmission with AChEIs, as well as suppression of the autoimmune response with corticosteroids (CSTs) or other immunosuppressive drugs (Table 7-31). At times of acute worsening ("myasthenic crisis"), the clinical situation can be improved temporarily by removing pathogenic anti-AChR antibodies using plasma exchange, or by modulation of the immune system with intravenous immunoglobulin (IVIg). Finally, given the presumed role of the thymus in the pathogenesis of MG, thymectomy is often performed in patients with early-onset disease, and variably in other subgroups. As with so many diseases, therapy must be individualized, balancing the clinical severity against the efficacy, rapidity of benefit, frequency of adverse effects, expense, and convenience. The ideal therapy—one that works quickly, is highly effective and permanent, has minimal toxicity, and is inexpensive—is not yet available. As the immunopathogenesis of MG is clarified further, the prospects for a treatment fulfilling these criteria increase (Nicolle et al. 1994).

#### *Symptomatic treatment with acetylcholinesterase inhibitors*

Acetylcholinesterase inhibitors have been used widely since the first successful treatment of MG with physostigmine (Walker 1934). By inhibiting acetylcholinesterase at the neuromuscular junction, AChEIs prolong the duration of action of acetylcholine, increasing the probability that ACh will interact with remaining functioning AChRs. Some AChEIs may have additional direct effects on the AChRs (Taylor 1996). These agents are symptomatic treatments only and do not influence the underlying immune process (Genkins et al. 1987; Sanders and Scoppetta 1994). Their efficacy depends on the availability of functional AChRs at the muscle endplate, which may explain the lack of efficacy in some patients who might have muscle endplate destruction or antibodies blocking the cholinergic binding site.

There is no evidence that any of the available agents are superior (Rowland 1980). Pyridostigmine and neostigmine are more commonly used in North America. Pyridostigmine has a longer duration of action and, unlike physostigmine, does not cross the blood–brain barrier (Taylor 1996; Massey 1997), and may have fewer muscarinic adverse effects than neostigmine (Verma and Oger

Table 7-31 Common Therapies in the Management of Myasthenia Gravis

| THERAPY | ROUTE REGIMEN | AVERAGE COST[a] (PER DAY) | COMMON ADVERSE EFFECTS | ONSET OF BENEFIT | PEAK BENEFIT |
|---|---|---|---|---|---|
| *Symptomatic* | | | | | |
| AChEI (e.g., pyridostigmine) | Oral or parenteral<br>Variable, titrate to clinical response (e.g., 30 mg PO q6h to 120 mg PO q3h) | \$0.20–1.60 | Muscarinic cholinergic<br>Nicotinic chlolinergic (see text) | < 1 hour | 1–3 hours |
| *Immunosuppressive* | | | | | |
| Corticosteroids (e.g., prednisone) | Oral or parenteral<br>Variable (e.g., 0.3 mg/kg qod, 1 mg/kg per day)<br>Taper slowly after improvement | \$0.01–0.09 | Many, see Table 7-32<br>NB, early worsening in up to 48% (see text) | 2–4 weeks | 3–6 months |
| Azathioprine | Oral<br>Variable (e.g., 2–3.5 mg/kg per day) | \$1.72–2.29 | Gastrointestinal<br>Idiosyncratic flu-like<br>Bone marrow suppression<br>Hepatitis<br>Infections | 3 months | 6–12 months |
| Cyclosporine | Oral<br>Variable (e.g., start at 2–5 mg/kg per day as bid dose and adjust to keep trough serum level at 100–150 ng/mL) | \$5.68–13.08 | Many but especially nephrotoxicity, hypertension, headache | 1–2 months | 3–6 months |
| *Temporary* | | | | | |
| Plasma exchange | Intravenous<br>3–5 exchanges of 50 mL/kg each over 6–10 days | \$1000 per exchange or \$5000 per course of 5 exchanges | Hypotension<br>Vascular access | 2–10 days | 8–16 days |
| Intravenous immunoglobulin | Intravenous<br>2 g/kg over 2–5 days | \$4200 per 2-g course | Many minor, see Table 7-33 | 4 days | 8–15 days |
| *Surgical* | | | | | |
| Thymectomy | Operative (see text) | | Perioperative morbidity | 6 months–2 years | 2–10 years |

[a]Costs estimated by section author based on local pharmacy costs of drug only (converted to US from Can\$), or as indicated for IVIg and PE.

1992; Weinberg et al. 1994; Taylor 1996). The short duration of action of edrophonium, used parenterally for the diagnosis of MG, precludes any therapeutic applications (Taylor 1996). Although there is reasonably good correlation in an individual patient between the dose of pyridostigmine and its concentration in plasma, the correlation is poor between patients (Rowland 1980; Massey 1997). Even in the same patient on a constant dose, plasma concentrations may vary considerably (Massey 1997). Absorption of both pyridostigmine and neostigmine is poor, with bioavailability estimated at 10 to 20 and 1 to 2% respectively (Aquilonius and Hartvig 1986). After absorption, AChEIs are rapidly hydrolyzed in the plasma. Peak plasma levels occur at 1.7 hours, and can be later if it is taken with food (Aquilonius and Hartvig 1986). The half-life is approximately 84–200 minutes for pyridostigmine and 54 minutes for neostigmine (Hartvig et al. 1990). Neither pyridostigmine nor neostigmine significantly bind to serum proteins and drug interactions are rare (Aquilonius and Hartvig 1986). Pyridostigmine, and to a lesser extent neostigmine, is excreted mainly by renal tubular secretion, necessitating a reduction of dosage in patients with severe renal failure (Aquilonius and Hartvig 1986; Hartvig et al. 1990).

A corollary of the pharmacologic properties of AChEIs is that the optimal dose is highly variable. This necessitates an initial empirical choice of dose, followed by a careful titration against clinical response. A common practice is to start at 30 mg orally four times a day, and to gradually titrate upward. Only rarely are doses above 120–180 mg PO every 3–4 hours beneficial, and the risk of a "cholinergic crisis" is increased at these doses. After appropriate education, many patients are able to adjust the timing and dosage themselves. This is done by adjusting the dose in 15- to 30-mg increments, and the dosing interval by 30–60 minutes, every several days. Some patients benefit from small doses of AChEI on an as-needed basis before times of increased muscular effort. The benefit with pyridostigmine begins within 30–45 minutes, with peak effects at 1–2 hours (Massey et al. 1989). Thus, timing medications appropriately before meals may improve swallowing (Massey et al. 1989). The variation in the duration of action after a given dose is large, commonly 3–6 hours for pyridostigmine and 2–4 hours for neostigmine (Taylor 1996). Either insufficient or excess AChEIs can result in weakness, the latter because of desensitization of the acetylcholine receptors (Hartvig et al. 1990). The requirements for AChEIs may change over time, and when immunosuppression is added, the same dose of pyridostigmine may have an increased effect (Dalakas 1990). At this stage, AChEIs can often be reduced, or even discontinued. Changes in the dose or interval should be based on the cumulative pattern of recent subjective and objective observations of the patient and physician. Results of the edrophonium test are of little use in adjusting the dose (Rowland 1980).

In addition to the regular 60-mg tablets of pyridostigmine, a long-acting preparation (Mestinon Supraspan 180 mg) is available for bedtime use for patients with significant morning weakness (Taylor 1996). Its absorption is even more variable, and its use during the day is discouraged (Genkins et al. 1987; Sanders and Scoppetta 1994). Pyridostigmine may also be prepared as a syrup (60 mg/5 mL), useful in the pediatric patient. Innovative methods of delivery include the use of pyridostigmine or neostigmine as an aerosol, or as a continuous parenteral infusion, which are especially useful in patients with significant dysphagia. Pyridostigmine is also available for parenteral infusion (IM or IV) as a 5 mg/mL solution (equivalent dose approximately 1/30 of oral dose) (Verma and Oger 1992). Neostigmine is available in 15-mg tablets, or in solution for parenteral use (0.5, 1, or 2.5 mg/mL; dose approximately 1/30–1/60 of oral pyridostigmine) (Verma and Oger 1992).

There are no controlled trials of AChEI use in MG, although there is abundant anecdotal evidence of their efficacy. A few small studies demonstrated improved respiratory function or the reversal of electrophysiologic abnormalities immediately after administration of an AChEI (Rowland 1980; Aquilonius and Hartvig 1986; Goti et al. 1995). A consequence of the latter observation is that it might be reasonable to withhold AChEIs before diagnostic electrophysiologic investigations (Massey et al. 1989). Although effective, AChEIs are often not sufficient alone and are generally even less effective in ocular MG (Evoli et al. 1988; Verma and Oger 1992; Weinberg et al. 1994; Kupersmith et al. 1996). Thus treatment with CSTs or other immunosuppressives is eventually required in many patients (Rowland 1980; Weinberg et al. 1994; Massey 1997).

Adverse effects occur in about one-third of patients treated with AChEIs (Beekman et al. 1997). They reflect stimulation of muscarinic AChRs at autonomic ganglia and include abdominal cramps, diarrhea, sialorrhea, bronchorrhea, sweating, lacrimation, bradycardia, bronchoconstriction, and blurred vision. These are rarely disabling and can often be ameliorated by blocking muscarinic AChRs with diphenoxylate, loperamide, glycopyrrolate, ipratropium, propantheline, or scopolamine (Sanders and Scoppetta 1994). Bradycardia and hypotension are uncommon with oral preparations and are seen only occasionally with parenteral use, usually in patients with preexisting cardiac disease (Arsura et al. 1987; Sanders and Scoppetta 1994). Stimulation of nicotinic AChRs produces muscle fasciculations and cramps, or if severe, a cholinergic crisis (Massey 1997). With increasing weakness in the setting of a recent increase in AChEI dose and significant muscarinic adverse effects, this should be considered, although whether a true "cholinergic crisis" exists is debatable (Rowland 1980). It is noteworthy that anticholinergics may mask the muscarinic-mediated symptoms of a cholinergic crisis, making a clinical diagnosis difficult. AChEIs are often discontinued in a myasthenic crisis, as the muscarinic effects of AChEIs may complicate the management of a ventilated patient with significant swallowing difficulties. Although the chronic administration of high-dose pyridostigmine to animals damaged the neuromuscular junction, there is no evidence of this in humans (Rowland 1980; Sanders and Scoppetta 1994).

**PRINCIPLE When a drug is used to counter the adverse effects of another, the clinician will be severely challenged for dose adjustments of each agent even when the endpoint desired is immediate and easily monitored.**

**SUMMARY**
**Acetylcholinesterase inhibitors are useful for the symptomatic management of MG. They do not have significant long-term adverse effects. Their utility is limited by wide variations in the dose and interval required both within and between patients, by muscarinic adverse effects, and by their limited efficacy for ocular symptoms. Moreover, they have no effect on the underlying pathogenic immune process in MG.**

***Immunosuppressive treatments***

Similar efficacy is produced by most of the available immunosuppressive agents when used to treat MG; 70 to 90% of patients are significantly improved or put into remission (Cornelio et al. 1987; Drachman 1987; Massey 1997). Therefore, the choice of agents is dictated by how quickly a response is needed, by likely acceptability of the adverse effects, and by expense (Table 7-31). There may also be synergism with combinations of immunosuppressives (Cornelio et al. 1987).

**CORTICOSTEROIDS** Adrenocorticotropic hormone (ACTH) was first used in MG decades before the recognition that MG was an autoimmune disorder (Verma and Oger 1992). Over the next 30 years, the use of CSTs was limited by the frequent occurrence of significant early deterioration in strength and by concerns about efficacy (Rowland 1980; Arsura et al. 1985). In the early 1970s, prednisone became available, and success with the use of CSTs improved. Although commonly used in MG since, their benefits must be balanced against a significant risk of adverse effects.

Although the precise mechanism of CSTs in reversing MG is unknown, they likely have multiple effects on both the cellular and humoral immune responses (Arsura et al. 1985; Dalakas 1990; Verma and Oger 1992). A gradual decrease in AChR antibody levels after CST administration, concurrent with clinical improvement, is commonly seen (Arsura et al. 1985; Komiya and Sato 1987; Verma and Oger 1992). Animal studies suggest that CSTs may also directly facilitate or inhibit neuromuscular transmission (Wilson et al. 1974; Miller et al. 1986). These pharmacologic effects are seen within hours of administration and may explain the early worsening produced by high-dose CSTs (see below), as well as the fluctuation of clinical signs with alternate-day therapy (Seybold and Drachman 1974; Wilson et al. 1974; Sghirlanzoni et al. 1984; Miller et al. 1986). CSTs may stabilize the muscle membrane and may induce expression and availability of AChRs (Sghirlanzoni et al. 1984; Dalakas 1990; Kaplan et al. 1990). Prednisone and prednisolone are used for the outpatient therapy of myasthenia gravis, with hydrocortisone reserved for parenteral use (Dalakas 1990). High-dose intravenous methylprednisolone or dexamethasone may also be effective (Sghirlanzoni et al. 1984; Arsura et al. 1985). CSTs are given in a single, morning oral dose, with peak concentration occurring 1–3 hours after taking prednisone, or 7–10 hours after taking it with meals (Dalakas 1990). After absorption, most of the drug is transported in serum bound to either albumin or transcortin, with the unbound form being active (Dalakas 1990). Prednisone is metabolized in the liver to prednisolone. Drugs that stimulate hepatic microsomal enzymes increase CST metabolism, leading to an increased requirement for CST. Conversely, the effects of CSTs may be increased with cyclosporine or oral contraceptives (Dalakas 1990).

There are several possible ways of beginning CSTs in patients with myasthenia gravis (Genkins et al. 1987; Dalakas 1990). Starting with a daily high dose (1–1.5 mg/kg per day) of CSTs will likely result in relatively rapid improvement, but also will carry an increased risk of causing early worsening and adverse effects (Seybold and Drachman 1974; Sghirlanzoni et al. 1984; Dalakas 1990; Weinberg et al. 1994). Beginning with low-dose, alternate-day CST (e.g., 15–25 mg on alternate days), followed by gradual increases until improvement is seen, lessens the risk of early worsening and the incidence of adverse effects, but prolongs the latency until clinical improvement becomes apparent (Seybold and Drachman 1974; Massey 1997). The benefits of each of these strategies must be weighed against the risks and the urgency of the situation. Once CSTs are started, patients must be monitored closely for early worsening (see below) even though the dose is continued until clinical improvement is seen (Cornelio et al. 1987). In one study, the mean dose needed for benefit was 68 mg on alternate days (Grob et al. 1981), although patients with ocular MG may respond to lower doses. After significant improvement, CSTs are gradually tapered, initially to alternate-day therapy, and then with the intention of discontinuation (Dalakas 1990). Alternate-day therapy is thought to minimize adverse effects, or even to reverse them (Table 7-32) (Dalakas 1990) (see also Chapter 10, Connective Tissue and Bone Disorders).

Retrospectively, the morbidity and mortality of MG have been reduced since the advent of CST therapy. However, despite their widespread use in MG, controlled studies documenting their efficacy are lacking. In the only randomized, controlled study of CST in MG, three out of seven placebo-treated MG patients and three out of six MG patients treated with alternate-day, high-dose corticosteroids improved at 6 months (Howard et al. 1976). The remaining unimproved patients in the placebo group improved with subsequent CST, for an overall improvement in seven out of ten steroid-treated patients. The numbers were too small to permit statistical analysis (Howard et al. 1976). In a recent randomized, unblinded trial, prednisone was compared with azathioprine, initially in combination with a short course of prednisone, and then alone (Myasthenia Gravis Clinical Study Group 1993). The time to the first deterioration was similar with both, but early treatment failures in the prednisone group were almost

Table 7-32 Adverse Effects of Corticosteroids

| ADVERSE EFFECT | MANAGEMENT[a] | COMMENT |
|---|---|---|
| *Gastrointestinal* | | |
| Dyspepsia | Take with food | Higher risk with concurrent use of NSAIDS. |
| Peptic ulcers | Concomitant use of anti-ulcer agent ($H_2$ blocker, proton pump inhibitor, cytoprotective agent), especially if previous history of ulcer, or taking NSAIDS | |
| *Body Habitus* | | |
| Cushingoid | Alternate-day dosage | Reversible after dose reduction or discontinuation. |
| Weight gain | Diet | |
| *Skin* | | |
| Acne | | Reversible after dose reduction or discontinuation. |
| Hirsutism | | |
| Striae | | |
| Alopecia | | |
| Easy bruising | | |
| Delayed wound healing | | |
| *Metabolic, Fluid and Electrolyte* | | |
| Peripheral edema | | Reversible after dose reduction or discontinuation. |
| Hypertension | Monitor BP regularly, reduce $Na^+$ intake, add diuretics | |
| Hypokalemia/muscle cramps | High $K^+$ diet, KCl supplementation | |
| Hyperglycemia | Oral hypoglycemic and/or insulin if necessary<br>CHO/calorie-restricted diet | |
| Menstrual changes | | |
| Adrenal suppression | Single morning dose and/or slow tapering<br>Alternate-day dosage | May be prolonged even after discontinuation requiring corticosteroid coverage at times of stress (surgery, illness, etc.). |
| *Muscle* | | |
| Cramps | High $K^+$ diet | Reversible after dose reduction or discontinuation, but may take up to a year. |
| Myopathy | Regular exercise | Suspect with weakness of proximal legs despite improving MG otherwise, and if neck flexion preserved. |
| *Behavioral* | | |
| Anxiety | Symptomatic treatment | More common with high dose, first time on steroids?<br>Reversible after dose reduction or discontinuation.<br>Psychosis not a contraindication to another trial of CST. |
| Insomnia | | |
| Psychosis | | |
| Mania | | |
| Depression | | |
| *Bone* | | |
| Osteoporosis | Alternate-day dosage<br>Monitor bone mineral density in high-risk patients<br>Prophylaxis with calcium/biphosphonates/vitamin D if long-term use looks likely | |

Table 7-32 **Adverse Effects of Corticosteroids (Continued)**

| Adverse Effect | Management[a] | Comment |
|---|---|---|
| | Consider withdrawing steroids | |
| Avascular necrosis | Alternate-day dosage | |
| | Prompt investigation of hip pain with plain radiographs, MRI, etc. | |
| *Ocular* | | |
| Blurred vision | | ? Secondary to fluid, electrolyte changes, check for hyperglycemia. |
| Cataracts | Regular slit-lamp examination with long-term use | |
| Glaucoma | Check intraocular pressure | |
| *Growth* | | |
| Growth retardation | Alternate-day dosage | In children |
| *Infection* | | |
| | Monitor for symptoms and signs of infection | Immunosuppression reversible after dose reduction or discontinuation. |

[a]For all, use the lowest dose/duration possible to minimize adverse effects.
Abbreviations: BP, blood pressure; CHO, carbohydrate; CST, corticosteroids; MRI, magnetic resonance imaging.

three times more common than in the azathioprine group (Myasthenia Gravis Clinical Study Group 1993). At 3 years, 67% and 64% were in remission or minimally symptomatic with prednisone or azathioprine, respectively. In the remaining reports, all of which were uncontrolled and retrospective, improvement was seen in 65 to 100% of CST-treated MG patients (Seybold and Drachman 1974; Sghirlanzoni et al. 1984; Arsura et al. 1985; Cornelio et al. 1987; Myasthenia Gravis Clinical Study Group 1993; Sanders and Scoppetta 1994; Kupersmith et al. 1996; Massey 1997). Disparate schedules of administration and outcome measures make comparisons of these studies difficult. In individuals not responding to CSTs, the addition of azathioprine may be helpful (Cornelio et al. 1987; Myasthenia Gravis Clinical Study Group 1993). Limited evidence suggests that patients with late-onset disease are more likely to respond to CSTs (Sghirlanzoni et al. 1984; Cornelio et al. 1987), whereas CSTs are less beneficial in juvenile MG (Badurska et al. 1992). In ocular MG, CSTs are more effective than AChEIs (Weinberg et al. 1994; Kupersmith et al. 1996), and may decrease the chances of subsequent generalization of the disease (Sommer et al. 1997).

The onset of benefit after starting CST may take 1–3 weeks, with significant improvement not occurring for 3–6 months, and maximal benefit in 4–9 months (Rowland 1980; Sghirlanzoni et al. 1984; Anonymous 1993). Accordingly, a trial of at least 6 months of CST is recommended (Sghirlanzoni et al. 1984). AChEI requirements may decline as improvement secondary to CST treatment begins (Seybold and Drachman 1974; Arsura et al. 1985). When CSTs are tapered, relapses are less likely when the taper rate is slow (5 mg/day or less each month), the target dose is high, and azathioprine is also utilized (Dalakas 1990). It may take several attempts before CSTs can be tapered successfully (Miano et al. 1991), and frequently, discontinuation of treatment is impossible, as low-dose CSTs are needed for long periods (Sghirlanzoni et al. 1984; Dalakas 1990). Corticosteroid-resistant cases may be a result of particularly severe disease, suboptimal doses, noncompliance, overly aggressive tapering, or the wrong diagnosis. When the starting dose of CST is high, early clinical worsening is seen in up to 48% of patients. This worsening is especially likely in more severely affected patients. In <10%, the worsening is severe (Seybold and Drachman 1974; Wilson et al. 1974; Arsura et al. 1985; Kupersmith et al. 1996). Beginning treatment with low dose, alternate-day CST may prevent worsening, as may plasma exchange (Seybold and Drachman 1974; Wilson et al. 1974; Fornasari et al. 1985; Sanders and Scoppetta 1994; Massey 1997). Worsening generally occurs within 4–5 days (range 1–21 days) of starting therapy, and lasts 4–7 days (range 1–20) even when therapy continues (Wilson et al. 1974; Arsura et al. 1985). Electrophysiologic evidence of decreased neuromuscular transmission may be seen within hours of CST administration. This early worsening likely reflects a pharmacologic effect of CST at the neuromuscular junction, although a transiently increased immune response to the AChR is also possible (Arsura et al. 1985; Miller et al. 1986; Verma and Oger 1992). Consequently, in severely weak patients, especially if there is significant bulbar or respiratory involvement, the initial stages of CST therapy should be performed either in the hospital or under close outpatient supervision (Massey 1997).

The adverse effects of CSTs are frequent, occurring in 20–80% of MG patients and are more likely with prolonged high-dose CST therapy and in the elderly (Donaldson et al. 1990). More common adverse effects include the development of a cushingoid appearance and weight gain (14 to 56%), infections (up to 50%), osteoporosis (3 to 30%), hypertension (3–12%), and cataracts (8–26%) (Table 7-32) (Sghirlanzoni et al. 1984; Arsura et al. 1985; Cornelio et al. 1987; Donaldson et al. 1990; Anonymous 1993; Beekman et al. 1997). As long-term therapy is frequently required, strategies to reduce these risks must be used (Table 7-32) (Dalakas 1990; Verma and Oger 1992; Sanders and Scoppetta 1994; Massey 1997). To avoid infections and delayed wound healing, thymectomy is performed when possible before high-dose CST administration. However, the risks of operating on a poorly controlled myasthenic are significant. If there are significant bulbar or respiratory symptoms the patient should first be stabilized with CST, to minimize the morbidity from subsequent thymectomy.

**SUMMARY**
**Extensive experience with CSTs in MG suggests that they are effective, often in a relatively short therapeutic regimen and are inexpensive. Their use is limited by the frequent occurrence of relapses after the dose is reduced, necessitating long-term use and leading to a high rate of adverse effects.**

**AZATHIOPRINE** A relatively weak immunosuppressive drug (Matell 1987; Massey 1997), azathioprine inhibits purine synthesis (Matell 1987; Diasio and LoBuglio 1996). It is metabolized by xanthine oxidase to 6-mercaptopurine (6-MP), which may cause most of its toxicity, while azathioprine itself is a more effective immunosuppressant (Matell 1987; Diasio and LoBuglio 1996). To minimize gastrointestinal toxicity, treatment is initiated using 50 mg/day and then increased by 50 mg every 3–7 days until the therapeutic dose (2–3.5 mg/kg per day given as a single dose) is reached (Massey 1997). It is well absorbed, with peak concentrations appearing in plasma at 1–2 hours (Matell 1987; Diasio and LoBuglio 1996). The drug and its metabolites are excreted in the urine (Diasio and LoBuglio 1996). Allopurinol inhibits xanthine oxidase, necessitating a reduction in the azathioprine dose to avoid excessive toxicity (Matell 1987; Sanders and Scoppetta 1994; Diasio and LoBuglio 1996). As with other immunosuppressives, azathioprine has multiple effects on both cellular and humoral arms of the immune system including a decrease in AChR antibody levels and suppression of T-helper lymphocyte responses to the AChR (Matell 1987; Mantegazza et al. 1988; Kuks et al. 1991).

Two randomized controlled trials have compared azathioprine with CST in MG (Myasthenia Gravis Clinical Study Group 1993; Bromberg et al. 1997). In the first, there was a much lower rate of treatment failure with azathioprine (Myasthenia Gravis Clinical Study Group 1993). The rates of remission or significant improvement at 3 years were similar in both azathioprine- and prednisone-treated groups (64 and 67%), although azathioprine had a more favorable adverse-effect profile (Myasthenia Gravis Clinical Study Group 1993). Conversely, in a more recent but much smaller study, there was an unusually high dropout rate in the azathioprine group and a poor response in the remaining patients (Bromberg et al. 1997). In uncontrolled trials, 70 to 90% of patients achieve a significant improvement or remission, similar to that with CSTs (Rowland 1980; Cornelio et al. 1987; Genkins et al. 1987; Matell 1987; Mantegazza et al. 1988; Kuks et al. 1991; Sanders and Scoppetta 1994). Compared with conservative treatment, the advent of azathioprine therapy has apparently reduced the mortality in MG (Matell 1987). The long latency before onset of clinical benefit frequently precludes the use of azathioprine as a first-line drug (Mantegazza et al. 1988), so that it is generally combined with CSTs with which it might have synergism (Cornelio et al. 1987; Genkins et al. 1987; Mantegazza et al. 1988; Sanders and Scoppetta 1994). Azathioprine has a steroid-sparing effect, allowing a more rapid rate of tapering and lower dose of CSTs (Matell 1987; Mantegazza et al. 1988; Kuks et al. 1991; Miano et al. 1991; Massey 1997). Azathioprine may have a selective advantage in thymoma-associated MG (Niakan et al. 1986; Matell 1987), and like other immunosuppressive agents, also in late-onset MG (Sghirlanzoni et al. 1984; Cornelio et al. 1987; Matell 1987; Donaldson et al. 1990; Kuks et al. 1991; Verma and Oger 1992). The effects of azathioprine may take 2–10 months to develop; maximal benefit is seen at 6–24 months (Rowland 1980; Genkins et al. 1987; Matell 1987; Kuks et al. 1991; Massey 1997). This long latency limits the use of azathioprine in an acutely deteriorating patient.

Slow tapering over 12–24 months after stable remission is achieved may decrease the risk of relapse (Matell 1987; Kuks et al. 1991).

Adverse effects of azathioprine occur in about one-third (10 to 54%) of MG patients (Cornelio et al. 1987; Genkins et al. 1987; Matell 1987; Donaldson et al. 1990; Kuks et al. 1991; Sanders and Scoppetta 1994; Beekman et al. 1997). About 10 to 25% of patients are unable to continue azathioprine because of gastrointestinal, hematological, or hepatic toxicity (Cornelio et al. 1987; Beekman et al. 1997). As with all immunosuppressives, susceptibility to infections is increased (Matell 1987). Transient gastrointestinal upset, common initially, can usually be ameliorated by a transient reduction of dose, by taking it with food or by dividing the dose (Cornelio et al. 1987; Matell 1987; Mantegazza et al. 1988; Beekman et al. 1997). Hepatic toxicity is also relatively common (Kuks et al. 1991). To a certain extent, bone marrow suppression is a desired and dose-related consequence of therapy with azathioprine, and increases in the red blood cell (RBC) mean corpuscular volume may correlate with benefit (Matell 1987; Massey 1997). However, excessive myelosuppression with neutropenia and thrombocytopenia must be avoided. Both hepatic and hematological toxicity must be checked for with frequent (e.g., once a week for 8 weeks and monthly thereafter) monitoring of liver enzymes and hematological indices. These adverse effects can occur at any time, and early in treatment they are usually reversible by decreasing or discontinuing the drug (Matell 1987). Angiotensin-converting enzyme inhibitors may increase the risk of bone marrow suppression caused by azathioprine (Gossmann et al. 1993). Some patients develop an early idiosyncratic reaction characterized by severe flu-like symptoms, which usually limits further use (Matell 1987; Verma and Oger 1992; Sanders and Scoppetta 1994; Massey 1997). Rarer adverse effects include skin rash, alopecia, and pancreatitis. Contrary to the use of azathioprine in renal transplant patients and perhaps patients with multiple sclerosis, there does not appear to be an increased risk of malignancy, specifically lymphoma, in MG patients caused by the drug (Matell 1987; Massey 1997). Despite warnings perpetuated in the literature, azathioprine is likely relatively safe in pregnancy (Ramsey-Goldman and Schilling 1997) (see Chapter 19).

SUMMARY

**Azathioprine is used as a primary therapy in MG when the clinical situation is not pressing, or when there are contraindications to CST use. It is also used to spare steroid dosage. It is effective and has fewer adverse effects than CSTs. However, its use requires monitoring for hepatic and hematological toxicity, it is expensive, and there is a long delay before benefit occurs.**

**CYCLOSPORINE** A fungal metabolite, cyclosporine is a potent immunosuppressive agent (Diasio and LoBuglio 1996). By binding to calcineurin and interfering with nuclear factor of activated T lymphocytes (NF-AT)-mediated transcription, interleukin-2 (IL-2) production, and IL-2 receptor upregulation (Tindall et al. 1993; Diasio and LoBuglio 1996), it inhibits the activation of T-helper lymphocytes. In MG, this presumably deprives B lymphocytes of the help required for production of AChR antibody.

The initial dose is 2–5 mg/kg (lean body weight) given as a divided dose every 12 hours. The dose is then adjusted to maintain a trough concentration in serum of 100–150 ng/mL (Verma and Oger 1992; Sanders and Scoppetta 1994; Massey 1997). Higher doses and serum levels may lead to earlier improvement, but at a risk of increased toxicity (Tindall et al. 1993). A newer preparation, Neoral has improved oral absorption and bioavailability (Diasio and LoBuglio 1996). Peak concentrations of drug occur 1.3–4 hours after oral administration, with most of the drug taken up in erythrocytes and leukocytes (Diasio and LoBuglio 1996). Metabolism occurs mainly in the liver, largely by the cytochrome P450 system, and excretion occurs via bile into the bowel (Diasio and LoBuglio 1996).

Cyclosporine is ordinarily used in MG patients who are intolerant of, or unresponsive to, CSTs or azathioprine (Tindall et al. 1993; Bonifati and Angelini 1997). After the successful results of several small, open trials in MG (Antonini et al. 1990; Bonifati and Angelini 1997), an RCT assessed cyclosporine in MG patients on AChEIs only. Although a favorable response was seen, its use was limited by significant toxicity (Tindall et al. 1987). A second RCT in MG patients who had failed CST therapy was also positive (Tindall et al. 1993). Improvement was seen as early as 1–2 months and was significant at 3–5 months, with most patients improved and on lower doses of CSTs by 6 months. Maximal benefit occurred at 12 months (Tindall et al. 1993; Sanders and Scoppetta 1994), and AChR antibody titers were reduced in parallel to clinical improvement (Tindall et al. 1987; Tindall et al. 1993). Unfortunately, patients often relapsed after discontinuation of cyclosporine (Tindall et al. 1993). There was some suggestion that ocular and bulbar involvement might be preferentially improved (Tindall et al. 1993).

Dose-related adverse effects, especially nephrotoxicity and hypertension, limit the utility of cyclosporine in MG (Tindall et al. 1987, 1993; Diasio and LoBuglio 1996). Others include hepatotoxicity, hirsutism, nausea, gingival hyperplasia, tremor, headache, neuropathy, and psychiatric changes (Diasio and LoBuglio 1996). Preexisting renal failure, poorly controlled hypertension, or significant hepatic dysfunction are relative contraindications to cyclosporine, as they increase the risk of adverse effects. Frequent monitoring of renal function, blood pressure, and serum trough cyclosporine levels is necessary. Lower trough levels (100–150 ng/mL) reduce the risk of adverse effects, but may also reduce and/or delay the onset of clinical benefit (Tindall et al. 1987, 1993; Sanders and Scoppetta 1994). A number of medications affect cyclosporine metabolism, requiring close monitoring of blood levels (Diasio and LoBuglio 1996).

SUMMARY
**Cyclosporine is one of the few agents shown by RCT data to be of benefit in MG, with a latency to benefit of several months. It is expensive, has considerable toxicity, and requires close monitoring of trough drug levels and renal function (Table 7-31). For these reasons, it is used mainly in situations of severe MG not responding to CST and azathioprine.**

CYCLOPHOSPHAMIDE An alkylating nitrogen mustard, cyclophosphamide interferes with DNA synthesis, and as it may preferentially suppress B lymphocytes, is theoretically advantageous for humorally mediated disorders like MG (Diasio and LoBuglio 1996). It has been used in small numbers of MG patients who have become refractory to other immunosuppressive agents (Sanders and Scoppetta 1994; Massey 1997). Doses of 1.5–5 mg/kg per day orally are used for MG patients, although intermittent monthly intravenous injections also have been used (Perez et al. 1981; Sanders and Scoppetta 1994). Peak plasma concentrations occur 1 hour after oral dosing, with a half-life of 7 hours.

In an animal model of MG, cyclophosphamide reduced AChR antibody levels and increased junctional AChR levels (but only at very high doses). The high doses also produced the need for subsequent bone marrow transplantation (Pestronk et al. 1983). In human MG, open trials show a benefit in 70 to 86% of small numbers of patients (Perez et al. 1981; Niakan et al. 1986; Badurska et al. 1992). The initial response often was seen within a month, and most improvement took a year. Those who achieved remission did so within 3–4 years (Perez et al. 1981). There was a relationship between improvement and cumulative dose (Perez et al. 1981). Relapse after discontinuation occurred in 38%, with recovery following reinitiating (Niakan et al. 1986).

Although potentially effective, cyclophosphamide is impressively toxic (Matell 1987). Its adverse effects include hepatotoxicity, alopecia, pancytopenia, nausea and vomiting, arthralgia, dizziness, susceptibility to infections, and hemorrhagic cystitis (Perez et al. 1981; Niakan et al. 1986; Matell 1987; Diasio and LoBuglio 1996). The cystitis is less likely with sufficient pre- and postdose hydration, and may be prevented with the use of the sulfhydryl agent MESNA. Mucosal ulcerations, dizziness, cardiotoxicity, and interstitial pulmonary fibrosis may also be seen. Regular monitoring should include a complete blood count (CBC) and differential, evaluation of liver enzymes, and urinalysis. It is teratogenic, and long-term use may decrease fertility (Matell 1987; Ramsey-Goldman and Schilling 1997).

SUMMARY
**Although based entirely on uncontrolled evidence, there is some indication that cyclophosphamide may be effective in patients with severe MG who are resistant to CST and azathioprine, but it is significantly more toxic.**

**PRINCIPLE Case reports, uncontrolled studies, and open studies may provide some legitimacy for hypothesis generation, but they do not set clear legitimacy for routine treatment. For that, blinding and controls usually are required.**

### *Thymectomy*

Thymectomy plays a central role in the treatment of MG, yet it too (like some of the above) remains a very controversial topic. The scientific rationale for thymectomy in MG is as follows. First, the thymus is involved in the education of immature lymphocytes to recognize nonself (foreign) antigens and to tolerate self antigens. Second, it contains potentially antigenic AChR sequences either on myoid cells or in thymic epithelial cells (Hohlfeld and Wekerle 1994). Third, pathologic involvement of the thymus, either hyperplasia or thymoma, is frequent in MG (Hohlfeld and Wekerle 1994), and the hyperplastic thymus in MG contains both AChR-reactive T and B lymphocytes and is the source of considerable AChR antibody production (Willcox and Vincent 1988; Hohlfeld and Wekerle 1994). However, although there is widespread acceptance for thymectomy in the treatment of MG, the precise indications and optimal approach to the thymus remain controversial (Rowland 1980; Lanska 1990). Some of the unresolved issues include which subgroups benefit from thymectomy (early or late onset, seropositive or seronegative, males or females, ocular or generalized), whether thymectomy late in the course of MG is worthwhile, how it should be performed (transcervical or transsternal), and whether the outcome relates to the pathology (hyperplastic, thymoma, normal, or atrophic) (Lanska 1990).

Although more than 700 papers have been published with reference to thymectomy in MG, none involve controlled trials. Before the use of AChEIs and effective immunosuppression, thymectomy reduced the mortality from MG to one-third of that seen in patients who did not have surgery (Verma and Oger 1992) and increased the rates of remission (Oosterhuis 1981). It is generally agreed that thymectomy is beneficial when done promptly in the course of an early-onset generalized myasthenia patient, and that it should also be performed in patients with a thymoma (Lanska 1990; Mantegazza et al. 1990; Verma and Oger 1992). In the early-onset generalized group, approximately 30 to 40% achieve a lasting drug-free remission and 40 to 50% are significantly improved, for an overall rate of improvement of up to 90% (Mante gazza et al. 1990; Verma and Oger 1992; Weinberg et al. 1994), whereas 10 to 30% are unchanged. Improvements in myasthenic symptoms are less after the removal of a thymoma (Rowland 1980; Oosterhuis 1981). The mortality and morbidity of the procedure is minimal (Rowland 1980). Even if only equivalent to medical therapy, the avoidance of the considerable adverse effects of long-term CSTs and immunosuppression is a compelling indication.

Debate continues as to the optimal surgical approach (Jaretzki 1997). Ectopic thymic tissue is found in 10 to 40% of thymus resections, often in the anterior mediastinal fat or neck (Ashour 1995; Jaretzki 1997). This ectopic tissue may be missed with a cervical approach, and its presence may explain a poor outcome from thymectomy and the need for reoperation, even when repeat imaging does not show residual thymic tissue (Miller et al. 1991; Ashour 1995). There is a trend toward increased remission rates with more aggressive approaches (Jaretzki 1997). More controversial is whether thymectomy is effective in nonthymomatous late-onset myasthenia, when the thymus is often atrophic and the rationale for thymectomy seemingly weaker (Olanow et al. 1982; Lanska 1990).

Improvement after thymectomy may not be seen for 2–10 years (Oosterhuis 1981; Mantegazza et al. 1990; Verma and Oger 1992). Given this long latency before benefit, thymectomy should not be performed in an unstable patient. For this reason, preoperative plasma exchange is often performed in patients with significant bulbar or respiratory involvement to minimize perioperative complications. There is no evidence of deleterious immunosuppression or of an increased risk of malignancy after thymectomy (Verma and Oger 1992).

SUMMARY
**Although there is considerable uncontrolled evidence suggesting benefit in selected subgroups, a randomized controlled trial is needed to settle many of the controversies about the role of thymectomy in MG.**

PRINCIPLE **When a disease is rare and sporadic, open and uncontrolled observations have great and perpetual influence that may never be justified.**

### *Temporary treatments*

PLASMA EXCHANGE The initial success of plasma exchange (PE) in resistant MG was encouraging (Pinching et al. 1976), as was the utility of PE in other disorders where a humoral pathogenesis seemed likely (Thornton and Griggs 1994). In MG, the rationale is that PE removes pathogenic humoral factors, confirmed by reductions in anti-AChR antibodies by 50 to 70% (Komiya and Sato 1987; Seybold 1987; Goti et al. 1995; Cornblath et al. 1996), temporarily improving neuromuscular transmission and resulting in clinical improvement (Genkins et al. 1987; Cornblath et al. 1996). Each exchange removes approximately 60% of serum components, so that a course of three to five exchanges removes 93 to 99% of serum IgG, along with other serum factors (Thornton and Griggs 1994). The non-IgG components, with a shorter half-life, are quickly replaced, but IgG with a half-life of 21 days returns at a much slower rate (Thornton and Griggs 1994). AChEIs are not significantly removed during plasma exchange (Verma and Oger 1992). Although there is no evidence to support any particular regimen, a common schedule consists of three to five exchanges, each exchanging 5% of body weight (50 mL/kg), over 3–10 days (Sanders and Scoppetta 1994). However, in one study two exchanges were as effective as more intensive therapy (Antozzi et al. 1991). PE is used primarily at times of significant worsening with respiratory and bulbar involvement, as well as before a surgical procedure to reduce postoperative complications (Pinching et al. 1976; d'Empaire et al. 1985; Seybold 1987). It is effective in seronegative MG (Rowland 1980; Miller et al. 1981; Genkins et al. 1987; Seybold 1987), but not in the congenital myasthenic syndromes (Pinching et al. 1976). It is debatable whether PE is useful to prevent or manage the early worsening seen with CSTs (Fornasari et al. 1985).

After beginning PE, electrophysiologic improvement in neuromuscular transmission may be seen within 24 hours (Konishi et al. 1981), although clinical benefit is usually delayed for 2–10 days (Massey 1997), and is maximal at 8–16 days (Gajdos et al. 1997). The duration of improvement ranges from 2 to 8 weeks (Seybold 1987; Massey 1997). Before thymectomy, it is useful to warn the patient that improvements after PE may be followed by a return to baseline before the benefits of thymectomy occur. To sustain the effects of PE, immunosuppression is required (Dau 1981; Milner-Brown and Miller 1982). PE does not modify the disease more than immunosuppression alone does, so that there is no role for repeated PE in the long-term management of MG (Dau 1981; Milner-Brown and Miller 1982; Thornton and Griggs 1994). In uncontrolled trials 60 to 88% of MG patients improve (Fornasari et al. 1985; Seybold 1987; Gajdos et al. 1997). Patients with severe disease are less likely to respond, and there is no correlation between AChR antibody levels and response. Significant complement-mediated endplate damage might explain this variation in response between patients. Despite the dearth of controlled studies of PE in MG, given the compelling rationale for its use and considerable evidence from uncontrolled observations, use of PE in MG is generally accepted (NIH Consensus Development [Conference] 1986; Cornblath et al. 1996). In one uncontrolled study, although both plasma exchange and pyridostigmine produced benefit, PE was superior with improvement that occurred on day 2–4 (Goti et al. 1995). In another retrospective series, patients given prethymectomy PE required less mechanical ventilation and had shorter stays in the ICU than patients who did not have PE (d'Empaire et al. 1985). Although there are no prospective studies comparing PE to placebo, an RCT comparing PE to intravenous immunoglobulin (IVIg) in worsening MG demonstrated similar benefit from both, although IVIg had fewer adverse effects (Gajdos et al. 1997). PE is generally well tolerated (Cornblath et al. 1996). More common side effects occur in 12 to 40% and require the discontinuation of 2 to 10% of exchanges (Antozzi et al. 1991; Gajdos et al. 1997). They include difficulties with venous access, hypotension, fever, chills, nausea, vomiting, citrate-induced hypocalcemia, hypoalbuminemia, changes in clotting with thrombocytopenia, and bleeding (Thornton and Griggs 1994; Cornblath et al. 1996; Massey 1997).

**PRINCIPLE** **Piling uncontrolled observations upon one another really does not generate rationale for therapy with or without "academic endorsement." But if the response is like that from giving an appropriate antibiotic to pneumococcal pneumonia patients and if the effect is in major disease, the intervention is justified. In such settings, evidence-based medical approaches to justify continued practice are mandatory.**

**SUMMARY**
**There is a good rationale for the use of PE in MG, and considerable evidence from uncontrolled studies to support its use. Limited controlled studies suggest that PE is equivalent to IVIg. PE, as with IVIg, is expensive, produces temporary improvement, and is not advisable for the long-term management of MG (Table 7-31). Because of the rapid benefit in comparison with other therapies, it is useful in a deteriorating patient. As their indications in MG are similar, PE is often used interchangeably with (but not immediately after) IVIg, although further study is needed to clarify the roles of these two therapies in MG.**

**INTRAVENOUS IMMUNOGLOBULIN** Although IVIg was employed successfully with ACTH in MG in the 1970s (Genkins et al. 1987), it was not until after promising results treating patients with idiopathic thrombocytopenic purpura (ITP) (NIH Consensus Conference 1990) that IVIg use appeared favorable in two small series of MG patients (Fateh-Moghadam et al. 1984; Gajdos et al. 1984). A course of IVIg consists of either 0.4 g/kg per day for 5 days or 1 g/kg per day for 2 days. These regimens were extrapolated from those used in ITP, without any evidence to favor a specific treatment schedule (Gajdos et al. 1997). IVIg is prepared from the plasma of 3000–15,000 human donors (Misbah and Chapel 1993). Although there are several immunologically active proteins in IVIg, the principal active component is likely IgG (Thornton and Griggs 1994). After infusion, the half-life of IgG is approximately 21 days (range 12–45) (Thornton and Griggs 1994). The mechanism of action of IVIg likely differs depending on the disease being treated, and in MG there are several possible subgroups perhaps mediated by different mechanisms (Ferrero et al. 1993). A moderate decrease in AChR antibody levels is often, but not always, seen after IVIg (Fateh-Moghadam et al. 1984; Gajdos et al. 1984; Ferrero et al. 1993; Gajdos et al. 1997).

In a series of open trials, 50 to 87% of MG patients improved with IVIg (Fateh-Moghadam et al. 1984; Gajdos et al. 1984; Ferrero et al. 1993; Edan and Landgraf 1994; Gajdos et al. 1997). In the only RCT published to date, IVIg was compared with PE (although only three exchanges were used). Only 61% of patients improved with IVIg, fewer than in many of the uncontrolled trials, although this was perhaps a consequence of more rigorous clinical analysis. Although IVIg was as effective as PE, it was better tolerated (Thornton and Griggs 1994; Gajdos et al. 1997). The onset of benefit occurred within 4 days of beginning the infusion (Ferrero et al. 1993; Misbah and Chapel 1993; Edan and Landgraf 1994) and was optimal at 8–15 days (Misbah and Chapel 1993; Gajdos et al. 1997). It lasted a median of 40–106 days (Misbah and Chapel 1993; Edan and Landgraf 1994). The peak benefit with IVIg may be slightly delayed in comparison with that of PE (Gajdos et al. 1997).

The frequency of adverse effects with IVIg is variable, ranging from 0 to 80% (Fateh-Moghadam et al. 1984; Gajdos et al. 1984; Anonymous 1990; Misbah and Chapel 1993; Brannagan et al. 1996; Gajdos et al. 1997). When surveyed specifically in patients with neurologic diseases including MG, the adverse effects were more common than in patients without neurologic abnormalities, occurring in 59 to 81% of patients (Brannagan et al. 1996). The more common adverse effects (Table 7-33) are mild, occur during or shortly after infusion, and can be minimized by decreasing drug delivery rates or by using appropriate symptomatic therapy (Anonymous 1990; Misbah and Chapel 1993; Edan and Landgraf 1994; Brannagan et al. 1996). To minimize the risks of more serious adverse effects, special attention is warranted in the presence of certain risk factors (Table 7-33) (Misbah and Chapel 1993; Brannagan et al. 1996). Screening for IgA deficiency before IVIg therapy is often recommended, although anaphylaxis in IgA-deficient individuals is likely an extremely rare occurrence (Thornton and Griggs 1994; Sandler et al. 1995). With modern preparation techniques, the risk of transmitting known infectious agents is negligible (Misbah and Chapel 1993).

SUMMARY

**Both uncontrolled and limited RCT data support the efficacy of IVIg in MG. The indications for IVIg are similar to those for PE. Further information is needed on the optimal treatment schedules, and on the role of IVIg in comparison to less expensive conventional therapies for the long-term management of MG. Practically, IVIg is more convenient to obtain and administer than PE and has fewer serious adverse effects than PE. However, supplies of IVIg are increasingly limited, and as with PE, the expense is considerable (Table 7-31).**

## SPECIAL ISSUES

### Ocular Myasthenia Gravis

Many MG patients (30 to 50%) present with isolated ptosis and diplopia (Genkins et al. 1987; Oosterhuis 1989; Sanders and Scoppetta 1994; Weinberg et al. 1994; Beek-

**Table 7-33 Adverse Effects of Intravenous Immunoglobulin G**

| |
|---|
| *Common, mild, early, reversible and related to infusion rate* |
| Abdominal pain, arthralgia, backache, myalgia |
| Chest tightness, wheezing, dyspnea |
| Fever, chills |
| Headache |
| Nausea, vomiting |
| Presyncopal sensations |
| Rash, pruritus, skin flushing |
| Vasomotor/cardiovascular—changes in BP and HR |
| *Rare, potentially more severe, delayed* |
| Alopecia |
| Aseptic meningitis |
| Cerebral thrombosis/stroke, reversible cerebral vasospasm |
| Coagulopathy, deep vein thrombosis |
| Erythema multiforme |
| Hemolytic anemia (anti-blood group A or rhesus D contained in IVIg) |
| Hypersensitivity/anaphylaxis (? more likely in IgA-deficient recipients) |
| Leukopenia, neutropenia (transient) |
| Renal failure, proteinuria |
| Transient increase in liver transaminases |
| Transmission of infection (hepatitis C) |
| *Risk factors* |
| Concurrent infection (antibody in IVIg binding to infectious agent) |
| High infusion rates/volumes especially with preexisting cardiac or vascular disease |
| Recipient IgA deficiency, may increase risk for anaphylaxis |
| Immobility (and increased risk of venous thrombosis) |
| Increased age |
| Increased serum viscosity—paraproteinemia, dehydration |
| Migraine (increased risk of headache and aseptic meningitis) |
| Renal failure (high solute load in IVIg or immune complex formation) |

ABBREVIATIONS: BP, blood pressure; HR, heart rate; IVIg, intravenous immunoglobulin G.

man et al. 1997) and most of the remaining patients have ocular symptoms along with generalized disease. In 15–20% of cases, the disease remains restricted to the EOM, the remainder having developed generalized weakness, often within the first 2–3 years (Evoli et al. 1988; Oosterhuis 1989; Weinberg et al. 1994). Most ocular MG patients respond poorly to AChEIs but do well on low-dose CSTs, with some evidence suggesting that early CST use in ocular MG may reduce subsequent generalization of the disease (Weinberg et al. 1994; Kupersmith et al. 1996; Sommer et al. 1997). However, as ocular MG is a relatively benign form of MG, it is particularly prudent to balance these benefits against the risks of CSTs. Following the logic of reducing risks of subsequent generalization of the disease, perhaps thymectomy should also be offered to patients with sufficiently severe ocular MG, although ocular symptoms may respond less well to thymectomy.

## Seronegative Myasthenia Gravis

In 21 to 71% of ocular MG and 6 to 25% of generalized MG, anti-AChR antibodies are not detected (Beekman et al. 1997; Sanders et al. 1997). However, seronegative MG is also humorally mediated (Mossman et al. 1986; Drachman et al. 1987), and its treatment including PE is similar to that for seropositive disease (Drachman et al. 1987; Birmanns et al. 1991; Sanders et al. 1997). Thymic hyperplasia may be less frequent in seronegative patients (Willcox et al. 1991), and the role for thymectomy less certain (Willcox et al. 1991).

## Pregnancy

The effects of pregnancy are equally likely to be neutral, beneficial, or deleterious to the course of MG, and the pregnancy itself is usually unaffected by MG so that cesarean section should be performed only if there are other obstetrical indications. Deterioration is more likely during the postpartum period (Plauché 1991). Many drugs used in the management of MG may be relatively safely continued during pregnancy, including AChEI, CSTs, and azathioprine (Sanders and Scoppetta 1994; Ramsey-Goldman and Schilling 1997). The irregular absorption of AChEIs may be worsened during pregnancy (Plauché 1991). The risks of uncontrolled MG during pregnancy probably outweigh a possible increase in the occurrence of cleft lip and palate with CST (Plauché 1991). Plasma exchange is possible, although hypotension must be avoided (Plauché 1991). Myasthenic mothers are more sensitive to neuromuscular blockade, should an anesthetic be required (Genkins et al. 1987). Magnesium, used to treat eclampsia, can impair neuromuscular transmission by interfering with presynaptic voltage-gated calcium channels, and should be avoided (Bashuk RG and Krendel 1990; Plauché 1991). AChEIs appear safe in breast-feeding mothers, with only 0.1% of the maternal dose appearing in breast milk (Aquilonius and Hartvig 1986; Plauché 1991).

## Neonatal Myasthenia Gravis

In 10 to 20% of pregnancies in myasthenics, especially those with severe disease, the transplacental passage of anti-AChR antibodies produces transient weakness in the neonate (Plauché 1991). Neonatal MG may also occur in seronegative MG mothers (Mier and Havard 1985). Appearing within the first several days, the weakness may last several weeks before resolving, and does not recur. Neonatal MG can be treated with pyridostigmine until the weakness resolves.

## Drugs and Myasthenia Gravis

A number of drugs may worsen neuromuscular transmission (Table 7-34) (Wittbrodt 1997). However, many myasthenics take one or more of these medications without any obvious ill effect, and in some cases the evidence implicating individual drugs as a cause of worsening MG is feeble. Part of the management of patients with myasthenia gravis is to educate them and their general physicians about this possibility, and to consider these medications as a cause of otherwise unexplained worsening.

**PRINCIPLE All too often worsening of a disease is attributed to factors beyond control and not to physician-introduced determinants.**

## Juvenile Myasthenia Gravis

In 10% of myasthenics, the onset is before age 18. Juvenile MG is more frequently ocular and seronegative, especially with prepubertal onset, but is otherwise clinically similar to the adult disease (Andrews et al. 1994). The first step in management is to rule out a congenital myasthenic syndrome, as immunosuppression or thymectomy has no role in the management of these disorders. The management of juvenile MG is similar to that for the adult disease in all respects, although growth retardation from long-term CST must be considered. Thymectomy is safe in children after the first year (Rowland 1980), with

**Table 7-34 Drugs That May Worsen Myasthenia Gravis[a]**

| |
|---|
| *Antibiotics* |
| Aminoglycosides[a] |
| Macrolides (erythromycin, clarithromycin) |
| Fluoroquinolones (norfloxacin, ofloxacin, pefloxacin) |
| Polymixin B sulfate, colistin sulfate |
| Tetracyclines, oxytetracyclines |
| Lincomycin HCl and clindamycin (HCl and phosphate) |
| Ampicillin |
| *Cardiovascular* |
| β-Adrenergic blockers (including topical/ocular)[a] |
| Quinidine[a] (quinidines: gluconate, polygalacturonate, sulfate) |
| Procainamide HCl[a] |
| Verapamil HCl and perhaps other calcium channel blockers |
| *CNS active* |
| Diphenylhydantoin/phenytoin sodium[a] |
| Trimethadione |
| Lithium carbonate |
| Chlorpromazine HCl, promazine HCl |
| Trihexyphenidyl HCl |
| Morphine sulfate? |
| Amantadine HCl |
| *Antirheumatic and immunosuppressive* |
| Chloroquine[a] (HCl and phosphate) |
| D-Penicillamine[a] |
| Prednisone[a] (high doses may produce early worsening in MG) |
| *Anesthetic agents* |
| Nondepolarizing agents (pancuronium bromide, vecuronium bromide, atracurium besylate) —increased sensitivity in MG |
| Depolarizing agents (succinylcholine chloride)—decreased effect in MG, increased if on pyridostigmine |
| *Miscellaneous* |
| Procaine HCl and lidocaine HCl (IV)[a] |
| Magnesium[a] |
| Bretylium tosylate |
| Topical ophthalmic drugs (timolol, betaxolol HCl, echothiophate iodide) |
| Quinine sulfate |
| Lactate |
| Iodinated contrast agents |
| Citrate anticoagulant |
| Diphenhydramine HCl |
| Aprotinin (Trasylol) |
| Emetine |
| D,L-Carnitine |

[a]Drugs that are most consistently reported as causing problems in MG.

an efficacy similar to that in the adult disease, and noevidence for long-term adverse effects such as malignancies or immunodeficiencies (Youssef 1983).

## Late-onset Myasthenia Gravis and Thymoma

There are a few differences in the management of late-onset MG. The response to CST and azathioprine may be better in late-onset MG (Sghirlanzoni et al. 1984; Cornelio et al. 1987; Matell 1987; Donaldson et al. 1990; Kuks et al. 1991; Verma and Oger 1992). Because of the normal involution of the thymus in later life, thymectomy in this age group is more controversial (Lanska 1990). The removal of a thymoma, much more common in the elderly, is generally accepted as an absolute indication for thymectomy to avoid local growth and infiltration of adjacent mediastinal structures (Lanska 1990), yet has less effect on myasthenic symptoms than does removal of a hyperplastic thymus (Rowland 1980; Oosterhuis 1981; Mantegazza et al. 1990). However, in an elderly individual with a small thymoma and/or increased operative risk, close clinical and radiological follow-up is an option (Sanders and Scoppetta 1994). If extension through the thymus capsule occurs grossly or microscopically, postoperative radiotherapy reduces the chance of subsequent recurrence (Sanders and Scoppetta 1994; Regnard et al. 1996).

## Myasthenic Crisis

Precipitants for a myasthenic crisis include infections, aspiration, pregnancy, drugs, or withdrawal of medications in a treated patient, although in many cases no cause is found (Thomas et al. 1997). The management consists of intubation and respiratory support in the intensive care unit if lung volumes and partial pressure of oxygen ($P_{O_2}$) are decreasing. Identified causes should be treated, and a pattern of AChEI use and symptoms that might suggest a cholinergic crisis should be explored. Generally, AChEIs are withheld initially. Plasma exchange or IVIg is initiated, and CSTs are started to sustain the response, with careful monitoring for early worsening (Dau 1981; Milner-Brown and Miller 1982). There is no agreement as to whether edrophonium injection allows the distinction between a myasthenic or cholinergic crisis (Rowland 1980).

## Other Issues

Several other issues may affect outcome. In seronegative patients who do not respond to treatment, other diagnoses should be considered. In seropositive nonresponders, concurrent diseases such as polymyositis, thyroid disease, or steroid myopathy may limit the response to therapy. Immunization for influenza is advisable, and vaccines that are inactivated are safe, while attenuated vaccines such as oral polio vaccine should not be given. Patient education about the disease and its treatment is an important part of the therapy of MG. This improves compliance with therapies that in the short term may have significant adverse effects, but which in the long term can be extremely effective.

**PRINCIPLE Toxicity, though not life-threatening, may lead to noncompliance with efficacious therapy unless the patient is motivated to overcome the desire to stop treatment.**

**SUMMARY**

**More is known about the pathogenesis of MG than many of the other autoimmune disorders. Partly as a result of this, the treatment of MG is successful, although the frequency of adverse effects is often a limiting factor. The lack of standard measures of disease severity or outcome makes comparison of results from retrospective and uncontrolled studies difficult. Hence, there are many opportunities for randomized controlled trials of therapy in MG, although these are practically difficult because of the rarity and considerable clinical and immunologic heterogeneity of MG, and because of the apparent efficacy of currently employed therapies. Nevertheless, evidence-based data are emerging for some agents that confirm the efficacy seen in uncontrolled studies. Managing a patient with MG usually is a rewarding experience, with most patients responding to treatment and achieving significant improvement in their symptoms, although the adverse effects of long-term treatment can be severe. The future goals will be to devise less toxic immunosuppressive agents, and to elucidate the immunopathogenesis so that truly antigen-specific immunotherapies can be devised (Nicolle et al. 1994).**

## REFERENCES


Andrews PI, Massey JM, Howard JF, et al. 1994. Race, sex, and puberty influence onset, severity, and outcome in juvenile myasthenia gravis. *Neurology* **44**:1208–14.

Antonini G, Bove R, Filippini C, et al. 1990. Results of an open trial of cyclosporine in a group of steroid-dependent myasthenic subjects. *Clin Neurol Neurosurg* **92**:317–21.

Antozzi C, Gemma M, Regi B, et al. 1991. A short plasma exchange protocol is effective in severe myasthenia gravis. *J Neurol* **238**:103–7.

Aquilonius SM, Hartvig P. 1986. Clinical pharmacokinetics of cholinesterase inhibitors [review]. *Clin Pharmacokinet* **11**:236–49.

Arsura E, Brunner NG, Namba T, et al. 1985. High-dose intravenous methylprednisolone in myasthenia gravis. *Arch Neurol* **42**: 1149–53.

Arsura EL, Brunner NG, Namba T, et al. 1987. Adverse cardiovascular effects of anticholinesterase medications. *Am J Med Sci* **293**: 18–23.

Ashour M. 1995. Prevalence of ectopic thymic tissue in myasthenia gravis and its clinical significance. *J Thorac Cardiovasc Surg* **109**:632–5.

Badurska B, Ryniewicz B, Strugalska H. 1992. Immunosuppressive treatment for juvenile myasthenia gravis. *Eur J Pediatr* **151**:215–7.

Bashuk RG, Krendel DA. 1990. Myasthenia gravis presenting as weakness after magnesium administration. *Muscle Nerve* **13**:708–12.

Beekman R, Kuks JBM, Oosterhuis HJGH. 1997. Myasthenia gravis: diagnosis and follow-up of 100 consecutive patients. *J Neurol* **244**:112–8.

Birmanns B, Brenner T, Abramsky O, et al. 1991. Seronegative myasthenia gravis: clinical features, response to therapy and synthesis of acetylcholine receptor antibodies in vitro. *J Neurol Sci* **102**: 184–9.

Bonifati DM, Angelini C. 1997. Long-term cyclosporine treatment in a group of severe myasthenia gravis patients. *J Neurol* **244**:542–7.

Brannagan TH, Nagle KJ, Lange DJ, et al. 1996. Complications of intravenous immune globulin treatment in neurologic disease. *Neurology* **47**:674–7.

Bromberg MB, Wald JJ, Forshew DA, et al. 1997. Randomized trial of azathioprine or prednisone for initial immunosuppressive treatment of myasthenia gravis. *J Neurol Sci* **150**:59–62.

Cornblath DR, Braine HG, Dyck PJ, et al. 1996. Assessment of plasmapheresis. *Neurology* **47**:840.

Cornelio F, Peluchetti D, Mantegazza R, et al. 1987. The course of myasthenia gravis in patients treated with corticosteroids, azathioprine, and plasmapheresis. *Ann N Y Acad Sci* **505**:517–525.

Dalakas M. 1990. Pharmacologic concerns of corticosteroids in the treatment of patients with immune-related neuromuscular diseases [review]. *Neurol Clin* **8**:93–118.

Dau PC. 1981. Response to plasmapheresis and immunosuppressive drug therapy in sixty myasthenia gravis patients. *Ann N Y Acad Sci* **377**:700–8.

d'Empaire G, Hoaglin DC, Perlo VP, et al. 1985. Effect of prethymectomy plasma exchange on postoperative respiratory function in myasthenia gravis. *J Thorac Cardiovasc Surg* **89**:592–6.

Diasio RB, LoBuglio AF. 1996. Immunomodulators: immunosuppressive agents and immunostimulants. In: Hardman JG, Limbird LE, editors. *Goodman & Gilman's The Pharmacological Basis of Therapeutics*. New York: McGraw-Hill. p 1289.

Donaldson DH, Ansher M, Horan S, et al. 1990. The relationship of age to outcome in myasthenia gravis. *Neurology* **40**:786–90.

Drachman DB. 1987. Present and future treatment of myasthenia gravis. *N Engl J Med* **316**:743–5.

Drachman DB, de Silva S, Ramsay D, et al. 1987. Humoral pathogenesis of myasthenia gravis [review]. *Ann N Y Acad Sci* **505**:90–105.

Edan G, Landgraf F. 1994. Experience with intravenous immunoglobulin in myasthenia gravis: a review. *J Neurol Neurosurg Psychiatry* **57**(Suppl.):S55–S6.

Evoli A, Tonali P, Bartoccioni E, et al. 1988. Ocular myasthenia: diagnostic and therapeutic problems. *Acta Neurol Scand* **77**: 31–5.

Fateh-Moghadam A, Wick M, Besinger U, et al. 1984. High-dose intravenous gammaglobulin for myasthenia gravis [letter]. *Lancet* **1**:848–9.

Ferrero B, Durelli L, Cavallo R, et al. 1993. Therapies for exacerbation of myasthenia gravis. The mechanism of action of intravenous high-dose immunoglobulin G. *Ann N Y Acad Sci* **681**:563–6.

Fornasari PM, Riva G, Piccolo G, et al. 1985. Short and long-term clinical effects of plasma-exchange in 33 cases of myasthenia gravis. *Int J Artif Organs* **8**:159–62.

Gajdos P, Chevret S, Clair B, et al. 1997. Clinical trial of plasma exchange and high-dose intravenous immunoglobulin in myasthenia gravis. Myasthenia Gravis Clinical Study Group. *Ann Neurol* **41**:789–96.

Gajdos P, Outin H, Elkharrat D, et al. 1984. High-dose intravenous gammaglobulin for myasthenia gravis [letter]. *Lancet* **1**:406–7.

Genkins G, Kornfeld P, Papatestas AE, et al. 1987. Clinical experience in more than 2000 patients with myasthenia gravis [review]. *Ann N Y Acad Sci* **505**:500–13.

Gossmann J, Kachel HG, Shoeppe W, et al. 1993. Anemia in renal transplant recipients caused by concomitant therapy with azathioprine and angiotensin-converting enzyme inhibitors. *Transplantation* **56**:585–9.

Goti P, Spinelli A, Marconi G, et al. 1995. Comparative effects of plasma exchange and pyridostigmine on respiratory muscle strength and breathing pattern in patients with myasthenia gravis. *Thorax* **50**:1080–6.

Grob D, Brunner NG, Namba T. 1981. The natural course of myasthenia gravis and effect of therapeutic measures. *Ann N Y Acad Sci* **377**:652–69.

Hartvig P, Wiklund L, Aquilonius SM, et al. 1990. Clinical pharmacokinetics of acetylcholinesterase inhibitors [review]. *Prog Brain Res* **84**:139–43.

Hohlfeld R, Wekerle H. 1994. The thymus in myasthenia gravis [review]. *Neurol Clin* **12**:331–42.

Howard FM Jr, Duane DD, Lambert EH, et al. 1976. Alternate-day prednisone: preliminary report of a double-blind controlled study. *Ann N Y Acad Sci* **274**:596–607.

Jaretzki A. 1997. Thymectomy for myasthenia gravis. Analysis of the controversies regarding technique and results. *Neurology* **48**(Suppl. 5):S52.

Kaplan I, Blakely BT, Pavlath GK, et al. 1990. Steroids induce acetylcholine receptors on cultured human muscle: implications for myasthenia gravis. *Proc Natl Acad Sci USA* **87**:8100–4.

Keesey JC. 1989. AAEE Minimonograph #33: Electrodiagnostic approach to defects of neuromuscular transmission. *Muscle Nerve* **12**:613–26.

Komiya T, Sato T. 1987. Long-term follow-up study of relapse in symptoms and reelevation of acetylcholine receptor antibody titers in patients with myasthenia gravis. *Ann N Y Acad Sci* **540**:605–7.

Konishi T, Nishitani H, Matsubara F, et al. 1981. Myasthenia gravis: relation between jitter in single-fiber EMG and antibody to acetylcholine receptor. *Neurology* **31**:386–92.

Kuks JBM, Djojoatmodjo S, Oosterhuis HJHG. 1991. Azathioprine in myasthenia gravis: observations in 41 patients and a review of literature [review]. *Neuromuscul Disord* **1**:423–31.

Kupersmith MJ, Moster M, Bhuiyan S, et al. 1996. Beneficial effects of corticosteroids on ocular myasthenia gravis. *Arch Neurol* **53**:802–4.

Lanska DJ. 1990. Indications for thymectomy in myasthenia gravis. *Neurology* **40**:1828–9.

Mantegazza R, Antozzi C, Peluchetti D, et al. 1988. Azathioprine as a single drug or in combination with steroids in the treatment of myasthenia gravis. *J Neurol* **235**:449–53.

Mantegazza R, Beghi E, Pareyson D, et al. 1990. A multicentre follow-up study of 1152 patients with myasthenia gravis in Italy. *J Neurol* **237**:339–44.

Massey JM. 1997. Treatment of acquired myasthenia gravis. *Neurology* **48**(Suppl. 5):S46

Massey JM, Sanders DB, Howard JF Jr. 1989. The effect of cholinesterase inhibitors of SFEMG in myasthenia gravis. *Muscle Nerve* **12**:154–5.

Matell G. 1987. Immunosuppressive drugs: azathioprine in the treatment of myasthenia gravis. *Ann N Y Acad Sci* **505**:588–94.

McEvoy KM. 1994. Diagnosis and treatment of Lambert-Eaton myasthenic syndrome [review]. *Neurol Clin* **12**:387–99.

Miano MA, Bosley TM, Heiman-Patterson TD, et al. 1991. Factors influencing outcome of prednisone dose reduction in myasthenia gravis. *Neurology* **41**:919–21.

Mier AK, Havard CWH. 1985. Diaphragmatic myasthenia in mother and child. *Postgrad Med J* **61**:725–7.

Miller RG, Filler-Katz A, Kiprov D, et al. 1991. Repeat thymectomy in chronic refractory myasthenia gravis. *Neurology* **41**:923–4.

Miller RG, Milner-Brown HS, Dau PC. 1981. Antibody-negative acquired myasthenia gravis: successful therapy with plasma exchange [letter]. *Muscle Nerve* **4**:255.

Miller RG, Milner-Brown HS, Mirka A. 1986. Prednisone-induced worsening of neuromuscular function in myasthenia gravis. *Neurology* **36**:729–32.

Milner-Brown HS, Miller RG. 1982. Time course of improved neuromuscular function following plasma exchange alone and plasma exchange with prednisone/azathioprine in myasthenia gravis. *J Neurol Sci* **57**:357–68.

Misbah SA, Chapel HM. 1993. Adverse effects of intravenous immunoglobulin [review]. *Drug Saf* **9**:254–62.

Mossman S, Vincent A, Newsom-Davis J. 1986. Myasthenia gravis without acetylcholine-receptor antibody: a distinct disease entity. *Lancet* **1**:116–9.

Myasthenia Gravis Clinical Study Group. 1993. A randomised clinical trial comparing prednisone and azathioprine in myasthenia gravis. Results of the second interim analysis. *J Neurol Neurosurg Psychiatry* **56**:1157–63.

Niakan E, Harati Y, Rolak LA. 1986. Immunosuppressive drug therapy in myasthenia gravis. *Arch Neurol* **43**:155–6.

Nicolle MW, Nag B, Sharma SD, et al. 1994. Specific tolerance to an acetylcholine receptor epitope induced in vitro in myasthenia gravis $CD4^+$ lymphocytes by soluble major histocompatibility complex class II-peptide complexes. *J Clin Invest* **93**:1361–9.

NIH Consensus Conference. 1990. Intravenous immunoglobulin. Prevention and treatment of disease. *JAMA* **264**:3189–93.

NIH Consensus Development [Conference]. 1986. The utility of therapeutic plasmapheresis for neurological disorders. *JAMA* **256**:1333–7.

Olanow CW, Lane RJM, Oses AD. 1982. Thymectomy in late-onset myasthenia gravis. *Arch Neurol* **39**:82–3.

Oosterhuis HJ. 1981. Observations of the natural history of myasthenia gravis and the effect of thymectomy. *Ann N Y Acad Sci* **377**:678–90.

Oosterhuis HJGH. 1989. The natural course of myasthenia gravis: a long term follow up study. *J Neurol Neurosurg Psychiatry* **52**:1121–7.

Oosterhuis HJGH, Limburg PC, Hummel-Tappel E, et al. 1983. Anti-acetylcholine receptor antibody in myasthenia gravis. Part 2. Clinical and serological follow-up of individual patients. *J Neurol Sci* **58**:371–85.

Perez MC, Buot WL, Mercado-Danguilan C, et al. 1981. Stable remissions in myasthenia gravis. *Neurology* **31**:32.

Pestronk A, Drachman DB, Teoh R, et al. 1983. Combined short-term immunotherapy for experimental autoimmune myasthenia gravis. *Ann Neurol* **14**:235–41.

Pinching AJ, Peters DK, Newsom-Davis J. 1976. Remission of myasthenia gravis following plasma-exchange. *Lancet* **2**:1373–6.

Plauché WC. 1991. Myasthenia gravis in mothers and their newborns [review]. *Clin Obstet Gynecol* **34**:82–99.

Ramsey-Goldman R, Schilling E. 1997. Immunosuppressive drug use during pregnancy [review]. *Rheum Dis Clin North Am* **23**: 149–67.

Regnard JF, Magdeleinat P, Dromer C, et al. 1996. Prognostic factors and long-term results after thymoma resection: a series of 307 patients. *J Thorac Cardiovasc Surg* **112**:376–84.

Rowland LP. 1980. Controversies about the treatment of myasthenia gravis. *J Neurol Neurosurg Psychiatry* **43**:644–59.

Sanders DB, Andrews PI, Howard JF, et al. 1997. Seronegative myasthenia gravis. *Neurology* **48**(Suppl. 5):S40.

Sanders DB, Scoppetta C. 1994. The treatment of patients with myasthenia gravis [review]. *Neurol Clin* **12**:343–68.

Sandler SG, Mallory D, Malamut D, et al. 1995. IgA anaphylactic transfusion reactions [review]. *Transfus Med Rev* **9**:1–8.

Seybold ME. 1987. Plasmapheresis in myasthenia gravis. *Ann N Y Acad Sci* **505**:584–7.

Seybold ME, Drachman DB. 1974. Gradually increasing doses of prednisone in myasthenia gravis: reducing the hazards of treatment. *N Engl J Med* **290**:81–4.

Sghirlanzoni A, Peluchetti D, Mantegazza R, et al. 1984. Myasthenia gravis: prolonged treatment with steroids. *Neurology* **34**:170–4.

Shillito P, Vincent A, Newsom-Davis J. 1993. Congenital myasthenic syndromes [review]. *Neuromusc Disord* **3**:183–90.

Sommer N, Sigg B, Melms A, et al. 1997. Ocular myasthenia gravis: response to long-term immunosuppressive treatment. *J Neurol Neurosurg Psychiatry* **62**:156–62.

Somnier FE. 1993. Clinical implementation of anti-acetylcholine receptor antibodies. *J Neurol Neurosurg Psychiatry* **56**:496–504.

Taylor P. 1996. Anticholinesterase agents. In: Hardman JG, Limbird LE, editors. *Goodman & Gilman's The Pharmacological Basis of Therapeutics*. New York: McGraw-Hill. p 161.

Thomas CE, Mayer SA, Gungor Y, et al. 1997. Myasthenic crisis: clinical features, mortality, complications, and risk factors for prolonged intubation. *Neurology* **48**:1253–60.

Thornton CA, Griggs RC. 1994. Plasma exchange and intravenous immunoglobulin treatment of neuromuscular disease [review]. *Ann Neurol* **35**:260–8.

Tindall RS, Phillips JT, Rollins JA, et al. 1993. A clinical therapeutic trial of cyclosporine in myasthenia gravis. *Ann N Y Acad Sci* **681**:539–51.

Tindall RSA, Rollins JA, Phillips TJ, et al. 1987. Preliminary results of a double-blind, randomized, placebo-controlled trial of cyclosporine in myasthenia gravis. *N Engl J Med* **316**:719–24.

Verma P, Oger J. 1992. Treatment of acquired autoimmune myasthenia gravis: a topic review [review]. *Can J Neurol Sci* **19**:360–75.

Vincent A, Newsom-Davis J. 1985. Acetylcholine receptor antibody as a diagnostic test for myasthenia gravis: results in 153 validated cases and 2967 diagnostic assays. *J Neurol Neurosurg Psychiatry* **48**:1246–52.

Walker M. 1934. Treatment of myasthenia gravis with physostigmine. *Lancet* **1**:1200.

Weinberg DA, Lesser RL, Vollmer TL. 1994. Ocular myasthenia: a protean disorder [review]. *Surv Ophthalmol* **39**:169–210.

Willcox N, Schluep M, Ritter MA, et al. 1991. The thymus in seronegative myasthenia gravis patients. *J Neurol* **238**:256–61.

Willcox N, Vincent A. 1988. Myasthenia gravis as an example of organ-specific autoimmune disease. In: Bird G, Calvert JE, editors. *B Lymphocytes in Human Disease*. Oxford: Oxford Univ. Press. p 469.

Wilson RW, Ward MD, Johns TR. 1974. Corticosteroids: a direct effect at the neuromuscular junction. *Neurology* **24**:1091–5.

Wittbrodt ET. 1997. Drugs and myasthenia gravis: an update [review]. *Arch Intern Med* **157**:399–408.

Youssef S. 1983. Thymectomy for myasthenia gravis in children. *J Pediatr Surg* **18**:537–41.

# Drug-Induced Neurologic Disorders

B. M. Demaerschalk, P. E. Cooper

*Chapter Outline*



Drugs commonly affect the nervous system to produce clinically significant adverse effects. In this chapter, we highlight the more common or more serious drug-induced neurologic disorders and in doing this, we have chosen to organize our discussion in an anatomical manner.

## CEREBRAL CORTEX

### Seizures

Only 0.08% of patients in the Boston Collaborative Surveillance Program experienced drug-induced seizures (Boston Collaborative Drug Surveillance Program 1972). Factors that contribute to drug-induced seizures have been divided into those related to the drug itself: *intrinsic epileptogenicity, serum levels, and CNS levels;* and those related to the patient: *preexisting epilepsy, underlying neurologic abnormality, reduced drug elimination, and blood–brain barrier breakdown.* Of these, the most important factor is the intrinsic epileptogenicity of the drug.

The drugs that most commonly caused seizures are listed in Table 7-35. If there is an underlying neurological disorder, particularly if the patient has idiopathic epilepsy, then drugs that might only occasionally cause a seizure in normal patients can have a more profound effect. Drugs such as phenobarbital and benzodiazepines, when withdrawn rapidly from the dependent patient, can cause seizures and even status epilepticus. A similar effect can be seen with withdrawal from ethanol.

### Cerebral Vascular Disease

#### *Ethanol*

Ethanol may predispose to both ischemic and hemorrhagic stroke by affecting the heart, the vascular system, platelets, coagulation cascade, and cerebral metabolism. The proposed pathophysiologic mechanisms are outlined in Table 7-36 (Gorelick 1990).

#### *Street drugs*

Use of drugs of abuse such as cocaine, amphetamines, heroin, PCP, LSD, and marijuana has been associated with increased risk of stroke, via different pathophysiologic mechanisms (Gorelick 1990).

Levine (1991) proposed several mechanisms for cocaine-related ischemic stroke: vasoconstriction of pial vessels, vasospasm following subarachnoid hemorrhage, vasculopathy, vasculitis, and reduction in cerebral blood flow. For cocaine-related intracerebral hemorrhage, mechanisms may include acute hypertension, thrombocytopenia, and venular vasospasm.

Both intracerebral hemorrhage (ICH) and cerebral infarction are associated with amphetamine use (Cahill 1981; Rothrock 1988). Hemorrhagic and ischemic strokes result from a direct toxic or immunologic induction of a necrotizing angiitis of the cerebral vasculature. Amphetamine compounds also potentiate stroke by inducing hypertension and vasoconstriction (Bowen 1983). Phenylpropanolamine (PPA) and ephedrine are sympathomimetic amines, structurally similar to amphetamines, and are contained in many over-the-counter appetite suppressants and decongestants. Cerebral ischemia and hemor-

**Table 7-35 Drugs That Can Cause Seizures When Used at Therapeutic Doses in Normal Patients**

| COMMONLY | OCCASIONALLY | RARELY OR NEVER |
|---|---|---|
| Meperidine | General anesthetics | Antidepressants |
| Phenothiazines | β-Lactams | Anticonvulsants |
| Clozapine | Isoniazid | Lidocaine |
| Contrast agents | Theophylline | Narcotics (other than meperidine) |
| Flumazenil[a] | Alkylating agents | Quinolones |
| Vaccines[b] | Butyrophenones | Acyclovir |
| β-Blockers | | |

From Garcia and Alldredge 1994, with permission.
[a]In patients taking benzodiazepines or drug overdoses.
[b]Febrile seizures.

rhages have been associated with their use as well (Kase 1987).

Phencyclidine (PCP), "angel dust," is a synthetic drug chemically related to phenothiazines (Ellenhorn 1988; Bryson 1989) and may cause strokes by inducing hypertension or vasospasm (Eastman 1975).

Lysergic acid diethylamide (LSD) also induces intracerebral vasospasm (Sobel 1971). Marijuana associated alterations in blood pressure and vasospasm are proposed causes of cerebral infarction (Zachariah 1991).

Other drugs of abuse may cause strokes as well (Gorelick 1990).

**Table 7-36 Pathophysiologic Mechanisms Linking Alcohol Consumption to Stroke**

*Ischemic Stroke*
- Cardiovascular disorders
  - "Holiday heart" syndrome (cardiac rhythm disturbances, including atrial fibrillation, which may follow weekend or holiday drinking sprees)
  - Alcoholic cardiomyopathy
  - Induced hypertension
- Coagulation and platelet disorders
  - Decreased fibrinolytic activity, factor VII-related antigen, and factor VIII ristocetin cofactor
  - Shortened bleeding time
  - "Rebound thrombocytosis" and platelet hyperaggregability following alcohol withdrawal
  - Increased platelet reactivity to adenosine diphosphate and thromboxane $B_2$ formation after acute ingestion of alcohol
- Cerebral blood flow and metabolic disorders
  - Decreased regional cerebral blood flow related to toxic effects of alcohol on cerebral metabolism or alcohol-induced vasospasm
  - Hemoconcentration

*Hemorrhagic Stroke*
- Cardiovascular disorders (induction of hypertension)
- Coagulation disorders
  - Decrease in circulating levels of clotting factors produced by liver
  - Excessive fibrinolysis
  - Qualitatively abnormal fibrinogens
  - Disseminated intravascular coagulation

Reprinted with permission from Gorelick 1990.

**SUMMARY**

**Drugs of abuse may increase risk of stroke by various mechanisms:**

| *Drug* | *Mechanism* |
|---|---|
| **Cocaine** | **Hypertension, vasospasm, vasculitis, platelet aggregation** |
| **Amphetamines** | **Necrotizing angiitis, hypertension, vasoconstriction** |
| **Phencyclidine** | **Hypertension, vasospasm** |
| **LSD** | **Vasospasm** |
| **Marijuana** | **Change in blood pressure, vasospasm** |
| **Heroin** | **Angiitis, infective endocarditis, foreign body emboli** |
| **T's and Blues (pentazocine and tripelennamine)** | **Infective endocarditis, foreign body emboli, vasculopathy** |

***Anticoagulant, antiplatelet, and thrombolytic therapy***

Intracerebral hemorrhage and hemorrhagic infarction are recognized complications of anticoagulation. Medical factors that are associated with a higher risk of hemorrhagic complications in patients taking warfarin include advanced age, hypertension, and excessive anticoagulation (Wintzen 1984; Kase 1985). Heparin is also associated with ICH and hemorrhagic infarction. Low-molecular-weight heparin is believed to be safer in this regard than standard heparin (Massey 1990). Patients receiving heparin can also develop thromboembolism and hemorrhage in association with heparin-induced thrombocytopenia (Becker 1989).

Although antiplatelet agents reduce the incidence of myocardial infarction (MI), transient ischemic attack, cerebral infarction, and vascular death, clinical trials have found an increased incidence of hemorrhagic stroke (Antiplatelet Trialists' Collaboration 1988).

Intracerebral hemorrhage is an infrequent but definite complication of streptokinase and tissue plasminogen activator used to treat acute myocardial infarct and cerebral infarction.

#### *Oral contraceptives and anabolic steroids*

Steroid hormones may increase the incidence of ischemic and hemorrhagic stroke by affecting blood pressure, carbohydrate metabolism, lipid metabolism, platelet function, and the coagulation cascade. Although oral contraceptive use continues to be a risk factor for stroke, the risk is substantially lower with more recent products that contain lower amounts of estrogen (Porter 1985). Stroke has also been reported in association with anabolic steroid use (Frankel 1988).

#### *Antineoplastic agents*

Antineoplastic agents may lead to stroke by causing thrombocytopenia secondary to bone marrow suppression and by impairing coagulation factor synthesis secondary to hepatotoxicity.

#### *Antibiotics*

Antibiotic-associated ICH may result from inhibition of platelet aggregation, inhibition of vitamin K synthesis by microbes in the GI tract, and thrombocytopenia (Fass 1987).

## Cognitive Impairment

Meador (1998) reviewed the cognitive adverse effects of medications. He cautions the reader about the multitude of methodological problems that make the literature difficult for the clinician to use as a guide in this regard.

Delirium and pseudodementia are the two most common cognitive adverse effects. Meperidine, benzodiazepines, and anticholinergics are the most common causes of drug-induced postoperative delirium (Meador 1998). Risk of delirium is increased in the elderly and in patients with co-morbid conditions such as severe illness, sepsis, renal failure, and electrolyte disturbance.

Drug-induced pseudodementia is most commonly caused by sedative-hypnotics and antihypertensives. Other drugs that may cause this problem include neuroleptics, analgesics, cimetidine, insulin, amoxapine, and amantadine. Polypharmacy increases the risk with the relative odds increased from 2.7 with two to three drugs, to 9.3 with four to five drugs, and to 13.7 with more than six drugs (Meador 1998).

## Syncope

Syncope is defined as the transient loss of consciousness with loss of postural tone, and presyncope is characterized as syncopal symptoms without full loss of consciousness. Approximately 13% of patients with syncope have been found to have drug-induced syncope (Hanlon 1990). Drugs used for the treatment of hypertension including $\alpha$-adrenergic receptor blocking agents, $\beta$-adrenergic receptor blockers, calcium channel blockers, angiotensin converting-enzyme (ACE) inhibitors, and nitrates can produce syncope or presyncope related to an excessive fall in blood pressure, especially when prescribed in excessive doses. Diuretics, which can cause volume depletion, can produce marked orthostatic changes resulting in syncopal symptoms as well. A number of drugs used primarily to treat psychiatric disorders have $\alpha$-receptor blocking effects that also cause orthostatic hypotension. Tricyclic antidepressants, phenothiazines, and monoamine oxidase inhibitors all potentially induce a significant drop in blood pressure that can be symptomatic (Goldberg 1984).

## Headache

Headache is one of the most common neurologic symptoms. It is said to have a one-day point prevalence in men of 11 and 22% in women (Rassmussen et al. 1991). Most reports in the literature of medication-related headache refer to adverse drug reactions in single patients or to anecdotal data. Of course, such associations do not prove causation.

Patients with a preexisting tendency to headache, especially migraine, are more likely to experience drug-related headache. Silberstein recently reviewed this topic in depth (1998).

Classically, vasodilators (e.g., nitroglycerin) are known to produce headache. Headache is reported as a common adverse effect of $\beta$-adrenergic receptor blockers, dihydroperidine calcium channel blockers (especially nifedipine), ACE inhibitors, and methyldopa. The mechanism of action of these medications is uncertain and even the association is unclear because propranolol and verapamil are both effective in the prophylaxis of migraine. Some nonsteroidal anti-inflammatory drugs (NSAIDs), especially indomethacin, cause headache through what is believed to be compensatory vasodilation. Other NSAIDs, especially ibuprofen, have been found to cause aseptic meningitis.

Estrogen withdrawal, synthetic progestin use, and drugs that interfere with estrogen action (e.g., tamoxifen) may trigger migraine. Ethanol can induce migraine in susceptible individuals. Intrathecal methotrexate and diaziquone can produce aseptic meningitis and headache, as can intravenous immune globulin. Methodichlorophen, $\beta$-interferon, and interleukin-2 have been associated with headache, as have the immunomodulating drugs cyclosporine, FK-506, thalidomide, and antithymocytic globulin. Amphotericin, griseofulvin, tetracycline, and sulfonamides have been associated with headache.

Medication overuse by headache-prone patients, especially the use of codeine and caffeine-containing compounds, may produce a drug-induced rebound headache.

Intracranial hypertension accompanied by headache, often referred to as pseudotumor cerebri, has been associated with minocycline, isotretinoin, nalidixic acid, tetracycline, trimethoprim-sulfamethoxazole, cimetidine, prednisolone, methylprednisolone, tamoxifen, beclomethasone, and methylprednisolone.

## CRANIAL NERVES

### Smell and Taste

Aminoglycosides are reported to cause anosmia. Vasoconstrictor nose drops, intranasal cocaine, and diltiazem have also been implicated (Berman 1985).

Transient ageusia or dysgeusia may occur with captopril therapy, particularly when there is co-administration of thiazides or $\beta$-adrenergic receptor blockers (Vlasses 1979). Other drugs that are reported to cause ageusia or dysgeusia include penicillamine, carbimazole, clofibrate, lithium, griseofulvin, gold preparations, levodopa, ethambutol, and acetylsalicylic acid (ASA) (Diamond 1981).

### Vision

Anticholinergic agents, antidepressants, and antihistamines can all act on the parasympathetic nervous system, particularly the ciliary muscles, and cause blurred vision through lack of accommodation (Dickey 1990).

Chloroquine, which has affinity for melanin in the retinal pigment layer, is the most common cause of serious drug-induced retinopathy. Quinine in toxic concentrations, phenothiazines, indomethacin, digoxin, and tamoxifen also cause retinopathy. Nicotinic acid and diuretics, including hydrochlorothiazide and acetazolamide, can cause macular edema. Estrogens may cause retinal artery occlusion and retinal vein thrombosis. Retinal hemorrhages are associated with nonsteroidal anti-inflammatory drugs (NSAIDs) and sulfonamides. Optic neuritis has occurred with use of the antituberculous drugs ethambutol and isoniazid. Toxic amblyopia has been associated with ibuprofen, sulfonylureas, salicylates, phenylbutazone, ergotamine, and quinidine. Disulfiram may cause optic neuritis. Recently, Krauss et al. (1998) reported four patients with evidence of retinal cone dysfunction associated with treatment with the anticonvulsant vigabatrin.

Sildenafil, the cyclic guanosine monophosphate (cGMP) phosphodiesterase inhibitor for the treatment of impotence, can cause transient blue visual discoloration or increased sensitivity to light. The pathophysiology of this is thought to be inhibition of phosphodiesterase type 6 in the retina.

### Extraocular Movements

Drug-induced diplopia is most commonly caused by weakening of fixation reflexes (Dickey 1990). Ophthalmoplegia can occur with drug-induced myasthenia gravis and may also occur in drug-induced increased intracranial pressure. Ophthalmoplegia is also reported in association with reserpine, cardiac glycosides, quinine, chloroquine, imipramine, monoamine oxidase inhibitors, diazepam, sulfonamides, vincristine, barbiturates, and phenytoin. Nystagmus may be seen in patients receiving therapeutic doses of antiepileptic drugs, benzodiazepines, and antipsychotics. At higher drug levels, more severe nystagmus and even ataxia may occur.

### Hearing and Balance

The vestibulocochlear apparatus and its central connections to brainstem and cerebellum are all vulnerable to direct toxic effects of drugs. Antibiotic-induced ototoxicity is probably the most common and serious. Streptomycin, gentamicin, and tobramycin are predominantly vestibulotoxic, causing vertigo and ataxia, whereas neomycin, kanamycin, and amikacin are predominantly cochleotoxic. Ototoxicity is caused by topical as well as parenteral aminoglycosides. Vancomycin and erythromycin are also implicated in ototoxicity. Loop diuretics and acetazolamide are ototoxic. Chloroquine, quinine, and quinidine may also cause hearing impairment. NSAIDs and

ASA are responsible for dose-related tinnitus, and in rare instances, have been associated with deafness.

## BASAL GANGLIA

Drug-induced movement disorders may be either acute (e.g., dystonia, choreoathetosis, akathisia, tics), subacute (e.g., parkinsonism, tremor), or chronic (e.g., levodopa-induced dyskinesia in Parkinson's disease, or tardive dyskinesia). This subject has been reviewed recently by Diederich and Goetz (1998).

### Dystonia

Acute drug-induced dystonias affect mainly the musculature of the face and neck. It is often painful and frightening to the patient and may initially be thought to be hysterical. Young adults are especially prone to develop this complication. The syndrome is caused most commonly by drugs that block dopamine receptors in the CNS—e.g., phenothiazines, butyrophenones, and metoclopramide. Drugs with affinity for different subtypes of the serotoninergic (5-hydroxytryptamine, 5-HT) receptor, including buspirone and sumatriptan, have been reported to cause this problem as well. The cause of this syndrome is unclear, and there is evidence both for relative dopaminergic understimulation and overstimulation (Diederich and Goetz 1998).

### Choreoathetosis

These bizarre movements affect mainly the extremities. Contraceptive-induced chorea can be seen in women with a past history of Sydenham's chorea, rheumatic fever, or cyanotic congenital heart disease. Cocaine, by potentiation of dopaminergic transmission, can cause chorea. Choreoathetotic movements have been reported in patients receiving phenytoin, carbamazepine, felbamate, and gabapentin. They can also be seen in mild or moderate lithium intoxication where the chorea may be accompanied by myoclonus.

### Akathisia

This inability to keep the legs still, and inability to remain seated (e.g., "the jitters"), is usually accompanied by the sensation of restlessness and may be confused with agitation and hyperactivity. It is an adverse effect of most dopamine receptor blockers and has been reported to occur with the use of selective serotonin reuptake inhibitors (SSRIs) as well.

### Tics

Drug-induced tics, indistinguishable from those seen in patients with Gilles de la Tourette's syndrome, have been reported in patients receiving methylphenidate, pemoline, and amphetamines. Sertraline, an SSRI, can aggravate tics as well.

### Drug-Induced Parkinsonism

Symptoms of drug-induced parkinsonism (DIP) develop in up to 90% of patients treated with dopamine receptor-blocking agents for 3 months or more (Silberstein 1998). The most commonly implicated drugs are the piperazine class of phenothiazines and the butyrophenones. The calcium channel blockers flunarizine and cinnarizine have piperazine-like properties and can cause DIP, especially in the elderly. Fluoxetine, and less commonly, paroxetine and fluvoxamine, may induce DIP either alone or in combination with cimetidine or selegiline. Valproic acid has also been associated with DIP symptoms accompanied by cognitive impairment and hearing loss (Armon et al. 1996). The dopamine depleters reserpine and tetrabenazine can cause DIP.

Isolated case reports implicate many other drugs as potentially causing DIP. This literature is very hard to interpret. A careful history of drug treatment and use from patients presenting with parkinsonism is essential, and observation after withdrawal of suspected offending compounds is indicated.

### Tremor

Sympathomimetics, thyroxine (in excess), tricyclic antidepressants, theophylline, and lithium can all cause tremor in some patients. Sodium valproate will cause tremor in as many as 25% of patients taking over 750 mg per day (Karas et al. 1982). Cyclosporin may cause a cerebellar tremor that resolves with time. Postural tremor can be seen in over half of patients receiving amiodarone, and this drug may be associated with ataxia and peripheral neuropathy as well (Charness et al. 1984). A flapping, almost myoclonic-like tremor can be seen in patients treated with carbamazepine, clozapine, and lithium.

### Levodopa-Induced Dyskinesias in Parkinson's Disease

These choreic or dystonic movements are seen in patients with Parkinson's disease after longer-term therapy. They are thought to be due to hypersensitivity of striatal dopamine neurons and are seen most commonly when doses of L-dopa peak in the bloodstream. Less commonly, they occur toward the end of the dosing interval.

### Tardive Dyskinesias

All types of dopamine receptor blockers have been associated with the development of tardive dyskinesia (TD). New or atypical antipsychotic agents appear to carry less risk, and to date, there have been no convincing cases of tardive dyskinesia reported with clozapine (Diederich and Goetz 1998). Elderly patients can develop TD following prolonged treatment with metoclopramide. Some case reports also have implicated antihistamines/decongestants, fluoxetine, and amoxapine; however, the confounding effect of concomitant drug use and other factors cannot be excluded.

### Neuroleptic Malignant Syndrome

A strict definition of this syndrome requires the presence of severe rigidity and fever (without other causes) accompanied by 2 of 10 minor features including diaphoresis, dysphagia, tremor, incontinence, altered mentation, mutism, tachycardia, elevated or labile blood pressure, leukocytosis, and elevated creatine phosphokinase levels (DSM-IV). This condition develops most commonly a few days after initiation of a neuroleptic drug (50% of cases), but it can develop immediately, or after the patient has been taking the drug for many months (Addonizio et al. 1987).

The syndrome can occur following exposure to any dopamine receptor-blocking drug (e.g., metoclopramide), and it has been reported to occur in Parkinson's disease patients following the abrupt withdrawal of dopaminergic medications (Keyser and Rodnitzky 1991). Treatment includes prompt recognition, ruling out predisposing factors (e.g., acute infection), general support (e.g., cooling), muscle relaxants (e.g., dantrolene), and central dopamine agonists (e.g., bromocriptine).

SUMMARY

**Drugs can cause the following types of acute or chronic movement disorders:**

- **Acute dystonias**
- **Tremor**
- **Choreoathetoid movements**
- **Levodopa-induced dyskinesia**
- **Akathisia**
- **Tardive dyskinesia**
- **Tics**
- **Neuroleptic malignant syndrome**
- **Drug-induced parkinsonism**

## CEREBELLUM

The most common cause of a cerebellar syndrome due to drug toxicity is that associated with antiepileptic medications, particularly phenytoin. Transient ataxia, dysarthria, and nystagmus usually develop when serum concentrations of phenytoin, carbamazepine, or barbiturates are above the therapeutic range. Ethanol intoxication also causes acute cerebellar dysfunction. "Worm wobble" is a reversible cerebellar syndrome that occurs in children taking piperazine for threadworm infection. High-dose administration of 5-fluorouracil or cytosine arabinoside also causes reversible cerebellar ataxia. The acute encephalopathy of lithium toxicity is accompanied by a cerebellar deficit that may not be totally reversible (Bradley 1996).

## SPINAL CORD

High-dose intravenous or intrathecal methotrexate can cause transverse myelitis, or stroke-like symptoms with encephalopathy, that usually resolves without treatment (Machkhas and Harati 1998).

## PERIPHERAL NERVES

Many pharmaceutical agents can cause a peripheral polyneuropathy that is generally reversible when the offending drug is discontinued. A careful history of drug treatment and use should be obtained in every patient presenting with polyneuropathy. Only drugs that consistently or commonly produce peripheral neuropathy (motor, sensory, or both) are listed in Table 7-37.

## NEUROMUSCULAR JUNCTION

Under normal circumstances, there is a high margin of safety for neuromuscular transmission, and drug-induced neuromuscular blockade is rarely a problem. In patients with myasthenia gravis, Lambert–Eaton syndrome, electrolyte disturbances, or following the administration of muscle relaxants during general anesthesia, a drug-induced myasthenic syndrome may occur. Drugs that are most consistently reported to affect neuromuscular transmission under these circumstances include aminoglycosides, $\beta$-adrenergic receptor blockers, quinidine, procainamide, phenytoin, chloroquine, D-penicillamine, prednisone, procaine, lidocaine, and magnesium (see sections in this chapter "Neurologic Disorders" and "Myasthenia Gravis").

Table 7-37 **Drugs That May Cause Peripheral Neuropathy**

| DRUG | ACTION/INDICATION | NEUROPATHY |
|---|---|---|
| Almitrine | Chemoreceptor antagonist used in chronic obstructive pulmonary disease | Painful distal symmetrical sensory neuropathy |
| Amiodarone | Antiarrhythmic | Sensorimotor polyneuropathy |
| Amphetamines | Multiple mononeuropathies due to necrotizing hypersensitivity | Angiitis |
| Chloramphenicol | Antibiotic | Painful sensorimotor polyneuropathy with optic neuropathy—especially in children and young adults on prolonged, high dose therapy |
| Chloroquine | Antimalarial, also used in treatment of some collagen vascular diseases | Sensorimotor axonal polyneuropathy |
| *cis*-Platinum | Treatment of ovarian, bladder, and testicular malignancies and squamous cell carcinoma | Dose-dependent, predominantly large-fiber polyneuropathy |
| Colchicine | Treatment of gout | Subacute proximal weakness and mild distal axonal polyneuropathy |
| Dapsone | Treatment of leprosy, HIV, and skin disorders | Motor polyneuropathy with high doses |
| ddC and ddI | Treatment of AIDS | Dose-limiting dysesthetic sensory neuropathy[a] |
| Disulfiram | Treatment of alcoholism | Sensorimotor distal axonopathy |
| Gold | Treatment of rheumatoid arthritis | Polyneuropathy resembling Guillain-Barré syndrome, rarely a dose-related distal axonal polyneuropathy |
| Heroin | Narcotic | Nontraumatic plexopathy in brachial or lumbosacral distribution |
| Hydralazine | Antihypertensive | Sensory polyneuropathy (rare) |
| Isoniazid | Antituberculous drug | Interferes with vitamin $B_6$-dependent coenzymes, polyneuropathy in 2% of patients on conventional doses |
| Metronidazole | Treatment of protozoal and anaerobic bacterial infections and inflammatory bowel disease | Sensory polyneuropathy with prolonged treatment |
| Nitrofurantoin | Broad-spectrum antimicrobial used to treat urinary tract infections | Sensorimotor polyneuropathy and may be associated with distal axonal type |
| Nitrous oxide | Inhalational anesthetic | Sensory polyneuropathy |
| Phenytoin | Antiepileptic | Asymptomatic polyneuropathy |
| Pyridoxine | Vitamin $B_6$ | Severe sensory polyneuropathy when used in excess |
| Taxol | Treatment of ovarian cancer and some other solid neoplasms | Sensory neuropathy |
| Thalidomide | Treatment of leprosy and rare skin conditions | Polyneuropathy when used at high doses or with chronic administration |
| L-Tryptophan | Amino acid | Severe axonal sensorimotor polyneuropathy may be a feature of the eosinophilia-myalgia syndrome (EMS) seen in individuals taking L-tryptophan (probably due to a contaminant and not the amino acid itself) |
| *Vinca* alkaloids | Antineoplastic agents | Vincristine causes a sensorimotor polyneuropathy. |

[a]Berger 1993.

## MUSCLE

Several distinct clinical syndromes of drug-induced myopathy have been described (Dickey 1990).

### Rhabdomyolysis

This is the most severe form of myopathy, presenting with diffuse muscle pain, tenderness, swelling, elevated serum creatine kinase (CK), and myoglobinuria. It has been reported in association with ethanol abuse, amphetamines, phencyclidine, cytotoxic agents, amphotericin B, barbiturates, diazepam, and theophylline.

### Acute/Subacute Painful Proximal Myopathy

Three drug-induced syndromes, clinically indistinguishable but with distinct histological abnormalities, have been defined—necrotizing myopathy, inflammatory myositis, and hypokalemic myopathy. *Necrotizing myopathy* can be caused by any drug that produces rhabdomyolysis. It has also been associated with ε-aminocaproic acid, emitine, colchicine, clofibrate, gemfibrozil, and with inhibitors of hydroxymethylglutaryl-coenzyme A (HMG-CoA) used to treat hyperlipidemia (e.g., lovastatin and simvastatin). Usually such rhabdomyolysis is associated with creatine phosphokinase levels more than 3 times normal. Isolated reports also implicate salbutamol, terbutaline, danazol, amiodarone, lithium, propranolol, and labetalol. Intravenous hydrocortisone is also reported to cause an acute necrotizing myopathy. *Inflammatory myositis*, a polymyositis-like syndrome, has been described in association with penicillamine. Hydralazine, phenytoin, and procainamide also cause a myositis. *Hypokalemic myopathy* may occur in association with diuretics, purgatives, and amphotericin B, or other potassium-losing status (e.g., ingestion of large amounts of licorice, containing glycyrrhizinic acid).

### Subacute/Chronic Painless Myopathy

This is the most common form of drug-induced muscle disease, associated with steroid use. Many cases are subclinical or misdiagnosed as simply representing progression of the disease being treated, such as polymyositis. Any steroid may be responsible, but potent fluorinated steroids such as triamcinolone are most commonly implicated. Muscle weakness is proximal and progressive. Chloroquine is able to produce a myopathy clinically indistinguishable from that caused by steroids. Rifampin also causes a painless myopathy.

### Myotonia

In patients with myotonic disorders, such as myotonia congenita and myotonic dystrophy, the condition may be unmasked or exacerbated by $\beta$-adrenergic receptor blockers (including pindolol and propranolol), barbiturates, and depolarizing muscle relaxants.

## AUTONOMIC NERVOUS SYSTEM

Many classes of drugs besides the obvious atropine derivatives antagonize muscarinic receptors at multiple sites. Elderly patients may be at greater risk for this effect. The most common symptoms include dry mouth, visual problems, delirium, heat stroke, ileus, constipation, tachycardia, loss of bladder detrusor tone, and acute urinary retention (especially in elderly men with prostatic enlargement). The phenothiazines, tricyclic antidepressants, antiemetics, and antihistamines are the largest classes of drugs with undesired anticholinergic properties. Benztropine, trihexyphenidyl, tropicamide, propantheline, scopolamine, ipratropium and tincture of belladonna all have this effect.

A variety of sympathomimetic drugs, often taken as nasal decongestants or as "diet pills," can cause patients to develop tachycardia, hypertension, nervousness, tremor, or palpitations. Phenylpropanolamine, ephedrine, caffeine, or dextro-amphetamine may produce such effects. Drugs such as these may often be obtained in over-the-counter formulations or even soft drinks, and patients may forget to mention them to the physician.

**PRINCIPLE Drug adverse effects as a cause of neurologic dysfunction may not be readily apparent at first. It is important, therefore, that a careful drug history be obtained from every patient and that a search is made for neurologic adverse effects of a patient's medications when patients present with neurologic problems.**

## REFERENCES

Addonizio G, Susman VL, Roth SD. 1987. Neuroleptic malignant syndrome: review and analysis of 115 cases. *Biol Psychiatry* **22**: 1004–20.

Antiplatelet Trialists' Collaboration. 1988. Secondary prevention of vascular disease by prolonged antiplatelet treatments. *Br Med J (Clin Res Ed)* **296**:320–31.

Armon C, Shin C, Miller P, et al. 1996. Reversible parkinsonism and cognitive impairment with chronic valproate use. *Neurology* **47**:626–35.

Becker PS, Miller VT. 1989. Heparin-induced thrombocytopenia. *Stroke* **20**:1449–59.

Berger AR, Arezzo JC, Schaumberg HH, et al. 1993. 2′,3′-Dideoxycytidine (ddC) toxic neuropathy: a study of 52 patients. *Neurology* **43**:358–62.

Berman JL. 1985. Dysosmia, dysgeusia, and diltiazem. *Ann Intern Med* **102**:717.

Boston Collaborative Drug Surveillance Program. 1972. Drug-induced convulsions. *Lancet* **2**(7779):677–9.

Bowen JS, Davis GB, Kearney TE, et al. 1983. Diffuse vascular spasm associated with 4-bromo-2.5-dimethoxy amphetamine ingestion. *JAMA* **249:**1477–9.

Bryson PD. 1989. *Comprehensive Review in Toxicology*. 2nd ed. Rockville, MD: Aspen Publishers.

Cahill DW, Knipp H, Mosser J. 1981. Intracranial hemorrhage with amphetamine abuse. *Neurology* **31**:1058–9.

Charness ME, Morady F, Scheinman MM. 1984. Frequent neurologic toxicity associated with amiodarone therapy. *Neurology* **34**: 669–71.

Diamond C. 1981. Ear, nose, and throat disorders. In: *Textbook of Adverse Drug Reactions*, pp 11–34. DM Davies, (ed) Oxford, England: Oxford Univ Press.

Diederich NJ, Goetz CG. 1998. Drug-induced movement disorders. *Neurol Clin North Am* **16**:125–39.

Eastman JW, Cohen SN. 1975. Hypertensive crisis and death associated with phencyclidine poisioning. *JAMA* **231**:1270–1.

Ellenhorn MJ, Barceloux DG. 1988. *Medical Toxicology: Diagnosis and Treatment of Human Poisoning*. New York: Elsevier.

Fass RJ, Copelan EA, Brandt JT, et al. 1987. Platelet-mediated bleeding caused by broad-spectrum penicillins. *J Infect Dis* **155**:1242–8.

Frankel MA, Eichberg R, Zachariah SB. 1988. Anabolic androgenic steroids and a stroke in an athlete: case report. *Arch Phys Med Rehabil* **69**:632–3.

Garcia PA, Alldredge BK. 1994. Drug-induced seizures. *Neurol Clin North Am* **12**:85–99.

Goldberg LI. 1984. Dopamine receptors and hypertension. Physiologic and pharmacologic implications. *Am J Med* **77**(4A):37–44.

Gorelick PB. 1990. Stroke from alcohol and drug abuse: a current social peril. *Postgrad Med* **88**:171–8.

Hanlon JT, Linzer M, MacMillan JP, et al. 1990. Syncope and presyncope associated with probable adverse drug reactions. *Arch Int Med* **150**:2309–12.

Karas BJ, Wilder BJ, Hammond EJ, et al. 1982. Valproate tremors. *Neurology* **32**:428–32.

Kase CS, Robinson RK, Stein RW, et al. 1985. Anticoagulant intracerebral hemorrhage. *Neurology* **35**:943–8.

Keyser DL, Rodnitzky RL. 1991. Neuroleptic malignant syndrome in Parkinson's disease after withdrawal or alteration of dopaminergic therapy. *Arch Int Med* **151**:794–6.

Krauss GL, Johnson MA, Miller NR. 1998. Vigabatrin-associated retinal cone system dysfunction: electroretinogram and ophthalmologic findings. *Neurology* **50**:614–8.

Levine SR, Brust JCM, Futrell N, et al. 1991. A comparative study of the cerebrovascular complications of cocaine: alkaloidal versus hydrochloride—a review. *Neurology* **41**:1173–7.

Machkhas H, Harati Y. 1998. Side effects of immunosuppressant therapies used in neurology. *Neurol Clin North Am* **16**:171–88.

Massey EW, Biller J, Davis JN, et al. 1990. Large-dose infusions of heparinoid ORG 10172 in ischemic stroke. *Stroke* **21**:1289–92.

Meador KJ. 1998. Cognitive side effects of medications. *Neurol Clin North Am* **16**:141–55.

Porter JB, Hunter JR, Jick H, et al. 1985. Oral contraceptives and nonfatal vascular disease. *Obstet Gynecol* **66**:1–4.

Rasmussen BK, Jensen R, Schroll M, et al. 1991. Epidemiology of headache in a general population—a prevalence study. *J Clin Epidemiol* **44**:1147–57.

Rothrock JF, Rubenstein R, Lyden PD. 1988. Ischemic stroke associated with methamphetamine inhalation. *Neurology* **38**:589–92.

Silberstein SD. 1998. Drug-induced headache. *Neurol Clin North Am* **16**:107–23.

Sobel J, Espinas OE, Friedman SA. 1971. Carotid artery obstruction following LSD capsule ingestion. *Arch Intern Med* **127**:290–1.

Stroke Prevention in Atrial Fibrillation Investigators. 1991. Stroke prevention in atrial fibrillation: final results. *Circulation* **84**:527–39.

Vlasses PH, Ferguson RK. 1979. Temporary ageusia related to captopril [letter]. *Lancet* **2**:526.

Wintzen AR, Dejonge H, Loeliger EA, et al. 1984. The risk of intracerebral hemorrhage during oral anticoagulant treatment: a population study. *Ann Neurol* **16**:553–8.

Zachariah SB. 1991. Stroke after heavy marijuana smoking. *Stroke* **22**:406–9.

CHAPTER

# 8 TREATMENT OF PSYCHIATRIC DISORDERS

Leo E. Hollister

### *Chapter Outline*



## AN OVERVIEW OF PSYCHIATRIC DISORDERS

### Problems with Psychiatric Diagnosis and Nosology

Diagnosis of psychiatric disorders remains the most clinically based system in medicine. Unlike other medical disciplines, which enjoy an abundance of diagnostic tools or eventually the priceless feedback from the autopsy room, psychiatry has few tests that validate diagnosis. Not surprisingly, expert opinion may vary considerably about the most appropriate diagnosis for any particular patient.

Sources of data are limited and highly subjective. We must rely on what patients tell us (sometimes not very reliably), what others tell us about the patient (possibly a bit better), and clinical observation of the patient's behavior. From these, we draw inferences about the diagnosis. Psychological testing usually confirms the clinical diagnosis but in difficult situations, it is often couched in such vague and comprehensive terms as to rival horoscopes. No specific electroencephalographic (EEG) patterns have been adduced for most psychiatric disorders; abnormalities usually lead to investigations of organic causes. A similar situation applies in the case of brain scans, where an abundance of minor abnormalities of unknown significance have been reported in patients with various diagnoses. Whether these are the cause or the result of the disorder is uncertain, but in any case, their sensitivity and specificity have been remarkably low. The ability to measure regional cerebral blood flow and metabolism, or to image the distributions of various neurotransmitter receptors, may ultimately provide a totally new way of categorizing psychiatric disorders; at present, none of the reported abnormalities have been well established.

To compensate for these deficiencies, increasing efforts have been made to define psychiatric diagnoses in terms of presenting symptoms and signs, the natural history of the disorder, and various exclusionary criteria. The *Diagnostic and Statistical Manual of the American Psychiatric Association* has been revised for a fourth edition (DSM-IV 1994). As desirable as a more precise definition of terms may be, one should recognize the defects of such a system. First, the definitions represent only the prevailing opinions of a group of experts at some period of time and are constantly changing. Second, definitions expounded by one group (DSM) may not be congruent with those of another, say, the International Classification of Disease (ICD 10 1993). Third, a variety of so-called research diagnostic criteria have been proposed for defining diagnoses. Many of these do not agree either with DSM or ICD criteria, or, for that matter, with each other (Overall and Hollister 1979). Fourth, renaming an old disorder somehow carries the magical implication that by so doing one gains more insight into its cause and treatment. Today's fashionable diagnosis of panic disorder was called an acute anxiety attack 30 years ago. Fifth, old rubrics may be discharged (homosexuality and neurosis), while new ones may be added (late luteal phase dysphoria, a fancy name for premenstrual tension).

Considering these difficulties, psychiatrists do much better than might be expected. It is still possible to form a working diagnosis and to try what might be construed as the best treatments for it. When diagnosis is less certain, it becomes possible to entertain a number of possibilities, in order of presumed certitude, and to try a number of different treatments successively. Thus, it should not be surprising that some patients initially diagnosed as having generalized anxiety disorder may ultimately respond to an antidepressant, or someone initially thought to be schizophrenic might respond best to a drug useful for treating mania.

**PRINCIPLE In the field of psychiatry, with uncertainty of diagnosis and nonspecificity of action of many drugs, the careful therapeutic trial with close observation of results assumes even greater importance.**

## Schizophrenia

By any kind of reckoning, schizophrenia is the most severe mental disorder. It is found worldwide in almost all cultures and countries (although not always with the same name).

The 6-month prevalence rate for schizophrenia in three urban U.S. samples ranged from 0.6 to 1.1% for schizophrenia, and from 0.1 to 0.2% for schizophreniform disorders (Myers et al. 1984). Lifetime prevalence rates were 1.0 to 1.9% and 0.1 to 0.3%, respectively (Robins et al. 1984). Such estimates are close to those made earlier, which suggested that about 1 to 2% of the population is susceptible to developing a schizophrenia-like psychosis at some time in their lives. Similar rates of prevalence have been obtained from other countries. The burden of schizophrenia far outweighs its prevalence. The disorder tends to occur early in adult life and may last an entire lifetime. The cost in economic terms of supporting and treating patients is huge. The cost in personal tragedy, not only for the affected person but also for friends and family, is incalculable.

### *Nature of schizophrenia*

Modern concepts of schizophrenia were developed at the beginning of this century. Kraepelin (1905) considered significant hallmarks of the disorder to be negativisms, mannerisms, stereotypes, disturbances of volition, disruption of judgment, discrepancy between mood and the general reaction, peculiar attention and thinking disorders, and a deterioration of a differentiation between the real and the unreal. Whether schizophrenia is a single disorder with multiple degrees of severity and manifestations, or whether it is a syndrome whose clinical manifestations represent a number of disorders of differing etiologies, is still a matter of some debate.

### *Classification of schizophrenia*

Over the years, various attempts have been made to subtype variations of schizophrenia. The older subtypes (paranoid, catatonic, disorganized, undifferentiated, and residual) are still used in DSM-IV. All these, as well as other classifications, are based primarily on the presence of clusters of symptoms and signs. Emphasis placed on negative symptoms over the past two decades led to a somewhat broader classification: psychomotor poverty (decreased speech, movement and blunted affect, a negative symptom complex), reality distortion (delusions and hallucinations), disorganization (formal thought disorder), depression, and psychomotor agitation (Liddle et al. 1994). Despite the growing emphasis on negative symptoms, a survey of several hundred patients with a diagnosis of schizophrenia indicated that positive symptoms were much more specific for making the diagnosis (Klosterkotter et al. 1995). Still another possible classification alludes to Kraepelinian schizophrenia, based on a deteriorating longitudinal course of the illness.

Schizophrenia might also be considered as a spectrum, with milder forms being called schizophreniform disorder, or even milder, schizotypal personality. If affective symptoms are present, a diagnosis of schizoaffective disorder may be made, although this diagnosis is going out of style. Although not all patients suffer a chronic, deteriorating course, one makes the diagnosis with some trepidation because of the generally poor prognosis (Bleuler 1950).

### *Possible pathogenesis*

The postulated mechanisms for producing schizophrenia have been numerous, as is usually the case in conditions that are poorly understood. The wide ranges of postulated disorders are summarized in Table 8-1. None has been established or conclusively refuted. The dopaminergic hypothesis, which postulates that for one reason or another dopaminergic activity is increased in the mesolimbic system of the brain, is the bedrock on which drug therapy is founded (McKenna 1987). Evidence has been circumstantial: schizophrenia-like disorders have followed use of drugs that work through dopaminergic mechanisms (amphetamine psychosis); all effective antipsychotic drugs

**Table 8-1 Some Postulated Mechanisms for Schizophrenia**

| |
|---|
| Dopaminergic overactivity |
| ?Increased dopamine receptors found at postmortem and demonstrated in vivo with PET scans |
| ?Improvement with dopamine-receptor blocking drugs |
| Other catecholamine abnormalities |
| ?β-Phenethylamine increased in CSF |
| ?Improvement with β-adrenoreceptor blocking drugs |
| Indolealkylamine abnormalities |
| Improvement with serotonin-receptor blocking drugs |
| Genetic factors |
| Concordance in 50% of identical twins |
| Concordance in 20% of first-degree relatives |
| Viral disease |
| Season of birth, increased during winter |
| ?Viral particles in CSF, cells of brain |
| Autoimmune disorders |
| ?Anti-brain antibodies |
| Structural and metabolic abnormalities |
| Variable brain atrophy on CT and MRI scans |
| Variable decrease in brain metabolism on PET scans |
| Environment |
| Stress and emotional factors |
| Parental influences |

Abbreviations: CSF, cerebrospinal fluid; CT, computed tomography; MRI, magnetic resonance imaging; PET, positron emission tomography.

seem to act by blocking postsynaptic dopamine D2 receptors; schizophrenia may be aggravated by dopamine precursors, (e.g., levodopa), by dopamine releasers (e.g., amphetamines), and by dopamine-receptor agonists (e.g., apomorphine). Direct links to a dopaminergic abnormality have been more difficult to establish.

Recent neuropathologic studies have suggested that schizophrenia might result from neurodevelopmental abnormality in which migrating axons fail to make proper connections in the brain, that is, the wiring is distorted. On the other hand, evidence that a morphologic change in the brain, enlarged ventricles, continues during the course of schizophrenia suggests that a degenerative process might also be present. If such pathogenetic mechanisms are correct, it does not bode well for attempts to treat the disorder.

#### *Unsolved problems*

An appraisal of the major public health problems in the United States at mid-century listed schizophrenia along with alcoholism, hypertension, arteriosclerosis, and cancer. It is rather disappointing that four decades later so little progress has been made in understanding the cause of schizophrenia and in advancing its treatment. Although in the 1950s one out of every four hospital beds was occupied by a schizophrenic patient, that problem has been "solved" by returning many psychiatric patients back to the community; the numbers still hospitalized have decreased by 80 to 90%.

One of the great hopes is that molecular genetic approaches may identify a gene or genes associated with schizophrenia and that by finding ways to counter the gene products treat the disorder more rationally. Thus far, attempts to establish genetic linkages have been controversial. Part of the problem has been the difficulty in finding strongly affected families, both due to the comparative rarity of the condition and the disruption and dispersal of such families caused by the illness. Another problem relates to the unreliability of the clinical diagnoses of the phenotype.

## Manic-Depressive (Bipolar) Disorder

#### *Nature and prevalence*

An elevated, expansive, or irritable mood is the primary characteristic of mania. Such elevations of mood may on other occasions be replaced by depressed mood, although the sequences between mania and depression may vary from one patient to another. The older name *manic-depressive disorder* was much more descriptive than the recent term, *bipolar mood disorder*. The diagnosis is established by the presence of a manic episode.

The term "bipolar disorder" does not truly describe the course of the illness. Rather than having episodes of mania and depression separated by a period of normal mood, some patients show simultaneously symptoms and signs of both mania and depression, so-called mixed mania. Such patients are usually more difficult to treat and more likely to commit suicide. The terms "primary" and "secondary" have been used to differentiate classical manic-depressive disorder from episodes of mania that seem to be triggered by drugs, brain injuries, and other nonspecific causes. It seems more reasonable to assume that anyone who develops mania, regardless of the presumed cause, has the classical disorder. Thus, a depressed patient without a previous episode of mania who becomes manic after treatment with an antidepressant, is best considered to have been misdiagnosed and should be properly diagnosed henceforth as a manic-depressive patient.

The affliction occurs in slightly $< 1\%$ of the general population. Onset may be at any age but is most common in the third decade of life. Episodes are almost always recurrent with considerable morbidity and an appreciable mortality.

Patients with mania often present with psychotic symptoms, manifested by paranoia and delusions of grandeur. Consequently, diagnostic confusion often occurs between the diagnosis of manic-depressive disorder and paranoid schizophrenia. Such diagnostic confusion vexed Bleuler and has persisted until the present, when diagnosis in individual patients may vary from one to the other during successive episodes. In some patients, episodes assume a crescendo pattern with increased frequency and shorter symptom-free intervals. This pattern, as well as the response of some patients to anticonvulsants, has led to the "kindling" hypothesis (induction of seizures by repeated subthreshold stimuli). However, it has been impossible to actually demonstrate this mechanism for the disorder (Post 1987).

***Possible mechanism of manic-depressive disorder***

Because the disorder tends to run in families, a number of investigations have attempted to identify a genetic locus. Genetic linkage studies have reported an association with the X chromosome as well as two loci on chromosome 11 (Mendlewicz et al. 1987; Baron et al. 1987; Egeland et al. 1987). However, other studies have failed to identify a genetic marker. Consequently, the issue is unresolved, or perhaps cannot be readily resolved if the disorder is heterogeneous. A number of neurotransmitters have been implicated in mania, but none is paramount. Neuroleptics, which block dopamine receptors, are usually somewhat effective, pointing to involvement of dopamine. As mania has been induced by tricyclic antidepressants, which increase noradrenergic or serotonergic activity, these transmitters may also be involved. Increasing cholinergic activity has also been found to alleviate mania. A variety of disturbances of circadian rhythms have been noted, but whether these are primary or secondary to the disorder remains uncertain.

Because of the more serious import and prognosis of manic disorder, it is likely that such patients should be referred to a biologically minded psychiatrist for management. Many episodes require hospitalization; even during periods of remission, patients require close clinical monitoring.

## Depressive Disorders

***Prevalence***

Serious depressive disorders should be referred for psychiatric care, as the morbidity is great and mortality, by suicide, is appreciable. Many depressed patients are seen by general physicians. A host of complaints mask the true disorder. Patients with many vague, unexplainable symptoms, affecting multiple organ systems, as well as those considered to be "crocks" with visits to many clinics, should be suspected of being depressed.

An epidemiologic survey of three communities found major depression to vary over a 6-month period from 2.2 to 3.5%, with minor depression (dysthymia) ranging between 2.1 and 3.8%. The lifetime prevalence of each was estimated as between 3.7 and 6.7%, and 2.1 and 3.8%, respectively (Myers et al. 1984, Robins et al. 1984).

A somewhat higher prevalence was found in a survey conducted in six European countries. The 6-month prevalence of major depression was 6.9% and for minor depression, 1.8%. Patients in both groups considered their working or social lives impaired. Another 8.3% of depressed patients had no substantial impairment (Lepine et al. 1997).

***Etiologic considerations***

**Heterogeneity** Depressions may have two major bases, one psychologic and the other genetic-biochemical. Psychologically, most depressions involve a feeling of loss. Anger engendered by the loss may be directed inward, with feelings of worthlessness and guilt, or outward, with expressions of hostility. Some psychological treatments are directed at helping patients express this repressed rage.

The depression evoked by reserpine suggested that depression may have a biochemical basis. Reserpine reduces stores of biogenic amines and produces depression. Therefore, depression is thought to be associated with reduced biogenic amines. This simple syllogism was the basis for the amine hypothesis of depression.

**PRINCIPLE Unwanted effects of drugs may sometimes provide clues to the pathogenesis of naturally occurring disorders. Another example would be the parkinsonian syndrome induced by some antipsychotic drugs.**

These two mechanisms also suggest the possibility of interaction. Patients with a genetic predisposition for depression may develop clinical manifestations mainly when experiencing psychological stress. The biochemical basis may be a necessary but not sufficient condition for the phenotypic expression of depression.

**AMINE HYPOTHESIS** The idea that deficient concentrations of biogenic amines in the CNS may be related to depression was given additional support by the action of depressant drugs (Green 1987). Many antidepressants inhibit the reuptake of these amines, especially serotonin and norepinephrine. Monoamine oxidase (MAO) inhibitors block their catabolism. Sympathomimetics also increase the availability of catecholamines at synapses.

Thus, all three possible treatments, in differing ways, increase the amount of neurotransmitter available at CNS synapses. The secondary effect of such increase is a compensatory decrease, or "*down-regulation,*" of postsynaptic receptors (Byerley et al. 1988). Nonetheless, direct confirmation of the amine hypothesis has been difficult, and, despite its heuristic value, it is still not established.

**OTHER POSSIBILITIES** Many basic bodily rhythms involving hunger, sleep, sexual desire, and motor activity are altered in depression. This has suggested that depression might be caused by alteration of usual diurnal rhythms. Attempts have been made to treat depression by advancing the phase of sleep–wake cycles with variable success.

The fact that some patients seem to experience depression associated with seasonal changes also suggests some disturbance of bodily rhythms. Winter depression is more common than summer depression. It is believed to be due to more darkness during the winter months and has been treated with exposure to bright light.

**PRINCIPLE When N=1, do not be too quick to attribute any positive or negative event in the patient to the drug or procedure you are providing at the time.**

**BIOLOGICAL CORRELATES OF DEPRESSION** A number of biological abnormalities have been found in depressed patients, but their importance in the etiology is uncertain. These include 1) nonsuppression of cortisol by dexamethasone, 2) hypersecretion of corticotropin-releasing factor, 3) decreased latency of the first episode of rapid eye-movement of sleep, and 4) immunologic changes. Each of these has low sensitivity and specificity for the diagnosis, but their presence may strengthen a clinical diagnosis.

### *Nosology of depression*

An abundance of dichotomies has given a variety of names to depressive syndromes. The one most widely used is the division of unipolar and bipolar depression, the latter being diagnosed by the presence of mania. A functional distinction has been made between major and minor depressions. The former, which used to be called "endogenous," are more often diagnosed but that may be because they are more evident. The latter include the diagnosis of dysthymia (often called "characterological depression" in the past), recurrent brief depressions, and subsyndromal depression. When depression is not totally remittent, so that patients may alter between episodes of major and minor depression, a diagnosis of "double depression" may be made. The term "atypical depression" is also often used, although its meaning has varied. If one thinks of a spectrum of depressive disorders, then these various terms make more sense, ranging from the most serious to the least impairing, all manifestations of the same underlying disorder (Judd 1997).

The distinction between unipolar and bipolar depression has been difficult. Clinically, they appear to be similar. This resemblance has led to the hypothesis that both types of depression, as well as manic-depressive disorder, are related to each other. Controversy about this formulation abounds.

A depressed mood is less often the patient's chief complaint than are somatic symptoms. Consequently, many depressed patients are first seen by general physicians rather than psychiatrists. Depression and anxiety are often inextricably intertwined, leading often to the misdiagnosis of one of the anxiety disorders. Somatic complaints, besides those due to disturbed bodily rhythms, may affect multiple organ systems. Guilt is almost unique to depression. Depressed mood is, of course, the major diagnostic manifestation. Until the advent of AIDS, depression was well on its way to supplant syphilis and tuberculosis as the "great imitator."

## Anxiety Disorders

### *Prevalence*

Surveys of the frequency of anxiety disorders have led to variable rates of prevalence. The most comprehensive was the Epidemiologic Catchment Area (ECA) Survey sponsored by the National Institute of Mental Health. The 6-month prevalence of anxiety disorders ranged from 6.6 to 14.9% with lifetime prevalence rates varying between 10.4 and 25.1% (Myers et al. 1984; Robins et al. 1984).

Oddly enough, only four subclasses of anxiety disorders were distinguished: phobias, panic disorder, obsessive-compulsive disorder, and somatization. Generalized anxiety disorder, which for years has been thought to be clinically the most frequent and which has been the basis for the approval of almost all antianxiety drugs, was omitted from the list of subtypes.

**PRINCIPLE The way questions are framed often determines the answers.**

A more recent survey focusing on panic disorder found a variation in lifetime prevalence rates from 0.4 to 2.9% among various countries (Weissman et al. 1997). These rates were similar to those found earlier, which ranged from 1.4 to 1.5%. In any case, anxiety disorders were the most frequently encountered over a 6-month period and were exceeded only by a small margin in lifetime prevalence by disorders caused by substance abuse. Thus, anxiety is very common in the general population; no wonder that drugs for treating anxiety have found such a ready market.

Fear, panic, and anxiety have many qualitative similarities; the big differences are the severity of clinical manifestations and the natural course (Table 8-2). In a sense, fear-anxiety may be considered one of the body's major defense mechanisms, and like so many others, operates through redundant mechanisms.

### *Possible mechanisms of anxiety disorder*

**SYMPATHOMIMETIC MODEL** Physiologic changes associated with fear-anxiety resemble those associated with stimulation of the sympathetic nervous system. Walter Cannon interpreted these as indicating that the organism is prepared for "fight or flight," implying the defensive function of fear-anxiety. Sympathomimetic compounds, such as epinephrine, often induce a sensation of anxiety, although the psychological changes may be less a model than the physiologic changes. The use of drugs that block the sympathetic nervous systems, such as $\beta$-adrenoreceptor blocking drugs, alleviate some aspects of fear-anxiety (Ananth and Lin 1986).

**LOCUS CERULEUS, $\alpha$-ADRENORECEPTOR MODEL** The locus ceruleus, a blue streak of cells at the base of the fourth ventricle, is the origin of most of the norepinephrine innervation of the brain. Electrical stimulation of this area in animals mimics anxiety, but lesions prevent fearful behavior. $\alpha$-Adrenoreceptor antagonists, such as yohimbine and piperoxan, increase the firing of these cells and elicit some symptoms of anxiety. Drugs that act as $\alpha$ agonists, such as clonidine, decrease firing and alleviate anxiety. Locus ceruleus cells also have inputs from other neurotransmitters, including serotonin, acetylcholine, $\gamma$-aminobutyric acid (GABA), and several neuropeptides (Charney and Heninger 1986). Nonetheless, the role of the locus ceruleus in mediating fear-anxiety in humans is still uncertain.

**GABA-BENZODIAZEPINE-RECEPTOR MODEL** The discovery of a macromolecular complex with binding sites for GABA, benzodiazepines, barbiturates and other sedative-hypnotics, and some convulsants, such as picrotoxin, has stimulated much speculation about its physiologic functions (Martin 1987). This complex regulates an ion channel for chloride ions, whose entry into the cell hyperpolarizes it. GABA-benzodiazepine binding sites are selectively distributed in the human brain and occur in animals far down the phylogenetic line. This complex has the peculiar property of accommodating three conformations: agonist, antagonist, and inverse agonist (Costa 1991). The latter has been especially provocative, as the action may often mimic the effects of fear-anxiety. Whether or not endogenous inverse agonists exist is still under investigation. One might speculate that the major function of this complex would be to serve as a fear-anxiety mechanism, activated by endogenous inverse agonists. Persons with anxiety disorders might have an exaggerated mechanism that makes them more prone to become anxious than the general run of people.

**PRINCIPLE It is tempting to assume that when a drug alleviates a manifestation its mechanisms of action provide clues to the origin of the manifestation. Deductions about pathogenesis based on the action of drugs must always be considered shaky or at best incomplete because all of the important actions of drugs take decades to be understood.**

**OTHER NEUROTRANSMITTERS** The relatively new anxiolytic drug buspirone apparently exerts its major action by blocking serotonin receptors of the 5-$HT_{1A}$ type

**Table 8-2 Clinical Differences Between Fear, Panic, and Anxiety**

| PARAMETER | FEAR | PANIC | ANXIETY |
|---|---|---|---|
| Onset | Sudden, unanticipated | Sudden, unanticipated | Insidious, may be anticipated |
| Duration of signs or symptoms | Insidious, may be anticipated | Brief, spontaneous subsidence | Long-lived |
| Severity of manifestation | Very severe | Moderate to severe | Mild to moderate |
| Participant | External, recognized | Unknown, unrecognized | Unknown, unrecognized |
| Course | Single episode, self-limiting | Single episode, self-limiting | Chronic with varying remission |
| Other psychiatric disorders | None | Other anxiety disorders, depression | Other anxiety disorders, depression |

(Palmer 1988). Thus, buspirone represents the first of this new class of anxiolytic drugs. The possible role of serotonin has been considerably strengthened by the fact that selective serotonin reuptake inhibitors (SSRIs), most often used for depression, are also effective as treatments for panic disorder, social phobia, and post-traumatic stress disorder.

### *Problems from the broadened concept of anxiety disorders*

Formerly, virtually all anxiety disorders were encompassed by the term *anxiety neurosis*. However, the most recent classification of these disorders has broadened the concept. Most people would have no difficulty reconciling the inclusion of panic disorder in the group; some would insist that it always was included. The various phobias may deserve a place (the root of *phobia* is the Greek word for fear). But should obsessive-compulsive disorder be included? Recent work suggests that its pathogenesis might be considerably different from that of other forms of fear-anxiety (Rapoport 1988). Thus, to the extent that the concept of anxiety disorders is broadened, so will the potential pathogenetic mechanisms.

## Sleep Disorders

### *Prevalence*

Difficulty in initiating or maintaining sleep (insomnia) is a common complaint. Approximately 36% of the American population complains of poor sleep, which is chronic in 25% of this group. Insomnia produces difficulty in concentrating, decreased memory, and inability to cope with minor irritations. Fatigue-related automobile accidents are also 2.5 times as likely in poor sleepers (Mendelson and Jain 1995). Among the increasing number of elderly, more than half who live at home suffer from some disturbance of sleep; even more living in nursing homes suffer the same problems. It is estimated that probably no more than 15% of insomniacs are treated, either with drugs or with other means.

### *Biology of sleep*

The functions of sleep are unknown. Few people can postpone it for much more than a few days. Sleep-wake rhythms are locked into the diurnal cycle, although when free-running, the rhythms do not always follow a 24-hour periodicity (Moore-Ede et al. 1983).

Sleep is a complex, nonhomogeneous state. Rapid eye movement (REM) sleep occurs periodically during the night (about 20% of total sleep time) and is often associated with dreaming. The remainder of sleep is non-REM sleep, which is arbitrarily divided into four stages based on slowing of waves of the EEG. Even a normal night of sleep may be punctuated by brief awakenings.

Serotonin seems to be involved in function of non-REM sleep and acetylcholine in REM sleep, but the exact role of either of these, or other neurotransmitters, is not known. Peptides have been isolated from the brain that appear to induce sleep and that accumulate with sleep deprivation, which is the most important determinant of sleep (Krueger et al. 1986).

### *Classification of sleep disorders*

A number of classification systems have been proposed or are under revision. Two broad categories have been mentioned, the dyssomnias and the parasomnias. Dyssomnias include insomnia, hypersomnia, and disorders of sleep–wake cycle. Parasomnias include aberrations of sleep, such as nightmares, sleep terror, and sleepwalking. Insomnia is the most frequent complaint about sleep; either the patient does not sleep long enough or does not feel rested. The clinical diagnosis of insomnia is justified when inadequate sleep occurs several times a week for at least 1 month. When it is more than 3 months in duration, insomnia is said to be chronic. Diagnosis relies heavily on the history, including one taken from a bed partner. Physical examination may reveal sources of pain that might interfere with sleep. Ordinary laboratory workup is usually noncontributory. Sleep laboratory studies are expensive and are not required for evaluation of transient or chronic insomnia. They are indicated for the evaluation of suspected sleep-related breathing disorders and periodic limb movement disorders, both of which can contribute to a complaint of insomnia (American Sleep Disorders Association 1995). About 35% of insomnia is thought to be associated with other psychiatric disorders, mainly anxiety and depression. An undetermined amount is due to drug taking, either social drugs such as alcohol or caffeine or a variety of medications with stimulant properties.

Sleep apnea and periodic movements of sleep are unusual causes of insomnia. Both may be suspected on the basis of testimony from a bed partner. Sleep apnea may cause hundreds of minor awakenings through the night. Even though patients may not be fully aware of being awake, they feel excessively fatigued the following day. The bed partner may describe periods in which the patients snores loudly followed by rapid breathing and then a period of quiet with barely noticeable respiration. Two types are recognized. Obstructive apnea is due to excessive laxity of the soft palate, which may fall back and occlude the airway. Surgical revision of the palate, placement of a permanent tracheostomy, or continual positive pressure oxygen are the proper treatments for this cause.

Central apnea is due to a lack of adequate respiratory drive. After a period of apnea in which the $CO_2$ tension increases, breathing resumes with a start, followed by a brief period of hyperventilation. Drugs that stimulate respiration, such as almitrine, acetazolamide, and medroxyprogesterone have been used successfully in such patients (DeBacker 1995). Sleep apneas are more frequent in elderly patients and those who are obese. Generally, any drug that can depress respiratory drive, which would include the benzodiazepines, should be avoided in such patients. The diagnosis may be suspected on clinical grounds: daytime sleepiness or the need for napping; snoring or uneven respirations, as noted by a bed partner; headaches and hypertension; or marked obesity. Sleep laboratory studies are usually definitive.

Periodic movements of sleep occur throughout the night. Restless legs disturb sleep not so much by causing awakenings but by reducing the depth of sleep. This diagnosis, too, may be suspected from the testimony of a bed partner. Sleep laboratory studies establish the diagnosis. Although clonazepam has been specifically recommended as treatment, quite likely any benzodiazapine would suffice. Many other drugs have been reported to be helpful; levodopa or dopamine agonists, clonidine, carbamazepine, and opiates (Wetter and Pollmacher 1997).

Sleepwalking, sleep terrors, and enuresis occur during slow-wave sleep. Enuresis has been satisfactorily treated with tricyclic antidepressants. The other conditions may respond to drugs that tend to eliminate or reduce slow-wave sleep, which would include most benzodiazepines.

Many larger medical centers have a sleep laboratory. The normal architecture of sleep has been well described so that patients with sleep problems may be compared with the norm to determine the nature of the disturbance. Some patients are found to have a normal amount of sleep and normal sleep architecture despite a subjective complaint of poor sleep. The effects of drugs on the architecture of sleep can also be studied in sleep laboratories. In general, most hypnotic drugs reduce the amount of REM and slow-wave sleep and increase total sleep time.

## Childhood and Adolescent Disorders

### *Nature and prevalence*

Diagnosis of psychiatric disorders in children and adolescents is complicated by the fact that one is dealing with a developing person. Furthermore, the manifestations of such disorders in these age groups may be somewhat different from those of adult disorders. Finally, clinicians are much less keen about using definitive diagnostic terms in young persons because the mere fact of labeling may affect the future development of the person.

Because of these difficulties, no precise estimates of the prevalence of childhood disorders have been made. Although a surprising number of children and adolescents are hospitalized in psychiatric institutions at any given point in time, it is difficult to tell how many of them have true psychiatric disorders as opposed to problems in living. The best data probably pertain to the various forms of mental retardation, which are most clearly diagnosable even though the cause of the majority of instances remains obscure.

### *Disorders in common with adults*

So far as one can tell, most of the common psychiatric disorders of adults can also be found in children and adolescents. Thus, one can make a diagnosis of anxiety disorders, depression, mania, and schizophrenia. However, these diagnoses are made far less commonly in children for the reasons mentioned previously. Anxiety in childhood may be manifested by a variety of behaviors, possibly labeled initially with the rather nonspecific term *conduct disorder*. Depression is more apparent in adolescence, being manifested tragically by the fact that suicide is a major cause of death in this age group. Schizophrenia characteristically tends to become evident in late adolescence and early adult life; earlier on, it may be mistaken for anxiety disorders. Mania may occur in children but is more likely first to be misdiagnosed as attention deficit/hyperactivity disorder (ADHD).

### *Disorders peculiar to children and adolescents*

Attention deficit/hyperactivity disorder usually becomes evident in the early school years. The pathogenesis is uncertain, but it is highly amenable to treatment. Empiric therapy can be proven efficacious without knowledge of the mechanism of action of the drug. Longer-term follow-up studies indicate that it may persist during adult life.

**PRINCIPLE One does not have to understand the cause of a disorder to treat it effectively.**

Autism used to be considered to be a form of childhood schizophrenia but is now considered to be entirely separate. It may or may not be associated with mental retardation. A variety of other conditions have also been described. Conduct disorder is a diagnosis made frequently (about 4% of boys), but its boundaries are not clear; it may often be a "wastebasket" diagnosis. Enuresis is mainly found in children and declines with advancing years. Anorexia and bulimia are most likely to become evident during adolescence. Tourette's syndrome, the "barking tic," usually first becomes recognized in adolescence. Narcolepsy can be recognized in adolescents, although its diagnosis may be deferred until adult life.

***Unsolved problems***

Children and adolescents have been referred to as "therapeutic orphans." Few psychiatric drugs are tested in children as they are in adults. As a result, the package label usually states "no evidence is available to direct the use of this drug in children and adolescents." This deficiency has led to a proposal that all new drugs should be tested in children and adolescents as well as adults before being licensed (Vitiello and Jensen 1997). Obviously this proposal, though seemingly sensible, would cause more expense and delay in getting new drugs to the market. Perhaps a better solution would be to provide contingent approval of new drugs without this information, the contingency being that within a reasonable period, suitable data should be made available to make recommendations about the drug's use in this population. At this writing, the issue has not been resolved.

## Disorders in Old Age

***Nature and prevalence***

Projections of an increasing population of aged persons in developed countries have been interpreted by some as indicating an impending "silent epidemic" of Alzheimer's disease. This disease, also sometimes called *primary degenerative dementia* or *senile dementia of the Alzheimer type*, has become a major focus of inquiry into both its causes and its treatment. Some evidence suggests that the disease may be heterogeneous. Early-onset forms (age below 58 years) are known to occur and seem to follow an autosomal-dominant mode of transmission. Later onset forms, which may affect 10% or more of the population over 85 years of age, may be blamed on both a genetic predisposition and environmental influences (Davies 1986). The progression of the disease may also vary from rapid to slow. The association of Alzheimer's neuropathologic change with Down syndrome has pointed a finger of suspicion at chromosome 21, which is triplicate in Down syndrome. This chromosome seems to be the locus of the $\beta$-amyloid gene, and amyloid deposits are a prominent part of the neuropathologic lesions, but whether the Alzheimer gene is located on this chromosome is unknown.

The only secure diagnosis of Alzheimer's disease is neuropathologic, which hardly suffices for the clinician. Error rates for the clinical diagnosis of probable Alzheimer's disease have varied from 5 to 25%, depending on the series. A number of potentially reversible causes of dementias of old age have been reported, which creates a problem in determining how much medical workup is required. If one is unable to live with uncertainty, the possible workup can be extensive (Arnold and Kumar 1993). However, a quantitative review of studies from 1972 to 1994 indicated wide variations in frequency of reversible dementia, from 0% to as high as 23%. Most instances of reversible dementias were accountable by misdiagnosis; depression and drug intoxication were most frequent, followed by metabolic and neurosurgical disorders. In the latest four studies, the prevalence of reversible dementia had fallen to <1% (Weytingh et al. 1995).

In general, most reversible causes are found in younger patients; an insidious onset of dementia in older patients is almost always due to Alzheimer's disease. The two psychiatric states most likely to be confused with dementia are delirium and depression. Delirium is almost always associated with concurrent drugs or concomitant medical illness (Francis et al. 1990). Depression may create a pseudodementia, but close inquiry into cognitive functions shows a disparity between the degree of social withdrawal and the cognitive impairment.

***Other psychiatric disorders of old age***

Multi-infarct dementia may occur after a succession of small strokes that do not present with customary major neurologic impairments. Mental disturbances may be episodic with declines following each episode of infarct; these may be temporary or become stable until the next episode. The renewed realization that vascular disorders co-exist with Alzheimer's disease has increased interest in attempts to treat the vascular component. Some elderly patients with little history of prior psychiatric disorder develop a paranoid state. If other signs of schizophrenia are present, one may be dealing with a late-onset form of paranoid schizophrenia, so called paraphrenia. On the other hand, one may be dealing with an affective disorder if mood changes predominate. Elderly patients may also become highly hypochondriacal, becoming so obsessed with some bodily function as to appear somewhat psychotic. Usually, however, this problem is not difficult to recognize, although it may be difficult to treat.

***Unsolved problems***

An extensive search for peripheral biologic markers of Alzheimer's disease has not yet established any as clinically useful. Present investigations focus around peripheral deposits of amyloid around small blood vessels, such as might be examined by a skin biopsy, or the presence of a unique protein in the cerebrospinal fluid. As it is unlikely that any treatment possible in the near term could reverse the pathologic lesions of well-established Alzheimer's disease, earlier detection might allow a potential treatment to show a greater effect. Ultimately, we should like to know better the pathogenetic mechanisms by which the degeneration of neurons occurs.

## DRUG THERAPY OF PSYCHIATRIC DISORDERS

It is somewhat paradoxical that serendipity has played a significant role in the drug treatment of psychiatric disorders. The first exemplars of almost every class of drug had their beginnings more or less by chance. Reserpine, chlorpromazine, imipramine, iproniazid (the first monoamine oxidase inhibitor), lithium, and the benzodiazepines were all the result of good clinical observations or unanticipated chemical reactions.

**PRINCIPLE Pasteur's injunction that "chance favors the prepared mind" has been shown repeatedly to be true in the discovery of psychotherapeutic drugs.**

### Multiple Drugs

As each new class of drugs was discovered, many chemical homologs were synthesized. Therapeutic effects were similar, but sometimes potency was increased or a modified array of side effects was achieved. Probably more than 100 phenothiazines with antipsychotic effects are known throughout the world. The pharmacologic properties of the original member, chlorpromazine, led to a battery of screening tests and the discovery of new chemicals but old drugs. A minor modification of the side chain of phenothiazines resulted in the thioxanthene group. Haloperidol, the first of a variety of butyrophenones, was somewhat different, not only in being highly potent but also in having narrower pharmacologic actions. A similar multiplication occurred among other classes of drugs. The number of tricyclic antidepressants or related compounds increased dramatically. Most were discovered because they blocked uptake of aminergic neurotransmitters, such as norepinephrine or serotonin. Nowhere has the multiplicity of homologs been more evident than in the class of benzodiazepines. Just when one thinks that no more can possibly be found that are different, a drug such as midazolam, which is ultrashort-acting and water-soluble, appears on the scene. Whether the benzodiazepine era is at an end, to be supplanted by drugs of the buspirone type, remains to be seen. Buspirone, which has a structure resembling that of a butyrophenone, was synthesized as a potential antipsychotic. After it failed that use, its antianxiety effects were discovered.

The past decade has seen a remarkable explosion of new antipsychotics and antidepressants. The former were heralded by the "atypical" antipsychotic, clozapine. A number of other atypical antipsychotics have reached the market or are about to: risperidone, olanzapine, sertindole, Seroquel, ziprasodone and others. A new class of antidepressants were named "selective serotonin reuptake inhibitors" (SSRI) to denote a greater specificity of action of these from former drugs. Fluoxetine was the first, followed quickly by paroxetine, sertraline, mirtazepine, and fluvoxamine.

In addition, some new drugs were variations on an older theme: moclobemide was a reversible monoamine oxidase inhibitor (MAOI), nefazodone was a sibling of trazodone, and venlafaxine had mixed effects on aminergic neurotransmitters similar to imipramine and amitriptyline. Lithium remains the basic drug for treating mania, but carbamazepine is now considered to be a suitable alternative. The latter drugs were discovered on the simplistic notion that because both mania and seizures are episodic, an anticonvulsant drug might have antimanic action. This concept has been incorporated into the kindling hypothesis of mania. Another anticonvulsant, divalproex sodium (valproic acid), has also become available.

**PRINCIPLE Less-than-convincing hypotheses often lead to discovery of new drugs or indications whose mechanisms can remain totally obscure.**

These developments have had the consequence that clinicians now have an abundance of drugs from which to choose for treating various psychiatric disorders. The advantages of having such a wide choice are several. First, patients may respond to one drug better than to another; the clinician can successively try drugs to determine which best meets the patient's need. Unfortunately, there is no way to predict in advance which drug may be best for a given patient. Second, some patients are better able to tolerate the side effects of one drug than another, even though the drugs may be equally effective. This wide choice allows attempts not only to find the most effective drug for an individual patient, but also to identify the one best tolerated. A disadvantage is that physicians may be overwhelmed by the sheer number of these drugs; it is difficult even for those in the field to remember the generic and trade names, the doses, and the dosage forms of so many compounds.

**PRINCIPLE Whenever there is an abundance of drugs more or less equivalent for treating an illness, it may be better to learn to use a few well than to attempt to use them all at the risk of doing so poorly. In using this principle, learn the pharmacology of those drugs with a different mechanism of action so that one can exploit fully the pharmacologic differences between agents.**

### Limitations of Current Drugs

No therapeutic area has ideal drugs; psychiatric disorders are no exception. Antipsychotic drugs have revolutionized the treatment of psychotic persons, perhaps too much so. The reduction in the number of state hospital beds during the 1960s in the United States had a consequence recognized during the 1980s of producing a plethora of homeless, mentally ill persons on the streets of our major cities. Even under the best conditions, antipsychotic drugs benefit only 60 to 65% of patients, and remissions are far from complete. Antidepressants, too, are effective in only 65 to 70% of patients and seldom lead to complete recovery. The efficacy of these drugs in large groups of patients is roughly equivalent, with no substantial increase during the past 30 years. All have major side effects that limit their acceptance by patients; noncompliance with treatment is the major cause for relapse.

Many antidepressants are potentially lethal in overdose, a consideration of importance for depressed patients. It is generally agreed that benzodiazepines are effective for alleviating anxiety, but spontaneous fluctuations in this disorder have often led to relatively few demonstrable differences from placebo in comparative studies. The problems of dependence when these drugs are abused was recognized early in their use, but the new concept of *therapeutic-dose dependence* has put some desirable limitations on the amount of exposure to these drugs. Buspirone may mitigate this problem, but the lack of overt sedation, rather than being an advantage, seems to be a disadvantage for patients who have sleep problems.

**PRINCIPLE When multiple drugs are available for the same indication, using the pharmacologic nuances between them can create the best choice of drug for a specific individual.**

Lithium has been relatively safe but also is not effective in all patients. Carbamazepine is no more effective overall but may help patients unresponsive to lithium. Since keeping patients on medication is a most difficult problem with manic patients, the fact that neither of these drugs is available in any long-acting IM preparation limits their utility. The number of available psychotherapeutic drugs has increased markedly during the past 35 years. However, increased efficacy has been difficult to attain, and reduction in side effects has been difficult to achieve. The ideal drug still remains elusive.

## ANTIPSYCHOTICS

Most general physicians prefer to have a psychiatrist make the diagnosis of schizophrenia or other psychoses. Many patients are very clearly psychotic, but because "craziness" comes in many guises, it is well to have a diagnosis made by a specialist. Once the patient is started on drug treatment, the primary responsibility for follow-up may fall on the primary care physician.

Another situation is that of the patient who has been hospitalized for an acute psychosis but is discharged from the mental hospital taking maintenance medication. If a psychiatrist is not available for follow-up or is not willing to undertake it, the responsibility becomes that of the general physician. An adequate record of the patient's illness should be forwarded, and a physician at the hospital should be available for consultation or re-referral. The main goal of the follow-up care of these patients is to ensure that they continue to function adequately, and to be alert to the development of any complications of treatment, especially tardive dyskinesia (abnormal movements that resemble those of Huntington disease, which appear late in the course of treatment).

### Drug Classes

A number of different chemical structures have been found to possess the spectrum of pharmacologic actions that indicate utility as an antipsychotic drug. A battery of screening tests was derived from the actions of the first of these drugs, chlorpromazine, and then applied to others as they were synthesized. The phenothiazine group of compounds, exemplified by the three subfamilies based on different side chains (aliphatic-chlorpromazine, piperidine-thioridazine, piperazine-fluphenazine), have been the most developed. A relatively minor molecular change produced the thioxanthenes, in which chlorprothixene is the homolog of chlorpromazine. Other classes, suc butyrophenones (e.g., haloperidol), the indoles (e.g., molindone), the dibenzoxazepines (e.g., loxapine), and the dibenzodiazepines (e.g., clozapine), have somewhat different chemical structures. Clinical consensus has been that the differences among these classes are substantial enough to merit this proliferation.

**PRINCIPLE Always ask whether a new chemical is really a new drug and whether or not it has enough advantages over previous drugs to merit widespread adoption.**

Atypical antipsychotics are the fastest growing group and are probably now the most widely prescribed drugs. The term "atypical" refers to several putative properties of these drugs: 1) a much decreased predilection for producing various extrapyramidal motor syndromes; 2) decreased rates of other side effects that result in more patients staying in treatment for longer periods of time; 3) a long-term potential for greater social rehabilitation of patients, possibly due to less cognitive impairment; 4) increased improvement in so-called negative symptoms, such as emotional withdrawal, poverty of speech and movement, anhedonia, and loss of initiative. These reputed advantages are sufficient for making many physicians now consider them to be first-line treatments, despite an increase in cost of as much as 100-fold compared with older antipsychotic drugs.

## Pharmacodynamics

Virtually all effective antipsychotic drugs block postsynaptic D2 dopamine receptors. Positron emission tomography (PET) scanning techniques have shown that clinically effective doses of these drugs block central $D_2$ dopamine receptors with an occupancy of 65 to 85%. Blockade persisted for many days after the drug repository forms of haloperidol were withdrawn (Farde et al. 1988). Postsynaptic dopamine-receptor block in the mesolimbic dopamine system has been considered to be the primary mechanism for the antipsychotic action, a desired effect. A similar block of receptors in the nigrostriatal dopamine system leads to the parkinsonian syndrome and other unwanted neurologic effects. Blockade of dopamine receptors in the tuberoinfundibular system leads to elevated serum prolactin concentrations and sexual side effects.

Although atypical antipsychotics also block $D_2$ dopamine receptors, they are often more potent in blocking $D_1$ and $D_4$ dopamine receptors and serotonin (5-$HT_2$) receptors. Efforts to explain the different actions of the atypical drugs have centered on the role of these receptors, in accounting for either superior antipsychotic action or decreased extrapyramidal side effects. To date, no evidence exists that blockade of these other receptors by itself has any ameliorative effect on schizophrenia or on extrapyramidal syndromes.

Another way of looking at the atypical drugs is to consider them as weak $D_2$ receptor blocking agents. The first atypical drug was the phenothiazine derivative, thioridazine, which was so weak in blocking $D_2$ receptors (as compared with other antipsychotics then available) that many pharmacologists expressed doubts that it would be an effective antipsychotic agent. The other criterion that makes thioridazine comparable to the atypical drugs is that it had very little predilection for producing extrapyramidal motor reactions. At the time, this beneficial action was considered related to the strong intrinsic antimuscarinic actions of the drug.

A consideration of the spectrum of pharmacologic actions of haloperidol (which had for a time long replaced chlorpromazine as the reference drug for typical antipsychotics), thioridazine, and the atypical drugs (as shown in Table 8-3) reveals the similarities and differences between them. All, without exception, block $D_2$ receptors. Other than that, few have the same spectrum of pharmacodynamic effects. How then to explain the clinical differences? First, blockade of $D_2$ receptors as measured by PET accounts for all $D_2$ receptors, mostly from the nigrostriatal system. Perhaps a weaker dopamine blocking action is adequate for therapeutic degrees of blockade in the mesolimbic system but not enough in the nigrostriatal system to evoke extrapyramidal motor syndromes. As the latter are often difficult to distinguish from negative symptoms, perhaps a specific action on the latter is more apparent than real. Nonetheless, a decrease in such disabling symptoms might lead to increased social rehabilitation. On the other hand, the lack of strong effects on muscarinic, $\alpha$-adrenergic, and $H_1$ histamine receptors no doubt decreases many of the side effects of traditional drugs, which patients found disagreeable and led to problems in compliance.

**PRINCIPLE Just because a drug has some pharmacodynamic action does not mean that this action contributes to its therapeutic effect.**

Because of their growing clinical and theoretical importance of the atypical neuroleptics, it seems reasonable to consider some of these in some detail.

Table 8-3 **Relative Strength of Antagonist Effects of Typical and Atypical Neuroleptics on a Variety of CNS Receptors**

| | Receptor | | | | | | | |
|---|---|---|---|---|---|---|---|---|
| **Drug** | **$D_2$** | **$D_3$** | **$D_4$** | **$D_1$** | **5-$HT_2$** | **Musc** | **$H_1$** | **$\alpha_1$-Adr** |
| Typical | | | | | | | | |
| Chlorpromazine | ++ | + | | | ++ | ++ | + | ++ |
| Haloperidol | +++ | | | ± | + | ± | ± | + |
| Atypical | | | | | | | | |
| Thioridazine | + | ± | | ± | + | +++ | ++ | +++ |
| Clozapine | + | | ++ | + | ++ | ++ | ++ | ++ |
| Risperidone | ++ | | | ± | ++ | | | |
| Olanzapine | + | | | + | ++ | ++ | ++ | ++ |
| Sertindole | ++ | | | + | ++ | 0 | 0 | ++ |
| Quetiapine | + | | | ± | + | 0 | + | + |
| Ziprazodone | ++ | ++ | 0 | + | + | | | |

Atypical drug definition: Low propensity for inducing extrapyramidal motor reactions versus antipsychotic effects; relatively less induction of catalepsy in animal studies; increased efficacy for negative symptoms? Receptors: $\alpha_1$-Adr, $\alpha_1$-adrenergic; $D_{1-4}$, dopamine; $H_1$, histamine; 5-$HT_2$, serotonin; Musc, muscarinic.

### *Clozapine*

Clozapine has had a checkered history. Synthesized in 1969, it was first tested clinically in Europe. All seemed to be going well when, in 1975 in Finland, it created the worst epidemic of drug-induced agranulocytosis in medical history. As one of the early complications of treatment with clozapine is fever, and as in Finland aminopyrine is often used for symptomatic treatment, the most reasonable conclusion was that agranulocytosis occurred because of an additive depression of leukopoiesis. All use of the drug was stopped except for some "compassionate" cases in which the drug appeared to have been far better than preceding treatments. In the early 1980s, the drug company organized a study in which patients previously refractory to chlorpromaline were treated with clozapine or chlorpromazine. The results were fairly conclusive that clozapine offered new hope for refractory patients (Kane et al. 1988). Therefore, it was reintroduced into the market but with strict controls for monitoring leukocyte counts.

**PRINCIPLE A drug may survive in spite of a life-threatening adverse effect if it is perceived as offering a significant advantage for a serious disorder.**

Although it is possible that monitoring leukocyte counts need not be so strict after the first few months of treatment, use of clozapine has declined with the advent of other atypical drugs without this serious complication. Because of the substantially higher cost of clozapine, a pharmacoeconomic study compared clozapine with haloperidol in hospitalized patients with schizophrenia. Over a 1-year period, clozapine-treated patients required less time in the hospital, so that despite an almost 10-fold difference in average wholesale price of the drugs (which in any event was a small proportion of the total cost of care), the total costs of treatment were similar (Rosenheck et al. 1997).

### *Risperidone*

This drug has become the most widely prescribed atypical antipsychotic. A meta-analysis of controlled trials comparing risperidone with typical antipsychotics revealed a similar efficacy but less need for treatment of extrapyramidal syndromes, fewer dropouts, and more response of negative symptoms (Song 1997). Doses of the drug appear to be critical; doses larger than 4 to 6 mg/day have been associated with extrapyramidal syndromes of all types.

### *Olanzapine*

This drug is a homolog of clozapine that lacks the complication of agranulocytosis. It has become the major competitor of risperidone among the atypical drugs. A drug company-sponsored comparison of olanzapine with risperidone showed the former drug to have some advantages: better response of negative symptoms; longer lasting benefit; and less extrapyramidal movement disorder, hyperprolactinemia, and sexual dysfunction. Both were equally effective and safe (Tran et al. 1997). Another company-sponsored study in which it was compared with haloperidol showed that olanzapine produced a greater response rate, fewer extrapyramidal motor reactions, less effect on prolactin levels, and decreased negative sy- toms (Tollefson et al. 1997).

***Sertindole***

This drug is believed to have a selective action on $D_2$ receptors in the mesolimbic system. A drug company-sponsored study comparing sertindole with haloperidol found comparable efficacy, but sertindole produced fewer extrapyramidal side effects and was significantly better than placebo in managing negative symptoms (Zimbroff et al. 1997). After being approved for marketing, the drug has temporarily been withdrawn because of its tendency to increase Q–T interval on the EKG.

***Quetiapine***

This drug has some chemical resemblance to clozapine, with a similar pharmacologic profile. A collaborative trial of the drug in 286 patients compared two doses, 250 and 750 mg/day, versus placebo. Of 280 patients in whom efficacy of treatment was evaluated, 42% of those receiving high doses, 57% of those receiving low doses, and 59% of those receiving placebo withdrew before completion of the 6-week study, primarily because of treatment failure. The high-dose group showed some significant changes in total symptom improvement, especially with positive symptoms. No clear effect was noted on negative symptoms. The drug did not induce extrapyramidal motor reactions or increase serum prolactin levels (Small et al. 1997). These results would seem to have damned the drug with faint praise, but they resulted in no adverse regulatory actions.

## Pharmacokinetics

All these drugs are membrane-active lipid-soluble agents with consequent high volumes of distribution. They are readily but incompletely absorbed. Protein binding is around 90 to 95%. Very little unchanged drug is excreted in the urine; the majority of elimination is by metabolism through a variety of hepatic pathways. Elimination half-lives vary from 10 to 24 hours, but clinical duration of action seems to be much longer.

Although extensive studies have attempted to define a range of therapeutic plasma concentrations, the data are unclear for most of these agents. Therefore, monitoring of plasma concentrations is not done in clinical practice.

## Indications

The primary indication for antipsychotics is schizophrenia. Although the drugs are by no means curative and in fact have many deficiencies, they are the best-established treatment of this serious disorder. Patients with a diagnosis of schizoaffective disorder may also benefit from the use of these drugs to treat their psychotic symptoms. Acute mania may not respond to lithium alone; the judicious and temporary use of antipsychotics may be extremely helpful. Psychoses of old age are best managed with antipsychotics, although such treatment is entirely symptomatic. Some acute brain syndromes, such as the "recovery or intensive care unit syndrome," respond to antipsychotics. Tourette's's syndrome responds well to some antipsychotics, notably haloperidol, pimozide, and risperidone. While not a primary treatment for depression, antipsychotics may have an adjunctive role in patients with psychotic or agitated depressions. Efforts to persuade physicians to use these drugs in small doses for treating anxiety or other minor emotional disorders have, fortunately, not met with much success.

## Dosing Guidelines

This group of drugs has a very wide range of doses that have been used clinically (Table 8-4). Because of the desire to limit total exposure to these drugs because of concern about tardive dyskinesia, the doses currently used are fairly conservative, usually at the lower end of customary dose ranges. Such modest doses seem overall to be as effective as the larger doses formerly used.

Initial doses are usually divided over the day, although some of the atypical drugs may be given as a single daily dose. By the time most patients are in the maintenance phase of treatment, a single daily dose given at bedtime is desirable.

Most often, these drugs are given orally, either as tablets or as liquid concentrates. Intramuscular dosage forms of some of the high-potency drugs are also available. Fluphenazine and haloperidol are also available as decanoate esters, to serve as intramuscular depot preparations for maintenance therapy.

These drugs may be combined safely with almost any other psychotherapeutic drug. Combinations of two or more antipsychotics make little sense. The most frequent drugs used in combination with an antipsychotic drug are the anti-Parkinson agents. Those of the anticholinergic type, such as trihexyphenidyl and benztropine mesylate, are most commonly used. The anticholinergic action may cause some impairment of mental function, or possibly mild delirium, so that they should be used cautiously. Amantadine reduces these problems, but it is a far more expensive treatment.

**PRINCIPLE The cost of drugs is becoming an important consideration in choice. It is far better to have a patient purchase and take an older drug that may have fewer advantages, than it is to prescribe a more expensive agent and never have the prescription filled.**

**Table 8-4 Equipotent Doses and Usual Daily Doses of Common Antipsychotic Drugs**

| Drug | Equipotent Dose (mg) | Dose Range (mg/day) | Dose (mg) | Average Wholesale Price (per month) |
|---|---|---|---|---|
| Chlorpromazine HCl | 100 | 50–800 | 50 bid | Generic $12<br>Thorazine $62 |
| Thioridazine HCl | 100 | 50–800 | 100 bid | Generic $5<br>Mellaril $35 |
| Clozapine | 100 | 12.5–900 | 100 bid | Clozaril $205 |
| Loxapine succinate | 10 | 15–160 | 25 tid | Generic $81<br>Loxitane $139 |
| Perphenazine | 10 | 40–160 | 16 tid | Generic $60<br>Trilafon $129 |
| Sertindole | 4 | 20–24 | | NA |
| Thiothixene | 2 | 6–20 | 5 tid | Generic $16<br>Navane $63 |
| Fluphenazine HCl | 2 | 2–20 | 5 bid | Generic $25<br>Prolixin $91 |
| Haloperidol | 2 | 2–20 | 5 bid | Generic $2<br>Haldol $77 |
| Risperidone | 2 | 4–6 | 2 bid | Generic NA<br>Risperdal $190 |

Source of drug costs is *Mosby's GenR*$_x$ 1998, on the basis of the price calc. (calculation) dose. Current prices may vary from those quoted, but comparative prices among products are expected to be similar. The reader should check on local prices at the time of prescribing. NA, not available.

Schizophrenia can be one of the most chronic mental illnesses known. It is highly likely that many patients will require treatment over much of their lives. Because the course is variable and unpredictable, many clinicians terminate drug treatment after the first episode has been treated successfully, to see how long the patient stays in remission. If relapse occurs soon thereafter, maintenance treatment probably will be needed. Presently, two approaches have been recommended. If the patient is under close supervision by knowledgeable family or custodians, it may be possible to treat intermittently as each relapse occurs. The consequence of such "as needed" treatment is to reduce the total amount of exposure to drug, and to decrease many of the unpleasant side effects. If such close supervision is not available, or if it fails, the alternative strategy is continual treatment with the lowest possible dose required to sustain remission. Compliance in taking medication is a problem because these drugs tend to become unpleasant as the patient improves. Use of the depot preparations may circumvent the problem of compliance by producing such low concentrations of drug as to make it better tolerated.

## Adverse Effects

The wide range of effects on other receptor systems accounts for many relatively less severe adverse reactions. Antimuscarinic blockade accounts for the dry mouth, blurred vision, constipation, and urinary hesitancy often experienced by patients. In extreme cases, patients may become confused. $\alpha_1$-Adrenoreceptor blockade may produce orthostatic hypotension. Most of these side effects can be managed by adjustments of dose.

### *Extrapyramidal motor reactions*

Extrapyramidal motor reactions include acute dystonias, akathisia, and parkinsonian syndrome. These have become less of a concern now that the doses of conventional antipsychotics have been lowered and the atypical drugs increasingly used. They are usually managed with anti-Parkinson drugs.

### *Neuroleptic malignant syndrome*

*Neuroleptic malignant syndrome* is a rare (< 1/1000) and most severe type of antipsychotic-induced movement disorder (Addonizio et al. 1987). Muscle rigidity is the key finding; the increased muscle activity increases heat production. If the excess heat can be lost by sweating, the appearance of fever may be delayed. The patient may be stiff as a board and drenched with sweat. When the mechanism for dissipation of heat becomes inadequate, the body temperature may rise to hyperpyretic levels. It should be emphasized that fever is not required to make the diagnosis; one could argue that by the time it appears, the diagnosis has been delayed. Patients usually manif altered consciousness and autonomic dysregulati characteristic laboratory abnormality is an elevation of muscle-derived creatine phosphokinase (CPK). Other laboratory abnormalities, such as leukocytosis, are stress-related. The combination of high fever and leukocytosis has occasionally raised the question of sepsis, but the neurologic state should be a ready tip-off. Although earlier cases were sometimes fatal, more recent series have been without fatalities, probably because of both earlier recognition and better management.

Peripheral treatment includes mechanical cooling and use of skeletal muscle relaxants, such as dantrolene sodium, baclofen, or diazepam. Central approaches attempt to restore the disturbed dopamine system by use of direct agonists (e.g., bromocriptine), uptake inhibitors (e.g., amantadine), or precursors (e.g., levodopa). This approach is based on the assumption that the mechanism of this disorder is a too-rapid depletion of CNS dopaminergic activity due to the blockade of receptors. Many of these patients are severely dehydrated with high serum potassium concentrations from muscle damage; fluid and electrolytes must be carefully managed. For reasons that are not clear, a few patients have been reported to have responded to electroconvulsive therapy (ECT).

***Tardive dyskinesia***

*Tardive dyskinesia*, as the name implies, consists of abnormal movements that appear late in the course of treatment. The abnormal movements begin insidiously, usually affecting first the mouth, tongue, and face. Choreoathetoid movement of the extremities may follow, and in advanced cases, truncal dyskinesias are observed. The mechanism of tardive dyskinesia is thought to be supersensitivity of dopamine neurons in the basal ganglia induced by prolonged pharmacologic blockade. If this is the case, then three points of pharmacologic treatment come to mind. First, reducing dopaminergic activity would be desirable, possibly by gradually eliminating antipsychotic drugs and allowing supersensitive receptors to become desensitized. Clozapine or other atypical drugs might make such a course more feasible, as many patients cannot be left totally without treatment. Increasing cholinergic activity would also be reasonable but is not easily done clinically. Eliminating anticholinergic drugs, such as antiparkinsonian or tricyclic antidepressants, eliminates potential aggravating factors. Finally, increasing efferent GABA activity with benzodiazepines has been useful. Despite these eminently sensible pharmacologic approaches, tardive dyskinesia remains difficult to treat, sometimes being thought to be "irreversible."

Clinicians who use antipsychotic drugs for patients in long-term treatment should be constantly on the alert for the early signs of the disorder. The patients or family members should be informed about the risk of developing this problem when antipsychotic drugs are begun. Tardive dyskinesia not handled in this way has become a major source of malpractice actions.

### Drug Interactions

Most interactions of antipsychotics are pharmacodynamic, representing the additive sedative, anticholinergic, or $\alpha$-adrenergic blocking effects of these drugs when combined with others having similar properties. The quinidine-like effect of thioridazine, when combined with similar effects from tricyclic antidepressants, may enhance cardiotoxicity. Pharmacokinetic interactions have been described, but most are trivial and of no real clinical significance.

### Overdoses

Suicidal overdoses of these drugs are less common than with tricyclic antidepressants. In general, the same supportive measures are used. Except for thioridazine and mesoridazine, life-threatening cardiac arrhythmias are not a problem.

## ANTIDEPRESSANTS

Not all patients with depression need drug therapy. Many patients become depressed as a reaction to temporary adverse circumstances. The *reactive* depressions usually subside with time; only when the depression is out of proportion to the problem or when it persists beyond resolution of the problem, need drug therapy be considered.

Psychotherapy may be useful for all types of depression. Several specific types have been devised for treating depression, the cognitive-behavioral type being most widely used. Severely depressed patients may not be able to benefit from such treatment until after some alleviation of depression by drug therapy.

Drug therapy has been most effective for patients with *endogenous* depression. Such patients are characterized by having the disturbances of bodily rhythms mentioned earlier. They tend to have repeated episodes of depression throughout life; a family history of depression also supports the diagnosis. Often these depressions are autonomous, in that they may be precipitated, sometimes abruptly, without any evident psychosocial stressor. Drug therapy has been useful for both minor and major depressions. The less severe states are called dysthymia or subsyndromal depression. The presence of persisting and disabling depressive symptoms, regardless of the severity, may therefore constitute an indication for drug therapy.

There has been much concern that individuals with depression are seriously undertreated. The consequences are long-lasting personal suffering, occupational and family/social impairments, and suicide. Patients may not recognize symptoms or may underestimate the degree of their severity. Mental health workers may not be attuned to the subtleties of diagnosis. The present health care system may not be willing, mainly for economic reasons, to deal with the problem adequately (Hirschfeld et al. 1997).

A number of guidelines have been published to help physicians in the better management of depressed patients (American Psychiatric Assn. 1993; U.S. Dept. Health Human Services 1993). Obviously, much more effort must be made to find ways to treat depressed patients better.

## Classes of Antidepressants

Over the years, several distinct classes of drugs have been used as antidepressants. Those currently in each class are shown in Table 8-5. In order of appearance in the clinic, they are the following.

### *Tricyclics*

Tricyclics, as the name implies, are drugs with three rings in their structure. Promazine, like other phenothiazine derivatives, has a 6-6-6 three-ring structure, each ring having six members. A minor modification of this tricyclic structure to 6-7-6 was thought to preserve its antipsychotic action. Quite unexpectedly, the first clinical study indicated that this new drug, imipramine, was not very effective as an antipsychotic but relieved depression in affected schizophrenics. Subsequently, its antidepressant action was confirmed in depressed patients.

**PRINCIPLE Minor alterations in chemical structure may cause profound changes in the pharmacology and clinical indications of a drug.**

Both imipramine and amitriptyline have active monodemethylated side-chain metabolites (desipramine and nortriptyline, respectively), which have been marketed as separate entities. Doxepin and protriptyline differ from the

**Table 8-5 Pharmacokinetic Parameters of Various Antidepressants (and Their Active Metabolites)**

| Drug (Active Metabolite) | Plasma $T_{1/2}$ (h)[a] | Protein-Binding (%) | $V_d$ (L/kg) | Therapeutic Plasma Levels (ng/mL)[a] | Usual Daily Dose Range (mg) |
|---|---|---|---|---|---|
| *Tricyclics* | | | | | |
| Imipramine | 6–20 | 88–93 | 20–30 | > 180 total | 50–300 |
| (Desipramine) | 14–30 | 70–90 | 22 | 145 | 50–200 |
| Amitriptyline | 19–31 | 82–96 | 15 | > 200 total | 50–300 |
| (Nortriptyline) | 18–28 | 93 | 21–57 | 50–1550 | 50–300 |
| *Second-generation* | | | | | |
| Amoxapine | 8–30 | | | 200–400 | 200–300 |
| Maprotiline HCl | 21–40 | 89 | 52 | 200–300 | 75–225 |
| Bupropion | 11–14 | 85 | | 25–110 | 200–300 |
| *SSRIs* | | | | | |
| Fluoxetine HCl | 1–3 days | 94 | 12–97 | 73–453 mg/mL | 20–60 |
| (Norfluoxetine) | 7–15 days | | | | NA |
| Sertraline | 25 | 94 | 20 | | 50–200 |
| (Desmethylsertraline) | 66 | | | | NA |
| Paroxetine | 7–65 | 95 | 8–28 | 0.9–573 mg/mL | 10–50 |
| Fluvoxamine maleate | 15 | 77 | >5 | 20–417 mg/mL | 100–300 |
| Citalopram | 33 | 82 | 12–16 | 38–288 mg/mL | 30–60 |
| (Desmethylcitalopram) | 33 | 74 | | 10–105 mg/mL | NA |
| Trazodone HCl | 4–7 | 5–11 | 1.04 | 240–4900 | 150–600 |
| Venlafaxine HCl | | | | | |
| (Desmethyl-venlafaxine) | 5<br>11 | 27 | 7.5 | | 75–350<br>NA |
| Mirtazapine | 20–40 | 85 | | | 15–45 |

Adapted from Baumann, 1996; van Harten, 1993; Lane, 1996.
[a]Except as indicated.
Abbreviations: SSRI, selective serotonin reuptake inhibitors, $t_{1/2}$, elimination half-life; $V_d$, volume of distribution.

**Table 8-6 Effects of Antidepressants on Receptors and Neurotransmitters**

| DRUG | RECEPTOR | | | | | |
|---|---|---|---|---|---|---|
| | 5-HT$_2$ | NOR | D$_2$ | $\alpha_1$-ADR | MUSC | H$_1$ |
| *Tricyclics* | | | | | | |
| Imipramine | ++ | ++ | + | +++ | ++ | ++ |
| Amitriptyline | ++ | + | + | +++ | +++ | +++ |
| Desipramine | 0 | +++ | + | ++ | + | + |
| *Second-generation* | | | | | | |
| Amoxapine | ++ | ++ | ++ | +++ | + | ++ |
| Bupropion | ± | ± | ++ | 0 | 0 | ± |
| *SSRIs* | | | | | | |
| Fluvoxamine maleate | +++ | + | 0 | | ± | ± |
| Sertraline | +++ | ± | ± | 0 | 0 | 0 |
| Paroxetine | +++ | ± | 0 | 0 | 0 | 0 |
| Fluoxetine HCl | ++ | 0 | 0 | 0 | 0 | 0 |
| Venlafaxine HCl | ++ | ++ | ± | 0 | 0 | 0 |
| Mirtazapine | ++ | ++ | 0 | 0 | 0 | ++ |
| Nefazodone HCl/ Trazodone HCl | ++ | 0 | ± | ++ | 0 | 0 |

Receptors: $\alpha_1$-Adr, $\alpha_1$-adrenergic; D$_2$, dopamine; H$_1$, histamine; 5-HT$_2$, serotonin reuptake; Musc, muscarinic; Nor, norepinephrine reuptake.

other tricyclics only in minor modifications of the tricyclic ring structure. Clomipramine differs from imipramine only in having a chlorine atom at the 3 position of the tricyclic moiety.

***Monoamine oxidase inhibitors***

When patients with pulmonary tuberculosis were first treated with iproniazid, they became euphoric. Shortly afterward, liver toxicity caused iproniazid to be replaced by isoniazid. The latter drug was used to exploit the euphoriant action in depressives but to no avail. It was only after iproniazid was found to be a potent inhibitor of the enzyme MAO and isoniazid a very weak inhibitor that it became apparent that enzyme inhibition was the key factor in any antidepressive action of iproniazid. Several older MAOIs were used in medical practice, the most popular being phenelzine. During the past decade, a new class of short-acting, reversible MAO inhibitors, exemplified by moclobemide, have taken over the field.

***Heterocyclic or "second-generation" antidepressants***

This group of drugs was introduced about 1980. They are distinguished by having a fourth ring in their structure, leading to the term "heterocyclic." They were also referred to as "second generation" drugs using the analogy with antibiotics. They never became very popular, as few offered any significant advantages over tricyclics.

***Selective serotonin reuptake inhibitors (SSRIs)***

This group, introduced largely in the 1990s, have become the most important and widely used antidepressants. Although no evidence indicates that they are more effective overall than earlier drugs, their side-effect profile is quite different, making them better tolerated by patients. Furthermore, unlike tricyclics and heterocyclics, they are remarkably safe in overdoses.

## Pharmacodynamics

***Tricyclics***

The effects of various antidepressants on neurotransmitters and transporters are summarized in Table 8-6. Tricyclics are rather nonspecific in their pharmacologic actions. The principal action by which the antidepressant effects are thought to be mediated, is their ability to block uptake of biogenic amine neurotransmitters (Richelson 1994). Amitriptyline and imipramine, by virtue of their active metabolites, have a mixed action in blocking uptake of both serotonin and norepinephrine. Only desipramine is specific for blocking uptake of norepinephrine. To the extent that the action of this neurotransmitter is increased, mild sympathomimetic effects may appear.

Sedation may be due to a combination of antihistaminic and $\alpha_1$-adrenoreceptor blocking actions. Anticholinergic action produces numerous side effects, such as dry mouth, blurred vision, urinary hesitancy, and constipation. Adrenoreceptor blockade also contributes to orthostatic hypotension. Most tricyclics are membrane-active local anesthetics, which may contribute to both an antiarrhythmic and an arrhythmogenic potential. Slight variations occur in this spectrum of pharmacologic actions among various tricyclics (Table 8-5). Although reuptake of released neurotransmitters can be blocked by the very first doses of these drugs, the subsequent downregulation of receptors may take longer. This delay in the ultimate consequence of these drugs has been adduced as an explanation for delays in clinical response (Sulser 1987). However, a delayed response has been questioned on the basis of two independent, multicenter double-blind studies. No evidence was found for a delayed onset of action of various antidepressants. An early response was predictive of ultimate improvement; 70% of patients who improved at 14 days became responders (Stassen et al. 1996). Previous recommendations of waiting 6 to 12 weeks to assess response may have prolonged the agony for some patients. When these drugs have been given intensively, either with large initial oral doses or following parenterally administered loading doses, clinical responses may occur within a few days. Therefore, the relative contributions of pharmacodynamics and pharmacokinetics to the rate of clinical response to these drugs are still uncertain.

***Monoamine oxidase inhibitors***

The enzyme MAO works presynaptically to catabolize monoamine neurotransmitters (dopamine, norepinephrine, serotonin). Blocking this enzyme presumably allows more neurotransmitter to accumulate and become available for release at the synapse. Increased neurotransmitter at synapses leads to downregulation of postsynaptic receptors, the same endpoint attained with tricyclics (Pare 1985). Consequently, both MAO inhibitors as well as tricyclics achieve the goals predicted by the amine hypothesis of depression: they remedy the presumed deficiency of neurotransmitter at the synapse.

***Heterocyclics***

This group of drugs also acts primarily by blocking uptake of aminergic neurotransmitters. Amoxapine (a metabolite of the antipsychotic, loxapine) retains some of the dopamine receptor-blocking action of the latter drug. It has been proposed as especially useful for psychotic depressives, although extemporaneous combinations of antipsychotic and antidepressants might be more flexible. Maprotiline, which bears some chemical resemblance to desipramine, acts like the latter drug, largely blocking uptake of norepinephrine. Trazodone is the most peculiar drug of this group, working in a complex way against serotonin receptors. Not only does it block these receptors but it also blocks the reuptake of serotonin, two apparently opposing actions. It also has $\alpha_1$-adrenergic blocking activity. Trazodone promotes sleep, and often is used as a hypnotic for depressed patients, especially in those who have sleep disturbances induced by other antidepressants, such as SSRIs. It has the advantage of relatively few side effects. Because of its primary effects on serotonin, it is often linked with the specific serotonin reuptake inhibitors.

Bupropion is not a heterocyclic, but, because it appeared along with the others of this group, is often linked with them. Its structure resembles that of the amphetamines and it might be considered a "tamed down" amphetamine. Its primary actions are through dopamine and norepinephrine, similar to the amphetamines, yet it has no clinical effects resembling the latter drugs. Side effects are few; the most serious complication is seizures, which are dose-related, appearing mainly with doses in excess of 600 mg/day. It has the advantage of having little adverse effect on sexual function (Ascher et al. 1995).

***Selective serotonin reuptake inhibitors (SSRIs)***

This class of drugs appeared during the past decade and have been proliferating ever since, now virtually dominating the antidepressant market. Several drugs are relatively specific in acting on serotonin while others have mixed affects on other neurotransmitters. The ones currently available are as follows.

**FLUOXETINE** Fluoxetine was the first drug in this class and quickly became a phenomenal commercial success. Although there was little evidence to suggest that this drug was more effective than the older tricyclics, it had a different, and less noxious, pattern of side effects, making it more acceptable to patients. The absence of affinity for muscarinic, histamine, $\alpha$-adrenergic, $\beta$-adrenergic, and dopamine receptors produced many fewer side effects, with nausea and headache being most common.

**SERTRALINE** This SSRI has a somewhat different pharmacologic profile than fluoxetine, yet its primary modes of action seem to be similar. Like the other SSRIs, it has been proven in many studies to be more effective than placebo and as effective as a number of tricyclics (Reimherr et al. 1990, Zimbroft et al. 1997).

**PAROXETINE** Although structurally dissimilar to the other SSRIs (as they are to each other), this drug also acts primarily by blocking reuptake of serotonin. It has been shown to be superior to placebo and comparable in efficacy to tricyclics. Withdrawal from treatment due to side effects was less frequent than with the latter drugs (Dechant and Clissold 1991). However, a meta-analysis of discontinuation rates between SSRIs and other antidepressants indicated that the largest differences in favor of the SSRIs were in comparisons with imipramine and amitriptyline, but that such differences were less apparent when comparisons were made with newer tricyclics or heterocyclics.

**FLUVOXAMINE** Although technically only approved in the United States for treatment of obsessive-compulsive disorder, this drug has proven antidepressant activity comparable to comparison drugs (Palmer and Benfield 1994). One of the few published comparisons of two SSRIs studied fluvoxamine (50–200 mg/day) versus paroxetine (20–30 mg/day) in 120 patients with major depression treated for 6 weeks. Similar improvement was found in both groups on all rating instruments. Severe adverse effects were less commonly reported with paroxetine (13%) than with fluvoxamine (28%), resulting in less frequent discontinuation of treatment with the former drug (Ansseau et al. 1994).

**NEFAZODONE** This drug is a sibling of trazodone. It resembles the latter drug structurally and in its pharmacodynamic actions. Like trazodone, it has a favorable side-effects profile but a spotty record as an antidepressant. It has been shown to have more favorable aspects on the sleep architecture and quality of sleep than does fluoxetine (Armitage et al. 1997). This finding is not surprising, as trazodone has often been used empirically as a hypnotic in depressed patients. Nefazodone, like trazodone, has the disadvantage of a short span of action requiring multiple daily doses.

**VENLAFAXINE** This novel phenethylamine structure not only inhibits serotonin reuptake but also affects norepinephrine similarly. Combined with the lack of effects on other receptors, it would be predicted to be equivalent to tricyclics, such as imipramine and amitriptyline, but with far fewer side effects (Schweizer et al. 1994). A comparison with imipramine in 234 outpatients with major depression showed the two drugs to be equally effective, but venlafaxine had a lower attrition rate due to side effects. Nonetheless, side effects are numerous, including asthenia, anorexia, nausea, dry mouth, dizziness, and nervousness, and, in men, abnormal ejaculation, abnormal orgasm, and impotence.

**MIRTAZAPINE** Mirtazapine is not, strictly speaking, an SSRI. Rather, it enhances both serotonergic and noradrenergic neurotransmission by different mechanisms. Noradrenergic activity is increased by blockade of $\alpha_2$ presynaptic adrenoreceptors, while serotonin activity is increased by two mechanisms: an increase in 5-HT$_1$-mediated cell firing, and $\alpha$-2 adrenoceptor blockade. 5-HT$_2$ and 5-HT$_3$ receptors are also blocked (Holm and Marchan 1999). A meta-analysis of trials with amitriptyline and mirtazapine in severely depressed patients showed these drugs to be equally effective with no differences in time course (Kasper et al. 1997).

### *Hypericum (St. John's wort)*

This herbal remedy has been used clinically in Germany for several years. It is not available in the United States as an approved prescription drug, but it is available in health food stores and herbal shops. Some 1757 patients with mild to moderate depression had been treated in randomized clinical trials. Hypericum was more effective than placebo and about equally effective as standard drugs, although doses of the latter were low (Linde et al. 1996). The current high public attention regarding natural products has made most of us somewhat suspicious of new miracle herbs. Historically, many of our most important drugs have started as natural products, from digitalis, aspirin, and quinine to the *Vinca* alkaloids and tamoxifen. These products gained wider acceptance following purification of the active agent, and subsequent rigorous clinical testing. However, the efficacy and place, if any, for hypericum in the treatment of depression is uncertain.

**PRINCIPLE An open mind is warranted when the experience of history indicates the possibility of something new.**

### *Reversible inhibitors of monoamine oxidase (RIMA)*

Older MAOIs have the disadvantage that their action is nonspecific and irreversible; that is, once enzyme inhibition is achieved, it lasts for days. Failure to regenerate monoamine oxidase-A promptly accounted for the many interactions for which older drugs (e.g., phenelzine) are noted. Moclobemide is a new reversible inhibitor of MAO, which mitigates these interactions. A multicenter clinical trial that compared moclobemide, imipramine, and placebo found the two active drugs to be equally effective. Moclobemide was better tolerated in regard to side effects (UK Moclobemide Study Group 1994). Similar results have been obtained in comparisons with SSRIs and older nonselective MAOIs. Unlike SSRIs, moclobemide seems to have no adverse effect on sexual functioning (Fulton and Benfield 1996).

### *Miscellaneous drugs*

Pindolol, a $\beta$-adrenoceptor blocker with properties as a 5-HT$_1$ receptor antagonist, has been used in combination with SSRIs to shorten treatment response latency in newly treated patients, or to cause additional improvement in treatment-resistant patients. The rationale is that the initial increase in extracellular serotonin stimulates inhibitory 5-

$HT_{1A}$ autoreceptors that diminish extracellular serotonin. By blocking this inhibitory action, pindolol is thought to improve response rates (Artigas et al. 1996). Clinical results of such combined treatment have been somewhat contradictory, so it remains to be seen whether this approach, as logically founded as it is, will become part of clinical practice.

Sympathomimetics have long been out of favor as antidepressants, although occasional good results are reported in older patients, many of whom are poorly tolerant of other antidepressants. Lithium is seldom used for unipolar depressions, unless it is highly treatment-resistant and then only as an adjunct; it is properly used for treating depression that is part of manic-depressive disorder.

## Pharmacokinetics

Most older antidepressants, such as the tricyclics and heterocyclics, have moderately long half-lives that allow for once-daily dosing. A very long duration of action is intrinsic to the irreversible MAO inhibitors, which requires a waiting period of a week or two before treatment is started with other antidepressants. Such is not the case with the newer, reversible MAO inhibitors. The SSRIs are highly protein-bound with a large volume of distribution. Most have moderately long half-lives, but fluoxetine is atypical in that it, as well as its active metabolite, have very long half-lives (Table 8-5). This drug also has the property of inhibiting some drug-metabolizing enzymes, thereby creating problems of interactions with other agents (Van Horten 1993). The pseudo-SSRIs, such as trazodone and nefazodone, are characterized by short half-lives that make it necessary to divide doses during the day (Bauman 1996).

Although attempts have been made to establish a range of therapeutic plasma concentrations for the newer drugs, it has been difficult to say with any certainty that these are clinically useful. Although such ranges have been better established for older drugs, such as the tricyclics, determinations of plasma concentrations are seldom required, except for unusual circumstances, mainly those concerning compliance of patients in taking medication.

## Guidelines for Clinical Use

The plethora of antidepressants makes the choice of drug more perplexing for clinicians. An old rule that still seems worth following is: Use the drug the patient has best responded to before. These may include tricyclics and heterocyclics. If the best response was from an MAO inhibitor, it would be better to use the newer reversible inhibitors, exemplified by moclobemide. If it comes down to a choice between the newer SSRIs and other drugs, no clear guidelines are available. The SSRIs vary not only in their pharmacology, pharmacokinetics, and side-effect profile, but also in the clinical responses elicited in individual patients. Thus, the choice among these drugs is largely empiric (Devane 1995). Many young and middle-aged men are poorly compliant with SSRIs because of their ability to dampen libido and potency. For them, the best choice might be bupropion, which has the least adverse effects on sexual functioning. On the other hand, patients with anxiety and sleeplessness and poor toleration of any side effects might best be treated first with trazodone, the best tolerated of these drugs, even though the therapeutic effects are less certain.

**PRINCIPLE One must try to make the shoe fit the foot.**

The goal of treatment should be complete remission of depression. This goal is likely, more often than not, to be only partially realized. Many strategies have been suggested for managing treatment-resistant patients, including increasing the dose to the maximum tolerated, increasing the duration of treatment, trying another drug, or even considering nondrug treatment, which in severe cases might be electroconvulsive therapy. Lithium is often recommended in a combination with other drugs. However, using two drugs that might increase serotonergic activity might produce an alarming "serotonin reaction." Combinations of tricyclics and MAO inhibitors have been studied over the years with some reports of increasing benefit from such combinations. Enough significant hazards are present with any combinations to make them somewhat experimental. They require close attention by a knowledgeable person.

Besides their use in treating depression, a number of other uses have been described for antidepressants. They are well established for treating bulimia. The SSRIs have virtually replaced clomipramine as treatment for obsessive-compulsive disorders and have a growing use in the treatment of social phobias. Trazodone has been recommended as a hypnotic for patients with and without concurrent depression. Several antidepressants have been found useful for treating premenstrual tension. Tricyclics are often used for treating chronic pain, especially of neuropathic causes, along with conventional analgesics.

**PRINCIPLE Drugs are often given restrictive labels or rubrics that do not fully describe the entire range of their uses.**

### Pharmacoeconomic Considerations

Traditionally, physicians have prescribed drugs with little thought about their cost. Because many of the older psychotherapeutic drugs are now available as generics, and because the newer ones are usually quite expensive, a huge gap in price exists between new drugs and old. This increased drug cost raises the question of whether the newer ones are really cost effective. Two recent surveys have looked at this problem with respect to antidepressants. Both were published in British journals, perhaps signifying a greater concern about drug costs in these countries. One study performed a meta-analysis on 63 controlled trials comparing SSRIs with tricyclics and related drugs. No difference in efficacy or drop-out rates was found. Slightly more patients on tricyclics dropped out for lack of efficacy (19%) as compared with treatment with SSRIs (16%). Routine use of an SSRI as first-line treatment was thought to greatly increase cost with only questionable benefit (Song et al. 1993). Another similar study found no evidence that SSRIs were more cost effective than tricyclics, but attributed this conclusion to a dearth of prospective studies in primary care situations (Hotopf et al. 1997).

It has long been known that undertreatment of many hypertensive patients has been due to prescriptions not being filled; the tendency of physicians to use the latest drug leads to underutilization of older, equally effective, and much cheaper drugs. Physicians should at least inquire of their patients how the prescriptions will be paid for, and acquaint themselves with the formularies of many insurance plans, some of which limit reimbursement for the more expensive drugs. Such concerns are by no means unique to psychotherapeutic drugs. It is difficult, because of a multi-tier pricing system for drugs, to make exact comparisons of costs. The average wholesale price of a drug to a retail pharmacist is much more than it would be to a large HMO. In the glossary of this chapter, we have, by the use of dollar signs, indicated the relative costs of various drugs from inexpensive (usually generic, $) to expensive ($$$). The same considerations plague interpretations of pharmacoeconomic studies.

## MOOD STABILIZERS

Although it is tempting to term all drugs used for treating mania *antimanic*, most are not especially effective for acute mania. Antipsychotics are more effective for such symptoms. Rather, drugs specific for mania might be construed as *mood stabilizers*, affecting the cycles of both mania and depression. At the moment, three drugs are widely used as mood stabilizers: lithium, carbamazepine, and valproic acid. As each works by somewhat different mechanisms, it is often logical and desirable to combine these in patients who do not respond to a single drug.

### Lithium

#### *Pharmacodynamics*

The discovery of lithium's efficacy was serendipitous. It was used in animals as lithium urate, the urate being thought to counter a nonexistent toxic substance in the urine. Fortuitously, it was noted that the lithium component had a calming effect in the animals. When the first trial in humans with lithium carbonate was undertaken, an amazingly fortunate choice of dose (600 mg 3 times daily) confirmed its efficacy (Amdisen 1987).

For a simple cation, lithium has a complicated set of actions on the cell that probably play some role in its pharmacodynamic effects. The relative importance of each is still in doubt. The most favored molecular explanation of its action is that it blocks the phosphatidylinositol second messenger system. Blockade of the conversion of inositol diphosphate to the monophosphate interferes with the recycling process of membrane phosphoinositides. Consequently, two major signaling chemicals are depleted in the brain: free inositol and diacylglycerol. Other possible mechanisms include effects on serotonin, norepinephrine, dopamine, acetylcholine, and $\gamma$-aminobutyric acid. In addition, effects on G proteins and protein kinase C may also be important. Some of these effects may be secondary to the blockade of the inositol recycling system. The complexity of these mechanisms may also explain the dual action of lithium in ameliorating both mania and depression (Lenox and Manji 1995).

#### *Pharmacokinetics*

Lithium is a cation and has very simple kinetics, as outlined in Table 8-7. Two methods have been used to predict the proper loading dose to attain therapeutic serum levels. One uses a 24-hour determination of lithium concentration following a test dose (both the size of the test doses and the frequencies of obtaining concentrations have been varied) to make a prediction. The other, which is far simpler, is based on body weight. A dose of 0.5 mEq/kg (one 300-mg dose unit = 8 mEq) is adequate to produce initial concentrations in the therapeutic range. A simple calculation [(body weight in kg)/16 = number of 500-mg dose units of lithium carbonate/day] can be used to estimate proper initial doses (Groves et al. 1991).

Monitoring of serum lithium concentrations is considered mandatory because the therapeutic margins of this

**Table 8-7 Pharmacokinetic Parameters of Mood Stabilizers**

| Parameter | Lithium Carbonate | Carbamazepine | Divalproex Sodium |
|---|---|---|---|
| Bioavailability (%) | 100 | | |
| Protein binding (%) | 0 | 70–80 | 80–90 |
| $V_d$ (L/kg) | 0.7 | 1.2 | |
| Plasma $t_{1/2}$ (h) | 20 | 31–35 | 9–16 |
| Metabolite | None | 10,11-Epoxide | None |
| Renal excretion | 20% of creatine clearance | None | None |
| Therapeutic levels | 0.5–1.4 mEq/L | 4–12 $\mu$g/mL | 50–100 $\mu$g/mL |

Abbreviations: $t_{1/2}$, elimination half-life; $V_d$, volume of distribution.

drug are small. Generally a range of 0.5–1.4 mEq/L has been recommended for acute treatment as well as for prophylaxis.

Because lithium must enter the cell to act, its onset of action is often slow, so that it may be a week or so before therapeutic effects are noted. Similarly, it may take a while for relapse to occur following its discontinuation. In severely manic patients, it is often necessary to initiate treatment with antipsychotics, alone or combined with sedative-hypnotics, to control agitated behavior.

***Indications***

The principal indication for lithium is for management of manic-depressive disorder. The drug is more effective against the manic than against depressive symptoms. Its major value has been its ability to prevent subsequent recurrent episodes of both mania and depression. Although it has been reported to be useful in unipolar depressions (that is, without mania), other antidepressants are preferred. In schizoaffective disorders, lithium may be combined with antipsychotics to good effect. Its use in addition to antipsychotics in treatment-resistant schizophrenia, or antidepressants in treatment-resistant depression, has been helpful.

***Doses and duration of treatment***

If doses are related to body weight, extremes of 600–2400 mg/day may be considered. The majority of patients do well with doses of 1500–1800 mg/day. More important is monitoring of serum concentrations to keep patients within the therapeutic range. The first determination may be done 1 week after starting treatment with a fixed dose, when the patient should have reached steady state. A simple arithmetic adjustment of dose can be made to fine-tune the therapeutic concentration. Once that is attained, measurement of serum concentration is needed only when signs of toxicity or changes in the status of the patient (an intercurrent illness, starting another medication) develop.

Treatment of an acute manic episode is measured in weeks or months; prophylaxis against recurrent episodes is measured in months or years. Usually, two or more episodes during the span of a year is considered an indication for prophylactic treatment. Serum concentrations during this phase of treatment may be lower than those during acute treatment (Consensus Development Conference 1984a).

***Drug interactions***

Thiazide diuretics decrease renal clearance of lithium by about 25%, so that doses need to be reduced; inexplicably, furosemide apparently does not have such an action. A similar reduction in renal clearance has followed use of several newer NSAIDs; again, inexplicably, aspirin and ibuprofen do not do this.

***Adverse effects***

Tremor is relatively frequent when lithium reaches therapeutic doses and is usually of little clinical consequence. Other neurologic abnormalities, such as ataxia, dysarthria, neuromuscular irritability, and choreoathetosis, may herald toxicity. Appearance of any new neurologic or psychiatric symptoms during treatment is reason to stop the drug and to assess serum concentrations. Gastrointestinal symptoms, such as anorexia, nausea, or vomiting may also herald toxicity, but diarrhea is common even at therapeutic concentrations.

Because lithium inhibits activation of adenyl cyclase in the distal nephron, the action of antidiuretic hormone is attenuated. Mild symptoms are merely those of increased water turnover, but when excretion reaches 3.5 L/day or more, the patient is presumed to have nephrogenic diabetes insipidus. Amiloride is acceptable treatment (Battle et al. 1985). Chronic interstitial nephritis has been reported but the finding is controversial.

Thyroid impairment is thought to be common, but is rarely of clinical significance. About 10 to 20% of patients develop a mild goiter during long-term treatment, with clinical hypothyroidism in a smaller number. Levothyroxine treats both goiter and hypothyroidism (Maarbjerg et al. 1987).

Dysmorphogenesis, characterized mainly by an increase in cardiac malformations, has been associated with lithium treatment. Therefore, it is contraindicated during pregnancy or, if the fetus has been inadvertently exposed, the woman should be counseled about possible choices. Lithium excretion decreases after parturition and postpartum toxicity has occurred if doses are not decreased. The ion readily enters the breast milk and can contribute to lethargy and poor reflexes in the neonate. Other adverse effects of lithium that are frequent but of little clinical concern include edema, acneiform eruptions, and leukocytosis. The last is due to a direct effect on leukopoiesis and not simply recruitment from the marginal pool. Lithium has actually been employed as a treatment for drug-induced and other forms of granulocytopenia. Abnormal T waves are seen in the ECG, but exacerbations of the sick sinus syndrome are more serious; this condition would also constitute a contraindication to use of the drug.

### *Overdoses*

Many overdoses are iatrogenic and occur during therapy with the drug. Intentional overdoses are life-threatening and may produce permanent neurologic residua (Sansone and Ziegler 1985). Both peritoneal and hemodialysis are useful for eliminating the small lithium ion. Concentrations in serum should be reduced to well below the therapeutic range before dialysis is stopped (Simard et al. 1989).

## Carbamazepine

Carbamazepine was first used to treat manic-depressive disorder in 1971, based on a hypothesized similarity between the rhythmic mood alterations of manic-expressive disorder and epileptiform discharges. Although the rationale for using it was weak, the drug has been proved effective in several blinded, controlled studies. It is now considered to be equivalent to lithium and a suitable alternative to that drug.

### *Pharmacodynamics*

Like lithium, carbamazepine has a multitude of pharmacologic actions, which vary according to whether administration is acute or chronic administration. Carbamazepine interacts with sodium and potassium channels, dampening the influx of these ions into neurons. Because this action would have a stabilizing effect on synaptic transmission, its efficacy as an anticonvulsant and in the treatment of trigeminal neuralgia may be based on these effects. As one would expect with any tricyclic, carbamazepine blocks the reuptake of norepinephrine, although it has only 25% the activity of imipramine. This action may contribute to its efficacy as an anticonvulsant, as the destruction of norepinephrine neurons blocks the anticonvulsant effects of carbamazepine. Moreover, this action may well explain its antidepressant effects in both bipolar and unipolar depression. Carbamazepine is a competitive adenosine antagonist. However, whether this pharmacologic action is related to efficacy in manic-depressive illness awaits elucidation of adenosine's functions as a neurotransmitter. The clinical course of manic-depressive illness is often characterized by an increasing number of episodes over time. Such sensitization is analogous to kindling in epileptics. Consequently, it has been proposed that its major action in treating manic-depression is to decrease kindling, although kindling has never been demonstrated in humans (Post et al. 1992).

### *Pharmacokinetics*

The absorption of carbamazepine from the GI tract is slow. The attainment of peak serum concentrations can be highly variable (2–12 hours); the drug's half-life is relatively long (31–35 hours). Protein binding is approximately 70 to 80%. Achieving stable therapeutic serum concentrations of carbamazepine can be complicated by the fact that the drug can induce its own metabolism by hepatic enzymes. The relationship between dose and plasma concentrations is poor. It may take several days before one can select a daily dose that maintains therapeutic serum concentrations (4–12 $\mu$g/L). Pharmacokinetic parameters are summarized in Table 8-7. Metabolism of carbamazepine occurs as oxidation, first to a 10,11-epoxide metabolite that has anticonvulsant activity and then to the 10,11-dihydroxide. One-third of the 10,11-dihydroxide is then conjugated as the glucuronide and eliminated, while two-thirds is eliminated in the free form. The drug is excreted in both the urine and feces.

### *Indications*

The primary indication for carbamazepine has been seizures. It is also useful for treating trigeminal neuralgia. The fact that lithium and carbamazepine have similar overall rates of efficacy in manic-depressive patients should not be construed to mean that they are interchangeable in individual patients. The clinical profile of the patient who benefits from carbamazepine may differ from that of a lithium responder. It makes good clinical sense that patients who do not respond adequately to lithium should be tried on carbamazepine. In some cases of mania, concurrent administration of carbamazepine and lithium may be superior to treatment with either agent alone.

**PRINCIPLE When drugs with different mechanisms of action are found to be efficacious for the same indication, their use in sequence or in combination is rational and often useful.**

***Dosing guidelines***

Clinical use of carbamazepine for manic-depressive illness follows guidelines similar to those for its use for epilepsy. One should begin treatment with carbamazepine with a dosage schedule of 200 mg/day until a daily dose of 600–800 mg/day is achieved. Serum concentrations should be assessed 5–6 days after this dose has been reached, and additional dose increments can be made as required. Most patients require a dose of no more than 1200 mg/day. As noted previously, carbamazepine may induce its own metabolism; consequently, the daily dose may require further adjustment over the course of several days. In the treatment of manic-depressive disorder, it has been difficult to show a correlation between serum concentrations and the degree of the clinical anti-manic response. Some experts recommend that the daily dose of carbamazepine should be increased without regard to serum concentrations until intolerable side effects are encountered or until the dose reaches 1200 mg/day.

As with lithium, patients who have responded to carbamazepine but who are thought to require prophylactic treatment may be continued on carbamazepine for months or even years (Kishimoto et al. 1983). For patients who do not seem to need long-term treatment, the drug can be gradually discontinued after remission has been maintained for 3–4 months.

***Interactions***

Clinically significant interactions between carbamazepine and other drugs are few. The one of greatest concern is a pharmacodynamic interaction in which the combination of carbamazepine with lithium increases neurotoxicity.

***Adverse effects***

Approximately one-third of patients treated with carbamazepine experience adverse effects. The most commonly encountered adverse effects are related to the CNS, namely, sedation, nausea, weakness, ataxia, diplopia, and mild nystagmus. These effects are dose-dependent and may be avoided or reversed by reducing the dose. Subtle interference with a variety of cognitive processes, such as memory or attention, also may occur, even when clearcut sedation is absent. Carbamazepine is known to induce leukopenia. In many cases the extent of this side effect is mild and spontaneously reversible and should not constitute an absolute contraindication for further therapy. In other cases, leukopenia may be irreversible and life-threatening. The drug should be discontinued immediately in these cases. Since leukopenia usually occurs early in treatment, a reasonable precaution is to obtain leukocyte counts weekly for the first 4 weeks of treatment, and to discontinue treatment if a steadily progressive decrease in the leukocyte count occurs, or if the leukocyte count falls below 4000/$\mu$L per cubic millimeter on any occasion.

***Overdoses***

Carbamazepine overdose is potentially life-threatening. The initial symptoms are drowsiness and ataxia, associated with plasma concentrations of 11–15 $\mu$g/L. As plasma concentrations rise to 15–25 $\mu$g/L, combativeness, hallucinations, and choreiform movements may follow. Concentrations above 25 mg/L are associated with severe disturbance of consciousness, often coma. Coma usually lasts less than 24 hours. Although neurotoxic effects predominate, cardiotoxicity may include prolonged conduction and repolarization times. Cardiopulmonary arrest is a potential cause of death.

The kinetics of the drug change during massive overdose. Half-life is prolonged, and the epoxide metabolite increases, presumably contributing to toxicity. The usual methods are used in trying to rid the body of drug, including gastric lavage followed by repeated administration of charcoal. Although the drug has a large volume of distribution, charcoal hemoperfusion may be considered. Supportive measures should include close cardiac monitoring and management of electrolyte abnormalities. Seizures may be treated with diazepam or phenytoin. In short, many of the same principles of management are used as with overdoses of tricyclic antidepressants.

## Valproic Acid

Another anticonvulsant that has been useful in treating manic-depressive disorders is valproic acid. As valproic acid is now available as an inexpensive generic, an enterprising drug company has created a dimer known as divalproex sodium. The new name masks the old drug. The dimer is alleged to cause less gastrointestinal and other side effects, possibly because it is released more slowly.

***Pharmacodynamics***

The mode of action in manic-depressive disorder is not really known. The drug acts primarily by checking the spread of focal epileptic seizures and also has anti-kindling action. Thus, it might abort episodes and subsequently decrease their frequency. It is also possible that it might work by increasing activity of the inhibitory neurotransmitter, GABA.

***Pharmacokinetics***
The drug is highly available, protein-bound, and metabolized. A large number of metabolites, both inactive and active, are formed. A correlation between plasma concentrations and clinical effects, either in epilepsy or manic-depression, is poor, so there is little reason to monitor plasma concentrations.

***Indications***
Valproate has become one of the most widely used anticonvulsants and is rapidly growing in use as a mood stabilizer. A large collaborative study sponsored by the manufacturer compared lithium and divalproex in manic patients. Both were significantly more effective than placebo and comparable with each other in many respects. Doses were monitored by plasma concentrations (Bowden et al. 1994). A meta-analysis of lithium compared with valproic acid and carbamazepine revealed that the efficiency of the three treatments was virtually identical. A slight tendency towards greater tolerance and fewer side effects was noted for the anticonvulsants (Emilien et al. 1996).

***Dosing guidelines***
A loading dose of 20 mg/day of divalproex was compared with haloperidol 0.2 mg/kg/day in acute manic patients. Both produced equally rapid control of symptoms, although adverse effects were lower with divalproex (McElroy et al. 1996). Although doses in investigative studies have been monitored by plasma concentrations, such monitoring is not practicable for clinical use. The initial dose is usually 750 mg/day, with increments as required to attain control or reach limiting side effects. Maximum doses are 60 mg/kg/day. As with other mood stabilizers, long-term treatment is probably required, either through the present episode or prophylactically.

***Adverse reactions***
Nausea, vomiting, dizziness, somnolence, and increased accidents have been the most common adverse effects found in clinical trials. Overdoses can be fatal but rarely are. The fraction of unbound drug in overdoses is higher than with therapeutic doses, allowing the use of hemodialysis to remove the excess drug.

### Other Drugs

A number of other anticonvulsants are being investigated in the treatment of mania. Lamotrigine, which acts via GABA, proved useful as an adjunct in refractory manic-depressives (Kusumakar and Yatham 1997). Calcium channel blockers, especially verapamil, have been reported to be effective adjuncts. The most compelling controlled study indicated lithium to be superior as a single treatment (Walton et al. 1996). Antipsychotics must be used in some instances where mania is not controlled. Haloperidol has been most widely used; the neurologic complications reported from combinations with lithium were clearly due to lithium intoxication. Recently, newer antipsychotics, such as clozapine and risperidone, have also been used with some success.

Reports of inducing manic episodes by treatment with tricyclic antidepressants during the depressed phase of manic-depression have raised concerns about the best treatment of this problem. Current feeling is that adequate treatment with mood stabilizers is the best solution. If antidepressants must be used, tricyclics are preferred to SSRIs. Electroconvulsive treatment is the most effective treatment for both mania and depression but is used only as a last resort due to its difficulty and expense.

## ANTIANXIETY DRUGS

For practical purposes, only two types of drugs are used for treating anxiety. One might be called "sedating" and includes principally the benzodiazepines and all of their predecessors; the other might be termed "non-sedating" and is exemplified by buspirone. Other conditions classified as anxiety states, such as panic disorder, social phobia, and obsessive-compulsive disorder, have also been treated with SSRIs.

### Pharmacodynamics

The discovery of the GABA–benzodiazepine–receptor complex has provided a new basis for the understanding of the mode of action of these drugs, as well as others in the sedative-hypnotic group. The complex, a tetramer or pentamer, surrounds a channel for the passage of chloride ions. Binding of GABA opens the chloride channel and allows chloride ions to hyperpolarize the cell, reducing the likelihood of its firing. Benzodiazepines, which bind at a different locus on the complex, merely facilitate the physiologic action of GABA (Tallman et al. 1980). Although other potential mechanisms of action have been described for the benzodiazepines, either as a group or for individual drugs, this mechanism seems to be the most pertinent to their usual therapeutic uses. It is possible that barbiturates and other conventional sedative-hypnotics operate through a similar mechanism.

Buspirone represents a novel drug, both chemically and pharmacologically. Its structure is reminiscent of a butyrophenone, and its first clinical application was as an antipsychotic. It has no overt sedative, hypnotic, or autonomic actions. Its major proposed mechanism of action is by blocking 5-$HT_1$ receptors; it also has weak dopamine $D_2$-receptor blocking action (Taylor 1988). Because of its lack of sedative effects, it has not been abused, and withdrawal reactions are unknown.

The separation of sedation from antianxiety action might represent a pharmacologic "Holy Grail." Paradoxically, many patients, especially if they have previously been treated with benzodiazepines, prefer the latter drugs. The onset of action is quicker than with buspirone and the sedative effects, rather than being a bane, might assist an accompanying sleep disorder. The efficacy of buspirone in treating anxiety has raised the question of the role of the 5-$HT_{1A}$ receptor in its pathogenesis. Other drugs of the same class, such as gepirone and ipsapirone, are being tested as potential antidepressants.

## Pharmacokinetics and Metabolism

Although various benzodiazepines are promoted for differing uses (sedative, hypnotic, antipanic, antidepressant, muscle relaxant, anticonvulsant, anesthetic), much of the selectivity is based on commercial considerations. Although a few pharmacodynamic differences have been reported, especially for alprazolam, clonazepam, and lorazepam, these are neither particularly compelling nor of any demonstrated clinical significance. Pharmacokinetic parameters are summarized in Table 8-8. Pharmacokinetic differences are more pronounced (Greenblatt and Shader 1985). Benzodiazepines can be classified, on the basis of plasma half-life, as very short acting (midazolam), short-acting (alprazolam), intermediate-acting (diazepam), long-acting (prazepam), and very long acting (flurazepam). These differences in plasma half-life do not always accurately define the clinical span of action of these drugs, but can be used as guides.

Differences in metabolism have dubious clinical importance. Drugs that require only glucuronide formation (oxazepam, lorazepam) are said to be safer in patients

**Table 8-8 Pharmacokinetic Parameters and Doses of Commonly Used Antianxiety Drugs**

| Drug | Plasma $T_{1/2}$ (h) | $V_d$ (L/kg) | Protein-binding (%) | Active Metabolite | Plasma $T_{1/2}$ (h) | Therapeutic Concentration (ng/mL) | Dose (mg) |
|---|---|---|---|---|---|---|---|
| *Very Short Acting* | | | | | | | |
| Buspirone (BuSpar) | 2.5–3.0 | | | 1-Pyrimidinylpiperazine (1-PP) | | | 5–40 |
| *Short Acting* | | | | | | | |
| Alprazolam (Xanax) | 6–20 | 0.7–0.8 | | | | | 0.75–4 |
| Lorazepam (Ativan) | 9–22 | 0.7–1.0 | 85 | None | | | 2–6 |
| Oxazepam (Serax) | 6–24 | 0.6–1.6 | 86 | None | | | 30–180 |
| *Intermediate Acting* | | | | | | | |
| Chlordiazepoxide (Librium) | 10–29 | 0.3–0.6 | 93 | Nordiazepam | 10–18 | | 15–100 |
| | | | | Demoxepam | 28–63 | | |
| | | | | Desoxydemoxepam | 39–61 | | |
| Clonazepam (Klonopin) | 19–42 | | | | | | 1–3 |
| Diazepam (Valium) | 14–61 | 0.7–2.6 | 98 | Nordiazepam | 36–200 | 400–1200 | 4–40 |
| Halazepam (Paxipam) | 9–28 | 0.1–1.3 | 98 | Nordiazepam | 36–200 | | 20–160 |
| *Long Acting* | | | | | | | |
| Clorazepate dipotassium (Tranxene) | | 1.0–1.3 | 98 | Nordiazepam | 36–200 | 430 | 15–60 |
| Prazepam (Centrax) | | 1.0–1.3 | 98 | Nordiazepam | 36–200 | 430 | 15–30 |

Abbreviations: $t_{1/2}$, elimination half-life; $V_d$, volume of distribution.

whose drug-metabolizing capacity may be diminished, such as the elderly or those with extensive liver damage. On the other hand, a traditional way of handling these situations is to use a slightly smaller dose and to increase the dosing interval. Many of these drugs have active metabolites, nordiazepam being the major one for diazepam, chlordiazepoxide, clorazepate, prazepam, and halazepam. In fact, the last three drugs are best considered as prodrugs for nordiazepam. When diazepam is given chronically, its active metabolite, nordiazepam, becomes more prevalent than the parent drug. As nordiazepam has a rather long half-life, whereas the half-life of diazepam is relatively briefer, the net result is that diazepam becomes a long-acting drug, even though its half-life is only about 24 hours. This example indicates why determination of half-life alone is not always a good indicator of duration of action. Pharmaceutical preparations may influence the uses of these drugs. Midazolam is water-soluble and is easily administered IV. Combined with its short duration of action, this property allows its exploitation as an IV anesthetic. Some drugs (diazepam, chlordiazepoxide), because of the diluent required, are not highly available when given IM. On the other hand, lorazepam is both well tolerated and highly available when given by that route.

Buspirone has a rather short half-life. Consequently, several divided doses each day are recommended. Whether this dosage schedule is really required has not been tested.

## Therapeutic Indications

The extended concept of anxiety disorders has widened the scope of drugs useful for treating them. For most, antianxiety drugs will be the main treatment.

### *Generalized anxiety disorder*

Formerly, virtually all anxiety was included under this diagnosis. Since the current fad for the diagnosis of panic disorder began, even the existence of generalized anxiety disorder has been questioned; it was not included as a possible diagnosis in the ECA Survey. General physicians will probably recognize this diagnosis more often and will tend to use either benzodiazepines or buspirone to treat it. If a benzodiazepine is to be used, the physician should choose whichever one the patient previously found to be effective. Other than that guideline, there is little reason to choose among those indicated for anxiety.

### *Panic disorder*

*Panic* is the name that has been given to acute anxiety attacks that border on fear. It has existed under a variety of names over the past century, most recently as "neurocirculatory asthenia." The attacks can be quite frightening as well as embarrassing. Consequently, some patients develop a secondary agoraphobia. Imipramine was found in the mid-1960s to be useful in treating this disorder. Later phenelzine, an MAO inhibitor, also was found to be effective. Alprazolam has been extensively studied as a treatment, and it is effective (treatment response about 65 to 70% vs. 30 to 35% for placebo). The doses used have been quite high, sometimes enough to place the patient at risk of dependence. Weaning patients away from this drug is not easy, and relapse of panic attacks is frequent (Fyer et al. 1987). It now appears that an antipanic action is not unique to alprazolam but may be shown with other benzodiazepines, such as lorazepam and clonazepam, given in equivalent doses.

### *Phobia*

Fear of public places is the most common phobia. Previously, agoraphobia was considered to be of psychological origin. Now it is more often considered to be secondary to acute anxiety. The same drugs mentioned for treating panic disorder may be useful, as well as behavioral techniques aimed at desensitizing the fear.

Fear of scrutiny by others is often associated with generalized anxiety disorder, which might be treated as indicated above. Or one may choose to use benzodiazepines in an ad hoc manner for situations that are likely to provoke this phobia. Fear of specific stimuli, such as snakes, dogs, and others, is effectively treated with behavioral techniques.

### *Obsessive-compulsive disorder*

Intrusive thoughts or a compelling urge to repeat meaningless rituals can be highly disabling. Whether this diagnosis belongs under the anxiety rubric may be questioned. It is currently believed to represent some sort of dysfunction of the basal ganglia. Usual antianxiety drugs have been of little help. A tricyclic antidepressant, clomipramine, has demonstrated efficacy (Clomipramine Study Group 1991). Because this drug works primarily through serotonin, it now is believed that this neurotransmitter plays some role (Rapoport 1988). Other selective serotonin-uptake inhibitors, such as fluoxetine and fluvoxamine, have also been helpful.

### *Other indications*

**MUSCLE SPASM** Whether drugs can relieve muscle spasm by a central action other than sedation has always been questioned. The GABA-ergic action of benzodiazepines provides some rationale for their use, as GABA decreases the firing of motor neurons in the spinal cord via presynaptic inhibition.

**ALCOHOL WITHDRAWAL** Benzodiazepines are cross-tolerant with alcohol as well as being effective anticonvulsants. They have now replaced older sedatives for alleviating alcohol withdrawal. Although other types of drugs, such as clonidine or carbamazepine have some benefit, benzodiazepines remain generally preferred.

**UNCONTROLLED SEIZURES** Intravenously administered benzodiazepines afford prompt relief with less respiratory depression than other sedatives. Because of their brief duration of effect, they are usually followed with loading doses of phenytoin. Diazepam used to be the preferred drug for this indication, but lorazepam and midazolam are better tolerated when given by vein.

**INTRAVENOUS ANESTHETIC** A short-acting IV anesthetic is useful for induction of general anesthesia, and for endoscopies, reduction of minor fractures, electric cardioversion, or dental surgery. Lorazepam and midazolam are now the preferred agents.

**CONTROL OF AGITATION IN PSYCHOTIC PATIENTS** The combination of a sedative-hypnotic drug with an antipsychotic has long been used for this purpose. Either IM lorazepam or sodium phenobarbital may be used (Garza-Trevino et al. 1989).

## Principles of Use

Use of benzodiazepines has declined in recent years. Part of the decline has been the removal of these drugs from some publicly funded formularies. Such mandated restrictions have had the unintended effect of increasing the use of antipsychotics and tricyclics, which are far less effective and safe. Buspirone has not been as widely accepted as was hoped; if patients are willing to give the drug a fair trial, some may find it to be effective. General principles of use of antianxiety drugs are as follows.

- Use only when symptoms are disabling or discomforting.
- Consider nonpharmacologic treatments.
- Try intermittent treatment courses.
- Adjust doses on the basis of clinical response and side effects.
- Monitor treatment closely; failure to respond may signify a misdiagnosis.
- Avoid taking the drugs before undertaking potentially dangerous activities.
- Do not discontinue their use suddenly.
- Use with care or not at all in patients with addictive problems.

After almost 30 years of extensive use, benzodiazepines have proved to be remarkably safe. Toxicity involving any of the major organ systems is rare. Virtually all problems have been related to the action on the CNS.

Buspirone seems to have relatively few side effects. Some patients have experienced anxiety, restlessness, insomnia, and manic-like symptoms. Digestive complaints are also more common with this drug.

## Adverse Effects

Most patients recognize when they are oversedated and spontaneously reduce the dose. Tolerance develops to this effect over time, so that the same dose that produced overt sedation initially may not after chronic use.

Both physical and psychic dependence may occur with chronic use of benzodiazepines. Dependence, tolerance, and withdrawal from sedatives is discussed in chapter 17, Substance Abuse: Dependence and Treatment.

## Other Effects

Probably all benzodiazepines have some degree of amnesic effect. Amnesia could be an advantage when they are used as anesthetic agents. Triazolam has been most troublesome in this respect, although such instances are rare. Alprazolam has provoked mania, which has been adduced as evidence for an antidepressant effect. As the drug is widely used in depressed patients, it seems more likely that patients with manic-depressive disorder may have been erroneously treated with this drug. Hip fractures, especially in the elderly, are increased in patients taking sedatives of any type. Dysmorphogenesis remains an unresolved issue. One would have thought that if it were a major risk, it would have become evident by now.

Overdoses of benzodiazepines are remarkably safe. Supportive treatment usually suffices. Respiratory support is rarely needed unless other depressants, such as alcohol, have been ingested. If clinically desired, all the sedative effects can be reversed by a specific benzodiazepine antagonist, flumazenil. Buspirone is also quite safe.

# HYPNOTICS

For almost 30 years benzodiazepines have been the hypnotics of choice. During the past few years, nonbenzodiazepine hypnotics have also entered the field. Zolpidem is an imidazopyridine, chemically different from the benzodiazepines, but it works through one of the benzodiazepine receptors. Only three benzodiazepines have been marketed specifically as hypnotics, but because all benzodiazepines share many common properties, virtually any may be used as such.

## Pharmacodynamics

Presumably the same mechanism of action accounts for the hypnotic effects as it does for the antianxiety effect. The GABA-benzodiazepine receptor complex is a pentamer composed of three different subunits, thus affording the possibility for multiple receptors. However, one subunit in particular seems to be required for the sedative-hypnotic actions. It has been speculated that drugs acting specifically on certain receptors may separate antianxiety from hypnotic effects, mitigate withdrawal reactions, and isolate other possible therapeutic actions, such as muscle relaxation. The GABA-benzodiazepine complex is not the only mechanism by which sleep may be induced. Blockade of histamine $H_1$ receptors is known to produce sleepiness, which explains the use of antihistamines as OTC hypnotics. Blockade of $\alpha_1$-adrenoreceptors also helps sleep. Sleepiness is also induced by melatonin, the secretion of which is induced by darkness. It would be surprising if such an important function as sleep did not have redundant mechanisms for its induction.

## Pharmacokinetics

Paradoxically, the three benzodiazepines marketed as hypnotics virtually span the range of plasma half-lives (Table 8-9). Triazolam is short-acting, with a plasma half-life measured in a few hours, while flurazepam, via its active metabolite desalkylflurazepam, has a half-life measured in days. Temazepam has a half-life that is intermediate. Following single doses of each drug, differences are not especially apparent. Triazolam has been said to produce rebound insomnia or anxiety even within a single night, but this contention is controversial (Mendelson and Jain 1995). On the other hand, the long half-life of flurazepam opens the possibility of cumulative oversedation if doses are too high and the drug is taken chronically. Once again, the clinical importance of pharmacokinetic differences seems not to be of major consequence. Zolpidem has a short half-life in the order of that of triazolam. It is said not to cause rebound insomnia or to have abuse liability. However, abuse of hypnotics is rare in any case.

## Therapeutic Indications

Treatment of sleep disorders should logically follow a diagnosis (Consensus Development Conference 1984b). Unfortunately, the majority of cases of insomnia do not fit usual diagnoses. The major consideration is not to miss an underlying psychiatric disorder, physical cause, or insomnia due to drugs. Most cases of insomnia must be considered to be "primary," that is, of unknown cause. It is possible that persistent insomnia may herald the later appearance of depression. If so, early recognition and treatment might conceivably prevent future psychiatric disorders (Ford and Kamerow 1989).

Transient sleep disturbances are ideal for drug treatment. These include sleeping in strange quarters, or moving through several time zones, or sleeping at a different time of day because of altered work schedules. Accommodation occurs quickly, and drugs may be needed for only a few days. A bigger problem is recurrent insomnia with no obvious cause. In this case, the possibility exists that drugs may be overused. Nonetheless, the greatest use of hypnotics is probably in patients with so-called primary insomnia.

Sleep apnea consists of irregular breathing with alternating periods of apnea followed by hyperventilation. Clinically, it may be suspected by the report of a bed partner of episodes of loud snoring, or by the patient's complaints of daytime sleepiness requiring frequent naps, morning headache, and a finding of hypertension. Polysomnography is definitive for making the diagnosis (American Sleep Disorders Association 1995). The importance of making this diagnosis is that any drug that depresses respiratory drive will accentuate the problems. Care should also be taken when using these drugs in alcoholics in whom the combination of high plasma con-

**Table 8-9 Pharmacokinetic Parameters of Hypnotic Drugs**

| Drug | $C_{max}$ (h) | Protein-binding (%) | Metabolite | Active plasma $T_{1/2}$ (h) |
|---|---|---|---|---|
| Flurazepam HCl | 1–3 | 96 | Desalkyl | 40–114 |
| Temazepam | 2–3 | 96 | None | 9.5–12.4 |
| Triazolam | 0.7–2 | 80 | None | 1.3–3.9 |
| Zolpidem tartrate | 1.6 | 92 | None | 1.4–4.5 |

Abbreviations: $C_{max}$, maximum plasma concentration of drug; $t_{1/2}$, elimination half-life.

centrations of alcohol and high doses of hypnotics may result in unintentional suicide.

## Principles of Use

### *Choice of drug*

Assuming that benzodiazepines will be used, how should one choose among them? The best criterion for making a choice is the preference of the patient. Triazolam is the current favorite, possibly because its short plasma half-life may minimize daytime hangover. Flurazepam has been used the longest; its long half-life might provide an advantage when some degree of daytime sedation is required for attendant anxiety. Temazepam has a half-life similar to that of lorazepam. Diazepam, when given in single doses, is a relatively short-acting drug, as its action is terminated largely by redistribution. Thus, almost any benzodiazepine used for treating anxiety might be equally suitable for treating insomnia. Clinical trials have shown that usually recommended equipotent doses of zolpidem and triazolam do not differ in any major way. As zolpidem is considerably more expensive than the generic benzodiazepines, its use will be limited to patients with expensive tastes (Lobo and Greene 1997).

### *Dosing guideline*

The proper dose is one that facilitates, rather than enforces, sleep. Therefore, one should start out with a small dose and increase it only as needed. For drugs that come as capsules, such as flurazepam and temazepam, one is limited to the dose contained in each capsule. A scored tablet, like triazolam, permits one to reduce the dose unit by cracking the tablet. For many persons, a dose of 0.125 mg of triazolam (one-half of a 0.25-mg tablet) is sufficient. Maximum doses have been proposed for hypnotics: 0.5 mg for triazolam and 60 mg for either temazepam or flurazepam.

### *Frequency of use*

Most preferred uses of hypnotics are patterns of short duration, affording relief from temporary disturbances of sleep. Unfortunately, most cases of primary insomnia tend to be chronic. Patients will tend to ignore instructions to use these drugs only intermittently and, being apprehensive of the deleterious effects of fretful sleep on daytime functioning, take these drugs routinely. Despite a high frequency of such chronic use, it is surprising that virtually no adverse effects have been described. One might wish to recommend to such patients that they try to avoid taking hypnotics on weekends, even suffering a night or two of poor sleep while avoiding daytime naps, so that a minor degree of sleep deprivation may allow resumption of a more normal pattern.

The concept of sleep deprivation as the driving force for sleep explains several phenomena. First, even if hypnotics were not available, people with insomnia would eventually sleep. Second, oversleeping, by reducing the degree of deprivation, may be followed by insomnia. These constructs are important in educating insomniac patients about the physiology of sleep.

## Adverse Effects

Although a few instances of dependence on benzodiazepines have been attributed to their use as hypnotics, closer inspection reveals that almost all involved gross misuse of the drugs. Small doses and infrequent administration (even when a single dose is taken each night) protect against dependence. Psychic dependence may be found among patients who feel that they simply must take a hypnotic every night.

Rebound anxiety and insomnia have been reported from use of short-acting hypnotics, mainly triazolam. However, others deny their existence. One could make a case that any insomnia the night following use of a hypnotic may simply reflect some degree of "oversleeping," with a subsequent reduced drive for sleep.

Too large a dose of hypnotic might result in daytime lethargy simply due to hangover effects. Accumulation of long-acting drugs, such as flurazepam, might result in mild intoxication.

One of the great advantages of benzodiazepines has been less respiratory depression than from older hypnotics. Depression of respiration is a common precipitant of respiratory failure in patients with chronic obstructive pulmonary disease. Nonetheless, small doses of triazolam were well tolerated, so long as patients did not have hypoxemia or carbon dioxide retention during the waking state (Timms et al. 1988).

Despite the failed memory of patients up to 36 hours following the dose, anterograde amnesia rarely follows use of triazolam. Whether amnesia is made more likely by a large dose or concomitant alcohol indigestion, is uncertain.

Because insomnia may be a symptom of more severe psychiatric illness, mainly depression, patients may attempt suicide with their hypnotics. Benzodiazepines are much safer than barbiturates and other drugs; it is virtually impossible to commit suicide with their use alone.

## Nondrug Treatments

A meta-analysis of non-pharmacologic approaches to treating insomnia found that controlling external stimuli that might disturb sleep and sleep restriction were the most effective single therapy measures. Treated patients were substantially more improved than those not treated, with lasting benefit (Morin et al. 1994). The effects of a warm bath, massage, or relief of sexual tension for promoting sleep are well known. Bedtime rituals may provide a conditioning aspect for promoting sleep. Exercise during the day, enough to produce a moderate degree of fatigue, is helpful. Preferably, it should not occur too close to the time of retiring. A patient who customarily awakes too early in the morning might well be advised to delay his or her bedtime. It must always be remembered that the primary drive for sleep comes from being sleep deprived. Someone who has overslept the night before may find it difficult to court sleep the following night.

**PRINCIPLE Effects of drugs can often lead to extensions of their indications: hypnotics to insomnia; antibiotics to other infections; antiarrhythmics to arrhythmias, etc.**

## DRUGS FOR TREATING MENTAL DISORDERS OF OLD AGE

### Alzheimer's Disease

The problems in evaluating drug therapy in Alzheimer's disease are considerable, for one is often dealing with a complex interplay of psychosocial, neurologic, and general physical disorders. Some of these factors may fluctuate, while others are progressive. The contribution of each of these multiple factors to the total degree of disability is difficult to gauge. Many studies to evaluate drug therapy are performed in patients with such advanced dementia that it would be very difficult to show much positive benefit. In any case, gains are likely to be small and may take time to become apparent.

#### *Drug treatment*

Vasodilating agents were used for many years for treating Alzheimer's disease because the pathogenesis was assumed to be inadequate brain perfusion. This pharmacologic approach was exemplified by ergoloid mesylates (Hydergine) that, for a while, was the only approved treatment although its presumed benefit was unclear. During the 1970s and 1980s, attention was focused on the role of acetylcholine. Then, Alzheimer's disease was considered to be caused by a central cholinergic deficiency analogous to the dopamine deficiency hypothesis of Parkinson's disease. Attempts were made to increase cholinergic activity by use of precursors of acetylcholine (e.g., lecithin, choline), by receptor agonists (e.g., muscarine) and by cholinesterase inhibitors (e.g., physostigmine, tetrahydroaminacrin, and donepezil). During the past 5 years, the inflammatory aspects of the disease have aroused much interest, leading to trials with nonsteroidal anti-inflammatory agents and vitamin E (to alleviate oxidative stress). In addition, other drugs have been proposed based on other hypotheses or on empirical evidence (American Psychiatric Association Guidelines 1997).

**ERGOLOID MESYLATES (HYDERGINE)** Evidence to support use of this combination has been scanty, and their use remains controversial after 40 years. The strongest evidence of efficacy is in treating vascular dementia. With the recent appreciation (long known to neuropathologists) that Alzheimer's disease and vascular dementia often coexist, there now seems to be more rationale for ergoloids. In all likelihood, previous recommended doses were too small; doses should be at least 6 mg/day or higher (Schneider and Olin 1994).

**TACRINE** This cholinesterase inhibitor (tetrahydro-9-acridinamine monohydrochloride monohydrate) was suggested for use after a few clinical trials had shown modest efficacy for physostigmine. While relatively new to the United States, this drug had been widely used in Australia since the 1960s, chiefly by anesthesiologists as a waking agent. Following the introduction of tacrine as the first drug specifically approved by the U.S. Food and Drug Administration (FDA) for Alzheimer's disease, a similar compound, velnacrine, also was studied. Two studies of tacrine led to somewhat divergent views. A controlled comparison of tacrine with placebo in 486 patients using maximum doses of 60 mg/day found that the magnitude of the treatment effect was clinically important, and that the effects were recognizable by the physician (Farlow et al. 1992). However, about 25% of patients developed asymptomatic reversible elevations of liver enzymes.

A separate study found that 215 of 632 eligible patients showed some response to tacrine during preliminary exposure. These 215 patients were then randomly assigned to treatment with tacrine (doses to 80 mg/day) or placebo. After 6 weeks of treatment, tacrine reduced the decline in cognitive function to a statistically significant degree. However, this reduction was not large enough to be detected by the study physicians' global assessments of the patients (Davis et al. 1992). Neither study reported on the number of dropouts, which have been fairly high in clinical practice. Despite the poor odds of success, tacrine is widely used.

**PRINCIPLE When an important disease has little or no positive interventions, even sophisticated physicians grasp at straws. These are situations where thinking of doing no harm becomes quite important.**

DONEPEZIL This cholinesterase inhibitor has also been found to slow the rate of decline of patients with Alzheimer's disease as compared with placebo. A company-sponsored controlled trial in 160 patients with mild-to-moderate Alzheimer's disease compared daily doses of 1, 3, or 5 mg/day versus placebo. Modest improvements were noted (Rogers et al. 1996). The drug has been marketed for a short time and clinical experience is still limited. Like tacrine, donepezil is expensive, costing about $4–5/day.

OTHER DRUGS Preliminary studies suggest possible beneficial effects of vitamin E and the MAO-B enzyme inhibitor, selegiline. The roles of aspirin, NSAIDs, warfarin, and estrogens are still under investigation. An herbal remedy, extract of *Gingko biloba* (EGb) has been approved in Germany for treatment of dementia. A controlled trial by a North American group found that doses of 120 mg/day of the extract were effective in stabilizing cognitive performance in 202 of the 309 patients who completed a 1-year trial. The results, though modest, were appreciated by caregivers as well as shown on rating scales. It is believed that this extract acts as a free radical scavenger (Le Bars et al. 1997). It will be interesting to follow its progress.

SYMPTOMATIC TREATMENTS The use of these drugs is simply to control behavioral symptoms. Small doses of traditional antipsychotics have been helpful in improving self-care and, in combination with benzodiazepines, in restoring a normal sleep cycle. Whether the atypical antipsychotics offer any advantages remains to be seen. Depression may coexist with Alzheimer's disease, but choice of the best antidepressant is obscure.

## Multi-infarct Dementia

The availability of sensitive imaging techniques should make this diagnosis easier to establish. Cognitive performance correlates with impairments of cerebral blood flow (Judd et al. 1986).

Arteriosclerotic changes rarely exist alone (only about 10% of senile dementias) but may accompany Alzheimer's disease (25% or more). Thus, it should be possible to identify patients with this disorder when it occurs alone or complicates other disorders.

### *Drug treatment*

The brain damaged by a lacunar infarct cannot be restored, but it may be possible to prevent future damage. Control of hypertension, therapy of carotid artery disease, and antiembolic therapy may be important interventions.

## Depression

Depression is more common in elderly persons for a variety of reasons. So-called pervasive depression was found in 13% of a sample of elderly persons in London, and 10% in a simultaneously examined New York group (Garland et al. 1985). Suicide is also more common in the elderly, although it does not rank high among causes of death. Depression may also present in a somewhat atypical fashion in older persons. Social withdrawal, mental confusion, delusions of persecution, hostile behavior, and severe hypochondriasis add to the diagnostic problem. Whether the diagnostic difficulty results in many patients not being recognized and treated with serious consequences is uncertain.

### *Drug treatment*

Although antidepressants have been shown to be effective in elderly patients, the choice among drugs is more critical than for younger persons (Thompson et al. 1983). Tricyclics with anticholinergic effects may increase mental confusion; desipramine is perhaps the safest drug of this class to use to avoid this adverse effect. The MAO inhibitors are more likely to produce orthostatic hypotension and falls when used in the elderly. Some of the newer antidepressants, such as bupropion or fluoxetine, may prove to be more acceptable.

## Other Disorders

Late-onset schizophrenic-like psychosis (paraphrenia) is a difficult and uncertain diagnosis. As one can deduce, psychotic symptoms can be present during depression, as well as in patients with Alzheimer's disease. If psychotic symptoms occur in the context of mood changes, the patient may best be treated with a combination of antipsychotic and antidepressant. In the absence of mood changes, the antipsychotic should be tried first. Doses of antipsychotics should be small, at least initially. Severe hypochondriasis may be thought to be a manifestation of psychosis. The patient becomes almost pathologically fixated on some complaint or set of complaints. One should be sure that the complaints do not signify the somatic complaints so often found in depression in order not to miss the chance to treat a reversible disorder. Even if the patient is not depressed, low doses of a sedative antidepressant, such as trazodone, might be helpful. Benzodiazepines may also be useful in patients who are anxious or have insomnia.

## DRUGS FOR DISORDERS IN CHILDREN AND ADOLESCENTS

The diagnosis of psychiatric disorders in children and adolescents is much more difficult than in adults. The onset is more subtle, the manifestations more variable, and the course more unpredictable. Furthermore, it is much easier to identify problems in the life of the child, either with peers or with family, that suggest a psychological approach to treatment.

For these reasons, formal studies of the effects of drugs on various disorders of children and adolescents, with a few exceptions, are neither abundant nor terribly convincing. The reluctance to use drugs, coupled with the uncertainty about diagnosis, create a situation in which children in fact become "therapeutic orphans." The usual dictum on the drug label that "experience with children under the age of 12 years is limited" continues to be true. In recent years, interest in using drug treatments in children has increased, but even now, < 20% of psychotherapeutic drugs have been specifically tested for safety and efficacy in children. Three recently published reviews have summarized data regarding the use of psychotherapeutic drugs in children and adolescents (Mirza et al. 1994; Kaplan and Hussain 1995; Carrey et al. 1996).

It is helpful to consider treatment of psychiatric disorders in terms of those that children and adolescents share with adults and those that are more specific to the youngsters.

### Disorders Shared by Children or Adolescents and Adults

#### *Anxiety disorders*

Specific anxiety disorders for children and adolescents have been denoted in the current diagnostic system. These include: 1) separation anxiety, 2) avoidance disorder, and 3) overanxious disorder. The validity of these syndromes, as well as the use of antianxiety drugs for testing them, remains largely unexplored. The prevalence of other anxiety disorders such as panic states, phobias, and obsessive-compulsive disorders is not known, but each occur in children. Obsessive-compulsive disorder has attracted recent attention; the manifestations are too bizarre and too typical to be attributed to something in the child's environment.

A beneficial effect of benzodiazepines on anxiety has been difficult to show clearly in this group. Nonetheless, clinicians often find these drugs "useful." Although an early report suggested that a form of separation anxiety, social phobia, responded to imipramine, a later study by the same group failed to replicate these findings (Klein et al. 1992).

Obsessive-compulsive disorder responded better to clomipramine than placebo in a large multicenter trial (DeVaugh-Geiss et al. 1992). A controlled trial of fluoxetine also showed a similar superiority (Riddle et al. 1992). Whether these findings can be extended to other SSRIs is not known. A follow-up study of the 54 patients 2–4 years after an initial response to the clomipramine revealed that the effects were generally sustained (Leonard et al. 1993).

#### *Sleep disorders*

Insomnia is not a common complaint and is usually of less significance in young persons than in adults faced with daily responsibilities. A thorough investigation should be made to rule out psychiatric disorders. Sedating antihistamines, such as hydroxyzine, were promoted for this use in the past; once again it is difficult to understand why a more dangerous drug should be preferred to benzodiazepines.

**PRINCIPLE Old drugs may be slow to die, even when evidence strongly suggests that they should, because of continued prescribing based on habit or routine.**

Sleepwalking and sleep terror are parasomnias that occur in younger age groups. As they characteristically occur during deep slow-wave sleep, benzodiazepines, which reduce or eliminate this type of sleep, are most useful.

Enuresis has a long history of responding to tricyclic antidepressants. Usually single doses of 25–50 mg of imipramine given at bedtime suffice. The mechanism for efficacy is unclear, but clinical proof of efficacy has been substantial. Benefits last only as long as the drug is given; some patients may lose benefits during prolonged treatment. Thus, other non-pharmacologic measures to deal with the problem should also be used.

#### *Depression*

Depressed children and adolescents are much less easily diagnosed than depressed adults, but depression does occur. Suicide is a major cause of death among adolescents.

Drug treatment is seldom considered to be a primary treatment for depression. First efforts are usually made to identify sources of stress in interpersonal relationships or frustrations in achieving goals. A few studies of treatment of depression with tricyclic antidepressants have produced results not nearly as convincing as in adults. Possibly the small sample sizes and high rate of spontaneous remission may have created negative bias.

A comparison of fluoxetine with placebo showed the former drug to be superior on most clinical measures but not significantly so. Once again, despite the lack of evidence from controlled trials, clinicians have found antidepressants to be helpful in some cases. Virtually no experience exists in regard to use of MAO inhibitors.

#### *Manic-depressive (bipolar) disorder*

This disorder may start at any epoch of life, from before the age of 10 years to after the age of 80 years. When it appears in children, it is most commonly misdiagnosed as ADHD. Treatment with stimulants, ordinarily useful in the latter condition, makes manic-depressive disorder worse, suggesting the proper diagnosis.

Lithium carbonate has been as effective in the younger patients as it has been in adults. Thirty of 46 patients, aged 3–19 years, responded to such treatment (Youngerman and Canino 1978). Serum lithium concentrations should be monitored exactly the same way as for adults. Uncontrolled studies have suggested some utility of carbamazepine and valproate as well.

#### *Schizophrenia*

Little doubt exists about the occurrence of schizophrenia in children and adolescents. The peak age of onset is late adolescence. Characteristically, schizophrenia develops insidiously, and the first symptoms may not suggest a psychosis. Only when symptoms become fairly obvious is drug treatment started. The favored drugs of the past were low potency antipsychotics such as chlorpromazine or thioridazine. However, little experience is available for atypical antipsychotics.

A summary of the use of drug treatments for children and adolescents is shown in Table 8-10.

## Disorders Peculiar to Children and Adolescents

#### *Attention deficit/hyperactivity disorder (ADHD)*

ADHD is a well-established psychiatric diagnosis, although making the diagnosis may be difficult, as many conditions may mimic it. When it is successfully treated, no one is happier than the family with such a child. Most often the disorder is discovered in school-age children who are restless and inattentive in class. Although no symptoms of the disorder are unique to it, a constellation of symptoms often ensures the diagnosis. In extreme cases, the child resembles a "whirling dervish," constantly moving about and poking into things.

The efficacy of treatment with stimulant drugs, such as dextroamphetamine, has been known for more than 50 years. Such drugs are still the mainstay of treatment. The use of stimulants in children who already appear to be overstimulated seems paradoxical. However, hyperactivity is probably a manifestation of poor attention; stimulants are believed to focus attention. The actions of amphetamines are complex, involving not only increased release of catecholaminergic neurotransmitters, but also inhibition of their uptake, as well as a mild degree of inhibition of MAO activity. The net effect is to increase dopaminergic, and to a lesser extent noradrenergic, receptor stimulation. Methylphenidate, now the preferred stimulant, seems to act in a similar fashion but has been far less well studied. Pemoline, another such drug, seems to work solely through dopamine.

Recently a mixture of salts of the two isomers of amphetamines have been marketed, in doses of 2.5–10 mg/day. The plasma half-life is longer than dextroamphetamine but duration of action is not a problem with stimulants, other than it being too long. Most drugs are given early in the day when they are less likely to interfere with sleep.

Doses of dextroamphetamine and methylphenidate vary from 2.5–40 mg/day for the former drug, or 5–80 mg/day for the latter. Dextroamphetamine is rapidly absorbed, with peak plasma concentrations at 3–4 hours; its plasma half-life is about 6–7 hours. Methylphenidate is more rapidly absorbed, with peak concentrations being attained at 1 hour; its plasma half-life is about 2–4 hours. Thus, both these drugs are commonly given in divided daily doses with dosing limited to the early hours of the day. Magnesium pemoline has an appreciably longer elimination half-life, so that single doses (37.5–112.5 mg) can be given in the morning.

The expected side effects of sympathomimetic stimulants are encountered. Insomnia indicates a need for change in the dose or dosing schedule. Weight loss and growth retardation may occur during treatment. Both adverse effects are reversed when the drug is discontinued, as it usually is during the summer vacation months. Most children attain their predicted stature despite treatment (Klein et al. 1988). The concern that exposure to stimulant drugs early in life might predispose to later abuse of these drugs has been ill-founded.

ADHD may persist into adult life. Treatment with stimulants remains the choice for such cases, although results may be less favorable than for children.

**Table 8-10 Summary of the Use of Psychotherapeutic Drugs in Children or Adolescents**

| | | |
|---|---|---|
| *Anxiolytics or Hypnotics* | | |
| Indications: | anxiety, isomnia, night terror, sleepwalking | |
| Doses: | unexplored | |
| *Antidepressants* | | |
| Indications: | depression, phobias, separation anxiety, enuresis, anorexia-bulimia, autism, obsessive-compulsive disorder, Tourette's syndrome | |
| Doses: | imipramine HCl | 2.5 mg/kg/day |
| | clomipramine HCl | 75–100 mg/day |
| | fluoxetine maleate | 10–20 mg/day |
| *Mood Stabilizers* | | |
| Indications: | manic-depressive, aggressive behavior, conduct disorder | |
| Doses: | lithium carbonate to concentration of 0.6–1.2 mEq/L | |
| *Antipsychotics* | | |
| Indications: | schizophrenia, mania, mental retardation, autism, Tourette's syndrome, conduct disorder | |
| Doses: | thioridazine HCl | 1.5–3.0 mg/kg/day |
| | haloperidol | 0.1–0.5 mg/kg/day |
| | pimozide | 0.05–0.2 mg/kg/day (Tourette's) |
| *Stimulants* | | |
| Indications: | ADHD, narcolepsy | |
| Doses: | dextroamphetamine sulfate | 2.5–40 mg/day |
| | methylphenidate | 5–80 mg/day |
| | pemoline | 37.5–112.5 mg/day |

Abbreviations: ADHD, attention-deficit hyperactivity disorder.

### *Autism*

This disorder, which used to be considered a form of childhood schizophrenia, is now considered to be a separate entity. It may or may not occur with concomitant mental retardation. The outcome is variable, so that some children may ultimately lead rather normal lives while others are handicapped for life. The major symptoms are a lack of awareness or feeling for others, difficulties in communication, and stereotyped behaviors, with an onset in infancy or childhood.

Antipsychotic drugs have been used with only modest success in curbing some of the worst of the behaviors; sometimes they have possibly enhanced ability to learn. The finding of an elevated level of platelet serotonin in such children became the basis for trying the serotonin-depleting drug fenfluramine. Results have been variable, but a controlled trial using doses of 1.5–20 mg/day showed no benefit from the drug compared with placebo (Campbell 1988).

To test the serotonin hypothesis further, clomipramine (a partial serotonin uptake inhibitor) was compared with desipramine (a norepinephrine uptake inhibitor) and placebo in a cross-over, double-blind study. Clomipramine was superior to both other treatments on ratings for stereotypies, ritualized behaviors, and anger; no differences were found between desipramine and placebo. Both tricyclics were superior to placebo for amelioration of hyperactivity (Gordon et al. 1993). As drug treatment seems to offer little, the major therapeutic approaches have been behavioral modification techniques and efforts at education.

### *Tourette's syndrome*

This tic syndrome usually starts in adolescence, being characterized by barking sounds and motor tics. It has a familial predisposition with an apparent relationship to obsessive-compulsive disorder. Symptoms may wane spontaneously as the patient approaches the fourth decade of life. Although antipsychotics that block dopamine $D_2$ receptors, such as pimozide and haloperidol, have been used for many years, recent genetic studies suggest that tic disorders are part of a continuum with obsessive-compulsive disorders, both being ascribed to a deficiency of serotonin in basal ganglia. Accordingly, current approaches to treatment tend to focus on SSRIs, which may be combined with antipsychotics as needed. Such combinations may be particularly pertinent when Tourette's syndrome coexists with obsessive-compulsive disorder.

### *Anorexia-bulimia*

Eating disorders are epidemic, or so it would seem. These disorders, which primarily affect adolescent girls, have been effectively managed with both tricyclic antidepressants and MAO inhibitors, even in the absence of clinical depression. Doses of 60–90 mg/day of phenelzine have been used (Walsh et al. 1984).

More recently, other antidepressants have also been used. Tricyclics, such as desipramine, have shown some promise (McCann and Agras 1990). However, current favorites are various SSRIs. Psychological treatments are also worth considering, although the recent emphasis on childhood sexual abuse may be misplaced.

### *Narcolepsy*

Paroxysmal attacks of sleep or catalepsy are also more frequent in recent years. Stimulants, such as dextroamphetamine, have been used to prevent sleep attacks. Imipramine mitigates the cataleptic seizures. Newer stimulants, such as modanafil, may also be useful (Nishino and Mignot 1997). Guidelines for the use of stimulants in narcolepsy have been published (American Sleep Disorders Association 1994).

### *Conduct disorders*

This "wastepaper diagnosis" of boys is manifested mainly by highly aggressive and explosive behavior. Doses of haloperidol from 1–6 mg/day or lithium from 500–2000 mg/day were better than placebo (Campbell et al. 1984).

Since conduct disorders frequently co-exists with other disorders such as ADHD, mood disorders, substance abuse, and oppositional defiant disorder, attempts to treat these conditions might be well placed. Otherwise, treatment is symptomatic and empirical.

**Glossary of Drugs (Generic and Trade Names) Mentioned in Chapter 8**

| Drug | Cost |
|---|---|
| *Antipsychotic* | |
| Chlorpromazine[a] (Thorazine) | $ |
| Clozapine[a] (Clozaril) | $$$ |
| Fluphenazine (Prolixin) | $$ |
| Haloperidol[a] (Haldol) | $$ |
| Loxapine (Loxitane) | $$$$ |
| Molindone (Moban) | $$$$ |
| Olanzapine (Zyprexa) | $$$$ |
| Perphenazine[a] (Trilafon) | $$ |
| Quetiapine (Seroquel) | $$$$ |
| Risperidone (Risperdal) | $$$$ |
| Sertindole (removed from market) | |
| Thioridazine[a] (Mellaril) | $ |
| Thiothixene[a] (Navane) | $$ |
| *Antidepressants* | |
| Amitriptyline[a] (Elavil) | $ |
| Amoxapine[a] (Asendin) | $$ |
| Bupropion (Wellbutrin) | $$ |
| Citalopram (not yet marketed) | |
| Clomipramine[a] | $$ |
| Desipramine[a] (Norpramin) | $$ |
| Fluoxetine (Prozac) | $$$$ |
| Fluvoxamine (Luvox) | $$$$ |
| Imipramine[a] (Tofranil) | $ |
| Iproniazid (no longer marketed) | |
| Maprotiline (Ludiomil) | $$$ |
| Mirtazapine (Pemeron) | $$$$ |
| Moclobemide | |
| Nefazodone (Serzone) | $$$ |
| Nortriptyline[a] (Pamelor) | $$ |
| Sertraline (Zoloft) | $$$$ |
| Phenelzine (Nardil) | |
| Trazodone[a] (Desyrel) | $ |
| Paroxetine (Paxil) | $$$$ |
| Venlafaxine (Effexor) | $$$$ |
| *Antianxiety Drugs* | |
| Alprazolam[a] (Xanax) | $$ |
| Buspirone (Buspar) | $$$$ |
| Chlordiazepoxide[a] (Librium) | $ |
| Clonazepam[a] (Klonopin) | $$$ |
| Clorazepate[a] (Tranxene) | $$ |
| Diazepam[a] (Valium) | $ |
| Lorazepam[a] (Ativan) | $ |
| Oxazepam (Serax) | $$ |
| *Hypnotics* | |
| Flurazepam[a] (Dalmane) | $ |
| Temazepam[a] (Restoril) | $ |
| Triazolam[a] (Halcion) | $$$ |
| Zolpidem (Ambien) | $$$$ |
| *Mood Stabilizers* | |
| Carbamazepine[a] (Tegretol) | $ |
| Divalproex sodium (Depakote) | $$$ |
| Lithium (Eskalith) | $ |
| Valproic acid[a] (Depakene) | $ |
| *Disorders of Old Age* | |
| Donepezil (Aricept) | $$$$ |
| Ergoloid mesylates (Hydergine) | $$ |
| Tacrine (Cognex) | $$$$ |
| *Disorders of children* | |
| Dextroamphetamine[a] (Dexedrine) | $$ |
| Pemoline (Cylert) | $$$ |
| Methylphenidate[a] (Ritalin) | $$ |
| Pimozide (Orap) | $$$$ |

[a]Generic equivalents available.

## REFERENCES

Addonizio G, Susman VL, Roth SD. 1987. Neuroleptic malignant syndrome: review and analysis of 115 cases. *Biol Psychiatry* **22**: 1004–20.

Amdisen A. 1987. The history of lithium. *Biol Psychiatry* **22**:522–3.

American Psychiatric Association. 1993. Practice guidelines for major depressive disorder in adults. *Am J Psychiatry* **150** (Suppl):1–26.

American Psychiatric Association. 1997. Practice guidelines for the treatment of patients with Alzheimer's disease and other dementias of late life. *Am J Psychiatry* **154** (Suppl):18–27.

American Sleep Disorders Association. 1994. Practice parameters for the use of stimulants in the treatment of narcolepsy. *Sleep* **4**:348–51.

American Sleep Disorders Association. 1995. Practice parameters for the use of polysomnography in the evaluation of insomnia. *Sleep* **8**:55–7.

Ananth J, Lin KM. 1996. Propranolol in psychiatry: therapeutic uses and side effects. *Neuropsychobiology* **15**:20–7.

Ansseau M, Gabriels A, Loyens J, et al. 1994. Controlled comparison of paraoxetine and fluvoxamine in major depression. *Hum Psychopharmacol* **9**:329–36.

Armitage R, Yonkers K, Cole D, et al. 1997. A multicenter, double-blind comparison of the effects of nefazodone and fluoxetine on sleep architecture and quality of sleep in depressed outpatients. *Clin Psychopharmacol* **17**:161–8.

Arnold SE, Kumar A. 1993. Possible reversible dementias. *Med Clin North Am* **77**:215–30.

Artigas F, Romero L, de Montigny C, et al. 1996. Acceleration of the effect of selected antidepressant drugs in major depression by $5HT_{1A}$ antagonists. *Trends Neurosci* **19**:378–83.

Ascher JA, Cole JO, Noel-Colin J, et al. 1995. Buproprion: a review of its mechanism of antidepressant activity. *J Clin Psychiatry* **56**: 395–401.

Baron M, Risch N, Hamburger R, et al. 1987. Genetic linkage between X-chromosome markers and bipolar affective illness. *Nature* **326**:289–92.

Battle DC, von Riotte AB, Gaviniril M, et al. 1985. Amelioration of polyuria by amiloride in patients receiving long-term lithium therapy. *N Engl J Med* **312**:408–14.

Baumann P. 1992. Clinical pharmacokinetics of citalopram and other selective serotonin reuptake inhibitors (SSRI). *Int Clin Psychopharmacol* **6** (Suppl 5):13–20.

Baumann S. 1996. Pharmacodynamics and pharmacokinetics of citalopram and other SSRIs. *Int Clin Psychopharmacol* (Suppl 1):5–11.

Bleuler E. 1950. *Dementia Praecox or the Group of Schizophrenias.* New York: International Universities Press.

Bowden CL, Brugger AM, Swann A, et al. 1994. Efficacy of divalproex vs lithium and placebo in mania. The Depakote Mania Study Group. *JAMA* **271**:918–24.

Byerley WF, McConnell EJ, McCabe RT, et al. 1988. Decreased beta-adrenergic receptors in rat brain after chronic administration of the selective serotonin uptake inhibitor, fluoxetine. *Psychopharmacology* **94**:141–3.

Campbell M. 1988. Fenfluramine treatment of autism. *J Child Psychol Psychiatry* **29**:1–10.

Campbell M, Small AM, Green WH, et al. 1984. Behavioral efficacy of haloperidol and lithium carbonate: a comparison in hospitalized aggressive children with conduct disorder. *Arch Gen Psychiatry* **41**:650–6.

Carrey NJ, Wiggins DM, Milin RP. 1996. Pharmacological treatment of psychiatric disorders of children and adolescents: focus on guidelines for primary care practitioners. *Drugs* **51**:750–9.

Charney DS, Heninger GR. 1986. Abnormal regulation of noradrenergic function in panic disorders. *Arch Gen Psychiatry* **43**:1042–54.

Clomipramine Study Group. 1991. Clomipramine in the treatment of patients with obsessive-compulsive disorder. *Arch Gen Psychiatry* **48**:730–8.

Consensus Development Conference. 1984a. Mood Disorder: Pharmacologic Prevention of Recurrences. Vol. 5, No. 4. Bethesda, MD: National Institutes of Health.

Consensus Development Conference. 1984b. Drugs and insomnia: the use of medications to promote sleep. *JAMA* **251**:2410–4.

Costa E. 1991. The allosteric modulation of GABA receptors: seventeen years of research. *Neuropsychopharmacology* **4**:225–35.

Davies P. 1986. The genetics of Alzheimer's disease: a review and a discussion of the implications. *Neurobiol Aging* **7**:459–65.

Davis KL, Thal LJ, Gamuz ER, et al. 1992. A double-blind, placebo-controlled multicenter study of tacrine for Alzheimer's disease. The Tacrine Collaborative Study Group. *N Engl J Med* **327**: 1253–9.

DeBacker WA. 1995. Central sleep apnea, pathogenesis and treatment: an appraisal and perspective. *Eur Respir J* **8**:1372–83.

Dechant KL, Clissol SP. 1991. Paroxetine: a review of its pharmacodynamic and pharmacokinetic properties and therapeutic potential in depressive illness. *Drugs* **41**:225–53.

Devane CL. 1995. Comparative safety and tolerability of selective serotonin reuptake inhibitors. *Hum Psychopharmacol* **10**: S185–93.

[DSM-IV]. 1994. *Diagnostic and Statistical Manual, Fourth Edition* (DSM-IV). Washington, DC: American Psychiatric Press. p 886.

Egeland JA, Gerhard DS, Pauls DL, et al. 1987. Bipolar affective disorders linked to DNA markers on chromosome 11. *Nature* **325**:783–7.

Emilien G, Maloteaux JM, Seghers A, et al. 1996. Lithium compared with valproic acid in the treatment of mania: a statistical meta-analysis. *Eur Neuropsychopharmacol* **6**:245–52.

Farde L, Wiesel FA, Halldin C, et al. 1988. Central $D_2$-dopamine receptor occupancy in schizophrenic patients treated with antipsychotic drugs. *Arch Gen Psychiatry* **45**:71–6.

Farlow M, Gracon SI, Hershey LA, et al., for the Tacrine Study Group. 1992. A controlled trial of tacrine for Alzheimer's disease. *JAMA* **268**:2523–9.

Ford DE, Kamerow DB. 1989. Epidemiologic study of sleep disturbances and psychiatric disorders: an opportunity for prevention? *JAMA* **262**:1479–84.

Francis J, Martin D, Kapoor WN. 1990. A prospective study of delirium in hospitalized elderly. *JAMA* **263**:1097–101.

Fulton B, Benfield P. 1996. Moclobemide: an update on its pharmacologic properties and therapeutic uses. *Drugs* **52**:450–74.

Fyer AJ, Liebowitz MR, Gorman JG, et al. 1987. Discontinuation of alprazolam treatment in panic patients. *Am J Psychiatry* **144**: 303–8.

Garland BJ, Wilder DE, Copeland J. 1985. Concepts of depression in the elderly: Signposts to future mental health needs. ln: Gaitz CM, Samorajski T, editors. *Aging 2000: Our Health Care Destiny*. New York: Springer-Verlag. pp 443–51.

Garza-Trevino E, Hollister LE, Overall JE, et al. 1989. Efficacy of combination of intramuscular antipsychotics and sedative-hypnotics for control of psychotic agitation. *Am J Psychiatry* **146**:1598–1601.

Gordon CT, State RC, Nelson JE, et al. 1993. A double-blind comparison of clomipramine, desipramine and placebo in the treatment of autistic disorder. *Arch Gen Psychiatry* **50**:441–7.

Green AR. 1987. Evolving concepts on the interactions between antidepressant treatments and monamine neurotransmitters. *Neuropharmacology* **26**:815–22.

Greenblatt DJ, Shader RI. 1985. Clinical pharmacokinetics of the benzodiazepines. In: Smith DE, Wesson DR, editors. *The Benzodiazepines: Current Standards of Medical Practice.* Lancaster, UK: MTP Press. p 43–50.

Groves EG, Clothier JL, Hollister LE. 1991. Predicting lithium doses by the body-weight method. *Int J Clin Psychopharmacol* **6**: 19–23.

Hirschfeld RMA, Keller MB, Panico S, et al. 1997. The National Depressive and Manic Depressive Association consensus statement on the undertreatment of depression. *JAMA* **277**:333–40.

Holm KJ, Marchan A. 1999. Mirtazapine. A review of its use in major depression. *Drugs* **57**:607–31.

Hotopf MW, Hardy R, Lewis G. 1997. Discontinuation rates of SSRIs and tricyclic antidepressants: a meta-analysis and investigation of heterogeneity. *Br J Psychiatry* **170**:120–7.

[ICD 10]. 1993. *The ICD-10 Classification of Mental and Behavioral Diseases.* Geneva: World Health Organization.

Judd BW, Meyer JS, Rogers RL, et al. 1986. Cognitive performance correlates with cerebrovascular impairments in multi-infarct dementia. *J Am Geriatr Soc* **34**:355–60.

Judd LL. 1997. Pleomorphic expressions of unipolar depressive disease: summary of the 1996 CINP president's workshop. *J Affective Disord* **45**:106–19.

Kane J, Honigfeld G, Singer J, et al. 1988. Clozapine for the treatment-resistent schizophrenic: a double-blind comparison with chlorpromazine. *Arch Gen Psychiatry* **45**:789–96.

Kaplan AA, Hussain S. 1995. Use of drugs in child and adolescent psychiatry. *Br J Psychiatry* **166**:291–8.

Kasper S, Zivkor M, Roes KC, et al. 1997. Pharmacological treatment of severely depressed patients: a meta-analysis comparing efficacy of mirtazapine and amitriptyline. *Eur Neuropsychopharmacol* **7**:115–24.

Kishimoto A, Ogura C, Hazama H, et al. 1983. Long-term prophylactic effects of carbamazepine in affective disorder. *Br J Psychiatry* **143**:327–31.

Klein RG, Koplewicz HS, Kanner A. 1992. Imipramine treatment of children with separation anxiety. *J Am Acad Child Adolesc Psychiatry* **31**:21–8.

Klein RG, Landa B, Mattes JA, et al. 1988. Methylphenidate and growth in hyperactive children: A controlled withdrawal study. *Arch Gen Psychiatry* **45**:1127–33.

Klosterkotter J, Albers M, Steinmeyer EM, et al. 1995. Positive or negative symptoms—which are more appropriate as diagnostic criteria for schizophrenia? *Acad Psychiatric Scand* **92**:321–6.

Kraepelin F. 1905. *Lectures on Clinical Psychiatry.* New York: William Wood.

Krueger JM, Karaszewski JW, Davenne D, et al. 1986. Somnogenic muramyl peptides. *Fed Proc* **45**:2552–5.

Kusumakar V, Yatham LN. 1997. An open study of lamotrigine in refractory bipolar depression. *Psychiatry Res* **72**:145–8.

Lane RM. 1996. Pharmacokinetic drug interaction potential of selective serotonin reuptake inhibitors. *Int Clin Psychopharmacol* **11**(Suppl 5):31–61 [Published erratum appears in *Int Clin Psychopharmacol.* 1997. **12**(2):126].

LeBars PL, Katz MM, Berman N, et al. 1997. A placebo-controlled, double-blind, randomized trial of an extract of *Gingko biloba* for dementia. *JAMA* **278**:1327–32.

Lenox RH, Manji HK. 1995. Lithium. In: Schatzberg AF, Nemeroff CB, editors. *Textbook of Psychopharmacology.* Washington, DC: American Psychiatric Press. p 303–19.

Leonard HL, Swedo SE, Lenana MC, et al. 1993. A 2–4 year followup of 54 obsessive-compulsive children and adolescents. *Arch Gen Psychiatry* **50**:429–39.

Lepine JR, Gastpar M, Mendlewicz J, et al., on behalf of the DEPRES steering committee. 1997. Depression in the community: the first pan-European study DEPRES (Depression Research in European Society). *Int J Clin Psychopharmacol* **12**:19–29.

Liddle P, Carpenter WT, Crow T. 1994. Syndromes of schizophrenia: classic literature. *Br J Psychiatry* **165**:721–7.

Linde K, Ramirez G, Mulrow CD, et al. 1996. St. John's wort for depression—an overview and meta-analysis of randomized clinical trials. *Br Med J Clin Res* **313**:253–8.

Lobo EL, Green WL. 1997. Zolpidem: distinct from triazolam? *Ann Pharmacother* **11**:625–32.

Maarbjerg K, Vestergaard P, Schou M. 1987. Changes in serum thyroxine (T4) and serum thyroid-stimulating hormone (TSH) during prolonged lithium treatment. *Acta Psychiatr Scand* **75**:217–21.

Martin IL. 1987. The benzodiazepines and their receptors: 25 years of progress. *Neuropharmacology* **26**:957–70.

McCann UD, Agras WS. 1990. Successful treatment of compulsive binge-eating with desipramine: a double-blind, placebo-controlled study. *Am J Psychiatry* **147**:1509–13.

McElroy SL, Keck PE, Stanton SP, et al. 1996. A randomized com parison of divalproex oral loading dose versus haloperidol in the initial treatment of acute psychotic mania. *J Clin Psychiatry* **57**: 142–6.

McKenna PJ. 1987. Pathology, phenomenology and the dopamine hypothesis of schizophrenia. *Br J Psychiatry* **151**:288–301.

Mendelson WB, Jain BA. 1995. Assessment of short-acting hypnotics. *Drug Saf* **13**:257–70.

Mendlewiez J, Simon P, Sevy S, et al. 1987. Polymorphic DNA marker on X-chromosome and manic depression. *Lancet* **1**:1230–4.

Mirza KAH, Michael A, Dinan TG. 1994. Recent advances in paediatric psychopharmacology: a brief overview. *Hum Psychopharmacol* **9**:13–24.

Moore-Ede MC, Czeisler CA, Richardson GS. 1983. Circadian timekeeping in health and disease. *N Engl J Med* **309**:469–536.

Morin CM, Culbert JP, Schwartz SM. 1994. Nonpharmacological interventions for insomnia: a meta-analysis of treatment efficacy. *Am J Psychiatry* **151**:1172–80.

Myers JK, Weissman MM, Tischler GL, et al. 1984. Six-month prevalence of psychiatric disorders in three communities: 1980 to 1982. *Arch Gen Psychiatry* **41**:959–67.

Nishino S, Mignot E. 1997. Pharmacological aspects of human and canine narcolepsy. *Prog Neurobiology* **52**:27–78.

Overall JE, Hollister LE. 1979. Comparative evaluation of research diagnostic criteria for schizophrenia. *Arch Gen Psychiatry* **36**:1198–1205.

Palmer DP. 1988. Buspirone, a new approach to the treatment of anxiety. *Fed Am Soc Exp Biol J* **2**:2445–52.

Palmer KJ, Benfield P. 1994. Fluvoxamine: an overview of its pharmacological properties and review of its therapeutic potential in non-depressive states. *CNS Drugs* **1**:57–87.

Pare CMP. 1985. The present status of monamine oxidase inhibitors. *Br J Psychiatry* **146**:576–84.

Post RM. 1986. Mechanisms of action of carbamazepine and related anticonvulsants in affective illness. In: Meltzer HY, editor. *Psychopharmacology: The Third Generation of Progress.* New York: Raven Press. pp 567–84.

Post RM, Weiss SRB, Chuang DM. 1992. Mechanisms of action of anticonvulsants in affective disorders: comparison with lithium. *Int J Psychopharmacol* **12**:23S–35S.

Rapoport JL. 1988. The neurobiology of obsessive-compulsive disorder. *JAMA* **260**:2888–90.

Reimherr GW, Chouinard G, Hohn CK, et al. 1990. Antidepressant efficacy of sertraline: a double-blind, placebo and amitriptyline-controlled multicenter comparison study in outpatients with major depression. *J Clin Psychiatry* **51** (Suppl B):18–27.

Richelson E. 1994. The pharmacology of antidepressants at the synapse: focus on newer drugs. *J Clin Psychiatry* **55**:34–9.

Riddle MA, Scahill L, King RS, et al. 1992. Double-blind crossover trial of fluoxetine in children and adolescents with obsessive-compulsive disorder. *J Am Acad Child Adolesc Psychiatry* **31**: 106–9.

Robins LN, Helzer JE, Weissman MM, et al. 1984. Lifetime prevalence of specific psychiatric disorders in three sites. *Arch Gen Psychiatry* **41**:949–58.

Rogers SL, Friedhoff LT, Apter JT, et al. 1996. The efficacy and safety of donepezil in patients with Alzheimer's disease: results of a US multi-center, randomized double-blind, placebo-controlled trial. *Dementia* **7**:293–303.

Rosenheck R, Cramer J, Weichun X, et al. 1997. A comparison of clozapine and haloperidol in hospitalized patients with refractory schizophrenia. Department of Veterans Affairs Cooperative Study Group on Clozapine in Refractory Schizophrenia. *N Engl J Med* **337**:809–15.

Schweitzer E, Feighner J, Mandos LA, et al. 1994. Comparison of venlafazine and imipramine in the acute treatment of major depression in outpatients. *J Clin Psychiatry* **55**:104–8.

Schneider LS, Olin CT. 1994. Overview of clinical trials of hydergine in dementia. *Arch Neurolog* **51**:787–98.

Small JC, Hirsch SR, Arvanitis LA, et al., and the Seroquel Study Group. 1997. Quetiapine in patients with schizophrenia: a high- and low-dose double-blind comparison with placebo. *Arch Gen Psychiatry* **54**:549–57.

Sansome ME, Ziegler DK. 1985. Lithium toxicity: a review of neurologic complications. *Clin Neuropharmacol* **8**:242–8.

Simard M, Gumbiner B, Lee A, et al. 1989. Lithium carbonate intoxication. A case report and review of the literature. *Arch Int Med* **49**:36–46.

Song F. 1997. Risperidone in the treatment of schizophrenia: a meta-analysis of randomized controlled trials. *J Psychopharmacol* **11**:65–71.

Song F, Freemantle N, Sheldon TA, et al. 1993. Selective serotonin reuptake inhibitors: meta-analysis of efficacy and acceptability. *BMJ* **306**:683–7.

Stassen HH, Angst J, Delini-Stula A. 1996. Delayed onset of action of antidepressant drugs? Survey of results of Zurich meta-analyses. *Pharmacopsychiatry* **29**:87–96.

Sulser F. 1987. Serotonin-norepinephrine receptor interactions in the brain: implications for the pharmacology and pathophysiology of affective disorders. *J Clin Psychiatry* **48** (Suppl):12–8.

Tallman JF, Paul SM, Skolnick P, et al. 1980. Receptors for the age of anxiety: pharmacology of the benzodiazepines. *Science* **207**:274–81.

Taylor DP. 1988. Buspirone, a new approach to the treatment of anxiety. *FASEB J* **2**:2445–52.

Thompson TL, Moran MG, Nies AS. 1983. Psychotropic drug use in the elderly. *N Engl J Med* **308**:134–8, 194–9.

Timms RM, Dawson A, Hajdukovic RM, et al. 1988. Effect of triazolam on sleep and arterial oxygen saturation in patients with chronic obstructive pulmonary disease. *Arch Intern Med* **149**:2159–63.

Tollefson GD, Beasley CM Jr, Tran PV, et al. 1997. Olanzapine versus haloperidol in the treatment of schizophrenia and schizoaffective and schizophreniform disorders: results of an international collaborative trial. *Am J Psychiatry* **154**:457–65.

Tran PV, Hamilton SH, Kuntz AJ, et al. 1997. Double-blind comparison of olanzapine versus risperidone in the treatment of schizophrenia and other psychotic disorders. *J Clin Psychopharmacol* **17**: 407–18.

UK Moclobemide Study Group. 1994. A multicenter comparative trial of moclobemide, imipramine and placebo in major depressive disorder. *Int J Clin Psychopharmacol* **9**:109–13.

U.S. Department of Health and Human Resources. 1993. *Depression in Primary Care*. Vol. 1. *Detection and Diagnosis*, and Vol. 2. *Treatment of Major Depression*. Clinical Practice Guideline Number 5. AHCPR Publication Nos. 93-0550 and 93-0551. Rockville, MD: Agency for Health Care Policy and Research.

Vitiello B, Jensen PS. 1997. Medication development and testing in children and adolescents: current problems, future directions. *Arch Gen Psychiatry* **54**:871–6.

Van Harten J. 1993. Clinical pharmacokinetics of selective serotonin reuptake inhibitors. *Clin Pharmacokinet* **24**:203–20.

Walton SA, Berk M, Brook S. 1996. Superiority of lithium over verapamil in mania. *J Clin Psychiatry* **57**:543–6.

Walsh BR, Stewart JW, Roose SP, et al. 1984. Treatment of bulimia with phenelzine: a double-blind, placebo-controlled study. *Arch Gen Psychiatry* **41**:1105–9.

Weissman MM, Bland RC, Canino GJ, et al. 1997. The cross-national epidemiology of panic disorder. *Arch Gen Psychiatry* **54**:303–9.

Wetter TC, Pollmacher T. 1997. Restless legs and periodic leg movements in sleep disorder. *J Neurol* **244** (Suppl 1):S37–45.

Weytingh MD, Bossuyt PM, van Crevel R. 1995. Reversible dementia: more than 10% or less than 1%: a quantitative review. *J Neurol* **242**:466–71.

Youngerman J, Canino I. 1978. Lithium carbonate use in children and adolescents. *Arch Gen Psychiatry* **35**:216–24.

Zimbroff DL, Kane JM, Tamminga CA, et al, and the Sertindole Study Group. 1997. Controlled dose-response study of sertindole and haloperidol in the treatment of schizophrenia. *Am J Psychiatry* **154**:782–91.

CHAPTER

# 9 ENDOCRINE AND METABOLIC DISORDERS

# Diabetes Mellitus

Jeffrey W. Miller, Fredric B. Kraemer

*Chapter Outline*



## PHYSIOLOGY OF THE ENDOCRINE PANCREAS

The endocrine pancreas and related hormones orchestrate the delivery of fuel substrates for use and storage during fed (absorptive) periods, as well as mobilization of fuel stores during fasting (postabsorptive) periods. Maintenance of blood glucose homeostasis is critical for the function of many organs, particularly the brain. During the absorptive period after a meal, rising blood glucose concentrations, and food-related stimuli, acting via enteric hormones and the autonomic nervous system, stimulate insulin release from the $\beta$-cells in the pancreatic islets of Langerhans. Insulin enters the portal circulation where it initially acts on the liver to suppress gluconeogenesis and fatty acid oxidation. Insulin is subsequently distributed systemically where it promotes glucose uptake into many cells by translocation of glucose transporters from endosomal compartments to the plasma membrane. The overall effect of insulin is to coordinate tissue glucose uptake, glycogen synthesis, fatty acid storage, and protein synthesis.

### Insulin Action

Insulin is secreted from $\beta$-cells in the pancreatic islets by a $Ca^{2+}$-mediated signaling pathway. An ATP-sensitive $K^+$ channel, which regulates voltage-dependent $Ca^{2+}$ influx, is the molecular target of the sulfonylurea class of hypoglycemic agents. Insulin binds to insulin receptors on the surface of many cells; these receptors have tyrosine kinase activity in their intracellular carboxy-terminal domain and initiate a series of phosphorylation/dephosphorylation reactions. Although the intracellular signaling pathways of the insulin receptor are not completely understood, they are likely to include transcription of genes that regulate the utilization of energy substrates. Nuclear transcription factors such as PPAR-$\gamma$ may be stimulated by pharmacologic agents such as thiazolidinediones, and they improve insulin sensitivity in insulin-resistant patients.

### Counterregulatory Response to Hypoglycemia

During postabsorptive periods, glucose concentrations decline, and insulin release is suppressed. Decreases in plasma glucose concentrations to a critical degree elicit multiple neurohormonal responses aimed at restoring glucose into the normal range; these responses include pancreatic glucagon release, sympathetic nervous system activation, and hypothalamic–pituitary–adrenal release of growth hormone, cortisol, and epinephrine. The counterregulatory hormones all act to increase glycogenolysis and to inhibit insulin release. The prodromal symptoms of hypoglycemia are caused by adrenergic stimulation (nervousness, tachycardia, tremor, sweating). Failure of the counterregulatory response is seen in diabetic autonomic neuropathy, adrenal insufficiency, and panhypopituitarism and may result in neuroglycopenic symptoms (changes in mental status) without prodromal hyperadrenergic symptoms. Counterregulatory hormones mediate two hyperglycemic phenomena that commonly occur during the treatment of diabetes: the "dawn" phenomenon of early morning hyperglycemia and the Somogyi phenomenon of rebound hyperglycemia following excessive insulin action.

# DIABETES MELLITUS

## Classification of Diabetes Mellitus

The prevalence of diabetes mellitus is approximately 5% in industrialized countries, and approximately 85% of cases are so-called *type 2 diabetes.* Type 2 diabetes defines a syndrome that is constituted by several different disease processes including glucose transporter defects, desensitization of insulin receptors, toxic effects of hyperglycemia, and the metabolic demands of obesity. A large portion of nondiabetic adults in industrialized countries demonstrate impaired insulin-mediated glucose uptake, which is qualitatively similar to that seen in type 2 diabetes; this abnormality is termed *insulin resistance.* Unlike other hormone resistance syndromes, insulin resistance is very rarely due to abnormalities of insulin binding or the insulin receptor. Although many insulin-resistant people maintain glucose homeostasis during their lifetime, progressive loss of glucose homeostasis, due to an inability to maintain elevated rates of insulin secretion, in a portion of this population leads to impaired glucose tolerance and frank diabetes mellitus. Insulin resistance is also seen in approximately 40% of patients with primary hypertension, and the syndrome of hypertension, insulin resistance, truncal obesity, and dyslipidemia has been termed *syndrome X* or the *metabolic syndrome*.

The classification of diabetes mellitus as juvenile-onset and adult-onset, or insulin-dependent and non-insulin-dependent, has recently been simplified to reflect the two major clinical syndromes of chronic diabetes—type 1 and type 2 (Table 9-1). *Type 1 diabetes mellitus* is a syndrome of absolute insulin deficiency. It is characterized by predisposition to recurrent ketoacidosis in the absence of insulin therapy, and most cases are due to autoimmune destruction of pancreatic β-cells. Most type 1 diabetics are diagnosed before the age of 35; however, the incidence of type 2 diabetes at younger ages has increased. For this reason, the age of onset does not define the type of diabetes in teenagers and young adults. The requirement for insulin may also confuse the proper classification of diabetes mellitus, since many type 2 diabetics require insulin therapy for optimal blood glucose control. Type 1 diabetic patients require insulin therapy to prevent recurrent ketoacidosis. Many type 1 patients presenting with ketoacidosis have a "honeymoon" period of residual β-cell function in which intensive insulin therapy is not required. This period may last up to one year or longer, after which ketoacidosis develops routinely when insulin therapy is interrupted. In contrast, a variant of type 2 diabetes termed *maturity onset diabetes of the young* (MODY) can present with acute hyperglycemia and ketoacidosis in teenagers, but may be managed by diet and oral agents for many years without recurrent ketoacidosis. MODY was initially described as an autosomal dominant syndrome in African Americans in the southern United States, but should also be considered in young adults with a strong family history of early-onset type 2 diabetes.

The occurrence of impaired glucose tolerance during pregnancy in a woman without a previous history of diabetes is termed *gestational diabetes mellitus* (GDM). GDM is seen in approximately 4% of all pregnancies in the United States and is associated with an increased risk of fetal abnormalities, adverse birth outcomes, and increased lifelong maternal risk of chronic diabetes. Insulin resistance is normal in pregnancy and results, in part, from high progesterone concentrations. Glucose tolerance is most impaired during the third trimester, and oral glucose tolerance testing is recommended between weeks 24 and 28 of gestation. The treatment of GDM focuses on tight control of blood glucose to improve perinatal outcomes, as well as behavioral interventions to minimize the risk of type 2 diabetes later in life.

## Diagnostic Criteria

The diagnostic criteria for diabetes mellitus (Table 9-2) were revised in a 1997 Expert Committee Report (Report of the Expert Committee on the Diagnosis and Classification of Diabetes Mellitus 1997b). In these guidelines, the criteria for interpretation of the 75 g oral glucose tolerance test (OGTT) have been retained, but the fasting

Table 9-1 **Classification of Diabetes Mellitus**

| TYPE | ETIOLOGY |
|---|---|
| Type 1 diabetes mellitus | Autoimmune, ketoacidosis-prone |
| Type 2 diabetes mellitus | Insulin resistance or relative insulin secretory defect |
| Gestational diabetes mellitus | New-onset glucose intolerance in pregnancy |
| Other specific types | Exocrine pancreas diseases, genetic syndromes, endocrinopathies, other autoimmune syndromes, drug-induced diabetes |

**Table 9-2 Diagnostic Criteria for Diabetes Mellitus**

1. Randomly obtained plasma glucose concentration ≥200 mg/dL, which is accompanied by symptoms of diabetes (polydipsia, polyuria, weight loss), or
2. Fasting blood glucose >126 mg/dL, or
3. Plasma glucose >200 mg/dL at 2 h after 75 g glucose administration.

blood glucose criterion has been lowered to 126 mg/dL (7 mmol/L). This level of fasting hyperglycemia correlates with the point of increased risk for diabetic retinopathy and renal disease defined in epidemiological studies. This threshold for fasting blood glucose is also highly predictive of patients who will demonstrate abnormal OGTT results. Fasting plasma glucose concentrations of 110–126 mg/dL (6–7 mmol/L) reflect impaired fasting glucose regulation and may warrant behavioral interventions to reduce the risk of developing type 2 diabetes. Measurements of glycosylated hemoglobin concentrations are not used diagnostically because of poor standardization among clinical laboratories, but are useful in therapeutic monitoring when performed at a consistent laboratory.

The high prevalence of type 2 diabetes mellitus, and the proven efficacy of diabetic therapy in reducing disease-related complications, warrant an active approach to case finding and adherence to evidence based therapeutic guidelines. The development of clinical symptoms in type 2 diabetes (polyuria, polydipsia, unexplained weight loss) often occurs after the onset of microvascular complications. Current American Diabetes Association guidelines (American Diabetes Association 1997a) recommend screening all adults over 45 years of age with a fasting blood glucose measurement every 3 years, and a more aggressive approach for adults with other risk factors (Table 9-3). Screening for type 1 diabetes is not recommended, as the incidence of this disease is low, and there are no current therapeutic measures that are of proven benefit before initial symptom presentation.

**Table 9-3 Risk Factors for Type 2 Diabetes Mellitus**

- Obesity (BMI >27 kg/m$^2$)
- ≥1 First degree relative with type 2 diabetes
- African-American, Hispanic, or Native American ethnic background
- Personal history of gestational diabetes mellitus or delivery of a baby weighing >9 lb
- Hypertension
- HDL cholesterol ≤ 35 mg/dL and/or fasting triglyceride concentration ≥250 mg/dL
- Personal history of impaired fasting glucose or impaired glucose tolerance

## Therapeutic Guidelines

Although type 1 diabetic patients are usually treated with insulin following their initial presentation, the initial therapy for all patients with type 2 diabetes mellitus is a program that combines dietary modification and exercise. Since most patients with type 2 diabetes mellitus are overweight, dietary modifications generally entail caloric restriction, reduction in the intake of saturated fat, and a relative increase in complex carbohydrates in their diet. Specific dietary recommendations, and the scientific bases on which they are founded, are beyond the scope of this chapter. The reader is referred to recent reviews on this topic (Franz et al. 1994; Ha and Lean 1998) for further information. If patients are asymptomatic and have glucose values <300 mg/dL, a period of 3–6 months of dietary intervention should be undertaken before pharmacologic therapy is considered; however, for symptomatic patients or patients with glucose values >300 mg/dL, initiating drug therapy concurrently with dietary intervention is warranted. Exercise is an important adjunct to dietary treatment and is associated with improvements in glucose control independent of changes in body weight in both type 1 and type 2 diabetes.

Based on the results of major prospective therapeutic trials in diabetes (discussed in this section), the goal for glycemic control in both type I and type II diabetes is to achieve preprandial blood glucose of 80–120 mg/dL, postprandial (1.5–2 hours) blood glucose <180 mg/dL, and bedtime blood glucose of 100–140 mg/dL. In addition to optimal glycemic control, patients with type 1 and type 2 diabetes benefit from expectant management of diabetic complications (Weir et al. 1994). Treatment of blood pressure >140/90 mmHg to achieve blood pressure <130/85 mmHg reduces the incidence of diabetes-related morbidity and mortality. Angiotensin-converting enzyme (ACE)-inhibitor therapy in patients who have demonstrated elevated urinary albumin on at least two occasions (by timed collection or urinary albumin/creatinine ratio) reduces the progression of diabetic nephropathy in type 1 diabetes and the progression of proteinuria in type 2 diabetes. Since cardiovascular disease is the leading cause of mortality in diabetes, aggressive treatment of modifiable risk factors (smoking, hypertension, dyslipidemia) is warranted. Diabetic patients have demonstrated mortality benefits from hydroxymethylglutaryl coenzyme A (HMG-CoA) reductase therapy in the secondary prevention of coronary disease (Sacks et al. 1996). Although a definitive primary prevention study has not been conducted in diabetic patients, reduction of low-density lipoprotein (LDL) cholesterol to <130 mg/dL is recommended in the current (US) National Cholesterol Education Program guidelines for management of dyslipidemia (Second Report of the Expert Panel on Detection, Evaluation, and Treatment of High Blood Cholesterol in Adults (Adult Treatment Panel II) 1993b), with an ideal goal <100 mg/dL suggested by the American Diabetes Association (American Diabetes Association 1997a). Annual ophthalmological examination, with laser therapy of proliferative lesions, reduces the progression of diabetic retinopathy. Patient education for foot care and early identification and treatment of foot ulcers reduces the rate of amputation in patients with diabetic neuropathy. Since diabetic women are at increased risk for adverse pregnancy outcomes, contraceptive measures and optimization of glycemic control before pregnancy planning are warranted.

## INSULIN THERAPEUTICS

### History of Insulin

The development of insulin as a therapeutic agent for type 1 diabetes mellitus is one of the great success stories of allopathic medicine. Although the syndrome of glucosuria and polydipsia was described in antiquity, the role of the pancreas in diabetes mellitus was elucidated by nineteenth century physicians and experimental physiologists. Surgical removal of the pancreas and pancreatic duct ligation (which leads to atrophy of the exocrine pancreas) identified the islets of Langerhans as the source of a hormone that controlled glucose metabolism. Multiple attempts to extract this hormone resulted in documentation of the hypoglycemic effects of pancreatic extracts in animals in 1921 by N.C. Paulesco in Romania (Paulesco 1924). Banting, Best, and Collip in Toronto improved the method of extraction and administered a preparation of beef insulin to a diabetic patient for the first time in 1922 (Banting 1926). Commercial production of insulin was under way in 1922. The purity of animal insulins was gradually improved in subsequent years. In the 1930s and 1940s, it was recognized that crystallization of insulin with zinc and combination with the cationic protein protamine resulted in prolongation of insulin action, leading to the commercial availability of intermediate-acting insulins. Human insulin, prepared by chemical modification of porcine insulin and by recombinant DNA technology, became commercially available by 1980. In the 1990s, attempts to modify the pharmacokinetics of insulin by targeted modification of key amino acids led to the production of insulin analogs such as lispro and aspart insulin. In addition to advances in insulin synthesis, technical improvements in insulin delivery have led to continuous subcutaneous insulin infusion (CSII) and convenient pen-style multiple-dose injection devices.

### Insulin Pharmacology

Human insulin is a protein containing 51 amino acids; it consists of A and B chains linked by disulfide bonds. The two chains are produced along with C-peptide from a single proinsulin molecule. C-peptide can be measured clinically as an indicator of endogenous insulin production in diabetic patients. Porcine insulin differs by one amino acid and bovine insulin by three amino acids from human insulin, although the three-dimensional structure is very similar in a variety of species. As predicted by amino acid homology, bovine insulin is more immunogenic than porcine insulin when used therapeutically.

A large portion of the insulin in the portal circulation is degraded in the liver before reaching the peripheral circulation. Exogenously administered insulin is not selectively delivered to the liver; hence, hepatic effects, such as suppression of gluconeogenesis, are achieved at doses that expose systemic tissues to relatively higher insulin concentrations. This may explain why hepatically mediated insulin therapeutic effects, such as suppression of very low density lipoprotein (VLDL) synthesis, may be incomplete at doses that achieve relative euglycemia. The rate of absorption of subcutaneously administered insulin is modified by a variety of factors: the physical properties of the insulin, species of insulin, volume of injection, site of injection, and concentration of the dose. Even when insulin dose and administration technique are tightly controlled, the rate of absorption of insulin varies by 50% from day to day in healthy subjects (Galloway et al. 1981). Human insulin is absorbed more rapidly than porcine insulin, and both are absorbed more rapidly than bovine insulin. Pharmacologic insulin preparations consist of insulin hexamers and dimers; these complexes are absorbed more slowly than monomeric insulin. Insulin circulates in the blood stream in monomeric or dimeric forms, which are not associated with a natural binding protein. Autoantibodies to insulin, common in insulin-treated patients, may act as binding proteins. Most insulin autoantibodies have no effect on insulin action, but high-avidity or high-titer antibodies may prolong the time course of insulin action by decreasing insulin clearance, leading to a prolonged hypoglycemic response. Systemically administered insulin is degraded by proteases in the kidney and liver, and by receptor-mediated clearance at sites of insulin action. Subcutaneous degradation of injected insulin rarely accounts for more than 5% loss of the administered dose.

## Formulations

### *Regular insulin*

Insulin formulations are displayed in Table 9-4. Soluble (regular, Semilente) insulins are noncrystallized insulins that are formulated with zinc and buffered at physiologic pH. Regular insulin is predominantly dimeric and hexameric. These insulins are often termed *short-acting* or *rapid-acting insulins* to distinguish them from crystalline insulin formulations, but the recent development of rapid-acting monomeric insulin analogs has rendered these terms obsolete. Their duration of action is shorter than crystallized insulin formulations, but longer than that of meal-related endogenous insulin release. Onset of action begins approximately 0.5 hours after injection; consequently, patients are instructed to administer the dose 30–45 minutes before eating. Peak insulin concentrations are achieved approximately 90 minutes after subcutaneous injection. The duration of action of a single injection of regular insulin varies according to dose. In healthy subjects, a dose of 6 units of regular insulin elevates plasma insulin concentrations for approximately 6 hours. Regular insulin is the only form of insulin available for intravenous or intramuscular administration, and it is the only insulin formulated at concentrations greater than 100 units/mL (Insulin U–500). Although refrigerated storage is recommended, the formulations of soluble insulin are stable at 25°C. With prolonged storage or heat, visible insulin aggregates are formed by covalent aggregation (fibrillation). These high-molecular-weight insulin aggregates are highly immunogenic; hence, regular insulin should never be injected if it appears cloudy. Fibrillation, in addition to binding soluble insulin to plastic surfaces, may contribute to episodes of diabetic ketoacidosis in patients using subcutaneous insulin pump (CSII) regimens.

**Table 9-4 Insulin Formulations**

| Insulin | Marketed Name | Dispensing Information | Time of Onset | Peak Effect | Cost Index |
|---|---|---|---|---|---|
| *Soluble insulin* | | | | | |
| Human recombinant | Humulin, Novolin | 100 U/mL 10-mL bottles, or 1.5-mL cartridges | 45 min | 1.5–4 h | 2.5 (bottle) (cartridge) |
| Semisynthetic human | Velosulin | 100 U/mL 10-mL bottles, or 1.5-mL cartridges | 45 min | 1.5–4 h | 2.5 (bottle) (cartridge) |
| Regular concentrated | Iletin II U-500 | 500 U/mL, 10-mL bottles | 45 min | 1.5–4 h | 1 |
| *Monomeric insulin analog* | | | | | |
| Insulin lispro | Humalog | 100 U/mL 10-mL bottles, or 1.5-mL cartridges | 15 min | 1–2.5 h | 2 (bottle) 3 (cartridge) |
| *Intermediate-acting insulins* | | | | | |
| Human Lente insulin | Humulin L Novolin L | 100 U/mL 10-mL bottles | 1.5 h | 6–14 h | 1.5 |
| Pork Lente insulin | Iletin II, Lente L | 100 U/mL 10-mL bottles | 1.5 h | 7–15 h | 1.8 |
| Isophane (NPH) insulin | Novolin N Humulin N | 100 U/mL 10-mL bottles, or 1.5-mL cartridges | 1 h | 4–12 h | 1.5 |
| *Insulin mixtures* | | | | | |
| 70/30 | Humulin 70/30 Novolin 70/30 | 100 U/mL 10-mL bottles, or 1.5-mL cartridges | | | 1.5–2 |
| 50/50 | Humulin 50/50 | 100 U/mL 10-mL bottles | | | 2 |
| *Long-acting Insulin* | | | | | |
| Beef Ultralente | Ultralente U | 100 U/mL 10-mL bottles | 4 h | 12–24 h | 1.1 |
| Human Ultralente | Humulin U Ultralente | 100 U/mL 10-mL bottles | 3 h | 8–16 h | 1.8 |

***Monomeric insulin analogs***

Insulin lispro is a monomeric soluble insulin analog in which the order of the amino acids lysine and proline at positions 28 and 29 of the B chain have been reversed. Recently, a similar rapid-acting insulin analog (insulin aspart) has been approved by regulatory agencies. Onset of action of insulin lispro begins within several minutes after subcutaneous injection; consequently, the dose can be administered immediately before eating. In healthy subjects, an injection of 10 units of insulin lispro elevates insulin concentrations for approximately 4 hours, compared with 7 hours for 10 units of regular human insulin (Figure 9-1). Clinical trials comparing insulin lispro (Humalog) to regular human insulin demonstrate a reduction in postprandial glucose excursions and a lower incidence of late postprandial hypoglycemia with insulin lispro (Anderson et al. 1997a, 1997b). The relative reduction in hypoglycemia is due to the shorter duration of action, which more closely matches the absorptive period.

***Zinc-protamine insulin suspension or isophane insulin suspension (NPH)***

Addition of the basic protein protamine to insulin with zinc produces a crystalline insulin (neutral protamine Hagedorn [NPH] or isophane insulin) that is absorbed more slowly than soluble insulin. Protamine, a DNA binding protein from fish sperm, stabilizes the insulin hexamers in the crystals. Zinc is incorporated into the crystals in a fixed ratio and is not free in solution. The onset of action of human NPH insulin occurs within 1 hour, and peak insulin concentrations are achieved at approximately 4 hours after subcutaneous injection. Intermediate-acting insulins produce a gradual increase in insulin concentrations over time; hence, acute hypoglycemia is uncommon. The duration of action is dose-dependent. In healthy volunteers, 20 units of human NPH insulin elevates insulin concentrations for 18–24 hours. Protamine-zinc crystallized insulin (PZI), which has a delayed absorption pattern, comparable to Ultralente insulin, is now rarely used.

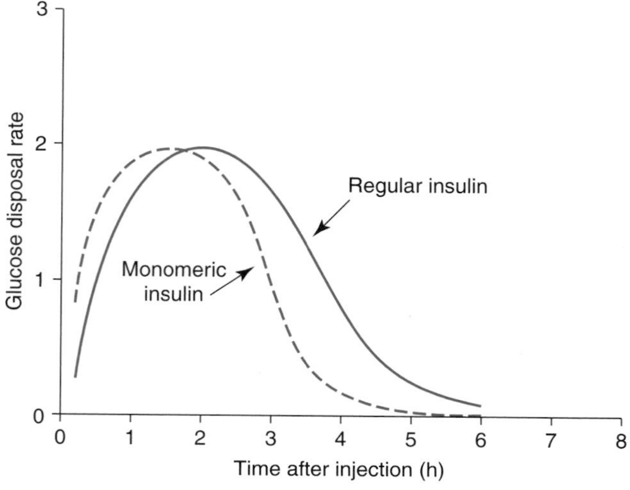


**FIGURE 9-1 Time course of insulin lispro versus regular insulin.**

***Zinc crystallized intermediate insulin suspension (Lente)***

Precipitation of insulin by higher concentrations of zinc also produces crystalline insulin with delayed absorption kinetics (Lente insulins). At neutral pH, an amorphous insulin precipitate is produced that demonstrates moderately delayed absorption; whereas, at acid pH a crystalline precipitate is formed that is absorbed even more slowly. Commercially available Lente insulin is a 7:3 ratio of crystalline to amorphous insulin aggregates. The onset of action of Lente insulin is similar to that of NPH, although the duration of action is slightly longer. Lente demonstrates less of a peak in insulin concentrations than NPH insulin. Because zinc is present in solution, mixture of Lente insulin with soluble insulin may alter the absorption of the soluble insulin. For this reason, Lente insulin is not suitable for formulation of fixed mixtures of rapid-acting and intermediate-acting insulins. Lente insulin can, however, be mixed with regular insulin before injection without significantly delaying the absorption of the regular insulin.

***Long-acting insulin (Ultralente)***

A preparation of 100% acid-crystallized insulin demonstrates even more delayed absorption than Lente insulin. The onset of action of human Ultralente insulin occurs in approximately 3 hours. Maximal hypoglycemic effects are seen at 20 hours after subcutaneous injection of 20 units in healthy volunteers. Human Ultralente demonstrates a peak hypoglycemic effect between 16 and 24 hours. For this reason, human Ultralente may need to be administered twice daily to achieve a steady insulin profile. Steady-state insulin concentrations are achieved only after 3 days of therapy. Bovine Ultralente has superior pharmacokinetic properties as a long-acting insulin, but is also more immunogenic and is now not widely used.

***Insulin mixtures***

Mixtures of NPH and rapid-acting insulin have been developed as a convenient insulin preparation for patients on mixed insulin regimens. A variety of NPH to regular insulin ratios (90:10, 80:20, 70:30, 50:50) have been developed, although not all forms are marketed in all countries. In countries such as the United States, where only 70:30 and 50:50 mixtures are available, these preparations may not provide the optimal amounts of rapid-acting and intermediate-acting insulin. These preparations are useful for patients with physical impairments (visual or manual) that make preparation of an insulin injection from two vials difficult.

## Delivery Technology

In addition to interest in development of new insulin analogs with superior pharmacokinetics, the route of delivery of insulin is an area of active research. Pulmonary, nasal, and implantable administration methods are in varying stages of clinical development. Insulin syringes are currently the most widely used method of insulin administration. "Lo-Dose" insulin syringes can deliver 0.3 or 0.5 mL (30 or 50 units) of insulin and allow insulin dosage to be measured more accurately than conventional 100-unit syringes. Recently a convenient "pen injector" has been introduced, which allows repeated administration of insulin from cartridges containing 1.5 mL of regular, monomeric, or fixed mixture (70:30) insulins. This device simplifies multiple daily injection regimens for patients with active lifestyles. The continuous subcutaneous insulin infusion (CSII, insulin pump) has been in use for nearly 20 years. CSII was originally hailed as the most physiologic method of insulin therapy, because of its ability to deliver mealtime boluses of rapid-acting insulin superimposed on a continuous basal level of infusion. For several reasons, however, this method is not clearly preferable to multiple daily injection therapy. Because of its reliance on rapid-acting insulin, CSII does not provide the body with a "depot" of subcutaneous insulin waiting to be absorbed. Because of this, the patient is vulnerable to occasional interruptions of insulin delivery due to depletion of the insulin reservoir, blockage of the tubing, or displacement of the subcutaneous needle, and may lapse rapidly into diabetic ketoacidosis. Inflammation and occasional infection of the skin may also complicate CSII therapy.

## Factors Influencing Efficacy

Prevention of diabetes-related morbidity and mortality requires integrated pharmacologic and behavioral management. In order to design an optimal therapeutic regimen, a number of factors must be considered (Table 9-5). The dose and timing of pharmacologic agents is only one part of a comprehensive therapeutic regimen. Therapeutic success requires realistic goal-setting; design of a diet, drug, and activity regimen suited to these goals; and therapeutic monitoring at appropriate intervals. Even with optimal behavioral management, insulin therapy faces the challenge of maintaining energy homeostasis under constantly changing physiologic conditions. Successful insulin therapy of type 2 diabetes requires caloric restriction; whereas, successful insulin therapy of type 1 diabetes often requires regularity in timing and amount of ingested calories.

## Pharmacokinetics

Estimates of the time of onset and duration of action of insulin formulations (Table 9-4) have been derived in studies of healthy volunteers under standardized conditions (see Owens 1986 and Binder and Brange 1997 for review). A number of factors may lead to error in extrap-

**Table 9-5 Factors Influencing Therapeutic Goals in Diabetes**

| | |
|---|---|
| Behavioral issues | Is the patient willing and able to monitor blood sugar?<br>Is the patient willing/able to adhere to a diet regimen?<br>Is the patient's lifestyle stable, or does the therapeutic regimen need to accommodate high day-to-day variability? |
| Caloric intake | What is the patient's daily meal schedule?<br>What amount of calories is being ingested at each meal? |
| Activity | Are there episodes of activity that preempt scheduled food or insulin?<br>Are there activities that may alter insulin absorption (exercise) or pose increased risk of hypoglycemia? |
| Insulin injection method | Are insulin injection sites free of scars and rotated regularly?<br>Is there consistency in the use of abdominal or limb sites?<br>If limb sites are used, does the patient exercise after injection?<br>Is the injection technique consistent? |
| Intrinsic variability | Is there high variability in blood sugar control that is seemingly unrelated to other variables? |

olation of mean pharmacokinetic parameters to clinical practice in diabetic patients (Table 9-6). Doses of insulin that have significant pharmacologic effects in lean type 1 diabetics may be ineffective in insulin-resistant type 2 diabetic patients. Even among patients with the same type of diabetes, differences in diet, activity, insulin absorption, insulin resistance, and therapeutic compliance result in variable responses to insulin treatment.

Because of the complexity of insulin therapeutics, therapeutic (blood glucose) monitoring is the cornerstone of insulin therapy. For patients in whom tight glycemic control is feasible, changes in insulin regimen should be assessed by collection of a seven-point glycemic profile on several occasions (Figure 9-2). Optimal glycemic control is defined as fasting blood glucose of 80–120 mg/dL, with 2-hour postprandial glucose concentrations <180 mg/dL. If fasting euglycemia is achieved without adequate control of meal-related glucose excursion, monomeric insulin analogs may be preferred to regular insulin. In addition to the daily glucose profile, patients should check 2:00–3:00AM glucose concentrations on several occasions after any adjustment in the insulin regimen. After the patient achieves optimal glucose control on a stable insulin regimen, only fasting and premeal glucose measurements are required, in order to select the dose of short-acting insulin to be administered with each meal. Common scenarios requiring adjustment of the insulin regimen are depicted in Table 9-7.

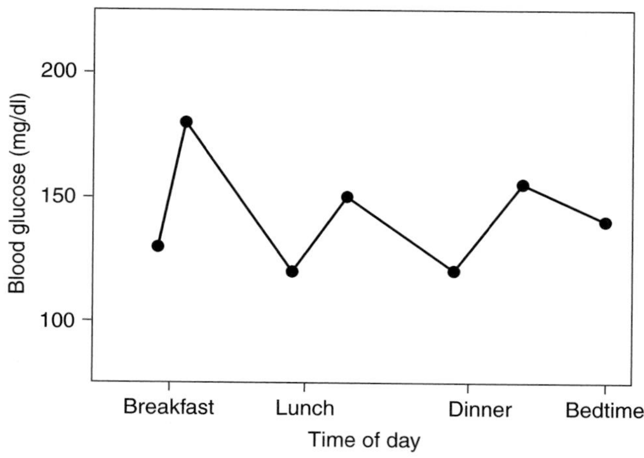


FIGURE 9-2 **The seven-point glycemic profile.**

## Adverse Effects

Insulin therapy is associated with manageable adverse effects (Table 9-8). Primary among these is hypoglycemia, which is managed by optimal insulin dosing, blood glucose monitoring, and education of patients and family members. All insulin-treated diabetic patients and family members should be instructed in the recognition of hypoglycemia, the use of sugar or glucose tablets (when the patient is conscious), and the Glucagon Emergency Kit (when the patient is unconscious or uncooperative). The occurrence of episodes of hypoglycemia, at present, is an inevitable event in patients whose diabetic control is adequate to forestall serious diabetic complications. In patients who can recognize the symptoms of hypoglycemia and are trained to respond appropriately, insulin therapy should not lead to restrictions in job or daily activities. Fear of hypoglycemia should not be allowed to interfere with the goals of optimal blood glucose control.

Other adverse effects of insulin therapy are rarely encountered. Lipohypertrophy is a benign proliferation of subcutaneous adipose tissue that occurs at injection sites because of an anabolic effect of insulin. It is rarely disfiguring and usually remits after injections are rotated to other sites of injection. Lipoatrophy is a cosmetically dis-

Table 9-6 **Factors Influencing the Efficacy of Insulin Therapy**

| VARIABLE | CLINICAL RELEVANCE |
|---|---|
| Insulin sensitivity | Insulin is less potent in insulin-resistant patients |
| Endogenous insulin | A dose of insulin has less incremental impact when insulin concentrations are high before dosing (e.g., insulin-resistant type 2 patients, or patients treated with large doses of long-acting insulin) |
| Absorption site | Insulin is more rapidly absorbed from the abdomen than from limb injection sites |
| Skin perfusion | Exercise increases skin perfusion and absorption rate, especially from limb injection sites. Dehydration (e.g., diabetic ketoacidosis or hyperosmolar crisis) decreases absorption rate. |
| Insulin antibodies | May prolong the time course of insulin action by acting as binding proteins and reducing clearance |
| Caloric intake | The therapeutic effect of insulin varies with the amount and rate of delivery of calories |
| GI function | Autonomic neuropathy may produce irregular delivery of calories despite standard meal size |

Table 9-7 Clinical Scenarios in Adjustment of Insulin Therapy

| GLUCOSE DATA | CAUSE | THERAPEUTIC OPTIONS | GOAL |
|---|---|---|---|
| Fasting morning hyperglycemia | Inadequate morning insulin | Increase dose of evening NPH, Lente, or Ultralente<br>Take insulin at bedtime | Fasting morning BG 80–120 |
| Fasting morning euglycemia with hypoglycemia early in the day | Inadequate breakfast calories<br>Protracted effect of bedtime insulin dose | Shift lunch or dinner calories to breakfast. Decrease PM insulin dose | |
| Nocturnal or fasting morning hypoglycemia | Excessive nocturnal insulin | Reduce PM NPH, Lente<br>Bedtime snack<br>Change PM insulin from dinner to bedtime | Bedtime BG 100–140 mg/dL |
| Fasting morning euglycemia with daytime hyperglycemia | Inadequate daytime or meal-related insulin | Increase morning NPH/Lente<br>"Split-mixed" regular/monomeric insulin + NPH/Lente/Ultralente twice per day<br>Multiple daily injection with rapid-acting insulin (at each meal) and Ultralente (morning and/or bedtime) | Preprandial BG 80–120 mg/dL before lunch and dinner; 2-hour postprandial BG <180 mg/dL |
| Fasting morning euglycemia with daytime or evening hypoglycemia | Excessive daytime insulin due to "peak effect" of NPH, Lente or human Ultralente, or protracted action of regular insulin | Administer smaller doses of long-acting insulin twice per day<br>Reduce regular insulin or change to monomeric insulin | |
| Preprandial euglycemia with daytime hypoglycemia | Excessive effect of rapid-acting insulin at meals | Decrease rapid-acting insulin<br>Check timing of regular insulin administration<br>Replace regular with monomeric insulin | |

ABBREVIATIONS: BG, blood glucose; NPH, Neutral protamine Hagedorn.

figuring atrophy of subcutaneous tissues that is largely due to immunologic response to impurities in insulin preparations. It is rarely encountered with human insulin. Autoantibodies to insulin were frequently encountered during the era of animal insulins and were rarely of clinical significance. The rare occurrence of a high titer of antibodies with high avidity may reduce the bioavailability of injected insulin and require higher doses. In rare cases of immunologically mediated insulin resistance requiring very high doses of insulin to control blood glucoses, only human insulin should be used, and antibody titers usually decline in several months with prolonged exposure to insulin. Dissociation of insulin from binding autoantibodies during postabsorptive periods may cause hypoglycemia. Delayed hypersensitivity skin reactions to insulin are rarely encountered with human insulin and are diagnosed by skin testing. These reactions abate over time with continued exposure to human insulin.

Table 9-8 Adverse Effects of Insulin Therapy

| |
|---|
| Hypoglycemia |
| Lipohypertrophy |
| Insulin allergy |
| Insulin antibodies |
| Lipoatrophy |

## The Role of Insulin Therapy in Type 1 Diabetes

Insulin therapy in type 1 diabetes prevents hyperglycemic symptoms, prevents ketoacidosis, and reduces the incidence of microvascular and neuropathic complications of diabetes. The prospective, randomized Diabetes Control and Complications Trial (DCCT), conducted in the 1980s, has demonstrated that maintenance of near-normal blood glucose concentrations in type 1 diabetics by intensive insulin regimens is associated with approximately 50% reductions in the risk of retinopathy, nephropathy, and neuropathy, when compared with twice-daily insulin administration (The Diabetes Control and Complications Trial Research Group 1993a). This study was conducted in relatively young patients, where the incidence of macrovascular disease was too low to assess the impact of tight glucose control on cardiovascular endpoints. Fasting blood glucose concentrations and glycosylated hemoglobin $A_{1c}$ (Hb $A_{1c}$) concentrations in the control group were approximately 200 mg/dL and 9% compared with 140 mg/dL and 7% in the intensively treated group in the DCCT trial.

## Insulin Regimens in Type 1 Diabetes

The DCCT trial has demonstrated that the insulin regimen of choice in type 1 diabetes should be the most intensive regimen to which the patient will adhere. Unless the patient is unwilling or unable to pursue optimal glycemic control, insulin should be administered in multiple daily injections (MDI), that is, three or more injections per day. There are a variety of different regimens that can be used to provide an intensive insulin program consisting of three or more injections per day. These regimens can consist of regular or monomeric insulin before each meal along with intermediate- or long-acting insulin once (generally at bedtime) or twice per day, or regular or monomeric insulin before breakfast and dinner along with intermediate- or long-acting insulin twice per day (usually given before breakfast and bedtime). Nonobese type 1 diabetic patients typically require replacement of endogenous daily insulin production (approximately 0.5–1.0 units/kg of body weight) in divided insulin doses. Approximately 0.4–0.5 units/kg will be required in the form of intermediate- or long-acting insulin ("basal" insulin). When patients are taking regular or monomeric insulin before each meal, intermediate- or long-acting insulin can generally be administered at bedtime in order to achieve fasting euglycemia and to provide basal insulin needs. However, because human NPH or Lente insulin does not always provide adequate 24-hour basal insulin replacement, they sometimes must be given twice daily. When patients are not taking regular or monomeric insulin before each meal, intermediate- or long-acting insulin should be administered in order to provide the greatest effect during the hours of peak caloric consumption. With this type of regimen human NPH or Lente insulin should be administered twice daily with approximately two-thirds of the daily dose at the beginning of the day. Dose adjustments of intermediate- or long-acting insulin with these regimens should be made to achieve fasting morning and predinner euglycemia.

Regular or monomeric (lispro or aspart) insulin should be provided before each meal in doses sufficient to achieve 2-hour postprandial blood glucose concentrations <180 mg/dL. For patients following an intensive regimen with regular or monomeric insulin before each meal, it is useful for the patient to be able to calculate his or her required dose based on predefined relationships between the amount of insulin needed per amount of carbohydrate ingested to prevent significant postprandial hyperglycemia and the amount of additional insulin needed to correct any preprandial hyperglycemia that may exist. Regular insulin should be administered 30–45 minutes before eating, whereas monomeric insulin may be administered immediately before meals. In patients who are unable to assess postprandial blood glucose concentrations, adjustment of the morning dose of short-acting insulin should be based on prelunch glucose concentrations, adjustment of the lunch time dose of short-acting insulin should be based on predinner glucose concentrations, whereas adjustment of the evening dose of short-acting insulin should be based on prebedtime glucose concentrations. Although twice-daily "split-mixed" injections are a convenient form of insulin therapy, they do not constitute an intensive insulin regimen and may not control postprandial hyperglycemia at lunchtime. Afternoon hyperglycemia may be managed by reduction in midday caloric intake or the addition of short-acting insulin before lunch. The pharmacokinetic profile of different insulin regimens is presented in Figure 9-3. CSII is a suitable alternative to multiple daily injections for some type 1 diabetic pa-

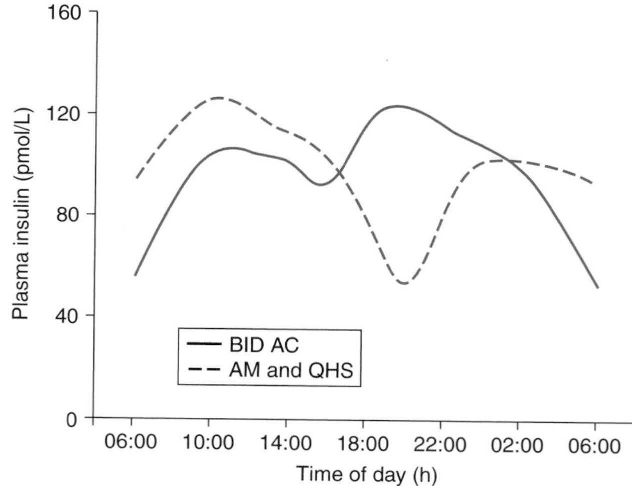


**FIGURE 9-3 The pharmacokinetic profile of different insulin regimens.**

tients. A period of inpatient monitoring is sometimes required to define the basal rate of insulin infusion. The size of meal-related insulin bolus doses can be adjusted as an outpatient under conditions of normal diet and activity. Meal-related insulin bolus doses should be calculated by the patient based on established requirements of the amount of insulin needed per amount of carbohydrate ingestion to prevent significant postprandial hyperglycemia and on the amount of insulin needed to correct any preprandial hyperglycemia that may exist.

### The Role of Insulin Therapy in Type 2 Diabetes

As with type 1 diabetes, the goal of insulin therapy in type 2 diabetes is to achieve near euglycemia. Therapeutic goals in type 2 diabetes have been assessed in several prospective clinical trials. The University Diabetes Group Program Trial (UDGP) in the 1960s failed to demonstrate a beneficial effect of insulin or oral hypoglycemic agents on morbidity and mortality in type 2 diabetes (Knatterud et al. 1978). Among several shortcomings of this study, the lack of home blood glucose monitoring at the time of this study limits its extrapolation to the current practice of insulin therapy. In a recent US Veteran's Hospital prospective study of intensive blood glucose control in type 2 diabetes (Abraira et al. 1997), approximately one-quarter of the participants experienced a major cardiovascular event (myocardial infarction, bypass surgery, coronary intervention, or cerebrovascular accident) during mean follow-up of 27 months, underscoring the importance of cardiovascular prevention in the therapeutic goals for type 2 diabetes. The United Kingdom Prospective Diabetes Study (UKPDS) has demonstrated the therapeutic benefit of improved glycemic control on microvascular endpoints in approximately 4000 type 2 diabetic patients followed for 10 years (United Kingdom Prospective Diabetes Study (UKPDS) Group 1998b). In contrast to the wide difference between conventional and intensive therapy in the DCCT, the UKPDS study achieved a smaller difference in glycemic control between treatment groups (0.9% difference in Hb $A_{1c}$), and the median Hb $A_{1c}$ was approximately 8.1% in the "intensively" treated group during the final years of the study. This study used relatively low doses of insulin and did not routinely implement multiple daily injections in insulin-treated patients. Despite the suboptimal glycemic control achieved in the UKPDS, treatment with insulin and/or sulfonylurea drugs resulted in a 25% reduction in the incidence of microvascular endpoints. The incidence of myocardial infarction was reduced by 16% in the intensively treated patients, although this was of borderline statistical significance. Insulin therapy was not significantly more efficacious than sulfonylurea agents, although this study utilized an "intention-to-treat" analysis, which may have minimized the differences in efficacy of specific therapies.

### Insulin Regimens in Type 2 Diabetes

One important observation in the UKPDS is that unless therapeutic interventions are escalated, glycemic control worsens with time in type 2 diabetes. Insulin therapy is the only treatment modality that can be increased to compensate for this time-related therapeutic failure; consequently, insulin is likely to be required in the optimal therapy of many patients with type 2 diabetes. Patients who have had type 2 diabetes for many years may not have sufficient residual $\beta$-cell function to respond to oral hypoglycemic agents, particularly sulfonylurea drugs. Approximately 10% of adult patients diagnosed with type 2 diabetes have a slowly progressive autoimmune destruction of the pancreatic islets and may develop weight loss and ketosis at some point. These patients are likely to require intensive insulin management similar to that of type 1 diabetes. In patients with inadequate glycemic control by other measures, insulin therapy may be initiated by administering 15–20 units of Ultralente, NPH, or Lente insulin at bedtime. The dose may be increased at weekly intervals to achieve fasting euglycemia in the morning. Daytime administration of metformin or other oral hypoglycemic agents may be continued, but if glycemic control deteriorates during the day, intermediate-acting or combined short-and intermediate-acting insulin should be administered twice daily, and the oral hypoglycemic agent should be discontinued. If a twice-a-day regimen of split-mixed insulin (regular or monomeric insulin combined with NPH or Lente) fails to achieve euglycemia, then an MDI schedule of basal and preprandial insulin (similar to type 1 regimens) should be used. The approach to interpretation of daily blood glucose monitoring and insulin dose adjustments is similar to that used in type 1 diabetes (Table 9-7).

## ORAL AGENTS

The initial therapy for all patients with type 2 diabetes mellitus is a program that combines dietary modification and exercise. Since most patients with type 2 diabetes mellitus are overweight, dietary modifications generally entail caloric restriction, which incorporates a reduction in the intake of saturated fat along with an increase in complex carbohydrates. Specific dietary recommendations, and the scientific bases on which they are founded, are beyond the scope of this chapter. The reader is referred to recent reviews on this topic (Franz et al. 1994; Ha and Lean 1998) for further information. Exercise is an important adjunct to dietary treatment and is associated with improvements in glucose control independent of changes in body weight. If patients are asymptomatic and have glucose values <300 mg/dL, a period of three to six months of dietary intervention should be undertaken before pharmacologic therapy is considered; however, for symptomatic patients or patients with glucose values ≥300 mg/dL, initiating drug therapy concurrently with dietary intervention is warranted. There are currently four different classes of oral agents, along with insulin, that can be considered for patients with type 2 diabetes mellitus. Because of their low cost and long history, sulfonylureas were long considered the first agents selected for use; however, results of recent long-term, randomized prospective studies suggest that metformin (biguanides) should be the preferred agent for initial therapy (see "Biguanides"). Nonetheless, it is important to realize that at present no specific guidelines exist for selecting oral agents.

## Sulfonylureas (Insulin Secretagogues)

### *History*

Sulfonylureas were the first oral drugs to be developed for use as hypoglycemics. The hypoglycemic activity of sulfonylureas was discovered during World War II when a French clinician, Marcel Janbon, noted that hypoglycemia developed in several patients in whom he was using a sulfonamide derivative to treat typhoid fever (Loubatières 1969). The effects of malnutrition and disease as potential causes of the hypoglycemia were excluded when the "sulfonylurea" was shown by Loubatières to induce hypoglycemia in normal dogs. Loubatières also noted that the sulfonylurea had no effect in pancreatectomized animals, leading him to hypothesize that the drug worked via increasing insulin secretion. Following these observations, thousands of derivatives of sulfonylureas were produced and studied in animals. The first sulfonylurea available for clinical use (carbutamide) was produced in 1955 in Germany. Shortly thereafter, several sulfonylureas became available for use in the United States, including tolbutamide, chlorpropamide, tolazamide, and acetohexamide. In 1984 glyburide and glipizide, "second-generation" sulfonylureas, were released, followed by glimepiride in the 1990s. Recently, a new insulin secretagogue, repaglinide, which is a non-sulfonylurea of the meglitinide class, has become available (Figure 9-4).

### *Mechanism of action*

Sulfonylureas and repaglinide lower glucose concentrations by stimulating the release of insulin from pancreatic $\beta$-cells. The mechanisms regulating insulin secretion are highly complex, with numerous factors influencing insulin secretion. Glucose is the most important secretagogue, but other substrates, such as amino acids, ketone bodies, and free fatty acids, also may increase insulin secretion. In addition, several hormones, such as glucagon, GLP-1 (glucagon like peptide-1), GIP (gastric inhibitory peptide), acetylcholine, and cholecystokinin, are potentiators of insulin secretion, whereas somatostatin and epinephrine inhibit insulin secretion. A simplified scheme depicting how insulin secretion is coupled to glucose and the step where sulfonylureas act is shown in Figure 9-5. Glucose is transported across the plasma membrane by GLUT2 glucose transporters and phosphorylated by glucokinase, the rate-limiting enzyme in glycolysis. The metabolism of glucose results in an increase in ATP concentrations. ATP then binds to a specific potassium channel decreasing its permeability (i.e., closing the channel). These ATP-sensitive potassium channels are the binding sites (sulfonylurea receptors) for sulfonylureas and repaglinide, although sulfonylureas and rapaglinide appear to bind to different regions of the sulfonylurea receptor. The interaction of these drugs with the sulfonylurea receptor also causes the potassium channels to close. The resulting change in potassium causes the membrane to depolarize, activating voltage-dependent calcium channels. The resulting influx of calcium ions raises the cytosolic concentration of calcium and triggers the exocytosis of insulin. Although a variety of extrapancreatic effects, such as alterations in several steps in the insulin signaling cascade, have been attributed to sulfonylureas, these effects appear to occur secondary to improvements in glucose control brought about by the primary action of sulfonylureas on pancreatic insulin secretion.

### *Pharmacokinetics*

Sulfonylureas and repaglinide are oral medications that are efficiently absorbed from the GI tract with peak blood concentrations occurring 1–4 hours after ingestion. All of the sulfonylureas and repaglinide are highly protein bound (90–99%). The metabolic elimination pathways differ among the drugs, giving rise to differences in half-lives. All of these agents are extensively metabolized by the liver, but have negligible hepatic first-pass metabolism. Tolbutamide has a half-life of 6–8 hours and is converted

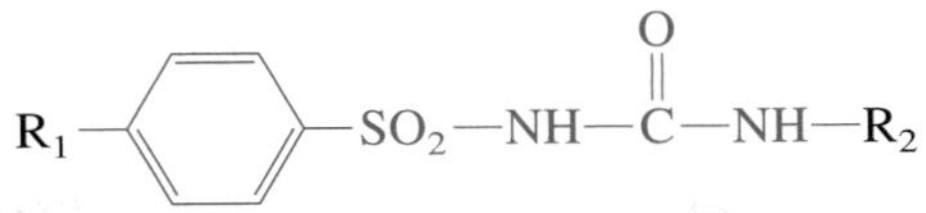

**Sulfonylurea**

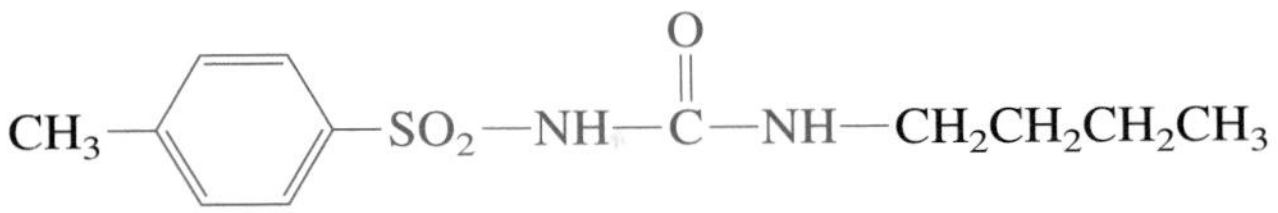

**Tolbutamide**

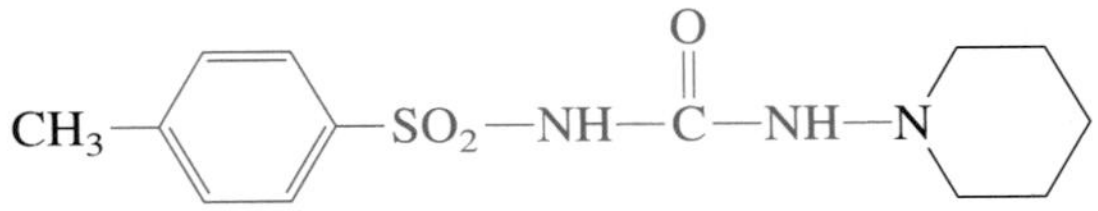

**Tolazamide**

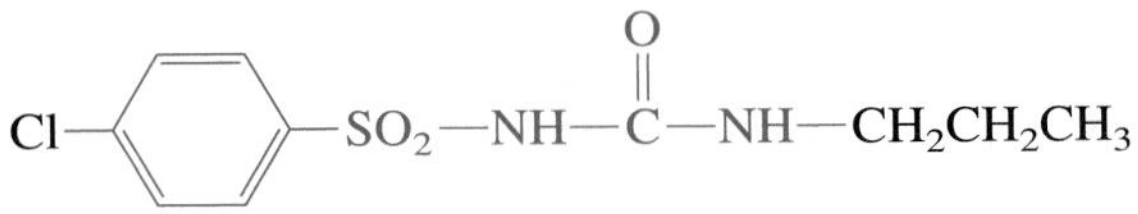

**Chlorpropamide**

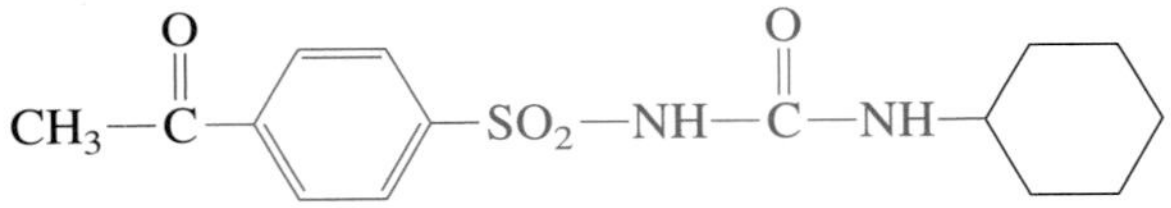

**Acetoheximide**

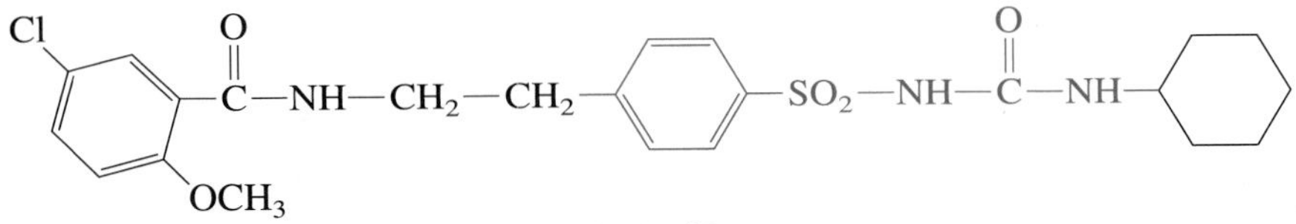

**Glyburide**

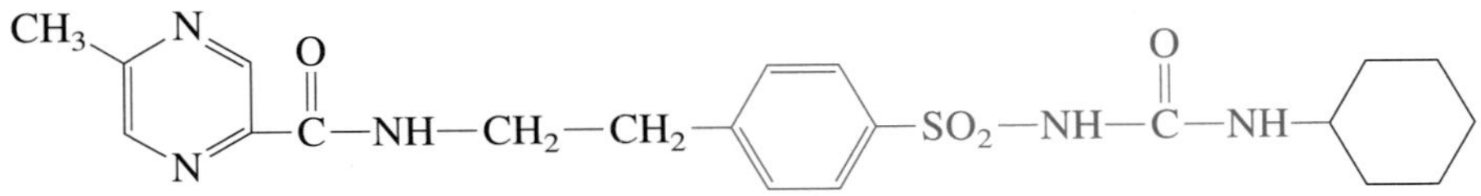

**Glipizide**

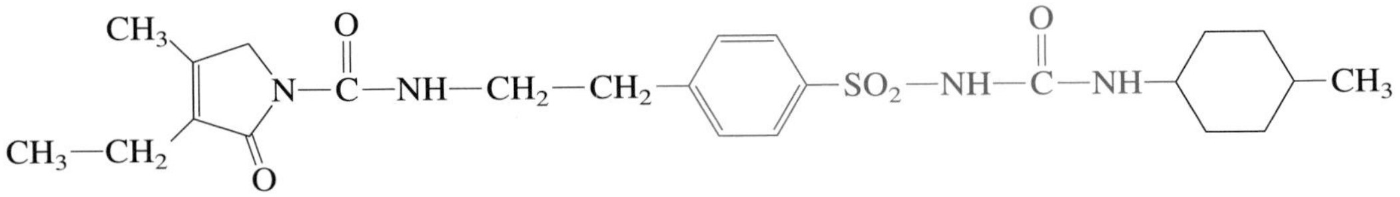

**Glimepiride**

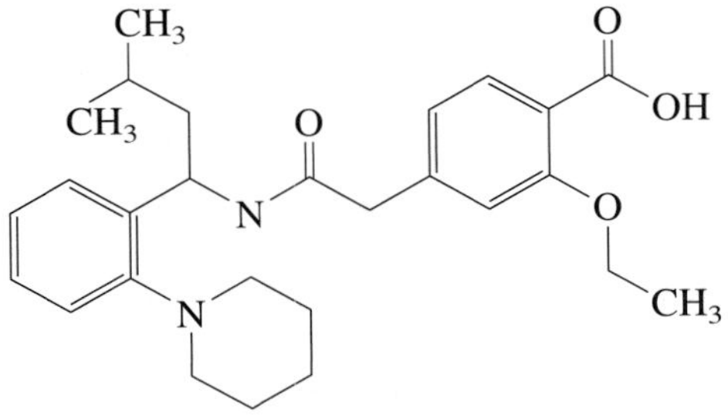

**Repaglinide**

FIGURE 9-4 **Chemical structure of insulin secretagogues.**

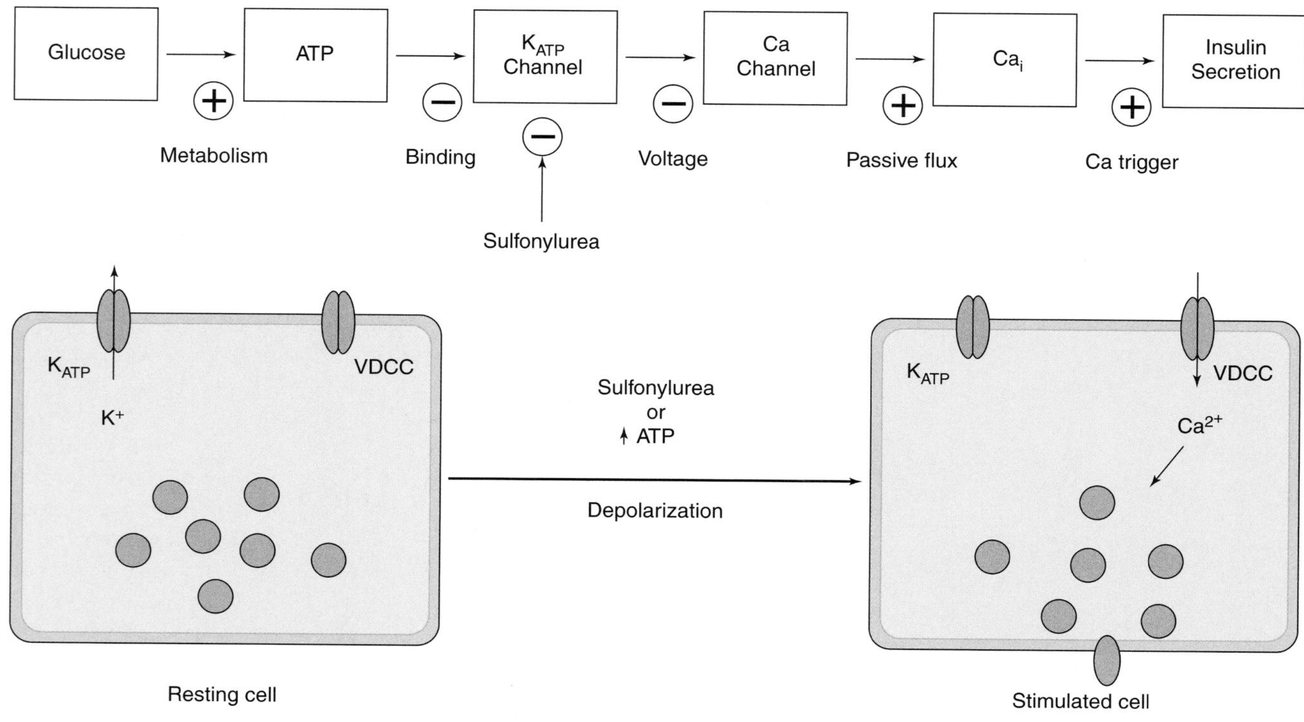


FIGURE 9-5 **Mechanism of insulin secretion.**

to inactive metabolites that are excreted by the kidneys; it has a dose range of 500–3000 mg per day divided into two or three doses. Tolazamide is metabolized to inactive metabolites. Tolazamide's half-life is ~6 hours. It has a dose range of 100–750 mg per day divided into two or three doses. Acetohexamide has a half-life of ~1.5 hours; however, its major metabolite hydroxyhexamide is two and a half times as potent as the parent compound and has a half-time of elimination of ~6 hours. Acetohexamide has a dose range of 500–1500 mg per day divided into two or three doses. Chlorpropamide has a half-life of 36 hours or longer, with 20% of the drug excreted in the urine unchanged; it has a dose range of 100–500 mg and is taken once per day. Glyburide is metabolized to inactive compounds that are excreted equally in bile and in urine. Glyburide's half-life is ~10 hours; however, its glucose-lowering effects can last up to 24 hours. Glyburide's dose range is 1.25–20 mg per day; it is taken once daily or divided into two doses for doses greater than 10 mg. Glipizide is predominantly metabolized to inactive compounds (10% excreted unchanged in the urine) and has a half-life of 2–4 hours, but can exhibit glucose-lowering effects for up to 24 hours; it has a dose range of 2.5–40 mg per day, with amounts greater than 15 mg taken in two daily doses. Glimepiride is completely metabolized to inactive compounds that are excreted in both urine and bile and has a half-time of elimination of 5–9 hours, but glucose-lowering effects are maintained for 24 hours. Glimepiride has a dose range of 1 to 12 mg; it is taken once per day. Repaglinide is completely converted to inactive metabolites that are eliminated by the kidneys. It has a half-life of 1 hour and a dose range of 0.5 to 4 mg preprandially, up to a maximum daily dose of 16 mg. In general, dose adjustments for sulfonylureas can be made every 1–2 weeks on the basis of glucose values.

### *Indications and efficacy*

Sulfonylureas and repaglinide are indicated in the treatment of patients with type 2 diabetes who do not respond adequately to a program of dietary modification and exercise. Although there are a large number of studies demonstrating the short-term efficacy of these agents in improving glucose control, there are few long-term randomized trials. One of the important randomized trials involving sulfonylureas was the University Group Diabetes Program (UGDP), which was conducted in the 1960s and early 1970s, in which patients with recent-onset (<1 year) type 2 diabetes were randomized to receive either placebo, tolbutamide at a fixed dose of 1500 mg daily, phenformin at 100 mg per day (see below), insulin at a fixed dose of 15 units daily, or insulin at a variable dose. UGDP was conducted before the advent of home glucose monitoring or glycosylated hemoglobin measurement; consequently, glucose control was assessed on the basis of fasting glucose values obtained 4 times per year. The primary endpoints examined by the UGDP were mortality and cardiovascular events. Tolbutamide initially decreased glucose values 24% compared with 13% for placebo (diet alone); however, after 4 years, glucose values had steadily risen to 7% higher than baseline as compared with 11.6% above baseline for the placebo group. The tolbutamide arm of the study was terminated early because of the observations that tolbutamide treatment appeared to be associated with an increase in cardiovascular mortality (12.7 vs. 4.9% placebo) and that it did not appear to be any more effective than diet therapy in controlling glucose values (The University Group Diabetes Program 1970; The University Group Diabetes Program 1976). Following the results of UGDP there was a decline in the use of sulfonylureas; however, a number of criticisms of the results and interpretation of UGDP emphasized the fact that the results should not be generalized to other drugs or to type 2 diabetics at large. As a consequence the use of sulfonylureas increased following the introduction of second-generation sulfonylureas.

Clinical data are clearly needed from a controlled trial that goes well beyond the serious limitations of the original UGDP study. The United Kingdom Prospective Diabetes Study (UKPDS) is an ongoing trial in which more than 4000 patients with newly diagnosed diabetes who had fasting glucoses 110–270 (mean Hb $A_{1c}$ 9.1% that fell to 7.2% after 3 months of diet before randomization) were randomized to diet alone, chlorpropamide, glyburide, insulin, or metformin (for obese patients, see below). After 3 years of therapy, similar improvements in Hb $A_{1c}$ were seen with chlorpropamide, glyburide, insulin, and metformin when compared with diet alone; however, there was evidence for greater deterioration and worsened control in obese as compared with nonobese patients no matter which therapy was assigned (United Kingdom Prospective Diabetes Study Group 1995a). By 6 years of follow-up, there was continued deterioration in glucose control with Hb $A_{1c}$ rising to 7.1% in the patients treated with either sulfonylurea or insulin, but this remained lower than the 8.0% in the conventionally treated group (United Kingdom Prospective Diabetes Study Group 1995b; Turner et al. 1996; United Kingdom Prospective Diabetes Study Group 1998a). In other words, treatment of patients with type 2 diabetes with sulfonylureas is associated with improvements in glucose control, but there is a tendency for glucose control to worsen over time no matter what therapy is used. It is interesting that when clinical outcomes were evaluated after 10 years of follow-up, patients assigned intensive management with chlorpropamide, glyburide, or insulin had statistically significant reductions in diabetes-related endpoints primarily because of a 25% reduction in microvascular endpoints, such as retinopathy and neuropathy (United Kingdom Prospective Diabetes Study Group 1998b). In contrast to the results of the UGDP study, there was no increase in mortality in sulfonylurea-treated patients; rather, there was a reduction in diabetes-related and all-cause mortality that did not reach statistical significance. No differences in glucose control or in outcomes were observed among patients assigned chlorpropamide, glyburide, or insulin; however, patients assigned insulin gained significantly more weight. Therefore, UKPDS has shown that sulfonylureas are safe and effective agents for treating patients with type 2 diabetes, reducing the development of complications without statistically impacting mortality.

In addition to their use as monotherapy, sulfonylureas can be used in combination with a variety of other hypoglycemic agents. For example, the combination of a sulfonylurea with metformin (see below) is more effective in lowering glucose values below those achieved with either agent alone (Hermann et al. 1994; DeFronzo et al. 1995). Likewise, the use of a sulfonylurea in combination with an $\alpha$-glucosidase inhibitor (see "$\alpha$-Glucosidase inhibitors") or with a thiazolidinedione (see "Thiazolidinediones") has been shown to be more effective than either agent given alone in lowering glucose values (Chiasson et al. 1994; Iwamoto et al. 1996). In addition, sulfonylureas have been used in combination with insulin, although only glimepiride is currently approved by the US Food and Drug Administration (FDA) for use in combination with insulin. Most studies that have examined the efficacy of the combination of a sulfonylurea with insulin have found that combined insulin-sulfonylurea therapy leads to similar or slightly improved glucose control compared with insulin alone (Pugh et al. 1992; Ykijarvinen et al. 1992; Clauson et al. 1996). This comparable degree of glucose control is achieved at lower doses of insulin and usually with the convenience of a single daily injection of insulin and with less weight gain.

Sulfonylureas have not been studied in women during pregnancy. Although studies in animals have shown no teratogenicity of sulfonylureas, sulfonylureas are not recommended during pregnancy. Since sulfonylureas are excreted in breast milk, they should not be used during lactation. In addition, the safety and effectiveness of sulfonylureas have not been studied in children, and their use in children should be avoided.

***Adverse effects and drug interactions***

Sulfonylureas are very well tolerated medications, with a generally low incidence of adverse effects. The second-generation and newer agents tend to have a lower incidence of adverse effects. The most common adverse effect observed with sulfonylureas is hypoglycemia, which occurs in 1–3% of patients treated with sulfonylureas. Mild hypoglycemia can be treated with oral glucose and adjustment of the dose of the sulfonylurea; however, severe hypoglycemia, which is defined as neurologic impairment with or without coma or seizures, requires emergency treatment. Emergency treatment of severe hypoglycemia usually consists of one to two ampules of 50% glucose solution, followed by a continuous infusion of 5–10% glucose for 24–48 hours or longer as required, given the long half-lives of the sulfonylureas. The hypoglycemic action of the sulfonylureas is potentiated by a variety of agents that are also highly protein bound, such as nonsteroidal anti-inflammatory agents, salicylates, warfarin, probenecid, monoamine oxidase inhibitors, and sulfonamides. As opposed to potentiating the hypoglycemic actions of sulfonylureas, many drugs may tend to cause hyperglycemia, such as corticosteroids, thyroid hormone, estrogens, phenytoin, niacin, and isoniazid. Withdrawal of any of these hyperglycemic agents can be associated with the development of hypoglycemia in patients treated with sulfonylureas.

Gastrointestinal adverse effects associated with sulfonylureas include cholestatic jaundice, nausea, vomiting, diarrhea, and anorexia. These occur in less than 1–5% of patients treated with sulfonylureas. Similarly, allergic reactions or skin rashes are observed in <1% of subjects. Although seen with several different sulfonylureas, the syndrome of inappropriate antidiuretic hormone with hyponatremia and a disulfiram-like reaction to alcohol are primarily observed with chlorpropamide.

## Biguanides

***History***

Although sulfonylureas were the first drugs commercially developed as oral hypoglycemic agents, biguanides or their parent compound, guanidine, found in the plant *Galega officinalis* (goat's rue or French honeysuckle), have been used since medieval times for the treatment of diabetes in southern and eastern Europe (Bailey and Day 1989). Guanidine was shown to be the active chemical responsible for the hypoglycemic properties of the French lilac in the early part of the twentieth century, but guanidine proved too toxic to give to humans. Several guanidine derivatives and biguanides were synthesized and evaluated in the 1920s, but not pursued (Bailey 1992). Following the development of sulfonylureas in the 1950s, two active biguanides were developed in the late 1950s, phenformin or phenethylbiguanide and metformin or dimethylbiguanide (Figure 9-6). Phenformin was the only biguanide initially available in the United States; however, it was withdrawn from clinical use in the 1970s after the UGDP study reported an increase in the incidence of lactic acidosis and an excess all-cause and cardiovascular mortality in patients treated with phenformin (The University Group Diabetes Program 1971). Although available and widely used in Europe, metformin did not become available in the United States until 1995 and is the only biguanide currently used in clinical practice.

***Mechanism of action***

In contrast to sulfonylureas, metformin exerts its glucose-lowering actions independent of any effects on insulin secretion. Indeed, serum insulin concentrations are unchanged or decreased by metformin. Because its effects are not mediated by increases in insulin secretion, a wide variety of mechanisms have been proposed to explain the glucose-lowering effects of metformin (Bailey and Turner 1996). Most of the action of metformin in decreasing plasma glucose values appears to be due to an inhibition of basal hepatic glucose production, which is abnormally elevated in patients with type 2 diabetes mellitus. The

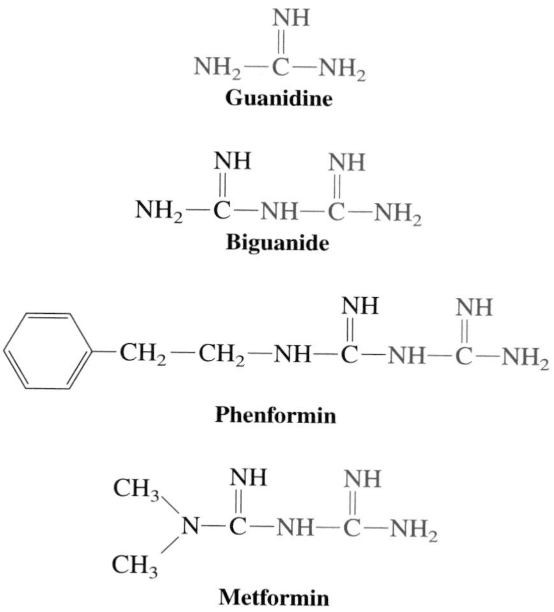

$NH_2—C(=NH)—NH_2$

**Guanidine**

$NH_2—C(=NH)—NH—C(=NH)—NH_2$

**Biguanide**

$C_6H_5—CH_2—CH_2—NH—C(=NH)—NH—C(=NH)—NH_2$

**Phenformin**

$(CH_3)_2N—C(=NH)—NH—C(=NH)—NH_2$

**Metformin**

FIGURE 9-6 **Chemical structure of biguanides.**

molecular mechanism through which metformin lowers hepatic glucose production is not understood. In addition to its effects on hepatic glucose production, metformin has been reported to improve peripheral sensitivity to insulin, that is, insulin-mediated glucose uptake, in muscle and adipose tissue in some, but not all, studies (Bailey 1992; Inzucchi et al. 1998). This improvement in insulin sensitivity is of a smaller magnitude than the reduction in hepatic glucose production, and, although several steps in the insulin signaling cascade—including increases in insulin receptors and improvements in post receptor events—have been shown to be favorably affected by metformin (Bailey 1992), it is not clear whether these changes are direct effects of metformin on the tissues or whether they are secondary to improvements in glucose control. Metformin also slows the rate of glucose absorption from the intestine, although overall absorption of glucose is not altered, an action that may contribute to the effects of metformin on lowering postprandial glucose values. Free fatty acid concentrations and fatty acid oxidation are decreased by metformin; these changes could also contribute to its glucose-lowering effects by means of the glucose–fatty acid cycle.

***Pharmacokinetics***

Metformin is an oral medication that is 50–60% bioavailable following a single oral dose. Although its absorption is decreased when it is administered with food, the clinical relevance of this effect is unclear since administration with food is often able to overcome some of the adverse gastrointestinal events associated with metformin (see below). Steady-state plasma concentrations of metformin are achieved in 24–48 hours. Metformin has a half-life in plasma of ~6 hours and a half-life in blood of ~17 hours; this longer elimination time from blood reflects the distribution of metformin into red blood cells. Metformin is negligibly bound by plasma proteins and does not undergo any hepatic metabolism or biliary excretion. It is excreted unchanged by the kidneys, where its clearance is 3–4 times that of the glomerular filtration rate, suggesting the involvement of renal tubular secretion and providing a basis for the development of adverse effects associated with renal impairment (see below). Metformin is supplied as 500 mg, 850 mg, and 1000 mg tablets, and is administered twice or three times daily with meals up to a maximal dose of 2.55 g per day. Dose adjustments of metformin should not be made more frequently than every 2 weeks.

***Indications and efficacy***

Metformin is indicated in the treatment of patients with type 2 diabetes who do not respond adequately to a program of dietary modification and exercise. Although there are a large number of studies demonstrating the short-term efficacy of metformin and biguanides in improving glucose control, there are few long-term randomized trials. One of the important randomized trials involving biguanides was the University Group Diabetes Program (UGDP) in which patients with recent onset (<1 year) type 2 diabetes were randomized to receive a placebo, tolbutamide at a fixed dose of 1500 mg daily (see above), phenformin at 100 mg per day, insulin at a fixed dose of 15 units daily, or insulin at a variable dose. The phenformin arm of the trial was terminated early because of an observed increase in the incidence of lactic acidosis and an excess all-cause and cardiovascular mortality in patients treated with phenformin (The University Group Diabetes Program 1971). Clearly, the results of UGDP led to dramatic changes in the treatment of type 2 diabetes in the United States and the removal of phenformin from clinical use. Likewise, the results of the recently reported United Kingdom Prospective Diabetes Study (UKPDS) will probably alter the way in which type 2 diabetes is managed. Among the patients in UKPDS, ~1700 were overweight and were randomized to diet alone, metformin, glyburide, chlorpropamide, or insulin. Similar improvements in Hb $A_{1c}$ were seen with chlorpropamide, glyburide, insulin, and metformin when compared with diet alone; however, there was evidence for deterioration and worsened control over time in all patients no matter which therapy was assigned (United Kingdom Prospective Diabetes Study (UKPDS) Group 1995a). Although patients allocated to metformin showed no statistically significant impact on microvascular endpoints, patients initially allocated to metformin had a highly significant 42% reduction in diabetes-related mortality and a 36% reduction in all-cause mortality when compared with conventional (diet) therapy or to sulfonylurea or insulin therapy (United Kingdom Prospective Diabetes Study (UKPDS) Group 1998c). These results of UKPDS suggest that metformin should be considered to be the initial oral agent selected for the treatment of patients with type 2 diabetes who do not respond adequately to a program of dietary modification and exercise.

In addition to its use as monotherapy, metformin can be used in combination with a variety of other hypoglycemic agents. The combination of metformin with a sulfonylurea (see above) is more effective in lowering glucose values below that achieved with either agent alone (Hermann et al. 1994; DeFronzo et al. 1995). Nonetheless, it should be noted that in UKPDS the early addition of metformin to patients who had inadequate therapeutic responses to sulfonylureas was associated with an increase in diabetes-related mortality compared with sulfonylurea therapy alone; however, the clinical significance of this finding is unclear since no increased diabetes-related mortality was observed when an analysis of all patients within UKPDS who received a combination of metformin and sulfonylurea was performed (United Kingdom Prospective Diabetes Study (UKPDS) Group 1998c). The use of metformin in combination with an $\alpha$-glucosidase inhibitor (see "$\alpha$-Glucosidase Inhibitors") or with a thiazolidinedione (see "Thiazolidinediones") has been shown to be more effective than either agent given alone in lowering glucose values (Chiasson et al. 1994; Inzucchi et al. 1998). Although not currently approved by the FDA, metformin can be used in combination with insulin, with a reduction in insulin requirements and improved glucose control.

Besides its favorable effects on glucose control, metformin therapy results in improvements in plasma lipid and lipoprotein concentrations. Metformin results in reductions in total cholesterol, LDL cholesterol, and triglyceride values, along with favorable increases in high-density lipoprotein (HDL) cholesterol concentrations that are not observed with sulfonylurea therapy (DeFronzo et al. 1995). Metformin is not associated with weight gain, as is often seen with sulfonylureas, thiazolidinediones or insulin; rather, weight loss may occur.

Metformin has not been studied in women during pregnancy. Although studies in animals have shown no teratogenicity, it is not recommended during pregnancy. Since metformin is excreted in breast milk, it should not be used during lactation. In addition, the safety and effectiveness of metformin has not been studied in children, and its use in children should be avoided. Because of concerns and a propensity for the development of lactic acidosis (see below), metformin is contraindicated in patients with renal insufficiency (serum creatinine $\geq$1.5 mg/dL) and in patients who are predisposed to develop lactic acidosis, such as patients with severe congestive heart failure, patients with hepatic dysfunction, and patients who ingest excessive amounts of alcohol. Metformin is not indicated in the treatment of type I diabetes or in patients with diabetic ketoacidosis.

#### *Adverse effects and drug interactions*

Metformin is generally a well-tolerated medication. As opposed to sulfonylureas, metformin monotherapy is not associated with the development of hypoglycemia; however, when used in combination with other hypoglycemic agents, such as sulfonylureas, thiazolidinediones, and insulin, the incidence of hypoglycemia is increased by metformin. The most serious adverse effect associated with metformin therapy is lactic acidosis. The incidence of lactic acidosis associated with metformin is rare and is estimated to be ~0.03 per 1000 patient-years, which is 1/10 to 1/20 that seen with phenformin (Bailey and Turner 1996). When lactic acidosis develops in association with metformin, it has a mortality of ~50%. Most cases of lactic acidosis associated with metformin therapy have occurred in patients who have had significant renal insufficiency, or tissue hypoperfusion associated with severe congestive heart failure, myocardial infarction, respiratory failure, sepsis, dehydration, or surgery, or other serious conditions such as hepatic failure or alcohol intoxication. For these reasons metformin should be discontinued whenever there is an intervening serious illness. In addition, since metformin is exclusively excreted by the kidneys and renal dysfunction predisposes to lactic acidosis, metformin should be withheld before and for 48 hours after any intravenous dye studies or surgical procedures. If lactic acidosis develops in the setting of metformin therapy, metformin can be removed efficiently by hemodialysis (Gan et al. 1992).

Gastrointestinal symptoms, such as nausea, vomiting, anorexia, abdominal pain, and diarrhea, are the most common adverse effects with metformin, occurring in <5% of patients. The incidence of GI symptoms can be reduced by taking metformin with meals and initiating therapy at low doses, starting with a test dose of 500 mg with breakfast for 3 days and then increasing to 500 mg twice daily. Approximately 3% of patients develop a metallic taste while taking metformin. The incidence of allergic reactions or skin rashes is similar to placebo. Serum concentration of vitamin $B_{12}$ is reduced in ~9% of patients treated with metformin; but the development of anemia is very rare.

Because metformin is eliminated via renal tubular secretion, there is a theoretical possibility that other drugs that are secreted in a similar fashion, such as amiloride, cimetidine, ranitidine, triamterene, and trimethoprim, could interfere with the elimination of metformin; however, this does not appear to occur when examined directly, although studies are limited.

### $\alpha$-Glucosidase Inhibitors

#### *History*

Dietary carbohydrate requires enzymatic digestion by $\alpha$-glucosidases into monosaccharides within the gastrointestinal tract in order to be able to be absorbed. Since dietary carbohydrate ingestion results in postprandial hyperglycemia in patients with diabetes, investigators at Bayer AG began to search for inhibitors of $\alpha$-glucosidases in the late 1960s in an attempt to delay carbohydrate absorption and to mimic the effects of dieting on glucose control (Puls et al. 1977). The first active α-glucosidase inhibitor was isolated from wheat flour and, although it potently inhibited pancreatic α-amylase, it had little effect on carbohydrate absorption of cooked starch or a mixed meal. Following this, several other α-glucosidase inhibitors were isolated from microbial sources; these agents were found to have more potent effects on carbohydrate absorption, because they inhibited not only pancreatic α-amylase, but also brush border enzymes such as glucoamylase, dextrinase, maltase, and sucrase. The first compound found to have these actions and developed for clinical use was acarbose (Figure 9-7), a pseudotetrasaccharide isolated from *Actinoplanes utanhensis.* The second α-glucosidase inhibitor available for clinical use in the United States was miglitol, a deoxynojirimycin derivative, that is structurally related to monosaccharides.

### *Mechanism of action*

Since acarbose is structurally similar to oligosaccharides derived from starch digestion, it reversibly binds with high affinity to α-glucosidases, α-amylase, glucoamylase, dextrinase, maltase, and sucrase; however, the C-N linkage in acarbose cannot be cleaved by the α-glucosidase enzymes. Although structurally different from acarbose, miglitol displays similar enzyme kinetics except it has no effects on α-amylase. Acarbose and miglitol are reversible, competitive inhibitors of oligosaccharide digestion, primarily in the upper small intestine (Bischoff 1994). Undigested oligosaccharides are, however, digested in the distal ileum, as miglitol is absorbed proximally and acarbose is broken down by gut bacteria leading to less capacity to inhibit glucosidases in the distal ileum. Therefore, acarbose and miglitol result in a delay in the digestion of complex carbohydrates and a reduction in the rate of complex carbohydrate-derived glucose absorption. Acarbose has no effects on lactase activity; however, miglitol does inhibit lactase. Neither acarbose nor miglitol affects the absorption or transport of glucose by the intestine.

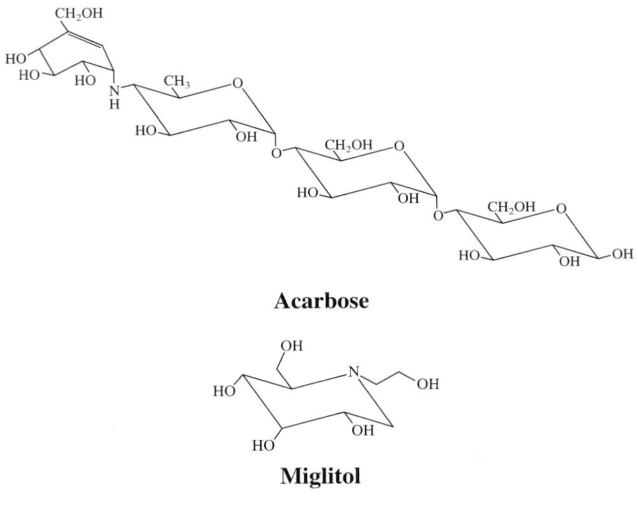

**FIGURE 9-7 Chemical structure of α-glucosidase inhibitors.**

### *Pharmacokinetics*

Acarbose (Precose) and miglitol (Glyset) exert their actions entirely within the intestinal tract. Acarbose displays very poor bioavailability; less than 2% of an oral dose of acarbose is absorbed from the gastrointestinal tract with peak plasma values attained at approximately 1 hour. In contrast, miglitol is completely absorbed at low doses with peak plasma values at 2–3 hours. Miglitol is not metabolized while acarbose is metabolized within the gastrointestinal tract by bacteria and intestinal enzymes to multiple products, at least one of which is metabolically active. Miglitol, nonmetabolized acarbose, and metabolic products that are absorbed are excreted entirely by the kidneys and have a half-time of elimination from plasma of ~2 hours. Therefore, serum concentrations of acarbose and miglitol will rise in patients with severe renal impairment. Acarbose and miglitol are supplied as 25-, 50-, and 100-mg tablets. The usual initial dose is 25 mg at the start of each meal, three times daily. The dose should be adjusted every 4–8 weeks up to a maximum of 100 mg with each meal.

### *Indications and efficacy*

α-Glucosidase inhibitor are indicated in the treatment of patients with type 2 diabetes who do not respond adequately to a program of dietary modification and exercise. No long-term trials examining diabetes outcomes have been conducted with α-glucosidase inhibitors; however, studies as long as one year in duration have been conducted to examine the efficacy of α-glucosidase inhibitors on glucose control (Chiasson et al. 1994; Hoffmann and Spengler 1997; Johnston et al. 1998). These studies have shown that use of inhibitors of α-glucosidase results in significant decrements in postprandial glucose excursions and reductions in fasting glucose and Hb $A_{1c}$ values; however, the improvement in Hb $A_{1c}$ values is generally of a smaller magnitude than seen with either sulfonylurea or metformin therapy. No effects of α-glucosidase inhibitors are observed on serum lipids or insulin concentrations. Because hypoglycemia is not associated with α-glucosidase inhibitor therapy, it has been suggested that α-glucosidase inhibitors might be preferable for use in elderly patients in whom the risk of complications from hypoglycemia is high. Nonetheless, based on available long-term intervention trials, $\alpha$-glucosidase inhibitors appear to be secondary agents for treating type 2 diabetics. $\alpha$-Glucosidase inhibitors are effective adjuvant therapy when used in combination with either a sulfonylurea, metformin, or insulin, resulting in further improvements in glucose control in patients not adequately controlled on their initial agent (Chiasson et al. 1994).

$\alpha$-Glucosidase inhibitors have not been studied in women during pregnancy. Although studies in animals have shown no teratogenicity, they are not recommended during pregnancy. Miglitol is excreted in breast milk and should not be used during lactation. In addition, the safety and effectiveness of $\alpha$-glucosidase inhibitors have not been studied in children, and their use in children should be avoided. $\alpha$-Glucosidase inhibitors are not indicated for use in patients with type 1 diabetes or with cirrhosis. In addition, they are contraindicated in patients with inflammatory bowel disease, partial intestinal obstruction, colonic ulcerations, or in patients with marked disorders of digestion or absorption.

#### *Adverse effects and drug interactions*

When given as monotherapy, $\alpha$-glucosidase inhibitors do not result in hypoglycemia; however, when administered in combination with other hypoglycemic agents, there is an increased potential for hypoglycemia. Furthermore, because of the mechanism of action of acarbose and miglitol to inhibit the hydrolysis of complex carbohydrates, neither complex carbohydrates nor sucrose are effective for treating episodes of hypoglycemia that occur in patients undergoing $\alpha$-glucosidase inhibitor therapy. However, since they have no effects on glucose transport in the intestine, they do not alter the absorption of dietary glucose. The most common adverse effects with $\alpha$-glucosidase inhibitors are gastrointestinal symptoms, including abdominal pain, diarrhea, and flatulence, with an incidence up to ~30% seen at the highest doses. An increase in serum transaminase values has been observed at doses higher than 100 mg three times daily, but the incidence of these abnormalities is not different from placebo at dosages within the recommended range. $\alpha$-Glucosidase inhibitors have not been described to interfere with the absorption of any other medications; however, the concomitant ingestion of intestinal enzymes will reduce the effectiveness of acarbose and miglitol.

## Thiazolidinediones

#### *History*

In searching for new compounds to enhance sensitivity to insulin, Fujita and colleagues synthesized a large number of hindered phenolic compounds with a thiazolidine ring, one of which, ciglitazone, was shown to improve insulin sensitivity and glucose and triglyceride concentrations in insulin-resistant rats and dogs (Fujita et al. 1983). Although ciglitazone was not further developed for clinical use because of unacceptable adverse effects, additional phenolic compounds with a thiazolidine ring were examined. One of these compounds, troglitazone (Figure 9-8), was synthesized to contain an $\alpha$-tocopherol moiety in order to combine an ability to inhibit lipid peroxidation with the hypolipidemic and hypoglycemic actions of the thiazolidine ring (Yoshioka et al. 1989). Troglitazone, rosiglitazone, and pioglitazone are currently available for clinical use in the United States.

#### *Mechanism of action*

Thiazolidinediones act as ligands for the peroxisomal-proliferator-activated receptor $\gamma$ (PPAR$\gamma$), a subtype of PPARs that comprise the family of thyroid/steroid hor-

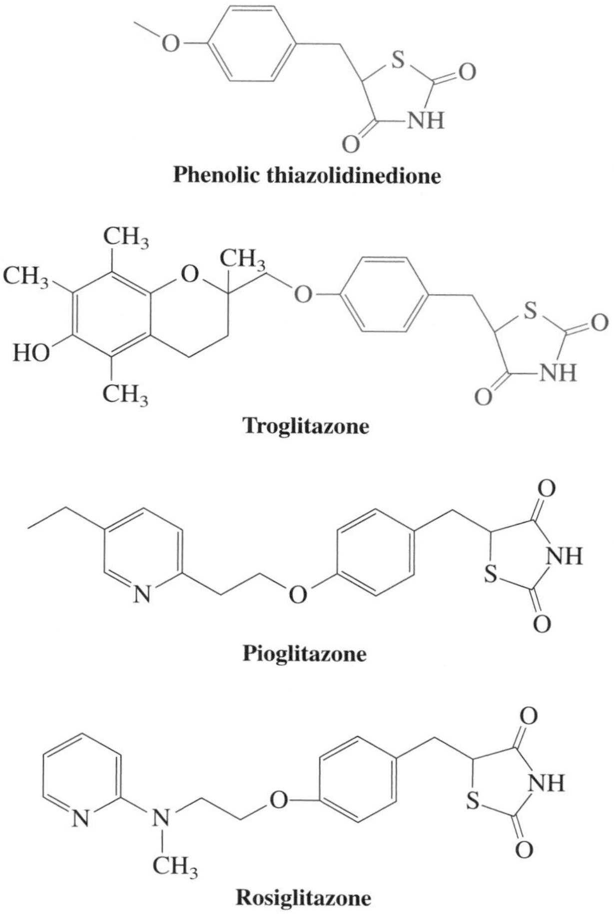

Phenolic thiazolidinedione

Troglitazone

Pioglitazone

Rosiglitazone

FIGURE 9-8 **Chemical structure of thiazolidinediones.**

mone receptors that act as nuclear transcription factors (Forman et al. 1996). Although the details are beyond the scope of this chapter, thiazolidinediones influence multiple steps in lipid and glucose metabolism by affecting the transcription of a variety of genes through activation of PPAR$\gamma$ in adipose tissue (Brun et al. 1997) and skeletal muscle. The major action of troglitazone is to enhance insulin sensitivity in peripheral tissues (Inzucchi et al. 1998; Henry 1997). It has no effects on glucose metabolism in the absence of insulin, and it does not affect insulin release by the pancreas. Thiazolidinediones do not appear to influence hepatic glucose production (Inzucchi et al. 1998).

***Pharmacokinetics***

Troglitazone is rapidly absorbed following oral administration, reaching a peak plasma concentration within 2–3 hours. The extent of absorption is increased by 30–85% when it is taken with food; consequently, it is recommended that troglitazone be taken with a meal to enhance drug availability. Steady-state plasma concentrations of troglitazone are achieved in 3–5 days, with a half-time of elimination from plasma of 16–34 hours. Troglitazone is highly bound by serum albumin (>99%) and is extensively metabolized by the liver (85%), accounting for the majority of metabolites of troglitazone being excreted in bile and recoverable in feces. Small amounts (3%) of metabolites are excreted by the kidneys, but excretion is not affected by changes in renal function. Troglitazone is supplied as tablets of 200, 300, and 400 mg. The usual initial dose for monotherapy is 400 mg per day, although 200 mg per day is recommended as the starting dose when troglitazone is being added as combination therapy. Dose adjustments can be made every 2–4 weeks up to a maximum daily dose of 600 mg.

Rosiglitazone is well absorbed with peak plasma concentrations appearing within one hour. Rosiglitazone may be administered without regard to meals. The usual starting dose is 4 mg per day. Therapeutic effects with twice daily dosing are similar to those with once daily dosing. Improvement in blood glucose values is slower than that observed with sufonylurea drugs. An increase to the maximum daily dose of 8 mg should be considered after 3–4 months if glycemic control is inadequate.

Pioglitazone is well absorbed with peak plasma concentrations appearing approximately 2 hours after dosing. Pioglitazone may be administered without regard to meals. Pioglitazone is extensively metabolized by cytochrome p450 pathways including CYP 3A4. The elimination half-lives of active metabolites of pioglitazone range from 16 to 24 hours. Pioglitazone and its metabolites are predominantly eliminated in the feces and renal impairment does not require dose adjustment. The usual starting dose of pioglitazone is 15–30 mg administered once daily. An increase to the maximum daily dose of 45 mg should be considered after 3–4 months if glycemic control is inadequate.

***Indications and efficacy***

Thiazolidinediones are indicated in the treatment of patients with type 2 diabetes who do not respond adequately to a program of dietary modification and exercise. Rosiglitazone and pioglitazone are indicated as monotherapy and as an additive therapy for patients poorly controlled with other hypoglycemic agents. In view of troglitazone's potential toxicity, it should be reserved for patients who have not responded adequately to other medications. No long-term trials examining diabetes outcomes have yet been reported with thiazolidinediones; however, studies lasting as long as 1 year have been conducted to examine the efficacy of troglitazone on glucose and lipid control (Inzucchi et al. 1998; Fonseca 1998). These studies have shown that use of troglitazone as monotherapy results in significant decrements in fasting glucose and Hb $A_{1c}$ values that are comparable to those seen with either sulfonylurea or metformin therapy. Placebo-controlled clinical trials conducted with rosiglitazone and pioglitazone in patients with poorly controlled diabetes report a mean maximal decrease in Hb $A_{1c}$ of 1.4 to 1.6% at the maximum doses. These changes correspond to mean decreases in fasting blood glucose of approximately 60 mg/dL. Efficacy may be slightly greater in monotherapy of patients who have not failed other therapies. Troglitazone therapy is also associated with a significant decrease in serum triglycerides and small increases in HDL, LDL, and total cholesterol concentrations. Serum insulin concentrations are decreased during thiazolidinedione therapy. In addition to their use as monotherapy, thiazolidinediones can be used in combination with other hypoglycemics, such as sulfonylureas, metformin, and insulin. In fact, troglitazone was originally approved for use only in patients with type 2 diabetes who were taking more than 30 units of insulin per day. When given to patients who are not adequately controlled with insulin, troglitazone therapy is associated with an improvement in Hb $A_{1c}$ values that occur while the daily dose of insulin is decreased (Schwartz et al. 1998). Similarly, a greater improvement in glucose control, as assessed by a fall in Hb $A_{1c}$ values, is observed when troglitazone is given in conjunction with either metformin (Inzucchi et al. 1998) or a sulfonylurea (Horton et al. 1998).

Thiazolidinediones have not been studied in women during pregnancy. Although studies in animals have shown no teratogenicity of thiazolidinediones, they are not recommended during pregnancy. It is not known whether thiazolidinediones are excreted in human breast milk; nonetheless, they should not be used during lactation. In addition, the safety and effectiveness of thiazolidinediones have not been studied in children, and their use in children should be avoided. Thiazolidinediones are not indicated for use in patients with type 1 diabetes. In addition, they are contraindicated in patients with hepatic dysfunction or active hepatic disease manifest by clinical or laboratory abnormalities of transaminases elevated above 3 times normal. Since troglitazone is associated with an increase in plasma volume (see below) and has been associated with cardiac enlargement in rodents, its use in patients with severe congestive heart failure is not recommended unless there is substantial evidence that its potential benefit would outweigh its risks.

In addition to their use in treating patients with type 2 diabetes, thiazolidinediones have been used and studied in patients with insulin resistance who do not have clinical diabetes mellitus. A particular group of insulin-resistant subjects who have been studied is women with polycystic ovary disease, who are characterized by menstrual irregularities with anovulation, androgen excess with hirsutism, hyperinsulinemia, and insulin resistance. The use of troglitazone in short-term trials in patients with polycystic ovary disease has resulted in significant improvements in insulin sensitivity with reductions in fasting hyperinsulinemia and serum androgen concentrations, and, in some women, a resumption of ovulatory cycles (Sattar et al. 1998). Therefore, women with polycystic ovary disease may constitute another indication for thiazolidinedione therapy. Furthermore, premenopausal women who are treated with thiazolidinediones should be cautioned regarding contraception because of the possibility of enhanced fertility.

***Adverse effects and drug interactions***

During controlled trials, the incidence of adverse symptoms associated with troglitazone was similar to that with placebo; however, 2.2% of patients treated with troglitazone were noted to have elevations in serum transaminases above three times normal compared to 0.6% of placebo treated patients. Several postmarketing cases of troglitazone-induced hepatic failure leading to liver transplantation or death have been reported. These cases appear to result from an idiosyncratic drug reaction causing severe hepatocellular injury. These reports led to the withdrawal of troglitazone from the market in the United Kingdom, although it continues to be an approved agent in the United States. Nonetheless, because of the concern for severe hepatic injury, it is recommended that patients begun on troglitazone have serum transaminases measured before therapy, monthly for the first 6 months of therapy, every 2 months for the next half year, and then periodically thereafter. Anyone taking troglitazone who develops signs or symptoms of hepatic dysfunction, nausea, vomiting, loss of appetite, or jaundice should have his or her liver function assessed. Troglitazone should be discontinued in anyone developing jaundice or displaying an elevation of serum transaminases above three times normal. In clinical trials, rosiglitazone and pioglitazone have not demonstrated rates of transaminase elevations which are greater than placebo. While severe hepatic injury has not been reported for these agents, the extent of clinical experience with these newer thiazolidinediones is less than that of troglitazone. The hypothesis that the lack of transaminase-elevating effects is predictive of overall hepatic safety remains to be confirmed. In addition to hepatic injury, thiazolidinediones may increase plasma volume 6–8%, which can be associated with edema, worsened congestive heart failure, and weight gain. A small decline in hemoglobin concentration and hematocrit can also be seen. When given as monotherapy, thiazolidinediones do not result in hypoglycemia; however, when administered in combination with other hypoglycemic agents, there is an increased potential for hypoglycemia.

Studies have suggested that troglitazone might induce the metabolism of other drugs by the 3A4 isozyme of the hepatic cytochrome P450 system. Agents that are metabolized by this metabolic pathway include amiodarone, astemizole, erythromycin, lansoprazole, omeprazole, loratadine, terfenadine, theophylline, cisapride, statins, steroids, and cyclosporine. Although troglitazone has only been shown to decrease plasma concentrations of terfenadine and oral contraceptives, it is likely that troglitazone could alter the effectiveness of any of these agents. Thus, in individuals receiving any of these agents, troglitazone should be prescribed cautiously. Rosiglitazone does not interact with the CYP 3A4 pathway; however, pioglitazone is metabolized by the CYP 3A4 pathway and its potential for adverse drug interaction via this metabolic pathway is not currently known.

## REFERENCES

Abraira C, Colwell J, Nuttall F, et al. 1997. Cardiovascular events and correlates in the Veterans Affairs Diabetes Feasibility Trial. Veterans Affairs Cooperative Study on Glycemic Control and Complications in Type II Diabetes. *Arch Int Med* **157**:181–8.

Anderson JH Jr, Brunelle RL, Keohane P, et al. 1997a. Mealtime treatment with insulin analog improves postprandial hyperglycemia and hypoglycemia in patients with non-insulin-dependent diabetes mellitus. Multicenter Insulin Lispro Study Group. *Arch Intern Med* **157**:1249–55.

Anderson JH Jr, Brunelle RL, Koivisto VA, et al. 1997b. Reduction of postprandial hyperglycemia and frequency of hypoglycemia in IDDM patients on insulin-analog treatment. Multicenter Insulin Lispro Study Group. *Diabetes* **46**:265–70.

American Diabetes Association. 1997a. Clinical practice recommendations 1997. *Diabetes Care* **20**(Suppl. 1):S1–70.

Bailey CJ. 1992. Biguanides and NIDDM. *Diabetes Care* **15**:755–72.

Bailey CJ, Day C. 1989. Traditional plant medicines as treatments for diabetes. *Diabetes Care* **12**:553–64.

Bailey CJ, Turner RC. 1996. Metformin. *N Engl J Med* **334**:574–9.

Banting FG. 1926. Diabetes and insulin. Nobel Prize Lecture, Stockholm 1925. *Can Med Assoc J* **16**:221–32.

Binder C, Brange J. 1996. Insulin chemistry and pharmacokinetics. In: Porte D, Sherwin RS, editors. *Ellenberg and Rifkins's Diabetes Mellitus: Theory and Practice.* Stamford, CT: Appleton & Lange. p 698–708.

Bischoff H. 1994. Pharmacology of α-glucosidase inhibition. *Eur J Clin Invest* **24**(Suppl. 3):3–10.

Brun RP, Kim JB, Hu E, et al. 1997. Peroxisome proliferator-activated receptor gamma and the control of adipogenesis. *Curr Opin Lipidol* **8**:212–18.

Chiasson JL, Josse RG, Hunt JA, et al. 1994. The efficiacy of acarbose in the treatment of patients with non-insulin-dependent diabetes mellitus. A multicenter controlled trial. *Ann Int Med* **121**:928–35.

Clauson P, Karlander S, Steen L, et al. 1996. Daytime glibenclamide and bedtime NPH insulin compared to intensive insulin treatment in secondary sulfonylurea failure: a 1-year follow-up. *Diabet Med* **13**:471–7.

DeFronzo RA, Goodman AM, et al. 1995. Efficacy of metformin in patients with non-insulin-dependent diabetes mellitus. Multicenter Metformin Study Group. *N Engl J Med* **333**:541–9.

Fonseca VA, Valiquett TR, Huang SM, et al. 1998. Troglitazone monotherapy improves glycemic control in patients with type 2 diabetes mellitus: a randomized, controlled study. The Troglitazone Study Group. *J Clin Endocrinol Metab* **83**:3169–76.

Forman BM, Chen J, Evans RM. 1996. The peroxisome proliferator-activated receptors: ligands and activators. *Ann N Y Acad Sci* **804**:266–75.

Franz MJ, Horton ES Sr, Bantle JP, et al. 1994. Nutrition principles for the management of diabetes and related complications. *Diabetes Care* **17**:490–518.

Fujita T, Sugiyama Y, Taketomi S, et al. 1983. Reduction of insulin resistance in obese and/or diabetic animals by 5-[4-(1-methylcyclohexylmethoxy)benzyl]-thiazolidine-2,4-dione (ADD-3878, U-63,287, ciglitazone), a new antidiabetic agent. *Diabetes* **32**:804–10.

Galloway JA, Spradlin CT, Nelson RL, et al. 1981. Factors influencing the absorption, serum insulin concentration, and blood glucose responses after injections of regular insulin and various insulin mixtures. *Diabetes Care* **4**:366–76.

Gan SC, Barr J, Arieff A, et al. 1992. Biguanide-associated lactic acidosis: case report and review of the literature. *Arch Int Med* **152**:2333–6.

Ha TK, Lean ME. 1998. Recommendations for the nutritional management of patients with diabetes mellitus. *Eur J Clin Nutr* **52**:467–81.

Henry RR. 1997. Thiazolidinediones. *Endocrinol Metab Clin North Am* **26**:553–73.

Hermann LS, Scherstén B, Bitzén P-O, et al. 1994. Therapeutic comparison of metformin and sulfonylurea, alone and in various combinations. *Diabetes Care* **17**:1100–9.

Hoffmann J, Spengler M. 1997. Efficacy of 24-week monotherapy with acarbose, metformin, or placebo in dietary-treated NIDDM patients: the Essen-II Study. *Am J Med* **103**:483–90.

Horton ES, Whitehouse F, Ghazzi MN, et al. 1998. Troglitazone in combination with sulfonylurea restores glycemic control in patients with type 2 diabetes. The Troglitazone Study Group. *Diabetes Care* **21**:1462–9.

Inzucchi SE, Maggs DG, Spollett GR, et al. 1998. Efficacy and metabolic effects of metformin and troglitazone in type II diabetes mellitus. *N Engl J Med* **338**:867–72.

Iwamoto Y, Kosaka K, Kuzuya T, et al. 1996. Effect of combination therapy of troglitazone and sulfonylureas in patients with type 2 diabetes who were poorly controlled by sulfonylurea therapy alone. *Diabet Med* **13**:365–70.

Johnston PS, Lebovitz HE, Coniff RF, et al. 1998. Advantages of α-glucosidase inhibition as monotherapy in elderly type 2 diabetic patients. *J Clin Endocrinol Metab* **83**:1515–22.

Knatterud GL, Klimt CR, Levin M, et al. 1978. Effects of hypoglycemic agents on vascular complications in patients with adult-onset diabetes. VII. Mortality and selected nonfatal events with insulin treatment. *JAMA.* **240**:37–42.

Loubatières A. 1969. The discovery of hypoglycemic sulfonamides and particularly of their action mechanism. *Acta Diabetol Lat* **6**(Suppl. 1):20–56.

Owens DR. 1986. *Human Insulin: Clinical Pharmacological Studies in Normal Man.* Lancaster, England: MTP Press Ltd.

Paulesco NC. 1924. Traitement du diabete. *La Presse Med* **32**:202–4.

Pugh JA, Wagner ML, Sawyer J, et al. 1992. Is combination sulfonylurea and insulin therapy useful in NIDDM patients?—a meta-analysis. *Diabetes Care* **15**:953–9.

Puls W, Keup U, Krause HP, et al. 1977. Glucosidase inhibition: a new approach to the treatment of diabetes, obesity and hyperlipoproteinemia. *Naturwissenschaften* **64**:536–7.

Report of the Expert Committee on the Diagnosis and Classification of Diabetes Mellitus. 1997b. *Diabetes Care* **20**:1183–97.

Sacks FM, Pfeffer MA, Moye LA, et al. 1996. The effect of pravastatin on coronary events after myocardial infarction in patients with average cholesterol levels. The Cholesterol and Recurrent Events Trial Investigators. *N Engl J Med* **335**:1001–9.

Sattar N, Hopkinson ZEC, Greer LA. 1998. Insulin-sensitising agents in polycystic-ovary syndrome. *Lancet* **351**:305–7.

Schwartz S, Raskin P, Fonseca V, et al. 1998. Effect of troglitazone in insulin-treated patients with type II diabetes mellitus. The Troglitazone and Exogenous Insulin Study Group. *N Engl J Med* **338**:861–6.

Second Report of the Expert Panel on Detection, Evaluation, and Treatment of High Blood Cholesterol in Adults (Adult Treatment Panel II). 1993b. Bethesda, MD, National Institutes of Health, National Heart, Lung, and Blood Institute. NIH Publication No. 93-3095, 180 pp.

The Diabetes Control and Complications Trial Research Group. 1993. The effect of intensive treatment of diabetes on the development and progression of long-term complications in insulin-dependent diabetes mellitus. *N Engl J Med* **329**:977–86.

The University Group Diabetes Program. 1970. A study of the effects of hypoglycemic agents on vascular complications in patients with adult-onset diabetes. II. Mortality results. *Diabetes* **19**:789–830.

The University Group Diabetes Program. 1971. Effects of hypoglycemic agents on vascular complications in patients with adult-onset diabetes. IV. A preliminary report on phenformin results. *JAMA* **217**:777–84.

The University Group Diabetes Program. 1976. A study of the effects of hypoglycemic agents on vascular complications in patients with adult-onset diabetes. VI. Supplementary report on nonfatal events in patients treated with tolbutamide. *Diabetes* **25**:29–53.

Turner R, Cuu C, Holman R. 1996. United Kingdom Prospective Diabetes Study (UKPDS). 17: a 9-year update of a randomized, controlled trial on the effect of improved metabolic control on complications in non-insulin-dependent diabetes mellitus. United Kingdom Prospective Diabetes Study Group. *Ann Int Med* **124**:136–45.

United Kingdom Prospective Diabetes Study (UKPDS) Group. 1995a. United Kingdom Prospective Diabetes Study (UKPDS). 13: Relative efficacy of randomly allocated diet, sulfonylurea, insulin, or metformin in patients with newly diagnosed non-insulin dependent diabetes followed for three years. *BMJ* **310**:83–8.

United Kingdom Prospective Diabetes Study (UKPDS) Group. 1995b. United Kingdom Prospective Diabetes Study (UKPDS). 16: overview of 6 years' therapy of type II diabetes: a progressive disease. *Diabetes* **44**:1249–58.

United Kingdom Prospective Diabetes Study (UKPDS) Group. 1998a. United Kingdom Prospective Diabetes Study (UKPDS) 24: a 6-year, randomized, controlled trial comparing sulfonylurea, insulin, and metformin therapy in patients with newly diagnosed type 2 diabetes that could not be controlled with diet. *Ann Int Med* **128**:165–75.

United Kingdom Prospective Diabetes Study (UKPDS) Group. 1998b. United Kingdom Prospective Diabetes Study (UKPDS). 33: Intensive blood-glucose control with sulfonylureas or insulin compared with conventional treatment and risk of complications in patients with type 2 diabetes (UKPDS 33). *Lancet* **352**:837–53.

United Kingdom Prospective Diabetes Study (UKPDS) Group. 1998c. Effect of intensive blood-glucose control with metformin on complications in overweight patients with type 2 diabetes (UKPDS 34). *Lancet* **352**:854–65.

Weir GC, Nathan DM, Singer DE. 1994. Standards of care for diabetes. *Diabetes Care* **17**:1514–22.

Ykijarvinen H, Kauppila M, Kujansuu E, et al. 1992. Comparison of insulin regimens in patients with non-insulin-dependent diabetes-mellitus. *N Engl J Med* **327**:1426–33.

Yoshioka T, Fijita T, Kanai T, et al. 1989. Studies on hindered phenols and analogues. 1. Hypolipidemic and hypoglycemic agents with ability to inhibit lipid peroxidation. *J Med Chem* **32**:421–8.

# Dyslipidemias

**Fredric B. Kraemer, Jeffrey W. Miller**

*Chapter Outline*



Lipoprotein and lipid abnormalities are disorders that commonly occur in the general population. There has been longstanding interest in lipid and lipoprotein metabolism since lipoproteins were first detected as constituents of normal plasma in the early twentieth century. This interest was further fueled by evidence suggesting an association between elevated cholesterol and risk of developing atherosclerosis. There have been many advances over the past 40 years in the understanding of the pathophysiologic bases of lipoprotein abnormalities. Results from epidemiological and interventional studies in humans linking hyperlipidemia to atherosclerosis have moved the treatment of lipid and lipoprotein disorders to the forefront in strategies of preventive medicine. This chapter reviews normal lipoprotein metabolism and the pathophysiology of lipoprotein disorders. Then, each class of drugs available for treatment of lipoprotein disorders is discussed in terms of its pharmacology and indications, with particular emphasis on efficacy demonstrated in clinical trials involving primary or secondary prevention of disease.

## THE LIPOPROTEINS

Lipoproteins are macromolecules that are responsible for transporting lipids (cholesteryl esters and triglycerides) from their sites of synthesis to their sites of utilization

(Scanu and Landsberger 1980) (see Fig. 9-9). All classes of lipoproteins share the same general structure, consisting of a core of nonpolar lipids (cholesteryl esters and triglycerides) surrounded by a monolayer of phospholipids, unesterified cholesterol, and various apolipoproteins. The apolipoproteins are essential for maintaining the structure of the lipoproteins and for directing the metabolism of the particle. The amphipathic properties (hydrophobic and hydrophilic orientation) of the phospholipid and apolipoprotein surface components allow the otherwise water-insoluble lipids to be transported in plasma.

Although the overall structure of lipoproteins is similar, differences in the chemical and apolipoprotein compositions of the particles result in the various classes of lipoproteins. Classification of lipoproteins is generally based on their physical properties and can be viewed as a continuous spectrum of particles with a progressively changing pattern of lipid and protein composition. Lipoproteins are conventionally separated by their densities during ultracentrifugation but also can be separated by electrophoresis or by size.

## Chylomicrons

Chylomicrons are derived from dietary lipids and are usually found in postprandial plasma only and not in the plasma of fasting normal subjects. Chylomicrons float in the cold without centrifugation, having a density <0.94 g/mL, and remain at the origin during electrophoresis (Table 9-9). They are the largest lipoproteins, ranging in diameter from 70 to 120 nm and larger.

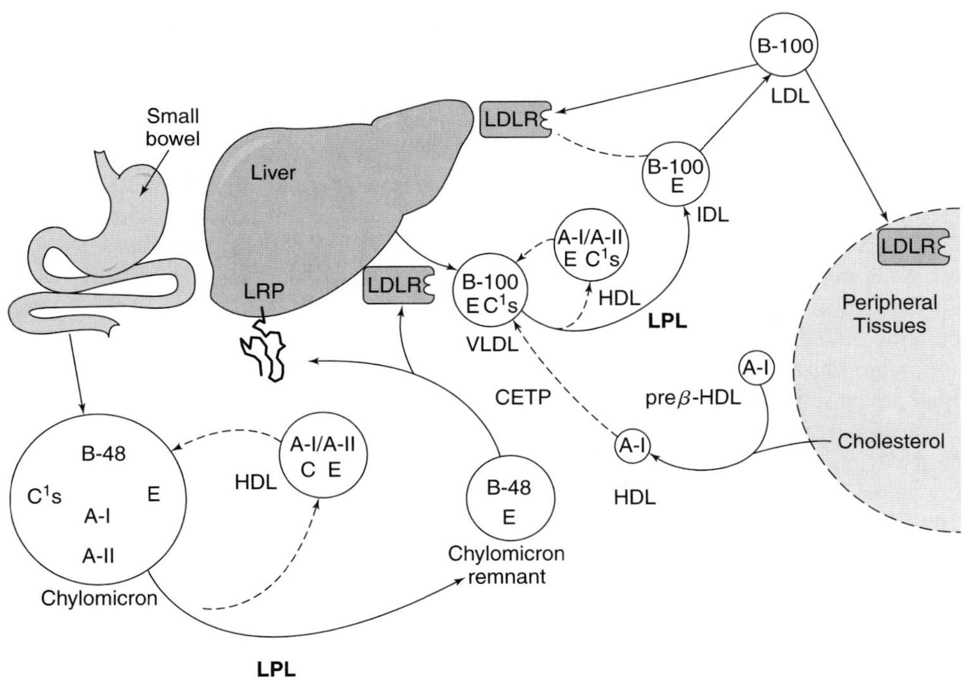


**FIGURE 9-9 Lipid metabolism.** ABBREVIATIONS: **A-I, A-II, apolipoproteins A-I and A-II; B-100, apolipoprotein B-100; B-48, apolipoprotein B-48; CETP, cholesteryl ester transfer protein; Cs, apolipoprotein Cs; E, apolipoprotein E; HDL, high-density lipoprotein; IDL, intermediate-density lipoprotein; LDL, low-density lipoprotein; LDLR, low-density lipoprotein receptor; LPL, lipoprotein lipase, LRP, low-density lipoprotein receptor-related protein; VLDL, very low density lipoprotein.**

Table 9-9 Lipoprotein Classification

| CLASS | ULTRACENTRIFUGAL DEFINITION | ELECTROPHORETIC DEFINITION | SIZE (NM) |
|---|---|---|---|
| *Major* | | | |
| Chylomicrons | $d < 0.94$ | Remain at origin | 70–120 |
| Very low density lipoproteins (VLDL) | $d < 1.006$ | pre-$\beta$ mobility | 30–70 |
| Intermediate-density lipoproteins (IDL) | $d = 1.006–1.019$ | $\beta$ mobility | 23–30 |
| Low-density lipoproteins (LDL) | $d = 1.019–1.063$ | $\beta$ mobility | 18–23 |
| High-density lipoproteins (HDL) | $d = 1.063–1.215$ | $\alpha$ mobility | 5–12 |
| *Minor* | | | |
| Lipoprotein(a) | | pre-$\beta$ mobility | 23–26 |
| $\beta$-Very low density lipoproteins ($\beta$-VLDL) | | $\beta$ mobility | 30–70 |

Chylomicrons are formed in the intestinal epithelial cells. Following hydrolysis of dietary lipids in the intestinal lumen, the absorbed fatty acids and cholesterol are reesterified in these cells to triglycerides and cholesterol esters and then packaged with polar lipids and structural apolipoproteins (B-48, AI, AII). Apolipoprotein B-48 is produced in the intestines and is found only in lipoproteins of intestinal origin in humans. Chylomicrons are lipoproteins that are very rich in triglycerides, consisting of 90 to 95% triglycerides and small amounts of cholesterol esters, unesterified cholesterol, phospholipids, and apolipoproteins (Table 9-10). Chylomicrons are initially secreted into lymph and then enter the peripheral circulation, where they acquire apolipoproteins E and C from circulating high-density lipoproteins (HDL). In the peripheral circulation, chylomicrons are acted on by lipoprotein lipase, an enzyme located on the surface of capillary endothelium. Lipoprotein lipase is activated by apolipoprotein CII and hydrolyzes the triglycerides of the chylomicrons, liberating free fatty acids.

During hydrolysis of the triglycerides, phospholipids and apolipoprotein C are lost from chylomicrons. The resulting particles (chylomicron remnants) are smaller, poor in triglycerides and apolipoprotein C, and rich in cholesteryl ester and apolipoprotein E, because other apolipoproteins and cholesteryl esters are not lost during hydrolysis by lipoprotein lipase. Chylomicron remnants are rapidly cleared from the circulation by parenchymal cells of the liver via recognition of apolipoprotein E by specific receptors (Cooper 1997).

## Very Low Density Lipoproteins

Whereas chylomicron production occurs in the intestine and depends on dietary fat intake, very low density lipoproteins (VLDL) are triglyceride-rich lipoproteins that are produced by the liver. VLDL are smaller than chylomicrons (range 30 to 70 nm), have a density <1.006 g/mL (the density of plasma), and exhibit pre-$\beta$ mobility on electrophoresis (Table 9-9). Although they are triglyceride-rich lipoproteins (50 to 60% triglyceride by weight), VLDL contain significant amounts of cholesteryl esters (15 to 20%), with the remainder consisting of phospholipid and apolipoproteins (Table 9-10).

Very low density lipoprotein production depends on the availability of substrate for triglyceride synthesis by the liver, that is, circulating free fatty acids or chylomicron triglyceride uptake. The newly synthesized triglycerides are packaged with cholesterol, phospholipids, and apolipoprotein B-100 (a large molecular weight apolipo-

Table 9-10 Composition of Lipoproteins

| LIPOPROTEIN | CHYLOMICRONS (%) | VLDL (%) | LDL (%) | HDL (%) |
|---|---|---|---|---|
| Triglyceride | 80–90[a] | 45–65 | 4–8 | 2–7 |
| Cholesteryl esters | 2–4 | 16–22 | 45–50 | 15–20 |
| Free cholesterol | 1–3 | 4–8 | 6–8 | 3–5 |
| Phospholipid | 3–6 | 15–20 | 18–24 | 26–32 |
| Protein | 1–2 | 6–10 | 18–22 | 45–55 |
| Apolipoprotein species | B-48, AI, AIV, CI, CII, CIII, E | B-100, CI, CII, CIII, E | B-100 | AI, AII, CI, CII, CIII, D, E |

[a]Percent by weight.

protein B synthesized exclusively by the liver in humans), apolipoprotein C, and apolipoprotein E. Following secretion, VLDL can be directly removed by the liver via low density lipoprotein (LDL) receptors (see below); alternatively, VLDL can acquire more C apolipoproteins from HDL, enabling hydrolysis in the peripheral circulation by lipoprotein lipase, as occurs for chylomicrons.

As the triglycerides of VLDL become depleted, VLDL remnants or intermediate density lipoproteins (IDL) (density = 1.006 − 1.019 g/mL, $\beta$ mobility) are formed that are poor in triglycerides and apolipoprotein C and rich in cholesterol and apolipoprotein E. IDL are metabolized by one of two different pathways: They are either removed from the circulation by the liver via receptor recognition of apolipoprotein E or converted to LDL by a processing mechanism involving hepatic lipase. Under normal conditions, approximately half of the IDL is removed by the liver and half is converted to LDL. A decreased expression of hepatic LDL receptors results in less clearance of IDL by the liver and greater conversion to LDL. Conversely, with increased expression of hepatic LDL receptors, more IDL is removed by the liver and less converted to LDL. Therefore, an inverse relationship exists between the amount of IDL converted to LDL (i.e., LDL production) and the number of LDL receptors expressed by the liver.

## Low-Density Lipoproteins

Low-density lipoproteins, the major cholesterol-carrying lipoproteins in humans (responsible for about 70% of total cholesterol in plasma), are the catabolic product of VLDL. LDL have a density of 1.019–1.063 g/mL and exhibit $\beta$ mobility on electrophoresis. Approximately 50% of the mass of LDL consists of cholesteryl esters, and the remainder comprises equal amounts of phospholipids and apolipoproteins, with apolipoprotein B-100 the predominant (>95%) species.

LDL provide cholesterol to extrahepatic cells for membrane synthesis in dividing cells and for steroid hormone production in the adrenals and gonads. Although all nucleated cells are capable of de novo synthesis of cholesterol, cholesterol derived from LDL is preferentially utilized when available. Approximately 60 to 80% of LDL catabolism occurs through uptake by the liver and the remainder by extrahepatic tissues. LDL are primarily catabolized via specific cell surface receptors (LDL receptors) that recognize apolipoprotein B-100 and apolipoprotein E. In general, the number of LDL receptors expressed by cells is inversely related to intracellular cholesterol content.

## High-Density Lipoproteins

High-density lipoproteins (HDL) are a heterogeneous group of small lipoprotein particles (range 5 to 12 nm) with densities of 1.063 to 1.215 g/mL and $\alpha$ mobility on electrophoresis (Table 9-9). Although considered cholesterol-rich lipoproteins, HDL are predominantly composed of phospholipids and apolipoproteins, with 20% of the mass consisting of cholesteryl esters (Table 9-10). Apolipoprotein AI (70%) and apolipoprotein AII (20%) account for most of the protein of HDL, with small amounts of apolipoprotein C, apolipoprotein D, and, in the lighter density HDL particles, apolipoprotein E, composing the remainder.

Along with their physical and compositional heterogeneity, HDL are metabolically heterogeneous. HDL are derived from two major pathways: direct secretion from the liver and intestine and formation from excess surface components produced during hydrolysis of chylomicrons and VLDL by lipoprotein lipase. Intact HDL are probably not secreted or formed directly, but HDL are first found as discoidal phospholipid-apolipoprotein bilayers that acquire unesterified cholesterol on efflux from peripheral cells. The unesterified cholesterol is then converted to cholesteryl esters in the HDL core by the plasma enzyme lecithin: cholesterol acyltransferase, which is activated by apolipoprotein AI. The cholesteryl esters in HDL can then be transferred to "acceptor" lipoproteins, for example, chylomicron remnants, VLDL and LDL, by a process requiring lipid transfer proteins. Thus, HDL plays an important role in transporting cholesterol from peripheral tissues to the liver, the process of "reverse cholesterol transport."

## Other Lipoproteins

In addition to the major classes of lipoproteins, several other minor lipoproteins are important in normal or disease states. Of these, lipoprotein(a) has received particular attention, owing to the association of increased concentrations of lipoprotein(a) with increased risk of coronary heart disease (Scanu et al. 1991). Lipoprotein(a) has a density of 1.050 to 1.08 g/mL, a composition relatively similar to LDL but with slightly more protein and less cholesterol, and pre-$\beta$ mobility on electrophoresis. The apolipoproteins in lipoprotein(a) are apolipoprotein B-100 and a unique apolipoprotein, apolipoprotein(a), that displays structural homology to plasminogen. Lipoprotein(a) is produced by the liver and catabolized through as yet poorly understood mechanisms. There is no apparent metabolic interconversion of lipoprotein(a) with any other lipoproteins.

Another lipoprotein of importance is $\beta$-VLDL, occurring in patients with familial dysbetalipoproteinemia, diabetes mellitus, or uremia (Mahley 1982). $\beta$-VLDL have a density <1.006 g/mL, similar to normal VLDL, but migrate on electrophoresis with $\beta$ mobility. $\beta$-VLDL resemble "remnant" particles, being both rich in cholesterol and apolipoprotein E and poor in triglycerides and apolipoprotein C.

## LIPOPROTEIN ABNORMALITIES

### Lipoprotein Abnormalities as Risk Factors

#### *Cholesterol*

Diagnosis of a lipoprotein abnormality is based, for the most part, on the results of laboratory testing. However, unlike other conditions where a diagnosis depends solely on the results of laboratory tests, the range of normal values for serum lipids and lipoproteins is not defined by the 90 to 95% confidence limits of a normal reference population.

**PRINCIPLE When an identifiable parameter of health places an entire population or a significant percentage of that population at increased risk for a disease, the definition of "abnormal" should be adjusted to include all individuals at risk.**

Normal or, more appropriately, desirable lipid and lipoprotein levels have been established on the basis of experimental and epidemiological studies demonstrating relationships between particular lipid concentrations and the risk of developing specific diseases such as atherosclerosis. This is best illustrated by a large number of epidemiological studies that document a strong, positive relationship between serum LDL cholesterol values and the incidence of atherosclerotic coronary heart disease (Jacobs et al. 1992).

The Multiple Risk Factor Intervention Trial (MRFIT) has the greatest discriminatory power of these studies because it is the largest, having evaluated more than 350,000 middle-aged men over a period of 6 years (Neaton et al. 1992). The results from MRFIT display a nonlinear, continuously graded rise of mortality from coronary heart disease with increasing levels of serum LDL cholesterol, without evidence of a threshold phenomenon. An ever-increasing relative risk was observed, beginning with LDL cholesterol levels of 150 mg/dL (Fig. 9-10). Even though

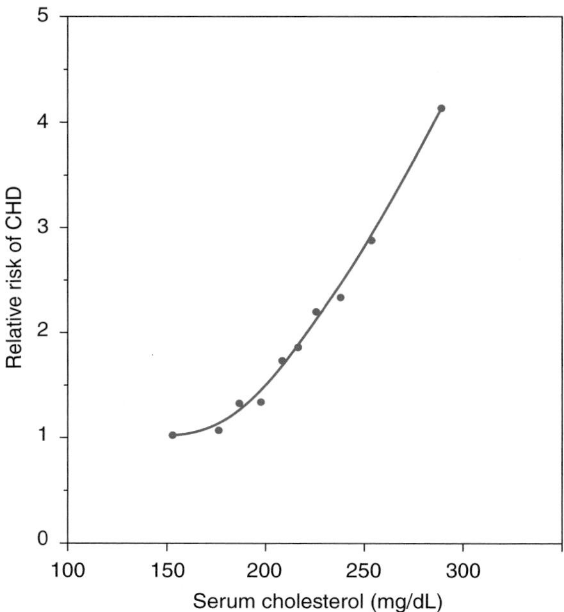


**FIGURE 9-10 Relationship between serum LDL cholesterol concentration and relative risk of death from coronary heart disease over 6 years. (Adapted from data from the Multiple Risk Factor Intervention Trial, Neaton et al. 1992.)**

fewer studies have examined cohorts that do not consist of middle-aged men, it appears that the relationship between serum LDL cholesterol and coronary heart disease also holds in women (National Cholesterol Education Program Expert Panel 1994a) and older individuals (Manolio et al. 1992; Kronmal et al 1993), at least up to about age 75.

As opposed to the strong positive relationship between LDL cholesterol and coronary heart disease, HDL cholesterol levels have been found to be inversely related to coronary heart disease rates in a number of epidemiological studies (NIH Consensus Development Conference 1993). This has led to the proposal that HDL cholesterol levels <35 mg/dL are a positive risk factor for coronary heart disease and that levels ≥60 mg/dL are a negative risk factor.

#### *Triglyceride*

Although there is reasonable unanimity of opinion regarding the relationship between serum LDL cholesterol and coronary heart disease, the relationship between triglyceride values and coronary heart disease is much more controversial (Austin 1991). Some large epidemiological studies have found a strong correlation between triglyceride values and coronary heart disease, but others have been unable to detect such a relationship. Part of this controversy stems from the fact that the statistical significance of the correlation between serum triglyceride levels and coronary heart disease is often lost when examined by multivariant analysis. This is particularly true when HDL cholesterol values are considered, because HDL cholesterol values are, in general, inversely related to serum triglyceride concentrations.

**PRINCIPLE When variables are physiologically interrelated, whether one variable (triglycerides) is mechanistically involved with the disease process (atherogenesis) may be less important than its clinical value as a marker or predictor of that disease.**

Nonetheless, whether elevations of triglycerides directly contribute to the development of atherosclerosis or simply reflect other, possibly unmeasured, contributory factors, it appears that triglyceride levels do correlate with the incidence of coronary heart disease in some well-defined settings. Specifically, the incidence of coronary heart disease in patients with diabetes mellitus appears to be related strongly to elevations in serum triglycerides (Fontbonne et al. 1991). Because the relationship of hypertriglyceridemia to coronary heart disease has not been definitively established, agreement on a definition of hypertriglyceridemia has been difficult to reach (NIH Consensus Development Conference 1993). Nonetheless, all available evidence substantiates a strong relationship between triglyceride values greater than 1000 mg/dL and development of acute pancreatitis.

## Screening Guidelines

***Primary prevention***

On the basis of the above analyses, the National Cholesterol Education Program (NECP) and the American College of Physicians (ACP) have developed slightly different recommendations for individuals without known vascular disease. Current NCEP recommendations propose a screening measurement of serum total cholesterol and HDL cholesterol in all adults over the age of 20 every 5 years (National Cholesterol Education Program Expert Panel 1994a), whereas the ACP recommends measurement only of serum total cholesterol in men 35 to 65 years old and in women 45 to 65 years old (ACP 1996) (Table 9-11).

The ACP does not recommend screening men aged ≤35 or women aged ≤45 unless a history suggests a familial lipoprotein disorder or two or more other cardiovascular risk factors are present. Other cardiovascular risk factors include age ≥45 years for men, age ≥55 years for women or premature menopause not on estrogen replacement, a family history of premature coronary heart disease (defined as sudden death or definite myocardial infarction in a male first-degree relative before age 55 or in a female first-degree relative before age 65), current cigarette smoking, hypertension (BP ≥140/90 mm Hg), a low HDL cholesterol (≤35 mg/dL), and diabetes mellitus (Table 9-12). An HDL cholesterol ≥60 mg/dL is considered a negative risk factor. The ACP neither encourages nor discourages screening men and women aged 65 to 75 years and does not recommend screening men and women aged >75.

If the cholesterol value obtained on screening is elevated, the serum total cholesterol should be reassessed, along with measurement of plasma triglyceride and HDL

Table 9-11 Guidelines for Screening

| PRIMARY PREVENTION—ADULTS | SECONDARY PREVENTION | PRIMARY PREVENTION—CHILDREN |
|---|---|---|
| National Cholesterol Education Program<br>All adults >20 years | All patients with known CV disease | Age >2 years with one of the following: several CV risk factors; a family history of early CV disease; or a parent with a cholesterol >240 mg/dL |
| American College of Physicians<br>Men 35–65 years<br>Women 45–65 years<br>Men <35 years and women <45 years only with a family history of CV disease or ≥2 other CV risk factors | | |

ABBREVIATIONS: CV, cardiovascular.

**Table 9-12 Other Cardiovascular Risk Factors**

*Positive*
- Men ≥45 years
- Women ≥55 years
- Family history of premature CV disease or sudden death (first-degree relative, men <55 years, women <65 years)
- Current smoking
- Hypertension
- HDL cholesterol <35 mg/dL
- Diabetes mellitus

*Negative*
- HDL cholesterol ≥60 mg/dL

ABBREVIATIONS: CV, cardiovascular; HDL, high density lipoprotein.

cholesterol, in order to define the lipoprotein abnormality present and to determine the concentration of LDL cholesterol, which is calculated according to the formula LDL cholesterol = total cholesterol − HDL cholesterol − (triglycerides ÷ 5) (Friedewald et al. 1972). This calculation is reasonably accurate provided triglyceride levels do not exceed 300 mg/dL and the patient does not have type III (dysbetalipoproteinemia) hyperlipoproteinemia (see below). For screening children, the NCEP [National Cholesterol Education Program (NCEP) 1992a] and the American Academy of Pediatrics (American Academy of Pediatrics, Committee on Nutrition 1992b) recommend individualizing the process so that a serum total cholesterol, triglyceride, HDL cholesterol, and a calculated LDL cholesterol are obtained only in children over the age of 2 who have one of the following risk factors: 1) a family history of a parent or grandparent with coronary or peripheral vascular disease before age 55, 2) a parent with a total cholesterol >240 mg/dL, or 3) several cardiovascular risk factors (hypertension, diabetes mellitus, smoking, obesity, physical inactivity) and the family history is not obtainable.

### *Secondary prevention*

All patients with known coronary heart disease or other vascular disease should have a lipid analysis that includes total cholesterol, HDL cholesterol, and triglyceride, with LDL cholesterol calculated from these values.

## Treatment Goals

### *Cholesterol*

The established goal (Table 9-13) for primary prevention is to decrease LDL cholesterol to <190 mg/dL in men <35 years old and premenopausal women without other cardiovascular risk factors who have LDL cholesterol values >220 mg/dL after dietary therapy. Other individuals with fewer than two other cardiovascular risk factors and LDL cholesterol values ≥190 mg/dL who do not respond to diet therapy are advised to undergo treatment with lipid-lowering drugs with a goal of reducing LDL cholesterol below 160 mg/dL. Individuals with LDL cholesterol ≥160 mg/dL who have two or more additional cardiovascular risk factors are advised to be treated with hypocholesterolemic agents to achieve an LDL cholesterol <130 mg/dL if an adequate response is not observed with diet.

The therapeutic goal for patients who have known coronary artery or vascular disease is an LDL cholesterol level ≤100 mg/dL. In addition, patients without known vascular disease, but with significant additional cardiovascular risk factors such as diabetes mellitus also should have a goal of LDL cholesterol ≤100 mg/dL.

**PRINCIPLE Therapy should be more aggressive in individuals who manifest a disease than in individuals in whom treatment is instituted as a potential preventive measure.**

**Table 9-13 Treatment Goals**

| STRATEGY | TARGET CONCENTRATION |
|---|---|
| *Primary prevention* | |
| Men <35 years and premenopausal women | LDL cholesterol <190 mg/dL |
| Men >35 years and women >45 years with <2 other CV risk factors | LDL cholesterol <160 mg/dL |
| Adults with ≥2 other CV risk factors | LDL cholesterol <130 mg/dL |
| Adults with diabetes mellitus or a strong family history of early CV disease | LDL cholesterol ≤100 mg/dL |
| *Secondary prevention* | LDL cholesterol ≤100 mg/dL |

ABBREVIATIONS: CV, cardiovascular; LDL, low-density lipoprotein.

***Triglycerides***
Based on the variability of triglyceride measurements, a triglyceride level >500 mg/dL is considered high and warrants therapy for prevention of pancreatitis (NIH Consensus Development Conference 1993). Patients with triglyceride values between 250 and 500 mg/dL should be considered for therapy in light of the presence or absence of other cardiovascular risk factors (see above). If known vascular disease or significant cardiovascular risk factors are present in addition to hypertriglyceridemia, hypolipidemic therapy is probably indicated. Although this approach is a compromise, it emphasizes that therapeutic decisions need to be individually determined and with respect to the patient as a whole.

**PRINCIPLE Not just one, but all relevant factors should be considered when deciding to initiate preventive therapy for a disease.**

## SPECIFIC LIPOPROTEIN ABNORMALITIES

### Hypertriglyceridemia

Hypertriglyceridemia occurs when there are elevations in plasma values of triglyceride-rich lipoproteins, that is, chylomicrons, VLDL, or both chylomicrons and VLDL. The excessive accumulation of these lipoprotein particles can result from increased production, decreased removal, or both.

***Chylomicronemia***
Chylomicrons are not usually present in normal fasting plasma. Fasting hyperchylomicronemia or type I hyperlipoproteinemia in the Fredrickson classification (Fredrickson et al. 1967) is caused by deficiency in lipoprotein lipase or, even more rarely, deficiency of apolipoprotein CII, the cofactor that activates lipoprotein lipase. In either case there is a severe defect in the catabolism of chylomicrons. Chylomicronemia is a rare disorder with homozygous affected individuals occurring with a frequency of about 1:1,000,000 in the general population. Type I hyperlipoproteinemia usually presents in childhood with pancreatitis, hepatosplenomegaly, eruptive xanthoma, and lipemia retinalis.

Because chylomicrons are derived entirely from dietary fat, treatment consists of a marked reduction of dietary fat to 5 to 15% of total calories, which generally leads to a highly efficacious therapeutic response. No hypolipidemic agents are generally indicated in the therapy of this disorder, although triglyceride-lowering agents are sometimes used to blunt the hypertriglyceridemic response to carbohydrate or the hypertriglyceridemia that occurs with pregnancy. Although not generally thought to increase the risk for atherosclerosis, chylomicronemia in some patients has been reported to contribute to atherosclerosis (Benlian et al. 1996).

***Increased VLDL or increased VLDL and chylomicrons***
Hypertriglyceridemia caused by elevations of VLDL of normal composition (type IV hyperlipoproteinemia) is the most common lipid abnormality observed in the general population. When VLDL values increase to triglyceride values greater than 500 mg/dL, chylomicrons also begin to accumulate in plasma, because VLDL and chylomicrons share and compete for similar removal mechanisms. Differentiation between type IV hyperlipoproteinemia and accumulation of increased amounts of VLDL, and hyperchylomicronemia (type V hyperlipoproteinemia), is determined by the absence or presence of chylomicrons. This reflects the severity of the hypertriglyceridemia or of the patient's diet more than differences in the underlying pathophysiology.

Types IV and V hyperlipoproteinemia are heterogeneous disorders that may occur secondarily owing to a number of diseases or polygenetic causes. Secondary causes of hypertriglyceridemia include diabetes mellitus, uremia, nephrotic syndrome, alcohol abuse, estrogen use, glucocorticoid excess (endogenous or exogenous), metabolic stress (including trauma, burns, infections, and sepsis), glycogen storage disease, dysglobulinemia, pregnancy, and lipodystrophies. Individuals without evidence of secondary etiologies have familial or sporadic hypertriglyceridemia. The hypertriglyceridemia in these individuals (excluding type I insulin dependent diabetes mellitus and uremia) is caused by increased production of VLDL, along with variable defects in removal of VLDL.

The factors leading to the increased production of VLDL are probably multiple; however, most patients are overweight and characterized by insulin resistance, hyperinsulinemia, and increased free fatty acid flux (Reaven 1988). It is vital that initial therapy in these patients be directed toward decreasing free fatty acid flux and insulin resistance by weight loss and/or correction of the underlying disease before pharmacological intervention is considered.

### Hypercholesterolemia

Hypercholesterolemia, in the absence of elevated triglycerides, is caused by elevations in LDL concentrations (type IIa hyperlipoproteinemia). The one important exception to this generalization is the individual with hyperalphalipoproteneimia who has normal values of LDL cholesterol but increased values of HDL (Glueck et al. 1975). In contrast to the typical hypercholesterolemic patients, these individuals are not at increased risk for coronary heart disease and, consistent with the definition of hypercholesterolemia as an elevated LDL cholesterol (see above), do not require therapy to lower their total cholesterol levels. This lipoprotein pattern is more common among women; hence, the simple measurement of total cholesterol may be less predictive of coronary risk among women than men. Patients with type IIa hyperlipoproteinemia constitute a heterogeneous group consisting of several different monogenetic and polygenetic abnormalities.

The best studied of these abnormalities is called "familial hypercholesterolemia," a monogenetic disorder in which defects in the LDL receptor lead to elevations of LDL cholesterol. Familial hypercholesterolemia is an autosomal recessive disorder with heterozygotes constituting approximately 1 out of 500 in the population and homozygotes about 1 in 1 million people. These people are characterized by hypercholesterolemia, tendon xanthomas, and an increased risk of coronary heart disease. A number of different molecular defects at the genetic level lead to abnormal expression of LDL receptors (Hobbs et al. 1990). The decreased expression of LDL receptors results in defective catabolism of LDL from plasma. In addition, because LDL receptors also mediate the removal of VLDL and VLDL remnants from plasma, there is a concomitant increase in the production of LDL secondary to an increased conversion from uncleared VLDL and VLDL remnants. Consequently, elevated LDL concentrations occur because of a combination of increased production and decreased removal of LDL.

A mutation in apolipoprotein B-100, termed "familial defective apolipoprotein B-100" (Innerarity et al. 1990), is a genetic abnormality causing hypercholesterolemia in which LDL receptors are normal. In these patients, the mutation in apolipoprotein B-100 diminishes the affinity of LDL for its receptor, leading to decreased catabolism of LDL; in these individuals, there is a normal LDL production rate, since apolipoprotein-E mediated removal of VLDL and VLDL remnants remains normal.

Even though genetic defects in LDL receptors or apolipoprotein B-100 have been studied extensively, the majority of patients with type IIa hyperlipoproteinemia do not have these highly specific genetic defects. Some patients have hypercholesterolemia that occurs secondarily to an underlying disease, such as hypothyroidism, nephrotic syndrome, dysglobulinemia, glucocorticoid excess, hepatic cholestasis, anorexia nervosa, or acute intermittent porphyria; evaluation of these possibilities should be pursued in the appropriate clinical setting. However, most patients have an array of metabolic (polygenetic) causes characterized by an increased rate of LDL production in some and by a decreased rate of LDL removal without apparent defects in LDL receptors or apolipoprotein B-100 in others (Vega et al. 1991).

## Combined Hypercholesterolemia and Hypertriglyceridemia

Not infrequently, hypercholesterolemia and hypertriglyceridemia coexist in the same individual or within the same family. When this occurs, it can be secondary to an underlying disease (e.g., diabetes mellitus, nephrotic syndrome, use of corticosteroids) or caused by a genetic abnormality. Patients with combined hypercholesterolemia and hypertriglyceridemia fall into two classifications: type IIb hyperlipoproteinemia and type III hyperlipoproteinemia.

### *Familial combined hyperlipidemia or type IIb hyperlipoproteinemia*

Patients with type IIb hyperlipoproteinemia, also known as "familial combined hyperlipidemia (or dyslipidemia)" or "hyperapobetalipoproteinemia," represent a heterogeneous group of subjects (Grundy et al. 1987). This disorder is a very common abnormality in which patients display multiple lipoprotein phenotypes, with individuals or family members having hypertriglyceridemia, hypercholesterolemia, or both hypertriglyceridemia and hypercholesterolemia at any given time. Consequently, patients with familial combined hyperlipidemia are often erroneously classified as type IV or type IIa hyperlipoproteinemia. As opposed to patients with type IV hyperlipoproteinemia, where the relationship to atherosclerosis is controversial, individuals with familial combined hyperlipidemia (whether hypertriglyceridemic, hypercholesterolemic, or both) are at increased risk for coronary heart disease (Goldstein et al. 1973). Independent of the prevailing lipoprotein phenotype, patients with familial combined hyperlipidemia are characterized by elevated levels of apolipoprotein B, with an increased rate of VLDL apolipoprotein B and VLDL triglyceride production in hypertriglyceridemic individuals and an increased production rate of LDL apolipoprotein B seen in all of these patients. Rates of removal of LDL are normal. The genetic basis for familial combined hyperlipidemia is unknown, but its phenotypic expression is influenced by factors such as age, obesity, and diabetes mellitus.

### *Type III hyperlipoproteinemia or dysbetalipoproteinemia*

Type III hyperlipoproteinemia, or familial dysbetalipoproteinemia, is a rare disorder caused by the accumulation of cholesterol-rich VLDL in plasma that results in elevations of triglycerides and cholesterol. This disorder cannot be detected using routinely performed lipid analyses but rather requires direct analysis of VLDL composition using ultracentrifugation or apolipoprotein E phenotyping. The diagnosis of familial dysbetalipoproteinemia should be considered in any patient with marked elevations of both cholesterol and triglyceride values. However, particular attention should be directed at those patients with both hypercholesterolemia and hypertriglyceridemia who have evidence of accelerated atherosclerosis or a strong family history of atherosclerosis and hyperlipidemia. The cholesterol-rich VLDL, or $\beta$-VLDL, that accumulate in these patients are remnant particles that are not cleared normally by the liver (Mahley et al. 1991). This defect in removal is because of the presence of apolipoprotein E-2, one of three isoforms of apolipoprotein E, which possesses a markedly decreased affinity for binding to both LDL and chylomicron remnant receptors, compared with the other isoforms. Although 1% of the population is homozygous for apolipoprotein E-2, fewer than 5% of homozygous individuals are hyperlipidemic, suggesting that an additional abnormality is required in order to develop type III hyperlipoproteinemia (Walden and Hegele 1994). The additional abnormality can include metabolic disorders (e.g., noninsulin dependent diabetes mellitus, hypothyroidism, nephrotic syndrome, use of glucocorticoids and estrogens, or obesity) or inherited disorders (e.g., familial hypertriglyceridemia or familial combined hyperlipidemia). The common feature of these disorders is an increase in VLDL production.

## THERAPY OF LIPOPROTEIN ABNORMALITIES

The therapeutic approach to an individual with hyperlipidemia is predicated on establishing the type of lipid abnormality the patient has and then tailoring therapy toward altering the underlying pathophysiology. Establishing a patient's lipoprotein abnormality entails determining not only which lipoprotein classes are elevated but also whether the lipid abnormality is primary (genetic, environmental) or secondary to another underlying disorder.

**PRINCIPLE Therapy directed toward an underlying disease should be maximized prior to initiating treatment of a symptom or sign of a secondary lipoprotein abnormality.**

If an underlying disease is uncovered that can contribute to the hyperlipidemia, therapy should be directed at correcting the causative disorder before a specific therapy for the lipid abnormality is instituted. This is particularly important if hypothyroidism or diabetes mellitus is discovered, because these relatively common disorders dramatically affect lipoprotein metabolism and can be directly treated effectively. Indeed, achievement of euthyroidism and normalization or improvement in glucose control frequently results in correction or marked improvement of the hyperlipidemia in these instances.

Once secondary etiologies of hyperlipidemia are excluded or properly treated, initial therapy for all patients with hyperlipidemias should be dietary modification. Dietary modifications generally entail a reduction in total fat intake, particularly reduction in saturated fat, decrease in dietary cholesterol, and frequently caloric restriction in overweight patients. Specific dietary recommendations, and the scientific bases on which they are founded, are beyond the scope of this chapter. The reader is referred to recent reviews on this topic for further information (National Cholesterol Education Program Expert Panel 1994a). A period of 3 to 6 months of dietary intervention should be undertaken before pharmacologic therapy is considered for primary prevention; however, initiating drug therapy concurrently with dietary intervention is warranted for secondary prevention (patients with known vascular disease). Because the rationale for treatment is to lower the risk of development and progression or to increase the regression of atherosclerosis by decreasing atherogenic lipoproteins, therapy is planned to continue for many years. Therefore, it is essential to consider risks and benefits carefully when prescribing hypolipidemic agents.

**PRINCIPLE When drug therapy is planned to extend over the lifetime of a patient for the purpose of preventing a serious disease, the cumulative risk (morbidity, mortality, and quality of life) of the treatment itself must be carefully weighed against the effectiveness of the intervention.**

If hypercholesterolemia persists after dietary restrictions, present recommendations for primary prevention are to treat with bile acid sequestrants, followed, in order, by trials of niacin, HMG CoA reductase inhibitors (statins), and gemfibrozil, whereas statins are the drugs of choice for secondary prevention (National Cholesterol Education Program Expert Panel 1994a). However, given their efficacy, statins are also becoming the agents of choice for primary prevention. If marked hypertriglyceridemia persists after dietary restriction, gemfibrozil and niacin are the drugs of choice, with statins having utility in some clinical settings. The use of each of these agents, singly or in combination, is discussed in the following sections.

## Bile Acid Sequestrants

### *History*

The bile acid sequestrants were the first agents successfully developed for the treatment of hyperlipidemia. Based on findings in the early 1950s that feeding ferric chloride could attenuate the hypercholesterolemia induced by dietary cholesterol in chickens through its ability to precipitate bile acids in the gastrointestinal tract (Siperstein et al. 1953), nontoxic agents that bound bile acids were sought. Cholestyramine, a nonabsorbable anion exchange resin that avidly binds bile acids, was developed in 1960 (Tennet et al. 1960). Later, a second bile acid binding resin with a different structure (colestipol) was developed (Parkinson et al. 1970).

### *Mechanism of action*

To understand the mechanism of action of bile acid sequestrants, it is necessary first to review bile metabolism briefly (Packard and Shepherd 1982). Bile secreted by the liver consists of bile acids, phospholipids, and unesterified cholesterol (biliary cholesterol) solubilized by the detergent effects of bile acids and phospholipids. Bile acids are the principal oxidative product of hepatic cholesterol metabolism. The two major bile acids, cholic and chenodeoxycholic acid, are produced from 7$\alpha$-hydroxycholesterol, which is formed from cholesterol by the action of cholesterol 7$\alpha$-hydroxylase, the rate-limiting enzyme in bile acid synthesis. Bile acid synthesis is under feedback regulation, with cholic and chenodeoxycholic acids inhibiting the activity of cholesterol 7$\alpha$-hydroxylase. In humans, approximately 30% of the bile acids and 20% of the biliary cholesterol are derived from newly synthesized cholesterol, the vast majority being derived from lipoprotein cholesterol. After bile is secreted into the intestine, the bile acids undergo further metabolism by the bacterial flora. Normally, 95% of the bile acids secreted into the intestine are reabsorbed by the terminal ileum and returned to the liver through the portal system where they are reutilized. Nonetheless, the bile acids and biliary cholesterol that are not reabsorbed represent the major route of removal of cholesterol from the body.

Through their ability to bind bile acids and form an insoluble complex, cholestyramine and colestipol interrupt the enterohepatic circulation of bile acids and promote sterol excretion in the feces. As bile acids are sequestered by bile acid resins, the feedback inhibition of cholesterol 7$\alpha$-hydroxylase activity is released, leading to a 3- to 10-fold increase in bile acid synthesis. This increase in bile acid synthesis allows a new steady state to be reached so that the total bile acid pool is not significantly depleted by bile acid sequestrant therapy. The increased diversion of cholesterol into bile acid synthesis causes an apparent decrease in the pool of intracellular cholesterol. Depletion of intracellular, unesterified cholesterol removes the feedback inhibition on HMG CoA reductase activity and LDL receptor expression, resulting in increased cholesterol synthesis and increased LDL uptake mediated by means of LDL receptors (Goldstein and Brown 1990). In parallel, an increase in triglyceride synthesis in some, but not all, subjects results from complex integration of sterol metabolism through bile acid and cholesterol synthesis with triglyceride production. Consequently, a fall in plasma LDL concentration occurs due to a greater catabolism of LDL by the liver; however, this effect is attenuated in part by the compensatory increases in cholesterol and triglyceride syntheses that give rise to increases in VLDL production.

### *Pharmacokinetics*

Cholestyramine (Questran) is the chloride salt of a quartenary ammonium anion exchange resin in which the basic groups are attached by carbon bonds to a styrene-divinyl benzene copolymer skeleton (Fig. 9-11). Colestipol (Colestid) is an anion exchange resin that is a copolymer of diethylenetriamine and 1-chloro-2,3-epoxypropane. Neither cholestyramine nor colestipol is soluble in water, nor is either absorbed from the intestine to any appreciable degree ($<$0.02%). Cholestyramine is available both as a powder and as a "granola" bar (Cholybar), which some patients find more palatable. No matter what formulation, both agents must be taken with water or a suitable liquid. The dose of cholestyramine ranges from 8 to 24 g/day, and the dose of colestipol from 15 to 30 g/day; however, some patients display adequate therapeutic responses to lower doses. The bile acid sequestrants should be taken with meals so as to coincide with the times of maximum bile acid secretion.

Although cholestyramine has a slightly higher capacity on a weight-per-weight basis (4 g cholestyramine are

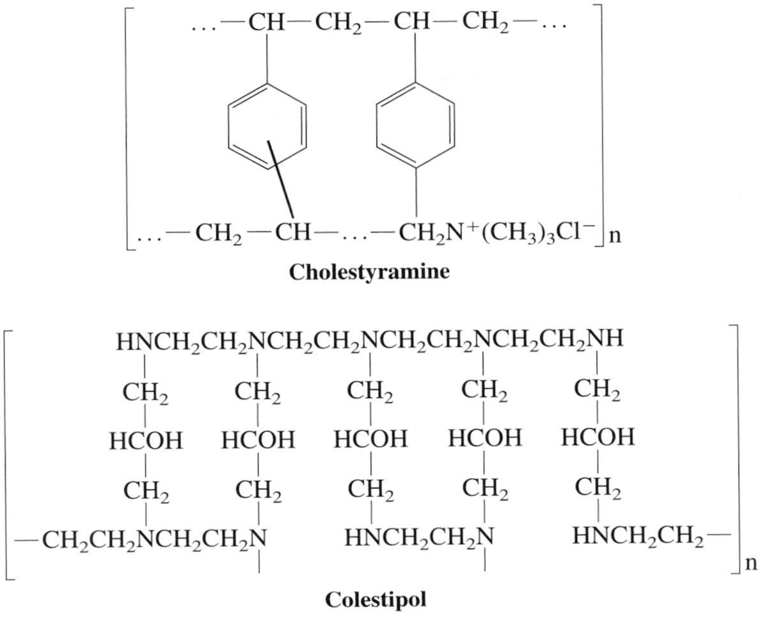

...—CH—CH$_2$—CH—CH$_2$—...

...—CH$_2$—CH—...—CH$_2$N$^+$(CH$_3$)$_3$Cl$^-$ n

**Cholestyramine**

HNCH$_2$CH$_2$NCH$_2$CH$_2$NCH$_2$CH$_2$NCH$_2$CH$_2$NH

CH$_2$ CH$_2$ CH$_2$ CH$_2$ CH$_2$

HCOH HCOH HCOH HCOH HCOH

CH$_2$ CH$_2$ CH$_2$ CH$_2$ CH$_2$

—CH$_2$CH$_2$NCH$_2$CH$_2$N HNCH$_2$CH$_2$N HNCH$_2$CH$_2$— n

**Colestipol**

FIGURE 9-11 **Chemical structures of bile acid sequestrants.**

roughly equivalent to 5 g colestipol), both agents bind bile acids similarly to form insoluble complexes. The bile acid sequestrants have a greater affinity for chenodeoxycholate than cholate. This increased affinity for chenodeoxycholate, combined with the greater induction of cholic acid synthesis than chenodeoxycholic acid synthesis, causes a marked alteration in bile composition. Although these changes in the species of bile acids occur, there are no alterations in the ratio of total bile acids to biliary cholesterol or phospholipid; thus, the lithogenicity of bile remains unchanged (chapter 4, Hepatic Disorders and the Influence of Liver Function on Drug Disposition).

### *Indications and efficacy*

Bile acid sequestrants are indicated in the treatment of hypercholesterolemia caused by elevations in LDL concentrations (type II hyperlipoproteinemia). A large number of controlled trials have established the safety and efficacy of bile acid sequestrants for this indication. Findings of these studies have shown that treatment with bile acid sequestrants results in a 15 to 35% reduction in serum cholesterol levels caused entirely by a reduction in LDL cholesterol. In parallel to the reduction in LDL cholesterol, there is a fall in apolipoprotein B values. Plasma triglyceride values are generally unchanged or increased, and no consistent alterations in HDL cholesterol values have been observed with bile acid sequestrants. Similarly, no changes in lipoprotein(a) concentrations occur.

The largest randomized controlled trial to examine the efficacy of bile acid sequestrants was the Lipid Research Clinics Primary Prevention Trial (Lipid Research Clinics Program 1984a,b), which showed that cholestyramine monotherapy produced a 12% reduction in LDL cholesterol levels and a 19% reduction in coronary artery disease compared with placebo, when given to 3800 middle-aged men with serum cholesterols ≥265 mg/dL and serum triglycerides ≤300 mg/dL over 7 years. However, total mortality was unchanged owing to an increased number of accidental and violent deaths in the group receiving cholestyramine. Similarly, the NHLBI Type II Coronary Intervention Study found a lower incidence of progression of coronary artery lesions by angiography in patients treated with cholestyramine (Brensike et al. 1984; Levy et al. 1984). Based on the efficacy demonstrated in these studies and on the absence of long-term adverse effects, bile acid sequestrants have traditionally been the drugs of first choice for initiation of therapy of hypercholesterolemia after failure of dietary restriction for primary prevention (National Cholesterol Education Program Expert Panel 1994a).

**PRINCIPLE The ideal agent for life-long primary prevention should be effective and have no systemic adverse effects. Unfortunately, few are found.**

The cholesterol-lowering effects of the bile acid sequestrants are synergistic with other hypolipidemic agents. A variety of drug combinations involving bile acid sequestrants are efficacious and discussed in later sections. Patients with homozygous familial hypercholesterolemia who are LDL-receptor-negative do not respond to bile acid sequestrants. Because the bile acid sequestrants are not absorbed, they are probably safe for use by pregnant and nursing women and are the only agents recommended for use in children. However, these groups of patients have not been extensively studied, and attention to the nutritional availability of fat-soluble vitamins is warranted in these subjects. The bile acid sequestrants are contraindicated in patients with marked elevations in plasma triglyceride values, because these drugs may accentuate the hypertriglyceridemia. However, bile acid sequestrants can be used in these patients if initial use of a triglyceride-lowering agent leads to elevations in LDL cholesterol.

In addition to their effects as hypocholesterolemic agents, bile acid sequestrants are effective in reducing pruritis in patients with partial biliary obstruction, by depleting the bile acid pool.

### *Adverse effects and drug interactions*

Because the bile acid sequestrants are not absorbed from the gastrointestinal tract, there are no appreciable systemic adverse effects. However, a small but statistically significant increase in the levels of aspartase aminotransaminase (SGOT) and alkaline phosphatase and a small decrease in the level of serum carotene were noted in the Lipid Research Clinics Primary Prevention Trial (Lipid Research Clinics Program 1984a). The major adverse effects of bile acid sequestrants are confined to the gastrointestinal system. Constipation is the primary problem, with an incidence reported between 10% and 50% that increases at higher doses and in patients over 60 years of age. In addition, minor to severe complaints of flatulence, abdominal discomfort, nausea, vomiting, and poor palatability are encountered. There is no evidence for any increased risk for gastrointestinal or other malignancies.

Because the total bile acid pool is not significantly depleted during therapy, fat malabsorption is unusual but may be seen at the highest doses. Similarly, concentrations of fat-soluble vitamins are not usually disturbed and do not require supplementation unless maximum doses are utilized. However, vitamin-K-responsive hypoprothrombinemia has been reported at submaximal doses. Because the bile acid sequestrants are anion exchange resins, it is possible for increases in chloride absorption to predispose to hyperchloremic metabolic acidosis, particularly in children. Furthermore, the resins are capable of binding acidic and basic substances in addition to bile acids and, thus, impairing the absorption of many drugs. Although the interaction of the bile acid sequestrants with a few drugs has been assessed, the number of drugs studied is limited (Table 9-14). Therefore, it is prudent to assume that the bile acid sequestrants will interfere with another drug's absorption and to give other drugs at least 1 hour before or 4 hours after the dose of the bile acid sequestrant.

**PRINCIPLE Once a fundamental mechanism of drug interactions has been demonstrated with an index drug and several other drugs, burden of proof as to whether it more broadly applies lies with the physician, not with the "system" or the industry.**

## Statins (HMG CoA Reductase Inhibitors)

### *History*

From the time elevations in serum cholesterol were first associated with the development of atherosclerosis in experimental animals and, later, in epidemiological studies in humans, many efforts have been directed toward developing inhibitors of cholesterol synthesis as a strategy for lowering serum cholesterol and preventing or reversing atherosclerosis. Initial efforts in this direction were undertaken at a time prior to the full understanding of cholesterol and lipoprotein metabolism that exists today. The early compounds successfully developed as inhibitors of cholesterol synthesis proved to cause serious metabolic adverse effects (many of which are now understandable based on the present knowledge of cholesterol metabolism).

In the early 1950s, $\Delta^4$-cholestenone was noted to act through an unknown mechanism as a potent inhibitor of

**Table 9-14 Reduced Drug Bioavailability Reported with Bile Acid Sequestrant Therapy**

| CARDIOVASCULAR DRUGS | CNS DRUGS |
|---|---|
| Digoxin | Imipramine HCl |
| Furosemide | Phenytoin |
| Gemfibrozil | **Antimicrobials** |
| Niacin | Clindamycin HCl |
| Thiazides | Penicillin G |
| Warfarin sodium | Tetracycline |
| **Nonsteroidal analgesics** | **Endocrine agents** |
| **Aspirin** | Glipizide |
| **Vitamins A, D, E, K, folate** | Thyroid hormone |
| | Raloxifene |

cholesterol biosynthesis (Tomkins et al. 1953). However, it was clear that cholestenone was not clinically useful because it caused the accumulation of dihydrocholesterol, a compound that was as atherogenic as cholesterol (Steinberg et al. 1958). In 1959, the first compound that had a known site of action was developed—Triparanol, or MER-29 (Blohm and MacKenzie 1959). Triparanol blocked the final step in cholesterol synthesis, conversion of desmosterol to cholesterol (Avigan et al. 1960). Triparanol caused significant reductions in concentrations of serum cholesterol in humans, but there were reciprocal elevations of desmosterol (Steinberg et al. 1961) that proved to be associated with development of accelerated atherosclerosis in rabbits, and cataracts in humans (Avigan and Steinberg 1962; Laughlin and Carey 1962). These experiences led investigators to be wary of inhibitors of cholesterol synthesis and to search for compounds that would inhibit an early step of cholesterol biosynthesis before the formation of sterol intermediates.

**PRINCIPLE By inhibiting an early step in a biosynthetic pathway, the accumulation of toxic intermediates can be avoided; however, the possibility for inhibiting other products that have important cellular functions is increased.**

While searching for potential inhibitors of cholesterol synthesis among products of microorganisms, Endo and colleagues (Endo et al. 1976a, 1976b) reported the isolation of several metabolites from *Penicillium citrinum* that inhibited HMG CoA reductase, the rate-limiting step in cholesterol biosynthesis. One of the metabolites, ML-236B, was termed compactin, because it was also isolated from the fungus *Penicillium brevicompactin* (Brown et al. 1976). Compactin lowered serum cholesterol values effectively in several animals and in humans (Yamamoto et al. 1980). Shortly after the discovery of compactin, a closely related compound was isolated from *Aspergillus terreus* (mevinolin) and from *Monascus ruber* (monacolin K) (Endo 1979; Alberts et al. 1980). Mevinolin differs from compactin by the substitution of a methyl group for a hydrogen at carbon 6; this structural difference is associated with a twofold increase in affinity for HMG CoA reductase. After early clinical trials, compactin was never developed for the marketplace (the reasons for this decision were not revealed). However, mevinolin (lovastatin) was approved in 1987 for sale in the United States. Several newer agents (simvastatin, pravastatin, and atorvastatin) have been produced by chemical modifications of mevinolin and compactin or by de novo synthesis (fluvastatin and cerivastatin) (Fig. 9-12).

***Mechanism of action***

These agents act as competitive inhibitors of HMG CoA reductase, the rate-limiting enzyme in cholesterol biosynthesis; this enzyme catalyzes the conversion of HMG CoA to mevalonate (Fig. 9-13). HMG CoA, the natural substrate of the enzyme, has a $K_m$ of ~10 $\mu$M, whereas lovastatin has a $K_i$ of ~1 nM, or approximately 10,000 times the affinity for the enzyme. This very high affinity of the inhibitors for HMG CoA reductase results from their binding to two separate sites on the enzyme (Nakamura and Abeles 1985). By inhibiting HMG CoA reductase, synthesis of cholesterol and other polyisoprenoid products (compounds containing multiple copies of the 5-carbon isopentenyl pyrophosphate) of mevalonate metabolism (Fig. 9-13) can be inhibited in vitro. However, at the doses used in vivo, no significant suppression of noncholesterol polyisoprenoids was expected or found, because much higher doses and more complete inhibition of HMG CoA reductase are required to suppress noncholesterol polyisoprenoids (Brown and Goldstein 1980).

**PRINCIPLE If an agent is developed to inhibit an early step in a biosynthetic pathway, depletion of other, nontargeted, products of the pathway can potentially cause adverse effects.**

In vivo studies using sterol balance or urinary excretion of mevalonate to assess total body cholesterol synthesis have found that maximal reduction of serum lipoprotein values was associated with only modest suppression of total body cholesterol synthesis, suggesting that mechanisms other than inhibition of cholesterol synthesis are involved in the lipoprotein-lowering effects of these drugs (Grundy and Bilheimer 1984; Parker et al. 1984). The modest reduction in cholesterol synthesis produced by statins can be explained, in part, by the fact that these competitive inhibitors induce the expression of HMG CoA reductase in vitro and in vivo, which tends to attenuate their inhibitory effects (Brown et al. 1978; Stone et al. 1989).

The mechanism whereby a modest suppression of cholesterol synthesis causes a large reduction of lipoprotein values appears to be due to normal homeostatic responses, where suppression of cholesterol synthesis results in a fall in intracellular cholesterol concentration, which then triggers an increase in the expression of LDL receptors (Ma et al. 1986). The enhanced expression of LDL

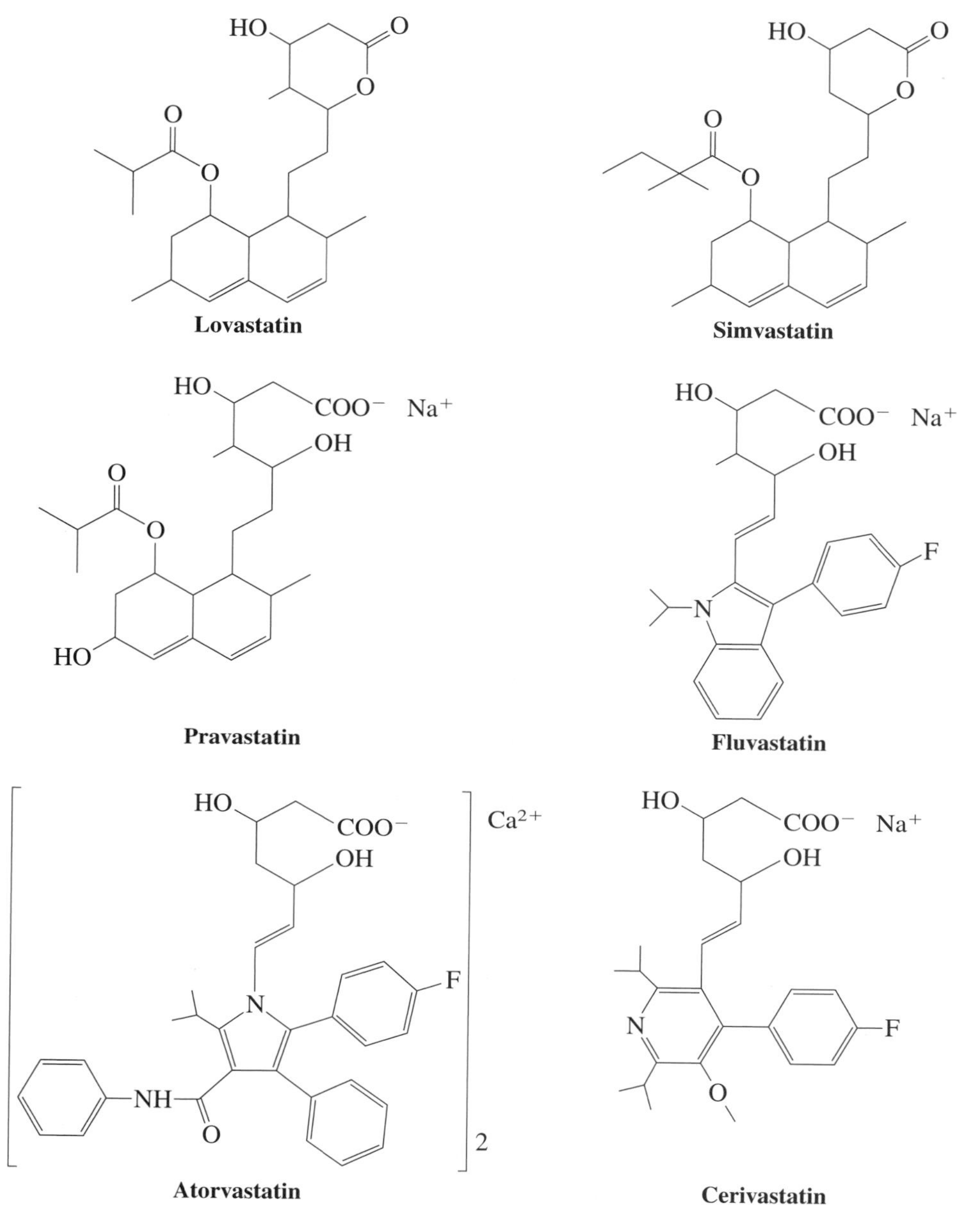

Lovastatin

Simvastatin

Pravastatin

Fluvastatin

Atorvastatin

Cerivastatin

FIGURE 9-12 **Chemical structures of hydroxymethylglutaryl coenzyme A (HMG-CoA) reductase inhibitors (statins).**

receptors by the liver causes an increased catabolic clearance of LDL and a fall in plasma LDL values (Bilheimer et al. 1983). Some studies have failed to observe an increase in catabolism of LDL but, instead, have found a decrease in LDL production (Grundy and Vega 1985). This finding is compatible with an enhanced expression of LDL receptors increasing the receptor-mediated clearance of VLDL and IDL (VLDL remnants), resulting in reduction both of triglyceride values and of the rate of production of LDL. In addition, it appears that statins directly inhibit hepatic formation of lipoproteins, which might be the mechanism responsible for most of the cholesterol-lowering activity (Ginsberg et al. 1987). The statins do not consistently alter bile metabolism and, therefore, are not associated with any consistent changes in net excretion of sterol from the body.

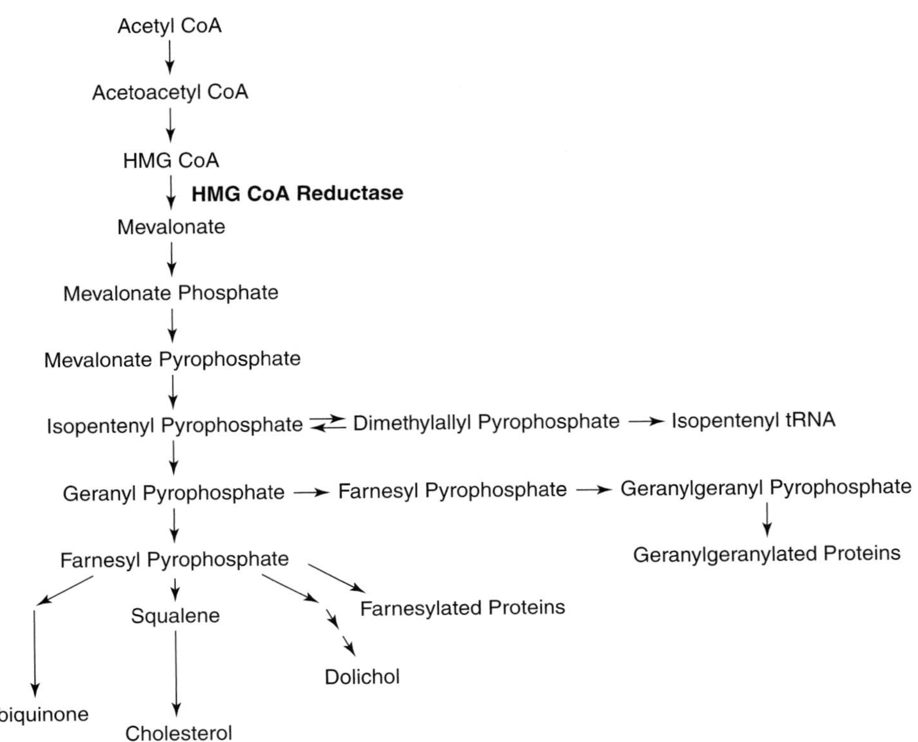


FIGURE 9-13 **Pathway of cholesterol and polyisoprenoid synthesis from acetate.**

***Pharmacokinetics***

All the statins are given orally. Lovastatin and simvastatin are prodrugs containing a lactone ring that is metabolized by the liver to a pharmacologically active β-hydroxyacid form. The lactone moiety of lovastatin and simvastatin allows the active forms of the drugs to be targeted to the liver, where the majority of drug is metabolized during its first pass. In contrast, pravastatin, fluvastatin, atorvastatin, and cerivastatin are delivered as active drug. Although gastrointestinal absorption varies from 12% (atorvastatin) to >90% (fluvastatin), all the statins except cerivistatin undergo extensive first-pass extraction in the liver with very low amounts of active drug found in extrahepatic tissues. High first-pass hepatic metabolism is the main mechanism by which pharmacological effects are targeted to the liver.

**PRINCIPLE A high first-pass effect may be a marked advantage for a drug whose action is intended to be targeted to the liver itself.**

After oral administration, approximately 10 to 20% of statins are excreted in the urine and the remainder found in feces, representing unabsorbed drug and hepatically metabolized drug that is excreted in bile. Statins have no effect on antipyrine kinetics. Statins are highly protein bound (50 to 99%) and display a variable ability to cross both the blood–brain barrier and the placenta. Protein binding has been proposed to limit the systemic bioavailability of statins, but adverse drug reactions do not differ between highly bound (fluvastatin, atorvastatin) and weakly bound (pravastatin) drugs. Plasma concentrations of drug and metabolites peak between 1 and 4 hours after an oral dose and return toward baseline by 24 hours. The elimination half-life of atorvastatin (14 hours) is longer than other statins (<4 hours), but it is not clear whether this accounts for the greater intrinsic efficacy of atorvastatin compared with other statins. Steady-state concentrations are achieved by 2 to 3 days; however, because lipoprotein values do not stabilize for 2 to 4 weeks, adjustments of dose should not be made more frequently than every 4 weeks.

Plasma drug concentrations may increase or decrease when statins are administered with meals; however, plasma concentrations of drug do not correlate well with lipid lowering, because the actions of the statins are mediated in the liver where most drug is removed during first pass. Most statins can be given once per day, but twice-a-day dosing is required at higher doses of lovastatin and fluvastatin. The dosage range for atorvastatin is 10 to 80 mg/day, for cerivastatin 0.2 or 0.3 mg/day, for fluvastatin 20 to 80 mg/day, for lovastatin 20 to 80 mg/day, for pravastatin 10 to 40 mg/day, and for simvastatin 10 to 80 mg/day.

### *Indications and efficacy*

Statins are indicated in the treatment of all types of hypercholesterolemia because they are, as a class, the effective agents for lowering cholesterol. They are the agents of choice for secondary prevention and, although they have not been generally recommended as initial therapy for primary prevention, they are increasingly being used as the first-line agents for primary prevention.

Statins are indicated in patients with elevations of LDL due to heterozygous familial hypercholesterolemia (type II hyperlipoproteinemia), as well as polygenic forms of hypercholesterolemia. Given as a single agent, statins may decrease LDL cholesterol values up to 60%. Average LDL reductions with most statins are approximately 25 to 35%. In addition, consistent decreases in VLDL cholesterol concentrations and reductions in triglyceride levels range between 10% and 30%, and generally increases in HDL cholesterol of 2 to 15% are seen. The decline in LDL and VLDL levels is paralleled by reduction of LDL and VLDL apolipoprotein B values. No changes in lipoprotein(a) levels occur. A limited number of controlled trials have directly compared the efficacy of some of the statins. Table 9-15 lists the reported effects of each of the statins on total cholesterol, LDL cholesterol, HDL cholesterol, and triglyceride levels.

When statins are combined with bile acid sequestrants, further reductions in LDL cholesterol values are observed. Similar falls in LDL cholesterol values are seen when statins are combined with niacin; however, this combination should be used cautiously because of potential enhanced adverse effects (see below). Additional reductions of LDL cholesterol values can be obtained when statins are combined with bile acid sequestrants and niacin. Consequently, statins are an important part of therapeutic regimens designed to normalize severely and moderately elevated values of LDL cholesterol.

**Table 9-15 Effect of Statins on Serum Lipid Concentrations at Commonly Used Daily Doses**

| | Percent Change | | | |
|---|---|---|---|---|
| Drug | Total cholesterol | LDL cholesterol | Triglycerides | HDL cholesterol |
| Atorvastatin calcium | | | | |
| 10 mg | −29 | −39 | −19 | +6 |
| 20 mg | −33 | −43 | −26 | +9 |
| 40 mg | −37 | −50 | −29 | +6 |
| 80 mg | −45 | −60 | −37 | +5 |
| Cerivastatin | | | | |
| 0.2 mg | −17 | −25 | −10 | +10 |
| 0.3 mg | −19 | −28 | −12 | +10 |
| Fluvastatin sodium | | | | |
| 20 mg | −17 | −22 | −7 | +4 |
| 40 mg | −21 | −24 | −9 | +6 |
| 80 mg | −27 | −32 | — | — |
| Lovastatin | | | | |
| 10 mg | −16 | −21 | −10 | +5 |
| 20 mg | −17 | −24 | −10 | +7 |
| 40 mg | −22 | −30 | −14 | +7 |
| 80 mg | −29 | −40 | −19 | +9 |
| Pravastatin sodium | | | | |
| 10 mg | −16 | −22 | −15 | +7 |
| 20 mg | −24 | −32 | −11 | +2 |
| 40 mg | −25 | −34 | −24 | +12 |
| Simvastatin | | | | |
| 5 mg | −17 | −24 | −10 | +7 |
| 10 mg | −24 | −33 | −10 | +9 |
| 20 mg | −25 | −33 | −19 | +11 |
| 40 mg | −28 | −40 | −19 | +12 |

Patients with homozygous familial hypercholesterolemia who are LDL-receptor-negative (i.e., do not express LDL receptors) do not respond to statins; however, a therapeutic response may be seen in some individuals who have decreased expression of LDL receptors (Stein 1989). Because the statins have been teratogenic in animals, they should not be used in premenopausal women unless the probability of pregnancy is very low. In addition, nursing mothers should not be treated with statins because the drugs are excreted in milk. To date, there have been no extensive studies in children, but it may be appropriate to use statins in severely hypercholesterolemic children and adolescents.

**PRINCIPLE When drugs tested in adults are used in children, the need for extraordinary surveillance of these children is obvious. Most important, the clinician must be willing to consider the development of any unexpected event as caused by the drug until proved otherwise.**

In addition to their primary indications for patients with elevated concentrations of LDL, statins are very effective in other lipoprotein abnormalities. Statins markedly decrease both triglyceride and cholesterol values in patients with type III hyperlipoproteinemia (dysbetalipoproteinemia) by increasing the catabolism and decreasing the production of $\beta$-VLDL (Vega et al. 1988). Furthermore, conditions where both VLDL and LDL concentrations are raised (e.g., familial combined hyperlipidemia, diabetic dyslipidemia, and nephrotic syndrome) appear to respond well to statins. Treatment of patients with familial combined hyperlipidemia with statins results in substantial reductions in cholesterol and triglyceride levels. Hyperlipidemic patients with noninsulin dependent diabetes mellitus have responded to statins with a 15 to 35% and 30% reduction of cholesterol and triglyceride levels, respectively (Gylling and Miettinen 1997); patients with nephrotic syndrome have shown a 30 to 35% reduction of cholesterol and triglycerides levels (Massy et al. 1995). Because hypertriglyceridemia frequently predominates in these conditions, characterized by both elevated VLDL and LDL concentrations, gemfibrozil or niacin is commonly used initially. Addition of an HMG CoA reductase inhibitor may yield further benefit, but these combinations should be used cautiously (see below).

Several very large randomized controlled studies have established the effectiveness of statins in modifying clinically significant endpoints. In fact, the primary and secondary prevention trials with statins have provided the strongest and most convincing evidence that lowering cholesterol produces beneficial clinical outcomes. The two largest primary prevention trials have been the West of Scotland Coronary Prevention Study (WOSCOP) (Shepherd et al. 1995) and the Air Force/Texas Coronary Atherosclerosis Prevention Study (AFCAPS) (Downs et al. 1998). In WOSCOP, 6500 men with cholesterol >250 mg/dL and without known cardiovascular disease were randomized to pravastatin (40 mg/day) or placebo (Shepherd et al. 1995). Pravastatin resulted in 20% lower total cholesterol, 26% lower LDL cholesterol, 10% lower triglycerides, and 5% higher HDL cholesterol values compared with the placebo group. Drug treatment led to statistically and clinically significant reductions of 31% in the combined endpoints of death from myocardial infarction or definite myocardial infarction and 32% in death from all cardiovascular causes. There was a 22% reduction in mortality from all causes, which was of borderline statistical significance.

AFCAPS randomized 5600 men and 1000 women who were at high risk (total cholesterol/HDL cholesterol ratio >5) but without clinical evidence of atherosclerotic disease to lovastatin (20–40 mg/day) or placebo (Downs et al. 1998). The lovastatin group had 19% lower total cholesterol, 27% lower LDL cholesterol, 12% lower triglyceride, and 5% higher HDL cholesterol values compared with the group receiving placebo. These reductions were associated with statistically significant reductions of 37% in the combined endpoints of unstable angina, fatal and nonfatal myocardial infarction, or sudden cardiac death. However, there were too few deaths from cardiovascular causes to analyze the results, and there were no differences in mortality from all causes.

The two largest secondary prevention trials with statins have been the Scandinavian Simvastatin Survival Study (4S) (Scandinavian Simvastalin Survival Study Group 1994b) and the Cholesterol and Recurrent Events (CARE) trial (Sacks et al. 1996). The 4S trial randomized 4444 men and women with known coronary artery disease and serum cholesterol values of 212 to 309 mg/dL to simvastatin (20 or 40 mg/day) or placebo. Active treatment led to 25% lower total cholesterol, 35% lower LDL cholesterol, 10% lower triglyceride, and 8% higher HDL cholesterol values. These lipid changes were also associated with highly statistically significant reductions of 42% in mortality from coronary heart disease and 30% in mortality from all causes. The CARE trial randomized 4159 men and women who had had a myocardial infarction and a total cholesterol <240 mg/dL to pravastatin (40 mg/day) or placebo and showed 20% reduction in total cholesterol, 28% reduction in LDL cholesterol, 14% reduction in triglycerides, and 5% increase in HDL cholesterol values (treatment versus placebo groups). There was a statistically significant decrease in fatal or definite myocardial infarction in the pravastatin group but no statistically significant change in all-cause mortality. Interestingly, the CARE trial did not see any benefit in coronary events in those patients who had LDL cholesterol values <125 mg/dL at entry into the study, whereas significant reductions in events were observed in those with LDL cholesterol values >125 mg/dL at entry.

When the above three intervention trials are combined with other trials utilizing statins (Hebert et al. 1997), a reduction in risk of overall mortality of 28% and 21% is seen in primary and secondary trials, with a reduction of cardiovascular mortality of 37% and 26%, respectively. In addition, the compilation of the interventions using statins was associated with a 29% reduction in nonfatal strokes, without a difference from placebo in fatal strokes. Consequently, the use of statins appears to result in an overall reduction of cardiovascular mortality of 28% and a reduction in total mortality of 22%, without any evidence for an increase in noncardiovascular deaths.

> **Key Point:** Statins are the most efficacious agents available for lowering LDL cholesterol and have proven efficacy in primary and secondary prevention trials. Statins are the only lipid-lowering agents shown to reduce mortality from all causes.

#### *Adverse effects and drug interactions*

Statins are very well tolerated medications with few adverse side effects. The major adverse effect necessitating discontinuation of therapy has been elevation of liver transaminases. Increases in transaminases to values greater than three times the upper limits of normal occur in less than 2% of patients. The hepatotoxicity of statins is dose-dependent and is observed with both fungus-derived and synthetic HMG-CoA reductase inhibitors. In the majority of patients with increases in transaminases, the changes have occurred within 48 weeks of initiation of therapy. Typically, these changes have returned to normal upon discontinuation of therapy. In addition to increases in transaminases, reversible symptomatic hepatitis manifested by cholestatic or hepatocellular changes has been reported in some patients. Consequently, it is important to follow liver function tests on a regular basis.

A potentially severe adverse effect of statins is myopathy, which is defined by diffuse muscle pain or weakness with elevations of creatine kinase greater than 10 times the upper limits of normal. This develops in <0.2% of treated patients. Frank rhabdomyolysis with renal failure has been described. Most, but not all, of the patients developing severe myopathy have received concomitant therapy with cyclosporine, gemfibrozil, niacin, erythromycin, or imidazole antifungals. The mechanisms for the possible increased risks associated with combination therapy are not clear. Renal insufficiency may increase the risk. The association of myopathy with the combination of gemfibrozil and statins appears to be due to the myopathic effects of each agent and not to any effects of gemfibrozil on the kinetics of statins. Because approximately 5% of patients taking this combination develop myopathy, it should be used with particular caution.

Retrospective analysis of coronary prevention trials has documented cases of myopathy and rhabdomyolysis in patients receiving niacin and a statin, along with other medications. The underlying mechanism for this interaction is unclear because niacin does not affect statin metabolism and is not associated with myopathy when given as a single agent. Several prospective clinical trials combining niacin with either pravastatin or lovastatin have suggested reduced risk of CPK elevations during combined therapy with less than 2 g/day niacin therapy (Gardner et al. 1996). Nonetheless, levels of creatine kinase should be regularly evaluated in patients taking statins, particularly when those patients are on additional medications that might predispose to myopathy.

Lovastatin, simvastatin, and atorvastatin are metabolized by the 3A4 isozyme of the hepatic cytochrome P450 system. By inhibiting this metabolic pathway, some drugs (Table 9-16) may cause reduced first-pass metabolism of statins and possible subsequent higher systemic exposure.

Other, less serious, adverse effects include skin rash in <0.3%, with hypersensitivity reactions presenting as anaphylaxis, lupus-like syndromes, or urticaria reported in a few patients. Gastrointestinal complaints in <0.3%, with constipation the major manifestation, and insomnia in 0.1% are potential adverse effects. There are possible interactions of lovastatin with warfarin, because elevated prothrombin times have been reported in some patients. Lenticular opacities were reported in early clinical trials of lovastatin, but subsequent clinical followup has revealed no ocular toxicity of lovastatin or other drugs in this class.

## Nicotinic Acid (Niacin)

#### *History*

Nicotinic acid was first produced in 1867 from the oxidation of nicotine, derived from the leaves of the plant nicotinia, which had been introduced into France from

Table 9-16 Commonly Used Drugs That Can Inhibit CYP3A4 or Are Substrates of CYP3A4

| Class | Inhibitors of CYP3A4 | Substrates for CYP3A4 |
|---|---|---|
| Antidepressants | Fluoxetine HCl | |
| Antifungals | Ketoconazole, itraconazole | |
| Antihistamines | | Astemizole |
| Anti-infectives | Erythromycin, ciprofloxacin, clarithromycin | |
| Benzodiazepines | | Various |
| Calcium channel blockers | | Various |
| Cardiac agents | Amiodarone HCl | Quinidine sulfate or gluconate |
| Chemotherapeutic agents | Various | |
| Gastrointestinal agents | Cimetidine | Cisapride monohydrate |
| Hormonal agents | | Estrogen, tamoxifen, prednisone |
| Immunosuppressants | Cyclosporine | Cyclosporine |
| Protease inhibitors | Indinavir, ritonavir, saquinavir mesylate | |
| Miscellaneous | Grapefruit juice, cannabinoids | Cocaine HCl |

America by Count Nicotin (Altschul 1964). In the early twentieth century, nicotinic acid (Fig. 9-14) was directly isolated from foodstuffs and suggested to be a nutrient; however, it was not until the mid-1930s that nicotinic acid was shown to be a vitamin and to cure pellagra. At that time, nicotinic acid and its amidated form, nicotinamide, were identified as components of nicotinamide adenine dinucleotide (NAD) and nicotinamide adenine dinucleotide phosphate (NADP) and, thus, important cofactors in a variety of metabolic pathways utilizing oxidative processes.

In 1942, nicotinic acid was renamed niacin (**ni**cotinic **ac**id vitam**in**) in order to avoid confusion with nicotine in food labeling. Based on niacin's involvement in oxidative processes and on an earlier observation that an increased oxygen tension could lower serum cholesterol, Altschul et al. (1955) gave large doses of niacin in an attempt to decrease serum cholesterol concentrations by increasing its oxidation. A decline in total cholesterol of up to 21% was observed in subjects with cholesterol levels >250 mg/dL treated with nicotinic acid, but no effects were seen with nicotinamide. This led to niacin becoming the first agent to be used widely for decreasing concentrations of cholesterol in serum. Later, niacin's ability to lower triglyceride levels was observed (Carlson and Oro 1962), leading to one of its major therapeutic indications.

### *Mechanism of action*

Even though niacin has been used as a hypolipidemic agent for more than 40 years, its mechanisms of action in reducing lipoprotein values are not fully understood. The major action of niacin is to decrease the hepatic production of VLDL without affecting its catabolism (Grundy et al. 1981). This decrease in VLDL production is due principally to a fall in production of triglycerides, leading to a decrease in the triglyceride content of VLDL; however, a decrease in apolipoprotein B production also appears to occur with a decline in the number of VLDL particles. Furthermore, the rate of production of LDL, but not its catabolism, is also reduced (Levy and Langer 1972). Niacin exerts its primary effect in adipose tissue, where it causes a rapid suppression of lipolysis, leading to a decreased concentration of circulating free fatty acids (Carlson and Oro 1962). Interestingly, nicotinamide, which is ineffective as a hypolipidemic agent, does not suppress lipolysis. The decrease in free fatty acid flux lowers the amount of precursor (fatty acids) available to the liver for triglyceride synthesis (reesterification) and VLDL production. Since VLDL are the precursors of LDL, a fall in

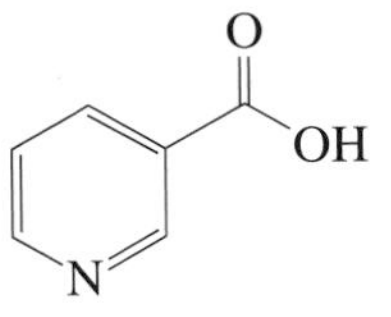

O
OH
N
**Niacin (Nicotinic acid)**

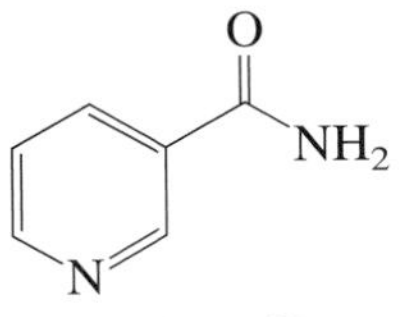

O
$NH_2$
N
**Niacinamide**

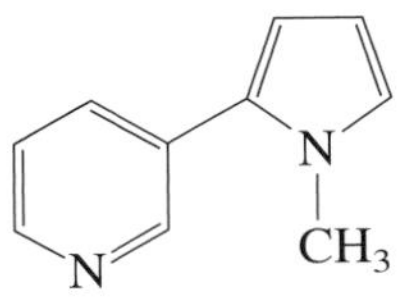

N
N
$CH_3$
**Nicotine**

FIGURE 9-14 **Chemical structures of niacin (nicotinic acid), niacinamide (nicotinamide), and nicotine.**

VLDL production then leads to a subsequent decline in LDL production.

This model might explain the actions of niacin on lipoprotein metabolism, but it is not the sole explanation for niacin's effects, because there is escape from the suppression of free fatty acids by niacin over time. In fact, daylong values of free fatty acids are not significantly lower in patients treated chronically with niacin. Consequently, a direct effect of niacin on inhibition of VLDL (triglyceride) synthesis by the liver has been proposed. Indeed, nicotinic acid has been reported to decrease hepatic synthesis of cholesterol by an uncertain mechanism (Miettinen 1968). Niacin increases the concentration of HDL cholesterol and apolipoprotein AI by decreasing apolipoprotein AI catabolism (Shepherd et al. 1979); however, the underlying mechanism for this effect also is not known. Niacin does not appear to have any consistent effects on fecal sterol excretion or on the composition of bile.

### *Pharmacokinetics*

Niacin is part of the water-soluble vitamin B complex. It is rapidly and completely absorbed from the intestine following oral administration. Time-released preparations of niacin have a delayed absorption and lower peak serum concentrations. Although 15 mg is the daily requirement of niacin as a vitamin, hypolipidemic effects are not seen until daily doses greater than 1 g of crystalline niacin are reached. Up to 6.5 g may be needed for full therapeutic effects. No additional benefit is seen at even higher doses.

After absorption, niacin is cleared by first-pass hepatic metabolism. However, because hepatic metabolism of niacin is saturable, a greater percentage of unaltered niacin enters the systemic circulation with increasing doses (Weiner and Van Eys 1983). The half-life of niacin in plasma is approximately 45 minutes. It distributes to all tissues in the body, where it acts as a vitamin cofactor. Niacin is first amidated to niacinamide, which is active as a vitamin but not as a hypolipidemic agent. Niacinamide is further metabolized by N-methylation and 2-pyridone derivatization (Bicknell and Prescott 1953). The major metabolic derivative of niacin is nicotinuric acid, its glycine conjugate. The amounts of unaltered niacin and of nicotinuric acid appearing in the urine increase progressively at higher doses. When niacin therapy is initiated, dosing should begin at 100 mg given three times daily and increase progressively every 5 to 7 days until a therapeutic effect is achieved.

### *Indications and efficacy*

Niacin is indicated as a first-line agent in the treatment of all forms of hypertriglyceridemia and hypercholesterolemia. Once therapeutic doses are achieved (3 to 6.5 g/day), niacin generally decreases plasma triglyceride (VLDL) values by 20 to 80%, with the greatest decreases seen in subjects with the greatest initial values. In parallel, cholesterol levels decrease 10 to 40% due to decrements in VLDL cholesterol and LDL cholesterol; HDL cholesterol concentrations increase 10 to 30%. The decline in VLDL cholesterol is greater in patients with hypertriglyceridemia and is primarily responsible for the decrement in serum cholesterol levels in these patients. In normotriglyceridemic subjects, the decline in VLDL is relatively small, and most of the fall in serum cholesterol occurs in the LDL fraction.

In concert with these changes in lipid values, niacin causes a decrease in apolipoprotein B values, reflecting fewer circulating VLDL and LDL particles, and causes an increase in apolipoprotein AI, reflecting an increase in HDL. Interestingly, niacin is the only agent reported to lower lipoprotein(a) values. Since its major action is to decrease VLDL production, niacin is particularly effective in patients with type IV and type V hyperlipoproteinemia, as well as type III. Furthermore, since niacin effectively lowers VLDL and LDL levels, it is useful as a single agent in patients where both VLDL and LDL concentrations are raised, e.g., familial combined hyperlipidemia, diabetic dyslipidemia, and nephrotic syndrome. However, its use in diabetes has been associated with worsened glucose control in some patients (Garg and Grundy 1990), and its use in the nephrotic syndrome has not been thoroughly evaluated.

Although no studies have been conducted to evaluate the long-term efficacy of niacin in patients with hypertriglyceridemia, the Coronary Drug Project (The Coronary Drug Project Research Group 1975) compared niacin with placebo in men who had previously had a documented myocardial infarction. These men had multiple risk factors including hypertension, cigarette smoking, glucose intolerance, and hyperlipidemia; as a group, hypertriglyceridemia was the most prevalent abnormality with serum cholesterol averaging about 250 mg/dL and serum triglyceride averaging about 550 mg/dL. After 5 years of followup, serum cholesterol fell 10% and serum triglyceride 26% with niacin therapy. These changes were associated with a 27% reduction in nonfatal myocardial infarction, but no differences in overall mortality (compared with placebo). However, 15-year followup revealed an 11% reduction in overall mortality with niacin (Canner et al. 1986).

**PRINCIPLE Absence of a positive "long-term" effect when the drug has been given for a reasonably brief period does not exclude the long-term effect when studies are sufficiently lengthened.**

Although niacin produces only modest decreases in cholesterol and LDL levels when given as a single agent, it is very effective when used in combination with other hypolipidemic agents. Bile acid sequestrants increase LDL catabolism, but their actions are attenuated by an increase in VLDL production. The ability of niacin to suppress VLDL production results in a synergistic effect. Indeed, a combination of bile acid sequestrant and niacin can normalize LDL cholesterol values in patients with heterozygous familial hypercholesterolemia.

A combination of colestipol and niacin was compared with placebo in the Cholesterol-Lowering Atherosclerosis Study to examine the effects of cholesterol lowering on progression of atherosclerosis in men who have had coronary artery bypass surgery (Blankenhorn et al. 1987). At entry these men were principally hypercholesterolemic with mean cholesterol values of 246 mg/dL and triglyceride values of 151 mg/dL. After 2 years, the treatment group experienced a 26% decrease in cholesterol, a 43% decrease in LDL cholesterol, a 22% decrease in triglycerides, and a 47% increase in HDL cholesterol. These changes were associated with significantly less progression and greater regression of atherosclerotic lesions on coronary angiography.

In another randomized secondary prevention trial, the Stockholm Ischaemic Heart Disease Secondary Prevention Study, niacin was used in combination with clofibrate in men with previous myocardial infarctions (Carlson and Rosenhamer 1988). After 5 years of followup, serum cholesterol and triglyceride decreased 13% and 19%, respectively, from initial values of approximately 230 and 210 mg/dL, respectively. These changes were associated with a decrease in mortality from ischemic heart disease of 36% and in overall mortality of 26%. Thus, niacin has been shown to be a very effective agent, singly and in combination, for reducing triglyceride and cholesterol levels in a variety of hyperlipoproteinemias. Unfortunately, its usefulness as a hypolipidemic agent is frequently limited by its adverse effects.

***Adverse effects and drug interactions***

At the large doses used to produce hypolipidemic effects, niacin has a considerable number of adverse effects that are not observed at the low doses taken as a vitamin (Hotz 1983). The most obvious and dramatic adverse effect is an intense cutaneous flush, with or without pruritus, that occurs within minutes to hours after an oral dose. This cutaneous flush is part of a generalized vasodilatory effect of niacin that appears to be mediated via prostaglandins. Aspirin (325 mg) is effective in preventing the flush and can be given 30 minutes preceding a dose to prevent symptoms. However, aspirin is often not required, since tachyphylaxis develops to the vasodilatory effects of the drug, with diminution of the symptoms over time while the same doses are continued. Other skin changes such as dryness, hyperpigmentation, and acanthosis nigracans occur occasionally. Additionally, the incidence of atrial fibrillation and ventricular ectopy may be increased by niacin.

The most serious adverse effect of niacin is hepatic dysfunction with elevations of alkaline phosphatase and transaminases commonly occurring at doses greater than 3 g/day. Occasionally, symptomatic hepatitis with jaundice is seen. The hepatic abnormalities are reversible upon discontinuation of the drug; however, hepatic fibrosis has been reported. An inhibitory effect of the high doses of niacin on normal NAD synthesis is the presumed mechanism of the hepatotoxicity. Time-released preparations of niacin are associated with less cutaneous flushing but appear to produce greater incidence of elevation of liver function tests (Knopp et al. 1985). Niacin increases gastric acid secretion and is contraindicated in patients with peptic ulcer disease. It also is associated with other gastrointestinal effects, such as abdominal discomfort, nausea, and diarrhea.

Another adverse effect is deterioration of glucose tolerance, which generally occurs in patients with preexisting impaired glucose tolerance. Prospective trials have documented increases in hemoglobin Alc of $<0.5\%$ in diabetic and nondiabetic subjects when treated with low doses of niacin in combination with pravastatin (Tsalamandris et al. 1994; Gardner et al. 1997). However, increases in hemoglobin A1c of $>1\%$ were seen in diabetics treated with niacin 4.5 g/day (Garg and Grundy 1990). Hyperuricemia secondary to increases in purine metabolism and decreases in renal clearance may occur, occasionally with precipitation of gouty arthritis. The possible interaction between niacin and statins in terms of risk of muscle injury is described above. Decreased levels of total thyroxine due to low thyroxine binding globulin have been observed in patients on the combination of colestipol and niacin, even though thyroid function tests are normal on either agent alone.

Niacin has been formulated in sustained-release preparations using polygel or wax matrix excipients, which results in reduced cutaneous symptoms and the convenience of once-per-day dosing. Sustained-release niacin is the major form of niacin available as a nonprescription preparation, and formulation and bioavailability have not been standardized among available preparations. Prescription formulations of sustained-release niacin include Nicobid, Slo-Niacin, and Niaspan. The pharmacological effects of crystalline and sustained-release niacin are different. Sustained-release niacin is more efficacious in LDL lowering but less efficacious in raising HDL and lowering triglycerides. Daily doses of sustained-release niacin of 1.5 g demonstrate LDL-lowering effects similar to 3 g/day of crystalline niacin (approximately 20% reduction). At this dose of sustained-release niacin, 25 to 33% reductions in triglycerides and 6 to 12% increases in HDL have been reported (Gray et al. 1994; McKenney et al. 1994). Unlike crystalline niacin, which has triglyceride and HDL effects at doses lower than those required for LDL reduction, sustained-release niacin does not demonstrate preferential effects on HDL and triglyceride. Clinical trials with Niaspan in approximately 300 patients, once-daily bedtime dosing of 1.5 g, demonstrated LDL reduction of 13%, HDL elevation of 18%, and TG lowering of 25% compared with placebo.

Sustained-release niacin has hepatotoxicity at lower doses than found for crystalline niacin. In one clinical trial with 46 patients, mean transaminase concentrations were elevated twofold at doses over 1.5 g/day (McKenney et al. 1994). In a retrospective analysis of 969 patients treated with 1.5 g/day of sustained release niacin (Slo-Niacin), approximately one-half of patients discontinued therapy due to cutaneous symptoms, worsened hyperglycemia, or increased transaminases (Gray et al. 1994). In this population, 4.7% of subjects experienced transaminase elevations that were probably or possibly related to niacin therapy. Clinical trials with Niaspan have demonstrated increased transaminases in less than 2% of 245 subjects during 17 weeks of therapy with doses of 0.5 to 3 g/day. Sustained-release niacin may be useful in patients with combined hyperlipidemia who do not tolerate crystalline niacin, but liver function should be monitored carefully.

## Fibric Acids

### *History*

In screening chemicals for hypolipidemic activity, a series of aryloxyisobutyric acid compounds were found to lower cholesterol levels in rats; the most potent of these was ethyl 2-(p-chlorophenoxy)-2-methyl-isobutyrate (CPIB) (Thorp and Waring 1962). Originally, CPIB, or clofibrate as it was later named, was thought to exert its action through a synergistic effect with the adrenal steroid androsterone. Therefore, the first formulation included clofibrate in combination with androsterone (Atromid). However, when it became apparent that the hypolipidemic effects of Atromid were due solely to the actions of clofibrate, androsterone was deleted from the preparation, and it was renamed Atromid-S. After successful introduction of clofibrate as a hypolipidemic agent, several other analogues were produced. Of these "fibric acids," gemfibrozil, a substituted xylyloxy-valeric acid, and fenofibrate, a substituted propanoic acid, are available in the United States, while bezafibrate and others are in use in Europe or are in clinical development (Fig. 9-15).

### *Mechanism of action*

Although the fibric acids have been in use for more than 30 years, their mechanism of action has only recently been determined and is not yet fully understood. Fibric acids act as ligands for the peroxisomal proliferator activated receptor (PPAR), a member of the family of thyroid/steroid hormone receptors that act as nuclear transcription factors (Forman et al. 1996). Although the details are beyond the scope of this chapter, fibric acids influence multiple steps in lipid and lipoprotein metabolism by modi-

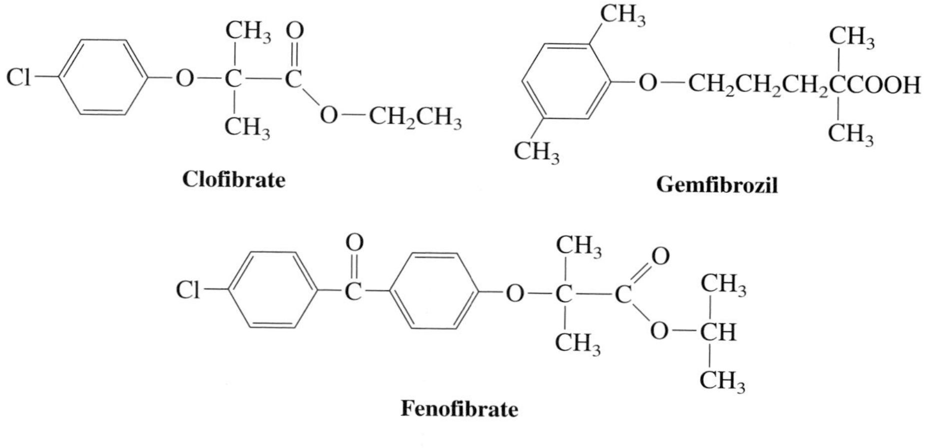

FIGURE 9-15 Chemical structures of fibric acids.

fying the transcription of a variety of genes through activation of PPAR (Schoonjans et al. 1996). The major action of the fibric acids is to decrease VLDL concentrations by increasing the rate of catabolism of VLDL (Kesaniemi and Grundy 1984). The fibric acids appear to promote catabolism of VLDL by stimulating lipoprotein lipase activity. Whereas an increase in catabolism of VLDL explains most of the reduction in concentrations of VLDL, fibric acids also decrease VLDL triglyceride and apolipoprotein B production. The explanation for the decline in production of VLDL is not fully understood, but has been attributed to several mechanisms of the fibric acids: inhibition of hepatic acetyl CoA carboxylase (an important enzyme in triglyceride synthesis) and suppression of lipolysis and free fatty acid flux.

The effects of the fibric acids on LDL metabolism are variable. In patients with hypertriglyceridemia, fibric acids frequently increase LDL values by decreasing LDL catabolism with no change or small decreases in production of LDL (Vega and Grundy 1985). This alteration probably is not a direct effect of fibric acids but occurs secondarily to the enhanced catabolism of VLDL and the resultant down-regulation of LDL receptors in the liver induced by increased clearance of VLDL and VLDL remnants (IDL). In patients with hypercholesterolemia and normal triglycerides, fibric acids have been reported to increase receptor-mediated catabolism of LDL slightly, without affecting production of LDL (Stewart et al. 1982); however, no direct effects of fibric acids on cholesterol synthesis have been observed. The fibric acids raise HDL cholesterol and apolipoprotein AI values by increasing the production rate of apolipoprotein AI (Saku et al. 1985). All of the fibric acids increase biliary cholesterol and decrease bile acid secretion, leading to a saturated or lithogenic state that predisposes to formation of gallstones (Palmer 1987).

### *Pharmacokinetics*

The fibric acids presently available in the United States are clofibrate, gemfibrozil (Lopid), and micronized fenofibrate (Tricor). They are prescribed in doses of 0.5 to 1 g bid, 300 to 600 mg bid, and 67 mg qd to tid, respectively. Because clofibrate is generally less efficacious and usually associated with more adverse effects (see below), it is not frequently recommended. Fibric acids are readily absorbed from the gastrointestinal tract. Clofibrate and fenofibrate are very highly protein bound (90 to 95%) and have a plasma half-life of 7 to 8 hours and 20 hours, respectively, whereas gemfibrozil has a half-life of only 1.5 hours. Elimination of clofibrate and fenofibrate occur through conjugation with subsequent renal excretion. In contrast, gemfibrozil undergoes hydroxylation and conjugation before renal excretion.

### *Indications and efficacy*

Although fibric acids have been used as hypocholesterolemic agents for more than 30 years, they are primarily indicated in the treatment of patients with various forms of hypertriglyceridemia, since their major effect is to lower VLDL values. In general, the fibric acids produce a 25 to 60% decrease in triglycerides, while lowering cholesterol values 5 to 25%. HDL cholesterol usually increases 10 to 20% with fibric acids; however, the LDL cholesterol response is quite variable, with decreases of 10 to 20% occurring in some patients, and increases of 5 to 20% occurring in others. The response of LDL cholesterol appears to depend on the underlying hyperlipidemia being treated. Increases in LDL cholesterol generally occur in patients with primary hypertriglyceridemia (type IV hyperlipoproteinemia), and modest decreases in LDL cholesterol occur in patients with hypercholesterolemia (type II hyperlipoproteinemia) or in patients with combined hypertriglyceridemia and hypercholesterolemia (type IIb hyperlipoproteinemia). Apolipoprotein values usually parallel the lipid changes observed; apolipoprotein B values either decrease or remain unchanged, and apolipoprotein AI values usually increase.

Because fibric acids will decrease both triglyceride and cholesterol levels in patients with type IIb hyperlipoproteinemia, they are useful in other patients with elevations of VLDL and LDL, such as diabetic dyslipidemia and nephrotic syndrome. Indeed, fibric acids might improve glucose tolerance; however, their use in nephrotic syndrome should be undertaken with caution, since renal insufficiency predisposes to some of their adverse effects (see below). Additionally, fibric acids are very effective in patients with type III hyperlipoproteinemia (dysbetalipoproteinemia) because of their ability to lower VLDL.

Fibric acids have been used in combination with other hypolipidemic agents, including bile acid sequestrants, statins (see above), and niacin (see above). These combinations are generally considered when patients with type IV or type IIb hyperlipoproteinemia have a good hypotriglyceridemic response to a fibric acid, but an increase in LDL cholesterol is observed. While these combinations can be effective, an increase in adverse effects may be seen when used with statins (see above) but not when used with bile acid sequestrants.

Fibric acids have not been studied in women during pregnancy or lactation. Studies in animals have shown no teratogenicity of fibric acids, but embryotoxicity and carcinogenesis have been observed at high doses. Consequently, fibric acids are not routinely recommended during pregnancy but can be used cautiously in women with severe hypertriglyceridemia that is exacerbated by pregnancy.

Fibric acids have been employed in several long-term primary and secondary prevention trials. In the largest primary prevention trial, sponsored by the World Health Organization (WHO), 10,000 men with moderate hypercholesterolemia (mean cholesterol ~270 mg/dL) were randomized to clofibrate or placebo (Committee of Principal Investigators 1978). After 5 years of followup, clofibrate reduced cholesterol levels by 9% and decreased nonfatal myocardial infarction by 25%; however, no differences in fatal myocardial infarction were noted. Most disturbing, clofibrate use was associated with a 25% increase in overall mortality, due primarily to diseases of the gastrointestinal tract (see below). Following discontinuation of therapy, the excess mortality in the clofibrate-treated group did not continue (Committee of Principal Investigators 1984).

In a secondary prevention trial of men with previous myocardial infarctions (the Coronary Drug Project), 1100 men were randomized to clofibrate (The Coronary Drug Project Research Group 1975). These men had multiple risk factors including hypertension, cigarette smoking, glucose intolerance, and hyperlipidemia. As a group, hypertriglyceridemia was the most prevalent abnormality, with serum cholesterol averaging ~250 mg/dL and serum triglyceride averaging ~550 mg/dL. After 5 years of followup, serum cholesterol fell 6.5% and serum triglycerides fell 22% with clofibrate; however, no differences in myocardial infarction (fatal or nonfatal) or in overall mortality were noted. On the contrary, clofibrate use was associated with an increased incidence of thromboembolic disease, arrhythmias, claudication, and the development of angina.

On the basis of the results of the WHO and the Coronary Drug Project studies, the use of clofibrate has declined, and its use cannot be generally recommended. In contrast to the results with clofibrate, the findings of a primary prevention trial with gemfibrozil were more encouraging (Frick et al. 1978). More than 4000 men with a variety of lipoprotein abnormalities (mean total cholesterol 289 mg/dL, mean triglyceride 178 mg/dL), and all with non-HDL cholesterol values ≥200 mg/dL, were randomized to gemfibrozil or placebo for 5 years. At the completion of the study there were 10% and 35% declines in cholesterol and triglyceride levels, with an 11% increase in HDL (Manninen et al. 1988). These changes were associated with a 34% reduction in the incidence of coronary heart disease, but no differences in overall mortality due to an increase in accidental and violent deaths. The improvement in the incidence of coronary heart disease was greatest for patients with type IIb hyperlipoproteinemia and correlated best with the extent of increase of HDL. In a recent secondary prevention trial with gemfibrozil (Veterans Affairs Cooperative Studies Program High-Density Lipoprotein Cholesterol Intervention Trial—VA-HIT), ~2500 men with coronary heart disease, HDL cholesterol ≤40 mg/dL, and LDL cholesterol ≤140 mg/dL were randomized to placebo or 1200 mg of gemfibrozil daily for 5 years (Rubins et al. 1999). Active treatment lead to a 6% increase in HDL cholesterol (34 vs. 32 mg/dL), a 4% reduction in total cholesterol (170 vs. 177 mg/dL), a 31% reduction in triglycerides (115 vs. 166 mg/dL), and no differences in LDL cholesterol (113 mg/dL). These lipid changes were associated with a statistically significant 22% reduction in death from coronary heart disease or nonfatal myocardial infarction; however, no statistically significant effects on all-cause mortality were seen. Thus, with the results of the various intervention trials to date, gemfibrozil can be recommended as a first line agent for the treatment of hypertriglyceridemia and as a secondary agent for the treatment of several other hyperlipidemias.

**PRINCIPLE Before using a surrogate endpoint as the sole measure of efficacy, the clinician must be assured that the surrogate correlates very well with the ultimate efficacy being sought.**

### *Adverse effects and drug interactions*

The number and incidence of reported adverse effects is more extensive with clofibrate than gemfibrozil or fenofibrate. The most common adverse effects with fibric acids involve the gastrointestinal tract. Abdominal pain, diarrhea, nausea, and vomiting are seen in some patients, with reversible elevations in hepatic transaminases also observed. Therefore, liver function should be routinely evaluated in patients taking fibric acids and their use is contraindicated in patients with pre-existing liver disease. The most serious adverse effect is an approximate twofold increase in gallstones with clofibrate (Committee of Principal Investigators 1978; The Coronary Drug Project Research Group 1977). This incidence of gallstones has not been observed with gemfibrozil; however, gemfibrozil and fenofibrate do alter the lithogenicity of bile as does clofibrate, and a trend toward a greater prevalence of gallstones has been observed. Fibric acids should be avoided in patients with cholelithiasis. Other complications observed during long-term therapy include an increased incidence of thromboembolic events and a trend toward an increased mortality from gastrointestinal disease, particularly with clofibrate (as described above). The syndrome of inappropriate antidiuretic hormone with hyponatremia has been reported with clofibrate. Furthermore, fibric acids are associated with myositis and rhabdomyolysis, which are more likely to develop in patients with renal insufficiency possibly since the fibric acids are cleared primarily by the kidneys. In addition, the combination of fibric acids with statins appears to predispose to a greater incidence of myositis (see above). Finally, major interactions of the fibric acids with other drugs occur, specifically with oral anticoagulants. Fibric acids potentiate the action of oral anticoagulants, necessitating close monitoring of the prothrombin time and adjustment of doses to achieve appropriate anticoagulation.

**PRINCIPLE The most important interactions on which to focus involve one or more drugs with narrow therapeutic indices.**

### Other Drugs

Several other drugs have been used as hypolipidemic agents, but they should be considered as alternative therapy; some drugs that have been used as hypolipidemic agents in the past cannot be recommended for use at the present time. Such drugs include probucol, neomycin, activated charcoal, psyllium hydrophilic mucilloid, $\beta$-sitosterol, and D-thyroxine.

## COST AND PRACTICAL CONSIDERATIONS IN HYPOLIPIDEMIC THERAPY

Hypolipidemic agents vary widely with respect to efficacy, ease of dosing, drug–disease interactions, and cost of therapy. For these reasons, individualization of the therapeutic regimen requires consideration of multiple factors. A major therapeutic distinction must be made between primary and secondary prevention of cardiovascular disease. NCEP treatment guidelines for primary prevention emphasize stepped care, beginning with diet and progressing to niacin or bile acid sequestrant therapy. Although this regimen effectively decreases LDL cholesterol values, primary prevention of coronary disease has demonstrated a significant mortality benefit only for hypercholesterolemic middle-aged men treated with a HMG-CoA reductase inhibitor (Shepherd et al. 1995).

Statin therapy is more convenient and results in a higher percentage of patients achieving therapeutic LDL goals but is significantly more expensive than stepped care (Oster et al. 1996). For patients requiring mild to moderate LDL reduction, fluvastatin is the most cost-effective HMG-CoA reductase inhibitor (Spearman et al. 1997). Due to a plateau in the dose-response curve for statins, increasing to maximal doses significantly worsens the cost-effectiveness of statin therapy (Perreault et al. 1998). Combination therapy with low-dose statin and either niacin or bile acid sequestrants may be more cost-effective if patient compliance is satisfactory (Heudebert et al. 1993). Using a multivariate model of cardiovascular risk, the cost of lovastatin therapy in middle-aged women is approximately 3 to 5 times higher than that in men (Perreault et al. 1998). Hypolipidemic therapy for primary coronary prevention is not highly cost-effective in low-risk populations.

Due to the high rate of recurrent cardiovascular events in patients with known coronary disease, hypolipidemic therapy demonstrates greater cost-effectiveness in secondary prevention. Cost per year of life saved in clinical trials using pravastatin or simvastatin is in the range of commonly accepted health interventions (Ashraf et al. 1996; Johannesson et al. 1997). When indirect costs such as lost economic productivity are considered, secondary prevention in young patients has a positive economic impact. In the secondary prevention population, vigorous management of hyperlipidemia is justified, but other practical considerations may affect the choice of therapy. For instance, a retrospective analysis of the CARE study has demonstrated that dyslipidemic patients with LDL <125 mg/dL derive no mortality benefit from statin therapy for secondary prevention; however, this floor effect was not observed in the 4S trial. Although short-term mortality benefit has best been demonstrated for statins, the most common lipoprotein disorder, combined hyperlipidemia, is not always satisfactorily treated by HMG-CoA reductase inhibitors alone. Hypertriglyceridemic patients with low HDL cholesterol demonstrate a high total cholesterol/HDL ratio, which is a more powerful predictor of coronary risk than LDL cholesterol alone. The VA-HIT secondary prevention trial appears to support the clinical benefit of raising HDL and lowering triglycerides.

Due to aggressive therapeutic goals in secondary prevention (LDL <100 mg/dL), dose-dependent risk of hepatotoxicity and myopathy, and marginal costs of high-dose statin therapy, combination hypolipidemic therapy should be considered in patients who do not achieve therapeutic goals with low-to-moderate doses of statins. For patients with isolated LDL elevation, statins and bile acid sequestrants are safe in combination and produce >40% reductions in LDL. For patients with combined hyperlip-

Table 9-17 Drug Costs

| AGENT | USUAL DAILY DOSE | COST ($/MONTH)AWP | ADVERSE EFFECTS | MAY BE COMBINED WITH |
|---|---|---|---|---|
| *Statins* | | | Hepatitis, myopathy, drug interactions | Bile acid sequestrants, niacin, or fibrates; requires monitoring |
| Lovastatin | 10–80 mg | Mevacor (20 mg) $70 | | |
| Pravastatin sodium | 10–40 mg | Pravachol (20 mg) $68 | | |
| Simvastatin | 5–80 mg | Zocor (20 mg) $114 | | |
| Atorvastatin calcium | 10–80 mg | Lipitor (10 mg) $66 | | |
| Cerivastatin | 0.2–0.3 mg | Baycol (0.2 mg) $40 | | |
| Fluvastatin sodium | 20–40 mg | Lescol (40 mg) $38 | | |
| *Fibrates* | | | Myopathy, GI | Bile acid sequestrants, niacin |
| Gemfibrozil | 600–1200 mg | Generic (1.2 g) $11, Lopid (1.2 g) $72 | | |
| Clofibrate | 1–2 g | Generic (2 g) $31, Atromid-S (2 g) $107 | | |
| Fenofibrate | 67–201 mg | Tricor (201 mg) $62 | | |
| *Niacin* | | | Flushing, pruritus, hepatic, hyperglycemia, hyperuricemia | Bile acid sequestrants, fibrates, statins (low dose with monitoring) |
| Crystalline | 1.5–6 g | Generic (3 g) $5, Nicolar (3 g) $115 | | |
| Slow release | 1–2 g | Generic (1 g) $25 | | |
| *Bile acid sequestrants* | | | Constipation, reduced drug Absorption | Statins, fibrates, niacin May reduce absorption |
| Cholestyramine | 4–24 g | Questran (16 g) $76 | | |
| Colestipol | 5–30 g | Colestid (20 g) $147 | | |

ABBREVIATIONS: AWP, average wholesale price; NA, not applicable.
SOURCE: Source of drug prices is 1999 *Redbook*. Current prices may vary from those quoted, but comparative prices among products are expected to be similar. The reader should check on local prices at the time of prescribing.

idemia that is not well controlled on monotherapy, therapeutic options are problematic. Atorvastatin and high doses of other statins demonstrate 20 to 30% triglyceride-lowering effects but are often not adequate as monotherapy in combined hyperlipidemia. Low-dose immediate-release niacin (1.5 g/day) combined with a statin appears to be safe and well tolerated but requires monitoring of hepatic function and glucose tolerance. Combination therapy with statins and fibrates is effective but poses increased risk of myopathy. The costs and therapeutic considerations for hypolipidemic agents are presented in Table 9-17.

## REFERENCES


Alberts AW, Chen J, Kuron G, et al. 1980. Mevinolin: A highly-potent competitive inhibitor of hydroxymethylglutaryl-coenzyme A reductase and a cholesterol agent. *Proc Natl Acad Sci USA* **77**:3957–61.

Altschul R. 1964. Influence of nicotinic acid (niacin) on hypercholesterolemia and hyperlipemia and on the course of atherosclerosis. In: Altschul R, editor. *Niacin in Vascular Disorders and Hyperlipemia.* Springfield, IL: Charles C. Thomas, pp 3–135.

Altschul R, Hoffer A, Stephen JD. 1955. Influence of nicotinic acid on serum cholesterol in man. *Arch Biochem Biophys* **54**:558–9.

American Academy of Pediatrics. Committee on Nutrition. 1992b. Statement on cholesterol. *Pediatrics* **90**:469–73.

American College of Physicians (ACP). 1996. Guidelines for using serum cholesterol, high-density lipoprotein cholesterol, and triglyceride levels as screening tests for preventing coronary heart disease in adults. *Ann Intern Med* **124**:515–7.

Ashraf T, Hay JW, Pitt B, et al. 1996. Cost-effectiveness of pravastatin in secondary prevention of coronary artery disease. *Am J Cardiol* **78**:409–14.

Austin MA. 1991. Plasma triglyceride and coronary heart disease. *Arterioscler Thromb* **11**:2–14.

Avigan J, Steinberg D. 1962. Deposition of desmosterol in the lesions of experimental atherosclerosis. *Lancet* **1**:572.

Avigan J, Steinberg D, Vroman HE, et al. 1960. Studies of cholesterol biosynthesis. I: The identification of desmosterol in serum and tissues of animals and man treated with MER-29. *J Biol Chem* **235**:3123–6.

Benlian P, De Gennes JL, Foubert L, et al. 1996. Premature atherosclerosis in patients with familial chylomicronemia caused by mutations in the lipoprotein lipase gene. *N Engl J Med* **335**:848–54.

Bicknell F, Prescott F. 1953. Nicotinic acid. In: *The Vitamins in Medicine.* New York: Grune & Stratton. p 333–89.

Bilheimer DW, Grundy SM, Brown MS, et al. 1983. Mevinolin and colestipol stimulate receptor-mediated clearance of low density lipoprotein from plasma in familial hypercholesterolemia heterozygotes. *Proc Natl Acad Sci USA* **80**:124–8.

Blankenhorn DH, Nessim SA, Johnson RL, et al. 1987. Beneficial effects of combined colestipol-niacin therapy on coronary atherosclerosis and coronary venous bypass grafts. *JAMA* **257**: 3233–40.

Blohm TR, MacKenzie RD. 1959. Specific inhibition of cholesterol biosynthesis by a synthetic compound (MER-29). *Arch Biochem Biophys* **85**:245–9.

Brensike JF, Levy RI, Kelsey SF, et al. 1984. Effects of therapy with cholestyramine on progression of coronary arteriosclerosis: Results of the NHLBI type II coronary intervention study. *Circulation* **69**:313–24.

Brown AG, Smale TC, King TJ, et al. 1976. Crystal and molecular structure of compactin, a new antifungal metabolite from *Penicillum brevicompactum. J Chem Soc Perkin* **1**:1165–70.

Brown MS, Faust JR, Goldstein JL, et al. 1978. Induction of 3-hydroxy-3-methylglutaryl coenzyme A reductase activity in human fibroblasts incubated with compactin (ML-236B), a competitive inhibitor of the reductase. *J Biol Chem* **253**:1121–8.

Brown MS, Goldstein JL. 1980. Multivalent feedback regulation of HMG CoA reductase, a control mechanism coordinating isoprenoid synthesis and cell growth. *J Lipid Res* **21**:505–17.

Canner PL, Berge KG, Wenger NK, et al. 1986. Fifteen year mortality in Coronary Drug Project patients: long-term benefit with niacin. The Coronary Drug Project Research Group. *J Am Coll Cardiol* **8**:1245–55.

Carlson LA, Oro L. 1962. The effect of nicotinic acid on plasma free fatty acids: Demonstration of a metabolic type of synapthicolysis. *Acta Med Scand* **172**:641–5.

Carlson LA, Rosenhamer G. 1988. Reduction of mortality in the Stockholm Ischaemic Heart Disease Secondary Prevention Study by combined treatment with clofibrate and nicotinic acid. *Acta Med Scand* **223**:405–18.

Committee of Principal Investigators. 1978. A co-operative trial in the primary prevention of ischaemic heart disease using clofibrate. *Br Heart J* **40**:1069–118.

Committee of Principal Investigators. 1984. WHO cooperative trial on primary prevention of ischaemic heart disease with clofibrate to lower serum cholesterol: Final mortality follow-up. *Lancet* **2**:600–4.

Cooper AD. 1997. Hepatic uptake of chylomicron remnants. *J Lipid Res* **38**:2173–92.

Downs JR, Clearfield M, Weis S, et al. 1998. Primary prevention of acute coronary events with lovastatin in men and women with average cholesterol levels: results of AFCAPS/TexCAPS. *JAMA* **279**:1615–22.

Endo A, Monakolin K. 1979. A new hypocholesterolemic agent produced by a *Monascus* species. *J Antibiot* **32**:852–4.

Endo A, Kuroda M, Tanzawa K. 1967a. Competitive inhibition of 3-hydroxy-3-methylglutaryl coenzyme A reductase by ML-236A and ML-236B, fungal metabolites having hypocholesterolemic activity. *FEBS Lett* **72**:323–6.

Endo A, Kuroda M, Tsujita Y. 1976b. ML-236A, ML-236B, and ML-236C, new inhibitors of cholesterologenesis produced by *Penicillium citrinum. J Antibiot* **29**:1346–8.

Fontbonne A, Charles MA, Thibult N, et al. 1991. Hyperinsulinaemia as a predictor of coronary heart disease mortality in a healthy population. The Paris Prospective Study, 15-year follow-up. *Diabetologia* **34**:356–61.

Forman BM, Chen J, Evans RM. 1996. The peroxisome proliferator-activated receptors: ligands and activators. *Ann NY Acad Sci* **804**:266–75.

Fredrickson DS, Levy RI, Lees RS. 1967. Fat transport in lipoproteins: an integrated approach to mechanism and disorders. *N Engl J Med* **27**:34–43, 94–103, 148–56, 215–24, 273–81.

Frick MH, Elo O, Haapa K, et al. 1987. Helsinki Heart Study: primary prevention trial with gemfibrozil in middle-aged men with dyslipidemia: Safety of treatment, changes in risk factors, and incidence of coronary heart disease. *N Engl J Med* **317**:1237–45.

Friedewald WT, Levy RI, Frederickson DS. 1972. Estimation of the concentration of low density lipoprotein cholesterol in plasma, without use of the preparative ultracentrifuge. *Clin Chem* **18**:499–502.

Gardner SF, Marx MA, White LM, et al. 1997. Combination of low-dose niacin and pravastatin improves the lipid profile in diabetic patients without compromising glycemic control. *Ann Pharmacother* **31**:677–82.

Gardner SF, Schneider EF, Granberry MC, et al. 1996. Combination therapy with low-dose lovastatin and niacin is as effective as higher-dose lovastatin. *Pharmacotherapy* **16**:419–23.

Garg A, Grundy SM. 1990. Nicotinic acid as therapy for dyslipidemia in non-insulin-dependent diabetes-mellitus. *JAMA* **264**:723–6.

Ginsberg HN, Le N-A, Short MP, et al. 1987. Suppression of apolipoprotein B production during treatment of cholesteryl ester storage disease with lovastatin: Implications for regulation of apolipoprotein B synthesis. *J Clin Invest* **80**:1692–7.

Glueck CJ, Fallat RW, Millett F, et al. 1975. Familial hyper-alphalipoproteinemia: Studies in eighteen kindreds. *Metabolism* **24**:1243–65.

Goldstein JL, Brown MS. 1990. Regulation of the mevalonate pathway. *Nature* **343**:425–30.

Goldstein JL, Schrott HG, Hazard WR, et al. 1973. Hyperlipidemia in coronary heart disease. II: Genetic analysis of lipid levels in 176 families and delineation of a new inherited disorder, combined hyperlipidemia. *J Clin Invest* **52**:1544–68.

Gray DR, Morgan T, Chretien SD, et al. 1994. Efficacy and safety of controlled-release niacin in dyslipoproteinemic veterans. *Ann Int Med* **121**:252–8.

Grundy SM, Bilheimer DW. 1984. Inhibition of 3-hydroxy-3-methylglutaryl-CoA reductase by mevinolin in familial hypercholesterolemia heterozygotes: effects on cholesterol balance. *Proc Natl Acad Sci USA* **81**:2538–42.

Grundy SM, Chait A, Brunzell JD. 1987. Familial Combined Hyperlipidemia Workshop. *Arteriosclerosis* **7**:203–7.

Grundy SM, Mok HYI, Zech L, et al. 1981. Influence of nicotinic acid on metabolism of cholesterol and triglycerides in man. *J Lipid Res* **22**:24–36.

Grundy SM, Vega GL. 1985. Influence of mevinolin on metabolism of low density lipoproteins in primary moderate hypercholesterolemia. *J Lipid Res* **26**:1464–75.

Gylling H, Miettinen TA. 1977. Treatment of lipid disorders in non-insulin-dependent diabetes mellitus. *Curr Opin Lipidol* **8**: 342–7.

Hebert PR, Gaziano JM, Chan KS, et al. 1997. Cholesterol lowering with statin drugs, risk of stroke, and total mortality: An overview of randomized trials. *JAMA* **278**:313–21.

Heudebert GR, Van Ruiswyk J, Hiatt J, et al. 1993. Combination drug therapy for hypercholesterolemia: The trade-off between cost and simplicity. *Arch Int Med* **153**:1828–37.

Hobbs HH, Russell DW, Brown MS, et al. 1990. The LDL receptor locus in familial hypercholesterolemia: Mutational analysis of a membrane protein. *Annu Rev Genet* **24**:133–70.

Hotz W. 1983. Nicotinic acid and its derivatives: A short survey. *Adv Lipid Res* **20**:195–217.

Innerarity TL, Mahley RW, Weisagraber KH, et al. 1990. Familial defective apolipoprotein B-100: A mutation of apolipoprotein B that causes hypercholesterolemia. *J Lipid Res* **31**:1337–49.

Jacobs D, Blackburn H, Higgins M. 1992. Report of the Conference on Low Blood Cholesterol: mortality associations. *Circulation* **86**:1046–60.

Johannesson M, Jonsson B, Kjekshus J, et al. 1997. Cost effectiveness of simvastatin treatment to lower cholesterol levels in patients with coronary heart disease. Scandinavian Simvastatin Survival Study Group. *N Engl J Med* **336**:332–6.

Kesaniemi YA, Grundy SM. 1984. Influence of gemfibrozil on metabolism of cholesterol and plasma triglycerides in man. *JAMA* **251**:2241–6.

Knopp RH, Ginsberg J, Albers JJ, et al. 1985. Contrasting effects of unmodified and time-release forms of niacin on lipoproteins in hyperlipidemic subjects: Clues to mechanism of action of niacin. *Metabolism* **34**:642–50.

Kronmal RA, Cain KC, Ye Z, et al. 1993. Total serum cholesterol levels and mortality risk as a function of age: A report based on the Framingham data. *Arch Intern Med* **153**:1065–73.

Laughlin RC, Carey TF. 1962. Cataracts in patients treated with triparanol. *JAMA* **181**:339–40.

Levy RI, Brensike JF, Epstein SI, et al. 1984. The influence of changes in lipid values induced by cholestyramine and diet on progression of coronary artery disease: results of the NHLBI type II Coronary Intervention Study. *Circulation* **69**:325–37.

Levy RI, Langer T. 1972. Hypolipidemic drugs and lipoprotein metabolism. *Adv Exp Med Biol* **27**:155–63.

Lipid Research Clinics Program. 1984a. The Lipid Research Clinics Coronary Primary Prevention Trial results. I: reduction in incidence of coronary heart disease. *JAMA* **251**:351–64.

Lipid Research Clinics Program. 1984b. The Lipid Research Clinics Coronary Primary Prevention Trial results. II: The relationship of reduction in incidence of coronary heart disease to cholesterol lowering. *JAMA* **251**:365–74.

Ma PTS, Gil G, Sudhof TC, et al. 1986. Mevinolin, an inhibitor of cholesterol synthesis, induces mRNA for low density lipoprotein receptor in livers of hamsters and rabbits. *Proc Natl Acad Sci USA* **83**:8370–4.

Mahley RW. 1982. Atherogenic lipoproteins: the cellular and molecular biology of plasma lipoproteins altered by dietary fat and cholesterol. *Med Clin North Am* **66**:375–402.

Mahley RW, Weisgraber KH, Innerarity TL, et al. 1991. Genetic defects in lipoprotein metabolism: elevation of atherogenic lipoproteins caused by impaired catabolism. *JAMA* **265**:78–83.

Manninen V, Elo O, Frick H, et al. 1988. Lipid alterations and decline in the incidence of coronary heart disease in the Helsinki Heart Study. *JAMA* **260**:641–51.

Manolio TA, Pearson TA, Wenger NK, et al. 1992. Cholesterol and heart disease in older persons and women: review of an NHBLI workshop. *Ann Epidemiol* **2**:161–76.

Massy ZA, Ma JZ, Louis TA, et al. 1995. Lipid-lowering therapy in patients with renal disease. *Kidney Int* **48**:188–98.

McKenney JM, Proctor JD, Harris S, et al. 1994. A comparison of the efficacy and toxic effects of sustained- vs immediate-release niacin in hypercholesterolemic patients. *JAMA* **271**:672–7.

Miettinen TA. 1968. Effect of nicotinic acid on catabolism and synthesis of cholesterol in man. *Clin Chim Acta* **20**:43–51.

*Mosby's GenR$_x$ 1998: The Complete Reference for Generic and Brand Drugs.* 8th ed. St. Louis: Mosby-Year Book.

Nakamura CE, Abeles RH. 1985. Mode of interaction of 3-hydroxy-3-methylglutaryl coenzyme A reductase with strong inhibitors: Compactin and related compounds. *Biochemistry* **24**:1364–76.

National Cholesterol Education Program (NCEP). 1992a. Highlights of the Report of the Expert Panel on Blood Cholesterol Levels in Children and Adolescents. *Pediatrics* **89**:495–500.

National Cholesterol Education Program Expert Panel. 1994a. Report of the National Cholesterol Education Program Expert Panel on Detection, Evaluation, and Treatment of High Blood Cholesterol in Adults. *Circulation* **89**:1329–445.

Neaton JD, Blackburn H, Jacobs D, et al. 1992. Serum cholesterol level and mortality findings for men screened in the Multiple Risk Factor Intervention Trial. *Arch Intern Med* **152**:1490–500.

NIH Consensus Development Conference. 1993. Triglyceride, high-density lipoprotein, and coronary heart disease. *JAMA* **269**:505–10.

Oster G, Borok GM, Menzin J, et al. 1996. Cholesterol-Reduction Intervention Study (CRIS): A randomized trial to assess effectiveness and costs in clinical practice. *Arch Int Med* **156**:731–9.

Packard CJ, Shepherd J. 1982. The hepatobiliary axis and lipoprotein metabolism: Effects of bile acid sequestrants and ileal bypass surgery. *J Lipid Res* **23**:1081–98.

Palmer RH. 1987. Effects of fibric acid derivatives on biliary lipid composition. *Am J Med* **83**(Suppl 5B):37–43.

Parker TS, McNamara DJ, Brown CD et al. 1984. Plasma mevalonate as a measure of cholesterol synthesis in man. *J Clin Invest* **74**:795–804.

Parkinson TM, Gundersen K, Nelson NA. 1970. Effects of colestipol (U-26, 597A), a new bile acid sequestrant, on serum lipids in experimental animals and man. *Atherosclerosis* **11**:531–7.

Perreault S, Hamilton VH, Lavoie F, et al. 1998. Treating hyperlipidemia for the primary prevention of coronary disease. Are higher dosages of lovastatin cost-effective? *Arch Int Med* **158**:375–81.

Reaven GM. 1988. Role of insulin resistance in human disease. *Diabetes* **37**:1595–608.

Rubins HB, Robins SJ, Collins D, et al. 1999. Gemfibrozil for the secondary prevention of coronary heart disease in men with low levels of high-density lipoprotein cholesterol. Veterans Affairs High-Density Lipoprotein Cholesterol Intervention Trial Study Group. *N Engl J Med* **341**:410–418.

Sacks FM, Pfeffer MA, Moye LA, et al. 1996. The effect of pravastatin on coronary events after myocardial infarction in patients with average cholesterol levels. The Cholesterol and Recurrent Events Trial Investigators. *N Engl J Med* **335**:1001–9.

Saku K, Gartside PS, Hynd BA, et al. 1985. Mechanism of action of gemfibrozil on lipoprotein metabolism. *J Clin Invest* **75**:1702–12.

Scandinavian Simvastatin Survival Study Group. 1994b. Randomised trial of cholesterol lowering in 4444 patients with coronary heart disease: The Scandinavian Simvastatin Survival Study (4S). *Lancet* **344**:1383–9.

Scanu AM, Landsberger FR. 1980. Lipoprotein structure. *Ann NY Acad Sci* **348**:1–434.

Scanu AM, Lawn RM, Berg K. 1991. Lipoprotein(a) and atherosclerosis. *Ann Intern Med* **115**:209–18.

Schoonjans K, Stael B, Auwerx J. 1996. Role of the peroxisome proliferator-activated receptor (PPAR) in mediating the effects of fibrates and fatty acids on gene expression. *J Lipid Res* **37**:907–25.

Shepherd J, Cobbe SM, Ford I, et al. 1995. Prevention of coronary heart disease with pravastatin in men with hypercholesterolemia. *N Engl J Med* **333**:1301–7.

Shepherd J, Packard CJ, Patsch JR, et al. 1979. Effects of nicotinic acid therapy on plasma high density lipoprotein distribution and composition and on apolipoprotein A metabolism. *J Clin Invest* **63**:858–67.

Siperstein MD, Nichols CW Jr, Chaikoff IL. 1953. Effects of ferric chloride and bile on plasma cholesterol and atherosclerosis in the cholesterol-fed bird. *Science* **117**:386–9.

Spearman ME, Summers K, Moore V, et al. 1997. Cost-effectiveness of initial therapy with 3-hydroxy-3-methylglutaryl coenzyme A reductase inhibitors to treat hypercholesterolemia in a primary care setting of a managed-care organization. *Clin Ther* **19**:582–602.

Stein EA. 1989. Treatment of familial hypercholesterolemia with drugs in children. *Arteriosclerosis* **9**(Suppl 1):I. 145–51.

Steinberg D, Avigan J, Feigelson EB. 1961. Effects of triparanol (MER-29) on cholesterol biosynthesis and on blood sterol levels in man. *J Clin Invest* **40**:884–93.

Steinberg D, Fredrickson DS, Avigan J. 1958. Effects of Δ4-cholestenone in animals and in man. *Proc Soc Exp Biol* **97**:784–90.

Stewart JM, Packard CJ, Lorimer AR, et al. 1982. Effects of bezafibrate on receptor-mediated and receptor-independent low density lipoprotein catabolism in type II hyperlipoproteinemic subjects. *Atherosclerosis* **44**:355–65.

Stone BG, Evans CD, Prigge WF, et al. 1989. Lovastatin treatment inhibits sterol synthesis and induces HMG-CoA reductase activity in mononuclear leukocytes of normal subjects. *J Lipid Res* **30**:1943–52.

Tennent DM, Siegel H, Zanetti ME, et al. 1960. Plasma lowering action of bile acid binding polymers in experimental animals. *J Lipid Res* **1**:469–73.

The Coronary Drug Project Research Group. 1975. Lofibrate and niacin in coronary heart disease. *JAMA* **231**:360–81.

The Coronary Drug Project Research Group. 1977. Gallbladder disease as a side effect of drugs influencing lipid metabolism: experience in the Coronary Drug Project. *N Engl J Med* **296**:1185–90.

Thorp JM, Waring WS. 1962. Modification of metabolism and distribution of lipids by ethyl chlorophenoxyisobutyrate. *Nature* **194**:948–9.

Tomkins GM, Sheppard H, Chaikoff IL. 1953. Cholesterol synthesis by liver. IV: Suppression by steroid administration. *J Biol Chem* **203**:781–6.

Tsalamandris C, Panagiotopoulos S, Sinha A, et al. 1994. Complementary effects of pravastatin and nicotinic acid in the treatment of combined hyperlipidaemia in diabetic and non-diabetic patients. *J Cardiovasc Risk* **1**:231–9.

Vega GL, Denke MA, Grundy SM. 1991. Metabolic basis of primary hypercholesterolemia. *Circulation* **84**:118–28.

Vega GL, East C, Grundy SM. 1988. Lovastatin therapy in familial dysbetalipoproteinemia: effects on kinetics of apolipoprotein B. *Atherosclerosis* **70**:131–43.

Vega GL, Grundy SM. 1985. Gemfibrozil therapy in primary hypertriglyceridemia associated with coronary heart disease: effects on metabolism of low-density lipoproteins. *JAMA* **253**:2398–403.

Walden CC, Hegele RA. 1994. Apolipoprotein E in hyperlipidemia. *Ann Intern Med* **120**(12):1026–35.

Weiner M, van Eys J. 1983. *Nicotinic Acid: Nutrient-Cofactor-Drug.* New York: Marcel Dekker.

Yamamoto A, Sudo H, Endo A. 1980. Therapeutic effects of ML-236B in primary hypercholesterolemia. *Atherosclerosis* **35**:259–66.

# Adrenal Steroids

Jeffrey W. Miller

### *Chapter Outline*



## PHYSIOLOGY OF THE HYPOTHALAMIC–PITUITARY–ADRENAL AXIS

### Classification of Adrenal Steroids

The adrenal cortex produces families of steroid hormones classified as glucocorticoids, mineralocorticoids, and adrenal androgens. Glucocorticoids have varied biologic effects including appetite regulation, fuel mobilization, nervous system arousal, suppression of inflammation, and blood pressure homeostasis. These effects mediate the response to physiologic stress and, along with the autonomic nervous system, are the mechanisms of the "fight or flight" physiologic response that Hans Selye termed the "general adaptation syndrome" (Selye 1956). Mineralocorticoids, in contrast, appear to serve a single role of regulating electrolyte homeostasis by effects on the kidney, brain, and other tissues. Adrenal androgens, which are weak agonists for the androgen receptor, have a poorly defined role as substrates for conversion to more potent androgenic and estrogenic steroids. The clinical significance of normal adrenal steroid production is best seen in

Addison disease, which is characterized by weight loss, hypotension, poor tolerance of severe illness, and reduced reproductive function.

Agents from each of the three classes of adrenal steroids are used therapeutically for replacement of normal adrenal function and pharmacotherapy of nonadrenal diseases. The glucocorticoids are among the most widely used classes of drugs, and their role in the therapy of pulmonary, inflammatory, dermatologic, and oncologic diseases are described in Chapters 2, 10, 11, and 13, respectively. Endocrinologic uses of glucocorticoids include the treatment of adrenal insufficiency as well as suppression of excessive androgen and mineralocorticoid synthesis. Mineralocorticoid agonists and antagonists are used in the therapy of blood pressure and electrolyte disorders. The adrenal androgen dehydroepiandrosterone (DHEA) is a frequently used nonprescription health supplement. This chapter reviews the pharmacologic properties of natural and synthetic steroids, their therapeutic role in abnormalities of adrenal function, and the pharmacotherapy of excess adrenal steroid production.

***Shared features of adrenal steroids***
Adrenal steroids have several common features, including biosynthesis and mechanisms of receptor activation. Biosynthetic functions are regionally segregated in the adrenal cortex by localized expression of genes for specific steps of steroid biosynthesis (Table 9-18). The common feature of all zones of the adrenal cortex is the ability to convert cholesterol, (which is derived from lipoprotein particles, or synthesized de novo) into steroid precursors (Figure 9-16). Many of the enzymes involved in steroid biosynthesis are cytochrome P450 enzymes, which are susceptible to inhibition by agents such as imidazole-containing antifungal drugs.

In addition to biosynthetic similarities, steroid hormones share a common mechanism of cellular action. Steroid hormone binding to the ligand binding domains of intracellular receptors leads to translocation of the ligand–receptor complex to the nucleus, with binding to hormone-specific regulatory regions in the 5′ regions of target genes (Figure 9-17). Steroid receptors do not show the degree of subtype differentiation that is seen with many transmembrane bound receptor families. Tissue specificity of steroid hormone action is achieved by tissue-specific expression of steroid receptors and transcription factors.

## GLUCOCORTICOIDS

### Regulation of Endogenous Cortisol

Cortisol is synthesized and released acutely from the adrenal zona fascicularis in a diurnal pattern under control by adrenocorticotropic hormone (ACTH). ACTH release from the corticotroph cells of the anterior pituitary is mediated by hypothalamic corticotropin-releasing hormone (CRH), and to a lesser extent by vasopressin. The early morning rise in cortisol levels occurs in concert with other hypothalamic and pituitary hormones, beginning at approximately 4 AM for subjects in a conventional sleep cycle (Figure 9-18). The gluconeogenic effects of several of these hormones (cortisol, growth hormone, and epinephrine) contribute to the "dawn phenomenon" of early morning hyperglycemia in diabetes. Cortisol concentrations wane during the day; hence, elevated AM cortisol and lower PM cortisol concentrations are hallmarks of normal pituitary–adrenal function. The ability of synthetic glucocorticoids (e.g., dexamethasone 1 mg) administered at night to suppress AM cortisol levels to below 5 $\mu$g/dL (140 nM/L) is an important screening test for Cushing syndrome.

***Cortisol distribution and metabolism***
Approximately 80% of circulating cortisol is bound by cortisol-binding globulin (CBG), with high affinity ($K_d$ = 30 nM) in a 1:1 stoichiometric ratio. CBG concentrations are usually sufficient to bind 25 $\mu$g/dL of cortisol; hence,

Table 9-18 Synthetic Enzymes and Regulation of Adrenal Steroidogenesis

| Steroid Class | Adrenal Region | Active Steroid | Key Structure | Synthetic Enzymes | Hormonal Regulation |
|---|---|---|---|---|---|
| Mineralocorticoid | Zona glomerulosa | Aldosterone | 21-carbon<br>18-aldo | CMO I and II | Ang II, $K^+$, ACTH (minor) |
| Glucocorticoid | Zona fasciculata | Cortisol | 21-carbon<br>17-hydroxy<br>11-$\beta$-hydroxy | 21-, 17$\alpha$- and 11-$\beta$-hydroxylases | ACTH |
| Adrenal androgen | Zona reticularis | Dehydroepiandrosterone | 19-carbon | 17,20-lyase | Uncertain, ACTH (permissive) |

Abbreviations: Ang II, angiotensin II; ACTH, adrenocorticotrophic hormone; CMO, corticosteroid methyloxidase.

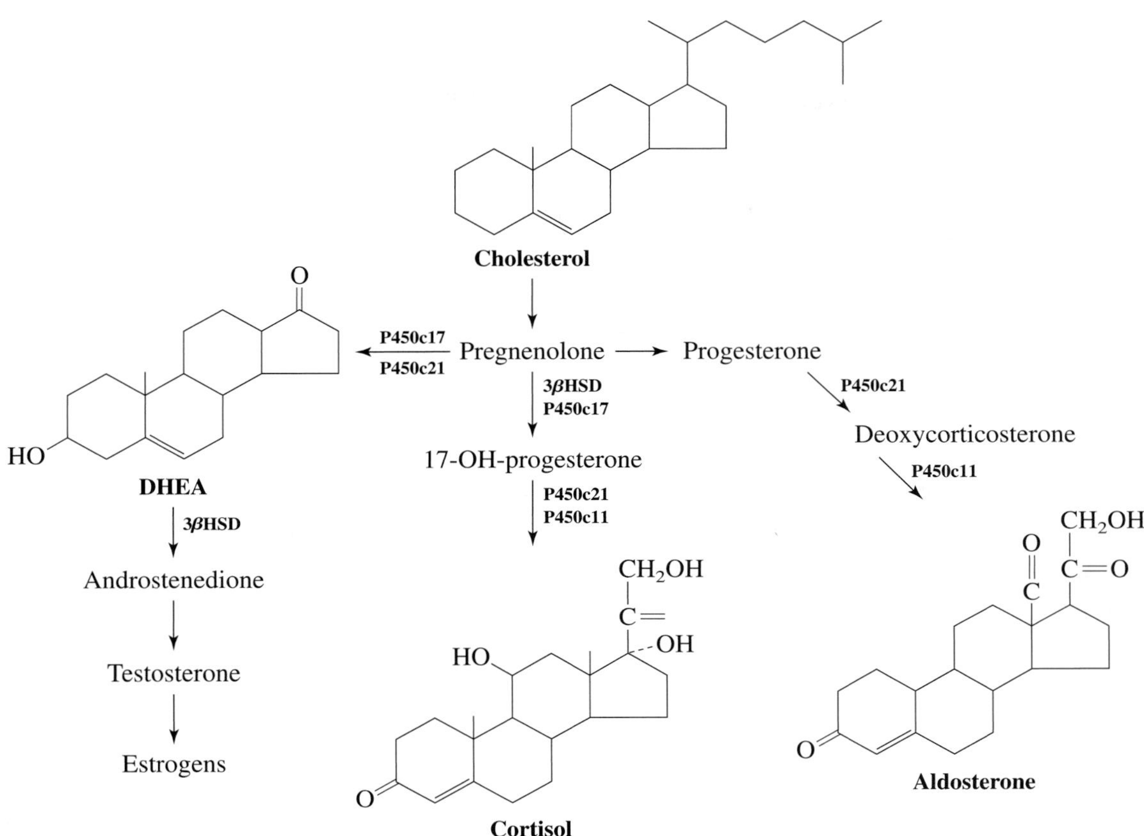


FIGURE 9-16 **Adrenal steroid biosynthesis. The side chain cleavage enzyme produces 21-carbon steroids from cholesterol for entry into steroidogenic pathways. Glucocorticoids are 21-carbon steroids with hydroxylations at 21-, 17-, and 11-carbon sites. The 11-β-hydroxylation is key to GCR and MR binding affinity. Mineralocorticoids are 21-carbon steroids in which an 18-keto group has been added by the angiotensin II regulated isoform of p450c11. Adrenal androgens are 17-carbon steroids which undergo 17-hydroxylation to form testosterone, and subsequent aromatization to form estrogens.**

CBG saturation occurs only at peak cortisol concentrations under normal physiologic conditions. Approximately 10% of cortisol is weakly bound to albumin, but albumin-bound cortisol may diffuse freely into tissues. Most synthetic glucocorticoids have low affinity for CBG and are more bioavailable to target tissues. Progesterone is also bound by CBG, but its plasma concentration is lower than that of cortisol; hence, it does not alter the bound: free ratio of cortisol under normal conditions. Hepatic synthesis of CBG is increased by estrogen and thyroxine.

Daily cortisol production is approximately 10 mg (Esteban et al. 1991; Kerrigan et al. 1993) in healthy adults. Glucocorticoids are metabolized by oxidative and conjugative enzymes in the liver prior to renal excretion of most metabolites. Less than 1% of plasma cortisol is excreted unchanged in the urine under normal conditions. During hypercortisolemia, a greater proportion of cortisol is free or weakly bound; hence, urinary cortisol excretion may increase significantly. This phenomenon underlies the utility of 24-hour, urine free cortisol measurement in the diagnosis of Cushing syndrome.

In addition to conventional hepatic metabolism and renal excretion, cortisol is metabolized by a unique mechanism that regulates local concentrations of cortisol in target tissues (Frey et al. 1994). The enzyme 11-β-hydroxysteroid dehydrogenase (11βHSD) catalyzes the reversible interconversion of 11-β-hydroxy and 11-ketosteroids, and is expressed in mineralocorticoid target tissues. The 11-ketosteroids have low affinity for the glucocorticoid or mineralocorticoid receptors. Since 11-β-hydroxysteroids (i.e., cortisol) have high affinity for the mineralocorticoid receptor (MR), 11βHSD is an important mechanism by which mineralocorticoid effects such as renal sodium retention are protected from excessive stimu-

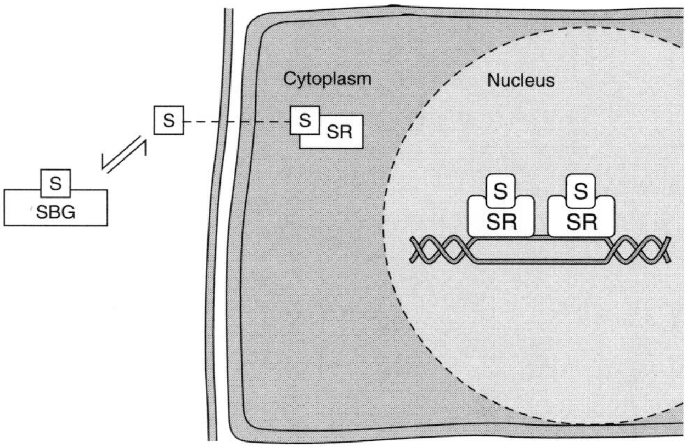

**FIGURE 9-17 Steroid receptor action. Most steroid hormones circulate in association with binding globulins or albumin. Free steroid diffuses across plasma membrane and binds to intracellular steroid receptors. These receptors may associate with other transcription factors or heat shock proteins. Ligand-bound receptors are translocated to the nucleus and bind to regulatory sites of target genes in dimeric forms.**

lation by circulating glucocorticoids in the kidney. The interconversion of 11-hydroxy and 11-keto steroids is reversible and accounts for the conversion of the "prodrugs" cortisone and prednisone to their pharmacologically active forms, cortisol and prednisolone, respectively.

***Mechanism of glucocorticoid action***

Glucocorticoids are lipid-soluble cholesterol derivatives that diffuse across plasma membranes where they bind to intracellular glucocorticoid receptors (GCR) (Figure 9-19). Classical glucocorticoid responses involve receptor binding by ligand, transport to the nucleus, dimerization of ligand bound receptor, binding to regulatory elements in target genes, and transcriptional regulation of responsive genes. Although many glucocorticoid responses are mediated by dimerization of ligand bound GCR, the glucocorticoid receptor can also heterodimerize with other transcription factors such as AP-1 and NF-κB. This alternate pathway of glucocorticoid action mediates many of the inhibitory effects of glucocorticoids on cellular responses (Bamberger et al. 1996). The half-life of glucocorticoid effects such as pituitary suppression exceeds that of its elimination from plasma by at least twofold (Meikle et al. 1977).

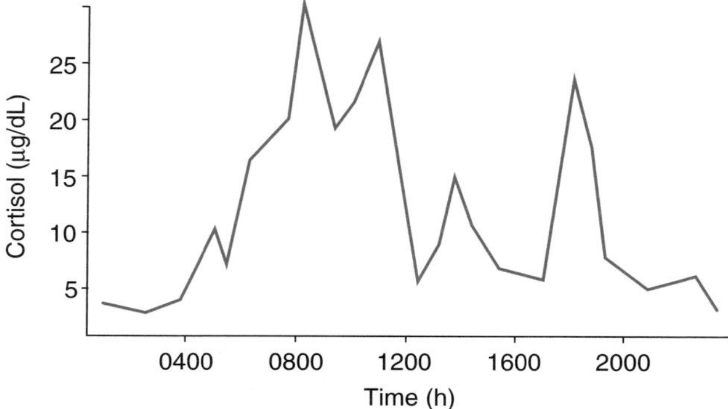


**FIGURE 9-18 Diurnal cortisol profile. Pulsatile secretion of cortisol is greatest in the early morning. Lesser cortisol peaks follow meal ingestion later in the day.**

## Synthetic Glucocorticoids

***Development of synthetic glucocorticoids***

The first synthetic glucocorticoids were developed for oral and parenteral administration in the late 1940s. These molecules included the natural glucocorticoids hydro-fjcortisone (cortisol) and cortisone as well as analogs of cortisol such as prednisolone, 9-$\alpha$-fluorohydrocortisone (fludrocortisone), and dexamethasone (Figure 9-20). Experience with these compounds demonstrated that synthetic molecules

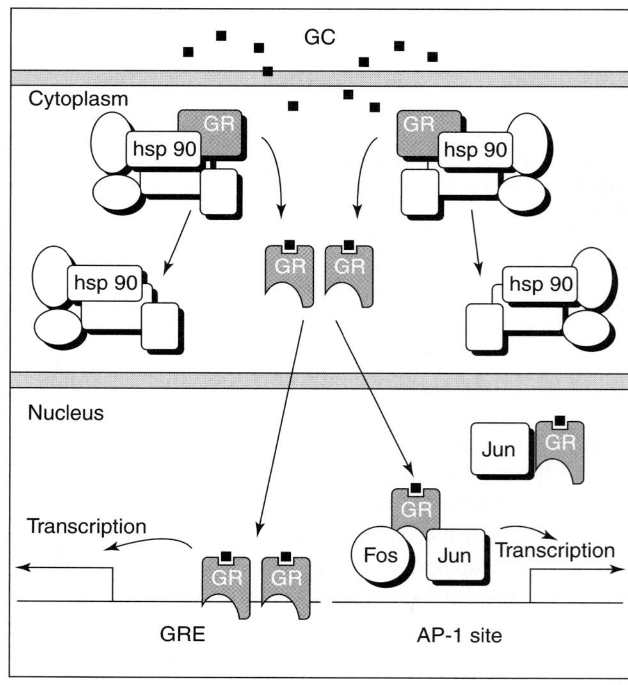


**FIGURE 9-19 Glucocorticoid signaling. Glucocorticoids act by classical GCR dimerization and upregulation of gene transcription. GCR association with the Fos and Jun proteins exerts negative gene regulation by the AP-1 promoter site. (From Bamberger et al. 1996 with permission.)**

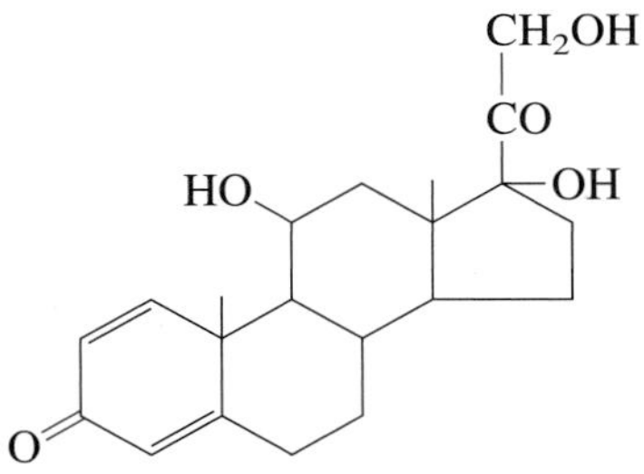

**Prednisolone**

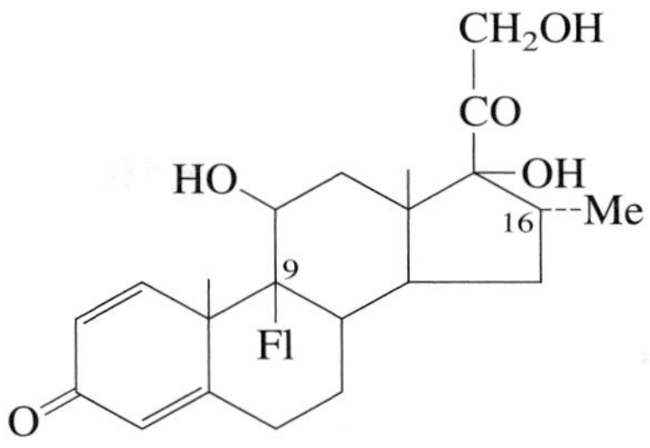

**Dexamethasone**
**(16α-Methyl-9α-fluoroprednisolone)**

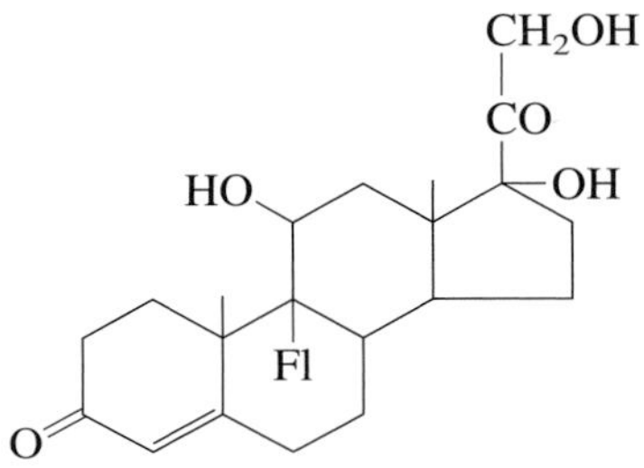

**Fludrocortisone**
**(9α-Fluorocortisol)**

**FIGURE 9-20 Early synthetic corticosteroids. Cortisol analogs from the early 1950s achieved greater potency by modifications of the A-ring of the steroid nucleus, addition of fluoride group at the 9-carbon site, and methylation of the 16-carbon site.**

could be more potent than the endogenous ligand cortisol (Ballard et al. 1975), and that glucocorticoid and mineralocorticoid activity could be dissociated. The receptor binding affinities of these molecules have revealed the importance of the 11-hydroxyl group to GCR binding affinity. After the early era of synthetic glucocorticoids, new formulations and routes of delivery were developed as strategies for achieving a high therapeutic index in the treatment of dermatologic, respiratory, and articular inflammatory conditions. Highly potent glucocorticoids have been developed for dermatologic and respiratory diseases that employ more complex structures at the 16 and 17 carbon sites of the steroid nucleus (Figure 9-21).

***Relative potency of synthetic glucocorticoids***

Natural and synthetic glucocorticoids display varied receptor-binding affinities and pharmacokinetic features (Table 9-19). Although potency in various in vitro systems correlates well with GCR binding affinity (Luzzani et al. 1984), it does not predict potency in vivo. Several factors determine the in vivo potency of corticosteroids including bioavailability, route of administration, protein binding, lipophilicity, GCR binding affinity, and elimination half-life. The relative potency of different glucocorticoids has generally been defined on the basis of pituitary ACTH suppressive effects on the morning following single doses of commonly used oral glucocorticoids (Meikle et al. 1977). The relative potency of these agents in pituitary suppression varies according to the time point of assessment after single-dose administration. Although the intrinsic potency of dexamethasone is only 17 times that of cortisol, it is 150 times as potent as cortisol at 14 hours after a single dose given at 6 PM. For this reason, this relative potency assessment is appropriate for assessing the likelihood of pituitary suppression of daily doses of glucocorticoids, but cannot be extrapolated to multiple daily dose regimens, or to other pharmacologic endpoints, such as anti-inflammatory or antitumor effects. The only reliable method of determining the relative potency of different glucocorticoids is by controlled clinical trials that compare the effects of different dose regimens on relevant clinical endpoints (Kobberling and Rotenberger 1992; Toogood et al. 1989).

***Strategies to reduce adverse effects of glucocorticoid therapy***

TISSUE SELECTIVITY Because of the frequent and troubling adverse effects of systemic glucocorticoid therapy, agents with novel pharmacologic profiles have been sought. Deflazacort is a potent anti-inflammatory glucocorticoid that has been reported to have diminished effects on calcium and glucocorticoid metabolism (Pagano et al.

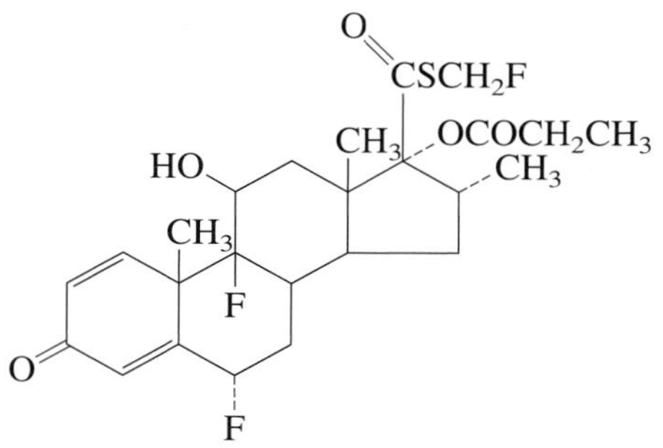

**Fluticasone propionate**

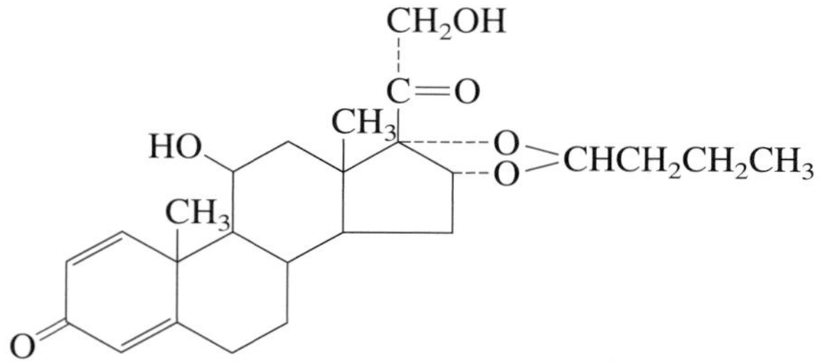

**Budesonide**

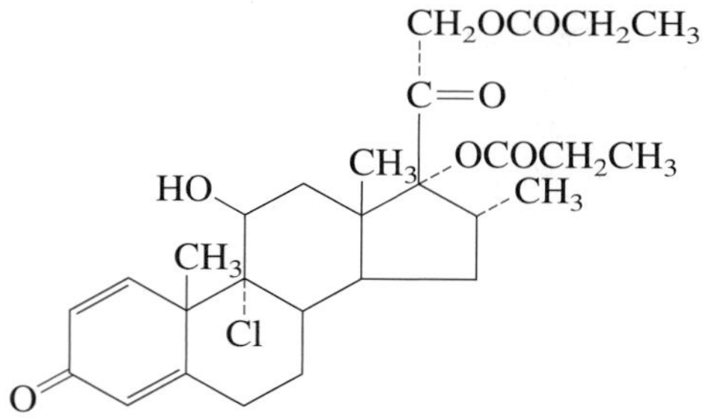

**Beclomethasone dipropionate**

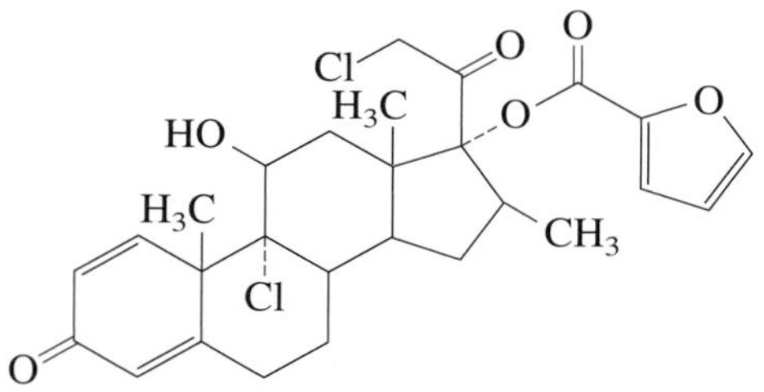

**Mometasone**

**FIGURE 9-21 High potency glucocorticoids. Later synthetic glucocorticoids achieved greater potency by more complex substitution of the cortisol structure. Complex structures at the 16- and 17-carbons sites are prone to rapid metabolism, which may be advantageous for topically delivered glucocorticoids.**

1989; Imbimbo et al. 1984). Critical review of available data suggests that when deflazacort is compared with equieffective doses of other glucocorticoids, it actually displays no difference in adverse effects (Kobberling and Rotenberger 1992; Lund et al. 1987). None of the currently available synthetic glucocorticoids displays tissue selectivity in its effects.

**ALTERNATE DAY THERAPY** The dependency of pharmacologic effect on dose interval has been demonstrated in studies of alternate day steroid therapy. Glucocorticoid administration on alternate mornings produces less ACTH and cortisol suppression than the same dose administered in divided doses each day (Harter et al. 1963; Ackerman and Nolsn 1968).

Pituitary suppression is also more likely when glucocorticoids are administered in the evening. This observation has led to "alternate day" glucocorticoid regimens for the treatment of inflammatory diseases. Since alternate day glucocorticoid administration produces less continuous pharmacologic effects on the pituitary, it may also lead to less continuous therapeutic effects. Widespread clinical use of this strategy has demonstrated the ability to maintain disease remission and reduce adverse effects in some patients, although alternate day glucocorticoid therapy is not devoid of dose-dependent adverse effects such as bone loss and impaired glucose tolerance (Walton et al. 1970; Gluck et al. 1981).

**TRANSDERMAL, AEROSOLIZED, AND PARENTERAL GLUCOCORTICOIDS** Another important strategy to maintain an advantageous therapeutic index in glucocorticoid therapy is the use of local delivery systems such as topical, aerosolized, depot injections, and ophthalmologic preparations (Table 9-20). In the case of aerosolized glucocorticoids for pulmonary disease, agents such as fluticasone demonstrate high potency (requiring relatively small amounts of drug to be delivered) and rapid systemic metabolism (limiting the systemic exposure of drug absorbed through the respiratory tract). Topical agents such as triamcinolone are rapidly metabolized after dermal absorption but must be absorbable into the dermis. Acetonide and other structures at the 17-hydroxy sites of lipophilic steroids such as hydrocortisone and triamcinolone improve dermal penetration of these agents. For depot injection in arthritic conditions, crystalline formulations with slow systemic absorption such as triamcinolone hexacetonide are used to maintain a high local concentration near the site of injection and a low rate of delivery to other tissues.

Table 9-19 **Pharmacologic Features of Systemically Administered Glucocorticoids**

| Compound | Receptor Affinity | Pharmacokinetic $T_{1/2}$ (min) | Pharmacodynamic $T_{1/2}$ (h) | Relative MR Affinity | Equivalent Daily Dose | Cost per Day[a] |
|---|---|---|---|---|---|---|
| Hydrocortisone | 1 | 80–110 | 8–12 | ++ | 20 mg | $0.09 |
| Cortisone[b] | | | | | 25 mg | $0.12 |
| Prednisone[b] | 2 | 200 | 18–36 | + | 5 mg | $0.03 |
| Methylprednisolone | 15 | 214 | 18–36 | – | 4 mg | $0.52 |
| Dexamethasone | 8 | 200 | 36–54 | – | 0.75 mg | $0.08 |

Adapted from Swartz and Dluhy 1978.
[a]Cost based on generic formulations only.
[b]Low intrinsic activity, but display pharmacologic characteristics of 11-β-hydroxy forms (cortisol, prednisolone) after conversion by 11βHSD enzyme.
Abbreviation: MR, mineralocorticoid receptors.
SOURCE: *Redbook* 1998.

## Glucocorticoid Replacement in Adrenal Insufficiency

### *Etiology and diagnosis*

Adrenal insufficiency is a glucocorticoid-deficient state that may or may not be associated with mineralocorticoid deficiency. Primary adrenal insufficiency is due to intrinsic adrenal disease and is associated with elevated concentrations of ACTH and other proopiomelanocortin (POMC)-derived peptides. The melanocyte stimulating effect of POMC derivatives leads to hyperpigmentation of mucosal membranes, extensor surfaces, and skin in primary adrenal insufficiency. Destruction of the adrenal cortex may occur by a variety of mechanisms (Table 9-21) including autoimmune mechanisms (Addison disease). Mineralocorticoid synthesis by the zona glomerulosa may be impaired to varying degrees in these conditions. Glucocorticoid deficiency is diagnosed by characteristic signs and symptoms, elevated ACTH concentration, and a plasma cortisol concentration of less than 20 μg/dL within one hour after intravenous or intramuscular administration of 0.25 mg of synthetic ACTH.

Secondary adrenal insufficiency is a glucocorticoid deficiency state without associated mineralocorticoid deficiency, and is due to hypothalamic and/or pituitary dysfunction. The most common cause of secondary adrenal deficiency is iatrogenic adrenal insufficiency following the therapeutic use of glucocorticoids. Prolonged glucocorticoid therapy suppresses both pituitary ACTH release in response to CRF (Schlaghecke et al. 1992) and adrenal responses to ACTH (Graba et al. 1965). Normal adrenal function may require up to 9 months after discontinuation of glucocorticoid therapy to return to normal. In addition to iatrogenic causes, secondary adrenal insufficiency may result from intrinsic pituitary disease. Secondary adrenal insufficiency is diagnosed by the same criteria of cortisol responses to ACTH stimulation. Other tests of cortisol secretory capacity such as insulin induced hypoglycemia and synthetic CRH stimulation may be useful in cases of

Table 9-20 **Characteristics of Glucocorticoid Preparations for Localized Delivery**

| Route of Administration | Key Features | Pharmacology and Formulation | Example |
|---|---|---|---|
| Intravenous | Aqueous solubility | $Na^+$ succinate salts | Hydrocortisone $Na^+$ succinate (Solu-Cortef) |
| Periarticular injection | Long action | Insoluble, crystalline | Triamcinolone hexacetonide, methylprednisolone acetate (Depo-Medrol) |
| Pulmonary inhalation | High potency, limited systemic effect | Rapid first pass metabolism | Fluticasone |
| Dermal | High potency, limited systemic effect | Lipophilic | Hydrocortisone acetate, triamcinolone acetonide |

**Table 9-21 Causes of Adrenal Insufficiency**

| | |
|---|---|
| Vascular | Adrenal infarction (sepsis, coagulopathy) |
| Inflammatory/infectious | Granulomatous disease |
| | Viral (CMV in HIV states) |
| Neoplastic | Metastatic adenocarcinoma |
| Drugs | Ketoconazole, Etomidate |
| Congenital/genetic | Enzymatic defects, glucocorticoid resistance |
| Autoimmune | Addison disease |
| Iatrogenic | Glucocorticoid suppression |

Abbreviations: CMV, cytomegalovirus; HIV, human immunodeficiency virus.

borderline ACTH stimulation results; however, these tests have not been correlated with clinical outcomes in a large number of patients (Christy 1992).

***Replacement therapy***

The goal of glucocorticoid replacement therapy in primary adrenal disease is to reproduce the physiologic pattern of endogenous cortisol. Although endogenous cortisol production is approximately 10 mg per day, most adrenally insufficient patients require 15–30 mg/day in oral replacement regimens. Orally administered cortisol (hydrocortisone) is approximately 80% bioavailable; hence, daily glucocorticoid concentrations are higher than normal in patients on glucocorticoid replacement regimens which exceed 20 mg/day of cortisol (Figure 9-22). At conventionally used replacement doses, ACTH concentrations may be elevated in adrenally insufficient patients even when treated with supraphysiologic glucocorticoid doses (Feek et al. 1981), suggesting that the hypothalamic–pituitary axis may become resistant to glucocorticoid action. Controlled trials using psychological questionnaires demonstrate that patients with adrenal insufficiency feel better when the daily steroid dose is given in divided doses of which approximately two thirds is given in the morning (Riedel et al. 1993; Groves et al. 1988). One problem with glucocorticoid replacement therapy is the lack of objective tests of adequate glucocorticoid dose. ACTH concentrations are highly variable and are not as clinically useful as, for example, TSH monitoring of thyroid hormone replacement. Glucocorticoid dose is adjusted empirically to correct symptoms of weight loss and fatigue. Mineralocorticoid replacement therapy is usually administered in primary adrenal insufficiency (see below), although hydrocortisone alone has mineralocorticoid activity at usual doses. Maximum daily cortisol output is approximately 250 mg, which serves as the basis for administering 50–100 mg of hydrocortisone intravenously 4 times per day in the treatment of adrenal insufficiency crisis.

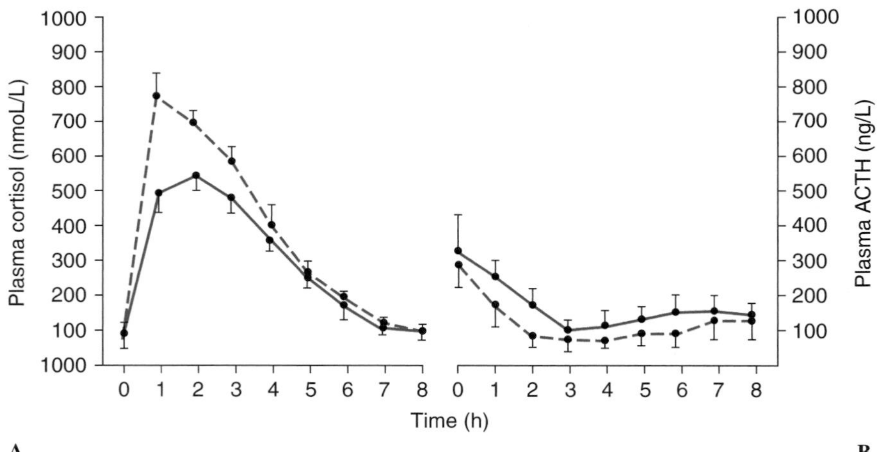


**FIGURE 9-22 Relative bioavailability of hydrocortisone and cortisone. At dosages used in adrenal steroid replacement which are commonly thought to be equivalent, hydrocortisone achieves higher peak cortisol concentrations. (From Feek et al. 1981 with permission.)**

**ADVERSE EFFECTS OF GLUCOCORTICOID REPLACEMENT THERAPY** Glucocorticoids are associated with a large number of adverse effects (Table 9-22). Most of these occur in the setting of high-dose glucocorticoid therapy or pathological cortisol excess; hence, their relevance to glucocorticoid replacement therapy may be questioned. Patients treated with glucocorticoids for Addison disease demonstrated lower bone mineral density (Valero et al. 1994), although deficiency of sex steroids may be partly responsible. Patients treated with hormone replacement therapy for panhypopituitarism demonstrate excess cardiovascular morbidity (Rosen and Bengtsson 1990), although growth hormone deficiency may be partly responsible. Excess cardiovascular morbidity is seen in patients on glucocorticoid replacement therapy after bilateral adrenalectomy for Cushing syndrome (Welbourn 1985; Hamberger et al. 1982), and in steroid-treated patients with rheumatoid arthritis (Ichikawa et al. 1977; Kalbak 1972). Although clinical experience with glucocorticoid replacement therapy has been favorable, it is prudent to manage adrenally insufficient patients with the lowest acceptable dose of glucocorticoids.

**GLUCOCORTICOID DOSAGE DURING STRESS** Management of glucocorticoid dosage during illness and surgery poses a challenge in the therapy of all forms of adrenal insufficiency. The early era of glucocorticoid replacement in the 1950s led to case reports of glucocorticoid-treated patients experiencing cardiovascular collapse during surgery and other severe illness. The use of "stress dose" steroid regimens has become widespread since that time. No clinical trial has been published to support the common clinical practice of doubling the daily glucocorticoid dosage during minor ambulatory illnesses. Small clinical trials of perioperative "stress dose" glucocorticoid regimens in patients with iatrogenic secondary adrenal insufficiency demonstrate no difference in outcomes between patients maintained on the usual daily dose of glucocorticoids, and those treated with high doses of hydrocortisone (Glowniak and Loriaux 1997; Kehlet and Binder 1973). A systematic review of perioperative steroid management studies suggests that the usual dose of glucocorticoid should be continued during surgery, and that, if used, high-dose steroids do not need to be tapered slowly during convalescence (Salem et al. 1994).

## Pharmacologic Management of Cushing Syndrome

### *Steroid synthesis inhibitors*

Drug therapy has a small role to play in the treatment of endogenous glucocorticoid excess (Cushing syndrome) (Miller and Crapo 1993). This condition is due to pituitary hypersecretion of ACTH (Cushing disease) in approximately 70% of cases, and due to paraneoplastic ACTH secretion, adrenal cancer, and adrenal adenoma in approximately 10% each of cases. Cushing disease is usually treated by transsphenoidal adenomectomy or hypophysectomy, which is curative in approximately 70% of cases. Surgical therapy is also highly effective in benign adrenal tumors. In cases of Cushing disease that have failed surgical resection and in ectopic ACTH syndrome, medical therapy may be undertaken to control cortisol excess. Several agents are available that reduce cortisol synthesis in the adrenal cortex, including ketoconazole, aminoglutethimide, and metyrapone. Ketoconazole, an imidazole antifungal agent, inhibits a variety of cytochrome P450 enzymes, including the side chain cleavage enzyme that converts cholesterol to the 21-carbon steroid structure. Because of the multiple sites of steroidogenic inhibition, ketoconazole and aminoglutethimide do not lead to build up of pharmacologically active precursors such as 11-deoxycortisol. Metyrapone predominantly inhibits the 11-hydroxylase enzyme, and its use may result in excessive mineralocorticoid effects of 11-deoxycortisol.

**Table 9-22 Adverse Effects of Glucocorticoid Therapy**

| | |
|---|---|
| Neurologic | Insomnia, agitation, withdrawal syndrome |
| Infectious | Increased infections, opportunistic infections |
| Vascular | Increased atherosclerotic risk |
| Skin | Atrophy |
| Skeletal | Reduced calcium absorption, osteoporosis, avascular necrosis (hip) |
| Muscular | Myopathy |
| Metabolic | Obesity, dyslipidemia, glucose intolerance |
| Reproductive | Hypogonadism |
| GI | Peptic ulcer |
| Ocular | Cataracts |

Uncontrolled trials of ketoconazole therapy of Cushing disease suggest that cortisol concentrations may be decreased in most patients. The dose range employed, 600–1200 mg/day, is higher than the dose commonly used for fungal infections. Gastrointestinal distress or elevated liver transaminases are seen in approximately 30% of patients (Sonino et al. 1991). Although gonadal sex steroid synthesis is not usually affected, adrenal androgen production is reduced and gynecomastia has been reported. Ketoconazole inhibits the CYP3A4 drug metabolism pathway and may lead to adverse drug interactions with a variety of other drugs due to inhibition of their metabolism.

#### *Mitotane*

Mitotane is a steroidogenic inhibitor that produces atrophy of adrenal tissue. This "adrenolytic" effect has led to its use in adrenal cancer. Although its mechanism of action is not well understood, mitotane appears to impair the ability of ACTH to increase cAMP in adrenal cells. Mitotane is widely used in metastatic adrenal carcinoma, but its effect on survival is modest (Hutter and Kayhoe 1998). Mitotane has been used in Cushing disease, where trials have demonstrated disease-free remission after 1–2 years of therapy with doses of 4–12 g/day. Response rate is increased with external beam pituitary radiation. Gastrointestinal upset is a frequent dose-limiting adverse effect.

#### *Glucocorticoid receptor antagonism*

RU486 (mifepristone) is a nonsteroidal antagonist of progesterone and glucocorticoid receptors. It is not currently licensed in the US but has been used in small clinical studies of normal subjects and patients with Cushing syndrome (Nieman et al. 1985; Bertagna et al. 1984). Mifepristone leads to hormonal changes consistent with glucocorticoid antagonism (increased ACTH and cortisol concentrations). Its use may produce hypoadrenalism in the setting of high ACTH and cortisol concentrations.

## Mineralocorticoid Pharmacology

#### *Mineralocorticoid physiology*

Aldosterone and other 18-hydroxy or 11-hydroxy 21-carbon steroids are synthesized in the anadrenal zona glomerulosa under the dual regulation of angiotensin II and ACTH. Angiotensin II, controlled by the renin system of the kidney, is the primary regulator of mineralocorticoid synthesis; ACTH appears to play a permissive role only. Mineralocorticoid synthesis from 21-carbon precursors is achieved by tissue-specific regulation of a multifunctional steroidogenic enzyme, P450c11, which catalyzes the terminal steps in aldosterone synthesis. The gene for the P450c11 enzyme responsible for aldosterone synthesis, also known as corticosteroid methyloxidase (CMO), contains angiotensin II responsive elements in its promoter region. In the zona fasciculata, a highly homologous P450c11 gene produces the 11-$\beta$-hydroxylase enzyme, which synthesizes cortisol under ACTH regulation. Glucocorticoid suppressible hyperaldosteronism is a rare disorder in which the ACTH responsive element of the 11-$\beta$-hydroxylase enzyme is translocated to the CMO enzyme and results in excess aldosterone synthesis during normal daily ACTH release.

Aldosterone synthesis is increased when the renal juxtaglomerular apparatus senses insufficient circulatory volume and stimulates renin release and subsequent angiotensin II formation. This may occur in true volume-deficient states, or in diseases where renal perfusion is impaired, such as renal artery stenosis, congestive heart failure, and hypoalbuminemic states. Restoration of normal renal perfusion leads to suppression of renin release and reduced aldosterone synthesis. Aldosterone circulates at plasma concentrations of 1–3 nM/L, in contrast to average cortisol concentrations of 100–300 nM/L; aldosterone is not significantly protein bound. Mineralocorticoids bind specific cytosolic mineralocorticoid receptors (MR) and regulate MR responsive genes in a fashion analogous to other steroids. Target genes include ion transport and cellular respiration enzymes in the distal collecting duct of the nephron (Figure 9-23). Mineralocorticoid receptors are also expressed in the gut, sweat glands, brain, and vascular smooth muscle. Physiologic functions in the kidney include increased sodium retention by the $Na^+/K^+$ and $Na^+/H^+$ ion exchange systems.

#### *Mineralocorticoid excess*

Mineralocorticoid excess occurs in primary (adrenal) and secondary (renin–angiotensin-mediated) forms (Table 9-23). Primary mineralocorticoid excess is commonly due to aldosterone-producing adrenal adenomas (APA) or idiopathic hyperaldosteronism (IHA). IHA is usually a state of bilateral hyperplasia of the zona glomerulosa that is not cured by surgery. Other causes of mineralocorticoid excess include adrenal carcinoma, severe hypercortisolism, 11-$\beta$-hydroxysteroid dehydrogenase deficiency, and glucocorticoid-suppressible hyperaldosteronism. The diagnostic strategy to identify surgically correctable hyperaldosteronism focuses on identifying autonomous aldosterone production by the failure of plasma aldosterone to suppress below 10 ng/dL after sodium loading (Bravo et al. 1983; Weinberger et al. 1979).

Pharmacologic therapy of mineralocorticoid hypertension includes the use of the mineralocorticoid receptor antagonist spironolactone, or other diuretics that antago-

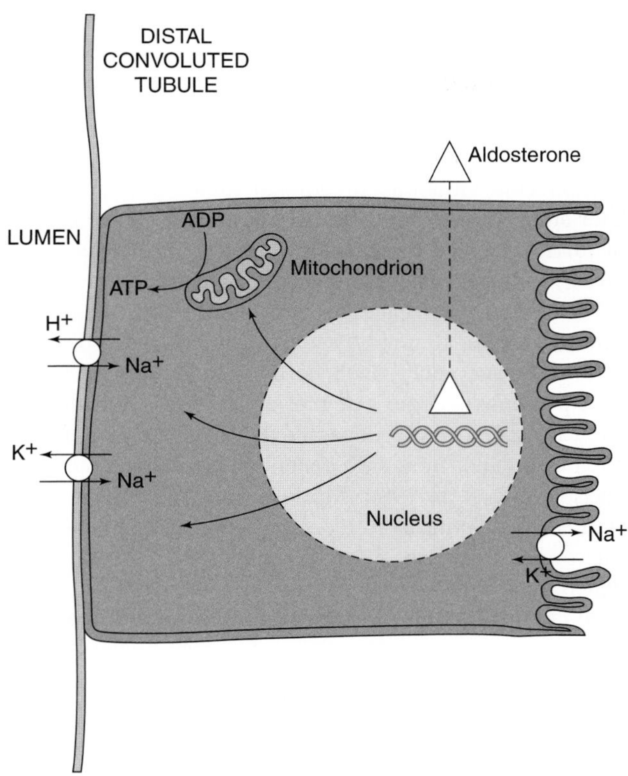


FIGURE 9-23 **Mineralocorticoid action. Mineralocorticoid receptors upregulate the transcription of genes involved in cellular respiration and electrolyte exchange in the distal nephron.**

nize $Na^+$ exchange in the distal nephron (e.g., amiloride, triamterene). Spironolactone is a modified steroid derivative with antagonist affinity for both the mineralocorticoid and androgen receptors. In studies of hypertensive patients with low or normal plasma renin activities, spironolactone demonstrated efficacy comparable to that of other antihypertensive agents (Brest 1986). Antihypertensive efficacy increases over the dose range from 50 to 400 mg/day. At higher doses, antiandrogenic effects in males such as gynecomastia are common. Spironolactone may cause hyperkalemia and hyperchloremic metabolic acidosis.

***Treatment of mineralocorticoid deficiency***

Primary mineralocorticoid deficiency occurs in Addison disease, destructive neoplasms, and other adrenal disease. The hallmarks of this condition are hyperkalemia, hyponatremia, and postural hypotension associated with low plasma aldosterone and elevated plasma renin activity. Glucocorticoid deficiency symptoms such as nausea, weight loss, asthenia, and hyperpigmentation usually accompany mineralocorticoid deficiency when it is due to adrenal disease. Secondary mineralocorticoid deficiency is commonly seen in older patients and results from reduced renin release due to age-related renal insufficiency (hyporeninemic hypoaldosteronism). This condition is usually diagnosed by low plasma renin activity in the setting of postural hypotension and electrolyte abnormalities.

**FLUFOROHYDROCORTISONE** Although hyporeninemic hypoaldosteronism may often be managed with dietary sodium supplementation, primary mineralocorticoid deficiency often requires orally administered synthetic mineralocorticoids. Aldosterone is rapidly metabolized by the liver and is not used for mineralocorticoid replacement. 9-$\alpha$-Fluorohydrocortisone (fludrocortisone) is the most commonly used synthetic mineralocorticoid because of its long half-life and selectivity for mineralocorticoid effects. 9-$\alpha$-Fluorohydrocortisone is a potent glucocorticoid agonist, but has approximately 10 times the affinity for the MR as for the GCR. At the low doses used in mineralocorticoid replacement (0.05–0.2 mg/day), the glucocorticoid agonist effect of fludrocortisone is negligible. Postural blood pressure responses and plasma renin activity are used to assess the adequacy of mineralocorticoid replacement in patients with Addison disease. Because of the long pharmacodynamic half-life of fludrocortisone (18–36 hours), many patients may require only

Table 9-23 **Mineralocorticoid Excess and Deficiency**

| | |
|---|---|
| Primary mineralocorticoid excess | Aldosterone-producing adrenal adenoma<br>Idiopathic hyperaldosteronism (bilateral hyperplasia)<br>Glucocorticoid suppressible hyperaldosteronism |
| Secondary mineralocorticoid excess | Renovascular hypertension |
| Enhanced tissue sensitivity | Syndrome of apparent mineralocorticoid excess (11-$\beta$HSD impairment) |
| Primary mineralocorticoid deficiency | Adrenal disease |
| Secondary mineralocorticoid deficiency | Hyporeninemic hypoaldosteronism |

ABBREVIATIONS: 11-$\beta$HSD, 11-$\beta$-hydroxysteroid dehydrogenase.

alternate-day fludrocortisone therapy. Hypertension and hypokalemia may develop on fludrocortisone therapy. Patients who develop hypertension on fludrocortisone should have the dose reduced or dose interval prolonged. Use of fludrocortisone in the treatment of autonomic insufficiency is described in chapter 1, Cardiovascular Disorders.

## DEHYDROEPIANDROSTERONE AND ADRENAL ANDROGENS

### Endocrinology of Adrenal Androgens

Adrenal androgens are produced by conversion of 21-carbon steroids to 19-carbon steroids by the 17,20-lyase enzyme in a fashion similar to gonadal steroidogenesis. The major adrenal steroids are dehydroepiandrosterone (DHEA) and androstenedione. DHEA is rapidly conjugated to DHEA sulfate, which forms the predominant circulating form of this androgen. DHEA sulfate is pharmacologically inactive, but may be converted to DHEA. Adrenal androgen production is partially regulated by ACTH and shows some diurnal variation. ACTH regulation does not account for changes over the lifespan in which circulating androgen concentrations rise at puberty and decline in later adult years. Nor do adrenal androgens exert feedback regulation of ACTH secretion, which is controlled by cortisol. DHEA and androstenedione are weak agonists for the androgen receptor. In the gonads and other sites, androstenedione is converted to testosterone by the 17-ketosteroid reductase enzyme. In women, a large portion of plasma testosterone is derived from adrenal androgens, whereas the contribution of adrenal androgens to total testosterone in men is small. Testosterone may be converted to estradiol by the action of the aromatase enzyme on the A ring of the steroid nucleus.

### Clinical Disorders of Adrenal Androgens

No unique receptor for adrenal androgens has yet been identified; hence, the physiologic effects of adrenal androgens are presumed to occur by conversion to more potent sex steroids. Girls and women with impairment of the 21-hydroxylase and 11-hydroxylase steroidogenic enzymes produce excessive amounts of adrenal androgens and may develop hirsutism and masculinization. This state of steroidogenic excess is ACTH driven and is treated by administration of long-acting glucocorticoid agonists at night, in order to suppress adrenal steroid production. Boys with androgen excess may demonstrate secondary sexual characteristics suggestive of premature puberty, although adrenal androgen excess does not activate pituitary gonadotropin secretion.

***Dehydroepiandrosterone therapy***

Plasma concentrations of adrenal androgens decline in later adult years. Some, but not all, epidemiologic studies of DHEA have demonstrated a correlation between low DHEA sulfate concentrations and increased cardiovascular disease in men (Nafziger et al. 1991). The age-related decline in adrenal androgens, as with age-related declines in testosterone and growth hormone, has been proposed as a pathophysiologic event in aging. Most, but not all, clinical studies of high-dose DHEA (1600 mg/day) therapy have demonstrated no beneficial effects on lean body mass (Welle et al. 1990; Mortola and Yen 1990; Nestler et al. 1988). Serum HDL concentrations in postmenopausal women decrease by approximately 10% at this dose which may reflect an androgenic effect of DHEA. A placebo-controlled study of DHEA administration in elderly subjects, using doses that achieved plasma DHEA concentrations typical of young adults (50 mg/day), failed to show significant effects on lean body mass, cholesterol, or insulin sensitivity parameters. DHEA administration (50 mg/day) did result in slightly higher androstenedione concentrations and higher scores on a psychological well-being questionnaire (Morales et al. 1994).

DHEA therapy has been proposed for a variety of autoimmune and immune deficiency syndromes but has not been tested in placebo-controlled trials in most cases. One controlled trial of 28 patients with systemic lupus erythematosus demonstrated improved symptom scores and reduced frequency of disease flares during 3 months of treatment with 200 mg/day of DHEA (van Vollenhoven et al. 1995); however, a longer trial was inconclusive due to a high dropout rate during the study (van Vollenhoven et al. 1998). Controlled trials of DHEA during influenza vaccination have demonstrated no enhancement of the immune response in elderly subjects (Danenberg et al. 1997).

## REFERENCES


Ackerman GL, Nolsn CM. 1968. Adrenocortical responsiveness after alternate-day corticosteroid therapy. *N Engl J Med* **278**:405–9.

Ballard PL, Carter JP, Graham BS, et al. 1975. A radioreceptor assay for evaluation of the plasma glucocorticoid activity of natural and synthetic steroids in man. *J Clin Endocrinol Metab* **41**:290–304.

Bamberger CM, Schulte HM, Chrousos GP. 1996. Molecular determinants of glucocorticoid receptor function and tissue sensitivity to glucocorticoids. *Endocr Rev* **17**:245–61.

Bertagna X, Bertagna C, Luton JP, et al. 1984. The new steroid analog RU 486 inhibits glucocorticoid action in man. *J Clin Endocrinol Metab* **59**:25–8.

Bravo EL, Tarazi RC, Dustan HP, et al. 1983. The changing clinical spectrum of primary aldosteronism. *Am J Med* **74**:641–51.

Brest AN. 1986. Spinolactone in the treatment of hypertension: a review. *Clin Ther* **8**:568–85.

Christy NP. 1992. Pituitary-adrenal function during corticosteroid therapy. Learning to live with uncertainty. *N Engl J Med* **326**:266–7.

Danenberg HD, Ben-Yehuda A, Zakay-Rones Z, et al. 1997. Dehydroepiandrosterone treatment is not beneficial to the immune response to influenza in elderly subjects. *J Clin Endocrinol Metab* **82**: 2911–4.

Esteban NV, Loughlin T, Yergey AL, et al. 1991. Daily cortisol production rate in man determined by stable isotope dilution/mass spectrometry. *J Clin Endocrinol Metab* **72**:39–45.

Feek CM, Ratcliffe JG, Seth J, et al. 1981. Patterns of plasma cortisol and ACTH concentrations in patients with Addison's disease treated with conventional corticosteroid replacement. *Clin Endocrinol* **14**:451–8.

Frey FJ, Escher G, Frey BM. 1994. Pharmacology of 11 beta-hydroxysteroid dehydrogenase. *Steroids* **59**:74–9.

Glowniak JV, Loriaux DL. 1997. A double-blind study of perioperative steroid requirements in secondary adrenal insufficiency. *Surgery* **121**:123–9.

Gluck OS, Murphy WA, Hahn TJ, et al. 1981. Bone loss in adults receiving alternate day glucocorticoid therapy. A comparison with daily therapy. *Arthritis Rheum* **24**:892–8.

Graba AL, Ney RL, Nicholson WE, et al. 1965. Natural history of pituitary-adrenal recovery following long term suppression with corticosteroids. *J Clin Endocrinol Metab* **25**:11–16.

Groves RW, Toms GC, Houghton BJ, et al. 1988. Corticosteroid replacement therapy: twice or thrice daily? *J R Soc Med* **81**: 514–6.

Hamberger B, Russell CF, van Heerden JA, et al. 1982. Adrenal surgery: trends during the seventies. *Am J Surg* **144**:523–6.

Harter JG, Reddy WJ, Thorn GW. 1963. Studies on an intermittent corticosteroid dose regimen. *N Engl J Med* **296**:591–6.

Hutter AM, Kayhoe DE. 1998. Adrenal cortical carcinoma: results of treatment with o, p′-DDD in 138 patients. *Am J Med* **41**:581–92.

Ichikawa Y, Toguchi T, Kawagoe M, et al. 1977. ECG abnormalities in steroid-treated rheumatoid patients. *Lancet* **2**:82.

Imbimbo B, Tuzi T, Porzio F, et al. 1984. Clinical equivalence of a new glucocorticoid, deflazacort and prednisone in rheumatoid arthritis and S.L.E. patients. *Adv Exp Med Biol* **171**:241–56.

Kalbak K. 1972. Incidence of arteriosclerosis in patients with rheumatoid arthritis receiving long-term corticosteroid therapy. *Ann Rheum Dis* **31**:196–200.

Kehlet H, Binder C. 1973. Adrenocortical function and clinical course during and after surgery in unsupplemented glucocorticoid-treated patients. *Br J Anaesth* **45**:1043–8.

Kerrigan JR, Veldhuis JD, Leyo SA, et al. 1993. Estimation of daily cortisol production and clearance rates in normal pubertal males by deconvolution analysis. *J Clin Endocrinol Metab* **76**:1505–10.

Kobberling J, Rotenberger J. 1992. Problems in evaluating dose equivalences of glucocorticoids. *Int J Clin Pharmacol Ther Toxicol* **30**:434–6.

Lund B, Egsmose C, Jorgensen S, et al. 1987. Establishment of the relative antiinflammatory potency of deflazacort and prednisone in polymyalgia rheumatica. *Calcif Tissue Int* **41**:316–20.

Luzzani F, Barone D, Galliani G, et al. 1984. Ex vivo binding to thymic glucocorticoid receptors: correlation with biological responses. *Adv Exp Med Biol* **171**:313–20.

Meikle AW, Tyler FH. 1977. Potency and duration of action of glucocorticoids. Effects of hydrocortisone, prednisone and dexamethasone on human pituitary-adrenal function. *Am J Med* **63**:200–7.

Miller JW, Crapo L. 1993. The medical treatment of Cushing's syndrome. *Endocr Rev* **14**:443–58.

Morales AJ, Nolan JJ, Nelson JC, et al. 1994. Effects of replacement dose of dehydroepiandrosterone in men and women of advancing age. *J Clin Endocrinol Metab* **78**:1360–67.

Mortola JF, Yen SS. 1990. The effects of oral dehydroepiandrosterone on endocrine-metabolic parameters in postmenopausal women. *J Clin Endocrinol Metab* **71**:696–704.

Nafziger AN, Herrington DM, Bush TL. 1991. Dehydroepiandrosterone and dehydroepiandrosterone sulfate: their relation to cardiovascular disease. *Epidemiol Rev* **13**:267–293.

Nestler JE, Barlascini CO, Clore JN, et al. 1988. Dehydroepiandrosterone reduces serum low density lipoprotein levels and body fat but does not alter insulin sensitivity in normal men. *J Clin Endocrinol Metab* **66**:57–61.

Nieman LK, Chrousos GP, Kellner C, et al. 1985. Successful treatment of Cushing's syndrome with the glucocorticoid antagonist RU 486. *J Clin Endocrinol Metab* **61**:536–40.

Pagano G, Bruno A, Cavallo-Perin P, et al. 1989. Glucose intolerance after short-term administration of corticosteroids in healthy subjects. Prednisone, deflazacort, and betamethasone. *Arch Intern Med* **149**:1098–101.

Riedel M, Wiese A, Schurmeyer TH, et al. 1993. Quality of life in patients with Addison's disease: effects of different cortisol replacement modes. *Exp Clin Endocrinol* **101**:106–11.

Rosen T, Bengtsson BA. 1990. Premature mortality due to cardiovascular disease in hypopituitarism. *Lancet* **336**:285–8.

Salem M, Tainsh RE Jr, Bromberg J, et al. 1994. Perioperative glucocorticoid coverage. A reassessment 42 years after emergence of a problem. *Ann Surg* **219**:416–25.

Schlaghecke R, Kornely E, Santen RT, et al. 1992. The effect of long-term glucocorticoid therapy on pituitary-adrenal responses to exogenous corticotropin-releasing hormone. *N Engl J Med* **326**:226–30.

Selye H. 1956. *The Stress of Life*. New York: McGraw-Hill.

Sonino N, Boscaro M, Paoletta A, et al. 1991. Ketoconazole treatment in Cushing's syndrome: experience in 34 patients. *Clin Endocrinol* **35**:347–52.

Swartz SL, Dluhy RG. 1978. Corticosteroids: clinical pharmacology and therapeutic use. *Drugs* **16**:238–55.

Toogood JH, Baskerville J, Jennings B, et al. 1989. Bioequivalent doses of budesonide and prednisone in moderate and severe asthma. *J Allergy Clin Immunol* **84**:688–700.

Valero MA, Leon M, Ruiz Valdepenas MP, et al. 1994. Bone density and turnover in Addison's disease: effect of glucocorticoid treatment. *Bone Mineral* **26**:9–17.

van Vollenhoven RF, Engleman EG, McGuire JL. 1995. Dehydroepiandrosterone in systemic lupus erythematosus. Results of a double-blind, placebo-controlled, randomized clinical trial. *Arthritis Rheum* **38**:1826–31.

van Vollenhoven RF, Morabito LM, Engleman EG, et al. 1998. Treatment of systemic lupus erythematosus with dehydroepiandrosterone: 50 patients treated up to 12 months. *J Rheumatol* **25**: 285–9.

Walton J, Watson BS, Ney RL. 1970. Alternate-day vs shorter-interval steroid administration. *Arch Intern Med* **126**:601–7.

Weinberger MH, Grim CE, Hollifield JW, et al. 1979. Primary aldosteronism: diagnosis, localization, and treatment. *Ann Int Med* **90**:386–95.

Welbourn RB. 1985. Survival and causes of death after adrenalectomy for Cushing's disease. *Surgery* **97**:16–20.

Welle S, Jozefowicz R, Statt M. 1990. Failure of dehydroepiandrosterone to influence energy and protein metabolism in humans. *J Clin Endocrinol Metab* **71**:1259–64.

# Thyroid Disease

Jeffrey W. Miller

*Chapter Outline*



## PHARMACOLOGY OF THE HYPOTHALAMIC–PITUITARY–THYROID AXIS

### Regulation of Thyroid and Thyroid-Stimulating Hormone Secretion

The hypothalamic–pituitary–thyroid (HPT) axis modulates metabolic rate by regulating transcription of genes involved in cellular respiration, ATP hydrolysis, and ion exchange. Thyroid hormone binds intracellular receptors that are closely related to the c-*erb* oncogene product. Thyroid hormone receptors are expressed in virtually all tissues; hence, thyroid dysfunction is a multisystem clinical syndrome. The secretion of thyroid hormones tetraiodothyronine (*l*-thyroxine, $T_4$) and triiodothyronine (liothyronine, $T_3$), stimulated by thyroid-stimulating hormone (TSH), is regulated at secondary (pituitary) and tertiary (hypothalamic) levels (Fig. 9-24). Thyroid hormone, particularly $T_3$, exerts negative feedback at both secondary and tertiary levels. Hypothalamic release of TSH-releasing hormone (TRH) is under neuroregulatory control, including inhibition by dopamine, somatostatin, and glucocorticoids. TRH travels by the portal venous system of the pituitary to stimulate TSH release from the thyrotroph cells of the anterior pituitary. TSH acts on the thyroid gland to increase iodine uptake and release preformed thyroid hormones. Although the HPT axis shows some diurnal activity, TSH concentrations do not vary significantly during the day (Fig. 9-25). Unlike the growth hormone and glucocorticoid axes, randomly obtained thyroid hormone and TSH concentrations are adequate for diagnosis of most thyroid conditions. Despite this apparent simplicity, commonly encountered clinical events, such as acute illness or use of numerous drugs or other hormones, complicate the accurate measurement of thyroid hormone status by causing changes that may mimic alterations found in thyroid disease.

### Thyroid Gland and Hormone Production

Thyroid-stimulating hormone stimulates release of preformed thyroid hormones from the thyroid gland; hence, the synthesis and storage of thyroid is an important pharmacological target in thyroid disease. Thyroid epithelial cells are unique in their ability to actively transport and accumulate iodide ($I^-$). Iodide is subsequently oxidized and covalently attached to the 3 and 5 positions on the aromatic ring of tyrosine amino acid residues on thyroglobulin. This "organification" is catalyzed by the multifunctional enzyme thyroid peroxidase (TPO). Iodine excess and thioamide drugs inhibit the action of this enzyme. This enzyme also catalyzes the coupling of mono- and diiodotyrosine moieties to form triiodo- and tetraiodothyronine. Iodination of thyroglobulin occurs in exocytotic

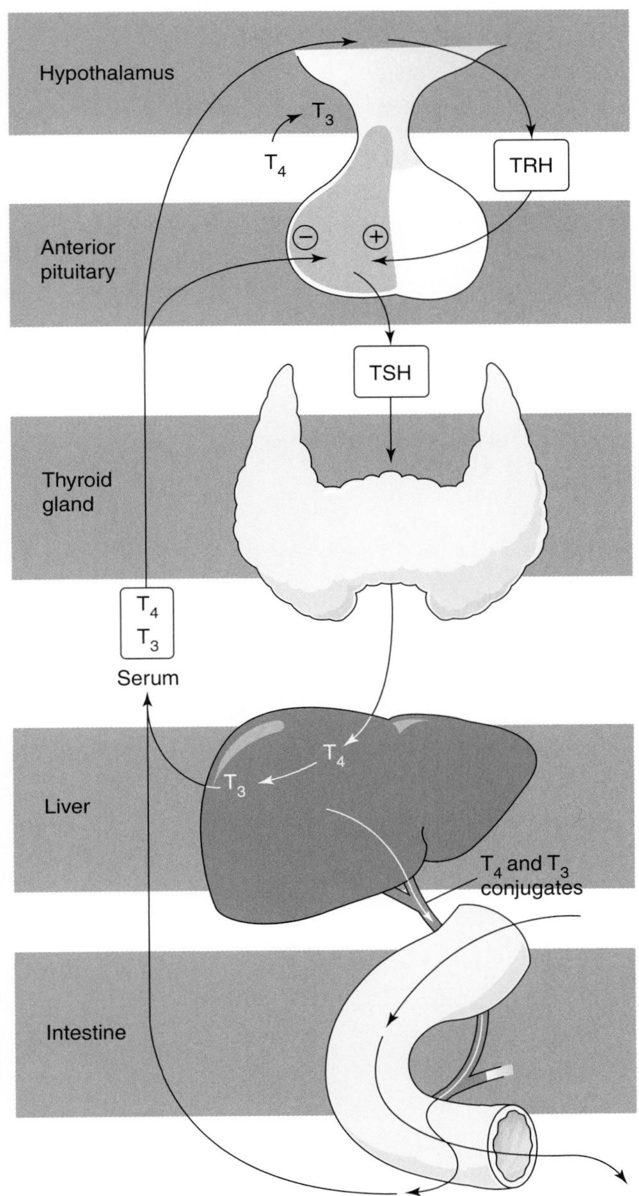


FIGURE 9-24 **Regulation and secretion of thyroid hormones. (From Surks, 1995).**

vesicles that secrete hormone-laden thyroglobulin into the interior follicles of the thyroid gland.

## Release, Distribution, and Metabolism of Thyroid Hormones

In addition to synthesis and storage, other processes such as release, transport, peripheral conversion of $T_4$ to $T_3$, and metabolism of thyroid hormones influence thyroid hormone action. Stimulation by TSH causes endocytosis of thyroglobulin from follicular stores, proteolysis in pinocytotic vesicles, and release of thyroid hormone into the circulation. This process is inhibited by iodine excess. The release of thyroid hormone occurs by a cAMP-mediated signaling pathway and may be inhibited by lithium therapy.

Tetraiodothyronine is the predominant hormone released by the thyroid gland; however, $T_3$ is 10 times as potent in binding to the thyroid receptor. $T_4$ is converted to $T_3$ by 5′-deiodinase enzymes in the liver and throughout the body that remove iodide from the 5′ position on the outer benzene ring. $T_4$-to-$T_3$ conversion may be inhibited by a number of drugs used in the therapy of hyperthyroidism.

Both $T_4$ and $T_3$ are largely protein-bound in the plasma to thyroid-binding globulin, albumin, and prealbumin. Thyroid-binding globulin (TBG) is produced by the liver under hormonal regulation by estrogens, androgens, and glucocorticoids. $T_4$ is the predominant circulating form of thyroid hormone and is greater than 99% protein-bound. $T_3$, which circulates in lower concentrations than $T_4$, is also extensively bound but dissociates more readily from binding proteins. Approximately 70% of $T_4$ is bound to TBG, whereas 20% is bound to thyroid-binding prealbumin (transthyretin), and 10% is bound to albumin.

Tetraiodothyronine and $T_3$ are rendered pharmacologically inactive by deiodination at other positions. $T_4$ may be deiodinated at the 5 position of the inner benzene ring to produce reverse $T_3$ ($rT_3$) (Fig. 9-26). In addition to deiodination, thyroid hormone may be hydrolyzed by oxidative enzymes in the liver. These enzymes may be induced by commonly used medications (e.g., antiseizure

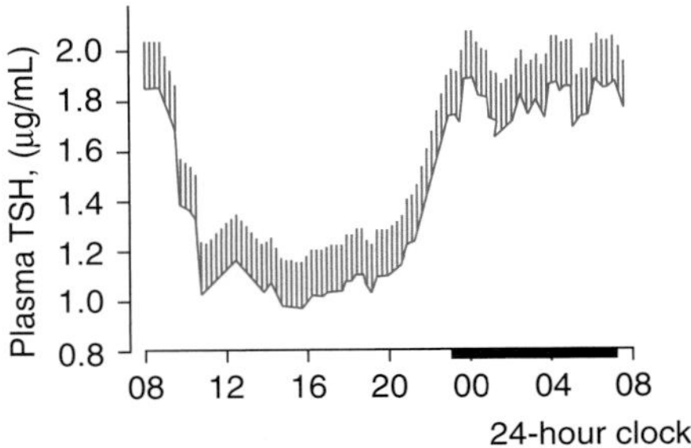


FIGURE 9-25 **Diurnal variation in plasma thyroid-stimulating thyroid concentrations. TSH may be measured at any time of day, but has a diurnal pattern similar to other pituitary hormones. X-axis represents time of day with the black bar depcting the normal sleep cycle. (Reproduced with permission of S. Karger AG, Basel from Vancouver 1990.)**

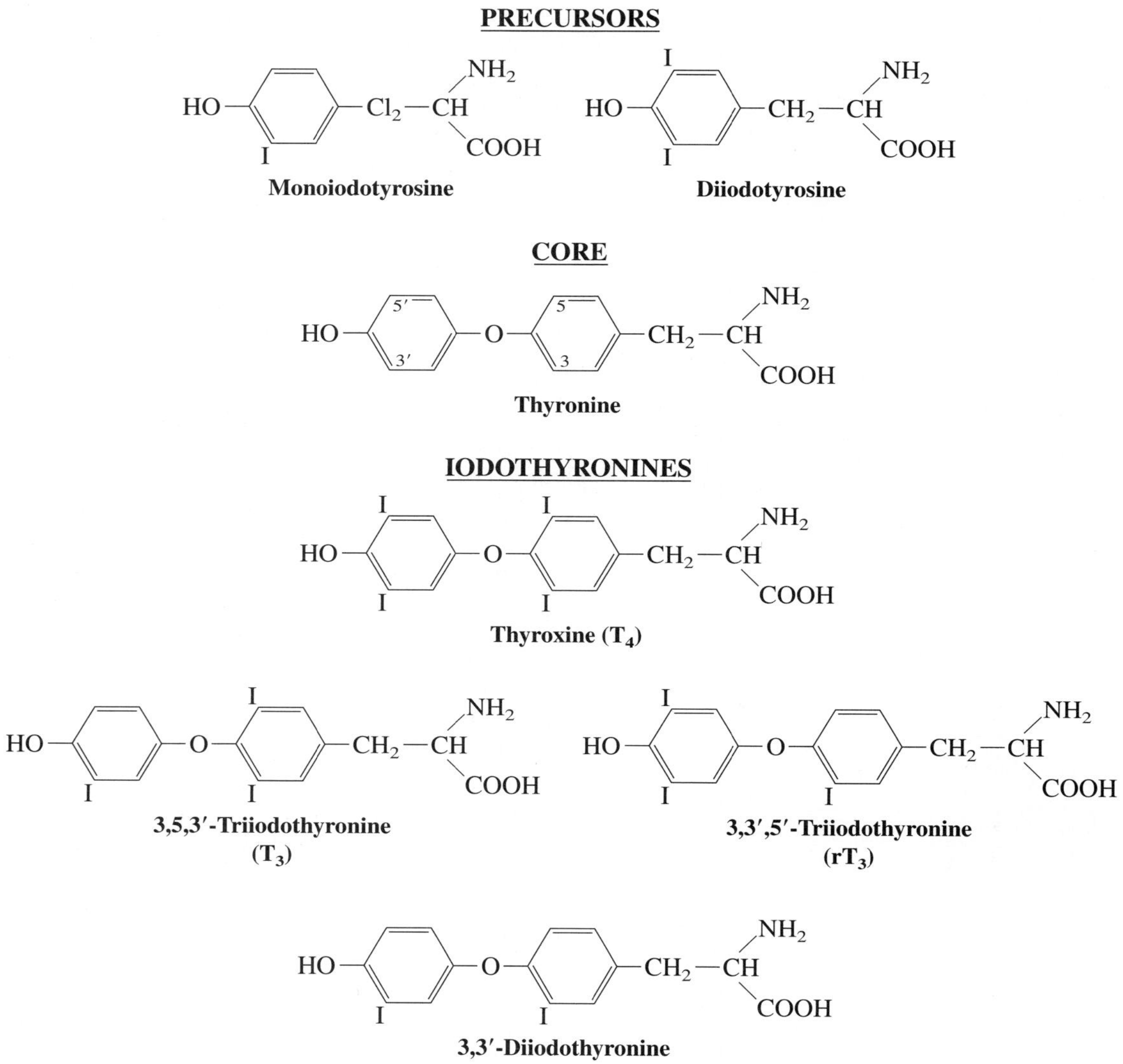

**PRECURSORS**

**Monoiodotyrosine**

**Diiodotyrosine**

**CORE**

**Thyronine**

**IODOTHYRONINES**

**Thyroxine ($T_4$)**

**3,5,3′-Triiodothyronine ($T_3$)**

**3,3′,5′-Triiodothyronine ($rT_3$)**

**3,3′-Diiodothyronine**

FIGURE 9-26 **Structures of thyroid hormones.**

medications). Intact thyroid hormone and metabolites are excreted in the bile and urine. Biliary excretion of thyroid hormones leads to enterohepatic recirculation, which may be interrupted by cholestasis or various medications.

## Differential Regulation of Central and Peripheral Thyroid Activity

Conversion of $T_4$ to $T_3$ occurs in the liver and in target tissues throughout the body. The 5′-deiodinase that produces $T_3$ in the brain (type II) is different from the peripheral (type I) 5′-deiodinase. These enzymes are differentially regulated. Physiological conditions such as starvation and nonspecific illness reduce the peripheral (type I) 5′-deiodinase activity, thereby decreasing systemic $T_3$ concentrations. This change in $T_3$ decreases peripheral consumption of energy substrates as a homeostatic response to catabolic stress. The type II 5′-deiodinase expressed in the central nervous system is not inhibited under these conditions; hence, $T_4$ to $T_3$ conversion continues at the normal rate in the hypothalamus. Locally produced $T_3$ in the brain provides the normal negative feedback to the HPT axis, which prevents the lower systemic $T_3$ concentrations from increasing TSH secretion and overcoming the reduction in peripheral metabolic rate in non-specific illness.

## Clinical Assessment of Thyroid Hormone Status

Proper interpretation of thyroid tests is critical to appropriate therapy of thyroid disease. Historically, a confusing array of tests has been used, but diagnosis has now been simplified by widespread availability of accurate and sensitive TSH and free thyroid hormone assays. TSH is measured by immunometric assay methods that are now sufficiently sensitive to distinguish normal from suppressed levels of TSH.

The most widely used assays for free thyroid hormone concentrations now rely on either radioimmunoassay (RIA) or enzyme-linked immunosorbent assay (ELISA) with the use of a radiolabeled analog of $T_4$. The free $T_4$ assay, by either method, allows measurement of thyroid hormone and correction for protein binding, so it accurately quantifies free $T_4$ or $T_3$ in most cases. Free $T_4$ is more commonly measured than free $T_3$, as it circulates at higher concentrations and has stable protein-binding kinetics. Measurement of free $T_4$ or $T_3$ by equilibrium dialysis is the most accurate method but is costly to perform.

In addition to measurements of thyroid hormone concentration, assessment of thyroid $^{125}I$ uptake and scanning are widely used diagnostic tests in suspected hyperthyroidism. In the absence of definitive abnormalities of thyroid hormone concentrations, $^{125}I$ uptake is not useful in diagnosing hyper- or hypothyroidism. An elevated $^{125}I$ uptake with a diffuse distribution on thyroid scanning in the hyperthyroid patient is usually diagnostic of Graves disease. A low $^{125}I$ uptake is the hallmark of thyroiditis or iodine excess, and regionally localized $^{125}I$ uptake is usually indicative of hyperfunctioning adenomas. Tests of antithyroid antibodies are not highly sensitive and are not necessary for the proper diagnosis of most thyroid disease.

## Interpretation of Thyroid-Stimulating Hormone and Free Thyroid Hormone Tests

The most commonly used diagnostic strategy utilizes measurement of both TSH and free thyroid hormone (e.g., $FT_4$). An elevated concentration of TSH with a low concentration of $FT_4$ is diagnostic of hypothyroidism, whereas a low TSH concentration with a high $FT_4$ concentration is diagnostic of hyperthyroidism. Since these two independent tests may be discordant, a variety of differential diagnoses must be considered (Table 9-24).

The effects of nonthyroidal illness on the HPT axis (euthyroid sick syndrome) is a common cause of discordant thyroid tests. Otherwise healthy patients who take thyroid hormone in an irregular pattern may have discordant thyroid hormone and TSH concentrations, rendering hormone measurements misleading. Assessment of the clinical setting and degree of abnormality of thyroid test results are critical to proper interpretation of discordant thyroid hormone tests.

**PRINCIPLE Even with the availability of modern, sensitive, and specific assays, proper diagnosis is the key to rational management of thyroid disease. Therapy should be initiated cautiously or not at all in the case of discordant thyroid tests, unless a definitive diagnosis has been made to account for the pattern of test results.**

Table 9-24 **Differential Diagnosis of Discordant Thyroid-Stimulating Hormone and Free Levothyroxine Measurements**

| TEST RESULTS | DIAGNOSIS | CLINICAL RELEVANCE |
|---|---|---|
| Low FT4, low TSH | Secondary hypothyroidism | Assess pituitary function |
| Low FT4, normal TSH | 1) Drug effect<br>2) Subclinical thyroiditis with high $T_3/T_4$ ratio<br>3) Abnormal binding protein interference with FT4 assay<br>4) Secondary hypothyroidism | 1) Check FT3<br>2) Consider equilibrium dialysis FT4<br>3) Assess pituitary function |
| Normal FT4, low TSH | Mild or subclinical hyperthyroidism | Thyroid exam consider need for thyroid scan and treatment |
| Normal FT4, high TSH | Mild or subclinical hypothyroidism | Consider need for treatment |
| High FT4, normal TSH | Thyroid hormone resistance | Clinically euthyroid, assess family history |
| High FT4, high TSH | 1) Thyroid hormone resistance<br>2) TSH-secreting pituitary adenoma | 1) Clinically euthyroid, assess family history<br>2) Clinically hyperthyroid, assess pituitary function |

ABBREVIATIONS: FT3, free liothyronine ($T_3$); FT4, free levothyroxine ($T_4$); TSH, thyroid-stimulating hormone.

# HYPOTHYROIDISM

## Diagnosis of Hypothyroidism

Thyroid insufficiency commonly results from autoimmune destruction of the thyroid gland, and it presents as a multisystem disorder of reduced metabolic rate. The most common clinical findings are weight gain, lethargy, constipation, cold intolerance, and dry skin. Because of the protean nature of these symptoms, which can often be elicited from even healthy patients, mild hypothyroidism is difficult to diagnose with certainty on clinical grounds alone.

The most common etiology of hypothyroidism is chronic autoimmune thyroiditis (Hashimoto disease). Physical and iatrogenic causes of thyroid gland destruction, such as head and neck surgery or $^{131}I$ administration for Graves disease, are usually clinically evident. Iodine deficiency and congenital defects in iodine metabolism are rare. Pituitary insufficiency, usually due to compressive tumors of the anterior pituitary, is a less common cause of hypothyroidism and is usually associated with loss of gonadal function and other hormonal deficits.

## Treatment of Hypothyroidism

***Thyroid hormone preparations***

Both $T_4$ (levothyroxine) and $T_3$ (liothyronine) are available separately as synthetic drugs and in a fixed 4:1 combination (liotrix). The fixed combination preparation mimics the natural ratio of endogenous thyroid hormones but has no clinical advantage compared with *l*-thyroxine in thyroid hormone replacement. Thyroid hormone extracts derived from animal thyroid glands (e.g., Armour Thyroid) were used extensively in the past but are now obsolete.

Synthetic $T_4$ and $T_3$ differ in pharmacological potency and in pharmacokinetic features. The two agents are contrasted in Table 9-25. $T_4$ is the preferred agent for chronic replacement therapy, because its long elimination half-life contributes to stable plasma concentrations and minimizes the effect of missed doses. The average daily $T_4$ replacement dose is 1.7 $\mu$g per kilogram of body weight but generally should be closer to 1.0 $\mu$g/kg in elderly or obese patients. Since $T_4$ and $T_3$ are metabolized by similar mechanisms, the difference in half-life between the two is largely due to more avid protein binding of $T_4$. Agents with long half-lives are advantageous for chronic therapy, because the impact of an occasional missed dose on the steady-state drug concentration is small. One drawback, however, is that a period of 4 to 5 half-lives is required to reach steady state; hence, prompt symptomatic relief is more difficult to achieve when using *l*-thyroxine.

Thyroid testing to determine whether the dose is adequate should not be performed earlier than 5 weeks after initiation of therapy with *l*-thyroxine. In all cases of hypothyroidism due to pituitary impairment, a normal TSH concentration is the appropriate goal for therapeutic monitoring of thyroid replacement in patients who take $T_4$ on a regular schedule (Helfand and Crapo 1990). Patients who take $T_4$ in an intermittent schedule may show discordant thyroid tests. One common scenario is that of the noncompliant patient whose $T_4$ concentrations are low until an upcoming doctor's appointment motivates compliance or even overcompensation with the thyroid regimen. In this case serum TSH may remain high, but $T_4$ concentrations may be normal or even elevated owing to doses of $T_4$ taken within a few days of the lab test. Although this pattern of thyroid hormone tests may suggest the rare condition of thyroid hormone resistance, this diagnosis cannot be made unless medication compliance is strictly monitored. In patients with pituitary insufficiency, a dose should be identified that relieves hypothyroid symptoms and results in a free $T_4$ concentration that is typically in the middle of the normal range.

**Table 9-25 Thyroid Hormone Preparations**

| DRUG | TYPICAL DOSE | COST PER DAY (AWP) | HALF-LIFE | PROTEIN BINDING AFFINITY | MARKETED NAMES |
|---|---|---|---|---|---|
| *l*-Thyroxine ($T_4$) | 75–200 $\mu$g (1–1.7 $\mu$g/kg/d) | $0.10 | 7 days | Very high | Cytomel, Generic |
| Liothyronine ($T_3$) | 25–75 $\mu$g/d | $0.29 | 1–2 days | High | Various, generic |
| Liotrix ($T_4$:$T_3$ = 4:1) | 60–180 mg (1–3 gr) | $0.50 | | | Thyrolar, euthyroid |
| Desiccated thyroid | 60–180 mg (1–3 gr) | | | | Armour Thyroid, generic |

ABBREVIATION: AWP, average wholesale price.
SOURCE: *The Red Book*. 1997. Average wholesale price.

**Table 9-26 Thyroid Hormone Replacement in Special Medical Settings**

| Clinical scenario | Considerations |
|---|---|
| Neonatal and pediatric use | Neonatal diagnosis, weight-adjusted dosing |
| Catabolic illnesses, nephrotic syndrome | Reduced protein binding (decrease dose) |
| General medical or psychiatric illness | Reassess abnormal tests after convalescence |

### *Thyroid Hormone Replacement in Special Medical Settings*

In the adult patient, the appropriate dose for hormone replacement is determined empirically with attention to physiological conditions that may alter thyroid economy. The dose of thyroid hormone replacement may require adjustment in special clinical settings (Table 9-26).

Congenital hypothyroidism is a common and treatable disease that can lead to lifelong cognitive impairment. Treatment of this condition requires appropriate dose adjustment throughout childhood growth (Table 9-27). During adulthood, thyroid hormone requirements may change with significant changes in body weight. Adequate thyroid hormone replacement does not prevent obesity; hence, weight gain should not be treated by increased thyroid hormone dose, unless biochemical testing confirms the insufficiency of the replacement dose.

Women on a stable dose of thyroid hormone who become pregnant, or who begin estrogen replacement therapy or oral contraceptives, may experience increases in protein binding of $T_4$ to thyroid-binding globulin. This increase in protein binding of $T_4$ may increase total $T_4$ concentrations. Free $T_4$ concentrations should remain unchanged after equilibration at higher levels of protein binding.

Patients experiencing catabolic illnesses or hypoalbuminemia may require reduction in dose. Patients with prior thyroid disease are susceptible to drug-induced changes in thyroid economy; hence, dosage should be reevaluated when medications that interact with the thyroid axis (see below and Table 9-31) are initiated in a patient on a previously stable thyroid-replacement regimen.

Elderly patients may be at risk for cardiac complications of thyroid hormone replacement therapy. Initiation of thyroid hormone replacement has been widely reported to precipitate or exacerbate angina pectoris, although no controlled study to support this claim has been done. In one retrospectively analyzed series, angina pectoris was reported in 6% of approximately 1500 patients treated for hypothyroidism at the Mayo Clinic (Keating et al. 1961). Of the 90 patients with angina in this cohort, 23% reported increased angina within 1 year of initiating thyroid hormone replacement, 23% reported decreased angina, 28% reported no change, and 26% developed angina after 1 year of thyroid replacement. Although thyroid hormone increases cardiac contractility, heart rate, and myocardial oxygen demand, it also leads to reduced peripheral vascular resistance and improved diastolic cardiac function.

In contrast to the adverse effects on anginal symptoms, uncontrolled clinical studies have reported reduced progression of angiographic coronary lesions and improved left ventricular function in hypothyroid patients treated with full replacement doses of *l*-thyroxine (Bernstein et al. 1991; Perk and O'Neill 1997). The recommended regimen for thyroid hormone replacement in patients at risk for coronary disease is to initiate *l*-thyroxine at 25 μg/day and increase in 25-μg increments every 4 weeks. This regimen has not been studied prospectively.

In addition to angina pectoris, thyroid hormone therapy is associated with atrial fibrillation, an important risk factor for stroke in the elderly. A prospective study of more than 2000 clinically euthyroid elderly subjects demonstrated a threefold relative risk of developing atrial fibrillation during 10 years of followup when TSH levels were suppressed to less than 0.1 mIU/L (Sawin et al. 1994). Patients taking a thyroid hormone replacement were among those with suppressed TSH concentrations who developed atrial fibrillation, suggesting that this may be a complication of excessive thyroid hormone replacement.

#### *Treatment of subclinical hypothyroidism*

With the widespread use of thyroid tests, it is now possible to identify many subjects with normal $T_4$ and $T_3$ concentrations but mildly elevated TSH concentrations (5 to 10 mIU/L). Because of biological variability, many healthy people have TSH concentrations above the upper limit of normal. In the setting of significant nonthyroidal illness, the normal range of TSH values is wider; hence, a greater percentage of acutely ill patients may have apparently elevated TSH concentrations.

**Table 9-27 Pediatric Dosing of *l*-Thyroxine**

| Age | Dose per day (μg) | Daily dose per kg (μg) |
|---|---|---|
| 0–6 mo | 25–50 | 8–10 |
| 6–12 mo | 50–75 | 6–8 |
| 1–5 yr | 75–100 | 5–6 |
| 6–12 yr | 100–150 | 4–5 |
| 12–18 yr | 100–150 | 2–3 |

Appropriate management of patients with mild TSH elevation requires accurate diagnosis. The term *subclinical* or *asymptomatic* TSH elevation should be applied when the patient does not present with clear symptoms of hypothyroidism. Since a healthy pituitary is capable of large increases in TSH concentration (10 to 100 times normal concentrations), TSH elevations of 2 to 3 times normal rarely reflect significant deficiency of thyroid hormone. Thyroxine supplementation in this population has not been assessed in large clinical trials, but a small, placebo-controlled trial suggests little clinical benefit (Cooper et al. 1984). Patients with subclinical hypothyroidism who demonstrate significantly increased cholesterol levels, body weight, or neuropsychiatric symptoms may benefit from a trial of thyroxine supplementation. Approximately one-third of patients with subclinical hypothyroidism will progress to unequivocal hypothyroidism in subsequent years (Tunbridge et al. 1981), suggesting the need for appropriate follow-up of untreated patients.

## HYPERTHYROIDISM

### Clinical Features of Hyperthyroidism

Thyroid excess is a multisystem clinical syndrome with predominantly metabolic and cardiovascular symptoms and signs. Distinctive features are weight loss in the setting of hyperphagia, tremor, nervousness, and atrial tachyarrhythmias (sinus tachycardia or atrial fibrillation). Many symptoms and signs of hyperthyroidism are shared by overactivity of the autonomic nervous system, including $\beta$-adrenergic (tachycardia, tremor), sympathetic cholinergic (increased sweating), and parasympathetic (increased GI motility) symptoms. Elderly and chronically ill patients may demonstrate a paucity of symptoms or even paradoxically reduced neuropsychiatric status (i.e., apathetic hyperthyroidism) (Lahey 1931) and commonly present with isolated atrial fibrillation.

### Etiologies of Hyperthyroidism

Hyperthyroidism occurs by either TSH receptor-dependent or receptor-independent thyroid hormone release. The most common hyperthyroid syndrome, Graves disease, results from autoantibodies (thyroid-stimulating antibody [TSAb] or long-acting thyroid stimulator [LATS]) that activate the TSH receptor. TSH-dependent hyperthyroidism is almost invariably associated with diffuse goiter. The other major hyperthyroid syndromes result from TSH receptor-independent release of thyroid hormone. Nodular goiters, both multinodular and solitary hyperfunctioning adenomas, are benign neoplasias of the thyroid gland that are autonomous from normal TSH regulation. Multinodular changes in the thyroid gland are common with increasing age.

As long as autonomous thyroid hormone release is less than the daily requirement, this condition remains clinically silent because of proportionate suppression of TSH secretion. Palpation of the thyroid gland may not reveal significant goiter. If autonomous thyroid hormone release exceeds daily requirements or is stimulated by dietary or medicinal iodine ingestion, clinical hyperthyroidism may ensue. The multinodular thyroid gland is also susceptible to a variety of drug actions that may alter thyroid economy in patients who lack pituitary control over thyroid hormone release.

### Radioiodine and Surgical Treatment of Hyperthyroidism

#### *Graves disease*

Graves disease is definitively diagnosed by hyperthyroidism associated with clear ocular findings (scleritis, proptosis, diplopia) or a diffusely increased uptake pattern on radionuclide scanning. In most cases, the disease follows a chronic or relapsing clinical course. Curative treatment options include subtotal thyroidectomy or $^{131}I$ ablative therapy. Although no randomized prospective trials have compared these two treatment modalities, both are highly effective. Subtotal thyroidectomy is associated with an approximately 1 to 2% rate of permanent hypoparathyroidism or recurrent laryngeal nerve damage, as well as a recurrence rate of approximately 15% (Sugino et al. 1995). $^{131}I$ therapy, in contrast, is associated with few adverse effects but may not render the patient euthyroid for 2 to 6 months after treatment. $^{131}I$ therapy may induce radiation thyroiditis, but this is rarely clinically detectable in patients appropriately treated with $\beta$-adrenergic receptor antagonists ("beta-blockers") and antithyroid medications during the first 6 weeks after treatment.

In one prospective trial, approximately 15% of hyperthyroid patients with mild or no ophthalmopathy at baseline experienced worsened eye symptoms after $^{131}I$ treatment. Two-thirds of these patients improved spontaneously, but 5% of patients with Graves disease experienced persistent eye changes. Concurrent treatment with prednisone 30 mg/day for 3 months after $^{131}I$ therapy prevented the progression of ophthalmopathy in this study (Bartalena et al. 1998). In another prospective trial, daily doses of 20 to 60 mg of prednisone resulted in ophthalmological improvement in 61% of patients with severe Graves ophthalmopathy (Prummel et al. 1989). Other studies have found thyrotropin receptor autoantibodies to be increased with $^{131}I$ therapy compared with medical or surgical therapy of Graves disease (Tallstedt et al. 1992). As a consequence, it has been hypothesized that radiation-induced thyroiditis increases the autoimmune response, which shows cross-reactivity with antigens in the ocular muscles.

***Toxic multinodular goiter or solitary adenoma***

Hyperthyroidism due to multinodular thyroid disease is usually diagnosed by multiple areas of increased activity with suppression of other thyroid tissue on $^{131}$I thyroid scan, a pattern rarely seen in Graves disease. Occasionally, multinodular thyroid glands that receive increased iodine exposure may respond with increased hormone production, mimicking the hyperthyroidism produced by iodine therapy of iodine-deficient goiters (Jodbasedow phenomenon). For this reason, recent exposure to radiocontrast agents and other sources of iodine should be considered in evaluating the elderly patient with hyperthyroidism.

Surgery may be desirable if the multinodular goiter has local compressive effects. $^{131}$I radioiodine therapy may reduce the mass of autonomous tissue without harming the normally functioning thyroid tissue, where iodine uptake is reduced because of low TSH levels. Therapeutic considerations for a single hyperfunctioning nodule are similar. Thyroid cancer is rarely, if ever, hyperfunctioning and is not considered in the differential diagnosis of toxic goiter.

## Pharmacological Therapy of Hyperthyroidism

***Antithyroid drugs***

The thioamide drugs propylthiouracil, methimazole, and carbimazole (a prodrug form of methimazole) are thiourea derivatives that inhibit the activity of the enzyme thyroid peroxidase (TPO). The primary effect of these drugs is to inhibit formation of new thyroid hormone. Release of preexisting thyroid hormone is not affected; hence, the thyroid hormone concentrations are not lowered until existing supplies in the gland are depleted. In healthy people, the amount of thyroid hormone stored in thyroid follicles is sufficient for 6 weeks. Stores of thyroid hormone are more rapidly depleted in hyperthyroid patients, but the therapeutic effect of these drugs may require several weeks to become evident. In one prospective study of 509 patients, approximately two-thirds of patients treated with high doses of methimazole were rendered euthyroid within 3 weeks, whereas more than 90% of patients were in remission after 6 weeks (Benker et al. 1995). In addition to inhibition of hormone synthesis, propylthiouracil inhibits peripheral conversion of $T_4$ to $T_3$.

Despite their general similarity, thiourea derivatives (e.g., propylthiouracil [PTU]) and thiocarbamides (e.g., methimazole) have different pharmacokinetic and pharmacological properties, summarized in Table 9-28. Initial treatment of hyperthyroidism with PTU requires dosing three or four times per day, whereas methimazole may be given once or twice daily (Kallner et al. 1996). In a large, prospective European study, initial treatment with 40 mg/day of methimazole produced euthyroidism more rapidly than 10 mg/day; the larger dose was slightly more efficacious (91.6% versus 84.9% of patients rendered euthyroid) (Reinwein et al. 1993). Single daily doses of methimazole are as effective as divided doses (Shiroozu et al. 1986). When clinical response is evident (usually within 6 weeks), the dose may be reduced to 5 to 10 mg of methimazole to maintain euthyroidism. Single daily doses of 30 to 40 mg of methimazole result in increased adverse drug reactions (25% of patients) compared with doses of 10 to 15 mg (15% of patients) (Reinwein et al. 1993; Mashio et al. 1997). Administration of higher doses of methimazole in conjunction with thyroid replacement therapy for 12 to 18 months does not reduce the 36 to 58% rate of relapse during 6 to 12 months of followup after discontinuation of antithyroid medications (Reinwein et al. 1993; Rittmaster et al. 1998).

***Adverse effects***

Many toxicities are shared by methimazole and PTU (see Table 9-28) including skin rashes, granulocytopenia, and hepatic injury. Skin rashes are the most frequent side effect and may diminish with continued treatment. Dermal reaction to one agent may not recur with retreatment after a drug holiday or after change to a different antithyroid drug. Dermal reactions do not increase the probability of adverse hepatic or bone marrow effects. Granulocytopenia is uncommon and usually reversible after discontinuation of the medication. There are very few reported cases of fatal or irreversible bone marrow suppression with these agents. All patients treated with this class of drugs must be advised of this risk and counseled to seek medical attention in the event of fever, pharyngitis, or other symptoms of infection. The incidence of adverse reactions increases with dose and age; hence, use of high doses (30 mg/day methimazole or 300 mg/day PTU) in elderly subjects should be carefully justified and monitored.

***Clinical use***

Outcomes of surgical, medical, and radiotherapy of Graves disease have not been compared in large prospective trials, but more than 90% of patients achieve remission by each of these modalities. The risk/benefit ratio of antithyroid drug therapy, and comparison to surgical or $^{131}$I therapy alternatives, must be considered on an indi-

Table 9-28 **Antithyroid Drugs**

| FEATURE | PROPYLTHIOURACIL | METHIMAZOLE |
|---|---|---|
| Serum half-life | 1–2 h | 6–12 h |
| Initial dose | 100–200 mg, tid to qid | 10–20 mg, qd, bid |
| Chronic dose | 50–200 mg, qd to bid | 5–20 mg qd |
| Pharmacological effects | TPO inhibition, suppresses thyroid autoimmunity, inhibits $T_4$ to $T_3$ conversion | TPO inhibition, suppresses thyroid autoimmunity |
| Shared adverse effects | Rash, arthralgia, fever (2–5%), agranulocytosis (0.2%) | Rash, arthralgia, fever (2–5%), agranulocytosis (0.2%) |
| Other adverse effects | Anticoagulant effect, dysgeusia | Neonatal scalp aplasia |
| Rare adverse effects | Hepatocellular hepatitis, vasculitis, interstitial pneumonitis | Cholestatic jaundice, hypoglycemia (insulin autoantibodies) |
| Protein binding | High | Low |
| Transplacental passage and breast milk distribution | Low | High |
| Dose strengths available | 50 mg | 5, 10 mg |
| Wholesale cost per day | $0.18 (100 mg) | $0.43 (10 mg) |
| Other uses | Treatment of hepatic cirrhosis | None |

ABBREVIATIONS: $T_3$, liothyronine; $T_4$, levothyroxine; TPO, thyroid peroxidase.
SOURCE: *The Red Book*. 1997. Average wholesale price.

vidual basis. Conditions such as severe Graves disease and toxic multinodular goiter are likely to require long-term therapy with potentially toxic drugs. $^{131}$I therapy may be preferable in these settings. In patients who are severely symptomatic from hyperthyroidism, or who are not likely to tolerate radiation-induced transient increases in thyroid hormone, antithyroid drugs may be used for 1 to 3 months before definitive $^{131}$I therapy. A diagnostic thyroid uptake and scan should be performed before initiating therapy with antithyroid medications.

Treatment with methimazole 10 to 20 mg four times per day, or propylthiouracil 50 to 100 mg four times per day should be initiated. Treatment should be reevaluated in 4 to 6 weeks. Antithyroid drugs, which reduce iodide trapping in the thyroid gland, should be discontinued 1 week before $^{131}$I therapy and may be resumed 2 weeks after $^{131}$I therapy in severely symptomatic patients. Serum TSH may remain suppressed for up to 3 months after restoration of euthyroidism. Free $T_4$ levels should be maintained at the upper end of the normal range during chronic medical therapy, in order to minimize the risk of dose-related toxicity of antithyroid medications.

### *Adjunctive pharmacotherapy*

Severe hyperthyroidism requires adjunctive medical therapy in addition to antithyroid medications. Beta-adrenergic receptor antagonists are useful due to their rapid onset of action and specificity for many of the symptomatic complaints of hyperthyroidism (tremor, tachycardia, and agitation). Beta blockers are not adequate as monotherapy for thyrotoxicosis (Mazzaferri et al. 1976), and their clinical benefit may be small in patients adequately treated with antithyroid drugs (Jones et al. 1981; Kvetny et al. 1981). Propranolol provides greater symptomatic relief than selective $\beta_1$-adrenergic receptor antagonists such as atenolol (McDevitt and Nelson 1978). In contrast to the undesirable CNS depressant effects of propranolol in hypertensive patients, hyperthyroid patients may benefit from CNS penetration of more lipophilic beta blockers. Other nonselective beta blockers (nadolol, timolol) have not been studied in controlled trials but may be considered. In the initial treatment of hyperthyroidism, propranolol should be given four times per day or in a sustained release preparation (Jones et al. 1981), at doses that eliminate tachycardia. Propranolol, but not other $\beta$-adrenergic receptor antagonists, has been shown to inhibit peripheral $T_4$ to $T_3$ conversion (Nilsson et al. 1979). Beta blockers may be continued during $^{131}$I therapy.

### *Iodide*

In severe Graves disease, or thyroiditis with cardiovascular instability or hyperthermia (thyroid storm), iodide should be administered. Iodide is a uniquely effective agent in the acute management of hyperthyroidism. The dominant pharmacological effects of iodide are to inhibit release of thyroid hormone (Wolff-Chaikoff block) and reduce peripheral conversion of $T_4$ to $T_3$. Marked falls in thyroid hormone concentrations in Graves disease are typically achieved within 4 days (Roti et al. 1988). In patients with autoimmune or nodular thyroid disease, the thyroid gland is incapable of overcoming this effect; hence, therapeutic effect may be maintained for prolonged periods. Because of loading of the thyroid gland with iodide, iodide trapping is reduced; therefore, radionuclide imaging or therapy is not possible for several months after discontinuation of iodide treatment. See Table 9-29 for sources and doses of iodide in pharmaceutical and radiological preparations.

***Hyperthyroidism during pregnancy***

Because of the high incidence of autoimmune thyroid disease in young women, management of Graves disease in pregnancy is a common clinical problem. Uncontrolled hyperthyroidism in pregnant women is associated with low-birth-weight infants and peripartum maternal complications (Momotani et al. 1984). Hyperthyroidism does not affect cognitive development of the infant.

$^{131}$I therapy is contraindicated in pregnancy, where fetal thyroid tissue is at risk after its development in the tenth week; hence, antithyroid drug therapy is often indicated. Scalp aplasia has occurred in babies born to mothers treated with methimazole. Methimazole crosses the placenta and is excreted in breast milk to a greater extent than PTU (Marchant et al. 1977). Despite its inconvenient dosing frequency, PTU is the antithyroid drug of choice for pregnant and postpartum patients. The clinical experience with the use of antithyroid drugs in pregnancies is extensive. Retrospectively analyzed cohort studies suggest that maternal and fetal outcomes are improved with antithyroid drug therapy in pregnancy (Momotani et al. 1984). Therapy with PTU should be initiated at 50 to 100 mg four times per day. FT4 should be followed and maintained at or slightly above the upper limit.

Autoimmune thyroid disease often improves during the second trimester; hence, the PTU dose may be reduced or eliminated at term. Patients should be monitored for exacerbation in the postpartum period. The risk of hypothyroidism and goiter in the infant in carefully monitored therapy of pregnant patients is very low. Infants born to mothers with Graves disease may have goiter and hyperthyroidism due to maternal autoantibodies; this condition usually remits within several months.

## CONFOUNDING DIAGNOSES IN THYROID ASSESSMENT

A number of thyroidal and nonthyroidal conditions may confound the diagnosis and treatment of chronic thyroid disease (see Table 9-30).

### Painless Thyroiditis

Painless thyroiditis is a transient form of autoimmune thyroiditis that may occur in up to 10% of normal women in the postpartum period. Although it may occur in both men and women in other clinical settings, it is an important diagnostic consideration in postpartum depression. Thyroid hormone levels are often elevated for several months after onset and subsequently drop to subnormal levels for several months (see Fig. 9-27) (Woolf 1985). Thyroid tests may be normal or discordant (e.g., low TSH with normal FT4) during this transition period; hence, tests should be repeated in patients with persistent symptoms. Although most patients spontaneously remit within 6 months, severely symptomatic patients may benefit from a 3- to 6-month course of low doses of *l*-thyroxine.

### Subacute Thyroiditis

Subacute thyroiditis is an autoimmune form of thyroiditis that typically follows a recent upper respiratory illness. Clinical findings include a history of thyroid pain, which may be referred to the ears, a firm goiter, and transient

**Table 9-29 Iodide Sources in Pharmacological Preparations**

| Feature | Iodine Content | Dose in Thyrotoxicosis | Other Uses | Dispensed |
|---|---|---|---|---|
| Lugol's solution (10%, KI, 5% $I_2$) | 8 mg/drop | 2 drops/day in juice | Sweet syndrome (rare) | 120-mL bottle |
| Supersaturated potassium iodide solution (SSKI) | 50 mg/drop | 1 drop/day | Expectorant (300–600 mg PO qid) | 30-mL bottle |
| Potassium iodide tablets | 130 mg/tablet | ? tab per day | | |
| Iodinated glycerol | 6–25 mg/mL<br>15 mg/tablet | | Expectorant (30 mg PO qid) | |
| Radiopaque contrast agents (10–60% $I_2$) | | | Cholecystography, urography, angiography, computed tomography | |

**Table 9-30 Self-Limited Thyroid Disease, Nonthyroidal Illness, and Rare Thyroid Diseases**

| CONDITION | CLINICAL FEATURES |
|---|---|
| *Common thyroid conditions* | |
| Painless thyroiditis | Common self-limiting thyroid dysfunction in postpartum women |
| Subacute thyroiditis | Rock-hard goiter with local pain after upper respiratory illness |
| Acute suppurative thyroiditis | Tender inflamed thyroid abscess |
| *Common nonthyroidal conditions* | |
| Systemic medical illness | Euthyroid sick syndrome |
| Acute psychiatric illness | Self limiting thyroid lab test abnormalities |
| Factitious hyperthyroidism | Overuse of thyroid hormone (especially as weight control agent) |
| Familial dysalbuminemia, other serum protein abnormalities | Abnormal serum binding proteins alter $T_4$ measurements; TSH is normal |
| *Rare thyroid conditions* | |
| Pituitary disease | Hypopituitarism (common), TSH-secreting adenoma (rare) |
| Thyroid hormone resistance | Rare syndrome of increased free $T_4$, normal TSH, goiter |
| Paraneoplastic thyroid syndromes | hCG-secreting gonadal tumors, struma ovarii, teratoma |

ABBREVIATIONS: hCG, human chorionic gonadotropin; $T_3$, liothyronine; $T_4$, levothyroxine; TSH, thyroid-stimulating hormone.

increases and/or decreases in thyroid hormone concentrations. Radionuclide thyroid uptake is low, as is the case with all forms of thyroiditis other than Graves disease. Hypothyroidism is not a prominent feature of this syndrome, and the usual therapeutic course is to refrain from thyroid hormone replacement. Rarely, patients with subacute thyroiditis may progress to chronic hypothyroidism with anti-TPO antibodies, which suggests immunological overlap with Hashimoto thyroiditis.

## Euthyroid Sick Syndrome

Perhaps more than any other commonly performed clinical laboratory test, the normal range of thyroid tests differs in patients with concurrent medical illness from that in a healthy ambulatory population. Under conditions of systemic illness, the HPT axis undergoes adaptations that serve to reduce metabolic rate and conserve energy. The main mechanism for this homeostatic response is down-

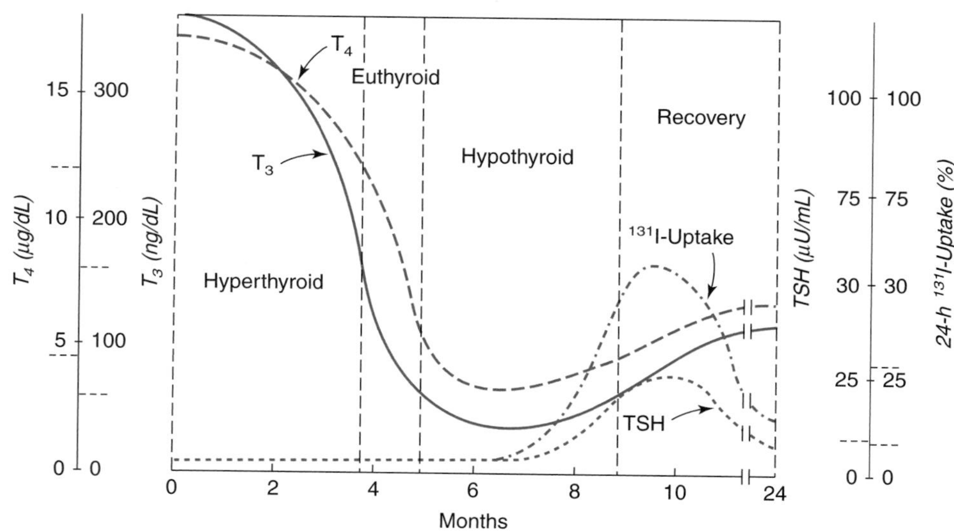


**FIGURE 9-27 The time course of changes in $T_4$ and TSH concentrations following painless thyroiditis. Not all subjects experience a hypothyroid phase prior to recovery of normal thyroid function. (From Woolf 1980.)**

regulation of peripheral 5′-deiodinase activity, which leads to decreased circulating $T_3$ concentrations. As a consequence, a greater amount of circulating $T_4$ is converted by a different deiodinase (5′-deiodinase) to reverse-$T_3$ ($rT_3$), which is inactive at the thyroid hormone receptor. In addition to decreased $T_3$ concentrations and elevated $rT_3$ concentrations, the normal range of TSH and $T_4$ concentrations is wider during nonthyroidal illness; hence, these values may be found to be high or low.

One prospective observational study documented abnormal thyroid hormone tests in 88% of patients admitted to a medical intensive care unit (Koh et al. 1996). The unreliability of thyroid tests in the critically ill patient creates diagnostic and therapeutic dilemmas. There are no controlled studies of clinical outcomes in critically ill patients treated with thyroid hormone. Administration of thyroid hormone to patients undergoing cardiac bypass surgery does not result in improved outcomes (Klemperer et al. 1995).

## Acute Psychiatric Illness

Another common condition that impairs the reliability of thyroid hormone testing is acute psychiatric illness. Central nervous system regulation of the HPT axis may be altered during acute psychosis. In two series that analyzed thyroid hormone tests in psychiatric inpatients, 27 to 49% of patients demonstrated abnormal thyroid tests that were not attributed to thyroid disease (Roca et al. 1990; Levy et al. 1981). Repeat thyroid tests and assessment of objective signs of thyroid illness (goiter, tremor, ocular changes, reflex relaxation rate) are usually sufficient to identify patients with true thyroidal illness (Griffin 1985).

## Drugs and the Thyroid Hormone System

In addition to the significant changes in thyroid physiology and thyroid hormone concentrations induced by medical and psychiatric illness, the HPT axis is affected by a wide variety of drugs (Table 9-31). The clinical impact of these drug effects often depends on the presence of preexisting thyroid disease, which may often be clinically occult. As a general rule, a healthy HPT axis will overcome drug effects on protein binding, $T_4$ to $T_3$ conversion, and thyroid hormone metabolism by homeostatic feedback to modulate hormone release. For this reason, the myriad drug effects on thyroid hormone concentrations are rarely of significance in healthy people. In clinical settings of preexisting thyroid disease and significant concurrent medical conditions, the compensatory reserve of the HPT may be unable to compensate sufficiently.

Because of the high prevalence of autoimmune thyroid disease and nodular goiter, elderly women are particularly susceptible to drug effects on thyroid function. Antithyroid antibodies are seen in approximately one-fifth of nursing home residents (Szabolcs et al. 1995). In addition to the effects of severe nonthyroidal illness on the HPT axis, agents commonly used in the critical care setting such as glucocorticoids and dopamine reduce TSH secretion.

## Goitrogens

In addition to dietary goitrogens found in vegetables of the cabbage, turnip, and kale families, lithium commonly induces goiter. Lithium reduces thyroid hormone release, which leads to increased TSH secretion. Thyroid hormone concentration is not significantly reduced, but TSH con-

**Table 9-31 The Effect of Drugs on Thyroid Function and Thyroid Tests**

| PHARMACOLOGICAL EFFECT | DRUGS | CLINICAL RELEVANCE |
|---|---|---|
| Reduce TSH secretion | Dopamine, glucocorticoids, octreotide | Critical care setting |
| Reduced thyroid hormone release | Iodine containing agents, amiodarone, lithium | Numerous products<br>Goitrogen |
| Reduce absorption or enterohepatic cycling | Bile acid binding resins, sucralfate, ferrous sulfate | Need to administer at separate times of day |
| Increase serum binding proteins | Estrogens, tamoxifen, raloxifene, heroin, methadone, 5-fluorouracil | Hepatic estrogenic effects |
| Reduce serum binding proteins | Androgens, glucocorticoids, anabolic steroids | |
| Displacement from binding proteins | Salicylates (>4 g/day) furosemide (high dose IV) | |
| Increase metabolism of $T_3$, $T_4$ | Phenobarbital, phenytoin, carbamazepine, rifampin | Induction of hepatic enzymes |
| Reduced $T_4$ to $T_3$ conversion | Amiodarone, iodine, glucocorticoids, $\beta$-adrenergic antagonists | |

ABBREVIATIONS: $T_3$, liothyronine; $T_4$, levothyroxine; TSH, thyroid-stimulating hormone.
SOURCE: Adapted from Surks 1995.

centrations may remain elevated and lead to trophic effects on the thyroid gland. In one cohort study, mean TSH concentrations rose from 3.3 to 5.3 μU/mL during the first 3 months of lithium therapy, whereas elevated TSH concentrations were observed in 8% of subjects on chronic lithium therapy (Emerson et al. 1973). Because subclinical autoimmune thyroid disease is very common, patients on lithium should be monitored for hypothyroidism.

## Thyroid-Binding Globulin Effects and Dysalbuminemic States

Numerous drugs and medical conditions affect the binding of thyroid hormones to the circulating thyroid-binding proteins such as thyroid-binding globulin, albumin, and prealbumin. These conditions alter the partitioning of total and free thyroid hormone but do not impair the maintenance of euthyroidism per se. Hormonal effects on hepatic synthesis of binding proteins are notable: Estrogen agonists and pregnancy increase TBG, whereas glucocorticoids and androgens reduce TBG concentrations. Nephrosis and hepatic failure may also affect TBG and albumin. Other drugs may alter $T_4$–TBG binding affinity (phenytoin, heparin, furosemide, sulfonylureas). These effects may be significant in patients on exogenous thyroid hormone replacement whose dosage may need to be adjusted if TSH concentrations become abnormal.

## Metabolism of Thyroid Hormones

Numerous drugs alter thyroid hormone metabolism. Drugs that induce drug-metabolizing enzymes in the liver such as carbamazepine, phenobarbital, and rifampin increase the rate of elimination of thyroid hormone. Cholestyramine and colestipol lower thyroid hormone concentrations by inhibiting absorption and enterohepatic circulation of conjugated thyroid hormones. These effects become clinically significant in patients whose compensatory reserve is limited (e.g., thyroid hormone replacement).

## Amiodarone and Iodinated Contrast Agents

Amiodarone is an iodinated compound that acts similarly to dietary iodide (Fig. 9-28). The iodide load of amiodarone may cause hypothyroidism in patients with underlying abnormalities of the thyroid gland. Subjects with even subclinical thyroid autoimmunity may not overcome the blockade of iodide uptake by iodine-containing agents. Rarely, the amiodarone-mediated iodide load may cause hyperthyroidism, especially in patients with multinodular goiter.

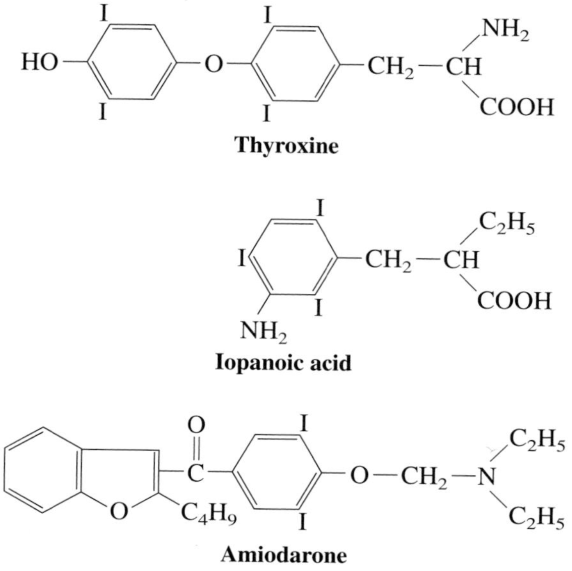

**Thyroxine**

**Iopanoic acid**

**Amiodarone**

FIGURE 9-28 **Structures of thyroxine, iopanoic acid, and amiodarone.**

Amiodarone also impairs $T_4$ to $T_3$ conversion. Amiodarone has a very long half-time of elimination; hence, supportive therapy may be required after the diagnosis of amiodarone-related thyroid disease. In addition to amiodarone, most radiographic contrast agents contain large amounts of iodide, which may produce similar effects in patients with subclinical thyroid abnormalities (Table 9-29).

# THYROID CANCER AND THYROID NODULES

## Classification and Prognosis

Thyroid cancers may be categorized as well-differentiated tumors or clinically aggressive tumors (see Table 9-32). Well-differentiated thyroid carcinomas demonstrate a

Table 9-32 **Classification of Thyroid Cancer**

| |
|---|
| *Well differentiated* |
| Papillary |
| Follicular |
| Hürthle cell and papillary-follicular variants |
| *Clinically aggressive* |
| Anaplastic thyroid carcinoma |
| Medullary thyroid carcinoma |
| Thyroid lymphoma |

wide spectrum of clinical behavior. In patients with favorable prognostic features, 10-year mortality is less than 1% (Mazzaferri and Young 1981; DeGroot et al. 1990). In some cases, however, papillary or follicular carcinoma may be as unresponsive to treatment as poorly differentiated thyroid carcinoma. One cohort study of 1355 patients with papillary or follicular thyroid carcinoma documented an 8% cancer death rate during median followup of 15.7 years (Mazzaferri and Jhiang 1994). Several prognostic scales have been proposed for clinical staging, most of which contain the prognostic factors listed in Table 9-33. $^{131}$I therapy following total or near-total thyroidectomy has not been studied in a prospective randomized fashion. Retrospective analysis of large series of well-differentiated thyroid cancers demonstrate a significant effect of $^{131}$I ablation on cancer survival (Samaan et al. 1983), including both metastatic cancers and thyroidal tumors greater than 1.5 cm in diameter (Mazzaferri and Jhiang 1994). Clinical benefit of $^{131}$I therapy, in addition to surgery and thyroxine therapy, for nonmetastatic papillary or follicular cancers less than 1.5 cm in diameter, has not been demonstrated.

## Thyroxine Suppression Therapy

Because the prognosis for papillary and follicular carcinoma is generally favorable, thyroid hormone therapy is used to maintain remission for prolonged periods after surgical resection. Thyroxine replacement therapy is used in patients with medullary carcinoma, anaplastic carcinoma, and thyroid lymphoma only to restore euthyroidism when surgery has rendered the patient hypothyroid. In retrospective analyses, thyroxine suppression therapy improves long-term survival in papillary and follicular carcinoma (Simpson et al. 1988) and has now become standard therapy.

The goal of thyroxine therapy in well-differentiated carcinoma is to reduce the trophic effect of TSH on neoplastic thyroid tissue, by suppressing TSH concentrations. Thyroxine suppression therapy is typically initiated approximately 4 to 6 weeks after near-total thyroid resection and ablative $^{131}$I therapy. In select cases of low-risk patients (well differentiated papillary or follicular carcinoma, small tumor size, absence of metastases, age 18 to 45) surgery alone, followed by thyroxine suppression, may be performed (Crile et al. 1985).

Therapeutic goals are determined by the patients risk factors for recurrence and the results of periodic $^{131}$I imaging studies and serum thyroglobulin measurements. In patients with known metastases, detectable thyroglobulin concentrations, or adverse prognostic features, TSH concentrations should be reduced to below 0.1 $\mu$U/mL, without producing symptomatic hyperthyroidism. Retrospective analysis of cohort studies has suggested that disease-free survival is increased with greater suppression of TSH (Pujol et al. 1996). The usual suppressive dose of $T_4$ is approximately 2.5 $\mu$g/kg daily. In more favorable clinical settings, TSH concentrations between 0.1 and 0.5 $\mu$U/mL may be acceptable. Suppressive *l*-thyroxine therapy should be continued indefinitely, unless contraindicated by other medical conditions (e.g., atrial fibrillation, psychiatric disease) where the dose may need to be reduced.

**Table 9-33 Prognostic Factors in Thyroid Carcinoma**

| FAVORABLE PROGNOSTIC FACTORS IN WELL-DIFFERENTIATED THYROID CARCINOMA |
|---|
| Age 18–45 years |
| Well-encapsulated tumors (complete resection) |
| No metastases |
| Tumor size <4 cm |

## Periodic Assessment of Cancer Recurrence

Thyroglobulin measurements may be obtained during thyroxine therapy, and should be assessed serially over the first year after surgery. Thyroglobulin concentrations greater than 10 ng/mL in patients who have undergone postoperative thyroid ablation indicate recurrence of cancer (Schlumberger 1986). Within 6 to 12 months after surgery and $^{131}$I ablation, *l*-thyroxine therapy should be stopped, and total-body $^{131}$I scanning should be performed under hypothyroid conditions. Four to 6 weeks are usually required to achieve a TSH concentration greater than 25 $\mu$U/mL, which is intended to enhance $^{131}$I uptake. During temporary discontinuation of *l*-thyroxine therapy, hypothyroid symptoms such as fatigue, leg cramps, and cold sensitivity are likely to develop. In severely symptomatic patients, thyroxine may be administered at half the usual dose for 5 weeks, or longer if needed, to achieve the target TSH concentration (Guimaraes and DeGroot 1996).

Another therapeutic option is to replace *l*-thyroxine dosing with oral administration of the lowest dose of liothyronine ($T_3$) that suppresses hypothyroid symptoms (25 to 75 $\mu$g/day), then discontinue this 3 weeks before $^{131}$I scanning. In patients with no evidence of metastasis or recurrence, scanning should be performed annually for up to 3 years and at later time points as indicated by thyroglobulin measurements. Thyroglobulin concentrations should be measured at the time that TSH is elevated.

Low thyroglobulin concentrations under these conditions may confirm the lack of disease recurrence.

## Thyroxine Suppressive Therapy for Benign Thyroid Nodules

Clinically detectable thyroid nodules occur in approximately 5% of the adult population, and higher prevalence is reported with thyroid ultrasonography and in autopsy studies. Approximately 95% of thyroid nodules in adults are benign. Despite its widespread use, the use of thyroxine to suppress the growth of benign goiters and nodules is not efficacious (Gharib and Mazzaferri 1998). Significant reduction in nodule size is observed in only 10 to 20% of cases, and this rate may not exceed the rate of spontaneous shrinkage of thyroid nodules.

Nodule shrinkage following thyroxine therapy does not exclude the possibility of malignancy, and adequate fine-needle aspiration cytology should be obtained in all cases of euthyroid ("warm") or hypofunctioning ("cold") nodules. Recurrence of thyroid nodules after resection of a benign nodule is not prevented by thyroxine therapy.

## Adverse Effects of Thyroxine Suppression Therapy

In addition to causing symptoms of hyperthyroidism, thyroxine suppression therapy may promote atrial fibrillation and osteoporosis in vulnerable patients. Atrial fibrillation is a major risk factor for stroke, and hyperthyroidism is a common cause of this dysrhythmia. Thyroxine-induced atrial fibrillation may occur in elderly patients without associated signs of hyperthyroidism.

Hyperthyroidism is a known risk factor for osteoporosis. Studies of patients treated for thyroid cancer suggest that bone mineral density reduction is proportionate to the degree of TSH suppression. At mild levels of TSH suppression, premenopausal women are not likely to experience clinically significant effects (Faber and Galloe 1994). In postmenopausal women, this effect may lead to clinically significant acceleration of postmenopausal bone loss.

## REFERENCES

Bartalena L, Marcocci C, Bogazzi F, et al. 1998. Relation between therapy for hyperthyroidism and the course of Graves' ophthalmopathy [see comments]. *N Engl J Med* **338**:73–8.

Benker G, Vitti P, Kahaly G, et al. 1995. Response to methimazole in Graves' disease. The European Multicenter Study Group [see comments]. *Clin Endocrinol* **43**:257–63.

Bernstein R, Muller C, Midtbo K, et al. 1991. Cardiac left ventricular function before and during early thyroxine treatment in severe hypothyroidism. *J Intern Med* **230**:493–500.

Cooper DS, Halpern R, Wood LC, et al. 1984. L-Thyroxine therapy in subclinical hypothyroidism. A double-blind, placebo-controlled trial. *Ann Int Med* **101**:18–24.

Crile G Jr, Antunez AR, Esselstyn CB Jr, et al. 1985. The advantages of subtotal thyroidectomy and suppression of TSH in the primary treatment of papillary carcinoma of the thyroid. *Cancer* **55**:2691–7.

DeGroot LJ, Kaplan EL, McCormick M, et al. 1990. Natural history, treatment, and course of papillary thyroid carcinoma. *J Clin Endocrinol Metab* **71**:414–24.

Emerson CH, Dysno WL, Utiger RD. 1973. Serum thyrotropin and thyroxine concentrations in patients receiving lithium carbonate. *J Clin Endocrinol Metab* **36**:338–46.

Faber J, Galloe AM. 1994. Changes in bone mass during prolonged subclinical hyperthyroidism due to L-thyroxine treatment: A meta-analysis. *Eur J Endocrinol* **130**:350–6.

Gharib H, Mazzaferri EL. 1998. Thyroxine suppressive therapy in patients with nodular thyroid disease [review][68 refs]. *Ann Int Med* **128**:386–94.

Griffin JE. 1985. The dilemma of abnormal thyroid function tests—is thyroid disease present or not? [review][60 refs]. *Am J Med Sci* **289**:76–88.

Guimaraes V, DeGroot LJ. 1996. Moderate hypothyroidism in preparation for whole body $^{131}$I scintiscans and thyroglobulin testing [see comments]. *Thyroid* **6**:69–73.

Helfand M, Crapo LM. 1990. Monitoring therapy in patients taking levothyroxine [see comments]. *Ann Int Med* **113**:450–4.

Jones GR, Lazarus JH, Wynford TD. 1981. A study of long acting propranolol in the early management of hyperthyroidism. *Br J Clin Pharmacol* **12**:825–8.

Kallner G, Vitols S, Ljunggren JG. 1996. Comparison of standardized initial doses of two antithyroid drugs in the treatment of Graves' disease. *J Intern Med* **239**:525–9.

Keating FRJ, Parkin TW, Selby JB, et al. 1961. Treatment of heart disease associated with myxedema. *Prog Cardiovasc Dis* **3**:364.

Klemperer JD, Klein I, Gomez M, et al. 1995. Thyroid hormone treatment after coronary-artery bypass surgery [see comments]. *N Engl J Med* **333**:1522–7.

Koh LK, Eng PH, Lim SC, et al. 1996. Abnormal thyroid and adrenocortical function test results in intensive care patients. *Ann Acad Med Singapore* **25**:808–15.

Kvetny J, Frederikesen PK, Jacobsen JG, et al. 1981. Propranolol in the treatment of thyrotoxicosis. A randomized double-blind study. *Acta Med Scand* **209**:389–92.

Lahey FH. 1931. Non-activated (apathetic) type of hyperthyroidism. *N Engl J Med* **204**:747–8.

Levy RP, Jensen JB, Laus VG, et al. 1981. Serum thyroid hormone abnormalities in psychiatric disease. *Metab Clin Exp* **30**:1060–4.

Marchant B, Brownlie BE, Hart DM, et al. 1977. The placental transfer of propylthiouracil, methimazole and carbimazole. *J Clin Endocrinol Metab* **45**:1187–93.

Mashio Y, Beniko M, Matsuda A, et al. 1997. Treatment of hyperthyroidism with a small single daily dose of methimazole: A prospective long-term follow-up study. *Endocr J* **44**:553–8.

Mazzaferri EL, Jhiang SM. 1994. Long-term impact of initial surgical and medical therapy on papillary and follicular thyroid cancer [published erratum appears in *Am J Med* **98**:215; 1995]. *Am J Med* **97**:418–28.

Mazzaferri EL, Reynolds JC, Young RL, et al. 1976. Propranolol as primary therapy for thyrotoxicosis. *Arch Intern Med* **136**: 50–6.

Mazzaferri EL, Young RL. 1981. Papillary thyroid carcinoma: A 10-year follow-up report of the impact of therapy in 576 patients. *Am J Med* **70**:511–18.

McDevitt DG, Nelson JK. 1978. Comparative trial of atenolol and propranolol in hyperthyroidism. *Br J Clin Pharmacol* **6**:233–7.

Momotani N, Ito K, Hamada N, et al. 1984. Maternal hyperthyroidism and congenital malformation in the offspring. *Clin Endocrinol* **20**:695–700.

Nilsson OR, Karlberg BE, Kagedal B, et al. 1979. Non-selective and selective beta-l-adrenoceptor blocking agents in the treatment of hyperthyroidism. *Acta Med Scand* **206**:21–5.

Perk M, O'Neill BJ. 1997. The effect of thyroid hormone therapy on angiographic coronary artery disease progression [see comments]. *Can J Cardiol* **13**:273–6.

Prummel MF, Mourits M, Berghout A, et al. 1989. Prednisone and cyclosporine in the treatment of severe Graves' ophthalmopathy. *N Engl J Med* **321**:1353–9.

Pujol P, Daures JP, Nsakala N, et al. 1996. Degree of thyrotropin suppression as a prognostic determinant in differentiated thyroid cancer. *J Clin Endocrinol Metab* **81**:4318–23.

Reinwein D, Benker G, Lazarus JH, et al. 1993. A prospective randomized trial of antithyroid drug dose in Graves' disease therapy. European Multicenter Study Group on Antithyroid Drug Treatment. *J Clin Endocrinol Metab* **76**:1516–21.

Rittmaster RS, Abbott EC, Douglas R, et al. 1998. Effect of methimazole, with or without L-thyroxine, on remission rates in Graves' disease. *J Clin Endocrinol Metab* **83**:814–8.

Roca RP, Blackman MR, Ackerley MB, et al. 1990. Thyroid hormone elevations during acute psychiatric illness: Relationship to severity and distinction from hyperthyroidism. *Endocr Res* **16**:415–47.

Roti E, Robuschi G, Gardini E, et al. 1988. Comparison of methimazole, methimazole and sodium ipodate, and methimazole and saturated solution of potassium iodide in the early treatment of hyperthyroid Graves' disease. *Clin Endocrinol* **28**:305–14.

Samaan NA, Maheshwari YK, Nader S, et al. 1983. Impact of therapy for differentiated carcinoma of the thyroid: An analysis of 706 cases. *J Clin Endocrinol Metab* **56**:1131–38.

Sawin CT, Geller A, Wolf PA, et al. 1994. Low serum thyrotropin concentrations as a risk factor for atrial fibrillation in older persons [see comments]. *N Engl J Med* **331**:1249–52.

Shiroozu A, Okamura K, Ikenoue H, et al. 1986. Treatment of hyperthyroidism with a small single daily dose of methimazole. *J Clin Endocrinol Metab* **63**:125–8.

Simpson WJ, Panzarella T, Carruthers JS, et al. 1988. Papillary and follicular thyroid cancer: Impact of treatment in 1578 patients. *Int J Radiat Oncol Biol Phys* **14**:1063–75.

Sugino K, Mimura T, Ozaki O, et al. 1995. Early recurrence of hyperthyroidism in patients with Graves' disease treated by subtotal thyroidectomy. *World J Surg* **19**:648–52.

Surks S. 1995. Drug therapy: Drugs and thyroid function. *N Engl J Med* **333**:1688–94.

Szabolcs I, Bernard W, Horster FA. 1995. Thyroid autoantibodies in hospitalized chronic geriatric patients: Prevalence, effects of age, nonthyroidal clinical state, and thyroid function. *J Am Geriatr Soc* **43**:670–73.

Tallstedt L, Lundell G, Torring O, et al. 1992. Occurrence of ophthalmopathy after treatment for Graves' hyperthyroidism. The Thyroid Study Group [see comments]. *N Engl J Med* **326**:1733–8.

Tunbridge WM, Brewis M, French JM, et al. 1981. Natural history of autoimmune thyroiditis. *BMJ* **282**:258–62.

Woolf PD. 1980. Transient painless thyroiditis and hyperthyroidism: A variant of lymphocytic thyroiditis? *Endocr Rev* **1**:411–20.

Woolf PD. 1985. Thyroiditis. *Med Clin N Am* **69**:1035–48.

# Reproductive Steroids

Jeffrey W. Miller

## Chapter Outline



In contrast to other endocrine systems that typically maintain physiologic variables within a narrow homeostatic range, the hypothalamic–pituitary–gonadal (HPG) axis regulates the major nonhomeostatic function shared by all eukaryotic organisms, sexual reproduction. The regulation of human sexual function at different life stages requires age-specific regulation of sex hormones during puberty, maturity, and aging. The hormones and drugs that modulate the HPG axis may show activity unique to the stage in sexual development and the specific disorder (Table 9-34). Although a variety of pharmacologic agents are used to treat reproductive health disorders, this section reviews the pharmacology of estrogen, progesterone, and testosterone. The clinical use of agonists and antagonists of sex steroids spans the fields of gynecology, endocrinology, and oncology. By reviewing these areas of therapeutics in light of the HPG axis, an attempt is made to emphasize the pharmacologic features and physiologic effects of a broad array of agents. For further information on the hormonal therapy of osteoporosis and cancer, the reader is referred to chapter 10, Connective Tissue and Bone Disorders, and chapter 13, Oncologic Disorders.

## PHYSIOLOGY AND PHARMACOLOGY OF THE HYPOTHALAMIC–PITUITARY–GONADAL AXIS

### Sex Steroids Before Puberty

Human infants, male and female, are born with high plasma estrogen concentrations (>1000 pg/mL) that are dependent on both maternal and infant steroidogenesis. Gynecomastia

**Table 9-34 Pharmacotherapy of Sex Steroids by Gender and Age**

| Age and disease or condition | Therapeutic class |
|---|---|
| *Adolescence* | |
| Precocious puberty | GnRH agonists |
| Hypogonadism | Estrogens, androgens |
| *Menarchal women* | |
| Contraception | Estrogens, progestins |
| Endometriosis | GnRH agonists, progestins |
| Infertility | Antiestrogens, gonadotropins, GnRH agonists |
| Polycystic ovary syndrome | Estrogens, progestins, antiandrogens, GnRH agonists |
| *Postmenopausal women* | |
| Osteoporosis, climacteric symptoms | Estrogens, progestin, antiestrogens |
| Breast cancer | Antiestrogens, progestins, aromatase inhibitors |
| *Men* | |
| Prostate cancer | Antiandrogens, GnRH agonists, estrogens |
| Benign prostatic hyperplasia | 5-$\alpha$-Reductase inhibitor |

ABBREVIATIONS: GnRH, gonadotropin-releasing hormone.

is common among male infants, but these estrogen concentrations have no harmful long-term effects on newborn infants. In contrast, androgen exposure in utero from drugs or congenital adrenal hyperplasia may lead to ambiguous genital development in female infants. HPG axis activity and concentrations of sex steroids decline over the first year of life to low values (estradiol <10 pg/mL in girls, testosterone <20 ng/dL in boys) until the onset of puberty. Increased adrenal androgen synthesis (adrenarche) is one of the earliest events in puberty. Before puberty, adrenergic, dopaminergic, and opioid mechanisms maintain gonadotropin-releasing hormone (GnRH) activity in a quiescent state. The stimulus for the onset of puberty is poorly understood but involves the onset of pulsatile GnRH secretion from the hypothalamus. GnRH stimulates luteinizing hormone (LH) and follicle-stimulating hormone (FSH) secretion from the anterior pituitary, which in turn act on gonadal cells to stimulate steroidogenesis and gamete maturation. Normal GnRH release is episodic, and GnRH receptors downregulate following continuous ligand exposure. This phenomenon underlies the paradoxical effect of therapeutic GnRH agonists to suppress the HPG axis by continuous stimulation of GnRH receptors.

## Sex Steroids in Women

The onset of menses begins a pattern of cyclic estrogen and progesterone synthesis (Fig. 9-29). At the time of menses an increase in pulsatile FSH secretion promotes the growth of selectable ovarian follicles that begin steroidogenesis during the early follicular phase (Gougeon 1996). Androstenedione is synthesized by thecainterstitial cells under the influence of LH, whereas FSH induces the aromatase enzyme in granulosa cells, which converts androgen to estrogen. Although androgens may have cosmetic and behavioral effects in women, they function primarily as precursors for estrogen synthesis. By the end of the follicular phase, plasma estradiol concentrations typically increase tenfold to approximately 300 pg/mL (1.1 nmol/L). Estrogen exerts negative feedback in the pituitary and hypothalamus, and FSH secretion declines during the luteal phase. Estrogen antagonists such as clomiphene augment FSH secretion and increase follicular selection. The midcycle LH surge precedes ovulation by approximately 24 hours. At the time of ovulation, the follicle forms the corpus luteum and increases progesterone production. Estrogen concentrations decline during the 14-day luteal phase. By a poorly understood process, the corpus luteum undergoes lysis at the end of the luteal phase, and menses occurs 14 days after the LH surge, following the decline in plasma progesterone concentrations. This pattern is mimicked by the "progesterone withdrawal" treatment for irregular menses, in which progestin is administered for approximately 12 days in order to induce subsequent menstrual bleeding.

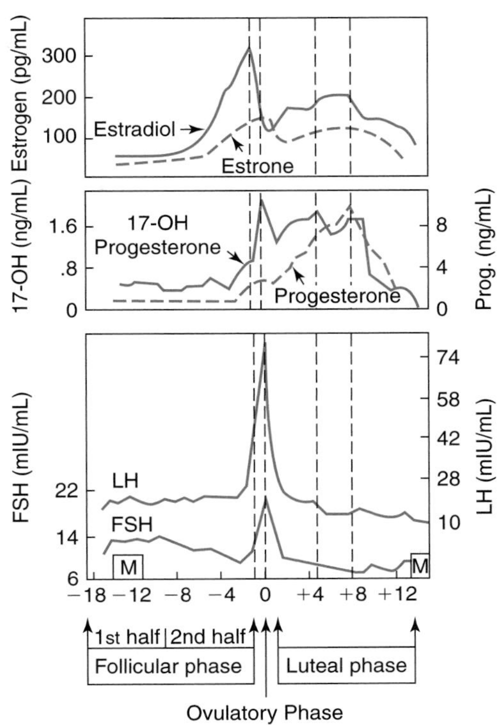


**FIGURE 9-29 Hormonal profile of the menstrual cycle. During the normal menstrual cycle, follicle-stimulating hormone (FSH) secretion increases during menses and stimulates follicular development. Rising estrogen concentrations augment FSH and luteinizing hormone (LH) secretion at midcycle. The midcycle LH surge stimulates ovulation, at which time progesterone concentrations rise. Progesterone secretion from the corpus luteum declines in the late luteal phase and results in menses 14 days after the LH surge. ABBREVIATIONS: Prog., progesterone; 17-OH, 17β-hydroxy. (From Yen SSC, Jaffe RB, editors. 1986. *Reproductive Endocrinology,* 2nd ed. Philadelphia: WB Saunders.)**

## The Postmenopausal Hormonal Milieu

At the time of menopause, the ovary is largely depleted of selectable follicles, and gonadotropin concentrations rise without stimulating further ovarian steroidogenesis. Adrenal androgens are converted to estrogens by aromatase in adipose tissue and other sites. The relative estrogen deficiency of menopause is accompanied by increased bone resorption and increased risk for coronary artery disease. The therapeutic use of estrogen for these conditions is considered in chapter 10, Connective Tissue and Bone Disorders. The postmenopausal years are the period of peak incidence of breast cancer; many of these tumors grow more quickly in the presence of estrogens. Progesterone, which counteracts some estrogen effects in reproductive tissues in the premenopausal years, is not secreted in appreciable amounts in postmenopausal women.

### Androgens in the Life Cycle

At the onset of puberty, LH-stimulated testicular steroidogenesis becomes the major source of circulating androgen in men. Testosterone is both a potent androgen and a precursor for another androgen (dihydrotestosterone) and also for estrogens in men. Adult male plasma testosterone concentrations are more than 10 times prepubertal values. In women, testosterone concentrations are comparable to those of prepubertal boys. Adrenal and testicular androgen synthesis declines gradually with age. The decline in testosterone synthesis is due to both reduced GnRH secretion and reduced LH responsiveness of the testes with age (Vermeulen and Kaufman 1995). Progesterone plays no known physiologic role in men, although synthetic progesterone agonists such as megestrol acetate may suppress the HPG axis in men.

## ESTROGEN

### Estrogen Biosynthesis

Endogenous estrogens are produced by aromatization of the A ring of the 19-carbon androgenic steroids. The aromatase enzyme that catalyzes this step also removes carbon 19, producing the 18-carbon estrane nucleus shared by all endogenous estrogens (Fig 9-30). The aromatase enzyme, expressed in the ovaries, in adipose and other tissues, leads to estrogen production from adrenal or ovarian androgens. Estradiol (E2) is the most potent endogenous estrogen and is readily converted to the less potent estrogen estrone (E1) by the 17$\beta$-hydroxysteroid dehydrogenase (CYP17) enzyme. Hydroxylation at other sites further reduces estrogen receptor (ER) binding affinity. Estrogens bind in target tissues and may be metabolized locally in a manner that alters the tissue concentrations of different estrogen metabolites. CYP17 is present in reproductive tissues where it may diminish estrogen action by conversion of estradiol to estrone (Cortes et al. 1975; Mehta et al. 1987). Estrone is the major circulating estrogen in postmenopausal women.

HO

**Cholesterol**

↓

$CH_3$
C
O

**Progesterone ($C_{21}$)**

↓

O
O

**Androgens ($C_{19}$)**

↓

O
HO

**Estrogens ($C_{17}$)**

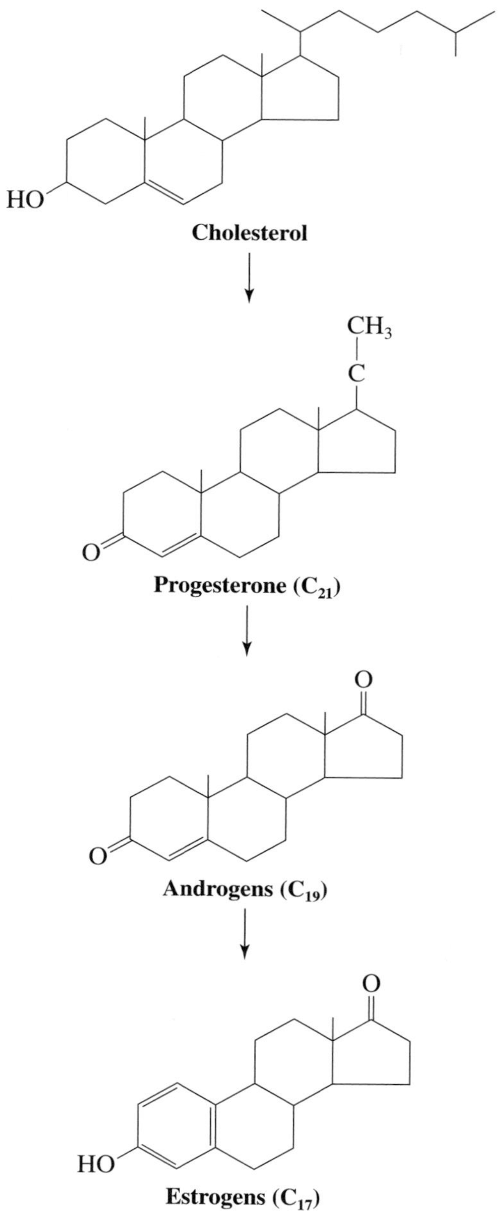

**FIGURE 9-30 Biosynthesis of sex steroids. Cholesterol conversion to progesterone (21-carbon) structures is the initial step in the biosynthesis of all steroid hormones. Androgens (19-carbon molecules) are formed from progestins by oxidative cleavage of carbons 20 and 21. Estrogens are produced from androgens by aromatization of the A ring of the androgen nucleus, with removal of the carbon 19 methyl group. Different natural estrogens and androgens vary by the arrangement of hydroxyl and ketone structures at carbons 3 and 18.**

## Estrogen Distribution, Metabolism, and Elimination

More than 99% of estrogen is bound to circulating albumin and sex-hormone-binding globulin (SHBG); free estrogen concentrations are about 1 to 10 pmol/L. The functional significance of plasma protein binding is controversial. Since free estradiol concentrations are too low to maximally occupy estrogen receptors, tissue concentrations of estrogen may be important in determining target organ effects. SHBG and albumin binding of estrogens may facilitate, rather than limit, the bioavailability of estrogens by allowing estrogen to dissociate throughout the microcirculation of target organs (Pardridge 1988; Rosner 1990).

The primary metabolism of estrogens is by phase 1 hepatic oxidation reactions. Induction of hepatic cytochrome P450 enzymes by drugs such as phenytoin, phenobarbital, and rifampin may enhance metabolism of endogenous and therapeutically administered estrogens. All the natural estrogens are further metabolized to pharmacologically inactive sulfate and glucuronide conjugates. Substantial amounts of conjugated estrogens are excreted in bile and may be reabsorbed after deconjugation by bacterial enzymes (enterohepatic circulation). Conjugation of estrogens is reversible, since oral and intravenous administration of estrogen conjugates leads to increased plasma concentrations of unconjugated estrogens. Estrogens are freely filtered by the kidney but are readily reabsorbed unless rendered more polar by hydroxylation and conjugation.

## Mechanisms of Estrogen Action

Plasma estrogen dissociates from serum proteins and binds cytosolic estrogen receptors, which dimerize and translocate to the cell nucleus to regulate estrogen-responsive genes. Two estrogen receptor genes, alpha and beta, have been identified (Mosselman et al. 1996) that share similar patterns of ligand binding affinity (Kuiper et al. 1997). The functional difference of these two receptor subtypes is unclear at present. The classical pathway of estrogen action involves DNA binding of the estrogen response element (ERE) of estrogen responsive genes by ligand-bound, dimerized ER. The binding of estrogen agonists to cytosolic and nuclear receptors correlates closely with functional estrogen responses (Katzenellenbogen 1984). Some estrogen effects may be mediated by non-ERE-mediated signaling pathways. The partial estrogen agonist, raloxifene, as well as several estrogen metabolites, elicit biochemical responses in osteoclasts with relative potency that is different from other estrogenic responses (Yang et al. 1996). Estrogen also has posttranscriptional effects such as reducing the stability of albumin mRNA, leading to decreased albumin synthesis (Riegel et al. 1986). Estrogen may also have acute pharmacologic effects such as regulation of calcium flux and vasomotor responses (Jiang et al. 1992).

## Physiologic and Pharmacologic Effects

Estrogen receptors are widely distributed and mediate numerous physiologic actions, chiefly the maintenance of female sexual function, secondary sexual characteristics, and skeletal development (Table 9-35). In addition to the effects of ovarian estrogens, orally administered estrogens demonstrate hepatically mediated effects such as decreasing LDL cholesterol concentrations, elevating plasma VLDL and HDL concentrations, and increasing the synthesis of several plasma proteins. Lipoprotein effects are due in part to inhibition of hepatic lipase activity and may be a pharmacologic effect of exposing the liver to high estrogen concentrations following absorption of orally administered estrogens. Estrogen administration alters the plasma concentrations of several hemostatic proteins such as factor VII, fibrinogen, and plasminogen activation inhibitor 1 (PAI-1). Observational studies have suggested that postmenopausal estrogen administration prevents car-

Table 9-35 Estrogen Physiologic Effects

| ORGAN SYSTEM | EFFECT |
|---|---|
| Uterus | Endometrial proliferation, cervical mucus maturation |
| Genitourinary | Epithelial maturation |
| Breast | Glandular development |
| Skeletal | Pubertal skeletal growth, epiphyseal closure, antiresorptive effects |
| Hepatic | Binding globulins, lipoproteins, coagulant proteins, IGF-binding proteins |
| Behavioral | Libido, mood |
| CNS | Hypothalamic and pituitary feedback, vasomotor stability |

ABBREVIATIONS: CNS, central nervous system; IGF, insulin-like growth factor.

diovascular disease, but prospective studies have not confirmed this hypothesis (Fig. 9-31) (Bush and Barrett-Conner 1985; Hulley et al. 1998).

## Therapeutic Estrogen Agonists

### *Natural estrogens*

The endogenous estrogens, 17$\beta$-estradiol (E2), estrone, and estriol (Fig. 9-32) are poorly bioavailable when orally administered; hence, their clinical use is limited to the relatively low estrogen doses required for postmenopausal hormone replacement. A microcrystalline formulation of E2 (Estrace) displays greater oral bioavailability and is used clinically in postmenopausal hormone replacement therapy at relatively high doses (1 to 2 mg daily). Micronization may increase estradiol absorption in a manner that reduces the capacity of the liver for first-pass metabolism of estradiol. Transdermal delivery that bypasses hepatic first-pass metabolism is an effective method of administering E2. When given in doses that produce comparable systemic effects to oral estrogen, transdermal estrogen produces smaller changes in hepatically mediated parameters (e.g., lipoproteins, coagulation factors, binding globulins) (Chetkowski et al. 1986).

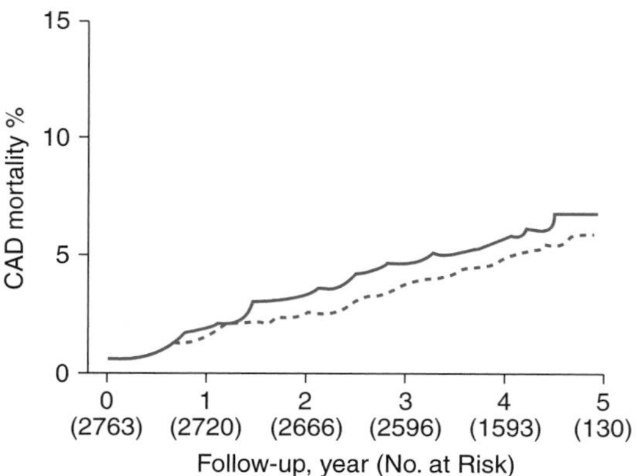


**FIGURE 9-31 Estrogen use and death from coronary artery disease in women. The results of a controlled clinical trial of estrogen/progestin therapy in secondary prevention of coronary disease show no benefit of combined hormone replacement therapy on coronary mortality (estrogen/progestin, solid line; placebo, dashed line). These results contrast with the significant reduction in coronary mortality predicted on the basis of observational studies and stress the importance of randomized clinical trials to test hypotheses derived from epidemiological studies. The number at risk is under the x-axis in parentheses. (From Hulley et al. 1998). CAD = coronary artery disease.**

### *Conjugated estrogens*

Therapeutically administered estrogens are readily interconverted between the three major forms of endogenous estrogens, such that the highest circulating estrogen concentration following oral administration of micronized estradiol is that of estrone (Yen et al. 1975). Estrogen preparations extracted from the urine of pregnant mares (conjugated equine estrogens, CEE, Premarin) consists of multiple types of conjugated estrogen metabolites. After oral CEE administration, endogenous sulfatase activity increases the serum concentrations of estradiol and estrone in postmenopausal women.

### *Synthetic steroidal estrogen agonists*

The poor oral bioavailability of natural estrogens may be overcome by addition of an ethinyl group to the carbon 17 of the estrane nucleus, producing the two most widely used synthetic estrogen agonists: ethinyl estradiol (EE) and mestranol. The latter compound is a prodrug of EE, containing a methylether substitution on the A ring of the steroid nucleus, which slows hepatic metabolism. Oral administration of both of these compounds results in elevation of plasma estradiol and estrone concentrations due to hepatic metabolism. Mestranol (50 $\mu$g) produces elevations in circulating estrogens and pharmacologic effects that are comparable to 20 to 35 $\mu$g of EE (Bhavnani 1998).

### *Relative potency of estrogen agonists*

Clinical studies of the relative potency of estrogens have utilized either hepatically mediated effects such as hormone-binding globulin concentrations or effects of systemically distributed estrogen such as vaginal cytology, gonadotropin suppression, or uterine effects. By these standards, 10 $\mu$g of ethinyl estradiol and 1.25 mg of CEE are approximately equivalent oral estrogen doses (Geola et al. 1980; Mandel et al. 1982). Effects on vaginal cytology have been used to assess the relative potency of transdermal estradiol and oral estrogens. By this approach, 50 $\mu$g/day of transdermal estradiol is approximately equipotent to 0.625 of CEE (Chetkowski et al. 1986).

### *The nonsteroidal estrogen agonist diethylstilbestrol*

Estrogens are the only class of steroid hormones where nonsteroidal agonists have been developed for therapeutic use. Before the synthesis of orally active steroidal estrogens, diethylstilbestrol (DES) was discovered to be a potent oral estrogen agonist. DES was used widely for gynecologic conditions before the observation of congenital and developmental anomalies in the offspring of DES-treated pregnant women (Hatch et al. 1998). DES expo-

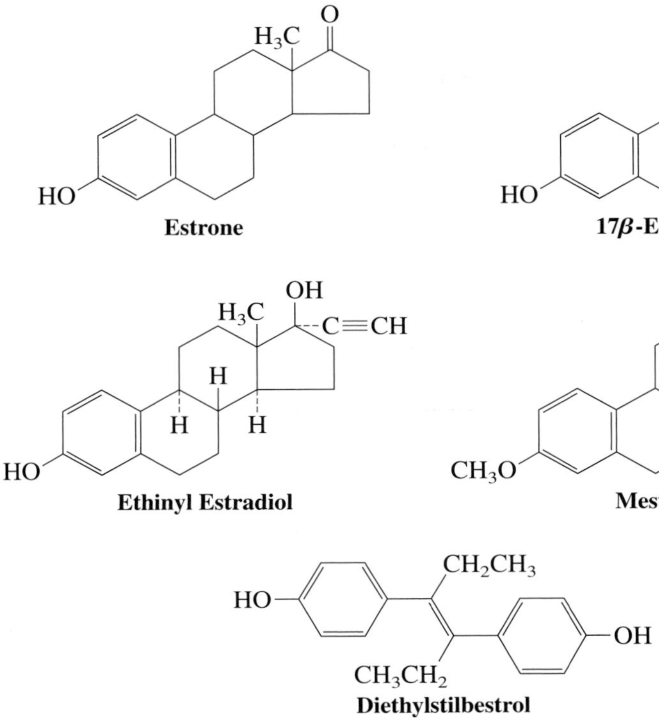

FIGURE 9-32 **Estrogens and estrogen agonists. Natural estrogens include 17$\beta$-estradiol and estrone, which are interconverted by the CYP17 enzyme in many target tissues. Synthetic steroidal estrogens have improved bioavailability owing to alkyl groups at carbon 17 and methyl ether substitutions at carbon 3. Diethylstilbestrol (DES) was the first nonsteroidal steroid receptor agonist developed for clinical use.**

sure in utero has been associated with an increased incidence of congenital uterine abnormalities in female offspring, an increased lifetime risk of clear cell adenocarcinoma of the vagina and cytological abnormalities (vaginal adenosis) of the cervix. DES has been used in the hormonal therapy of male prostate cancer and in palliation of metastatic breast cancer.

***Other estrogen preparations and estrogenic substances*** Estradiol conjugates with benzoate, valerate, and dipropionate are used in parenteral and oral estrogen formulations. These preparations are useful for oil-based formulations, which demonstrate delayed absorption characteristics, but are not widely used. Some skin creams and cosmetic products contain estrogens, which may have pharmacologic effects with sustained use. At high doses cardiac glycosides display estrogenic effects and may cause gynecomastia in men. Dietary and plant sources contain phytoestrogens with weak estrogen agonist activity. The role of dietary and phytoestrogens in human health is unclear at present (Tham et al. 1998).

## PROGESTERONE

### Progesterone Biosynthesis, Distribution, and Metabolism

Progesterone is an early step in the biosynthetic pathway for all steroids and is synthesized in large quantities by the adrenal gland and ovary. Most progesterone in the adrenal gland is readily converted to other steroids; hence, adrenally produced progesterone does not circulate in significant concentrations. Progesterone is produced in the mature ovarian follicle, corpus luteum, and placenta. Metabolic elimination pathways for progesterone include numerous sites of hydroxylation and conjugation.

### Mechanism of Progesterone Action

Progesterone shares the general mechanism of action of other steroid compounds. Two isoforms of the progesterone receptor (PR) are generated by alternate splicing of mRNA from the PR gene. Functional differences between these two forms of the progesterone receptor are unknown. Expression of the progesterone receptor is induced by estrogen, whereas progesterone inhibits expression of the estrogen receptor. These effects help orchestrate the menstrual cycle in which follicular phase estrogen precedes the progesterone-dominant luteal phase, and progesterone action during the luteal phase interrupts the estrogenic stimulus to uterine proliferation. PR is highly homologous to the mineralocorticoid, glucocorticoid, and androgen receptors, and high progesterone concentrations during pregnancy may antagonize mineralocorticoid effects in the kidney. Natural progesterone has little affinity for the androgen receptor, although many synthetic progestins are partial androgenic agonists.

## Physiological and Pharmacologic Effects

Progesterone is the steroid hormone that sustains pregnancy and inhibits menstrual cycling during pregnancy. Major sites of action are the uterus (endometrium and cervical mucus), the breast (glandular development), and the pituitary (gonadotropin suppression). Progesterone acts on the hypothalamus to increase basal body temperature and increase respiratory drive. Progesterone is also responsible, in part, for the impaired glucose tolerance of pregnancy. Progesterone administration during postmenopausal estrogen replacement reduces the incidence of endometrial hyperplasia, demonstrating an antiestrogenic effect in the uterus (The Writing Group for the PEPI Trial 1996a). Progesterone does not, however, antagonize estrogenic effects on bone and vasodilatory symptoms. Orally administered progestins may antagonize the LDL and HDL cholesterol effects of concomitantly administered estrogen (The Writing Group for the PEPI Trial 1995b) but do not independently produce adverse effects on lipoprotein parameters at doses used in current therapeutic preparations (Wolfe and Huff 1993).

## Therapeutic Progestational Agonists

### *19-Nortestosterone derivatives*

Like natural estrogens, progesterone is poorly bioavailable following oral administration. Practical oral progestin therapy became possible after the discovery that removal of the carbon 19 of testosterone produced a substantially progestational steroid 19-nortestosterone. Addition of the 17-ethylene structure, which had been used to increase the bioavailability of estrogen, led to the first useful synthetic progestin 19-norethisterone (Fig. 9-33). Synthetic progestins are commonly synthesized from a plant steroid, diosgenin, extracted from the wild yam *Dioscorea,* native to Central America. Other 19-nortestosterone derivatives

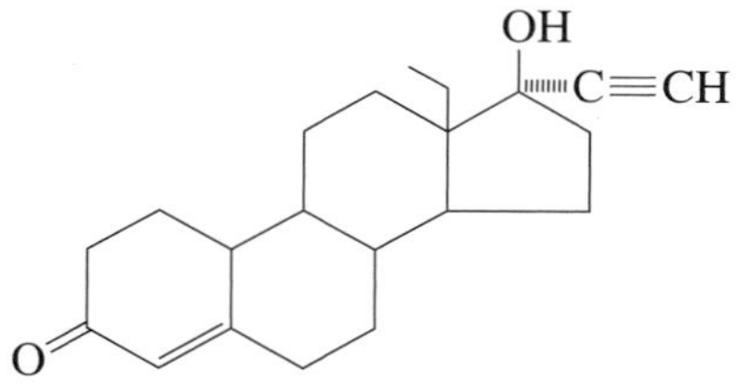

OH C≡CH O

**Levonorgestrel**

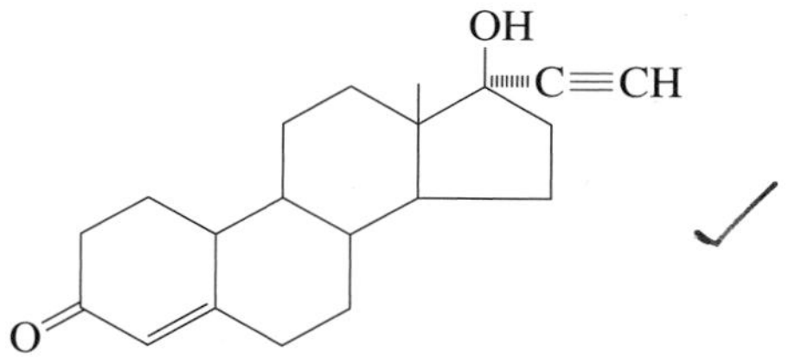

OH C≡CH O

**Norethisterone (Norethindrone)**

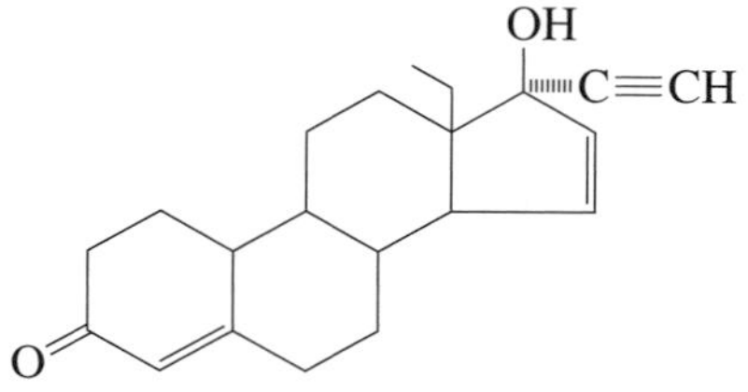

OH C≡CH O

**Gestodene**

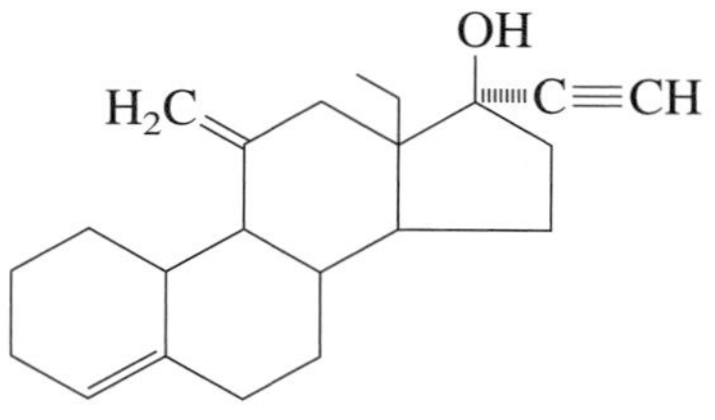

OH C≡CH $H_2C$

**Desogestrel**

FIGURE 9-33 **New-generation progestins. Removal of the carbon 19 methyl group from testosterone (19-nortestosterone) produces potent progesterone agonists with reduced androgenicity. Bioavailability of these compounds is enhanced by 17-alkylation. Newer-generation progestins have greater potency as progestational agonists, allowing them to be used at doses with relatively less androgenic stimulation.**

have been developed that differ in potency and in androgenic effects. Several "new generation" synthetic progestins (i.e, desogestrel, norgestimate, gestodene) have been developed to reduce androgenic effects. These agents are also 19-nortestosterone derivatives, and their affinity for the androgen receptor is similar to that of older compounds. Compared to levonorgestrel, the newer progestins have higher affinity for the progesterone receptor; hence, at doses that are equipotent in progestational effect, these compounds produce relatively less androgenic effect (van der Vange et al. 1990).

***Pregnane derivatives***
Another approach to the development of oral progestins has been to modify the native progesterone structure. Medroxyprogesterone (MPA) contains a methyl group at carbon 6 that improves bioavailability by reducing first-pass hepatic metabolism. MPA is used in 2.5 to 10 mg doses, compared with 100 μg doses for potent 19-nortestosterone derivatives. Micronized progesterone (Prometrium) is administered in relatively large doses (100 to 200 mg) in combined hormone replacement therapy.

## GYNECOLOGIC THERAPEUTICS

### Combined Contraceptive Agents

***Progesterone and estrogen contraceptive pharmacology***
Although ovarian extracts were observed to reduce the fertility of laboratory animals in the 1930s, the combined oral contraceptive (COC) was first marketed in 1961. Progestins administered alone are effective contraceptives; progestins suppress gonadotropin secretion, inhibit the midcycle LH surge, and block ovulation. Progestins also induce atrophy of endometrial glands, thickening of cervical mucus, and decreases in tubal motility, which reduce fertility. The significance of these last-mentioned effects is seen in progestin-only contraceptive agents, which are clinically effective because of cervical and endometrial effects at doses that suppress ovulation in only two-thirds of cycles (Fraser et al. 1998). When added to progestins in the COC, estrogens decrease the required dosage of the progestational component and have added direct contraceptive effects. Estrogen induces progesterone receptors, thereby increasing tissue sensitivity to progestins. Estrogens suppress FSH to a greater degree than progesterone, thereby providing additional ovarian suppression. Estrogens also reduce the incidence of breakthrough menstrual bleeding from the atrophic endometrium that results from progestin therapy. The COC is an example of a powerfully effective combined therapeutic agent.

***Dose of estrogen agonists in COC***
Ethinyl estradiol and its prodrug mestranol have been used widely, but recently ethinyl estradiol has become the only estrogen used in development of new COC agents (Table 9-36). Early COCs used ≥100 μg/day of EE. Following the recognition of adverse thrombotic events in COC users (Inman and Vessey 1968), doses of EE have been progressively decreased. Most COC preparations since 1970 have contained 50 or 35 μg/day of EE. Multiphasic COCs utilize lower doses of estrogen during the later phase of the cycle, mimicking the natural menstrual pattern. Doses of EE as low as 20 μg/day have been used in COCs. At this dose the rate of breakthrough bleeding is increased slightly in comparison to preparations containing 35 μg/day of EE (Archer et al. 1997; Endrikat et al. 1997).

***Synthetic progestins in COCs***
In contrast to the limited pharmacopoeia of estrogen agonists, numerous synthetic progestins have been utilized in COCs. Pregnane derivatives such as medroxyprogesterone acetate have been used in parenteral progestin-only contraception (Depo-Provera), but the more potent 19-nortetosterone derivatives such as norethisterone and levonorgestrel have been used primarily in COCs. Early COCs containing large doses of levonorgestrel or norethisterone were implicated in some epidemiological analyses of adverse cardiovascular events (Inman et al. 1970; Meade et al. 1980). Recently COCs containing "new generation" progestins (e.g., desogestrel, gestodene, norgestimate) have been in wide clinical use. These formulations also employ lower estrogen dosages that, independently of progesterone content, have resulted in reduced incidence of myocardial infarction in COC users. COCs containing new generation progestins have not resulted in lower rates of venous thromboembolism in COC users (World Health Organization Collaborative Study of Cardiovascular Disease and Steroid Hormone Contraception 1995a; Jick et al. 1995).

***Adverse effects of COCs***
Numerous adverse effects have been observed with COCs (Table 9-37). The vascular complication of COCs were first observed in large observational studies from the United States and Britain at a time when COCs contained higher doses of estrogen and progestin, and concomitant cardiovascular risk factors (e.g., smoking, age, and hypertension) were not routinely considered to be contraindications to COCs. Based on these studies, cigarette-smoking COC users over 35 years of age were observed

**Table 9-36 Available Combined Oral Contraceptive Preparations**

| BRAND | PROGESTIN | ESTROGEN | COMPANY |
|---|---|---|---|
| *Norethindrone* | | | |
| Nor-QD | Norethindrone 0.35 mg | None | Syntex |
| Micronor | Norethindrone 0.35 mg | None | Ortho |
| Ovcon 35 | Norethindrone 0.4 mg | Ethinyl estradiol 35 μg | Mead Johnson |
| Brevicon | Norethindrone 0.5 mg | Ethinyl estradiol 35 μg | Syntex |
| Genora 0.5/35 | Norethindrone 0.5 mg | Ethinyl estradiol 35 μg | Rugby |
| Modicon | Norethindrone 0.5 mg | Ethinyl estradiol 35 μg | Ortho |
| Norinyl 1+35 | Norethindrone 1.0 mg | Ethinyl estradiol 35 μg | Syntex |
| Norethin 1/35 | Norethindrone 1.0 mg | Ethinyl estradiol 35 μg | Schiapparelli Searle |
| Norcept-E 1/35 | Norethindrone 1.0 mg | Ethinyl estradiol 35 μg | GynoPharma |
| Ortho-Novum 1/35 | Norethindrone 1.0 mg | Ethinyl estradiol 35 μg | Ortho |
| Genora 1/35 | Norethindrone 1.0 mg | Ethinyl estradiol 35 μg | Rugby |
| Ovcon 50 | Norethindrone 1.0 mg | Ethinyl estradiol 50 μg | Mead Johnson |
| Genora 1/50 | Norethindrone 1.0 mg | Mestranol 50 μg | Rugby |
| Ortho-Novum 1/50 | Norethindrone 1.0 mg | Mestranol 50 μg | Ortho |
| Norethin 1/50 | Norethindrone 1.0 mg | Mestranol 50 μg | Schiapparelli Searle |
| Norinyl 1+50 | Norethindrone 1.0 mg | Mestranol 50 μg | Syntex |
| Ortho-Novum 1/80 | Norethindrone 1.0 mg | Mestranol 80 μg | Ortho |
| Ortho-Novum 2 mg | Norethindrone 2.0 mg | Mestranol 100 μg | Ortho |
| Tri-Norinyl | Norethindrone 0.5 mg | Ethinyl estradiol 35 μg (X7d) | Syntex |
| | Norethindrone 1.0 mg | Ethinyl estradiol 35 μg (X9d) | |
| | Norethindrone 0.5 mg | Ethinyl estradiol 35 μg (X5d) | |
| Ortho-Novum 7/7/7 | Norethindrone 0.5 mg | Ethinyl estradiol 35 μg (X7d) | Ortho |
| | Norethindrone 0.75 mg | Ethinyl estradiol 35 μg (X7d) | |
| | Norethindrone 1.0 mg | Ethinyl estradiol 35 μg (X7d) | |
| Ortho-Novum 10/11 | Norethindrone 0.5 mg | Ethinyl estradiol 35 μg (X10d) | Ortho |
| | Norethindrone 1.0 mg | Ethinyl estradiol 35 μg (X11d) | |
| *Norethindrone Acetate* | | | |
| Loestrin 1/20 | Norethindrone acetate 1.0 mg | Ethinyl estradiol 20 μg | Parke-Davis |
| Loestrin 1.5/30 | Norethindrone acetate 1.5 mg | Ethinyl estradiol 30 μg | Parke-Davis |
| *Ethynodiol Diacetate* | | | |
| Demulin 1/35 | Ethynodiol diacetate 1.0 mg | Ethinyl estradiol 35 μg | Searle |
| Demulin 1/50 | Ethynodiol diacetate 1.0 mg | Ethinyl estradiol 50 μg | Searle |
| *Norgestrel* | | | |
| Lo/Ovral | Norgestrel 0.3 mg | Ethinyl estradiol 30 μg | Wyeth-Ayerst |
| Ovral | Norgestrel 0.5 mg | Ethinyl estradiol 50 μg | Wyeth-Ayerst |
| Ovrette | Norgestrel 0.075 mg | None | Wyeth-Ayerst |
| *Levonorgestrel* | | | |
| Nordette | Levonorgestrel 0.15 mg | Ethinyl estradiol 30 μg | Wyeth-Ayerst |
| Levelen | Levonorgestrel 0.15 mg | Ethinyl estradiol 30 μg | Berlex |
| Tri-Levelen | Levonorgestrel 0.05 mg | Ethinyl estradiol 30 μg (X6d) | Berlex |
| | Levonorgestrel 0.075 mg | Ethinyl estradiol 40 μg (X5d) | |
| | Levonorgestrel 0.125 mg | Ethinyl estradiol 30 μg (X10d) | |
| Tri-Phasil | Levonorgestrel 0.05 mg | Ethinyl estradiol 30 μg (X6d) | Wyeth-Ayerst |
| | Levonorgestrel 0.075 mg | Ethinyl estradiol 40 μg (X5d) | |
| | Levonorgestrel 0.125 mg | Ethinyl estradiol 30 μg (X10d) | |

**Table 9-37 Adverse Effects of Combined Oral Contraceptives**

| Organ system | Effect | Association |
|---|---|---|
| Reproductive | Breakthrough bleeding | Common during initial therapy |
| | Postpill amenorrhea | Small or no increased risk |
| | Mastalgia | Dose adjustment possibly beneficial |
| | Breast cancer | No increased risk |
| | Cervical cancer | Causal association unlikely |
| | Developmental toxicity | No increased risk with early exposure in pregnancy |
| Cardiovascular | Deep venous thrombosis | 4-fold increased risk |
| | Stroke | 2-fold relative risk, small absolute risk |
| | Myocardial infarction | No increased risk with current formulations; smokers >35 yo at increased risk |
| CNS | Migraine | No controlled studies to quantify risk |
| Hepatic | Adenomas and peliosis | Rare with current formulations |
| | Cholestasis | Small or no increased risk |
| Metabolic | Glucose intolerance | Risk increased with prior glucose intolerance |
| | Hypertriglyceridemia | Risk increased with prior hypertriglyceridemia |

to have an increased risk of myocardial infarction and stroke. The association was strongest for doses of estrogen ≥50 μg of ethinyl estradiol. In more recent epidemiological studies, the incidence of myocardial infarction with low-dose COCs is not elevated (Vessey et al. 1989; Sidney et al. 1996). Observational studies of past estrogen use, such as the Nurses Health Study (Bush and Barrett-Conner 1985), show no long-term increased risk of atherosclerotic disease attributable to past COC use. The low-dose pill (<50 μg ethinyl estradiol) is associated with a two- to threefold increased risk of stroke (World Health Organization Collaborative Study of Cardiovascular Disease and Steroid Hormone Contraception 1996b), which occurs at an absolute rate of approximately 11/100,000 woman years in premenopausal women (Petitti et al. 1996). The relative risk of deep venous thrombosis is increased approximately fourfold in COC users (World Health Organization Collaborative Study of Cardiovascular Disease and Steroid Hormone Contraception 1995a).

### *COC failure and postpill amenorrhea*

COC failure rate for compliant patients is lower than any other nonsurgical contraceptive method. COC failure is greatest during the first year of use. Despite the known developmental toxicities of estrogen agonists, COC use is not associated with an increased risk of developmental abnormalities in children born after COC failure (Bracken 1990). After stopping COC use, resumption of fertility is delayed when compared with barrier contraceptive methods, but pregnancy rates return to normal within 2 years. The rate of secondary amenorrhea after COC use, termed *postpill amenorrhea,* is not significantly greater than that in comparable control populations (Furuhjelm and Carlstrom 1973; Berger et al. 1977; Hull et al. 1981).

### *Cancer risk and COC use*

The risk of gynecologic cancer with COC use has been examined in large epidemiological studies. The risk of ovarian and endometrial cancer is reduced approximately 40% in women who have used COCs for at least 3 years. Because of the long-term followup required for these studies, the COC use that has been assessed to date includes preparations containing ≥50 μg of EE. Studies that examine the cancer risk of newer low-dose COCs are not definitive at this time. Oral contraceptive use is not associated with a significant increased risk of developing breast cancer. The incidence of cervical neoplasms is increased in COC users but may be biased by the increased number of sexual partners and exposure to infectious agents among COC users.

### *Individualization of COC therapy*

Although multiphasic COCs minimize total estrogen and progestin dose and appear to mimic the physiology of the menstrual cycle, no clinical studies have reported greater efficacy or reduced adverse effects when compared with monophasic COCs containing ≤50 μg of ethinyl estradiol. For these reasons, low-dose monophasic or multiphasic COCs may be considered clinically equivalent. Individualization of therapy may be based on other considerations. Breakthrough bleeding that persists after the first two cycles may improve with a higher progestin content COC. Nausea and weight gain are primarily progestin-related adverse effects that may be minimized with lower-dose preparations. Patients with hirsutism or acne may benefit from a higher dose of estrogen or new generation progestational preparation.

## Progestin-Only Contraceptives

Both parenteral and oral forms of progestin-only contraceptives have been developed. Intramuscular medroxyprogesterone acetate (Depo-Provera) and implantable levonorgestrel (LNG, Norplant) provide long-acting contraceptive efficacy with greater ease of compliance than oral preparations. Implantable LNG is effective for up to 5 years. During the first year after administration, LNG concentrations are high and menses are irregular in most patients. In the later phase of implantable LNG use, daily LNG dose is approximately 30 μg, and menstrual cycling is normal in most patients. Progestin-only contraceptives are associated with an increased incidence of ovarian cysts, headache, and weight gain (Fraser et al. 1998). Oral progestin-only preparations utilize doses of progestin (e.g., 300 μg levonorgestrel) relatively larger than those used in COCs. Method failure rates of progestin-only pill are approximately 3 times those of COCs but compare favorably to other contraceptive methods (Trussell et al. 1990).

## Postcoital Contraception

***Postcoital hormonal contraceptive regimens***
Estrogens and estrogen–progestin combinations effectively reduce the rate of pregnancy after insemination (Glasier 1997). The use of combined estrogen and progestin was initially proposed by Yuzpee and Lancee (1977). The regimen of 100 μg of ethinyl estradiol and 500 μg of levonorgestrel administered twice within 72 hours of intercourse is difficult to achieve with most current OCP formulations, which contain proportionately less estrogen. The U.S. Food and Drug Administration (FDA) has recommended the postcoital use of several commonly available COCs (Table 9-38). Postcoital contraception, termed *interception* or the *"morning after pill,"* acts by several possible mechanisms depending on the timing relative to ovulation. Fertilization may occur following insemination during a time window beginning 5 days before ovulation until approximately 24 hours after ovulation. Prior to ovulation, high concentrations of estrogen and progestin may inhibit gonadotropin secretion, blunt the LH surge, and prevent ovulation. Progestin administration may advance the luteal phase changes in the endometrium and cervical mucus, decreasing sperm longevity and impairing implantation, even if ovulation has occurred. Because of the precipitous nature of this therapy, few controlled clinical studies have been performed with postcoital contraception, but it seems likely that this is largely a contraceptive, rather than abortifacient, therapy. An estimated efficacy rate of 74% has been based on historical comparison to expected pregnancy rates (Glasier 1997). Nausea is a common adverse effect of this regimen.

***The progesterone antagonist RU486 (mifepristone)***
The nonsteroidal progesterone receptor antagonist mifepristone is a competitive antagonist of both progesterone and glucocorticoid receptors. Short-term administration in humans may result in symptoms of adrenal insufficiency in the setting of high plasma cortisol and ACTH concentrations (Laue et al. 1990). In pregnant women, progesterone receptor antagonism results in decreased viability of the embryo and ripening of the cervix. Mifepristone in doses of 100 to 600 mg/day is an effective abortifacient and is often administered with a prostaglandin analog (Brogden et al. 1993). In single doses, mifepristone (600 mg) is also a highly effective postcoital contraceptive agent (Webb et al. 1992). Mifepristone is not currently licensed in the United States.

## Estrogen Therapy in Female Hypogonadism

***Turner syndrome***
Turner syndrome is a form of gonadal dysgenesis resulting from loss of part or all of one X chromosome (45XO karyotype). Women with Turner syndrome are hypoestrogenic because they lack functioning ovaries. Associated symptoms and signs include short stature, web neck, congenital

Table 9-38 **Postcoital Contraceptive Regimens**

| Estrogen content | Progestin content | Proprietary names | No. pills per dose[a] |
|---|---|---|---|
| Ethinyl estradiol 50 μg | Norgestrel 0.5 mg | Ovral | 2 |
| Ethinyl estradiol 30 μg | Norgestrel 0.3 mg | Lo/Ovral | 4 |
| Ethinyl estradiol 30 μg | Levonorgestrel 150 μg | Nordette, Levlen | 4 |
| Ethinyl estradiol 30 μg | Levonorgestrel 125 μg | Trilevlen, Triphasil | 4 |

[a]First dose to be taken within 72 hours of intercourse, second dose 12 hours later.

aortic and renal abnormalities, and a predisposition to hypothyroidism. Growth hormone therapy has recently become the therapy of choice for the short stature of Turner syndrome, because of positive effects on final adult height (Van den Broeck et al. 1995; Rosenfeld et al. 1998). Although premature estrogen therapy may induce epiphyseal closure and reduction of final height, appropriate estrogen supplementation should begin in adolescence. A regimen of gradually escalating estrogen therapy beginning at 10 to 12 years of age provides developmental, cosmetic, and psychological benefits to adolescent girls with Turner syndrome (Ross et al. 1996). Estrogen and progestin replacement therapy is continued on a lifelong basis.

#### *Ovarian failure*

Premature ovarian failure is defined as the onset of hypogonadism before age 40 that is not due to a correctable cause of secondary amenorrhea. Most patients with ovarian failure experience oligomenorrhea with intermittent ovulation for months or years before cessation of ovarian activity. Estrogen therapy does alter the course of ovarian failure (Taylor et al. 1996) but may be indicated for treatment of menopausal symptoms or prevention of osteoporosis. Because of intermittent ovulation and potential fertility, other contraceptive methods should be considered if estrogen therapy is initiated.

## PARTIAL AND TISSUE-SELECTIVE ESTROGEN AGONISTS

### Classes of "Antiestrogens"

Despite their structural similarity to DES, compounds such as MER-25 (the first triphenylethylene antiestrogen), clomiphene, and tamoxifen were found to have antiestrogenic effects in the treatment of infertility and breast cancer (Fig. 9-34). Although these agents are widely described as antiestrogens, they are best characterized pharmacologically as partial estrogen agonists. The estrogenic or antiestrogenic effects of these agents depend on the level of endogenous estrogen and the target organ affected (Fig. 9-35). In the estrogen-replete premenopausal hormonal milieu, these agents display antiestrogen effects such as augmentation of ovarian folliculogenesis, inhibition of endometrial proliferation, vasodilatation ("hot flushes"), and increased bone resorption. In estrogen-deficient postmenopausal women, tamoxifen displays agonist effects on endometrial proliferation, bone resorption, and plasma lipoproteins. In both premenopausal and postmenopausal women, tamoxifen demonstrates an antiestrogenic effect on breast cancer, suggesting that its estrogen antagonist effects may be tissue specific. Toremifene is another triphenylethylene compound with pharmacology similar to tamoxifen. The benzothiophene compound, raloxifene, displays a pattern of agonist and antagonist effects different from that of triphenylethylene derivatives. The nonsteroidal estrogen agonists may be termed *tissue-specific estrogen agonists,* or *selective estrogen receptor modulators* (SERMs).

### Clomiphene

#### *Clinical pharmacology of clomiphene*

Clomiphene was initially developed as a contraceptive because of observed antifertility effects in rodents but subsequently was found to augment ovarian folliculogenesis in humans (Clark and Markaverich 1981). The dose and time dependency of clomiphene effects has been studied in nonhuman primates. Administration of clomiphene during the mid-follicular phase increases follicular development and ovarian steroidogenesis. FSH elevations are modest (Littman and Hodgen 1985). Doses of up to 250 mg/day have been tested in women and found to be not significantly more effective than 50 mg (Shalev et al. 1989). Clomiphene is administered in single daily doses of 50 to 150 mg/day for 5 days, starting 3 to 5 days after the onset of menses. The endometrium displays a partial antiestrogenic effect (Eden et al. 1989), and cervical mucus may be adversely affected (Randall and Templeton 1991). The pharmacokinetics of clomiphene have not been well characterized. Clomiphene is excreted for several weeks after dosing; hence, it may have prolonged antiestrogenic effects on the uterus. The LH surge is also blunted with clomiphene, and the duration to the onset of the next menstrual cycle may be prolonged (Marut and Hodgen 1982).

#### *Clinical use of clomiphene in infertility*

Clomiphene is a first-line agent in the treatment of female infertility that is not due to hypopituitarism or hyperprolactinemia (Collins and Hughes 1995). Multiple gestations are observed in approximately 8% of clomiphene-induced pregnancies. Hot flushes are reported by approximately 10% of patients. Clomiphene is less effective in patients with hyperandrogenic ovulatory dysfunction. Clomiphene use for longer than 12 months has been associated with a threefold increased risk of ovarian cancer (Rossing et al. 1994). Ovarian hyperstimulation syndrome has been reported (Holtz et al. 1982) but is rare with appropriate hormonal and ultrasound monitoring of follicular development.

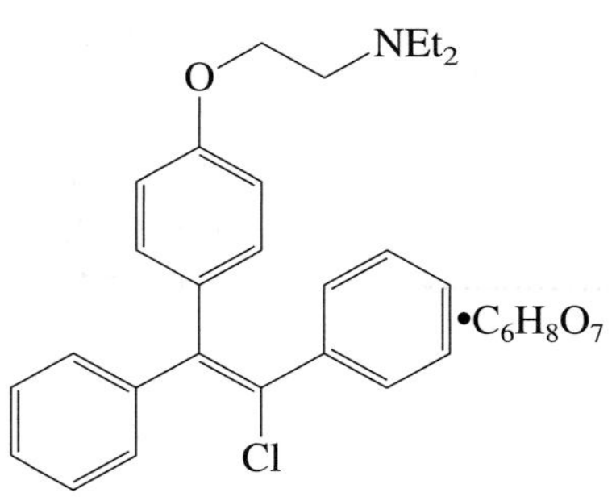

Clomiphene citrate

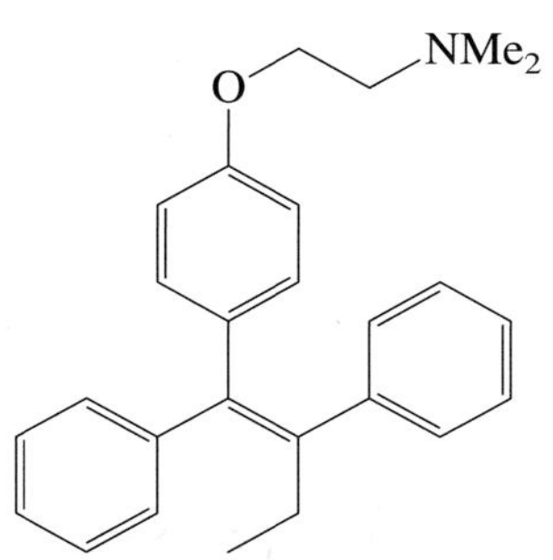

Tamoxifen

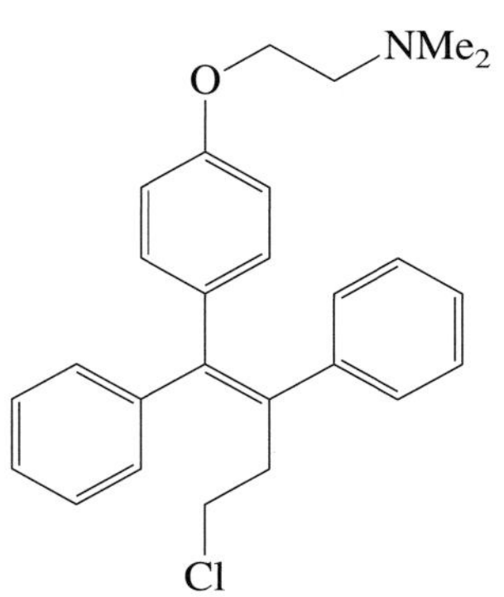

Toremifene

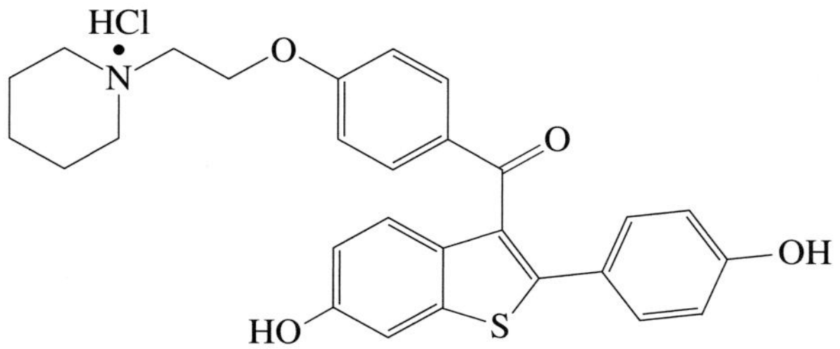

Raloxifene hydrochloride

FIGURE 9-34 **Partial and tissue-selective estrogen agonists. Triphenylethylene derivatives are used in cancer and infertility therapy because of antagonism of estrogen action on the hypothalamic–pituitary–gonadal (HPG) axis and breast. These compounds are partial estrogen agonists on the uterus, bone resorption, and hepatic parameters (binding globulins, lipoproteins, coagulation factors). Benzothiophene derivatives are antiestrogenic in the pituitary, breast, and uterus but are partial estrogen agonists for bone resorption and hepatic parameters.**

## Tamoxifen

### *Clinical pharmacology of tamoxifen*

Tamoxifen was initially developed as a fertility agent, and has been used for this indication in some countries. In the early 1970s tamoxifen was found to be an effective treatment of breast cancer and has since become a primary therapy for metastatic breast cancer (see chapter 13, Oncologic Disorders). Tamoxifen and its active metabolites are competitive antagonists of estradiol binding to estrogen receptors. Tamoxifen is metabolized by phase 1 hydroxylation reactions. The metabolite 4-OH-tamoxifen is a potent ER antagonist that circulates at nanomolar concentrations during chronic tamoxifen therapy. Tamoxifen has a long elimination half-time of approximately 4 to 7 days, whereas its major circulating metabolite, *N*-desmethyl-tamoxifen, has an elimination half-life of 7 to 14 days. Tamoxifen binds to plasma albumin, but not SHBG, and is extensively bound in tissues such as the liver, uterus, and breast. Although several hypotheses of tamoxifen's mechanism of action have been proposed, the primary effect of tamoxifen is to inhibit estrogen binding to the ER (for a review see Furr and Jordan 1984).

### *Clinical use of tamoxifen*

Tamoxifen is used in the treatment of metastatic breast cancer in doses of 20 to 40 mg/day. Tamoxifen is indicated in the adjuvant therapy of metastatic breast tumors, in combination with surgery and local irradiation. ER- and PR-containing tumors are more likely to respond, but receptor status does not uniformly predict clinical response. Tamoxifen is also indicated for the secondary prevention of breast cancer in carefully selected high-risk patients (Fisher et al. 1998).

### *Adverse effects of tamoxifen therapy*

Tamoxifen has adverse effects that are consistent with its pharmacologic classification as a partial estrogen agonist. Chronic tamoxifen treatment leads to endometrial thickening in the majority of postmenopausal breast cancer patients (Lindahl et al. 1997) and has been associated with an increased risk of endometrial cancer (Fisher et al.

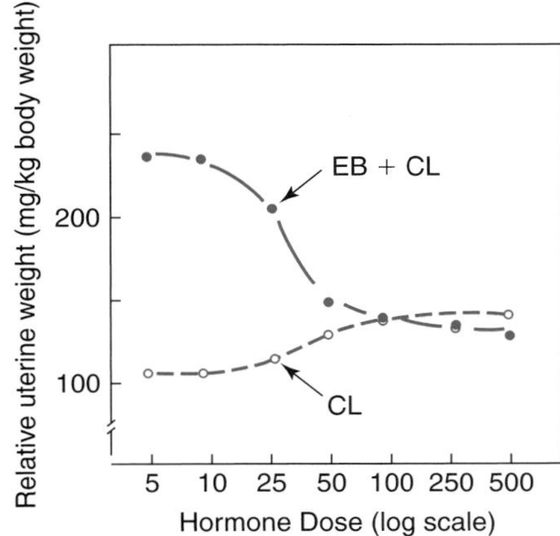


**FIGURE 9-35 Partial agonist properties of antiestrogens. The pharmacological effect of a partial agonist depends on the level of stimulation with the endogenous ligand. The effect of clomiphene (CL) on uterine weight in the ovariectomized rat is predominantly antiestrogenic in the presence of estrogen (EB), but weakly agonistic in the absence of estrogen. (From Clark and Markaverich 1981, with permission from Elsevier Science.)**

1998). Tamoxifen also shows partial estrogen agonist effects on lipoprotein concentrations, bone mineral density, and vaginal epithelial cytology in postmenopausal women. Tamoxifen causes increased venous thromboembolic events and shows alterations in plasma hemostatic parameters that are similar to estrogen hormone replacement therapy (Mannucci et al. 1996). Tamoxifen use has been associated with an increased incidence of ovarian cysts in both premenopausal and postmenopausal women (Shushan et al. 1996). In premenopausal women, tamoxifen produces modest decreases in bone mineral density and causes hot flushes. At clinically used doses, tamoxifen does not inhibit menstrual cycling in premenopausal women; hence, fertile women may be at risk for teratogenic effects.

## Raloxifene

Raloxifene differs from triphenylethylene estrogen agonists in its lack of agonist effect on reproductive tissues. Raloxifene is used for the prevention and treatment of postmenopausal osteoporosis (see chapter 10, Connective Tissue and Bone Disorders). In postmenopausal, estrogen-deficient women, raloxifene demonstrates no endometrial thickening (Delmas et al. 1997) but has partial agonist effects on bone resorption and plasma lipoproteins (Kauffman et al. 1997). Raloxifene has not been associated with increases in breast or uterine cancer during osteoporosis clinical trials but may increase the frequency of postmenopausal hot flushes. Raloxifene is extensively conjugated by hepatic first-pass metabolism and the mode of elimination is primarily in the bile and feces. The elimination half-time is approximately 30 hours, shorter than that of clomiphene or tamoxifen.

# OTHER ESTROGEN-LOWERING THERAPIES

The actions and metabolism of sex-steroid-lowering therapies are shown in Fig. 9-36.

## Gonadotropin-Releasing Hormone Agonists

### *Gonadotropin-releasing hormone pharmacology*

Normal pulsatile GnRH secretion stimulates LH and FSH release and may be reproduced by subcutaneous GnRH pump therapy in the treatment of infertility (for the pharmacotherapy of infertility, see Collins and Hughes 1995). (See also "Hypothalamic Hormone Therapy") Prolonged GnRH stimulation, however, produces reduction in gonadotropin secretion (Fig. 9-37) by receptor desensitization. The decapeptide GnRH (gonadorelin) and analogs of GnRH (leuprolide, nafarelin, goserelin, histrelin) are available for parenteral or intranasal administration (Table 9-39). The GnRH agonists (GnRH-A) are peptide analogs with amino acid modifications to increase GnRH receptor-binding affinity. In addition to increased potency, the synthetic analogs have elimination half-lives (3 to 4 hours) that are longer than native GnRH (10 to 40 minutes). GnRH agonists are used therapeutically in the treatment of estrogen- and androgen-dependent diseases and to suppress premature hypothalamic activity in precocious puberty. Administration of a GnRH-A is followed by a transient rise in gonadotropin secretion, which may temporarily exacerbate steroid-dependent diseases such as prostate cancer. After 2 to 4 weeks, gonadotropin concentrations are suppressed, and sex steroid concentrations decline to castrate levels.

### *Clinical use of gonadotropin-releasing hormone agonists*

Gonadotropin-releasing hormone agonists (GnRH-A) are effective in the treatment of precocious puberty (Comite et al. 1981), where they may be used continuously until the child reaches a suitable age to enter puberty. GnRH-A have also been used therapeutically to produce hypo-

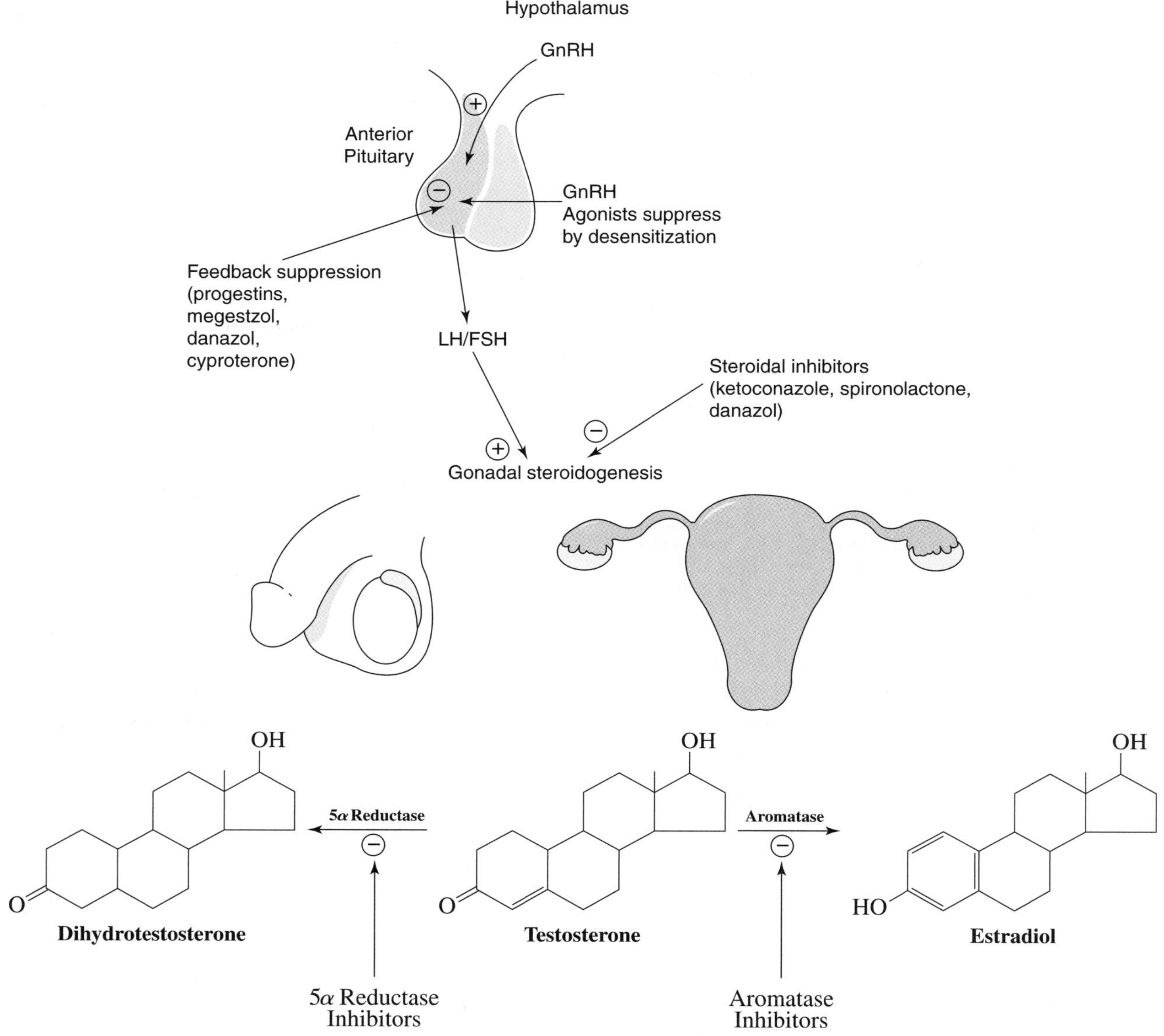


**FIGURE 9-36** **Sex-steroid-lowering therapies. Pharmacological strategies to lower sex-steroid concentrations are employed in the treatment of gynecological disorders, prostate disease, and reproductive cancers. LH and FSH secretion from the anterior pituitary may be reduced through the natural negative feedback mechanism by progestin, androgen, and estrogen agonists. Desensitization of LH and FSH release occurs when natural pulsatile GnRH secretion is replaced by long-acting GnRH agonists. Several compounds in clinical use inhibit steroidogenic enzymes, including the production of estrogens and dihydrotestosterone.**

gonadism in steroid responsive gynecologic disorders such as endmetriosis (Wheeler et al. 1992; Rock et al. 1993), uterinefibroids (Lumsden et al. 1994), and polycystic ovary syndrome (PCOS) (Goni et al. 1994). Symptoms of endometriosis are improved after 3 to 6 months of GnRH-A therapy, but recur in a large portion of patients within 1 year. GnRH-A have not been shown to improve infertility in patients with endometriosis (Fedele et al. 1992). GnRH-A therapy of benign uterine myomata has not been shown to produce long-term benefit, and use is limited to 3 months of preoperative therapy to reduce blood loss associated with surgery (Lumsden et al. 1994). In premenopausal women, GnRH-A produces premature menopause with accelerated bone resorption, genitouri-

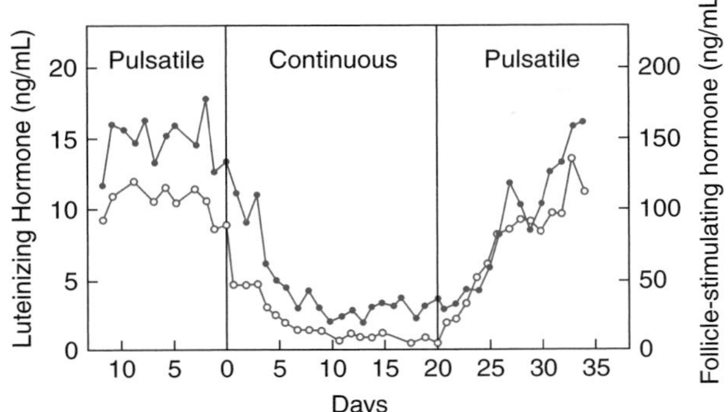


**FIGURE 9-37 Pulsatile versus sustained gonadotropin-releasing hormone administration. The pharmacological effects of GnRH administration in pulsatile or continuous patterns (filled circles) is demonstrated by the LH secretion profile (open circles) in GnRH-deficient monkeys. (From Belchetz et al. 1978, American Association for the Advancement of Science.)**

nary atrophy, and hot flushes. Loss of bone mineral density (BMD) is greatest during the first 12 months after GnRH-A treatment in premenopausal women, and long-term BMD reduction after a single course of GnRH-A therapy is minimal (Orwoll et al. 1994). Because of osteoporotic risk, GnRH agonist therapy of gynecologic conditions is limited to short courses of therapy. Concurrent treatment with hormone replacement regimens minimizes the adverse effects of GnRH-A therapy (Moghissi et al. 1998), but the impact of "add-back therapy" on the long-term efficacy of GnRH-A has not been fully assessed at this time. GnRH-A are also used in the treatment of prostate cancer in men (see chapter 13, Oncologic Disorders).

## Aromatase Inhibitors

Although antiestrogens display partial or tissue-selective estrogen agonist effects and GnRH-A reduce only gonadal sex steroids, aromatase inhibitors provide an alternate pharmacologic approach to inhibiting estrogen action. Inhibition of the aromatase enzyme reduces estrogen synthesis from both adrenal and gonadal androgens (Table 9-40). A number of inhibitors of the aromatase enzyme, including aminoglutethimide, testolactone, and 4-OH-androstenedione, have been used in small clinical studies over many years. These agents are either weak aromatase inhibitors or have nonspecific effects on other steroidogenic enzymes. Recently, highly specific, nonsteroidal aromatase inhibitors such as anastrozole and letrozole have been shown to reduce endogenous estrogen concentrations by approximately 85% in postmenopausal women. Anastrozole and letrozole demonstrate efficacy comparable to progestin therapy of metastatic breast cancer (Buzdar et al. 1997; Dombernowsky et al. 1998; see chapter 13, Oncologic Disorders). These agents are gen-

**Table 9-39 Gonadotropin-Releasing Hormone Agonists**

| AGENT | INDICATED USE | DOSAGE | FEATURES |
|---|---|---|---|
| Gonadorelin acetate | Hypothalamic/pituitary infertility | Subcutaneous pulsatile infusion | Ovarian hyperstimulation, multiple gestation |
| Leuprolide acetate | Endometriosis | Depot 3.75 mg every month for 6 doses | Hot flushes, genitourinary atrophy, reduced libido |
| | Metastatic prostate cancer | 1 mg every day SC<br>Depot 7.5 mg every month<br>Depot 22.5 mg every 3 months | |
| | Uterine fibroid (preoperative Rx) | Depot 3.75 mg every month for 3 doses | Hot flushes, genitourinary atrophy, reduced libido |
| | Central precocious puberty | 50 μg/kg per day SC injection | |
| Nafarelin acetate | Endometriosis | 200 μg (1 spray intranasal) bid for 6 months | Hot flushes, genitourinary atrophy, reduced libido |
| | Central precocious puberty | 1600 μg/day, divided tid | |
| Goserelin acetate | Endometriosis | 3.6 mg SC implant every month | Hot flushes, genitourinary atrophy, reduced libido |
| | Metastatic prostate cancer | 3.6 mg SC implant every month<br>10.8 mg SC implant every 3 months | |
| | Metastatic breast cancer | 3.6 mg SC implant every month | |
| Histrelin acetate | Central precocious puberty | 10 μg/kg per day | |

Table 9-40 Inhibitors of Sex Steroid Synthesis

| CLASS AND AGENT | INDICATED USE | DOSAGE |
|---|---|---|
| *Aromatase inhibitors* | | |
| Anastrozole | Metastatic breast cancer | 1 mg every day PO |
| Letrozole | Metastatic breast cancer | 2.5 mg every day PO |
| *5-α-Reductase inhibitor* | | |
| Finasteride | Benign prostatic hypertrophy | 5 mg every day PO |
| | Male pattern balding | 1 mg every day PO |

erally well tolerated in postmenopausal women but may produce hot flushes and genitourinary atrophy.

## Nonclassical Progestins

### *Danazol*

In contrast to the increased progestin/androgen selectivity of new generation progestins, danazol is an androgenic 17-alkylated 19-nortestosterone derivative with atypical pharmacologic effects (Barbieri and Ryan 1981) (Fig. 9-38). Danazol suppresses ovarian steroidogenesis in a fashion similar to other progestins (Telimaa et al. 1990). Danazol displays androgenic effects such as reduced HDL cholesterol (Telimaa et al. 1989), acne, and hirsutism. Although danazol is more androgenic than pregnane derivatives such as medroxyprogesterone acetate, its adverse effect profile is similar to that of other 19-nortestosterone derivatives. Danazol directly inhibits steroidogenic enzymes and binds to SHBG and cortisol-binding globulin (Barbieri and Ryan 1981), although the relative importance of these effects, compared with progestational activity, is unclear. Danazol (400 mg t.i.d.) has been used clinically in the treatment of endometriosis, where it provides moderate symptomatic relief without improving infertility (Telimaa 1988; Wheeler et al. 1992), as well as in fibrocystic breast disease (50 to 100 mg t.i.d). Danazol has also been studied for a variety of immunologic disorders. Danazol reduces immunoglobulin concentrations and alters serum complement activity in patients with hereditary angioedema, IgA nephropathy, and cholinergic urticaria (Gelfand et al. 1976; Tomino et al. 1987; Wong et al. 1987).

### *Megestrol acetate*

Megestrol is a pregnane derivative that differs from medroxyprogesterone by an acetyl group substitution at carbon 17. Megestrol has been described as an antiandrogen, but it does not antagonize androgen receptor binding (Poyet and Labrie 1985). Its primary antiandrogenic effect is by suppression of LH release. Megestrol reduces androgen concentrations and alters androgen metabolism in the prostate (Geller et al. 1976), although it is not clear whether this is due to direct effects on androgen metabolic pathways. Megestrol suppresses ovulation (Weiner and Johansson 1976) and antagonizes estrogen-induced endometrial hypertrophy in postmenopausal women in a fashion similar to other progestins (Kauppila et al. 1983). Megestrol has been used widely as an estrogen-lowering therapy in breast cancer where its efficacy is similar (Stuart et al. 1996; Buzdar et al. 1997) or inferior (Dombernowsky et al. 1998) to other therapies. Like other progestins, megestrol stimulates appetite and weight gain. Daily doses of 400 to 800 mg result in moderate weight

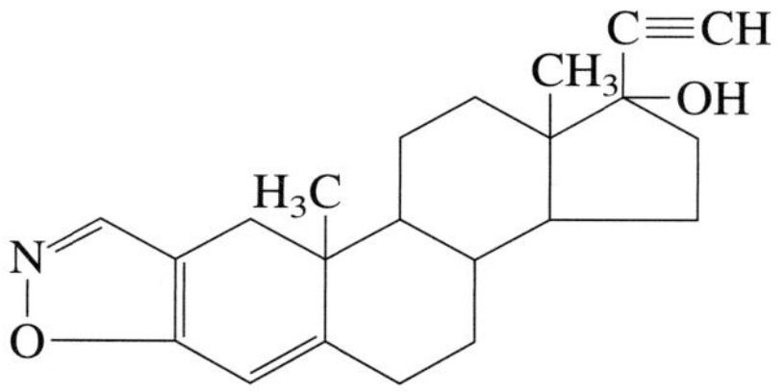

C≡CH
$CH_3$
OH
$H_3C$
N
O
**Danazol**

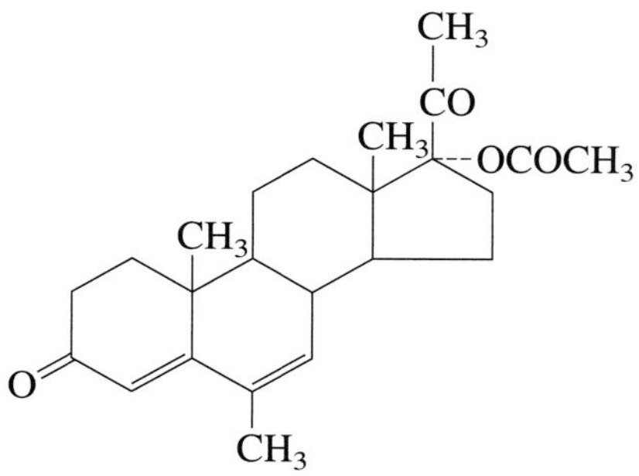

$CH_3$
CO
$CH_3$
OCOCH$_3$
$CH_3$
O
$CH_3$
**Megestrol Acetate**

FIGURE 9-38 Nonclassical progestin. Danazol has been widely used in the treatment of gynecological diseases, where it reduces endogenous estrogen concentrations and has mildly androgenic effects. Megestrol acetate is a progestin used in cancer therapy to reduce endogenous sex steroids and to stimulate appetite.

gain without improvement in performance status in patients with AIDS (Strang 1997) and advanced breast cancer (Vadell et al. 1998).

# ANDROGEN PHARMACOLOGY

## Testosterone Synthesis and Distribution in Men

Testosterone is synthesized by testicular Leydig cells in response to LH stimulation. Testosterone synthesis is intermittent, in response to episodic LH secretion, but plasma concentrations are relatively stable because of plasma protein binding. Approximately half of circulating testosterone is bound with high affinity ($K_d$ = 1.6 nM) by SHBG, which limits the bioavailability of testosterone. Most of the remainder is weakly bound by albumin ($K_d$ = 400 $\mu$M) or unbound (~2%) and constitutes the pool of readily bioavailable testosterone. SHBG concentrations rise with age and may contribute to the decline in androgen action with increasing age in men. Plasma concentrations of SHBG in men are decreased in obesity, glucocorticoid excess, and hypothyroidism; hence, total testosterone concentrations may be low in men with these conditions who are physiologically eugonadal.

## Testosterone Metabolism

### *Dihydrotestosterone*

Testosterone is metabolized by the enzyme 5-$\alpha$-reductase to produce dihydrotestosterone (DHT), an androgen agonist with approximately five times the binding affinity to the AR of testosterone. 5-$\alpha$-Reductase is distributed in tissues such as the skin, prostate, kidney, and brain where local generation of dihydrotestosterone may produce tissue-specific androgenic effects, such as male pattern baldness, beard growth, and prostate hyperplasia.

### *Estrogens in men*

Testosterone, like other androgens, may be converted to estrogen by the aromatase enzyme. Adult male plasma concentrations of estradiol are comparable to those of women in the early follicular phase of the menstrual cycle. Estrogen suppresses gonadotropin secretion in men. Estrogen resistance has been reported in men and is associated with delayed epiphyseal closure, low bone mineral density, and insulin resistance (Smith et al. 1994). The increase in growth velocity following administration of testosterone to male adolescents with constitutional growth delay may be partly due to aromatization to estrogen (Keenen et al. 1993). These findings suggest that estrogen may have important phyiologic roles in men. Oral estrogens decrease plasma LDL cholesterol concentrations in men, although at high doses (5 mg/day of conjugated equine estrogens or DES) estrogen therapy produces excess cardiovascular deaths in men (The Coronary Drug Project 1970) and excess venous thromboembolism (Chang et al. 1996).

### *Metabolic elimination*

Testosterone and DHT are also metabolized by oxidation and conjugation reactions. Hepatic extraction of plasma testosterone is approximately 50%, and orally administered testosterone is poorly bioavailable. Testosterone is predominantly excreted in the urine in the form of conjugated metabolites.

## Androgen Action

Testosterone and DHT bind the androgen receptor (AR), which, like other steroid receptors, is a ligand-dependent transcription factor. Androgens produce physiologic effects that are related to male sexual differentiation (Table 9-41), including increase in muscle mass, maintenance of positive nitrogen balance, and behavioral effects. The an-

**Table 9-41 Physiologic Effects of Androgens**

| ORGAN SYSTEM | EFFECT |
|---|---|
| Urogenital | Development of epididymis, vas deferens, seminal vesicles<br>Prostate and external genital development (DHT) |
| Skin and hair | Pubic, facial, and body hair<br>Sebaceous glands and acne<br>Male pattern balding (DHT) |
| Muscular | Anabolic effect |
| Larynx | Male voice |
| Bone marrow | Hematopoiesis |
| CNS | Behavior and aggression |

ABBREVIATIONS: DHT, dihydrotestosterone.

abolic and behavioral effects of androgens are the basis for the widespread abuse of synthetic androgens. The term *anabolic steroid* has been coined to denote dissociable anabolic and androgenic effects, but the pharmacologic basis for tissue specificity is unclear. DHT has been reported to have an AR binding affinity in prostate tissue higher than that in skeletal muscle, which may be mediated by tissue differences in metabolic elimination (Saartok et al. 1984). Transcription factors are involved in AR-mediated transcriptional effects (Scarlett and Robins 1995) and these may be differentially expressed in different tissues (Zhang et al. 1990). Although pharmacologic interaction with these mechanisms is possible, it is not known whether currently used androgen agonists have tissue-specific effects. Clinical trials of androgen therapy of eugonadal men suggest that supraphysiologic androgen therapy shows anabolic effects on lean body mass (LBM) and muscle strength (Bhasin et al. 1996) but that these effects are of small magnitude (Friedl et al. 1991; Young et al. 1993). Incremental effects on secondary sexual characteristics in men may be less clinically evident, giving a clinical impression of anabolic selectivity with androgen treatment.

***Androgen deficiency in men***

Male hypogonadism results from testicular disease, in which plasma gonadotropin concentrations are elevated (hypergonadotropic hypogonadism), or hypothalamic–pituitary dysfunction. Hypogonadism is a syndrome of diminished secondary sexual characteristics (e.g., beard growth), reduced libido, infertility, and reduced lean body mass. Use and abuse of exogenous androgens causes infertility with maintained secondary sexual characteristics due to androgenic suppression of LH secretion. Obesity, diabetes, and erectile dysfunction are common clinical findings in middle-aged men that may be associated with low-normal serum total testosterone concentrations. Relatively low testosterone concentrations in these eugonadal states may be due to low SHBG concentrations, and, in most cases, bioavailable testosterone ("free and weakly bound" testosterone) and gonadotropin concentrations are normal. The diagnosis of male hypogonadism is based on appropriate symptoms, subnormal testicular volume, and low testosterone concentrations associated with high gonadotropin concentrations (primary hypogonadism) or pituitary dysfunction (secondary hypogonadism) (Table 9-42). In contrast to the small magnitude of pharmacologic effect in healthy men, hypogonadal men typically experience clinically significant benefits with return to eugonadal testosterone concentrations (Davidson et al. 1979).

## Androgens in Women

The role of testosterone and other androgens in women's health is not well understood. Adrenal androgens decline with age and gonadal androgens decline at menopause. Small observational studies have documented loss of libido and psychological well-being in women associated with low androgen levels in older women (Davis and Burger 1996). Methyltestosterone has been combined with estrogen for the treatment of menopausal symptoms. Combined estrogen/androgen therapy has favorable effects on bone mineral density and libido but adverse effects on HDL cholesterol (Devor et al. 1992). Androgens do not antagonize estrogenic effects on the endometrium; hence, progestin therapy is required for long-term use in nonhysterectomized women. Elevated androgen concentrations are a hallmark of the polycystic ovary syndrome (PCOS) and may be associated with insulin resistance, menstrual dysregulation, and infertility.

## Therapeutic Androgen Agonists

***Testosterone preparations***

Because of poor oral bioavailability, testosterone is administered parenterally or transdermally (Table 9-43). Intramuscular preparations are testosterone esters in oil-based matrix that result in prolonged absorption with less irritation than aqueous testosterone formulations. For sev-

**Table 9-42 Diagnostic Findings in Male Hypogonadism**

| SYMPTOMS | SIGNS | LABORATORY FINDINGS |
|---|---|---|
| Decreased exercise tolerance<br>Decreased libido<br>Reduced shaving frequency<br>Impaired olfaction (Kallman syndrome) | Reduced testicular volume<br>Decreased lean body mass<br>Diminished secondary sexual characteristics<br>Eunuchoid proportions (arm span > height)<br>Baldness, cataracts, temporal wasting (myotonic dystrophy) | Low bioavailable testosterone concentrations<br>Gonadotropins increased or normal |

Table 9-43 **Testosterone Formulations for Hormone Replacement**

| DRUG FORMULATION | DAILY DOSE | SPECIFIC ADVERSE EFFECTS[a] |
|---|---|---|
| *Intramuscular preparations* | | |
| Testosterone enanthate | 200 mg (1 mL) IM every 2 wk | Injection discomfort and cost |
| Testosterone cypionate | 200 mg (1 mL) IM every 2 wk | Injection discomfort and cost |
| Testosterone propionate | 200 mg (2 mL) IM every 2 wk | Greater discomfort due to large volume or more frequent injection |
| *Transdermal preparations* | | |
| Scrotal application system | 4- or 6-mg patch once daily | Increased DHT concentrations, skin irritation |
| Nonscrotal application system | 2 patches (2.5 mg) applied once daily | Skin irritation |

[a]Adverse effects of erythrocytosis, priapism, prostate hypertrophy, gynecomastia, acne and sleep apnea syndrome are shared by all testosterone preparations.
ABBREVIATIONS: DHT, dihydrotestosterone.

eral days following IM injection, serum testosterone concentrations are supraphysiological; acute effects such as priapism are infrequently reported. It is likely that androgen receptors are saturated at these concentrations and that higher hormone concentrations do not produce additional effects. Transdermal testosterone preparations yield serum testosterone concentrations that are closer to the physiologic range. Transdermal testosterone applied to the scrotum is subject to metabolism by 5-$\alpha$-reductase to produce DHT at concentrations that exceed those in normal eugonadal men (Korenman et al. 1987). The long-term implications for prostate hyperplasia and balding are not known. Transdermal application to nongenital sites is not associated with high plasma DHT concentrations.

***Treatment of male hypogonadism***

Testosterone therapy is beneficial in hypogonadal conditions related to testicular or pituitary dysfunction. The usual doses for treatment of male hypogonadism is 200–400 mg of oil-based IM preparations administered every 2 to 4 weeks. Transdermal testosterone systems are applied daily. Testosterone therapy has been shown to improve lean body mass and symptom scores in AIDS-related hypogonadal cachexia (Grinspoon et al. 1998). Testosterone replacement in glucocorticoid treated men has demonstrated improvement in lean body mass and bone mineral density during 12 months of therapy (Reid et al. 1996), although long-term effects of androgen therapy on glucocorticoid-induced osteoporosis have not been studied. Although testosterone therapy improves libido in hypogonadal men, no clinical trial has demonstrated a benefit of testosterone therapy in men with erectile dysfunction and low-normal total testosterone concentrations.

***Andropause and testosterone replacement in aging***

Total and free testosterone concentrations decline gradually with age (Vermeulen and Kaufman 1995), because of both hypothalamic/pituitary and testicular mechanisms. Despite coinage of the term *andropause,* men do not display a programmed reduction in fertility similar to that of women. The decline in plasma androgen concentrations have been proposed to contribute to age-related changes in muscle strength, lean body mass, and athletic performance. Large-scale controlled trials of testosterone supplementation in normal aging men have not been published. Small clinical trials of testosterone therapy of elderly men with low-normal testosterone concentrations show mild clinical benefits in lean body mass and markers of bone resorption, but significant potential adverse effects such as erythrocytosis (Sih et al. 1997) and increased PSA concentrations (Tenover 1992).

***Synthetic steroidal androgens***

Several synthetic androgens have been developed for oral and parenteral therapy (Table 9-44). Although chemical modifications improve oral bioavailability relative to testosterone, these compounds are still subject to high first-pass hepatic metabolism. Alkylated testosterone derivatives (methyltestosterone, fluoxymesterone) achieve greater oral bioavailability, but are associated with adverse hepatic effects. Several steroidal androgen agonists (so called "anabolic steroids") suitable for oral therapy are weak AR agonists (stanozolol, oxymetholone, oxandrolone). Nandrolone is a parenteral androgen agonist with potency comparable to testosterone.

***Clinical use of synthetic androgens ("anabolic steroids")***

Synthetic androgens have been tested in small clinical studies in several cachexic states. Oxandrolone (5 to 15

Table 9-44 Synthetic Androgen Agonists

| DRUG | INDICATED USE | DOSAGE | ADVERSE EFFECTS[a] |
|---|---|---|---|
| Methyltestosterone | Male hypogonadism<br>Cryptorchidism<br>Reduction of postpartum breast engorgement<br>Breast cancer palliation | 10–50 mg every day PO<br>5–25 mg buccal<br>75 mg/day for 5 days<br>50–200 mg/day PO<br>25–100 mg buccal | Hepatic adenoma, peliosis hepatis, abnormal transaminases, infertility, erythrocytosis |
| Fluoxymestrone | Male hypogonadism<br>Reduction of postpartum breast engorgement<br>Breast cancer palliation | 5–20 mg every day PO<br>5–10 mg for 5 days<br>10–40 mg every day PO | Fluid retention reduction of HDL cholesterol |
| Nandrolone decanoate | Anemia of renal failure | 50–200 mg IM every week | |
| Oxandrolone | Cachexia | 5–20 mg divided in 2–4 daily doses | |
| Oxymetholone | Anemia of bone marrow failure | 50–150 mg every day PO | |
| Stanozolol | Hereditary angioedema | 2 mg PO tid acutely, 2 mg PO daily for maintenance of remission | |

[a]Adverse effects are shared by all androgens, although hepatic effects may be diminished in parenteral and buccal formulations.

mg/day) increases lean body mass and symptom scores in AIDS-related cachexia during 16 weeks of treatment (Berger et al. 1996). Stanozolol (12 mg/day) increased lean body mass in chronic obstructive pulmonary disease (COPD)-related cachexia, although pulmonary function was not improved (Ferreira et al. 1998). Nandrolone decanoate (25 to 50 mg every 2 weeks IM) in conjunction with nutritional supplementation showed similar mild benefit in COPD-related cachexia (Schols et al. 1995). Oxandrolone (10 mg bid) improves weight gain and physical performance during the recovery phase following major burns (Demling and DeSanti 1997).

#### *Adverse effects of therapeutic androgens*

Oral androgens have been associated with an increased incidence of blood-filled hepatic cysts (peliosis hepatis) as well as hepatic neoplasms. Oral methyltestosterone and fluoxymesterone may produce cholestatic jaundice. Oral androgens also show increased hepatic metabolic effects such as lowering of SHBG concentrations and reduction in plasma HDL cholesterol. Other adverse effects of androgen therapy are shared by parenteral testosterone including priapism, erythrocytosis, prostate hyperplasia, and gonadotropin suppression. Although atherosclerotic disease is more prevalent in men, adverse lipid effects are seen predominantly with high dose or oral androgen therapy. These include reduction in HDL cholesterol and minor effects on LDL cholesterol. Androgens suppress lipoprotein(a), an independent risk factor for coronary disease in men (Zmunda et al. 1996) (see also chapter 1, "Cardiovascular Disorders").

### Antiandrogens

#### *Steroidal antagonists in hyperandrogenic women*

Dysregulation of the luteal phase of the menstrual cycle is characteristic of the polycystic ovarian syndrome (PCOS), which is a common cause of infertility and secondary amenorrhea (Table 9-45). One frequent finding in PCOS is an abnormally high LH : FSH concentration ratio and increased ovarian androgen production. Ovarian androgens inhibit follicular development, and insufficient aromatization may contribute to follicular atresia and polycystic histology. Antiandrogens are commonly used to treat the cosmetic effects of hyperandrogenism in women. Androgen receptor antagonists include steroidal and nonsteroidal molecules. Steroidal antiandrogens in clinical use, such as spironolactone and cyproterone, have added pharmacologic effects beyond AR antagonism.

#### *Spironolactone*

Spironolactone is a mineralocorticoid and androgen receptor antagonist that is used as a potassium-sparing diuretic in the treatment of hypertension (Karim 1978). Spironolactone antagonizes androgen receptor binding and also impairs the synthesis of androgens. In contrast to the testosterone-elevating effects of nonsteroidal AR antagonists, spironolactone therapy results in lower plasma tes-

Table 9-45 Clinical Features of Polycystic Ovary Syndrome

| SYSTEM | ABNORMALITY |
|---|---|
| Gynecological | Multiple atretic ovarian follicles and cysts, thecal cell hypertrophy and androgen excess, ovulatory dysfunction and infertility, oligomenorrhea |
| Metabolic | Insulin resistance, obesity |
| Skin and hair | Acanthosis nigricans, acne, hirsutism |
| Hormonal | Increased LH:FSH concentration ratio, increased androgens, mild hyperprolactinemia glucose intolerance |

ABBREVIATIONS: FSH, follicular-stimulating hormone; LH, luteinizing hormone.

tosterone concentrations. Spironolactone has been used widely for the treatment of hirsutism at doses of 50 to 200 mg/day, although well-controlled studies are lacking. Doses greater than 200 mg/day do not achieve greater efficacy (Messina et al. 1983). Therapeutic effects of antiandrogen treatment of hirsutism require approximately 6 months to appear, because of the rate of turnover of androgen-dependent terminal hair. Hyperkalemia is uncommon in patients with normal renal function who do not receive concurrent potassium supplements or ACE inhibitors. Hirsutism without signs of virilization is a benign cosmetic disorder present in approximately 25% of women, for which patient education and mechanical hair removal methods may be preferable to pharmacologic therapy.

***Cyproterone***

Cyproterone acetate is an androgen receptor antagonist with progestational agonist effects (Klebe et al. 1983). Like spironolactone, cyproterone antagonizes androgen receptors while reducing plasma concentrations of testosterone. Cyproterone does not directly inhibit androgen biosynthesis but decreases gonadal androgen synthesis by its progestational effect to suppress gonadotropins. In one small clinical trial, cyproterone acetate 100 mg/day and spironolactone 100 mg/day were equally efficacious in reducing the need for cosmetic hair removal in hirsute women (O'Brien et al. 1991). Cyproterone acetate has been used in combination with ethinyl estradiol in COC in some countries but has not been registered in the United States. As a COC, the ethinyl estradiol/cyproterone acetate pill represents an attempt to further minimize the androgenic effects of the progestational component of the COC. The cyproterone-containing COC is an effective contraceptive agent that produces no reduction in HDL cholesterol, exacerbation of acne, or hirsutism. The antiandrogenic efficacy of the cyproterone COC is similar to that of COCs containing new generation progestins, which do not antagonize androgen receptors (Charoenvisal et al. 1996). COCs with antiandrogenic effects may be useful for premenopausal women with polycystic ovarian disorder (PCOS) (Greenwood et al. 1985; Falsetti and Galbignani 1990). Cyproterone acetate in combination with estrogen for postmenopausal hormone replacement may not exert the negative effect on HDL cholesterol that is seen with more androgenic progestins (Jensen et al. 1987).

## Nonsteroidal Androgen Receptor Antagonists in Prostate Cancer

The most common indications for antiandrogen therapy are prostate cancer, benign prostatic hyperplasia, and male pattern baldness. In the treatment of prostate cancer, nonsteroidal, selective AR antagonists (Table 9-46) have been used to a greater extent than the less potent steroidal agents (see chapter 13, Oncologic Disorders). In contrast to steroidal agents such as spironolactone and cyproterone, nonsteroidal AR antagonists do not demonstrate gonadotropin suppression or steroidogenic inhibition. Selective AR antagonists were expected to have added efficacy because of the ability to antagonize adrenal androgens that are not significantly reduced by orchiectomy or gonadotropin suppression. When used alone in the treatment of prostate cancer, however, AR antagonists are less efficacious than gonadotropin suppressive therapies (DES or GnRH-A) (Chang et al. 1996). AR antagonists produce compensatory rises in testosterone synthesis because of loss of negative feedback to the HPG axis, which may overcome the effects of competitive AR antagonists. Flutamide, nilutamide, and bicalutamide differ in AR-binding affinity and pharmacokinetic properties. Although the short elimination half-life of flutamide requires multiple

Table 9-46 Androgen Receptor Antagonists

| Drug | Indicated use | Dose | Adverse effects |
|---|---|---|---|
| Flutamide | Prostate cancer (adjunct to GnRH-A) | 250 mg tid PO | Hot flashes, hypogonadism, gynecomastia, transaminase elevations |
| Bicalutamide | Prostate cancer (adjunct to GnRH-A) | 50 mg every day PO | Hot flashes, hypogonadism, gynecomastia, transaminase elevations |
| Nilutamide | Prostate cancer (adjunct to castration) | 300 mg every day PO for 1 month after castration, then 150 mg every day PO | Interstitial pneumonitis, hepatitis, hot flashes, gynecomastia |
| Spironolactone | Hirsutism (off label) | 50–200 mg every day PO | Hyperkalemia, gynecomastia, increased BUN |

ABBREVIATIONS: BUN, blood urea nitrogen; GnRH-A, gonadotropin-releasing hormone A.

daily doses, its active metabolite OH-flutamide is the most potent of the nonsteroidal AR antagonists (Simard et al. 1997). Recent trials in prostate cancer have employed AR antagonists in combination with gonadotropin suppression therapy or orchiectomy. AR antagonists antagonize the transient increase in testosterone during initiation of GnRH-A therapy (Kuhn et al. 1989) and modestly improve clinical outcomes compared with GnRH-A or orchiectomy alone (Lunglmayr 1990; Janknegt 1993). Despite pharmacokinetic differences, the nonsteroidal AR antagonists appear to have similar clinical efficacy (Schellhammer et al. 1996; Mahler et al. 1998).

## Efficacy and Adverse Effects in Benign Prostatic Hyperplasia and Hirsutism

In the treatment of prostate cancer, AR antagonists have fewer adverse effects than other androgen-lowering therapies (Chang et al. 1996; Mahler et al. 1998). In the treatment of benign hyperandrogenic conditions such as benign prostatic hyperplasia (BPH) or hirsutism, however, the adverse effects of AR antagonists are more clinically evident. AR antagonists produce hot flashes, gynecomastia, and loss of libido in men. Nonsteroidal AR antagonists lead to increases in plasma androgens, which are then converted to estrogens, contributing to an increased incidence of gynecomastia. Small clinical trials of AR antagonists for the treatment of benign prostate hyperplasia have demonstrated no significant benefit (Caine et al. 1975; Erin and Tveter 1993). AR antagonists have been studied in small trials without placebo controls for the treatment of hirsutism. In women with PCOS, AR antagonism results in reductions in plasma androgen concentrations and improvement in hirsutism (Falsetti et al. 1997; De Leo et al. 1998).

## 5-$\alpha$-Reductase Inhibitors

The sensitivity of Wolffian-duct-derived structures to DHT has led to the use of selective inhibition of DHT biosynthesis as a treatment for prostate disease (see Table 9-40). 5-$\alpha$-Reductase has two isoforms in humans, type I and type II. Inhibition of the type 1 isoform reduces plasma DHT concentrations by approximately 30%. Finasteride preferentially inhibits the type II isoform and administration of 5 mg/day reduces plasma DHT concentrations by 70% in men (Schwartz et al. 1996). Intraprostatic DHT concentrations are reduced by 90% (Norman et al. 1993). Finasteride (5 mg/day) produces a moderate decrease in prostate size, increase in urinary flow rate, and improvement in prostate hyperplasia symptom scores (Marberger 1998; McConnell et al. 1998). Finasteride may be less efficacious than $\alpha_1$-adrenergic receptor antagonists in the treatment of BPH (Lepor et al. 1996). Finasteride has not been shown to be effective in the treatment of prostate cancer. Finasteride (1 mg/day) is also effective for the treatment of male pattern baldness in men. Finasteride is not registered for use in women but has been used in small trials without placebo controls for the treatment of hirsutism (Wong et al. 1995; Erenus et al. 1997), where it appears to have efficacy similar to that of spironolactone.

## REFERENCES

Archer DF, Maheux R, DelConte A, et al. 1997. A new low-dose monophasic combination oral contraceptive (Alesse) with levonorgestrel 100 micrograms and ethinyl estradiol 20 micrograms. North American Levonorgestrel Study Group (NALSG). *Contraception* **55**:139–44.

Barbieri RL, Ryan KJ. 1981. Danazol: Endocrine pharmacology and therapeutic applications. *Am J Obstet Gynecol* **141**:453–63.

Belchetz PE, Plant TM, , Nakai Y, et al. 1978. Hypophysical response to continuous and intermittent delivery of hypothalamic gonadotropin-releasing hormone. *Science* **202**:631–3.

Berger GS, Taylor RN, Jr, Treloar AE. 1977. The risk of post-pill amenorrhea: A preliminary report from the Menstruation and Reproduction History Research Program. *Int J Gynaecol Obstet* **15**: 125–7.

Berger JR, Pall L, Hall CD, et al. 1996. Oxandrolone in AIDS-wasting myopathy. *AIDS* **10**:1657–62.

Bhasin S, Storer TW, Berman N, et al. 1996. The effects of supraphysiologic doses of testosterone on muscle size and strength in normal men. *N Engl J Med* **335**:1–7.

Bhavnani BR. 1998. Pharmacokinetics and pharmacodynamics of conjugated equine estrogens: Chemistry and metabolism. *Proc Soc Exp Biol Med* **217**:6–16.

Bracken MB. 1990. Oral contraception and congenital malformations in offspring: A review and meta-analysis of the prospective studies. *Obstet Gynecol* **76**:552–7.

Brogden RN, Goa KL, Faulds D. 1993. Mifepristone. A review of its pharmacodynamic and pharmacokinetic properties, and therapeutic potential [published erratum appears in *Drugs* 46:268; 1993]. *Drugs* **45**:384–409.

Bush TL, Barrett-Conner E. 1985. Noncontraceptive estrogen use and cardiovascular disease. *Epidemiol Rev* **7**:89–104.

Buzdar AU, Jones SE, Vogel CL, et al. 1997. A phase III trial comparing anastrozole (1 and 10 milligrams), a potent and selective aromatase inhibitor, with megestrol acetate in postmenopausal women with advanced breast carcinoma. Arimidex Study Group. *Cancer* **79**:730–9.

Caine M, Perlberg S, Gordon R. 1975. The treatment of benign prostatic hypertrophy with flutamide (SCH: 13521): A placebo-controlled study. *J Urol* **114**:564–68.

Chang A, Yeap B, Davis T, et al. 1996. Double-blind, randomized study of primary hormonal treatment of stage D2 prostate carcinoma: Flutamide versus diethylstilbestrol. *J Clin Oncol* **14**:2250–7.

Charoenvisal C, Thaipisuttikul Y, Pinjaroen S, et al. 1996. Effects on acne of two oral contraceptives containing desogestrel and cyproterone acetate. *Int J Fertil Menopausal Studies* **41**:423–9.

Chetkowski RJ, Meldrum DR, Steingold KA, et al. 1986. Biologic effects of transdermal estradiol. *N Engl J Med* **314**:1615–20.

Clark JH, Markaverich BM. 1981. The agonistic-antagonistic properties of clomiphene: A review. *Pharmacol Ther* **15**:467–519.

Collins JA, Hughes EG. 1995. Pharmacological interventions for the induction of ovulation. *Drugs* **50**:480–94.

Comite F, Cutler GB, Jr, et al. 1981. A preliminary report. *N Engl J Med* **305**:1546–50.

Cortes-Gallegos V, Gallegos AJ, Basurto CS, et al. 1975. Estrogen peripheral levels vs estrogen tissue concentration in the human female reproductive tract. *J Steroid Biochem* **6**:15–20.

Davidson JM, Camargo CA, Smith ER. 1979. Effects of androgen on sexual behavior in hypogonadal men. *J Clin Endocrinol Metab* **48**:955–8.

Davis SR, Burger HG. 1996. Clinical review 82: Androgens and the postmenopausal woman. *J Clin Endocrinol Metab* **81**:2759–63.

De Leo V, Lanzetta D, D'Antona D, et al. 1998. Hormonal effects of flutamide in young women with polycystic ovary syndrome. *J Clin Endocrinol Metab* **83**:99–102.

Delmas PD, Bjarnason NH, Mitlak BH, et al. 1997. Effects of raloxifene on bone mineral density, serum cholesterol concentrations, and uterine endometrium in postmenopausal women. *N Engl J Med* **337**:1641–7.

Demling RH, DeSanti L. 1997. Oxandrolone, an anabolic steroid, significantly increases the rate of weight gain in the recovery phase after major burns. *J Trauma* **43**:47–51.

Devor M, Barrett-Connor E, Renvall M, et al. 1992. Estrogen replacement therapy and the risk of venous thrombosis. *Am J Med* **92**:275–82.

Dombernowsky P, Smith I, Falkson G, et al. 1998. Letrozole, a new oral aromatase inhibitor for advanced breast cancer: Double-blind randomized trial showing a dose effect and improved efficacy and tolerability compared with megestrol acetate. *J Clin Oncol* **16**: 453–61.

Eden JA, Place J, Carter GD, et al. 1989. The effect of clomiphene citrate on follicular phase increase in endometrial thickness and uterine volume. *Obstet Gynecol* **73**:187–90.

Endrikat J, Muller U, Dusterberg B. 1997. A twelve-month comparative clinical investigation of two low-dose oral contraceptives containing 20 micrograms ethinylestradiol/75 micrograms gestodene and 30 micrograms ethinylestradiol/75 micrograms gestodene, with respect to efficacy, cycle control, and tolerance. *Contraception* **55**:131–7.

Erenus M, Yucelten D, Durmusoglu F, et al. 1997. Comparison of finasteride versus spironolactone in the treatment of idiopathic hirsutism. *Fertil Steril* **68**:1000–3.

Erin LM, Tveter KJ. 1993. A prospective, placebo-controlled study of the antiandrogen Casodex as treatment for patients with benign prostatic hyperplasia. *J Urol* **150**:90–4.

Falsetti L, De Fusco D, Eleftheriou G, et al. 1997. Treatment of hirsutism by finasteride and flutamide in women with polycystic ovary syndrome. *Gynecol Endocrinol* **11**:251–7.

Falsetti L, Galbignani E. 1990. Long-term treatment with the combination ethinyl estradiol and cyproterone acetate in polycystic ovary syndrome. *Contraception* **42**:611–9.

Fedele L, Parazzini F, Radici E, et al. 1992. Buserelin acetate versus expectant management in the treatment of infertility associated with minimal or mild endometriosis: A randomized clinical trial. *Am J Obstet Gynecol* **166**:1345–50.

Ferreira IM, Verreschi IT, Nery LE, et al. 1998. The influence of 6 months of oral anabolic steroids on body mass and respiratory muscles in undernourished COPD patients. *Chest* **114**:19–28.

Fisher B, Constantino JP, Wickerham DL, et al. 1998. Tamoxifen for prevention of breast cancer: Report of the national surgical adjuvant breast and bowel project P-1 study. *J Natl Cancer Inst* **90**:1371–88.

Franchimont P, Legros JJ, Meurice J. 1972. Effect of several estrogens on serum gonadotropin levels in postmenopausal women. *Horm Metab Res* **4**:288–92.

Fraser IS, Tiitinen A, Affandi B, et al. 1998. Norplant consensus statement and background review. *Contraception* **57**:1–9.

Friedl KE, Dettori JR, Hannan CJ, et al. 1991. Comparison of the effects of high dose testosterone and 19-nortestosterone to a replacement dose of testosterone on strength and body composition in normal men. *J Steroid Biochem Mol Biol* **40**:607–12.

Furr BJ, Jordan VC. 1984. The pharmacology and clinical uses of tamoxifen. *Pharmacol Ther* **25**:127–205.

Furuhjelm M, Carlstrom K. 1973. Amenorrhea following use of combined oral contraceptives. *Acta Obstet Gynecol Scand* **52**:373–9.

Gelfand JA, Sherins RJ, Alling DW, et al. 1976. Treatment of hereditary angioedema with danazol. Reversal of clinical and biochemical abnormalities. *N Engl J Med* **295**:1444–8.

Geller J, Albert J, Geller S, et al. 1976. Effect of megestrol acetate (Megace) on steroid metabolism and steroid-protein binding in the human prostate. *J Clin Endocrinol Metab* **43**:1000–8.

Geola FL, Frumar AM, Tataryn IV, et al. 1980. Biological effects of various doses of conjugated equine estrogens in postmenopausal women. *J Clin Endocrinol Metab* **51**:620–5.

Glasier A. 1997. Emergency postcoital contraception. *N Engl J Med* **337**:1058–64.

Goni M, Markussis V, Tolis G. 1994. Efficacy of chronic therapy with the gonadotrophin releasing hormone agonist decapeptyl in patients with polycystic ovary syndrome. *Hum Reprod* **9**:1048–52.

Gougeon A. 1996. Regulation of ovarian follicular development in primates: Facts and hypotheses. *Endocr Rev* **17**:121–55.

Greenwood R, Brummitt L, Burke B, et al. 1985. Acne: double blind clinical and laboratory trial of tetracycline, oestrogen-cyproterone acetate, and combined treatment. *Br Med J Clin Res Ed* **291**: 1231–5.

Grinspoon S, Corcoran C, Askari H, et al. 1998. Effects of androgen administration in men with the AIDS wasting syndrome. A randomized, double-blind, placebo-controlled trial. *Ann Intern Med* **129**:18–26.

Hatch EE, Palmer JR, Titus-Ernstoff L, et al. 1998. Cancer risk in women exposed to diethylstilbestrol in utero. *JAMA* **280**:630–4.

Holtz G, Kling OR, Miller DD, et al. 1982. Ovarian hyperstimulation syndrome caused by clomiphene citrate. *South Med* **75**:368–9.

Hull MG, Bromham DR, Savage PE, et al. 1981. Post-pill amenorrhea: a causal study. *Fertil Steril* **36**:472–6.

Hulley S, Grady D, Bush T, et al. 1998. Randomized trial of estrogen plus progestin for secondary prevention of coronary heart disease in postmenopausal women. Heart and Estrogen/progestin Replacement Study (HERS) Research Group. *JAMA* **280**:605–13.

Inman WH, Vessey MP. 1968. Investigation of deaths from pulmonary, coronary, and cerebral thrombosis and embolism in women of child-bearing age. *Br Med J* **2**:193–9.

Inman WH, Vessey MP, Westerholm B, et al. 1970. Thromboembolic disease and the steroidal content of oral contraceptives. A report to the Committee on Safety of Drugs. *Br Med J* **2**:203–9.

Janknegt RA. 1993. Total androgen blockade with the use of orchiectomy and nilutamide (Anandron) or placebo as treatment of metastatic prostate cancer. Anandron International Study Group. *Cancer* **72**:3874–7.

Jensen J, Riis BJ, Christiansen C. 1987. Cyproterone acetate, an alternative progestogen in postmenopausal hormone replacement therapy? Effects on serum lipids and lipoproteins. *Br J Obstet Gynaecol* **94**:136–41.

Jiang C, Poole-Wilson PA, Sarrel PM, et al. 1992. Effect of 17 beta-oestradiol on contraction, $Ca^{2+}$ current and intracellular free $Ca^{2+}$ in guinea-pig isolated cardiac myocytes. *Br J Pharmacol* **106**:739–45.

Jick H, Jick SS, Gurewich V, et al. 1995. Risk of idiopathic cardiovascular death and nonfatal venous thromboembolism in women using oral contraceptives with differing progestagen components. *Lancet* **346**:1589–93.

Karim A. 1978. Spironolactone: disposition, metabolism, pharmacodynamics, and bioavailability. *Drug Metab Rev* **8**:151–88.

Katzenellenbogen BS. 1984. Biology and receptor interactions of estriol and estriol derivatives in vitro and in vivo. *J Steroid Biochem* **20**:1033–7.

Kauffman RF, Bensch WR, Roudebush RE, et al. 1997. Hypocholesterolemic activity of raloxifene (LY139481): pharmacological characterization as a selective estrogen receptor modulator. *J Pharmacol Exp Ther* **280**:146–3.

Kauppila A, Kivinen S, Leinonen P, et al. 1983. Comparison of megestrol acetate and clomiphene citrate as supplemental medication in postmenopausal oestrogen replacement therapy. *Arch Gynecol* **234**:49–58.

Keenan BS, Richards GE, Ponder SW, et al. 1993. Androgen-stimulated pubertal growth: The effects of testosterone and dihydrotestosterone on growth hormone and insulin-like growth factor-I in the treatment of short stature and delayed puberty. *J Clin Endocrinol Metab* **76**:996–1001.

Klebe U, Moltz L, Pickartz H. 1983. Effects of cyproterone acetate and ethinyl estradiol on endometrial histology. *Arch Gynecol* **234**:113–120.

Korenman SG, Viosca S, Garza D, et al. 1987. Androgen therapy of hypogonadal men with transscrotal testosterone systems. *Am J Med* **83**:471–8.

Kuhn JM, Billebaud T, Navratil H, et al. 1989. Prevention of the transient adverse effects of a gonadotropin-releasing hormone analogue (buserelin) in metastatic prostatic carcinoma by administration of an antiandrogen (nilutamide). *N Engl J Med* **321**:413–8.

Kuiper GG, Carlsson B, Grandien K, et al. 1997. Comparison of the ligand binding specificity and transcript tissue distribution of estrogen receptors alpha and beta. *Endocrinology* **138**:863–70.

Laue L, Lotze MT, Chrousos GP, et al. 1990. Effect of chronic treatment with the glucocorticoid antagonist RU 486 in man: toxicity, immunological, and hormonal aspects. *J Clin Endocrinol Metab* **71**:1474–80.

Lepor H, Williford WO, Barry MJ, et al. 1996. The efficacy of terazosin, finasteride, or both in benign prostatic hyperplasia. Veterans Affairs Cooperative Studies Benign Prostatic Hyperplasia Study Group. *N Engl J Med* **335**:533–9.

Lindahl B, Andolf E, Ingvar C, et al. 1997. Endometrial thickness and ovarian cysts as measured by ultrasound in asymptomatic postmenopausal breast cancer patients on various adjuvant treatments including tamoxifen. *Anticancer Res* **17**:3821–4.

Littman BA, Hodgen GD. 1985. A comprehensive dose-response study of clomiphene citrate for enhancement of the primate ovarian/menstrual cycle. *Fertil Steril* **43**:463–70.

Lumsden MA, West CP, Thomas E, et al. 1994. Treatment with the gonadotrophin releasing hormone-agonist goserelin before hysterectomy for uterine fibroids. *Br J Obstet Gynaecol* **101**:438–42.

Lunglmayr G. 1990. A multicenter trial comparing the lutenizing hormone releasing hormone analog Zoladex, with Zoladex plus flutamide in the treatment of advanced prostate cancer. The Inter national Prostate Cancer Study Group. *Eur Urol* 18 Suppl **3**: 38–9.

Mahler C, Verhelst J, Denis L. 1998. Clinical pharmacokinetics of the antiandrogens and their efficacy in prostate cancer. *Clin Pharmacokinet* **34**:405–17.

Mandel FP, Geola FL, Lu JK, et al. 1982. Biologic effects of various doses of ethinyl estradiol in postmenopausal women. *Obstet Gynecol* **59**:673–9.

Mannucci PM, Bettega D, Chantarangkul V, et al. 1996. Effect of tamoxifen on measurements of hemostasis in healthy women. *Arch Intern Med* **156**:1806–10.

Marberger MJ. 1998. Long-term effects of finasteride in patients with benign prostatic hyperplasia: A double-blind, placebo-controlled, multicenter study. PROWESS Study Group. *Urology* **51**:677–86.

Marut EL, Hodgen GD. 1982. Antiestrogenic action of high-dose clomiphene in primates pituitary augmentation but with ovarian attenuation. *Fertil Steril* **38**:100–4.

McConnell JD, Bruskewitz R, Walsh P, et al. 1998. The effect of finasteride on the risk of acute urinary retention and the need for surgical treatment among men with benign prostatic hyperplasia. Finasteride Long-Term Efficacy and Safety Study Group. *N Engl J Med* **338**:557–3.

Meade TW, Greenberg G, Thompson SG. 1980. Progestogens and cardiovascular reactions associated with oral contraceptives and a comparison of the safety of 50- and 30-microgram oestrogen preparations. *Br Med J* **280**:1157–61.

Mehta RR, Valcourt L, Graves J, et al. 1987. Subcellular concentrations of estrone, estradiol, androstenedione and 17 beta-hydroxysteroid dehydrogenase (17-beta-OH-SDH) activity in malignant and nonmalignant human breast tissues. *Int J Cancer* **40**:305–8.

Messina M, Manieri C, Biffignandi P, et al. 1983. Antiandrogenic properties of spironolactone. Clinical trial in the management of female hirsutism. *J Endocrinol Invest* **6**:23–27.

Moghissi KS, Schlaff WD, Olive DL, et al. 1998. Goserelin acetate (Zoladex) with or without hormone replacement therapy for the treatment of endometriosis. *Fertil Steril* **69**:1056–62.

Mosselman S, Polman J, Dijkema R. 1996. ER beta: identification and characterization of a novel human estrogen receptor. *FEBS Lett* **392**:49–53.

Norman RW, Coakes KE, Wright AS, et al. 1993. Androgen metabolism in men receiving finasteride before prostatectomy. *J Urol* **150**:1736–9.

O'Brien RC, Cooper ME, Murray RM, et al. 1991. Comparison of sequential cyproterone acetate/estrogen versus spironolactone/oral contraceptive in the treatment of hirsutism. *J Clin Endocrinol Metab* **72**:1008–13.

Orwoll ES, Yuzpe AA, Burry KA, et al. 1994. Nafarelin therapy in endometriosis: Long-term effects on bone mineral density. *Am J Obstet Gynecol* **171**:1221–5.

Pardridge WM. 1988. Selective delivery of sex steroid hormones to tissues in vivo by albumin and by sex hormone-binding globulin. *Ann N Y Acad Sci* **538**:173–92.

Petitti DB, Sidney S, Bernstein A, et al. 1996. Stroke in users of low-dose oral contraceptives. *N Engl J Med* **335**:8–15.

Poyet P, Labrie F. 1985. Comparison of the antiandrogenic/androgenic activities of flutamide, cyproterone acetate and megestrol acetate. *Mol Cell Endocrinol* **42**:283–8.

Randall JM, Templeton A. 1991. Cervical mucus score and in vitro sperm mucus interaction in spontaneous and clomiphene citrate cycles. *Fertil Steril* **56**:465–8.

Reid IR, Wattie DJ, Evans MC, et al. 1996. Testosterone therapy in glucocorticoid-treated men. *Arch Intern Med* **156**:1173–7.

Riegel AT, Martin MB, Schoenberg DR. 1986. Transcriptional and post-transcriptional inhibition of albumin gene expression by estrogen in *Xenopus* liver. *Mol Cell Endocrinol* **44**:201–9.

Rock JA, Truglia JA, Caplan RJ. 1993. Zoladex (goserelin acetate implant) in the treatment of endometriosis: A randomized comparison with danazol. The Zoladex Endometriosis Study Group. *Obstet Gynecol* **82**:198–205.

Rosenfeld RG, Attie KM, Frane J, et al. 1998. Growth hormone therapy of Turner's syndrome: beneficial effect on adult height. *J Pediatr* **132**:319–24.

Rosner W. 1990. The functions of corticosteroid-binding globulin and sex hormone-binding globulin: Recent advances. *Endocr Rev* **11**:80–91.

Ross JL, McCauley E, Roeltgen D, et al. 1996. Self-concept and behavior in adolescent girls with Turner syndrome: potential estrogen effects [published erratum appears in *J Clin Endocrinol Metab* 81:2191; 1996]. *J Clin Endocrinol Metab* **81**:926–31.

Rossing MA, Daling JR, Weiss NS, et al. 1994. Ovarian tumors in a cohort of infertile women. *N Engl J Med* **331**:771–6.

Saartok T, Dahlberg E, Gustafsson JA. 1984. Relative binding affinity of anabolic-androgenic steroids: Comparison of the binding to the androgen receptors in skeletal muscle and in prostate, as well as to sex hormone-binding globulin. *Endocrinology* **114**:2100–6.

Scarlett CO, Robins DM. 1995. In vivo footprinting of an androgen-dependent enhancer reveals an accessory element integral to hormonal response. *Mol Endocrinol* **9**:413–23.

Schellhammer PF, Sharifi R, Block NL, et al. 1996. A controlled trial of bicalutamide versus flutamide, each in combination with luteinizing hormone-releasing hormone analogue therapy, in patients with advanced prostate carcinoma. Analysis of time to progression. CASODEX Combination Study Group. *Cancer* **78**:2164–9.

Schols AM, Soeters PB, Mostert R, et al. 1995. Physiologic effects of nutritional support and anabolic steroids in patients with chronic obstructive pulmonary disease. A placebo-controlled randomized trial. *Am J Respir Crit Care Med* **152**:1268–74.

Schwartz JI, Van Hecken A, De Schepper PJ, et al. 1996. Effect of MK-386, a novel inhibitor of type 1 5 alpha-reductase, alone and in combination with finasteride, on serum dihydrotestosterone concentrations in men. *J Clin Endocrinol Metab* **81**:2942–7.

Shalev J, Goldenberg M, Kukia E, et al. 1989. Comparison of five clomiphene citrate dosage regimens: Follicular recruitment and distribution in the human ovary. *Fertil Steril* **52**:560–3.

Shushan A, Peretz T, Uziely B, et al. 1996. Ovarian cysts in premenopausal and postmenopausal tamoxifen-treated women with breast cancer. *Am J Obstet Gynecol* **174**:141–4.

Sidney S, Petitti DB, Quesenberry CP Jr, et al. 1996. Myocardial infarction in users of low-dose oral contraceptives. *Obstet Gynecol* **88**:939–44.

Sih R, Morley JE, Kaiser FE, et al. 1997. Testosterone replacement in older hypogonadal men: A 12-month randomized controlled trial. *J Clin Endocrinol Metab* **82**:1661–7.

Simard J, Singh SM, Labrie F. 1997. Comparison of in vitro effects of the pure antiandrogens OH-flutamide, Casodex, and nilutamide on androgen-sensitive parameters. *Urology* **49**:580–6; discussion 586–9.

Smith EP, Boyd J, Frank GR, et al. 1994. Estrogen resistance caused by a mutation in the estrogen-receptor gene in a man [published erratum appears in *N Engl J Med* **332**:131; 1995.] *N Engl J Med* **331**:1056–61.

Strang P. 1997. The effect of megestrol acetate on anorexia, weight loss and cachexia in cancer and AIDS patients (review). *Anticancer Res* **17**:657–62.

Stuart NS, Warwick J, et al. 1996. A randomised phase III cross-over study of tamoxifen versus megestrol acetate in advanced and recurrent breast cancer. *Eur J Cancer* **32A**:1888–92.

Taylor AE, Adams JM, Mulder JE, et al. 1996. A randomized, controlled trial of estradiol replacement therapy in women with hypergonadotropic amenorrhea. *J Clin Endocrinol Metab* **81**:3615–21.

Telimaa S. 1988. Danazol and medroxyprogesterone acetate inefficacious in the treatment of infertility in endometriosis. *Fertil Steril* **50**:872–5.

Telimaa S, Apter D, Reinila M, et al. 1990. Placebo-controlled comparison of hormonal and biochemical effects of danazol and high-dose medroxyprogesterone acetate. *Eur J Obstet Gynecol Reprod Biol* **36**:97–105.

Telimaa S, Penttila I, Puolakka J, et al. 1989. Circulating lipid and lipoprotein concentrations during danazol and high-dose medroxyprogesterone acetate therapy of endometriosis. *Fertil Steril* **52**: 31–5.

Tenover JS. 1992. Effects of testosterone supplementation in the aging male. *J Clin Endocrinol Metab* **75**:1092–8.

Tham DM, Gardner CD, Haskell WL. 1998. Clinical review 97: Potential health benefits of dietary phytoestrogens: A review of the clinical, epidemiological, and mechanistic evidence. *J Clin Endocrinol Metab* **83**:2223–35.

The Coronary Drug Project. 1970. Initial findings leading to modifications of its research protocol. *JAMA* **214**:1303–13.

The Writing Group for the PEPI Trial. 1995b. Effects of estrogen or estrogen/progestin regimens on heart disease risk factors in postmenopausal women. The Postmenopausal Estrogen/Progestin Interventions (PEPI) Trial. *JAMA* **273**:199–208.

The Writing Group for the PEPI Trial. 1996a. Effects of hormone replacement therapy on endometrial histology in postmenopausal women. The Postmenopausal Estrogen/Progestin Interventions (PEPI) Trial. *JAMA* **275**:370–5.

Tomino Y, Sakai H, Hanzawa S, et al. 1987. Clinical effect of danazol in patients with IgA nephropathy. *Jpn J Med* **26**:162–6.

Trussell J, Hatcher RA, Cates W, et al. 1990. Contraceptive failure in the United States: An update. *Studies in Family Planning* **21**:51–4.

Vadell C, Segui MA, Gimenez-Arnau JM, et al. 1998. Anticachectic efficacy of megestrol acetate at different doses and versus placebo in patients with neoplastic cachexia. *Am J Clin Oncol* **21**:347–51.

Van den Broeck J, Massa GG, Attanasio A, et al. 1995. Final height after long-term growth hormone treatment in Turner syndrome. European Study Group. *J Pediatr* **127**:729–35.

Van der Vange N, Blankenstein MA, Kloosterboer HJ, et al. 1990. Effects of seven low-dose combined oral contraceptives on sex hormone binding globulin, corticosteroid binding globulin, total and free testosterone. *Contraception* **41**:345–52.

Vermeulen A, Kaufman JM. 1995. Ageing of the hypothalamo-pituitary-testicular axis in men. *Horm Res* **43**:25–8.

Vessey MP, Villard-Mackintosh L, McPherson K, et al. 1989. Mortality among oral contraceptive users: 20 year follow up of women in a cohort study. *Br Med J* **299**:1487–91.

Webb AM, Russell J, Elstein M. 1992. Comparison of Yuzpe regimen, danazol, and mifepristone (RU486) in oral postcoital contraception. *Br Med J* **305**:927–31.

Weiner E, Johansson ED. 1976. Contraception with megestrol acetate implants. Megestrol acetate levels in plasma and the influence on the ovarian function. *Contraception* **13**:685–95.

Wheeler JM, Knittle JD, Miller JD. 1992. Depot leuprolide versus danazol in treatment of women with symptomatic endometriosis. I. Efficacy results. *Am J Obstet Gynecol* **167**:1367–71.

Wolfe BM, Huff MW. 1993. Effects of low dosage progestin-only administration upon plasma triglycerides and lipoprotein metabolism in postmenopausal women. *J Clin Invest* **92**:456–61.

Wong E, Eftekhari N, Greaves MW, et al. 1987. Beneficial effects of danazol on symptoms and laboratory changes in cholinergic urticaria. *Br J Dermatol* **116**:553–6.

Wong IL, Morris RS, Chang L, et al. 1995. A prospective randomized trial comparing finasteride to spironolactone in the treatment of hirsute women. *J Clin Endocrinol Metab* **80**:233–8.

World Health Organization Collaborative Study of Cardiovascular Disease and Steroid Hormone Contraception. 1995a. Effect of different progestagens in low estrogen oral contraceptives on venous thromboembolic disease. *Lancet* **346**:1582–8.

World Health Organization Collaborative Study of Cardiovascular Disease and Steroid Hormone Contraception. 1996b. Ischaemic stroke and combined oral contraceptives: Results of an international, multicentre, case-control study. *Lancet* **348**:498–505.

Yang NN, Venugopalan M, Hardikar S, et al. 1996. Identification of an estrogen response element activated by metabolites of 17$\beta$-estradiol and raloxifene [published erratum appears in *Science* 275:1249; 1997]. *Science* **273**:1222–5.

Yen SS, Martin PL, Burnier AM, et al. 1975. Circulating estradiol, estrone and gonadotropin levels following the administration of orally active 17beta-estradiol in postmenopausal women. *J Clin Endocrinol Metab* **40**:518–21.

Young NR, Baker HW, Liu G, et al. 1993. Body composition and muscle strength in healthy men receiving testosterone enanthate for contraception. *J Clin Endocrinol Metab* **77**:1028–32.

Yuzpe AA, Lance WJ. 1977. Ethinylestradiol and *dl*-norgestrel as a postcoital contraceptive. *Fertil Steril* **28**:932–6.

Zhang YL, Parker MG, Bakker O. 1990. Tissue-specific differences in the binding of nuclear proteins to a CCAAT motif in the promoter of the androgen-regulated C3 gene. *Mol Endocrinol* **4**:1219–25.

Zmunda JM, Thompson PD, Dickenson R, et al. 1996. Testosterone decreases lipoprotein(a) in men. *Am J Cardiol* **77**:1244–47.

# Hypothalamic Hormone Therapy

Steven A. Lieberman, Andrew R. Hoffman

*Chapter Outline*



The discovery of hypothalamic peptides that are released into the hypothalamic-hypophyseal portal circulation has greatly enlarged our understanding of endocrine control mechanisms and the means through which the central nervous system can communicate to the anterior pituitary and peripheral endocrine system. In addition, analogs of these hormones have been synthesized and are now used as pharmaceutical agents for a wide variety of illnesses. This chapter will discuss the pharmacologic effects of gonadotropin-releasing hormone (GnRH) and somatostatin. No significant therapeutic use has been found for thyrotropin-releasing hormone or corticotropin-releasing hormone. The use of growth hormone-releasing hormone and growth hormone-releasing peptides for the treatment of idiopathic growth hormone deficiency is being investigated.

## GONADOTROPIN-RELEASING HORMONE AND ITS ANALOGS

### Physiology of Gonadotropin-Releasing Hormone

The pituitary hormones responsible for regulation of gonadal function are the glycoprotein heterodimers luteinizing hormone (LH) and follicle-stimulating hormone (FSH). In the male, LH stimulates the Leydig cell of the testes to synthesize testosterone. FSH stimulates the Sertoli cells to synthesize inhibin and other proteins (including androgen-binding protein) and, in conjunction with high intratesticular concentrations of testosterone, initiates and maintains spermatogenesis. In females, LH interacts primarily with the theca cells to stimulate androgen synthesis, and FSH increases aromatase (estrogen synthase) activity and inhibin synthesis in the granulosa cells. Both LH and FSH are released from the gonadotrope cells of the anterior pituitary in response to the hypothalamic decapeptide hormone GnRH also known as LH-releasing hormone (LHRH).

Gonadotropin-releasing hormone is synthesized in the medial preoptic region of the hypothalamus in neurons whose projections go to the median eminence, where they abut capillaries of the hypothalamic-hypophyseal portal circulation. While high concentrations of GnRH are present in the portal circulation, very little hormone escapes into the peripheral circulation. In the systemic circulation, GnRH has a half-life of <10 minutes, as it is rapidly degraded, with initial proteolysis catalyzed by an endopeptidase between amino acids 6 and 7, and subsequently catalyzed by a carboxyamide peptidase between amino acids 9 and 10 (Handelsman and Swerdloff 1986).

Gonadotropin-releasing hormone is necessary for normal pubertal development and for the initiation and maintenance of fertility. In mice with a deletional mutation of the gene encoding GnRH, gonadotropin secretion is low, and gonadal maturation does not progress (Mason et al. 1986). Physiologic GnRH deficiency also occurs in humans, manifesting as congenital or acquired hypogonadotropic hypogonadism.

When GnRH was initially isolated, characterized, and chemically synthesized, several groups decided to treat men with idiopathic hypogonadotropic hypogonadism (IHH) and other hypothalamic lesions by GnRH replacement therapy. Since most peptides are degraded when ingested orally, GnRH was administered by intravenous or subcutaneous injection. Although large boluses of hormone were injected several times daily for months, gonadotropin and testosterone concentrations in plasma rarely increased into the normal range. In general, infrequent injections of native synthetic GnRH could not induce or maintain pubertal development in these patients. The reasons for this therapeutic failure were not readily apparent, but it was suggested that native GnRH had too short a half-life to be an effective therapeutic agent (Hoffman 1985).

Within several years of the discovery of GnRH, numerous potent, long-acting GnRH analogs were synthesized. In designing analogs, a strategy of substituting a bulky, hydrophobic D-amino acid at position 6 was employed to inhibit proteolysis; in many cases, the terminal amino acid was truncated with the addition of ethylamide to the proline at position 9. These synthetic peptides have a longer duration of action and a greater affinity for pituitary GnRH receptors than the native peptide (Karten and Rivier 1986). Several investigators used these analogs in an attempt to induce puberty in men with IHH. While serum gonadotropin concentrations rose initially, the increase in hormone secretion could not be maintained for more than several months, even when the dose of analog or the frequency of its administration was increased.

This failure of GnRH and its analogs to induce and maintain pubertal changes led to a reexamination of the normal physiology of the control of gonadotropin secretion. It had long been recognized that LH is secreted into the circulation in discrete pulses and not in a continuous manner. Knobil and his colleagues (Belchetz et al. 1978) reasoned that the pulsatile secretion of LH reflects episodic release of GnRH from the hypothalamus, and they demonstrated that only pulsatile administration of GnRH results in normal gonadotrope responsiveness. These workers studied castrated rhesus monkeys whose GnRH neurons had been stereotactically ablated. When these monkeys received IV boluses of GnRH, gonadotropin concentrations increased and remained elevated. A continuous infusion of GnRH, however, could not sustain this increase in gonadotropin secretion. When the timing of GnRH administration was altered from the known physiologic pulsatile frequency, the increased gonadotropin concentrations were not maintained. Subsequent studies demonstrated that continuous infusions of native GnRH ultimately inhibit LH secretion in normal persons by desensitizing the pituitary gonadotrophs.

**PRINCIPLE Cells may respond in a physiologic manner to intermittent exposure to an agonist but fail to respond to more frequent or continuous exposure to the same agent. Desensitization is more likely to occur during constant exposure to an agonist. Therapeutic advantage of such observations may be taken either by mimicking the natural release patterns to reproduce the effect of native substances or by deliberately desensitizing the receptors if inhibition of the effect of the native substance becomes desirable.**

These studies provided an explanation for the previous failure to induce puberty using GnRH and its analogs and suggested a rational basis for designing drug schedules for GnRH replacement therapy. On a long-term basis, the gonadotrope-producing cells respond only to pulsatile exposure to GnRH and not to a continuous infusion of the peptide. Moreover, the GnRH pulses must be delivered in a near-physiologic frequency in order for the pituitary to recognize the stimulatory signal. As a consequence, infrequent boluses of native GnRH cannot induce normal pubertal development, because they do not lead to sufficient LH secretion to maintain testicular secretion.

The pituitary is programmed to respond best to approximately 60- to 120-minute interpulse intervals of this hypothalamic hormone. Because of their long serum half-lives and greater duration of binding to the GnRH receptor, the GnRH analogs provide, in effect, a continuous, nonfluctuating level of GnRH bioactivity: A bolus injection of a long-acting agonist is pharmacodynamically similar to a constant infusion of the short-acting native hormone. In normal persons, the potent GnRH analogs initially stimulate gonadotropin secretion; however, by 4 weeks, gonadotrope function is suppressed, serum LH and FSH concentrations fall, and gonadal function declines markedly. This pharmacologic induction of hypogonadotropic hypogonadism has been termed a "medical castration," and, as described below, the GnRH analogs have become extremely useful agents for lowering sex steroid concentrations in clinical settings.

**PRINCIPLE All hormones are secreted in a pulsatile manner. However, in order for the receptor to experience pulsatile, intermittent exposure to an agonist, the interval between two pulses of hormone secretion (or drug administration) must be substantially longer than the half-life of the agonist.**

## Gonadotropin-Releasing Hormone Replacement Therapy

### *Induction of puberty in males with idiopathic hypogonadotropic hypogonadism*

After appreciating the implications of pulsatile hormone delivery in the hypothalamic–pituitary–gonadal network, it became possible to design treatment schedules for replacement of GnRH. Frequent, round-the-clock administration of hormone is achieved with the use of a portable infusion pump that can be programmed to deliver subcutaneous boluses of GnRH. Men with IHH are treated with 25 to 300 ng of GnRH per kilogram of body weight every 2 hours. On this treatment regimen, distinct pulses of GnRH are evident in the patient's serum. Pulsatile LH and FSH secretion is induced, testosterone concentrations reach the normal range for adult males, testicular size increases, and spermatogenesis ensues in most individuals (Hoffman and Crowley 1982). The success in restoring normal gonadal function in these men by administering GnRH at a physiologic frequency provides further evidence that IHH is in fact a disease of aberrant GnRH synthesis or secretion. Native GnRH has also been shown to be effective in the treatment of cryptorchidism (Pyorala et al. 1995).

***Induction of ovulation in women with hypothalamic amenorrhea***

Abnormalities or deficits in GnRH synthesis or secretion have been implicated in the menstrual disturbances and infertility associated with hypothalamic tumors, IHH, hyperprolactinemia, anorexia nervosa, "stress-" and weight-loss-associated amenorrhea, athletes' amenorrhea, and some forms of the polycystic ovarian disease syndrome. In a series of elegant experiments, Knobil (1980) and his associates demonstrated that pulsatile GnRH administration can induce ovulation in immature rhesus monkeys. Crowley and McArthur (1980) replicated this finding in women with IHH, inducing normal ovulatory cycles by administering a fixed dose of GnRH subcutaneously at a frequency of every 2 hours. In normal women, the frequency of gonadotropin secretion varies throughout the menstrual cycle. By altering the interval between doses of GnRH given to women with hypothalamic amenorrhea, it is possible to induce a menstrual cycle with daily sex steroid concentrations similar to those seen in a natural cycle. When the doses are given by IV or subcutaneous route via a portable infusion pump, ovulation and fertility can be achieved.

## Clinical Applications of GnRH Agonist Analogs

After an initial stimulatory phase, longer-acting GnRH analogs suppress the pituitary–gonadal axis by desensitizing the gonadotrope, downregulating GnRH receptors, and inhibiting postreceptor events. In addition, the ratio of bioactive to immunoreactive LH declines with chronic administration of long-acting GnRH agonists. A variety of GnRH analogs with agonist properties have been used in clinical studies, and preparations have been developed that can be administered by subcutaneous injection and nasal spray; long-acting implants are also available (Table 9-47). Efficacious dosing schedules are dependent on the particular analog and the route of administration.

***Central precocious puberty***

In normal children, puberty is heralded by the appearance of nocturnal gonadotropin secretion. Although it is not known what CNS events initiate the pubertal process, activation of GnRH-secreting neurons is believed to be the final neural pathway leading to sexual maturation. The diagnosis of idiopathic precocious puberty is made when puberty begins before the age of 8 in children who lack other obvious causes (e.g., hypothalamic lesions or gonadotropin-independent adrenal or gonadal hypersecretion). The early onset of pubertal levels of sex steroids may lead to premature closure of the epiphyses and ultimate short stature; also the adolescent behavior triggered

**Table 9-47 Gonadotropin-Releasing Hormone Agonist Analogs**

| STRUCTURE | GENERIC NAME | COMMERCIALLY AVAILABLE |
|---|---|---|
| *9-amino acid analogs* | | |
| [D-Trp$^6$, Pro$^9$ Net] GnRH | — | |
| [D-Trp$^6$, NMeLeu$^7$ Pro$^9$ Net] GnRH | Lutrelin | |
| [D-Leu$^6$, Pro$^9$ Net] GnRH | Leuprolide | yes |
| [D-His(Bzl)$^6$, Pro$^9$ Net] GnRH | Histerelin | |
| [D-Ser(tBut)$^6$, Pro$^9$ Net] GnRH | Buserelin | |
| *10-amino acid analogs* | | |
| Native GnRH[a] | Gonadorelin | yes |
| [D-Naphthyl-Ala (2)$^6$] GnRH | Nafarelin | yes |
| [D-Ser(tBut)$^6$, AzaGly$^{10}$] GnRH | Goserelin | yes |
| [D-Trp$^6$] GnRH | Tryptorelin | |

[a]Pyro-Glu-His-Trp-Ser-Tyr-Gly-Leu-Arg-Pro-Gly-$NH_2$
1 2 3 4 5 6 7 8 9 10.

by the hormonal changes can cause profound social difficulties for the child, the family, and the school.

Attempts to suppress the pubertal process, including inhibiting gonadotropin release with medroxyprogesterone, were met with limited success. Long-acting GnRH analogs, however, have been extremely effective in desensitizing the gonadotropes in patients with idiopathic precocious puberty. Within several weeks of therapy, gonadotropin concentrations fall and sex steroid concentrations decline into the prepubertal range. Menses may cease in girls, and boys may experience a decrease in testicular size. The abnormally accelerated rate of skeletal growth may also return to that appropriate for the child's chronological age. Striking amelioration of behavioral difficulties has also been reported. Children can be treated with a GnRH analog for several years, and, when its use is discontinued, normal puberty begins (Merke and Cutler 1996).

***Prostate cancer***

Since prostatic carcinoma is generally an androgen-dependent tumor, attempts to ablate testicular function have long been used for palliative therapy. Both castration and high-dose diethylstilbestrol (a potent estrogen that suppresses the hypothalamic–pituitary–testicular axis) are effective in the majority of patients with metastatic disease. However, castration is not acceptable to many men, and treatment with pharmacologic amounts of estrogens is associated with gynecomastia, thromboembolism, and an increased risk for coronary ischemic events. The use of a GnRH analog to inhibit gonadotrope function has been shown to be as effective a therapy as estrogen (The Leuprolide Study Group 1984; Bolla et al. 1997). Although GnRH analogs do not cause feminizing adverse effects, patients treated with these agents complain of hot flashes, diminished libido, and, in some cases, male erectile dysfunction. Incidentally, these drugs diminish sexual fantasies and desires, and they have been successfully used to treat men with deviant sexual behavior, such as paraphilia (Rosler and Witztun 1998).

During the first week of therapy, GnRH analogs stimulate the pituitary, and, as a result, testosterone concentrations transiently increase before falling to values seen in castrated men (approximately 5 to 10% of normal adult concentrations) by 1 month. This initial, transient rise is associated with a flare in bone pain and other symptoms in approximately 10% of patients with prostate cancer treated with the GnRH analogs alone. Furthermore, adrenal androgen secretion, which is not inhibited by GnRH analogs, continues, providing significant stimulation to the prostatic cancer. Therefore, in order to inhibit androgen action during the initial stimulatory phase of GnRH analog action, and to ablate the effects of adrenal androgens, the antiandrogen flutamide (a nonsteroidal compound that competes with testosterone for binding to the androgen receptor) is often added to the regimen (Crawford et al. 1989). Drugs that inhibit steroid synthesis may also be used.

**PRINCIPLE Desensitization caused by an agonist is preceded by agonist activity. Often, independent pharmacologic measures not dependent upon desensitization must be instituted to treat the disease until receptor desensitization is completed.**

***Gynecologic disease***

Gonadotropin-releasing hormone analogs can also be used to inhibit menstrual function and to produce a marked hypoestrogenic state. Endometriosis is an ectopic proliferation of endometrial tissue that results in pain and infertility. Since endometrial tissue is estrogen-dependent, medical castration induced by the GnRH analogs has proved to be an effective treatment that allows avoidance of both surgery and the use of androgenic steroids that can cause virilization (Moghissi et al. 1998). Uterine fibroids are also dependent on estrogen and may shrink with GnRH analog therapy (Healy et al. 1986).

The GnRH analogs are also used to inhibit secretion of endogenous gonadotropins before the start of exogenous gonadotropin therapy in some women with infertility who are undergoing in vitro fertilization (Damario et al. 1997). GnRH analogs are useful agents for the treatment of severe hirsutism, for which they can be used in conjunction with sex steroids to diminish androgen-dependent hair growth (Rittmaster 1995). The symptoms of the premenstrual syndrome may also abate with the use of GnRH analogs (Schmidt et al. 1998).

As with men, chronic use of the analogs causes hot flashes in women. In addition, prolonged hypoestrogenemia may result in osteoporosis, vaginal dryness, and dyspareunia. Since all GnRH agonist analogs briefly stimulate pituitary gonadotropin secretion before causing desensitization, sex-hormone-dependent diseases may flare during the initial treatment period.

## SOMATOSTATIN AND OCTREOTIDE

### History and Chemistry

Somatostatin is a phylogenetically ancient peptide that is found in all vertebrate classes, many invertebrates, and even protozoa (Berelowitz et al. 1982). Its name derives from the fact that it was initially discovered as an inhibitor of growth hormone (GH) secretion by the anterior pituitary; however, further study has revealed a wide range of biologic functions. The first evidence of its existence came in 1968 during the search for a GH-releasing factor (Krulich et al. 1968). Isolation and purification yielded a cyclic tetradecapeptide (14 amino acids) whose ring structure is the result of a disulfide bond between the third and fourteenth residues from the amino terminus (Fig. 9-39A). Other naturally occurring forms have been discovered, the most common of which, somatostatin-28, contains a 14-amino acid extension at the amino terminus. The relative amounts of these forms secreted varies from tissue to tissue.

## Anatomy

Somatostatin is widely distributed in the body, in concordance with its multiple physiologic roles. In addition to its hypothalamic role in the regulation of GH secretion, somatostatin is a neurotransmitter at multiple sites in the central and peripheral nervous systems (Lamberts et al. 1996). Regulation of multiple aspects of gastrointestinal function is the other major role of somatostatin. It is secreted by delta cells in the intestinal epithelium, pancreatic islets, and visceral autonomic nervous system, where it inhibits gut peptide secretion (e.g., secretion of secretin, gastrin, cholecystokinin), pancreatic endocrine secretion (e.g., insulin, glucagon), pancreatic exocrine secretion (e.g., bicarbonate, digestive enzymes), absorption of nutrients, and smooth muscle contraction.

**PRINCIPLE Somatostatin operates in several modes, functioning as an autocrine, paracrine, or endocrine factor or as a neurotransmitter, while playing regulatory roles in several organ systems.**

Five subtypes of somatostatin receptors have been identified. These membrane-bound receptors, which are coupled to G proteins, utilize a variety of intracellular second messenger systems to affect target cell function. Both the types of somatostatin receptors and the signal transduction mechanisms vary from tissue to tissue.

**PRINCIPLE Through variations in hormone structure, receptor affinity, and post-receptor-signaling events, a hormone related drug can help to regulate a wide range of physiologic functions to varying degrees in different organs.**

H-Ala-Gly-Cys-Lys-Asn-Phe-Phe-Trp-Lys-Thr-Phe-Thr-Ser-Cys-OH

**A**

H-(D)Phe-Cys-Phe-(D)Trp-Lys-Thr-Cys-Thr-ol acetate

**B**

FIGURE 9-39 A. **Primary structure of somatostatin-14.** B. **Primary structure of octreotide.**

## Physiology

Administration of exogenous somatostatin inhibits the secretion of a wide variety of peptide hormones (see Table 9-48). In the anterior pituitary, somatostatin suppresses GH secretion in response to virtually all known stimuli including GHRH, insulin-induced hypoglycemia, arginine infusion, and exercise (Hall et al. 1973; Prange-Hansen et al. 1973). In the pancreas, somatostatin suppresses glucagon secretion more potently than insulin secretion, although the effect on insulin secretion is of greater duration. Consequently, administration of somatostatin-14 in humans produces mild but transient hyperglycemia (Rizza et al. 1979).

In addition to its effects on endocrine organs, somatostatin inhibits many other physiologic activities, including gastric acid secretion, gastric motility, gall bladder emptying, pancreatic enzyme and bicarbonate secretion, visceral blood flow, and intestinal absorption of glucose, amino acids, triglycerides and water. This multitude of effects suggests therapeutic potential for somatostatin in a wide variety of diseases.

However, a number of characteristics of the native hormone make somatostatin unsuitable for clinical use. First, its elimination half-time of 1 to 3 minutes necessitates continuous infusion to sustain its effects. Second, rebound hypersecretion by target organs tends to follow the initial suppression of hormone release following a bolus dose. Because of these limitations, development of analogs with longer durations of action, lack of rebound effect, and narrowed spectra of action is under way.

## Octreotide—A Long-Acting Somatostatin Analog

One somatostatin analog, octreotide, is currently approved by the Food and Drug Administration for clinical use in the United States. Octreotide is a cyclic octapeptide

Table 9-48 **Hormones Inhibited by Somatostatin**

| SOURCE | HORMONE |
|---|---|
| Hypothalamus | GHRH |
| Anterior pituitary | GH |
| | TSH |
| Pancreas | Insulin |
| | Glucagon |
| | Gastrin |
| | Cholecystokinin (CCK) |
| | Secretin |
| | Pepsin |
| | Motilin |
| | Pancreatic polypeptide (PP) |
| | Gastrointestinal peptide (GIP) |
| | Vasoactive intestinal polypeptide (VIP) |
| Kidney | Renin |

with the structure shown in Fig. 9-39B. When administered intravenously, it has a volume of distribution of 18 to 30 L, a distribution half-life of 9 to 14 minutes, and an elimination half-life of 72 to 98 minutes (Kutz et al. 1986). Octreotide is rapidly and completely absorbed following subcutaneous injection, with peak concentrations occurring in 30 to 60 minutes. Its half-life following subcutaneous administration is 88 to 113 minutes. Thirty percent to 40% of the drug is metabolized by the liver, 11% is excreted unchanged in the urine, and less than 2% is excreted in the feces (Kutz et al. 1986; Longnecker 1988). The remainder of the peptide appears to undergo proteolytic degradation in the bloodstream and other tissues.

Octreotide produces almost all the effects of the native hormone, although to varying degrees. In comparison with somatostatin-14, the inhibitory effect of octreotide is 45 times greater on GH secretion, 11 times greater on glucagon secretion, and 1.3 times greater on insulin secretion (Bauer et al. 1982). As with the native hormone, both spontaneous and induced GH pulses are inhibited; however, there is no rebound phenomenon. Glucagon secretion is rapidly suppressed, as are basal and postprandial concentrations of insulin. Placebo-controlled studies in normal volunteers demonstrated a delayed and heightened postprandial peak in blood glucose that persisted for 4 hours after the meal. The delay in blood glucose elevation is attributed to slowing of nutrient absorption from the gut, whereas insulin suppression accounts for the exaggerated peak (Fuessl et al. 1987). Postprandial secretion of pancreatic polypeptide, gastrointestinal peptide, and motilin are inhibited to a greater degree than gastrin. The latter shows a rebound hypersecretion 3 to 4 hours postprandially (Fuessl et al. 1987).

***Treatment of acromegaly***

Chronic hypersecretion of GH produces the clinical syndrome of acromegaly: enlargement of the hands, feet, and jaw, sweating, hypertension, glucose intolerance, arthropathy, and paraesthesias. The vast majority of cases are caused by benign pituitary adenomas. If diagnosed early, resection of the tumor can be curative. However, the insidious onset of this disease often prevents early detection, requiring additional nonsurgical therapy in many cases.

Octreotide has been studied in a large number of acromegalic patients, with generally favorable results. Many symptoms, including fatigue, sweating, headaches, and paresthesias respond within days. The characteristic soft-tissue changes respond more slowly. Octreotide effectively suppresses levels of GH and insulinlike growth factor I (IGF-I), a protein hormone that modulates many of the effects of GH, in the vast majority of patients. In doses of 300 to 600 $\mu$g/day, octreotide lowers GH and IGF-I concentrations in 90% of patients, with normal IGF-I in 70% and GH levels $<5$ $\mu$g/L in most patients. Reversible shrinkage of the pituitary tumor occurs in up to half of patients (Lamberts et al. 1996). No desensitization to its GH-inhibiting effect has been noted with long-term continuous administration. Although octreotide is not first-line therapy for acromegaly, it is a useful adjunct in patients who are not cured by surgery or who are awaiting the slow effects of pituitary irradiation. Octreotide is also important in the management of acromegaly in older patients and others who have high surgical risks.

**PRINCIPLE Unlike the gonadotroph, the somatotroph is not routinely desensitized in vivo by chronic exposure to its trophic or inhibiting hormones.**

### *Treatment of other hormone-secreting tumors*

Because of the suppressive effects of somatostatin on neuroendocrine cells of the gastroenteropancreatic system, octreotide is useful in controlling hormone secretion by tumors arising from these cells. Such tumors secrete a variety of hormones and can cause a variety of endocrine syndromes. Many of these tumors arise in portions of the gastrointestinal tract drained by the portal vein. Because many of the secretory products are inactivated by the liver, the tumors may not produce symptoms until hepatic metastases are present. As a result, therapy in many cases is necessarily medical and palliative. Tumor hypersecretion of insulin, gastrin, glucagon, vasoactive intestinal polypeptide (VIP), or other products (e.g., as seen in patients with carcinoid syndrome) is usually suppressed by octreotide, although growth of subsets of tumor cells not expressing somatostatin receptors may produce secondary failure. Tumor shrinkage is uncommon.

**PRINCIPLE The degree of clinical improvement is frequently greater than the suppression of hormone levels, implicating direct effects of octreotide that are not mediated by hormone(s).**

### *Treatment of upper gastrointestinal hemorrhage*

Somatostatin has many effects on the gastrointestinal system that are unrelated to suppression of hormone secretion. Its suppression of splanchnic blood flow and inhibition of gastric acid secretion make it a potentially useful therapy in upper gastrointestinal hemorrhage due to esophageal varices or other causes.

Although variable short-term effects on portal and intravariceal pressure have been reported, controlled studies in patients with acute variceal hemorrhage have shown improved bleeding control rates and lower complication rates with continuous infusion of somatostatin or octreotide compared with vasopressin analogs (Imperiale and Birgisson 1995). Compared with endoscopic sclerotherapy (the standard treatment for variceal hemorrhage), continuous infusion of somatostatin or octreotide is equally effective in controlling hemorrhage acutely (Avgerinos et al. 1995). However, sclerotherapy is more effective than somatostatin or octreotide in preventing rebleeding (Avgerinos et al. 1995) and therefore remains the treatment of choice. Nonetheless, when emergent sclerotherapy is contraindicated or unavailable, infusion of octreotide is a useful adjunct.

In patients with nonvariceal hemorrhage, infusion of somatostatin or octreotide decreases the risk of continued bleeding or rebleeding by approximately 50% compared with placebo or histamine 2 receptor antagonists (Imperiale and Birgisson 1995). There are also trends toward lower blood transfusion requirements and less need for surgical intervention among patients treated with somatostatin or octreotide. These benefits appear to be most pronounced for patients with hemorrhage due to peptic ulcer rather than for other causes of nonvariceal bleeding (e.g., hemorrhagic gastritis) (Imperiale and Birgisson 1995).

### *Treatment of miscellaneous gastrointestinal disorders*

Identification of somatostatin's effects on numerous functions in the gastrointestinal tract has led to trials of somatostatin or octreotide in a variety of gastrointestinal disorders. In patients with pancreatic fistulas, suppression of pancreatic bicarbonate and enzyme secretion by octreotide diminishes the volume of fistula output, a necessary step in the spontaneous closure of such fistulas (Bassi et al. 1996). However, beneficial effects on actual closure rates or on the need for surgery have not been conclusively established (Bassi et al. 1996). Two large randomized studies have demonstrated decreased postoperative development of pancreatic fistulas in patients undergoing elective pancreatic surgery, suggesting a prophylactic role for octreotide in these patients.

Somatostatin inhibits gastrointestinal motility and intestinal secretion and increases absorption of water and electrolytes, which suggests utility in a variety of diarrheal disorders. As described previously, octreotide is effective in controlling several neuroendocrine tumors associated with diarrhea, including the carcinoid syndrome and VIP-secreting tumors. Octreotide also appears to be effective in patients with chemotherapy-induced diarrhea (Farthing 1996). In patients with short bowel syndrome, statistically significant but clinically modest effects have been found. There is only transient improvement in a minority (up to 20 to 30%) of patients with refractory AIDS-related diarrhea (Farthing 1996).

### *Adverse effects of octreotide*

In accordance with its multiple physiologic effects, a variety of generally mild and transient gastrointestinal adverse effects may occur with octreotide therapy, including abdominal cramping, bloating, nausea, diarrhea, steatorrhea, and flatulence. Pain at the site of subcutaneous injection is also a common complaint. Despite suppression of insulin and glucagon secretion, there is little overall effect on glucose tolerance or glucose levels in diabetic and nondiabetic subjects. Inhibition of cholecystokinin secretion and gall bladder contraction by octreotide promotes bile stasis and the formation of gallstones in 20 to 30% of patients, although symptomatic cholecystitis develops in only 1% per year (Lamberts et al. 1996).

**PRINCIPLE Further work is needed to find analogs of somatostatin with narrowed spectra of action to produce specific targeted actions while minimizing effects on other physiologic functions.**

## REFERENCES

Avgerinos A, Armonis A, Raptis S. 1995. Somatostatin and octreotide in the management of acute variceal hemorrhage. *Hepato Gastroenterol* **42**:145–50.

Bassi C, Falconi M, Caldiron E, et al. 1996. Somatostatin analogs and pancreatic fistulas. *Digestion* **57**(Suppl 1): 94–6.

Bauer W, Briner U, Doepfner W, et al. 1982. SMS 201-995: a very potent and selective octapeptide analog of somatostatin with prolonged action. *Life Sci* **31**:1133–40.

Belchetz PET, Plant TM, Nakai Y, et al. 1978. Hypophyseal responses to continuous and intermittent delivery of hypothalamic gonadotropin-releasing hormone. *Science* **202**:631–3.

Berelowitz M, LeRoith D, Von Schenk H. 1982. Somatostatin-like immunoreactivity and biological activity is present in *Tetrahymena pyriformis,* a ciliated protozoan. *Endocrinology* **110**:1939–44.

Bolla M, Gonzalez D, Warde P, et al. 1997. Improved survival in patients with locally advanced prostate cancer treated with radiotherapy and goserelin. *N Engl J Med* **337**:295–300.

Crawford ED, Eisenberger MA, McLeod DG, et al. 1989. A controlled trial of leuprolide with and without flutamide in prostatic carcinoma. *N Engl J Med* **321**:419–24.

Crowley WF Jr, McArthur JW. 1980. Stimulation of the normal menstrual cycle in Kallmann's syndrome by pulsatile administration of luteinizing hormone-releasing hormone (LHRH). *J Clin Endocrinol Metab* **51**:173–5.

Damario MA, Moomjy M, Tortoriello D, et al. 1997. Delay of gonadotropin stimulation in patients receiving gonadotropin-releasing hormone agonist (GnRH-a) therapy permits increased clinic efficiency and may enhance in vitro fertilization (IVF) pregnancy rates. *Fertil Steril* **68**:1004–10.

Farthing MJG. 1996. The role of somatostatin analogues in the treatment of refractory diarrhea. *Digestion* **57**(Suppl 1):107–13.

Fuessl HS, Burrin JM, Williams G, et al. 1987. The effect of a long-acting somatostatin analog SMS 201–995) on intermediary metabolism and gut hormones after a test meal in normal subjects. *Alimentary Pharm Ther* **1**:321–30.

Hall R, Schally AV, Evered D. 1973. Action of growth hormone release inhibitory hormone in healthy men and acromegaly. *Lancet***2**: 581–4.

Handelsman DJ, Swerdloff RS. 1986. Pharmacokinetics of gonadotropin-releasing hormone and its analogs. *Endocr Rev* **7**:95–105.

Healy DL, Lawson SR, Abbott M, et al. 1986. Toward removing uterine fibroids without surgery: Subcutaneous infusion of a luteinizing hormone-releasing hormone agonist commencing in the luteal phase. *J Clin Endocrinol Metab* **63**:619–25.

Hoffman AR. 1985. Fertility induction in hypothalamic hypogonadism, pp 643–646. In: Cutler GB Jr, moderator. Therapeutic applications of luteinizing-hormone-releasing hormone and its analogs. *Ann Intern Med* **102**:643–57.

Hoffman AR and Crowley WF Jr. 1982. Induction of puberty in men by long-term pulsatile administration of low dose gonadotropin-releasing hormone. *N Engl J Med* **307**:1237–41.

Imperiale TF, Birgisson S. 1997. Somatostatin or octreotide compared with H2 antagonists and placebo in the management of acute non-variceal upper gastrointestinal hemorrhage: a meta-analysis. *Ann Intern Med* **127**:1062–71.

Imperiale TF, Teran JC, McCullough AJ. 1995. A meta-analysis of somatostatin versus vasopressin in the management of acute esophageal variceal hemorrhage. *Gastroenterology* **109**:1289–94.

Karten MJ, Rivier JE. 1986. Gonadotropin-releasing hormone analog design. Structure-function studies toward the development of agonists and antagonists: rationale and perspective. *Endocr Rev* **7**:44–66.

Knobil E. 1980. The neuroendocrine control of the menstrual cycle. *Recent Prog Horm Res* **36**:53–88.

Krulich L, Dhariwal APS, McCann SM. 1968. Stimulatory and inhibitory effects of purified hypothalamic extracts on growth hormone release from rat pituitary in vitro. *Endocrinology* **83**:783–90.

Kutz K, Nuesch E, Rosenthaler J. 1986. Pharmacokinetics of SMS 201–995 in healthy subjects. *Scand J Gastroenterol* **21**(Suppl 119):65–72.

Lamberts SWJ, vanderLely A-J, deHerder WW, et al. 1996. Octreotide. *N Engl J Med* **334**:246–254.

Longnecker SM. 1988. Somatostatin and octreotide: Literature review and description of therapeutic activity in pancreatic neoplasia. *Drug Intell Clin Pharm* **22**:99–106.

Mason AJ, Hayflick JS, Zoeller RT, et al. 1986. A deletion truncating the gonadotropin-releasing hormone gene is responsible for hypogonadism in the *hpg* mouse. *Science* **234**:1366–1371.

Merke DP, and Cutler GB Jr. 1996. Evaluation and management of precocious puberty. *Arch Dis Child* **75**:269–71.

Moghissi KS, Schlaff WD, Olive DL, et al. 1998. Goserelin acetate (Zoladex) with or without hormone replacement therapy for the treatment of endometriosis. *Fertil Steril* **69**:1056–62.

Prange-Hansen A, Orskov H, Seyer-Hansen K, et al. 1973. Some actions of growth hormone release inhibiting factor. *Br Med J* **3**:523–524.

Pyorala S, Huttunen NP, Uhari M. 1995. A review and meta-analysis of hormonal treatment of cryptorchidism. *J Clin Endocrinol Metab* **80**:2795–9.

Rittmaster RS. 1995. Gonadotropin-releasing hormone (GnRH) agonists and estrogen/progestin replacement for the treatment of hirsutism: Evaluating the results. *J Clin Endocrinol Metab* **80**:3403–5.

Rizza R, Verdonk C, Miles J. 1979. Somatostatin does not cause sustained fasting hyperglycemia in man. *Horm Metab Res* **11**:643–644.

Rosler A, Witztum E. 1998. Treatment of men with paraphilia with a long-acting analogue of gonadotropin-releasing hormone. *N Engl J Med* **338**:416–22.

Schmidt PJ, Nieman LK, Danaceau MA, et al. 1998. Differential behavioral effects of gonadal steroids in women with and in those without premenstrual syndrome. *N Engl J Med* **338**:209–16.

The Leuprolide Study Group. 1984. Leuprolide versus diethylstilbestrol for metastatic prostate cancer. *N Engl J Med* **311**:1281–6.

CHAPTER

# 10 CONNECTIVE TISSUE AND BONE DISORDERS

## Rheumatic Disorders

Richard Day, David Quinn, Kenneth Williams, Malcolm Handel, Peter Brooks

*Chapter Outline*



## PATHOGENESIS OF THE RHEUMATIC DISORDERS

Musculoskeletal disorders are the most common reason for disability. Surveys indicate that about 30% of individuals have a musculoskeletal condition at any time, and one-quarter of these have suffered for more than 6 months (Brooks 1996). Arthritis and back pain are the conditions most often reported, and the prevalence of these conditions will increase dramatically with our aging population (Badley and Crotty 1995) (Table 10-1). These conditions can be inflammatory or noninflammatory. The noninflammatory conditions such as soft-tissue pain syndromes and osteoarthritis (OA) are most prevalent and affect older people. The inflammatory conditions such as rheumatoid arthritis (RA) are more threatening because of higher rates of disability and death. An important principle underpinning good management of these conditions is the value of a multidisciplinary approach, with team members contributing to relevant physical, social, psychologic, and educational factors, as well as the pharmacologic issues.

### Soft-Tissue Rheumatic Disorders and Regional Pain Syndromes

These conditions are surprisingly common and include rotator cuff tears of the shoulder joint, frozen shoulder, tennis and golfer's elbows, Achilles tendonitis, heel spurs, and metatarsalgia of the forefoot to name just a few. A careful history and examination usually reveal the injury, overuse, malalignment or other factors leading to the problem (de Jager 1996).

### Back and Neck Pain

Low back and neck pain are very prevalent; up to 85% of the population develops this symptom, and one in six primary care consultations is for this problem. The common variety of low back pain is associated with decreased spinal movement and is considered to be mechanical in origin. Radiation of pain into the thigh and leg in the lower lumbar and sacral nerve distributions is also common. It is common to have the initial episode in middle age, and about 90% of patients recover spontaneously. However, recurrence occurs in 20 to 60%. A small proportion of the latter will go on to chronic back pain, which is a difficult condition to manage and has massive direct and indirect financial costs for society (Borenstein and Weisel 1989; Frymoyer and Cats-Baric 1991; Cohen 1996; Borenstein 1997).

A careful history and examination will generally suggest important but unusual causes such as secondary malignancy, infection, or an inflammatory process such as ankylosing spondylitis (Table 10-2). Otherwise the exact cause of pain in the common variety of transient lower back or neck pain is uncertain. It is important to ascertain whether there is significant impingement on lumbar or sacral nerves manifest by muscle wasting, saddle and lower limb anesthesia and loss of muscle power, and diminished or absent knee or ankle reflexes. The possible need to decompress involved nerves is thereby raised. Much more commonly, associated leg pain is referred from nonneural structures such as zygapophyseal joints. There is much overinvestigation of simple back pain re-

Table 10-1 The Major Rheumatic Disorders

| GROUP | NAME | COMMENT ON CAUSES |
|---|---|---|
| Soft-tissue rheumatism and some regional pain syndromes | Strains and sprains | Trauma |
| | Fibrositis | Overuse |
| | Tissue and tendon injuries | Trauma |
| | Fibromyalgia syndrome | Unknown cause; younger patients |
| Spinal pain | Back and neck pain | Mechanical |
| Cartilage degenerative | Osteoarthritis | Multifactorial causes leading to loss of cartilage |
| Inflammatory arthritis | Rheumatoid arthritis | Inflammatory synovitis of unknown cause |
| | Spondyloarthropathies | |
| | –ankylosing spondylitis | Sacroiliac joints and back involved |
| | –psoriatic arthritis | Back and joints variously involved |
| | –reactive, e.g., Reiter syndrome | Postinfectious |
| | –associated with inflammatory bowel disease | Ulcerative colitis and Crohn disease |
| | –undifferentiated spondyloarthropathy | Features typical of spondyloarthropathies |
| Systemic connective tissue diseases | Systemic lupus erythematosus | Autoimmune, immune complex mediated |
| | Systemic sclerosis (progressive systemic sclerosis; scleroderma) | Autoimmune; limited and generalized varieties |
| | Dermato- and polymyositis | Autoimmune |
| Vasculitis syndromes | Polyarteritis nodosa | Autoimmune, renal failure common |
| | Wegener granulomatosis | Autoimmune; lung and kidney involved; rapidly fatal without immunosuppressive treatment |
| | Polymyalgia rheumatica | Autoimmune; diagnosis often missed |
| | Giant cell arteritis | Autoimmune; often associated with polymyalgia rheumatica |
| | Churg-Strauss | |
| Crystal-induced arthritis | Gout | Sodium urate monohydrate crystals in joints |
| | Calcium pyrophosphate deposition disease (CPPD) | Calcium pyrophosphate crystals in joints |

Table 10-2 Clinical Approach to Evaluation of Neck and Back Pain

| STEPS | COMMENT |
|---|---|
| Is the problem mechanical? | This explains most spinal pain—painful, limited spinal movements in the absence of systemic disease. Tenderness is diffuse. |
| What is the anatomic origin of the mechanical pain? | Inferred from location of tenderness and referred limb pain, by firm palpation over spinous processes and para-spinal structures. |
| Is associated limb pain (if present) radicular or somatic referred? | Important distinction for investigation and management. Radicular pain may require surgical intervention. Radicular pain is located to defined sclerotomes, is dysesthetic (shooting, burning, etc.) and accompanied by myotomal weakness or sclerotomal hyper or hypoesthesia; somatic referred pain is diffuse, poorly localized, dull and aching in nature and with no accompanying signs. |
| What are the psychosocial components? | Major contributors to chronicity following the acute disorder (Merskey 1993; Weiser and Cedraschi 1992). When distress appears in excess of any somatic contribution, behavioral, affective, and cognitive factors should be sought by simple inquiry of the patient (Cohen 1996). |

sulting in unnecessary high cost and, in some cases, promotion of behavior associated with illness and the development of the chronic pain syndrome. Avoidance of the latter by good management of the acute painful neck or back is a primary objective.

## Fibromyalgia Syndrome

There has been some controversy concerning the fibromyalgia syndrome, which is characterized by widespread musculoskeletal pain and abnormal soft-tissue tenderness commonly localized to identified tender points (Littlejohn 1998) (Table 10-3). The condition has no readily discernible cause on examination or investigation. Fibromyalgia is a disorder of the functioning of the pain system, perhaps owing to central sensitization of the pain-transmitting neurones of uncertain cause. It is prevalent, affecting 3 to 5% of the community; the female-to-male ratio is 6 to 1. This condition can be a cause of major disability for an individual and her or his family. It is important to make a confident diagnosis based on a good history and examination. There are no diagnostic laboratory findings.

## Osteoarthritis

Osteoarthritis (OA) is the most prevalent of the rheumatic disorders and affects about 10% of the population with a steep increase with age. Cartilage is lost from joints; the hips and knees are commonly affected along with the distal and proximal finger joints and the base of the thumb. The condition is more prevalent in women. Symptoms initially are pain and stiffness after inactivity, but as cartilage is lost, so also is function, for example, the ability to walk up and down stairs. Bony enlargement of affected joints is observed, which is a reaction to the loss of cartilage, and the joint has a reduced range of movement. Low-level inflammation can be observed and may be due to cartilage debris released into the joint, although this is disputed (March 1997).

The cartilage is composed of ground substance (glycosaminoglycans) held in place by a network of type II collagen fibers with chondrocytes embedded in the matrix responsible for synthesis and turnover of the cartilage components. The etiology of the loss of cartilage in OA is not fully understood, but the biochemical lesion is likely to be multifactorial in origin including genetic, traumatic, and developmental factors with the eventual result of joint failure.

## Rheumatoid Arthritis

Rheumatoid arthritis is primarily an inflammatory condition of the synovium of the joints, which leads to pain and morning stiffness and ultimately to joint damage and disability. The natural history and intensity of disease varies from mild and transient to inexorably progressive with multisystem involvement and general symptoms such as anemia, fever, weakness, and anorexia. Most individuals have a fluctuating, but progressive course with 50% chance of inability to work within 10 years and a short-

**Table 10-3 Features of the Fibromyalgia Syndrome**

| FEATURES | COMMENT |
|---|---|
| Chronic pain | Generalized or local |
| Low pain threshold | Generalized or local; tender points—18 "classic points" which are highly predictive for the condition |
| Allodynia | Pain in response to normally nonnoxious stimuli such as light touch |
| Dermatographia | Observed after palpating skin |
| Tiredness | Can be profound |
| Abnormal sleep | Sense of disturbed and inadequate sleep |
| Psychologic distress | Depression, anxiety, low self-esteem etc. |
| Associated features | Irritable bowel syndrome, morning stiffness or gel, subjective swelling of limbs, headaches, dysesthesias (pins and needles, numbness), Raynaud phenomenon |
| Can occur in conjunction with other rheumatic conditions such as OA, RA, and SLE | |
| Pain changes with various factors including weather, stress, physical activity | Large variations in patterns of pain |

ABBREVIATIONS: OA, osteoarthritis; RA, rheumatoid arthritis; and SLE, systemic lupus erythematosus.
SOURCE: Adapted from Littlejohn 1996.

ened life expectancy similar to those with Hodgkin disease or three-vessel coronary heart disease (Pincus 1988). About 1% of the world's population is affected. Women are three times more likely than men to acquire RA, and the disease can present at any age, although 25–50 years of age is most common. Commonly RA manifests with symmetrical polyarthritis of the small joints of the hands and feet and with one or more of the large joints such as knees or shoulders. There are symptoms and signs of inflammation such as morning stiffness of the limbs and tiredness, swelling, and tenderness of affected joints. Typical deformities of the hands and feet follow from the involvement of tendon sheaths and ligamentous laxity (Ahern and Smith 1997).

There is a genetic disposition to RA linked to histocompatibility antigens HLA DR 1 and 4. This genetic susceptibility has been related to a 5-amino acid sequence on the third hypervariable region of the HLA DR molecule, critical in presentation of antigen to T lymphocytes. Prominent synovial features are marked synovial lining cell hyperplasia, T-lymphocyte infiltration, and vascular proliferation of the synovium, as well as aggressive, inflammatory tissue at the attachment to bone known as pannus. The neutral proteinase enzymes collagenase and stromelysin along with superoxide and other free radical species are secreted into the joint. There is activation of the cellular and humoral immune responses and major involvement of chemokines, cell adhesion molecules, and cytokines, in particular tumor necrosis factor alpha (TNF$\alpha$) and interleukin 1 (IL-1). Extra-articular manifestations including vasculitis, peripheral neuropathy, and rheumatoid nodules occur in more severe cases.

The result of this intense process is loss of cartilage, bony erosions around the margins of the joint, and, ultimately, destruction of the joint. We know now that bone erosions appear within 2 years of onset and surmise that cartilage lesions occur even earlier (Emery 1994).

## Spondyloarthropathies

Spondyloarthropathies form a group of conditions (Table 10-4) that manifest as inflammation in the spine and peripheral joints, but are distinct from rheumatoid arthritis, particularly in the absence of rheumatoid factor in the serum. The members of this group share a number of features (Table 10-4), and there are many variations on the features exhibited by an individual (Edmonds 1997).

## Polymyalgia Rheumatica

The diagnosis of polymyalgia rheumatica is important to make because substantial distress and disability remain unrelieved. Second, there is a significant danger of sudden blindness due to concurrent giant cell arthritis unless appropriate treatment is instituted (Zilko 1996; Hunder 1997; Swannell 1997). The condition is characterized by pain and often intense stiffness around the shoulder and pelvic girdles, more so in the morning. The condition occurs in elderly (>65 years) individuals who become unwell often quite rapidly. There may be night sweats. The erythrocyte sedimentation rate (ESR) is usually elevated and is often very high. The clinician's main task is to exclude other conditions including malignancy, infections, and other connective tissue disorders such as RA or systemic lupus erythematosus (SLE). The condition is exquisitely sensitive to glucocorticosteroid therapy. It is associated with giant cell arteritis, which is a vasculitic condition affecting arteries arising from the arch of the aorta. Visual disturbances and unusual headaches along with feelings of malaise with a high ESR are typical of this condition, which may present independent of polymyalgia rheumatica. Scalp tenderness and jaw claudication on chewing are characteristic. The temporal arteries may be nodular, tender, and generally thickened. A temporal artery biopsy is recommended for diagnostic purposes.

## Systemic Lupus Erythematosus

Systemic lupus erythematosus is a multisystem, inflammatory, chronic connective tissue disorder most common in women of child-bearing age (Mills 1994). Clinical manifestations most commonly seen are arthralgia, a typical rash (facial malar rash), nephritis, cytopenias, mucositis, and cerebritis (Table 10-5). Precipitating factors identified include ultraviolet (UV) light, drugs, and possibly pregnancy. Susceptibility is increased in individuals with HLA-DR2 or HLA-DR3 or with certain complement component deficiencies, namely, C2 and C4. Immunologically, B-lymphocyte overactivity is evident with high titers of antinuclear autoantibodies with a homogenous appearance and the presence of anti-double-stranded DNA and Sm autoantibodies, which have high diagnostic sensitivity and specificity (Tan et al. 1982). Immune complexes are likely to account for some of the manifestations of this disease, in particular glomerulonephritis (Mills 1994).

## Progressive Systemic Sclerosis

Progressive systemic sclerosis is a rare connective tissue disorder characterized by fibrosis of the skin and visceral organs along with a microvascular disorder and is four

Table 10-4 **Features of the Spondyloarthropathies**

| Spondyloarthropathies (Can have any of the features listed in next column) | Features of the spondyloarthropathies | Comment about feature |
|---|---|---|
| Ankylosing spondylitis | Enthesopathy | Inflammatory reaction at site of insertion of ligaments, e.g., Achilles tendon insertion into heel |
| Reactive arthritis (includes Reiter syndrome) | Synovitis | Usually asymmetric involvement and often lower limb joints |
| Psoriatic arthritis and spondylitis | Sacroiliitis | Inflammation of sacroiliac joint that is usually bilateral |
| Enteropathic arthritis and spondylitis (ulcerative colitis, Crohn disease) | Spondylitis | Inflammation of the spine—inflammation of zygapophyseal joints and enthesitis at ligament attachments |
| Late onset, pauciarticular juvenile rheumatoid arthritis | Dactylitis | Sausage-shaped digits; asymmetric joint involvement contrasts with rheumatoid arthritis |
| Undifferentiated spondyloarthropathy | Extra-articular inflammation | Iritis (ankylosing spondylitis), psoriasis and psoriasiform rashes; nail changes (pitting); bowel inflammation, e.g., ulcerative colitis or Crohn disease; urethritis or diarrhea (Reiter syndrome or reactive arthritis) |
| | Presence of HLA B27 | Ranges from 90% of ankylosing spondylitis, 70% of reactive arthritis, and 50% of psoriatic arthritis patients |
| | Family history | Often different types of spondyloarthropathies in one family |

times more common in women (Systemic sclerosis 1996c; Rasaratnam and Ryan 1997b). The etiology is unknown. Related disorders have been linked to exposure to L-tryptophan, vinyl chloride, and other environmental agents. Clinical features can include Raynaud's phenomenon, polyarthralgia, and polyarthritis, and most characteristically, skin thickening over the fingers, hands, extensor aspects of the forearms, around the mouth and nose and around the throat. Rates of progression are extremely variable. Skin involvement can be limited to the distal extremities or widespread. The CREST (calcinosis, Raynaud's phenomenon, esophageal dysmotility, sclerodactyly, telangectasia) variant manifests limited skin involvement and gradual involvement of other organs such as lungs, kidneys, esophagus, and heart. Renal failure is the major cause of death and is more common in the diffuse variety of the disease.

## Polymyositis and Dermatomyositis

Polymyositis and dermatomyositis are conditions most common in younger women and in Blacks (Dalakas 1991). Autoimmune mechanisms are suspected, with the presence of autoantibodies, such as antinuclear antibody, and biopsy findings of muscle fibers that are attacked by CD8 receptor-positive lymphocytes and macrophages. The skin involvement is characteristic with a macular, erythematous rash over face and upper trunk; a bluish discoloration on the upper eyelid (the so-called *heliotrope rash*); and marked, raised erythema over the knuckles

Table 10-5 **Clinical Features of Systemic Lupus Erythematosus**

| System (% involvement) | Features |
|---|---|
| Musculoskeletal (95%) | Arthralgia, arthritis, myopathy |
| Skin and mucosa (80%) | Malar rash, photosensitivity, alopecia, vasculitis, oral ulcers |
| Hematologic (95%) | Anemia (chronic disease variety), leukopenia, thrombocytopenia |
| Renal | Abnormal renal biopsy in all, nephritis, renal failure |
| Cardiopulmonary (60%) | Pericarditis, pleurisy, pleural effusion |
| Neurologic (60%) | Cognitive disorders, organic brain syndrome, seizures |
| Constitutional (95%) | Fever, fatigue, weight loss, malaise |
| Immunologic | Infections, positive antinuclear antibodies, and autoantibodies: anti-double-stranded DNA, anti-Sm antibodies |

SOURCE: From Rasaratnam and Ryan 1997.

(Gottron's sign). In both conditions there is symmetric proximal muscle weakness, with about half the patients noting muscle tenderness. Other features include oropharyngeal involvement causing dysphagia and interstitial lung involvement, leading to dyspnea and myocarditis. Concomitant malignancy should be considered in cases of adult dermatomyositis. The diagnosis is confirmed by significantly elevated levels of plasma creatinine phosphokinase (CPK) and a characteristic electromyographic pattern and muscle biopsy (Day and Pearson 1981).

### Vasculitis

Vasculitis encompasses those conditions characterized by inflammation of blood vessel walls (Allen and Bressler 1997; Gross 1997; Jennette and Falk 1997). It can be a primary disorder such as polyarteritis nodosa or Wegener's granulomatosis or part of a multisystem disease such as Systemic lupus erythematosis (SLE) (Danning et al. 1998). The condition is classified also by the size of blood vessels involved and the various clinical syndromes associated with it (Table 10-1) (Fries, Hunder, et al. 1990). Typically, vasculitis is caused by immune-complex deposition in blood vessel walls, leading to an inflammatory reaction (Nowack et al. 1998; Sneller and Fauci 1997). Early and aggressive therapy is important for survival in a number of these conditions (Allen and Bressler 1997; Gross 1997).

### Gout and Calcium Pyrophosphate Deposition Disease

An attack of gout results from intense inflammation in joints, which in turn results from the precipitation of monosodium urate monohydrate into needle-shaped crystals. Phagocytes are disrupted, leading to release of metalloproteinase enzymes such as collagenase, superoxide, and other free radicals and various other proinflammatory mediators. A first attack usually reflects a substantial number of years of hyperuricemia, which may be primary (reduced renal clearance or excessive synthesis of uric acid) or secondary (drug-induced such as low-dose aspirin or thiazide diuretics, renal impairment, dietary and alcohol excess). Urate may also deposit in other tissues such as the renal tubules leading to renal calculi and as tophi commonly found around extensor surfaces such as the elbow.

Calcium pyrophosphate deposition disease (CPPD) manifests in a number of ways, but most dramatic is an acute inflammatory reaction in joints, reminiscent of acute gout, hence the name *acute pseudogout*. CPPD can also resemble OA, but is one of the reasons for apparently premature or accelerated OA. Radiographs of affected joints, such as the wrists or various finger joints, commonly show calcification of cartilage. The condition may sometimes resemble RA. The cause of the pain and inflammation is the formation of calcium pyrophosphate crystals in joints leading to an acute reaction with recruitment of large numbers of polymorphs. CPPD is associated rarely with hemachromatosis, Wilson's disease, hyperparathyroidism, and other unusual conditions.

### Drug-Induced Rheumatic and Immune Disease

Drug-induced lupus erythematosus is generally less severe than the spontaneous variety, but fever, rashes, and pleuritic involvement are often more intense. The condition reverses when the causative drug is withdrawn, but sometimes corticosteroid therapy is needed. Antinuclear antibody is positive, double-stranded DNA and Sm autoantibodies are not found, and antihistone antibodies are often detected. The common drugs causing this problem are listed in (Table 10-6). A number such as procainamide and hydralazine rely on hepatic acetylation for detoxification, and slow acetylators who have defective acetylation enzymes are prone to drug-induced lupus (Alarcon-Segovia and Kraus 1991).

Serum sickness reactions are common with antibiotics such as sulfur-containing antibiotics leading to arthralgias and arthritis along with skin rashes. Dramatic reactions can follow immunization against influenza and rubella, and they often require moderate doses of corticosteroids to control.

Numerous drugs have been suspected of causing painless or painful myopathies, often with concomitant drug-induced neuropathy (Le Quintrec and Le Quintrec 1991).

## DRUGS USED TO TREAT RHEUMATIC DISEASES

### Nonopioid Analgesics

Acetaminophen is a valuable analgesic and antipyretic and is effective when given in appropriate doses. The drug has no appreciable anti-inflammatory action in humans. It is a very weak inhibitor of cyclooxygenase and will inhibit this enzyme only if there are high concentrations of peroxides present, such as may be found in inflammatory lesions (Marshall et al. 1987). There is still uncertainty regarding the mechanism of its analgesic action (Graham

Table 10-6 Drug-Induced Musculoskeletal Disorders

| CONDITION | DRUGS | COMMENTS |
|---|---|---|
| Drug-induced lupus | Procainamide HCl, hydralazine HCl, INH, quinidine sulfate or gluconate, phenytoin, chlorpromazine HCl | Slow acetylators have greatest risk |
| Arthritis and arthralgias | Sulfonamides, INH, pyrazinamide, ethionamide, oral contraceptives, corticosteroids, quinidine sulfate or gluconate, rubella and influenza vaccine | Serum sickness reaction common with sulfonamides; withdrawal of corticosteroids associated with arthralgias |
| Acute gout | Low-dose aspirin, diuretics, alcohol, cytotoxic drugs, pyrazinamide | Aspirin and diuretics inhibit renal excretion of urate; cytotoxic drugs cause breakdown of nucleoproteins |
| Muscle pain; cramps | HMG-CoA reductase inhibitors, diuretics, clofibrate, corticosteroids, estrogen and oral contraceptives, succinylcholine chloride | |
| Aseptic necrosis | Corticosteroids | Especially pulse-steroid regimens |
| Bone growth inhibition | Corticosteroids, tetracyclines | Children |
| Osteoporosis | Corticosteroids, heparin, methotrexate sodium | Methotrexate osteoporosis seen prepubertally |
| Painless myopathy: nonneuropathic | Corticosteroids, $\beta$-adrenergic receptor blockers | |
| Painless myopathy: neuropathic | Colchicine, chloroquine HCl, hydroxychloroquine sulfate | |
| Painful myopathy; nonneuropathic | Penicillamine, cimetidine, penicillin, sulfonamides, propylthiouracil, quinolone antibiotics, clofibrate, HMG-CoA reductase inhibitors, cyclosporine, enalapril maleate, etretinate, metoprolol succinate, minoxidil, zidovudine | |
| Painful myopathy; neuropathic | Tryptophan (eosinophilic myalgia syndrome); vincristine sulfate, amiodarone HCl | |

ABBREVIATIONS: HMG-CoA, hydroxymethylglutaryl-coenzyme A; INH, isoniazid.
SOURCE: From Brooks 1997.

et al. 1998). Its antipyretic actions are considered to be due to prostaglandin synthesis inhibition in the hypothalamus. Peak analgesic actions are observed about 2.5 hours after oral dosing, and data conflict on the time course of loss of analgesic activity (Graham et al. 1998).

Acetaminophen is as effective as NSAIDs administered in anti-inflammatory doses when given to patients with OA (Bradley et al. 1991). This holds true even in those OA patients exhibiting the features of inflammation (Bradley et al. 1992). Because of the availability of acetaminophen over the counter (OTC), many people (and physicians) need reassurance that the drug is efficacious as an analgesic. Again this relates to adequate and sustained dosing. Unfortunately, patients have commonly tried 1 to 2 acetaminophen tablets or capsules occasionally and have prematurely discontinued the drug because of disappointment with the result.

The plasma half-life is 1 to 3 hours, and thus dosing is usually every 6 hours, with a maximum daily dose of 4 g in otherwise healthy adults. This dose produces peak plasma concentrations of about 15 mg/L. The drug is not protein-bound. A major advantage for acetaminophen is its lack of gastrointestinal toxicity, especially ulceration and bleeding. Hepatotoxicity is mostly seen with drug overdose but can occur rarely in patients with liver disease who have taken the drug in high dose. The daily dose should be carefully monitored in these situations. Regular high-dose acetaminophen is reputed to enhance the effect of warfarin, but the degree of effect and level of evidence for a significant interaction is low (Bartle and Blakely 1991). Background use of acetaminophen with NSAIDs can reduce the daily dose of NSAIDs in RA and OA patients without loss of overall analgesic efficacy, with a reduction in the risk for upper GI toxicity (Seideman and Melander 1988; Seideman et al. 1993).

## Opioid Analgesics in Rheumatic Diseases

The appropriate use of opioids in the management of the musculoskeletal disorders is a contentious and evolving issue (Graziotti and Goucke 1997). On the one hand, short-term use for acute problems of short duration such as acute mechanical back pain is appropriate. However, opioid use in chronic pain patients is much more problematic. This is because many of the patients are elderly, and adverse effects become very important. Thus constipation, cognitive impairment, drowsiness, risk of falling, and dependence all become critical issues.

The opioids most commonly used in the treatment of the rheumatic diseases are codeine and dextropropoxyphene, usually in combination with aspirin or acetaminophen. With the availability of slow-release morphine and other opioid formulations such as fentanyl came increasing use in patients with chronic pain problems. It has been surprisingly difficult to show incremental efficacy by adding codeine to acetaminophen. It appears that a minimum of 20 mg of codeine added to acetaminophen in a regular dosing regimen is needed to show any increment in pain relief over the usual dose of acetaminophen alone. This translates to a daily intake of between 120 and 240 mg codeine for treating a chronic condition. This dosage of codeine can be achieved by formulations that combine codeine at 15 to 30 mg with acetaminophen at 500 mg (Kjaersgaard-Andersen et al. 1990; de Craen et al. 1996).

Codeine has a first-pass metabolism of about 60% and a half-life of 2 to 4 hours. It is an extremely weak ligand for opioid receptors. About 10% of codeine is metabolized by cytochrome P450 2D6 to morphine, which is the active metabolite of codeine. Genetic polymorphisms of CYP 2D6 mean that about 8 to 10% of individuals will be unable to transform codeine to morphine, and the drug will be ineffective. Morphine is metabolized by glucuronidation largely in the liver. Morphine 6-glucuronide is an active metabolite with a longer half-life than morphine and is retained in renal impairment. Therefore, analgesic efficacy and careful monitoring for adverse effects is needed especially in the elderly.

Although dextropropoxyphene has been shown in some studies to add to the analgesic efficacy of acetaminophen in patients with rheumatic conditions, its use is not generally condoned in the chronic musculoskeletal disorders. The drug has been associated with some sudden and unpredictable cardiac deaths especially in overdose, but there is the suspicion that this may occur in elderly patients with coronary artery disease and renal impairment. Alcohol may contribute to this adverse effect. An oxidative metabolite, nor-dextropropoxyphene is considered to be cardiotoxic (Chan and Matzke 1987). The drug is dangerous in overdose when combined with acetaminophen.

Other opioids are used in the musculoskeletal disorders, notably oxycodone, if combination analgesics containing codeine have not been satisfactory, and, increasingly, oral slow-release morphine formulations and methadone are used by physicians specializing in treating chronic musculoskeletal pain.

## Nonsteroidal Anti-Inflammatory Drugs

Nonsteroidal anti-inflammatory drugs (NSAIDs) are widely used for their anti-inflammatory and analgesic properties, accounting for about 10% of all prescribing. NSAIDS are increasingly available over the counter. Up to 20% of elderly individuals take NSAIDs regularly, which raises important questions concerning community safety (Brooks and Day 1991). Of interest has been a recent worldwide decline in usage. In Australia there has been a 25% drop in usage, particularly in elderly OA patients, and this has been linked to educational programs and copayments for NSAIDs by patients (McManus et al. 1996). The indications for this class of drugs are broadening from the rheumatic diseases and various pain states such as cancer pain and biliary and renal colic to include possibly Alzheimer disease and colon cancer prevention. In addition, NSAIDs have antipyretic actions useful in pediatric practice in particular. Increasingly, NSAIDs are applied topically, and there is good evidence for their efficacy, in acute and chronic pain conditions, and their safety by this route (Moore et al. 1998). There is substantial interpatient variability in response to NSAIDs in the rheumatic diseases, which is still not fully understood.

**PRINCIPLE Some of the most useful indications for a drug become evident only after it is marketed.**

### *Mechanism of action*

NSAIDs are typically weak acids. They therefore sequester into cells found in acid environments such as the stomach, kidney, and inflamed joint, important sites of therapeutic and toxic actions of NSAIDs, through a process known as ion-trapping (Brune and Graft 1978). Inhibition of cyclooxygenase and the subsequent production of prostaglandins accounts for the therapeutic and toxic effects of NSAIDs (Vane 1971). Recently the discovery of two isoforms of cyclooxygenase, namely, COX-1 and COX-2, has revealed an important new rationale for the contrasts in effects between NSAIDs (Frolich 1995; Bahkle and Botting 1996). COX-1 is constitutive and responsible for normal physiologic function in platelets, the GI tract, and kidney. COX-2 is induced in inflammatory sites and has a limited distribution in brain, kidney, and testes (Fig. 10-1). The inhibitory potency against the two isoforms varies between NSAIDs (Luong et al. 1996). It would appear that an optimal NSAID for the rheumatic

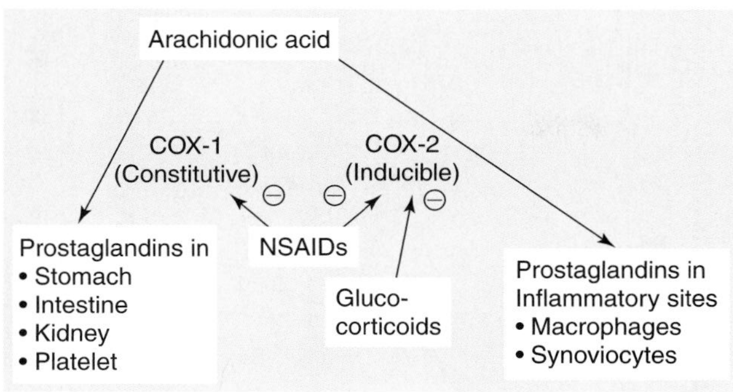


**FIGURE 10-1 Schema illustrating the metabolism of arachidonic acid by either the constitutive cyclooxygenase (COX-1) or the inducible form (COX-2). (From Needleman and Isakson 1997 with the permission of the publishers.)**

diseases will be a potent inhibitor of COX-2 but a weak or noninhibitor of COX-1. MK 966 and celecoxib are two such drugs now known as highly selective COX-2 inhibitors (Vane 1995), which are efficacious and appear substantially safer for the GI tract. NSAIDs are also reported to perturb a number of other processes important in inflammation, such as the production of the superoxide anion and intracellular transduction mechanisms in polymorphs, although there is no convincing confirmation of the significance of these effects for anti-inflammatory effect in vivo (Furst 1994). Contrasting mechanisms of action between NSAIDs, including ratios of COX-2/1 inhibitory efficacy, might result in interpatient differences in the response to NSAIDs, however (Brooks and Day 1991).

### *Pharmacokinetics*

Considerable interpatient differences in pharmacokinetic properties of NSAIDs have been observed. Also, relationships between plasma NSAID concentration and anti-inflammatory response have been demonstrated in RA (Fig. 10-2) and postoperative pain (Day et al. 1982; Laska et al. 1986; Dunagan et al. 1988). There is a clear relationship between NSAID daily dose and the risk of serious upper GI bleeding or perforation (Carson et al. 1987; Griffin et al. 1991; Langman et al. 1994). Dose and plasma concentrations of salicylates predict ototoxicity, and a linear relationship between plasma concentrations of salicylate and the intensity of tinnitus and degree of hearing loss has been demonstrated (Day et al. 1989). Thus pharmacokinetic factors do contribute to response variability in some patients, and some knowledge of the pharmacokinetics of these drugs will be useful in optimal selection and use of NSAIDs. NSAIDs are weak acids and characteristically exhibit low first-pass metabolism, good bioavailability, extensive binding to plasma albumin, and small volumes of distribution.

**PRINCIPLE Some but not necessarily all of a drug's effects may be linked to the drug's pharmacokinetic properties.**

**ABSORPTION** Bioavailability of NSAIDs is generally excellent. Exceptions are diclofenac with 54% bioavailability (Willis et al. 1979) and aspirin with 70% (Rowland et al. 1972). The rate of absorption of NSAIDs is slower when taken with meals than when fasting. However, it is recommended that the NSAIDs be taken with food to decrease gastric irritation. Dosing concurrent with antacids can also improve gastric tolerance but will not reduce the risk of serious complications such as bleeding. Generally, the extent of absorption is not affected by food or antacids (Day et al. 1987).

Aspirin is often administered as enteric or slow-release formulations, since plain or soluble forms cause too much gastric irritation. There may be considerable delay before enteric-coated tablets reach the small intestine where release and absorption occur. This is probably not significant at high, anti-inflammatory doses when the half-life of salicylate is about 15 hours. Although upper GI

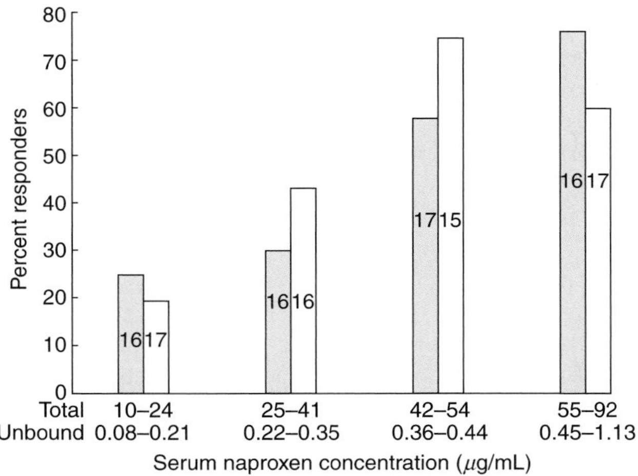


**FIGURE 10-2 Relationship between total (solid bars) and unbound (white bars) plasma concentrations of naproxen and response in patients with RA using a summed efficacy score. (From Day RO, Furst DE, Dromgoole SH, et al. 1982. Relationship of serum naproxen concentration to efficacy in rheumatoid arthritis. *Clin Pharmacol Ther* 31:733–40, with permission of the publisher, © Mosby.)**

symptoms are lessened, the risk of serious upper GI complications is not reduced (Kelly et al. 1996). Sustained-release tablets of NSAIDs with short half-lives have been developed to prolong their effect, but no therapeutic advantage has been demonstrated except that administration is less frequent. This may relate to the observation that synovial fluid concentration profiles remain essentially unchanged compared with the conventional immediate-release formulations. Thus, ketoprofen SR can be administered once daily versus twice to three times daily. There is uncertainty concerning the effect of sustained-release NSAIDs on the GI tract. Although Collins and coworkers (1988) found no difference on endoscopic examination between immediate and slow-release preparations of ketoprofen, it has been suggested that the greater relative risk for serious GI toxicity of ketoprofen compared with ibuprofen could be a function of the slow-release formulation (Henry et al. 1996).

**DISTRIBUTION AND PROTEIN BINDING** NSAIDs bind strongly to albumin in plasma, so that the volumes of distribution of the NSAIDs are low. Binding to plasma albumin is reversible, and an equilibrium exists between drug bound to albumin (bound drug) and unbound drug (free drug). Free drug diffuses across membranes and binds to the cyclooxygenase enzymes. The unbound fraction (free drug/free plus bound drug) is affected by many factors including plasma albumin concentrations, gender, age, pregnancy, drugs that compete for binding, and kidney and hepatic impairment. The unbound fraction of NSAIDs increases when plasma albumin is low from any cause and in renal failure. It is noteworthy that free drug concentrations of naproxen are found to be higher in the elderly and as RA activity increases, and this must be related to decreased clearance of free drug in these situations (van den Ouweland et al. 1987)

As dosages of naproxen, phenylbutazone, salicylate, and possibly ibuprofen increase, a less than proportional increase in total NSAID plasma concentrations is observed. This is because binding sites on albumin saturate. However, the unbound concentrations continue to increase linearly with dose. For example, total plasma concentrations of naproxen approach a plateau with increasing doses above 750 mg per day, but the unbound concentrations of naproxen increase in proportion with the dose (Fig. 10-3). An exception is seen with salicylate. Not only is there saturation of albumin binding, but the metabolism of salicylate is also saturable (zero order), so that unbound as well as total concentrations of salicylate increase disproportionately with dose (Furst et al. 1979; Bochner et al. 1987) (Fig. 10-4).

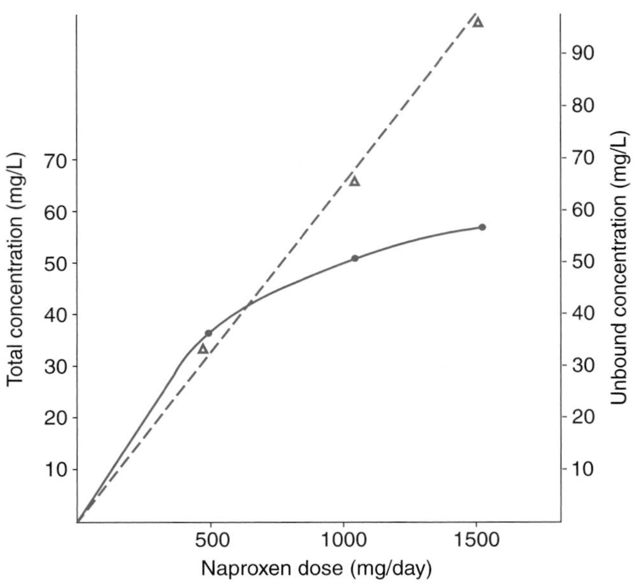


**FIGURE 10-3 Total (solid line) and unbound (dashed line) concentrations of naproxen in plasma versus daily dose of naproxen illustrating the linear increase in unbound concentrations with increasing dose. (From Dunagan FM, McGill PE, Kelman AW, et al. 1988. Naproxen dose and concentration: Response relationship in rheumatoid arthritis. *Br J Rheumatol* 27:48–53, with permission of the publishers.)**

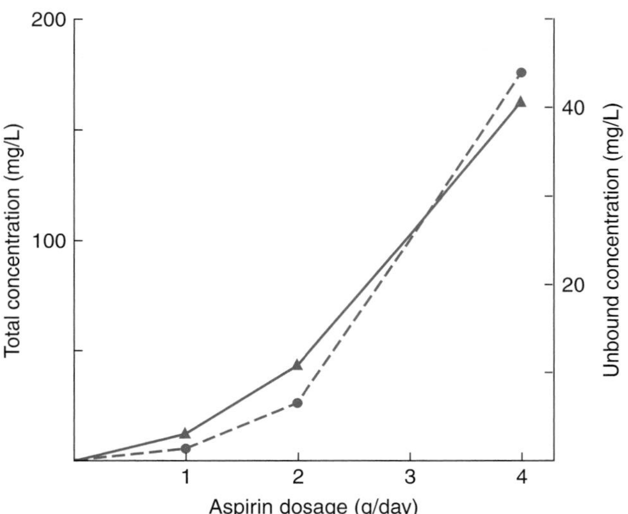


**FIGURE 10-4 Relationships between total (solid line) and unbound (dashed line) concentrations of salicylate and increasing daily dosage with aspirin. Note the more than proportional increase in total and unbound concentrations related to saturable metabolism and the relatively greater increase in unbound drug concentration. (Adapted from Bochner et al. 1987.)**

**HALF-LIFE** NSAIDs can be divided into those with short half-lives (<6 hours) and those with long half-lives (>12 hours) (Table 10-7) (Day and Brooks 1987). NSAIDs with long half-lives are usually given once or twice a day, which is good for compliance, and plasma concentrations will not fluctuate much during the dosage interval (Fig. 10-5). Drugs with long half-lives will accumulate in the body significantly after commencement of dosage as a function of half-life. Thus piroxicam with a half-life of about 60 hours will take about a week, that is, about three half-lives, to accumulate to close to 90% of its steady-state value. Naproxen with a half-life of about 14 hours (Table 10-7) will accumulate for about 2 days after commencement of treatment. Loading doses can be given to achieve high concentrations of long half-life NSAIDs quickly. A good example is the treatment of acute gout, where naproxen 500 to 750 mg is recommended as an initial dose, followed by 250 mg every 8 hours (Sturge et al. 1977).

The NSAIDs with short elimination half-lives are usually administered every 6 to 8 hours, an interval considerably longer than their half-lives in some instances. Despite substantial fluctuations in plasma concentrations, analgesic and anti-inflammatory activity is maintained well (Graham et al. 1984). Epidemiologic data suggest that NSAIDs with short half-lives are less likely to cause serious upper GI bleeding when used in usual doses (Henry et al. 1996).

Maximal effects of NSAID are achieved when plasma concentrations reach steady state. This is within a few days for NSAIDs with short half-lives (Huskisson et al. 1974; Aarons et al. 1983) and longer for NSAIDs with long half-lives. Pain seems to respond faster than joint swelling and heat (Aarons et al. 1983).

**SYNOVIAL FLUID CONCENTRATIONS** The major site of action of NSAIDs in inflammatory rheumatic conditions is probably in the synovial membrane. Synovial fluid concentrations give an indication of synovial membrane concentrations. All studies indicate that NSAIDs are transferred slowly between plasma and synovial fluid, but the pattern of synovial fluid NSAID concentrations relative to plasma concentrations is heavily influenced by the half-life of elimination of the NSAID from plasma. For NSAIDs with long elimination half-lives, the concentrations in synovial fluid are lower than, and parallel to, plasma concentrations. In contrast, NSAIDs that have short half-lives of elimination exhibit a characteristic crossover pattern with concentrations lower in synovial fluid than in plasma for the first 6 hours approximately, then higher than plasma concentrations subsequently (Fig. 10-5). Rapid clearance from plasma of short half-life NSAIDs and slow diffusion of short half-life NSAIDs into and out of synovial fluid explains this pattern (Graham, Williams, et al. 1988). Mean total concentrations (bound + unbound) of NSAIDs in synovial fluid over a dosage interval are approximately 60% of the mean total concentration in plasma (Day, Williams, et al. 1988; Day, Graham, et al. 1988; Graham et al. 1988), because of the lower levels of albumin and consequent lesser protein binding of NSAIDs in synovial fluid. By contrast, the mean unbound concentrations of NSAIDs in synovial fluid and plasma are very similar across a dosage interval (Day, Graham, et al. 1988; Day, Graham, et al. 1991).

**CLEARANCE** Interpatient differences in the metabolic clearances of individual NSAIDs may be quite marked; the result is considerable variation in steady-state concentrations of NSAIDs. The NSAIDs are cleared predominantly by hepatic metabolism, and the metabolites are generally inactive. However, several NSAIDs are inactive but have active metabolites (Table 10-7). Aspirin inhibits prostaglandin synthesis as seen in its antiplatelet activity, but salicylate, the metabolic product of aspirin hydrolysis, is an active anti-inflammatory agent and has a much longer half-life than its parent. Salsalate, which is a dimer of salicylic acid (salicylsalicylic acid) is inactive but is metabolized to salicylate. Another pro-drug that has no intrinsic activity until metabolized to 6-methoxy-2-naphthylacetic acid (6-MNA) is nabumetone, which has an elimination half-life of about 24 hours. Sulindac is metabolically reduced to a sulfide metabolite that has a long half-life (16 to 18 hours) and is responsible for the anti-inflammatory activity of sulindac. Sulindac is reduced to sulindac sulfide by microflora in the large intestine (Strong et al. 1985). It is important to note that the reduction of sulindac to its sulfide is reversible. Sulindac sulfide is metabolized back to sulindac in the kidney. This may explain the diminished effect of sulindac on renal function compared with other NSAIDs, although the importance of this contrast with other NSAIDs is debated (Sedor et al. 1984).

***Chirality*** Some NSAIDs have a center of asymmetry in their molecules and therefore exist as two optical isomers or enantiomers (Williams and Lee 1985) (Table 10-7). Sulindac has two enantiomers that have equal anti-inflammatory effect. The 2-arylpropionic acid NSAIDs including ibuprofen, ketoprofen, fenoprofen, naproxen, tiaprofenic acid, and flurbiprofen have two enantiomers each, but only the *S*-configured enantiomer of these NSAIDs inhibits cyclooxygenase (COX-1 and COX-2)

Table 10-7 **Pharmacokinetic Features of Nonsteroidal Anti-inflammatory Drugs (NSAIDs)**

| NSAID | Total daily dose range | Half-life (h) | Notes[a] |
|---|---|---|---|
| Aspirin | 4800 mg (bid, tid) | 0.25 | |
| Azapropazone | 1200 mg (bid, tid, qds) | 15 | Renal excretion unchanged drug 60%; reduce dose in renal impairment |
| Carprofen | 300 mg (bid) | 12 | Given as *R* and *S* isomers |
| Diclofenac | 50–150 mg (od, bid, tid) | 1–2 | World leader in sales |
| Diflunisal | 500–1000 mg (bid) | 7–15 | Decrease dose 50% in renal failure (creatinine clearance < 10 ml/min) |
| Etodolac | 400–600 mg (bid) | 7 | |
| Fenbufen | 900 mg (bid) | 11 | Given as *R* and *S* isomers |
| Fenoprofen calcium | 1200–2400 mg (bid) | 1–2 | *R* converted virtually completely to active *S* enantiomer |
| Flurbiprofen | 150–300 mg (bid) | 3–4 | *R* and *S* enantiomers; no inversion in humans |
| Ibuprofen | 1200–2400 mg (bid; tid) | 2–3 | About 60% *R* converted to active *S* enantiomer; safest NSAID for GI tract in low dose |
| Indomethacin | 25–200 mg (od, bid, tid) | 5 | Enterohepatic circulation; headaches, depersonalization reactions; suppositories for night pain |
| Ketoprofen | 100–300 mg (od; bid) | 1–4 | Commonly prescribed as slow release formulation; given as *R* and *S* isomers |
| Ketorolac tromethamine | 60 (elderly) to 90 (IM and IV); 30 (elderly) to 40 PO; (4–6 hourly for pain) | 4–6 | IM/IV and oral routes; 60% excreted unchanged in urine; used as an analgesic; great caution needed in postoperative situation and renal impairment |
| Meclofenamate sodium | 200–400 mg (bid) | 2.5 | Caution needed as it can prolong the bleeding time |
| Nabumetone | 1000–2000 mg (od) | 26 | Active metabolite is 6-methoxy-2-naphthylacetic acid) |
| Naproxen | 500–1000 mg (bid) | 12–15 | Administered as *S* isomer |
| Oxaprozin | 1200–1800 mg (od) | 49–60 | Hepatic metabolism |
| Phenylbutazone | 200–400 mg (od) | 29–140 | Avoid in general; avoid in renal and liver disease; reduce dose in elderly; monitor for pancytopenia |
| Piroxicam | 10–20 mg (od) | 30–86 | Decrease dose in liver disease |
| Salicylate | 2000–4000 mg (tid; qds) | 4–15 | Half-life increases with increasing dose; choline magnesium trisalicylate or salsalate well tolerated |
| Sulindac | 200–600 mg (bid) | 16–18 (sulfide) | Reduced to active sulfide. Enterohepatic circulation |
| Tenoxicam | 10–20 mg (od) | 60 | Hepatic metabolism |
| Tiaprofenic acid | 600 mg (bid; tid) | 3 | Given as *R* and *S* isomers; be alert for cystitis |
| Tolmetin | 1200–2000 mg (bid, tid, qds) | 1–1.5 | Renal excretion unchanged drug 17% |

[a]Decrease dose in renal and hepatic impairment and in the elderly for all NSAID.
ABBREVIATIONS: bid, twice a day; IM, intramuscular; IV, intravenous; od, optimal dose; PO, by mouth, orally; qds, to be taken four times a day; tid, three times a day.

and prostaglandin production. Naproxen was the first of this group to be marketed as the pure *S*-enantiomer. The remainder are available as racemic mixtures, namely equal amounts of the *R*- and *S*-enantiomers. Uniquely, the inactive *R*-enantiomers of ibuprofen and fenoprofen are metabolized to the active *S*-enantiomers in vivo and can be considered pro-drugs. About 60% of the inactive *R*-enantiomer of ibuprofen is converted to the active *S*-enantiomer, but the proportion is variable (Lee et al. 1985). Inversion of (*R*)- to (*S*)-fenoprofen is extensive (Rubin et al. 1985).

***Saturable Metabolism*** Steady-state or plateau plasma concentrations of NSAIDs are proportional to the dosage rate. Salicylate is an important exception as two of its metabolic pathways are saturable (Levy and Tsuchiya 1972; Levy G, et al. 1972). Thus, steady-state plasma concentrations of salicylate increase more than proportionally with dosage increases (Fig. 10-3), and its half-time of elimination increases from a few to about 15 hours. Salicylate is even more complicated because the drug induces its own metabolism. This leads to a significant decline in steady-state plasma salicylate concentra-

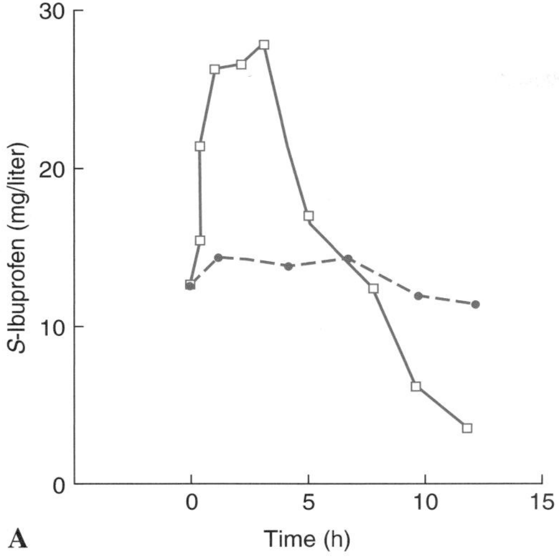


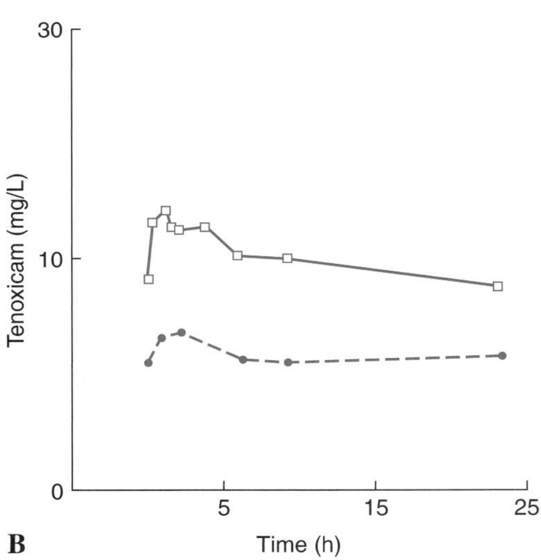


**F I G U R E 1 0 - 5 Total concentration of drug in plasma (square with dot) and synovial fluid (◆) after the administration of an NSAID with a short half-life (ibuprofen) and a long half-life (tenoxicam). Note the greater fluctuation in the plasma concentrations in the short–half-life ibuprofen and the cross-over in plasma and synovial fluid concentrations for that drug. (Adapted from Day et al. 1988 and Day et al. 1991, respectively.)**

tions between about 5 and 20 days after treatment commences (Muller et al. 1975; Day et al. 1983; Day, Furst, et al. 1988). Diflunisal, a salicylate derivative with a long half-life, is marketed as an analgesic (Table 10-7). Although it is not metabolized to salicylate, like salicylate its metabolism is saturable, and there is a disproportionate increase in plasma concentrations with increasing dosage (Meffin et al. 1983).

***Hepatic and Biliary Clearance*** Indomethacin and sulindac and their metabolites are subject to substantial enterohepatic cycling, which prolongs the effective half-life of indomethacin and sulindac sulfide (Dujovne et al. 1983). Plasma sulindac sulfide concentrations are increased about fourfold in alcoholic hepatic disease (Juhl et al. 1983). It is surprising that the clearance of azapropazone decreases as hepatic function deteriorates, as this NSAID is excreted predominantly unchanged in urine (Breuing et al. 1981). The clearance of ibuprofen (Juhl et al. 1983), diclofenac (Zimmerer et al. 1982), and salicylate (Roberts et al. 1983) is not affected by liver failure.

***Renal Clearance*** Only small proportions of the doses of most NSAIDs are excreted unchanged in urine; the only exception is salicylate. The renal clearance of salicylate is high when urinary pH is above 6.5, and plasma concentrations of salicylate can decrease (Levy and Leonards 1971). The clearance of several NSAIDs, including ketoprofen, naproxen, diflunisal, fenoprofen, and indomethacin decreases in patients with renal failure and in patients dosed concomitantly with probenecid. This seems surprising as only a fraction of these drugs is excreted unchanged in the urine. The explanation is that the acyl glucuronide metabolites of these drugs are retained in renal failure or when patients are dosed concomitantly with probenecid. The retained acyl glucuronides are hydrolyzed back to their parent NSAIDs, effectively decreasing their clearance and establishing a so-called *futile cycle*. (Meffin 1985). The effect is multiplied by the unidirectional inversion of some NSAIDs from inactive *R*- to active *S*-enantiomer as the (*R*)- and (*S*)-acylglucuronides are retained in renal impairment (Meffin et al. 1986). This mechanism is suspected in the benoxaprofen tragedy, when more than 60 generally elderly and renally impaired patients died of benoxaprofen-induced hepatic and renal failure. Also renal impairment is a risk factor for further impairment of kidney function induced by any NSAIDs in its own right, so these drugs should be used with great care in this setting (Clive and Stoff 1984).

***Age and NSAID Clearance*** NSAIDs are used most in the elderly who are also at greatest risk for adverse reactions to these drugs. Some of the increased risk most likely relates to reduced clearance of some NSAIDs with age. Naproxen (Upton et al. 1984; McVerry et al. 1986), ketoprofen (Advenier et al. 1983), azapropazone (Ritch et al. 1982), benoxaprofen (withdrawn), and salicylate (Roberts et al. 1983; Netter et al. 1985; Greenblatt et al. 1986) have reduced clearance in the elderly. The mechanism seems likely to be the reduced renal function in the elderly, and with naproxen, benoxaprofen, and ketoprofen in particular, the effect of retention of the acyl glucuronides and their ability to breakdown to their parent NSAID is likely to be important. Plasma concentrations of piroxicam have been found to vary widely in elderly patients, and even though toxicity has not been related to high plasma concentrations of the drug (Hobbs 1986), the possibility should be borne in mind. Although NSAID toxicity has not been correlated directly with impaired NSAID clearance in individual elderly patients, it is wise to commence with lower-than-usual doses of NSAIDs, which can be increased if necessary in the absence of adverse effects.

***Monitoring Plasma Concentrations of NSAIDs*** Salicylate plasma concentrations are maintained between 1.1 and 2.2 mmol/L (150 to 300 mg/L) for optimal anti-inflammatory effect, although formal validation is lacking (Needs and Brooks 1985). Measurement of plasma indomethacin concentrations in neonates given the drug in order to close a patent ductus arteriosus has been helpful (Brash et al. 1981).

***Responders and Nonresponders to NSAIDs: Relevance of Pharmacokinetics*** A classification of *responder* or *nonresponder* to particular NSAIDs has been applied to some patients with RA (Day and Brooks 1987). To test whether the difference is pharmacokinetic in origin, responders and nonresponders to a NSAID have been compared, but no pharmacokinetic contrasts have been discovered (Capell et al. 1977; Baber et al. 1979). In a study examining the relationship between naproxen dose and concentration and anti-inflammatory effect in RA, a proportion of patients did not respond to the highest dose of naproxen of 1500 mg per day. Most of the subjects in this study showed incremental anti-inflammatory effect with increasing dose of drug (Day et al. 1982). An explanation might be that an individual's lack of response to an NSAID, despite receiving maximal doses, is related to the balance of pathophysiologic mechanisms in that person showing lack of response to that particular drug's suite of mechanisms of action. A different NSAID may be effective because it has different mechanisms of action. For a proportion of RA and ankylosing spondylitis patients, preferences for particular NSAIDs have been found to be sustained for considerable periods (Wasner et al. 1981) and in trials involving blinded reexposure to drug (Preston et al. 1988; Walker et al. 1997). A number of investigators have found that RA patients who respond to NSAIDs are differentiated from the nonresponders by changes in markers of inflammation such as the acute-phase reactants usually not associated with NSAIDs (Cush et al. 1990; Walker et al. 1997).

### *Adverse effects*

Adverse reactions and effects from NSAIDs are the most commonly reported of any drug reaction to agencies around the world that are notified of adverse drug effects. Typically, 25% of all reports relate to NSAIDs. The elderly are more at risk for GI, renal, central nervous system, and hematologic adverse effects from NSAIDs in comparison with the young, and this might be due to a combination of reduced clearance of drug and increased tissue sensitivity. A more cautious approach to the use of NSAIDs, the dose of NSAIDs, and the duration of NSAID therapy is warranted because of these increased risks.

**GASTROINTESTINAL ADVERSE EFFECTS** NSAID-induced upper GI symptoms are common. They include dyspepsia, epigastric pain (heartburn), and less commonly nausea and would be expected in 20 to 30% of individuals taking NSAIDs regularly. Endoscopic lesions range from mucosal erythema through erosions to obvious peptic ulceration and are also found in 20 to 30% of subjects, but not necessarily those with upper GI symptoms. NSAID-induced gastric ulcers are found in the antral or prepyloric areas of the stomach. Duodenal injury is seen considerably less than gastric injury, although studies have shown protein and blood loss in the upper intestine in subjects taking NSAIDs (Bjarnason et al. 1993). The presence or absence of upper GI symptoms has not been shown to be a good predictor of the risk of serious bleeding from the upper GI tract, and this lack of correlation is more evident in the elderly. An interesting caveat comes from a study indicating that patients who knew less about the risks of NSAIDs and related upper GI symptoms were more likely to remain compliant with NSAID dosing instructions in the face of upper GI symptoms. These patients were significantly more likely to bleed (Wynne and Long 1996).

**PRINCIPLE The patient's full understanding of a drug could be a major determinant of its efficacy and toxicity in this person.**

The relative risk of serious complications of peptic ulcer disease, namely, hemorrhage and perforation, for an individual taking NSAIDs compared with a control patient not taking these drugs increases by about two- to sixfold. The absolute risk for NSAID-induced serious complications of peptic ulcer disease has been estimated to be about 3 to 6 per 1000 patient years of NSAID therapy from population-based studies. A rather higher estimate of 1 to 2% per annum comes from a large database of patients with RA (Fries et al. 1991a, 1991b). The relative risk increases in the elderly, those with a history of peptic ulcer or bleeding, if there is concomitant dosing with glucocorticosteroids, and notably with increasing dose of NSAID. The role of *Helicobacter pylori* in NSAID-induced upper GI complications remains uncertain (Yeomans et al. 1998). A recent study from Hong Kong suggested that identification of the organism before NSAID therapy was useful in reducing the incidence of complications, but confirmation is needed (Chan et al. 1997). It is interesting that omeprazole seems to be more effective as a prophylaxis against NSAID-induced gastric ulcer in patients infected with *H. pylori*, which suggests more research is needed (Hawkey et al. 1998). The high prevalence of usage of NSAIDs in the elderly is consistent with attribution of 20 to 30% of all serious ulcer complications to these drugs. This presents a major public health challenge, particularly as many of the patients have OA or soft-tissue rheumatic complaints and may not need NSAIDs at all (Jones et al. 1992).

Antacids, sucralfate, histamine H2-antagonists, prostaglandin analogs, and proton-pump inhibitors are used to treat NSAID-induced upper GI symptoms and to treat and prevent NSAID-induced peptic ulcers and their complications (Koch et al. 1996). Upper GI symptoms are reduced by taking NSAIDs with food and/or antacids. Histamine $H_2$ antagonists are widely used for treating dyspepsia induced by NSAIDs. Although there is little formal evidence of efficacy, available anecdotal evidence for benefit against dyspeptic symptoms is strong. All these therapies for NSAID gastropathy are effective in healing mucosal damage even if the NSAID is continued, although healing is slower in the face of concurrent NSAID therapy. It is widely perceived that $H_2$ antagonists protect against NSAID-induced gastric ulcers. However, only synthetic prostaglandin replacement therapy (misoprostol) and proton-pump inhibition with omeprazole have been shown to reduce the incidence of NSAID-induced gastroduodenal lesions significantly (Graham et al. 1988; Walt 1992; Elliott, Yeomans, et al. 1994; Hawkey et al. 1998; Yeomans et al. 1998). Recently, high doses of the $H_2$ antagonist famotidine were shown to do likewise, but the dose required and thus the cost seem to make this an impractical option (Taha et al. 1996). Misoprostol will reduce the incidence of gastric ulcers between 50% and 90%. Much more important, the incidence of serious bleeding and perforation is reduced significantly by misoprostol (Silverstein et al. 1995). Although omeprazole was only as effective as misoprostol in treating NSAID-induced gastric lesions, there was a lower rate of relapse and better tolerance compared with misoprostol (Hawkey et al. 1998). Misoprostol causes diarrhea in a small percentage of patients. However, studies of the cost-effectiveness of misoprostol and omeprazole in this setting have produced conflicting results. It seems clear that prophylactic therapy with misoprostol or omeprazole should be targeted toward individuals who truly need NSAID therapy, are using the safest NSAID at the lowest effective dose and for the shortest appropriate time, and have increased risks for serious upper GI adverse effects from NSAIDs. The availability of highly selective COX-2 inhibitors may have a profound effect on the need for prophylactic therapy.

**RENAL ADVERSE EFFECTS** NSAIDs affect the kidney in two broad ways—first by affecting the function of the kidney and second by causing tissue damage (Clive and Stoff 1984) (Table 10-8). Most important and prevalent are functional effects. Acute renal impairment and fluid and electrolyte disturbances are more likely to occur in the elderly, in patients with impaired kidney function, or when renal perfusion is reduced such as in situations of hypovolemia or cardiac failure. Tissue damage occurs much more rarely, and manifestations include acute interstitial nephritis with and without proteinuria in the nephrotic range, minimal change glomerulonephritis with nephrotic syndrome, papillary necrosis, acute tubular necrosis, and vasculitis. NSAID-induced interstitial nephritis is unusual. It occurs 2 weeks to 18 months after the patient starts NSAIDs and is frequently associated with protein-

Table 10-8 **Renal Adverse Drug Reactions to NSAIDs**

| TYPE | ADVERSE REACTION | FEATURES |
|---|---|---|
| Functional adverse effects | Decreased GFR<br>Sodium and water retention<br>Hyperkalemia | Most common; elderly and renally impaired at greatest risk; regular monitoring in at risk patients with plasma creatinine and electrolytes, weight and blood pressure |
| Pathologic adverse effects | | Rare; can happen with any NSAID |
| | Acute interstitial nephritis | With or without nephrotic syndrome; can happen with any NSAID; immunologic origin, possibly T-cell mediated |
| | Papillary necrosis | Incidence declining since removal of phenacetin-containing combination analgesics from the market |
| | Chronic renal failure | Mechanisms uncertain |

uria and renal failure; the patient slowly recovers over a year after NSAIDs are stopped. Prescribers should be aware that tiaprofenic acid can cause an intense interstitial cystitis, and a number of patients have been subject to needless investigation and surgery for this drug-induced problem (Crawford et al. 1997; O'Neill 1994).

Renal prostaglandins are important for maintaining renal function in situations of reduced renal perfusion such as hypovolemic states, ineffective circulatory volume (congestive heart failure, cirrhosis with ascites, or nephrotic syndrome), or primary renal disorders where vasoconstrictor hormones such as norepinephrine and vasopressin are secreted in response. Secretion of vasodilatory prostaglandins by the kidney is important in preventing excessive vasoconstriction of kidney blood vessels in this situation. Introduction of NSAIDs can disturb this balance by removing the modulatory prostaglandins, leading to a decrease of glomerular filtration rate (GFR) and renal blood flow that can progress to irreversible renal failure. Concurrent diuretic therapy is another risk factor. NSAID-induced renal impairment leads to a rise in plasma creatinine within days of commencement of NSAID therapy. In more severe cases serum potassium also rises, and weight gain is noted along with decreasing urine output. If identified early, cessation of the NSAID usually leads to rapid improvement. Careful monitoring of renal function is important, especially in the elderly or renally impaired (Johnson and Day 1991a, b).

Another adverse effect, NSAID-induced sodium and water retention with dependent edema, can occur in up to 25% of patients given NSAIDs, depending on the background health and age of the patient. Hyperkalemia can be marked: The risk factors are age, renal impairment, diabetes, and concurrent use of angiotensin-converting enzyme (ACE) inhibitors, potassium-sparing diuretics, and cyclosporine.

**HEMATOLOGIC ADVERSE EFFECTS** Chronic NSAID therapy can be associated with anemia secondary to blood loss from the GI tract, which is often unsuspected. Inflammatory disease per se and vitamin and nutritional deficiencies also commonly contribute to anemia in rheumatic disease patients. Elderly women have the greatest risk for phenylbutazone-induced aplastic anemia, at a rate of about 1 per 30,000 prescriptions. Excessive dosing in the face of reduced drug clearance is considered to be important in the etiology. Overall NSAID-induced bone marrow toxicity is rare. NSAIDs do inhibit the platelet COX-1, causing reduced platelet adhesiveness and prolonged bleeding time. Low-dose aspirin irreversibly acetylates COX-1, and bleeding time is prolonged for 10 to 12 days until new platelets are generated. NSAIDs other than aspirin reversibly inhibit COX-1, so bleeding time normalizes with elimination of the NSAID, usually within 24 hours of the last dose. Platelet function may take 72 hours to normalize after piroxicam is stopped because of its long half-life. Highly selective COX-2 inhibitors do not inhibit platelet function.

The incidence of NSAID-induced thrombocytopenia is rare, but because of the widespread use of NSAIDs in the community, the total number of cases reported is substantial. The thrombocytopenia is usually mild and reversible. However, serious bleeding and death have been reported, particularly with phenylbutazone and indomethacin.

**NEUROLOGIC ADVERSE EFFECTS** The antipyretic and probably part of the analgesic effect of NSAIDs are due to actions of the drugs in the central nervous system, so it is not surprising that there are other CNS effects (Ferreira et al. 1978). Clinicians need to be alert to the possibility of NSAID-induced CNS adverse effects, as these are often misdiagnosed in the elderly. NSAIDs are associated with various degrees of cognitive dysfunction, confusion, somnolence, behavioral disturbances, and dizziness (Goodwin and Regan 1982). These are extremely common problems in the elderly, and the possibility that NSAIDs cause these symptoms is commonly overlooked. Most of the reports have involved indomethacin, naproxen, and ibuprofen, but all NSAIDs should be considered capable of causing confusion and other CNS effects. Aseptic meningitis has been reported to occur as a result of therapy with ibuprofen and sulindac, particularly in individuals with SLE. Headache, often migraine-like and occurring more commonly in migraine sufferers, and other CNS symptoms are well-known adverse effects of indomethacin. Psychotic reactions have been reported with indomethacin and sulindac (O'Brien and Bagby 1985a, 1985b, 1985c, 1985d).

**LIVER DAMAGE AND NSAIDs** Serious hepatotoxicity is rare with therapeutic usage of NSAIDs. Anti-inflammatory dose aspirin causes mild, usually asymptomatic, reversible liver function abnormalities in 50% of patients, which become apparent within the first few weeks of therapy. Rarely, severe toxicity has occurred at lower salicylate concentrations, and the possibility of Reye syndrome in children has stopped the use of aspirin as an antipyretic in this age group. Phenylbutazone is associated with severe hepatotoxicity with a high fatality rate, another reason to reserve this drug as a second-line NSAID for problematic inflammatory disease.

Sulindac and diclofenac may be associated with a higher incidence of hepatotoxicity than other NSAIDs. Hepatotoxicity is more common in juvenile rheumatoid arthritis and patients with SLE. For most NSAIDs there is no consistent liver function or histopathologic abnormality in cases of liver injury. If an NSAID causes hepatotoxicity in an individual, it should not be readministered.

**CARDIOVASCULAR ADVERSE EFFECTS** Blood pressure should be carefully monitored in any patients with hypertension requiring NSAID therapy, as blood pressure can increase, the amount varying with the individual. Indomethacin is the most likely of the NSAIDs to elevate blood pressure and, when administered chronically, antagonizes the effect of antihypertensive drugs and significantly increases blood pressure in healthy elderly individuals (Johnson et al. 1994; de Leeuw 1996; de Leeuw 1997; Johnson 1997). NSAIDs inhibit vasodilatory prostaglandins that are secreted to counter the antihypertensive-induced secretion of vasoconstrictive hormones such as noradrenaline and angiotensin II. Whether NSAIDs precipitate cardiac failure has been controversial, but more recent case-control data suggest this might be a significant cause of morbidity and mortality (Henry et al. 1997).

**PULMONARY ADVERSE EFFECTS** Great care needs to be taken in prescribing NSAIDs to patients with a history of asthma. Asthma can be precipitated or exacerbated by aspirin or NSAIDs. Aspirin-induced bronchospasm can be acute and lethal, and the most severe forms occur in subjects with a history of aspirin allergy. Often these patients also have nasal polyps. All NSAIDs are contraindicated, but some of these patients are able to tolerate salicylic acid derivatives. Whether highly selective COX-2 inhibitors will be safe is unknown. Recent work suggests that excessive amounts of leukotriene $C_4$ accumulation in the face of prostaglandin synthesis inhibition may be the explanation for this dramatic and important adverse effect (Sampson et al. 1997).

**DERMATOLOGIC ADVERSE EFFECTS** Skin rashes are uncommon with NSAIDs, although serious reactions such as erythema multiforme are reported. Photosensitivity reactions are also reported.

**ADVERSE EFFECTS ON CARTILAGE** There is continuing suspicion that chronic, long-duration NSAID therapy may be associated with cartilage damage, although this is a controversial subject. Studies carried out in vitro and often using excessive concentrations of NSAIDs suggest that NSAIDs might have a deleterious effect on chondrocyte function. Confirmation that this is an important clinical effect has been harder to demonstrate, although one clinical study (Rashad et al. 1989) has suggested that deterioration of joints was more rapid in patients taking a more potent prostaglandin synthetase inhibitor (diclofenac) than those taking a relatively mild prostaglandin inhibitor (azapropazone). Recently, further in vitro work suggests that COX-2 is expressed in cartilage, and the highly selective COX-2 inhibitors may be more deleterious than the less-selective NSAIDs (Amin et al. 1997).

#### *NSAID drug interactions*

The elderly and patients with diabetes, cardiovascular, or renal disease are most at risk from drug interactions with NSAIDs, and consequently these patients require increased surveillance for drug interactions. The most important interactions of NSAIDs are pharmacodynamic, for example, the decreased activity of diuretics and antihypertensives in patients taking NSAIDs (Day et al. 1984; Johnson et al. 1993) (Table 10-9).

There are also some important pharmacokinetic interactions involving NSAIDs. NSAIDs generally have little effect on the hepatic clearance of other drugs; however, an exception is the inhibition of the metabolism of several drugs, including warfarin, phenytoin, and tolbutamide, by the pyrazole NSAIDs, phenylbutazone and azapropazone. It is preferable to use an alternative NSAID.

Although NSAIDs will displace other drugs from plasma albumin, potentiation of the pharmacologic effects of displaced drugs is unlikely (Sellers 1979; Rolan 1994). Warfarin is displaced from its albumin site by many NSAIDs, but increased anticoagulant activity has not been demonstrated. This is because steady-state, unbound concentrations of warfarin are unchanged. Phenytoin binding to plasma albumin is reduced by high-dose salicylate, but the effect of phenytoin is not potentiated (Paxton 1980). However, total plasma concentrations of phenytoin will be lower, and the therapeutic range should be adjusted accordingly, i.e., by approximately 25% to 30 to 60 mmol/L (7.5–15 mg/ml). In a similar way, high-dose aspirin leads to the fall in steady-state concentrations of a number of other NSAIDs, but there is no advantage to using such combinations (Day, Paull, et al. 1988).

The clearance of lithium is reduced by diclofenac (Reimann and Frolich 1981) and most likely other NSAIDs, as the probable mechanism is via inhibition of renal prostaglandin synthesis. Sulindac may be less likely to cause this interaction. Thus plasma lithium concentrations need to be monitored more frequently when NSAIDs are introduced or ceased.

Table 10-9 **Drug Interactions Involving NSAIDs**

| Drug affected | NSAID implicated | Effect of interaction | Management considerations |
|---|---|---|---|
| *Pharmacodynamic interactions* | | | |
| Antihypertensive drugs<br>β-Blockers<br>Diuretics<br>ACE inhibitors<br>Calcium channel blockers | Indomethacin; others less problematic; sulindac possibly least problematic | Blunting of antihypertensive effect | Avoid NSAID if possible<br>Increase monitoring; adjust dose of antihypertensive |
| Diuretics | Indomethacin (reversible renal failure has occurred with triamterene); others less problematic; sulindac possibly least problematic | Blunting of natriuretic and diuretic effects; cardiac failure worsened; increased risk of renal impairment; increased risk of hyperkalemia with potassium-sparing diuretics | Avoid NSAIDs; indomethacin and triamterene contraindicated<br>Increase clinical and laboratory monitoring<br>Adjust dose of diuretic; particular care with potassium-sparing diuretics |
| Anticoagulants | All | Inhibition of platelets; GI lesions a bleeding risk | Avoid NSAIDs; use low-dose, intermittent NSAID such as ibuprofen if needed |
| Hypoglycemic agents | Anti-inflammatory dose salicylate | Potentiates hypoglycemia; mechanism unknown | Avoid high-dose salicylate<br>Monitor blood glucose |
| *Pharmacokinetic interactions* | *NSAIDs that affect other drugs* | | |
| Warfarin sodium | Phenylbutazone; azapropazone | Inhibits metabolism of (*S*)-warfarin (more potent isomer) | Avoid combination; use another NSAID |
| Oral hypoglycemics, e.g., tolbutamide, glipizide | Phenylbutazone, azapropazone | Inhibits metabolism of oral hypoglycemic drugs | Avoid combination; use another NSAID |
| Phenytoin | Phenylbutazone; azapropazone | Inhibits metabolism of phenytoin and displaces phenytoin off albumin | Avoid combination;<br>Phenytoin requirements decreased; beware toxicity; monitor unbound phenytoin |
| Phenytoin | Other NSAIDs, e.g., ibuprofen and salicylates (high dose) | Displaces phenytoin from albumin, but unbound concentrations only rise if phenytoin metabolism is saturated or if folate depletion occurs | Monitor for phenytoin toxicity; unbound phenytoin concentrations may be helpful; may need phenytoin dose reduction |
| Methotrexate sodium | All | Risk of methotrexate toxicity; inhibition of renal excretion of methotrexate; not usually a problem; beware elderly, renally impaired; folate depleted | Be careful not to dose too heavily with methotrexate in the elderly and those with renal impairment; careful regular monitoring of blood count |
| Digoxin | All | NSAID-induced decrease in renal function leads to reduced clearance | Beware possible digoxin toxicity; monitor digoxin more closely |
| Aminoglycosides | All | Decreased renal function by NSAID increases aminoglycoside concentration and risk of nephrotoxicity | Close monitoring of aminoglycoside concentrations and renal function |

Table 10-9 Drug Interactions Involving NSAIDs (Continued)

| Drug affected | NSAID implicated | Effect of interaction | Management considerations |
|---|---|---|---|
| Lithium | All | Decreased renal function increases risk of lithium toxicity | Closer monitoring of lithium concentrations<br>Beware dehydration and concomitant illness |
| Valproic acid | Aspirin | Inhibition of valproate metabolism increasing valproate concentrations | Avoid aspirin<br>Monitor valproate concentrations more closely |
| Antacids | Salicylates | Alkalinization of urine increases renal clearance of salicylate and plasma concentrations fall | Monitor plasma salicylate concentrations more closely |
| Cholestyramine | All | Reduced absorption of NSAID | Avoid combination |
| Metoclopramide HCl | Aspirin; all | Increases absorption rate | Useful in migraine attacks |

ABBREVIATIONS: ACE, angiotensin-converting enzyme; β-blockers, β-adrenergic receptor blocking agents.

A dangerous interaction occurs between high-dose methotrexate, as used for treatment of malignancy, and NSAIDs. This has been demonstrated with salicylate, phenylbutazone, ketoprofen, and indomethacin, with resulting pancytopenia. The mechanism is thought to be inhibition of the proximal renal tubular secretion of methotrexate and is likely to occur with all NSAIDs (Liegler et al. 1969; Shen and Azarnoff 1978). Serious interactions between NSAIDs and methotrexate prescribed at doses appropriate for the treatment of inflammatory rheumatic diseases are uncommonly reported. However, great caution is needed in the elderly and those with renal impairment, even with low methotrexate doses, as the addition of an NSAID to the treatment could tip the balance, leading to methotrexate toxicity (Conaghan et al. 1995). Drugs that deplete folic acid such as antibiotics, trimethoprim, and various sulfonamides including sulfamethoxazole can be hazardous also in this situation.

### *Guidelines for NSAID usage*

If therapy with an NSAID is indicated for a rheumatic disease, most physicians commence with one of the newer NSAIDs rather than aspirin or indomethacin. Anti-inflammatory doses of aspirin cause deafness and tinnitus, whereas indomethacin is associated with a higher incidence of headaches and other CNS effects compared with newer NSAIDs. Indomethacin retains popularity for the short-term, high-dose treatment of acute gout. Phenylbutazone is no longer recommended for initial therapy of arthritic conditions because of the risk of bone marrow aplasia and hepatic damage. However, many patients with ankylosing spondylitis prefer phenylbutazone.

With these exceptions, selection of an NSAID is essentially a matter of the preference of an individual physician and patient. Selection might be based on a patient's previous experience with NSAIDs and the preferred dosing frequency and tempered by the league table for GI safety of NSAIDs (Henry et al. 1996) or overall safety and tolerance (Fries, Spitz, et al. 1990). Increasingly, the cost of prescriptions is influencing prescribing, and the costs of NSAID-induced adverse events are also being considered (Bloor and Maynard 1996). Selection might be based on relative safety and the lowest cost, and it has been associated with substantial savings in the United States (Smalley et al. 1995; Jones DL, et al. 1996). Once-daily dosing with piroxicam, tenoxicam, or slow-release formulations of ketoprofen or naproxen may be preferred to a twice or three times daily dosage with other NSAIDs such as ibuprofen and diclofenac. Some patients find that a nighttime NSAID suppository helps to control morning symptoms.

The dosage of an NSAID ought to be appropriate for the rheumatic condition and the age and general health of the patient. Bigger doses are indicated for inflammatory arthritis such as acute gout, whereas smaller doses are appropriate for OA. Particular care with dosing and monitoring is needed for the elderly, particularly those with low body weight, and patients with cardiac, renal, or liver impairment.

The dosage of NSAIDs should be adjusted according to clinical response, with the goal of using the minimal effective dose. If appropriate dosage increases do not deliver a satisfactory response or there is an unacceptable adverse reaction such as dyspepsia, then another NSAID can be substituted. Why this switch strategy sometimes is successful has not been elucidated. Unfortunately, NSAIDs are too commonly continued indefinitely, especially in the elderly with OA or nonspecific rheumatic symptoms, without proper review (Jones et al. 1992). The physician should review the status of patients on NSAID therapy regularly, taking particular note of GI symptoms, blood pressure, cardiac status, blood count, and renal function.

## Glucocorticosteroids

Glucocorticosteroids are used to treat all the inflammatory arthritides such as RA, vasculitis, and polymyalgia rheumatica but are also injected intra- and periarticularly in noninflammatory conditions such as OA and local soft-tissue conditions such as tennis elbow. Corticosteroids effectively and rapidly suppress systemic and local signs of synovitis in RA patients. Sometimes corticosteroids are used during the induction phase of therapy while the effect of disease-modifying antirheumatic drugs (DMARDs) is awaited. In RA low-doses of oral corticosteroids are used (usually 10 mg daily or less of prednisone or its active metabolite prednisolone) and are well-tolerated in the short term, but significant adverse effects occur with higher doses and long-term use. Patients with severe RA, vasculitis, or active SLE may require high-dose intravenous or oral corticosteroids (for example, 1 g methylprednisolone daily for a few days), and intravenous therapy is probably of no benefit over oral therapy outside of these settings (Hayball et al. 1992). Intra-articular corticosteroid injections with depot preparations of typically methylprednisolone acetate or triamcinolone hydrochloride are a very useful treatment for monoarticular inflammatory synovitis or for single joints that are difficult to control in the polyarthritis patient (Bird 1994). Improvement also occurs in noninjected joints for up to a week after injection. The long-term effects of intra-articular therapy are unclear, with animal studies suggesting both beneficial and detrimental effects on articular cartilage. Generally, an individual joint may be injected up to 3 to 4 times per year, but it is believed that exceeding this number in weight-bearing joints is unwise. Meticulous antisepsis is required, and patients should be clear about returning for urgent assessment if there is the possibility of infection in the joint after injection.

Corticosteroids are significantly better at relieving clinical symptoms in RA patients than is placebo, and they are superior to NSAIDs. The onset of effect is rapid. Corticosteroids have not traditionally been classified as DMARDs; however, an important recent placebo-controlled study in patients with early RA reported a reduced rate of joint destruction in the prednisone-treated group after 2 years (Kirwan 1995) as assessed radiologically. Further confirmation of this finding is needed. It is noteworthy that a study examining the effects of DMARDs, NSAIDs, and glucocorticosteroids on disability in patients with RA treated long-term revealed no effect of steroids in contrast to the positive effects of DMARDs (Fries et al. 1996). Pulse intravenous therapy is efficacious for at least several weeks; relatively few adverse effects are reported (Smith et al. 1990), although there is some concern regarding avascular necrosis of the hip.

### *Mechanism of action*

The glucocorticoid receptor is a transcription factor that is activated by glucocorticosteroids. The activated receptor enters the nucleus and binds to specific DNA sequences termed *glucocorticoid response elements* (GREs), resulting in transcription of genes bearing a GRE in their promoter region. This positive regulation of gene expression probably accounts for most of the metabolic and endocrine effects of glucocorticosteroids that, in excess, are recognized as Cushing syndrome. In this way, glucocorticosteroids enhance the expression of the protein lipocortin, which in turn downregulates phospholipase $A_2$ expression and leucocyte transmigration (Perretti et al. 1996; Getting et al. 1997; Bryant et al. 1998). An effect of lipocortin leading to decreased synthesis of proinflammatory prostaglandins and leukotrienes has also been demonstrated (Flower and Rothwell 1994; Getting et al. 1997; Bryant et al. 1998). In addition to their positive regulation of gene expression, glucocorticosteroids inhibit the expression of a wide variety of important proinflammatory genes that do not contain a recognizable GRE in their promoter regions (Heck et al. 1997).

Many of the important mediators of inflammation are proteins that are coded by genes containing promoter sites for the transcription factors AP-1 and NF-κB. Activated glucocorticosteroid receptors inhibit AP-1- and NF-κB-mediated transcription, and several mechanisms have been proposed (reviewed by Cato and Wade 1996). For example, glucocorticosteroids inhibit the NF-κB-mediated expression of adhesion molecules (ICAM-1, ELAM-1, E-selectin), cytokines (IL-2, IL-6, and IL-8), and enzymes (iNOS and COX-2) (Mitchell et al. 1993; Fessler et al. 1996; Youssef et al. 1996; Youssef et al. 1997; Bryant et al. 1998). Glucocorticosteroids also inhibit the AP-1-mediated expression of collagenases I and IV.

### *Pharmacokinetics*

The most widely used oral glucocorticosteroids in the treatment of the rheumatic diseases are prednisone and prednisolone (the active metabolite of prednisone). Prednisolone is well-absorbed, although there is some variation between formulations. The plasma half-life is short, on the order of 2 to 3 hours, but the half-life of its pharmacodynamic effect is longer, and prednisolone is administered once or twice a day. Protein binding in plasma is saturable. There has been little relationship demonstrated between plasma concentrations or pharmacokinetic variables and the important clinical effects of prednisolone. The widespread and intriguing variability between individuals in efficacy and adverse effects for given doses of prednisolone has not been explained to date. Thus, some individuals are more easily prone to the cushingoid effects of prednisolone.

### *Adverse effects*

Corticosteroid therapy is commonly associated with a broad range of adverse effects (Table 10-10). A daily dose equivalent to the physiologic requirements of cortisol, namely, 5.0 to 7.5 mg prednisolone per day, should not be exceeded if at all possible, as adverse effects increase with increasing dose (Sambrook and Jones 1995; Sambrook 1996). Dosing is best in the morning as it approximates the pattern of normal diurnal cortisol secretion, thereby reducing the inhibitory effect on ACTH secretion from the anterior pituitary and corticotrophin-releasing factor from the hypothalamus. Limiting daily dose to 7.5 mg in the morning is often possible in RA, but larger doses are often needed in other inflammatory rheumatic conditions such as the initial stages of polymyalgia rheumatica and various vasculitides. Longer-acting synthetic glucocorticosteroids such as dexamethasone are best avoided because they induce a more profound suppression of the hypothalamic–pituitary–adrenal axis and thus a greater risk of adverse effects. Also, prednisolone and prednisone are available in 1-mg tablet sizes, which allows gradual dose reduction. Concurrent therapy with NSAIDs is often used in the treatment of RA and SLE, but prescribers need to be aware that this significantly enhances the risk of NSAID-induced upper GI peptic ulceration and associated complications.

Bone loss is of considerable concern, especially in the elderly. Corticosteroids influence bone formation and resorption, leading to an increase in bone fracture rate. These catabolic effects are most pronounced in the first 6 to 12 months of therapy. There seems to be some reversibility of corticosteroid effect on bone after cessation of treatment, but there is a significant degree of individual variation. It is interesting that the osteoporotic effect of corticosteroids is less pronounced in RA patients than expected, perhaps because relief of the painful symptoms of RA allows more weight bearing-exercise to be undertaken, a factor that opposes bone demineralization (Sambrook and Jones 1995). Attention to prevention of glucocorticosteroid-induced osteoporosis is important if long-term therapy is envisaged and if doses are high. Studies have shown variable efficacy for estrogen, vitamin D analogs, and calcitonin, but recently alendronate has been shown to increase bone density in patients receiving corticosteroids accompanied by a small reduction in vertebral fracture rate (Saag et al. 1998).

Adrenal crisis, clinically manifest by hyponatremia and hyperkalemia, is a significant risk for patients who have received more than a few weeks' therapy with glucocorticosteroids (Claussen et al. 1992; LaRochelle et al. 1993; Bouachour et al. 1994). The period of vulnerability continues long after steroid therapy is stopped, for example, for up to 2 years depending on the dose and duration of corticosteroid treatment, but it is difficult to make predictions (Christy 1992; Schlaghecke et al. 1992). Adrenal crises are commonly precipitated by stressful situations including surgery, illness, or trauma. Managing the patient with extra corticosteroid will avoid the crisis (Salem et al. 1994; Lamberts et al. 1997). A common situation is that the patient having routine surgery is able to continue oral corticosteroid. The risk in this circumstance is probably small, but when there are perioperative complications or oral therapy has to be stopped, then there is a high risk (Salem et al. 1994; Friedman et al. 1995; Glowniak and Loriaux 1997; Lamberts et al. 1997). It is important not to taper chronic corticosteroid therapy too quickly after long-term therapy as this too will induce a form of adrenal crisis. The "withdrawal" syndrome can initially be difficult to diagnose, manifesting with fatigue, myalgia, arthralgia, anorexia, and weight loss (Dixon and Christy 1980). When the dose reduction achieves a daily dose of 10 to 15 mg/day of prednisone, the reduction schedule has to become more gradual.

## Methotrexate

Low-dose methotrexate given in doses up to 25 mg once weekly by the oral or intramuscular route is an established and effective DMARD for RA, psoriatic arthropathy, and other inflammatory connective tissue and joint diseases.

### *Efficacy*

Methotrexate is now the most widely used DMARD because of its favorable efficacy and toxicity profile and its rapid onset and offset of action. Also, patients are able to continue this drug longer than any other DMARDs. Data indicate that up to 75% of patients are still taking methotrexate 6 years after commencement of therapy (Buchbinder et al. 1993; Wolfe et al. 1994; Jobanputra et al. 1995; Wolfe 1995). Complete remission is rare, but sig-

Table 10-10 Adverse Effects of Glucocorticosteroids

| SYSTEM INVOLVED | ADVERSE EFFECT | COMMENT |
|---|---|---|
| Musculoskeletal | Osteoporosis | Risk increases with patient's age, increasing dose and duration of therapy |
| | Osteonecrosis | Occasionally seen with pulse steroid therapy |
| | Myopathy | |
| | Growth retardation | Major issue in juvenile rheumatoid arthritis |
| Endocrine and metabolic | Obesity | Fat redistributes into characteristic cushingoid pattern |
| | Glucose intolerance | Overt diabetes mellitus common |
| | Gluconeogenesis | Loss of subcutaneous, vascular wall, and bone protein |
| | Fat metabolism | Increase in plasma free fatty acids |
| | Electrolyte abnormalities | Tendency to hypokalemia |
| | Danger of adrenal insufficiency | Due to long-term suppression of endogenous cortisol production |
| Dermatologic | Striae | |
| | Bruising | |
| | Skin atrophy | |
| | Acne | |
| Neuropsychiatric | Psychosis | Usually at higher doses |
| | Depression | |
| | Benign intracranial hypertension | |
| Gastrointestinal | Peptic ulcer | When combined with NSAIDs |
| | Pancreatitis | |
| Immunity | Increased susceptibility to infections | Relates to anti-inflammatory actions |
| Ophthalmic | Cataract | Posterior subcapsular |

nificant improvement in pain and in the number of inflamed joints is seen in RA patients treated with methotrexate in comparison to placebo (Weinblatt et al. 1985; Williams et al. 1985; Tugwell et al. 1987). Methotrexate has been found to be superior to auranofin, injectable gold, penicillamine, azathioprine, and cyclosporine in RA (Felson et al. 1992; Willkens et al. 1995; Brooks 1997; O'Dell 1997). An important distinction from other DMARDs is that clinical improvement is seen within weeks of the start of methotrexate treatment. The effect of the drug generally stabilizes by 6 months, and a sustained response to methotrexate for over 7 years is not uncommon (Tugwell et al. 1987; Songsiridej and Furst 1990; Kremer 1997; Kremer and Lee 1988). An important feature is that methotrexate will allow the dose of concomitant corticosteroid to be reduced (Kremer 1989; Boers et al. 1997). Joint destruction may be retarded by methotrexate (Girgis et al. 1994), and progression of joint erosions and joint space narrowing was less pronounced in RA patients treated with methotrexate compared with patients receiving auranofin (Lopez-Mendez et al. 1993) or azathioprine (Jeurissen et al. 1991).

### *Mechanism of action*

Methotrexate (and its polyglutamate metabolites) competitively inhibits the enzyme dihydrofolate reductase (Tugwell et al. 1987). This inhibition results in reduction of the availability of reduced folate, an important requirement for the proliferation of cells. Methotrexate decreases production of several cytokines involved in RA, particularly IL-1, TNF$\alpha$, IL-6, and IL-8. Whether these effects are causal or simply epiphenomena remains unknown. At the molecular level, the inhibition of transmethylation reactions and methotrexate-induced increases in adenosine concentrations are possible mechanisms of anti-inflammatory and antirheumatic effects of this drug (Cronstein 1996, 1997) (see also chapter 13).

### *Pharmacokinetics*

The oral bioavailability of methotrexate is about 65% but varies significantly between individuals and moderately within the same individual over time (Bannwarth et al. 1996). The intramuscular or subcutaneous route can be used if excessive nausea occurs when the drug is taken orally and is not controlled by oral folic acid treatment or when the expected clinical response to increasing doses of oral methotrexate does not occur (Bannwarth et al. 1996; Hamilton and Kremer 1997). The plasma half-life is biphasic and possibly even triphasic; the initial half-life is short, of the order of 2 to 3 hours, followed by the dominant half-life of the order of 7 hours (Seideman et al. 1993). The drug is cleared partially by oxidation in the liver to an active metabolite, 7-hydroxymethotrexate. Methotrexate is transported actively into cells and is then polyglutamated. The half-life of the polyglutamated metabolite is substantially longer than that of methotrexate, and the polyglutamate is also a potent inhibitor of dihydrofolate reductase.

A substantial clearance route for methotrexate is through renal excretion of the unchanged drug, in large part via the weak acid secretory pathway in the proximal renal tubule, this route accounting for over half of the clearance of the drug (see also chapter 6). The drug is retained, therefore, in renal impairment. This is a very important factor for consideration by prescribers when selecting dosing regimens of this drug. In particular, great care needs to be taken in the elderly, who have reduced renal function as part of the aging process.

There are competitive excretion interactions at the weak acid secretory pathway in the proximal tubule particularly with high-dose aspirin and probenecid that can contribute to methotrexate toxicity. Concurrent use of methotrexate with drugs that may produce renal impairment such as cyclosporine and NSAIDs should be undertaken with caution and vigilance again especially in those with renal impairment and in the elderly (Quinn and Day 1995, 1997). Other drugs that interfere with the availability of reduced folate such as trimethoprim (also found in cotrimoxazole) can be hazardous in situations of renal impairment and relatively high methotrexate dosage.

#### *Adverse effects*

Adverse effects are the main reason for methotrexate discontinuation. Toxicity is common and may occur at any time in the course of the treatment but usually can be dealt with so that cessation of methotrexate is avoided (Conaghan et al. 1995). Gastrointestinal adverse effects such as anorexia, nausea, stomatitis, and diarrhea are the most frequent toxicities and occur in up to 60% of patients but are usually very mild. Dosage reduction, temporary drug discontinuation, or the use of folic or folinic acid concurrently are generally successful strategies (Alarcon and Morgan 1997). If the doses of the folate-repleting agents are too high, then the efficacy of the methotrexate will be lost (Cronstein 1996, 1997). Folate supplementation should be considered in all patients treated with methotrexate, and some prescribers routinely use supplementation. Folic acid is cheaper than folinic acid and most commonly used (Alarcon and Morgan 1997).

Renal function is very important in the selection of the dosage of methotrexate (Bannwarth et al. 1996). A lower dose or cessation of therapy should be considered in patients with renal impairment, or at times of volume depletion (such as perioperatively) or reduced renal perfusion (worsening heart failure) (Bridges and Moreland 1997). Older age predisposes to toxicity, specifically related to the renal impairment of aging.

Abnormal plasma liver enzyme levels are frequently seen with methotrexate use. However, with much cumulative experience it is apparent that clinically significant liver disease with fibrosis and cirrhosis is uncommon. Serious liver complications due to methotrexate may be more likely if there is concomitant use of alcohol or there is preexisting liver disease (West 1997). Cytopenias are reported in approximately 5% of methotrexate-treated patients, but severe myelosuppression, which is uncommon, is an extremely serious event (Conaghan et al. 1995; Gutierrez-Urena et al. 1996; Berthelot et al. 1997; Nygaard 1997). An elevated mean corpuscular volume may precede hematologic toxicity. There has always been concern about the possible increased risk for malignancy in patients treated with methotrexate, but investigators have been unable to establish risk levels, suggesting that any risk must be small. Recent case reports of Ebstein-Barr virus–related lymphomas in patients treated with methotrexate are cause for concern, particularly when combination of methotrexate with cyclosporine is considered (Ferraccioli et al. 1995; Moder et al. 1995; Bachman et al. 1996; Paul et al. 1997).

Interstitial pneumonitis is a serious and potentially fatal complication of methotrexate treatment, with occurrence rates reported to be from 0.3 to 11.6% (Conaghan et al. 1995; Kremer et al. 1997). Histologic findings range from lymphocytic interstitial infiltrates to interstitial fibrosis (Kremer et al. 1997). Many reported cases may have been due to infection, which must always be excluded (Aglas et al. 1995; Hilliquin et al. 1996). Methotrexate-induced pneumonitis is treated with methotrexate withdrawal and supportive care. Pregnancy is contraindicated during methotrexate usage because of the teratogenic potential of the drug (Sandoval et al. 1995; Buckley et al. 1997). Treatment with DMARDs and methotrexate can often be stopped during pregnancy as RA improves markedly during pregnancy, but unfortunately relapses post partum.

#### *Monitoring methotrexate therapy*

Methotrexate therapy should be avoided in patients with liver or lung disease. Abstinence from alcohol is recommended. The American Rheumatology Association (ARA) monitoring guidelines should be followed (American College of Rheumatology Ad Hoc Committee on Clinical Guidelines 1996a; American College of Rheumatology Ad Hoc Committee on Clinical Guidelines

1996b) (Table 10-11). Liver function tests are recommended every 4 to 8 weeks. Patients with persistently abnormal liver function tests should have methotrexate discontinued, and a liver biopsy should be considered (Kremer et al. 1994; Erickson et al. 1995; West 1997). The following baseline evaluations are recommended: a complete blood count, a chest radiograph, hepatitis B and C serology in high-risk patients, aspartate aminotransferase (AST), alanine aminotransferase (ALT), albumin, alkaline phosphatase, and creatinine. The complete blood count, AST, albumin, and creatinine should be monitored every 4 to 8 weeks in the course of the treatment (American College of Rheumatology Ad Hoc Committee on Clinical Guidelines 1996a).

## Sulfasalazine

Sulfasalazine is an effective and relatively safe antirheumatic drug in RA and is unique in that it has displayed efficacy in ankylosing spondylitis and HLA-B27–related arthropathies (Zwillich et al. 1988; Porter and Capell 1990). The drug also has efficacy in juvenile arthritis and psoriatic arthritis. Sulfasalazine consists of salicylic acid joined to sulfapyridine by an azo bond (Fig. 10-6). (See also inflammatory bowel disease in chapter 3, Gastrointestinal Disorders.)

### *Mechanism of action*

The mode of antirheumatic action of sulfasalazine is not known, but sulfasalazine and/or its metabolite sulfapyridine may suppress immunologic processes in the gut of relevance to the pathogenesis of RA and spondyloarthropathies (Day 1997). Possible mechanisms include scavenging proinflammatory reactive oxygen species; inhibition of the synthesis of leukotriene $B_4$ in polymorphs and thromboxane $A_2$ in platelets; and inhibition of synovial angiogenesis (Hoult and Moore 1980; Stenson and Lobos 1983; Porter and Capell 1990). Sulfasalazine reduces the

**Table 10-11 Monitoring Disease Modifying Antirheumatic Drugs (DMARDs) Therapy**

| Drug | Toxicity leading to monitoring | Baseline | Clinical monitoring | Laboratory monitoring |
|---|---|---|---|---|
| Hydroxychloroquine | Retinopathy | Ophthalmologic assessment | Ophthalmologic assessment every 6 months | |
| Sulfasalazine | Myelosuppression; hemolytic anemia; hepatotoxicity | CBC, urinalysis, liver and renal function tests | Symptoms and signs of myelosuppression | CBC, liver function tests every 2 weeks until dose stable, then every 1–3 months |
| Gold (IM) | Myelosuppression, nephrotic syndrome | CBC, urinalysis, plasma creatinine | Symptoms and signs of myelosuppression | CBC and urinalysis weekly for 1 month, then every 2–4 weeks for 20 weeks, then with each injection |
| Auranofin | Myelosuppression | CBC, urinalysis | Symptoms and signs of myelosuppression | CBC, urinalysis every 4–6 weeks |
| Penicillamine | Myelosuppression; nephrotic syndrome; immunologic disorders | CBC, urinalysis, plasma creatinine | Symptoms and signs of myelosuppression | CBC, urinalysis every 2 weeks until dose stable, then every 1–3 months |
| Methotrexate sodium | Bone marrow suppression; hepatic fibrosis; pulmonary fibrosis | CBC, renal function, liver function, chest radiograph | Cough and dyspnea; mouth ulcers; nausea and vomiting; myelosuppression | CBC, liver and renal function tests every 4–8 weeks (more frequent at outset) |
| Azathioprine | Myelosuppression; hepatotoxicity, lymphoproliferative disorders | CBC, plasma creatinine, liver function tests | Symptoms and signs of myelosuppression | CBC 1–3 months and within 1–2 weeks of any dose change |
| Cyclophosphamide | Myelosuppression; hemorrhagic cystitis; lymphoproliferative disorder | CBC, urinalysis, plasma creatinine, liver function tests | Symptoms and signs of myelosuppression and hemorrhagic cystitis | CBC 1–3 months; urinalysis and urine cytology every 6 months (and after cessation!) |
| Cyclosporine | Renal impairment; hypertension; anemia | BP, CBC, creatinine, uric acid | Edema, weight, BP | Blood pressure and plasma creatinine monthly |

ABBREVIATIONS: BP, blood pressure; CBC, complete blood count.
SOURCE: From American College of Rheumatology Ad Hoc Committee on Clinical Guidelines 1996a; Furst and Clements 1998.

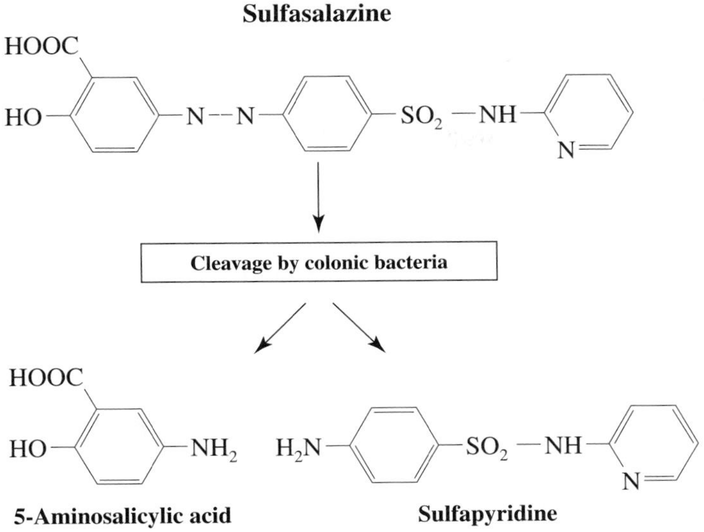

Sulfasalazine

HOOC, HO, N--N, $SO_2$ —NH, N

Cleavage by colonic bacteria

HOOC, HO, $NH_2$ $H_2N$ $SO_2$ —NH, N

5-Aminosalicylic acid Sulfapyridine

**FIGURE 10-6 The cleavage of sulfasalazine to its metabolites sulfapyridine and 5-aminosalicylate by colonic bacteria.**

number of activated lymphocytes circulating, and this is accompanied by significant falls in immunoglobulin IgM, rheumatoid factor, interleukins 1 and 6, and TNF$\alpha$ concentrations (Rhodes et al. 1981; Danis et al. 1992).

### *Pharmacokinetics*

There is little absorption of intact sulfasalazine (10 to 20%) as the drug is quite insoluble. Sulfapyridine and 5-aminosalicylic acid are liberated in the colon following bacterial reduction of the azo bond, and little sulfasalazine is found in stools (Taggart et al. 1986; Taggart et al. 1987; Rains et al. 1995). Sulfasalazine is highly protein bound (>95%), peak plasma concentrations occurring 3 to 5 hours after dosing, with an apparent plasma elimination half-life of 6 to 17 hours, probably reflecting the absorption half-life (Taggart et al. 1986; Taggart et al. 1987; Rains et al. 1995). About 50% of 5-aminosalicylic acid is found in the feces, whereas 30% is excreted in urine as the *N*-acetylation product. Sulfapyridine appears in plasma 4 to 6 hours after dosing and is metabolized extensively to ring hydroxylation and $N^4$-acetylation products; these are then subject to glucuronidation (Rains et al. 1995). Interindividual acetylation and oxidative capacities are quite variable because of genetic polymorphism, resulting in large contrasts in rates of metabolism and plasma concentrations of sulfapyridine (Das et al. 1973; Rains et al. 1995). It is suspected that sulfapyridine may be the antirheumatic component of sulfasalazine. 5-Aminosalicylic acid is the anti-inflammatory species in inflammatory bowel diseases such as ulcerative colitis (Neumann et al. 1986; Taggart et al. 1986). However, sulfasalazine could have important antirheumatic actions either in the gut or systemically in its own right. To date, no plasma concentration–response relationships for sulfapyridine have been discerned (Chalmers et al. 1990; Porter and Capell 1990; Rains et al. 1995).

### *Efficacy*

Sulfasalazine is about as effective as gold and D-penicillamine (Williams 1988) and is slightly more effective than antimalarials but works more rapidly. Efficacy is measurable at about 4 weeks (Neumann et al. 1986). Although sulfasalazine has fewer serious adverse effects than gold or D-penicillamine, discontinuation rates are similar to those of other DMARDs (Taggart et al. 1987; Day 1998). It is noteworthy that radiologic progression of RA was significantly less for sulfasalazine compared with hydroxychloroquine after 24 and 48 weeks, the contrast still apparent at 3 years (Brewer et al. 1986; van der Heijde et al. 1990), which supports other studies suggesting sulfasalazine retards radiologic progression in RA. Sulfasalazine is effective in juvenile arthritis (Grondin et al. 1988), ankylosing spondylitis (Ferraz et al. 1990), HLA-B27-associated asymmetrical, pavciarticular arthritis (Mielants et al. 1986), and psoriatic arthritis (Farr et al. 1990).

***Adverse effects***

Sulfasalazine ranks with antimalarials and auranofin as the best tolerated of the DMARDs. Thus, in a study of 774 RA patients followed for 1 to 11 years, there were no deaths or long-term adverse effects (Amos et al. 1986). Adverse effects are most common in the first 4 months of therapy (Sachar 1988; Scott and Dacre 1988; Donovan et al. 1990). The most common adverse effects involve the GI tract, hematologic system, liver function abnormalities, skin, and central nervous system. Dose reduction is often effective in treating these adverse effects. Despite the ranking of sulfasalazines as a relatively well tolerated drug, continuation rates range from 40 to 70% after 2 years; attrition is due to adverse effects and inadequate efficacy. After 5 years about 20% of patients were still taking sulfasalazine, similar to rates for gold and D-penicillamine.

Nausea and upper abdominal discomfort, often in association with headache and dizziness, are the most common adverse effects in the first months of therapy. These adverse effects are less likely if the dosage is increased gradually, and the enteric-coated formulation of sulfasalazine is used (Donovan et al. 1990). Neutropenia is most likely in the first 6 months of treatment but can occur at any time. Therefore there is a need for continued careful review, particularly because early recognition of neutropenia and dosage cessation or reduction leads to reversal in most cases. Glucose-6-phosphate dehydrogenase (G6PD) deficiency is a risk factor for hemolysis, and baseline enzyme level measurements are recommended. Baseline liver function tests are also recommended. Bodily secretions commonly become yellow, and this also affects plastic contact lenses. Sulfasalazine should be avoided at around the time of conception and early pregnancy, although no teratogenicity has been documented definitively. Sulfasalazine is considered safe for breast-feeding infants. Sulfasalazine can induce a reversible reduction in sperm count.

***Dosing and monitoring***

Usual adult dosage for the rheumatic diseases is 1 g twice a day of the enteric-coated formulation taken with meals. Tolerance is improved if dosing commences at 500 mg to 1 g/day increasing by 500 mg/day at minimum intervals of a week. Increases above 2 g/day are rarely helpful. Neutropenia is likely to occur suddenly, so that monitoring to avoid this is difficult. Many physicians order blood counts every 2 to 4 weeks during the first 3 months of therapy and then reduce the frequency (Table 10-11). It is important that patients understand that there is a possibility of serious hematologic effects and that they learn to recognize the important signs such as sore throat, fever, and significant malaise. Liver function tests are also undertaken, but less frequently than the blood counts.

## Hydroxychloroquine and Antimalarials

Hydroxychloroquine (HCQ) and chloroquine (Fig. 10-7) have been used to treat RA and SLE for almost 50 years. An important benefit is the absence of life-threatening toxicity. As this class of antirheumatic drug is considered to be somewhat less effective than other DMARDs, such as sulfasalazine or methotrexate, antimalarials are used more often to treat early, less intense RA and now, commonly, in combination regimens with other DMARDs.

***Mechanism of action***

Antimalarial drugs are basic and therefore concentrate in the acidic, lysosomal system of connective tissue and white blood cells, and this is considered a critical factor in their mechanism of action. The acidic lysosomal system is essential for a number of important cellular functions such as processing cell-surface receptors, protein glycosylation, and digestion of membrane lipids. Accumulation of antimalarials in lysosomes changes the pH from acid to alkaline, affecting the function of the lysosomal enzymes such as sphingomyelinase. These enzymes are important in the transduction of signal between cell surface TNF$\alpha$ receptors and activation of the nuclear transcription factor, NF-$\kappa$B, critical for proinflammatory gene expression (Wiegmann et al. 1994). Antimalarials may impair the antigen-processing function of monocyte/macrophages by their lysosomal actions and have been reported to inhibit the production of IL-1 and numerous enzymes of importance including phospholipase $A_2$ (Salmeron and Lipsky 1983).

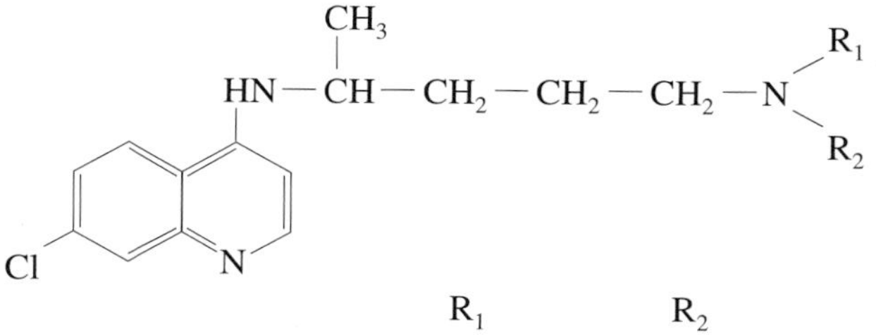

$HN-CH(CH_3)-CH_2-CH_2-CH_2-N(R_1)(R_2)$ (attached at position 4 of a 7-chloroquinoline ring; Cl, N)

| | $R_1$ | $R_2$ |
|---|---|---|
| **Chloroquine** | $CH_2CH_3$ | $CH_2CH_3$ |
| **Hydroxychloroquine** | $CH_2CH_3$ | $CH_2CH_2OH$ |

**FIGURE 10-7 Hydroxychloroquine and chloroquine.**

***Pharmacokinetics***

Bioavailability of antimalarials is likely to be an important contributor to variable outcomes with these drugs. This is because the bioavailability of HCQ varies considerably between individuals: The average is about 80%, but values may be as low as 20%. The bioavailability remains stable within an individual (McLachlan et al. 1994). HCQ ought to be administered with food, since bioavailability is unaffected, but GI adverse effects are reduced (Tett et al. 1990; McLachlan et al. 1993).

Antimalarials have exceptionally long half-lives of around 40 days, so that steady-state concentrations will not be achieved for some months. Some clinicians give a loading-dose regimen over the first week. The drugs concentrate in tissues and blood cells largely because of the lysosomal uptake (Tett et al. 1988). Dealkylation is the main metabolic pathway in the liver. There is substantial renal elimination of chloroquine (40%) and HCQ (25%), so the dose should be reduced in renal impairment.

In a retrospective study of patients with RA, higher blood concentrations of HCQ were associated with better disease control (Tett et al. 1993). As blood concentrations vary considerably between individuals, there is the possibility that blood concentration monitoring may improve outcomes, but this remains unproved.

***Efficacy***

Well-controlled, double-blind studies of HCQ and chloroquine have shown efficacy against placebo in patients with RA. Studies demonstrate efficacy in 60 to 80% of patients apparent over 4 to 6 months treatment in standard parameters of disease activity including functional class, joint count, pain, grip strength, morning stiffness, patient and observer's assessments, ESR, and hemoglobin, with a small proportion of patients achieving complete remission (Clark et al. 1993; The HERA Study 1995). Compared to sulfasalazine, HCQ has a slower onset of antirheumatic effect in RA, but there was no difference between these treatments at 48 weeks (Nuver-Zwart et al. 1989). Sulfasalazine was more effective than HCQ in slowing the progression of bony erosions around joints (van der Heijde et al. 1989). Indeed, antimalarials have not been proved to retard erosion formation, but appropriate studies have not been undertaken. Older studies indicated that HCQ 200 to 600 mg/day was as effective as chloroquine 250 to 500 mg/day in RA patients, with HCQ having a slight advantage with respect to fewer GI adverse effects. However, a meta-analysis revealed that chloroquine was more effective than HCQ at the usual dosing rates used for both drugs, a surprising finding that requires confirmation (Felson et al. 1990, 1992).

Children with juvenile RA were treated with HCQ 6 mg/kg per day for 12 months in a double-blind trial, but it showed little benefit compared with placebo (Brewer et al. 1986). A number of studies indicate considerable efficacy of HCQ and chloroquine in SLE with improvement in malaise and tiredness, disease flare-ups, skin rash, arthritis, and pleuritic pain. However, a recent double-blind, 48-week study showed a significant effect on joint pain only (Brewer et al. 1986). Moreover, in a double-blind, placebo-controlled study significant flares in disease activity occurred when HCQ was withdrawn from patients who had previously been stabilized on the drug (The Canadian Hydroxychloroquine Study Group 1991).

***Toxicity***

In contrast to other DMARDs, the majority of adverse effects of antimalarials are transient and not serious, and cessation of drug is generally unnecessary. HCQ in the usual doses used is less likely to be associated with adverse effects than chloroquine, and in the United States, Australia, and United Kingdom, HCQ is preferred.

Adverse reactions from antimalarials include rashes, GI upset, leukopenia, peripheral neuropathy, and a variety of ocular effects. Transient deterioration in vision with poor focusing may occur acutely at the start of therapy. Irreversible retinopathy characterized by progressive decrease in visual fields and irreversible blindness in combination with fundal changes that are characteristic have been reported in a number of patients taking chloroquine at higher daily doses than is now recommended. Very few reports incriminate HCQ, but in part this may reflect relative use of chloroquine and HCQ. Consensus opinion is that retinal toxicity correlates with daily dose of drug and that upper dosage limits for adults should be 4 mg base/kg daily for chloroquine and 6 mg base/kg daily for HCQ (Block 1998).

***Dosing and monitoring***

Dosage limits of less than or equal to 6 mg base/kg daily for HCQ or 4 mg base/kg daily of chloroquine should be adhered to. If clearly beneficial, antimalarial therapy should continue long-term. In the most common situation encountered, that is, partial response, adding a second DMARD is increasingly being considered, despite limited evidence from clinical trials (Paulus 1988).

Careful ophthalmologic screening at baseline and at 6-month intervals is currently recommended to identify retinal damage (Table 10-11). Although this is extremely uncommon, it is reversible if identified early. Examination should include fundoscopy and visual field charting by an ophthalmologist. Patients should be advised to report any visual symptoms, especially decreased night vision, loss of central or peripheral vision, and intolerance of glare. Full blood count and urinalysis can be performed at intervals coinciding with ophthalmologic review.

## Gold

Gold salts were first used in RA in the 1930s when Forestier reported a response rate of 75% in 550 patients with polyarthritis (Forestier 1935). Until the advent of methotrexate, gold salts were the preeminent DMARDs, but like other DMARDs, are now less popular than methotrexate. Aurothiomalate (ATM) and aurothioglucose (ATG) are approximately 50% gold by weight and are administered intramuscularly. They are essentially indistinguishable in terms of pharmacokinetics, biologic activity, and clinical efficacy. ATM is prepared in an aqueous solution, whereas ATG is prepared as a suspension in sesame seed oil that may reduce the incidence of rapid skin reactions such as flushing following injection.

### *Mechanism of action*

The mechanisms by which parenteral gold salts exert their effects are still to be delineated, although much has been learned recently. Gold salts are water-soluble, contain the monovalent aurous ion (oxidation state I) stabilized by attachment to a sulfur-containing ligand and generally exist as polymers (Fig. 10-8*A*). The polymeric gold is broken down to a monomeric form in vivo. This is achieved by the formation of monomeric aurocyanide from cyanide released during polymorph phagocytosis (Champion et al. 1990). Aurocyanide is lipid-soluble in contrast to the polymeric forms of ATM and ATG and therefore better able to penetrate cells. The sulfhydryl moiety is critical to distribution and therefore to the effects of these compounds. Gold enters cells by a sequence of ligand exchange reactions involving sulfhydryl groups on and within the cell (Snyder et al. 1986).

Gold salts may regulate gene expression by inhibiting the binding of critical transcription factors to their response elements in DNA. AP-1, a dimer of the protooncogenes *Jun* and *Fos*, and NF-κB are such critical transcription factors. Their binding to DNA is specifically inhibited by very low concentrations of gold at about 1 to 5mM (Handel et al. 1991; Handel et al. 1993; Handel et al. 1995; Yang et al. 1995) compatible with the concentration range seen in the serum of patients with RA treated with injectable gold salts. Reduced AP-1 transcriptional activity leads to reduced expression of a number of proinflammatory cytokines, metalloproteinases, and cell adhesion molecules (Koike et al. 1994).

Other potential mechanisms of action commonly require unrealistic concentrations of gold in vivo (Day 1998). Given this caveat, demonstrated effects in a variety of systems suggest a number of possible actions including inhibition of maturation and function of mononuclear phagocytes and of T cells with resulting diminution of the immune response as measured by antigen- or mitogen-induced lymphocyte proliferation (Lipsky and Ziff 1977; Danis et al. 1987; Danis et al. 1990; Handel et al. 1991; Handel et al. 1993; Handel et al. 1995), deactivation of superoxide free radicals (Corey et al. 1987), and reduction of immune globulins including rheumatoid factor (Gottlieb et al. 1975).

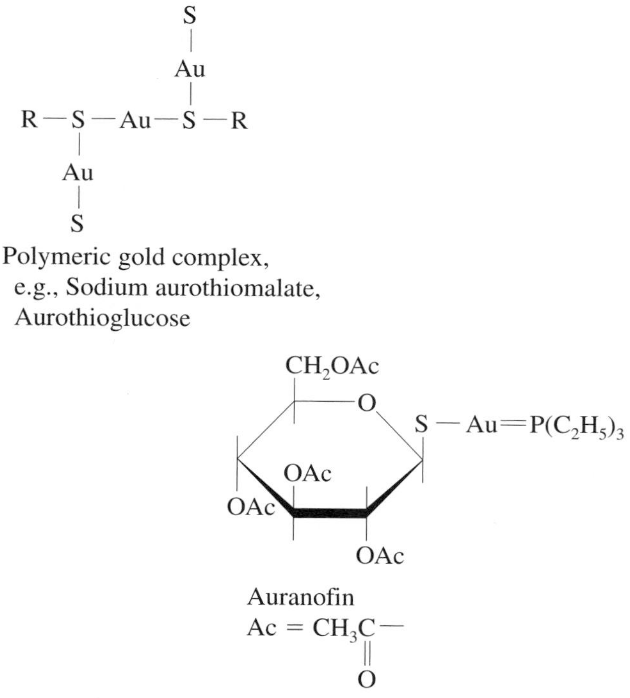

Auranofin (Fig. 10-8*B*) is monomeric, lipid-soluble, and partially absorbed following oral administration. It is substantially less effective than injectable gold salts. The pharmacodynamic properties of auranofin differ from those of parenteral gold salts as demonstrated in vitro, including reduction in extracellular release of lysosomal enzymes and interference with release of inflammatory mediators. Auranofin has particular effects on the activity of polymorphonuclear leukocytes not observed with the injectable gold salts (Rudkowski, Graham, et al. 1991; Rudkowski, Ziegler, et al. 1991). The reasons for this difference in described actions are unclear (Blocka and

S
|
Au
|
R—S—Au—S—R
|
Au
|
S

Polymeric gold complex,
e.g., Sodium aurothiomalate,
Aurothioglucose

$CH_2OAc$
O
S — Au=$P(C_2H_5)_3$
OAc
OAc
OAc

Auranofin
Ac = $CH_3C$— (with =O)

**FIGURE 10-8 Antiarthritic gold drugs (A) the general structure of the polymeric gold complexes, and (B) the monomeric gold complex, auranofin.**

Paulus 1987; Graham et al. 1993) but may relate to better cell penetration of auranofin in in vitro test systems as compared with the polymeric forms of ATM and ATG.

### *Pharmacokinetics*

After a single intramuscular injection of ATM (50 mg), peak serum concentration is reached within 2 hours (Gottlieb et al. 1974; Gottlieb and Gray 1981; Massarella et al. 1984). ATG has a slower rate of absorption and lower peak serum concentration because of its oil base. The serum concentration declines subsequently to half its peak over 7 days. With weekly administration, serum gold concentrations plateau at around 6 to 8 weeks.

Auranofin contains 29% gold by weight. Auranofin is more hydrophobic than the gold salts and is approximately 25% absorbed from the GI tract (Gottlieb and Gray 1981; Gottlieb 1982; Gottlieb 1983). Auranofin given orally at a dose of 6 mg/day produces steady-state serum gold concentration between 4 and 12 weeks after commencement (Champion et al. 1988). However, serum gold concentrations and tissue accumulation are significantly less than that of parenteral therapy with gold salts when compared over 6 months of therapy.

Gold is slowly eliminated in the urine and feces with an elimination half-life of 25 ± 5 days independent of whether it was administered parenterally or taken orally (Gottlieb and Gray 1981; Massarella et al. 1984). After a course of treatment, gold is often detectable in the serum a year after cessation (Gottlieb et al. 1974; Gottlieb and Gray 1981; Gottlieb 1982; Gottlieb 1983). Concurrent therapy with agents that also have a sulfhydryl group such as penicillamine and *N*-acetylcysteine increases gold excretion. The synovial fluid concentration of gold is about 50% of serum; gold selectively accumulates in the lysosomes of type A synovial cells and other macrophages (Ghadially et al. 1978).

### *Efficacy*

Gold therapy is of value in the treatment of RA, juvenile arthritis (rheumatoid factor positive, nonsystemic form), and psoriatic arthritis (nonspondylitic form). In relation to the clinical effectiveness of parenteral gold the following points are important (Brooks 1997; Day 1998):

- Dosages in the range 10 to 50 mg weekly for 1 to 2 years are superior to placebo, but no dose–response relationship has been established.
- A very good clinical response occurs in 10 to 35% of patients peaking at 12 months, but only half of these responders maintain their response after 12 months; long-term remission is rare.
- Gold compounds retard the development of erosions that occur in the majority of patients with rheumatoid arthritis within 2 years of developing the disease (Buckland-Wright et al. 1993).
- Even when dosage is reduced to maintenance levels, only approximately 20% of patients continue treatment after 4 years.
- As the incidence of toxicity declines, terminations of therapy because of loss of effectiveness continue to rise.
- Gold has efficacy similar to that of D-penicillamine, methotrexate, sulfasalazine, and azathioprine and is slightly more efficacious than antimalarials.

In relation to the clinical effectiveness of auranofin, the following points are important (Gofton et al. 1984; Heuer et al. 1985; Champion et al. 1988):

- Clinical improvement is not consistently present at dosages below 6 mg/day; auranofin is less effective than injectable gold and D-penicillamine, but causes less serious adverse effects than these drugs.
- Diarrhea limits the dose that can be given.
- At 45 months after the initiation of therapy approximately 35% of patients have ceased therapy because of lack of efficacy, whereas 15% have ceased because of toxicity.

### *Adverse effects*

The incidence of toxicity from gold compounds is high (Felson et al. 1990; Felson et al. 1992; Cash and Klippel 1994; Day 1998) (Figs. 10-9 and 10-10). Unfortunately, by 3 to 5 years after the start of gold most patients have stopped the drug because of lack of efficacy or adverse effects (Wolfe et al. 1990; Wolfe 1997). Approximately 40% of patients develop adverse effects, the most common complications observed including dermatitis (preceded by a skin itch) or stomatitis. The most serious adverse effect is bone marrow aplasia, which has a high mortality but is fortunately rare. At least these days this problem can be treated with colony-stimulating factors and transplantation. Transient mild proteinuria occurs in up to 50% of patients. Membranous nephritis with nephrotic syndrome occurs in 0.2 to 2.6% of patients but has a good prognosis (Silverberg et al. 1970). Vasomotor reactions may be seen in the 5 to 10 minutes subsequent to injection, whereas postinjection inflammatory reaction with transient arthralgias, myalgias, and other systemic symptoms may occur within 6 to 24 hours. Vasomotor and inflammatory reactions occur less commonly with ATG perhaps because of slower absorption from the oil base.

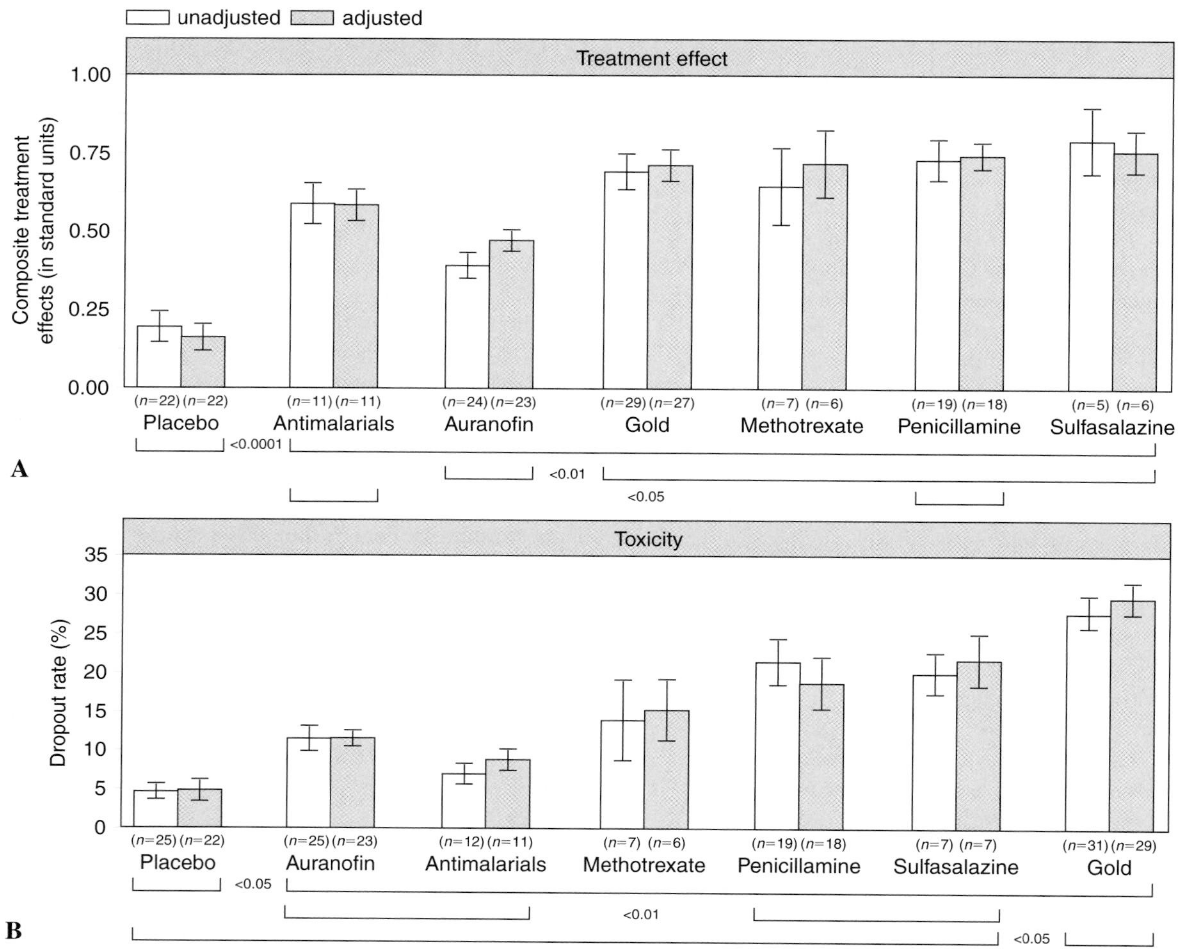


**FIGURE 10-9 A comparison between six DMARDs and placebo with respect to efficacy expressed as a composite treatment effect [(A) tender joint count, ESR, and grip strength] and toxicity [(B) expressed as relative dropout rate because of drug toxicity]. Rates were adjusted for 5 important covariates. Differences in outcomes between groups are shown below each figure. (From Felson et al. 1990 with permission of the publishers.)**

### *Dosing*

There is an important need to educate patients concerning efficacy, toxicity, and requirements for monitoring when injectable gold is to be used. Although ATG is less likely to cause postinjection reactions than ATM, a wider bore needle is required to inject ATG. Injection pain can be reduced by adding lidocaine to the syringe. A test dose (1 mg) is followed by 10 mg/week, then 10 to 50 mg/week, to a total dose of about 1 g or 6 month's therapy. A decision about continuing therapy can then be made, and monthly assessments of disease activity examining joint tenderness, morning stiffness, pain, global assessment of symptoms, ESR, and hemoglobin will indicate if improvement is occurring. Maintenance therapy is continued at 10 to 50 mg every 2 to 4 weeks and can be given indefinitely while there is perceived benefit. Concomitant NSAIDs are commonly taken and, increasingly, combinations with other DMARDs.

### *Monitoring*

Most adverse events induced by parenteral gold, if detected early, can be managed by discontinuing the drug. Evidence of toxicity should be evaluated before every injection. This should include checking for skin itch and mouth ulcers and regular monitoring of complete blood count and urinalysis (Table 10-11).

Mild or localized rashes may be managed with topical corticosteroids, but a generalized rash requires discontin-

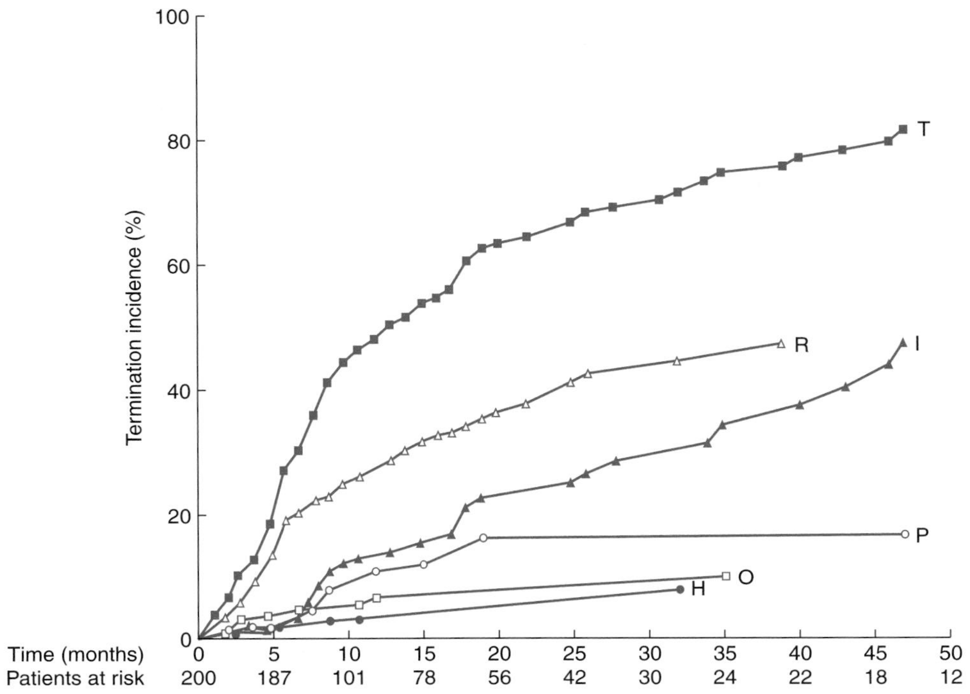


**FIGURE 10-10 Reasons for drop-outs from injectable gold therapy (Sambrook et al. 1982 with the permission of the publishers.) Hematologic, •—•; proteinuria, ○—○; inefficacy, ▲—▲I; rash, △—△R; other, □—□O; total, ■—■T.**

uation of therapy. Rashes will usually recede quite quickly; oral corticosteroids are needed rarely. Gold can be reintroduced once the reaction has been absent for some weeks, using extremely small doses of ATM or preferably ATG.

Full blood count weekly for the first month and then every 2 to 4 weeks for the next 5 months is the recommended monitoring regimen, with careful attention to downward trends in platelets or neutrophils. Such a trend requires increased surveillance and possible dosage reduction or cessation, at least temporarily. Blood count frequency may drop somewhat (e.g., 4 to 6 weekly) after 6 months according to dose and regimen selected and previous responses of the patient. Precipitous drops in white cells or platelets demand immediate cessation of gold injections. A flow sheet record of these laboratory values should be maintained for each patient. Intervention with high-dose corticosteroids, a chelating agent, and bone marrow transplantation significantly reduce the mortality associated with rare, gold-induced bone marrow aplasia (Adachi et al. 1987).

Urine testing for protein should be performed before each injection. Proteinuria of greater than 800 mg daily necessitates immediate cessation of gold therapy. Systemic corticosteroids may ameliorate nephrosis and pulmonary toxicity; the latter is a rare occurrence. The long half-life of gold after chronic administration means that many toxic effects may continue weeks to months after therapy has been ceased. Gold therapy should be avoided in individuals with a history of bone marrow depression or renal insufficiency. However, patients with RA and Felty syndrome with disease-induced neutropenia generally tolerate gold therapy without increased rates of toxicity.

Auranofin has a lower incidence of toxicity than parenteral gold compounds (Todd 1987). However, patients who develop serious toxicity from parenteral gold should not receive auranofin. The most common adverse effect is loose stools or diarrhea, which relates to the osmotic effects of gold left unabsorbed in the gut and which affects 40% of patients but leads to cessation in only 3% (Champion et al. 1988). Other common GI effects include nausea, vomiting, anorexia, and abdominal cramps. Rash, stomatitis, and conjunctivitis are common but rarely require cessation. Rare toxic effects include alopecia, proteinuria, microscopic hematuria, thrombocytopenia, leukopenia, metallic taste, aplastic anemia, cholestatic jaundice, and interstitial pneumonitis. In a retrospective review of 3082 patients, 11% discontinued auranofin because of adverse effects (Blodgett et al. 1984).

## D-Penicillamine

Penicillamine has been used since the 1960s to treat RA (Jaffe 1965), but its use is declining because of the superior efficacy to toxicity ratios of other DMARDs (Felson et al. 1990; Felson et al. 1992) (see Fig. 10-9). It is also used in other connective tissue disorders such as progressive systemic sclerosis and as a copper chelator in Wilson disease.

### *Chemistry and mode of action*

Structurally penicillamine is an analog of cysteine and is characterized by an amino, a carboxyl, and a sulfhydryl group (Fig. 10-11). The D-enantiomer of penicillamine is used because of the greater toxicity of the L-enantiomer. The sulfhydryl group is responsible for its biologic activity and pharmacokinetics (Joyce 1988, 1989, 1993; Joyce et al. 1988; Joyce and Murphy 1990). Although the mode of action of D-penicillamine in RA is uncertain, it seems likely that the drug could modulate the immune system via sulfhydryl exchange reactions in various immunologic cells. Through the sulfhydryl group D-penicillamine forms disulfide linkages with endogenous thiols and acts as a metal chelator, thereby modulating phagocyte oxyradical production, which should protect joints from oxygen radical damage (Joyce and Day 1990). Cysteine residues within the DNA-binding domains of proinflammatory transcription factors are potential targets for penicillamine. Penicillamine inhibits AP-1 DNA binding in nuclear extracts in the presence of free radicals, presumably by forming disulfide bonds with the cysteine residues in the DNA binding domains of Jun and Fos (Handel et al. 1996). Mutagenesis to remove cysteine residues in the DNA binding domains of these transcription factors results in loss of effect of penicillamine in experimental systems (Handel et al. 1996). Penicillamine has no cytotoxic effect (Joyce 1990). Penicillamine may also inhibit the crosslinkage of collagen (Joyce 1990).

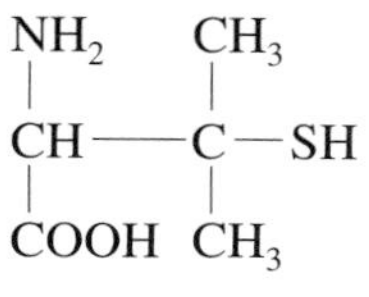

```
NH2     CH3
 |       |
CH ——— C — SH
 |       |
COOH    CH3
```

FIGURE 10-11 **The structure of penicillamine.**

### *Pharmacokinetics*

Penicillamine is rapidly absorbed, but net absorption is reduced by up to 50% if it is taken postprandially or coingested with iron supplements. Cholestyramine or antacids also diminish absorption (Perrett 1981; Osman et al. 1983; Tett 1993). Peak plasma concentrations occur 1.5 to 4 hours following ingestion with the terminal half-life of the drug between 1 and 7.5 hours. Penicillamine is highly bound by disulfide bonds to tissues and albumin with traces of drug evident for 3 months after dosing is ceased (Joyce and Day 1990; Tett 1993). The drug has a volume of distribution of 57 to 93L, with little uptake into cells, in keeping with its low lipid solubility. D-Penicillamine is cleared largely through oxidation to form disulfides with plasma albumin, L-cysteine, homocysteine, and D-penicillamine itself. D-Penicillamine albumin disulfide accumulates in the first weeks of therapy to concentrations 5 times those of D-penicillamine in plasma, making it a sink for D-penicillamine for a considerable period (Joyce 1990). *S*-Methyl-D-penicillamine and *N*-acetyl-D-penicillamine are minor urinary metabolites of D-penicillamine.

### *Efficacy*

In RA penicillamine improves clinical signs and corrects a number of laboratory parameters associated with RA and appears to be slightly more efficacious than hydroxychloroquine and auranofin (Felson et al. 1990, 1992, 1994; Brooks 1997). However, a crucial point is that penicillamine has not been shown to retard joint destruction in RA (Joyce 1990; Emery 1994), although this might relate to the lack of appropriate studies. An uncontrolled, open study with a 15-year follow-up in patients with progressive systemic sclerosis treated with penicillamine suggested a reduction in the degree of diseased skin involvement, and penicillamine has been shown to improve survival at 5 years (Steen et al. 1982; Steen et al. 1984; Steen and Medsger 1990; Jimenez and Sigal 1991). However, recent double-blind evidence did not support the hypothesis that D-penicillamine was effective in this disease (Clements et al. 1997).

### *Adverse effects*

Mild adverse effects such as rash, stomatitis, and metallic taste are common with D-penicillamine, whereas serious toxicity such as myelosuppression, proteinuria, nephrotic syndrome, and autoimmune syndromes (e.g., drug-induced lupus erythematosus; myasthenia gravis) are rare. Most adverse effects occur in the first 6 months after commencement of the drug, involving about 50% of patients and resulting in a significant drop-out rate from treatment. It has been suggested that patients who have poor sulfoxidation capacity and/or who express HLA DR3 or B8 antigens are at increased risk of adverse effects when treated with penicillamine (Stockman et al. 1986; Emery 1987; Seideman and Ayesh 1994) (Table 10-12).

***Dosing and monitoring***

Penicillamine treatment should be initiated with 125 mg daily for 4 to 8 weeks, then the dosage can be raised by the same amount until improvement is noticeable or a daily dose of 750 mg is achieved. The following baseline evaluations are recommended: complete blood cell count, creatinine, and urine dipstick for protein. A complete blood cell count and test for urinary protein should be checked every 2 weeks until a stable dosage is achieved. After that, these evaluations may be performed every 1 to 3 months (American College of Rheumatology Ad Hoc Committee on Clinical Guidelines 1996a) (Table 10-11). Once the disease has been controlled, penicillamine dosage may be reduced, but cessation usually results in exacerbation (Ahern et al. 1984).

## Cyclosporine

Cyclosporine, an immunomodulatory agent, is efficacious in patients with RA, but nephrotoxicity is a significant problem if doses are too high (Tugwell et al. 1990; Flipo and Reigneau 1996). Cyclosporine therapy in RA should be reserved for patients with refractory disease or severe extra-articular complications (Weinblatt et al. 1987; Yocum et al. 1988; McCune et al. 1994; Tugwell and Baker 1995).

***Mechanism of action***

Cyclosporine suppresses the immune response by inhibiting key signal transduction pathways (Yocum 1996). This is achieved by intracellular binding to immunophilin receptors, the complexes thus formed inhibiting calcineurin. Blocking the actions of calcineurin inhibits the nuclear translocation of cytosolic nuclear factor of activated T cells (NF-AT) with the result that genes influenced by this transcription factor such as IL-2 and IL-4 are not transcribed normally (Ho et al. 1996).

***Pharmacokinetics***

Oral cyclosporine has been recognized as having very variable bioavailability (Faulds et al. 1993) until the introduction recently of a capsule formulation containing a microemulsion of cyclosporine that provides better and more predictable bioavailability (Friman and Backman 1996). Cyclosporine has a low therapeutic index, and kidney damage has been shown to be more likely to occur in RA patients at dosing rates greater than 5 mg/kg daily (Yocum et al. 1988). The half-time of elimination is about 6 hours, but the drug is commonly administered twice daily. The drug is metabolized by the hepatic cytochrome P450 oxidase system (3A4 isoenzyme in particular) to multiple metabolites (Faulds et al. 1993). Its metabolism is inhibited by a range of drugs including ketoconazole and diltiazem and grapefruit juice and induced by others such as carbamazepine and phenytoin (Table 10-13; for a more complete review of clinically significant drug interaction see Campana et al. 1996).

***Efficacy***

Cyclosporine improves the clinical signs and symptoms of RA. Patients treated with cyclosporine show significant improvements in the number of active joints, pain, and functional status compared with controls (Tugwell et al. 1990). Low-dose cyclosporine is as effective as other DMARDs in controlling clinical symptoms (Yocum et al. 1988). There is evidence that low-dose cyclosporine retards further joint damage in previously involved joints and decreases the rate of new joint erosions in previously

**Table 10-12 Adverse Effects of D-Penicillamine**

| SYSTEM AFFECTED | COMMENT |
|---|---|
| Skin and mucous membranes | Itchy urticarial rash most common; oral ulcers and stomatitis; pemphigus |
| Blood | Thrombocytopenia (can occur rapidly and be profound); neutropenia; aplastic anemia |
| Kidney | Proteinuria (common); membranous or proliferative glomerulonephritis; more rarely nephrotic; rapidly progressive glomerulonephritis, e.g., Goodpasture syndrome or drug-induced SLE (beware hematuria) |
| Gastrointestinal | Nausea; metallic taste |
| Lungs | Bronchiolitis obliterans |
| Autoimmune | Drug-induced SLE; pemphigus; Goodpasture syndrome; myasthenia gravis; dermatopolymyositis |
| Reproduction | Teratogenic |

ABBREVIATIONS: SLE, systemic lupus erythematosus.
SOURCE: From Day 1998.

Table 10-13 Some Important Drug Interactions with Cyclosporine

| DRUGS THAT COULD INCREASE CYCLOSPORINE CONCENTRATIONS IN BLOOD | DRUGS THAT COULD DECREASE CYCLOSPORINE CONCENTRATIONS IN BLOOD | DRUGS THAT MAY CAUSE ADDITIVE NEPHROTOXICITY |
|---|---|---|
| Grapefruit juice | Phenytoin | NSAIDs |
| Amiodarone HCl | Phenobarbital | Trimethoprim (alone and when in combination with sulfonamides, e.g., co-trimoxazole) |
| Verapamil HCl | Carbamazepine | Aminoglycosides |
| Diltiazem HCl | Rifampicin | Enalapril maleate |
| Nicardipine HCl | Octreotide acetate | Melphalan |
| Allopurinol | Ciprofloxacin HCl | Ciprofloxacin |
| Doxycycline | Probucol | Colchicine |
| Erythromycin | | Amphotericin B |
| Fluconazole | | |
| Itraconazole | | |
| Miconazole | | |
| Ketoconazole | | |
| Metoclopramide HCl | | |
| Tacrolimus | | |
| Prednisolone | | |
| Oral contraceptive | | |
| Glipizide | | |
| Danazol | | |

SOURCE: See Campana et al. 1996; Quinn and Day 1997.

uninvolved joints, in patients with early RA (Pasero et al. 1996).

### *Adverse effects*

Nephrotoxicity is the principal adverse effect of cyclosporine (Faulds et al. 1993). This agent should be avoided in patients with preexisting renal disease. Careful dosing and monitoring are required when cyclosporine is used with other nephrotoxic agents (Table 10-13). If plasma creatinine increases by 30 to 50% above baseline, the dose should be reduced by 25 to 50%. Hypertension affects up to one-third of cyclosporine-treated RA patients. Hypertension can usually be controlled with $\beta$-adrenergic receptor antagonists ("beta-blockers") or ACE inhibitors, if one keeps a careful watch on renal function after introducing antihypertensive therapy. Less serious adverse effects such as nausea, vomiting, and loss of appetite are frequent. Elevated hepatic enzymes and bilirubin are usually associated with high doses of cyclosporine. Other adverse effects include anemia, gum hyperplasia, hirsutism, tremor, and paresthesias. Of concern are case reports of lymphoproliferative lesions and other malignancies developing in patients who have received cyclosporine therapy, but most of this experience has been in transplant patients and in combination with other immunosuppressing agents (Armitage et al. 1991; Opelz and Henderson 1993; Ferraccioli 1995; Hiesse et al. 1995).

### *Dosing and monitoring*

Cyclosporine should be initiated at doses of 2.5 mg/kg daily given in divided doses every 12 hours, increasing the dose 25 to 50% every 2 to 4 weeks until a maximum dose of 5 mg/kg daily is reached (Tugwell and Baker 1995). A complete blood count, creatinine, uric acid, and liver function tests, as well as the measurement of blood pressure, are recommended at baseline. At follow-up visits examination for edema and measurement of blood pressure are suggested every 2 weeks until the cyclosporine dosage is stable and monthly from then on. Plasma creatinine should be checked every 2 weeks until the dosage is stable. Periodic complete blood counts, plasma potassium, and liver function tests are suggested (Table 10-11). Plasma concentrations of cyclosporine should be monitored on starting or discontinuing any of the drugs listed in Table 10-11. Patients should be made aware of the interaction with grapefruit juice (Yee et al. 1995).

## Minocycline, Cotrimoxazole, and Antibiotics

The suspicion remains that RA is an infectious disease. Careful trials of various antibiotics, particularly of the tetracycline group, indicate efficacy, but mechanisms other than antimicrobial may explain these findings.

### *Mechanism of action*

Drugs from the tetracycline group have inhibitory activity against polymorphs, lymphocyte proliferation, cytokine release, and antibody production. Tetracyclines are also potent metalloproteinase inhibitors which could translate into inhibition of bone resorption in inflammatory rheumatic diseases (Kloppenburg, Dijkmans, et al. 1995; Kloppenburg et al. 1996).

### *Efficacy and toxicity*

Two well-conducted double-blind, randomized studies of 26 and 48 weeks' duration, respectively, have shown that minocycline 200 mg/day is more effective than placebo in clinical response and laboratory measures in RA (Kloppenburg, Breedveld, et al. 1994; Kloppenburg, Terweil, et al. 1994; Kloppenburg, Mattie, et al. 1995; Tilley et al. 1995). However, comparative efficacy and effect on erosions remains unknown. Nausea, light-headedness, dizziness, and photosensitive skin rashes are the most common adverse effects, and very rarely with tetracyclines there is the danger of severe liver damage. It is recommended that liver function tests and a full blood count are performed every 4 to 12 weeks.

## Azathioprine

Azathioprine is an immunosuppressive drug useful in the management of a number of inflammatory conditions including RA, SLE, and vasculitides (Luqmani et al. 1990; Hunter et al. 1975; Hamuryudan et al. 1997). It is normally reserved for patients failing to respond to first-line therapy with DMARDs. Azathioprine plays a useful role in allowing the dose of glucocorticosteroids to be decreased with reduction in potential for corticoid-induced adverse effects (Ginzler et al. 1975; Luqmani et al. 1990; McCarty et al. 1996). Azathioprine is slightly inferior to methotrexate in inducing clinical improvement and inhibiting progression of periarticular erosions in RA (Sambrook et al. 1986; Jeurissen et al. 1991; Willkens et al. 1995), but controlled studies and meta-analyses suggest that it has efficacy similar to that of other DMARDs apart from methotrexate (Wolfe 1995). The usual dose range is 1.25 to 3.0 mg/kg daily for RA. Small studies suggest efficacy in psoriatic arthritis, Reiter syndrome, Behçet syndrome, SLE, and polymyositis (Furst and Clements 1998).

### *Mode of action and pharmacokinetics*

Azathioprine probably exerts its immunosuppressive effects predominantly on B lymphocytes with resultant reduction in gamma-globulin and cytokine production and reduced lymphocyte proliferation (Levy J, et al. 1972; Yy et al. 1974; Luqmani et al. 1990). Azathioprine has an oral bioavailability of around 50% (Van Os et al. 1996). It is rapidly cleaved by a glutathione-dependent reaction in a wide variety of cells to 6-mercaptopurine that can be administered in its own right. The metabolite 6-mercaptopurine is metabolized intra-cellularly to active nucleotide metabolites notably 6-thioinosinate and 6-thiouric acid (Lin et al. 1980; Lennard 1992). This results in either direct inhibition of purine synthesis or conversion to thio-IMP which interferes with the salvage pathway of purine synthesis. Thio-IMP is also converted to thio-GTP that can be incorporated into DNA as a false nucleotide. Excretion of azathioprine and metabolites occurs principally in the urine (see also chapter 13).

### *Adverse effects*

The acute toxicity of azathioprine may be manifested by nausea and vomiting, dose-related marrow suppression or idiosyncratic reactions such as systemic hypersensitivity, skin rash, or hematoxicity (Singh et al. 1989; Luqmani et al. 1990; Morales 1996; Parnham et al. 1996; Fields et al. 1998). Increased bone marrow toxicity secondary to azathioprine is seen in patients with genetic deficiencies in the endogenous purine-metabolizing enzymes thiopurine methyltransferase or purine 5′-nucleotidase (Kerstens et al. 1995; Leipold et al. 1997; Snow and Gibson 1995; Vesell 1997; Yates et al. 1997). These patients comprise up to 15% of Caucasian populations (Weinshilboum 1989; Yates et al. 1997).

Coadministration of azathioprine or 6-mercaptopurine with allopurinol results in markedly increased toxicity of the antimetabolites because of the effect of allopurinol in inhibiting xanthine oxidase, which is a crucial enzyme in purine metabolism. The combination should be avoided if possible, or if essential, then the dose of azathioprine should be reduced by 75%. Use of the combination of azathioprine and methotrexate in the treatment of RA results in an acute febrile toxic reaction in 9% of patients; this abates rapidly with discontinuation (Blanco et al. 1996).

The use of azathioprine in rheumatic disorders has been limited to some extent by its potential for long-term adverse effects, especially malignancy (Opelz and Henderson 1993; Confavreux et al. 1996; Jones M, et al. 1996). The risk of malignancy increases with duration and cumulative dose of azathioprine, and this has been most apparent in the transplant setting. The relative risk for developing malignancy in RA with azathioprine therapy has been estimated at 1.3 and between 2.2 and 8.7 for lymphoproliferative disorders (Tsokos 1987; McKendry 1991).

### *Dosing and monitoring*

A gradual increase in dose is appropriate. It is good practice to commence with 25 to 50 mg daily and to increase by 0.5 mg/kg daily after a week. Increments of 0.5 mg/kg per day can continue at weekly or longer intervals until the total daily dose is between 2 and 3 mg/kg per day. Adjustments are made to obtain the best balance between efficacy and adverse effects. Monitoring requires full blood count every 2 weeks during dose alterations and then every 4 to 6 weeks, with liver function tests every 6 to 8 weeks (Table 10-11) (Furst and Clements 1998).

## Cyclophosphamide

### *Mechanism of action*

Alkylating agents are structurally diverse drugs that have in common reactive functional groups that are electron-deficient and bond covalently with electron-rich groups in nucleic acids, proteins, and other molecules (Brock 1996). Of these interactions, DNA binding is most important with the N-7 position on guanine as particularly important. Alkylation produces a number of effects including depurination, double- and single-strand breaks and inter- and intrastrand crosslinks, all of which may temporarily or permanently disrupt DNA replication and transcription, potentially resulting in reduction in protein and cytokine production, cell death, mutagenesis, or carcinogenesis. Lymphocytes are particularly susceptible to the effects of alkylating agents with the result that therapy induces immunosuppression by preventing proliferation and cytokine production (Cupps et al. 1982; Luqmani et al. 1990). B lymphocytes tend to recover more slowly from the effects of cyclophosphamide than T lymphocytes, and therefore immunosuppression tends to affect humoral immunity more than cellular (see also chapter 13).

### *Pharmacokinetics and metabolism*

When taken orally cyclophosphamide has a bioavailability of 60 to 90%. Cyclophosphamide is hydroxylated in the liver by the CYP2B group of P450 microsomal enzymes to its primary active metabolite, 4-hydroxycyclophosphamide (Chang et al. 1993). 4-Hydroxycyclophosphamide is actively taken up by cells where it decomposes spontaneously to another active alkylator, phosphoramide mustard. The elimination half-life of cyclophosphamide is around 8 hours, whereas that of its metabolite, phosphoramide mustard, is around 9 hours. All active metabolites are excreted renally (Grochow and Colvin 1979). Despite metabolism of cyclophosphamide by microsomal enzymes, inhibitors and inducers of these enzymes generally do not appear to have significant effects on the pharmacokinetics or toxicity of the drug. However, allopurinol and cimetidine have been identified as potential inhibitors of the metabolism of cyclophosphamide and therefore caution needs to be exercised if one is using either of these drugs with cyclophosphamide (Moore 1991).

### *Efficacy and dosing*

Cyclophosphamide is reserved for severe nonresponsive joint manifestations in RA, progressive vasculitis due to RA, SLE, primary vasculitides, or visceral involvement, particularly cerebral and renal involvement, in SLE (Townes et al. 1976; McCune et al. 1988; Boumpas et al. 1995; Neuwelt et al. 1995; Ciruelo et al. 1996; Cockwell 1997). Cyclophosphamide has significant efficacy in each of these situations, but its toxicity is considerable, and it should be commenced only after consultation with a clinician experienced in its use and after detailed discussion with the patient.

Doses of greater than 1.5 mg/kg daily are required for efficacy in RA, peak effectiveness is seen around 16 weeks, and there is limited evidence that cyclophosphamide will retard erosion formation. Cyclophosphamide is the most versatile alkylating agent. It is active if given intravenously in a pulse dose of 400 to 600 mg per meter squared every 3 to 4 weeks or on a chronic daily oral dosing schedule of 1.0 to 2.5 mg/kg per day for between 7 and 14 days in each month. Glucocorticosteroids are often coadministered with cyclophosphamide for therapeutic synergy (Gourley et al. 1996). It is the least carcinogenic of the alkylating agents, and studies suggest that pulse intravenous dosing results in a lower overall dose for response and may therefore have less carcinogenic and toxicity potential than when taken orally (Gourley et al. 1996).

### *Adverse effects*

Toxicities include nausea and vomiting, acute bone marrow suppression, acute and chronic infertility, pulmonary toxicity, and potential for carcinogenicity especially in the form of myelodysplastic syndromes, acute myeloid leukemia, bladder cancer, and non-Hodgkin lymphoma

(Baker et al. 1987; Gonzalez-Crespo et al. 1995; Radis et al. 1995; Fernandes et al. 1996; Jones M, et al. 1996; Malik et al. 1996; Rosenthal and Farhi 1996). Acrolein, a toxic metabolite of cyclophosphamide, may produce hemorrhagic cystitis. This adverse effect which can be avoided or minimized by maintenance of hydration before, during, and after therapy and by use of the urinary protective agent, mesna (see chapter 13, Oncologic Disorders) (Plotz et al. 1979; Hows et al. 1984; Talar-Williams et al. 1996; Ratliff and Williams 1998).

***Monitoring***

In monitoring patients on pulse intravenous cyclophosphamide, one should aim to avoid nadir neutrophil counts of less than 1000 because of the risk of infection, particularly from gram-negative bacteria (see chapter 14, Infectious Diseases) (Pryor et al. 1996). In patients on chronic oral cyclophosphamide schedules, weekly blood counts should be performed to monitor both the neutrophil count (>1000) and the total lymphocyte count to ensure it stays above 500, because below this the risk of complications from immunosuppression increases (Huynh-Do et al. 1995) (Table 10-11). Patients need to be warned about the risk of hemorrhagic cystitis and encouraged to consume large amounts of liquid around the time of therapy. Mesna (2-mercaptoethanesulfonate) should be administered if a pulse intravenous dose exceeds 750 mg per meter square of body surface area, or there has been previous hematuria following cyclophosphamide therapy. Patients need to be monitored clinically and by evaluation of appropriate laboratory parameters for response as well as toxicity.

## Biologic Agents and Bone Marrow Transplantation

An exciting era in the treatment of rheumatic diseases is upon us with the demonstration of good, sometimes remarkable efficacy in some individuals and short-term safety with a number of biologic agents (Koopman and Moreland 1998). Antibodies to TNF$\alpha$ (Elliott et al. 1994a, 1994b), recombinant human soluble receptors of TNF$\alpha$ (Moreland, Baumgartner, et al. 1997) and interleukin 1 (IL-I), and recombinant human IL-1 receptor antagonist (IL-1ra) (Campion et al. 1996) have shown rapid onset efficacy against the symptoms and signs of inflammation in RA such as joint swelling. TNF$\alpha$ blocking agents seem more active and have a rapid onset of action. IL-1ra may also have activity against bone erosions (Bresnihan 1997). Combinations of biologic therapies with conventional agents such as methotrexate are now starting to be explored in clinical trials, and these new agents are likely to have a major impact on the treatment of the inflammatory rheumatic diseases (Firestein and Zvaifler 1997; Moreland, Heck, et al. 1997; Skolnick 1997).

Stem cell transplantation is under investigation for the treatment of severe and unresponsive RA and other immunologic connective tissue disorders such as scleroderma. The hope is that the intensive immunosuppressive therapy possible with stem cell transplantation might eradicate disease. Mortality from this procedure is now around 1%, so that it may become an option for severe unremitting disease (Hamilton et al. 1995; Tyndall and Gratwohl 1996; Tyndall and Gratwohl 1997).

## Colchicine

Colchicine is a venerable drug used since antiquity that has proven efficacy in the relief of the pain and inflammation of acute gout. The drug does not lower plasma urate concentrations. Colchicine is efficacious also in the acute form of calcium pyrophosphate deposition disease (CPPD), or pseudogout, another crystal-induced acute inflammatory arthritis. Other indications include familial Mediterranean fever and amyloidosis, primary biliary cirrhosis, Behçet syndrome, and sarcoid arthritis.

***Mechanism of action***

It is an alkaloid of *Colchicum autumnale* (autumn crocus) that arrests dividing cells by binding to intracellular microtubules, thereby interfering with the mitotic process. Specifically, colchicine is thought to inhibit chemotaxis and the function of polymorphonuclear cells responsible for the acute inflammation in affected joints. The drug is not effective in other inflammatory arthritides such as RA, although polymorphs are usually abundant in the synovial fluid in those conditions.

***Efficacy and dosing***

The drug has fallen out of favor for the treatment of acute gout because NSAIDs are as effective without causing diarrhea, which is dose-limiting with colchicine (Conaghan and Day 1996). If NSAIDs are contraindicated (for example, because of a recent bleeding peptic ulcer), then colchicine remains an option, although short courses of prednisolone or intra-articular depot corticosteroids are often preferred.

Very careful dosing instruction is critical if the drug is to be used safely in the treatment of acute attacks of gout. At the first sign of an attack a dose of 0.5, 0.6, or 1 mg is administered. The drug is then administered in doses of 0.5 or 0.6 mg every 1 to 2 hours and is continued until relief is obtained or diarrhea or other GI adverse effect such as nausea or vomiting occurs. The maximum dose in a course should not exceed 6 mg orally, and the drug should not be restarted for at least 3 days.

Colchicine has a role in prevention of acute gout. The recurrence rate of attacks of acute gout can be reduced by low-dose, regular colchicine. A dose of 0.5 once or twice daily in association with lifestyle measures such as reduction of alcohol and seafood intake may avoid the need for lifelong hypouricemic therapy. The introduction of hypouricemic therapy with allopurinol or probenecid carries a substantial risk of inducing acute gout, the risk increasing with the severity and duration of hyperuricemia. Low-dose colchicine reduces this risk as does a gradual increase in the dose of the hypouricemic drug.

Colchicine is eliminated partially via the kidneys, and the dosage should be lowered in renal impairment. The drug is also metabolized in the liver, and, again, dosage reduction in hepatic disease is appropriate. The elderly are more sensitive to the drug, and dosing needs to be more conservative. Often bowel looseness or frank diarrhea indicates that dosage is excessive. The drug is lethal in overdose, inhibiting the replication of rapidly dividing cells in bone marrow and gut. Storage must be secure. Some work suggests that specific antibodies directed against the drug could be lifesaving in overdose (Baud et al. 1995). Occasionally the drug is used in low doses intravenously when the oral route is unavailable. Extravasation into the tissues can lead to severe damage, and loss of the limb and fatalities have occurred when the dose has been excessive. Intravenous colchicine should be avoided or used with extreme caution and only in exceptional circumstances.

## Allopurinol

Allopurinol is the most widely used hypouricemic drug and can prevent and reverse all the manifestations of gout. The drug was introduced as a potential cytotoxic drug by George Hitchings and Gertrude Elion (jointly 1988 Nobel laureates with James Black for his work on beta-blockers and $H_2$ antagonists).

### *Mechanism of action*

Allopurinol is an analog of the purine nucleoside metabolite hypoxanthine and competes with the latter for the enzyme xanthine dehydrogenase, the reduced form of xanthine oxidase. This enzyme catalyses the terminal steps of the purine metabolic pathway, namely, the sequential conversion of hypoxanthine to xanthine and xanthine to uric acid. In the process allopurinol is oxidized to its active metabolite oxypurinol, which is a potent, pseudo-irreversible inhibitor of xanthine oxidase (Fig. 10-12). Thus hypoxanthine and xanthine accumulate at the expense of uric acid. These purine metabolites are substrates for the purine salvage pathway and are thus able to inhibit the rate-limiting enzymatic step of the purine synthetic pathway.

### *Pharmacokinetics*

Allopurinol is well absorbed orally. Once absorbed it is quickly metabolized to oxypurinol; the half-life of elimination of allopurinol is about 1 to 3 hours. Although allopurinol is an effective reversible inhibitor of xanthine oxidase, it is its active metabolite that is the most important inhibitor of xanthine oxidase. Oxypurinol has an elimination half-life of about 16 hours, so that once-daily dosing is appropriate. Oxypurinol is cleared by the kidney, and the dosage of allopurinol needs to be reduced in renal impairment or in the elderly who have reduced renal function (Conaghan and Day 1996).

Allopurinol dose and plasma oxypurinol concentration–response relationships for plasma urate have been established. There is a linear relationship between allopurinol 50 to 900 mg daily and plasma oxypurinol concentrations; the plasma urate concentrations decrease exponentially as allopurinol dose and plasma oxypurinol concentrations increase (Graham et al. 1996).

### *Adverse effects*

Allopurinol is well-tolerated, but is hazardous if the dose is excessive in the face of renal impairment. In this situation serious skin, hepatic, and renal toxicity can occur with exfoliative dermatitis most feared. The drug can be reintroduced following a desensitization protocol commencing with very small doses (Meyrier 1976). The occurrence of acute gout following commencement of allopurinol is well-known, and the risk can be reduced by increasing the daily dose slowly, and covering the introduction with low-dose colchicine (see below).

An important interaction occurs with azathioprine and its metabolite 6-mercaptopurine. Because 6-mercaptopurine is detoxified by metabolism by xanthine oxidase, if the latter enzyme is inhibited by allopurinol, then fatal bone marrow suppression induced by 6-mercaptopurine can occur. The dose of azathioprine or 6-mercaptopurine needs to be reduced to about one-third if dosed concomitantly with allopurinol. Patients taking amoxicillin

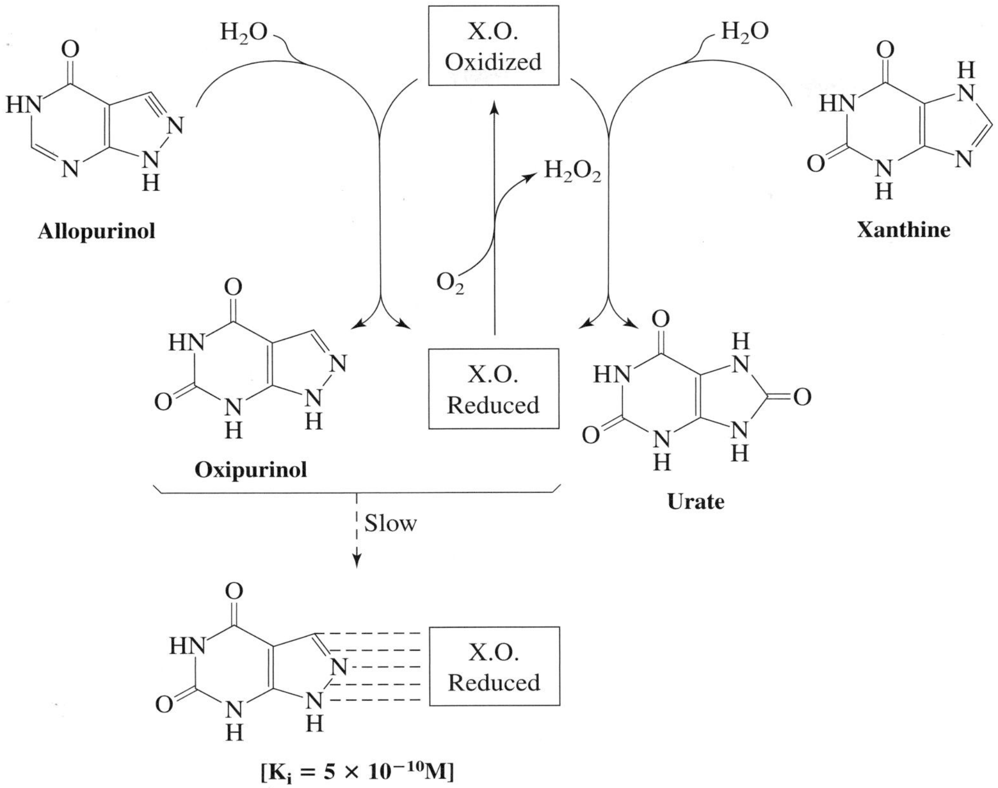

FIGURE 10-12 **The inhibition of xanthine oxidase (X.O.) by allopurinol and oxypurinol. (Reprinted from *Biochemical Pharmacology* 26, Spector T. Inhibition of urate production by allopurinol, pp 355–358, ©1977 with permission of Elsevier Science.)**

concurrent with allopurinol are likely to develop a maculopapular rash, the mechanism for which is not known.

## Uricosuric Drugs: Probenecid, Sulfinpyrazone, and Benzbromarone

Uricosuric drugs increase the renal clearance of urate and act from the renal tubule lumen by competing with urate for its transporter located in the brush border of the tubular epithelium. The bidirectional flux of urate across the tubular lumen results in opposing effects on urate transport by different doses of drugs active on this system. Thus, low doses of salicylate or phenylbutazone lead to urate retention, whereas high doses are uricosuric.

Probenecid is the most widely used uricosuric drug and is as effective in reducing plasma uric acid as allopurinol, but it is used much less than allopurinol these days. It is a weakly acidic drug that competes for the reuptake of uric acid from the ultrafiltrate in the renal tubule, thereby increasing the renal clearance of uric acid. It loses its efficacy in renal impairment. There is a danger that uric acid will precipitate in the renal tubules following initiation of therapy causing acute obstructive uropathy. This risk can be countered by a gradual introduction of the drug, keeping the patient well-hydrated during the early stages of therapy, and alkalinizing the urine with sodium bicarbonate. Sometimes the drug is used in combination with allopurinol in severe cases of tophaceous gout if renal function is satisfactory. The evidence for greater efficacy of the combination is anecdotal.

Another uricosuric drug that is used even less than probenecid is sulfinpyrazone. It is chemically related to phenylbutazone, which has uricosuric properties in high dosage, but there is not a measurable risk of aplastic anemia as is seen with phenylbutazone. Sulfinpyrazone was popular some years ago because of platelet inhibitory properties. Sulfinpyrazone is a metabolic inhibitor, and important interactions occur with oral hypoglycemic drugs (hypoglycemia) and warfarin (excessive anticoagulation).

Benzbromarone is also a uricosuric drug that is sometimes used in Europe in the management of hyperuricemia. This drug and its metabolites also inhibit urate reuptake in the proximal renal tubule. It is administered once daily and may retain activity in the face of renal impairment.

Probenecid and sulfinpyrazone both contain sulfur atoms and carry the risk of typical hypersensitivity reactions such as immune complex–mediated adverse effects.

## CLINICAL THERAPEUTICS OF THE RHEUMATIC DISORDERS

A substantial component of the management of the rheumatic and musculoskeletal disorders revolves around the management of chronic painful conditions that fluctuate in intensity. Accompanying the pain and sometimes stiffness are disability and distress; successful management of these complex dimensions of musculoskeletal diseases is essential. Improved results are achieved by taking a multidisciplinary approach involving a wide range of skills and including the patients and their families as active contributors to the program (Table 10-14).

The best results are achieved if a systematic approach is taken, for example, the POP approach: careful delineation of the problem (P); thorough evaluation of the costs and benefits of the available therapeutic options (O), pharmacologic and nonpharmacologic; a well-constructed plan (P) that is specific about goals, modalities of therapy e.g., physiotherapy and occupational therapy, individualization of drug regimens, appropriate surveillance for adverse effects of therapy (Table 10-15).

### Soft-Tissue Rheumatic Conditions

Managing the acute pain well reduces the risk of the development of chronic pain. Careful evaluation of the cause of the pain often reveals the remedy, for example, vigorous activity leading to shoulder or elbow pain suggests avoiding that activity in the short term. Often initial management is to follow the RICE acronym:

*R*est
*I*ce
*C*ompression
*E*levation

Once pain and swelling have started to recede, the goal should be a return to normal activity supported by a carefully graded program. Attention to activities of daily living, often with the help of an occupational therapist and a graded exercise regimen with the help of a physiotherapist, are important program components in many of these conditions. Acetaminophen taken regularly in appropriate dose (up to 4 g/day in a healthy adult) will provide effective analgesia in most cases. If there is considerable swelling and heat, as for example, with an acute ankle injury, and there are no contraindications, a short course of NSAIDs is reasonable. The use of topical analgesics (often NSAIDs, salicylates, or benzydamine) is rational, effective, and safe (Moore et al. 1998). The use of local injections of depot glucocorticosteroids may assist with conditions such as rotator cuff inflammation and tears, tennis elbow, trochanteric bursitis, etc. Good progress is expected over 2 to 3 weeks, and failure to improve requires careful reevaluation of the program as the specter of chronic pain begins to loom.

### Fibromyalgia Syndrome

Careful education concerning fibromyalgia syndrome is a helpful starting point and is often accompanied by relief for the patient that he or she is suffering from a defined condition that also affects others. A multidisciplinary and multifaceted approach to this chronic pain condition is essential (Table 10-16). Particular attention needs to be paid to the distress accompanying the syndrome, and psychologic counseling is very valuable for some. Generally, a graded exercise and activity program is useful, but this needs to be individualized to accommodate the particular problems and progress of the patient. Pharmacologic therapy is not dramatically efficacious, but tricyclic antidepressants proved effective and can assist with the sleep disturbance. Low-dose amitriptyline, increasing the dose gradually, for example, from 10 to 20 mg up to 50 to 75 mg each night, is used successfully in about 30% of patients. Careful coordination of the program is essential; an important goal is to promote a sound self-management approach. A supportive but realistic approach as described leads to a good outcome in most patients (Littlejohn 1996).

### Back and Neck Pain

Surprisingly, there is little controlled evidence for the efficacy of any interventions for the common mechanical origin lumbar and cervical neck pain (Teasell and White

Table 10-14 Multidisciplinary Approach to the Musculoskeletal and Rheumatic Disorders

| TEAM MEMBERS | NOTES |
|---|---|
| Patient | An educated, motivated individual who takes responsibility for his/her situation |
| Patient's family | Support patient's efforts to adhere to program and to maintain independence |
| General practitioner | Oversees medical therapy and may coordinate some services |
| Physical therapist | Helps develop program that will maintain strength and flexibility as well as relieve symptoms |
| Occupational therapist | Assists with coping with activities of daily living, strategies for dealing with pain |
| Psychologist | Helps to resolve conflicts, treat depression, deal with counterproductive psychologic patterns of thought and behavior |
| Podiatrist | Careful attention to correcting dysfunctional foot mechanics—overlooked too frequently |
| Social worker | Assists with occupational, social, family, and financial issues that are contributing to the distress of the disorder |
| Rheumatology nurse practitioner | Diagnostic role, helps manage therapy, coordinate program, oversees monitoring of drug therapy, educational input |
| Rheumatologist | Diagnostic role, establishes management plan, reviews progress in suppressing signs and symptoms of disease, coordination role |
| Orthopedic surgeon | Corrects deformities, replaces joints |
| Community arthritis group | Important role in promoting self-help attitude and skills |

1994a, 1994b; Hoffman et al. 1995) and lack of consensus about the efficacy of treatment options (Cherkin et al. 1995). However, the therapeutic goal is to treat the pain (and the distress associated) and the functional loss (disability) and to avoid chronicity (Table 10-17). Evidence is available that bed rest is not indicated, rather a graded return to activity and fitness is preferred, and this program will reduce deconditioning, muscle atrophy, and osteoporosis (Nicholas et al. 1992; Malmivaara et al. 1995). Dealing with obvious postural abnormalities and abnormal use patterns in the course of conditioning and fitness programs are beneficial. Adequate analgesia in the acute

Table 10-15 An Approach to the Management of the Rheumatic and Musculoskeletal Disorders

| PHASE OF PROGRAM | ELEMENTS | COMMENT |
|---|---|---|
| Problem | History, examination, investigation | Inflammatory or noninflammatory? Mechanical or not? |
| Options | Nonpharmacologic | Education, e.g., arthritis self-help groups |
| | | Coordinate physiotherapy, occupational therapy, podiatry, etc. |
| | Pharmacologic | Costs and benefits in light of goals of therapy, e.g., symptom control alone or disease suppression as well |
| Plan | Goals of therapy | Are there long-term considerations such as trying to delay onset of severe disability? |
| | Drug therapy regimens | Individualize on basis of age, organ function, progress |
| | Evaluation of therapy | What outcome measures will you record and rely on? |
| | Surveillance for safety and review of progress | Safety, progress, medication review |
| | Compliance | A well-informed, motivated, supported patient engaged in a comprehensive and well-constructed program is the best antidote to poor compliance |
| | Stop? | When can some of the therapeutic modalities be stopped, e.g., physiotherapy visits; corticosteroid dosing, etc.? |

Table 10-16 **Management Principles for Fibromyalgia Syndrome**

| PRINCIPLES | COMMENTS |
|---|---|
| Confident diagnosis | Avoid unnecessary investigations and unscientific explanations |
| Comprehensive education of patient and family | Engage well-established and well-constituted community organizations |
| Address psychologic factors that are contributing | Counseling; coping strategies; stress management; relaxation training; behavioral therapy |
| Exercise and physical program | Graded; realistic; regular review; attention to posture |
| Provide occupational and activities of daily living advice | Program gradual return to usual work, home and recreational activities |
| Address sleep disorder | Advise regarding optimizing sleep, e.g., review caffeine intake |
| Analgesia—simple, not NSAIDs or opioids | Rely on acetaminophen given in appropriate dose in time-contingent manner if effective |
| Prescribe "adjuvant" analgesia, i.e., tricyclic antidepressants | For example, amitriptyline 10–50 mg at night; will also assist with sleep; escalate dose slowly |
| Encourage self-management and discourage viewing illness as a disability | Key goals |

SOURCE: From Littlejohn 1998.

Table 10-17 **The Management of Mechanical Neck and Back Pain**

| PRINCIPLES | COMMENTS |
|---|---|
| Detailed education | Explain natural history, prognosis, and management principles |
| Recommend minimal bed rest | Rapid return to graded activity |
| Prescribe adequate analgesia for acute pain | Regular acetaminophen 1g qid *or if needed:* |
| | Regular acetaminophen 500 mg plus codeine phosphate 30 mg up to 2 tablets qid (some practitioners would use NSAIDs here if acetaminophen was unsatisfactory and there were no contraindications to NSAIDs) *or if needed:* |
| | Oxycodone 5 mg, 1–2 every 3–4 h regularly |
| For persistent or prolonged pain | As for acute pain *or if needed:* |
| | Sustained-release morphine bid (in consultation with specialist pain service) |
| Prescribe adjuvants to analgesics | Usually a tricyclic antidepressant, e.g., amitriptyline (10–50 mg) or doxepin (10–50 mg) at night *or if needed:* |
| | Membrane-stabilizing drugs, e.g., carbamazepine (100–200 mg bid) or sodium valproate (100–300 mg tid) |
| Correct abnormal posture and use-patterns of spine | Physical therapy assistance useful |
| Recommend active not passive physical therapy | Strength, flexibility, conditioning all helpful |
| Psychosocial factors | Important to address these; industrial origin with litigation concerns will prolong distress and disability |
| Consider neuro- or orthopedic surgery consultation | Flags include myelopathy, persistent radiculopathy, or loss of sphincter control |

SOURCE: From Cohen 1996.

stage will help the success of the program overall, as well as reduce the risk of chronicity. A rigorous double-blind study has established that in patients with chronic unresponsive cervical pain of mechanical origin, percutaneous radiofrequency neurotomy of nerves supplying the affected zygapophyseal joints is a successful procedure (Lord et al. 1996).

## Avoidance of Chronic Pain States in the Management of Musculoskeletal Conditions

Chronic musculoskeletal pain may be the result of an ongoing pathologic process such as RA but also can be the result of the evolution from an acute pain condition such as spinal pain or limb injury, to a chronic, neuropathic pain state. The simple recording of a noxious stimulus by the pain-recording neurons and brain centers characteristic of transient, mild trauma evolves into a neuropathic state because of sensitization of the central and peripheral nervous system involved in pain perception. The result is a fall in the threshold for activation and a lengthening of the duration of the pain response. Also stimuli normally not considered painful do induce pain (allodynia), and the response to normally painful stimuli is heightened (secondary hyperalgesia). When a common musculoskeletal pain condition of mechanical or traumatic origin does not resolve in the usual time (e.g., a few weeks), changes in pattern and quality as noted above, or increasing in severity, then the possibility of an emerging neuropathic or chronic pain state needs to be considered (Table 10-18). The best protection against this possibility is the effective management of the acute pain states as discussed under soft-tissue rheumatic conditions and neck and back pain. Also, awareness of so-called *flags* that designate patients at risk for the transition from acute to chronic pain states are useful to the clinician (Table 10-19).

## Osteoarthritis and Noninflammatory Rheumatic Conditions

Careful history and examination seeking the cause of pain and other symptoms will differentiate noninflammatory from inflammatory rheumatic conditions in most cases. In noninflammatory conditions such as OA and most back pain and soft-tissue conditions such as tennis elbow, simply making a confident diagnosis is often therapeutic. The use of nondrug options such as physical therapy, orthotics (inserts) for shoes, and assistance with joint protection at home and at work can be extremely effective (Table 10-20). Pharmacologic therapy for OA of the knee has been systematically reviewed using meta-analysis and gives useful guidance (Towheed and Hochberg 1997). Topical therapy with salicylate or NSAID-containing liniments or capsaicin (depletes substance P) is helpful and is safe (Altman et al. 1994). Drug therapy is symptomatic only, and acetaminophen in ample, time-contingent dosing regimens (up to 4 g daily in divided doses) may suffice and will not lead to gastric ulceration (Jones and Doherty 1992). If further pain relief is needed and there are no contraindications such as previous peptic ulcer or age greater than 65 years, commencement of low-dose NSAID such as ibuprofen or diclofenac is often useful. Acetaminophen may be continued and will allow smaller doses of NSAIDs to be used. The aim should always be to use the

**Table 10-18 Features of Chronic Musculoskeletal Pain**

| FEATURE | COMMENT |
|---|---|
| Persistence | Persists for longer than expected, e.g., acute mechanical back pain lasting longer than 3 weeks |
| Physical | Continuing gait and posture abnormalities |
| | Secondary hyperalgesia and allodynia |
| | Muscle wasting and weakness |
| Occupational and social | Substantial time away from work |
| | Income drop; burnout in career |
| | Dependence on benefits; insurance |
| | Relationship difficulties |
| | Contracting social contacts |
| Psychologic | Low self-esteem |
| | Anger and frustration |
| | Withdrawal |
| | Hopelessness and helplessness |
| | Depression; sleep disturbance |

Table 10-19 "Yellow flags" Signaling Potential Problems in the Management of Musculoskeletal Pain

| **Drug dependence or history of drug dependence** |
|---|
| Psychiatric illness or taking psychoactive medications for psychiatric condition |
| Work-related injury involving potential or actual litigation and the possibility of compensation |
| Liability for developing distress, depression, and social stress; poorly developed coping mechanisms and skills |
| History of alcohol abuse |

lowest dose of NSAID only for as long as needed. It is interesting that the presence of signs of inflammation such as effusions and heat over joints does not predict who will respond to acetaminophen. The judicious use of intra- and periarticular injections of depot glucocorticosteroids such as triamcinolone hydrochloride or methylprednisolone acetate can be effective if particular joints are painful and resistant to therapy. More recently, intra-articular injections of hyaluronic acid preparations have proved to have some benefit in OA of the knee (Puhl 1993; Jones et al. 1995).

## Rheumatoid Arthritis

A multidisciplinary approach to the patient is important, so that educational, physical, psychologic, social, sexual, occupational, and functional aspects are attended to along with pharmacologic therapy. The goal of therapy for RA is to suppress the synovitis. This is gauged by the regression of symptoms (pain, stiffness, tiredness), signs (swelling and tenderness), and abnormal laboratory tests (ESR or C-reactive protein, rheumatoid factor). Once RA is diagnosed, immediate commencement of DMARD therapy is required to reduce the rate of joint damage and ultimate disability (American College of Rheumatology Ad Hoc Committee on Clinical Guidelines 1996b). If response is unsatisfactory, aggressive modification of the DMARD regimen including consideration of cyclosporine and combination therapy is appropriate. Careful monitoring of patients for drug toxicity clinically and with blood and urine tests is mandatory (Table 10-11; American College of Rheumatology Ad Hoc Committee on Clinical Guidelines 1996a). Hydroxychloroquine and sulfasalazine are good options for milder disease, whereas methotrexate or gold intramuscularly is appropriate for more severely active disease. Low-dose prednisolone (10 mg/day or less) may be introduced if control is not satisfactory, although this should be avoided or the course and dosage limited as much as possible. Some practitioners use low-dose oral corticosteroid therapy during the early months of therapy to achieve faster control of the disease and then taper the dose as low as possible once other DMARDs have established their efficacy. The use of intra-articular injections of depot glucocorticosteroids is a very useful option for recalcitrant joints.

For rheumatoid arthritis, NSAIDs are symptomatic therapy only, and higher doses are needed than for the noninflammatory conditions. Inadequate effect or adverse effects are grounds for switching NSAIDs after 1 to 2 weeks. Upper GI symptoms are reduced by dosing concomitantly with food. $H_2$ antagonists are often used if dyspeptic symptoms are a problem; however, these drugs are not protective against NSAID-induced gastric ulceration. Only misoprostol has been shown to reduce the risk of NSAID-induced serious bleeding and misoprostol and omeprazole to protect against endoscopically proven NSAID-induced gastric ulcer.

Use of combinations of DMARDs is now commonplace, reflecting the appreciation of the need to suppress synovitis and disease activity early if the risk of erosions and later disability is to be reduced. There has been a lack of objective evidence of efficacy of combinations (Cash and Klippel 1994; Felson et al. 1994) until recently. The combination of methotrexate and sulfasalazine has been demonstrated to be superior to methotrexate alone (Haagsma et al. 1994), methotrexate, sulfasalazine, and HCQ better than a combination of sulfasalazine with HCQ or methotrexate alone, and cyclosporine improves the response in individuals not satisfactorily controlled by methotrexate alone (Cash and Klippel 1994; Tugwell and Baker 1995; Tugwell et al. 1995). Since the demonstration

Table 10-20 Stepped Approach to the Management of Osteoarthritis

| |
|---|
| Education, joint protection, weight loss, orthotics, stick if necessary, exercise program, activities of daily living support |
| Acetaminophen up to 4 g daily taken regularly when pain is persistent |
| Topical anti-inflammatory creams or capsaicin if needed |
| If pain relief is not sufficient, add ibuprofen (low dose) up to 400 mg qid if there are no contraindications |
| If pain relief is inadequate, consider full anti-inflammatory dose of NSAID. Consider prophylaxis for upper GI tract damage if patient is at risk. |
| If pain relief is inadequate or joints have reached end stage, consider referral for arthroscopy and possible débridement, osteotomy, or joint replacement |

SOURCE: Based on American College Guidelines for the Management of Osteoarthritis of Knee and Hip (Hochberg et al., 1995a, b).

of the antierosive effects of prednisone (Kirwan 1995), this drug has been used more in combinations. For example, a regimen of prednisone 60 mg/day reducing to 7.5 mg combined with methotrexate 7.5 mg/week has been shown to be superior to sulfasalazine over 1 year in patients who have early RA (Boers et al. 1997).

## Spondyloarthropathies

Ankylosing spondylitis and psoriatic arthritis are often lifelong problems, and in these conditions in particular the key to successful outcomes is excellent communication between doctor and patient with a high level of understanding on the part of the patient concerning the condition and its therapy (Edmonds 1997). The goals of the therapy are to relieve pain and stiffness; to maintain good posture, especially in those with spinal involvement; and to sustain the ability to undertake activities of daily living. High-dose NSAIDs are effective, and indomethacin 75 to 100 mg daily taken two or three times daily, sometimes with the addition of 100 mg per suppository at night, is most often preferred. Phenylbutazone is held in reserve because of its bone marrow toxicity, but can be considered if there is an unsatisfactory response to other NSAIDs and as long as appropriate safety monitoring is instituted. The spondyloarthropathies including Reiter syndrome respond to sulfasalazine or methotrexate if NSAIDs are insufficiently helpful (Creemers et al. 1994; Dougados et al. 1995; Clegg, Reda, Mejias, et al. 1996; Clegg, Reda, Weisman, et al. 1996a and b), although spinal stiffness does not seem to respond (Clegg, Reda, Weisman, et al. 1996a). Azathioprine has been shown to be efficacious in these conditions also. Sometimes local injections of corticosteroids are given into the sacroiliac joints under radiologic control or peripheral joints unresponsive to systemic therapy.

## Systemic Lupus Erythematosus

Good education of and communication with the patient is essential in this chronic, relapsing, inflammatory connective tissue disease (Mills 1994; Rasaratnam and Ryan 1997a; Rasaratnam and Ryan 1998). Involvement with lupus community self-help groups is invaluable. Avoidance of factors that cause flares, for example, excessive sunlight, and careful follow-up for disease and drug monitoring are vital concerns. The mainstays of drug therapy are NSAIDs, low-dose corticosteroids for uncontrolled disease flares for as short a period as possible, and antimalarial drugs, particularly hydroxychloroquine (The Canadian Hydroxychloroquine Study Group 1991; Bootsma et al. 1995). NSAIDs are more likely to cause renal impairment in SLE, so special care must be exercised. Also, CNS adverse effects such as meningitic reactions are more likely and can be confused with CNS involvement. There is a greater risk for osteonecrosis of the hip and atherosclerosis with corticosteroids in SLE. Immunosuppressive drugs, notably cyclophosphamide, are reserved for the treatment of resistant organ damage such as lupus nephritis, and there is good evidence of efficacy in slowing progression of renal scarring and the development of end-stage renal failure (Balow et al. 1984; Austin et al. 1986). Intravenous cyclophosphamide in combination with oral prednisolone is most effective for this condition (Balow et al. 1987; Boumpas et al. 1992).

## Progressive Systemic Sclerosis

Self-help groups are again of great value in this disorder (Rasaratnam and Ryan 1997b). Raynaud phenomenon is managed in the first instance by keeping the extremities very warm and avoiding smoking and beta-blocker drugs. As the attacks become longer and more severe, the pharmacologic options are calcium channel blockers such as nifedipine, topical nitrates, or ACE inhibitors. If attacks are extremely severe and unresponsive to drug therapy and there is a risk of gangrene, then infusions of prostaglandin $E_1$ or prostacyclin are indicated to save the limb (Wigley et al. 1994). Diffuse skin involvement has been treated with D-penicillamine 500 to 750 mg/day initially, then with a reduced dose, but despite promising early studies (Jimenez and Sigal 1991), there is no convincing double-blind evidence of efficacy to date (Clements et al. 1997). Skin inflammation secondary to calcium deposition can be treated with colchicine. Dry skin is common, so moisturizing creams and avoidance of excessive bathing and exposure to detergents is recommended. Musculoskeletal symptoms are controlled with NSAIDs (with caution because of the greater risk of renal toxicity) or low-dose corticosteroids. Maintaining joint range of motion in affected areas is important but extremely difficult. Hypertension needs to be treated aggressively with ACE inhibitors initially and then additional drugs such as calcium channel blockers as required (Steen et al. 1990). Esophageal reflux and dysphagia due to the involvement of the lower esophagus and gastroesophageal junction are managed successfully with prokinetic drug therapies including metoclopramide, domperidone, or cisapride. The proton-pump inhibitors such as omeprazole are efficacious against acid reflux. Pulmonary involvement with fibrosis is a grave development that may respond to D-penicillamine, corticosteroids, or cyclophosphamide.

## Polymyositis and Dermatomyositis

There is little double-blind evidence for the efficacy of pharmacologic therapy of these conditions, although experience indicates a marked effect of corticosteroids. Initial therapy is with prednisolone 1 mg/kg per day for 3 to 6 weeks tapering slowly, depending on muscle strength and muscle enzymes, to the lowest effective dose. If the condition is not controlled, or there is a need to reduce the dose of steroids, azathioprine and methotrexate have been used successfully. Only occasionally has plasmapheresis, cyclophosphamide, or cyclosporine been of apparent assistance (Rasaratnam and Ryan 1997b).

## Polymyalgia Rheumatica

This condition is exquisitely sensitive to corticosteroids at doses of around 20 mg of prednisolone daily, and if the response is not dramatic, then the diagnosis needs to be reconsidered. Initial dose should be 20 mg/day, and when a response has occurred, the dose can be very slowly reduced, for example, by 1 mg/day every 2 to 4 weeks depending on whether symptoms return and the movement of the ESR (Pountain and Hazleman 1995; Hunder 1997; Swannell 1997). The duration of the disorder is anywhere from 2 to 6 years, and the goal is to use the minimum dose of prednisolone in order to reduce the risk of adverse effects. If giant cell arteritis is present, as manifest by involvement of temporal or other arteries, then there is a risk of blindness due to involvement of the ophthalmic arteries. Prednisone 60 mg/day is indicated at the outset; the dose can be reduced once the disease is controlled. If steroid doses remain high for prolonged periods, consideration should be given to steroid-sparing therapy with methotrexate or azathioprine, as well as measures to protect against osteoporosis.

## Vasculitis

Therapy is determined by the extent and severity of the vasculitic syndrome (Allen and Bressler 1997; Luqmani et al. 1997; Valentini et al. 1998). Thus prednisolone in high dosage, e.g., 40 to 60 mg/day, is used to bring polyarteritis nodosa under control, but if the condition is still active or progressing, then a cytotoxic drug such as cyclophosphamide needs to be added (Allen and Bressler 1997; Langford et al. 1998; Richmond et al. 1998).

## Gout

***Asymptomatic hyperuricemia***

Treatment of asymptomatic hyperuricemia is not indicated in most circumstances, but some investigation of etiology is appropriate (Campion et al. 1987). Lifestyle adjustment including weight loss, reduction of intake of protein and purine-rich foods, for example, shell fish and whitebait, moderation of alcohol consumption, and attention to risk factors for cardiovascular disease is appropriate for patients with asymptomatic and symptomatic hyperuricemia.

***Acute gout***

An accurate diagnosis preferably confirmed by demonstration of negatively birefringent uric acid crystals in synovial fluid is important, particularly in atypical presentations accompanied by an elevated plasma uric acid. A short course of a high dose of an NSAID, for example, indomethacin 50 mg three times a day with food for 5 to 7 days, is standard. If NSAIDs are contraindicated, a course of prednisolone associated with prompt reductions of dose is reasonable, providing there are no contraindications. Colchicine remains an option, but the commonly resulting diarrhea has reduced the use of the drug for this indication.

***Recurrent acute gout and tophaceous gout***

Low-dose colchicine or indomethacin will reduce the rate of recurrence of attacks of acute gout. If recurrence is too frequent or disrupting or if tophaceous gout or urate nephropathy is present, then hypouricemic therapy with allopurinol or probenecid is indicated. Both drugs will effectively lower plasma urate, prevent new tophi from forming, and lead to the gradual diminution of tophi already present. Allopurinol is generally preferred, because there is no risk of acute obstructive uropathy on initiation of therapy. Also, probenecid is not effective in renal impairment.

Successful therapy with allopurinol requires very careful attention from the prescribing physician (Emmerson 1996). The need for lifelong therapy with the drug needs to be carefully established by the presence of recurrent acute gout or tophaceous gout. All other management options, notably the lifestyle adjustments of weight loss and reduction of alcohol and purine food consumption, in the early stages of recurrent attacks of acute gout need to be vigorously pursued. Allopurinol should be introduced at a starting daily dose in keeping with the patient's renal function (50 to 100 mg/day) increasing by 50 to 100 mg/day each week until a daily dose is reached that reduces the uric acid satisfactorily. This will avoid excessive dosing with allopurinol, particularly in the elderly, because the risk of serious adverse reactions relates to excessive dose rates in individuals with reduced renal function (Conaghan and Day 1996). Many elderly people can be managed on daily doses of <300 mg, for example, 100 to 200 mg daily, but unfortunately the most common daily dose remains 300 mg, largely through habit rather than defined need (Day, Miners, et al. 1988). Patients should be very well informed about the drug, particularly of the importance of meticulous compliance. Much reinforcement is required to help maintain compliance with the drug. The consequence of poor compliance is a substantial risk of inducing attacks of acute gout that will likely further worsen compliance. The risk of acute gout is reduced by the gradual increase of dose of allopurinol and prophylactic use of low-dose colchicine such as 0.5 mg twice daily or an NSAID such as indomethacin twice daily. Colchicine may be preferred to NSAIDs in this situation (Kot et al. 1993; Emmerson 1996), although some authors wonder whether prophylaxis against the acute attack is always necessary (Fam 1995). Hypouricemic therapy ought not to be started within 2 weeks of an acute attack of gout. Aspirin in lower doses causes urate retention and interferes with the actions of the uricosuric drugs, but this is a relative contraindication only, especially if the indication for aspirin use is important such as platelet inhibitory effects in vascular disease.

An important indication for allopurinol is the hyperuricemia associated with chemotherapy or radiotherapy used in cancer treatment. Prophylactic therapy with allopurinol is indicated in order to avoid acute obstructive uropathy from urate precipitating in the renal tubules consequent upon the breakdown of large numbers of cells with release of precursors of uric acid.

## Calcium Pyrophosphate Deposition Disease

Acute pseudogout is the most common cause of monoarthritis in elderly patients, usually involving the knee, shoulder, or wrist. Treatment is similar to that for acute gout, that is, NSAIDs, colchicine, or intra-articular glucocorticosteroids, although colchicine is less effective than in acute gout. Given the age of the patients, the intra-articular glucocorticosteroid option is often the best as long as the possibility of joint infection has been excluded. Chronic calcium pyrophosphate arthropathy that commonly involves knees, wrists, shoulders, elbows, hips, and mid-tarsal joints, also responds to NSAIDs or glucocorticosteroids.

## REFERENCES


Aarons L, Grennan DM, Rajapakse C, et al. 1983. Anti-inflammatory (ibuprofen) drug therapy in rheumatoid arthritis—rate of response and lack of time dependency of plasma pharmacokinetics. *Br J Clin Pharmacol* **15**:387–8.

Adachi JD, Bensen WG, Kassam Y, et al. 1987. Gold induced thrombocytopenia—12 cases and review of the literature. *Semin Arthritis Rheum* **16**:287–93.

Advenier C, Roux A, Gobert C, et al. 1983. Pharmacokinetics of ketoprofen in the elderly. *Br J Clin Pharmacol* **16**:65–70.

Aglas F, Rainer F, Hermann J, et al. 1995. Interstitial pneumonia due to cytomegalovirus following low-dose methotrexate treatment for rheumatoid arthritis. *Arthritis Rheum* **38**:291–2.

Ahern MJ, Hall NO, Case N, et al. 1984. D-Penicillamine withdrawal in rheumatoid arthritis. *Ann Rheum Dis* **84**:213.

Ahern MJ, Smith MD. 1997. Rheumatoid arthritis. *Med J Aust* **166**:156–61.

Alarcon GS, Morgan SL. 1997. Guidelines for folate supplementation in rheumatoid arthritis patients treated with methotrexate: Comment on the guidelines for monitoring drug therapy. *Arthritis Rheum* **40**:391.

Alarcon-Segovia D, Kraus A. 1991. Drug-related lupus syndromes and their relationship to spontaneously occurring systemic lupus erythematosus. *Bailliere's Clin Rheumatol* **5**:1–12.

Allen NB, Bressler PB. 1997. Diagnosis and treatment of the systemic and cutaneous necrotizing vasculitis syndromes. *Med Clin North Am* **81**:243–59.

Altman RD, Aven A, Holmburg CE, et al. 1994. Capsaicin cream 0.025% as monotherapy for osteoarthritis: A double-blind study. *Semin Arthritis Rheum* **23**(Suppl 3):25–33.

American College of Rheumatology Ad Hoc Committee on Clinical Guidelines. 1996a. Guidelines for monitoring drug therapy in rheumatoid arthritis. *Arthritis Rheum* **39**:723–31.

American College of Rheumatology Ad Hoc Committee on Clinical Guidelines. 1996b. Guidelines for the management of rheumatoid arthritis. *Arthritis Rheum* **39**:713–22.

Amin AR, Attur M, Patel RN, et al. 1997. Superinduction of cyclooxygenase-2 activity in human osteoarthritis-affected cartilage. Influence of nitric oxide. *J Clin Invest* **99**:1231–7.

Amos R, Pullar T, Capell H, et al. 1986. Sulphasalazine for rheumatoid arthritis: Toxicity in 774 patients monitored for one to 11 years. *Br Med J* **293**:420–23.

Armitage JM, Kormos RL, Stuart RS, et al. 1991. Posttransplant lymphoproliferative disease in thoracic organ transplant patients: Ten years of cyclosporine-based immunosuppression. *J Heart Lung Transplant* **10**:877–86; discussion 886–7.

Austin HAD, Klippel JH, Balow JE, et al. 1986. Therapy of lupus nephritis. Controlled trial of prednisone and cytotoxic drugs. *N Engl J Med* **314**:614–9.

Baber N, Halliday LD, van den Heuvel WJ, et al. 1979. Indomethacin in rheumatoid arthritis: Clinical effects of pharmacokinetics and platelet studies in responders and nonresponders. *Ann Rheum Dis* **38**:128–36.

Bachman TR, Sawitzke AD, Perkins SL, et al. 1996. Methotrexate-associated lymphoma in patients with rheumatoid arthritis: Report of two cases. *Arthritis Rheum* **39**:325–9.

Badley EM, Crotty M. 1995. An international comparison of the estimated effect of the aging of the population on the major cause of disablement musculoskeletal disorders. *J Rheumatol* **22**:1934–40.

Bahkle YS, Botting RM. 1996. Cyclooxygenase-2 and its regulation in inflammation. *Mediat Inflamm* **6**:765–8.

Baker GL, Kahl LE, Zee BC, et al. 1987. Malignancy following treatment of rheumatoid arthritis with cyclophosphamide. Long-term case-control follow-up study. *Am J Med* **83**:1–9.

Balow JE, Austin HAD, Muenz LR, et al. 1984. Effect of treatment on the evolution of renal abnormalities in lupus nephritis. *N Engl J Med* **311**:491–5.

Balow JE, Austin HAD, Tsokos GC, et al. 1987. NIH conference. Lupus nephritis. *Ann Intern Med* **106**:79–94.

Bannwarth B, Pehourcq F, Schaeverbeke T, et al. 1996. Clinical pharmacokinetics of low-dose pulse methotrexate in rheumatoid arthritis. *Clin Pharmacokinet* **30**:194–210.

Bartle WR, Blakely JA. 1991. Potentiation of warfarin anticoagulation by acetaminophen. *JAMA* **265**:1260.

Baud FJ, Sabouraud A, Vicaut E, et al. 1995. Brief report: Treatment of severe colchicine overdose with colchicine-specific Fab fragments. *N Engl J Med* **332**:642–5.

Berthelot JM, Maugars Y, Prost A. 1997. Pancytopenia secondary to methotrexate therapy in rheumatoid arthritis: Comment on the article by Gutierrez-Urena et al. *Arthritis Rheum* **40**:193–4; discussion 195–6.

Bjarnason I, Hayllar J, MacPherson AJ, et al. 1993. Side effects of nonsteroidal anti-inflammatory drugs on the small and large intestine in humans. *Gastroenterology* **104**:1832–47.

Blanco R, Martinez-Taboada VM, Gonzalez-Gay MA, et al. 1996. Acute febrile toxic reaction in patients with refractory rheumatoid arthritis who are receiving combined therapy with methotrexate and azathioprine. *Arthritis Rheum* **39**:1016–20.

Block JA. 1998. Hydroxychloroquine and retinal safety. *Lancet* **351**:771.

Blocka K, Paulus HE. 1987. The clinical pharmacology of gold compounds. In: Paulus HE, Furst DE, Dromgoole SH, editors. *Drugs for Rheumatic Disease.* New York: Churchill Livingstone, pp 49–83.

Blodgett RC Jr, Heuer MA, Pietrusko RG. 1984. Auranofin: A unique oral chrysotherapeutic agent. *Semin Arthritis Rheum* **13**:255–73.

Bloor K, Maynard A. 1996. Is there scope for improving the cost-effective prescribing of nonsteroidal antiinflammatory drugs? *PharmacoEconomics* **9**:484–96.

Bochner F, Graham GG, Polverino A, et al. 1987. Salicyl phenolic glucuronide pharmacokinetics in patients with rheumatoid arthritis. *Eur J Clin Pharmacol* **32**:153–8.

Boers M, Verhoeven AC, Markusse HM, et al. 1997. Randomised comparison of combined step-down prednisolone methotrexate and sulphasalazine with sulphasalazine alone in early rheumatoid arthritis. *Lancet* **350**:309–18.

Bootsma H, Spronk P, Derksen R, et al. 1995. Prevention of relapses in systemic lupus erythematosus. *Lancet* **345**:1595–9.

Borenstein DG. 1997. Epidemiology etiology diagnostic evaluation and treatment of low back pain. *Curr Opin Rheumatol* **9**:144–50.

Borenstein DG, Weisel SW. 1989. Low back pain: Medical diagnosis and comprehensive management (Philadelphia: Sanders).

Bouachour G, Tirot P, Varache N, et al. 1994. Hemodynamic changes in acute adrenal insufficiency. *Intensive Care Med* **20**:138–41.

Boumpas DT, Austin HAD, Fessler BJ, et al. 1995. Systemic lupus erythematosus: Emerging concepts. Part 1: Renal neuropsychiatric cardiovascular pulmonary and hematologic disease. *Ann Intern Med* **122**:940–50.

Boumpas DT, Austin HAD, Vaughn EM, et al. 1992. Controlled trial of pulse methylprednisolone versus two regimens of pulse cyclophosphamide in severe lupus nephritis. *Lancet* **340**:741–5.

Brady S, Day RO, Graham GG. 1999. Are intra-articular steroids effective? In: Bird, HA and Snaith, ML, editors. *Rheumatoid Arthritis.* Blackwell Science Ltd., Oxford, London, Edinburgh, Malden, Australia, France: pp 174–89.

Bradley JD, Brandt KD, Katz BP, et al. 1991. Comparison of an antiinflammatory dose of ibuprofen and an analgesic dose of ibuprofen and acetaminophen in the treatment of patients with osteoarthritis of the knee. *N Engl J Med* **325**:87–91.

Bradley JD, Brandt KD, Katz BP, et al. 1992. Treatment of knee osteoarthritis: Relationship of clinical features of joint inflammation to the response to a nonsteroidal antiinflammatory drug or pure analgesic. *J Rheumatol* **19**:1950–4.

Brash AR, Hickey DE, Graham TP, et al. 1981. Pharmacokinetics of indomethacin in the neonate. Relation of plasma indomethacin levels to response of the ductus arteriosus. *N Engl J Med* **305**:67–2.

Bresnihan B. 1997. Treatment of rheumatoid arthritis with recombinant human interleukin-1 receptor antagonist (IL-1ra). *J Rheumatol* **36**(Suppl 1):105.

Breuing KH, Gilfrich HJ, Meinertz T, et al. 1981. Disposition of azapropazone in chronic renal and hepatic failure. *Eur J Clin Pharmacol* **20**:147–55.

Brewer EJ, Giannini EH, Kuzmina N, et al. 1986. Penicillamine and hydroxychloroquine in the treatment of severe juvenile rheumatoid arthritis. Results of the U.S.A-U.S.S.R. double-blind placebo-controlled trial. *N Engl J Med* **314**:1269–76.

Bridges SL Jr, Moreland LW. 1997. Perioperative use of methotrexate in patients with rheumatoid arthritis undergoing orthopedic surgery. *Rheum Dis Clin North Am* **23**:981–93.

Brock N. 1996. The history of the oxazaphosphorine cytostatics. *Cancer* **78**:542–7.

Brooks PM. 1996. A template for diagnosis and management of musculoskeletal diseases. *Med J Aust* **165**:331.

Brooks PM. 1997. Rheumatic disorders. In: Speight GM, Holford NHG, editors. *Avery's Drug Treatment.* Auckland, NZ: Adis Int. pp 1113–62.

Brooks PM, Day RO. 1991. Nonsteroidal antiinflammatory drugs—differences and similarities. *N Engl J Med* **324**:1716–25.

Brune K, Graft P. 1978. Non-steroid anti-inflammatory drugs: Influence of extra-cellular pH on biodistribution and pharmacological effects. *Biochem Pharmacol* **27**:525–30.

Bryant CE, Perretti M, Flower RJ. 1998. Suppression by dexamethasone of inducible nitric oxide synthase protein expression in vivo: A possible role for lipocortin 1. *Biochem Pharmacol* **55**:279–85.

Buchbinder R, Hall S, Sambrook PN, et al. 1993. Methotrexate therapy in rheumatoid arthritis: A life table review of 587 patients treated in community practice. *J Rheumatol* **20**:639–44.

Buckland-Wright J, Graham S, Chikanza I, et al. 1993. Quantitative microfocal radiography detects changes in erosion area in patients with early rheumatoid arthritis treated with myocrisin. *J Rheumatol* **20**:243–7.

Buckley LM, Bullaboy CA, Leichtman L, et al. 1997. Multiple congenital anomalies associated with weekly low-dose methotrexate treatment of the mother. *Arthritis Rheum* **40**:971–3.

Campana C, Regazzi MB, Buggia I, et al. 1996. Clinically significant drug interactions with cyclosporin. An update. *Clin Pharmacokinet* **30**:141–79.

Campion EW, Glynn RJ, DeLabry LO. 1987. Asymptomatic hyperuricemia. Risks and consequences in the Normative Aging Study. *Am J Med* **82**:421–6.

Campion GV, Lebsack ME, Lookabaugh J, et al. 1996. Dose-range and dose-frequency study of recombinant human interleukin-1 receptor antagonist in patients with rheumatoid arthritis. The IL-1Ra Arthritis Study Group. *Arthritis Rheum* **39**:1092–101.

Capell HA, Konetschnik B, Glass RC. 1977. Anti-inflammatory analgesic drug responders and non-responders: A clinico-pharmacological study of flurbiprofen. *Br J Clin Pharmacol* **4**:623–4.

Carson JL, Strom BL, Soper KA, et al. 1987. The association of nonsteroidal anti-inflammatory drugs with upper gastrointestinal tract bleeding. *Arch Intern Med* **147**:85–8.

Cash JM, Klippel JH. 1994. Second-line drug therapy for rheumatoid arthritis. *N Engl J Med* **330**:1368–75.

Cato AC, Wade E. 1996. Molecular mechanisms of anti-inflammatory action of glucocorticoids. *Bioessays* **18**:371–8.

Chalmers I, Sitar D, Hunter T. 1990. A one-year open prospective study of sulfasalazine in the treatment of rheumatoid arthritis: Adverse reactions and clinical response in relation to laboratory variables drug and metabolite serum levels and acetylator status. *J Rheumatol* **17**:764–70.

Champion GD, Cairns DR, Bieri D, et al. 1988. Dose response studies and longterm evaluation of auranofin in rheumatoid arthritis. *J Rheumatol* **15**:28–34.

Champion GD, Graham GG, Ziegler JB. 1990. The gold complexes. *Bailliere's Clin Rheumatol* **4**:491–534.

Chan FK, Sung JJ, Chung SC, et al. 1997. Randomised trial of eradication of *Helicobacter pylori* before non-steroidal anti-inflammatory drug therapy to prevent peptic ulcers. *Lancet* **350**:975–9.

Chan GL, Matzke GR. 1987. Effects of renal insufficiency on the pharmacokinetics and pharmacodynamics of opioid analgesics. *Drug Intell Clin Pharm* **21**:773–83.

Chang TKM, Weber GF, Crespi CL, et al. 1993. Differential activation of cyclophosphamide and ifosphamide by cytochromes P-450 2B and 3A in human liver microsomes. *Cancer Res* **53**:5629–37.

Cherkin DC, Deyo RA, Wheeler K, et al. 1995. Physician views about treating low back pain. The results of a national survey. *Spine* **20**:1–9; discussion 9–10.

Christy NP. 1992. Pituitary-adrenal function during corticosteroid therapy. Learning to live with uncertainty. *N Engl J Med* **326**: 266–7.

Ciruelo E, de la Cruz J, Lopez I, et al. 1996. Cumulative rate of relapse of lupus nephritis after successful treatment with cyclophosphamide. *Arthritis Rheum* **39**:2028–34.

Clark P, Casas E, Tugwell P, et al. 1993. Hydroxychloroquine compared with placebo in rheumatoid arthritis. A randomized controlled trial. *Ann Intern Med* **119**:1067–71.

Claussen MS, Landercasper J, Cogbill TH. 1992. Acute adrenal insufficiency presenting as shock after trauma and surgery: Three cases and review of the literature. *J Trauma* **32**:94–100.

Clegg DO, Reda DJ, Mejias E, et al. 1996. Comparison of sulfasalazine and placebo in the treatment of psoriatic arthritis. A Department of Veterans Affairs Cooperative Study. *Arthritis Rheum* **39**: 2013–20.

Clegg DO, Reda DJ, Weisman MH, et al. 1996a. Comparison of sulfasalazine and placebo in the treatment of ankylosing spondylitis. A Department of Veterans Affairs Cooperative Study. *Arthritis Rheum* **39**:2004–12.

Clegg DO, Reda DJ, Weisman MH, et al. 1996b. Comparison of sulfasalazine and placebo in the treatment of reactive arthritis (Reiter's syndrome). A Department of Veterans Affairs Cooperative Study. *Arthritis Rheum* **39**:2021–7.

Clements PJ, Wong WK, Seibold JR, et al. 1997. High-dose (Hi-DPA) vs low-dose (LO-DPA) penicillamine in early diffuse systemic sclerosis trial: Analysis of trial [abstract]. In: *ARA National Scientific Meeting*. Washington DC: Arthritis and Rheumatism, p S173, abstract 854.

Clive DM, Stoff JS. 1984. Renal syndromes associated with nonsteroidal antiinflammatory drugs. *N Engl J Med* **310**:563–72.

Cockwell P. 1997. Systemic lupus erythematosus. *Br Med J* **314**: 292–5.

Cohen ML. 1996. Cervical and lumbar pain. *Med J Aust* **165**:504–8.

Collins AJ, Davies J, Dixon AS. 1988. A prospective endoscopic study of the effect of Orudis and Oruvail on the upper gastrointestinal tract in patients with osteoarthritis. *Br J Rheumatol* **27**:106–9.

Conaghan PG, Day RO. 1996. Management and prevention of gout. *Curr Therapeut* **1**:16–20.

Conaghan PG, Quinn DI, Brooks PM, et al. 1995. Hazards of low dose methotrexate. *Aust N Z J Med* **25**:670–3.

Confavreux C, Saddier P, Grimaud J, et al. 1996. Risk of cancer from azathioprine therapy in multiple sclerosis: A case-control study. *Neurology* **46**:1607–12.

Corey EJ, Mehrotra MM, Khan AU. 1987. Antiarthritic gold compounds effectively quench electronically excited singlet oxygen. *Science* **236**:68–9.

Crawford ML, Waller PC, Wood SM. 1997. Severe cystitis associated with tiaprofenic acid. *Br J Urol* **79**:578–84.

Creemers MC, van Riel PL, Franssen MJ, et al. 1994. Second-line treatment in seronegative spondylarthropathies. *Semin Arthritis Rheum* **24**:71–81.

Cronstein BN. 1996. Molecular therapeutics. Methotrexate and its mechanism of action. *Arthritis Rheum* **39**:1951–60.

Cronstein BN. 1997. The mechanism of action of methotrexate. *Rheum Dis Clin North Am* **23**:739–55.

Cupps TR, Edgar LC, Fauci AS. 1982. Suppression of human B lymphocyte function by cyclophosphamide. *J Immunol* **128**: 2453–7.

Cush JJ, Lipsky PE, Postlethwaite AE, et al. 1990. Correlation of serologic indicators of inflammation with effectiveness of nonsteroidal antiinflammatory drug therapy in rheumatoid arthritis. *Arthritis Rheum* **33**:19–28.

Dalakas MC. 1991. Polymyositis dermatomyositis and inclusion-body myositis. *N Engl J Med* **325**:1487–98.

Danis VA, Franic GM, Rathjen DA, et al. 1992. Circulating cytokine levels in patients with rheumatoid arthritis: results of a double blind trial with sulphasalazine. *Ann Rheum Dis* **51**:946–50.

Danis VA, Kulesz AJ, Nelson DS, et al. 1990. The effect of gold sodium thiomalate and auranofin on lipopolysaccharide-induced interleukin-1 production by blood monocytes in vitro: Variation in healthy subjects and patients with arthritis. *Clin Exp Immunol* **79**:335–40.

Danis VA, March LM, Nelson DS, et al. 1987. Interleukin-1 secretion by peripheral blood monocytes and synovial macrophages from patients with rheumatoid arthritis. *J Rheumatol* **14**:33–9.

Danning CL, Illei GG, Boumpas DT. 1998. Vasculitis associated with primary rheumatologic diseases. *Curr Opin Rheumatol* **10**: 58–65.

Das KM, Eastwood MA, McManus JP, et al. 1973. Adverse reactions during salicylazosulfapyridine therapy and the relation with drug metabolism and acetylator phenotype. *N Engl J Med* **289**: 491–5.

Day RO. 1997. Sulfasalzine. In: Kelly WN, Harris ED, Ruddy S, Sledge CB, editors. *Textbook of Rheumatology*, pp 741–6.

Day RO. 1998. SARDS. In: Klippel JH, Dieppe PA, editors. *Rheumatology*. St. Louis: Mosby, pp 8.1–10.

Day RO, Breit SN, Cairns D, et al. 1988. Aspects of the clinical trials of slow-acting anti-rheumatic drugs. *Agents Actions* **24**(Suppl):121–33.

Day RO, Brooks PM. 1987. Variations in response to non-steroidal anti-inflammatory drugs. *Br J Clin Pharmacol* **23**:655–8.

Day RO, Furst DE, Dromgoole SH, et al. 1982. Relationship of serum naproxen concentration to efficacy in rheumatoid arthritis. *Clin Pharmacol Therapeut* **31**:733–40.

Day RO, Furst DE, Dromgoole SH, et al. 1988. Changes in salicylate serum concentration and metabolism during chronic dosing in normal volunteers. *Biopharmaceut Drug Disposition* **9**:273–83.

Day RO, Graham GG, Bieri D, et al. 1989. Concentration-response relationships for salicylate-induced ototoxicity in normal volunteers. *Br J Clin Pharmacol* **28**:695–702.

Day RO, Graham GG, Champion GD, et al. 1984. Anti-rheumatic drug interactions. *Clin Rheum Dis* **10**:251–75.

Day RO, Graham GG, Williams KM. 1988. Pharmacokinetics of non-steroidal anti-inflammatory drugs. *Bailliere's Clin Rheumatol* **2**:363–93.

Day RO, Lam S, Paull P, et al. 1987. Effect of food and various antacids on the absorption of tenoxicam. *Br J Clin Pharmacol* **24**:323–8.

Day RO, Miners JO, Birkett DJ, et al. 1988. Allopurinol dosage selection: Relationships between dose and plasma oxipurinol and urate concentrations and urinary urate excretion. *Br J Clin Pharmacol* **26**:423–8.

Day RO, Paull PD, Lam S, et al. 1988. The effect of concurrent aspirin upon plasma concentrations of tenoxicam. *Br J Clin Pharmacol* **26**:455–62.

Day RO, Pearson CM. 1981. Primary inflammatory muscle diseases. *Compr Ther* **7**:22–30.

Day RO, Shen DD, Azarnoff DL. 1983. Induction of salicyluric acid formation in rheumatoid arthritis patients treated with salicylates. *Clin Pharmacokinet* **8**:263–71.

Day RO, Williams KM, Graham GG, et al. 1988. Stereoselective disposition of ibuprofen enantiomers in synovial fluid. *Clin Pharmacol Ther* **43**:480–7.

Day RO, Williams KM, Graham S, et al. 1991. The pharmacokinetics of total and unbound concentrations of tenoxicam in synovial fluid and plasma. *Arthritis Rheum* **34**:751–60.

de Craen AJ, Roos PJ, Leonard de Vries A, et al. 1996. Effect of colour of drugs: Systematic review of perceived effect of drugs and of their effectiveness. *Br Med J* **313**:1624–6.

de Jager JP. 1996. Problems with the shoulder, knee, ankle and foot. *Med J Aust* **165**:566–71.

de Leeuw PW. 1996. Nonsteroidal anti-inflammatory drugs and hypertension. The risks in perspective. *Drugs* **51**:179–87.

de Leeuw PW. 1997. Drug-induced hypertension. Recognition and management in older patients. *Drugs Aging* **11**:178–85.

Denton CP, Black CM, Korn JH, et al. 1996c. Systemic sclerosis: Current pathogenetic concepts and future prospects for targeted therapy. *Lancet* **347**:1453–8.

Dixon RB, Christy NP. 1980. On the various forms of corticosteroid withdrawal syndrome. *Am J Med* **68**:224–30.

Donovan S, Hawley S, MacCarthy J, et al. 1990. Tolerability of enteric coated sulphasalazine in rheumatoid arthritis: The results of a co-operative clinical study. *J Rheumatol* **29**:201.

Dougados M, vam der Linden S, Leirisalo-Repo M, et al. 1995. Sulfasalazine in the treatment of spondylarthropathy. A randomized multicenter double-blind placebo-controlled study. *Arthritis Rheum* **38**:618–27.

Dujovne CA, Pitterman A, Vincek WC, et al. 1983. Enterohepatic circulation of sulindac and metabolites. *Clin Pharmacol Ther* **33**: 172–7.

Dunagan FM, McGill PE, Kelman AW, et al. 1988. Naproxen dose and concentration: Response relationship in rheumatoid arthritis. *Br J Rheumatol* **27**:48–53.

Edmonds JP. 1997. Spondylarthropathies. *Med J Aust* **166**:214–9.

Elliott MJ, Maini RN, Feldmann M, et al. 1994a. Randomised double-blind comparison of chimeric monoclonal antibody to tumour necrosis factor alpha (cA2) versus placebo in rheumatoid arthritis. *Lancet* **344**:1105–10.

Elliott MJ, Maini RN, Feldmann M, et al. 1994b. Repeated therapy with monoclonal antibody to tumour necrosis factor alpha (cA2) in patients with rheumatoid arthritis. *Lancet* **344**:1125–7.

Elliott SL, Yeomans ND, Buchanan RR, et al. 1994. Efficacy of 12 months' misoprostol as prophylaxis against NSAID-induced gastric ulcers. A placebo-controlled trial. *Scand J Rheumatol* **23**: 171–6.

Emery P. 1987. Sulphoxidation ability and thiol status in rheumatoid arthritis patients. *Br J Rheumatol* **26**:163–5.

Emery P. 1994. The Roche Rheumatology Prize Lecture. The optimal management of early rheumatoid disease: The key to preventing disability. *Br J Rheumatol* **33**:765–8.

Emmerson BT. 1996. The management of gout. *N Engl J Med* **334**: 445–51.

Erickson AR, Reddy V, Vogelgesang SA, et al. 1995. Usefulness of the American College of Rheumatology recommendations for liver biopsy in methotrexate-treated rheumatoid arthritis patients. *Arthritis Rheum* **38**:1115–9.

Fam AG. 1995. Should patients with interval gout be treated with urate lowering drugs? *J Rheumatol* **22**:1621–3.

Farr M, Kitas GD, Waterhouse L, et al. 1990. Sulphasalazine in psoriatic arthritis: A double-blind placebo-controlled study. *Br J Rheumatol* **29**:46–9.

Faulds D, Goa KL, Benfield P. 1993. Cyclosporin. A review of its pharmacodynamic and pharmacokinetic properties and therapeutic use in immunoregulatory disorders. *Drugs* **45**:953–1040.

Felson DT, Anderson JJ, Meenan RF. 1990. The comparative efficacy and toxicity of second-line drugs in rheumatoid arthritis. Results of two metaanalyses. *Arthritis Rheum* **33**:1449–61.

Felson DT, Anderson JJ, Meenan RF. 1992. Use of short-term efficacy/toxicity tradeoffs to select second-line drugs in rheumatoid arthritis. A meta-analysis of published clinical trials. *Arthritis Rheum* **35**:1117–25.

Felson DT, Anderson JJ, Meenan RF. 1994. The efficacy and toxicity of combination therapy in rheumatoid arthritis. A meta-analysis. *Arthritis Rheum* **37**:1487–91.

Fernandes ET, Manivel JC, Reddy PK, et al. 1996. Cyclophosphamide associated bladder cancer—a highly aggressive disease: Analysis of 12 cases. *J Urol* **156**:1931–3.

Ferraccioli GF, Casatta L, Bartoli E, et al. 1995. Epstein-Barr virus-associated Hodgkin's lymphoma in a rheumatoid arthritis patient treated with methotrexate and cyclosporin A. *Arthritis Rheum* **38**:867–8.

Ferraz MB, Tugwell P, Goldsmith CH, et al. 1990. Meta-analysis of sulfasalazine in ankylosing spondylitis. *J Rheumatol* **17**:1482–6.

Ferreira SH, Lorenzetti BB, Correa FM. 1978. Central and peripheral antianalgesic action of aspirin-like drugs. *Eur J Pharmacol* **53**: 39–48.

Fessler BJ, Paliogianni F, Hama N, et al. 1996. Glucocorticoids modulate CD28 mediated pathways for interleukin 2 production in human T cells: Evidence for posttranscriptional regulation. *Transplantation* **62**:1113–8.

Fields CL, Robinson JW, Roy TM, et al. 1998. Hypersensitivity reaction to azathioprine. *South Med J* **91**:471–4.

Firestein GS, Zvaifler NJ. 1997. Anticytokine therapy in rheumatoid arthritis. *N Engl J Med* **337**:195–7.

Flipo RM, Reigneau O. 1996. The benefit/risk ratio of low dose cyclosporin A in rheumatoid arthritis. *J Rheumatol* **23**:404–5.

Flower RJ, Rothwell NJ. 1994. Lipocortin-1: Cellular mechanisms and clinical relevance. *Trends Pharmacol Sci* **15**:71–6.

Forestier J. 1935. Rheumatoid arthritis and its treatment with gold salts. *J Lab Clin Med* **20**:827–40.

Friedman RJ, Schiff CF, Bromberg JS. 1995. Use of supplemental steroids in patients having orthopaedic operations. *J Bone Joint Surg Am Vol* **77**:1801–6.

Fries JF, Hunder GG, Bloch DA, et al. 1990. The American College of Rheumatology 1990 criteria for the classification of vasculitis. Summary. *Arthritis Rheum* **33**:1135–6.

Fries JF, Spitz PW, Williams CA, et al. 1990. A toxicity index for comparison of side effects among different drugs. *Arthritis Rheum* **33**:121–30.

Fries JF, Williams CA, Bloch DA. 1991a. The relative toxicity of nonsteroidal antiinflammatory drugs. *Arthritis Rheum* **34**:1353–60.

Fries JF, Williams CA, Bloch DA, et al. 1991b. Nonsteroidal anti-inflammatory drug-associated gastropathy: Incidence and risk factor models. *Am J Med* **91**:213–22.

Fries JF, Williams CA, Morfeld D, et al. 1996. Reduction in long-term disability in patients with rheumatoid arthritis by disease-modifying antirheumatic drug-based treatment strategies. *Arthritis Rheum* **39**:616–22.

Friman S, Backman L. 1996. A new microemulsion formulation of cyclosporin: Pharmacokinetic and clinical features. *Clin Pharmacokinet* **30**:181–93.

Frolich JC. 1995. Prostaglandin endoperoxide synthetase isoenzymes: The clinical relevance of selective inhibition. *Ann Rheum Dis* **54**:942–3.

Frymoyer JW, Cats-Baric WL. 1991. An overview of the incidence and costs of low back pain. *Orthop Clin North Am* **22**:263.

Furst DE. 1994. Are there differences among nonsteroidal antiinflammatory drugs? Comparing acetylated salicylates, nonacetylated salicylates, and nonacetylated nonsteroidal antiinflammatory drugs. *Arthritis Rheum* **37**:1–9.

Furst DE, Clements PJ. 1998. Immunosuppressives. In: Klippel JH, Dieppe PA, editors. *Rheumatology*. St. Louis: Mosby, p 3, 9.1–9.10.

Furst DE, Tozer TN, Melmon KL. 1979. Salicylate clearance the resultant of protein binding and metabolism. *Clin Pharmacol Ther* **26**:380–9.

Getting SJ, Flower RJ, Perretti M. 1997. Inhibition of neutrophil and monocyte recruitment by endogenous and exogenous lipocortin 1. *Br J Pharmacol* **120**:1075–82.

Ghadially FN, DeCoteau WE, Huang S, et al. 1978. Ultrastructure of the skin of patients treated with sodium aurothiomalate. *J Pathol* **124**:77–83.

Ginzler E, Sharon E, Diamond H, et al. 1975. Long-term maintenance therapy with azathioprine in systemic lupus erythematosus. *Arthritis Rheum* **18**:27–34.

Girgis L, Conaghan PG, Brooks P. 1994. Disease-modifying antirheumatic drugs including methotrexate, sulfasalazine, gold, antimalarials, and penicillamine. *Curr Opin Rheumatol* **6**:252–61.

Glowniak JV, Loriaux DL. 1997. A double-blind study of perioperative steroid requirements in secondary adrenal insufficiency. *Surgery* **121**:123–9.

Gofton JP, O'Brien WM, Hurley JN, et al. 1984. Radiographic evaluation of erosion in rheumatoid arthritis: Double blind study of auranofin vs placebo. *J Rheumatol* **11**:768–71.

Gonzalez-Crespo MR, Gomez-Reino JJ, Merino R, et al. 1995. Menstrual disorders in girls with systemic lupus erythematosus treated with cyclophosphamide. *Br J Rheumatol* **34**:737–41.

Goodwin JS, Regan M. 1982. Cognitive dysfunction associated with naproxen and ibuprofen in the elderly. *Arthritis Rheum* **25**:1013–5.

Gottlieb NL. 1982. Comparative pharmacokinetics of parenteral and oral gold compounds. *J Rheumatol* **8**(Suppl):99–109.

Gottlieb NL. 1983. Comparison of the kinetics of parenteral and oral gold. *Scand J Rheumatol* **51**(Suppl):10–4.

Gottlieb NL, Gray RG. 1981. Pharmacokinetics of gold in rheumatoid arthritis. *Agents Actions* **8**(Suppl)**:**529–38.

Gottlieb NL, Kiem IM, Penneys NS, et al. 1975. The influence of chrysotherapy on serum protein and immunoglobulin levels, rheumatoid factor, and antiepithelial antibody titers. *J Lab Clin Med* **86**: 962–72.

Gottlieb NL, Smith PM, Smith EM. 1974. Pharmacodynamics of 197Au and 195Au labeled aurothiomalate in blood. Correlation with course of rheumatoid arthritis gold toxicity and gold excretion. *Arthritis Rheum* **17**:171–83.

Gourley MF, Austin HAD, Scott D, et al. 1996. Methylprednisolone and cyclophosphamide alone or in combination in patients with lupus nephritis. A randomized controlled trial. *Ann Intern Med* **125**: 549–57.

Graham DY, Agrawal NM, Roth SH. 1988. Prevention of NSAID-induced gastric ulcer with misoprostol: Multicentre double-blind placebo-controlled trial. *Lancet* **2**:1277–80.

Graham GG, Day RO, Champion GD, et al. 1984. Aspects of the clinical pharmacology of non-steroidal anti-inflammatory drugs. *Clin Rheum Dis* **10**:229–49.

Graham GG, Milligan MK, Day RO, et al. 1998. Therapeutic considerations from pharmacokinetics and metabolism: ibuprofen and paracetamol. In: Rainsford KD, Powanda MC, editors. *Safety and Efficacy of Non-Prescription (OTC) Analgesics and NSAIDs*. London: Kluwer Academic Publishers, pp 77–92.

Graham GG, Ziegler JB, Champion GD. 1993. Medicinal chemistry of gold. *Agents Actions* **44**(Suppl):209–17.

Graham S, Day RO, Wong H, et al. 1996. Pharmacodynamics of oxypurinol after administration of allopurinol to healthy subjects. *Br J Clin Pharmacol* **41**:299–304.

Graziotti PJ, Goucke CR. 1997. The use of oral opioids in patients with chronic non-cancer pain management strategies. *Med J Aust* **167**:30–4.

Greenblatt DJ, Abernethy DR, Boxenbaum HG, et al. 1986. Influence of age, gender, and obesity on salicylate kinetics following single doses of aspirin. *Arthritis Rheum* **29**:971–80.

Griffin MR, Piper JM, Daugherty JR, et al. 1991. Nonsteroidal antiinflammatory drug use and increased risk for peptic ulcer disease in elderly persons. *Ann Intern Med* **114**:257–63.

Grochow LB, Colvin M. 1979. Clinical pharmacokinetics of cyclophosphamide. *Clin Pharmacokinet* **4**:380–94.

Grondin C, Malleson P, Petty RE. 1988. Slow-acting antirheumatic drugs in chronic arthritis of childhood. *Semin Arthritis Rheum* **18**:38–47.

Gross WL. 1997. Systemic necrotizing vasculitis. *Bailliere's Clin Rheumatol* **11**:259–84.

Gutierrez-Urena S, Molina JF, Garcia CO, et al. 1996. Pancytopenia secondary to methotrexate therapy in rheumatoid arthritis. *Arthritis Rheum* **39**:272–6.

Haagsma CJ, van Riel PL, de Rooij DJ, et al. 1994. Combination of methotrexate and sulphasalazine vs methotrexate alone: A randomized open clinical trial in rheumatoid arthritis patients resistant to sulphasalazine therapy. *Br J Rheumatol* **33**:1049–55.

Hamilton JA, Biggs JC, Atkinson K, et al. 1995. Bone marrow transplantation in auto-immune disease. *Bailliere's Clin Rheumatol* **9**:673–87.

Hamilton RA, Kremer JM. 1997. Why intramuscular methotrexate may be more efficacious than oral dosing in patients with rheumatoid arthritis. *Br J Rheumatol* **36**:86–90.

Hamuryudan V, Ozyazgan Y, Hizli N, et al. 1997. Azathioprine in Bechet's syndrome: Effects on long-term prognosis. *Arthritis Rheum* **40**:769–74.

Handel ML, deFazio A, Watts CK, et al. 1991. Inhibition of DNA binding and transcriptional activity of a nuclear receptor transcription factor by aurothiomalate and other metal ions. *Mol Pharmacol* **40**:613–8.

Handel ML, Sivertsen S, Watts CK, et al. 1993. Comparative effects of gold on the interactions of transcription factors with DNA. *Agents Actions* **44**(Suppl):219–23.

Handel ML, Watts CK, deFazio A, et al. 1995. Inhibition of AP-1 binding and transcription by gold and selenium involving conserved cysteine residues in Jun and Fos. *Proc Natl Acad Sci U S A* **92**:4497–501.

Handel ML, Watts CK, Sivertsen S, et al. 1996. D-Penicillamine causes free radical-dependent inactivation of activator protein-1 DNA binding. *Mol Pharmacol* **50**:501–5.

Hawkey CJ, Karrasch JA, Szczepanski L, et al. 1998. Omeprazole compared with misoprostol for ulcers associated with nonsteroidal antiinflammatory drugs. Omeprazole versus Misoprostol for NSAID-Induced Ulcer Management (OMNIUM) Study Group. *N Engl J Med* **338**:727–34.

Hayball PJ, Cosh DG, Ahern MJ, et al. 1992. High dose oral methylprednisolone in patients with rheumatoid arthritis: Pharmacokinetics and clinical response. *Eur J Clin Pharmacol* **42**:85–8.

Heck S, Bender K, Kullmann M, et al. 1997. I kappaB alpha-independent downregulation of NF-kappaB activity by glucocorticoid receptor. *EMBO J* **16**:4698–707.

Henry D, Lim LL, Garcia Rodriguez LA, et al. 1996. Variability in risk of gastrointestinal complications with individual non-steroidal anti-inflammatory drugs: Results of a collaborative meta-analysis. *Br Med J* **312**:1563–6.

Henry D, Page J, Whyte I, et al. 1997. Consumption of non-steroidal anti-inflammatory drugs and the development of functional renal impairment in elderly subjects. Results of a case-control study. *Br J Clin Pharmacol* **44**:85–90.

Heuer MA, Pietrusko RG, Morris RW, et al. 1985. An analysis of worldwide safety experience with auranofin. *J Rheumatol* **12**:695–9.

Hiesse C, Kriaa F, Rieu P, et al. 1995. Incidence and type of malignancies occurring after renal transplantation in conventionally and cyclosporine-treated recipients: Analysis of a 20-year period in 1600 patients. *Transplant Proc* **27**:972–4.

Hilliquin P, Renoux M, Perrot S, et al. 1996. Occurrence of pulmonary complications during methotrexate therapy in rheumatoid arthritis. *Br J Rheumatol* **35**:441–5.

Ho S, Clipstone N, Timmermann L, et al. 1996. The mechanism of action of cyclosporin A and FK506. *Clin Immunol Immunopathol* **80**: S40–5.

Hobbs DC. 1986. Piroxicam pharmacokinetics: Recent clinical results relating kinetics and plasma levels to age sex and adverse effects. *Am J Med* **81**:22–8.

Hochberg MC, Altman RD, Brandt KD, et al. 1995a. Guidelines for the medical management of osteoarthritis. Part I. Osteoarthritis of the hip. American College of Rheumatology. *Arthritis Rheum* **38**:1535–40.

Hochberg MC, Altman RD, Brandt KD, et al. 1995b. Guidelines for the medical management of osteoarthritis. Part II. Osteoarthritis of the knee. American College of Rheumatology. *Arthritis Rheum* **38**:1541–6.

Hoffman LD, Turner JA, Clancy S, et al. 1995. Therapeutic trials for low back pain. *Spine* **19**:2068–75S.

Hoult JR, Moore PK. 1980. Effects of sulphasalazine and its metabolites on prostaglandin synthesis inactivation and actions on smooth muscle. *Br J Pharmacol* **68**:719–30.

Hows JM, Mehta A, Ward L. 1984. Comparison of mesna with forced diuresis to prevent cyclophosphamide-induced haemorrhage status in marrow transplantation—a prospective randomised study. *Br J Cancer* **50**:735–56.

Hunder GG. 1997. Giant cell arteritis and polymyalgia rheumatica. *Med Clin North Am* **81**:195–219.

Hunter T, Urowitz MB, Gordon DA, et al. 1975. Azathioprine in rheumatoid arthritis: A long-term follow-up study. *Arthritis Rheum* **18**:15–20.

Huskisson EC, Wojtulewski JA, Berry H, et al. 1974. Treatment of rheumatoid arthritis with fenoprofen: Comparison with aspirin. *Br Med J* **1**:176–80.

Huynh-Do U, Gantenbein H, Binswanger U. 1995. Pneumocystis carinii pneumonia during immunosuppressive therapy for antineutrophil cytoplasmic autoantibody-positive vasculitis. *Arch Intern Med* **155**:872–4.

Jaffe IA. 1965. The effect of penicillamine on the laboratory parameters in rheumatoid arthritis. *Arthritis Rheum* **8**:1064–79.

Jennette JC, Falk RJ. 1997. Small-vessel vasculitis. *N Engl J Med* **337**:1512–23.

Jeurissen ME, Boerbooms AM, van de Putte LB, et al. 1991. Influence of methotrexate and azathioprine on radiologic progression in rheumatoid arthritis. A randomized double-blind study. *Ann Intern Med* **114**:999–1004.

Jimenez SA, Sigal SH. 1991. A 15-year prospective study of treatment of rapidly progressive systemic sclerosis with D-penicillamine. *J Rheumatol* **18**:1496–503.

Jobanputra P, Hunter M, Clark D, et al. 1995. An audit of methotrexate and folic acid for rheumatoid arthritis. Experience from a teaching centre. *Br J Rheumatol* **34**:971–5.

Johnson AG. 1997. NSAIDs and increased blood pressure. What is the clinical significance? *Drug Saf* **17**:277–89.

Johnson AG, Day RO. 1991a. The problems and pitfalls of NSAID therapy in the elderly (Part I). *Drugs Aging* **1**:130–43.

Johnson AG, Day RO. 1991b. The problems and pitfalls of NSAID therapy in the elderly (Part II). *Drugs Aging* **1**:212–27.

Johnson AG, Nguyen TV, Day RO. 1994. Do nonsteroidal anti-inflammatory drugs affect blood pressure? A meta-analysis. *Ann Intern Med* **121**:289–300.

Johnson AG, Seideman P, Day RO. 1993. Adverse drug interactions with nonsteroidal anti-inflammatory drugs (NSAIDs). Recognition management and avoidance. *Drug Saf* **8**:99–127.

Jones AC, Berman P, Doherty M. 1992. Non-steroidal anti-inflammatory drug usage and requirement in elderly acute hospital admissions. *Br J Rheumatol* **31**:45–8.

Jones AC, Doherty M. 1992. The treatment of osteoarthritis. *Br J Clin Pharmacol* **33**:357–63.

Jones AC, Pattrick M, Doherty S, et al. 1995. Intra-articular hyaluronic acid compared to intra-articular triamcinolone hexacetonide in inflammatory knee osteoarthritis. *Osteoarthritis Cartilage* **3**: 269–73.

Jones DL, Kroenke K, Landry FJ, et al. 1996. Cost savings using a stepped-care prescribing protocol for nonsteroidal anti-inflammatory drugs. *JAMA* **275**:926–30.

Jones M, Symmons D, Finn J, et al. 1996. Does exposure to immunosuppressive therapy increase the 10 year malignancy and mortality risks in rheumatoid arthritis? A matched cohort study. *Br J Rheumatol* **35**:738–45.

Joyce DA. 1988. D-Penicillamine pharmacokinetics and action. *Agents Actions* **24**(Suppl):197–206.

Joyce DA. 1989. D-Penicillamine pharmacokinetics and pharmacodynamics in man. *Pharmacol Therapeut* **42**:405–27.

Joyce DA. 1990. D-Penicillamine. *Bailliere's Clin Rheumatol* **4**:553–74.

Joyce DA. 1993. Variability in response to D-penicillamine: Pharmacokinetic insights. *Agents Actions* **44**(Suppl):203–7.

Joyce DA, Day RO. 1990. D-Penicillamine and D-penicillamine-protein disulphide in plasma and synovial fluid of patients with rheumatoid arthritis. *Br J Clin Pharmacol* **30**:511–7.

Joyce DA, Forrest MJ, Brooks PM. 1988. D-Penicillamine metabolism in an in-vivo model of inflamed synovium. *Agents Actions* **25**: 336–43.

Joyce DA, Murphy BR. 1990. D-Penicillamine metabolism: The role of transformation in blood plasma. *Agents Actions* **31**:353–7.

Juhl RP, Van Thiel DH, Dittert LW, et al. 1983. Ibuprofen and sulindac kinetics in alcoholic liver disease. *Clin Pharmacol Ther* **34**: 104–9.

Kelly JP, Kaufman DW, Jurgelon JM, et al. 1996. Risk of aspirin-associated major upper-gastrointestinal bleeding with enteric-coated or buffered product. *Lancet* **348**:1413–6.

Kerstens PJ, Stolk JN, De Abreu RA, et al. A. 1995. Azathioprine-related bone marrow toxicity and low activities of purine enzymes in patients with rheumatoid arthritis. *Arthritis Rheum* **38**:142–5.

Kirwan JR. 1995. The effect of glucocorticoids on joint destruction in rheumatoid arthritis. The Arthritis and Rheumatism Council Low-Dose Glucocorticoid Study Group. *N Engl J Med* **333**:142–6.

Kjaersgaard-Andersen P, Nafei A, Skov O, et al. 1990. Codeine plus paracetamol versus paracetamol in longer-term treatment of chronic pain due to osteoarthritis of the hip. A randomised double-blind multi-centre study. *Pain* **43**:309–18.

Kloppenburg M, Breedveld FC, Terwiel JP, et al. 1994. Minocycline in active rheumatoid arthritis. A double-blind placebo-controlled trial. *Arthritis Rheum* **37**:629–36.

Kloppenburg M, Brinkman BM, de Rooij-Dijk HH, et al. 1996. The tetracycline derivative minocycline differentially affects cytokine production by monocytes and T lymphocytes. *Antimicrob Agents Chemother* **40**:934–40.

Kloppenburg M, Dijkmans BA, Breedveld FC. 1995. Antimicrobial therapy for rheumatoid arthritis. *Bailliere's Clin Rheumatol* **9**:759–69.

Kloppenburg M, Mattie H, Douwes N, et al. 1995. Minocycline in the treatment of rheumatoid arthritis: Relationship of serum concentrations to efficacy. *J Rheumatol* **22**:611–6.

Kloppenburg M, Terwiel JP, Mallee C, et al. 1994. Minocycline in active rheumatoid arthritis. A placebo-controlled trial. *Ann N Y Acad Sci* **732**:422–3.

Koch M, Dezi A, Ferrario F, et al. 1996. Prevention of nonsteroidal anti-inflammatory drug-induced gastrointestinal mucosal injury. A meta-analysis of randomized controlled clinical trials. *Arch Intern Med* **156**:2321–32.

Koike R, Miki I, Otoshi M, et al. 1994. Gold sodium thiomalate down-regulates intercellular adhesion molecule-1 and vascular cell adhesion molecule-1 expression on vascular endothelial cells. *Mol Pharmacol* **46**:599–604.

Koopman WJ, Moreland LW. 1998. Rheumatoid arthritis: Anticytokine therapies on the horizon. *Ann Intern Med* **128**:231–3.

Kot TV, Day RO, Brooks PM. 1993. Preventing acute gout when starting allopurinol therapy. Colchicine or NSAIDs? *Med J Aust* **159**:182–4.

Kremer JM. 1989. Methotrexate therapy in the treatment of rheumatoid arthritis. *Rheum Dis Clin North Am* **15**:533–56.

Kremer JM. 1997. Safety, efficacy, and mortality in a long-term cohort of patients with rheumatoid arthritis taking methotrexate: Followup after a mean of 13.3 years. *Arthritis Rheum* **40**:984–5.

Kremer JM, Alarcon GS, Lightfoot RW, et al. 1994. Methotrexate for rheumatoid arthritis: Suggested guidelines for monitoring liver toxicity. *Arthritis Rheum* **37**:316–28.

Kremer JM, Alarcon GS, Weinblatt ME, et al. 1997. Clinical laboratory radiographic and histopathologic features of methotrexate-associated lung injury in patients with rheumatoid arthritis: A multicenter study with literature review. *Arthritis Rheum* **40**:1829–37.

Kremer JM, Lee JK. 1988. A long-term prospective study of the use of methotrexate in rheumatoid arthritis. Update after a mean of fifty-three months. *Arthritis Rheum* **31**:577–84.

Lamberts SW, Bruining HA, de Jong FH. 1997. Corticosteroid therapy in severe illness. *N Engl J Med* **337**:1285–92.

Langford CA, Klippel JH, Balow JE, et al. 1998. Use of cytotoxic agents and cyclosporine in the treatment of autoimmune disease. Part 2: Inflammatory bowel disease systemic vasculitis and therapeutic toxicity. *Ann Intern Med* **129**:49–58.

Langman MJ, Weil J, Wainwright P, et al. 1994. Risks of bleeding peptic ulcer associated with individual non-steroidal anti-inflammatory drugs. *Lancet* **343**:1075–8.

LaRochelle GE Jr, LaRochelle AG, Ratner RE, et al. 1993. Recovery of the hypothalamic-pituitary-adrenal (HPA) axis in patients with rheumatic diseases receiving low-dose prednisone. *Am J Med* **95**:258–64.

Laska EM, Sunshine A, Marrero I, et al. 1986. The correlation between blood levels of ibuprofen and clinical analgesic response. *Clin Pharmacol Ther* **40**:1–7.

Lee EJ, Williams K, Day R, et al. 1985. Stereoselective disposition of ibuprofen enantiomers in man. *Br J Clin Pharmacol* **19**:669–74.

Leipold G, Schutz E, Haas JP, et al. 1997. Azathioprine-induced severe pancytopenia due to a homozygous two-point mutation of the thiopurine methyltransferase gene in a patient with juvenile HLA-B27-associated spondylarthritis. *Arthritis Rheum* **40**:1896–8.

Lennard L. 1992. The clinical pharmacology of 6-mercaptopurine. *Eur J Clin Pharmacol* **43**:329–39.

Le Quintrec JS, Le Quintrec JL. 1991. Drug-induced myopathies. *Bailliere's Clin Rheumatol* **5**:21–38.

Levy G, Leonards JR. 1971. Urine pH and salicylate therapy. *JAMA* **217**:81.

Levy G, Tsuchiya T. 1972. Salicylate accumulation kinetics in man. *N Engl J Med* **287**:430–2.

Levy G, Tsuchiya T, Amsel LP. 1972. Limited capacity for salicyl phenolic glucuronide formation and its effect on the kinetics of salicylate elimination in man. *Clin Pharmacol Ther* **13**:258–68.

Levy J, Barnett EV, MacDonald NS, et al. 1972. The effect of azathioprine on gammaglobulin synthesis in man. *J Clin Invest* **51**: 2233–8.

Liegler DG, Henderson ES, Hahn MA, et al. 1969. The effect of organic acids on renal clearance of methotrexate in man. *Clin Pharmacol Ther* **10**:849–57.

Lin SN, Jessup K, Floyd M, et al. 1980. Quantification of plasma azathioprine and 6-mercaptopurine levels in renal transplant patients. *Transplantation* **29**:290–4.

Lipsky PE, Ziff M. 1977. Inhibition of antigen- and mitogen-induced human lymphocyte proliferation by gold compounds. *J Clin Invest* **59**:455–66.

Littlejohn GO. 1996. Fibromyalgia syndrome. *Med J Aust* **165**:387–91.

Littlejohn GO. 1998. Fibromyalgia syndrome and disability: The neurogenic model. *Med J Aust* **168**:398–401.

Lopez-Mendez A, Daniel WW, Reading JC, et al. 1993. Radiographic assessment of disease progression in rheumatoid arthritis patients enrolled in the cooperative systematic studies of the rheumatic diseases program randomized clinical trial of methotrexate auranofin or a combination of the two. *Arthritis Rheum* **36**:1364–9.

Lord SM, Barnsley L, Wallis BJ, et al. 1996. Percutaneous radio-frequency neurotomy for chronic cervical zygapophyseal-joint pain. *N Engl J Med* **335**:1721–6.

Luong C, Miller A, Barnett J, et al. 1996. Flexibility of the NSAID binding site in the structure of human cyclooxygenase-2. *Nature Struct Biol* **3**:927–33.

Luqmani RA, Exley AR, Kitas GD, et al. 1997. Disease assessment and management of the vasculitides. *Bailliere's Clin Rheumatol* **11**:423–46.

Luqmani RA, Palmer RG, Bacon PA. 1990. Azathioprine cyclophosphamide and chlorambucil. *Bailliere's Clin Rheumatol* **4**:595–619.

Malik SW, Myers JL, DeRemee RA, et al. 1996. Lung toxicity associated with cyclophosphamide use. Two distinct patterns. *Am J Resp Crit Care Med* **154**:1851–6.

Malmivaara A, Hakkinen U, Aro T, et al. 1995. The treatment of acute low back pain—bed rest exercises or ordinary activity? *N Engl J Med* **332**:351–5.

March LM. 1997. Osteoarthritis. *Med J Aust* **166**:98–103.

Marshall PJ, Kulmacz RJ, Lands WE. 1987. Constraints on prostaglandin biosynthesis in tissues. *J Biol Chem* **262**:3510–7.

Massarella JW, Waller ES, Crout JE, et al. 1984. The pharmacokinetics of intramuscular gold sodium thiomalate in normal volunteers. *Biopharmaceut Drug Disp* **5**:101–7.

McCarty MJ, Lillis P, Vukelja SJ. 1996. Azathioprine as a steroid-sparing agent in radiation pneumonitis. *Chest* **109**:1397–400.

McCune WJ, Golbus J, Zeldes W, et al. 1988. Clinical and immunologic effects of monthly administration of intravenous cyclophosphamide in severe systemic lupus erythematosus. *N Engl J Med* **318**:1423–31.

McCune WJ, Vallance DK, Lynch JPR. 1994. Immunosuppressive drug therapy. *Curr Opin Rheumatol* **6**:262–72.

McLachlan AJ, Tett SE, Cutler DJ, et al. 1994. Bioavailability of hydroxychloroquine tablets in patients with rheumatoid arthritis. *Br J Rheumatol* **33**:235–9.

McLachlan AJ, Tett SE, Day RO, et al. 1993. Absorption and in vivo dissolution of hydroxychloroquine in fed subjects assessed using deconvolution techniques. *Br J Clin Pharmacol* **36**:405–11.

McManus P, Primrose JG, Henry DA, et al. 1996. Pattern of non-steroidal anti-inflammatory drug use in Australia 1990–1994. A report from the Drug Utilization Sub-Committee of the Pharmaceutical Benefits Advisory Committee. *Med J Aust* **164**:589–92.

McVerry RM, Lethbridge J, Martin N, et al. 1986. Pharmacokinetics of naproxen in elderly patients. *Eur J Clin Pharmacol* **31**:463–8.

Meffin PJ. 1985. The effect of renal dysfunction on the disposition of non-steroidal anti-inflammatory drugs forming acyl-glucuronides. *Agents Actions* **17**(Suppl):85–9.

Meffin PJ, Brooks PM, Bertouch J, et al. 1983. Diflunisal disposition and hypouricemic response in osteoarthritis. *Clin Pharmacol Ther* **33**:813–21.

Meffin PJ, Sallustio BC, Purdie YJ, et al. 1986. Enantioselective disposition of 2-arylpropionic acid nonsteroidal anti-inflammatory drugs. I. 2-Phenylpropionic acid disposition. *J Pharmacol Exp Ther* **238**:280–7.

Merskey H. 1993. Psychological consequences of whiplash. In: Teasell RW, et al. editors. *Cervical Flexion-Extension/Whiplash Injuries*. Philadelphia: Hanley and Belfus, pp 471–80.

Meyrier A. 1976. Desensitisation in a patient with chronic renal disease and severe allergy to allopurinol. *Br Med J* **2**:458.

Mielants H, Veys EM, Joos R. 1986. Sulphasalazine (Salazopyrin) in the treatment of enterogenic reactive synovitis and ankylosing spondylitis with peripheral arthritis. *Clin Rheumatol* **5**:80–3.

Mills JA. 1994. Systemic lupus erythematosus. *N Engl J Med* **330**: 1871–9.

Mitchell JA, Akarasereenont P, Thiemermann C, et al. 1993. Selectivity of nonsteroidal antiinflammatory drugs as inhibitors of constitutive and inducible cyclooxygenase. *Proc Natl Acad Sci U S A* **90**:11693–7.

Moder KG, Tefferi A, Cohen MD, et al. 1995. Hematologic malignancies and the use of methotrexate in rheumatoid arthritis: a retrospective study. *Am J Med* **99**:276–81.

Moore MJ. 1991. Clinical pharmacokinetics of cyclophosphamide. *Clin Pharmacokinet* **20**:194–208.

Moore RA, Tramer MR, Carroll D, et al. 1998. Quantitative systematic review of topically applied non-steroidal anti-inflammatory drugs. *Br Med J* **316**:333–8.

Morales JM. 1996. Drug-induced hepatotoxicity. *N Engl J Med* **334**:864.

Moreland LW, Baumgartner SW, Schiff MH, et al. 1997. Treatment of rheumatoid arthritis with a recombinant human tumor necrosis factor receptor (p75)-Fc fusion protein. *N Engl J Med* **337**:141–7.

Moreland LW, Heck LW Jr, Koopman WJ. 1997. Biologic agents for treating rheumatoid arthritis. Concepts and progress. *Arthritis Rheum* **40**:397–409.

Muller FO, Hundt HKL, de Kock AC. 1975. Decreased steady state salicylic acid plasma levels associated with chronic aspirin ingestion. *Curr Med Res* **3**:417–22.

Needleman P, Isakson PC. 1997. The discovery and function of COX-2. *J Rheumatol* **24**(Suppl 49):6–8.

Needs CJ, Brooks PM. 1985. Clinical pharmacokinetics of the salicylates. *Clin Pharmacokinet* **10**:164–77.

Netter P, Faure G, Regent MC, et al. 1985. Salicylate kinetics in old age. *Clin Pharmacol Ther* **38**:6–11.

Neumann VC, Taggart AJ, Le Gallez P, et al. 1986. A study to determine the active moiety of sulphasalazine in rheumatoid arthritis. *J Rheumatol* **13**:285–7.

Neuwelt CM, Lacks S, Kaye BR, et al. 1995. Role of intravenous cyclophosphamide in the treatment of severe neuropsychiatric systemic lupus erythematosus. *Am J Med* **98**:32–41.

Nicholas MK, Wilson PH, Goyen J. 1992. Comparison of cognitive-behavioral group treatment and an alternative non-psychological treatment for chronic low back pain. *Pain* **48**:339–47.

Nowack R, Flores-Suarez LF, van der Woude FJ. 1998. New developments in pathogenesis of systemic vasculitis. *Curr Opin Rheumatol* **10**:3–11.

Nuver-Zwart IH, van Riel PL, van de Putte LB, et al. 1989. A double blind comparative study of sulphasalazine and hydroxychloroquine in rheumatoid arthritis: Evidence of an earlier effect of sulphasalazine. *Ann Rheum Dis* **48**:389–95.

Nygaard H. 1997. Pancytopenia secondary to methotrexate therapy in rheumatoid arthritis: comment on the article by Gutierrez-Urena et al. *Arthritis Rheum* **40**:194–5; discussion 195–6.

O'Brien WM, Bagby GF. 1985a. Rare adverse reactions to nonsteroidal antiinflammatory drugs. *J Rheumatol* **12**:347–53.

O'Brien WM, Bagby GF. 1985b. Rare adverse reactions to nonsteroidal antiinflammatory drugs. *J Rheumatol* **12**:13–20.

O'Brien WM, Bagby GF. 1985c. Rare adverse reactions to nonsteroidal antiinflammatory drugs. 3. *J Rheumatol* **12**:562–7.

O'Brien WM, Bagby GF. 1985d. Rare adverse reactions to nonsteroidal antiinflammatory drugs. 4. *J Rheumatol* **12**:785–90.

O'Dell JR. 1997. Methotrexate use in rheumatoid arthritis. *Rheum Dis Clin North Am* **23**:779–96.

O'Neill GF. 1994. Tiaprofenic acid as a cause of non-bacterial cystitis. *Med J Aust* **160**:123–5.

Opelz G, Henderson R. 1993. Incidence of non-Hodgkin lymphoma in kidney and heart transplant recipients. *Lancet* **342**:1514–6.

Osman MA, Patel RB, Schuna A, et al. 1983. Reduction in oral penicillamine absorption by food antacid and ferrous sulfate. *Clin Pharmacol Ther* **33**:465–70.

Parnham AP, Dittmer I, Mathieson PW, et al. 1996. Acute allergic reactions associated with azathioprine. *Lancet* **348**:542–3.

Pasero G, Priolo F, Marubini E, et al. 1996. Slow progression of joint damage in early rheumatoid arthritis treated with cyclosporin A. *Arthritis Rheum* **39**:1006–15.

Paul C, Le Tourneau A, Cayuela JM, et al. 1997. Epstein-Barr virus-associated lymphoproliferative disease during methotrexate therapy for psoriasis. *Arch Dermatol* **133**:867–71.

Paulus HE. 1988. Antimalarial agents compared with or in combination with other disease-modifying antirheumatic drugs. *Am J Med* **85**:45–52.

Paxton JW. 1980. Effects of aspirin on salivary and serum phenytoin kinetics in healthy subjects. *Clin Pharmacol Ther* **27**:170–8.

Perrett D. 1981. The metabolism and pharmacology of D-penicillamine in man. *J Rheumatol* **7**(Suppl):41–50.

Perretti M, Croxtall JD, Wheller SK, et al. 1996. Mobilizing lipocortin 1 in adherent human leukocytes downregulates their transmigration. *Nat Med* **2**:1259–62.

Pincus T. 1988. Rheumatoid arthritis: Disappointing long-term outcomes despite successful short-term clinical trials. *J Clin Epidemiol* **41**:1037–41.

Plotz PH, Klippel JH, Decker JL, et al. 1979. Bladder complications in patients receiving cyclophosphamide for systemic lupus erythematosus or rheumatoid arthritis. *Ann Intern Med* **91**:221–3.

Porter DR, Capell HA. 1990. The use of sulphasalazine as a disease modifying antirheumatic drug. *Bailliere's Clin Rheumatol* **4**: 535–51.

Pountain G, Hazleman B. 1995. ABC of rheumatology. Polymyalgia rheumatica and giant cell arteritis. *Br Med J* **310**:1057–9.

Preston SJ, Arnold MH, Beller EM, et al. 1988. Variability in response to nonsteroidal anti-inflammatory analgesics: Evidence from controlled clinical therapeutic trial of flurbiprofen in rheumatoid arthritis. *Br J Clin Pharmacol* **26**:759–64.

Pryor BD, Bologna SG, Kahl LE. 1996. Risk factors for serious infection during treatment with cyclophosphamide and high-dose corticosteroids for systemic lupus erythematosus. *Arthritis Rheum* **39**: 1475–82.

Puhl W, Bernau A, Greiling H, et al. 1993. Intra-articular sodium hyaluronate in osteoarthritis of the knee: A multi-centre double-blind study. *Osteoarthritis Cartilage* **1**:233–41.

Quinn DI, Day RO. 1997. Clinically important drug interactions. In: Speight GM, Holford NHG, editors. *Avery's Drug Treatment.* Auckland, NZ: Adis Int, pp 301–338.

Quinn DI, Day RO. 1995. Drug interactions of clinical importance. An updated guide. *Drug Saf* **12**:393–452.

Radis CD, Kahl LE, Baker GL, et al. 1995. Effects of cyclophosphamide on the development of malignancy and on long-term survival of patients with rheumatoid arthritis. A 20-year followup study. *Arthritis Rheum* **38**:1120–7.

Rains CP, Noble S, Faulds D. 1995. Sulfasalazine: A review of its pharmacological properties and therapeutic efficacy in the treatment of rheumatoid arthritis. *Drugs* **50**:137–56.

Rasaratnam I, Ryan PF. 1997a. Systemic lupus erythematosus. *Med J Aust* **166**:266–70.

Rasaratnam I, Ryan PF. 1997b. Systemic sclerosis and the inflammatory myopathies. *Med J Aust* **166**:322–7.

Rasaratnam I, Ryan PF. 1998. Systemic lupus erythematosus (SLE): Changing concepts and challenges for the new millennium. *Aust N Z J Med* **28**:5–11.

Rashad S, Low F, Revell P, et al. 1989. Effect of non-steroidal anti-inflammatory drugs on course of osteoarthritis. *Lancet* **2**:1149.

Ratliff TR, Williams RD. 1998. Hemorrhagic cystitis chemotherapy and bladder toxicity. *J Urol* **159**:1044.

Reimann IW, Frolich JC. 1981. Effects of diclofenac on lithium kinetics. *Clin Pharmacol Ther* **30**:348–52.

Rhodes JM, Bartholomew TC, Jewell DP. 1981. Inhibition of leucocyte motility by drugs used in ulcerative colitis. *Gut* **22**:642–7.

Richmond R, McMillan TW, Luqmani RA. 1998. Optimisation of cyclophosphamide therapy in systemic vasculitis. *Clin Pharmacokinet* **34**:79–90.

Ritch AE, Perera WN, Jones CJ. 1982. Pharmacokinetics of azapropazone in the elderly. *Br J Clin Pharmacol* **14**:116–9.

Roberts MS, Rumble RH, Wanwimolruk S, et al. 1983. Pharmacokinetics of aspirin and salicylate in elderly subjects and in patients with alcoholic liver disease. *Eur J Clin Pharmacol* **25**:253–61.

Rolan PE. 1994. Plasma protein binding displacement interactions—why are they still regarded as clinically important? *Br J Clin Pharmacol* **37**:125–8.

Rosenthal NS, Farhi DC. 1996. Myelodysplastic syndromes and acute myeloid leukemia in connective tissue disease after single-agent chemotherapy. *Am J Clin Pathol* **106**:676–9.

Rowland M, Riegelman S, Harris PA, et al. 1972. Absorption kinetics of aspirin in man following oral administration of an aqueous solution. *J Pharm Sci* **61**:379–85.

Rubin A, Knadler MP, Ho PP, et al. 1985. Stereoselective inversion of (*R*)-fenoprofen to (*S*)-fenoprofen in humans. *J Pharm Sci* **74**:82–4.

Rudkowski R, Graham GG, Ziegler JB, et al. 1991. The effect of aurothiomalate on the oxidative burst of polymorphonuclear leukocytes varies with the quantity of drug in myocrisin ampoules. *J Rheumatol* **18**:666–71.

Rudkowski R, Ziegler JB, Graham GG, et al. 1991. Auranofin inhibits the activation pathways of polymorphonuclear leukocytes at multiple sites. *Biochem Pharmacol* **41**:1921–9.

Saag KG, Emkey R, Schnitzer TJ, et al. 1998. Alendronate for the prevention and treatment of glucocorticoid-induced osteoporosis. *N Engl J Med* **339**:292–299.

Sachar DB. 1988. The safety of sulfasalazine: The gastroenterologists' experience. *J Rheumatol* **16**(Suppl):14–6.

Salem M, Tainsh RE Jr, Bromberg J, et al. 1994. Perioperative glucocorticoid coverage. A reassessment 42 years after emergence of a problem. *Ann Surg* **219**:416–25.

Salmeron G, Lipsky PE. 1983. Immunosuppressive potential of antimalarials. *Am J Med* **75**:19–24.

Sambrook PN. 1996. Corticosteroid induced osteoporosis. *J Rheumatol* **45**(Suppl):19–22.

Sambrook PN, Browne CD, Champion GD, et al. 1982. Terminations of treatment with gold sodium thiomalate in rheumatoid arthritis. *J Rheumatol* **9**:932–4.

Sambrook PN, Champion GD, Browne CD, et al. 1986. Comparison of methotrexate with azathioprine or 6-mercaptopurine in refractory rheumatoid arthritis: A life-table analysis. *Br J Rheumatol* **25**: 372–5.

Sambrook PN, Jones G. 1995. Corticosteroid osteoporosis. *Br J Rheumatol* **34**:8–12.

Sampson AP, Cowburn AS, Sladek K, et al. 1997. Profound overexpression of leukotriene C4 synthase in bronchial biopsies from aspirin-intolerant asthmatic patients. *Int Arch Allergy Immunol* **113**:355–7.

Sandoval DM, Alarcon GS, Morgan SL. 1995. Adverse events in methotrexate-treated rheumatoid arthritis patients. *Br J Rheumatol* **34**:49–56.

Schlaghecke R, Kornely E, Santen RT, et al. 1992. The effect of long-term glucocorticoid therapy on pituitary-adrenal responses to exogenous corticotropin-releasing hormone. *N Engl J Med* **326**: 226–30.

Scott DL, Dacre JE. 1988. Adverse reactions to sulfasalazine: the British experience. *J Rheumatol* **16**(Suppl):17–21.

Sedor JR, Williams SL, Chremos AN, et al. 1984. Effects of sulindac and indomethacin on renal prostaglandin synthesis. *Clin Pharmacol Ther* **36**:85–91.

Seideman P, Ayesh R. 1994. Reduced sulphoxidation capacity in D-penicillamine induced myasthenia gravis. *Clin Rheumatol* **13**: 435–7.

Seideman P, Beck O, Eksborg S, et al. 1993. The pharmacokinetics of methotrexate and its 7-hydroxy metabolite in patients with rheumatoid arthritis. *Br J Clin Pharmacol* **35**:409–12.

Seideman P, Melander A. 1988. Equianalgesic effects of paracetamol and indomethacin in rheumatoid arthritis. *Br J Rheumatol* **27**: 117–22.

Seideman P, Samuelson P, Neander G. 1993. Naproxen and paracetamol compared with naproxen only in coxarthrosis. Increased effect of the combination in 18 patients. *Acta Orthop Scand* **64**:285–8.

Sellers EM. 1979. Plasma protein displacement interactions are rarely of clinical significance. *Pharmacology* **18**:225–7.

Shen DD, Azarnoff DL. 1978. Clinical pharmacokinetics of methotrexate. *Clin Pharmacokinet* **3**:1–13.

Silverberg DS, Kidd EG, Shnitka TK, et al. 1970. Gold nephropathy. A clinical and pathologic study. *Arthritis Rheum* **13**:812–25.

Silverstein FE, Graham DY, Senior JR, et al. 1995. Misoprostol reduces serious gastrointestinal complications in patients with rheumatoid arthritis receiving nonsteroidal anti-inflammatory drugs. A randomized double-blind placebo-controlled trial. *Ann Intern Med* **123**:241–9.

Singh G, Fries JF, Spitz P, et al. 1989. Toxic effects of azathioprine in rheumatoid arthritis. A national post-marketing perspective. *Arthritis Rheum* **32**:837–43.

Skolnick AA. 1997. Biological response modifiers may yield a new class of drugs to treat arthritis. *JAMA* **277**:276–8.

Smalley WE, Griffin MR, Fought RL, et al. 1995. Effect of a prior-authorization requirement on the use of nonsteroidal anti-inflammatory drugs by Medicaid patients. *N Engl J Med* **332**:1612–7.

Smith MD, Ahern MJ, Roberts-Thomson PJ. 1990. Pulse methylprednisolone therapy in rheumatoid arthritis: Unproved therapy unjustified therapy or effective adjunctive treatment? *Ann Rheum Dis* **49**:265–7.

Sneller MC, Fauci AS. 1997. Pathogenesis of vasculitis syndromes. *Med Clin North Am* **81**:221–42.

Snow JL, Gibson LE. 1995. The role of genetic variation in thiopurine methyltransferase activity and the efficacy and/or side effects of azathioprine therapy in dermatologic patients. *Arch Dermatol* **131**:193–7.

Snyder RM, Mirabelli C, Crooke S. 1986. Cellular association intracellular distribution and efflux of auranofin via sequential ligand exchange reactions. *Biochem Pharmacol* **35**:923–32.

Songsiridej N, Furst DE. 1990. Methotrexate—the rapidly acting drug. *Bailliere's Clin Rheumatol* **4**:575–93.

Spector T. 1977. Inhibition of urate production by allopurinol. *Biochem Pharmacol* **26**:355–8.

Steen VD, Costantino JP, Shapiro AP, et al. 1990. Outcome of renal crisis in systemic sclerosis: Relation to availability of angiotensin converting enzyme (ACE) inhibitors. *Ann Intern Med* **113**: 352–7.

Steen VD, Medsger TA Jr. 1990. Epidemiology and natural history of systemic sclerosis. *Rheum Dis Clin North Am* **16**:1–10.

Steen VD, Medsger TA Jr, Osial TA Jr, et al. 1984. Factors predicting development of renal involvement in progressive systemic sclerosis. *Am J Med* **76**:779–86.

Steen VD, Medsger TA Jr, Rodnan GP. 1982. D-Penicillamine therapy in progressive systemic sclerosis (scleroderma): A retrospective analysis. *Ann Intern Med* **97**:652–9.

Stenson WF, Lobos E. 1983. Inhibition of platelet thromboxane synthetase by sulfasalazine. *Biochem Pharmacol* **32**:2205–9.

Stockman A, Zilko PJ, Major GA, et al. 1986. Genetic markers in rheumatoid arthritis relationship to toxicity from D-penicillamine. *J Rheumatol* **13**:269–73.

Strong HA, Warner NJ, Renwick AG, et al. 1985. Sulindac metabolism: The importance of an intact colon. *Clin Pharmacol Ther* **38**: 387–93.

Sturge RA, Scott JT, Hamilton EB, et al. 1977. Multi-centre trial of naproxen and phenylbutazone in acute gout. *Adv Exp Med Biol* **76B**:290–6.

Swannell AJ. 1997. Polymyalgia rheumatica and temporal arteritis: diagnosis and management. *Br Med J* **314**:1329–32.

Taggart AJ, McDermott B, Delargy M, et al. 1987. The pharmacokinetics of sulphasalazine in young and elderly patients with rheumatoid arthritis. *Scand J Rheumatol* **64**(Suppl):29–36.

Taggart AJ, Neumann VC, Hill J, et al. 1986. 5-Aminosalicylic acid or sulphapyridine. Which is the active moiety of sulphasalazine in rheumatoid arthritis? *Drugs* **32**:27–34.

Taha AS, Hudson N, Hawkey CJ, et al. 1996. Famotidine for the prevention of gastric and duodenal ulcers caused by nonsteroidal antiinflammatory drugs. *N Engl J Med* **334**:1435–9.

Talar-Williams C, Hijazi YM, Walther MM, et al. 1996. Cyclophosphamide-induced cystitis and bladder cancer in patients with Wegener granulomatosis. *Ann Intern Med* **124**:477–84.

Tan EM, Cohen AS, Fries JF, et al. 1982. The 1982 revised criteria for the classification of systemic lupus erythematosus. *Arthritis Rheum* **25**:1271–7.

Teasell RW, White K. 1994a. Clinical approaches to low back pain. Part 1. Epidemiology diagnosis and prevention. *Can Fam Physician* **40**:481–5.

Teasell RW, White K. 1994b. Clinical approaches to low back pain. Part 2. Management sequelae and disability and compensation. *Can Fam Physician* **40**:490–5.

Tett S, Cutler D, Day R. 1990. Antimalarials in rheumatic diseases. *Bailliere's Clin Rheumatol* **4**:467–89.

Tett SE. 1993. Clinical pharmacokinetics of slow-acting antirheumatic drugs. *Clin Pharmacokinet* **25**:392–407.

Tett SE, Cutler DJ, Day RO, et al. 1988. A dose-ranging study of the pharmacokinetics of hydroxy-chloroquine following intravenous administration to healthy volunteers. *Br J Clin Pharmacol* **26**: 303–13.

Tett SE, Day RO, Cutler DJ. 1993. Concentration-effect relationship of hydroxychloroquine in rheumatoid arthritis—a cross-sectional study. *J Rheumatol* **20**:1874–9.

The Canadian Hydroxychloroquine Study Group. 1991. A randomized study of the effect of withdrawing hydroxychloroquine sulfate in systemic lupus erythematosus. *N Engl J Med* **324**:150–4.

The HERA Study. 1995. A randomized trial of hydroxychloroquine in early rheumatoid arthritis. *Am J Med* **98**:156–68.

Tilley BC, Alarcon GS, Heyse SP, et al. 1995. Minocycline in rheumatoid arthritis. A 48-week double-blind placebo-controlled trial. MIRA Trial Group. *Ann Intern Med* **122**:81–9.

Todd PA. 1987. Auranofin in rheumatoid arthritis. In: Gottlieb NL, editor. *Auranofin in Rheumatoid Arthritis*. Langhorne, PA: Adis Int, pp 78–106.

Towheed TE, Hochberg MC. 1997. A systematic review of randomized controlled trials of pharmacological therapy in osteoarthritis of the hip. *J Rheumatol* **24**:349–57.

Townes AS, Sowa JM, Shulman LE. 1976. Controlled trial of cyclophosphamide in rheumatoid arthritis. *Arthritis Rheum* **19**:563–73.

Tsokos GC. 1987. Immunomodulatory treatment in patients with rheumatic diseases: Mechanisms of action. *Semin Arthritis Rheum* **17**:24–38.

Tugwell P, Baker P. 1995. Guidelines for the use of cyclosporine in rheumatoid arthritis. *Clin Rheumatol* **14**:37–41.

Tugwell P, Bennett K, Gent M. 1987. Methotrexate in rheumatoid arthritis. Indications, contraindications, efficacy, and safety. *Ann Intern Med* **107**:358–66.

Tugwell P, Bombardier C, Gent M, et al. 1990. Low-dose cyclosporin versus placebo in patients with rheumatoid arthritis. *Lancet* **335**:1051–5.

Tugwell P, Pincus T, Yocum D, et al. 1995. Combination therapy with cyclosporine and methotrexate in severe rheumatoid arthritis. The Methotrexate-Cyclosporine Combination Study Group. *N Engl J Med* **333**:137–41.

Tyndall A, Gratwohl A. 1996. Haemopoietic stem and progenitor cells in the treatment of severe autoimmune diseases. *Ann Rheum Dis* **55**:149–51.

Tyndall A, Gratwohl A. 1997. Hemopoietic blood and marrow transplants in the treatment of severe autoimmune disease. *Curr Opin Hematol* **4**:390–4.

Upton RA, Williams RL, Kelly J, et al. 1984. Naproxen pharmacokinetics in the elderly. *Br J Clin Pharmacol* **18**:207–14.

Valentini RP, Smoyer WE, Sedman AB, et al. 1998. Outcome of antineutrophil cytoplasmic autoantibodies—positive glomerulonephritis and vasculitis in children: a single-center experience. *J Pediatr* **132**:325–8.

Van den Ouweland FA, Franssen MJ, van de Putte LB, et al. 1987. Naproxen pharmacokinetics in patients with rheumatoid arthritis during active polyarticular inflammation. *Br J Clin Pharmacol* **23**:189–93.

Van der Heijde DM, van Riel PL, Nuver-Zwart IH, et al. 1989. Effects of hydroxychloroquine and sulphasalazine on progression of joint damage in rheumatoid arthritis. *Lancet* **1**:1036–8.

Van der Heijde DM, van Riel PL, Nuver-Zwart IH, et al. 1990. Sulphasalazine versus hydroxychloroquine in rheumatoid arthritis: 3-year follow-up. *Lancet* **335**:539.

Van Os EC, Zins BJ, Sandborn WJ, et al. 1996. Azathioprine pharmacokinetics after intravenous oral delayed release oral and rectal foam administration. *Gut* **39**:63–8.

Vane JR. 1971. Inhibition of prostaglandin synthesis as a mechanism of action for aspirin-like drugs. *Nat New Biol* **231**:232–5.

Vane JR. 1995. NSAIDs, Cox-2 inhibitors, and the gut. *Lancet* **346**:1105–6.

Vesell ES. 1997. Therapeutic lessons from pharmacogenetics. *Ann Intern Med* **126**:653–5.

Walker JS, Sheather-Reid RB, Carmody JJ, et al. 1997. Nonsteroidal antiinflammatory drugs in rheumatoid arthritis and osteoarthritis: Support for the concept of "responders" and "nonresponders." *Arthritis Rheum* **40**:1944–54.

Walt RP. 1992. Misoprostol for the treatment of peptic ulcer and anti-inflammatory-drug-induced gastroduodenal ulceration. *N Engl J Med* **327**:1575–80.

Wasner C, Britton MC, Kraines RG, et al. 1981. Nonsteroidal anti-inflammatory agents in rheumatoid arthritis and ankylosing spondylitis. *JAMA* **246**:2168–72.

Weinblatt ME, Coblyn JS, Fox DA, et al. 1985. Efficacy of low-dose methotrexate in rheumatoid arthritis. *N Engl J Med* **312**:818–22.

Weinblatt ME, Coblyn JS, Fraser PA, et al. 1987. Cyclosporin A treatment of refractory rheumatoid arthritis. *Arthritis Rheum* **30**: 11–7.

Weinshilboum R. 1989. Methyltransferase pharmacogenetics. *Pharmacol Ther* **43**:77–90.

Weiser S, Cedraschi C. 1992. Psychosocial issues in the prevention of chronic low back pain—a literature review. *Bailliere's Clin Rheumatol* **6**:657–84.

West SG. 1997. Methotrexate hepatotoxicity. *Rheum Dis Clin North Am* **23**:883–915.

Wiegmann K, Schutze S, Machleidt T, et al. 1994. Functional dichotomy of neutral and acidic sphingomyelinases in tumour necrosis factor signaling. *Cell* **78**:1005–15.

Wigley FM, Wise RA, Seibold JR, et al. 1994. Intravenous iloprost infusion in patients with Raynaud phenomenon secondary to systemic sclerosis. A multicenter placebo-controlled double-blind study. *Ann Intern Med* **120**:199–206.

Williams HJ. 1988. Comparisons of sulfasalazine to gold and placebo in the treatment of rheumatoid arthritis. *J Rheumatol* **16**(Suppl): 9–13.

Williams HJ, Willkens RF, Samuelson CO Jr, et al. 1985. Comparison of low-dose oral pulse methotrexate and placebo in the treatment of rheumatoid arthritis. A controlled clinical trial. *Arthritis Rheum* **28**:721–30.

Williams KM, Lee EJD. 1985. Importance of drug enantiomers in clinical pharmacology. *Drugs* **30**:333–54.

Willis JV, Kendall MJ, Flinn RM, et al. 1979. The pharmacokinetics of diclofenac sodium following intravenous and oral administration. *Eur J Clin Pharmacol* **16**:405–10.

Willkens RF, Sharp JT, Stablein D, et al. 1995. Comparison of azathioprine methotrexate and the combination of the two in the treatment of rheumatoid arthritis. A forty-eight-week controlled clinical trial with radiologic outcome assessment. *Arthritis Rheum* **38**:1799–806.

Wolfe F. 1995. The epidemiology of drug treatment failure in rheumatoid arthritis. *Bailliere's Clin Rheumatol* **9**:619–32.

Wolfe F. 1997. Adverse drug reactions of DMARDs and DC-ARTs in rheumatoid arthritis. *Clin Exp Rheumatol* **15**:S75–81.

Wolfe F, Hawley DJ, Cathey MA. 1990. Termination of slow acting antirheumatic therapy in rheumatoid arthritis: A 14-year prospective evaluation of 1017 consecutive starts. *J Rheumatol* **17**:994–1002.

Wolfe F, Mitchell DM, Sibley JT, et al. 1994. The mortality of rheumatoid arthritis. *Arthritis Rheum* **37**:481–94.

Wynne HA, Long A. 1996. Patient awareness of the adverse effects of non-steroidal anti-inflammatory drugs (NSAIDs). *Br J Clin Pharmacol* **42**:253–6.

Yang JP, Merin JP, Nakano T, et al. 1995. Inhibition of the DNA-binding activity of NF-kappa B by gold compounds in vitro. *FEBS Lett* **361**:89–96.

Yates CR, Krynetski EY, Loennechen T, et al. 1997. Molecular diagnosis of thiopurine S-methyltransferase deficiency: Genetic basis for azathioprine and mercaptopurine intolerance. *Ann Intern Med* **126**:608–14.

Yee GC, Stanley DL, Pessa LJ, et al. 1995. Effect of grapefruit juice on blood cyclosporin concentration. *Lancet* **345**:955–6.

Yeomans ND, Tulassay Z, Juhasz L. 1998. A comparison of omeprazole with ranitidine for ulcers associated with nonsteroidal antiinflammatory drugs. Acid Suppression Trial: Ranitidine versus Omeprazole for NSAID-Associated Ulcer Treatment (ASTRONAUT) Study Group. *N Engl J Med* **338**:719–26.

Yocum DE. 1996. Cyclosporine FK-506: Rapamycin and other immunomodulators. *Rheum Dis Clin North Am* **22**:133–54.

Yocum DE, Klippel JH, Wilder RL, et al. 1988. Cyclosporin A in severe treatment-refractory rheumatoid arthritis. A randomized study. *Ann Intern Med* **109**:863–9.

Youssef PP, Haynes DR, Triantafillou S, et al. 1997. Effects of pulse methylprednisolone on inflammatory mediators in peripheral blood synovial fluid and synovial membrane in rheumatoid arthritis. *Arthritis Rheum* **40**:1400–8.

Youssef PP, Triantafillou S, Parker A, et al. 1996. Effects of pulse methylprednisolone on cell adhesion molecules in the synovial membrane in rheumatoid arthritis. Reduced E-selectin and intercellular adhesion molecule 1 expression. *Arthritis Rheum* **39**:1970–9.

Yy DT, Clements PJ, Peter JB, et al. 1974. Lymphocyte characteristics in rheumatic patients and the effect of azathioprine therapy. *Arthritis Rheum* **17**:37–45.

Zilko PJ. 1996. Polymyalgia rheumatica and giant cell arteritis. *Med J Aust* **165**:438–42.

Zimmerer J, Tittor W, Degen P. 1982. [Anti-rheumatic therapy in patients with liver diseases. Plasma levels of diclofenac and elimination of diclofenac and metabolites in urine of patients with liver disease.] *Fortschr Med* **100**:1683–8.

Zwillich SH, Comer SS, Lee E, et al. 1988. Treatment of the seronegative spondyloarthropathies with sulfasalazine. *J Rheumatol* **16**(Suppl):33–9.

# TREATMENT OF OSTEOPOROSIS

Robert Marcus

## *Chapter Outline*



Osteoporosis is a condition of low bone mass and disrupted skeletal microarchitecture that leads to fragile bones that fracture after minimal trauma. Common fracture sites include vertebral bodies, distal radius, and proximal femur, but porotic bone is diffusely fragile, and fractures throughout the skeleton are common. Osteoporosis is viewed to be of two broad categories, primary and secondary. Patients with secondary osteoporosis sustain bone loss because of systemic illness or medication use. Successful approach to the treatment of secondary osteoporosis requires prompt resolution of the underlying cause (for example, control of thyrotoxicosis). However, mechanisms of secondary osteoporosis all can be related in terms of disordered bone remodeling, so that the same therapeutic strategies may apply to those conditions as are appropriate for treatment of primary osteoporosis.

Primary osteoporosis has been divided by some authors into two types: type I osteoporosis, estrogen-dependent loss of trabecular bone at menopause; and type II osteoporosis, age-related loss of bone in men and women, reflecting long-term remodeling inefficiency, dietary inadequacy, and abnormal intestinal and renal function (Riggs et al. 1982). Compelling proof has not been presented that these two entities are truly separable. It has been assumed widely that osteoporosis must reflect excessive bone *loss*, but many patients have acquired less than usual bone during adolescence rather than undergoing excessive loss. Although many osteoporotic women have undoubtedly experienced substantial bone loss after menopause, it is preferable to consider osteoporosis the result of multiple physical, hormonal, and nutritional factors acting alone or in concert.

## SKELETAL ORGANIZATION AND REMODELING

The skeleton can be considered as two compartments, peripheral and central. The peripheral skeleton constitutes 80% of skeletal mass and is composed of compact plates of cortical bone organized about nutrient canals. The central, or axial skeleton, consists of trabecular bone contained within a thin cortical shell. Trabecular bone is a honeycomb of vertical and horizontal bars filled with red marrow and fat and is localized primarily in vertebral bodies, pelvis, and proximal femur. The increased surface area of trabecular bone accounts for the fact that changes in bone mass due to altered turnover are earlier and more impressive in the axial skeleton.

Bone remodeling is a continuous cycle of destruction and renewal that is carried out by individual, independent "bone remodeling units" (Fig. 10-13). Alterations in remodeling activity represent the final pathway through which diverse stimuli, such as dietary or hormonal insufficiency, affect the rate of bone loss. Remodeling begins on bone surfaces, when marrow precursor cells fuse to become multinucleated osteoclasts. These dig a cavity into the bone, which, in cortical bone, is a Haversian canal tunnel, and on trabecular surfaces is a scalloped area (Howship lacuna). Resorption leaves a cavity about 60 $\mu$m deep. Coupled to resorption, bone formation ensues when chemical mediators released from resorbed bone attract preosteoblasts into the resorption cavity. These mature into osteoblasts and secrete new collagen and matrix constituents that ultimately replace the missing bone. A complete remodeling cycle normally takes about 6 months. If replacement of resorbed bone were completely efficient, bone would be restored to its initial state on termination of a remodeling cycle. However, small bone deficits persist on completion of each cycle. The

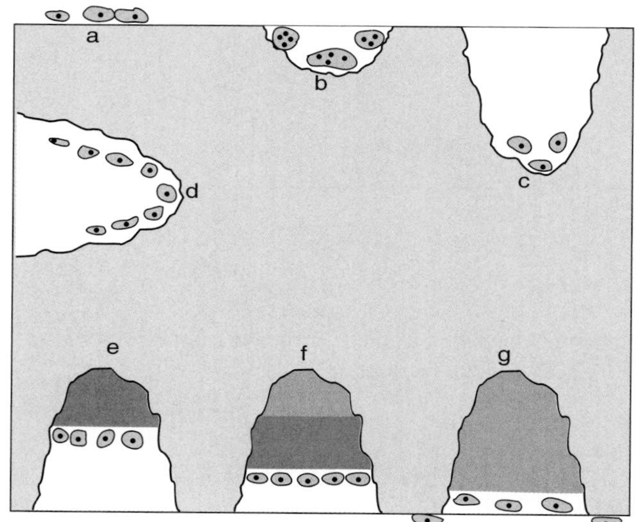


FIGURE 10-13 The bone remodeling cycle: (A) resting trabecular surface; (B) multinucleated osteoclasts dig a cavity of approximately 20 $\mu$m; (C) completion of resorption to 60 $\mu$m by mononuclear phagocytes; (D) recruitment of osteoblast precursors to the base of the resorption cavity; (E) secretion of new matrix by osteoblasts; (F) continued secretion of matrix, with initiation of calcification; and (G) completion of mineralization of new matrix. Bone has returned to quiescent state, but a small deficit in bone mass persists. (©1999 Robert Marcus, MD.)

consequence of this imbalance between resorption and formation is age-related bone loss, a normal phenomenon that is detected shortly after cessation of linear growth (Marcus 1987).

Bone density and fracture risk in later years are determined by the maximal bone mineral content at skeletal maturity (peak bone mass) and by subsequent rates of bone loss. Adolescent bone acquisition accounts for 60% of final adult levels. Peak bone mass is determined by genetic endowment and multiple environmental factors, such as physical activity, circulating estrogen and androgens, and diet.

Important regulators of bone mass during adult life are similar to those that affect bone acquisition in adolescence. In men and women, adult bone mass remains stable until about age 50, when progressive loss begins. Because of estrogen deficiency at menopause, women experience accelerated loss for several years, but subsequent rates of loss parallel those of men. Although the remainder of this chapter concerns pharmacologic management, all patients require an effective program of weight-bearing exercise and appropriate diet if therapy is to succeed.

**PRINCIPLE Pharmacologic therapy of chronic degenerative osteoporosis may be ineffective without "adjunctive" nonpharmacologic interventions.**

## GENERAL APPROACH TO OSTEOPOROSIS PREVENTION

A strategy to prevent bone loss follows from considerations outlined above. Regular physical activity of reasonable intensity is endorsed at all ages. Children and adolescents require adequate dietary calcium and vitamin D for optimal acquisition of peak bone mass. Attention to nutritional support may also be required in the seventh decade and beyond and might take the form of increased food calcium, or calcium and/or vitamin D supplementation.

For women at menopause, timely and sustained administration of estrogen is the most powerful intervention for preserving bone and minimizing fracture. Indeed, at any age, prevention or correction of hypogonadism is an important consideration. Details of hormone replacement therapy (HRT) are given below. Food and Drug Administration (FDA) approval has recently been granted to two different agents as alternatives for estrogen in osteoporosis prevention, raloxifene (Evista), a selective estrogen receptor modulator (SERM), and alendronate (Fosamax), a potent amino-bisphosphate. Both agents are discussed in detail below.

No therapy or combination of approaches can guarantee freedom from osteoporotic fracture. However, with appropriate lifelong attention to physical activity, nutritional state, and reproductive hormone status, important reductions in subsequent fracture risk can be achieved.

## PHARMACOLOGIC PREVENTION AND THERAPY OF OSTEOPOROSIS

Drugs available or under development for osteoporosis treatment fall into two groups. The first consists of agents that limit the rate of bone loss. These work by decreasing the rate of bone resorption and are called "antiresorptive" drugs. The second group consists of agents that promote bone formation. At present, FDA approval for this indication has been extended only to antiresorptive drugs (Table 10-21). Market forces driving the approval of these agents come largely from their application to women at or beyond menopause. To date, the attention of the phar-

**Table 10-21 Drugs Approved for Prevention or Treatment of Osteoporosis[a]**

| Drug | Indication | Daily Dose | Cost (AWP) (per month) |
|---|---|---|---|
| Calcium | OTC | 500–1500 mg | ~$3–12 |
| Vitamin D | OTC | 400–800 IU | <$2 |
| Estrogen | Prevention/ treatment | Conjugated estrogens 0.625 | $14[a] |
| | | Estrone sulfate 0.625/1.25 mg | $17–24 |
| | | Micronized estradiol 0.5–1.0 mg | $8–11 |
| | | Transdermal estradiol .05–.10 mg | $18–20 |
| SERMs | | | |
| Raloxifene | Prevention | 60 mg | $60[a] |
| Bisphosphonates | | | |
| —Alendronate | Prevention | 5 mg | $52 |
| | Treatment | 10 mg | $52 |
| Calcitonin | | | |
| Human (IM) | Treatment | 200 units (nasal spray) | $50[a] |
| Salmon (IM) | | 100 units (injectable) | $220–350 |

[a]Indications and doses are given only for FDA-approved uses as of March 1998. Dollar amounts reflect average wholesale drug prices for 30 days treatment, as reported in the *1997 Drug Topics Red Book*.
ABBREVIATIONS: OTC, over-the-counter sales, no prescription required; SERM, selective estrogen receptor modulator.

maceutical industry has been exclusively on the prevention and treatment of bone loss in postmenopausal women. Although small trials of these same agents in men with primary osteoporosis or in patients with secondary forms of osteoporosis indicate efficacy, adequate phase III clinical trials have not been reported in those settings. In the subsequent section, the term *established osteoporosis* refers to patients who have sustained at least one low-trauma fracture.

## Antiresorptive Agents

### *Calcium*

The use of calcium salts is properly considered a pharmacologic intervention, since mononutrient supplementation may produce effects that are not seen with dietary adjustments. The rationale for supplemental calcium differs with the time of life. For adolescents, adequate substrate calcium is necessary for bone accretion. Controlled trials of calcium in children and teens have clearly shown short-term improvement in bone mineral density (BMD), but whether this ultimately provides higher adult bone mass has not yet been shown.

Controversy surrounds the role of calcium during the early years after menopause. One frequently cited study claimed not to show efficacy of calcium administration, but the results actually indicated significant attenuation of cortical bone loss in calcium-treated women compared with a placebo group (Riis et al. 1987).

In the elderly, supplemental calcium reduces bone turnover and increases bone mass (Recker et al. 1977; Horowitz et al. 1984). Recent clinical trials indicate that administration of supplemental calcium to frail elders significantly decreases the incidence of fractures (Chapuy et al. 1992; Recker et al. 1996; Dawson-Hughes et al. 1997). Calcium supplementation, independent of other pharmacologic agents, should be an integral part of managing all patients with osteoporosis. A total daily calcium intake of 1500 mg is recommended for elderly men and women (NRC 1989).

Numerous calcium salts are available, the most frequently prescribed being the carbonate. Other preparations include lactate, gluconate, and citrate salts, as well as hydroxyapatite and powdered bone. Calcium citrate is more efficiently absorbed than other salts (Harvey et al. 1988), but the efficiency of absorption for most commonly prescribed calcium products is reasonable (Goddard et al. 1986; Sheikh et al. 1987), and the amount of calcium per pill is greater in high-dose calcium carbonate preparations, so the number of tablets required is less. For most patients, cost and palatability outweigh modest differences in absorption efficiency. The relative insolubility of calcium carbonate led to concern that individuals with poor gastric acidity will fail to absorb it, but Recker (1985) established that sufficient acidity is present in food to permit reasonable absorption even for achlorhydric patients.

Traditional dosing of calcium is about 1000 mg/day, nearly the amount present in a quart of milk. When added to the 400 to 500 mg of dietary calcium that typify the diet of elderly men and women, this provides a total daily intake of about 1500 mg. Heaney and Recker (1986) argued that more than this amount may be necessary to overcome endogenous intestinal calcium losses, but daily intakes of 2000 mg or more may be attended by constipation. Calcium supplements should be taken with meals.

### *Vitamin D*

The primary role of vitamin D is to increase the efficiency of intestinal calcium absorption. Vitamin D status is commonly marginal in elderly men and women (Omdahl et al. 1982; Chapuy et al. 1983). The mechanisms for this marginal status are multiple and include decreased exposure to sunlight, impaired cutaneous production of the vitamin, and inadequate renal production of calcitriol (1,25$(OH)_2$ vitamin D). Healthy, sunlight-replete men and women of all ages maintain blood 25-hydroxyvitamin D (calcifediol, 25-(OH)D) concentrations of 20 to 30 ng/ml. This metabolite is the most abundant circulating form of vitamin D and is the best overall reflection of vitamin D nutritional status. Levels below 8 ng/ml are associated with osteomalacia.

Intermediate values, 10 to 20 ng/ml, provide marginally adequate substrate for calcitriol production and promote compensatory hypersecretion of parathyroid hormone (PTH) to maintain blood calcium levels. Increased PTH supports calcium homeostasis at the expense of increased bone turnover and aggravated bone loss. The common occurrence of marginal vitamin D status in older men and women justifies a recommendation for a modest increase, perhaps to 1000 IU/day, in vitamin D intake for that population. In particular, frail elderly, individuals who live in northern latitudes, and nursing home residents would probably benefit from such a recommendation.

**PRINCIPLE Environmental variations may be determinants of dosage requirements that most often are neglected in advisories.**

Vitamin D is contained in many multivitamin preparations, usually in doses of 400 IU or less per tablet. Calcifediol (Calciferol) is also available by prescription. Gelatin capsules containing 400 IU vitamin D can be purchased at health food stores. In the United States, most bottled milk has been enriched in vitamin D with a nominal amount of 400 IU/quart, but the accuracy and consistency of milk supplementation has been challenged (Jacobus et al. 1992). Vitamin D is available as 50,000 IU capsules for intermittent use, such as once each week to once each month. At chronic doses exceeding 10,000 units/day, vitamin D leads to hypercalciuria and hypercalcemia. Doses of 50,000 to 100,000 IU/day are used to treat patients with hypo- and pseudo-hypoparathyroidism but are not indicated for treatment of osteoporosis.

**PRINCIPLE There are many instances in therapy where higher doses may produce a greater effect that becomes an adverse effect of the drug.**

### *Vitamin D metabolites*

Calcitriol and other polar vitamin D metabolites enjoy frequent use abroad, particularly Japan (Shiraki et al. 1985), but U.S. experience remains limited and mixed. Improved bone mass may be achieved at the cost of hypercalciuria and hypercalcemia (Aloia 1990; Gallagher and Goldgar 1990), necessitating close scrutiny and dose modifications. Vitamin D metabolites remain a promising avenue for future study, but their toxicity makes it premature to endorse them for widespread use.

### *Estrogen*

Various estrogen preparations have received FDA approval for both prevention and treatment of established osteoporosis. Estrogen suppresses bone resorption by regulating the maturation of osteoclast precursors and also the bone resorbing activity of mature osteoclasts. Substantial evidence establishes a major role for menopausal estrogen replacement in the conservation of bone mass and protection against fracture (Lindsay et al. 1976: Horsman et al. 1977; Recker et al. 1977; Nachtigall et al. 1979; Hutchinson et al. 1979; Lindsay et al. 1980; Weiss et al. 1980; Horsman et al. 1983; Civitelli et al. 1988a; Naessén et al. 1990). When estrogen is given as sole therapy, 0.625 mg/day of conjugated equine estrogens (Premarin) or its equivalent confer maintenance of BMD for approximately 95% of women (The Writing Group for the PEPI Trial 1996). Both oral and transdermal estrogen suppress bone turnover and conserve bone mass (Stevenson et al. 1990). The potential beneficial effects of estrogen on high-density lipoprotein (HDL) cholesterol are greater when oral estrogen is used, but in some women, metabolic features such as hypertriglyceridemia may make it advantageous to avoid the hepatic first-pass effect by administering transdermal estrogen.

Estrogen treatment for 5 years may be required to achieve protection against hip fracture (Weiss et al. 1980). Few if any of the clinical trials demonstrating the ability of estrogen to maintain BMD after menopause had adequate statistical power to demonstrate a reduction in rate of fractures. Thus, to date, most of the evidence supporting antifracture efficacy is epidemiologic in nature. However, the weight of evidence strongly indicates that women who take estrogen for 5 years or more will experience a reduction in risk for all fractures of about 60%. Cessation of estrogen leads rapidly to bone loss (Lindsay et al. 1978). Among women who had taken more than 10 years of postmenopausal estrogen, those still taking hormone replacement had a 75% decreased incidence in fractures during follow-up compared with women who had never received HRT. However, women whose total exposure to estrogen was identical to the "current users" but who had terminated treatment, showed no fracture protection compared with women who had never received HRT (Cauley et al. 1995).

Standard practice requires the cyclic or continuous administration of progestational drugs to women with an intact uterus, to reduce the risk of developing endometrial cancer. C-21 progestins (e.g., micronized progesterone or medroxyprogesterone acetate) do not diminish the beneficial skeletal effects of estrogen (The Writing Group for the PEPI Trial 1996). Certain 19-nortestosterone-derived progestins (e.g., norethindrone) may actually preserve or increase bone mass and provide added skeletal benefit when given with estrogen (Christiansen and Riis 1990). This effect reflects that norethindrone is itself a weak androgen and that it is transformed in the body to estrone.

The optimal time to institute estrogen replacement is in early menopause. The impact of initiating estrogen later on may be reduced, but skeletal benefit is achieved even where estrogen is prescribed for women in the seventh and eighth decades. For women without a uterus, therapy is continuous, relatively uncomplicated, and can be offered to women of any age. However, many women with an intact uterus will not accept cyclic bleeding or other anticipated or real side-effects of estrogen. Thus, initiation of estrogen therapy to elderly women, while rational, must be individualized.

From the foregoing, it can be seen that to achieve and maintain skeletal benefit, estrogen therapy, once initiated, must be very long-term, perhaps lifelong. Although discussion of the extraskeletal aspects of HRT is beyond the scope of this chapter, suffice it to say that a similar case can also be made for the importance of lifelong therapy to achieving cardiovascular benefits and reductions in total mortality (Grodstein et al. 1997). Such recommendations must be tempered by accounting for the potential adverse consequences of long-term HRT. These include the possibility, or even likelihood, of a 30% increase in breast cancer incidence (Colditz et al. 1995) as well as a small but real increase in risks for deep venous thrombosis and gall bladder disease. Thus, for an individual patient, adequate consideration must be given to her unique spectrum of cardiovascular, skeletal, breast, endometrial, and other health risks before a recommendation for or against HRT can be rationally made.

#### *Selective estrogen receptor modulators (SERMs)*

Despite its skeletal benefits, as well as those against coronary heart disease, estrogen has not been universally accepted by postmenopausal women. About one-third of women accept the recommendation to initiate estrogen, and of those who start HRT, 50% appear to have stopped medication 1 year later. Reasons given for stopping therapy include ongoing monthly vaginal bleeding and concerns about malignancy, particularly breast cancer. To meet this challenge, industry has begun to develop a series of compounds that act like estrogen on selected tissues but not on others. The first SERM to be developed was tamoxifen, which shows estrogen agonist activity on the liver, bone, and uterus, but is an antiestrogen in the breast and hypothalamus (Love et al. 1988; Turken et al. 1989). Another SERM, raloxifene (Evista), has estrogen agonist activities on liver and bone but does not stimulate the endometrium and antagonizes estrogen in the breast and brain (Delmas et al. 1998). Raloxifene (60 mg/day) is approved by the FDA for prevention of osteoporosis. Clinical trials of this drug for treatment of established osteoporosis are in progress.

#### *Calcitonin*

The peptide hormone calcitonin (CT) is a powerful inhibitor of osteoclastic bone resorption and modestly increases BMD in patients with osteoporosis (Gruber et al. 1984; Gonzales et al. 1986; Mazzuoli et al. 1986). Increases are most impressive (~15%) when the rate of bone turnover is high (Civitelli et al. 1988b). Because bone resorption and formation are coupled, CT eventually leads to a decrease in bone formation. Although CT clearly improves lumbar spine BMD, improvement elsewhere has been difficult to show, as has demonstration of antifracture benefit.

In the United States, salmon and human CTs are available for prescription. Both are given by injection, but a more convenient nasal spray form of salmon CT (Miacalcin), 200 IU/day, received FDA approval for treatment of osteoporosis. CT is not approved for prevention of osteoporosis, but patients requiring skeletal protection who are unable or unwilling to accept HRT and who cannot

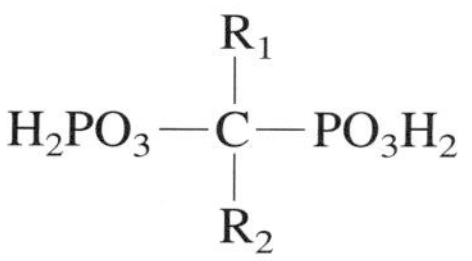

$$H_2PO_3-\underset{R_2}{\overset{R_1}{C}}-PO_3H_2 \qquad H_2PO_3-\underset{OH}{\overset{CH_3}{C}}-PO_3H_2$$

**Diphosphonate** 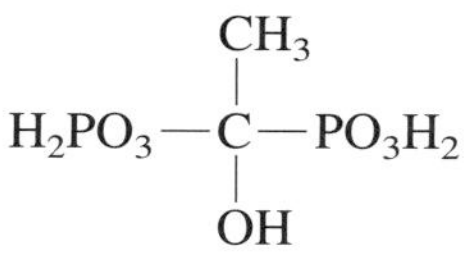 **Etidronate**

**FIGURE 10-14 Basic structure of bisphosphonates.**

tolerate bisphosphates may derive reasonable preservation of spine BMD from this agent (Reginster et al. 1987; MacIntyre et al. 1988).

***Bisphosphonates (geminal diphosphonates)***

These antiresorptive compounds, the bisphosphonates, have two phosphonic acid groups on the same carbon atom and mimic the structure of endogenous pyrophosphate. They differ from pyrophosphate in their resistance to hydrolysis by alkaline phosphatase. The general structure of bisphosphonates is shown in Fig. 10-14. In its simplest form the alkyl groups R1 and R2 are hydrogen. This agent, methylene diphosphonate, is widely used in technetium Tc 99m methylene diphosphonate scanning. Many bisphosphonates have been synthesized during the past 20 years. Those currently available in the United States are listed in Table 10-22.

Bisphosphonates have been used to treat Paget disease of bone for more than two decades. Early trials of these agents in osteoporosis involved etidronate, but only alendronate is currently approved by the FDA for treatment and prevention of osteoporosis. The mechanisms by which bisphosphonates inhibit bone resorption are not completely known. The drug is deposited on bone surfaces, and it is likely that osteoclasts ingest it during bone resorption, leading to profound inhibition of osteoclast function. This suppression of bone resorption makes bisphosphonates attractive for use in osteoporosis. However, for etidronate, another effect is inhibition of bone mineralization. Severe osteomalacia was observed in early trials where daily doses of 20 mg/kg were administered. Even at 5 to 10 mg/kg, focal osteomalacia is occasionally produced. Caution is therefore warranted in long-term use of etidronate. One attempt to avoid the mineralization defect involves intermittent drug administration. Two clinical trials (Storm et al. 1990; Watts et al. 1990) of intermittent etidronate (400 mg/day for 2 weeks, followed by 3 months without therapy) found that the drug increased bone mass over several years without evidence of osteomalacia and that these increases were associated with a reduction in vertebral fracture compared with the fracture rate in women assigned to placebo.

Interest in etidronate dissipated with the introduction of alendronate, an agent with a much higher ratio of antiresorptive to antimineralization potency, so that effective suppression of bone turnover occurs without risking osteomalacia. Given at 10 mg/day to elderly osteoporotic women, alendronate increased spine and hip BMD by 8% and ~3% over 3 years. In a very large clinical trial in women with existing vertebral fractures, alendronate lowered the incidence of single vertebral compression fractures by 50%, the incidence of multiple vertebral fractures by 90%, and, most important, the incidence of hip fracture by 50% (Black et al. 1996). Alendronate is currently ap-

**Table 10-22 Bisphosphonates Currently Approved in the United States[a]**

| AGENT | FDA APPROVED INDICATION | DAILY DOSE | DURATION |
|---|---|---|---|
| Technetium Tc 99m methylene diphosphonate | Skeletal imaging only | | Single use |
| Etidronate (Didronel) | Paget disease | 5 mg/kg | 6–12 months |
| | Osteoporosis[b] | 400 mg | Years |
| Alendronate (Fosamax) | Paget disease | 40 mg | 6–12 months |
| | Osteoporosis prevention | 5–10 mg | Years |
| | Osteoporosis treatment | 10 mg | Years |
| Pamidronate (injection) (Aredia) | Hypercalcemia of malignancy | 60–90 mg | As needed |
| | Paget disease | 60 mg/month | 4–6 months |
| Tiludronate (Skelid) | Paget disease | 400 mg | 6–12 months |
| Risedronate (Actonel) | Paget disease | 30 mg | 2 months |

[a]Indications and doses are given only for FDA approved uses as of April 1998.

[b]Although not approved by FDA for an osteoporosis indication, cyclic etidronate is occasionally administered to patients who cannot tolerate alendronate. Treatment is daily for 14 days every 3 months, with supplemental calcium alone during the intervening 76 days.

proved for osteoporosis treatment at 10 mg/day, whereas the approved prevention dose is 5 mg/day.

Absorption of oral bisphosphonates is poor. The drugs should be taken with a full glass of water following an overnight fast. Other liquids, such as coffee, tea, milk, or juices, substantially inhibit the absorption of bisphosphonates. If bisphosphonate residence in the stomach is prolonged, esophagitis may occur, even to a severe degree. Therefore, it is recommended that patients remain upright for at least 30 minutes following dosing. Taken as directed, alendronate-related esophageal complaints occur in fewer than 10% of patients.

Pamidronate (Aredia), another potent amino-bisphosphonate, has activity similar to that of alendronate and is approved for treatment of hypercalcemia of malignancy. Attempts to develop an oral form of pamidronate were unsuccessful because of severe esophagitis, so it is given by intravenous infusion, 60 to 90 mg over 4 hours. Patients with Paget disease or osteoporosis who cannot tolerate oral alendronate may respond to a series of monthly pamidronate infusions.

Although bisphosphonates constitute a major advance in therapeutics of osteoporosis, several important issues remain unresolved as of this writing. The optimal duration of therapy is not certain; long-term consequences of bisphosphonate administration are unclear; the impact of simultaneous use of bisphosphonate and HRT is not yet known; and their use in other than postmenopausal women (e.g., osteoporotic men, glucocorticoid-treated patients) has not been adequately studied. Clinical trials currently in progress should provide answers to these and other questions within a few years.

**PRINCIPLE It is far easier to demonstrate some efficacy of a drug in a chronic disease than to define its optimal use or its long-term effects.**

### *Thiazide diuretics*

Although not strictly antiresorptive, thiazides reduce urinary calcium excretion and help constrain bone loss in patients with hypercalciuria. Whether thiazides will prove useful in patients who are not hypercalciuric remains to be established, but recent epidemiologic data suggest that they provide significant protection against the risk for hip fracture (LaCroix et al. 1990).

## Bone-Forming Agents

### *Fluoride*

Sodium fluoride increases bone volume by increasing osteoblastic activity (Baylink et al. 1970; Briancon and Meunier 1981). In doses of 30 to 60 mg/day, fluoride increases spine BMD in many, but not all, patients. Fluoride may actually increase the risk for hip fracture (Hedlund and Gallagher 1989). Although fluoride increased spine BMD in two recent clinical trials, it did not confer protection against vertebral compression fracture in either one (Kleerekoper et al. 1989; Riggs et al. 1990). One study (Riggs et al. 1990) actually showed a significant increase in peripheral fractures with fluoride. These reports were criticized for using a very high fluoride dose (75 mg/day), and a trial in France (Mamelle et al. 1988) reported that 30 to 50 mg/day of sodium fluoride decreased fracture risk. However, the U.S. results clearly show that increased bone mass is not synonymous with improved bone strength and that if any dose of fluoride proves useful there is a fairly narrow therapeutic window.

Pak and colleagues (Pak et al. 1995) have reported antifracture efficacy (reduction in reported fractures) of a slow-release preparation of sodium fluoride. The critical feature of this agent is its pharmacokinetic profile, by which high and potentially toxic peak serum concentrations appear to be avoided. At present, slow-release fluoride has not received FDA approval.

**PRINCIPLE What may initially appear to be a logical surrogate endpoint for efficacy can turn out to be incorrect. This has happened so frequently that the FDA has become very cautious about accepting any surrogate endpoint for assessing drug efficacy.**

### *Androgens*

Testosterone deficiency is a major etiologic factor for osteoporosis in men, and replacement therapy significantly increases bone mass in such patients. Chronically administered, androgens improve bone mass in osteoporotic women, but therapy has been limited by the virilizing side-effects of the drugs. Norethindrone acetate (a progestin with androgenic properties, 5 mg/day with estrogen), and Nandrolone decanoate (an anabolic steroid with androgenic properties, 50 mg injection every 3 weeks) both increase bone mass with few bothersome side-effects in osteoporotic women (Need et al. 1989). Adequate data on the incidence of fracture are not yet available, so it is impossible to make a judgment on the therapeutic role for this therapy. However, in view of their potential benefits to muscle, as well as bone, in addition to their potential deleterious effects on lipoprotein metabolism and circulating HDL and LDL cholesterol, androgens clearly deserve additional careful study.

***Parathyroid hormone***

An anabolic effect of parathyroid hormone (PTH) on trabecular bone can be produced by intermittent administration of the hormone. PTH and its synthetic analogs increase axial bone mineral in patients with osteoporosis (Slovik et al. 1986; Reeve et al. 1990), although effects on cortical bone are disappointing. It seems likely that PTH will require concomitant administration of an antiresorptive drug to minimize loss of cortical bone (Lindsay et al. 1997). Phase III osteoporosis treatment trials using PTH are currently in progress.

## Nonpharmacologic Considerations

A number of hygienic measures may be of use in reducing the risk of fracture for osteoporotic patients. Proper instruction in lifting technique may reduce strain on the spine. Proper footwear and installation of safety features around the home may minimize the risk of falling. Such features include bathroom safety rails and night-lights, rails and lighting for stairways, and elimination of floor clutter and loose or slippery floor rugs. In most counties, home safety inspections by public health nurses can easily be arranged.

## REFERENCES


Aloia JF. 1990. Role of calcitriol in the treatment of postmenopausal osteoporosis. *Metabolism* **39**(Suppl):35–38.

Baylink DJ, Wergedal JE, Stauffer M, et al. 1970. Effect of fluoride on bone formation, mineralization, and resorption in the rat. In: Vischer TL, ed. *Fluoride and Medicine*. Bern: Hans Huber, pp 37–69.

Black D, Cummings SR, Karpf DB, et al. 1996. Alendronate reduces the risk of fractures in women with existing vertebral fractures: results of the Fracture Intervention Trial. The Fracture Intervention Trial Research Group. *Lancet* **348**:1535–1541.

Briancon D, Meunier PJ. 1981. Treatment of osteoporosis with fluoride, calcium and vitamin D. *Orthop Clin North Am* **12**:629–640.

Cauley JA, Seeley DG, Enstrud K, et al. 1995. Estrogen replacement therapy and fractures in older women. The Study of Osteoporotic Fractures Research Group. *Ann Intern Med* **122**:9–16.

Chapuy M-C, Arlot ME, Duboeuf F, et al. 1992. Vitamin $D_3$ and calcium to prevent hip fractures in elderly women. *N Engl J Med* **327**:1637–1642.

Chapuy M-C, Durr F, Chapuy P. 1983. Age-related changes in parathyroid hormone and 25 hydroxycholecalciferol levels. *J Gerontol* **38**:19–22.

Christiansen C, Riis BJ. 1990. 17$\beta$-Estradiol and continuous norethisterone: A unique treatment for established osteoporosis in elderly women. *J Clin Endocrinol Metab* **71**:836–841.

Civitelli R, Agnusdei D, Nardi P, et al. 1988a. Effects of one year treatment with estrogens on bone mass, intestinal calcium absorption, and 25-hydroxyvitamin D-1$\alpha$ hydroxylase reserve in postmenopausal osteoporosis. *Calcif Tissue Int* **42**:77–86.

Civitelli R, Gonnelli S, Zacchei F, et al. 1988b. Bone turnover in postmenopausal osteoporosis. Effect of calcitonin treatment. *J Clin Invest* **82**:1268–1274.

Colditz GA, Hankinson SE, Hunter DJ, et al. 1995. The use of estrogens and progestins and the risk of breast cancer in postmenopausal women. *N Engl J Med* **332**:1589–1593.

Dawson-Hughes B, Harris SS, Krall EA, et al. 1997. Effect of calcium and vitamin D supplementation on bone density in men and women 65 years of age or older. *N Engl J Med* **337**:670–676.

Delmas PD, Bjarnason NH, Mitlak BH, et al. 1998. Effects of raloxifene on bone mineral density, serum cholesterol concentrations, and uterine endometrium in postmenopausal women. *N Engl J Med* **337**:1641–1647

*1997 Drug Topics Red Book.*

Gallagher JC, Goldgar D. 1990. Treatment of postmenopausal osteoporosis with high doses of synthetic calcitriol. A randomized controlled study. *Ann Intern Med* **113**:649–655.

Goddard M, Young G, Marcus R. 1986. Short-term effects of calcium carbonate, lactate, and gluconate on the calcium-parathyroid axis in normal elderly men and women. *Am J Clin Nutr* **44**:653–658.

Gonzales D, Ghiringhelli G, Mautalen C. 1986. Acute antiosteoclastic effect of salmon calcitonin in osteoporotic women. *Calcif Tissue Int* **38**:71–75.

Grodstein F, Stampfer MJ, Colditz GA, et al. 1997. Postmenopausal hormone therapy and mortality. *N Engl J Med* **336**:1769–1775.

Gruber HE, Ivey JL, Baylink DJ, et al. 1984. Long-term calcitonin therapy in postmenopausal osteoporosis. *Metabolism* **33**:295–303.

Harvey JA, Zobitz MM, Pak CYC. 1988. Dose dependency of calcium absorption: A comparison of calcium carbonate and calcium citrate. *J Bone Miner Res* **3**:253–258.

Heaney RP, Recker RR. 1986. Distribution of calcium absorption in middle-aged women. *Am J Clin Nutr* **43**:299–305.

Hedlund LR, Gallagher JC. 1989. Increased incidence of hip fracture in osteoporotic women treated with sodium fluoride. *J Bone Miner Res* **4**:223–225.

Horowitz M, Need AG, Philcox JC, et al. 1984. Effect of calcium supplementation on urinary hydroxyproline in osteoporotic postmenopausal women. *Am J Clin Nutr* **39**:857–859.

Horsman A, Gallagher JC, Simpson M, et al. 1977. Prospective trial of oestrogen and calcium in postmenopausal women. *Br Med J* **2**:789–792.

Horsman A, Jones M, Francis R, et al. 1983. The effect of estrogen dose on postmenopausal bone loss. *N Engl J Med* **309**:1405–1407.

Hutchinson TA, Polansky SM, Feinstein AR. 1979. Post-menopausal oestrogens protect against fractures of hip and distal radius. A case-control study. *Lancet* **2**:705–709.

Jacobus CH, Holick MF, Shao Q, et al. 1992. Hypervitaminosis D associated with drinking milk. *N Engl J Med* **326**:1173–1177.

Kleerekoper M, Peterson E, Phillips E, et al. 1989. Continuous sodium fluoride therapy does not reduce vertebral fracture rate in postmenopausal osteoporosis [abstract]. *J Bone Miner Res* **4**(Suppl 1):S376.

LaCroix AZ, Wienpahl J, White LR, et al. 1990. Thiazide diuretic agents and the incidence of hip fracture. *N Engl J Med* **322**:286–290.

Lindsay R, Aitkin JM, Anderson JB, et al. 1976. Long-term prevention of postmenopausal osteoporosis by estrogen. Evidence for an increased bone mass after delayed onset of estrogen treatment. *Lancet* **1**:1038–1041.

Lindsay R, Hart DM, Forrest C, et al. 1980. Prevention of spinal osteoporosis in oophorectomised women. *Lancet* **2**:1151–1153.

Lindsay R, Hart DM, MacLean A. 1978. Bone response to termination of oestrogen treatment. *Lancet* **1**:1325–1327.

Lindsay R, Nieves J, Formica C, et al. 1997. Randomised controlled study of effect of parathyroid hormone on vertebral-bone mass and fracture incidence among postmenopausal women on oestrogen with osteoporosis. *Lancet* **350**:550–555.

Love R, Mazess R, Tormey D, et al. 1988. Bone mineral density in women with breast cancer treated with adjuvant tamoxifen for at least two years. *Breast Cancer Res Treat* **12**:297–301.

MacIntyre I, Stevenson JC, Whitehead MI, et al. 1988. Calcitonin for prevention of postmenopausal bone loss. *Lancet* **1**:900–901.

Mamelle N, Meunier PJ, Dusan R, et al. 1988. Risk-benefit ratio of sodium fluoride treatment in primary vertebral osteoporosis. *Lancet* **2**:361–365.

Marcus R. 1987. Normal and abnormal bone remodeling in man. *Annu Rev Med* **38**:129–141.

Mazzuoli GF, Passeri M, Gennari C, et al. 1986. Effects of salmon calcitonin in postmenopausal osteoporosis: A controlled double-blind study. *Calcif Tissue Int* **38**:3–8.

Nachtigall LE, Nachtigall RH, Nachtigall RD, et al. 1979. Estrogen replacement therapy I: A 10-year prospective study in the relationship to osteoporosis. *Obstet Gynecol* **53**:277–281.

Naessén T, Persson I, Adami H-O, et al. 1990. Hormone replacement therapy and the risk for first hip fracture. *Ann Intern Med* **113**:95–103.

Need AG, Horowitz M, Bridges A, et al. 1989. Effects of nandrolone decanoate and antiresorptive therapy on vertebral density in osteoporotic postmenopausal women. *Arch Intern Med* **149**:57–60.

[NRC] National Research Council. 1989. *Recommended Dietary Allowances*, 10th ed. Washington DC: National Academy Press, pp 174–184.

Omdahl JL, Garry PJ, Hunsaker LA, et al. 1982. Nutritional status in a healthy elderly population: vitamin D. *Am J Clin Nutr* **36**:1225–1233.

Pak CYC, Sakhaee K, Adams-Huet B, et al. 1995. Treatment of postmenopausal osteoporosis with slow-release sodium fluoride. *Ann Int Med* **123**:401–408.

Recker RR, Hinders S, Davies KM, et al. 1996. Correcting calcium nutritional deficiency prevents spine fractures in elderly women. *J Bone Miner Res* **11**:1961–1966.

Recker RR. 1985. Calcium absorption and achlorhydria. *N Engl J Med* **313**:70–73.

Recker RR, Saville PD, Heaney RP. 1977. Effect of estrogens and calcium carbonate on bone loss in postmenopausal women. *Ann Intern Med* **87**:649–655.

Reeve J, Davies UM, Hesp R, et al. 1990. Treatment of osteoporosis with human parathyroid peptide and observations on effect of sodium fluoride. *BMJ* **301**:314–318.

Reginster JY, Denis D, Albert A, et al. 1987. One-year controlled randomised trial of prevention of early postmenopausal bone loss by intranasal calcitonin. *Lancet* **2**:1481–1483.

Riggs BL, Hodgson S, O'Fallon WM, et al. 1990. Effect of fluoride treatment on the fracture rate in postmenopausal women with osteoporosis. *N Engl J Med* **322**:802–809.

Riggs BL, Wahner HW, Seeman E, et al. 1982. Changes in bone mineral density of the proximal femur and spine with aging. Differences between the postmenopausal and senile osteoporosis syndromes. *J Clin Invest* **70**:716–723.

Riis B, Thomsen K, Christianssen C. 1987. Does calcium supplementation prevent postmenopausal bone loss? A double-blind, controlled clinical study. *N Engl J Med* **316**:173–177.

Sheikh MS, Santa Ana CA, Nicar MJ, et al. 1987. Gastrointestinal absorption of calcium from milk and calcium salts. *N Engl J Med* **317**:532–536.

Shiraki M, Orimo H, Ito H, et al. 1985. Long-term treatment of postmenopausal osteoporosis with active vitamin D3, 1-alpha-hydroxycholecalciferol ($1\alpha OHD_3$) and 1,24-dihydroxycholecalciferol ($1{,}24(OH)_2D_3$). *Endocrinol Jpn* **32**:305–315.

Slovik DM, Rosenthal DI, Doppelt SH, et al. 1986. Restoration of spinal bone in osteoporotic men by treatment with human parathyroid hormone. (1-34) and 1,25-dihydroxyvitamin D. *J Bone Miner Res* **1**:377–381.

Stevenson JC, Cust MP, Gangar KF, et al. 1990. Effects of transdermal versus oral hormone replacement therapy on bone density in spine and proximal femur in postmenopausal women. *Lancet* **2**:265–269.

Storm T, Thamsborg G, Steiniche T, et al. 1990. Effect of cyclical etidronate therapy on bone mass and fracture rate in women with postmenopausal osteoporosis. *N Engl J Med* **322**:1265–1271.

The Writing Group for the PEPI Trial. 1996. Effects of hormone therapy on bone mineral density. Results from the Postmenopausal Estrogen/Progestin Interventions (PEPI) Trial. *JAMA* **276**:1389–1396.

Turken S, Siris E, Seldin D, et al. 1989. Effects of tamoxifen on spinal bone density in women with breast cancer. *J Natl Cancer Inst* **81**:1086–1088.

Watts NB, Harris ST, Genant HK, et al. 1990. Intermittent cyclical etidronate treatment of postmenopausal osteoporosis. *N Engl J Med* **323**:73–79.

Weiss NS, Ure CL, Ballard JH, et al. 1980. Decreased risk of fractures of the hip and lower forearm with postmenopausal use of estrogen. *N Engl J Med* **303**:1195–1198.

C H A P T E R

# 11 DERMATOLOGIC DISORDERS

Christopher M. Barnard, Marc E. Goldyne

*Chapter Outline*



Discussions about the therapy for cutaneous diseases are often introduced by citing the skin's role as a supportive interface between humans' external and internal milieu and as a barrier to potentially harmful agents in the environment. Because our knowledge regarding therapeutically relevant details of the skin's complex organization and functions are relatively limited, we must often satisfy ourselves with such introductory statements. Unfortunately, on a pharmacologic level, such statements are meaningless unless the barrier properties of the skin or the pathophysiologic events that lead to skin disease can be described in a way that assists therapeutic decisions. If the physician challenges the clichés regarding dermatologic therapy and attempts to understand how the skin may be interacting not only with the external milieu but with the internal milieu as well, he or she may begin to appreciate the need for actively thinking about the therapy for dermatologic diseases.

The fact that most dermatologic disorders are not life-threatening (but often significantly debilitating) should not lessen a physician's responsibility for having to make as correct a therapeutic decision as is currently possible. A lapse in this responsibility is exemplified by a fungal infection that is clinically misdiagnosed as eczema and inappropriately (and also ineffectually) treated with costly topical steroids and systemic antibiotics because of failure to perform a simple skin scraping and microscopic inspection for fungal hyphae. The risks of less-than-thorough evaluation of simple dermatologic problems apply when problems become more complex. In the specific case of identifying a malignant melanoma, for example, inappropriate evaluation or advising "let's watch it for a while" could cost a patient his or her life. Furthermore, when knowledge of the science of dermatology stops, the need to practice the art of medicine is as essential as ever. If the therapy causes more problems than the disease, the physician is not practicing good medicine. The message sounds self-evident, but ensuring its implementation can be challenging.

The drugs and the therapeutic principles reviewed in this chapter focus on five common dermatologic diagnoses for which a large number of drug prescriptions are written. In addition, a section is included on malignant melanoma, because it is the most consequential of skin cancers and its incidence continues to increase. The five other diagnoses addressed in this chapter are acne, eczema, impetigo, psoriasis, and drug-induced skin reactions. In the context of each diagnosis, relevant principles of dermatologic therapy are presented. To associate these principles with specific diseases may aid the clinician by putting them in context. In addition, Table 11-1 lists, in alphabetical order, the drugs that are mentioned in the text along with the dermatologic diseases for which they may be indicated and their relative costs.

## ACNE

### Pathogenesis of Acne

The specific genotype that permits the development of the disease called "acne" is unknown. The fact that acne provides a spectrum of clinical presentations suggests a com-

Table 11-1 **Drugs for Dermatologic Disorders and Their Relative Costs**

| MEDICATION | APPLICATION | INDICATION | RELATIVE COST PER MONTH |
|---|---|---|---|
| Adapalene | Topical | Acne | $$$ |
| Anthralin | Topical | Psoriasis | $$ |
| Azelaic acid | Topical | Acne | $$$ |
| Benzoyl peroxide | Topical | Acne | $ |
| Calcipotriene | Topical | Psoriasis | $$$$ |
| Clindamycin | Topical | Acne | $$ |
| Clobetasol propionate | Topical | Psoriasis, eczema | $$$ |
| Coal tar (crude) | Topical | Psoriasis | $ |
| Cyclosporine | Oral | Psoriasis | $$$$ |
| Dicloxacillin sodium | Oral | Impetigo | $$ |
| Erythromycin | Topical | Acne | $$ |
| Ethinyl estradiol/norgestimate | Oral | Acne | $$$ |
| Etretinate/acitretin | Oral | Psoriasis | $$$$ |
| Fluocinonide | Topical | Psoriasis, eczema | $$ |
| Hydroxyurea | Oral | Psoriasis | $$ |
| Isotretinoin | Oral | Acne | $$$$ |
| Methotrexate sodium | Oral | Psoriasis | $ |
| Methoxsalen + UVA (PUVA) | Oral | Psoriasis | $$ |
| Minocycline HCl | Oral | Acne | $$$ |
| Mupirocin | Topical | Impetigo | $$ |
| Tazarotene | Topical | Psoriasis | $$$$ |
| Tetracycline | Oral | Acne | $ |
| Tretinoin | Topical | Acne | $$$ |
| Triamcinolone | Topical | Psoriasis, eczema | $ |
| UVB | Topical | Psoriasis | $$ |

ABBREVIATIONS: UVA, ultraviolet A; UVB, ultraviolet B.

bination of endogenous and exogenous determinants. Nevertheless, knowledge of some of the factors that appear to contribute to each clinical presentation helps justify choosing a specific therapeutic protocol.

Acne is a disease of the pilosebaceous follicle. The interaction of three conditions appears essential to the evolution of acne: 1) altered keratinization of the infundibulum of the pilosebaceous duct (Knutson 1974; Plewig 1974), 2) overproduction of sebum by the sebaceous glands (Pochi and Strauss 1964), and 3) proliferation of the anaerobic diphtheroid *Propionibacterium acnes* within retained sebum (Leyden et al. 1975). Androgen excess or sebaceous gland hypersensitivity to normal androgen levels may be a fourth condition that contributes to the development of acne in certain individuals (Lucky et al. 1997). Follicular hyperkeratosis may be enhanced by androgens as well (Pochi 1991). Altered keratinization and desquamation of the ductal epithelium lead to impaction of the pilosebaceous duct with a mixture of sebum and keratin. The combination of ductal plugging and increased generation of sebum leads to distension of the follicular duct, which can be appreciated microscopically as a microcomedo. As the microcomedo expands, it forms either an open comedo (blackhead) if the follicular orifice dilates or a closed comedo if the orifice remains microscopic. The factors favoring the formation of closed versus open comedones are not known. The closed comedo has particular clinical significance because the escape channel for sebum is totally blocked. This condition sets the stage for inflammation.

Within the closed comedo, the lipid-rich sebum provides an ideal growth medium for the proliferation of *P. acnes,* an anaerobic diphtheroid normally found within the pilosebaceous duct. Data show that the lipase activity of *P. acnes* converts triglycerides in sebum to free fatty acids as well as free glycerol, which may function as a growth substrate for the bacteria (Rebello and Hawk 1978). The fatty acids themselves are comedogenic in animal models and may contribute to the chemotactic activity of sebum; they may also possess cytotoxic activity (Shalita 1974; Tucker et al. 1980).

The inflammation in acne is associated with the rupture of the closed comedo because of the continued secretion of sebum with resultant thinning of the follicular epithelium and because of release by *P. acnes* of low-molecular-weight chemotactic factors that diffuse through the thinned follicular wall and attract neutrophils that migrate through the follicular epithelium, ingest the *P. acnes,* and simultaneously release hydrolytic enzymes that attack the follicular epithelium, causing it to rupture (Webster et al. 1979a; Leyden and Webster 1980).

When the contents of the ruptured comedo enter the dermis, various inflammatory signals are triggered. Activation of the classic and alternate complement pathways by *P. acnes* leads to complement-derived (e.g., C5a) chemotactic factor generation (Webster et al. 1979b), and a foreign body response is generated by comedonal contents (Dalziel et al. 1984). Increased plasma total androgens in both men and women have been implicated in the stimulation of sebaceous gland production of sebum, and the fact that acne runs an inflammatory gamut from mild pustular comedones to large, multilocular, disfiguring cysts supports differences in individual host response to the factors so far described.

**PRINCIPLE The genotypic reasons for host differences are as yet unknown. However, the factors already implicated in the pathogenesis of acne provide a rational basis for current therapy.**

## Therapy for Acne

The treatment of acne is guided by knowledge of the factors contributing to the clinical presentation. The therapy can be divided into noninflammatory and inflammatory categories.

***Noninflammatory acne***

If noninflamed comedones, open or closed, constitute the majority of lesions, the abnormal keratinization and desquamation of the pilosebaceous orifice is the causative factor on which to focus. Therapy should accordingly be aimed at normalizing the altered keratinization and desquamation process. The drugs that appear to accomplish this best are topical tretinoin (Kligman et al. 1969) and a new topical retinoidlike compound, adapalene (Caron et al. 1997; Clucas et al. 1997).

Topical tretinoin (retinoic acid) is the acid form of vitamin A (retinol). It is applied as a cream (0.025, 0.05, and 0.1%), a gel (0.01 and 0.025%), a microsphere gel (0.1%), or a 0.05% solution to the affected skin once per day. Application is recommended at bedtime, since some animal data suggest that retinoic acid may enhance the tumorigenic potential of sunlight (Olsen 1982). Less than 10% of topically applied tretinoin is absorbed into the circulation, and it is metabolized in the liver and excreted in bile and in urine. The therapeutic efficacy of tretinoin as a comedolytic agent stems from its ability to decrease the cohesiveness of the follicular epithelium and to accelerate epithelial cell turnover (Wolff et al. 1975). These actions allow eventual expulsion of comedonal contents and prevention of new microcomedo formation.

Optimal treatment with tretinoin requires that the patient be informed about the potential side effects of therapy as well as the time frame in which the patient can expect to see improvement. A frequent cause of treatment failure is an uninformed patient who, experiencing some cutaneous irritation, stops therapy because of the fear that an allergic reaction to the medication has occurred or because 48 hours of therapy have not produced any improvement. Both these frequent compliance problems can be prevented by a physician's stressing the following points:

- Skin irritation may occur following initiation of tretinoin therapy; if this occurs, application should be stopped for 48 hours and then initiated again (alternatives are to lower the concentration of tretinoin, to change the vehicle—cream has the least potential for irritation—or to try initial alternate-day therapy).
- Exacerbation of lesions may occur during the first 2 to 3 weeks of therapy; this should not serve as an indication to stop application of tretinoin.
- Six to 12 weeks of therapy are required before maximal benefit and, therefore, clinical efficacy can be determined (Olsen 1982).
- Use of a sunscreen is strongly encouraged if prolonged exposure to ultraviolet light is contemplated, since tretinoin, at least in animal studies, appears to enhance the tumorigenic potential of ultraviolet light.

Another more recently introduced alternative is to switch to the microsize gel that incorporates the Microsponge technology (microscopic porous beads that entrap the active substance and serve as a carrier for delivery), thereby eliminating the irritation associated with organic solvents (Fedors 1997).

A new topical compound derived from naphthoic acid, adapalene gel 0.1%, which has the ability to bind specifically to retinoic acid nuclear receptors, is a less irritating alternative to topical tretinoin according to comparison studies with tretinoin gel 0.025% (Caron et al. 1997; Clucas et al. 1997). The proposed mechanism of action of adapalene is the normalization of follicular epithelial cell differentiation with a reduction on microcomedone formation (PDR 1998). Results from a study comparing the efficacy of adapalene 0.1% gel to retinoic acid 0.025% gel at 12 weeks reveal significantly better improvement in reducing both inflammatory and noninflammatory acne lesions with less irritation. No clinically significant hematologic, blood chemistry, or urinalysis abnormalities have been seen during treatment with adapalene (Shalita et al. 1996).

A patient must be told, repeatedly if necessary, that the aim of acne therapy is to control the disease; a cure, even with oral isotretinoin (to be described), cannot be guaranteed, but excellent control can be achieved with proper therapy and compliance.

**PRINCIPLE Inappropriate patient expectations can sabotage compliance with therapy and can preclude the possibility of a beneficial clinical response. The physician's obligations to the patient in this regard become obvious.**

### *Inflammatory acne*

The presence of inflammatory papules, pustules, and cysts should suggest not only that follicular plugging is present but also that the bacterial contribution to acne must be treated. This may be accomplished with a variety of topical or systemic antibiotics that are capable of controlling the proliferation of *P. acnes* and therefore the *P. acnes*-induced inflammatory stimuli reviewed above. The most frequently used agents include topical benzoyl peroxide, topical erythromycin or clindamycin, and systemic tetracycline or erythromycin.

Topical benzoyl peroxide is bactericidal for *P. acnes* as well as being mildly comedolytic (Burke et al. 1983). Its mechanism of action has not been established, whereas its clinical efficacy has been confirmed. When applied to the skin as a 2.5, 5, or 10% lotion, cream, or gel, less than 5% of the dose is absorbed through the skin over 8 hours (Nacht et al. 1981). Within the skin, it is completely metabolized to benzoic acid that enters the circulation as benzoate and is excreted by the kidneys unchanged (Yeong et al. 1983). Available data suggest that the drug is safe to use in pregnancy (Pochi and Rothman 1988). Because benzoyl peroxide can be potentially irritating, therapy should begin with the lowest concentration applied once daily to the affected areas of skin and progression to higher concentrations made if some therapeutic benefit is perceived.

Combining the use of topical tretinoin at night with the morning application of benzoyl peroxide can provide the benefits of both: the more potent comedolytic properties of the first agent and the antibacterial effects of the second agent. It is important to inform patients that when using both topical agents, the drugs should not be applied at the same time because the benzoyl peroxide will oxidatively inactivate the tretinoin (Hurwitz 1979). Benzoyl peroxide may induce allergic contact dermatitis after several weeks of use in up to 2.5% of patients (Haustein et al. 1985).

**PRINCIPLE The efficacy of combination drug regimens may depend crucially on timing and sequencing. While acne may not be life-threatening, cancers are, and the proper sequencing of drug therapy can make the difference between life and death.**

Topical clindamycin phosphate and erythromycin base are the two most frequently employed antibiotics for topical use in the treatment of mild acne when inflammatory papules and pustules, but not cysts, are the predominant lesions. Whereas topical benzoyl peroxide is bactericidal, clindamycin and erythromycin are bacteriostatic, functioning as competitive inhibitors of ribosomal protein synthesis. Use of these antibiotics is indicated when a patient cannot tolerate benzoyl peroxide because of irritation or contact allergy; they appear to be equally effective and are applied twice daily to all areas where acne lesions exist or where they have the potential to erupt (Shalita et al. 1984). The topical antibiotics are generally well tolerated with the major side effects being vehicle-related dryness and irritation. Because topical erythromycin and clindamycin are bacteriostatic, their use may result in development of resistant strains (Eady et al. 1989). Clinically this is suggested by the patient's complaint that an initial beneficial response to topical erythromycin or clindamycin is not continuing. In response to topical clindamycin there have been several cases of pseudomembranous colitis reported; however, this complication is rare (Milstone et al. 1981; Parry and Rha 1986). Nevertheless, any patient developing diarrhea while using topical clindamycin should be advised to stop treatment. Combination benzoyl peroxide 5% and erythromycin 3% gel has a more beneficial effect than topical erythromycin alone, with significant reduction of erythromycin-resistant, coagulase-negative staphylococcal and propionibacterial strains and shows significant clinical improvement in both inflammatory and comedonal acne lesions (Eady et al. 1996; Chu et al. 1997).

Azelaic acid is a naturally occurring compound that possesses anti-inflammatory, antibacterial, and antikeratizing properties and is well tolerated. For comparison,

20% azelaic acid cream has the same efficacy as benzoyl peroxide 5%, erythromycin 2%, or tretinoin 0.05% when used alone but is significantly more beneficial when combined with oral minocycline. Azelaic acid appears to maintain therapeutic benefit after discontinuation of the oral antibiotic (Graupe et al. 1996).

**PRINCIPLE Although we are accustomed to considering the skin as a barrier to the environment, we should not lose sight of the fact that many substances applied at high concentrations for prolonged periods will reach the systemic circulation. Expect systemic effects of topically applied drugs.**

If inflammatory lesions are the major clinical finding and an 8-week trial of a topical antibiotic, applied twice daily, fails to provide clinical improvement, systemic antibiotics should be considered.

Tetracycline hydrochloride and erythromycin base are the most frequently employed systemic antibiotics for acne. Studies show that both drugs significantly decrease bacterial counts of *P. acnes* and the levels of skin-surface free fatty acids (Strauss and Pochi 1966; Akers et al. 1975). In a controlled trial with 200 patients, both antibiotics have proved equally effective in treating papulopustular acne (Gammon et al. 1986). However, closed comedo counts did decrease more rapidly in patients treated with tetracycline. The initial quantity of antibiotic should be at least 1 g daily divided into either two or four doses. In more severe inflammatory acne, the benefit of doses of tetracycline >1 g daily (e.g., 2 g/day) has been documented (Baer et al. 1976). Other oral antibiotics such as minocycline (50 mg taken twice daily) have also shown efficacy in treating inflammatory acne, but because of higher cost, minocycline is often reserved for cases refractory to therapy with tetracycline or erythromycin.

**PRINCIPLE It is avoiding reality to believe that the cost of a prescription is not a factor in compliance and the eventual outcome of a therapeutic regimen.**

As with topical antibiotics, judgment of the clinical efficacy of systemic antibiotics should not be made until an 8-week treatment program has been completed. A major cause of apparent treatment failure is the physician's failure to inform the patient with acne that maximum improvement will not be seen for approximately 6 to 8 weeks. The anxious patient, expecting a 24-hour cure, stops the drug after a few days because improvement is not evident and then at a follow-up visit or, more likely, a visit to a new physician, the frustrated patient reports that systemic antibiotics failed to help and thereby eliminates an efficacious drug from further consideration. This problem can be avoided by proper instruction to the patient.

**PRINCIPLE When a physician is told that a particular therapy has failed, it is crucial to make sure that it was indeed the drug and not some other factor that caused the failure.**

If an adequate period of therapy does result in improvement, consideration can be given to decreasing the dose of systemic antibiotic to no less than 500 mg/day as long as improvement is maintained. It is essential to understand that it is not solely the antibiotic properties of these drugs that appear to provide therapeutic efficacy; for example, the oral antibiotics mentioned also appear to inhibit leukocyte chemotaxis and inhibit bacterial lipase activity without significantly affecting bacterial colony counts (Shalita and Wheatly 1970; Cunliffe et al. 1973; Esterly et al. 1978).

The inevitable question asked by the patient with acne is how long oral antibiotic therapy needs to be continued. Once therapeutic benefit is documented, the goal of subsequent therapy is to switch from a systemic to a topical antibiotic. The topical preparation should be introduced while the patient is still taking the minimum dose of the systemic antibiotic required for control of the acne. Then the systemic antibiotic can be withdrawn after a week's overlap to see whether topical therapy will suffice to maintain control. Other schedules can be tried with the ultimate criterion for change being the clinical response of the patient.

A concern often raised by physicians is how long one can safely maintain systemic antibiotic therapy. Studies have shown that treatment of acne with tetracycline for 3 to 4 years in otherwise healthy patients has not led to major morbidity from resistant organisms or opportunistic infections (Bjornberg and Roupe 1972; Akers et al. 1975; Gould and Cunliffe 1978; Adams et al. 1985).

The major side effect of systemic antibiotic therapy is modification of the GI flora; in roughly 5% of patients, this may lead to colic and/or diarrhea (Gould and Cunliffe 1978; Adams et al. 1985). In women, candida vaginitis may occur infrequently (Bjornberg and Roupe 1972; Gammon et al. 1986). Several cases of gram-negative folliculitis that resembled pustular acne but were unresponsive to continuing tetracycline therapy have also been documented (Fulton et al. 1968). There have also been several cases of benign intracranial hypertension reported in patients using oral tetracycline (Walters and Gubbay 1981).

**PRINCIPLE Maintain awareness of situations where a given drug can induce the very response it was designed to treat (e.g., infections in response to antibiotics, seizures in response to anticonvulsants, hypertension by antihypertensives, and arrhythmias by antiarrhythmic drugs).**

In regard to treating acne in pregnant women, tetracycline therapy is definitely contraindicated because of its association with maternal hepatic toxicity as well as with staining of deciduous teeth and with cataract formation in the developing fetus (Rothman and Pochi 1988).

In patients with severe nodulocystic acne involving the face and back, in patients with less severe inflammatory acne who have not responded to adequate therapeutic trials of the drugs heretofore discussed, or in patients suffering from significant dysmorphophobia in regard to their acne, systemic isotretinoin (13-*cis*-retinoic acid) therapy is the treatment of choice (Jones 1989). This derivative of vitamin A acid is well absorbed, is virtually totally protein-bound, and is excreted by both the kidneys and GI tract. Its elimination half-life is 10 to 20 hours. The majority of responding patients receive between 1 and 2 mg/kg of body weight per day b.i.d. over a period of 15 to 20 weeks. The remarkable effectiveness of isotretinoin (sold under the name Accutane) appears to stem from its influence on all the major etiologic factors associated with acne: 1) sebum secretion is reduced by 90% at 4 weeks (Jones et al. 1983), 2) pilosebaceous ductal cornification is normalized (Cunliffe et al. 1985), 3) microbial colonization of the skin is significantly reduced (King et al. 1982), and 4) inflammation is decreased (Camisa et al. 1982).

The major concern with isotretinoin therapy is its teratogenic potential in pregnant women (Lammer et al. 1985). Of 154 women inadvertently exposed to isotretinoin during the first trimester of pregnancy, 95 pregnancies ended in elective abortion and 12 ended in spontaneous abortion. Whereas 26 infants were born without major malformations noted at birth, 21 infants were born with major anomalies involving craniofacial structures, the heart, and the thymus. Therefore, isotretinoin must not be given to women of childbearing age unless the physician establishes by serum pregnancy testing that the female patient 1) is not pregnant before initiating therapy, 2) is using an effective form of birth control during therapy and for 1 month following cessation of therapy, and 3) understands the risks to a fetus should she become pregnant during therapy.

**PRINCIPLE We should be learning a lot about human nature when, in spite of the known toxicity of a highly efficacious drug, laxity in ensuring patient protection almost forced the FDA to remove this drug from the market. Consider the analogies with thalidomide.**

Other relatively common effects of isotretinoin therapy include dryness of the skin and mucous membranes (the latter sometimes leading to epistaxis) and elevation of serum triglyceride and high-density lipoprotein (HDL) concentrations. Hepatic transaminase concentrations in plasma are temporarily elevated in approximately 20% of patients taking isotretinoin. They return to normal despite continued therapy (DiGiovanna and Peck 1987). Less commonly seen are thinning of hair, muscle and joint pains, headache, corneal opacities, pseudotumor cerebri, inflammatory bowel disease, and anorexia. These problems are all reversible on discontinuation of therapy. Note that in the rare patient whose serum triglyceride concentrations increase to around 800 mg/dL, isotretinoin therapy should be stopped, because in such cases, acute hemorrhagic pancreatitis as well as eruptive xanthomas have been reported (Shalita et al. 1983). Consequently, pretreatment evaluation of liver function and of plasma lipid concentrations should be obtained, and then periodically reevaluated during the 15 to 20 weeks of therapy, and 2 weeks following cessation of therapy, to document normalization. In selected patients, a second course of therapy may be considered if, several weeks following an initial course, acne lesions begin to appear. The same precautions are indicated during retreatment. Need for retreatment appears to correlate with the use of less than a 1 g/kg dosage for initial therapy. Nevertheless, lower dosages are sometimes justified because an individual may find the adverse effects of the optimum dose too uncomfortable.

Women with elevated androgen levels or heightened sebaceous gland sensitivity to androgens may benefit from the use of oral estrogen preparations such as the triphasic, combination oral contraceptive (norgestimate-ethinyl estradiol) for treatment of acne (Lucky et al. 1997). Improvement in acne is significantly correlated with the normalization of biochemical hyperandrogenism as the free testosterone level falls and the sex hormone–binding globulin level increases during treatment (Mango et al. 1996; Redmond et al. 1997).

**PRINCIPLE Identification of, and directed therapeutic intervention for, the underlying processes that appear to be dominant in any given case of acne constitute the most expedient and effective approach to managing this disease.**

## ECZEMA

Eczema (derived from the Greek word *ekzein,* to boil out) is not a disease but a manifestation of a variety of skin diseases. Therefore, if the physician makes a diagnosis of eczema, he or she must still determine its underlying cause. The identification of the cause is the key to rational therapy.

Acute eczema presents either as a localized or as a more generalized condition, the severity of which may depend on the cause. The skin develops patches of erythema, papulation, and vesiculation with oozing of serous fluid, and crusting. Chronic eczema exhibits features of erythema, scaling, thickening of the skin with prominence of skin lines (lichenification), and hyper- or hypopigmentation. Vesiculation, weeping, and oozing are not features of chronic eczema.

### Pathogenesis of Eczema

Eczema is found most often in association with atopy, allergic contact dermatitis, or chemical and physical irritation of the skin. The common thread that appears to explain the clinically similar cutaneous manifestations of these different diseases is the disruption of the barrier function of the stratum corneum of the epidermis. Normally the lipid composition of this region serves to control transepidermal water loss (Elias and Finegold 1988). By excoriating the skin in response to the pruritus and/or inflammation induced by underlying disease, the patient disrupts the lipid barrier, leading to an increase in transepidermal water loss (to be differentiated from eccrine sweating). Through a yet-to-be-delineated mechanism, the abnormal transepidermal water loss lowers the threshold for pruritus, with the resultant initiation of an itch-scratch cycle.

#### *Atopy*

*Atopy* is the name applied to a symptom complex that may include asthma, hay fever, and eczema associated with the findings of elevated serum concentrations of the immunoglobulin IgE (80% of patients), suppressed in vitro mitogenic response of peripheral blood T cells, exaggerated leukocyte cyclic adenosine 3′,5′-cyclic phosphate (cAMP) responses to established stimuli, significantly increased incidence of skin colonization with *Staphylococcus aureus,* and increased susceptibility to cutaneous infections with herpes and vaccinia viruses (Leyden et al. 1974; Aly et al. 1977; Parker et al. 1977).

The eczema associated with atopy appears to result from the physical excoriation of the skin in response to the characteristically severe pruritus that is associated with the disease. The eczema appears in characteristic localizations from infancy (face, scalp, and extensor surfaces) through childhood (flexural folds of arms, legs, feet, and wrists, plus the skin of the eyelids and of the back and sides of the neck) to adulthood (more generalized to face, scalp, chest, neck, extremities, hands, and feet).

#### *Allergic contact eczema*

This form of eczema results from a delayed hypersensitivity reaction (cell-mediated or type IV hypersensitivity) to a low-molecular-weight (<1000) sensitizing agent that comes into contact with the skin (Roitt et al. 1985). The inciting molecules (haptens), which must be fat-soluble to traverse the stratum corneum of a susceptible patient, must become covalently or noncovalently bound to normal epidermal proteins to serve as antigenic determinants (epitopes) capable of eliciting T-cell recognition specific for the hapten-protein conjugate. Of central importance to this response is the epidermal Langerhans cell that serves as the Ia-bearing, antigen-presenting cell (Wolff and Stingl 1983). In contrast to tuberculin-type hypersensitivity that is primarily dermal in location, contact hypersensitivity is primarily epidermal.

The papulovesicles initially developing at sites of antigen contact most probably result from the T cell–mediated cytotoxicity and consequent edema occurring within the epidermis. The pruritus associated with this reactivity invites excoriation of the involved skin, leading to the clinical picture of acute eczema. Table 11-2 lists the most frequently implicated allergens encountered and their sources. Occasionally, a hapten will only become sensitizing following alteration by ultraviolet light; this type of reaction is suggested by a "photodistribution" of the eczema.

#### *Chemical and physical irritant eczema*

Occupational or recreational exposure to various solvents or detergents, or repeated hand washing, can alter the lipid

Table 11-2 **Allergic Contact Eczema Frequent Offenders**

| HAPTEN | SOURCES |
|---|---|
| Urushiol (pentadecylcatechol) | Poison oak, ivy, sumac oleoresin |
| *p*-Phenylenediamine | Hair dyes |
| Nickel | Earrings, necklaces, watchbands, zippers, metal buttons, coins |
| Ethylenediamine | Stabilizer in some topical corticosteroid creams; hardener for epoxy resins; may get drug eruption from aminophylline and ethylenediamine-related antihistamines |
| Dichromates | Leather dyes, preservatives, cement |
| Tetramethylthiuram monosulfide, mercaptobenzothiazole | Rubber materials |
| Neomycin sulfate | Topical antibiotic |
| Benzocaine | Topical anesthetic |
| Balsam Peru | Scented cosmetics; some suppositories |
| Parabens | Preservatives for some topical medicament creams |

barrier of the epidermis leading to both enhanced transepidermal water loss and enhanced penetration of potentially irritating substances. When this involves the hands, the induced pruritus and scratching in addition to continued contact with the offending agents can result in the generation of acute and chronic eczema commonly referred to as "hand" or "housewife's eczema." When other areas of skin are involved, both acute and chronic round (coin-shaped) patches of eczema can occur; this clinical presentation has been labeled *nummular* eczema from the Latin *numisma,* meaning coin. Some people develop a habit tic that involves the repeated excoriation of one skin site because of a perceived local pruritus that can be precipitated and propagated by stress. The resultant eczema, which is clinically distinct only because of its singular location, is referred to as localized neurodermatitis; this chronic lesion that often shows lichenification as a prominent feature is referred to as *lichen simplex chronicus.*

A unique form of hand and foot eczema that appears to be induced by stress in susceptible persons begins as an eruption of grouped tiny pruritic vesicles that have the appearance of tapioca kernels and erupt along the lateral margins of the fingers, and the thenar eminences. In more severe cases it can also involve the soles of the feet and the toes. Scratching of these pruritic vesicles leads to a clinical picture of acute eczema that with time may take on the features of chronic eczema. This condition has been given the name dyshidrotic eczema or pompholyx because of the misconception that the vesicles are the result of trapped eccrine sweat. The actual cause of the vesicles is unclear.

*Xerotic eczema* is the term used for eczema arising from pruritus-induced excoriation of dry skin. This disease is most frequently seen in elderly persons who, because of a presumed decline in surface lipids, demonstrate clinically dry skin due to increased transepidermal water loss. The episodes of eczema increase during the winter months (hence the term *winter eczema* is sometimes used) because of the increased drying of the skin that results from the drop in indoor humidity because of increased use of heating. The episodes of itching usually occur more frequently at night after clothing that has maintained higher local humidity of the covered skin is removed exposing the skin to a much lower humidity level. Combining this condition with hot soapy showers or baths that further delipidize the skin leads to increased dryness, concomitant pruritus, and excoriation. The result is a patient presenting with acute and chronic eczema who provides a history of increasingly itchy skin primarily involving the extremities that is more symptomatic at night.

## Therapy for Eczema

Therapy for eczema has to be approached from three aspects: suppression of inflammation, eradication of superinfection if present, and suppression and prevention of pruritus. The third aspect is conceptually the most important and most challenging to accomplish because if the physician does not achieve control of the pruritus, the patient will continue to scratch; the scratching will generate the eczema as the skin's response to repeated excoriation; and, in the case of atopic eczema, superinfection of the eczematized skin will more than likely occur.

***Suppression of inflammation***

Localized eczema that shows the acute signs of weeping, oozing, and crusting initially requires drying and debridement, since the serous fluid and epidermal debris can foster bacterial proliferation and, especially in atopic patients, infection with *S. aureus*. The first steps must be accomplished along with more specific anti-inflammatory therapy.

Drying of acute eczema is actually achieved through the application of water to the affected skin. By removing occlusive crusts and proteinaceous debris, as well as by delipidizing keratin, endogenous transepidermal water loss can be further enhanced at sites of eczema. The effect is drying. For localized eczema this is best achieved with cool or tepid tap water compresses with clean, closely woven cotton cloth (old bed sheets or T-shirts) for 20 to 30 minutes twice to three times a day. The use of dilute aluminum acetate solution (e.g., Domeboro powder or tablets dissolved in water) for use in compresses is a more effective astringent, and it also provides bacteriostasis. For more generalized eczema, drying of weeping lesions can be accomplished by tepid water baths to which can be added an oilated colloid (e.g., oilated oatmeal [Aveeno]). Once the weeping and oozing of acute eczema have been controlled, the physician needs to consider more specific suppression of inflammation.

The efficacy of topical corticosteroids in suppressing cutaneous inflammation is undisputed. The mechanism(s) involved have yet to be definitively established. Data show that corticosteroids 1) stabilize and prevent lysosomal enzyme release (Frichot and Zelickson 1972), 2) inhibit the synthesis of inflammatory mediators like prostaglandins and leukotrienes (eicosanoids) by inhibiting prostaglandin synthase type II, 3) deplete skin mast cells (Lavker and Schecter 1985), and 4) prevent intravascular margination of neutrophils and therefore their diapedesis into inflammatory sites (Allison et al. 1955).

The decisions that must be made by the physician in regard to topical corticosteroid therapy in eczema as well as in other topical steroid-responsive skin diseases are the potency of corticosteroid to use, the appropriate vehicle to use, the frequency of use, and the duration of treatment. By convention, the potency of various topical corticosteroid preparations (over 100 available) has been expressed in terms of relative capacity to constrict the dermal vessels of normal skin under given test conditions (Tan et al. 1986; Stoughton and Cornell 1987). Although there are inherent weaknesses in this system, it has provided acceptable correlation with clinical potency (Cornell and Stoughton 1985; Shah et al. 1989).

**PRINCIPLE Standardization of drugs by bioassay may not necessarily provide direct correlation with clinical potency.**

Table 11-3 lists some representative corticosteroids in the different potency categories along with average wholesale prices as listed in Medi-Span™ January 1999. The more recently introduced superpotent steroids (clobetasol propionate, betamethasone dipropionate, and diflurasone diacetate) are more than 1000 times more potent than hydrocortisone (Stoughton and Cornell 1987).

In treating eczema, the question of which potency of corticosteroid to use should be related to the extent and relative responsiveness to steroid of the particular form of eczema. For example, a localized plaque of neurodermatitis (lichen simplex chronicus), localized hand eczema, or localized allergic contact eczema could be most efficaciously treated with a superpotent topical corticosteroid, because the area of skin that is involved requires far less than the recommended upper limit of 50 g/week for therapy. Furthermore, the more potent the steroid in this setting, the more rapid should be the resolution. However, a patient with atopic dermatitis or xerotic eczema scattered over the arms and legs (roughly 54% of the adult body surface) requires roughly 30 g/day (see Fig. 11-1) of a steroid preparation. The wholesale cost to the pharmacist (not the patient) would amount to approximately $20 per day for a superpotent steroid versus approximately $4 per day for a generic intermediate-strength steroid such as triamcinolone acetonide.

**PRINCIPLE Consider the total surface area of treated skin and its severity of inflammation as an area of easily penetrated, leading to potential absorption of drug into the systemic circulation.**

Because of the more generalized nature of atopic dermatitis or xerotic eczema, use of the more potent steroid preparations can rapidly produce systemic concentrations that would significantly suppress pituitary–adrenal axis function. For example, studies using a superpotent topical corticosteroid showed that covering at least 30% of the body surface of adults with psoriasis or atopic dermatitis with 0.5% clobetasol dipropionate cream or ointment for one week resulted in depressed morning cortisol concentrations ($<5$ $\mu$g/dL) in 75% of patients receiving 7 g/day, 22% of patients receiving 3.5 g/day, and 11% of patients receiving 2 g/day (Olsen and Cornell 1986). Thus, some patients receiving the recommended maximum weekly dosage of 50 g/week demonstrated pituitary–adrenal axis suppression. However, it should also be noted that in all studies so far conducted, return of morning plasma cortisol concentrations to within normal limits occurred within 2 to 7 days. Nevertheless, it is important to re-

**Table 11-3 Topical Corticosteroids: Relative Potencies and Costs**

| | Cost (AWP) | | | |
|---|---|---|---|---|
| **Drug** | **Cream** | **Ointment** | **Lotion (Sol'n)** | **Gel** |
| *Low Potency* | | | | |
| Alclometasone dipropionate (Aclovate) | \$12.95 | \$12.95 | | |
| Hydrocortisone 2.5% (Hytone) | | \$23.46[a] | \$35.00[b] | |
| Desonide | | | | |
| (Desowen) | \$12.45 | \$12.45 | | |
| (Tridesilon) | \$15.88[c] | \$15.88[c] | | |
| *Medium Potency* | | | | |
| Fluticasone propionate (Cutivate) | \$14.34[d] | \$14.34[d] | | |
| Mometasone furoate (Elocon) | \$18.61[e] | \$18.61[e] | \$20.17[f] | |
| Hydrocortisone valerate 0.2% (Westcort) | \$14.59[g] | \$14.59[g] | | |
| Triamcinolone acetate 0.1% (Kenalog) | \$13.74[h] | \$13.73[h] | \$43.21[b] | |
| Prednicarbate 0.1%[i] (Dermatop) | \$14.10[h] | \$14.10[h] | | |
| *High Potency* | | | | |
| Clobetasol propionate (Temovate) | \$23.46 | \$23.46 | \$26.86[j] | \$23.46 |
| Augmented betamethasone dipropionate (Diprolene AF) | \$29.03 | \$29.03 | \$33.30[k] | \$29.03 |
| Diflorasone diacetate (Psorcon) | \$26.50 | \$31.63 | | |
| Halobetasol propionate (Ultravate) | \$23.82 | \$23.82 | | |
| Betamethasone dipropionate (Diprosone) | \$25.09 | \$25.09 | \$30.88[l] | |
| Fluocinonide (Lidex) | \$21.55 | \$21.55 | \$24.50[l] | \$21.55 |

NOTE: Prices listed are for 15-g tube unless otherwise indicated. Note that 30 g of a topical steroid is enough to cover the entire body once. Average wholesale prices (AWPs) are as listed in Medi-Span January 1999. Current prices may vary from those quoted, but comparative prices among products are expected to be similar. The reader should check on local prices at the time of prescribing.
[a]30 g. [b]60 mL. [c]Price depends on brand. [d] Daily dosing. [e]Dosing every day up to twice a day. [f]30 mL. [g]Dosing bid. [h]Dosing tid. [i]Limited to 3-week maximum use. [j]25 mL. [k]30 mL. [l]20 mL.
ABBREVIATIONS: sol'n, solution.

member that for a given period of application, the greater the surface area to be treated, the greater the probability for pituitary–adrenal axis suppression to occur with any topical corticosteroid.

It is helpful to remember, in a practical context, that the recommended use of superpotent topical steroids is for a maximum of 50 g/week of a 0.05% preparation (cream or ointment) for not longer than 2 weeks. Also, because of inherent regional variations in absorption of topically applied corticosteroids through the skin, certain sites (scrotal skin, facial skin, intertriginous skin) are more susceptible to beneficial therapy with lower-strength preparations than sites such as the palm or sole. Furthermore, eczematized skin or psoriatic skin even though clinically and histologically thicker shows enhanced penetration of topically applied corticosteroids.

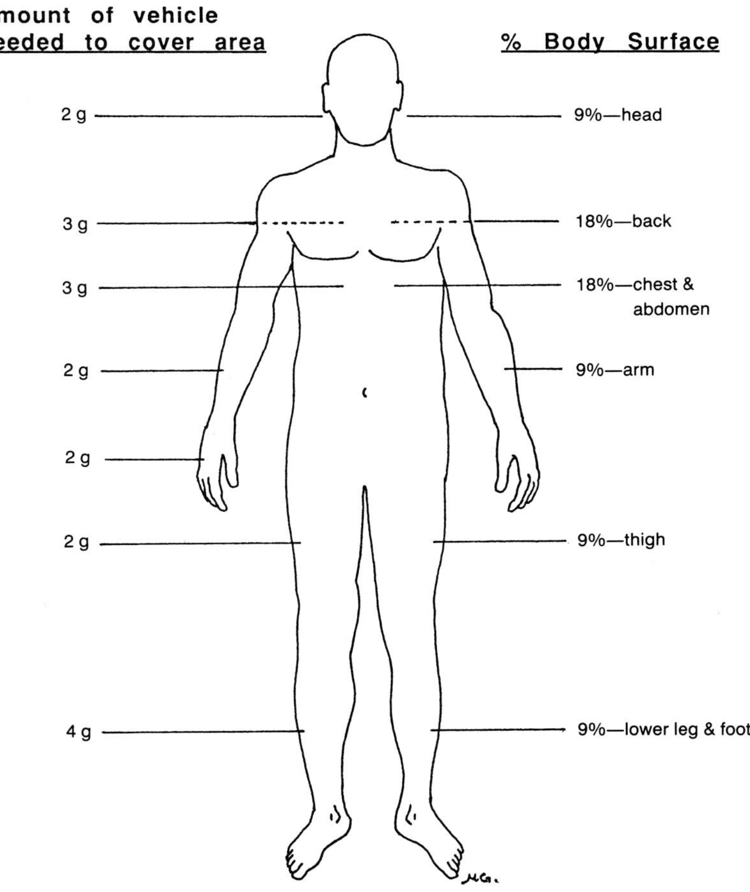


**FIGURE 11-1 Application of topical corticosteroids. Whole-body coverage requires approximately 30 to 60 g of cream or ointment or 120 mL of lotion per application.**

> **PRINCIPLE The fact that skin shows regional changes in anatomy, and therefore in drug absorptive properties, has been considered in the development of transdermal drug delivery systems. Be aware of this when such systems are used.**

In the specific case of allergic contact dermatitis, the discomfort produced by the acute eczematous response to widespread contact with an allergen (e.g., poison oak's oleoresin) may require systemic therapy with oral prednisone, especially if facial edema is present and pronounced. Systemic therapy in this case must be initiated by a high enough dose of prednisone (at least 60 to 80 mg/day single morning dose) and tapered over 21 days to avoid flare-up of the skin lesions when a shorter course of systemic therapy is followed. For more localized cases of allergic contact dermatitis, the superpotent topicals appear to be the most beneficial.

Several principles can guide the physician who is deciding on an appropriate vehicle for treating eczema: 1) use a cream or lotion on acute eczema, because the water base of the cream or lotion will not prevent the desired dehydration of weeping, oozing lesions, 2) use a cream on intertriginous skin because the apposition of skin surfaces in intertriginous areas already provides sufficient occlusion, and 3) use an ointment on very dry and thick eczema, since, by maximally hydrating the skin, it not only enhances penetration of the corticosteroid, but it helps alleviate the xerosis and accompanying pruritus.

The frequency of application of any topical steroid should not exceed three times per day. Most important, if the patient with eczema complains after a week of steroid therapy that his or her skin is still itchy and dry, the physician should not interpret this situation as an indication for more frequent use of a topical steroid or for a more potent steroid. Instead, the physician should increase the frequency of application of an appropriate emollient to increase hydration of the skin. This approach is supported by studies showing that applying a corticosteroid six times per day was not clinically more efficacious than a three-times-per-day schedule (Eaglestein et al. 1974). Furthermore, a study in monkeys by Wester et al. (1977) showed that a single application of [$^{14}$C]hydrocortisone (13.3 $\mu$g/cm$^2$) in acetone to a fixed area on the ventral surface of the forearm produced the same total percent absorption (based on radioactivity applied and recovered in the urine) as did three applications of this same dose to the same site at 6-hour intervals. However when 40 $\mu$g/cm$^2$ was applied, a substantial increase in percent absorption was seen compared to either the single or triple application of 13.3 $\mu$g/cm$^2$. These data suggest that there may be local effects induced by the initial application of a corticosteroid that significantly affect the absorption kinetics of a subsequent application to the same area if done within a specific time. In fact, acute tachyphylaxis to the vasoconstrictive and antimitotic effects of topically applied corticosteroids has been documented, which abates after 96 drug-free hours (de Vivier 1976). Consequently, in the patient with eczema, a single application of a topical steroid with adequately repeated application of an appropriate emollient may, in some instances, be as efficacious as use of the corticosteroid two or three times per day.

**PRINCIPLE Careful observation often reveals that more drug may not be needed or advantageous. Consider the case of continuous administration of nitroglycerin, or $\beta$-adrenergic agonists, and increasing doses and duration of administration of antibiotics, antiarrhythmics, phenothiazines, and tricyclic antidepressants. The example with corticosteroids illustrates how important it is to have a strategy to quantify the effects of therapy rather than simply "sitting back" and expecting a cure.**

Once the potency of, and vehicle for, the corticosteroid to be used has been determined, the physician is faced with the question of how long a given potency can be safely used before unwanted side effects occur (e.g., pituitary–adrenal axis suppression, skin atrophy, striae, steroid acne, allergic contact dermatitis to the corticosteroid itself [Reitamo et al. 1986]). This question cannot be answered easily because absorption and bioavailability of different preparations vary depending on the vehicle used, the absorption characteristics of different skin sites, and disease-related alterations in skin barrier function, all of which can significantly affect absorption of the drug (Jackson et al. 1989). Some studies indicate that outpatients treated for chronic skin disease over several years with daily application of potent fluorinated steroids showed little or no evidence of suppression of the pituitary–adrenal axis when occlusion therapy was avoided (occlusion of skin with impermeable plastic wrap can increase cutaneous absorption 10-fold) (Munro and Clift 1973; Wilson et al. 1973). However more recent studies on topical halcinonide, desoximetasone, and betamethasone valerate have documented depression of endogenous cortisol secretion (Cornell and Stoughton 1981). Furthermore, skin atrophy, the result of epidermal thinning, is evident histologically after one week of occlusive therapy with a potent fluorinated steroid ointment (Kirby and Monroe 1976). Since occlusion may enhance steroid penetration 10-fold, one might expect several weeks of nonocclusive topical therapy with a potent fluorinated steroid to be permissible. Consequently, one principle to be followed by the physician using potent or superpotent steroids in a patient for longer than 2 weeks is appropriate follow-up to document by inspection and appropriate laboratory work the absence of noticeable skin atrophy, steroid acne, or striae, as well as suppression of the pituitary–adrenal axis. Signs of skin atrophy, if found, often disappear within 6 months following discontinuation of the topical corticosteroid.

***Eradication of superinfection***

In eczema associated with atopy, there is both a higher-than-normal carriage rate and high lesional counts of *S. aureus* (Leyden et al. 1974; Aly et al. 1977). More recent studies have also documented increased colonization of nonatopic hand eczema with *S. aureus*. The reasons for altered bacterial flora in the forms of eczema studied are not well understood. Normal skin has efficient defense mechanisms that seem to discourage foreign organisms from colonizing. These mechanisms include desiccation, the antibacterial effect of certain skin-surface fatty acids, surface pH, and the presence of a resident microflora (Noble 1981). However, these mechanisms may be disturbed in eczema. For example, IgG and fibronectin may be present in the exudate associated with acute eczema, and the protein A in the cell wall of *S. aureus* has a high affinity for IgG and fibronectin (Ryden et al. 1983). Thus staphylococcal colonization could be propagated by these interactions.

For the physician confronting acute eczema, especially in the atopic patient, an important question is whether the lesions are not only pruritic but painful or tender. These latter two symptoms may signify superinfection of eczema even in the absence of frank pustulation. Under these circumstances empiric systemic antibiotic therapy should be considered part of the required therapy for the eczema. Many dermatologists initially treat all cases of acute atopic eczema with a 10-day course of erythromycin or a semisynthetic penicillinase-resistant penicillin (e.g., dicloxacillin). Culturing the lesions is encouraged only if an appropriate course of empirical therapy is ineffective, since initial culture of the lesions almost always grows out *S. aureus*. It should also be remembered that the presence of punched-out erosions at sites of eczema in atopic patients should raise the possibility of herpes simplex infection, and appropriate therapy (acyclovir) should be instituted based on viral culture.

The anti-inflammatory and immunosuppressive effects of corticosteroids sometimes become a theoretical cause for concern in treating eczema colonized with *S. aureus*. However, studies have shown that the application of superpotent clobetasol propionate to hand eczema in both atopic and nonatopic patients caused a significant reduction or complete elimination of *S. aureus* in association with eliminating the eczematous skin changes (Nilsson et al. 1986). The reasons for these findings have yet to be found. Thus, in acute nonatopic eczema, the use of bacteriostatic compresses (e.g., aluminum acetate) plus a potent topical steroid cream may be sufficient without the need for antibiotic therapy.

**PRINCIPLE Infection in the skin or elsewhere is not an automatic indication for antibiotic therapy.**

***Suppression and prevention of pruritus***

Since pruritus plays a pivotal role in the evolution and propagation of eczema, controlling or possibly eliminating it is the key to ultimate success in treating eczema. Unfortunately, despite a variety of approaches, this remains the most difficult aspect of eczema to treat.

Based on the premise that altered cutaneous-barrier function (with increased transepidermal loss of water) and endogenous release of histamine are contributing factors to pruritus, the use of various emollients and oral antihistamines constitutes the major therapeutic approach to managing pruritus.

The proper use of emollients in treating atopic eczema, xerotic eczema, nummular eczema, and localized neurodermatitis cannot be overemphasized. As previously mentioned, the acute stage of eczema should be handled with topical medications in creams or lotion vehicles, the dry eczema and associated dry skin should be handled with more frequent application of creams (e.g., Eucerin) or, if tolerated, very thinly applied ointments (e.g., white petrolatum). The physician must be specific in telling patients that frequency of application, not the brand of emollient, is the most crucial aspect of therapy.

Because so many cosmetics and OTC topical medicaments are used by society without any specific directions or cosmetic consequences, a less-than-attentive attitude on the part of the patient in regard to applying a topical emollient will only increase the chances of therapeutic failure. The patient needs to be told that when pruritus occurs, applying the appropriate emollient, not scratching, is the proper response. Furthermore, since bathing or showering, especially with soap, leads to increased dryness of the skin, especially in atopic but also nonatopic xerotic skin, washing should be minimized and when required should be accompanied by immediate application of an appropriate emollient to the still-wet skin followed by gentle pat drying.

**PRINCIPLE The clinician who focuses on the drug alone, ignoring so-called adjunctive measures, often creates impossible obstacles for the drug to overcome. Whereas therapeutic failure may easily be attributed to the drug, it is the doctor who really has failed and the patient who really pays.**

The use of oral antihistamines for pruritus may be effective only in so far as the associated sedation discourages the physical effort to scratch. While there is definite evidence that concentrations of free histamine are elevated in atopic skin and that histamine release may be more labile among atopic mast cells or basophils, the use of newer potent $H_1$ antagonists (e.g., astemizole, terfenadine) that have little or no sedative effect have not been shown to be efficacious in managing pruritus (Krause and Shuster 1983). Furthermore, $H_2$-receptor antagonists such as cimetidine do not provide any significant therapeutic benefit for pruritus associated with atopic dermatitis (Foulds and MacKie 1981). Since the sedative effect of the most widely used $H_1$ antagonists (e.g., diphenhydramine [Benadryl], hydroxyzine hydrochloride [Atarax]) appears to be the important property for combating pruritus associated with eczema, the patients must be warned about this drug effect if driving or working with dangerous machinery is part of their daily routine. Sometimes, suggesting that the patient take a leave of absence from work is most appropriate, since work-related stress may work against the best therapies for relieving severe pruritus related to eczema.

The chronic use of topical antihistamines (e.g., diphenhydramine, promethazine hydrochloride) available in OTC anti-itch preparations or the benzocaine-containing topical anesthetic ointments should be discouraged because of their potential to induce allergic contact dermatitis.

In summary, successful treatment of eczema fully depends on identifying its cause and then instituting appropriate topical and systemic therapies as outlined. Failure to respond should lead the physician to first document patient compliance with the prescribed therapy and then reevaluate the suspected cause. The most frequently missed diagnosis that may sometimes present as eczema is tinea corporis, which requires appropriate antifungal therapy. Diagnosis of tinea depends on the finding of typical hyphae on microscopic examination of scales (so-called potassium hydroxide or KOH preparation) as well as on culture for the fungus.

## IMPETIGO

*Impetigo* (from the Latin *impeto,* to assail) is the term applied to a rapidly expanding, highly contagious (especially in children) superficial skin infection. It has two characteristic presentations: 1) areas of extending, moist, honey-colored crusts or 2) short-lived flaccid bullae that collapse with the ensuing formation of quarter- to half dollar-sized annular, thin crusts sometimes giving the appearance of a fungal infection (relatively clear center with active border). The most common sites of involvement are the face, especially the perioral skin, arms, buttocks and legs, but any skin site may be involved. The highest incidence of bullous impetigo appears among preschool children.

### Pathogenesis of Impetigo

Whereas facial impetigo with honey-colored crusts was once thought to be primarily the result of streptococcal infection, most cases (about 70 to 90%) of impetigo, whether of the crusting or bullous presentation, appear to be caused by *S. aureus* (Brook et al. 1997). The bullae associated with bullous impetigo are caused by an exfoliative toxin most frequently associated with group II phage-type 71 strains of *S. aureus.* This toxin produces subcorneal cleavage in the epidermis leading to the formation of thin, evanescent bullae.

### Therapy for Impetigo

There are two approaches to therapy: topical antibiotic or systemic antibiotic. If lesions are relatively localized (e.g., below the nostrils and around the chin), topical 2% mupirocin ointment (Bactroban) can be applied three times a day for 10 days with good therapeutic results (Dagan and Bar-David 1992). If the lesions are more generalized, then oral antibiotics are preferred with semisynthetic penicillins such as dicloxacillin or cloxacillin being the drugs of choice. In the case of penicillin allergy, first-generation cephalosporins such as cephalexin (Keflex) and cefadroxil (Duricef) have good coverage of not only *S. aureus* but also *S. pyogenes* (Misko et al. 1997).

## MELANOMA

The incidence of melanoma appears to be increasing more rapidly than that of any other cancer both in the United States and internationally. According to the American Cancer Society, melanomas will account for 80% of the 9200 deaths expected in 1998 from skin cancer. Predictions estimate about 42,000 new cases of invasive melanoma, a 3% increase from 1997 (American Cancer Society 1998). Among Caucasians, the incidence of melanoma doubled between 1973 and 1991. It is the fifth most frequently occurring cancer in the United States. If current trends continue, by the year 2000, 1 in 75 Americans will have a lifetime risk of developing melanoma (compared with 1 in 150 in 1985 and 1 in 250 in 1980). And although the incidence of melanoma today is lower than that of other skin cancers, melanoma is more common than any nonskin cancer among people between 25 and 29 years of age and second only to breast cancer in women aged 30 to 34.

### Pathogenesis of Melanoma

The reasons offered for the rising incidence of melanoma include increased time spent in outdoor activities as well as increased surveillance, although the latter explanation does not appear to account for the increase (Rigel 1997). Whereas use of sunscreens that block the sunburn-producing ultraviolet B (UVB) rays are more widely used today, information that long-wave UVA can be carcinogenic has been increasing (Garland et al. 1993; Setlow and Woodhead 1994; Stern et al. 1997). Accordingly, traditional sunscreens that block primarily UVB may provide a false sense of security about protection from skin cancer. As a result, people who enjoy outdoor exercise (walkers, joggers, tennis players, golfers, windsurfers, skiers, rock climbers, hikers, cyclists, etc.) spend longer times in the sun exposed to UVA rays. Another contributor is the popularity of tanning parlors, which provide further exposure to UV.

Whereas the pathogenesis of melanoma is unclear, the following elements all have a statistically significant association with the incidence of melanoma:

- Red or blond hair
- A family history of melanoma (Novakovic et al. 1995)
- High freckle density on the upper back
- Overall number of pigmented nevi on the body (Bliss et al. 1995)
- Three or more blistering sunburns before the age of 20
- Three or more years of outdoor jobs while a teenager (Rigel 1995)

## Diagnosis of Melanoma

The diagnosis of melanoma is made by histopathologic examination of biopsy specimens. However, the decision to obtain a biopsy requires that the patient and/or the health care provider can recognize the skin properties associated with increased risk for melanoma, as well as the physical characteristics that help to differentiate melanomas from benign pigmented skin lesions. Since more than 90% of cutaneous melanomas can be recognized by the naked eye, the opportunity for early diagnosis is better than that for any other type of malignancy. The importance of this fact cannot be overemphasized, since the thickness of the tumor at the time of removal is one of the most useful prognostic parameters (Buzaid 1997); primary tumors less than 1.5 mm in thickness are associated with an 85% rate of 10-year survival, whereas those of greater than 4 mm are associated with a 44% rate of 5-year survival. In spite of an overall increased survival for patients with localized melanoma (50% in 1950s, about 90% in 1996), the absolute number of thicker melanomas is increasing as is the death rate; these facts support a real increase in incidence.

Furthermore, deficiencies in public awareness (and probably provider awareness) of melanoma risk factors, as well as significant public ignorance of the actual existence of melanoma have been documented (Miller et al. 1996). And since cost consciousness is becoming a more pervasive factor in health care, it is instructive to note that in 1997, the annual direct cost of treating new cases of melanoma is estimated to be around $600 million, 90% of which went to treating the 20% of patients with advanced disease (Tsao et al. 1998). For Medicare alone, the cost of melanoma therapy (assuming the current 6% annual increase in incidence) has been predicted to possibly exceed $5 billion by 2010 (Johnson et al. 1998). Thus early diagnosis and support programs that promote early diagnosis can have a major impact on health-care costs.

An "ABCD" acronym has been developed to assist in identifying potential melanomas. The A stands for asymmetry, B for border, C for color, and D for diameter. Melanomas tend to have ***A***symmetric shapes; irregular and sometimes focally indistinct ***B***orders; mottled ***C***olor including shades of blue-black, red, slate-gray, as well as brown and black; and a ***D***iameter greater than 6 mm. However, a very important, and frequently overlooked, aspect of evaluating any given pigmented lesion is whether the physical findings represent recent changes (weeks to months). A melanoma arising in a symmetrical, discrete, pigmented mole may initially show only a general deepening of color over a period of weeks. This is a more significant finding than a patient presenting with an 8-mm irregular brownish-black papule that has shown no change for 10 years. Although this comparison may appear simplistic, many dermatology consultations are requested based on the ABCD criteria without the provider ever documenting how long the lesion in question has been present.

**PRINCIPLE The history can be pivotal in deciding whether a biopsy should be taken of a lesion.**

## Therapy for Melanoma

Therapy for melanoma is initially surgical. If a practitioner suspects a melanoma, a total excisional biopsy, if at all possible, should be performed because of the prognostic importance of identifying the thickest portion of the tumor. Currently, a primary melanoma 1.0 mm or less in thickness can be excised with a 1.0-cm margin followed by a primary closure (Balch et al. 1993). This means that if a 1-cm margin was used in taking the biopsy, no further reexcision is required; if the biopsy margin was less than 1 cm (e.g., if the clinical diagnosis was not certain for melanoma), then a reexcision is done with both biopsy and reexcision margins totaling 1 cm. If the primary lesion was greater than 1.0 mm thick but less than 4.0 mm, a 2.0-cm excisional margin is safe, according to a randomized intergroup surgical trial. For thicker melanomas, a 3.0-cm margin is currently the maximum required. Since survival has not been shown to be improved by taking extra normal skin around a melanoma, a 1.0-cm margin or "that which can be closed primarily" may eventually be recognized as the excisional margin standard for all tumors.

Regional lymph node involvement is also a key element in prognosis and in guiding therapy. Recent studies have documented the value of sentinel lymph node biopsies identified by dye or radioisotope injection at the site of the primary melanoma followed by lymphoscintigraphy (Johnson et al. 1998). This technique is performed at the time of reexcision. Data suggest that few patients with negative sentinel nodes go on to develop lymph node metastases.

The therapy for metastatic melanoma is still in transition, with many clinical trials currently in progress. In a few cases where single organ involvement is documented, surgical resection can result in significant disease-free intervals. A detailed evaluation of the current approaches for metastatic disease is beyond the scope of this chapter. Suffice it to state that various experimental agents alone and in combination are being evaluated. These include tumor vaccines, biologic response modifiers (e.g., interferon $\alpha$-2b and interleukin 2 [IL-2]) and/or cytotoxic agents (e.g., dacarbazine [DTIC], carmustine [BCNU], lomustine [CCNU], and tamoxifen) (Johnson et al. 1998).

## PSORIASIS

Psoriasis is a skin disease characterized by a chronic relapsing eruption of scaling papules that so rapidly coalesce that the physician usually only finds erythematous, scaly plaques by the time the patient seeks consultation. It is estimated to affect roughly 7 million Americans with approximately 200,000 new cases occurring each year.

The classic predilection for plaques of psoriasis to appear symmetrically on the elbows and knees assists in the diagnosis. However, patients can present a broad clinical spectrum from only scalp involvement to scattered plaques on the trunk and extremities to, in the most serious cases, a generalized erythroderma accompanied by a rheumatoid factor–negative symmetric arthritis. In all these cases, the finding of very small pits in the nail plates of the hands and feet, the presence of gluteal "pinking" (erythema and slight scaling of the intergluteal cleft), and the occurrence of lesions conforming to specific sites of skin trauma (isomorphic response, or Koebner phenomenon) help secure a clinical diagnosis. A skin biopsy can help to confirm the diagnosis in cases in which lichen simplex chronicus, chronic nummular eczema, or severe seborrhea of the scalp may not be readily excluded on examination alone.

Acute guttate (Latin *gutta,* a drop) psoriasis is a unique presentation of the disease that follows a minor streptococcal infection; it presents as an eruption of small 1- to 3-mm erythematous, scaly papules in a generalized distribution that slowly enlarges to more closely resemble generalized plaque psoriasis (Whyte and Baughman 1964). Pustular psoriasis is another form of psoriasis that can become life-threatening with episodes of rapidly progressive flares involving more extensive surfaces of the body and the development of fever, chills, and leukocytosis, as well as fluid and electrolyte disturbances requiring immediate intensive therapy (Barnard 1997). Usually however, the pustular form of psoriasis is limited to the palms and soles and may be controlled with therapies discussed below. The multiple clinical presentations coupled with familial inheritance suggest that psoriasis is dominantly inherited with variable penetrance of the phenotype. Susceptibility to psoriasis appears to be linked to the class I and II, and, possibly, the class III major histocompatibility complex region on human chromosome 6. Other psoriasis susceptibility gene candidates are located at chromosomes 1, 4, and 17, lending further support to the concept that inheritance of psoriasis is polygenic (Henseler 1997).

### Pathogenesis of Psoriasis

The factors regulating the phenotypic expression of psoriasis are unclear. Although studies have explored alterations in cyclic nucleotide function, eicosanoid metabolism, polyamine synthesis, and a variety of other metabolic parameters, none of the alterations so far identified have been shown to be unique to involved psoriatic skin. Arachidonic acid and its metabolites are found in high levels in psoriatic lesions and may act as chemoattractants for neutrophils and have a vasodilatory effect as well. This in turn results in locally elevated levels of plasminogen activator recruiting further neutrophils via complement activation. Of particular interest is the fact that nonsteroidal antiinflammatory agents that inhibit cyclooxygenase may induce arachidonic acid accumulation, resulting in the exacerbation of preexisting psoriasis (Barnard et al. 1997). Studies have documented markedly accelerated in vivo turnover of epidermal cells in the involved skin of patients with psoriasis (approximately 4 days) versus normal epidermal cells (approximately 28 days) (Van Scott and Ekel 1963; Weinstein and Frost 1968) and consequently researchers have postulated an inherent epidermal defect.

However, there is a distinct possibility that the altered epidermal kinetics in psoriasis may, in fact, stem from pathologic stimulation of a normal epidermis by dermal fibroblasts (Saiag et al. 1985). Furthermore, the recent identification of a novel fibroblast-derived keratinocyte growth factor (KGF) that stimulates keratinocyte proliferation suggests that alterations in the production of such cytokines within the dermis could contribute to skin diseases characterized by a hyperproliferative epidermis (Rubin et al. 1989). Studies have shown that 1,25-dihydroxyvitamin $D_3$ (calcitriol/calcipotriene 0.005%) regulates calcium-induced keratinocyte differentiation and exerts a beneficial effect on psoriatic plaques (Bikle 1997). Clinical use of topical vitamin $D_3$ analogs is discussed below. A novel topical retinoid, tazarotene gel (0.05 and 0.1%), has been shown to be efficacious in controlling mild to moderate plaque-type psoriasis via mechanisms that include normalization of keratinocyte differentiation and interference with the antiproliferative and anti-inflammatory signal transduction pathways involved in psoriasis (Duvic et al. 1997).

It is interesting that β-adrenergic receptor blocking agents can exacerbate psoriasis (Gold et al. 1988). Whether this adverse effect is providing insight into the pathogenesis of psoriasis remains to be determined. Currently, however, the therapies that have evolved for psoriasis focus on the hyperproliferative epidermis.

**PRINCIPLE When a drug unexpectedly modulates a disease, think carefully about what follow-up you want in order to establish new understanding in regard to pathogenesis or to document drug efficacy. In this case, we would want to know whether the β-adrenergic antagonists are working by their blocking properties. If so, we might then expect to see studies on the effects of absorbable β-adrenergic agonists on the disease.**

## Therapy for Psoriasis

The treatment of psoriasis must be tailored to the type of clinical presentation that the physician encounters. Localized disease can be handled by a variety of topical therapies. More generalized disease may require different topical therapies with the additional consideration of systemic therapies in recalcitrant cases that cause serious morbidity for the patient (Greaves and Weinstein 1995).

### *Topical therapy*

For isolated hyperkeratotic plaques, the use of potent or superpotent topical corticosteroids probably is the most widely used initial treatment. The use of the superpotent clobetasol propionate 0.05% ointment has been shown to be superior to one of the high-potency steroid ointments both in terms of faster improvement and longer remission (Jacobson et al. 1986). If no more than the recommended 50 g/week of the superpotent topical corticosteroids is required, a 2-week course should be tried with these preparations (see previous section on use of topical corticosteroids). If less than 50 g/week is required over the initial 2 weeks, the physician can consider, especially for very thick plaques, alternate-day therapy first, with the superpotent corticosteroid alternating with a less potent corticosteroid (0.05% fluocinonide or 0.1% triamcinolone ointment on the off days). Another alternative is to apply a 1, 2, or 5% crude coal tar ointment to the lesions on the days when steroids are not administered. Some experienced clinicians feel that coal tar alone may have a steroid-sparing effect (Lowe 1988).

Once the lesions are flat and the erythema has significantly diminished, daily application of some of the commercially available coal tars can be used until the lesions are totally clear. Some of the available preparations include Estar Gel, psoriGel, Bakers PS and plus Gel, and T Derm Tar Oil. The reason for the therapeutic benefit of coal tar in psoriasis is unclear, even though it was introduced 65 years ago to treat psoriasis in combination with hot quartz (UVB) light therapy (Goeckerman 1925). Coal tar is a by-product of cooking ovens, and its specific composition depends on the type of coal burned, the temperature, and efficiency of the coking ovens (Gruber et al. 1970). One of the lingering concerns with using coal tar is its demonstrated carcinogenicity in laboratory animals (Rasmussen 1978). However, an international survey conducted in 1976 was able to identify only 3 out of 135,000 psoriatic patients who appeared to have skin cancer related to use of coal tar (Farber 1977). A more recent study of long-term use of topical coal tar in psoriasis was likewise unable to uncover an increased incidence of skin cancer (Pittlekow et al. 1981).

Another effective topical agent for use on isolated, noninflamed, thick plaques of psoriasis is anthralin (Dithranol). It is commercially available in different concentrations in both cream (Drithocreme 0.1, 0.25, 0.5, and 1.0%) and ointment (Anthra-Derm 0.1, 0.25, 0.5, and 1.0%) vehicles and is a coal tar derivative that appears to exert an antimitotic effect on the hyperproliferative epidermis (Swanbeck and Liden 1966). Because of its irritant effect on normal skin, most protocols employ a thick paste vehicle with the application of petrolatum around the involved skin to protect the normal skin. The drug is then left on the skin for the entire day. Although it is effective (daily application often produces clearing of plaques within an average period of 3 weeks), irritation of the normal skin as well as staining of clothing and bed sheets by anthralin can create problems with compliance of outpatients. More recent studies have demonstrated a more rapid absorption of anthralin through psoriatic epidermis and have therefore explored short exposure (10 to 30 minutes) of plaques to anthralin (Shaefer et al. 1980; Runne and Kunze 1982; Lowe et al. 1984). With short-term exposure, therapy takes an average of 4 to 6 weeks. The short exposure is efficacious in resolving localized plaques while minimizing the chance for skin irritation, especially if the physician begins with the lowest concentration of anthralin and increases the concentration as tolerated.

Calcipotriene 0.005% ointment is a vitamin $D_3$ derivative with modulatory effects on epidermal growth, keratinization, and inflammation that improves psoriatic plaques with topical application (Kragballe 1992; van de Kerkhof 1996). Calcipotriene 0.005% ointment (Dovonex) may be used in combination with high potency class I topical corticosteroid to prevent excessive irritation and minimize the risks associated with prolonged corticosteroid therapy alone (Lebwohl 1997). Calcipotriene applied twice daily is safe for up to 52 weeks at dosages below 100 g/week for maintenance and further clearing of psoriatic plaques (Poyner, et al. 1993; Ramsey 1997). Calcium homeostasis has been studied and appears to be minimally affected when the recommended dosages are used (Kragballe 1992), but hypercalcemia due to increased intestinal absorption of calcium is observed in patients receiving dosages as high as 360 g/week (Bourke et al. 1997). The new topical retinoid, tazorotene gel (0.05% and 0.1%) appears to offer another, more specific therapeutic approach for the treatment of mild to moderate plaque-type psoriasis in once daily dosing. Results with both concentrations are similar in reducing plaques as early as one week of treatment, and after 12 weeks of therapy, patients continue to have improvement for 12 additional weeks without treatment. Local irritation is the only reported adverse effect, and no significant drug-related systemic toxicity has been identified (Weinstein 1997).

For more generalized disease, the topical therapies reviewed above may become too cumbersome and lead to lack of patient compliance. Although these therapies may still be applied to localized sites where plaques may be especially hypertrophic, the most widely used therapy for generalized psoriasis is the combination of topical coal tar applications with UVB light (290- to 320-nm wavelength). This treatment, initiated by Goeckerman in the 1920s (still referred to as *Goeckerman therapy*), consists of combining topical coal tar treatment (in the form of ointments or tar solutions mixed into bathwater) three times per day with interspersed use of increasing exposures to UVB light to induce a mild erythema. In the 1950s the so-called Ingram method was introduced, replacing coal tar with anthralin (Ingram 1953). Both these therapies, while initially delivered in an inpatient setting, have, because of the increasing costs of inpatient care, been successfully transferred to the setting of so-called ambulatory psoriasis treatment centers, or psoriasis day-care centers (Bohm and Voorhees 1985).

***Systemic therapy***

For the population of psoriasis patients who suffer from generalized disease that is recalcitrant to the above therapies or for whom recurrence rates seriously interfere with occupational or other living demands, systemic therapies have been developed, again primarily based on suppressing the markedly increased epidermal cell proliferation. However, the increased risk of potentially adverse effects associated with these therapies can only be justified by the degree of morbidity that more extensive cases of psoriasis can occasionally produce. These systemic approaches include the following:

- Oral 8-methoxypsoralin combined with subsequent exposure to UVA light, so-called PUVA therapy (Melski et al. 1977)
- Oral or IM methotrexate, a folic acid antagonist that interferes with DNA, RNA, and protein synthesis (Roenigk et al. 1988) (see chapter 13, Oncologic Disorders)
- Oral hydroxyurea, a DNA-synthesis inhibitor (Leavell and Yarbro 1970) (see chapter 13)
- Oral etretinate, a vitamin A derivative that inhibits epidermal ornithine decarboxylase and thereby interferes with polyamine metabolism required for cell growth (Lowe et al. 1982; Kaplan et al. 1983)
- A combination of the retinoid etretinate and PUVA (so-called REPUVA) therapy that may shorten the required course of PUVA therapy, thereby decreasing its potential long-term hazards (Honigsmann and Wolff 1989)
- A new retinoid, acitretin, the active metabolite of etretinate but with a safer side effect profile
- Cyclosporin A, which, in addition to its immunosuppressive effects, appears to suppress keratinocyte DNA synthesis (Ellis et al. 1986; Furure et al. 1988; Meinardi and Bos 1988)

A detailed discussion of the systemic therapies is beyond the scope of this chapter. Needless to say, treatment of the more severe cases of psoriasis should be handled by clinicians experienced with the systemic therapies for psoriasis and their potential hazards, for example:

- Hepatotoxicity and hematologic side effects of methotrexate (O'Connor et al. 1989); macrocytic anemia, leukopenia, and thrombocytopenia associated with hydroxyurea therapy

- Teratogenicity, hyperlipidemia, skeletal hyperostoses, and hepatotoxicity associated with etretinate therapy (Matt et al. 1989)
- Cataracts and skin cancers associated with PUVA (Gupta and Anderson 1987)
- Nephrotoxicity with cyclosporin A (Picascia et al. 1988)

**PRINCIPLE From a therapeutic perspective, the best justification for subspecialization is to be found in the use of drugs that, because of the substantial toxicity that may accompany therapeutic efficacy, mandate special expertise in their delivery.**

## SKIN REACTIONS INDUCED BY SYSTEMIC MEDICATIONS

Drug-induced skin reactions may occur in approximately 2 to 3% of medical inpatients (60,000 to 90,000 reactions per year nationwide) (Shapiro et al. 1969). Roughly 1 in 44 inpatients may be expected to develop a morbilliform, urticarial, or other exanthem. The highest rates of reaction were noted for the combination of trimethoprim and sulfamethoxazole (59 per 1000 recipients) followed closely by ampicillin (52 per 1000 recipients) (Arndt and Jick 1976). With the exception of ampicillin and other semisynthetic penicillins (50% occur after one week of administration) cutaneous reactions usually occur within 1 week of beginning therapy with the offending drug.

### Pathogenesis of Skin Reactions to Systemic Medications

Untoward reactions of the skin to drugs administered systemically can be classified on the basis of etiology, if known, but clinical morphology still remains the basis for categorizing most cutaneous reactions to systemic medications. If an immunologic mechanism can be found that explains a skin reaction, the term *allergic drug reaction* is appropriate. However, nonimmunologic drug reactions can also be identified wherein a given drug can activate specific effector pathways without invoking participation of the immune system. An example of such nonimmunologic activation of effector pathways is the direct release of histamine and activation of complement in the absence of antibody by radiocontrast media (Lasser 1968; Arroyave et al. 1976). However, radiocontrast media themselves can produce a bullous skin reaction (Grunwald et al. 1985), as well as a necrotizing vasculitis (Kerdel et al. 1984). It thus becomes clear that any given systemically administered drug may be responsible for both immunologically and nonimmunologically mediated skin reactions depending on host factors yet to be accurately identified. Consequently, the following discussion will focus on morphologic patterns of skin response to drugs, those drugs most frequently associated with a given morphology, and approaches to therapy for drug reactions in the presence or absence of a defined etiology.

#### *Urticarial reactions*

Urticaria, sometimes accompanied by angioedema, probably is one of the most common cutaneous manifestations of an allergic drug reaction. In the vast majority of clinical cases of urticaria or angioedema, the cause cannot be identified (Champion et al. 1969). Urticaria or angioedema occurring within minutes of drug ingestion is termed an immediate reaction; a response manifesting itself 12 to 36 hours following drug exposure is termed an accelerated reaction. The term *chronic urticaria* is used to describe urticaria that lasts more than 6 weeks.

Urticaria can represent an IgE-mediated response in which drug or drug-metabolite–protein conjugates bind to hapten-specific IgE attached to Fc receptors ($Fc_{\varepsilon}R$) on the surface of mast cells or basophils. Bridging of these receptors through binding of antigen by the resident IgE molecules leads to mast cell or basophil degranulation. The released mediators can induce vasodilation, e.g., histamine, prostaglandin $D_2$, platelet-activating factor (PAF), and vascular permeability, e.g., leukotriene $C_4$, that are the pathophysiologic markers of urticaria.

Urticaria also can be a frequent manifestation of serum sickness and in this context occurs within 7 to 12 days following initial exposure to the offending drug. Accompanying fever, arthralgias, myalgias, and lymphadenopathy can help solidify the diagnosis. Data support IgG immune complex deposition in the cutaneous postcapillary venules with resultant complement activation and mast cell degranulation (Yancy and Lawley 1984) as an etiologic mechanism for the urticaria.

The drugs most frequently associated with urticaria or angioedema include penicillin and related derivatives that retain the 6-aminopenicillinic acid nucleus, sulfa drugs, barbiturates (especially phenobarbital), anticonvulsants, salicylates, allergy extracts, opiate analgesics, and, as mentioned, radiocontrast materials.

#### *Morbilliform reactions*

This is probably the most frequent type of skin reaction to systemically administered drugs and presents as a generalized fine maculopapular eruption resembling measles (hence morbilliform). It can be difficult to distinguish from viral exanthems. The mechanism underlying this type of reaction is unknown. It may be induced by a wide variety of drugs, penicillin and its derivatives being the most common inducers, with blood products (e.g., whole human blood, packed red blood cells, blood platelets) next highest in frequency (Arndt and Jick 1976).

***Erythema multiforme***
This skin eruption, erythema multiforme (EM), is characterized by the acute appearance of annular erythematous lesions, most having a central erythematous papule or bulla that gives the appearance of a marksman's target to the lesions (hence the term *target lesion*). Lesions are often generalized and can involve the palms and soles. *EM minor* is the term used for eruptions that involve the skin and/or one mucosal surface without systemic symptoms. Approximately 90% of these cases are associated with herpes simplex eruptions, and herpes simplex DNA has been identified in the erythema multiforme lesions of 75% of patients sampled in one study (Imafuku et al. 1997). There are, however, also reports of EM in response to drugs, with long-acting sulfonamides most frequently implicated (Carroll et al. 1966) and barbiturates, sulindac, and fenoprofen also frequent suspects (Hardie and Savin 1979). Whereas the pathogenesis of EM is not firmly established, an immune complex–mediated vasculitis may be implicated, based on studies on herpes simplex–associated and *Mycoplasma pneumoniae*–associated EM (Wuepper et al. 1980; Tonnesen et al. 1983).

The other type, *EM major* (Stevens–Johnson syndrome), is regarded by some as a more severe form of erythema multiforme characterized by erosive mucous membrane lesions (most prominent in the conjunctiva and mouth) as well as systemic symptoms of fever and malaise. However, the recent evidence linking most cases of EM with herpes simplex adds increasing support to regarding erythema multiforme as a separate entity from Stevens–Johnson syndrome (Roujeau 1997). The incidence of Stevens–Johnson syndrome ranges from 1.2 to 6 per million per year and carries about a 5% mortality (Wolkenstein and Revuz 1995). Sulfonamides, anticonvulsants, allopurinol, pyrazolone derivatives, oxicams, and chlormezanone are the drugs most frequently associated with Stevens–Johnson syndrome.

***Toxic epidermal necrolysis***
This severe cutaneous reaction, toxic epidermal necrolysis (TEN), is clinically seen as a more extensive form of Stevens–Johnson syndrome and is characterized by diffuse erythema with tenderness, fever, and malaise followed by widespread sloughing of the epidermis resembling a scalding injury. Mucous membranes show erythema, erosions, and bullae. The incidence of TEN ranges from 0.4 to 1.2 per million per year, but the disorder is fatal in about 30% of cases (Wolkenstein and Revuz 1995). Although TEN is associated with a variety of etiologic factors (Lyell 1967), drugs that are definitely implicated include sulfonamides, butazones, hydantoins, barbiturates, and penicillin (Hardie and Savin 1979).

Toxic epidermal necrolysis must be differentiated for both prognostic and therapeutic reasons from staphylococcal scalded skin syndrome (SSSS), which is caused by infection with specific strains of *S. aureus* and requires a different therapeutic approach (Elias et al. 1977). Clinically, SSSS may defy differentiation from TEN. An exfoliative cytology preparation obtained at the bedside and stained with Giemsa shows primarily nucleated squamous cells in SSSS but cell debris, leukocytes, and only occasional squamous cells in TEN. These differences are due to the fact that in SSSS the epidermal cleavage is attributable to a circulating bacterial epidermolytic exotoxin that attacks the epidermis at or below the stratum granulosum with little to be found as far as an inflammatory cell infiltrate; the bacteria are not present in the skin lesions but can be readily cultured from the nostrils. In drug-induced TEN, however, the full thickness of epidermis is destroyed in a reaction associated with numerous leukocytes (Amon and Diamond 1975).

***Other morphologic forms of cutaneous reactions to systemic drugs***
Although the cutaneous eruptions heretofore described represent the most common as well as clinically most consequential, a variety of other adverse cutaneous responses to systemic drugs would require far more space for complete discussion. These are covered in several references (Breathnach 1995a, 1995b).

## Therapy for Skin Reactions to Systemic Medications

The treatment of drug-induced skin reactions ultimately depends on identification and immediate cessation of therapy with the offending drug. If possible an alternate, structurally unrelated substitute should be found. In the case of a relatively asymptomatic morbilliform skin rash, the offending drug may be continued if it is absolutely essential. Resolution of morbilliform eruptions in the presence of continuing therapy has occurred. However, if evolution to a more symptomatic erythroderma appears possible by careful and repeated inspection by the physician, the offending drug should be immediately discontinued and every effort made to find adequate alternative therapy.

The therapy for urticarial drug reactions depends on the accompanying symptoms. In the extreme case of urticaria or angioedema as manifestations of an anaphylactic response, appropriate emergency procedures should be instituted including IM epinephrine, maintenance of airway, and other appropriate measures. When pruritus is the only symptom, treatment with $H_1$-antagonist antihistamines (e.g., hydroxyzine or diphenhydramine) may provide benefit if histamine is the major causative mediator. If pruritus is the major source of discomfort, these antihistamines may be beneficial through their sedative properties, even if the urticaria itself does not immediately respond.

In cases of chronic urticaria (>6 weeks) when there is a history of aspirin or NSAID sensitivity or penicillin sensitivity in the form of urticaria, chronic exposure to trace salicylates or penicillin derivatives present in various fruits, vegetables, and dairy products may be occurring. Attempts to remove potential dietary sources of these offending agents should be attempted. Studies have demonstrated that some of the long-acting nonsedating $H_1$ antihistamines provide benefit in chronic urticaria. Astemazole (Hismanal) may offer greater relief in chronic urticaria than the shorter-acting sedating antihistamines (Bernstein and Bernstein 1986).

The cutaneous reactions that carry a significant associated morbidity and mortality are Stevens–Johnson syndrome and TEN. The differentiation of TEN from SSSS is important, since the former reaction has a mortality rate of around 30% and is unaffected or possibly made worse if treated with an antibiotic that cross-reacts with the offending drug. Conversely, SSSS is associated with about a 4% mortality and responds to appropriate antistaphylococcal drugs; systemic corticosteroids are contraindicated (Elias et al. 1977). Because of the loss of significant areas of epidermis in EM major and TEN, treatment must focus on immediate cessation of therapy with the suspected drug, prevention of superinfection, and maintenance of fluid balance following the same procedures that one would for a burn patient. Patients with Stevens–Johnson syndrome or TEN should be managed in a hospital setting. The use of steroids in these patients remains controversial.

## REFERENCES


Adams SJ, Cunliffe WJ, Cooke MJ. 1985. Long-term antibiotic therapy for acne vulgaris: Effects on the bowel flora of patients and their relatives. *J Invest Dermatol* **85**:35–7.

Akers WA et al. 1975. Systemic antibiotics for treatment of acne vulgaris: Efficacy and safety. *Arch Dermatol* **111**:1630–6.

Allison F, Smith MR, Wood WB. 1955. Studies on the pathogenesis of acute inflammation: II. The action of cortisone on the inflammatory response to thermal injury. *J Exp Med* **102**:669–675.

Aly R, Maibach HI, Shinefeld HR. 1977. Microbial flora of atopic dermatitis. *Arch Dermatol* **113**:780–2.

American Cancer Society. 1999. Cancer Facts and Figures—1999.

Amon RB, Diamond RL. 1975. Toxic epidermal necrolysis: Rapid differentiation between staphylococcal- and drug-induced disease. *Arch Dermatol* **111**:1433–7.

Arndt KA, Jick H. 1976. Rates of cutaneous reactions to drugs. *JAMA* **235**:918–23.

Arroyave CM, Bhatt KN, Crown NR. 1976. Activation of the alternative pathway of the complement system by radiocontrast media. *J Immunol* **117**:1866–9.

Baer RL, Leshan SM, Shalita AR. 1976. High dose tetracycline therapy in severe acne. *Arch Dermatol* **112**:479–81.

Balch CM, Urist MM, Karakousis CP, et al. 1993. Efficacy of 2-cm surgical margins for intermediate-thickness melanomas (1 to 4 mm): results of a multi-institutional randomized surgical trial. *Ann Surg* **218**:262–7.

Barnard CM, Bauer EA, Kim YH. 1997. Psoriasis, lichen planus, and pityriasis rosea. In: Kelly WN editor. *Textbook of Internal Medicine*. 3d ed. Philadelphia: Lippincott-Raven, pp 1226–30.

Bernstein IL, Bernstein DI. 1986. Efficacy and safety of Astemizole, a long acting and nonsedating $H_1$ antagonist for the treatment of chronic idiopathic urticaria. *J Allerg Clin Immunol* **77**:37–42.

Bikle DD. 1997. Vitamin D. A calciotropic hormone regulating calcium-induced keratinocyte differentiation. *J Am Acad Dermatol* **37**: S42–S52.

Bjornberg A, Roupe G. 1972. Susceptibility to infections during long term treatment with tetracyclines in acne vulgaris. *Dermatologica* **145**:334–7.

Bliss JM, Ford D, Swerdlow AJ, et al. 1995. Risk of cutaneous melanoma associated with pigmentation characteristics and freckling: systematic overview of 10 case-control studies. The International Melanoma Analysis Group (IMAGE). *Int J Cancer* **62**(4):367–76.

Bohm ML, Voorhees JJ. 1985. Role of ambulatory psoriasis treatment center. *J Am Acad Dermatol* **12**:740–7.

Bourke JF, Mumford R, Whittaker P, et al. 1997. The effects of topical calcipotriol on systemic calcium homeostasis in patients with chronic plaque psoriasis. *J Am Acad Dermatol* **37**:929–34.

Breathnach SM. 1995a. Mechanisms of drug eruptions: Part I. *Australas J Dermatol* **36**:121–7.

Breathnach SM. 1995b. Management of drug eruptions: Part II. Diagnosis and treatment. *Australas J Dermatol* **36**:187–91.

Brook I, Frazier EH, Yeager JK. 1997. Microbiology of nonbullous impetigo. *Pediatr Dermatol* **74**:192–5.

Burke B, Eady EA, Cunliffe WJ. 1983. Benzoyl peroxide versus topical erythromycin in the treatment of acne vulgaris. *Br J Dermatol* **108**:199–204.

Buzaid AC, Ross MI, Balch CM, et al. 1997. Critical analysis of the current American Joint Committee on Cancer Staging System for Cutaneous Melanoma and proposal of a new staging system. *J Clin Oncol* **15**:1039–51.

Camisa C, Eisenstadt B, Ragoz A, et al. 1982. The effects of retinoids on neutrophil functions in vitro. *J Am Acad Dermatol* **6**:620–629.

Caron D, Sorba V, Kerrouche N, et al. 1997. Split-face comparison of adapalene 01% gel and tretinoin 0025% gel in acne patients. *J Am Acad Dermatol* **36**(6 Pt 2):S110–2.

Carroll OM, Bryan PA, Robinson RJ. 1966. Stevens-Johnson syndrome associated with long acting sulfonamides. *JAMA* **195**:691–693.

Champion RH, Roberts SOB, Carpenter RG, et al. 1969. Urticaria and angio-edema: A review of 554 patients. *Br J Dermatol* **81**: 88–97.

Chu A, Huber FJ, Plott RT. 1997. The comparative efficacy of benzoyl peroxide 5%/erythromycin 3% gel and erythromycin 4%/zinc 12% solution in the treatment of acne vulgaris. *Br J Dermatol* **136**(2):235–8.

Clucas A, Verschoore M, Sorba V, et al. 1997. Adapalene 01% gel is better tolerated than tretinoin 0025% gel in acne patients. *J Am Acad Dermatol* **36**(6 Pt 2):S116–8.

Cornell RC, Stoughton RB. 1981. Six month controlled study of effects of desoximethasone and betamethasone 17-valerate on the pituitary-adrenal axis. *Br J Dermatol* **105**:91–5.

Cornell RC, Stoughton RB. 1985. Correlation of the vasoconstriction assay and clinical activity in psoriasis. *Arch Dermatol* **121**:63–67.

Cunliffe WJ, Forster RA, Greenwood ND, et al. 1973. Tetracycline and acne vulgaris: A clinical and laboratory investigation. *Br Med J* **2**:332–5.

Cunliffe WJ, Jones DH, Pritlove J, et al. 1985. Long-term benefit of isotretinoin in acne. In: Saurat JH, editor. *Retinoids: New Trends in Research and Therapy*. Basel: Karger, pp 242–51.

Dagan R, Bar-David Y. 1992. Double blind study comparing erythromycin and mupirocin for treatment of impetigo in children: Implications of a high prevalence of erythromycin resistant *Staphylococcus aureus* strains. *Antimicrob Agents Chemother* **36**: 287–90.

Dalziel K, Dykes PJ, Marks R. 1984. Inflammation due to intracutaneous implantation of stratum corneum. *Br J Exp Pathol* **65**:107–15.

De Vivier A. 1976. Acute tolerance to effect of topical glucocorticoids. *Br J Dermatol* **94** (Suppl 12):25–32.

DiGiovanna JJ, Peck GL. 1987. Retinoid toxicity. *Prog Dermatol* **21**(3):1–8.

Duvic M, Nagpal S, Asano AT, et al. 1997. Molecular mechanism of tazarotene in psoriasis. *J Am Acad Dermatol* **37**:S18–S24.

Eady EA, Bojar RA, Jones CE, et al. 1996. The effects of acne treatment with a combination of benzoyl peroxide and erythromycin on skin carriage of erythromycin-resistant propionibacteria. *Br J Dermatol* **134**(1):107–13.

Eady EA, Cove JH, Holland KT, et al. 1989. Erythromycin resistant propionibacteria in antibiotic treated acne patients: Association with therapeutic failure. *Br J Dermatol* **121**:51–7.

Eaglestein WH, Farzad A, Capland L. 1974. Topical corticosteroid therapy: Efficacy of frequent application. *Arch Dermatol* **110**: 955–6.

Elias PM, Finegold K. 1988. Lipid-related barriers and gradients in the epidermis. *Ann N Y Acad Sci* **548**:4–13.

Elias PM, Fritsch P, Epstein EH Jr. 1977. Staphylococcal scalded skin syndrome: Clinical features, pathogenesis, and recent microbiological and biochemical developments. *Arch Dermatol* **113**:207–19.

Ellis CN, Gorsulowsky DC, Hamilton TA, et al. 1986. Cyclosporine improves psoriasis in a double blind study. *JAMA* **256**:3110–16.

Esterly NB, Furey NL, Flanagan LE. 1978. The effect of antimicrobial agents on leukocyte chemotaxis. *J Invest Dermatol* **70**:51–5.

Farber E (editor). 1977. *Coal tar survey. Int Psoriasis Bull* **4**(4):1–6.

Fedors PA. 1997. Ortho Pharmaceutical Corporation Medical Information, personal communication.

Foulds IS, MacKie RM. 1981. A double-blind trial of the H2 receptor antagonist cimetidine and the H1 receptor antagonist promethazine hydrochloride in the treatment of atopic dermatitis. *Clin Allergy* **11**:319–23.

Frichot BC III, Zelickson AS. 1972. Steroids, lysosomes and dermatitis. *Acta DermVenereol (Stockh)* **52**:311–19.

Fulton JE, Marples R, McGinley K, et al. 1968. Gram negative folliculitis in acne vulgaris. *Arch Dermatol* **98**:349–53.

Furure M, Gaspari A, Katz ST. 1988. The effect of cyclosporin A on epidermal cells: II. Cyclosporin A inhibits proliferation of normal and transformed keratinocytes. *J Invest Dermatol* **90**:796–800.

Gammon WR, Meyer C, Lantis S, et al. 1986. Comparative efficacy of oral erythromycin versus oral tetracycline in the treatment of acne vulgaris. *J Am Acad Dermatol* **14**:183–6.

Garland CF, Garland FC, Gorham ED. 1993. Rising trends in melanoma: An hypothesis concerning sunscreen effectiveness. *Ann Epidemiol* **3**:103–10.

Goeckerman WH. 1925. The treatment of psoriasis. *Northwest Med* **24**:2–9.

Gold MH, Holy AK, Roenigk HH. 1988. Beta-blocking drugs and psoriasis: A review of cutaneous side effects and retrospective analysis of their effects on psoriasis. *J Am Acad Dermatol* **19**:837–41.

Gould DJ, Cunliffe WJ. 1978. The long term treatment of acne vulgaris. *Clin Exp Dermatol* **3**:253–7.

Graupe K, Cunliffe WJ, Gollnick HP, et al. 1996. Efficacy and safety of topical azelaic acid (20 percent cream): An overview of trial results from European clinical trials and experimental reports. *Cutis* **5**(Suppl 1):20–35.

Greaves MW, Weinstein GD. 1995. Treatment of psoriasis. *N Engl J Med* **332**:581.

Gruber M, Klein R, Foxx M. 1970. Chemical standardization and quality assurance of whole crude coal tar USP utilizing GLC procedures. *J Pharm Sci* **59**(6):830–4.

Grunwald MH, David M, Feuerman EJ. 1985. Coexistence of psoriasis vulgaris and bullous diseases. *J Am Acad Dermatol* **13**:224–8.

Gupta AK, Anderson TF. 1987. Psoralen photochemotherapy. *J Am Acad Dermatol* **17**:703–34.

Hardie RA, Savin JA. 1979. Drug-induced skin diseases. *Br Med J* **1**:935–7.

Haustein UF, Tegetmeyer L, Ziegler V. 1985. Allergic and irritant potential of benzoyl peroxide. *Contact Dermatitis* **13**:252–7.

Henseler T. 1997. The genetics of psoriasis. *J Am Acad Dermatol* **37**:S1–S11.

Honigsmann H, Wolff K. 1989. Results of therapy for psoriasis using retinoid and photochemotherapy (REPUVA). *Pharmacol Ther* **40**:67–73.

Hurwitz S. 1979. Acne vulgaris: Current concepts of pathogenesis and treatment. *Am J Dis Child* **133**:536–44.

Imafuku S, Kokuba H, Aurelian L, et al. 1997. Expression of herpes simplex virus DNA fragments located in epidermal keratinocytes and germinative cells is associated with the development of erythema multiforme lesions. *J Invest Dermatol* **109**:550–6.

Ingram JT. 1953. The approach to psoriasis. *Br Med J* **2**:591–4.

Jackson DB, Thompson C, McCormack JR, et al. 1989. Bioequivalence (bioavailability) of generic topical corticosteroids. *J Am Acad Dermatol* **20**:791–6.

Jacobson C, Cornell RC, Savin RC. 1986. A comparison of clobetasol propionate 005 percent ointment and an optimized betamethasone dipropionate 005 percent ointment in the treatment of psoriasis. *Cutis* **37**:213–20.

Johnson TM, Yahanda AM, Chang AE, et al. 1998. Advances in melanoma therapy. *J Am Acad Dermatol* **38**:731–41.

Jones D, King K, Miller A, et al. 1983. A dose-response study of 13-*cis*-retinoic acid in acne vulgaris. *Br J Dermatol* **103**:333–43.

Jones DH. 1989. The role and mechanism of action of 13-*cis*-retinoic acid in the treatment of severe (nodulocystic) acne. *Pharmacol Ther* **40**:91–106.

Kaplan RP, Russell DH, Lowe NJ. 1983. Etretinate therapy for psoriasis: Clinical responses remission times epidermal DNA and polyamine responses. *J Am Acad Dermatol* **8**:95–102.

Kerdel FA, Fraker DL, Haynes HA. 1984. Necrotizing vasculitis from radiographic contrast media. *J Am Acad Dermatol* **10**:25–9.

King K, Jones DH, Daltry DC, et al. 1982. A double-blind study of the effects of 13-*cis*-retinoic acid on acne sebum excretion rate and microbial population. *Br J Dermatol* **107**:583–90.

Kirby JD, Monroe DD. 1976. Steroid induced atrophy in an animal and human model. *Br J Dermatol* **94**(Suppl 12):11–19.

Kligman AM, Fulton JE, Plewig G. 1969. Topical vitamin A acid in acne vulgaris. *Arch Dermatol* **99**:469–76.

Knutson DD. 1974. Ultrastructural observations in acne vulgaris: The normal sebaceous follicle and acne lesions. *J Invest Dermatol* **62**:288–307.

Kragballe K. 1992. Treatment of psoriasis with calcipotriol and other vitamin D analogues [review]. *J Am Acad Dermatol* **27**:1001–8.

Krause L, Shuster S. 1983. Mechanism of action of antipruritic drugs. *Br Med J* **287**:1199–200.

Lammer EJ, Chen DT, Hoar RM, et al. 1985. Retinoic acid embryopathy. *N Engl J Med* **313**:837–41.

Lasser EG. 1968. Basic mechanisms of contrast media reactions. *Radiology* **91**:63–65.

Lavker RM, Schecter N. 1985. Cutaneous mast cell depletion results from topical corticosteroid usage. *J Immunol* **135**:2368–73.

Leavell UW Jr, Yarbro JW. 1970. Hydroxyurea: A new treatment for psoriasis. *Arch Dermatol* **102**:144–50.

Lebwohl M. 1997. Topical application of calcipotriene and corticosteroids: Combination regimens. *J Am Acad Dermatol* **37**(Pt 2): S55–8.

Leyden JJ, Marples RR, Kligman AM. 1975. *Staphylococcus aureus* in the lesions of atopic dermatitis. *Br J Dermatol* **90**:525–30.

Leyden JJ, McGinley KJ, Mills O, et al. 1974. *Propionibacterium* levels in patients with and without acne vulgaris. *J Invest Dermatol* **65**:382–4.

Lowe NJ. 1988. Psoriasis. *Semin Dermatol* **7**(1):43–7.

Lowe NJ, Ashton RE, Koudsi H, et al. 1984. Anthralin for psoriasis: short-contact anthralin therapy compared with topical steroid and conventional anthralin. *J Am Acad Dermatol* **10**:69–72.

Lowe NJ, Kaplan R, Breeding J. 1982. Etretinate treatment for psoriasis inhibits epidermal ornithine decarboxylase. *J Am Acad Dermatol* **6**:697–698.

Lucky AW, Henderson TA, Olson WH, et al. 1997. Effectiveness of norgestimate and ethinyl estradiol in treating moderate acne vulgaris. *J Am Acad Dermatol* **37**:746–54.

Lyell A. 1967. A review of toxic epidermal necrolysis in Britain. *Br J Dermatol* **79**:662–671.

Mango D, Ricci S, Manna P, et al. 1996. Clinical and hormonal effects of ethinylestradiol combined with gestodene and desogestrel in young women with acne vulgaris. *Contraception* **53**(3):163–70.

Matt L, Lazarus VN, Lowe NJ. 1989. Newer retinoids for psoriasis—early clinical studies. *Pharmacol Ther* **40**:157–69.

Meinardi MM, Bos JD. 1988. Cyclosporine maintenance therapy in psoriasis. *Transplant Proc* **20**(3)(Suppl 4):42–9.

Melski JW, Tanenbaum L, Parrish JA, et al. 1977. Oral methoxsalen photochemotherapy for the treatment of psoriasis: A cooperative clinical trial. *J Invest Dermatol* **68**:328–35.

Miller DR, Geller AC, Wyatt SW, et al. 1996. Melanoma awareness and self-examination practices: Results of a United States survey. *J Am Acad Dermatol* **34**:962–70.

Milstone EB, McDonald AJ, Scholhamer CF. 1981. Pseudomembranous colitis after topical application of clindamycin. *Arch Dermatol* **117**:154–5.

Misko ML, Terracina JR, Diven DG, et al. 1997. Pediatric dermatology: Advances in therapy. *J Am Acad Dermatol* **36**:513–26.

Munroe DD, Clift DC. 1973. Pituitary-adrenal function after prolonged use of topical corticosteroids. *Br J Dermatol* **88**:381–5.

Nacht S, Young D, Beasley JN, et al. 1981. Benzoyl peroxide percutaneous penetration and metabolic disposition. *J Am Acad Dermatol* **4**:31–7.

Nilsson E, Henning C, Hjorleifsson M-L. 1986. Density of microflora in hand eczema before and after topical treatment with a potent corticosteroid. *J Am Acad Dermatol* **15**:192–7.

Noble WC. 1981. *Microbiology of Human Skin*. 2nd ed. London: Lloyd-Luke, pp 3–106.

Novakovic B, Clark WH Jr, Fears TR, et al. 1995. Melanocytic nevi, dysplastic nevi, and malignant melanoma in children from melanoma-prone families. *J Am Acad Dermatol* **33**:631–6.

O'Connor GT, Olmstead EM, Zug K, et al. 1989. Detection of hepatotoxicity associated with methotrexate therapy for psoriasis. *Arch Dermatol* **125**:1209–17.

Olsen EA, Cornell RC. 1986. Topical clobetasol-17-propionate: Review of its clinical efficacy and safety. *J Am Acad Dermatol* **15**: 246–55.

Olsen TG. 1982. Therapy of acne. *Med Clin North Am* **66**:851–71.

Parker CW, Kennedy S, Eisen AZ. 1977. Leukocyte and lymphocyte cyclic AMP responses in atopic eczema. *J Invest Dermatol* **68**:302–6.

Parry MF, Rha CK. 1986. Pseudomembranous colitis caused by topical clindamycin phosphate. *Arch Dermatol* **122**:583–4.

[PDR] 1998. *Physician's Desk Reference*. Montvale (NJ): Medical Economics Data Production Co.

Picascia DD, Garden JM, Freinkel RK, et al. 1988. Resistant severe psoriasis controlled with systemic cyclosporine therapy. *Transplant Proc* **20**(3)(Suppl 4):58–62.

Pittelkow MR, Perry HO, Muller SA, et al. 1981. Skin cancer in patients with psoriasis treated with coal tar: A 25-year follow-up study. *Arch Dermatol* **117**:465–8.

Plewig G. 1974. Follicular keratinization. *J Invest Dermatol* **62**:308–15.

Pochi PE, Strauss JS. 1964. Sebum production, casual sebum levels, titratable acidity of sebum, and urinary fractional 17-ketosteroid excretion in males with acne. *J Invest Dermatol* **43**:383–8.

Poyner Y, Hughes IW, Dass BK, et al. 1993. Long-term treatment of chronic plaque psoriasis with calcipotriol. *J Dermatol Treat* **4**: 173–7.

Ramsey CA. 1997. Management of psoriasis with calcipotriol used as monotherapy [review]. *J Am Acad Dermatol* **37**(Pt 2):S53–4.

Rasmussen JE. 1978. The crudeness of coal tar. *Prog Dermatol* **12**(5):23–9.

Rebello T, Hawk JLM. 1978. Skin surface glycerol levels in acne vulgaris. *J Invest Dermatol* **70**:352–4.

Redmond GP, Olson WH, Lippman JS, et al. 1997. Norgestimate and ethinyl estradiol in the treatment of acne vulgaris: A randomized, placebo-controlled trial. *Obstet Gynecol* **89**(4):615–22.

Reitamo S, Lauerma AI, Stubb S, et al. 1986. Delayed hypersensitivity to topical corticosteroids. *J Am Acad Dermatol* **14**:582–9.

Rigel DS. 1995. Identification of those at highest risk for development of malignant melanoma. *Adv Dermatol* **10**:151–70.

Rigel DS. 1997. Malignant melanoma: Incidence issues and their effect on diagnosis and treatment in the 1990s. *Mayo Clinic Proc* **72**(4):367–71.

Roenick HN Jr, Auerbach R, Maibach HI, et al. 1988. Methotrexate in psoriasis: revised guidelines. *J Am Acad Dermatol* **19**:145–56.

Roitt IM, Brostoff J, Male DK. 1985. *Immunology*. London: Gower Medical Publishing, pp 221–3.

Rothman KF, Pochi PE. 1988. Use of oral and topical agents for acne in pregnancy. *J Am Acad Dermatol* **16**:431–42.

Roujeau JC. 1997. Stevens-Johnson syndrome and toxic epidermal necrolysis are severity variants of the same disease which differs from erythema multiforme. *J Dermatol* **24**:726–9.

Rubin JS, Osada H, Finch PW, et al. 1989. Purification and characterization of a newly identified growth factor specific for epithelial cells. *Proc Natl Acad Sci USA* **86**:802–6.

Runne U, Kunze J. 1982. Short duration ("minutes") therapy with dithranol for psoriasis: A new outpatient regimen. *Br J Dermatol* **106**:135–9.

Ryden C, Rubin K, Speziale P, et al. 1983. Fibronectin in receptors from *Staphylococcus aureus*. *J Biol Chem* **258**:3396–401.

Saiag PB, Coulomb B, Lebreton C, et al. 1985. Psoriatic fibroblasts induce hyperproliferation of normal keratinocytes in a skin equivalent model in vitro. *Science* **230**:669–672.

Schaefer H, Farber EM, Goldberg L, et al. 1980. Limited application period for dithranol in psoriasis. *Br J Dermatol* **102**:571–3.

Setlow RB, Woodhead AD. 1994. Temporal changes in the incidence of malignant melanoma: Explanation from action spectra. *Mutat Res* **307**:365–74.

Shah VP, Peck CC, Skelly JP. 1989. "Vasoconstriction"—skin blanching—assay for glucocorticoids—a critique. *Arch Dermatol* **125**:1558–63.

Shalita AR. 1974. Genesis of free fatty acids. *J Invest Dermatol* **62**: 332–5.

Shalita AR, Cunningham WJ, Leyden JJ, et al. 1983. Isotretinoin treatment of acne and related disorders: An update. *J Am Acad Dermatol* **9**:629–38.

Shalita AR, Smith EB, Bauer E. 1984. Topical erythromycin v clindamycin therapy for acne: A multicenter double-blind comparison. *Arch Dermatol* **120**:351–5.

Shalita AR, Weiss JS, Chalker DK, et al. 1996. A comparison of the efficacy and safety of adapalene gel 01% and tretinoin gel 0025% in the treatment of acne vulgaris: A multicenter trial. *J Am Acad Dermatol* **34**(3):482–5.

Shalita AR, Wheatly V. 1970. Inhibition of pancreatic lipase by tetracycline. *J Invest Dermatol* **54**:413–6.

Shapiro S, Slone D, Siskind V, et al. 1969. Drug rash with ampicillin and other penicillins. *Lancet* **2**:969–72.

Stern R, Nichols K, Vakeva LH. 1997. Malignant melanoma in patients treated for psoriasis with methoxsalen (psoralen) and ultraviolet A radiation (PUVA). *N Engl J Med* **336**:1041–5.

Stoughton RB, Cornell RC. 1987. Review of super-potent topical corticosteroids. *Semin Dermatol* **6**(2):72–6.

Strauss JS, Pochi PE. 1966. Effect of orally administered antibacterial agents on titratable acidity of human sebum. *J Invest Dermatol* **47**:577–81.

Swanbeck G, Liden S. 1966. The inhibitory effect of dithranol (anthralin) on DNA synthesis. *Acta Derm Venereol (Stockh)* **66**:228–30.

Tan PL, Barnett GL, Flowers FP, et al. 1986. Current topical corticosteroid preparations. *J Am Acad Dermatol* **14**:79–93.

Tonnesen MG, Harrist TJ, Wintroub BU, et al. 1983. Erythema multiforme: Microvascular damage and infiltration of lymphocytes and basophils. *J Invest Dermatol* **80**:282–6.

Tsao H, Rogers GS, Sober AJ. 1998. An estimate of the annual direct cost of treating cutaneous melanoma. *J Am Acad Dermatol* **38**:669–80.

Tucker SB, Rogers RS, Winkelmann RK, et al. 1980. Inflammation in acne vulgaris leukocyte attraction and cytotoxicity by comedonal material. *J Invest Dermatol* **74**:21–5.

Van de Kerkhof PC. 1996. Reduction of epidermal abnormalities and inflammatory changes in psoriatic plaques during treatment with vitamin $D_3$ analogs [review]. *J Invest Dermatol Symp Proc.* **1**(Apr):78–81.

Van Scott EJ, Ekel TM. 1963. Kinetics of hyperplasia in psoriasis. *Arch Dermatol* **88**:373–80.

Walters BNJ, Gubbay SS. 1981. Tetracycline and benign intracranial hypertension: Report of five cases. *Br Med J* **282**:19–20.

Webster GF, Leyden JJ. 1980. Characterization of serum independent polymorphonuclear leukocyte chemotactic factors produced by *Propionibacterium acnes*. *Inflammation* **4**:261–9.

Webster GF, Leyden JJ, Nilsson UR. 1979. Complement activation in acne vulgaris: Consumption of complement by comedones. *Infect Immun* **26**:183–6.

Webster GF, Tsai CC, Leyden JJ. 1979. Neutrophil lysosomal release in response to *Propionibacterium acnes* [abstract]. *J Invest Dermatol* **72**:209.

Weinstein GD. 1997. Tazarotene gel: Efficacy and safety in plaque psoriasis. *J Am Acad Dermatol* **37**:S33–S38.

Weinstein GD, Frost P. 1968. Abnormal cell proliferation in psoriasis. *J Invest Dermatol* **50**:254–59.

Wester RC, Noonan PK, Maibach HI. 1977. Frequency of application on percutaneous absorption of hydrocortisone. *Arch Dermatol* **113**:620–2.

Whyte HJ, Baughman RD. 1964. Acute guttate psoriasis and streptococcal infection. *Arch Dermatol* **89**:350–6.

Wilson L, Williams DI, Marsh SD. 1973. Plasma corticosteroid levels in outpatients treated with topical steroids. *Br J Dermatol* **88**: 373–80.

Wolff HH, Plewig G, Braun-Falco O. 1975. Ultrastructure of human sebaceous follicles and comedones following treatment with vitamin A acid. *Acta Derm Venereol Suppl (Stockh)* **55**:90–110.

Wolff K, Stingl G. 1983. The Langerhans cell. *J Invest Dermatol* **80**(Suppl):17S–21S.

Wolkenstein P, Revuz J. 1995. Drug-induced severe skin reactions: incidence, management and prevention. *Drug Saf* **13**:56–68.

Wuepper KD, Watson PA, Kazmierowski JA. 1980. Immune complexes in erythema multiforme and the Stevens-Johnson syndrome. *J Invest Dermatol* **74**:368–71.

Yancy KB, Lawley TJ. 1984. Circulating immune complexes: Their immunochemistry, biology, and detection in selected dermatologic and systemic diseases. *J Am Acad Dermatol* **10**:711–31.

Yeong D, Nacht S, Bucks D, et al. 1983. Benzoyl peroxide: Percutaneous penetration and metabolic disposition: II. Effect of concentration. *J Am Acad Dermatol* **9**:920–4.

CHAPTER

# 12 HEMATOLOGIC DISORDERS

Richard Lin, Zhuo-Wei Hu

## Chapter Outline



## HEMATOPOIETIC ABNORMALITIES AND THEIR TREATMENT

### Overview of Hematopoiesis

Blood cells have one of the highest turnover rates of the many cell types in the human body. Red cells (erythrocytes) are subjected to mechanical and oxidant stresses that lead to their destruction as they travel through the circulation. Erythrocytes also need to be replaced following an episode of bleeding. Granulocytes are constantly needed to defend the body against invading microorganisms, especially in the gastrointestinal tract and skin. Granulocytes are destroyed during this process and need to be replaced continually. Lymphocytes perform complex immunologic functions that require selective amplification or downregulation of subsets of lymphocytes in response to physiologic demands. Finally, platelets are consumed during the process of coagulation and need to be replenished to maintain integrity of the vasculature.

Many hematologic diseases are caused by abnormalities in the hematopoietic process. Decreased or ineffective erythropoiesis leads to various anemias. Monoclonal proliferation of a myeloid progenitor cell in the myelopoietic process leads to myelogenous leukemias and myeloproliferative disorders. Monoclonal proliferation of a lymphoid progenitor cell leads to lymphocytic leukemias and lymphomas. Abnormalities in the megakaryocytic line can lead to either thrombocytopenia or thrombocythemia depending on the defect.

#### *Hematopoietic stem cells*

The bone marrow contains pluripotent stem cells that are present in very small numbers, capable of self-renewal, and able to differentiate into any one of the four blood cell lines, i.e., myeloid, lymphoid, erythroid, or megakaryocytic cell lines (Ogawa 1993). Hematopoiesis is a multistep differentiation process that directs the stem cell toward the production of one or more blood cell lineages (Fig. 12-1). The stem cells first give rise to hematopoietic progenitor cells. Compared with stem cells, these cells have decreased capacity for self-renewal and are more committed to differentiating into a particular blood cell type. With each generation, the descendants of progenitor cells differentiate into more mature cells with a limited life span and become restricted to a particular blood cell lineage. Ultimately, the process ends with mature cells, which have no further capacity to divide and give rise to red cells, leukocytes, and platelets.

Recently, murine stem cells have been experimentally separated from other cells in the bone marrow (Spangrude et al. 1991). During the early 1950s, it was discovered that shielding of murine spleen cells from irradiation or infusion of genetically identical bone marrow cells could protect mice from lethal irradiation. These initial studies indicated that viable cells from spleen or marrow could circulate in the blood and repopulate an ablated marrow and thus restore blood cell production. The recovery of marrow and blood counts of these irradiated animals after these transplants led to intensive investigation to identify the nature of hematopoietic stem cells.

The functional definition of a true hematopoietic stem cell is the ability to renew itself, to differentiate, and to restore all hematopoietic lineages following lethal irradi-

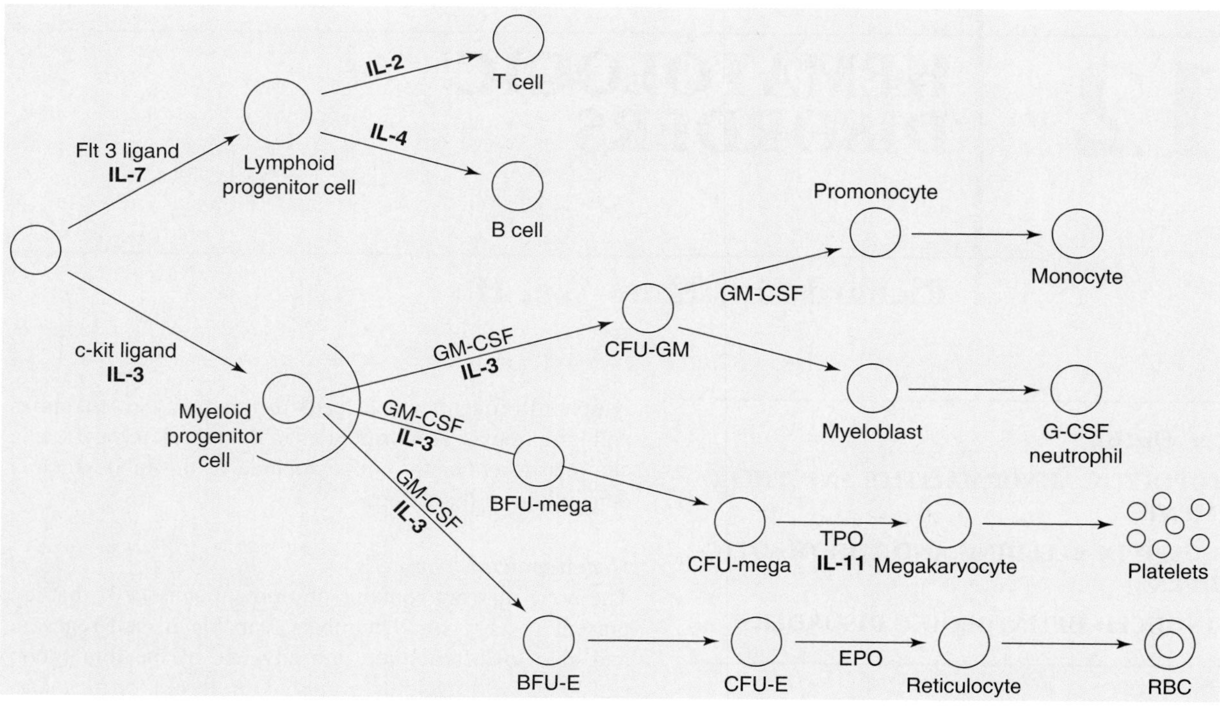


**FIGURE 12-1 Hematopoiesis and hematopoitic growth factors. The action of interleukins IL-2,3,4,7,11 and other hematopoietic growth factors is shown schematically. Abbreviations: BFU-E, burst-forming unit–erythroid; BFU-Mega, BFU-Megakaryocyte; CFU-E, colony-forming unit–erythroid; CFU-GM, colony-forming unit–granulocyte/macrophage; CFU-Mega, CFU-Megakaryocyte; EPO, erythropoietin; G-granulocyte; GM-, granulocyte/macrophage; M-, macrophage; GM-CSF, G-CSF, M-CSF colony-stimulating factors; RBC, red blood cell; TPO, thrombopoietin.**

ation. Incredibly small numbers of these stem cells, as few as 1 cell per mouse, can reconstitute a lethally irradiated recipient. It has been estimated that in the normal mouse, the number of pluripotent stem cells is between 1000 and 20,000, of which only about 20 stem cells are needed to support hematopoiesis at any one time. Based on these mouse experiments, the number of stem cells in humans is estimated to be between 25 and 500 million, and at any one time, only a small fraction of these cells are necessary to support hematopoiesis.

There are no distinctive morphologic features to identify a stem cell, because these are nondescript, small to medium-sized round mononuclear cells. The identification of stem cells was facilitated by the discovery of a surface antigen termed *CD34* that is common to stem cells. This antigen is expressed on all pluripotent stem cells and all committed hematopoietic progenitor cells. This discovery made it possible to rapidly identify a subset of CD34 cells that are murine stem cells. Although identification of stem cells is not as advanced in human studies, anti-CD34 antibody detection and flow cytometry have been used for enrichment of a population containing stem cells for transplantation following marrow ablative therapy.

Pluripotent stem cells can be harvested from peripheral blood as well as the bone marrow. This suggests that the stem cells may respond to environmental demands for differentiation and replication when circulating through the vasculature and also may wait in the bone marrow for humoral signals to respond. This stem cell circulation might also explain how infusions of bone marrow stem cells into the peripheral blood can lead to engraftment of the bone marrow during bone marrow transplantation and may also explain how leukemic cells are invariably found throughout the bone marrow.

Selective cultivation of bone marrow or peripheral blood in an appropriate medium can lead to the growth of discrete colonies containing cells having the morphology of phagocytes or of erythroid or megakaryocytic cells arising from particular committed stem cells. The relevance of these culture systems to hematopoiesis in humans and in experimental animals was evident from the fact that the presence, absence, or relative number of the

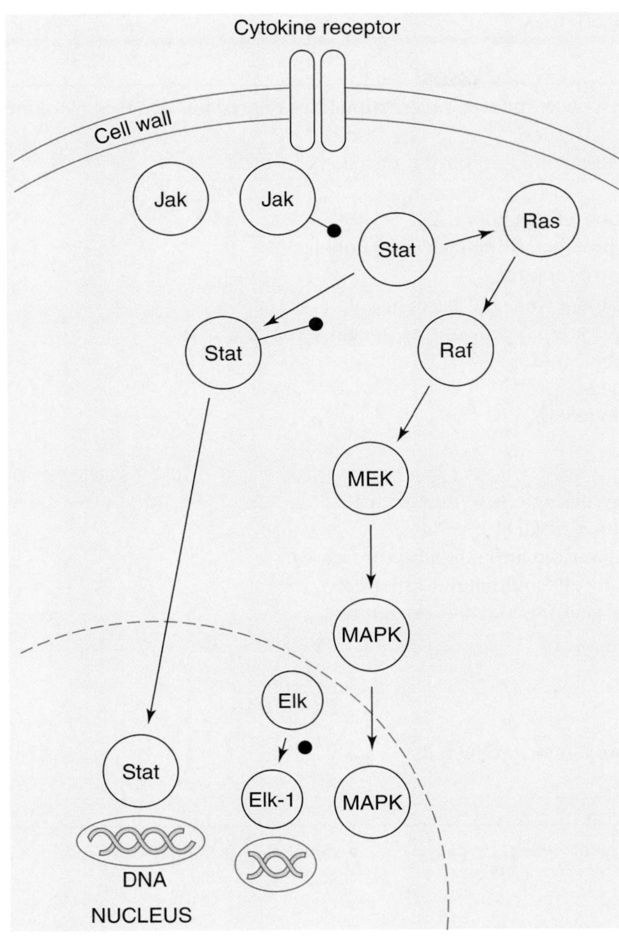


**F I G U R E 1 2 - 2 Cytokine signal transduction. Abbreviations: JAK, the Janus family of tyrosine kinase; MAPK, mitogen-activated protein; (MAP)kinase; MEK, Map-kinase kinase; STAT, protein, signal transducer and activator of transcription; within nucleus of cell; elk, elk-1, transcription factors of the ets family.**

colonies that can be obtained often changes in conjunction with alterations in the production of blood cells in the intact organism. Subsequently, humoral factors were isolated and shown to stimulate growth of particular blood cell colonies in vitro and later in animals. These humoral factors are named *hematopoietic growth factors*. Highly purified growth factors have been produced by recombinant molecular biology techniques, and their activity has been demonstrated in human studies.

### *Hematopoietic growth factors*

A hematopoietic growth factor is a molecule that regulates the proliferation or differentiation of hematopoietic cells. Some growth factors are now believed to act predominantly at early stages of hematopoiesis and others at later stages. Growth factors are also called *cytokines* (bioactive molecules secreted by cells). Although Fig. 12-1 depicts the growth factors acting on hematopoietic cells at a particular stage within a specific lineage, this represents the predominant effect of the particular hematopoietic growth factor. Physiologically, hematopoietic growth factors can have multiple effects on different hematopoietic progenitor cells, and there is also a great deal of redundancy and cross-regulation among these growth factors. Most hematopoietic cells are produced by many cell types including macrophages, fibroblasts, and lymphocytes. However, under physiologic conditions most growth factors are probably synthesized by marrow stroma cells.

A large number of cytokines and their receptors have been cloned and found to induce or inhibit the survival, proliferation, and differentiation of hematopoietic progenitors (Metcalf 1993). After binding to their receptors, cytokines increase cell proliferation by activating intracellular second messengers such as the Ras/MAPK or Jak/STAT signaling pathways (Fig. 12-2). These molecules then translocate to the nucleus and stimulate transcription of target genes and induce cell proliferation. Aside from cytokine-dependent signals, adhesive interactions between progenitors and stromal cells or extracellular matrix components also affect cell growth. Hematopoietic progenitors adhere to other stromal cells via cell surface-expressed adhesive ligands such as vascular cell adhesion molecule (VCAM-1) and adhere to extracellular components such as fibronectin via cell surface adhesion receptors such as $\beta_1$-integrins. Aside from anchoring progenitors in the microenvironment, the engagement of adhesion receptors also activates growth modulatory signals. It is now believed that the concerted action of cytokines and adhesive signals results in normal hematopoiesis (Coulombel et al. 1997).

### *Clinical use of hematopoietic growth factors: The colony-stimulating factors*

At least 20 hematopoietic growth factors have been cloned, and corresponding recombinant proteins have been produced (Table 12-1). All these factors can potentially be used in a therapeutic setting. At present, four recombinant growth factors have been approved for clinical use in humans; erythropoietin, granulocyte-colony-stimulating factor (G-CSF), granulocyte-macrophage colony-stimulating factors (GM-CSF), and interleukin-11 (IL-11). The clinical use of erythropoietin and IL-11 will be discussed later in this chapter. The FDA-approved indications for GM-CSF and G-CSF are relatively narrow; GM-CSF for marrow engraftment after bone marrow

Table 12-1 **Hematopoietic Growth Factors and Their Activities**

| FACTOR | ACTIVITIES AND EFFECTS |
|---|---|
| Interleukin-1 | Major regulator of inflammatory response, induces fever, stimulates expression of other cytokines. |
| Interleukin-2 | Stimulates T-cell proliferation and activation. |
| Interleukin-3 | Multilineage growth factor including myeloid erythroid, megakaryocytic. |
| Interleukin-4 | Costimulates B-cell proliferation. |
| Interleukin-5 | Stimulates proliferation and activation of eosinophils. |
| Interleukin-6 | Induces production of acute-phase proteins. Stimulates hematopoiesis. |
| Interleukin-7 | Stimulates lymphocyte progenitor proliferation. |
| Interleukin-8 | A chemokine for neutrophils, T lymphocytes, and basophils. |
| Interleukin-9 | Promotes growth of helper T cells, erythroid progenitors, megakaryocytes. |
| Interleukin-10 | An immunosuppressive factor, inhibits IL-2. |
| Interleukin-11 | Induces production of megakaryocytes. |
| Interleukin-12 | Has antitumor effects; inhibits angiogenesis. |
| Interleukin-13 | B-cell growth and differentiation. |
| Interleukin-14 | B-cell growth. |
| Interleukin-15 | A T-cell growth factor; shares many biologic activities with IL-2. |
| Interleukin-16 | Stimulates accumulation and activation of CD4+ cells. |
| Interleukin-17 | A T-cell-secreted factor involved in various inflammatory processes. |
| Interleukin-18 | Induces interferon-$\gamma$ production in T cells and natural killer cells. |
| GM-CSF | Multilineage growth factor, myeloid and monocytoid progenitors. |
| G-CSF | Neutrophil growth factor. |
| M-CSF | Monocyte growth factor. |
| Stem cell factor (c-kit ligand) | Stem cell proliferation. |
| Flt-3 ligand | Stem cell proliferation, lymphoid progenitor production. |
| Erythropoietin | Erythroid progenitor proliferation. |
| Thrombopoietin | A regulator of platelet production. |

Abbreviations: G-CSF, granulocyte colony-stimulating factor; GM-CSF, granulocyte-macrophage colony-stimulating factor; M-CSF, macrophage colony-stimulating factor.

transplantation and G-CSF for neutrophil recovery following myelosuppressive chemotherapy for nonmyeloid malignancies (Welte et al. 1996). However, both agents are actually widely used in a variety of settings (Table 12-2).

Pharmacologic doses of G-CSF and GM-CSF have dramatic stimulatory effects on neutrophil production. However, their specific physiologic roles in the normal regulation of myelopoiesis are not clearly defined. G-CSF and GM-CSF also enhance the functional responsiveness of mature neutrophils to inflammatory signals. G-CSF acts only on hematopoietic cells that are committed to become neutrophils, so it is relatively more lineage-specific than GM-CSF, which can also stimulate macrophages.

Both G-CSF and GM-CSF shorten the period of neutropenia after cytotoxic chemotherapy and bone marrow transplantation. This decreases the probability of infection, although this has been difficult to demonstrate in clinical trials. These growth factors decrease the length of hospital stays and probably reduce utilization of resources.

Recombinant G-CSF or GM-CSF administered intravenously or subcutaneously raises the absolute neutrophil count within 14 hours. When the drug is stopped, the absolute neutrophil count decreases by half within 24 hours and returns to baseline within 1 to 7 days. The response to these factors is decreased in patients who have been treated extensively with radiation or chemotherapy, because they have a reduced number of progenitor cells that can respond to growth factors.

Table 12-2 **Clinical Use of Colony-Stimulating Factors**

| FACTOR | CLINICAL USE |
|---|---|
| GM-CSF | Post-BMT hematopoietic reconstitution |
| | Postchemotherapy neutrophil recovery |
| | Aplastic anemia |
| | AIDS-related myelosuppression |
| | Myelodysplastic syndrome |
| G-CSF | Peripheral blood stem cell harvesting |
| | Cyclic neutropenia |

Abbreviations: BMT, bone marrow transplantation; G-CSF, granulocyte colony-stimulating factor; GM-CSF, granulocyte-macrophage colony-stimulating factor.

Granulocyte-CSF is usually better tolerated than GM-CSF. Although the administration of both may cause bone pain, GM-CSF therapy can rarely cause a pulmonary capillary leak syndrome with pulmonary edema and heart failure. Treatment with GM-CSF, unlike G-CSF, may also cause constitutional symptoms including fever, headache, and malaise.

## Hypoproliferative Anemia

Deficiencies in erythropoiesis can lead to anemia. At sea level, anemia should be suspected in an adult when the hematocrit is less then 41% in men and less than 37% in women. The absolute reticulocyte count is low in patients with hypoproliferative anemia. In contrast, hyperproliferative anemia is due to increased peripheral destruction of red blood cells (RBCs), and the absolute reticulocyte count is high. The most common cause of hypoproliferative anemia in the world is iron deficiency. Other causes of hypoproliferative anemia include folate or vitamin $B_{12}$ deficiency, chronic renal failure, cancer, inflammatory diseases such as rheumatoid arthritis, endocrine hormone deficiency, sideroblastic anemia, and bone marrow failure.

Treatment of anemia is often directed at addressing the underlying causative illness such as bleeding or an infection. However, three nutritional deficiencies and one hormonal deficiency can lead to the development of hypoproliferative anemia requiring specific pharmacologic intervention, i.e., iron, vitamin $B_{12}$, folate, and erythropoietin deficiency, respectively.

***Overview of erythropoiesis***

Erythrocytes are the oxygen-carrying cells of the blood. Like all blood cells, erythrocytes are derived from hematopoietic stem cells in the bone marrow. The earliest red cell progenitor is called the *burst-forming unit–erythroid* (BFU-E), which gives rise to a more differentiated progenitor cell, colony-forming unit–erythroid (CFU-E). These progenitor cells are not recognizable by conventional microscopy. The most primitive morphologically recognizable red cell precursor is the pronormoblast, which gives rise to the basophilic, polychromatophilic, and orthochromatic normoblasts, in order of maturation. Unlike its precursor cells, the orthochromatic normoblast cannot divide, and these cells further differentiate into reticulocytes, which have extruded their nucleus. However, the reticulocytes still contain residual RNA in their cytoplasm and can be distinguished from a mature red cell. It takes approximately 5 days for a pronormoblast to become a red cell and to enter the circulation. Once in the bloodstream, the red cell lives for about 4 months or 120 days.

Erythropoiesis is a tightly regulated process with the fraction of the blood volume occupied by red cells (hematocrit) maintained in the vicinity of 40% to 45%. Red cell production is controlled by several growth factors. However, once the stem cell has been committed to the red cell line, the erythroid progenitor cells are under the control of a glycoprotein hormone called *erythropoietin.*

***Erythropoietin***

The hormone erythropoietin is primarily produced by the peritubular capillary-lining cells in the kidney (Koury 1988) with a small fraction made by the liver. The production of erythropoietin is inversely related to renal oxygen tension. Hypoxia is the fundamental physiologic stimulus that causes a rapid increase in renal production of erythropoietin through an exponential increase in the number of erythropoietin-producing cells. However, factors other than tissue hypoxia might be involved in the regulation of erythropoietin production. Abnormally high erythropoietin levels have been observed in patients with aplastic anemia, and dramatic changes in serum levels have been described after chemotherapy and during vitamin $B_{12}$ or iron replacement therapy. These findings point to an inverse relationship between RBC precursor mass and serum erythropoietin level: the higher the number of RBC precursors, the lower the erythropoietin level.

Inflammatory cytokines may interfere with erythropoietin gene expression. Interleukin-1 (IL-1), tumor necrosis factor (TNF), and transforming growth factor (TGF) have been found to inhibit hypoxia-induced erythropoietin production in vitro. These cytokines also inhibit erythroid progenitor cell proliferation, thus playing a major role in the pathogenesis of the anemia of chronic inflammation (Rafael 1997). Increased plasma viscosity inhibits erythropoietin formation, thus contributing to anemia in both inflammation and monoclonal gammopathies.

Chemotherapeutic agents blunt the erythropoietin response. Cisplatin appears to be particularly toxic, causing a prolonged anemia. Cyclosporin A (cyclosporine) also attenuates the production of erythropoietin and may contribute to the anemia of patients undergoing organ transplantation. Finally, direct suppression of erythropoietin formation by human immunodeficiency virus (HIV) has been observed in vitro, suggesting that this may have a role in the pathogenesis of HIV-related anemia.

Erythropoietin exerts its effects by binding to a surface receptor present on erythroid progenitors and precursors (Fisher 1997). Although only a few receptors (<100/cell) are found on early BFU-Es, their number increases with differentiation and peaks at about 1100 receptors per cell on CFU-Es and pronormoblasts. Receptor expression then decreases with erythroid maturation, and almost undetectable levels are observed on reticulocytes. Evidence has shown that erythropoietin acts mainly as a survival factor. Recent studies on gene knockout mice have shown that erythropoietin is crucial in vivo for the proliferation and survival of CFU-Es, whereas it is not required for generation of BFU-Es and their differentiation to CFU-Es. Erythropoiesis can be substantially and steadily expanded only through preamplification of erythropoietin-dependent progenitor cells. Administering erythropoietin to normal individuals triggers premature expulsion of immature reticulocytes from the bone marrow into the circulation, followed by a slow increase in hemoglobin level.

These experimental results are highly relevant to the clinical use of recombinant erythropoietin. When endogenous erythropoietin levels are inappropriately low for the degree of anemia, administration of erythropoietin effectively increases the amount of hormone reaching the bone marrow, allowing survival of more red cell progenitors and output of more RBCs. Pharmacologic doses of the erythroid hormone can also expand erythropoiesis in normal individuals by preventing the programmed death of a few additional red cell progenitors. However, when the endogenous plasma level of erythropoietin is adequate for the degree of anemia, the amount of hormone circulating within the bone marrow may be saturated so that nearly all available marrow erythroid progenitors will survive. In this situation, it is very unlikely that pharmacologic doses of erythropoietin can further increase the exposure of erythroid progenitors to erythropoietin and expand erythropoiesis.

#### CLINICAL INDICATIONS FOR USE OF ERYTHROPOIETIN

The only disease in which a deficiency of a hematopoietic growth factor is clearly the cause is the anemia of renal failure. The kidneys do not produce adequate erythropoietin in these patients, and erythropoietin injections correct the anemia. Recombinant human erythropoietin is now a standard treatment for the anemia of chronic renal failure.

Erythropoietin, 150 units/kg of patient's body weight three times a week, will correct the anemia in 80% of patients with anemia of renal failure, and some of the unresponsive cases can benefit from higher doses. Treatment efficacy should be assessed by measuring hemoglobin and reticulocyte counts after 4 weeks. After 4 weeks of treatment, if the hemoglobin increase is less than 1 g/dL or reticulocyte count is $<40 \times 10^9$/L, the dosage should be increased (e.g., it may be doubled). When the desired response is achieved, dose adjustments should be performed to maintain the hemoglobin within the optimal range for each individual patient, based on subjective and objective benefits and treatment costs.

Several clinical trials have shown that erythropoietin treatment can also be effective in patients with disease states other than uremia. Patients with anemia due to chronic inflammation such as rheumatoid arthritis, inflammatory bowel disease, chronic infection, and AIDS have been treated with erythropoietin with some success (Cazzola et al. 1997). Erythropoietin has been used also in patients with anemia due to cancer and chemotherapy. As discussed previously, treatment with erythropoietin is likely to be most effective when the endogenous plasma level of erythropoietin is inadequate for the degree of anemia. Therefore, assessment of endogenous erythropoietin levels is a critical step before making the decision to initiate recombinant erythropoietin therapy.

The serum erythropoietin level has become a routine diagnostic test with the availability of commercial immunoassays for serum erythropoietin. Serum erythropoietin levels in normal individuals are in the range of 5 to 30 mU/mL. However, levels found in anemic patients cannot be simply compared with normal values. In fact, as long as the erythropoietin-generating apparatus in the kidney is competent, serum levels increase exponentially as the hematocrit decreases (Fig. 12-3). Serum erythropoietin level must therefore be evaluated in relation to the degree of anemia. The definition of defective erythropoietin production relies on a low serum erythropoietin level com-

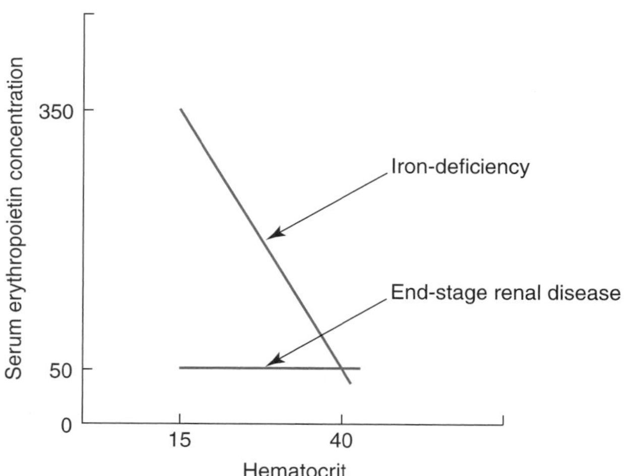


**FIGURE 12-3 Serum erythropoietin concentration correlates with hematocrit increase exponentially with decreasing hematocrit. The graphs are theoretical and not based on actual data points.**

pared with reference patients with similar hemoglobin levels. With the exception of patients with anemia due to renal failure, serum erythropoietin levels should be obtained from all anemic patients before erythropoietin therapy.

At present, the FDA has approved the use of erythropoietin in the treatment of anemia in HIV-infected patients with erythropoietin levels less than 500 mU/mL. A recent study suggests that erythropoietin treatment improves not only anemia associated with AIDS but also survival in these patients (Moore et al. 1998). Erythropoietin is also approved for treatment of anemia induced by chemotherapy of nonmyeloid malignancies. It is indicated for reduction of allogeneic blood transfusions in surgery patients at high risk for significant perioperative blood loss.

Recombinant erythropoietin is safe and effective in stimulating erythropoiesis and allowing preoperative donation of blood for autologous use in patients who were previously unable to deposit blood preoperatively because of anemia. The combined use of subcutaneous erythropoietin with intravenous iron is highly effective in autologous blood donation. One study has shown that erythropoietin with iron saccharate infusion facilitated the donation of autologous blood and reduced perioperative homologous blood transfusions in anemic patients with cancer (Braga et al. 1995).

A variety of dosages and administration schedules have been used for erythropoietin outside the uremia setting. Reported doses (from 150 to >1000 IU/kg per week) are clearly higher than those effective in renal anemia, indicating that erythropoietin is not just a replacement therapy in these situations. Besides endogenous erythropoietin levels, additional factors determine the amount of erythropoietin required to expand erythropoiesis. A major factor is residual marrow function, which can be estimated from the platelet count and transfusion requirement. Concomitant chemotherapy is also a crucial variable.

**ROUTE OF ADMINISTRATION AND DOSING INTERVAL FOR ERYTHROPOIETIN** There are substantial differences between intravenous and subcutaneous administration of recombinant erythropoietin. Subcutaneous administration of erythropoietin induces lower peak plasma erythropoietin concentrations, with an elimination half-life of about 19 to 22 hours versus the 4 to 5 hours with intravenous erythropoietin. Subcutaneous administration of smaller doses of erythropoietin more closely resembles the physiology of erythropoietin production and leads to greater efficacy than intravenous administration of larger doses. Therefore, erythropoietin should routinely be administered subcutaneously.

The optimal interval between erythropoietin doses has not been established. A recent report suggests that in normal subjects treated with intravenous iron, an interval of 72 hours between two doses of erythropoietin induces a higher reticulocyte response than a 24-hour interval (Breymann et al. 1996).

**ADVERSE EFFECTS OF ERYTHROPOIETIN** Erythropoietin is remarkably well tolerated. Adverse reactions have been described mainly in chronic renal failure, with development of hypertension and seizures. Outside of this clinical setting, there are no reports of significant adverse effects. Aggravation of splenomegaly has been occasionally observed in myeloproliferative disorders. Although erythropoietin may slightly increase platelet counts in occasional patients, no significant changes in any hemostatic variable can be shown in the vast majority of treated individuals.

### *Iron*

The developing red blood cell must make a large amount of hemoglobin. The synthesis of the hemoglobin molecule requires the production of four molecules of the oxygen-binding compound heme. The developing normoblast has everything required to make heme except iron. For the daily production of new erythrocytes, about 15 mg of iron is needed. The primary source of this iron requirement is met by recycling the iron from destroyed senescent red cells. However, a small but critical fraction is obtained from the diet. Daily excretion of iron primarily through the gastrointestinal tract is approximately 1 mg. Lack of iron for hemoglobin synthesis would limit erythropoiesis, because the availability of iron critically regulates the rate of red cell production.

To be available for hemoglobin synthesis, iron must be bound to the iron transport protein, transferrin. The iron–transferrin complex circulates in plasma and binds to transferrin receptors on the surface of developing erythroid cells in the bone marrow. Internalization of the iron–transferrin complex by receptor-mediated endocytosis is followed by cleavage of iron from the transferrin complex in acidic vesicles (endosomes) within the erythroid cell; the receptor subsequently returns the transferrin molecule to the cell surface, where it is released into the extracellular compartment. Within the erythroid cell, iron is either incorporated into heme or forms a complex with apoferritin to create ferritin. The latter mechanism is utilized when iron requirements for hemoglobin are exceeded. In patients with very high levels of transferrin saturation, such as those with iron overload or hemochromatosis, there is increased transfer of iron into parenchymal cells.

In individuals who do not have an active inflammatory disease, the plasma ferritin level reflects total-body iron stores. Ferritin production increases in response to increased cellular content of iron. In healthy males, the average plasma ferritin level is approximately 100 ng/mL. In healthy premenopausal females, it is approximately 30 ng/mL. This gender difference disappears after menopause. Iron-deficient patients will have low ferritin levels unless they have a concurrent process that can raise the serum ferritin level such as infection or liver disease. Iron-deficient patients also have a low serum iron level and a high total iron-binding capacity (TIBC). Microcytosis on the peripheral blood smear is a late finding. Clinically significant iron deficiency can occur before development of anemia. In a randomized clinical trial, iron replacement in young women with iron deficiency without anemia resulted in improved mental function (Bruner et al. 1996).

Oral iron should be administered in a fasting state and given with juice containing ascorbic acid to maximize absorption. Although vitamin C increases the absorption of dietary iron, it probably does not affect the absorption of pharmacologic doses of iron (Bendich and Cohen 1990), and therefore routine use of vitamin C supplement with iron treatment is not justified by the additional cost. At the acidic pH of the stomach, mucin binds to inorganic iron and enhances iron absorption. Consequently, antacids or other medications that reduce stomach acid production may interfere with optimal absorption of iron. Commercial preparations of ferrous sulfate usually contain 60 mg of elemental iron, and only 10 to 20% of ingested iron is absorbed by iron-deficient patients. The optimal dose is 180 mg of elemental iron per day. Patients optimally treated with 180 mg of elemental iron a day will increase hemoglobin concentration by about 1 g/dL per week. Iron supplementation should continue for 6 months after the hemoglobin level has normalized to replenish the body's iron stores.

The most common complaint by those taking iron is gastrointestinal irritation. Sometimes this can be very bothersome. If patients cannot tolerate ferrous sulfate tablets, using liquid iron preparations at a lower dose and gradually escalating the frequency of administration may be better tolerated. A polysaccharide–iron complex preparation is available that causes less gastrointestinal irritation but is more expensive. Parenteral iron is available if patients truly cannot tolerate oral iron.

Iron dextran is the intravenous form of iron available in the United States. Intravenous administration of iron dextran is preferable to the intramuscular route, which is often painful and may cause a discoloration at the injection site. Intravenous iron dextran needs to be administered slowly under close monitoring, because it may cause hypotension and anaphylactoid reactions. A test dose should be given before the administration of a therapeutic dose to make certain that an anaphylactoid reaction does not occur. Iron saccharate is approved in Europe, and this may be the preferred iron preparation (Sunder-Plassmann and Horl 1997). Allergic reactions to this preparation of intravenous iron are very rare.

Iron replacement causes a prompt rise in reticulocyte counts. The hemoglobin concentration of patients who are optimally treated with 180 mg/day of elemental iron increases by about 1 g/dL per week. If the reticulocyte count does not respond, the diagnosis of iron deficiency may be incorrect, or there may also be a concurrent process preventing the production of red cells.

***Functional iron deficiency during erythropoietin treatment***

Patients receiving erythropoietin should be closely monitored for possible iron-deficient erythropoiesis. Administration of erythropoietin in excess of functionally available iron will lead to iron-deficient erythropoiesis, diminished erythroid marrow response, and a waste of this costly drug.

Two different patterns of iron-deficient erythropoiesis may develop with erythropoietin administration. True iron deficiency may develop during chronic erythropoietin administration because of a progressive shift of iron from body stores to the red cells. The term *functional* or *relative iron deficiency* is used to define a situation in which the body iron stores are normal (or even increased) but the iron supply to the bone marrow is inadequate in active erythropoiesis. Functional iron deficiency, or iron-restricted erythropoiesis, appears in the initial phase of erythropoietin administration in subjects with normal iron stores. It is noteworthy that subjects with increased body iron stores and elevated transferrin saturation, particularly those with hereditary hemochromatosis, show no signs of functional iron deficiency and demonstrate a better response to erythropoietin. Functional iron deficiency has been found to be a frequent cause of poor response to erythropoietin.

An impaired iron supply to the erythroid marrow is indicated by a low transferrin saturation ($<20\%$). Serum ferritin levels less than 100 $\mu$g/L are generally associated with insufficient amounts of readily exchangeable iron in the reticuloendothelial cells and may be regarded as predictive of functional iron deficiency with erythropoietin treatment. Using an automated cell counter, it is possible to obtain the percentage of hypochromic RBCs (defined as an individual cell hemoglobin concentration $<28$ g/dL). These are normally lower than 2.5% of all RBCs. An increase to greater than 10% during erythropoietin therapy would indicate the development of functional iron deficiency and the need for more intensive iron supplementation. Any patient receiving erythropoietin treatment with transferrin saturation $<20\%$, serum ferritin $<100$ $\mu$g/L, or $>10\%$ hypochromic RBCs should be promptly considered for more aggressive intravenous iron supplementation therapy.

Iron supplementation should be administered routinely during the first 4 to 6 weeks of erythropoietin treatment to all patients except those with increased serum iron and transferrin saturation levels. Although iron absorption can increase severalfold when erythropoietin is used, oral iron supplementation may still be insufficient to match iron demands by the erythropoietin-expanded erythroid marrow. A randomized placebo-controlled trial showed that in iron-replete patients on hemodialysis treated with erythropoietin for anemia, concomitant treatment with intravenous iron significantly enhanced the hemoglobin response (Macdougall et al. 1996). In contrast, patients receiving oral ferrous sulfate, like the placebo-treated group, did not show improved hemoglobin response. This suggests that, even in iron-replete patients, supplementation with intravenous iron is better for maintaining iron balance, enhancing the hemoglobin response to erythropoietin, and lowering dosage requirements of erythropoietin when compared with oral iron and no iron supplementation.

***Megaloblastic anemia***

Deficiency of vitamin $B_{12}$ (cobalamin) and folate leads to megaloblastic anemia. Vitamin $B_{12}$ or folate deficiency leads to changes in RBCs and hypersegmented (more than five lobes) neutrophils. Both cobalamin and folate are critical cofactors in enzymatic reactions required for DNA synthesis.

The cobalamins are a group of molecules of similar structure that consists of a nucleotide (5,6-dimethylbenzimidazole) connected to a porphyrinlike corrin ring, which contains a central cobalt atom. A ligand is attached to this central cobalt atom, and the various cobalamins differ only in this ligand. Vitamin $B_{12}$ is the name of a specific cobalamin in which cyanide is the ligand attached to the cobalt (cyanocobalamin). Because vitamin $B_{12}$ is stable, it is the cobalamin that is used pharmaceutically. However, vitamin $B_{12}$ is not found naturally in the human body. The two cobalamins found in humans are methylcobalamin and adenosylcobalamin.

The cobalamins are required in two metabolic reactions. One is the conversion of homocyst(e)ine to methionine in which the methylcobalamin is the coenzyme for homocysteinemethionine methyltransferase, which transfers a methyl group from methyltetrahydrofolate to homocysteine to make methionine. Folate compounds are required for DNA synthesis as carbon donors in the conversion of deoxyuridine to deoxythymidine. This interdependency of cobalamin and methylfolate may explain the similarity of morphologic changes when either cobalamin or folate is deficient. The second is the conversion of methyl malonyl-coenzyme A to succinyl-coenzyme A in which the adenosylcobalamin is the coenzyme for methyl malonyl CoA mutase.

***Vitamin $B_{12}$ deficiency and pernicious anemia***

Vitamin $B_{12}$ is readily absorbed from the gastrointestinal tract with the aid of intrinsic factor secreted by parietal cells in the stomach. The intrinsic factor–cobalamin complex is absorbed via receptors on the ileal cell surface. The daily requirement of vitamin $B_{12}$ is 0.6 to 1.2 $\mu$g. Because vitamin $B_{12}$ is widely available in animal products, dietary deficiency is an uncommon cause of vitamin $B_{12}$ deficiency. Because the biologic half-life of vitamin $B_{12}$ stored in the liver is about 1 year, more than 2 years must pass after complete cessation of vitamin $B_{12}$ intake before clinical manifestations of cobalamin deficiency become apparent.

The most common cause of $B_{12}$ deficiency is pernicious anemia, a form of gastric secretory failure with gastric atrophy and consequent failure to secrete intrinsic factor. Autoimmune destruction is strongly suspected as the cause of this disorder. Anti-parietal cell and anti-intrinsic factor antibodies are detected in many patients with pernicious anemia. A two-stage test, initially with radiolabeled $B_{12}$ alone and then with radiolabeled $B_{12}$ with intrinsic factor (Shilling's test), can be performed to determine whether vitamin $B_{12}$ deficiency is due to pernicious anemia.

Treatment of vitamin $B_{12}$ deficiency should be initiated with parental cyanocobalamin. In maintenance treatment of pernicious anemia, the recommended therapy is monthly injections of 1 mg of cyanocobalamin. However, oral therapy with 1 mg of vitamin $B_{12}$ five times a week has been shown to be equally effective. Despite the lack of intrinsic factor, absorption by mass action still functions and can fulfill the daily requirement of 2 to 5 $\mu g$ (Lederle 1991). The application of a vitamin $B_{12}$ gel intranasally (ENER-B gel) has been approved by the FDA for dietary supplementation but not for treatment of pernicious anemia, although this application does consistently raise serum $B_{12}$ levels. Megaloblastic anemia due to folate deficiency may be corrected by supraphysiologic doses of vitamin $B_{12}$, and conversely, large doses of folic acid can reverse megaloblastic anemia due to vitamin $B_{12}$ deficiency. However, unlike folate deficiency, vitamin $B_{12}$ deficiency may also cause neurologic deficits, with paresthesias being the earliest sign progressing to loss of vibratory sense, ataxia, dementia, and coma. The neurologic disease caused by vitamin $B_{12}$ deficiency is not reversed by folate supplementation.

***Folic acid***

Folates are found in a wide variety of fresh foods. Folate is rapidly destroyed by heating during food preparation. Folic acid is widely distributed in nature as a conjugate with one or more molecules of glutamic acid. Naturally occurring folates must be reduced to mono- and deglutinates by conjugases in the stomach before they can be efficiently absorbed from the proximal small intestines. Folates are transported to the liver, where they are stored and transformed into 5-methyltetrahydrofolate, which is the form that enters tissue cells.

The normal daily requirement of folate is about 100 $\mu g$. Tissue stores of folate are estimated at 10 mg. Therefore inadequate dietary folate intake will lead to megaloblastic anemia much sooner than vitamin $B_{12}$ deficiency. During pregnancy, the need for folate is markedly increased, and folate deficiency during this period is associated with congenital neural tube defects. Folate supplementation is recommended for all pregnant women. Ethanol abuse is one common cause of folate deficiency anemia because of reduced folate intake and diminished folate absorption. Because the concentration of folate in bile is several times that of plasma, biliary diversion will lead to a fall in plasma concentration of folate. Patients with prolonged biliary drainage should be given oral folate supplementation.

Serum homocyst(e)ine level is inversely correlated with serum folate levels. There is increasing strong evidence that an elevated serum homocyst(e)ine level is an independent risk factor for atherosclerosis. Clinical studies have shown that folate treatment can reduce homocyst(e)ine levels and potentially lower the risk of cardiovascular diseases in these patients (Stein and McBride 1998). However, a recent prospective study did not find an association between elevated homocyst(e)ine level and coronary heart disease (Folsom et al. 1998). Prospective randomized clinical trials are needed to determine whether homocyst(e)ine level is truly a major, independent causative risk factor for atherosclerosis.

Folate deficiency can be diagnosed by measuring serum or RBC folate levels. Folate deficiency responds promptly to treatment with 1 mg of folate given orally daily. An injectable form is available for patients not able to take anything by mouth or incapable of enteric absorption. Folates may correct the megaloblastic anemia of vitamin $B_{12}$ deficiency but will not correct the neurologic damage due to lack of vitamin $B_{12}$. Therefore indiscriminate use of folate may mask the symptoms of vitamin $B_{12}$ deficiency and lead to irreversible neurologic deficits.

## Sickle Cell Anemia

Normal adult hemoglobin consists of identical half molecules, each containing two different polypeptide chains. These are called *alpha* and *beta chains*. Over 90% of the hemoglobin of normal adult is Hb A. Fetal hemoglobin, Hb F, like Hb A, has two alpha chains but differs by having two gamma chains instead of two beta chains. The production of alpha chains begins during early fetal life. The production of gamma chains drops off shortly before birth and is replaced by the increasing production of beta chains. At birth, Hb F still makes up about 75% of the total hemoglobin, but the level of Hb F drops to below 5% by age 6 months. Hb F constitutes less than 1% of normal adult hemoglobin.

Sickle cell disease is caused by a point mutation in the gene of the beta chain resulting in an amino acid substitution of glutamate for valine. Hb S consists of two normal alpha chains and two abnormal beta chains. In RBCs containing large amounts of Hb S, there is an increased tendency of intracellular polymerization and gelation of hemoglobin molecules. This tendency is increased with deoxygenation of RBCs, initiating the formation of rigid and deformed cells. Such cells, called *sickle cells*, have a markedly shortened survival time and are unable to navigate their way normally through the microcirculation, resulting in a chronic hemolytic anemia and painful vascular occlusive crises.

Individuals with sickle cell trait who have one mutated beta gene and one normal beta gene essentially have no resultant clinical disease. Although extensive deoxygenation will cause the RBCs to sickle in vitro, the degree of deoxygenation resulting from passage of blood through the microcirculation does not lead to clinically significant sickling in humans. Epidemiologic studies have related the frequency of Hb S in a population to the exposure to malaria. Apparently, heterozygosity for Hb S increases an individual's chance for survival in a malaria-endemic region. As homozygosity produces severe disease with a decreased likelihood of having children, this survival advantage in heterozygotes may explain the persistence of this gene in this population. Results from recent murine models of sickle cell disease developed using the gene knockout mouse technology further support the theory that Hb S protects against malaria in vivo (Ryan et al. 1997).

The red blood cells of the patient homozygous for the gene for Hb S undergo continuous sickling (Ballas and Mohandas 1996). Sickle cell patients have an unrelenting, severe hemolytic anemia that begins within weeks of birth as Hb S replaces Hb F and lasts throughout life. Masses of sickled RBCs repeatedly plug vessels in the microcirculation leading to painful vascular occlusive crises. Repeated episodes of ischemic necrosis lead to progressive organ damage, beginning with the spleen, whose function may be impaired even in infancy and which shrivels into a small remnant later in childhood as a result of repeated infarcts. Infections are frequent in infants and children. Five to 10 percent of children or young adults experience major cerebral vascular accidents: strokes or hemorrhage resulting from stenosis or aneurysmal dilatation of major cerebral arteries. Patients are also prone to attacks of an acute chest syndrome characterized by fever, pleural pain, and cough. Patients with sickle cell disease have a significantly reduced life span.

Treatment of sickle cell disease in the past has been primarily supportive with intravenous fluids, oxygen, and analgesics for pain. Blood transfusions including partial exchange transfusions to replace greater than 50% of the patient's RBCs with normal RBCs are indicated in some circumstances, such as after a stroke to prevent further cerebrovascular episodes (Vichinsky et al. 1995). Recent pharmacologic maneuvers to increase Hb F levels in patients with sickle cell disease have proved to be an effective strategy to lessen the clinical severity of this illness.

***Treatment of sickle cell disease with hydroxyurea***

Fetal hemoglobin levels presently have been shown to favorably modify the clinical manifestations of patients with sickle cell disease and related conditions. Recent advances in the understanding of molecular and cellular pathophysiology of sickle cell disease, coupled with new insights into the developmental regulation of human globin gene expression, have provided the scientific impetus and clinical rationale to augment the postnatal production of fetal hemoglobin.

Despite its apparent genetic simplicity, sickle cell disease has long been appreciated to exhibit a wide variability of clinical severity. Some individuals die in infancy or early childhood, whereas others display only a modest decrease in expected longevity and manifest minimal to moderate symptoms. Perhaps the best understood modifying factor of disease severity is the expression of fetal hemoglobin in patients with sickle cell disease. From the earliest observation of the protective effect of high levels of Hb F on the clinical manifestations of newborns with sickle cell disease in large epidemiologic studies of sickle cell patients from central India and the eastern province of Saudi Arabia, a clear inverse relationship has been established between the severity of clinical manifestations and levels of Hb F.

The biophysical basis for the observed improvement in symptoms among patients with high Hb F levels can be explained by at least two mechanisms. Hb F when present inside sickle erythrocytes does not enter into the deoxy Hb S polymer phase. This characteristic, together with the simultaneous decrease in intracellular Hb S concentrations as Hb F levels increase, has been termed the *sparing* effect and provides the biophysical basis of the mild clinical phenotype observed in newborns and older patients with persistent postnatal Hb F levels.

The possibility of ameliorating the clinical symptoms of sickle cell disease raises the possibility of finding pharmacologic agents that would manipulate the level of Hb F. It was found in baboons that 5-azacytidine, a potent inhibitor of DNA methylation, increased Hb F levels to as high as 70 to 80%. In patients with sickle cell disease and $\beta$-thalassemia, treatment with 5-azacytidine also leads to an increase in Hb F levels. However, because of its carcinogenic potential and anticipated chronic administration to maintain elevated Hb F levels in sickle cell patients, other cytotoxic agents were sought that may have better therapeutic profiles.

Hydroxyurea, a chemotherapeutic agent in phase I trials, was found to raise the population of reticulocytes containing Hb F (F reticulocytes) and to stimulate a small rise in the Hb F level. Subsequently, a multicenter randomized, double-blind, placebo-controlled trial convincingly demonstrated the efficacy of hydroxyurea in decreasing painful crises in severely affected adults with sickle cell anemia (Charache et al. 1995). However, not all patients benefited from treatment, and crises were not eliminated in most patients. No serious toxicity was seen in the multicenter trial. The dosage of hydroxyurea was escalated slowly, the aim being to achieve a dose just below that which would produce significant cytopenia. Most patients received a final dose of 10 to 20 mg/kg of body weight per day. Hydroxyurea has been used in a wide variety of hematologic disorders and it is relatively well-tolerated. However, the use of cytotoxic drugs in a nonmalignant condition raises questions about the long-term safety regarding carcinogenesis and teratogenesis.

The number of pain crises correlates with the percentage rise in Hb F levels. The increase in Hb F in patients treated with hydroxyurea was variable, but patients with the best response can achieve a mean Hb F level of 18%. There is evidence to suggest that noncompliance is a major factor in the variability of Hb F levels in sickle cell patients treated with hydroxyurea.

In a multivariate analysis of the data, a drop in the neutrophil count also correlated with clinical improvement of sickle cell symptoms (Charache et al. 1997). Smaller studies have shown a relation between higher leukocyte counts with higher mortality and a higher frequency of the acute chest syndrome. Neutrophils have a number of cytotoxic effects. Inflammatory agents released by neutrophils in a vasoocclusive event may contribute to the severity of disease. Hydroxyurea may ameliorate sickle cell symptoms by reducing the number of leukocytes.

#### *Allogeneic bone marrow transplantation to treat sickle cell disease*

The only curative therapy for sickle cell disease is allogeneic bone marrow transplantation. However, the immediate life-threatening risks of the procedure must be balanced against its potential benefits. The use of bone marrow transplantation for hemoglobinopathies was first proposed in thalassemia major and is now the therapy of choice for young patients affected by this disorder and having a suitable donor. The natural course of sickle cell disease is relatively unpredictable compared with thalassemia major patients. The median life span of patients with sickle cell disease is between 40 and 50 years. Because allogeneic transplantation is best performed at a younger age to decrease the risk of graft-versus-host disease, death due to the transplant procedure could potentially shorten the life span by 30 or more years.

Selection criteria for allogeneic bone marrow transplantation are difficult to establish and vary among medical teams and their patients' characteristics. Some of the factors playing a role in the decision process include genetic and environmental factors, features of the patient such as age or the presence of organ damage, and the possibility of using new alternative therapeutic approaches.

Results from a multicenter collaborative investigation of bone marrow transplantation for sickle cell disease showed promising results (Walters et al. 1997). Thirty-four children less than 16 years of age with severe sickle cell disease were given transplants of marrow allografts from HLA-identical siblings. Indications for transplantation included a history of stroke, recurrent acute chest syndrome or sickle pulmonary disease, and recurrent vasoocclusive crises. Of the 34 patients, 32 survived, with a median follow-up of 26.5 months (range, 0.2 to 66.9 months); 28 patients demonstrated stable engraftment of donor hematopoietic cells. Graft rejection or recurrence of sickle cell disease occurred in four patients, and two patients died of intracranial hemorrhage or graft-versus-host disease.

## Hematologic Malignancies and Their Treatment

#### *Overview of hematologic malignancies*

The hematologic malignancies include the leukemias, lymphomas, and monoclonal gammopathies. These malignancies are the result of monoclonal proliferation of an abnormal hematopoietic cell. Once started, proliferation continues unabated and a survival advantage allows the malignant clone to replace normal cell lines in the bone marrow or the lymphoid tissues. Indeed, contrary to commonly held belief, malignant cells do not necessarily multiply at a faster rate than normal hematopoietic stem cells. The harmful effects of hematopoietic malignancies are mainly due to the failure of the neoplastic cells to differentiate and enter the inevitable state following normal life span—death. Early in the disease, such immortal and immature malignant cells are suppressed by normal clones, but later, the normal cells die out leaving only the progeny of the malignant clone.

When the genetic defects leading to the malignant changes occur in early stem cells, the malignant transformation leads to diseases such as myelodysplastic syndromes and myeloproliferative disorders. The myeloid leukemias are disorders of progenitor cells further along in development toward the phagocytic (neutrophils and monocytes), erythroid, and megakaryocytic lineages. The lymphoid malignancies originating from lymphoid stem cells include the lymphocytic leukemias, lymphomas, and plasma cell neoplasms such as multiple myeloma.

#### *Cytotoxic drugs*

The treatment of hematologic malignancies is directed toward the destruction of malignant stem cells. The goal is to achieve selectivity, that is, the maximal destruction of tumor stem cells with minimal damage to healthy stem cells. It is fortunate that malignant stem cells are, for various reasons, more susceptible to damage than are normal stem cells. Although some biologic principles are useful in formulating the development and application of chemotherapy regimens, the accepted treatment combination is often discovered by a mixture of theoretical ideas and trial and error.

Since hematologic malignancies are usually disseminated at the time of diagnosis, surgical treatments are rarely applicable. Chemotherapeutic agents and occasionally radiation therapy are the mainstays of treatment for these diseases. Some properties of malignant cells affect their susceptibility to cytotoxic treatments and these properties vary at different stages of these cells' life cycle (Fig. 12-4). Resting cells are in $G_0$. In $G_1$, the cell prepares for replication of the genome by producing proteins and RNA needed for the replication. In S phase, the cell synthesizes DNA. In $G_2$, the cell synthesizes structural molecules needed for cell division. In M phase, mitosis and cellular division take place.

Most chemotherapeutic agents can be grouped according to whether their action depends on the malignant cell being in the cell cycle, i.e., not in the $G_0$ phase. It is important to note that most agents cannot be assigned to one category exclusively. Nonetheless, it is helpful for understanding drug activity and combinations by classifying these drugs using this approach.

Phase-specific drugs are most active against cells in a specific phase of the cell cycle. The limitation of these drugs is that there is a limited number of cells killed in a single drug exposure, because only those cells in the sensitive phase are killed. For more cells to be killed, treatment with these drugs needs to be prolonged or repeated to allow more cells to enter the sensitive phase of the cycle. Theoretically, a higher number of cells could be killed by a phase-specific drug if the malignant cells can be recruited into the sensitive phase.

Cell cycle-specific but not phase-specific drugs are effective while cells are actively in cycle but are not dependent on the cells being in a particular phase. This group includes most of the alkylating agents and antibiotics. Many of these agents also have some activity against cells that are in $G_0$, although not as much as when the cells are rapidly dividing. Drugs that are not specific to cells in an active phase of the cell cycle are effective even when cells are at rest, i.e., in the $G_0$ phase.

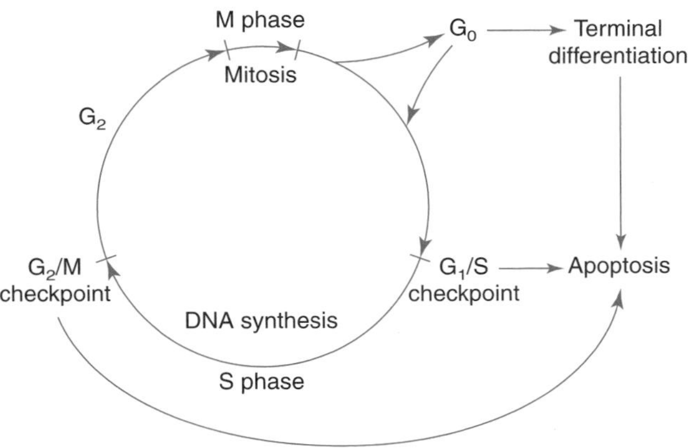


FIGURE 12-4 **Cell cycle.**

Cytotoxic agents kill a fixed fraction of tumor cells rather than a fixed number of cells, and the size of the fraction killed is proportional to the dose of treatment. This implies that treatment with a single cytotoxic agent given once will only be curative when the treatment dose is high and/or the tumor burden is small. This phenomenon partly explains why combination chemotherapy is more effective than single-drug treatment because each agent can reduce the tumor cell burden by a fraction until a sufficiently low level of cells is reached, below which their survival is no longer possible. Another reason favoring the use of treatment combinations is improved selectivity. A combination of agents acting against tumor cells by different mechanisms may be less toxic to normal cells than a higher dose of a single agent.

Cell differentiation usually takes cells out of the cell cycle. Tumor cells completely or partially fail to differentiate. Potentially, treatments can be devised that will induce tumor cells to overcome the differentiation block and to stop them from further division. An example of such a treatment is the use of all-*trans*-retinoic acid in acute promyelocytic leukemia and will be discussed later in this chapter.

**ANTHRACYCLINES** Anthracyclines, as a class, have the widest spectrum of activity against human cancers. These agents are widely used in the treatment of hematologic malignancies including lymphomas, acute myelogenous leukemia (AML), and acute lymphoblastic leukemias. Anthracyclines were isolated from a *Streptomyces* species from a soil sample collected from the grounds of the Castel del Monte, a twelfth-century castle in Andria, Italy (Di Marco 1964).

Anthracyclines interfere with DNA synthesis by their ability to intercalate between DNA base pairs. They also generate toxic oxygen metabolites and may thereby damage cells. The anthracyclines are toxic to rapidly growing cells, especially the bone marrow and hair follicles. Anthracyclines are very toxic to subcutaneous tissues and cause extensive necrosis if extravasation occurs during an intravenous infusion.

At present, four anthracyclines, namely daunorubicin, doxorubicin, idarubicin, and epirubicin, are widely used for treatment of hematologic malignancies. Daunorubicin was the first anthracycline discovered in the 1960s, and today it is still commonly used in the treatment of acute leukemias, both lymphoid and myeloid types. Doxorubicin (Adriamycin) differs from daunorubicin only by one hydroxyl group. Despite the minor difference in structure, antitumor activity differs greatly. Daunorubicin has little activity against carcinomas and sarcomas, whereas doxorubicin is one of the effective agents against these tumors. Among the hematologic malignancies, doxorubicin is mainly used in the treatment of lymphomas and multiple myeloma.

Idarubicin is also a daunorubicin analog and differs from daunorubicin at the C-4 position on one of its rings. Preclinical studies showed that idarubicin had greater antitumor activity than daunorubicin. However, results from clinical studies comparing idarubicin with daunorubicin in the treatment of AML are less clear. Two of the four major randomized trials comparing these two drugs, both used in conjunction with cytarabine, showed a statistically significant advantage for idarubicin in the treatment of AML, whereas two of the studies showed no difference. Moreover, the outcomes, including survival rate, for the idarubicin-treated group in these studies were not really superior to those achieved in another large study using daunorubicin and cytarabine (Mayer et al. 1994). Therefore, the potential superiority of idarubicin over daunorubicin remains unclear. Daunorubicin remains an essential component of treatment of acute lymphoblastic leukemia (ALL), and idarubicin also has activity in ALL, but no randomized trial has directly compared these two drugs in this disease.

Epirubicin is derived from a positional change of a hydroxyl group on the aminosugar moiety of doxorubicin. This compound was developed as a drug because it appears to have antitumor activity similar to that of doxorubicin but has less cardiotoxicity. In randomized trials, equimolar dosing of epirubicin was found to be less cardiotoxic than doxorubicin, while maintaining the same anticancer activity as doxorubicin (Robert 1993).

The most troublesome toxicity unique to anthracyclines is damage to the heart. The mechanisms for this relatively specific toxicity have not been established. This toxicity has lead to development of potential cardioprotective agents. The compound that has undergone the most evaluation is ICRF-187 (dexrazoxane). In clinical trials, the chronic cardiotoxicity of doxorubicin is significantly attenuated by chelation of iron by this compound (Venturini et al. 1996; Lopez et al. 1998). A greatly delayed type of doxorubicin cardiotoxicity has been recently found to occur in survivors of childhood cancers who were treated with doxorubicin without any immediate adverse effects but who develop chronic cardiomyopathy up to 15 years later. The pathogenesis of this type of toxicity remains to be determined.

**ALKYLATING AGENTS** Many chemotherapy agents are alkylating agents. Alkylating agents can substitute an alkyl group for a hydrogen atom on organic molecules including the bases of DNA. This results in a cross-linking of the strands of DNA that interferes with its replication and the transcription of RNA. Alkylating agents are not phase-specific, and some are not specific to the cell cycle. The differences between alkylating agents in clinical terms largely rests in their routes of administration, rates and onset of action, and mechanisms of elimination, which in some instances influence their toxicity.

The general toxicity of alkylating agents for normal cells involves inhibition of growth of relatively rapidly dividing cells in the bone marrow, skin (especially the hair follicles), and gastrointestinal tract. Consequently, their principal adverse effects are pancytopenia, hair loss, and ulceration of mucous membranes.

**VINCA ALKALOIDS** Vinca alkaloids, vincristine and vinblastine, inhibit tumor cell division by binding to the cell protein tubulin and inhibit the assembly of this protein into microtubules needed to form mitotic spindles. The vinca alkaloid molecule is composed of a large multiple ring structure called *catharanthine* and another multiple ring structure domain named *vindoline*. Recent data suggest that the catharanthine ring of the drug is responsible for binding to tubulin with the vindoline ring enhancing the binding to microtubules (Prakash 1991).

These agents are used in the treatment of lymphomas and acute lymphocytic leukemia. The primary toxicity of vinblastine is marrow suppression, whereas vincristine produces a dose-dependent neuropathy. The neuropathy is both sensory and motor and may be manifested initially by paresthesias in the toes, followed by loss of deep tendon reflexes in the ankles and difficulty walking. The neuropathy is reversed by cessation of treatment, although the resolution of symptoms may be slow.

**ANTIMETABOLITES** Compounds that block specific enzymes required for the survival of tumor cells are antimetabolites. They block DNA synthesis by inhibiting the function of enzymes required for normal purine or pyrimidine metabolism. Antimetabolites are used mainly in disorders with high proliferative rates in which many cells are in the S phase of growth cycle. The toxic complications of antimetabolites are generally very similar to those of alkylating agents.

**PYRIMIDINE ANALOGS** One of the most important agents used in the treatment of AML is cytosine arabinoside (ara-C). This agent is a pyrimidine analog that inhibits DNA synthesis by inhibiting DNA polymerase. Ara-C is rapidly deaminated in vivo to an inactive compound ara-U; consequently, rapid injections result in very short effective levels of ara-C. As a result, single doses of ara-C are generally ineffective for treating leukemia. The drug is usually given every 12 hours, because the S phase (DNA synthesis) of human AML cells last about 18 to 20 hours. If the drug is given every 24 hours, some cells that have not entered S phase when the drug is first administered would not be sensitive to its effect. Therefore these cells could pass all the way through the S phase before the next dose is administered and would completely escape any cytotoxic effect. However, when the drug is given every 12 hours, no cell in cycle would be able to escape the exposure to ara-C, as none would be able to get through one complete S phase without the drug's presence.

**PURINE ANALOGS** The specific site of action for purine analogs is less well defined than for most pyrimidine analogs, although it is well demonstrated that they interfere with normal purine interconversions and thus with DNA and RNA synthesis. 6-Thioguanine and 6-mercaptopurine are examples of this class of antimetabolites, and they are used in the treatment of acute lymphoblastic leukemia. Hydroxyurea is also an antimetabolite that acts by interfering with DNA synthesis, in part by inhibiting the enzymatic conversion of ribonucleotides to deoxyribonucleotides. It is one of the safest and best-tolerated myelosuppressive agents and is used in palliative treatment of chronic myelogenous leukemia (CML) and other myeloproliferative disorders. Hydroxyurea is also used in the treatment of sickle cell anemia as previously discussed.

Recently, inhibitors of the enzyme adenosine deaminase inhibitors have demonstrated efficacy and have become first-line treatments for lymphoid malignancies, including chronic lymphocytic leukemia (CLL) and hairy cell leukemia. Adenosine deaminase (ADA) converts adenosine to inosine and inhibition of ADA results in accumulation of deoxyadenosine triphosphate (dATP) intracellularly. High levels of dATP can potentially inhibit ribonucleotide reductase leading to depletion of other deoxynucleotides and inhibition of DNA synthesis. The three adenosine deaminase inhibitors are fludarabine, 2-chlorodeoxyadenosine, and deoxycoformycin.

Fludarabine phosphate is a purine nucleoside analog designed to be more water-soluble and resistant to deamination than adenosine arabinoside. Fluoridation of ara-A converts it to a compound resistant to inactivation by ADA. In plasma, the drug is rapidly dephosphorylated to fluoro-ara-A, which enters cells by a carrier-mediated nucleoside transport mechanism. Inside the cell, fluoro-ara-A is converted to fluoro-ara-A–ATP, which is incorporated into DNA and inhibits DNA synthesis. Although fludarabine is active mainly during the S phase, it is also toxic to nondividing cells, perhaps owing to activation of programmed cell death (apoptosis).

Fludarabine is highly active in treatment of CLL and low-grade non-Hodgkin lymphoma (Keating et al. 1996). In patients with alkylating-agent-resistant CLL, fludarabine produces complete remission in 4 to 20% of patients. In patients who have not previously received chemotherapy, fludarabine produces a 40 to 60% complete remission rate. Fludarabine has also produced responses in more than 50% of previously treated patients with low-grade non-Hodgkin lymphoma.

At the doses currently used for treatment of CLL and lymphoma, fludarabine has been well tolerated, with bone marrow suppression as the most common adverse effect. Other toxic effects include mild nausea, vomiting, diarrhea, and fatigue.

Another purine analog, 2-CdA, is also resistant to catabolism by adenosine deaminase. The drug inhibits DNA synthesis in replicating cells and causes accumulation of DNA strand breaks in nonreplicating cells. At present, a 7-day continuous infusion schedule at a dose of 0.1 mg/kg per day is used to treat hairy cell leukemia. The introduction of this drug has greatly improved the treatment of hairy cell leukemia. A single-course treatment with 2-CdA produces complete remission in 65 to 85% of patients regardless of prior treatment (Saven and Piro 1996). 2-CdA is also active against CLL and low-grade non-Hodgkin lymphoma, although few patients achieve complete remission. The toxicity of 2-CdA is mainly due to bone marrow suppression. Other toxic effects such as nausea, vomiting, mucositis, or neurologic dysfunction are rare.

Deoxycoformycin, a natural product isolated from *Streptomyces antibioticus*, is also a potent, irreversible inhibitor of adenosine deaminase and has been shown to have high levels of activity against hairy cell leukemia.

**METHOTREXATE** Methotrexate competes with dihydrofolate for the enzyme dihydrofolate reductase. This enzyme catalyzes the conversion of folic acid to tetrahydrofolate, which is an essential reaction for DNA synthesis. One unique feature of methotrexate treatment is that it is possible within a few hours after administration of the drug to give formyl tetrahydrofolate (leucovorin), which can circumvent the metabolic block and reverse the toxic effects of methotrexate. This strategy has been used in the treatment of acute lymphocytic leukemias.

**CORTICOSTEROIDS** Natural and synthetic glucocorticoids are used in the treatment of lymphocytic leukemias, multiple myeloma, and lymphomas. Their ability to kill lymphoid cells appears to be associated with their binding to cytoplasmic receptors, which then enter into the nucleus. The limiting factor in corticosteroid therapy is the myriad adverse effects associated with overproduction of glucocorticoids.

**INTERFERON-$\alpha$** There are at least five distinct types of interferons: alpha, beta, gamma, tau, and omega. These proteins were first discovered when chicken cells were incubated with a heat-inactivated influenza virus and found to secrete a substance that conferred resistance to viral infectivity. Subsequently, it was found that interferons also exhibited antiproliferative and immunomodulatory properties.

Alpha interferons are the most commonly used interferons in the treatment of hematologic malignancies. There are at least 13 subtypes of interferon-$\alpha$ (IFN-$\alpha$), all of which can bind to the type I interferon receptor on cell surfaces. IFN-$\alpha$ stimulates the cytotoxic activity of natural killer cells, lymphocytes, and macrophages. It enhances tumor-associated antigen and major histocompatibility antigen class I expression and inhibits the growth of a variety of tumor cell types (Pfeffer 1998). IFN-$\alpha$ is the treatment of choice for CML, and it also has activity against hairy cell leukemia and low-grade non-Hodgkin lymphomas.

Alpha interferon is the only agent that alters the survival curve of patients with CML. IFN-$\alpha$ has shown superiority over conventional chemotherapy in the treatment of chronic-phase chronic granulocytic leukemia to induce hematologic and cytogenetic remission. In three of four randomized trials comparing IFN-$\alpha$ with conventional chemotherapy, the IFN-$\alpha$-treated group showed prolonged survival and delayed progression to the blastic phase when compared with the hydroxyurea- or busulfan-treated group (The Italian Cooperative Study Group on Chronic Myeloid Leukemia 1994; Hehlmann et al. 1994; Allan et al. 1995; Ohnishi et al. 1995). IFN-$\alpha$ is also used in other myeloproliferative disorders including essential thrombocythemia and polycythemia vera, although clinical studies supporting this use are limited.

At therapeutic doses, IFN-$\alpha$ causes a host of dose-related toxicities. The occurrence and diversity of adverse reactions to IFN-$\alpha$ therapy vary depending on the dose, route, and duration of treatment and on the patient's underlying disease, age, and performance status. In general, patients tolerate lower doses in the range of 3 to 10 million IU/m$^2$ better than higher doses of 10 to 20 million IU/m$^2$. IFN-$\alpha$ can affect many different organ systems: the musculoskeletal system, causing joint pain and neuromuscular fatigue; the gastrointestinal tract, causing nausea and diarrhea; the cardiovascular system, causing orthostatic hypotension and tachycardia; the liver, causing hepatotoxicity; the hematologic system causing leukopenia and thrombocytopenia; the neuroendocrine system, causing fatigue and anorexia. One of the most prominent adverse reactions of IFN-$\alpha$ treatment is its effect on the central nervous system, causing depression, impaired concentration, hypersomnia, and anxiety.

The most common adverse reaction is a flulike syndrome with fever, chills, myalgia, and malaise associated with initial injections. These acute symptoms usually resolve with continued treatment and are manageable with acetaminophen. However, chronic symptoms, especially depression and fatigue, are the most difficult to manage and can become dose-limiting.

### *Therapeutics for specific hematologic malignancies*

**ACUTE LEUKEMIAS** The leukemias are classified by the lineage of the leukemic clone. The acute leukemias are divided into acute myelogenous leukemia (AML) and acute lymphoblastic leukemia (ALL). Most often the leukemic cell has markers in the white blood cell lineage, although occasionally it is of megakaryocytic or erythroid lineage. Classification into the AML or ALL form is usually based on the morphologic, histochemical, enzymatic, and immunologic characteristics of the blast cells. Recently, cytogenic and molecular techniques have also greatly aided in establishing the diagnosis.

The therapeutic objective in AML and ALL is to produce and maintain a complete remission (CR), which is defined as a morphologically normal bone marrow with fewer than 5% blasts, peripheral neutrophil count over 1000/$\mu$l, and platelet count over 100,000/$\mu$l without the need for red cell transfusions. With the possible exception of AML with t(15;17) cytogenic abnormality, intensive chemotherapy is required to achieve CR. Although the myelosuppressive treatment places patients at risk for fatal infections and hemorrhages, decreasing the dose of chemotherapy to decrease toxicity will reduce the CR rate. As these are potentially curable diseases, once the decision is made to proceed with curative rather than palliative intent, every effort should be made to use the maximally tolerated dose to maximize the chance of achieving a durable remission.

Treatment of acute leukemias occurs in stages. The first series of treatment to achieve CR is called *induction* chemotherapy. This is followed by *consolidation* or *intensification* chemotherapy, which refers to treatment after obtaining CR with combinations of drugs of comparable intensity to *induction* chemotherapy, usually given in repeated courses over several months. In ALL treatment, maintenance therapy is often used with lower doses given continuously for several years.

***Acute Myelogenous Leukemia*** Therapeutic responsiveness to chemotherapy varies greatly among patients with AML. Although, overall, only approximately 15% of unselected patients are cured, some subsets of patients are very responsive to treatment and have cure rates approaching 50% (Appelbaum and Kopecky 1997).

Cytogenetic classification appears to be the most prognostically useful classification scheme (Mrozek et al. 1997). Patients with inv(16), t(8:21) or t(15:17) have the best prognosis after treatment. The t(15:17) group is unique in that a noncytotoxic treatment is available to achieve CR. Patients with +8, and especially the −5 or 5q-chromosomal abnormalities have the worst prognosis. These groups of patients tend to be older and frequently have had myelodysplastic syndrome or have secondary AML following treatment for a previous malignancy. Patients with a normal karyotype or with other miscellaneous karyotypic abnormalities have intermediate prognosis.

The current recommended induction chemotherapy regimen includes an anthracycline with cytosine arabinoside (Bishop 1997). For patients who achieve CR, a few will stay in remission following this initial treatment, but most patients will relapse after a variable period (months to years). To decrease the likelihood of relapse, additional courses of chemotherapy (intensification), usually with very high doses of cytosine arabinoside, are given to kill small numbers of residual leukemic cells. This treatment strategy is recommended for AML patients with "favorable" cytogenetic abnormalities such as inv(16) and t(8:21).

At present, evidence suggests that for patients with poor risk cytogenetic abnormalities, if possible, allogeneic bone marrow transplantation from a histocompatible bone marrow sibling donor should be performed, because very few patients will stay in CR using conventional chemotherapy regimen. If a matched-donor is not available, autologous bone marrow or peripheral blood stem cell transplantation should be entertained as a possibility for these patients.

***All-trans-Retinoic Acid and Acute Promyelocytic Leukemia*** Although acute promyelocytic leukemia (APL) accounts for only a small percentage of patients with acute leukemia, recent advances in our understanding of the molecular etiology and treatment of APL have opened new perspectives for differentiation therapy in cancer. The use of all-*trans*-retinoic acid (etretinate) as induction therapy for APL has raised the complete remission rate to greater than 90%. Etretinate promotes differentiation of APL cells into mature neutrophils, which no longer have the capacity to divide.

Acute promyelocytic leukemia is characterized by an arrest of myeloid differentiation at the promyelocytic stage, a coagulopathy with disseminated intravascular coagulation, and the t(15:17) translocation. This chromosomal translocation results in fusion of the *pml* gene on chromosome 15 to the gene for the retinoic acid receptor alpha (RAR$\alpha$) gene on chromosome 17. RAR$\alpha$ is known to be involved in cellular differentiation, and PML is a phosphoprotein with growth-suppressive properties. This translocation results in expression of a chimeric PML/RAR$\alpha$ protein involved in both the leukemogenesis and the sensitivity to treatment by etretinate (Chen et al. 1997).

Several lines of research have provided strong evidence that the PML/RAR$\alpha$ protein is the cause of APL. The most convincing evidence came from studies of transgenic mice expressing PML/RAR$\alpha$. These animals developed leukemia resembling human APL, and their leukemia responded to etretinate treatment. In vitro, etretinate binds to PML/RAR$\alpha$, causing degradation of this fusion protein, whereas the wild-type RAR$\alpha$ remains intact (Raelson et al. 1996). This mechanism may explain why etretinate treatment resulted in restoration of terminal differentiation by APL cells.

Unfortunately, although etretinate is very effective in inducing CR in APL patients, alone it is not sufficient to maintain a disease-free survival, because most patients will develop resistance to etretinate. This is probably due to a change in metabolism of etretinate, because some investigators have found that APL cells from patients who have relapsed while undergoing etretinate treatment could still respond to etretinate in vitro. Induction of cytochrome P450 and of p170 may play a major role in the development of resistance. However, etretinate treatment is still beneficial, because it alleviates the need for induction chemotherapy, which often exacerbated the coagulopathy that is associated with this disease. Indeed, randomized clinical trials have shown that etretinate-induced CR followed by consolidation chemotherapy to eradicate the residual disease results in better disease-free survival than chemotherapy alone (Fenaux et al. 1993).

Etretinate treatment is associated with a potentially fatal capillary leak syndrome (retinoic acid syndrome), which is characterized by rising leukocyte counts, fever, and acute respiratory distress syndrome (ARDS). The progression of this syndrome can be aborted by treatment with high-dose corticosteroids and early initiation of consolidation chemotherapy.

***Acute Lymphoblastic Leukemia*** The current recommended treatment regimen for ALL consists of an anthracycline with vincristine, asparaginase, and prednisone (Levitt and Lin 1996). The use of this regimen resulted in a CR rate of 83% in a prospective randomized trial. Similar to AML chemotherapy regimens, ALL treatment also involves multiple cycles of "consolidative" chemotherapy after achieving CR. Unlike AML treatment, maintenance chemotherapy with low doses of oral methotrexate and mercaptopurine for 2 to 3 years following completion of intensive chemotherapy appears to be beneficial. Leukemic involvement of the central nervous system is more common with ALL (10%) than with AML. The treatment of CNS leukemia usually consists of intrathecal administration of methotrexate in combination with cranial irradiation. With adequate treatment, the presence of CNS leukemia at diagnosis does not appear to adversely influence survival rates in ALL patients.

Therapeutic responsiveness to treatment varies greatly among patients with ALL. Immunophenotyping of cell surface receptors on leukemic clones has been found to have greater prognostic value. The T-cell phenotype is associated with a better prognosis (5-year disease-free survival rate of more than 50%) than B-cell-lineage ALL (5-year disease-free survival rate of approximately 35%). Certain subgroups of B-cell-lineage ALL are found to have a lower survival rate following treatment. Cytogenetic abnormalities are also found in patients with ALL, and, in particular, patients with t(9;22) have dramatically reduced survival rates when treated with conventional chemotherapy regimens. Identification of these groups at high risk for relapse may allow the design of specific treatment regimens and consideration of experimental treatments including bone marrow transplantation in organized clinical studies.

**CHRONIC LEUKEMIAS** The leukemias are also classified according to the degree of cell differentiation. In chronic leukemias, the bone marrow infiltrate consists of a major proportion of differentiated cells. The chronic leukemias are also divided by the lineage of the leukemic clone.

***Chronic Myelogenous Leukemia*** In chronic myelogenous leukemia (CML), there is a malignant transformation of a pluripotent hematopoietic stem cell. A specific chromosomal translocation, named the *Philadelphia (Ph) chromosome*, is present in all myeloid cell lines, i.e., neutrophils, eosinophils, basophils, monocytes, erythroid precursors, and megakaryocytes. The Ph chromosome is also found in B lymphocytes; however, it is rarely found in peripheral T lymphocytes.

The Ph chromosome is a reciprocal balanced translocation of genetic material from the distal long arms of chromosomes 9 and 22, t(9;22)(q34;q11). The *c-abl* proto-oncogene is transposed from its normal location on chromosome 9 to the breakpoint cluster region (*BCR*) on chromosome 22. The new hybrid gene has oncogenic properties and is known as the *BCR-ABL* gene. It produces a 210-kDa fusion protein with tyrosine kinase activity, which is responsible for the cellular transformation. The Ph chromosome is also found in ALL. However, a majority of these patients have a breakpoint proximal to the *BCR* region, and the translocation results in a 190-kDa fusion protein.

The transformed CML stem cells give rise to an expanded pool of myelocytic stem cells and, as a consequence, an abnormal myelocytic overgrowth in the marrow that crowds out normal marrow elements. Because the abnormal cells retain their capacity for maturation, the marrow and blood contain mostly mature myeloid cells such as neutrophils, monocytes, eosinophils, and basophils. Platelet counts are often also increased early in the disease.

Chronic myelogenous leukemia is a biphasic or triphasic disease. In the initial (chronic) phase, the disease is manifested by an overproduction of relatively normal granulocytes, and it is readily controlled by chemotherapy. The duration of the chronic phase is approximately 3 to 5 years. Treatment with conventional chemotherapy, usually with hydroxyurea, does not change the survival curve of CML patients (Kantarjian et al. 1998). The disease invariably progresses to an accelerated phase and subsequent blastic phase. Survival time is less than 1.5 years in the accelerated phase and 3 to 6 months in the blastic phase, which is defined as a state of having 30% or more blasts in the marrow or blood.

Hydroxyurea is usually used in the treatment of CML because of its low toxicity profile. Busulfan is also effective in controlling the chronic phase of CML; however, it is associated with unpredictable prolonged myelosuppression and occasionally with organ fibrosis. Both busulfan and hydroxyurea result in hematologic remission in 70 to 80% of patients. However, the Ph chromosome persists in more than 90% of marrow metaphases.

As previously discussed, IFN-$\alpha$ has become the treatment of choice for CML. IFN-$\alpha$ induces complete hematologic remission in 70 to 80% of patients. But, more important, IFN-$\alpha$ can induce a significant cytogenetic response in CML patients: 40 to 60% of patients have some cytogenetic response, and 30 to 40% have major cytogenetic responses with suppression of Ph chromosome to $<$35%. In randomized trials, CML patients who have a major cytogenetic response to IFN-$\alpha$ have significantly prolonged survival compared with patients who did not have a significant cytogenetic response and with those treated with hydroxyurea (Kantarjian et al. 1998).

Allogeneic bone marrow transplantation is now the only proven cure for CML. Disease-free survival rates are significantly better in chronic than accelerated or blastic phases (Passweg et al. 1998). Younger patients with matched, related donors should be offered the option of bone marrow transplantation in the chronic phase, before disease transformation. Allogeneic bone marrow transplantation with matched, unrelated donors is now experimental. The procedure is associated with higher incidences of graft-versus-host disease and graft failure. Although there are some long-term survivors in some studies, the risk of the procedure must be carefully weighed against its benefits, particularly among older patients who experience major cytogenetic responses to IFN-$\alpha$.

***Chronic Lymphocytic Leukemia*** In chronic lymphocytic leukemia (CLL), the leukemic lymphocytes are morphologically indistinguishable from normal small lymphocytes. However, large numbers of these small lymphocytes infiltrate the marrow and circulate in the peripheral blood. CLL is considered a disease of advanced age, with a median age of diagnosis of 55 years. The median survival time for patients with newly diagnosed disease is between 4 and 5 years, but survival varies widely from a few months to more than 10 to 15 years in individual patients.

At present, CLL essentially remains an incurable disease. Consequently, conventional treatments should be initiated with palliative intent and not at the time of diagnosis. Studies have not demonstrated an improvement in survival with early intervention when compared with treating later in the course of disease. In general, treatment should begin when the patient becomes symptomatic or when there is evidence of frank progression of disease (Cheson et al. 1996). The use of bone marrow transplantation for CLL patients has been reported by several groups. Potentially, this treatment may be curative for certain patients. However, the follow-up of these studies is relatively short given the indolent nature of CLL, and durability of the initial response to this experimental therapy remains to be determined (Michallet et al. 1996).

The recommended treatment now is to use an alkylating agent such as chlorambucil because it is well-tolerated and clinical trials comparing it with other combination chemotherapy regimens failed to demonstrate a significant improvement in survival with these more toxic regimens. Recently, the advent of purine analogs, especially fludarabine, appears to be a promising first-line agent for this disease (Pott and Hiddemann 1997). Several large comparative clinical trials showed that treatment with fludarabine obtained a higher overall response rate than chlorambucil or alternative combination therapies (Byrd et al. 1998). However, the median survival of 5 years for CLL patients receiving fludarabine is not significantly different from historical results using an alkylating agent (Sorensen et al. 1997). These results suggest that purine analogs should be included in the list of drugs with proven efficacy in the initial treatment of patients with CLL, and although these drugs produce better responses, they do not cure CLL.

**LYMPHOMAS** The non-Hodgkin lymphomas are proliferative disorders of B or T lymphocytes of the peripheral lymphoid tissues. The distinction between a non-Hodgkin lymphoma and lymphocytic leukemia may become blurred when lymphoma diffusely infiltrates the bone marrow or when large numbers of lymphocytes enter the blood from tissues other than the bone marrow.

Hodgkin disease is fundamentally different from the non-Hodgkin lymphomas in that the malignant cells, the Reed-Sternberg cells and mononuclear neoplastic cells, constitute only a small fraction of the bulk of the tumor. The remaining abnormal cells are primarily normal reactive lymphocytes and/or fibrosis.

Lymphomas are also staged based on extent of the disease at presentation (Table 12-3). Staging is further subclassified to account for the poorer prognosis associated with systemic symptoms and extensive local tumor mass. If the patients experience systemic symptoms such as fever, drenching sweats, and weight loss, the stage is modified by a letter B. If the tumor is "bulky," defined as greater than one-third widening of mediastinum for a mediastinal mass, or greater than 10 cm in diameter for a nodal mass, the stage is modified by a letter *X*. If the patient has neither systemic symptoms nor bulky disease, the letter *A* is used. For example, if the patient has disease in two lymph node regions in the chest area but no systemic symptoms and the tumor mass is small, then the patient has stage IIA disease.

***Non-Hodgkin Lymphoma*** Although the histologic classification of non-Hodgkin lymphoma (NHL) is complex as in the Revised European American Lymphoma (REAL) classification system and at times the distinctions between different subtypes are subtle, there are only three clinically relevant subclassifications (Fig. 12-5). The low-grade or indolent lymphomas progress slowly and are in-

Table 12-3 **Lymphoma Staging (Modified Ann Arbor)**

| STAGE | DESCRIPTION |
|---|---|
| Stage I | Involvement of single lymphoid region |
| Stage II | Two or more lymphoid regions on the same side of the diaphragm |
| Stage III | Involvement on both sides of the diaphragm |
| Stage IV | Involvement of extranodal sites such as bone marrow, liver |
| B | Fever, night sweats, weight loss >10 lb |
| X | Bulky disease defined as mediastinal mass greater than one-third the widest interval diameter of thorax or >10-cm maximum dimension of nodal mass |

curable; the intermediate-grade lymphomas progress more rapidly but are also incurable with currently available chemotherapy; the high-grade lymphomas progress rapidly, but some patients are curable with treatment (Grogan et al. 1997).

The low-grade NHL group includes all the follicular lymphomas, both small and large cell, and the monocytoid B-cell types. The natural history of these diseases is that the survival curve has a constant and gentle slope, the illness has an indolent course, and it is not curable with available chemotherapy. Patients often present with stage III or IV disease, with only 10 to 20% having stage I to II disease. Although more than 90% of patients with stage I to II disease achieve a complete remission with radiation therapy, half will relapse and the actuarial progression-free survival is 40% at 20 years. There is a plateau on the survival curve suggesting that some patients are cured.

For advanced-stage (III to IV) disease, although CR can be achieved for a subgroup of the patients, conventional chemotherapy does not appear to alter the survival curve, with a median survival of no more than 5 years. There is no apparent advantage for multiple-agent chemotherapy regimens over a single alkylating agent. Like CLL, because of the incurable nature of disseminated disease and the inability to demonstrate a survival advantage with response to treatment, the approach has been to defer treatment until disease progression, unless the patient is involved in an experimental protocol (Horning and Rosenberg 1984). When the patient requires treatment, a single-agent alkylator such as chlorambucil or oral cyclophosphamide is usually used to minimize toxicity. Multiple randomized trials have shown that administration of more intensive therapy at the outset does not alter survival despite improving disease-free survival (Vose 1998). When patients become refractory to this low-intensity treatment, more intensive regimens such as CHOP (cyclophosphamide, doxorubicin, vincristine, prednisone) may be used. Recently, purine analogs are also being used to treat refractory indolent NHL. High-dose chemotherapy with bone marrow transplantation with either allogeneic or autologous transplantation also has been tried; however, the role of this treatment modality in this disease remains controversial.

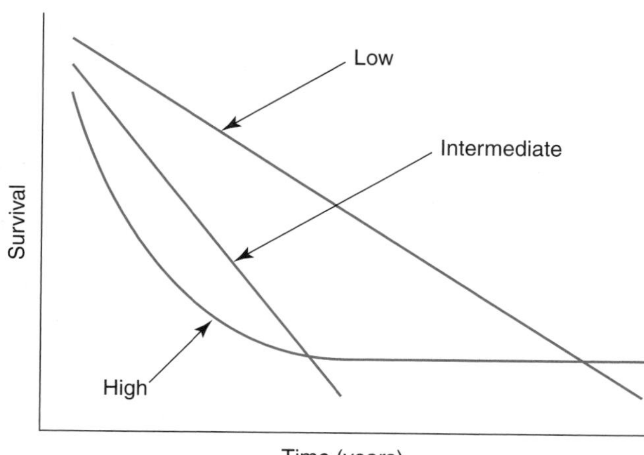


FIGURE 12-5 **Survival curve for patients with Non-Hodgkin lymphoma based on histologic grade.**

The intermediate-grade NHL group of lymphomas includes all histologic subtypes having a meaningful decrease in median survival as compared with low-grade NHL. Small lymphocytic, diffuse small-cleaved, mantle cell lymphomas and disseminated MALTomas [mucosa-associated lymphoid tissue (MALT)] can be classified in this group. These lymphomas are not indolent and cannot be cured with available chemotherapy. It is important to identify this group to recognize the poor prognosis and absence of curative potential and thus to allow for new or experimental therapeutic approaches.

The best therapeutic options for patients with these lymphomas have yet to be defined. It is unclear now whether an anthracycline-based regimen might improve survival compared with an alkylator-based regimen such as CVP (cyclophosphamide, vincristine, prednisone). In one randomized trial, no difference in outcome was found between CHOP and CVP treatment for patients with mantle cell lymphoma (Meusers et al. 1989).

The high-grade NHL group includes all histologic types having the worst initial prognosis, including all diffuse lymphomas. Although these lymphomas are rapidly progressive, they are highly responsive to chemotherapy regimens that include doxorubicin and are curable in approximately 40% of patients. The CHOP regimen is recognized as the standard treatment for patients with this group of lymphomas. In an attempt to improve these results, more intensive and complex regimens have been developed and have showed promise in single-institution trials. However, a large multicenter randomized trial comparing CHOP with three newer chemotherapy regimens showed no difference in survival among the four treatment groups (Fisher et al. 1993).

Important clinical factors that predict a patient's response to treatment include age, stage, lactate dehydrogenase (LDH) level, performance status, and number of extranodal sites involved. When patients are segregated based on these factors into low-, low-intermediate-, high-intermediate-, and high-risk groups, the predicted 5-year survival rates are 73%, 51%, 43%, and 26%, respectively. These prognostic factors may assist in an important way in identifying potential candidates for experimental treatments such as myeloablative radiation and chemotherapy followed by bone marrow transplantation.

For patients who are refractory to initial chemotherapy or who have relapses at a later time, high-dose chemotherapy followed by autologous and increasingly peripheral blood stem cell transplantation has become the gold standard, because relatively few patients are cured with conventional salvage chemotherapy.

***Hodgkin Lymphoma*** To date, the origin of the Reed-Sternberg cell remains unclear. The available evidence does not clearly designate the Reed-Sternberg cell as a B or T cell. Geographic clustering of cases of Hodgkin disease has suggested a possible viral cause. An association of Hodgkin disease with the Epstein-Barr virus (EBV) has been documented, with identification of EBV DNA in over half of the cases studied.

In distinct contrast to the non-Hodgkin lymphomas, which are generally widely disseminated at the time of diagnosis, Hodgkin disease is often localized and metastasizes through contiguous lymphatic node regions. Following a careful initial surgical pathologic evaluation, treatment is tailored according to the staging of the disease.

For patients with advanced stage disease (III to IV) and patients with early stage disease (I to II) but with B symptoms (fever, chills, night sweats, and weight loss) or bulky disease, combination chemotherapy is the primary initial treatment. The MOPP (nitrogen mustard, vincristine, procarbazine, and prednisone) chemotherapy regimen has the longest follow-up. Of 188 patients treated with this regimen for 6 cycles, 84% achieved a complete remission, and 54% have remained disease free for more than 10 years. Only 34% of patients who achieved a complete remission have relapsed. However, this regimen is associated with many toxicities including development of secondary AML, especially when combined with radiation therapy (5 to 7%). An alternative anthracycline-based regimen, ABVD (doxorubicin, bleomycin, vinblastine, and dacarbazine), has been found to be more effective and is associated with less than 1% risk of secondary AML. A randomized trial directly comparing MOPP with ABVD showed that relapse-free survival at 5 years was 50% for MOPP, 61% for ABVD, and 65% for a hybrid regimen combining the two regimens (Canellos 1992). Furthermore, the MOPP-containing regimens had more severe bone marrow toxicities, which resulted in higher incidence of infectious complications. These results indicate that the ABVD regimen should be the treatment of choice.

For early stage (stages I to II) disease without B symptoms, treatment with radiation can achieve disease-free survival and overall survival rates of 90% and 75%, respectively, at 20 years. However, treatment with radiation alone requires staging by laparotomy, which is not without risks. There is increased risk of late pneumococcal sepsis and possible increased risk for secondary leukemia in patients after splenectomy. A prospective randomized study comparing radiation therapy with MOPP for early-stage Hodgkin disease showed that chemotherapy was at least as effective as radiation therapy (Longo et al. 1991). Because exploratory laparotomy is not required for patients treated with chemotherapy (as the exact identification of disease location is not necessary), an ongoing trial is comparing ABVD with radiation therapy to determine whether chemotherapy may also be an appropriate first-line treatment of early-stage Hodgkin disease (Golomb 1998).

Patients who relapse after radiation therapy for early-stage Hodgkin disease can be treated effectively with chemotherapy. Because of the chance of secondary leukemias following MOPP, an anthracycline-based regimen such as ABVD is preferred. Patients who relapse following radiation therapy have 50 to 80% likelihood of long-term disease-free survival when treated with chemotherapy.

Approximately one-third of patients relapse following primary chemotherapy. However, if the recurrence is late, more than 12 months after a complete response, then it may be effectively treated again with combination chemotherapy. For patients who are refractory to initial chemotherapy or who have a brief initial complete response, salvage chemotherapy is often ineffective with a 5-year survival of only 10 to 25%, and patients are rarely cured. Similarly, for second relapses, the outlook is also poor, with a 5-year survival rate of less than 25%.

Myeloablative total-body radiation and high-dose chemotherapy followed by rescue with marrow or peripheral blood stem cells have been shown to be effective as a salvage treatment for Hodgkin disease patients who have failed conventional chemotherapy (Laport and Williams 1998). However, the precise role and optimal timing of high-dose chemotherapy and stem cell rescue in Hodgkin disease remain to be determined. The role of high-dose therapy as an adjuvant to standard treatment in patients at high risk for relapse is currently under investigation.

## Bone Marrow and Peripheral Blood Stem Cell Transplantation

The replacement of failed, abnormally functioning, or malignant bone marrow with normal marrow is a relatively recent achievement. Historically, restoration of bone marrow by transplanting a portion of bone marrow from another individual (allogeneic) was developed before saving a patient's own marrow stem cells and infusing them back at a later time (autologous), even though allogeneic transplantation is a much riskier and more difficult procedure. In allogeneic transplantation, it is necessary to overcome the problems of graft rejection and graft-versus-host disease (GVHD) to permit transplantation of marrow from another individual (Armitage 1994).

Bone marrow transplantation was first used to treat aplastic anemia and severe combined immune deficiencies. At present, HLA-matched related allogeneic stem cell transplantation has been used successfully as the treatment of choice in selected high-risk or recurrent hematologic malignancies, thalassemia major, marrow failure syndromes, severe congenital immunodeficiency states, and selected metabolic disorders (Armitage 1994). Breast cancer and other nonhematologic malignancies are increasingly becoming common indications for autologous bone marrow transplantation in order to achieve higher-intensity treatment, but the use of this treatment has been controversial.

Although the presence of true hematopoietic stem cells in peripheral blood has not been unequivocally demonstrated, there is convincing evidence that blood cell transplantation may indeed produce long-term sustained engraftment in the recipient after myeloablative regimens. The widespread use of these blood cell transplantations was hampered by the low frequency of circulating progenitors necessitating the need for multiple phereses, and by the inconsistent rate of hematopoietic recovery following infusion. A major advance was made with the discovery that peripheral blood stem cell levels can be markedly increased by mobilizing strategies based on hematopoietic growth factor administration and/or on the hematopoietic rebound effect that occurs following chemotherapy.

The use of myeloid growth factors such as GM-CSF and G-CSF may improve the reproducibility and the yield of peripheral blood stem-cell harvests. Conventional doses of these growth factors lead to a 20- to 50-fold increase in circulating CFU-GM and cells with the CD34 receptor ($CD34^+$ cells). Usually, a 7-day growth factor course is followed by leukopheresis on days 5, 6, and 7. The combination of myeloid growth factors with conventional or escalated-dose chemotherapy leads to the highest peripheral blood stem-cell collection yields (To 1997).

The use of peripheral blood stem cells resulted in enhanced neutrophil and platelet recovery compared with controls who received autologous bone marrow transplantation alone. A prospective, multicenter, randomized study in lymphoma and solid tumor patients, comparing engraftment after G-CSF-mobilized peripheral blood stem cells with autologous bone marrow transplantation, confirmed the beneficial effect of peripheral blood stem-cell transplant on neutrophil and platelet recovery (Hartmann et al. 1997). The accelerated hematologic recovery was associated with a number of clinical benefits including a reduction in platelet transfusion and shorter hospital stay, as well as lower total costs.

Single transplant studies in lymphoma, multiple myeloma, and breast cancer suggest that dose-intensification with peripheral blood stem-cell transplantation support can be applied safely to a wide range of patients. However, there are no prospective randomized trials yet available comparing long-term outcome after peripheral blood stem-cell versus bone marrow transplantation. Retrospective studies have shown that lymphoma patients who received peripheral blood-stem cell rather than bone marrow transplantation fared better when the disease involves the bone marrow (Vose et al. 1993).

Several investigators have developed systems for enriching the progenitor content of mononuclear cells using antibodies directed against the CD34 antigen. This technology enables a 1 log to 4 log reduction of cancer cells from marrow or peripheral blood harvest without compromising their engraftment potential and drastically reduces the infusion volume (Demuynck et al. 1995).

***Platelets***

Platelets are small, anucleate disc-shaped blood cells. Platelet counts in healthy human blood range from 150,000 to 450,000/$\mu$l. Platelets originate from giant polyploid cells called *megakaryocytes* in the bone marrow. However, the exact mechanism by which platelets form from these megakaryocytes is still unclear. This process is regulated by a hematopoietic growth factor termed *thrombopoietin* (TPO) and its receptors, and a proto-oncogene, named c-*mpl*, on megakaryocytes (Alexander and Begley 1998). The life span of a platelet is 7 to 10 days.

***Thrombocytopenia***

Thrombocytopenia is defined as having a platelet count of less than 150,000 cells/mm$^3$. The platelet count varies during the menstrual cycle and is also influenced by the patient's nutritional state. For example, severe iron, folic acid, and vitamin $B_{12}$ deficiency can also lead to a decrease in the platelet count. One of the following three mechanisms may cause thrombocytopenia:

- *Decreased bone marrow production.* Disorders that injure stem cells or prevent their proliferation in the bone marrow can lead to decreased production of megakaryocytes and, therefore, platelets. They usually affect multiple hematopoietic cell lines so that thrombocytopenia is accompanied by varying degrees of anemia and leukopenia.
- *Increased splenic sequestration.* Alteration in platelet distribution is another common mechanism responsible for thrombocytopenia. As one-third of platelets are normally sequestered in the spleen, splenomegaly is the most frequent cause of increased platelet sequestration.
- *Accelerated destruction of platelets in peripheral circulation.* Both immunologic and nonimmunologic causes may be responsible for accelerated destruction of platelets.

In addition, many commonly used drugs can cause thrombocytopenia.

**THROMBOPOIETIN** Thrombopoietin (TPO) is the major platelet growth factor responsible for stimulating platelet production under normal circumstances. Application of molecular cloning technology can now provide sufficient quantities of recombinant TPO for clinical use. TPO has been tested in several animals, including baboons, where its administration results in a marked increase in the platelet count. Recently, TPO has been used successfully in humans to stimulate platelet production in patients whose chemotherapy has caused low counts of blood platelets.

Recent data indicate that TPO levels correlate mainly with megakaryocyte mass, not with peripheral platelet count. Although TPO level is elevated in patients with idiopathic thrombocytopenia purpura (ITP), it is significantly less than TPO levels seen in patients with aplastic anemia-related or chemotherapy-induced thrombocytopenia (Hou 1998). These data support the hypothesis that megakaryocyte mass affects the plasma TPO concentration, and, in thrombocytopenic patients, a substantially increased plasma TPO implies deficient megakaryocyte numbers.

**INTERLEUKIN-11** The FDA has recently approved the use of recombinant human IL-11 to increase platelet counts and to decrease the need for platelet transfusions in patients with severe thrombocytopenia caused by chemotherapy for nonmyeloid malignancies. IL-11 is a cytokine that stimulates production of platelets by increasing the proliferation of hematopoietic stem cells and megakaryocyte progenitor cells and by promoting megakaryocyte maturation. In patients treated for cancer, the thrombopoietic effects of IL-11 begin 5 to 9 days after the first injection and last for up to 7 days after the last injection before returning to baseline. There is relatively little clinical experience with this growth factor, but the drug appears to be well-tolerated. The most common adverse effect is generalized edema due to sodium retention.

***Idiopathic thrombocytopenia purpura***

Idiopathic thrombocytopenia purpura (ITP) is a relatively common autoimmune bleeding disorder and the most frequent cause of isolated thrombocytopenia without accompanying anemia or neutropenia. ITP is an acquired disease in children and adults defined by a low platelet count in the absence of other clinically apparent causes of thrombocytopenia such as drug effect, HIV infection, systemic lupus erythematosus, and lymphoproliferative disorders.

Bleeding symptoms are rare in both children and adults unless the platelet count is very low ($<30 \times 10^9$/L). ITP is more common in children than in adults. However, in adults the disease is often chronic in nature, and spontaneous resolution is uncommon, whereas childhood ITP is acute in onset and often resolves spontaneously within several weeks to 6 months. However, the clinical course is not clearly defined for either children or adults. Deaths are rare, and when they occur, they are mostly a result of intracranial hemorrhage.

The lifespan of platelets is reduced from 7 to 10 days to a few hours in patients with ITP. Early observations that plasma infusions from patients with ITP cause acute and substantial thrombocytopenia in normal subjects suggest an autoimmune etiology. ITP is caused by the development of autoantibodies against platelet membrane antigens, leading to destruction of platelets by the reticuloendothelial system. It has been demonstrated that 50 to 80% of patients with ITP have elevated platelet-associated IgG levels against platelet surface glycoproteins.

The diagnosis of ITP is made by 1) excluding underlying systemic disorders that result in increased peripheral destruction or decreased production of platelets including hypersplenism, disseminated intravascular coagulation (DIC), drug-induced platelet lowering, infection, connective tissue disorders; 2) physical and peripheral blood smear examinations that reveal a normal-sized spleen with normal red and white blood cells; and 3) a normal bone marrow with an increase in number of megakaryocytes.

Indications for treatment of ITP depend on the severity of bleeding and degree of thrombocytopenia. Some adult ITP patients manifest mild disease with platelet counts $>50 \times 10^9$/L and no bleeding symptoms. These patients do not require specific treatment. Patients with bleeding symptoms or a platelet count $<30$ to $50 \times 10^9$/L should be treated. An initial treatment with prednisone (1 mg/kg daily for 2 to 4 weeks) or even lower dosages of prednisone (0.25 mg/kg daily) have been shown to produce a rise in the platelet count to $100 \times 10^9$/L within 1 to 4 weeks (Gillis 1996). However, corticosteroid therapy rarely induces a remission in chronic ITP. Patients who are refractory to corticosteroids or who are steroid-dependent should be referred for splenectomy. Splenectomy is the single most effective procedure in chronic ITP. Approximately 70% of patients will achieve a complete remission following splenectomy and will require no additional therapy. Other patients experience smaller increases, which are considered relatively "safe" in terms of bleeding complications.

A small but significant percentage of patients following splenectomy will still require ongoing therapy for severe, symptomatic thrombocytopenia. Although there are many types of treatment attempted for refractory ITP patients (Table 12-4) (McMillan 1997), none has proved to be satisfactory, and the management of these patients remains a challenge.

For patients who have not responded to splenectomy and require high doses of corticosteroids to control their disease, treatment with cytotoxic agents is a common next step. Cyclophosphamide or azathioprine is used presumably as an immunosuppressant and may be effective in one-third of patients with refractory ITP. However, these and other treatment options listed have not been compared with alternative treatments (or placebo) in controlled trials.

### *Thrombocytosis*

Thrombocytosis is defined as a platelet count greater than 400,000/mm$^3$. Elevated platelet counts may be reactive (secondary) to a variety of underlying conditions (solid tumors, infections or inflammatory disorders, postsplenectomy), or because of primary bone marrow disorder leading to an increase in production of platelets (myeloproliferative disorders). Elevated platelet counts in patients with reactive thrombocytosis are not associated with abnormal hemostasis and resolve with treatment of the underlying disorder. In contrast, thrombosis and bleeding are major complications of primary thrombocytosis, polycythemia vera (PV), and essential thrombocythemia (ET) and frequently require specific therapy. The reason for this clinical distinction is that platelet function is normal in reactive thrombocytosis, whereas platelets from patients with myeloproliferative disorders are qualitatively abnormal. A recent study reports that abnormalities of plasma von Willebrand factor (vWF) were detected in a group of six patients with essential thrombocythemia, suggesting a potential role for vWF in the pathogenesis of these hemostatic complications (van Genderen et al. 1997). Symptoms with essential thrombocythemia are generally associated with platelet counts of 1,000,000/mm$^3$ or greater.

**Table 12-4 Treatments Used in Refractory Idiopathic Thrombocytopenia Purpura**

| DRUG | DOSAGE |
|---|---|
| Dexamethasone | 40 mg/day for 4 days every 4 weeks |
| Vincristine sulfate | 1 to 2 mg/wk |
| Danazol | 200 mg qid |
| Colchicine | 0.6 mg tid |
| Dapsone | 100 mg/d |
| Staphylococcal-A immunoadsorption | 6 treatments |
| Cyclophosphamide | 150 mg/d |
| Azathioprine | 150 mg/d |
| Gamma-globulin | 0.5 to 1.0 g/kg |
| Cycloserine | 1.25 to 2.5 mg/kg bid |

Thrombocythemia may be associated with thrombosis (30%), bleeding (50%), or no hemostatic abnormalities (20%) (Silverstein 1996).

**TREATMENT OF ESSENTIAL THROMBOCYTHEMIA** Deciding whether to treat patients with ET is a difficult clinical problem. The importance of lowering platelet counts in asymptomatic patients has not been well demonstrated. Current recommendations suggest that only patients with prior or current thrombotic and bleeding complications should be treated. In patients with emergent hemorrhage or thrombosis associated with thrombocythemia, the treatment of choice—to lower the platelet count rapidly and to reduce symptoms—is plateletpheresis (Ravandi-Kashani and Schafer 1997).

Hydroxyurea (0.5 to 1.5 g/day) is effective in 90% of patients in controlling thrombocythemia, with responses that may persist even after discontinuation of treatment (Tatarsky and Sharon 1997). However, the teratogenic and leukemogenic potential of this drug has been of concern for long-term treatment in younger patients (Liozon et al. 1997; Tefferi, Elliott, et al. 1997). Therefore, long-term hydroxyurea therapy should be reserved for patients in whom the treatment benefits obviously outweigh the risk of inducing leukemia.

As previously discussed, IFN-$\alpha$ has antiproliferative effects on both hematopoietic and malignant stem cells, and it has been used successfully in another myeloproliferative disorder, CML. Interferon-$\alpha$ has also shown therapeutic activity in PV and ET, as demonstrated in multiple small studies and single-arm trials (Elliott and Tefferi 1997). Beneficial effects include the ability to control excessive erythrocytosis and thrombocytosis and such disease-related features as vasomotor symptoms, pruritus, and splenomegaly. Advantages over hydroxyurea include lack of known leukemogenic and teratogenic effects and the potential to alter the underlying course of disease. However, data allowing definitive therapeutic recommendations for the use of IFN-$\alpha$ in ET are still lacking, and randomized, controlled trials comparing IFN-$\alpha$ with standard therapy are needed.

Anagrelide hydrochloride (Agrelin) is an oral quinazoline derivative that is structurally similar to several prescription drugs such as ketanserin (an antiaggregant and antihypertensive), methaqualone (a CNS depressant), and metolazone (an antihypertensive saluretic). Anagrelide has anti-cyclic AMP phosphodiesterase activity and inhibits the release of arachidonic acid from phospholipase, possibly by inhibiting phospholipase $A_2$ ($PLA_2$). Based on these mechanisms, anagrelide was initially developed as a platelet antagonist. However, in initial human studies anagrelide unexpectedly induced a potent but reversible thrombocytopenia, which had not been observed in any antecedent animal studies *even* those involving nonhuman primates.

Anagrelide induced-thrombocytopenia is concentration-dependent, but the mechanism by which anagrelide reduces platelet counts remains obscure. At therapeutic concentrations, anagrelide may interfere with the maturation of megakaryocytes, and anagrelide reduces ploidy and cell diameter (Tefferi, Silverstein, et al. 1997). In a clinical trial involving 942 patients with essential thrombocythemia (58%) and other chronic myeloproliferative disorders who received therapeutic doses (<4 mg/day), anagrelide decreased platelet counts by 50% in 80% of patients within weeks of treatment (Silverstein et al. 1996). Treatment responses were durable, without loss of activity over time (median response duration, >2 years). Additional clinical trials indicated that the drug can reduce platelet counts in more than 90% of patients (Tefferi, Silverstein, et al. 1997). At therapeutic doses, anagrelide causes no significant changes in either white cell count or coagulation parameters, although it may have a clinically insignificant effect on red cell parameters.

Anagrelide is well absorbed from the gastrointestinal tract and has excellent bioavailability. When the drug is ingested without food, peak plasma levels occur in about 1 hour, and the plasma half-life is approximately 1.5 hours. Seventy-five percent of anagrelide is excreted in the urine, and a further 10% is excreted in the feces. Therapy with anagrelide starts at 0.5 mg four times daily or 1 mg twice daily for at least 1 week. Dose is then adjusted to reduce platelet counts to below 600,000/$\mu$L. The dose should be increased by no more than 0.5 mg/day in any one week; the total dose should not exceed 10 mg/day or 2.5 mg in a single dose.

Because anagrelide has a positive inotropic effect, it should be used with caution in older patients and patients with suspected heart disease. Platelet counts and other laboratory parameters must be monitored frequently during therapy. The most serious adverse effects include congestive heart failure, myocardial infarction, and other cardiovascular events. Frequent adverse effects include headache, palpitations, diarrhea, and asthenia. Although anagrelide has no demonstrable mutagenic activity, it is currently not recommended for pregnant patients.

**USE OF ANTIPLATELET DRUGS IN THROMBOCYTHEMIA** The use of aspirin and other antiplatelet agents in chronic myeloproliferative disorders has long been considered controversial (Mitus and Schafer 1990), because of the latent bleeding diathesis. However, treatment and prevention of thrombosis with aspirin has become an attractive therapy in essential thrombocythemia patients at high risk for developing thrombosis (Griesshammer et al. 1997). Low-dose aspirin (40 mg/day) has been demonstrated to be safe in a group of patients with high platelet counts (Landolfi and Patrono 1996). However, patients with bleeding associated with essential thrombocythemia should not receive antiplatelet agents because they may further increase the risk of bleeding. In contrast, patients with thrombocythemia associated with thrombotic events (gangrene, transient ischemic attacks) may benefit acutely from drugs that inhibit platelet formation, while other modalities are used concurrently to lower the platelet count.

## DRUGS USED IN BLEEDING AND THROMBOTIC DISORDERS

### Physiology of Normal Hemostasis

Normal hemostasis is a delicate balance among the hemostatic, anticoagulant, and fibrinolytic forces in the blood vessel. Damage to the blood vessel wall initiates a complex series of events involving platelets, endothelial cells, and coagulation proteins in the formation of a platelet-fibrin clot. Concurrently, the anticoagulation and the fibrinolytic systems are activated by the very products of the coagulation cascade to prevent formation of unwanted clots, i.e., thrombosis.

#### *Hemostatic role of platelets*

Platelets are involved in every aspect of hemostasis, from the initial adhesion of platelets to the vessel wall and spreading over the surface to form a platelet aggregate, to providing an activated lipid surface to accelerate coagulation and to stabilize the platelet aggregate by fibrin. When hemostasis is triggered by a pathologic stimulus (such as a ruptured atherosclerotic plaque), platelet activation can lead to the development of a pathologic vascular occlusion (thrombosis).

Platelets play a particularly important role in the arterial circulation where flow generates elevated wall shear stresses leading to damage of vascular endothelial cells. The sequence of events in hemostasis and pathologic thrombosis involves platelet adhesion and activation, platelet aggregation, and platelet secretion (Fig. 12-6).

Platelet adherence occurs through the interaction of integrin glycoprotein receptors with matrix proteins such as collagen. Following injury to arteries and arterioles, vWF binds to the exposed collagen matrix, and the matrix–vWF complex allows binding to platelets through the platelet membrane receptor gpIb–IX–V. Adhesion results in platelet activation, which in turn leads to the recruitment of other platelets to the site of injury. Platelet surfaces contain a wide variety of receptors that can be regulated by physiologic agonists to control platelet activation. The local production or release of agonists such as thrombin, ADP, and thromboxane $A_2$ ($TXA_2$) causes a conformational change in membrane gpIIb/IIIa receptors. These receptors then mediate the final and obligatory step in platelet aggregation, becoming functional receptors for adhesive molecules such as fibrinogen, fibronectin, vitronectin, and vWF. Platelet aggregates on the vessel wall accelerate the coagulation cascade by releasing its procoagulant granular contents and by providing phospholipid binding surfaces for enzyme complexes in the coagulation cascade. Activation of the coagulation system results in formation of thrombin that activates and recruits surrounding platelets to enlarge the platelet plug. he platelet plug is then reinforced by fibrin formed from activation of the coagulation cascade.

#### *Coagulation cascade*

In vivo, the tissue factor/factor VIIa complex plays a key role in initiating coagulation (Fig. 12-7). After vascular injury, factor VII binds to the exposed tissue factor and converts factor X to Xa, which in turn activates factor II (prothrombin) to IIa (thrombin). Thrombin then cleaves fibrinogen to fibrin, which stabilizes the primary platelet plug into a permanent plug. The tissue factor/factor VIIa complex also activates factor X indirectly by activating factor IX to IXa. Continued activation of factor X requires the factor IXa/factor VIIIa complex. This is why hemophiliacs with factor VIII or IX deficiency have a bleeding disorder.

#### *Physiologic anticoagulants*

Hemostasis is regulated by specific inhibitors of the activated factors (Fig. 12-7). The tissue factor/factor VIIa complex is inhibited by a protein called *tissue factor pathway inhibitor* (TFPI). TFPI first binds to factor Xa then inactivates tissue factor/factor VIIa by forming a quaternary complex. Administration of heparin releases endothelium-associated TFPI into the circulation.

Anticoagulant-activated protein C with its cofactor protein S, both vitamin K-dependent proteins, is the major inhibitor of factors Va and VIIIa. Thrombin activates the protein C pathway by first binding to thrombomodulin, which activates protein C on endothelial cell surfaces. Another physiologic anticoagulant is antithrombin III (ATIII). Heparin, as a cofactor for ATIII, greatly increases ATIII inactivation of factor Xa and thrombin. The physiologic relevance of ATIII, protein C, and protein S is

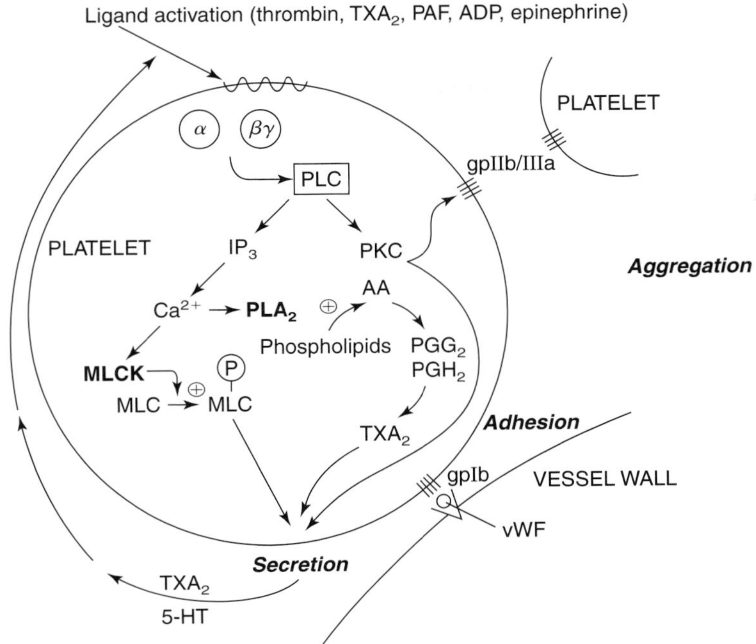


**FIGURE 12-6** Signaling mechanisms of platelet activation. Interactions among the platelet glycoprotein gpIb-ix-v complex, von willebrand factor (vWF), and other insoluble adhesive proteins lead to binding of adhesive receptors to collagen on the damaged vessel wall. Platelet adhesive interactions in turn initiate signals for platelet activation. Initiation signals and local or circulating activators of platelets stimulate membrane G protein-coupled receptors to generate second messengers $IP_3$ diacylglycerol (dag), which raise intracellular $CA^{2+}$ and activate protein kinase C, respectively. Increased intracellular $CA^{2+}$ stimulates formation of $TXA_2$ via a series of enzymatic reactions. Also, increased $CA^{2+}$ phosphorylates the myosin light chain. These responses finally lead to secreting platelet activators including adp, 5-HT, and epinephrine out of the platelets. These substances plus thrombin, which is formed on the surface of platelets, interact with the external receptors and thereby promote the platelet activation cycle. A major consequence of activation of these receptors is increase in expression of gpIIb/gpIIb/IIIa receptors into a high-affinity state for fibrinogen via a protein kinase C-dependent activation of protein p47. Interactions between activated gpIIb/IIIa and figbrinogen cause platelet aggregation. Abbreviations: AA, arachidonic acid; ADP, adenosine diphosphate; gpIIb/IIIa, glycoprotein IIb-IIa complex; 5-HT, serotonin; IP3, inositol-1,4,5-trisphosphate; MLC, myosin light chain; MLCK, myosin light chain kinase; MLC-P, phosphorylated myosin light chain; PAF, platelet-activating factor; $PGG_2$, prostaglandin $G_2$; $PGH_2$, prostaglandin $H_2$; PKC, protein kinase C; $PLA_2$, phospholipase $A_2$; PLC, phospholipase C; $TXA_2$, thromboxane $A_2$; vWF, von Willebrand Factor.

underscored by the greatly increased risk of venous thrombosis in patients deficient in these natural anticoagulants. Replacement therapy with recombinant ATIII is available to prevent thrombosis in hereditary or acquired (i.e., nephrotic syndrome) ATIII-deficient patients.

### *Fibrinolytic system*

In addition to the physiologic anticoagulant, the body uses the fibrinolytic system to regulate hemostasis by lysing established fibrin clots (Fig. 12-8). Fibrinolysis is regulated mainly by the enzyme tissue plasminogen activator (tPA). Circulating tPA is relatively inactive. Once incorporated into the fibrin clot, tPA actively converts fibrin-bound plasminogen to plasmin, which degrades the fibrin clot. Inhibitors of the fibrinolytic system include plasminogen activator inhibitor (PAI-1) and alpha$_2$-antiplasmin.

## Hemostatic Drugs

When bleeding is the consequence of a specific defect in the hemostatic system, the treatment is to correct that defect. A typical example is the replacement of factor VIII by transfusion in hemophilic patients. Specific treatment, however, may not be possible when bleeding is the result of multiple defects or no specific cause can be identified. In such situations, drugs that are not transfused and that help stop bleeding are indicated. These drugs may also be indicated for patients who refuse blood transfusions or for

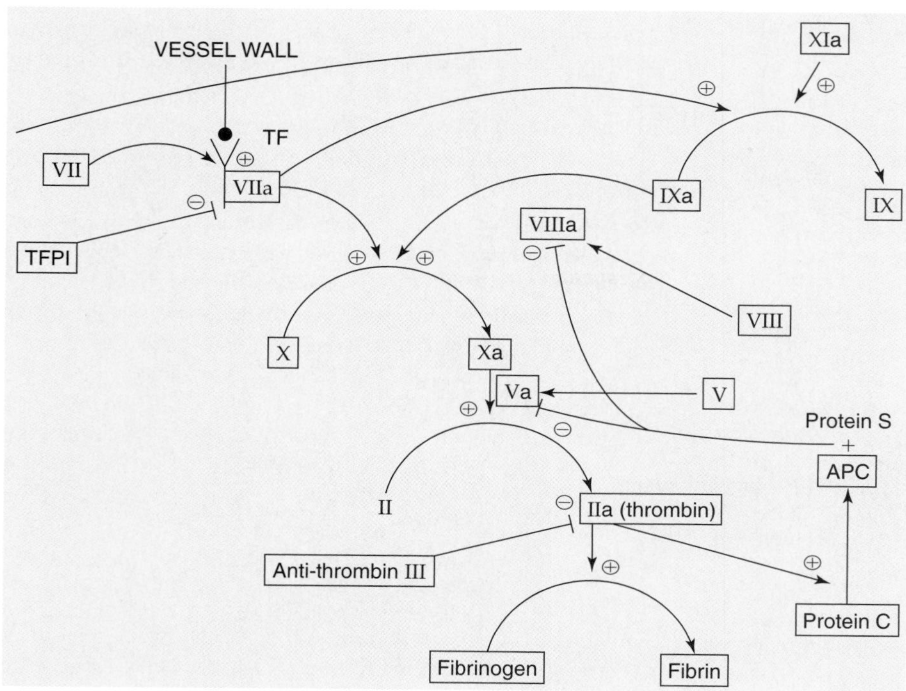


FIGURE 12-7 **Mechanisms of direct and indirect inhibition of thrombin. Direct thrombin inhibitors inhibit proteolytic activity of thrombin by binding to the active site of thrombin without requiring the presence of cofactors of antithrombin III (ATIII). Indirect thrombin inhibitors such as heparin enhance proteolytic activity of endogenous cofactor ATIII to inactivate thrombin. abbreviations: APC, activated protein C; TF, tissue factor; TFPI, tissue factor pathway inhibitor.**

those undergoing surgical procedures associated with large blood losses necessitating transfusions of donated blood.

Many hemostatic drugs that are not transfused have been evaluated, including antifibrinolytics, aprotinin, desmopressin, and conjugated estrogens, but only a few have proved to have clinical efficacy.

### *Antifibrinolytics*

Two synthetic derivatives of the amino acid lysine, 6-aminohexanoic acid (aminocaproic acid) and 4-(aminomethyl) cyclohexanecarboxylic acid (tranexamic acid), are used as antifibrinolytics. Both drugs bind reversibly to plasminogen and interfere with lysine-binding sites on plasminogen, thereby blocking the binding of plasminogen to fibrin and its activation and transformation to plasmin (Fig. 12-7).

Aminocaproic acid and tranexamic acid (which has a longer half-life) are effective even when bleeding is not associated with laboratory signs of excessive fibrinolysis. Because both drugs enter the extravascular space and accumulate in tissues, the basis for their efficacy is thought to be the inhibition of tissue fibrinolysis and the consequent stabilization of clots (see also the section on Cerebrovascular Diseases in chapter 7, Treatment of Neurologic Disorders).

Clinical indications for the use of antifibrinolytics follow.

**GASTROINTESTINAL BLEEDING** The gastrointestinal tract has a high concentration of fibrinolytic enzymes; therefore, treatment of GI bleeding with antifibrinolytics seems to be logical. A meta-analysis of studies involving 1267 patients with peptic ulcers, erosions, or other causes of bleeding found antifibrinolytics reduce recurrent bleeding by 20 to 30%, the need for surgery by 30 to 40%, and mortality by 40% (Henry and O'Connell 1989). Despite these results, antifibrinolytics are not widely used to treat patients with bleeding from the upper digestive tract because of the efficacy of other medical and endoscopic treatments.

**BLEEDING IN THE URINARY TRACT** The urinary tract also has a highly activated fibrinolytic system, and after

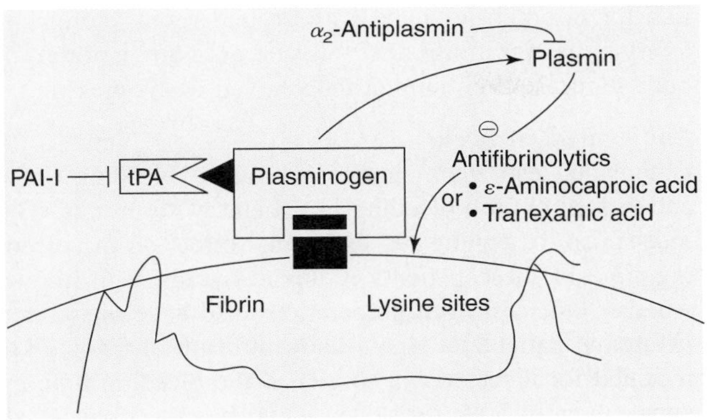


FIGURE 12-8 **Activation of plasminogen to promote plasmin inhibition by antifibrinolytics (inhibitors of the fibrinolytic system) at the lysing binding site on fibrin. Abbreviations: PAI-1, plasminogen activator inhibitor-1; TPA, tissue plasminogen activator.**

prostatectomy, hematuria can cause anemia. In clinical trials involving patients who had undergone prostatectomy, aminocaproic acid or tranexamic acid reduced blood loss by approximately 50%, as compared with placebo (Stefanini et al. 1990). The treatment is started intravenously immediately after surgery, followed by oral dosing until macroscopic hematuria ceases. However, these drugs are not known to reduce the need for transfusion or to decrease mortality after prostatectomy. These drugs are contraindicated in patients with bleeding from the upper urinary tract, because of the risk that clots will be retained in the ureter and the bladder.

**LIVER TRANSPLANTATION** Patients undergoing liver transplantation are at risk of developing severe bleeding, in part because of preexisting coagulopathy and intraoperative fibrinolysis. In a clinical study of 45 patients given high-dose tranexamic acid (20 to 30 mg/kg) or placebo during surgery, treated patients had half the intraoperative blood loss [original: 50% less intraoperative blood loss, 50% less not allowed] and required fewer transfusions (Boylan et al. 1996). Further studies are needed to confirm the efficacy of this antifibrinolytic to reduce bleeding and the need for blood products in this surgical procedure.

**CONTROL OF MUCOSAL BLEEDING IN HIGH-RISK PATIENTS** Antifibrinolytic drugs are useful for the control of bleeding after dental extractions in patients with hemophilia, patients who require dental extraction while receiving long-term oral anticoagulant therapy, and in patients with thrombocytopenia, because the oral mucosa and saliva are rich in plasminogen activators. Although the use of antifibrinolytics in these settings appears rational, prospective randomized clinical studies supporting this are lacking.

**ADVERSE EFFECTS OF ANTIFIBRINOLYTICS** The main risk involved with these drugs is the thrombotic complications resulting from inhibition of fibrinolysis, which is a natural mechanism of defense against the formation of thrombus. However, no striking increase in the risk of thrombosis has been observed when the drugs have been used during operations that are often complicated by venous and arterial thromboembolism, such as cardiac surgery and knee replacement. However, these studies were not designed to evaluate thrombotic complications, and most were too small to detect differences in outcomes with relatively low incidence, such as stroke, myocardial infarction, or coronary-bypass graft occlusion.

### *Desmopressin*

Plasma concentrations of factor VIII, the clotting factor that is deficient or defective in patients with hemophilia A, and vWF, the adhesive protein that is deficient or defective in patients with von Willebrand disease, can be increased for a short time by the administration of 1-deamino-8-D-arginine vasopressin (desmopressin), an analog of arginine vasopressin. These effects, which mimic replacement therapy with blood products, are the basis for the use of desmopressin in the treatment of patients with hemophilia A or von Willebrand disease, both of which are congenital bleeding disorders. The evidence of efficacy is so clear that no controlled clinical trials have been deemed necessary (Mannucci 1998).

Desmopressin has also been used in patients with other congenital and acquired bleeding disorders. In such patients, the effect of desmopressin may be mediated by the attainment of supranormal plasma concentrations of vWF or ultralarge multimers of vWF, which support platelet adhesion to the vascular subendothelium more actively than multimers of normal size. Increased hemostasis may also be mediated by high plasma concentrations of factor VIII, a rate-accelerating factor in the process of fibrin formation.

Clinical indications for the use of desmopressin follow.

**DEFICIENCY IN VON WILLEBRAND FACTOR AND FACTOR VIII** Desmopressin is the treatment of choice for patients with mild hemophilia A or type I von Willebrand disease who have spontaneous bleeding or who are scheduled to undergo surgery. Desmopressin shortens or normalizes the bleeding time in some patients with congenital defects of platelet function. Although the effect of desmopressin on a laboratory measure such as the bleeding time may not correspond to a hemostatic effect in patients, the results of a few well-studied cases suggest that desmopressin may be an alternative to blood products during or after surgery or childbirth in such patients.

The recommended intravenous or subcutaneous dose of desmopressin in patients with congenital bleeding disorders is 0.3 μg/kg, and the optimal intranasal dose is 300 μg in adults and 150 μg in children (Lethagen et al. 1987). Plasma concentrations of factor VIII and vWF are approximately doubled or quadrupled by the administration of desmopressin, reaching a peak 30 to 60 minutes after intravenous infusion and 60 to 90 minutes after subcutaneous or intranasal administration. These doses can be repeated as clinically necessary at intervals of 12 to 24 hours, but tachyphylaxis may occur after three or four doses.

Most patients with low plasma concentrations of normal vWF (that is, those with type I von Willebrand disease) respond to desmopressin with increases in factor VIII concentrations similar to or even greater than those in patients with mild hemophilia, and their bleeding time becomes normal. However, the bleeding time in patients with severe vWF deficiency (type III von Willebrand disease) or those with dysfunctional vWF (type II disease) is usually not shortened.

**ACQUIRED BLEEDING DISORDERS** Desmopressin has also been used in patients with uremia, who have complex abnormalities of hemostasis, reflected in part by a prolonged bleeding time. In a group of these patients who were given an intravenous infusion of desmopressin, the prolonged bleeding time normalized for 4 to 6 hours in about 75%.

At present, the clinical use of desmopressin in patients with uremia is based on the link between the degree of prolongation of the bleeding time and the patient's tendency toward excessive bleeding. Conjugated estrogens are an alternative to desmopressin for patients with uremia who have bleeding problems.

**ADVERSE EFFECTS OF DESMOPRESSIN** Common adverse effects include mild facial flushing and headache. Because of its potent antidiuretic effect, desmopressin can cause water retention and hyponatremia. In patients given more than one dose, plasma sodium and body weight should be measured daily and excessive administration of fluids avoided. Arterial thrombosis (sometimes causing fatal stroke or myocardial infarction) has occurred in a few patients treated with desmopressin. In patients at high risk for thrombosis (such as those undergoing coronary-artery bypass grafting), there was no excess rate of thrombotic complications among those given desmopressin.

### *Conjugated estrogens*

Conjugated estrogens shorten prolonged bleeding times and reduce or stop bleeding in patients with uremia. The mechanism of conjugated estrogens' effect on the bleeding time in these patients is unknown, nor is it known whether other estrogen preparations also have this effect. In uremic patients, a single daily infusion of 0.6 mg/kg, repeated for 4 to 5 days, shortened the bleeding time by approximately 50% for at least two weeks (Livio et al. 1986). A daily oral dose of 50 mg shortened the bleeding time after an average of 7 days of treatment (Shemin et al. 1990).

The chief advantage of conjugated estrogens over desmopressin is the longer duration of their effect on the bleeding time (10 to 15 days). Hence, conjugated estrogens should be given when long-lasting hemostasis is required. However, desmopressin should be given when an immediate effect on hemostasis is required. The two drugs can be given concurrently, thus utilizing the different timing of their maximal effects.

Conjugated estrogens are well tolerated, and adverse effects are negligible or absent. Because no more than five to seven daily doses are recommended, adverse effects due to estrogenic hormonal activity are usually avoided.

### *Aprotinin*

Aprotinin is an approximately 6.5-kDa protein purified from bovine lung. It inhibits the action of several serine proteases (such as trypsin, chymotrypsin, plasmin, and tissue and plasma kallikrein) through the formation of reversible enzyme-inhibitor complexes. Aprotinin inhibits kallikrein and therefore indirectly inhibits the formation of activated factor XII. Consequently, aprotinin inhibits the initiation of both coagulation and fibrinolysis induced by the contact of blood with a foreign surface. Aprotinin is administered intravenously. The enzymatic activity of the compound is expressed in kallikrein inactivation units (KIU). Plasma concentrations of 125 KIU/mL are necessary to inhibit plasmin, and concentrations of 300 to 500 KIU/mL are needed to inhibit kallikrein.

Clinical indications for the use of aprotinin follow.

**REDUCING BLOOD LOSS DURING CARDIAC SURGERY** During cardiac surgery, the exposure of blood to artificial surfaces in the extracorporeal oxygenator and enzymatic and mechanical injury to platelets and coagulation factors lead to a hyperproteolytic and hyperfibrinolytic state. The broad antiproteolytic action of aprotinin prompted its use in reducing blood loss in patients undergoing cardiac surgery. Double-blind studies have demonstrated the effectiveness of aprotinin in patients undergoing common operations such as valve replacement and coronary-artery bypass grafting (Lemmer et al. 1994). Aprotinin is less effective when given postoperatively than when given prophylactically.

**ADVERSE EFFECTS OF APROTININ** Because aprotinin is a heterologous protein, it can cause hypersensitivity reactions, particularly after repeated exposure. In one study of 240 patients given aprotinin two or more times, 7 had hypersensitivity reactions (ranging from skin flushing to severe circulatory depression). Most reactions occurred when aprotinin was administered a second time within 6 months after the first exposure but were not life-threatening.

Aprotinin can cause venous and arterial thrombosis and possible occlusion of coronary-bypass grafts (CBG) and other vascular grafts. However, in controlled studies with coronary angiography, aprotinin did not lead to an increased rate of early occlusion of saphenous-vein or internal-mammary-artery grafts. In prospective, placebo-controlled, randomized studies of aprotinin-treated patients who had undergone coronary artery bypass surgery (CABS), there was no increase in the occurrence of myocardial infarction (MI) or death. Pooled analysis of data from six studies of coronary artery bypass surgery (CABS), which evaluated a total of 861 patients assigned to receive aprotinin or placebo, found a lower prevalence of stroke among the patients treated with aprotinin (Mannucci 1998).

## Antithrombotic Drugs

Thrombosis is a major cause of death and disability resulting from the occlusion of arteries leading to myocardial infarction, stroke, and peripheral ischemia, or of veins causing deep venous thrombosis (DVT) and pulmonary embolism. Disabling or fatal thrombotic disease may stem from formation of thrombi within arteries at sites of arterial endothelial damage or in veins as a consequence of stasis or increased systemic coagulability. Thrombi may also form within the chambers of the heart, on damaged or prosthetic heart valves, or within the microcirculation as the result of DIC.

### *Arterial thrombosis*

In the high-flow rate of the arterial system, endothelial injury is the dominant cause in thrombogenesis. Arterial thrombi form only at sites with underlying arterial wall disease, caused by atherosclerosis, trauma following balloon angioplasty, or autoimmune vasculitis. Arterial thrombosis attributable to elevated homocysteine is also probably due to its toxic effect on endothelial cells and damage to the arterial wall.

### *Venous thromboembolism*

In contrast, the vessel wall is frequently intact in venous thrombosis. Stasis plays a more dominant role and permits the buildup of platelet aggregates and nascent fibrin in areas of sluggish flow. It has become clear that venous thrombosis is frequently attributable to a combination of environmental risk factors such as surgery and estrogen, with an underlying genetic predisposition owing to inherited deficiencies or abnormalities of the proteins in the natural anticoagulant pathway.

Activated protein C is the most potent endogenous anticoagulant. Resistance to this protein is considered to be present when challenge with activated protein C prolongs the partial-thromboplastin time in plasma to a lesser degree than in control subjects. In 1994, Svensson and Dahlback found a high prevalence of resistance to activated protein C among persons with a history of venous thrombosis. This resistance appeared to be inherited as an autosomal dominant trait. Soon thereafter, three groups simultaneously described the point mutation (the substitution of adenine for guanine) in the gene coding for coagulation factor V that is responsible for activated protein C resistance. Glutamine replaces arginine at position 506, thereby making activated factor V more difficult for activated protein C to cleave and inactivate. This is called the *factor V Leiden mutation*. In the Physicians' Health Study, the relative risk of venous thrombosis in men with the mutation was 2.7. When 24 populations were analyzed, the mutation appeared to be most common in Europe and least common in Africa and Southeast Asia. Factor V Leiden also appeared to increase the risk of recurrent pulmonary embolism after discontinuation of anticoagulation by a factor of 2 to 4.

Pregnancy and use of oral contraceptives increase the frequency of activated protein C resistance even in women without the factor V Leiden mutation. Women with factor V Leiden who use oral contraceptive agents have an estimated 35-fold increase in the risk of venous thromboembolism, as compared with women without the mutation.

Plasma hyperhomocysteinemia is usually caused by mild deficiencies of folate and is occasionally caused by inadequate intake of vitamin $B_6$ or $B_{12}$. In case-control studies from Padua, Italy, and the Netherlands, the risk of DVT among patients with homocysteinemia was 2 to 3 times that of subjects without homocysteinemia. In the Physicians' Health Study, homocysteinemia tripled, and the factor V Leiden mutation doubled the risk of venous thrombosis. However, the presence of both homocysteinemia and the factor V Leiden mutation increased the risk of any venous thrombosis by almost 10-fold and increased the risk of idiopathic venous thrombosis by a factor of 20.

Many patients with antiphospholipid antibodies or the lupus anticoagulant do not have systemic lupus erythematosus. This acquired abnormality may be associated with an increased risk of venous thrombosis, recurrent miscarriage, stroke, or pulmonary hypertension. In a case-control study, the lupus anticoagulant was detected in 8.5% of the 59 patients who had DVT confirmed by contrast venography but in none of the 117 with normal venography.

The routine laboratory workup for a hypercoagulable state in patients with pulmonary embolism previously included assays of antithrombin III, protein C, and protein S levels. The levels of all three of these coagulation-inhibiting proteins can be depressed during an acute thrombotic state. In addition, heparin depresses antithrombin III levels, and warfarin depresses protein C and protein S levels. Furthermore, pregnancy and the use of oral contraceptive agents cause protein S levels to decline. Overall, these proteins should not be measured routinely unless there is a strong suspicion because the results may be misleading, and deficiencies of antithrombin III, protein C, and protein S rarely occur. Genetic testing for the factor V Leiden mutation should be done because it is responsible for the most common hypercoagulable state, and the test is not affected by treatment. Testing for homocysteinemia is also recommended, because it can be readily treated with B vitamins.

Testing for the lupus anticoagulant is also helpful because its presence may indicate the need for more intensive anticoagulation. Laboratory diagnosis involves the detection of antibodies to cardiolipin or a lupus anticoagulant, or both. The latter causes in vitro a prolonged activated partial thromboplastin time and a prolonged dilute Russell's viper venom test, which corrects with excess phospholipids but is paradoxically associated in vivo with thrombosis. Lupus anticoagulants can also be induced by infections and drugs but are not usually associated with thrombosis in these circumstances.

### *Antiplatelet drugs*

Platelets play a central role in arterial thrombosis, which is implicated in pathogenesis of coronary arterial heart disease, stroke, and peripheral arterial disorders. Inhibition of platelet functions forms an essential part of antithrombotic therapy. Aspirin, the prototype antiplatelet agent, has been in clinical use as an antithrombotic for almost half a century. However, clinical trials have exposed the limitations of aspirin therapy, and there has been considerable recent progress in the development of more effective antiplatelet agents. These new agents are rationally based on interrupting specific steps in the platelet activation mechanism.

**BIOLOGICAL PROPERTIES OF PLATELETS** Platelet membrane represents the site of platelet interactions with the external environment and is ultimately involved in the control or generation of the many specialized functional properties of the cell. Platelet surface glycoprotein (gp) receptors play a particular important role in regulation of all these biologic processes (Andrews et al. 1997). The thrombus needed to arrest bleeding in injured vessels is poorly formed or absent in patients with abnormal platelet functions, resulting from congenital absence, reduction, or dysfunction of platelet glycoprotein receptors such as the gpIb–IX–V complex, or the gpIIb–IIIa or gpIa–IIa complex (Bray 1994; Clemetson 1997). Knowledge derived from the critical roles of the gpIb–IX–V complex in platelet adhesion, or gpIIb/IIIa in platelet aggregation, has resulted in the development of novel antiplatelet drugs directed against these receptors (Nurden 1996; Coller 1997a,b).

The platelet gpIb–IX–V complex is primarily activated by shear forces within the arterial circulation and interacts with vWF and other insoluble adhesive proteins to facilitate adherence of the platelet to collagen on the damaged vessel wall. Binding of insoluble adhesive proteins such as vWF to the gpIb–IX–V complex in turn leads to a $Ca^{2+}$ influx and $Ca^{2+}$-dependent activation of other glycoprotein receptors such as gpIIb/IIIa. The gpIb–IX–V complex is thus named the *initiating adhesion receptor* because it functions as a receptor for vWF and collagen and initiates signals that lead to platelet activation (Du and Ginsberg 1997).

The gpIIb–IIIa complex is expressed only in platelets (and their percussor megakaryocytes) at an extraordinary high density (80,000 copies spaced <200 Å apart). Furthermore, there is an additional internal pool of gpIIb/IIIa in the $\alpha$-granules that can be rapidly mobilized to the platelet surface. The gpIIb–IIIa complex binds to circulating fibrinogen, fibronectin, and vWF, allowing platelet aggregation, firm adhesion, and spreading during thrombus formation (Du and Ginsberg 1997). Although the mechanism for activation of gpIIb/IIIa is still unclear, the gpIb–IX–V complex and many other platelet activators such as ADP, epinephrine, and particularly thrombin are able to induce transformation of gpIIb/IIIa into a high-affinity state for fibrinogen. These may relate to protein kinase C-dependent activation of plekstrin, a cytoplasmic protein p47 (Fig. 12-6).

Platelets are a rich source of a wide range of biologically active materials that are capable of inducing or augmenting their primary roles in hemostasis and in the development of pathologic thrombosis and/or certain inflammatory responses. Such materials have been shown to be preformed mediators stored in either the dense bodies or $\alpha$-granules. The substances in dense bodies ($\delta$-granules) are ATP, ADP, $Ca^{2+}$, and serotonin. The substances in $\alpha$-granules include platelet-specific proteins: platelet factor 4, $\beta$-thromboglobulin and several growth factors such as platelet-derived growth factor (PDGF), endothelial cell growth factor (PD-ECGF), and transforming growth factor-$\beta$ (TGF$\beta$). Alpha granules also contain several hemostatic proteins, including fibrinogen, factor V, and vWF.

**REGULATORS OF PLATELET ACTIVATION** A wide variety of cell surface receptors on the platelet plasma membrane have recently been identified and characterized (Akkerman and Willigen 1996). These receptors mediate agonist-induced stimulation or inhibition of platelet activation. Pharmacologic agents could theoretically be developed to either stimulate or inhibit these receptors to regulate platelet function (Fig. 12-6).

The excitatory receptors are $\alpha_2$-adrenergic receptors for catecholamines; $P_2$-purinergic receptor ($P_{2T}$) for ADP, 5-$HT_2$ receptor for serotonin; platelet activation factor receptor, prostanoid receptor (TP) for $TXA_2$, vasopressin (VP), and thrombin receptors. The inhibitory receptors are $\beta_2$-adrenergic receptor, adenosine receptor, $PGD_2$, and $PGI_2$ receptors. They all belong to a superfamily of G-protein-coupled receptors and have seven transmembrane domains with a high degree of sequence analogy as demonstrated by molecular cloning.

Heterotrimeric G-proteins function as molecular switches linking intracellular effectors such as phospholipases, adenylyl cyclase, or ionic channels to the platelet surface receptors. Receptor-induced platelet activation is primarily mediated by several different signal transduction pathways that are involved in the isoforms of phospholipases. Activation of phospholipase C leads to the production of two second messengers, inositol 1,4,5-triphosphate (IP3) and diacylglycerol (DAG), which raise intracellular $Ca^{2+}$ and activate protein kinase C isoforms respectively, and is a major signal pathway for most platelet activators. Activation of phospholipase $A_2$ ($PLA_2$) releases arachidonate from membrane phospholipids, which is transformed into $TXA_2$ by a series of oxidative enzymatic reactions involving cyclooxygenase (COX) and thromboxane synthetase. However, platelet activation is regulated by inhibitory signals that attenuate or prevent agonist-stimulated responses. The major inhibitory signal pathway in platelets utilizes intracellular second messenger cAMP, which is produced by the action of adenylyl cyclase on ATP after antagonists bind to inhibitory receptors such as $PGI_2$ and $PGD_2$.

Thrombin, a very potent platelet activator, plays a particularly critical role in hemostasis and thrombosis. Prothrombin is converted to thrombin on the activated platelet surface because of the activation of blood coagulation systems. The local appearance of thrombin amplifies the reaction initiated by subendothelial collagen (Coughlin 1994) through the induction of a shift in platelet reactivity from adhesion and spreading on the vessel wall mediated by gpIb–IX–V /vWF to reactivity mediated by gpIIb/IIIa (Lu et al. 1993), which results in platelet aggregation and recruitment. Indeed, platelet recruitment in the formation of vascular thrombus is mediated primarily by thrombin, which not only activates membrane glycoprotein receptors and thrombin receptors leading to platelet aggregation but also converts fibrinogen to fibrin in the coagulation cascade. Moreover, thrombin is chemotactic for monocytes and mitogenic for lymphocytes and vascular smooth muscle cells, which play important roles in the development of inflammatory reactions in the blood vessel (Fenton et al. 1998).

The thrombin receptors on platelets are G-protein-coupled receptors with relatively large N-terminal extracellular domains. Following binding of thrombin to this domain, thrombin specifically cleaves the bond between Arg-41 and Ser-42, thereby releasing a 41-amino acid peptide and generating a new N-terminal that acts as a tethered ligand for the thrombin receptor itself and activates the G-protein coupled intracellular signal pathway leading to platelet activation. However, as platelets from the thrombin receptor gene knockout mice can still be activated by thrombin, this suggests the existence of a second thrombin receptor on platelets (Connolly 1997). This second platelet thrombin receptor, designated *protease-activated-receptor-3* (PAR-3), has recently been identified and characterized (Ishihara et al. 1997). This novel thrombin receptor is expressed in a variety of tissues, including megakaryocytes and platelets.

Adenosine diphosphate was the first platelet-aggregating agent to be recognized, but its receptor, $P_2$-purinergic receptor, was not identified until very recently (see review by Gachet et al. 1997). Although ADP is a less potent platelet activator than thrombin, it interacts with the $P_{2T}$ receptors to regulate a broad range of platelet functions such as platelet shape, accelerating fibrinogen binding, and aggregation. $P_{2T}$ receptors are expressed only in platelets and megakaryoblastic cells; the physiologic agonist of $P_{2T}$ receptors is ADP, and ATP functions as its antagonist (Gachet et al. 1995).

Thromboxane $A_2$, a major metabolite of arachidonic acid in human platelets, is a potent stimulator of platelet aggregation, vasoconstriction, and bronchoconstriction. Recently, there are two major advances in our understanding of $TXA_2$ formation and action. The first is the discovery of two cyclooxygenase (COX) isoforms in mammalian cells, COX-1 and COX-2 (Table 12-5) (Feng et al. 1993; O'Neill et al. 1993). It is now known that COX-1 is constitutively expressed in most cells (Vane and Botting 1997). In contrast, COX-2 is an inducible enzyme that is expressed after exposure to cytokines, immunologic stimuli, and growth factors (Vane et al. 1994; Masferrer et al. 1994). It is noteworthy that human platelets contain only COX-1 (Otto and Smith 1995). The second major advance is the identification by molecular cloning of the $TXA_2$ receptor facilitating its pharmacologic and biochemical characterization (Armstrong 1996).

Inhibitors of specific platelet agonist–receptor interactions include antithrombins, $TXA_2$ receptor antagonists, and ADP receptor blockers including ticlopidine and clopidogrel. Inhibitors of arachidonic acid metabolism and $TXA_2$ include omega-3 fatty acids, aspirin and other nonsteroidal anti-inflammatory drugs that inhibit cyclooxygenase, and thromboxane synthase inhibitors. The clinical efficacy of many of these agents may be limited by their actions, being restricted to a single, specific platelet receptor or metabolic pathway. Global interruption at the final step of platelet aggregation can be achieved with monoclonal antibodies and RGD (arginine-glycine-aspartic acid) analogs that block ligand binding to the platelet gpIIb/IIIa. Initial clinical trials with these novel agents have demonstrated superior efficacy in preventing reocclusion and restenosis following coronary angioplasty and atherectomy.

### *Drugs that interfere with thromboxane $A_2$ formation: Aspirin*

Acetylsalicylic acid (aspirin), the acetic acid ester of salicylic acid, was synthesized in 1897, more than 100 years ago. At that time and for the following 50 years, aspirin was used mainly as an anti-inflammatory, antipyretic, and analgesic drug. An increased bleeding tendency has been known for more than 40 years and was considered an unwanted side effect (Mueller and Scheidt 1994). Today, aspirin has become the "gold standard" for antiplatelet agents used in the prophylaxis and treatment of arterial thrombotic disorders such as angina pectoris, myocardial infarction, and stroke.

The main antiplatelet effect of aspirin results from its ability to block the synthesis of various prostanoids, and in platelets the particular prostanoid involved is $TXA_2$, a potent vasoconstrictor and platelet aggregate, via covalently acetylating a serine residue near the active site of the enzyme COX. As platelets do not synthesize new proteins, aspirin-blocked-$TXA_2$ synthesis from arachidonic acid in platelets is irreversible, and the resulting suppression of platelet secretion and aggregation lasts for the life of the platelet, approximately 7 to 10 days. Aspirin also blocks the synthesis of the platelet inhibitor prostacyclin in endothelial cells; however, this effect is shorter-lived than the effect on $TXA_2$ synthesis. The inhibitory effect of aspirin on platelet aggregation is demonstrated by prolonged bleeding times in patients taking aspirin.

Aspirin is a relatively selective inhibitor of the constitutive isoform COX-1 with a more potent inhibition of COX-1: approximately 150 to 200 times the inhibition of COX-1 compared to the inducible isoform COX-2 (Schror 1997). This explains the different dosage requirements for aspirin as an antithrombotic (involved in inhibition of COX-1) and an anti-inflammatory drug (involved in inhibition of COX-2) (Table 12-5). The antiplatelet action of aspirin is due to COX-1 inhibition, and COX-2 remains essentially unaffected at antithrombotic doses (<300 mg). The optimal dose of aspirin as an antithrombotic drug can differ in different organ circulations. Whereas 100 mg daily is sufficient for prevention of thrombus formation in the coronary circulation, higher doses may be required for the prevention of vascular events in the cerebral and peripheral circulation.

However, any effective dose of aspirin for antiplatelet treatment is associated with an increased risk of bleeding. The antithrombotic action of aspirin is probably mediated solely through its effect on prostaglandin synthesis. As a result, platelet activation caused by other factors remains unchanged and may result in resistance against inhibition of platelet function by aspirin during clinical use. This involves platelet activation by shear stress and ADP. In addition, there is no "sparing" of endothelial prostacyclin synthesis in clinical conditions of atherosclerotic endothelial injury. In this case, inhibition of COX-1 by aspirin will also reduce the amount of precursors needed for vascular prostacyclin synthesis provided, for example, from adhering platelets.

Aspirin is rapidly absorbed from the gastrointestinal tract. Aspirin is partially hydrolyzed to salicylate on the first pass through the liver and is widely distributed into

Table 12-5 **Properties of Cyclooxygenases 1 (COX-1) and 2 (COX-2)**

| PARAMETER | COX-1 | COX-2 |
|---|---|---|
| Gene expression | Constitutive | Inducible |
| Catalytic product | $PGG_2/PGH_2$ | $PGG_2/PGH_2$ |
| Tissue distribution | Ubiquitous | Limited |
| Expression in platelet | + | − |
| Stimulation by | All kinds of stimuli | Inflammatory factors such as cytokines and growth factors |
| Function | Homeostasis, hemostasis | Defense mechanism, inflammation, immune reaction, mitogenesis |
| Selective inhibition by aspirin | High | Low |

ABBREVIATIONS: COX-1, cyclooxygenase; COX-2, cyclooxygenase; $PGG_2$, prostaglandin $G_2$; $PGH_2$, prostaglandin $H_2$.
SOURCE: Data from Schror's review (1997).

most body tissues. Following oral administration, salicylate can be present in serum within 5 to 30 minutes, and peak serum concentrations are attained within 1 hour. Hemostasis returns to normal roughly 36 hours after the last dose of the drug, although 4 to 7 days is required for complete turnover of the platelet pool. Gastrointestinal irritation is the most common adverse effect. Tinnitus and central nervous system toxicity are uncommon with the low dosages used to achieve antithrombotic effects.

**ACUTE MYOCARDIAL INFARCTION** Aspirin therapy is now a standard treatment in the initial management strategy of patients with suspected AMI in the emergency room. Multiple, large, randomized trials have unequivocally demonstrated the efficacy of aspirin in improving the survival rate of patients with AMI and in reducing mortality by 20%. This reduction represents the avoidance of about 25 early deaths for every 1000 patients with suspected AMI who are treated with aspirin for 1 month. Furthermore, the early benefits of short-term treatment persist for at least several years. Assignment to 1 month of aspirin therapy in the ISIS-2 trial approximately halved patients' risk of repeat infarction and of stroke, typically preventing an additional 10 nonfatal repeat infarctions and 3 nonfatal strokes per 1000 treated patients. Moreover, continuation of aspirin therapy beyond the first month approximately doubled these early benefits, with about 40 further deaths, repeat infarctions, or strokes prevented per 1000 patients during the first few years of additional treatment.

A loading dose of 160 to 325 mg of aspirin is recommended for myocardial infarction (MI), because it may take several days to inhibit cyclooxygenase and to decrease $TXA_2$ production with a dose lower than 160 mg. In order to achieve therapeutic blood levels rapidly, chewed aspirin is recommended to promote buccal absorption rather than gastric mucosal absorption. Virtually complete inhibition of cyclooxygenase can be maintained indefinitely with a minimum dose of 75 mg per day.

**SECONDARY PREVENTION OF MYOCARDIAL INFARCTION** As indicated above, aspirin therapy should be continued following an acute cardiac event to prevent recurrence of MI. Many studies have demonstrated the efficacy of aspirin in preventing recurrence of myocardial infarction. Results from meta-analysis of multiple clinical trials indicated that 325 mg/day of aspirin reduced cardiovascular mortality by 13%, nonfatal repeat infarction by 31%, nonfatal stroke by 42%, and all significant vascular events by 25%. In clinical trials, doses of 75 to 325 mg daily were protective, with no clinical evidence of greater benefit from higher doses. Hence, the appropriate dose for long-term aspirin therapy appears to be the lowest dose in the range of 75 to 325 mg daily that is convenient to prescribe. The enteric-coated aspirin should be prescribed only if patients cannot tolerate the standard preparation of aspirin because of gastric toxicity. ***Given the definite and substantial benefits of aspirin therapy during and after AMI, including unstable angina, it should not be withheld from patients with only mild contraindication*** (Collins et al. 1997).

**PRIMARY PREVENTION OF MYOCARDIAL INFARCTION** Several larger clinical trials have shown that the use of aspirin for primary prevention of cardiovascular diseases has reduced cardiovascular events, on average, by 25%. Recent data suggest that the prophylactic effect of aspirin may be partly due to its anti-inflammatory effect and not just its anticoagulant properties. In a study of 543 apparently healthy men participating in the Physicians' Health Study in whom myocardial infarction, stroke, or venous thrombosis subsequently developed, prevention of the first MI was greatest among men with the highest baseline C-reactive protein concentration, which was measured as a marker for systemic inflammation, and this benefit diminished significantly with decreasing concentrations of this inflammatory marker (Antiplatelet Trialists' Collaboration 1994a).

**UNSTABLE ANGINA** The pathophysiology of unstable angina involves platelet activation and thrombus formation at the site of an active plaque. Several randomized clinical trials have shown that low-dose aspirin (30 mg to 325 mg/day) reduces the incidence of MI and death from cardiac causes by approximately 50% in patients with unstable angina. For the minority of patients with unstable angina when aspirin is contraindicated, ticlopidine is a suitable alternative.

**TRANSIENT ISCHEMIC ATTACKS AND STROKE** Aspirin is the primary treatment for prevention of stroke in patients with transient ischemic attacks (TIAs). In several randomized clinical trials, aspirin reduced the risk of developing subsequent TIAs, stroke, and death in patients with TIAs (ref). The Canadian Cooperative Study Group (1978) showed that 325 mg of aspirin four times daily for 26 months reduced the risk of subsequent TIA, stroke, and death by 19%; if only stroke and death endpoints were considered, aspirin reduced the risk of these events by 31%. The doses of aspirin used in prevention of TIA and stroke have ranged from 300 mg per day to 1.5 g per day. However, analysis of several clinical trials suggests that the lower doses (30 mg/day to 325 mg/day) of aspirin are just as effective as the higher doses (1.2 to 1.5 g/day) but have fewer adverse effects (UK-TIA Study Group 1988; The Dutch TIA Study Group 1988).

**PERIPHERAL VASCULAR DISEASE** Aspirin 330 mg/day plus dipyridamole 75 mg/day was effective in delaying the progression of arterial occlusive disease (Hess et al. 1985). Recent overviews of a number of randomized clinical trials demonstrated that aspirin alone or aspirin plus dipyridamole can significantly increase vascular patency in patients with peripheral arterial disease (Antiplatelet Trialists' Collaboration 1994b).

**VENOUS THROMBOSIS AND PULMONARY EMBOLISM** Although antiplatelet therapy has been used mainly in arterial thrombosis, recent data from a large number of clinical trials indicate that a few weeks of aspirin therapy can reduce the risk of developing DVT and pulmonary embolism (Antiplatelet Trialists' Collaboration 1994b). In these trials, aspirin also significantly reduced the number of deaths attributed to pulmonary embolism. These results indicate that antiplatelet therapy, in addition to other proven antithromboembolic agents (such as subcutaneous heparin) should be considered for prevention of venous thrombosis.

Although aspirin is a cost-effective drug in the prevention of arterial thrombosis, it is a relatively weak antiplatelet agent, as it does not inhibit platelet activation by $TXA_2$-independent pathways. For example, aspirin therapy does not affect formation of thrombin, which is believed to play a major role in platelet activation, particularly in acute ischemic syndromes.

The limitations of aspirin therapy have led to the development of multiple novel antiplatelet agents. However, one must ask, do these new antiplatelet agents add significant clinical benefits, when compared with aspirin, and at what cost? Indeed, the cost-effectiveness of any new antiplatelet agent should be carefully evaluated in comparison with this safe and very inexpensive drug.

Despite overwhelming evidence of the benefit of aspirin in patients with coronary heart disease, many, if not most, patients with established disease do not take aspirin. Reviewing the treatment of Medicare patients with acute myocardial infarction, the Cooperative Cardiovascular Project found that only 50% of patients received aspirin within 48 hours after the diagnosis of infarction (Ellerbeck et al. 1995). Moreover, the mortality rate at 6 months among patients not receiving aspirin was twice the rate among those receiving it (Krumholz et al. 1996). Physicians' misperceptions of the available data may be a substantial problem. A survey of internists found that only 55% believe that aspirin definitely improves the long-term prognosis after MI (Ayanian et al. 1994). The reasons for not prescribing effective therapies are complex and may involve cost considerations. In the case of aspirin, high cost is not a factor.

#### *Antagonists of membrane receptors for platelet activation: Ticlopidine and clopidogrel*

Ticlopidine hydrochloride and its chemical analog clopidogrel are acidic thienopyridine derivatives that are freely soluble in water. Both ticlopidine and clopidogrel strongly inhibit the primary and secondary phases of ADP-induced platelet aggregation. They also moderately inhibit platelet aggregation induced by collagen, epinephrine, thrombin, and platelet-activating factor by an indirect mechanism. The exact mechanism through which they affect these platelet functions is unknown. However, it is known that ticlopidine and clopidogrel interfere with the ADP-induced binding of fibrinogen to the platelet glycoprotein receptor gpIIb/IIIa without directly affecting the gpIIb/IIIa receptor. Consequently, platelet aggregation is inhibited and this inhibitory effect is irreversible.

Ticlopidine is rapidly and well absorbed through the gastrointestinal tract. Peak plasma concentration is achieved in about 2 hours, but the inhibitory effect on platelets is not reached until after approximately 4 days of regular dosing. Steady-state concentration is achieved in 2 to 3 weeks. Ticlopidine is extensively metabolized and excreted mainly through the kidney. As a result, renal impairment significantly increases plasma concentrations.

The bioavailability of clopidogrel is not affected by food or antacids. The plasma elimination half-life of clopidogrel is about 8 hours. Following oral administration, the time to peak concentration is about 1 hour.

Clinical indications for the use of ticlopidine and clopidogrel follow.

**MYOCARDIAL INFARCTION AND STROKE** Ticlopidine is primarily used in prevention of stroke in patients with cerebrovascular disease, nonfatal MI in patients with unstable angina, and graft occlusion in patients undergoing coronary artery bypass grafting (Flores-Runk and Raasch 1993). Evidence from clinical trials suggest that ticlopidine is more efficacious than aspirin. In a recent randomized trial, ticlopidine plus aspirin produced an 86% reduction in the risk of death, MI, or need for reintervention compared with conventional anticoagulant therapy (aspirin, heparin, and warfarin) (Schomig et al. 1996).

Clopidogrel was approved by the FDA in 1997 for the treatment of unstable angina and as a preventive measure against stroke. A recent clinical trial directly compared clopidogrel with aspirin in preventing ischemic events. Approximately 19,000 patients who had atherosclerotic disease were entered into a double-blind, randomized, multicenter trial. Patients received 75 mg of clopidogrel or 325 mg of aspirin. The measures of efficacy included ischemic stroke, MI, and death from other vascular causes. The relative risk reduction was 8.7% in favor of clopidogrel compared with aspirin. However, there was no significant difference in the percentage of fatal events. A favorable trend was noted for clopidogrel on each of the primary endpoints, with the greatest benefit seen for prevention of MI. The data suggest that clopidogrel may be able to prevent more major ischemic events than aspirin albeit at a significantly higher cost. It was also noted that clopidogrel significantly reduced the relative risk for primary ischemic events in patients with peripheral arterial disease (CAPRIE Steering Committee 1996).

**ADVERSE EFFECTS OF TICLOPIDINE AND CLOPIDOGREL** The most frequent (5%) and serious adverse effect of ticlopidine is bone marrow depression, especially leukopenia. Patients need to be closely monitored during the first 12 weeks of ticlopidine therapy. Additionally, ticlopidine therapy has been found to be infrequently associated with the development of thrombotic thrombocytopenic purpura (Bennett et al. 1998). Because these adverse effects are serious, ticlopidine is limited for use in patients intolerant or unresponsive to aspirin therapy.

The mechanism of action of clopidogrel is similar to that of ticlopidine, but clopidogrel appears to have minimal bone marrow suppressive effects (Verstraete 1995). The most frequently seen adverse effects of clopidogrel are gastrointestinal upset, bleeding disorders, rash, and diarrhea. A few patients needed to discontinue clopidogrel therapy because of gastrointestinal hemorrhage.

***Glycoprotein IIb/IIIa antagonists***

The binding of fibrinogen and, to a lesser extent, other ligands to the gpIIb/IIIa receptor represents the final common pathway of thrombus formation. Unlike other integrins, this receptor is platelet-specific and the most abundant receptor found on activated platelets.

The gp IIb/IIIa is a member of the integrin family of receptors. Its receptor has an $\alpha$ and $\beta$ subunit, $\alpha_{\text{IIb}}$ or gpIIb and $\beta_3$ or gpIIIa. The structure of the gpIIb/IIIa complex was mapped by electron microscopy and immunological studies. The gpIIIa subunit contains the binding site for the tripeptide sequence arginine-glycine-aspartic acid (RGD) found on fibrinogen, vWF, fibronectin, and vitronectin. The gpIIb subunit contains four repeating segments, which are the binding sites for $Ca^{2+}$ and required for receptor function.

Both subunits of gpIIb/IIIa must be present for platelet aggregation to occur. The two subunits are encoded by different genes on the long arm of chromosome 17. Dysfunction of either subunit results in Glanzmann's thrombasthenia, a condition in which platelet aggregation does not occur; gpIIb/IIIa is therefore a logical therapeutic target for management of arterial thrombotic diseases.

There are at least four pharmacologic inhibitors of gpIIb/IIIa receptors in use or under development, namely abciximab (c7E3Fab or ReoPro), eptifibatide (Integrilin), tirofiban (Aggrastat), and xemilofiban (SC-54684A). Abciximab has received FDA approval for prevention of post–coronary angioplasty occlusion (Coller 1997b).

**ABCIXIMAB** Abciximab is a monoclonal antibody that binds to gpIIb/IIIa receptors on platelets and megakaryocytes and blocks binding of fibrinogen and other ligands. Abciximab also binds to the vitronectin receptor, although the importance of this function is not yet fully understood.

Abciximab was developed from the murine immunoglobulin G1 monoclonal antibody m7E3. The Fc portion of the antibody was removed to avoid potential activation of complement and to minimize development of thrombocytopenia due to clearance of antibody-coated platelets. Because of concerns about the potential for immunogenicity from a murine antibody, the murine constant domain of the antibody was replaced with human constant domain sequences. Consequently, only the heavy- and light-chain variable regions are of murine origin.

A definite correlation exists between the percentage of receptors blocked and inhibition of platelet aggregation. When the number of unbound gpIIb/IIIa receptors is reduced to below 20,000 per platelet, platelet aggregation decreases and is sufficient to prevent thrombus formation. When the number of unbound receptors falls under 10,000 per platelet, bleeding time increases, which were more pronounced when there are fewer than 8,000 unbound gpIIb/IIIa receptors.

The dose of abciximab used in most clinical trials was a bolus of 250 $\mu$g/kg followed by an infusion of 10 $\mu$g/minute. Dosing regimens were determined by following ex vivo platelet aggregation studies and bleeding times. Fluorescence flow cytometry studies showed that platelets are uniformly coated with abciximab within 30 minutes of infusion. The half-life of unbound abciximab is very short, less than 10 to 30 minutes. Less than 5% of abciximab can be found in plasma 2 hours after a bolus injection. However, the bound antibody is cleared only with coated platelets, and it is interesting that surface-bound abciximab can be detected on platelets some 14 days after administration, which suggests that some antibodies are transferred to new platelets.

**EPTIFIBATIDE** This pharmacologic agent was discovered by screening for compounds contained in snake venom that inhibit platelet function via gpIIb/IIIa. One venom from the southeastern pygmy rattlesnake was found to be a specific inhibitor for gpIIb/IIIa. The 73-amino acid purified protein from the venom, named *barbourin*, contains a lysine-glycine-aspartic acid (KGD) peptide sequence rather than the RGD sequence in other gpIIb/IIIa binding compounds.

Eptifibatide is a cyclic heptapeptide synthesized by using the KDG peptide sequence as the template. It is a relatively small molecule with little, if any, antigenicity. Phase I trials showed complete inhibition of platelet aggregation at infusion rates of 1.0/1.5 $\mu$g/kg per minute, with only slight prolongation of bleeding times at higher infusion rates.

Eptifibatide has a short half-life of about 90 to 120 minutes. After discontinuing an infusion, bleeding times returns to normal in approximately 15 to 30 minutes, and platelet function returns to normal within 2 to 4 weeks. The short half-life and quick return of normal platelet function should decrease potential for bleeding from the use of this drug.

**TIROFIBAN AND LAMIFIBAN** These compounds are the two most studied nonpeptide gpIIb/IIIa inhibitors, with a relatively low-molecular-weight ($M_r$ <500 kDa). Both agents selectively bind to gpIIb/IIIa to inhibit platelet aggregation and are currently being studied in phase III clinical trials.

**XEMILOFIBAN** Xemilofiban is an oral gpIIb/IIIa inhibitor that is currently in phase III trials. It is an ethyl ester pro-drug that is readily absorbed. In clinical trials, 3 times per day administration at a dose of 2 to 25 mg inhibited platelet aggregation by 80%. Platelet inhibition usually peaks about 4 to 5 hours after a dose.

**CLINICAL INDICATIONS FOR THE USE OF GLYCOPROTEIN IIB/IIIA INHIBITORS**

***Post–Coronary Angioplasty Reocclusion*** Large clinical trials have demonstrated abciximab's efficacy at reducing post–coronary angioplasty restenosis. This is the first demonstration that clinical restenosis can be prevented by pharmacologic therapy. In one clinical trial, using composite endpoints (death, MI, emergency coronary artery bypass graft [CABG], emergency percutaneous transluminal coronary angioplasty [PTCA], stent placement, and intra-aortic balloon pump insertion), treatment benefit was present at all time points evaluated: 30 days, 6 months, and 3 years. Although abciximab did not affect patient survival, it did reduce the incidence of cardiac arrests and the need for emergency procedures, including coronary surgery.

***Unstable Angina*** The therapeutic role of gpIIb/IIIa inhibitors in this disease state is now unknown. In a double-blind study of 3232 patients with unstable angina who were already receiving aspirin, additional treatment with intravenous tirofiban for 48 hours appears to have some additional benefit when compared with aspirin and heparin. However, in another trial 1915 patients with unstable angina or non-Q-wave MI were randomly assigned to receive heparin, tirofiban plus heparin, or tirofiban alone. In addition, all patients received aspirin. The study was stopped prematurely in the tirofiban-alone group because of excess mortality at 7 days (4.6%, as compared with 1.1% for heparin alone and 1.5% for the combined therapy).

**COMPLICATIONS AND ADVERSE EFFECTS OF GLYCOPROTEIN IIB/IIIA ANTAGONISTS** Hemorrhagic risk is the major adverse effect of gpIIb/IIIa antagonists as with other antiplatelet agents. Data from several clinical trials indicate that anti-gpIIb/IIIa therapy was not associated with central nervous system bleeding or fatal bleeding but was associated with a two- to threefold increased risk of other major bleeding (Coller 1997a).

Drug-induced thrombocytopenia has been reported in about 5.2% (<100,000 platelets/mL) and 1.6% (<50,000 platelets/mL) of the patients. The thrombocytopenia can occur very rapidly and can be quite profound. Fresh platelet transfusions can reverse this effect.

Trials are ongoing to investigate the efficacy of gpIIb/IIIa inhibitors in other arterial thrombotic diseases such as unstable angina, acute myocardial infarction, and prevention of stent thrombosis during placement of intracoronary stents.

The various agents either in use or under development to inhibit platelet function and their mechanism of action are summarized in Table 12-6.

### *Thrombin inhibitors*

Thrombin plays a critical role in both the coagulation cascade and platelet activation. Agents that interfere with thrombin activity can therefore inhibit both arms of the hemostatic mechanism. Heparin, both unfractionated and low-molecular-weight preparations, activates antithrombin III to inactivate thrombin. Hirudin and its analog, hirulog, are direct thrombin inhibitors and do not require antithrombin III for their anticoagulant activity.

**INDIRECT THROMBIN INHIBITORS: HEPARIN** Heparin is a naturally occurring, highly sulfated glycosaminoglycan widely distributed in a variety of normal human tissues. Unfractionated heparin is commercially obtained from either bovine lung or porcine intestinal mucosa and consists of a heterogeneous mixture of polysaccharides with molecular masses ranging from 5000 to 30,000 kDa. As a result, the anticoagulant activity is variable, because the chain length of the molecules affects activity and the clearance of heparin.

The pharmacologic heterogeneity of heparin results from the variation of 1) the number of disaccharide resi-

**Table 12-6 Pharmacologic Classification of Agents That Interfere with Platelet Functions**

| MECHANISMS OF ACTION | REPRESENTATIVE AGENT(S) |
|---|---|
| 1. Drugs that interfere with $TXA_2$ formation | |
| • Phospholipase $A_2$ inhibition | Mepacrine HCl |
| • Cyclooxygenase inhibition | Aspirin |
| • Thromboxane synthetase inhibition | Dazoxibene, ozagrel |
| • $TXA_2$ receptor antagonism | Ridogrel, isbogrel, nidogrel |
| 2. Drugs that interfere with receptors for platelet activation | |
| • ADP ($P_{2T}$ purinergic) receptor antagonism | Ticlopidine, clopidogrel |
| • Thrombin receptor antagonism | Hirudin, hirulog and antithrombin receptor peptide |
| • PAF receptor antagonism | Gingkolides |
| • 5-HT receptor antagonism | Ketanserin, sarpogrelate |
| • $\alpha_2$-Adrenergic receptor antagonism | Yohimbine, dihydrocryptine |
| 3. Drugs that interfere with platelet adhesion receptors | |
| • GpIb–V–IX antagonism | GpIb antibody, antibody to vWF, inactive vWF fragments |
| • GpIIb–IIIa antagonism | C7E3Fab (abciximab), small peptides containing specific sequences |
| 4. Drugs that raise intracellular cAMP in platelets | |
| • Activation of adenylyl cyclase | $PGE_1$ |
| • Inhibition of phosphodiesterase | Dipyridamole, caffeine, theophylline |
| • Activation of guanylyl cyclase | Nitrate derivatives, NO |

ABBREVIATIONS: 5-HT, serotonin; cAMP, cyclic AMP; Gp or gp, glycoprotein; NO, nitric oxide; PAF, platelet-activating factor; $PGE_1$, prostaglandin $E_1$; $TXA_2$, thromboxane$_2$; vWF, von Willebrand factor.

dues, 2) which uronic acid is present, and 3) the extent and position of sulfate residues. Heparin consists of alternating residues of uronic acid and glucosamine that may be variably sulfated. The negative charge imparted by sulfation appears to be an important determinant of the anticoagulant effect of a given heparin preparation.

The anticoagulant function of heparin is mediated largely through its ability to bind to antithrombin III and catalyzes its anticoagulant activity. Antithrombin is a member of the serine protease inhibitor (SERPIN) family and regulates coagulation by inactivating activated coagulation proteases that have a serine residue at their enzymatically active centers by irreversible complex formation. These activated factors include factors IX, X, XI, XII, and thrombin. Binding of heparin to ATIII occurs through a specific pentasaccharide sequence containing a particular glucosamine unit that combines with lysine sites on the ATIII molecule, thereby producing a conformational change that exposes an arginine reactive site on the heparin–ATIII complex. This arginine site can then inhibit the active center on the serine site of the activated coagulant factors. In this mechanism, heparin acts as a catalyst and is not consumed in the reaction process.

In addition to its anticoagulant activity, at high concentrations heparin combines with the heparin cofactor II to inhibit thrombin directly. Other effects of heparin include interfering with the interaction of coagulation factors on the platelet surface; inhibiting platelet aggregation; increasing vessel-wall permeability; and inhibiting proliferation of vascular smooth muscle cells with modulation of angiogenesis (Levine, Hirsh, Salzman, et al. 1994; Hirsh et al. 1995). The significance of these effects is not clear, but most of these effects may contribute to heparin's potential to cause bleeding. Platelet activation may also be important in heparin-associated thrombocytopenia (discussed below).

***Pharmacokinetics of Heparin*** Heparin is a highly charged molecule and is therefore poorly transported across biologic membranes. Consequently, parenteral administration is recommended, either intravenously or subcutaneously. Use of the intramuscular route is discouraged, because it may produce large hematomas. Heparin avidly binds to plasma proteins after administration. This results in reduced bioavailability and variability of the anticoagulant response in different patients. The average half-life of an intravenous heparin dose is 1 to 1.5 hours. The half-life appears to be dose-dependent, as half-life increases with increasing dosage.

Given the variability of response to heparin administration, dosage adjustment is based on the anticoagulant response as measured by partial-thromboplastin times. Measurement of plasma concentrations of heparin is not done routinely. However, in patients who appear to have a resistance to heparin, arbitrarily defined as a requirement for more than 50,000 U of heparin per 24 hours, plasma heparin levels may be measured rather than partial thromboplastin times to avoid unnecessary dose escalation. Plasma heparin levels are also useful for titrating heparin concentrations in the presence of a prolonged partial thromboplastin time at baseline because of lupus anticoagulants. The total amount of heparin required to achieve the same degree of anticoagulant effect over the same time period does not appear to differ whether the heparin is administered intravenously or subcutaneously (Hirsh et al. 1995).

***Administration and Monitoring of Heparin*** Most investigators recommend using the activated partial thromboplastin time (aPTT), a global assessment of the intrinsic coagulation pathway, which is sensitive to the inhibitory effects of heparin on thrombin, factor Xa, and IXa, to monitor heparin anticoagulation. An initial dose of heparin is chosen, and subsequent dosage adjustments are guided by aPTT assays. For example, it is recommended that patients with proximal DVT be given a bolus loading dose of heparin of 5000 units intravenously followed by a continuous infusion of heparin on the order of 20 to 25 units/kg per hour. The goal is to rapidly achieve prolongation of the aPTT between 1.5 and 2.5 times the laboratory control aPTT. A prospective study of the relation between the degree of prolongation of the aPTT and recurrence of venous thromboembolism found that recurrence was rare if the aPTT was prolonged to 1.5 or more times the control values at all times, and if this prolongation was achieved within 24 hours.

It is important to rapidly achieve adequate anticoagulation, because the patient continues to be at risk for thrombus extension and/or embolization until the aPTT is therapeutically prolonged. Consequently, rigorous use of heparin therapy coupled with frequent monitoring of aPTT values (every 4 to 6 hours until the aPTT is within the therapeutic range, then daily) is mandatory. Patients with pulmonary emboli or massive venous thrombosis should be initially treated with a heparin bolus of 10,000 units intravenously, followed by a continuous infusion of heparin of 25 to 30 units/kg per hour. After successful anticoagulation is achieved, daily aPTT values should be obtained, because heparin requirements may diminish with cessation of the hypercoagulable state.

Although some physicians believe that intermittent intravenous heparin injections every 4 to 6 hours represent an acceptable alternative therapy, continuous intravenous infusion offers the advantages of consistent therapeutic anticoagulation and may decrease the rate of bleeding complications (Levine et al. 1992).

***Clinical Indications for the use of Heparin*** Two general indications for heparin administration are 1) using high-dose heparin for therapy of acute thrombotic diseases, and 2) using subcutaneous low-dose heparin for an effective and safe form of prophylaxis in patients who are at risk of thromboembolism. The basis for therapeutic high-dose heparin anticoagulation is that patients with established thrombotic disease require large doses to neutralize large amounts of thrombin generated during intravascular coagulation and thrombosis. In contrast, patients at risk but who have not yet developed thrombosis can avoid thrombosis with smaller doses of heparin.

*Deep Venous Thromboembolism and Pulmonary Embolism* Studies done before the introduction of routine anticoagulant therapy indicated that 20% of patients with untreated venous thrombosis died of pulmonary embolism. A controlled trial using heparin followed by an oral anticoagulant demonstrated a dramatic reduction in deaths from pulmonary embolism and in nonfatal recurrences in high-risk patients. These and other studies (summarized in Hirsh et al. 1995) provide convincing evidence that anticoagulants are very effective in preventing extension of venous thrombosis and pulmonary embolism in patients with documented venous thrombotic disease.

Current recommendations are to administer heparin for at least 5 days, because studies have shown that a 5-day course of heparin was as effective as a 10-day course in treating DVT (Pineo and Hull 1996). Warfarin can be safely started once a therapeutic aPTT level has been achieved. Initial therapy with warfarin without therapeutic levels of heparin may paradoxically intensify hypercoagulability and increase the frequency of recurrent venous thromboembolism.

*Acute Myocardial Infarction and Unstable Angina* Although intravenous heparin has been routinely used in the treatment of AMI and unstable angina, data supporting this therapeutic indication have not been conclusive. Studies of heparin therapy in patients who did not routinely receive aspirin (or fibrinolytic therapy) do indicate some net benefit from heparin, despite the occurrence of major bleeding in about 10 patients per 1000 treated. However, it is no longer relevant to assess heparin in the absence of aspirin, because aspirin has been found to have substantial value even when given with heparin. The key question is whether heparin should be added to aspirin. So far, the evidence is not compelling.

Among patients with unstable angina, there is also uncertainty about improvement in major clinical outcomes with the addition of intravenous heparin to aspirin, either in individual trials or in a formal meta-analysis (Oler et al. 1996; Collins et al. 1997).

In summary, the available (extensive) data do not provide any clear justification for routine heparin therapy in patients with suspected AMI (or unstable angina), because the benefit, if any, is small, and heparin therapy is associated with increased risk of bleeding and other complications.

*Transient Ischemic Attacks and Stroke* The efficacy of heparin in treating nonhemorrhagic cerebral vascular events remains unconfirmed. No large, randomized, placebo-controlled trials have been done to determine the efficacy of unfractionated heparin in the treatment of stroke. Three small trials have demonstrated a trend supporting the use of heparin. Low-dose heparin has been shown to be effective in lowering the risk of DVT and pulmonary embolism in stroke patients. Recently, promising results from a study using low-molecular-weight heparin suggest a role for anticoagulation in the treatment of stroke patients.

***Contraindications and Complications of Heparin Therapy*** Heparin use is contraindicated in patients with underlying thrombocytopenia or coagulopathy, trauma, CNS disease, or active bleeding. Heparin should be administrated with caution to patients who have recently undergone surgery, who have severe hypertension, and who have a recent or past history of cerebrovascular, gastrointestinal, or genitourinary hemorrhage or metastatic cancer. Heparin is thought to be safe for use in pregnancy (discussed below).

Numerous adverse effects have been described with heparin use. Bleeding is the most frequent complication, usually presenting as epistaxis, hematuria, melena, or ecchymosis. One large survey of drug-related deaths among medical inpatients found that heparin was the major drug responsible for drug-related deaths in patients considered to be reasonably healthy. Actual hemorrhage caused by heparin is usually associated with overdosage or misuse of the drug. Hemorrhage associated with heparin therapy has made many practitioners overly cautious with respect to its proper use. This may result in delays of initiating therapeutic anticoagulation and inadequate heparin dosage during initial anticoagulation.

**PRINCIPLE The fear of toxicity may be difficult to overcome when the administration of an efficacious drug is complicated. But the fear of toxicity is not an excuse for the inadequate administration of the drug.**

*Heparin-Induced Thrombocytopenia* Another adverse effect of heparin administration is thrombocytopenia, with or without thrombosis. Heparin-induced thrombocytopenia and thrombosis are serious complications of heparin treatment. The incidence, as previously reported, varies widely from 5% to 30%, but recent analysis indicates that the true incidence is less than 3% (Schmitt and Adelman 1993).

Heparin-induced thrombocytopenia causes venous thrombosis more often than arterial thrombosis. Although rapid loading of warfarin used to be recommended, this strategy may precipitate venous gangrene of the limbs, possibly as a result of a precipitous warfarin-mediated decline in protein C levels. Appropriate treatment approaches include use of a heparinoid or direct thrombin inhibitor such as hirudin (described below).

*Other Complications* Other complications caused by heparin are much less frequent and include heparin allergy and osteoporosis. Patients who exhibit hypersensitivity to one preparation of commercial heparin (e.g., bovine heparin) should receive another preparation (porcine heparin). The advent of low-molecular-weight heparin preparations should further diminish this adverse effect of heparin. Osteoporosis is seen only in the infrequent patients who receive large doses of heparin (>20,000 units per day) for longer than 6 months (Hirsh et al. 1995). This adverse effect results from increased bone resorption induced by heparin. Patients who receive adjusted-dose subcutaneous heparin prophylaxis for prolonged periods may also be at risk of experiencing this complication.

*Treatment of Heparin Overdosage* Patients who receive therapeutic doses of heparin, have aPTT values above the therapeutic range (>2.5-$\mu$l per baseline), and have little or no bleeding should have heparin infusion rates diminished or briefly curtailed. The short half-life of heparin (1 to 1.5 hour) ensures rapid correction of the prolonged aPTT. Care should be taken to avoid loss of therapeutic anticoagulation if heparin is temporarily discontinued.

Patients who sustain a major hemorrhage associated with heparin use are candidates for immediate reversal of heparin anticoagulation with protamine sulfate. The anticoagulant effect of heparin (strongly negatively charged) is promptly neutralized by protamine sulfate (strongly positively charged). Protamine is given by intravenous infusion; a loading dose is calculated using the assumption that 1 mg of protamine will neutralize about 100 units of heparin. Given the short half-life of heparin, an estimate of the quantity of heparin in the body at the time of the protamine infusion should be made so that excess protamine is not administered. Protamine sulfate should be infused slowly for over 10 minutes to avoid potential adverse reactions such as hypotension, dyspnea, and flushing.

Several studies suggest that patients allergic to fish or patients who receive insulin containing protamine are at increased risk of developing a true anaphylactic reaction to protamine infusion. In addition, positively charged proteins when infused rapidly may lead to mast cell degranulation; this histamine release may cause severe hypotension. Excess protamine administration should be avoided, because it can result in a "paradoxical" bleeding diathesis. The mechanism of paradoxical bleeding following excess protamine administration is drug-induced platelet aggregation and thrombocytopenia and interference with fibrin formation by protamine.

**INDIRECT THROMBIN INHIBITORS: LOW-MOLECULAR-WEIGHT HEPARINS** Low-molecular-weight heparins (LMWHs) have established their role as an important class of antithrombotic compounds (Weitz 1997). LMWHs have replaced unfractionated heparin for both prophylaxis and treatment of venous thromboembolic diseases in most parts of Europe but are only now finding their place in North America. However, application of LMWHs in arterial thrombotic disorders such as coronary arterial disease and ischemic stroke is just evolving.

Pharmaceutical heparin is commonly extracted from porcine intestinal mucosa or bovine lung. By the extraction procedure, the polysaccharides are degraded to a heterogeneous mixture of fragments exhibiting a molecular weight range of approximately 300 to 30,000 $K_d$ (unfractionated heparin). Now, these low-molecular-weight heparin preparations are obtained either by fractionation or by controlled depolymerization of unfractionated heparin achieved by using various technical procedures. It should be noted that the LMWHs produced by different methods are to be considered as individual pharmacologic compounds.

Both unfractionated heparin and LMWHs exert their anticoagulant activity by activating antithrombin III. Their interaction with antithrombin III is mediated by a unique pentasaccharide sequence that is randomly distributed along the heparin chains. Approximately one-third of the chains of unfractionated heparin, but only 15 to 25% of the chains of low-molecular-weight heparins, contain this pentasaccharide sequence.

The chief difference in the anticoagulatory mechanism between unfractionated heparin and low-molecular-weight heparins lies in their relative inhibitory activity against factor Xa and thrombin. Any pentasaccharide-containing heparin chain can inhibit the action of factor Xa simply by binding to antithrombin III and causing a conformational change. In contrast, to inactivate thrombin, heparin must bind to both antithrombin III and thrombin, thereby forming a ternary complex. This complex can be formed only by pentasaccharide-containing heparin chains composed of at least 18 saccharide units. Whereas most of the chains of unfractionated heparin are at least 18 saccharide units long, fewer than half of those of LMWHs are of sufficient length to bind to both antithrombin and thrombin. As a consequence, unlike unfractionated heparin, which has equivalent activity against factor Xa and thrombin, low-molecular-weight heparins have greater activity against factor Xa (Fig. 12-9).

Clinically, the principal advantages of LMWHs are their more predictable anticoagulant response and their ease of use without laboratory monitoring. LMWHs can be administered by once-daily subcutaneous injection without careful laboratory monitoring. This is due to the decreased propensity of LMWHs to bind to plasma proteins, endothelial cells, and macrophages (Weitz 1997). As a consequence, the bioavailability of LMWH is about 90%, whereas that of unfractionated heparin is only in the range of 20%.

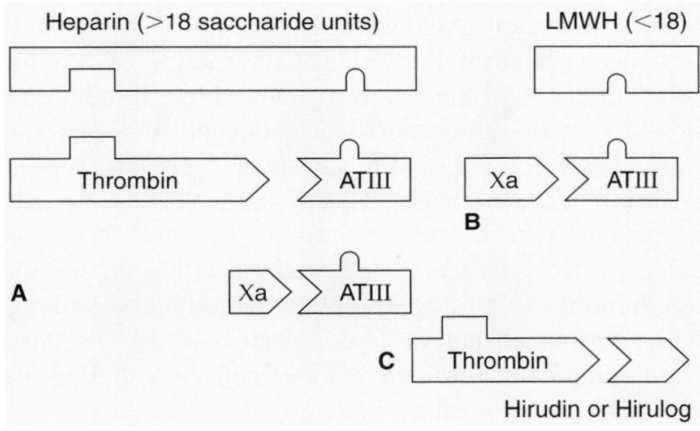


**F I G U R E 1 2 - 9 Relative inhibition of thrombin and factor Xa by heparin, LMWH, and hirudin. (*A*.) Formation of a ternary complex of heparin with both antithrombin and thrombin depends on pentasaccharide-containing heparin chains composed of at least 18 saccharide units, whereas formation of heparin/Xa complex does not require this size of heparin. (*B*.) LMWH molecules are of sufficient length to bind to antithrombin. Thus, unfractionated heparin has equivalent activity against factor Xa and thrombin but LMWHs have greater activity against factor Xa. (*C*.) Hirudin binds directly to ATIII. abbreviations: ATIII, anti-thrombin III; LMWHs, low-molecular-weight heparins.**

Evidence from clinical trials shows that there is no significant difference in the incidence of major bleeding when LMWHs are compared with unfractionated heparin (Thomas 1997). However, drug induced-thrombocytopenia and osteoporosis are less frequent with LMWHs compared with unfractionated heparin, when given for more than 1 month.

The plasma half-life of LMWH is about 2 to 4 hours after intravenous injection and from 3 to 6 after subcutaneous injection (Nurmohamed et al. 1997), two to four times as long as the half-life of unfractionated heparin. Maximum plasma levels after subcutaneous injections of LMWH are reached within 2 to 3 hours.

Clinical indications for the use of low-molecular-weight heparins follow.

***Deep Venous Thrombosis and Pulmonary Embolism*** LMWHs are effective in preventing DVT in orthopedic surgical patients, resulting in an approximately 75% risk reduction compared with untreated controls (Pini 1997). Once-daily administration is the norm, the first dose being given preoperatively. LMWHs have also been shown to provide effective prophylaxis when started postoperatively in high-risk orthopedic patients (Turpie 1997). LMWHs provide more effective prophylaxis than does fixed low-dose standard heparin, with an additional risk reduction of approximately 25% for DVT (Hirsh 1998). LMWHs appear to be particularly effective in preventing proximal DVT and pulmonary embolism and are emerging as the prophylactic method of choice for patients at high risk for DVTs.

A particular useful therapeutic use of LMWHs is that they can be used safely and effectively to treat patients with proximal DVT at home (Levine et al. 1996). In the treatment of acute DVT, LMWHs administered subcutaneously in a fixed dose per kilogram of body weight showed efficacy and safety equivalent to those from intravenous heparin in adjusted doses, and use of LMWHs allows home treatment in selected cases. In the treatment of DVT after the acute phase, LMWHs are as effective as and safer than oral anticoagulants.

Two recent studies indicate that unmonitored low-molecular-weight heparin is also as safe and effective as intravenous unfractionated heparin in patients with pulmonary embolism. The first study compared these agents in 1021 patients with venous thromboembolism, 26% of whom had pulmonary embolism, and reported similar rates of recurrent thromboembolism (5.3% and 4.9%, respectively) and major bleeding (3.1% and 2.3%). In the second study, 912 patients with pulmonary embolism were randomly assigned to receive unfractionated heparin or low-molecular-weight heparin. The incidence of death, recurrent venous thromboembolism, or major bleeding was essentially the same in both groups (2.9% and 3.0%, respectively). These findings may shift the management of venous thromboembolism from the inpatient to the outpatient setting.

***Acute Myocardial Infarction and Unstable Angina*** A number of LMWHs, dalteparin, enoxaparin, and nadroparin have been evaluated in unstable angina, and results from these studies are quite promising. Dalteparin has been evaluated in two large clinical trials in the management of unstable angina. The low-molecular-weight heparin (Fragmin) during Instability in Coronary Artery Disease trial [Fragmin during Instability in Coronary Artery Disease (FRISC) Study Group 1996] showed that dalteparin resulted in a 63% reduction in risk of death or acute MI compared with aspirin alone. The Fragmin in Unstable Coronary Artery Disease (FRIC) trial showed that dalteparin was as effective as intravenous heparin (Klein et al. 1997). Enoxaparin resulted in a statistically significant 16% reduction in the combined outcome of death, MI, and recurrence of angina in comparison with standard heparin in the Efficacy and Safety of Subcutaneous Enoxaparin in Non-Q-Wave Coronary Events (ESSENCE) trial (Mark et al. 1998).

***Stroke*** In acute ischemic stroke, preliminary results are promising, but the evidence of efficacy must be substantiated by other studies that are now in progress.

***Direct Thrombin Inhibitors: Hirudin and Hirulog*** Hirudin is a 7-kDa (65-amino acid) polypeptide originally found in the salivary glands of the leech, *Hirudo medicinalis*. Hirudin is a potent anticoagulant and shows promise as a novel antithrombotic agent (Markwardt 1994; Wallis 1996). Hirulog, a 20-amino-acid synthetic analog was designed using hirudin as a model and manufactured by standard solid-phase peptide methodologies. Both hirudin and hirulog are direct thrombin inhibitors and do not require antithrombin III for their anticoagulant effect.

***Pharmacology and Pharmacokinetics of Direct Thrombin Inhibitors*** The mechanism of hirudin-induced anti-thrombin action appears to be specific and unique. It reacts very rapidly with thrombin to form an inactive one-to-one complex with a high binding affinity and specificity for thrombin (dissociation constant, $K_i < 1$ pM). Unlike heparin, hirudin binds to the active site of thrombin and produces a direct inhibition of thrombin's proteolytic function without requiring the presence of endogenous cofactor antithrombin III (Fig. 12-9). In addition, because thrombin is a potent platelet activator as described in the previous section, hirudin prevents thrombin-induced platelet aggregation. Additionally, the binding of thrombin to thrombomodulin is also inhibited, which may result in a reduced activation of protein C.

Anticoagulant and antithrombotic effects of hirudin have been demonstrated in various animal models of experimental venous and arterial thrombosis, DIC, experimental angioplasty, cardiopulmonary bypass, thrombosis of arteriovenous shunts, and experimental hemodialysis (Markwardt 1994; Wallis 1996). It is of major significance that hirudin inhibits fibrin-bound thrombin, which is poorly accessible to the heparin–antithrombin III complex. This effect of hirudin may be particularly useful in preventing reocclusion after intravascular thrombosis (Weitz et al. 1998).

Preclinical studies in experimental animals and in healthy volunteers have shown that hirudin had no significant adverse effects after acute or chronic administration (Glusa 1998). Administration of hirudin intravenously or subcutaneously is well tolerated in humans. Of note, hirudin has little hemorrhagic effect at dosages used for antithrombotic therapy (Markwardt 1994).

There are several theoretical advantages of hirudin over heparin and other anticoagulants. First, hirudin and hirulog provide more consistent anticoagulation and antithrombosis without significant adverse effects such as heparin-induced bleeding. This is particularly important for patients with surgical procedures because the major adverse effect of heparin and warfarin is bleeding. Second, hirudin and hirulog can inhibit clot-bound thrombin, unlike unfractionated or low-molecular-weight heparin. Third, hirudin and hirulog are not associated with drug-induced thrombocytopenia.

Findings from animal and human studies indicate that, when administered intravenously, hirudin follows an open, two-compartment model with first-order pharmacokinetics. The elimination half-life of hirudin is 1 to 2 hours. Approximately 60% of a parenteral dose is eliminated unchanged via glomerular filtration. Therefore, the elimination of hirudin is decreased (15 to 50 hours) in patients with renal failure (Vanholder et al. 1997). Hirulog has a shorter half-life than hirudin and is eliminated through metabolic pathways and the urine.

***Clinical Studies of the Use of Hirudin and Hirulog*** Two recombinant hirudins, desulfatohirudin and HBW023, and a synthetic hirulog, bivalirudin, are available for clinical studies.

*Deep Venous Thrombosis and Pulmonary Embolism* Evidence from clinical trials demonstrates that hirudin or bivalirudin are more effective in the prevention of venous thromboembolic disease in patients undergoing orthopedic surgery than heparin or LMWH (Eriksson, Ekman, et al. 1997; Eriksson BI, Wille-Jorgensen, et al. 1997). Randomized placebo-controlled studies assessing subcutaneous hirudin, versus standard heparin or LMWHs, showed that hirudin is more efficacious than heparins at reducing the frequency of DVT and pulmonary embolism after hip surgery without significantly increasing the incidence of abnormal bleeding (Eriksson et al. 1996). Efforts are under way to develop orally bioavailable direct antithrombins for outpatient management of venous thromboembolism (Harker et al. 1997).

*Acute Coronary Syndromes* Clinical trials have also been carried out comparing hirudin with heparin in the following clinical situations: 1) coronary angioplasty; 2) unstable angina; and 3) acute myocardial infarction. Bivalirudin has been shown to increase the rate of TIMI grade 3 patency (from 35% to 48%, $P = 0.03$) at 90 minutes after streptokinase administration (White 1997). Data from the TIMI 9 and GUSTO II trials showed that hirudin therapy caused a 14% reduction in repeat infarction at 30 days, but there was no effect on mortality or on the combined end point of death and nonfatal MI (10.8% heparin versus 10.0% hirudin). In therapy of acute coronary artery syndromes, hirudin and bivalirudin have consistently produced more predictable and less variable levels of anticoagulation, which lead to reduction of adverse clinical events. However, results from clinical trials indicate that hirudin and bivalirudin have a narrow therapeutic window similar to heparin's. There is an increased risk for bleeding, including intracerebral hemorrhage, when aPTT levels are greater than 100 seconds during treatment. The major disappointment of direct thrombin inhibitors in treatment of coronary arterial disease has been the inability to sustain the short-term benefit. Further trials are necessary to determine whether there is a role for these agents in the treatment of acute coronary syndromes.

All the thrombin inhibitors need to be administered parenterally. However, anticoagulation often is needed for a prolonged period. At present, warfarin is the only inhibitor of the coagulation system that can be administered orally.

***Oral anticoagulant: Warfarin***

The discovery of warfarin dates back to the 1920s, when cattle fed spoiled sweet clover were found to develop a hemorrhagic disorder. Identification of the agent in clover by Campbell and Link in 1941 as bishydroxycoumarin (dicoumarol) led to the development of synthetic derivatives such as warfarin.

Warfarin is a member of a class of vitamin K antagonists derived from coumarin, and the structures of warfarin and vitamin K are shown in Fig. 12-10. Also shown is a summary of the vitamin K cycle that is essential to understanding the mechanism of warfarin activity. Warfarin acts as an inhibitor of epoxide reductase and vitamin K reductase (Fig. 12-10), two enzymes in the vitamin K cycle responsible for recycling oxidized vitamin K to the reduced form. Warfarin thereby prevents generation of the reduced form of vitamin K, which is a necessary cofactor for the carboxylation of glutamic acid residues to form $\gamma$-carboxylation of key coagulation factors and other proteins including factors II, VII, IX, and X and proteins C and S.

Warfarin treatment results in the production of inactive clotting factors, because they lack the $\gamma$-carboxyglutamyl side chains necessary for calcium binding and subsequent activity. The anticoagulant effects of warfarin are not observed until many hours or days after drug administration. The anticoagulant effect of warfarin results from disappearance of the normal $\gamma$-carboxylated coagulation factors from the blood. The rates of disappearance of these proteins are inversely related to their elimination half-lives. The decrease in concentrations of prothrombin and factors VII, IX, and X following administration of warfarin into the therapeutic range (about 20% of normal) requires 4 to 5 days. This is the basis for the recommendation that patients given warfarin should be anticoagulated with therapeutic heparin for at least 5 days until the full therapeutic effect of warfarin is achieved.

Warfarin is a racemic mixture of the enantiomers R- and S-warfarin, which have different drug interactions and different pharmacokinetic and pharmacodynamic properties. After oral administration, warfarin is rapidly absorbed, reaches peak blood concentrations after 90 minutes, and has a plasma half-life of approximately 40 hours with a bioavailability of close to 100%. Individual differences in absorption are not important as a cause of altered drug response. Warfarin binds extensively to plasma proteins, chiefly albumin. Hepatic metabolism converts war-

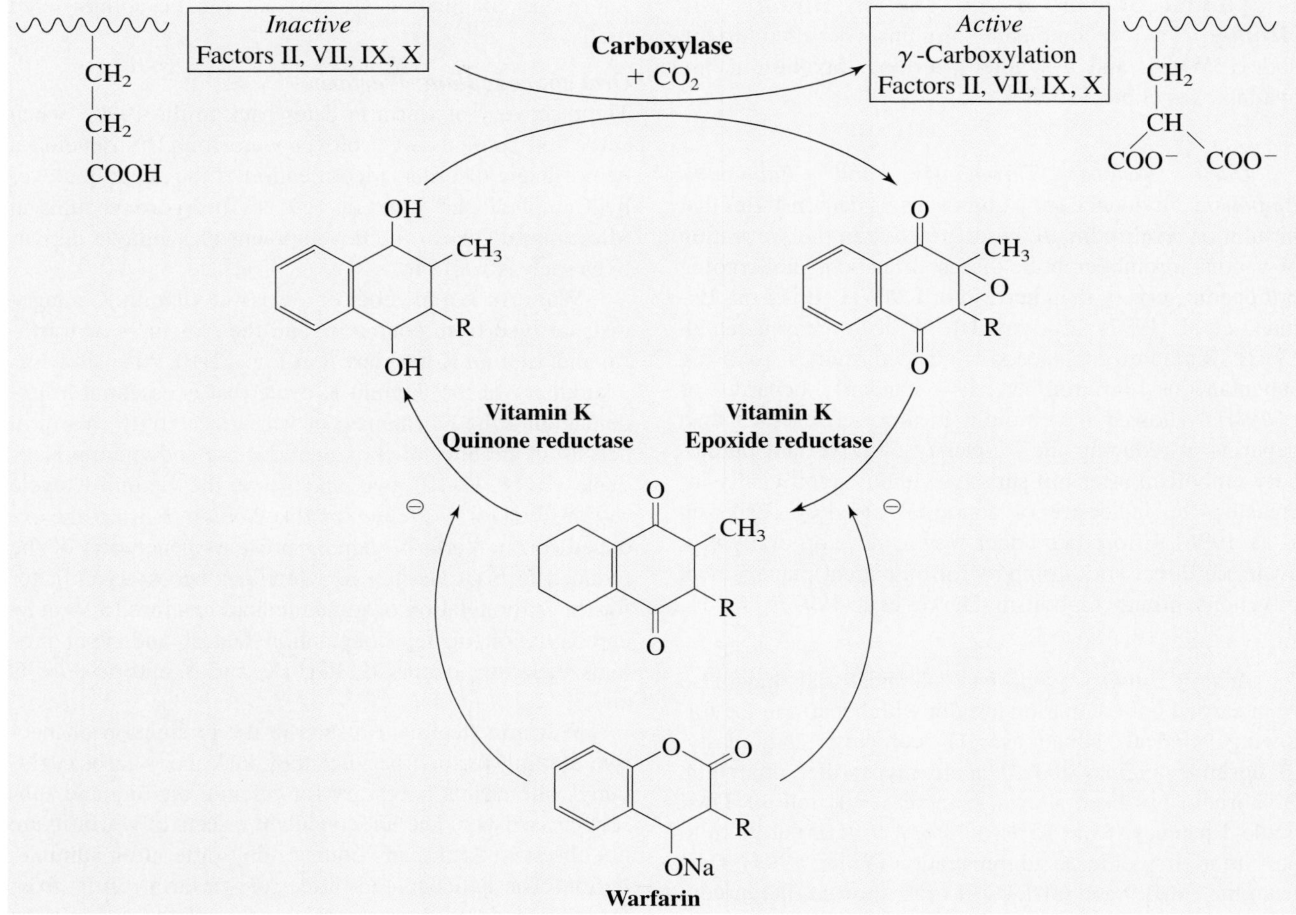


FIGURE 12-10 **Mechanism of action of warfarin. Warfarin shares similar chemical structures with vitamin K. Warfarin acts as a competitive inhibitor of epoxide reductase and vitamin K reductase to block the vitamin K cycle and thereby prevents formation of γ-carboxylation of key coagulation factors and other coagulant proteins. (Modified from Furie and Furie 1990.)**

farin to inactive products that are subsequently conjugated to glucuronic acid. These inactive metabolites undergo enterohepatic recirculation and are ultimately excreted in urine and stool. Liver disease is well known to enhance warfarin's anticoagulant effect, but renal disease does not increase the response to warfarin. Plasma concentrations of warfarin are about 2 mg/mL in patients who are adequately anticoagulated. As discussed below, monitoring of warfarin therapy is done using functional coagulation tests; obtaining plasma warfarin concentrations is reserved for the unusual patient who does not respond to standard warfarin therapy and in whom malabsorption, noncompliance, or inherited drug resistance is a possible explanation.

**MONITORING WARFARIN THERAPY** Crucial to the understanding of monitoring warfarin therapy is the concept of the international normalized ratio of prothrombin time (INR), a method that standardizes coagulation assays used to monitor patients taking warfarin. Variations in reagents used in the prothrombin time (PT) assay led to excessive warfarin anticoagulation and hemorrhagic complications in patients. Recognition of this important variable in warfarin therapy led to clinical trials using less intense warfarin therapy and the development of INR.

Current guidelines recommend INR levels of 2.0 to 3.0 for the prevention and treatment of venous thromboembolism and other thrombotic disorders (Table 12-7). However, there is evidence that a lower INR may be ef-

Table 12-7 Recommended Therapeutic Range for Oral Anticoagulant Therapy

| Clinical indications | INR |
|---|---|
| Treatment of venous thrombosis | |
| Treatment of pulmonary embolism | |
| Prevention of systemic embolism | |
| • Tissue heart valves | 2.0–3.0 |
| • Prevention of systemic embolism after acute MI | |
| • Valvular heart disease | |
| • Atrial fibrillation | |
| Mechanical prosthetic valves (high risk) | 2.5–3.5 |

NOTE: The optimal therapeutic range for oral anticoagulant therapy was recommended and reviewed by the Committee on Antithrombotic Therapy of the American College of Chest Physicians (ACCP) and the National Heart, Lung, and Blood Institute in 1992. This recommendation has been clarified and supported by many clinical trials (see Hirsh et al. 1995).

ABBREVIATIONS: INR, international normalized ratio of prothrombin time; MI, myocardial infarction.

fective in patients receiving primary prophylaxis (Levine, Hirsh, Gent, et al. 1994). Another consideration in using the INR to monitor warfarin therapy is that heparin therapy exerts an unpredictable effect on the INR. Therefore, the physician should measure the INR after heparin has been discontinued to ensure appropriate oral anticoagulant dosing.

Duration of warfarin therapy depends on whether risk factor(s) for thrombosis continue (i.e., inherited disorders, prolonged immobilization). If no continuing risk factors are identified, a 3-month course of warfarin therapy may be appropriate. Shorter treatment intervals may be as useful, but large-scale studies are necessary to demonstrate their effectiveness. Treatment duration for patients with venous thrombosis because of an inherited disorder is currently controversial. Some investigators have suggested that these patients should receive lifelong therapeutic warfarin (Hirsh 1995).

#### CLINICAL INDICATIONS FOR THE USE OF WARFARIN

***Venous Thromboembolism*** The primary use of warfarin is in the long-term prophylaxis against new or recurrent DVTs and pulmonary embolism. Numerous studies have documented warfarin's efficacy in this setting (Hirsh et al. 1995).

***Myocardial Infarction*** Warfarin has been shown to be effective in reducing mortality and morbidity following myocardial infarction. Warfarin can prevent reocclusion, thromboembolic phenomena associated with left ventricular aneurysm or atrial fibrillation, and venous thromboembolism in the postinfarction period. Analysis of pooled data from seven randomized trials published between 1964 and 1980 showed that oral anticoagulant (mainly warfarin) therapy during a 1- to 6-year treatment period reduced the combined endpoints of mortality and nonfatal repeat infarction by approximately 20% (Hirsh et al. 1995). A recent trial, Anticoagulants in the Secondary Prevention of Events in Coronary Thrombosis (ASPECT) [Anticoagulants in the Secondary Prevention of Events in Coronary Thrombosis (ASPECT) Research Group 1994], reported that warfarin therapy (INR 2.8 to 4.8) produces a greater than 50% reduction in repeat infarction and a 40% reduction in stroke.

Patients with anterior wall MI are at increased risk for thromboembolic events. Warfarin has been shown to prevent left ventricular thrombi and embolic events and aid in resolution of developed thrombi in this patient population. In addition, in post-MI patients who are at high risk for developing mural thrombi such as those with a large infarction zone or area of dyskinesia, congestive heart failure (CHF), and atrial fibrillation, treatment with 3 months of warfarin therapy is recommended.

The benefits of aspirin versus warfarin after MI remain controversial, as few trials have directly compared these two treatments. Overall, the data appear to favor the use of aspirin over warfarin in the post-MI period. However, there is some recent evidence that their combined use may have some added advantage over aspirin alone. In a trial investigating primary prevention of ischemic heart disease, low-intensity warfarin therapy (INR ~1.5) with aspirin was more effective at reducing all ischemic events than single treatment with aspirin or warfarin. In this trial, warfarin's beneficial effect is mainly due to the reduction of fatal events; in contrast, aspirin reduced mainly nonfatal events. In the Coumadin Aspirin Reinfarction Study (CARS) (CARS Investigators 1997), the use of a fixed dose (1 or 3 mg, INR 1.19) warfarin with low-dose aspirin

(80 mg) was no more effective than using 160 mg of aspirin for secondary prevention of myocardial infarction. This result may suggest a simple pharmacologic truism, drugs should be used at the minimum therapeutic dose needed to realize a therapeutic benefit.

***Stroke and Atrial Fibrillation*** Another important clinical indication for warfarin therapy is in patients with nonrheumatic atrial fibrillation. Numerous epidemiologic studies have shown that nonrheumatic atrial fibrillation is a strong risk factor for stroke, raising the risk of stroke fivefold and with the prevalence of stroke increasing with age (Wolf and Singer 1997). Stroke in these patients is thought to be due to thromboembolism arising from the fibrillating atria, although the dynamics of blood flow are such that intravascular thrombi and in situ thrombosis, in addition to intracardiac thrombi, could account for the cerebral event. In the last few years, six trials have been completed in patients with atrial fibrillation to test the efficacy of warfarin for preventing stroke. All six trials found that low-intensity anticoagulation (INR 1.4 to 2.8) is highly effective for preventing stroke in patients with atrial fibrillation. Each trial was stopped early because warfarin was so effective that continuing the study was regarded as unethical. Warfarin trials may have underestimated the efficacy of warfarin, because a large fraction of strokes counted in the warfarin-treated groups occurred in patients who were not actually taking warfarin at the time of the stroke. Indeed, nearly all the risk of stroke attributable to atrial fibrillation appears to be eliminated by warfarin therapy.

Warfarin has also proved to be remarkably safe, even in elderly patients. Intracranial bleeding, the most dreaded complication, was very rare (the rate was less than 0.5% per year), and the rate of major bleeding at other sites was also low. Unless there is a very strong contraindication, low-intensity warfarin therapy should be routinely initiated in patients with chronic atrial fibrillation, including elderly patients.

***Mechanical Heart-Valve Replacement*** Despite improvements in valve design, thromboembolism remains a serious complication after mechanical heart-valve replacement. It is generally agreed that lifelong anticoagulant therapy is indicated in all patients with mechanical valves and in patients with tissue valves (bioprosthesis) if there is associated atrial fibrillation or previous thromboembolism. Furthermore, relatively high-intensity anticoagulation (INR 3 to 4) is recommended for this prophylactic use. Despite the use of anticoagulants, major systemic embolism still occurs at a rate of about 2 to 3% per year. For patients with mechanical heart valves, the addition of aspirin to warfarin to prevent systemic embolism is still controversial. In a double-blind, randomized, placebo-controlled trial, the administration of 100 mg of aspirin per day in patients receiving anticoagulation therapy with warfarin for heart-valve replacement reduced the annual rate of the combined outcome of major systemic embolism and vascular death by 77%. Although there was an increased risk of bleeding in the combined treatment group, the net beneficial effect of aspirin was still considerable.

**COMPLICATIONS OF WARFARIN THERAPY** As with all anticoagulant therapy, the major complication when using warfarin is hemorrhage. Use of recommended low-intensity dosage regimens dramatically lowers the risk of bleeding (Saour et al. 1990). When bleeding occurs in patients with optimal INRs, this often results from warfarin-induced structural bleeding. In these cases, warfarin-associated bleeding is not diffuse hemorrhage, but rather is related to preexisting polyps, ulcers, carcinomas, and so forth. Therefore, patients receiving warfarin who develop genitourinary or GI bleeding while their INRs are optimal should be evaluated for occult disease.

Reversal of warfarin-induced bleeding depends on the severity of the bleeding and whether resumption of anticoagulation will be necessary following the bleeding episode. Patients receiving warfarin who develop bruising or other minor bleeding associated with INR values outside the therapeutic range should have their dosage tapered or withheld for a short time (3 days) until the INR value falls into the appropriate range. Patients with more emergent bleeding because of excessive warfarin anticoagulation and who are nearing completion of their period of anticoagulation can be easily treated by stopping their warfarin and administering vitamin K. Parenteral vitamin K can totally correct prolonged INR values due to warfarin within 12 to 24 hours. For such patients, 5 to 10 mg of vitamin K is given, preferably by the subcutaneous route. Administration by the intravenous route has been associated with rare but severe episodes of anaphylactoid reactions and has no advantage over the subcutaneous route of administration. The IM route may be associated with formation of hematoma, especially in patients who have a profound coagulopathy due to warfarin excess. For patients with life-threatening bleeding or for serious warfarin overdosage, the use of fresh-frozen plasma (2 to 4 units for a 70-kg patient) provides rapid reversal of anticoagulation in these patients.

Vitamin K–dependent proteins mediate events other than coagulation. Toxicity from this effect can be seen when pregnant mothers receive warfarin during the first trimester. An important bone matrix protein, osteocalcin, is vitamin K–dependent; during embryogenesis, vitamin K deficiency results in fetal bone malformations. Indeed, warfarin does cross the placenta and has been associated with the development of warfarin embryopathy, central nervous system anomalies, and fetal hemorrhage, although the true incidence of these events is not known (Bates and Ginsberg 1997). For this reason, warfarin therapy is contraindicated during the first trimester of pregnancy. In fact, most practitioners recommend adjusted-dose subcutaneous heparin for patients requiring anticoagulation during pregnancy. Women receiving warfarin should be informed of its teratogenic effect and should avoid becoming pregnant while taking the drug. Warfarin is not found in breast milk of nursing mothers taking the drug.

Warfarin-induced skin necrosis is an unusual but devastating complication of warfarin therapy, usually occurring within a week of initiating the drug. The basis for this complication is thought to be rapid reduction in plasma concentrations of proteins C or S in patients with deficiency of one of these vitamin K–dependent anticoagulant proteins. Ensuring that patients are therapeutically anticoagulated with heparin before initiation of warfarin therapy and that large loading doses of warfarin are not used can prevent this complication.

**INTERACTIONS OF WARFARIN WITH OTHER DRUGS AND MEDICAL CONDITIONS** Patients receiving warfarin frequently have underlying diseases (other than thrombosis) and take additional medications. More drug–drug interactions are reported with warfarin than with any other drug. Drugs may interact with warfarin through pharmacodynamic or pharmacokinetic mechanisms (Wells et al. 1994). Table 12-8 summarizes medical conditions and drugs that interact with warfarin to either enhance or reduce the anticoagulant effect, as well as the mechanisms involved in these interactions.

Few drugs have been shown to alter warfarin absorption; the importance of protein-binding displacement has been exaggerated, and, as warfarin is not eliminated to any extent unchanged by the kidney, the most important kinetic interactions are those due to inhibition or induction of its hepatic metabolism. Isomeric differences in metabolism form an important basis for stereoselective metabolic interactions, especially inhibition; this has been demonstrated with phenylbutazone, metronidazole, and co-trimoxazole. Enzyme induction, although recognized for many years, may still pose problems in therapeutics, usually on withdrawal of the inducing agent. Physician awareness of these interactions between warfarin and other medications or medical disorders will help the patient avoid excessive or inadequate anticoagulation (O'Reilly 1987).

Because of the numerous potential interactions, patients taking warfarin should be told to notify the physician when any other medication is begun or discontinued, or when a new illness occurs. If a potentially interacting drug must be added to or deleted from the patient's regimen, the dose of warfarin should be changed appropri-

**Table 12-8 Drugs and Other Factors That Potentiate or Inhibit the Anticoagulant Effect of Warfarin**

| LEVEL[a] | POTENTIATION OF WARFARIN | INHIBITION OF WARFARIN |
|---|---|---|
| | PHARMACODYNAMIC | |
| 1 | Clofibrate, low vitamin K intake | High vitamin K intake |
| 2 | Coagulopathies, hypermetabolic state, liver diseases, malabsorption | |
| | PHARMACOKINETIC | |
| | Increase warfarin level | Decrease warfarin level |
| 1 | Alcohol (with concomitant liver disease), cimetidine, cotrimoxazole, erythromycin, fluconazole, isoniazid, metronidazole, miconazole, omeprazole, phenylbutazone, piroxicam, propafenone HCl, propranolol HCl, sulfinpyrazone | Barbiturates, carbamazepine, cholestyramine, rifampin, griseofulvin |
| 2 | Disulfiram | Dextropropoxyphene |
| | MECHANISMS TO BE ESTABLISHED | |
| 1 | Isoniazid, propafenone HCl, propranolol HCl, piroxicam | Chlordiazepoxide, sucralfate |
| 2 | Acetaminophen, anabolic steroids, aspirin, chloral hydrate, ciprofloxacin HCl, itraconazole, quinidine sulfate, phenytoin, simvastatin, tamoxifen, tetracycline, influenza vaccine | Dicloxacillin sodium |

[a]Level 1 indicates a highly probable interaction, level 2 indicates a probable interaction (see Hirsh 1995).

ately, and the physician should closely monitor the INR to determine whether further adjustment of warfarin dosage is indicated.

### *Thrombolytic therapy*

Beside antiplatelet agents and anticoagulants described above, another approach to the treatment of thromboembolic disorders involves pharmacological dissolution of the blood clot by activating the fibrinolytic system. Intravenous administration of thrombolytic agents is an accepted efficacious therapy for acute myocardial infarction, stroke, and pulmonary embolism. These agents reestablish patency of vessels more quickly than heparin and LMWHs. The dosage and route of administration of these agents are specific for different clinical settings, and in some instances the agent is administered by selective infusion into the involved vessel.

**PHARMACOLOGY OF THROMBOLYTICS** The fibrinolytic system contains a proenzyme, plasminogen, which is converted to the active enzyme plasmin, a nonspecific proteolytic enzyme, by the action of plasminogen activators. The two physiologic plasminogen activators are tissue-type plasminogen activators (tPA) or urokinase-type plasminogen activators (uPA). Plasmin in turn lyses fibrin and hydrolyzes fibrinogen and other coagulation factors, leading to a systemic lytic state (Fig. 12-8) (Collen 1997). At present, four thrombolytic agents are commercially available for clinical use. All thrombolytic agents are plasminogen activators, and they are able either directly or indirectly to enhance the generation of plasmin from plasminogen. Pharmacologic and pharmacokinetic properties of these common thrombolytic agents are summarized in (Table 12-9).

***Streptokinase*** Streptokinase (SK) is a protein derived from group A $\beta$-hemolytic streptococci. It does not directly activate plasminogen but forms a complex with plasminogen, thereby enhancing the conversion of plasminogen to plasmin. Because SK is a bacterial protein, it can be very antigenic. Patients with anti-streptococcal antibodies can develop fever, allergic reactions, and therapeutic resistance. Most important, patients who have received SK previously should not be treated again with SK.

Anisoylated plasminogen–streptokinase activator complex (APSAC) is an equimolar complex of streptokinase and plasminogen. Purified human plasminogen is bound beforehand to an SK molecule that is acylated to protect the active site. APSAC is without enzymatic activity until its active site is deacylated following administra-

**Table 12-9 Pharmacological properties of thrombolytic agents**

| | SK | UK | APSAC | RTPA | RETEPLASE |
|---|---|---|---|---|---|
| Dose | 1.5 MU (30–60 min) | 3 MU in 45–90 min | 30 mg (5 min) | 15-mg bolus, then 50 mg/30 min, then 35 mg/30 min | 10-mg bolus, then 10-mg bolus again in 30 min |
| Circulating half-life (min) | 20 | 15–20 | 100 | 2–6 | 2–4 |
| Fibrinogen breakdown | 4+ | 3+ | 4+ | 1–2+ | 1–2+ |
| Duration of infusion | 60 or less | 5–15 | 2–5 | 180 or less | 30 min or less |
| Early heparin required | No | No | No | Yes | No |
| Source | Streptococcal culture | Mammalian tissue culture | Streptococcal culture | Mammalian tissue culture | Mammalian tissue culture |
| Antigenic | Yes | No | Yes | No | No |
| Allergic reactions | Yes | No | Yes | No | No |
| Intracerebral hemorrhage | 0.4% | 0.4% | 0.6% | 0.6% | N/A |
| Hypotension | Yes | No | Yes | No | No |
| Patency at 90 min | 53–65 (53) | 66 | 55–65 | 81–88 | 86–90 |
| Lives saved per 100 treated | 2.5 | 2.5 | 2.5 | 3.5 | N/A |
| Cost per dose (US$) | $300/1.5 MU | $2200/3 MU | $1200/30 mg | $2300/100 mg | $2500 /50 mg |

ABBREVIATIONS: APSAC, plasminogen–streptokinase activator complex; MU, million units; rtPA, recombinant tissue plasminogen activator; SK, streptokinase; UK, urokinase.

tion. Anistreplase has a half-life 4 to 5 times that of SK, and thus it can be given as a single bolus intravenously, which is its major advantage.

***Urokinase*** Urokinase (UK) is a direct plasminogen activator purified from cultured human fetal kidney cells. UK directly converts plasminogen to plasmin by cleaving the arginine-valine bond in plasminogen. Because UK is a human protein, it is not antigenic; however, UK is considerably more expensive than SK.

***Tissue Plasminogen Activator*** Recombinant tissue plasminogen activator (rtPA) (or alteplase) is a direct activator of plasminogen that is relatively fibrin-specific; rtPA preferentially cleaves plasminogen that is bound to fibrin rather than free plasminogen in the blood and theoretically should cause less systemic fibrinolytic activation. However, in clinical use, the therapeutic dosage of rtPA also induces a systemic lytic state and has an increased risk of bleeding similar to SK and UK treatments.

***Reteplase*** Reteplase is a modified tPA constructed by genetic engineering in an attempt to improve the lytic characteristics of rtPA without increasing its hemorrhagic potential. Reteplase is smaller than rtPA and retains only the kringle 2 and the protease domains of rtPA. Consequently, reteplase does not bind fibrin as tightly as rtPA, which allows the drug to diffuse more easily through the fibrin clot rather than binding only to the clot surface. The redesigned tPA does not compete with plasminogen for fibrin-binding sites even at high concentrations, thus allowing plasminogen at the site of the clot to be converted into plasmin. These two modifications may explain the faster reperfusion rates seen in patients receiving reteplase compared with those on alteplase.

Reteplase has a higher plasma clearance and shorter half-life (about 11 to 19 minutes) than rtPA. Reteplase undergoes renal (and some hepatic) clearance. The shorter half-life makes the drug ideal for double-bolus dosing (10-million-U bolus IV followed by a second 10-million-U bolus IV 30 minutes later). This is more convenient regimen than with rtPA therapy, which is given as a 15-mg bolus followed by a 90-minute intravenous infusion.

In the International Joint Efficacy Comparison of Thrombolytics (INJECT) (International Joint Efficacy Comparison of Thrombolytics 1995) study involving 6010 patients comparing reteplase with SK, 35-day mortality was similar for the two drugs (8.9% with reteplase versus 9.4% with SK). However, the number of patients with congestive heart failure and cardiogenic shock was significantly lower in the reteplase group. In the Reteplase and Alteplase Patency Investigation During Myocardial Infarction trial (RAPID-II) (Bode et al. 1996), significantly more patients had restored coronary blood flow after 90 minutes in the reteplase group than in the rtPA group. However, followup at 5 to 14 days did not show a significant difference in patency rates, mean ejection fraction, or regional wall motion.

All of these thrombolytic agents suffer from a number of inadequacies including resistance to reperfusion, occurrence of acute coronary reocclusion, and bleeding complications (see below). Several lines of research are being explored to improve the properties of these thrombolytic agents. Recombinant molecular biology techniques allow construction of plasminogen activator mutants, chimeras, and conjugates with other proteins. New molecules such as pro-urokinase, saruplase, K1K2Pu, and staphylokinase have shown some promise in animal models and in pilot clinical studies of AMI. However, more clinical trials are needed to determine whether these novel recombinant thrombolytic agents have improved efficacy and fibrin specificity with minimal bleeding tendencies (Reddy 1998).

#### CLINICAL INDICATIONS FOR THE USE OF THROMBOLYTIC THERAPY

***Acute Myocardial Infarction*** Thrombolytic therapy has been recognized as the most significant improvement in the management of AMI in the past decade. Indeed, to date, most clinical experience for use of thrombolytic agents has been gained from treating patients with acute myocardial infarction. These agents improve myocardial oxygen supply by dissolving the thrombus associated with acute myocardial infarction, thereby reestablishing blood flow to the ischemic myocardium. As a consequence, the extent of myocardial necrosis and infarct size is limited, and the likelihood of survival is significantly improved if thrombolysis is achieved in a timely fashion.

There is convincing evidence that thrombolytic therapy improves survival in patients with acute myocardial infarction. A randomized, 2 × 2 factorial design, placebo-controlled trial involving 417 hospitals in 16 countries and 17,187 patients between March 1985 and December 1987 assessed the effect of intravenous SK, one month of oral aspirin, or both, on long-term survival of patients with acute MI (Baigent 1998). Long-term follow up of these patients provided clear evidence that the early survival advantage produced by thrombolytic therapy in acute MI persists for many years (at least 10) after treatment. The early survival benefit produced by one month of aspirin treatment also persisted. Most important, the survival benefit of thrombolytic therapy was additive to that of aspirin therapy.

Another large trial (ISIS-3) showed that SK plus aspirin is as effective as rtPA or APSAC. However, a subsequent trial (GUSTO III) (GUSTO III Investigators 1997) showed a small advantage for rtPA when given with heparin over SK, although the rtPA regimen was associated with a significantly higher risk of hemorrhagic stroke. In summary, thrombolytic therapy in combination with aspirin is clearly beneficial in acute MI and should be administered to all eligible patients including the elderly. The survival advantages of appropriate use of these drugs undoubtedly transcends the minor clinical differences between the various agents.

***Stroke*** Thrombolytic agents are also used in the treatment of acute ischemic stroke. There is a therapeutic window of approximately 6 hours for thrombolytic therapy to be successful based on the pathophysiologic changes caused by cerebral ischemia and reperfusion. Effective interventions must be initiated as soon as possible after onset of symptoms to reduce the extent of tissue injury, infarct volume, and poststroke morbidity (Hamann 1997). Recently, FDA approved rtPA for selected patients with acute ischemic stroke when therapy is initiated within 3 hours after onset of symptoms (Fisher and Bogousslavsky 1998).

Five large clinical trials have evaluated thrombolytic therapy for the treatment of hyperacute (<6 hours) stroke. Three of these studies were negative, one was equivocal, and one was strongly positive. Failure to demonstrate efficacy in four of these trials may be related to a number of methodological factors, including the type and dose of drug administered, the timing of drug administered, and patient selection. The one positive trial (NINDS) showed that rtPA therapy has substantial benefits when administered within 3 hours of stroke onset when strict patient selection criteria were used. However, the risk of clinically significant bleeding is also increased. To achieve the favorable risk/benefit ratio demonstrated in the NINDS trial, patients must be screened by experienced clinicians, and the initial computer tomography (CT) brain scan must be carefully evaluated for radiographic features that are associated with increased risk of bleeding (Goldszmidt and Wityk 1998).

***Venous Thromboembolism*** SK is approved by FDA for the treatment of acute pulmonary embolism and DVT, and UK and rtPA are approved by FDA for treatment of acute pulmonary embolism.

Therapeutic indications for the use of thrombolytics include massive pulmonary embolism with or without hemodynamic compromise, submassive pulmonary embolism in patients who cannot tolerate further cardiopulmonary compromise, heparin treatment failures, and extensive proximal DVTs. Thrombolytic agents offer the greatest benefit to patients suffering from acute decompensation with hypotension and low cardiac output following pulmonary embolism.

**CONTRAINDICATIONS AND COMPLICATIONS OF THROMBOLYTIC THERAPY** Absolute contraindications to thrombolytic agents include acute pericarditis, possible aortic dissection, active internal bleeding, recent cerebrovascular accident and intracranial diseases such as neoplasm, arteriovenous fistulas, aneurysm, and hemorrhage. Relative contraindications include recent craniospinal surgery, major surgery within the preceding 10 days, pregnancy, bleeding diathesis, thrombocytopenia or coagulopathy, uncontrolled hypertension (diastolic BP > 110 mm Hg or systolic BP > 200 mm Hg), and prolonged cardiopulmonary resuscitation with evidence of resulting chest trauma.

It is no surprise that hemorrhage is the major complication associated with the use of thrombolytic agents. Major hemorrhagic complications occur in up to 15% of patients with thrombolytic therapy. Allergic reactions and fever are more commonly seen in patients receiving SK than patients receiving tPA or UK, although serious allergic reactions are rare. In addition, data from clinical trials indicated that an important complication of thrombolytic therapy for patients with AMI is reocclusion following treatment (Reddy 1998).

**DOSING OF THROMBOLYTIC AGENTS** For treatment of acute myocardial infarction, SK is given as intravenous infusion at 1.5 million units over 1 hour. UK is administered as a 3-million-unit intravenous infusion over 60 to 90 minutes. There are many dosing regimens for rtPA. The standard dose is 100 mg intravenously over 3 hours, with 60 mg during the first hour, then 40 mg over the next 2 hours; an accelerated dosing regimen used in the GUSTO trial for treatment of AMI consists of a bolus dose of 15 mg rtPA followed by an infusion of 0.75 mg/kg of body weight over a 30-minute period (not to exceed 50 mg), then 0.5 mg/kg (up to 35 mg) over the next 60 minutes. Reteplase is given as two boluses with the first

10 million units administered over 2 minutes, then a second 10 million units given 30 minutes later.

## DRUG-INDUCED HEMATOLOGIC DISORDERS

A wide variety of drugs that are well tolerated by the majority of patients occasionally induce hematologic disorders. The hematologic disorders induced by drugs include neutropenia, thrombocytopenia, hemolytic anemia, and aplastic anemia in that order of frequency (Lubran 1989; Patton and Duffull 1994). Although they account for only a minor fraction of adverse drug reactions (ADRs), these reactions have a relatively high morbidity and mortality compared with other ADRs. Basic knowledge of drug-induced hematologic disorders is therefore essential for all physicians who may be faced with a potentially life-threatening condition. Some of the drugs associated with drug-induced hematologic disorders are listed in Table 12-10.

The diagnosis of drug-induced hematologic disorders is often complicated for the following reasons (Heimpel 1996). First, drug-induced hematologic disorders are an uncommon adverse effect, and a practicing physician cannot be expected to have sufficient personal experience with similar cases. The incidence of drug-induced hematologic disorders depends on a number of factors including the cell line affected, the specific drug, dose of the drug, and possibly genetic predisposition.

The exact incidence of drug-induced hematologic disorders is difficult to estimate. Recent studies in several countries including the United States (Kaufman et al. 1996), Sweden (Wiholm 1996), France (Mary et al. 1996), and Thailand (Issaragrisil et al. 1996) reported an incidence of approximately 0.01% for drug-induced agranulocytosis to 0.06% of drug-induced aplastic anemia. It is often difficult to establish a temporal relationship between the initiation of the drug and the onset of symptoms, because patients are often taking a number of different medications when the hematologic disorders occur. The time between exposure to the drug and the onset of the hematologic disorders depends on the hematologic disorder induced and the drug itself. For agranulocytosis, hemolytic anemia, and thrombocytopenia, it is usually less than 4 weeks and a longer period of time in aplastic anemia.

Mechanisms by which drugs induce hematologic disorders vary with the different drugs. Generally, the mode of action of drugs leading to hematologic disorders can be divided into two categories. The first is a dose-dependent, predictable toxicity on hematopoietic cells, as caused by agents used for antineoplastic, immunosuppressive or antiviral therapy. Whether suppression of hemopoiesis is regarded as a desirable or undesirable effect depends on the condition being treated. The second category of drug-induced hematologic disorders belongs to so-called idiosyncratic reactions. *Idiosyncrasy* describes an individual hypersusceptibility of any type. The category of idiosyncratic reactions can be further divided into two subtypes, namely, immunological (Claas 1996; Winkelstein and Kiss 1997) or metabolic (Jacobasch and Rapoport 1996), based on their pathophysiological mechanisms, which may be inborn or acquired. However, in most cases, the mechanisms are not understood, and the categorization as idiosyncratic is based solely on clinical observations.

### Drug-Induced Aplastic Anemia

Drug-induced aplastic anemia is one of the few life-threatening reactions to drugs. Aplastic anemia can be defined as a pancytopenia (a decrease in all the cellular components of peripheral blood) with a hypocellular bone marrow and no significant evidence of increased peripheral blood cell destruction. A diagnosis of aplastic anemia can be made if the patient meets two of the following criteria: a white blood cell count of 3500/mm$^3$ or less, a platelet count of 50,000/mm$^3$ or less, or a hemoglobin value of 10.0 g/dL or less with a reticulocyte count of 30,000/mm$^3$ or less. The bone marrow must be free of neoplastic infiltration or significant myelofibrosis. There also must be no history of exposure to antineoplastic agents or radiation treatment.

The onset of drug-induced aplastic anemia is usually insidious with symptoms appearing on the average about 6.5 weeks after initiation of the offending drug. The symptoms often appear after the drug has been discontinued. The incidence of drug-induced aplastic anemia in patients taking medications is approximately 2 to 4 per million and is higher in patients taking such drugs as indomethacin and phenylbutazone. Table 12-10 lists a number of drugs that have been associated with drug-induced aplastic anemia. The association of most drugs with aplastic anemia is based on case reports rather than epidemiological studies that provide quantitative estimates of the risk.

The pathophysiological basis of drug-induced aplastic anemia is based on damage to the hematopoietic stem cell. The earlier the stem cell is affected in the maturation process, the greater the likelihood that the drug-induced aplastic anemia will be long-term. There is no evidence

Table 12-10 **Drugs Associated with Hematologic Disorders**

| Aplastic anemia | Hemolytic anemia | Agranulocytosis | Thrombocytopenia |
|---|---|---|---|
| Acetazolamide | *Immune mechanism*: | Acetaminophen | Acetazolamide |
| Antihistamines | Acetaminophen | Acetazolamide | Acetylsalicylic acid |
| Carbamazepine | *p*-Aminosalicylic acid | Acetylsalicylic acid | Allopurinol |
| Chloramphenicol | Antihistamines | Allopurinol | Aminoglutethimide |
| Chloroquine HCl | Cephalosporins | *p*-Aminosalicylic acid | Aminosalicylic acid |
| Chlorothiazide | Chlorpropamide | Benzodiazepines | Amrinone lactate |
| Felbamate | Chlorpromazine HCl | $\beta$-Lactam antibiotics | Cephalothin sodium |
| Furosemide | Diclofenac | Brompheniramine maleate | Chlorothiazide |
| Gold salts | Hydralazine HCl | Captopril | Cimetidine |
| Indomethacin | Ibuprofen | Carbamazepine | Desipramine HCl |
| Interferon (alpha) | Isoniazid | Ceftriaxone sodium | Diazepam |
| Methimazole | Levodopa | Chloramphenicol | Digitoxin |
| Oral antidiabetics | Mefenamic acid | Chlorpropamide | Furosemide |
| Oxyphenbutazone | Melphalan | Cimetidine | Hydrochlorothiazide |
| Penicillamine | Methadone HCl | Clindamycin HCl | Hydroxychloroquine sulfate |
| Pentoxifylline | Methyldopa | Clomipramine HCl | Interferon |
| Phenobarbital | Methysergide maleate | Clozapine | Isoniazid |
| Phenothiazines | Nomifensine | Dapsone | Meclofenamate sodium |
| Phenytoin | Omeprazole | Desipramine HCl | Morphine sulfate |
| Propylthiouracil | Penicillins | Doxycycline | Penicillin |
| Quinidine | Probenecid | Ethacrynic acid | Phenylbutazone |
| Sulfonamides | Procainamide HCl | Ethosuximide | Phenytoin |
| Ticlopidine HCl | Quinidine | Fenoprofen calcium | Procainamide HCl |
| | Quinine sulfate | Flucytosine | Quinidine |
| | Rifampin | Ganciclovir | Quinine sulfate |
| | Sulfonamides | Gentamicin sulfate | Rifampin |
| | Streptomycin | Gold salts | Sulfisoxazole |
| | Tetracycline | Griseofulvin | Trimethoprim |
| | Tolbutamide | Hydralazine HCl | |
| | Triamterene | Hydroxychloroquine sulfate | |
| | | Ibuprofen | |
| | *Metabolic mechanism*: | Imipramine HCl | |
| | Ascorbic acid | Indomethacin | |
| | Aspirin | Isoniazid | |
| | Benzocaine | Levamisole HCl | |
| | Chloramphenicol | Levodopa | |
| | Chloroquine HCl | Lincomycin HCl | |
| | Dapsone | Meprobamate | |
| | Diazoxide | Methazolamide | |
| | Menadiol sodium diphosphate | Methimazole | |
| | Methylene blue | Methyldopa | |
| | Nitrofurantoin | Metronidazole | |
| | Nitrofurazone | Nitrofurantoin | |
| | Phenazopyridine | Oxyphenbutazone | |
| | Salazosulfapyridine | Penicillamine | |
| | | Phenothiazines | |
| | | Phenylbutazone | |
| | | Phenytoin | |
| | | Phenazocine | |
| | | Primidone | |
| | | Procainamide HCl | |
| | | Propranolol HCl | |

Table 12-10 Drugs Associated with Hematologic Disorders (Continued)

| APLASTIC ANEMIA | HEMOLYTIC ANEMIA | AGRANULOCYTOSIS | THROMBOCYTOPENIA |
|---|---|---|---|
| | | Propylthiouracil | |
| | | Pyrimethamine | |
| | | Quinine sulfate | |
| | | Rifampin | |
| | | Streptomycin | |
| | | Sulfa antibiotics | |
| | | Thiazide diuretics | |
| | | Tocainide HCl | |
| | | Tolbutamide | |
| | | Vancomycin | |
| | | Zidovudine | |

that drug-induced aplastic anemia occurs because of the destruction of the microenvironment of the bone marrow.

Three mechanisms have been proposed as causes of drug-induced aplastic anemia. One mechanism is drug-induced idiosyncratic reactions. This includes individual variations in the pharmacokinetics of the suspected drug or hypersensitivity of hematopoietic stem cells to the implicated drug. The second mechanism relates to the fact that some drugs have dose-dependent toxic effects on hematopoietic stem cells. The third mechanism is a drug- or drug-metabolite-induced immune reaction that is specific to the stem cell population. More than one mechanism can be involved in a particular case.

Clinical observations and laboratory studies have supported an immune basis for most acquired aplastic anemias, with the majority of patients responding to immunosuppressive therapy. The mechanism by which chemical and biological agents incite an immune response remains unclear. Whatever the initial events, immune system destruction of hematopoiesis plays a central role in the development of acquired aplastic anemia (Young 1996, 1997).

The prognosis of drug-induced aplastic anemia is similar to that of idiopathic aplastic anemia, because these patients respond to bone marrow transplantation or immunosuppressive therapy in a manner similar to patients with idiopathic aplastic anemia. The 5-year survival rate for patients who develop drug-induced aplastic anemia is approximately 60%. As with all cases of drug-induced hematologic disorders, the suspected offending agent must be removed. Early withdrawal of the agent may allow for reversal of the disease. Patients with drug-induced aplastic anemia need to be treated symptomatically for infection and bleeding. Antithymocyte globulin, cyclosporine, and corticosteroids have been employed to treat this condition.

## Drug-Induced Hemolytic Anemia

### *Immunologically mediated anemia*

Drug-induced hemolytic anemia is a disorder that causes peripheral erythrocyte destruction. The causes of drug-induced hemolytic anemia can be divided into two categories: immune and metabolic. The first category results from production of autoantibodies, and the second involves the induction of hemolysis by metabolic abnormalities in the erythrocytes. Patients with drug-induced hemolytic anemia can present with signs of intravascular or extravascular hemolysis. The onset of drug-induced hemolytic anemia is variable and depends on the drug and mechanism of hemolysis. Table 12-10 lists a group of drugs that have been associated with drug-induced hemolytic anemia.

Acquired drug-related hemolytic anemia is induced mainly by immune mechanism or microvascular lesion. Three mechanisms of drug-induced immunologic injury to RBCs are recognized (Jefferies 1994). These mechanisms are injury by hapten or drug adsorption, by ternary or drug–antibody–target cell complex, and by autoantibodies.

For the drug adsorption or hapten mechanism, penicillin has long been known as the prototypic drug by which this mechanism causes hemolytic anemia. High concentrations of penicillin (10 to 20 million U/day) may lead to production of IgG antibodies that recognize the benzylpenicilloyl determinant or other metabolite of penicillin that is bound to the RBC membrane. Penicillin-induced immune hemolysis is mild and promptly ceases after discontinuation of the antibiotic therapy. Similar reactions have been seen with the semisynthetic penicillins and cephalosporins.

A second mechanism that leads to drug-induced hemolysis occurs when drugs or drug metabolites bind to antidrug antibodies in the patient's serum. The drug–antibody complex then initiates complement activation on the RBC membrane surfaces that leads to intravascular hemolysis. Quinidine is a classic example of this type of drug-induced hemolysis. The hemolysis often begins abruptly and can be quite severe.

The third mechanism relates to the development of autoantibodies that react with intrinsic RBC antigens and do not react with the drug in vitro; $\alpha$-Methyldopa is an example of drugs that may induce hemolysis through this mechanism. About 20% of patients treated with $\alpha$-methyldopa developed a positive direct Coombs' test, whereas 0.5% of patients developed hemolytic anemia. The clinical course and prognosis of patients who develop this type of drug-induced hemolytic anemia are similar to those of patients who have idiopathic hemolytic anemia.

The treatment of drug-induced hemolytic anemia includes the removal of the offending medications and supportive therapy. Intravenous immune globulin have been tested for treatment of this anemia.

***Metabolically mediated anemia***

Drug-induced oxidation of hemoglobin is a hereditary condition most often associated with a glucose-6-phosphate dehydrogenase (G6PD) enzyme deficiency but can occur because of other enzyme defects (Jacobasch and Rapoport 1996).

Red blood cells can only fulfill their functions over the normal lifespan of approximately 120 days if they withstand external and internal stresses. This requires ATP and redox equivalents, which have to be permanently regenerated by energy and redox metabolism. These pathways are necessary to maintain the biconcave shape of the cells, their specific intracellular cation concentrations, the reduced state of hemoglobin with a divalent iron and the sulfhydryl groups of enzymes, and glutathione and membrane components. If an enzyme deficiency of one of these metabolic pathways limits the ATP and/or NADPH production, distinct membrane alterations result in removal of damaged cells by the reticuloendothelial system. Hereditary enzyme deficiencies of all these pathways have been identified.

Glucose-6-phosphate dehydrogenase deficiency is by far the most common enzyme deficiency that can lead to oxidant-induced hemolytic anemia. The highest gene frequency has been found among Kurdish Jews (0.7%). G6PD deficiency is also prevalent among Africans, African-Americans, and populations of Mediterranean countries and South East Asia. G6PD deficiency is a heterogenous disease, as there are many G6PD variants. Among the G6PD-deficient Africans and African-Americans, the condition is usually asymptomatic until they are exposed to oxidant drugs or develop a serious infection. In G6PD-deficient patients from the Mediterranean, the hemolytic anemia is usually more severe when they are exposed to oxidant stress.

## Drug-Induced Agranulocytosis

Drug-induced neutropenia is probably the most common cause of isolated neutropenia. Drug-induced profound neutropenia, termed *agranulocytosis*, is a rare, potentially fatal idiosyncratic reaction that can occur unpredictably with a wide variety of drugs when taken in conventional dosages. Drug-induced agranulocytosis can be defined as a drug-mediated reduction in the granulocytes in the blood to less than $0.5 \times 10^9$/L.

The overall mortality rate in agranulocytosis is 16%, and the mortality rate in the patients with agranulocytosis increases when the patient develops bacteremia or renal failure. The symptoms can appear rapidly, within 7 to 14 days after initiation of the offending agent, or in the case of phenothiazine-induced agranulocytosis, patients can be asymptomatic at the time of diagnosis, probably because of a milder form of the disorder. In the large majority of cases, the drug-induced agranulocytosis will resolve over time. Table 12-10 provides a list of medications that have been reported to cause drug-induced agranulocytosis. As with drug-induced aplastic anemia, relatively few controlled epidemiological studies have been done to establish which drugs cause agranulocytosis.

Hematopoietic growth factors such as G-CSF have been used in the treatment of drug-induced agranulocytosis. Mani et al. (1993) summarized the effect of G-CSF in five patients with this disorder who presented to Yale-New Haven Hospital during 1990 through 1992. Three patients treated with G-CSF and two patients treated with routine care were studied for relevant clinical outcomes. Treatment with G-CSF was associated with a shorter duration of neutropenia and decreased hospital stay, consistent with recent case reports. Despite the high cost of the drug, treatment with GCSF was found to be cost-effective for patients with uncomplicated drug-induced agranulocytosis.

Accelerated myeloid recovery following G-CSF therapy can have unexpected consequences. Three patients, two with a severe infection and one with preexisting pulmonary infiltrates, developed worsening of their respiratory status during neutrophil recovery, resulting in clinical manifestations of the adult acute respiratory distress syndrome (ARDS). This may be due to the release of toxic substances from the newly produced neutrophils in response to the underlying infection.

## Drug-Induced Thrombocytopenia

Drug-induced thrombocytopenia is a relatively common and potentially serious problem. Mechanisms of drug-induced thrombocytopenia are either a dose-dependent toxic effect of drugs directly on platelet production or an immune-mediated reaction that leads to platelet destruction. The most common drugs that have direct toxic effects on platelet production are primarily cancer chemotherapy agents. In addition, organic solvents, pesticides, and amrinone have also been implicated in drug-induced thrombocytopenia. Several agents such as chloramphenicol, phenylbutazone, and gold may also cause aplastic anemia with a decrease in platelet counts. Although most drugs that reduce platelet production also inhibit hematopoietic stem cells causing pancytopenia, some agents, such as alcohol, primarily inhibit megakaryocyte production and lead to isolated thrombocytopenia.

Many commonly used drugs such as heparin can cause thrombocytopenia via an immunological mechanism (Table 12-10). In one study, the median length of exposure to the offending drug before the development of thrombocytopenia was 21 days. The median platelet count was $11 \times 10^9$/L, and 74% of the patients had clinical hemorrhage with a mortality rate of 3.6% (Pedersen-Bjergaard et al. 1997).

Bone marrow examination in this type of drug-induced thrombocytopenia usually shows hyperplastic reactive changes and a variable number of megakaryocytes. The majority of cases have a complete and relatively rapid recovery when the drug is withdrawn. Although treatment with corticosteroids probably does not alter the clinical course, severe symptomatic cases of drug-induced thrombocytopenia should be treated with corticosteroids as in idiopathic thrombocytopenic purpura because of the difficulty of differentiating the two conditions upon initial presentation.

## REFERENCES

Alexander WS, Begley CG. 1998. Thrombopoietin in vitro and in vivo. *Cytokines Cell Mol Ther* **4**:25–34.

Allan NC, Richards SM, Shepherd PC. 1995. UK Medical Research Council randomised, multicentre trial of interferon-alpha n1 for chronic myeloid leukaemia: Improved survival irrespective of cytogenetic response. The UK Medical Research Council's Working Parties for Therapeutic Trials in Adult Leukaemia. *Lancet* **345**:1392–7.

Akkerman JW, van Willigen G. 1996. Platelet activation via trimeric GTP-binding proteins. *Haemostasis* **26**(Suppl 4):199–209.

Andrews RK, Lopez JA, Berndt MC. 1997. Molecular mechanisms of platelet adhesion and activation. *Int J Biochem Cell Biol* **29**:91–105.

Anticoagulants in the Secondary Prevention of Events in Coronary Thrombosis (ASPECT) Research Group. 1994. Effect of long-term oral anticoagulant treatment on mortality and cardiovascular morbidity after myocardial infarction. *Lancet* **343**:499–503.

Antiplatelet Trialists' Collaboration. 1994a. Collaborative overview of randomised trials of antiplatelet therapy. I. Prevention of death, myocardial infarction, and stroke by prolonged antiplatelet therapy in various categories of patients. *BMJ* **308**:81–104.

Antiplatelet Trialists' Collaboration. 1994b. Collaborative overview of randomised trials of antiplatelet therapy. II. Maintenance of vascular graft or arterial patency by antiplatelet therapy. *BMJ* **308**:159–68.

Appelbaum FR, Kopecky KJ. 1997. Long-term survival after chemotherapy for acute myeloid leukemia: The experience of the Southwest Oncology Group. *Cancer* **80**(Suppl 11):2199–2204.

Armitage J., Vose JM, Bierman PJ, et al. 1994. Salvage therapy for patients with lymphoma. *Seminar Oncology* Aug:**21**(4 Suppl 7):82–85.

Armstrong RA. 1996. Platelet prostanoid receptors. *Pharmacol Ther* **72**:171–91.

Ayanian JZ, Hauptman PJ, Guadagnoli E, et al. 1994. Knowledge and practices of generalist and specialist physicians regarding drug therapy for acute myocardial infarction. *N Engl J Med* **331**:1136–42.

Baigent C, Collins R, Appleby P, et al. 1998. ISIS-2: 10 year survival among patients with suspected acute myocardial infarction in randomised comparison of intravenous streptokinase, oral aspirin, both, or neither. *BMJ* **316**:1337–43.

Ballas SK, Mohandas N. 1996. Pathophysiology of vaso-occlusion. *Hematol Oncol Clin North Am* **10**:1221–39.

Bates SM, Ginsberg JS. 1997. Anticoagulants in pregnancy: Fetal effects. *Baillieres Clin Obstet Gynaecol* **11**:479–88.

Bendich A, Cohen M. 1990. Ascorbic acid safety: Analysis of factors affecting iron absorption. *Toxicol Lett* **51**:189–201.

Bennett CL, Weinberg PD, Rozenberg-Ben-Dror K, et al. 1998. Thrombotic thrombocytopenic purpura associated with ticlopidine. A review of 60 cases. *Ann Intern Med* **128**:541–4.

Bishop JF. 1997. The treatment of adult acute myeloid leukemia. *Semin Oncol* **24**:57–69.

Bishop JF. 1998. Approaches to induction therapy with adult acute myeloid leukaemia. *Acta Haematol* **99**:133–7.

Bode C, Smalling RW, Berg G, et al. 1996. Randomized comparison of coronary thrombolysis achieved with double-bolus reteplase (recombinant plasminogen activator) and front-loaded, accelerated alteplase (recombinant tissue plasminogen activator) in patients with acute myocardial infarction. The RAPID II Investigators. *Circulation* **94**:891–8.

Boylan JF, Klinck JR, Sandler AN, et al. 1996. Tranexamic acid reduces blood loss, transfusion requirements, and coagulation factor use in primary orthotopic liver transplantation. *Anesthesiology* **85**:1043–48.

Braga M, Gianotti L, Vignali A, et al. 1995. Evaluation of recombinant human erythropoietin to facilitate autologous blood donation before surgery in anaemic patients with cancer of the gastrointestinal tract. *Br J Surg* **82**:1637.

Bray PF. 1994. Inherited diseases of platelet glycoproteins: Considerations for rapid molecular characterization. *Thromb Haemost* **72**:492–502.

Breymann C, Bauer C, Major A, et al. 1996. Optimal timing of repeated rh-erythropoietin administration improves its effectiveness in stimulating erythropoiesis in healthy volunteers. *Br J Haematol* **92**:295.

Bruner AB, Joffe A, Duggan AK, et al. 1996. Randomised study of cognitive effects of iron supplementation in non-anaemic iron-deficient adolescent girls. *Lancet* **348**:992–6.

Byrd JC, Rai KR, Sausville EA, et al. 1998. Old and new therapies in chronic lymphocytic leukemia: Now is the time for a reassessment of therapeutic goals. *Semin Oncol* **25**:65–74.

Canadian Cooperative Study Group 1978. A randomized trial of aspirin and sulfinpyrazone in threatened stroke. Canadian Cooperative Study Group. *N Engl J Med* **299**:53–9.

Canellos GP. 1992. Chemotherapy of advanced Hodgkin's disease with MOPP, ABVD or MOPP alternating with ABVD. *NEJM* **327**:1478–84.

CAPRIE Steering Committee. 1996. A randomised, blinded, trial of clopidogrel versus aspirin in patients at risk of ischaemic events (CAPRIE). *Lancet* **348**:1329–39.

CARS Investigators. 1997. Randomised double-blind trial of fixed low-dose warfarin with aspirin after myocardial infarction. *Lancet* **350**:389–96.

Cazzola M, Mercuriali F, Brugnara C. 1997. Use of recombinant human erythropoietin outside the setting of uremia. *Blood* **89**:4248–67.

Charache S. 1997. Mechanism of action of hydroxyurea in the management of sickle cell anemia in adults. *Semin Hematol* **34**:15–21.

Charache S, Terrin ML, Moore RD, et al. 1995. Effect of hydroxyurea on the frequency of painful crises in sickle cell anemia. *N Engl J Med* **332**:1317–22.

Chen Z, Wang ZY, Chen SJ. 1997. Acute promyelocytic leukemia: Cellular and molecular basis of differentiation and apoptosis. *Pharmacol Ther* **76**:141–9.

Cheson BD, Bennett JM, Grever M, et al. 1996. National Cancer Institute-sponsored Working Group guidelines for chronic lymphocytic leukemia: Revised guidelines for diagnosis and treatment. *Blood* **87**:4990–7.

Claas FH. 1996. Immune mechanisms leading to drug-induced blood dyscrasias. *Eur J Haematol* **60**(Suppl):64–8.

Clemetson KJ. 1997. Platelet GPIb-V-IX complex. *Thromb Haemost* **78**:266–70.

Collen D. 1997. Thrombolytic therapy. *Thromb Haemost* **78**:742–6.

Coller BS. 1997a. GPIIb/IIIa antagonists: Pathophysiologic and therapeutic insights from studies of c7E3 Fab. *Thromb Haemost* **78**:730–5.

Coller BS. 1997b. Platelet GPIIb/IIIa antagonists: The first anti-integrin receptor therapeutics. *J Clin Invest* **100**(Suppl):S57–S60.

Collins R, Peto R, Baigent C, et al. 1997. Aspirin, heparin, and fibrinolytic therapy in suspected acute myocardial infarction. *N Engl J Med* **336**:847–60.

Connolly AJ, Ishihara H, Kahn ML, et al. 1997. Role of the thrombin receptor in development and evidence for a second receptor. *Nature* **381**:516–9.

Coughlin SR. 1994. Molecular mechanisms of thrombin signaling. *Semin Hematol* **31**:270–7.

Coulombel L, Auffray I, Gaugler MH, et al. 1997. Expression and function of integrins on hematopoietic progenitor cells. *Acta Haematol* **97**(12):13–21.

Council for International Organizations of Medical Sciences[CIOMS]. 1991. Standardization of definitions and criteria of causality assessment of adverse drug reactions. Drug-induced cytopenia. *Int J Clin Pharmacol Ther Toxicol* **29**:75–81.

Demuynck H, Delforge M, Zachee P, et al. 1995. An update on peripheral blood progenitor cell transplantation. *Ann Hematol* **71**:29–33.

Demuynck H, Zachee P, Verhoef GE, et al. 1995. Risks of rhG-CSF treatment in drug-induced agranulocytosis. *Ann Hematol* **70**:143–7.

Di Marco A, Silverstrini R, Di Marco S, et al. 1965. Inhibiting effect of the new cytotoxic antibiotic daunomycin or nucleic acids and mitotic activity of HeLa cells. *J Cell Biol* **27**:545–50.

Du X, Ginsberg MH. 1997. Integrin alpha IIb beta 3 and platelet function. *Thromb Haemost* **78**:96–100.

Dutch TIA Study Group 1988. Alternative reference for Dutch TIA Trial but in 1991: [Anonymous]. 1991a. A comparison of two doses of aspirin (30 mg vs 283 mg a day) in patients after transient ischemic attack or minor ischemic stroke. The Dutch TIA Trial Study Group. *N Engl J Med* **325**:1261–6.

Ellerbeck EF, Jencks SF, Radford MJ, et al. 1995. Quality of care for Medicare patients with acute myocardial infarction: A four-state pilot study from the Cooperative Cardiovascular Project. *JAMA* **273**:1509–1914.

Elliott MA, Tefferi A. 1997. Interferon-alpha therapy in polycythemia vera and essential thrombocythemia. *Semin Thromb Hemost* **23**:463–72.

Eriksson BI, Ekman S, Kalebo P, et al. 1996. Prevention of deep-vein thrombosis after total hip replacement: Direct thrombin inhibition with recombinant hirudin, CGP 39393. *Lancet* **347**:635–9.

Eriksson BI, Ekman S, Lindbratt S, et al. 1997. Prevention of thromboembolism with use of recombinant hirudin. Results of a double-blind, multicenter trial comparing the efficacy of desirudin (Revasc) with that of unfractionated heparin in patients having a total hip replacement. *J Bone Joint Surg Am* **79**:326–33.

Eriksson BI, Wille-Jorgensen P, Kalebo P, et al. 1997. A comparison of recombinant hirudin with a low-molecular-weight heparin to prevent thromboembolic complications after total hip replacement. *N Engl J Med* **337**:1329–35.

Fenaux P, Le Deley MC, Castaigne S, et al. 1993. Effect of all-*trans*-retinoic acid in newly diagnosed acute promyelocytic leukemia. Results of a multicenter randomized trial. European APL 91 Group. *Blood* **82**:3241–9.

Feng L, Sun W, Xia Y, et al. 1993. Cloning two isoforms of rat cyclooxygenase: Differential regulation of their expression. *Arch Biochem Biophys* **307**:361–8.

Fenton JW II, Ofosu FA, Brezniak DV, et al. 1998. Thrombin and antithrombotics. *Semin Thromb Hemost* **24**:87–91.

Fisher JW. 1997. Erythropoietin: Physiologic and pharmacologic aspects. *Proc Soc Exp Biol Med* **216**:358–69.

Fisher M, Bogousslavsky J. 1998. Further evolution toward effective therapy for acute ischemic stroke. *JAMA* **279**:1298–1303.

Fisher RI, Gaynor ER, Dahlberg S, et al. 1993. Comparison of a standard regimen (CHOP) with three intensive chemotherapy regimens for advanced non-Hodgkin's lymphoma. *N Engl J Med* **328**:1002–06.

Flores-Runk P, Raasch RH. 1993. Ticlopidine and antiplatelet therapy. *Ann Pharmacother* **27**:1090–8.

Folsom AR, Nieto FJ, McGovern PG, et al. 1998. Prospective study of coronary heart disease incidence in relation to fasting total homocysteine, related genetic polymorphisms, and B vitamins: The Atherosclerosis Risk in Communities (ARIC) study. *Circulation* **98**:204–10.

Fragmin during Instability in Coronary Artery Disease (FRISC) Study Group. 1996. Low-molecular-weight heparin during instability in coronary artery disease. *Lancet* **347**:561–8.

Furie B, Furie BC. 1990. Molecular basis of vitamin K-dependent gamma-carboxylation. *Blood* **75**:1753–62.

Gachet C, Cattaneo M, Ohlmann P, et al. 1995. Purinoceptors on blood platelets: Further pharmacological and clinical evidence to suggest the presence of two ADP receptors. *Br J Haematol* **91**:434–44.

Gachet C, Hechler B, Leon C, et al. 1997. Activation of ADP receptors and platelet function. *Thromb Haemost* **78**:271–5.

Gillis S. 1996. The thrombocytopenic purpuras. Recognition and management. *Drugs* **51**:942–53.

Glusa E. 1998. Pharmacology and therapeutic applications of hirudin, a new anticoagulant. *Kidney Int* **64**(Suppl):S54–S6.

Goldszmidt A, Wityk RJ. 1998. Recent advances in stroke therapy. *Curr Opin Neurol* **11**:57–64.

Golomb HM. 1998. Management of early-stage Hodgkin's disease: A continuing evolution. *Semin Oncol* **25**:476.

Griesshammer M, Bangerter M, van Vliet HH, et al. 1997. Aspirin in essential thrombocythemia: Status quo and quo vadis. *Semin Thromb Hemost* **23**:371–7.

Grogan TM, Miller TP, Fisher RI. 1997. A Southwest Oncology Group perspective on the Revised European-American Lymphoma classification. *Hematol Oncol Clin North Am* **11**:819–46.

GUSTO III Investigators. 1997. A comparison of reteplase with alteplase for acute myocardial infarction. *N Engl J Med* 337:1118–23.

Hamann GF. 1997. Acute cerebral infarct: Physiopathology and modern therapeutic concepts. *Radiologe* **37**:843–52.

Harker LA, Hanson SR, Kelly AB. 1997. Antithrombotic strategies targeting thrombin activities, thrombin receptors and thrombin generation. *Thromb Haemost* **78**:736–41.

Hartmann O, Le Corroller AG, Blaise D, et al. 1997. Peripheral blood stem cell and bone marrow transplantation for solid tumors and lymphomas: Hematologic recovery and costs. A randomized, controlled trial. *Ann Intern Med* **126**:600–7.

Hehlmann R, Heimpel H, Hasford J, et al. 1994. Randomized comparison of interferon-alpha with busulfan and hydroxyurea in chronic myelogenous leukemia. The German CML Study Group. *Blood* **84**:4064–77.

Heimpel H. 1996. When should the clinician suspect a drug-induced blood dyscrasia, and how should he proceed? *Eur J Haematol* **60**(Suppl):11–15.

Henry DA, O'Connell DL. 1989. Effects of fibrinolytic inhibitors on mortality from upper gastrointestinal haemorrhage. *BMJ* **298**:1142–6.

Hess H, et al. 1985. *Lancet* 1(8426):415–19.

Hirsh J. 1995. Optimal intensity and monitoring warfarin. *Am J Cardiol* **75**:39B–42B.

Hirsh J. 1998. Low-molecular-weight heparin for the treatment of venous thromboembolism. *Am Heart J* **135**(Suppl):S336–42.

Hirsh J, Raschke R, Warkentin TE, et al. 1995. Heparin: Mechanism of action, pharmacokinetics, dosing considerations, monitoring, efficacy, and safety. *Chest* **108**(Suppl):258S–75S.

Horning SJ, Rosenberg SA. 1984. The natural history of initially untreated low-grade non-Hodgkin's lymphomas. *N Engl J Med* **311**:1471–5.

Hou M, Andersson PO, Stockelberg D, et al. 1998. Plasma thrombopoietin levels in thrombocytopenic states: Implication for a regulatory role of bone marrow megakaryocytes. *Br J Haematol* **101**:420–4.

International Joint Efficacy Comparison of Thrombolytics. 1995. Randomised, double-blind comparison of reteplase double-bolus administration with streptokinase in acute myocardial infarction (INJECT): Trial to investigate equivalence. [Published erratum appears in *Lancet* **346**:980 1995]. *Lancet* **346**:329–36.

Ishihara H, Connolly AJ, Zengl D, et al. 1997. Protease-activated receptor 3 is a second thrombin receptor in humans. *Nature* **386**: 502–6.

Issaragrisil et al. 1996. *Eur J Haematol Suppl* **60**:31–4.

Jacobasch G, Rapoport SM. 1996. Hemolytic anemias due to erythrocyte enzyme deficiencies. *Mol Aspects Med* **17**:143–70.

Jefferies LC. 1994. Transfusion therapy in autoimmune hemolytic anemia. *Hematol Oncol Clin North Am* **8**:1087–104.

Kakkar AK, Williamson RCN. 1997. Prevention of venous thromboembolism in cancer using low-molecular-weight heparins. *Haemostasis* **27**(Suppl):32–7.

Kantarjian H, Estey E. Clinical experience with fludarabine in hemato-oncology. *Hematol Cell Ther* **38**(Suppl 2):S83–91.

Kantarjian HM, Giles FJ, O'Brien SM, et al. 1998. Clinical course and therapy of chronic myelogenous leukemia with interferon-alpha and chemotherapy. *Hematol Oncol* **12**:31–80.

Keating MJ, O'Brien S, McLaughlin P, et al. 1996. Clinical experience with fludarabine in hemato-oncology. *Hematol Cell Ther* **38**(Suppl 2):S83–91.

Klein W, Buchwald A, Hillis WS, et al. 1997. Fragmin in unstable angina pectoris or non-Q-wave acute myocardial infarction (the FRIC study). Fragmin in Unstable Coronary Artery Disease. *Am J Cardiol* **80**:30E–4E.

Koury ST, Bondurant MC, Koury MJ. 1988. Localization of erythropoietin synthesizing cells in murine kidneys by in situ hybridization. *Blood* **71**:524–7.

Krumholz HM, Radford MJ, Ellerbeck EF, et al. 1996. Aspirin for secondary prevention after acute myocardial infarction in the elderly: Prescribed use and outcomes. *Arch Intern Med* **124**:292–8.

Landolfi R, Patrono C. 1996. Aspirin in polycythemia vera and essential thrombocythemia: Current facts and perspectives. *Leuk Lymphoma* **22**(Suppl 1):83–6.

Laport GF, Williams SF. 1998. The role of high-dose chemotherapy in patients with Hodgkin's disease and non-Hodgkin's lymphoma. *Semin Oncol* **25**:503.

Lederle FA. 1991. Oral cobalamin for pernicious anemia. Medicine's best kept secret? *JAMA* **265**:94–5.

Lemmer JH Jr, Stanford W, Bonney SL, et al. 1994. Aprotinin for coronary bypass operations: Efficacy, safety, and influence on early saphenous vein graft patency. A multicenter, randomized, double-blind, placebo-controlled study. *J Thorac Cardiovasc Surg* **107**:543–51.

Lethagen S, Harris AS, Sjorin E, et al. 1987. Intranasal and intravenous administration of desmopressin: Effect on F VIII/vWF, pharmacokinetics and reproducibility. *Thromb Haemost* **58**:1033.

Levine MN, Gent M, Hirsh J, et al. 1996. A comparison of low-molecular-weight heparin administered primarily at home with unfractionated heparin administered in the hospital for proximal deep-vein thrombosis. *N Engl J Med* **334**:677–81.

Levine MN, Hirsh J, Gent M, et al. 1994. Double-blind randomised trial of a very-low-dose warfarin for prevention of thromboembolism in stage IV breast cancer. *Lancet* **343**:886–9.

Levine MN, Hirsh J, Landefeld S, et al. 1992. Hemorrhagic complications of anticoagulant treatment. *Chest* **102**(Suppl 4):352S–63S.

Levine MN, Hirsh J, Salzman EW. 1994. Side effects of antithrombotic therapy. In: Colman et al. *Hemostasis and Thrombosis: Basic Principles and Clinical Practice*. 3rd ed. Philadelphia: Lippincott, pp 936–55.

Levitt L, Lin R. 1996. Biology and treatment of adult acute lymphoblastic leukemia. *West J Med* **164**:143–55.

Liozon E, Brigaudeau C, Trimoreau F, et al. 1997. Is treatment with hydroxyurea leukemogenic in patients with essential thrombocythemia? An analysis of three new cases of leukaemic transformation and review of the literature. *Hematol Cell Ther* **39**:11–18.

Livio M, Mannucci PM, Vigano G, et al. 1986. Conjugated estrogens for the management of bleeding associated with renal failure. *N Engl J Med* **315**:731–5.

Longo DL, Glatstein E, Duffey PL, et al. 1991. Radiation therapy versus combination chemotherapy in the treatment of early-stage Hodgkin's disease: seven-year results of a prospective randomized trial. *J Clin Oncol* **9**:906–17.

Lopez M, Vici P, Di Lauro K, et al. 1998. Randomized prospective clinical trial of high-dose epirubicin and dexrazoxane in patients with advanced breast cancer and soft tissue sarcomas. *J Clin Oncol* **16**:86–92.

Lu H, Menashi S, Garcia I, et al. 1993. Reversibility of thrombin-induced decrease in platelet glycoprotein Ib function. *Br J Haematol* **85**:116–23.

Lubran MM. 1989. Hematologic side effects of drugs. *Ann Clin Lab Sci* **19**:114–21.

Macdougall IC, Tucker B, Thompson J, et al. 1996. A randomized controlled study of iron supplementation in patients treated with erythropoietin. *Kidney Int* **50**:1694–9.

Mani S, Barry M, Concato J. 1993. Granulocyte-colony stimulating factor therapy in drug-induced agranulocytosis. *Arch Intern Med* **153**:2500–1.

Mannucci PM. 1998. Hemostatic drugs. *N Engl J Med* **339**:245.

Mark DB, Cowper PA, Berkowitz SD, et al. 1998. Economic assessment of low-molecular-weight heparin (enoxaparin) versus unfractionated heparin in acute coronary syndrome patients: results from the ESSENCE randomized trial. Efficacy and Safety of Subcutaneous Enoxaparin in Non-Q wave Coronary Events [unstable angina or non-Q-wave myocardial infarction]. *Circulation* **97**:1702–7.

Markwardt F. 1994. The development of hirudin as an antithrombotic drug. *Thromb Res* **74**:1–23.

Mary JY, et al. *Eur J Hematol Suppl* **60**:35–4.

Masferrer JL, Zweifel BS, Manning PT, et al. 1994. Selective inhibition of inducible cyclooxygenase 2 in vivo is antiinflammatory and nonulcerogenic. *Proc Natl Acad Sci USA* **91**:3228–32.

Mayer RJ, Davis RB, Schiffer CA, et al. 1994. Intensive postremission chemotherapy in adults with acute myeloid leukemia. Cancer and Leukemia Group B. *N Engl J Med* **331**:896–903.

McMillan R. 1997. Therapy for adults with refractory chronic immune thrombocytopenic purpura. *Ann Intern Med* **126**:307–14.

Metcalf D. 1993. Hematopoietic regulators: Redundancy or subtlety? *Blood* **82**:3515–23.

Meusers P, Engelhard M, Bartels H, et al. 1989. Multicentre randomized therapeutic trial for advanced centrocytic lymphoma: Anthracycline does not improve the prognosis. *Hematol Oncol* **7**:365–80.

Michallet M, Archimbaud E, Bandini G, et al. 1996. HLA-identical sibling bone marrow transplantation in younger patients with chronic lymphocytic leukemia. European Group for Blood and Marrow Transplantation and the International Bone Marrow Transplant Registry. *Ann Intern Med* **124**: 311–15.

Mitus AJ, Schafer AL. 1990. Thrombocytosis and thrombocythemia. *Hematol Oncol Clin North Am* **4**:157–178.

Moore RD, Keruly JC, Chaisson RE. 1998. Anemia and survival in HIV infection. *J Acquir Immune Defic Syndr Hum Retrovirol* **19**:29–33.

Mrozek K, Heinonen K, de la Chapelle A, et al. 1997. Clinical significance of cytogenetics in acute myeloid leukemia. *Semin Oncol* **24**:17–31.

Mueller RL, Scheidt S. 1994. History of drugs for thrombotic disease. Discovery, development, and directions for the future. *Circulation* **89**:432–49.

Nurden AT. 1996. New thoughts on strategies for modulating platelet function through the inhibition of surface receptors. *Haemostasis* **26**(Suppl 4):78–88.

Nurmohamed MT, ten Cate H, ten Cate JW. 1997. Low molecular weight heparin(oid)s. Clinical investigations and practical recommendations. *Drugs* **53**:736–51.

Ogawa M. 1993. Differentiation and proliferation of hematopoietic stem cells. *Blood* **81**: 2844–53.

Ohnishi K, Ohno R, Tomonaga M, et al. 1995. A randomized trial comparing interferon-alpha with busulfan for newly diagnosed chronic myelogenous leukemia in chronic phase. *Blood* **86**:906–16.

Oler A, Whooley MA, Oler J, Grady D. 1996. Adding heparin to aspirin reduces the incidence of myocardial infarction and death in patients with unstable angina. A meta-analysis. *JAMA* **276**:811–5.

O'Neill GP, Ford-Hutchinson AW. 1993. Expression of mRNA for cyclooxygenase-1 and cyclooxygenase-2 in human tissues. *FEBS Lett* **330**:156–60.

O'Reilly RA. 1987. Warfarin metabolism and drug-drug interactions. *Adv Exp Med Biol* **214**:205–12.

Otto JC, Smith WL. 1995. Prostaglandin endoperoxide synthases-1 and -2. *J Lipid Mediat Cell Signal* **12**:139–56.

Passweg JR, Rowling PA, Horowitz MM. 1998. Related donor bone marrow transplantation for chronic myelogenous leukemia. *Hematol Oncol* **12**:81–92.

Patton WN, Duffull SB. 1994. Idiosyncratic drug-induced haematological abnormalities. Incidence, pathogenesis, management and avoidance. *Drug Safety* **11**:445–62.

Pedersen-Bjergaard U, Andersen M, Hansen PB. 1996. Thrombocytopenia induced by noncytotoxic drugs in Denmark 1968–91. *J Intern Med* **239**:509–15.

Pedersen-Bjergaard U, Andersen M, Hansen PB. 1997. Drug-induced thrombocytopenia: Clinical data on 309 cases and the effect of corticosteroid therapy. *Eur J Clin Pharmacol* **52**:183–9.

Pfeffer LM, Dinarello CA, Herberman RB, et al. 1998. Biological properties of recombinant alpha-interferons: 40th anniversary of the discovery of interferons. *Cancer Res* **58**:2489–99.

Physicians' Health Study. Ridker PM, Hennekens CH, Lindpaintner K, et al. 1995. *N Engl J Med* **332**:912–17.

Pineo GF, Hull RD. 1996. Prevention and treatment of venous thromboembolism. *Drugs* **52**:71–92.

Pini M. 1997. Low molecular weight heparin. *Recent Prog Med* **88**:594–602.

Pott C, Hiddemann W. 1997. Purine analogs in the treatment of chronic lymphocytic leukemia. Leukemia **11**(Suppl 2):S25–8.

Prakash V, Tomasheff SN 1991. Mechanism of interaction of vinca alkaloids with tubulin: catharanthine and vindolin. *Biochemistry* **30**:873–80.

Raelson JV, Nervi C, Rosenauer A, et al. 1996. The PML/RAR alpha oncoprotein is a direct molecular target of retinoic acid in acute promyelocytic leukemia cells. *Blood* **88**:2826–32.

Rafael JL. 1997. Iron, infections, and anemia of inflammation. *Clin Infect Dis* **25**:888–95.

Ravandi-Kashani F, Schafer AI. 1997. Microvascular disturbances, thrombosis, and bleeding in thrombocythemia: Current concepts and perspectives. *Semin Thromb Hemost* **23**:479–88.

Reddy DS. 1998. Newer thrombolytic drugs for acute myocardial infarction. *Indian J Exp Biol* **36**:1–15.

Robert J. 1993. Epirubicin. Clinical pharmacology and dose-effect relationship. *Drugs* **45**(Suppl 2):20–30.

Ryan TM, Ciavatta DJ, Townes TM. 1997. Knockout-transgenic mouse model of sickle cell disease. *Science* **278**:873–6.

Saour JN, Sieck JO, Mamo LA, et al. 1990. Trial of different intensities of anticoagulation in patients with prosthetic heart valves. *N Engl J Med* **322**:428–32.

Saven A, Piro LD. 1996. 2-Chlorodeoxyadenosine: A potent antimetabolite with major activity in the treatment of indolent lymphoproliferative disorders. *Hematol Cell Ther* **38**(Suppl 2):S93–101.

Schmitt BP, Adelman B. 1993. Heparin-associated thrombocytopenia: A critical review and pooled analysis. *Am J Med Sci* **305**:208–15.

Schomig A, Neumann FJ, Kastrati A, et al. 1996. A randomized comparison of antiplatelet and anticoagulant therapy after the placement of coronary-artery stents. *N Engl J Med* **334**:1084–9.

Schror K. 1997. Aspirin and platelets: The antiplatelet action of aspirin and its role in thrombosis treatment and prophylaxis. *Semin Thromb Hemost* **23**:349–56.

Shemin D, Elnour M, Amarantes B, et al. 1990. Oral estrogens decrease bleeding time and improve clinical bleeding in patients with renal failure. *Am J Med* **9**:436–40.

Smalling RW, Bode C, Kalbfleisch J, et al. 1995. More rapid, complete, and stable coronary thrombolysis with bolus administration of reteplase compared with alteplase infusion in acute myocardial infarction. RAPID Investigators. *Circulation* **91**:2725–32.

Sorensen JM, Vena DA, Fallavollita A, et al. 1997. Treatment of refractory chronic lymphocytic leukemia with fludarabine phosphate via the group C protocol mechanism of the National Cancer Institute: Five-year follow-up report. *J Clin Oncol* **15**:458–65.

Spangrude GJ, Smith L, Uchida N, et al. 1991. Mouse hematopoietic stem cells. *Blood* **78**:1395–1402.

Stefanini M, English HA, Taylor AE. 1990. Safe and effective, prolonged administration of epsilon aminocaproic acid in bleeding from the urinary tract. *J Urol* **143**:559–61.

Stein JH, McBride PE. 1998. Hyperhomocysteinemia and atherosclerotic vascular disease: Pathophysiology, screening, and treatment of. *Arch Intern Med* **158**:1301–6.

Sunder-Plassmann G, Horl WH. 1997. Safety aspects of parenteral iron in patients with end-stage renal disease. *Drug Safety* **17**:241–50.

Svensson PJ, Dahlbäck B. 1994. Resistance to activated protein C as a basis for venous thrombosis. *N Engl J Med* **330**:517–22.

Tatarsky I, Sharon R. 1997. Management of polycythemia vera with hydroxyurea. *Semin Hematol* **34**:24–8.

Tefferi A, Elliott MA, Solberg LA Jr, et al. 1997. New drugs in essential thrombocythemia and polycythemia vera. *Blood Rev* **11**:1–7.

Tefferi A, Silverstein MN, Petitt RM, et al. 1997. Anagrelide as a new platelet-lowering agent in essential thrombocythemia: Mechanism of actin, efficacy, toxicity, current indications. *Semin Thromb Hemost* **23**:379–83.

The Italian Cooperative Study Group on Chronic Myeloid Leukemia. 1994. Interferon alfa-2a as compared with conventional chemotherapy for the treatment of chronic myeloid leukemia. *N Engl J Med* **330**:820–5.

Thomas DP. 1997. Does low-molecular-weight heparin cause less bleeding? *Thromb Haemost* **78**:1422–5.

To LB, Haylock DN, Simmon PJ, et al. 1997. The biology and clinical uses of blood stem cells. *Blood* **89**:2233–58.

Turpie AG, Gent M, Laupacis A, et al. 1993. A comparison of aspirin with placebo in patients treated with warfarin after heart valve replacement. *N Engl J Med* **329**:524.

Turpie AG. 1997. Low-molecular-weight heparin: From the bench to the orthopedic patient. *Orthopedics* **20**(Suppl):10–13.

UK-TIA Study Group 1988. Alternative reference for UK-TIA Study but in 1991: [Anonymous]. 1991b. The United Kingdom transient ischemic attack (UK-TIA) aspirin trial: Final results. UK-TIA Study Group. *J Neurol Neurosurg Psychiatry* **54**:1044–54.

Van Genderen PJ, Leenknegt H, Michiels JJ. 1997. The paradox of bleeding and thrombosis in thrombocythemia: Is von Willebrand factor the link? *Semin Thromb Hemost* **23**:385–9.

Vane JR, Botting RM. 1997. Mechanism of action of aspirin-like drugs. *Semin Arthritis Rheum* **26**(Suppl 1):2–10.

Vane JR, Mitchell JA, Appleton I, et al. 1994. Inducible isoforms of cyclooxygenase and nitro-oxide synthase in inflammation. *Proc Natl Acad Sci USA* **91**:2046–50.

Vanholder R, Camez A, Veys N, et al. 1997. Pharmacokinetics of recombinant hirudin in hemodialyzed end-stage renal failure patients. *Thromb Haemost* **77**:650–5.

Venturini M, Michelotti A, Del Mastro L, et al. 1996. Multicenter randomized controlled clinical trial to evaluate cardioprotection of dexrazoxane versus no cardioprotection in women receiving epirubicin chemotherapy for advanced breast cancer. *J Clin Oncol* **14**:3112–20.

Verstraete M. 1995. New developments in antiplatelet and antithrombotic therapy. *Eur Heart J* **16**(Suppl L):16–23.

Vichinsky EP, Haberkern CM, Neumayr L, et al. 1995. A comparison of conservative and aggressive transfusion regimens in the perioperative management of sickle cell disease. *N Engl J Med* **333**:206–13.

Vose JM, Anderson JR, Kessinger A, et al. 1993. High-dose chemotherapy and autologous hematopoietic stem-cell transplantation for aggressive non-Hodgkin's lymphoma. *J Clin Oncol* **11**:1846–51.

Vose JM. 1998. Current approaches to the management of non-Hodgkin's lymphoma. *Semin Oncol* **25**:483–91.

Wallis RB. 1996. Hirudins: From leeches to man. *Semin Thromb Hemost* **22**:185–96.

Walters MC, Patience M, Leisenring W, et al. 1997. Collaborative multicenter investigation of marrow transplantation for sickle cell disease: Current results and future directions. *Biol Blood Marrow Transplant* **3**:310–15.

Weitz JI. 1997. Low-molecular-weight heparins. [Published erratum appears in *N Engl J Med* **337**:1567 1997]. *N Engl J Med* **337**:688–98.

Weitz JI, Leslie B, Hudoba M. 1998. Thrombin binds to soluble fibrin degradation products where it is protected from inhibition by heparin-antithrombin but susceptible to inactivation by antithrombin-independent inhibitors. *Circulation* **97**:544–52.

Wells PS, Holbrook AM, Crowther NR, et al. 1994. Interactions of warfarin with drugs and food. *Ann Intern Med* **121**:676–83.

Welte K, Gabrilove J, Bronchud MH, et al. 1996. Filgrastim (r-metHuG-CSF): The first 10 years. *Blood* **88**:1907–29.

White HD. 1997. Clinical trials of direct thrombin inhibitors in acute ischaemic syndromes. *Thromb Haemost* **78**:364–6.

Wiholm 1996. *Eur J Haematol Suppl* **60**:42–6.

Winkelstein A, Kiss JE. 1997. Immunohematologic disorders. *JAMA* **278**:1982–92.

Wolf PA, Singer DE. 1997. Preventing stroke in atrial fibrillation. *Am Fam Physician* **56**:2242–50.

Young NS. 1996. Immune pathophysiology of acquired aplastic anaemia. *Eur J Haematol* **60**(Suppl):55–9.

CHAPTER

# 13 ONCOLOGIC DISORDERS

Joseph R. Bertino, Owen A. O'Connor

*Chapter Outline*



The modern era of antineoplastic pharmacology began with the demonstration by C. Huggins and C.U. Hodges in 1941 that prostate cancer regressed when treated with diethylstilbestrol (Huggins et al. 1941). Soon after, the report that nitrogen mustard, a derivative of sulfur mustard used to kill or incapacitate soldiers during World War I, could cause regressions in patients with lymphoma, stimulated a search for other cancer chemotherapeutics (Gilman and Phillips 1946; Gilman 1963). During the 1950s and 1960s, the evaluation of chemicals using inhibition of tumor growth as an experimental assay resulted in the discovery of additional agents that were subsequently found to be of value in the treatment of patients with cancer. The understanding of a drug's mechanism of action and the molecular basis for drug resistance, attributed in great part to the advances in gene cloning, began only 20 years ago. The past decade has been one of truly remarkable progress in our understanding of the pathogenesis of cancer. Although this knowledge has not yet led to a significant improvement in the treatment of patients with cancer, there is every expectation that the next decade will see a large number of new and effective therapies introduced into the clinic.

It is now clear that cancer is primarily a degenerative disease of aging that results from accumulated genetic damage. This damage is thought to result from multiple endogenous and exogenous factors that lead to inactivation of tumor suppressor genes or activation of growth-promoting oncogenes. In a relative minority of cases, inactivation of normal DNA repair mechanisms becomes manifest as a hereditary or familial predisposition to cancer. Evolving therapeutic strategies are likely to target these molecular defects, holding the promise of enhanced tumor selectivity. It is also clear from the elegant work of Vogelstein and his colleagues that many human cancers, especially those of epithelial origin, arise after multiple genetic changes (Fearon and Vogelstein 1990; Fearon 1995). Since the previous edition of this volume, several new drugs have been approved by the Food and Drug Administration (FDA) for the treatment of cancer patients, and more treatment options are available today than ever before.

Despite the progress and optimism for the future, our present antineoplastic drugs can cure only a few types of disseminated malignancies (Table 13-1). Lymphoid malignancies (acute lymphocytic leukemia [ALL], Hodgkin disease, high-grade or intermediate-grade non-Hodgkin lymphoma), germ-cell tumors, choriocarcinoma, and several childhood solid tumors (e.g., Wilms tumor) are potentially curable with existing drugs. The introduction of new "supportive" agents that can decrease the acute toxicities due to chemotherapy (i.e., nausea and vomiting), and reduce drug-induced marrow toxicity (granulocyte and granulocyte-macrophage colony-stimulating factors [G-CSF and GM-SCF]), have made treatment administration safer and more tolerable (Gabrilove et al. 1988).

Table 13-1 Responsiveness of Cancer to Chemotherapy

I. *Cure (>30%) of Advanced Disease*
  - Choriocarcinoma
  - Acute lymphocytic leukemia (childhood)
  - Malignant lymphoma (Hodgkin disease, diffuse high-grade or intermediate-grade non-Hodgkin lymphoma
  - Hairy cell leukemia
  - Germ cell tumors
  - Childhood solid tumors (embryonal rhabdomyosarcoma, Ewing sarcoma, Wilms tumor)
  - Acute myelocytic leukemia
  - Promyelocytic leukemia

II. *Significant Palliation, Some Cures of Advanced Disease (5–30%)*
  - Ovarian cancer
  - Bladder cancer
  - Small cell lung cancer
  - Gastric cancer

III. *Palliation, Probably Increases in Survival*
  - Breast cancer
  - Multiple myeloma
  - Head and neck cancer

IV. *Adjuvant Treatment Leading to Increased Cure*
  - Breast cancer
  - Colon cancer
  - Osteogenic sarcoma
  - Early-stage large cell lymphoma

These improvements in chemotherapy administration have allowed for a modest increase in dose intensity when used in conjunction with bone marrow or peripheral blood progenitor cell transplants. However, long-term toxicities due to combination chemotherapy in cured patients are still observed (sterility, secondary malignancies), and efforts to eliminate these adverse effects through the substitution of less toxic drugs are in progress (Table 13-2). Long-term remissions are also observed after treatment of patients with other malignancies, for example, acute myeloid leukemia (AML), small-cell lung cancer, and bladder cancer. However, cure rates are low (10- to 30%), and attempts to intensify treatment to improve curability are not yet definitive. Some tumors commonly respond to chemotherapy with no prospect for cure, although others seem oblivious to the therapy imposed (Table 13-1).

Despite the fact that chemotherapy is rarely curative in some cancers, it is clear that its integration into the multimodality treatment of localized disease, where the frequency of occult micrometastases is known to be high, can render patients disease-free. This strategy has proved to be important in the management of diseases such as breast and colon cancer (Table 13-1).

## DISCOVERY OF ANTICANCER DRUGS

Although there is no animal model or in vitro test that predicts with certainty the anticancer activity of a drug in the clinic, cell lines derived from human cancers, rodent tumors, and human xenografts propagated in rodents have been used with some success to evaluate new compounds. Although of limited value, in vitro sensitivity tests using fresh human tumors are also used, where an index of cell death or clonogenicity (i.e., the ability of cells to form colonies in a "clonogenic assay") are used as the principle endpoints. In vitro culture conditions, especially for solid tumors, are limited by their inability to mimic conditions of tumor growth in vivo and obviously fail to provide information regarding host toxicity. Some useful information may be obtained from these assays with regard to the resistance of tumors to various drugs. When the mechanism of action of a drug is known, the effect of a drug on that target may be measured in vitro, using a sample of the patient's tumor cells, and related to a prediction of drug resistance or sensitivity. For example, levels of thymidylate synthase mRNA expression in gastrointestinal tumors may be predictive of response to fluorouracil, a chemotherapeutic agent that is converted to fluorodeoxyuridylate, a potent inhibitor of this enzyme (Lenz et al. 1996; Gorlick et al. 1998). Although screening of random compounds (from natural products or chemical libraries) still continues, modern drug discovery uses rational design based on structures of key targets elucidated by x-ray crystallography and nuclear magnetic resonance.

## EVALUATION OF NEW DRUGS IN THE CLINIC

New drugs entering the clinic are first tested in patients who have advanced cancer and are refractory to conventional treatment regimens in a phase I trial. Phase I trials are designed to answer questions of toxicity and to determine a maximum tolerated dose (MTD) of the drug. The starting dose for phase I trials is usually one-tenth the toxic dose ($LD_{10}$) in the most sensitive animal species (usually mice or dogs). Subsequent patients are treated with increasing doses, initially by doubling the dose, then with smaller increments of dose escalation until toxicity is observed and a MTD is determined. The MTD is defined as the dose that produces life-threatening toxicity in two or more of six patients treated at that dose level. Phase II trials are designed to address questions of antitumor efficacy in a variety of tumor types. The dose used

Table 13-2 Long-Term Toxicities Associated with Cancer Treatment

| MEDICAL CONDITION | AGENTS |
|---|---|
| *Pulmonary fibrosis/pulmonary insufficiency* | Bleomycin<br>Cyclophosphamide<br>Carmustine<br>Radiotherapy to lung fields |
| *Coronary artery disease/valvular heart disease* | Radiation therapy |
| *Cardiomyopathy* | Anthracyclines<br>• Doxorubicin<br>• Mitoxantrone<br>Mitomycin C (especially when used in conjunction with anthracyclines) |
| *Secondary malignancies* | Most alkylating agents<br>• Procarbazine/Dacarbazine (leukemia)<br>• Mechlorethamine (leukemias)<br>• Melphalan<br>• Cyclophosphamide (leukemia, bladder)<br>Etoposide/Teniposide (11q translocations)<br>Tamoxifen (endometrial cancer)<br>Radiation therapy (lung and breast cancer, leukemia) |
| *Gonadal dysfunction (Infertility)* | Most alkylating agents<br>• Mechlorethamine<br>• Cyclophosphamide<br>• Chlorambucil<br>• Procarbazine<br>• Busulfan<br>Cisplatin<br>Radiation therapy to gonads |

for subsequent phase II trials is usually one dose level lower than the MTD. If encouraging antitumor effects are produced in one or more phase II trials, then a phase III trial is warranted. Phase III trials are designed to determine whether the new drug is more effective or has less toxicity with equal effectiveness compared with the present standard of care. If these criteria are met, then the drug may be approved by the FDA and marketed.

As most disseminated tumors are now treated with combination chemotherapy, evaluation of a new drug in a previously treated patient with a large tumor burden can represent a significant obstacle to new drug development. In general, these patients have a lower probability of response compared with patients not previously treated. In advanced cancers not curable by chemotherapy (e.g., non-small-cell lung cancer), evaluation of a new drug in a phase II trial before using a standard regimen has been accepted as a way of addressing this problem and has been shown not to adversely affect patient outcome (Simon 1997).

## DETERMINANTS OF TUMOR RESPONSE TO DRUGS

The treatment objective in cancer management is tumor regression without serious or lethal toxicity, leading to an increase in disease-free survival of the patient and possibly cure. It is now clear that tumor cell death as a consequence of chemotherapy is due to apoptosis, or programmed cell death. Apoptosis is an active process, generated by intracellular signals that activate proteases that lead to degradation of intracellular contents forming small apoptotic bodies, which are eventually phagocytized. This process is different from nonapoptotic cell death or necrosis, which results in spilling of nuclear contents and an inflammatory response.

Tumor cells, especially epithelial cancers, are malignant because they have mutations that result in stimulated growth (lack of tumor suppressor genes or oncogene activation) coupled with genetic changes that prevent cell death. In general, drugs can induce apoptosis in cancer cells by activating enzymes, receptors, or other target molecules that promote programmed cell death, or by inhibiting target molecules that tend to prevent apoptosis. In the case of drug "sensitive" tumors such as lymphoid malignancies and testicular cancer, these cells rapidly die after the drug achieves a sufficient concentration to inactivate its molecular target. In the case of drug "refractory" tumors such as pancreatic cancer and sarcoma, "drug failure" may be due to pharmacokinetic and/or pharmacodynamic properties or intrinsic cellular biology. For example, the inability of a drug to achieve the required cytotoxic concentration or duration of exposure required to modify the target molecule would produce a "refractory" state. Conversely, the refractory nature of the malignancy may be secondary to that tumor's expression of antiapoptotic proteins, which allow cell survival and proliferation despite various cytotoxic agents.

This chapter emphasizes the principles of chemotherapy of malignant diseases. Because this field is rapidly changing, detailed information on drug usage is not provided. Instead, generalizations regarding classes of drugs and principles of their use are stressed. Examples of therapeutic programs for specific cancers are given in other references (DeVita et al. 1997; Holland et al. 1997).

## THEORETICAL CONSIDERATIONS

### Tumor and Normal Stem Cell Kinetics

The growth rate of a tumor is a function of the number of stem or clonogenic cells present (the so-called growth fraction), the generation of these cells, and the rate of cell loss. In tissues that normally renew themselves frequently (e.g., mucosa, bone marrow, hair follicles), the rate of cell production is exquisitely balanced by the rate of cell loss. This balance results in a steady state with no net growth of the tissue or organ. Tumors increase in size when these variables in the steady state are shifted out of balance. Such is the case when the proliferative rate of the malignant cells exceeds their death rate, or the death rate declines with an otherwise stable proliferative rate. It also follows that the growth rate of a tumor, usually expressed as the doubling time, does not provide insight into the dynamics of tumor growth. For example, a "slow-growing" tumor may have a high growth fraction and a short generation time but may be balanced by a high rate of cell loss (Schackney and Ritch 1982).

### Cell-Kill Hypothesis

In experimental tumor systems, especially transplanted mouse tumors (e.g., the L1210 leukemia), most available chemotherapeutic agents increase the survival of tumor-bearing mice by killing a proportion of stem cells (Skipper et al. 1964; Skipper 1967). In the L1210 system, a single cell can eventually cause death at a predictable time when a critical tumor size is reached (about $10^9$ cells). The increase in survival that occurs when animals bearing a known tumor burden are treated is therefore related to the number of tumor cells left after treatment. The use of this model system has made it possible to show that a given treatment will produce a relatively constant and predictable "cell kill," regardless of the number of tumor cells initially present. For example, if $10^5$ cells could be killed by a given treatment, cure is possible if $10^4$ cells are present but will not occur if $10^6$ cells or greater are present.

Because most chemotherapy is nonselective, it tends to kill a fraction of normal cell populations (e.g., bone marrow, gut epithelium) as well as abnormal cells. The challenges in chemotherapy administration therefore are twofold: 1) attain as large a difference as possible in cell kill between malignant and normal cell populations (i.e., increase the therapeutic window), and 2) manage all complications that arise from the destruction of normal cells.

How do we obtain "selective" cell kill? To cure the mice bearing the L1210 tumor as discussed above, up to $10^9$ cells must be eradicated (Skipper et al. 1964). It has been estimated that a 20-kg child dying of acute lymphoblastic leukemia has approximately $10^{12}$ malignant cells (Frei 1984). Assuming that the smallest detectable tumor weighs roughly 1 g, which contains approximately $10^9$ cells, chemotherapy must eradicate the entire malignant population of $10^{12}$ cells. This obviously must be accomplished without producing an intolerable loss of normal cells, such as bone marrow precursors and gut epithelium. An estimate of the "logs of kill" that these normal cell compartments can withstand has been obtained (Bruce and Bergsagel 1967). In humans, 450 rad of whole-body irradiation is probably lethal, although about 600 rad is considered the lethal dose in mice. A dose of 600 rad produces a 2 log reduction in murine hemopoietic stem cells. Extrapolating a similar response in humans from the lethal dose, it is assumed that a 450-rad dose of radiation in humans produces a 2 log reduction in stem cells (Alexander 1965). With intense supportive therapy, perhaps another log of normal stem cells can be killed without fatal adverse effects on the patient. Therefore, a successful treatment program must eradicate 9 to 12 logs of tumor cells (whether by surgery, x-ray, drugs, and/or immunotherapy), although decreasing normal stem cells by only 2 to 3 logs. Dose-limiting myelotoxicity can be circumvented through the use of autologous peripheral blood stem cells, which are infused back into the patient following high-dose chemotherapy. In these cases, dose-limiting toxicities are often dictated by organs other than the bone marrow.

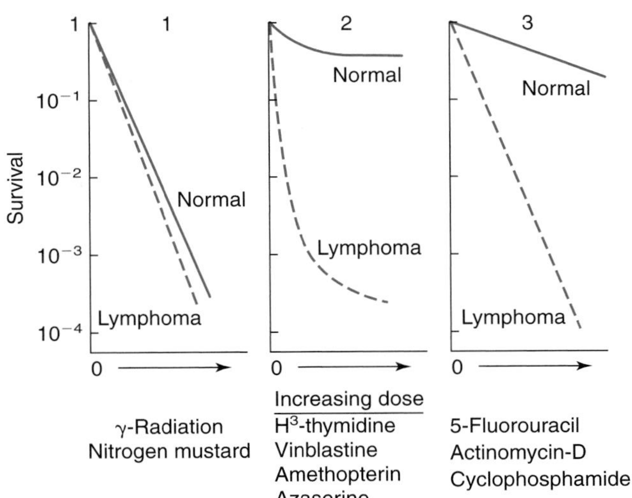


**FIGURE 13-1 Dose–survival curves for nine different anticancer agents tested (24-hour exposure) against normal hemopoietic and lymphoma colony-forming cells. Class 1 are *non-cycle-active* drugs; class 2 and 3 agents are considered to be *cycle-active* agents. (From Bruce et al., 1966.)**

## Cycle-Specific and Non-Cycle-Specific Drugs

To approach the problem of selectivity, a model system in an experimental animal was devised to quantify the effects of chemotherapeutic agents on both normal and malignant cells (Bruce et al. 1966). This study demonstrated a linear relationship between the number of hemopoietic stem cells injected into irradiated mice and the macroscopic colonies produced in the spleen (Till and McCulloch 1961). Similarly, transplantable AKR lymphoma cells produced macroscopic colonies in the spleens of syngeneic mice in direct relationship to the number of cells inoculated (Bruce et al. 1966). This assay allows for the measurement of effects of dose and duration of drug treatment on both tumor and hemopoietic stem cell proliferation. On the basis of differential effects on these two compartments of cells, drugs were classified into one of three groups (Bruce et al. 1966). The first group of drugs (which included nitrogen mustard, 1,3-bis-2-chloroethyl-1-nitrosourea (BCNU), and x-ray [see Fig. 13-1]) completely eradicated both the normal hemopoietic stem cells and tumor cells to the same extent. However, the second and third classes of drugs, also given over a similar 24-hour period, eradicated the tumor population to a much greater extent than the normal stem cells. When some of the drugs in the third class were given at high doses, they killed as much as 10,000 times the number of lymphoma cells than normal stem cells. This class included drugs such as cyclophosphamide (Fig. 13-1), dactinomycin, and 5-fluorouracil (5-FU). The remaining drugs tested (methotrexate, vinblastine, azaserine, 6-mercaptopurine, and high-specific-activity tritiated thymidine [$^3$H]TdR) still achieved a marked differential cell kill (500-fold), but the differences diminished as the dose of drugs increased.

The selectivity of the agents in the last two classes was attributed to a differential effect of the agents on proliferating versus nonproliferating cells. Hematopoietic stem cells are typically in a state of low proliferative activity compared with lymphoma cells. However, the susceptibility of the normal stem cells to agents of the second and third class increased when their proliferative activity increased (e.g., after sublethal irradiation or drug treatment) and reverted to usual only when this increased rate of proliferation returned to baseline levels (Valeriote and Bruce 1967; Bruce et al. 1969). Bruce (1967) suggested that class II and III agents were capable of killing cells only if the drug was present when these cells were engaged in active proliferation (DNA synthesis and mitosis). The cells that were not killed by therapy were considered quiescent during the time of drug exposure. On implantation into animals however, these cells actively proliferated and produced splenic colonies. The proliferating cells killed by the class II and III agents were said to be in "cycle." The *cell cycle* refers to the orderly and strictly regulated phases of cell growth, and consists of four phases that include $G_1$ (gap 1), S (DNA synthesis), $G_2$ (gap 2), and M (mitosis) phase (Fig. 13-2). The interval between each cell division is termed the *$G_0$ phase*. Agents

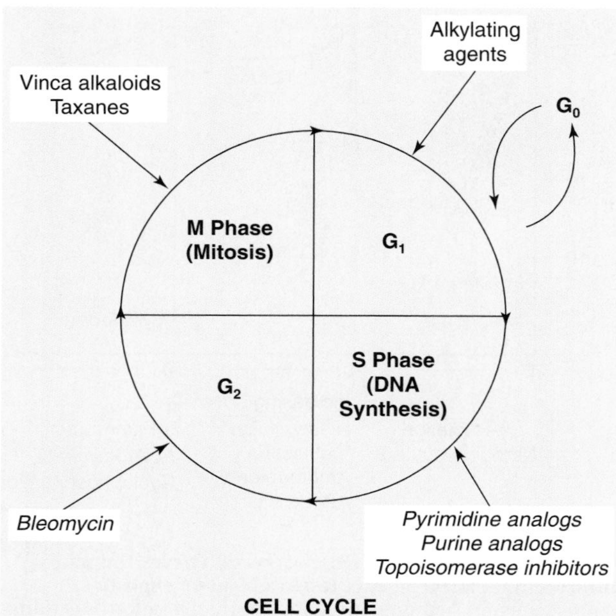


FIGURE 13-2 **Conceptual scheme of the cell cycle, depicting the phases of growth that both normal and neoplastic cells follow. The relative proportion of time spent in any given phase varies. Typically, for any particular cell, the greatest amount of time is spent in $G_1$ (or $G_0$, the resting phase), whereas M phase (mitosis), is the shortest phase. Cell-cycle-specific agents include drugs that act in S phase (DNA synthesis) or M phase; drugs that are not cell-cycle-specific act in $G_1$ or $G_2$.**

that killed both the normal and tumor cells irrespective of their proliferative state (class I) have been referred to as *non-cycle-specific agents*, and agents of the second and third class have been called *cycle-specific agents*. Cycle-specific agents may be further characterized in some instances on the basis of studies of cell killing that used synchronous populations of cells. Some agents (e.g., methotrexate, cytosine arabinoside, hydroxyurea) kill cells in the S phase of the cell cycle, during which DNA synthesis occurs. Other agents such as bleomycin, paclitaxel, and the vinca alkaloids affect cells during the $G_2$–M phase of the cycle as they undergo mitosis (Fig. 13-2).

The classification of chemotherapeutic agents into cycle-specific or non-cycle-specific subgroups has been useful in terms of certain generalizations that may be made concerning the properties of these drugs (Table 13-3).

**PRINCIPLE Cycle-active agents are "schedule dependent," that is, antitumor and toxic results are dependent more on the duration of exposure than the dose.**

Very large doses of cycle-active drugs may be given if the duration of exposure is short and the interval between retreatment is sufficiently long. For example, in high-dose methotrexate (MTX) regimens, 20 g/m$^2$ of MTX is safe and effective against acute lymphocytic leukemia (ALL) if the duration of exposure is kept to 36 hours or less by using leucovorin rescue, and the treatment is not repeated more than weekly or biweekly (Ackland and Schilsky 1987; Chu and Allegra 1996). In contrast, 20 mg/m$^2$ per day of MTX is highly toxic to normal bone marrow and gastrointestinal (GI) mucosa if given as a 5-day continuous infusion. The explanation for this difference in relative toxicity is that short-term exposure to antimetabolites spares bone marrow stem cells. Stem-cell proliferation subsequently leads to replenishment of the decimated proliferating and differentiating cells, although longer exposures to antimetabolites (48 hours or longer) begin to kill stem cells that have been recruited into cycle.

**PRINCIPLE It follows that agents that can excessively damage or stress the bone marrow (e.g., previous radiation therapy, protracted chemotherapy, or infection) can compromise the recruitment of stem cells into cycle, which may predispose patients to myelosuppression with antimetabolites.**

As a consequence, treatment of patients with ALL using high intermittent-pulse dosing of antimetabolite regimens may be safe as well as effective if instituted while the patient is in bone marrow remission, although similar treatment of patients with infection or who are in bone marrow relapse may cause serious marrow toxicity.

In contrast to the relative selectivity that may be obtained with antimetabolites in the treatment of rapidly proliferating malignancies, non-cycle-active agents have a steeper dose response and less of a selective action in relation to marrow toxicity.

**PRINCIPLE Total dose, rather than dose schedule, is important for non-cycle-active agents.**

The choice of schedule used with non-cycle-active agents may depend more on other adverse side effects rather than bone marrow toxicity. For example, doxorubicin delivered as a continuous infusion (over 48- to 96 hours) or as a pulse (every 3 weeks) has similar marrow toxicity at the same total dose, but continuous infusions of doxorubicin may be less cardiotoxic (Legha et al. 1982).

Table 13-3 Examples of Cycle-Specific and Non-Cycle-Specific Chemotherapeutic Agents

| CELL-CYCLE-SPECIFIC (CCS) AGENTS | NON-CELL-CYCLE-SPECIFIC (NCCS) AGENTS |
|---|---|
| *S-phase-specific agents* | *Non-phase-specific agents* |
| Antimetabolites (methotrexate [MTX], 5-fluorouracil/FUdR, cytarabine, gemcitabine) | Alkylating agents (nitrogen mustards, nitrosoureas, alkyl sulfonates, ethylenimines, nonclassical) alkylating agents) |
| Hydroxyurea | Platinum analogs |
| Topoisomerase I inhibitors (irinotecan, topotecan) | Actinomycin D/Mitomycin C |
| Topoisomerase II inhibitors (etoposide, teniposide, anthracyclines) | |
| *$G_2$–M-phase-specific agents* | |
| Vinca alkaloids (vincristine, vinblastine) | |
| Taxanes (paclitaxel, docetaxel) | |
| Bleomycin | |

ABBREVIATIONS: FUdR, 5-fluorodeoxyuridine; MTX, methotrexate.

## Effect of Size on Growth Rate of a Tumor

The concepts developed thus far have assumed that the rate of tumor growth is constant. However, in most circumstances, as the size of the tumor increases, its rate of growth slows. This may be due to an increase in the generation time of the tumor, a decrease in the growth fraction of the tumor, and/or an increase in the death rate of the tumor cells (Steel 1967). These changes may result from overcrowding and decreased nutrition of the tumor; the process at present is poorly understood. In this phase of growth the tumor population may not be in a state of active proliferation. Both tumor and normal cells may be in a resting state, thus compromising the differential cell kill of the cycle-specific agents (Table 13-3). In fact, if marrow involvement with tumor or infection is present, the normal cells of the marrow may be in a more active proliferative state phase than the tumor cells. In this setting, even greater toxicity than usual may be produced with drug therapy.

DNA synthesis in cells in the plateau phase of growth is less sensitive to the action of cycle-specific drugs than are cells in the logarithmic phase of growth (Hryniuk et al. 1969). Therefore, when tumors are large and growth has reached a plateau, attempts to decrease tumor size by the use of non-cycle-active agents, surgery, or x-ray therapy should be considered. The use of a non-cycle-active agent is of value if recovery of the normal tissues are more rapid than recovery of the malignant tissue. Because the dose–response curve of these agents is steep, a maximum dose should be administered to kill as may cells as possible, keeping in mind the narrow therapeutic index of this class of antineoplastic compounds. If sufficient tumor kill of cells is obtained, the logarithmic phase of tumor growth may be reestablished, and the cycle-specific agents may regain their value.

## Compartmentalization of Cells

Not all tumor-bearing compartments of the body are affected to the same degree by a course of chemotherapy (Skipper 1965). In model animal systems, as well as in humans, cells in the central nervous system (CNS) are least affected by chemotherapy, owing to failure of most drugs to pass readily through the blood–brain barrier. This failure to achieve a substantial cell kill in the CNS may account for relapses in leukemia. Intrathecal administration of chemotherapeutic agents is necessary in patients with documented CNS involvement. In contrast, similar cells in the blood are more sensitive to the effects of antimetabolites (at least when methotrexate is used) (Hryniuk and Bertino 1969b). Furthermore, sensitivity of tumor cells in different organs (e.g., leukemia cells in the spleen, kidney, or liver) may vary depending on the drug used. Organ-specific differences in tumor sensitivity may be related to binding or metabolism of the drug in the different tissues or to biochemical influences of the organ on growth or metabolism of the neoplastic cells.

## Drug Resistance

Tumors may be intrinsically resistant to certain drugs or may acquire resistance following an initial period of drug sensitivity. Intrinsic drug resistance is considered to reflect the genetic makeup of the tumor. Specifically, intrinsic drug resistance mechanisms may compromise the ability of a drug to achieve intracellular concentrations required to inactivate the drug target or may impair the cell's response to correct the molecular damage. For example, cells that lack p53, despite inhibition of the target enzyme (e.g., dihydrofolate reductase by methotrexate), may not arrest at the $G_1$/S phase checkpoint and undergo apoptosis but may continue to progress through S phase and the remaining cell cycle, generating clones with multiple genetic abnormalities.

Most drug resistance is considered to result from the high spontaneous mutation rate of cancer cells (genetic instability), which leads to the development of heterogeneous subpopulations, some of which exhibit resistance to a variety of drugs. An important form of resistance is multidrug resistance (MDR), mediated by a cell membrane glycoprotein (P-glycoprotein). P-glycoprotein is thought to function as an energy-dependent efflux pump that actively extrudes a variety of cytotoxic agents from cells (Beck 1987; Endicott and Ling 1989), including natural products such as plant alkaloids (vincas, podophyllotoxins, paclitaxel), anthracyclines (doxorubicin, daunorubicin), and some synthetic agents (e.g., mitoxantrone). P-glycoprotein is normally expressed in tissues such as the lining of the gut, the brush border of the kidney, and the choroid plexus, perhaps to deal with toxic products in the environment. Studies performed on tumor biopsy specimens have documented that P-glycoprotein-positive tumors usually exhibit resistance to doxorubicin. Tumor types such as sarcoma, neuroblastoma, malignant lymphoma, and myeloma are usually P-glycoprotein-negative at the time of diagnosis but are frequently positive for P-glycoprotein when the patient relapses from chemotherapy (Wallner et al. 1991; Grogan et al. 1993). A series of noncytotoxic drugs have been identified that reverse drug resistance mediated by P-glycoprotein (e.g., verapamil, cyclosporine). Several other potential reversal agents are now being tested in the clinic in an effort to identify more effective and less toxic agents that may enhance the cytotoxicity of the MDR-effluxed agents. Other mechanisms of multidrug resistance have also been identified, including multidrug-related proteins (MRP), which also facilitate efflux of certain chemotherapeutic agents from cells (Deeley and Cole 1997). Mutations in topoisomerase II also give rise to resistance to multiple drugs that target these enzymes, in particular anthracyclines and etoposide.

Specific resistance mechanisms in human tumors for drugs not involving the multidrug-resistance mechanisms described above have also been elucidated in recent years. For example, intrinsic or natural resistance of patients with acute myelogenous leukemia to methotrexate is attributed to lack of retention of this drug by leukemic blasts. These cells form low levels of methotrexate polyglutamates, the drug metabolite that is retained by cells. In contrast, acute lymphocytic leukemia blasts (pre-B, not T-cells) convert methotrexate to its polyglutamates efficiently and are sensitive to treatment with this drug. In those 20% of patients with pre-B acute lymphocytic leukemia not cured by combination chemotherapy, acquired resistance has been found to be associated with impaired uptake due to abnormalities in the reduced folate carrier transport protein or to low-level amplification of the dihydrofolate reductase gene, the molecular target for methotrexate (Gorlick et al. 1996, 1997). Table 13-4 lists some mechanisms of acquired resistance that have been found to occur in human tumors.

## Pharmacokinetic Considerations

Although intrinsic drug sensitivity appears to be the most critical determinant of response to chemotherapy, pharmacokinetic factors related to the route of administration, bioavailability, metabolism, and elimination are of great importance in cancer therapy. Many cytotoxic agents exhibit a steep dose–response curve with a narrow therapeutic index. In other words, low doses of a drug may have little to no antineoplastic activity, although higher doses may produce prohibitive host toxicity. Because of the steep dose–response relationship, doses of most cytotoxic agents are calculated in relation to body surface area, a more accurate method than dose calculations based on body weight. Although patients may prefer the oral route of drug administration, marked variations in bioavailability, plus inconsistent patient compliance, can compromise attainment of the required therapeutic serum levels. For example, with the alkylating agent melphalan, more than a 10-fold variation in plasma levels has been documented after standard oral dosing (Alberts et al. 1979a). When plasma assays are not available, the occurrence of myelosuppression following drug administration should be used to ensure optimal dosage for those drugs in which myelotoxicity is dose limiting. For patients presenting with hypercalcemia or other complications of myeloma, oral melphalan would be considered undesirable, as these patients need to achieve effective plasma levels immediately. Similar difficulties are encountered with oral administration of fluorouracil, methotrexate, and 6-mercaptopurine. Bioavailability is adequate after oral administration of agents such as tamoxifen and low doses of cyclophosphamide (<500 mg/day).

The intravenous route of drug administration is preferable for most cytotoxic drugs, as it assures producing adequate plasma levels with minimal compliance problems. For some agents, continuous intravenous drug administration for 4 days or longer provides better results

Table 13-4 Some Mechanisms of Resistance to Antineoplastic Drugs

| DRUG | MECHANISMS OF RESISTANCE |
|---|---|
| Methotrexate | Impaired transport<br>Amplification of dihydrofolate reductase |
| Cytosine arabinoside | Decreased deoxycytidine kinase<br>Increase in cytidine deaminase |
| 5-Fluorouracil | Increased thymidylate synthase<br>Increased nucleoside salvage<br>Increased dihydropyrimidine dehydrogenase |
| Cisplatin | Decreased uptake<br>Increased DNA repair |
| Taxol and vinca alkaloids | Multidrug resistance (MDR) phenotype<br>Mutations in tubulin resulting in decreased binding |
| Doxorubicin | MDR expression<br>Decrease of alterations in topoisomerase II |
| Irinotecan and topotecan | Decrease in topoisomerase I |

and less toxicity than do bolus or short-duration infusions. This is because tumor response for many agents can be related to the "area-under-the-plasma-disappearance curve" (AUC) for the drug, whereas toxicity is generally a function of the peak plasma concentrations rather than the AUC. With the advent of vascular access devices such as subcutaneous ports, external catheters, and infusion pumps, outpatient continuous infusion chemotherapy can now be used for stable drugs such as fluorinated pyrimidines, anthracyclines, and vinca alkaloids. Subcutaneous administration can be used effectively with drugs such as cytarabine, interferon-$\alpha$, G-CSF, GM-SCF, and erythropoietin. Depot intramuscular formulations are available for a variety of endocrine agents used in the treatment of breast and prostate cancer.

## CLINICAL PHARMACOLOGY OF DRUGS USED IN CANCER TREATMENT

### Antimetabolites

#### *Folate antagonists: Aminopterin and methotrexate*

**HISTORY** The folate antagonist aminopterin, an antimetabolite analog of folic acid, was the first drug shown to induce complete remissions in children with ALL (Farber et al. 1947). It was soon appreciated that these remissions were short-lived, as resistance inevitably developed following administration of the aminopterin. In the 1950s MTX supplanted aminopterin in the clinic, based on studies of mouse tumors that showed that it had an improved therapeutic index compared with aminopterin. The structures of folic acid (the vitamin), aminopterin, MTX, and trimetrexate are shown in Fig. 13-3.

**MECHANISM OF ACTION** The major mechanism of action of MTX is through the potent inhibition of the enzyme dihydrofolate reductase (DHFR). This enzyme catalyzes the reduction of dihydrofolate to tetrahydrofolate, the coenzyme form of folic acid (Gorlick et al. 1996; Chu and Allegra 1996). As a consequence of this inhibition, the levels of intracellular folate coenzymes are rapidly depleted. Because folate coenzymes are required for thymidylate biosynthesis as well as purine biosynthesis, DNA synthesis is blocked and cell replication stops (Fig. 13-4). In addition, MTX blocks uptake of reduced folates, and thus restoration of folate stores is also impaired. Recent work has shown that MTX is retained in certain cells for extended periods. The intracellular retention of MTX is a consequence of the enzymatic reaction (folylpolyglutamate synthetase [FPGS]) that adds additional glutamates (up to five) to the antifolate (for a review, see Chu and Allegra 1996). This process is an important determinant of MTX selectively, because cells capable of the reaction (e.g., lymphoblasts) may be more susceptible to cell kill-

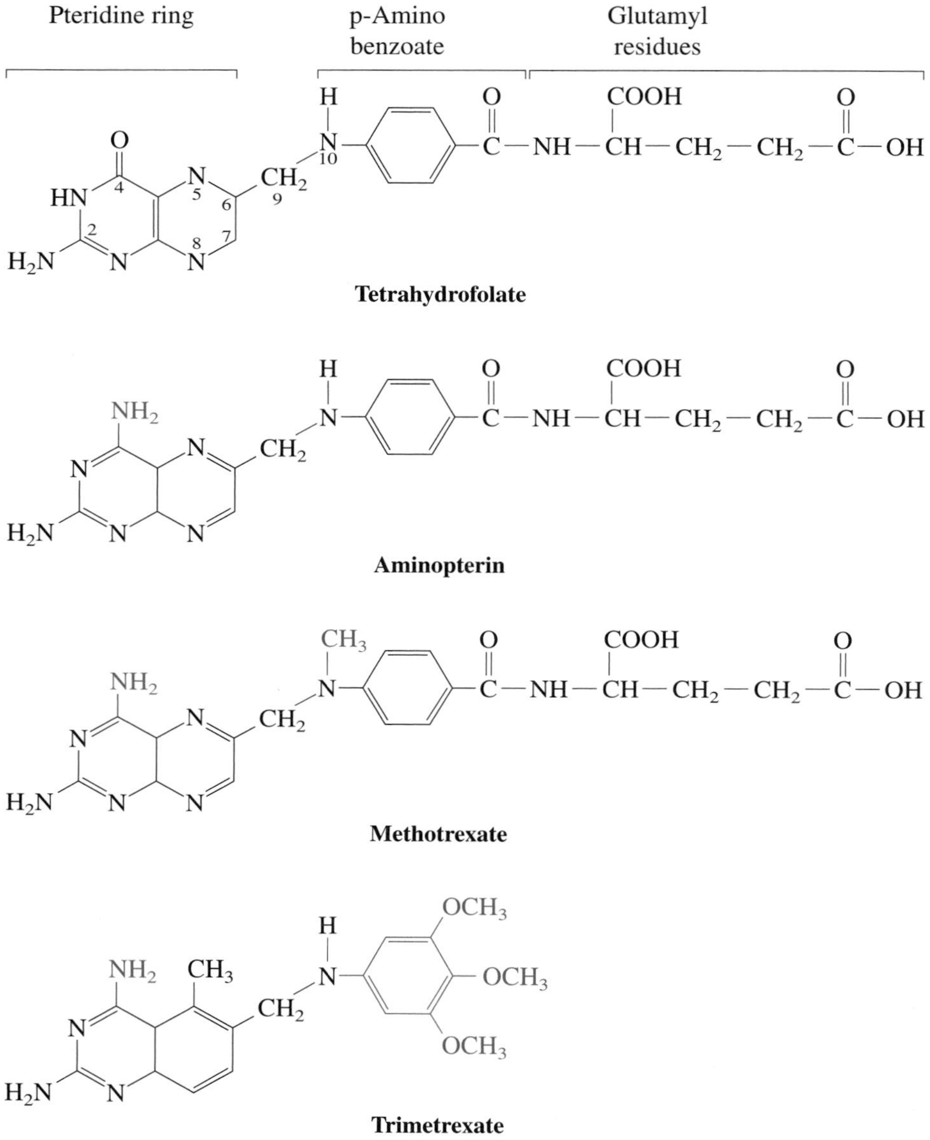

Pteridine ring p-Amino benzoate Glutamyl residues

**Tetrahydrofolate**

**Aminopterin**

**Methotrexate**

**Trimetrexate**

FIGURE 13-3 **Chemical structures of tetrahydrofolate (the reduced form of folic acid), aminopterin, methotrexate, and trimetrexate.**

ing by MTX (Whitehead et al. 1987). Acquired resistance to MTX in patients with leukemia has been shown to be due to one or more mechanisms including increased concentrations of DHFR as a consequence of gene amplification or impaired drug uptake (for a review, see Gorlick et al. 1996).

**CLINICAL PHARMACOLOGY** When administered orally in low doses (5 to 10 mg), MTX is well absorbed (see Table 13-5). However, when doses exceeding 30 mg are given, oral bioavailability decreases, with significant interpatient variation (Henderson et al. 1965). Therefore, doses of MTX of 30 mg or greater should be administered IV, IM, or subcutaneously. After IV injection, the disappearance of MTX from the plasma is triphasic. Typically, the distribution phase ($\alpha$ $t_{1/2}$) is 30 to 45 minutes, the renal clearance phase ($\beta$ $t_{1/2}$) is 3 to 4 hours, and the terminal half-life is considered to be 6 to 20 hours.

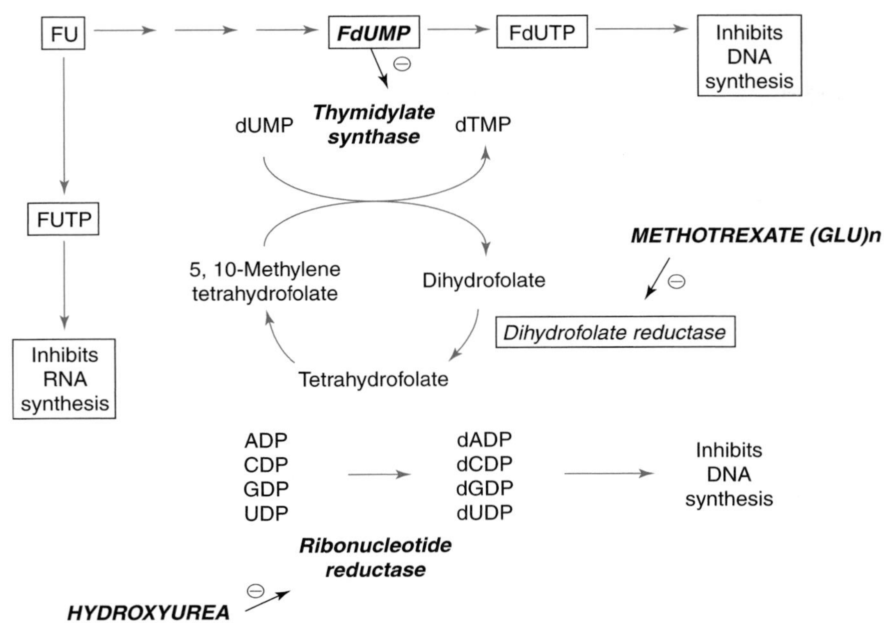


**FIGURE 13-4** Schematic depiction of the metabolic interconversions that occur with antineoplastic drugs known to inhibit key enzymes required for DNA synthesis, including thymidylate synthase (TS), ribonucleotide reductase, and dihydrofolate reductase (DHFR). Abbreviations: FdUMP, fluorodeoxyuridine monophosphate; FdUDP, fluorodeoxyuridine diphosphate; FU, 5-fluorouracil; FUDP, fluorouridine diphosphate; FUTP, fluorouridine triphosphate; ADP, CDP, GDP, and UDP represent the diphosphate nucleotides of adenine, cytosine, guanine, and uracil; "d" refers to the deoxyribose form of that sugar.

Methotrexate is excreted primarily unchanged by the kidneys by both glomerular filtration and active tubular secretion. With larger doses, a significant amount of the drug (7 to 30%) is excreted in the urine as the major metabolite 7-hydroxymethotrexate, formed principally in the liver by the action of the enzyme aldehyde oxidase. A small amount of 2,4-diamino-$N^{10}$-methylpteroic acid has also been noted in plasma and urine, presumably because of cleavage of the peptide bond by intestinal microflora. Patients with renal impairment ordinarily should not be treated with MTX, because the prolonged plasma concentrations that result may lead to increased hematologic and GI toxicity. In some patients, renal toxicity may result from MTX treatment, especially high-dose regimens, and thus the excretion of the drug may be delayed. In this circumstance leucovorin (folinic acid, $N^5$-formyl tetrahydrofolate) should be administered until concentrations of MTX decrease to nontoxic values ($<1 \times 10^{-8}$ M). In the presence of effusions, MTX may accumulate in this third space, acting as a storage depot, potentially increasing toxicity by maintaining plasma concentrations over longer periods.

**ADVERSE EFFECTS** The dose-limiting toxicities of MTX are myelosuppression and gastrointestinal toxicity (Table 13-5). These adverse effects usually occur 7 to 10 days after treatment. An early sign of MTX toxicity to the GI tract is mucositis, involving the oral mucosa. Severe toxicity may be manifest as diarrhea due to small-bowel irritation, which can progress to ulceration and bleeding.

Less common toxic effects caused by MTX include skin rash, pleuritis, and hepatitis. Hepatitis, usually manifest as an increase in serum transaminase, is reversible in most patients, but low-dose chronic administration may lead to fibrosis and cirrhosis of the liver in a small percentage of patients. Renal toxicity is uncommon with conventional doses of MTX but has been a problem with high-dose regimens ($>0.5$ g/m$^2$) in adults. Alkalinization (with $NaHCO_3$) and hydration, as well as monitoring of MTX serum concentrations, are important prophylactic measures to avoid serious nephrotoxicity (Bertino et al. 1989; Chu and Allegra 1996). Leucovorin, the antidote used to treat potential toxic effects of MTX overdose, is also used as part of high-dose MTX regimens as a planned

Table 13-5 **Clinical Pharmacology of Antimetabolites: Pyrimidine Analogs and Antifolates**

| PHARMACOLOGIC PARAMETER | 5-FLUORO-URACIL | FLUORODEOXY-URIDINE | CYTARABINE | DIFLUORODE-OXYCYTIDINE | METHOTREXATE |
|---|---|---|---|---|---|
| *Plasma half-life*[a] | $t_{1/2}$ = 8–14 min | $t_{1/2}$ = 25 min | $t_{1/2\alpha}$ = 7–20 min<br>$t_{1/2\beta}$ = 2 h | $t_{1/2}$ = 42–79 min | $t_{1/2\alpha}$ = 2–3 h<br>$t_{1/2\beta}$ = 8–10 h |
| *Routes of elimination* | 90% undergoes hepatic metabolism, <10% excreted unchanged in urine<br>DPD* rate limiting | Converted to 5-FU, only 10–13% excreted unchanged | Hepatic deamination by cytosine deaminase | 75% excreted in urine within 24 h, 98% in 1 week; metabolized to inactive uridine derivative | Undergoes 7-hydroxylation in liver, excreted unchanged in urine |
| *Routes of administration* | IV | IV and Hepatic IA | IV and IT | IV | IV and IT |
| *Major toxicities* | • Diarrhea<br>• BMS<br>• Ulcerative stomatitis | • Aphthous stomatitis | • BMS<br>• Mucositis<br>• N/V | • BMS | • BMS<br>• Mucositis<br>• Renal tubular obstruction |
| *Less common toxicities* | • Dermatologic (HFS)<br>• Cardiac<br>• Neurological (cerebellar)<br>• Ocular | • Biliary sclerosis (>with hepatic artery infusion)<br>• BMS | • Cerebellar/ high doses<br>• Cerebral dysfunction<br>• Conjunctivitis | • Flulike syndrome<br>• Elevated transaminases<br>• Hypotension | • Hepatotoxicity<br>• Pneumonitis<br>• Hypersensitivity reactions |
| *Major indications* | • Colon<br>• Breast<br>• Head and neck<br>• Pancreatic<br>• Gastric<br>• Esophagus | • Hepatic metastasis from colon cancer<br>• Hepatocellular | • AML<br>• Intermediate- or high-grade NHL | • Non-small-cell lung<br>• Colon (salvage)<br>• Pancreatic<br>• Small cell lung | • ALL<br>• Breast<br>• Trophoblastic<br>• Head and neck<br>• Bladder<br>• Intermediate- or high-grade NHL |
| *Comments* | • DPD deficiency >risk of toxicity | • Used primarily in hepatic artery infusions | | | |

[a]Pharmacokinetic data summarized from Kristenson et al. 1975; Chabner et al. 1978; Breithaupt et al. 1982; McDermott et al. 1982; Slevin et al. 1983; Muggia et al. 1991; Shipley et al. 1992; Bouffard et al. 1993.
ABBREVIATIONS: ALL, acute lymphoblastic leukemia; AML, acute myelogenous leukemia; BMS, bone marrow suppression; DPD, dihydropyrimidine dehydrogenase; IA, intra-arterial; HFS, hand-foot syndrome; IT, intrathecal; IV, intravenous; NHL, non-Hodgkin lymphoma; N/V, nausea and vomiting.

"rescue" (i.e., administered 24 to 36 hr after MTX). Table 13-6 describes some high-dose MTX regimens used in the clinic and guidelines for monitoring these patients.

**PRINCIPLE Monitoring of MTX serum concentrations in patients receiving high-dose therapy is "essential" for safe use of this agent.**

**THERAPEUTIC USES** Methotrexate continues to be a key drug in combination regimens used to treat ALL and is used widely in combination therapy of intermediate-grade and high-grade lymphomas, breast cancer, cancer of the head and neck, osteogenic sarcoma, and bladder cancer (Table 13-5). It is also used intrathecally to treat meningeal involvement by leukemia or carcinomas. Meth-

**Table 13-6 High-Dose (>0.5 $g/m^2$) Methotrexate Treatment**

**I. PREHYDRATION AND ALKALINIZATION OF URINE**

Approximately 8 to 12 h before treatment with methotrexate, begin IV hydration with normal saline or 5% glucose amended with 100 mEq of $HCO_3$ and 20 mEq KCl/L at a rate of 1.5 L/$m^2$. Continue until urine pH is 7.0 or greater at time of MTX administration.

**II. MTX ADMINISTRATION**

*Regimen*

1. 0.5–3.0 $g/m^2$ MTX as 20- to 30-min bolus. Begin leucovorin at the 24th hour at a dose of 15 $mg/m^2$, every 6 h for a total of 6 doses.
2. Jaffe regimen: 1.2–6 $g/m^2$ over 6 h IV infusion, with continued IV hydration for an additional 18 h. Begin leucovorin 2 h after MTX infusion at a dose of 15 $mg/m^2$, every 6 h for a total of 7 doses.
3. 36-h infusion: Give MTX, 50 $mg/m^2$ as bolus, followed by an infusion of MTX over 36 h at a dose of 1.5 $g/m^2$. Start leucovorin rescue at the end of infusion, administering 200 $mg/m^2$ over 12 h as an infusion, then 25 $mg/m^2$ IM every 6 h for a total of 6 doses.

**III. DRUG MONITORING**

Monitor MTX concentrations at 24 h for regimen no. 1, or 48 h for regimens 2 and 3. Determine serum creatinine concentrations before treatment, and at 24 h and 48 h.

For regimen 1, 24-h concentrations of MTX of greater than $1 \times 10^{-6}$ M require additional leucovorin rescue; for regimens 2 and 3, 48-h MTX concentrations above $5 \times 10^{-7}$ should receive additional leucovorin rescue. The dose of leucovorin should be increased to 100 $mg/m^2$ q6h for blood concentrations of $1 \times 10^{-6}$ to $5 \times 10^{-6}$ M, and patients with concentrations above $5 \times 10^{-6}$ M should receive doses of 200 $mg/m^2$ or higher. MTX concentrations should be monitored daily and leucovorin continued (in decreasing doses as the blood concentration of MTX falls) until the plasma concentration of MTX is below $1 \times 10^{-8}$ M.

otrexate in low doses is also used to treat many nonmalignant diseases, including psoriasis, rheumatoid arthritis, autoimmune disease, as an abortifacient, and to prevent graft vs. host disease in cancer patients receiving allogeneic transplants after high-dose chemotherapy treatments.

### *Pyrimidine antagonists: 5-fluorouracil and 5-fluorodeoxyuridine*

**HISTORY** The development of 5-FU as an antitumor drug is an example of the rational design of drugs (Heidelberger et al. 1957). The observation that uracil was salvaged more efficiently by certain malignant cells than by normal tissues led to the synthesis of a uracil analog, 5-FU, and its deoxy- and ribose nucleosides (Fig. 13-5).

**MECHANISM OF ACTION** 5-FU exerts its cytotoxic effects through the inhibition of thymidylate synthesis, and/or by incorporation into RNA, thus inhibiting RNA processing and function, and/or by incorporation directly into DNA (Fig. 13-4). The active metabolite of 5-FU, 5-fluorodeoxyuridylate (5-FdUMP), interrupts DNA synthesis through the potent inhibition of thymidylate synthase. Recent studies have led to the suggestion that when intermittent high "pulse" doses of 5-FU are used, the mechanism of action is predominantly via incorporation into RNA. When this drug is given by continuous infusion over several days, the mechanism of cell kill is primarily by inhibition of thymidylate synthase (Sobrero et al. 1997).

**"MODULATION" OF 5-FU ACTION** The cytotoxicity of 5-FU can be modulated in a number of different ways, several of which are shown in Table 13-7. For example, the ternary complex formed by FdUMP, the bioactive folate $N^5$,$N^{10}$-methylenetetrahydrofolate, and thymidylate synthase has been noted to dissociate slowly, with a half-life of several hours. The presence of excess bioactive folate ensures maximal ternary-complex formation and retards the dissociation of FdUMP from the complex. On the basis of this understanding, recent clinical trials have used high doses of folinic acid ($N^5$-formyltetrahydrofolate, also called leucovorin), followed by 5-FU administration, in the hope of maximizing ternary-complex formation, impaired DNA synthesis in malignant cells, and ultimately cell death (Mini et al. 1990).

Methotrexate or trimetrexate pretreatment may increase 5-FU cytotoxicity by increasing 5-phosphoribosyl-

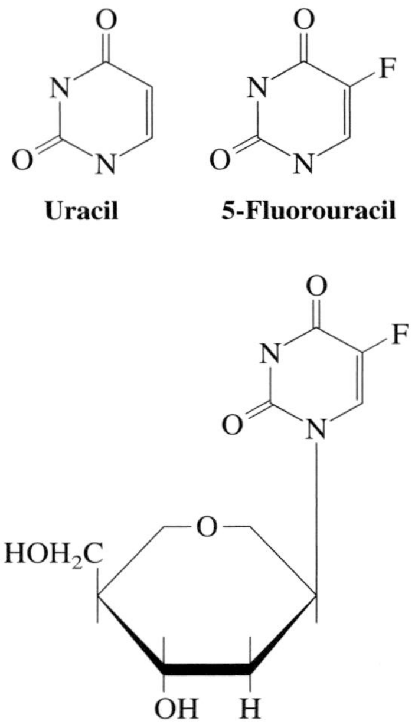

Uracil

5-Fluorouracil

5-Fluorodeoxyuridine

FIGURE 13-5 **Chemical structures of uracil, its antimetabolite 5-fluorouracil, and the nucleoside 5-fluorodeoxyuridine (5-FUdR).**

1-pyrophosphate (PRPP) concentrations in cells, thus increasing 5-FU nucleotide formation (Cadman et al. 1979, 1981). Increased PRPP concentrations are a consequence of the ability of MTX to inhibit purine biosynthesis. In addition, inhibition of dihydrofolate reductase by MTX leads to an increase in dihydrofolate polyglutamates in cells, thereby enhancing FdUMP binding to thymidylate synthase (Fernandez and Bertino 1980). The use of MTX followed by 5-FU has led to an increase in response rate in certain solid tumors, notably colon cancer (Bertino 1997). Other strategies to modulate 5-FU cytotoxicity are also being tested in the clinic. These include pretreatment with trimetrexate, also a dihydrofolate reductase inhibitor, pretreatment with inhibitors of thymidylate synthase (e.g., raltitrexed) (Dragnev et al. 1998), and coadministration of nucleoside transport inhibitors like dipyridamole, nitrobenzylmercaptopurine riboside (NBMPR or nitrobenzylthioinosine), and draflazine.

**CLINICAL PHARMACOLOGY** 5-FU is absorbed erratically after oral administration and is therefore administered IV (see Table 13-4). Several 5-FU prodrugs, like capecitabine, an oral fluoropyrimidine carbamate, are more efficiently absorbed following parenteral dosing and are now in clinical trial (Budman et al. 1998; Sawada et al. 1998). 5-FU has a short plasma half-life (10 to 15 minutes), and, after a pulse exposure with conventional doses (600 mg/m$^2$), cytotoxic concentrations ($>1$ $\mu$M) are maintained in the blood for only 6 hours or less. Cytotoxicity of 5-FU depends on many factors, including: 1) the efficiency of conversion of 5-FU to its active metabolites, FdUMP and FUTP; 2) the concentrations of the competing substrate, dUMP; 3) the concentrations of the folate coenzyme, $N^5$,$N^{10}$-methylenetetrahydrofolate; 4) the concentration of the target enzyme, thymidylate synthase in the malignant cell; and 5) the extent of incorporation

Table 13-7 **Modulation of 5-Fluorouracil Activity in Cells**

| MODULATING AGENT | MECHANISM OF ACTION |
|---|---|
| Folinic acid (leucovorin) pretreatment | Increases folate cofactor in cells, increasing ternary complex formation |
| PALA treatment | Blocks de novo pyrimidine synthesis, increasing 5-FU nucleotide formation |
| Thymidine | Enhances 5-FU incorporation into RNA; delays 5-FU catabolism |
| MTX pretreatment | Increases PRPP, thus increasing FU nucleotide formation; increases dihydrofolate polyglutamates in cells |
| Uridine posttreatment | Protects normal cells from 5-FU toxicity; mechanism not entirely clear |
| Dideoxynucleosides (e.g., AZT) | May synergize with drugs that inhibit de novo thymidylate biosynthesis; affinity of DNA polymerase for such drugs increased under conditions of relative thymidine depletion |
| Nucleoside transport inhibitors (e.g., NBMPR, dipyridamole, draflazine) | Inhibits thymidine salvage following inhibition of de novo thymidylate synthesis |

ABBREVIATIONS: AZT, zidovudine; 5-FU, 5-fluorouracil; NMBPR, nitrobenzylmercaptopurine riboside (nitrobenzylthioinosine); PALA, *N*-(phosphonacetyl)-L-aspartate; PRPP, 5-phosphoribosyl-1-pyrophosphate.

of 5-FU into RNA. Various dosage schedules of 5-FU have been investigated, including daily bolus treatment for 5 days once a month, weekly bolus treatment, and continuous infusions of 5-FU lasting 24, 48, 120 hours or longer.

When continuous infusions of 5-FU are administered, the major dose-limiting toxicity is gastrointestinal (i.e., mucositis), although bolus treatment usually produces leukopenia and thrombocytopenia as the dose-limiting toxicity. The drug distributes freely into third spaces (e.g., cerebrospinal fluid [CSF], ascites, pleural effusions). The major catabolic pathway involves hepatic dihydropyrimidine dehydrogenase, producing dihydrofluorouracil. Additional breakdown products include fluoroureidoproprionic acid and $CO_2$. The hepatic metabolism of 5-FU has been exploited in hepatic artery infusions and intraperitoneal administration of the drug. This method achieves high local concentrations with decreased systemic toxicity. 5-Fluorodeoxyuridine (5-FUdR) is even more rapidly metabolized by the liver than 5-FU. Administration of this drug into the intrahepatic artery is used to treat isolated hepatic metastases from colon cancer with high response rates (Kemeny et al. 1989).

**ADVERSE EFFECTS** The major dose-limiting toxicities of 5-FU and 5-FUdR are myelosuppression and GI toxicity (Table 13-5). Stomatitis and diarrhea usually occur 4 to 7 days after treatment. Further treatment is typically withheld until the normal host tissues have recovered. The nadir of leukopenia and thrombocytopenia usually occurs 7 to 10 days after a single dose or a 5-day course of the drug, and recovery usually takes place in 14 days. The dose-limiting toxicity of infusions of 5-FUdR via the hepatic artery is transient liver toxicity, occasionally resulting in biliary sclerosis.

Less common toxicities noted with 5-FU after systemic administration include skin rash, cerebellar symptoms (with single-pulse doses greater than 800 mg/m$^2$), conjunctivitis, and tearing. Myocardial infarction and cardiac vasospasm have also been reported in patients receiving 5-FU.

**CLINICAL USES** Both 5-FU and 5-FUdR have antitumor activity against solid tumors, most notably colon cancer, breast cancer, and head and neck cancer (Table 13-5). A topical preparation containing 5-FU is also used topically to treat skin hyperkeratosis and superficial basal cell carcinomas.

### *Cytosine arabinoside*

**HISTORY** Cytosine arabinoside (ara-C,1-$\beta$-D-arabino-furanosylcytosine) is an antimetabolite analog of deoxycytidine (Fig. 13-6). The difference between deoxycytidine and ara-C is that the -OH group at the 2′ position of the sugar moiety is in the arabinose configuration in ara-C. This compound was first isolated from the sponge *Cryptothethya crypta*.

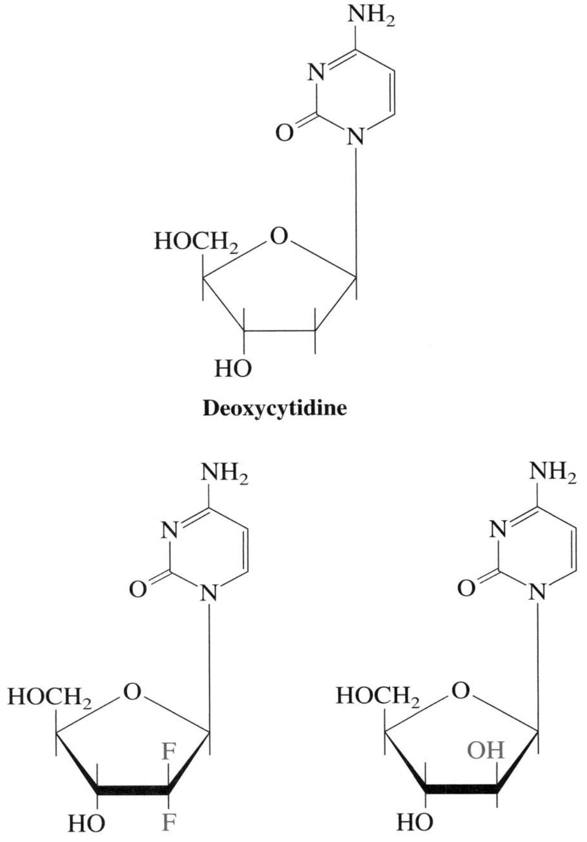

**FIGURE 13-6 Chemical structures of deoxycytidine and the antimetabolites cytosine arabinoside (ara-C) and gemcitabine (2′,2′-difluoro-deoxycytidine).**

**MECHANISM OF ACTION** Cytosine arabinoside is converted to the nucleotide triphosphate (ara-CTP) intracellularly. This latter compound is an inhibitor of DNA polymerase and is incorporated directly into DNA (Kufe et al. 1984). The latter event is considered to be lethal, as incorporation into DNA results in defective elongation of newly synthesized fragments of DNA.

Both ara-C and its mononucleotide may be inactivated by two intracellular enzymes, cytidine deaminase and deoxycytidylate deaminase, respectively (Chabner 1996). The ara-U (uracil arabinoside) formed from ara-C deamination is more slowly cleared from plasma than ara-C and may slow subsequent metabolism of ara-C in high-dose regimens (Capizzi et al. 1985).

**RESISTANCE** Although several mechanisms for acquired resistance to ara-C have been elucidated in experimental tumor systems, an explanation for the acquired resistance in leukemia cells of patients is still not complete (Tattersall et al. 1974). Decreased uptake and an increase in nucleotidase activity appear to be the major mechanism of resistance (Fig. 13-4). Other explanations include a decrease of deoxycytidine kinase activity, an increased pool size of CTP, and increased activity of cytidine deaminase, primarily in ara-C-resistant cell lines (Chabner 1996). The level of intracellular ara-CTP formation achieved after drug administration has been reported to be useful in monitoring drug efficacy (Liliemark et al. 1985).

**CLINICAL PHARMACOLOGY** Because it is poorly absorbed orally, ara-C is administered IV as a pulse dose or as a continuous infusion. The drug distributes rapidly into body water. In high concentrations, roughly 50% of the plasma concentration can be detected in the CSF 2 hours after IV administration. Ara-C disappears rapidly from plasma with a $t_{1/2}$ of 7 to 20 minutes. With higher doses, plasma half-life is longer, presumably because of inhibition of metabolism of ara-C by ara-U. The formation of ara-U also occurs in plasma, liver, granulocytes, and other tissues of the body (Pallavincini 1984; Capizzi et al. 1985). Most cytarabine is excreted in the urine in the form of the inactive metabolite, ara-U. As in the case of MTX, single-bolus infusions of doses as high as 5 g/m$^2$ (given over 1 to 3 hours) produce little bone marrow toxicity because of its rapid clearance, although doses of 1 g/m$^2$ given IV over 48 hours or longer may produce severe marrow toxicity (Capizzi et al. 1985).

**ADVERSE EFFECTS** In conventional doses (100 to 200 mg/m$^2$ per day for 5 to 10 days), the dose-limiting toxicity of ara-C is myelosuppression. Although mild nausea and vomiting can be seen with these doses, this adverse side effect increases markedly when higher doses are used. Repeated administration of the drug can result in some tolerance to the nausea and vomiting. Although leukopenia and thrombocytopenia nadirs occur around day 10, the bone marrow suppression is rapidly reversible. In addition to increased nausea and vomiting, neurological, GI, and hepatotoxicity have been observed when high-dose ara-C regimens are used (Rudnick et al. 1979; Spriggs et al. 1988). The severity of these effects increases with increasing duration of therapy. High doses (2 to 3 g/m$^2$) given every 12 hours for a total of 6 doses may be as effective as 12 doses. Lower doses of ara-C (0.5 to 1 g/m$^2$) given over 2 hours every 12 hours may be as effective as higher doses.

**CLINICAL USES** Cytosine arabinoside remains the drug of choice for the treatment of acute myelogenous leukemia (AML). When used together with an anthracycline drug (i.e., daunomycin, idarubicin, mitoxantrone), remissions may be achieved in 60 to 80% of patients with AML. This drug is also used in combination to treat other hematologic malignancies, but its exact role in the treatment of these neoplasms is less well defined. Cytosine arabinoside is also used intrathecally to treat meningeal leukemia. Intrathecal ara-C is usually well tolerated, but adverse neurological effects, such as seizures and alterations in mental status, have been reported.

### *Gemcitabine (Gemzar)*

**HISTORY** Gemcitabine (2′,2′-difluorodeoxycytidine; dFdC) is a novel pyrimidine nucleoside analog with structural similarities to cytosine arabinoside (Fig. 13-6). Both drugs are catabolized by cytidine deaminase and require intracellular phosphorylation by deoxycytidine kinase for activation. Although the drug was only recently approved for the treatment of advanced pancreatic carcinoma, it has shown promising activity in a wide range of experimental tumor cell lines (Michael and Moore 1997). For example, some studies have shown gemcitabine to be more potent against human leukemia cells in comparison with cytarabine, and nude mouse models have demonstrated activity in other solid tumors including lung, ovarian, colon, and breast cancer (Hertel et al. 1990; Bouffard et al. 1991).

**MECHANISM OF ACTION AND CLINICAL PHARMACOLOGY** As mentioned, gemcitabine is phosphorylated in a stepwise fashion to 2′,2′-difluorodeoxycytidine monophosphate (dFdCMP), diphosphate (dFdCDP), and triphosphate (dFdCTP) derivatives (Bouffard et al. 1993). This drug's principle mechanism of action has been attributed to its incorporation into DNA and disruption of DNA chain elongation. In addition, gemcitabine has been shown to inhibit DNA polymerases involved in DNA repair (dFdCTP), to inhibit ribonucleotide reductase (dFdCDP), and to be incorporated into RNA. Although its mechanism of action is similar to cytarabine, it differs in the fact that gemcitabine is less efficient at DNA chain termination, and its dFdCTP metabolite has a longer half-life than araCTP (Heinemann et al. 1990; Bouffard et al. 1991).

**ADVERSE EFFECTS** The major dose-limiting toxicity of gemcitabine is myelosuppression, which is dramatically influenced by dosing schedule. For example, an intravenous infusion of 800 to 1250 mg/m$^2$ over 30 minutes every week for 3 out of 4 weeks results in trilineage myelosuppression with a favorable adverse effects profile. Administration of the drug on a twice weekly regimen markedly reduces the tolerated dose to 65 mg/m$^2$ when given over a 30-minute infusion. Protracted weekly infusions of up to 24 hours have also been shown to reduce the maximally tolerated dose to approximately 180 mg/m$^2$, resulting in leukopenia and lethargy. Other notable adverse effects include transient elevations in liver transaminases, a flulike syndrome, severe hypotension, bronchospasm and skin rashes (Clavel et al. 1989; Michael and Moore 1997) (Table 13-8).

**CLINICAL USES** At present, gemcitabine is approved for the treatment of pancreatic cancer, where it has been shown to improve disease-related symptoms in approximately 25% of patients, with a modest increase in survival, when compared with 5-FU. Several phase II trails are underway to explore the utility of gemcitabine as first-line therapy for patients with other solid tumors.

### *Purine antagonists: 6-Mercaptopurine and 6-thioguanine*

**HISTORY** The purine analogs 6-mercaptopurine (6-MP) and 6-thioguanine (6-TG) (Fig. 13-7) were synthesized by Elion et al. (1952) and introduced into the clinic by Burchenal et al. (1953). Other purine analogs are also used clinically, including azathioprine, a 6-MP prodrug and potent immunosuppressive agent; allopurinol, an inhibitor of xanthine oxidase, which has proved useful in the prevention of uric acid nephropathy and acute gouty arthritis; and antiviral compounds such as ara-A (adenine arabinoside) (Flowers and Melmon 1997).

**MECHANISM OF ACTION** Both 6-MP and 6-TG have a thiol group substitution for the 6-hydroxy moiety found in hypoxanthine and guanine, respectively (Fig. 13-7). Both compounds are converted to nucleotides by the enzyme hypoxanthine-guanine phosphoribosyl transferase (HGPRT). Following oral administration, 6-MP undergoes extensive intestinal and hepatic metabolism. HGPRT catalyzes the formation of 6-MP ribose monophosphate, which inhibits de novo purine biosynthesis. The triphosphate derivatives of 6-MP are generally assimilated into DNA and RNA. Catabolism and excretion of 6-MP typically involves oxidation by xanthine oxidase to 6-thiouric acid, or S-methylation by thiopurine methyltransferase (TPMT) to produce 6-methylmercaptopurine. It is interesting that polymorphisms in TPMT have been noted in up to 10% of the general population and may be important in patients with protracted myelosuppression and perhaps even relapse (Lennard et al. 1983, 1989). In contrast, 6-TG is converted by HGPRT to the active metabolite 6-thioguanylic acid (TGMP). Although some of these intermediates can ultimately be found in RNA, the critical cytotoxic lesion is thought to involve direct incorporation into DNA. Unlike 6-MP though, 6-TG is not inactivated by xanthine oxidase. Rather, 6-TG undergoes deamination by guanase to form 6-thioinosine. Because xanthine oxidase is not a critical enzyme in the elimination of 6-TG, inhibitors of this enzyme such as allopurinol do not alter its adverse effects profile as noted for 6-MP.

In experimental tumor cells, resistance to 6-TG and 6-MP are most commonly attributed to a decrease in the activity of the activating enzyme HGPRT (Brockman 1963). In human ALL for example, resistance has been associated with an increase in activity of membrane bound alkaline phosphatase, which is capable of degrading the nucleotides of the 6-thiopurines (Rosman et al. 1974; Scholar and Calabresi 1979). Absence of HGPRT activity is a rare cause of resistance in patients with AML. An alteration of this enzyme leading to decreased thiopurine binding to this enzyme has been found in the blast cells of some patients (Rosman and Williams 1973).

**CLINICAL PHARMACOLOGY** Both 6-MP and 6-TG are given orally, although absorption is erratic and variable (LePage and Whitecar 1971) (see Table 13-8). The clinical benefit may be related to the serum concentrations of drug, suggesting a benefit for dose adjustment in individual patients (Koren et al. 1990).

**PRINCIPLE Monitoring blood concentrations of potent anticancer agents may be required to ensure that adequate dose intensity is achieved.**

Because 6-MP is metabolized primarily by xanthine oxidase to 6-thiouric acid, a reaction that is inhibited by allopurinol, a dosage reduction of 75% is recommended when allopurinol is used in conjunction with 6-MP. In general, no dose reduction is necessary when 6-TG and allopurinol are administered together (Table 13-8).

**ADVERSE REACTIONS** Except for less GI toxicity from 6-TG compared with 6-MP, presumably because 6-TG is metabolized by the GI mucosa, both drugs have equivalent dose-limiting toxicity with respect to myelosuppression (see Table 13-8). A mild reversible increase in hepatic transaminases may be noted after treat-

**Table 13-8 Clinical Pharmacology of Antimetabolites: Purine Analogs**

| Pharmacologic Parameter | Fludarabine | Cladribine | Pentostatin | 6-Mercaptopurine | 6-Thioguanine |
|---|---|---|---|---|---|
| *Plasma half-life*[a] | $t_{1/2\alpha}$ = 5 min<br>$t_{1/2\beta}$ = 1 h<br>$t_{1/2\gamma}$ = 7–12 h | $t_{1/2\alpha}$ = 8 min<br>$t_{1/2\beta}$ = 66 min<br>$t_{1/2\gamma}$ = 6.3 h | $t_{1/2\gamma}$ = 2.6–15 h | $t_{1/2}$ = 50 min | $t_{1/2}$ = 90 min |
| *Routes of elimination* | Rapid dephosphorylation followed by intercellular phosphorylation. | Renal excretion | Minimal metabolism, majority (80%) excreted unchanged in urine. | Hepatic xanthine oxidase converts drug to 6-thiouric acid, then renal excretion. | Hepatic metabolism to 6-thioxanthine by guanase. |
| *Routes of administration* | IV | IV and PO | IV | IV and PO | IV and PO |
| *Major toxicities* | • BMS | • BMS | • BMS | • BMS | • BMS; |
| *Less common toxicities* | • N/V<br>• Neurotoxicity syndrome (cortical blindness, encephalopathy, seizures) | • Fever<br>• Renal failure at high doses<br>• Motor weakness and paraparesis | • Photosensitivity<br>• Nephrotoxicity | • N/V<br>• Hepatotoxicity | • N/V<br>• Hepatotoxicity |
| *Major indications* | • CLL<br>• Low grade lymphomas | • CLL<br>• Low-grade lymphoma | • CLL<br>• PLL<br>• Low-grade lymphoma | • ALL and AML | • ALL and AML |
| *Comments* | • Causes prolonged immunosuppression | | | • Dose reduction when used with allopurinol | • No dose reduction required with allopurinol |

[a]Pharmacokinetic data summarized from Loo et al. 1968; Kontis et al. 1982; Smyth et al. 1986; Malspeis et al. 1990; Liliemark and Juliusson 1991.
ABBREVIATIONS: ALL, acute lymphoblastic leukemia; BMS, bone marrow suppression; CLL, chronic lymphocytic leukemia; N/V, nausea and vomiting; PLL, prolymphocytic leukemia.

ment with either of these compounds; cirrhosis has been observed in patients treated with these drugs over long periods.

**CLINICAL USE** Both 6-MP and 6-TG are used for the treatment of ALL and AML as part of combination regimens; 6-MP and MTX are used as part of the maintenance therapy administered after remission is achieved in patients with ALL (Table 13-8).

**FLUDARABINE** Fludarabine (Fludara, 5-fluoroadenosine monophosphate) is an analog of adenosine that inhibits DNA polymerase and ribonucleotide reductase (Fig. 13-8). Fludarabine is the single most active agent available for the treatment of chronic lymphocytic leukemia (CLL) and also exhibits some antitumor activity in other indolent lymphomas and in macroglobulinemia. Fludarabine is usually given intravenously in a dose of 25 mg/m$^2$ daily over 30 minutes for 5 days every 4 weeks. The major toxicity is myelosuppression (Table 13-8). Higher doses administered in early trials in patients with acute nonlymphocytic leukemia (AML) occasionally produced cortical blindness. In the lower dosage schedule

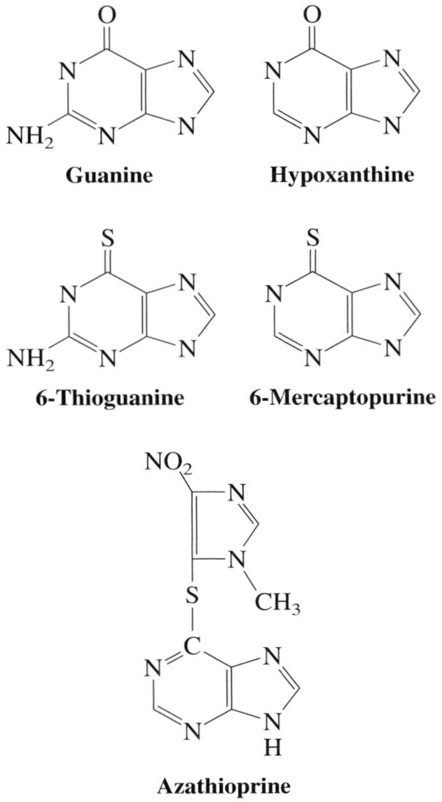

Guanine Hypoxanthine

6-Thioguanine 6-Mercaptopurine

Azathioprine

FIGURE 13-7 **Chemical structures of the purines guanine and hypoxanthine (a metabolic product of purine oxidation, and precursor to uric acid, formed by xanthine oxidase) and the purine antimetabolites 6-mercaptopurine (6-MP), 6-thioguanine (6-TG), and azathioprine.**

used in chronic lymphocytic leukemia and other lymphoid neoplasms, adverse effects are usually mild and reversible. Combinations of fludarabine with cyclophosphamide and mitoxantrone are currently being evaluated for the treatment of low-grade lymphomas.

Additional purine antagonists include deoxycoformycin (DCF) and 2-chlorodeoxyadenosine (2-CDA). Deoxycoformycin, or pentostatin (Fig. 13-8), is a purine analog that was originally isolated from *Streptomyces.* It is a potent inhibitor of adenosine deaminase, which results in accumulation of the cytotoxic product deoxyadenosine (Smyth et al. 1980). Pentostatin has been found to be a useful agent in the treatment of T-cell malignancies as well as hairy cell leukemia (HCL). Both DCF and 2-CDA are extremely active agents in the treatment of hairy cell leukemia and can produce prolonged remissions after a single course of treatment (Piro et al. 1990). Pentostatin schedules of 0.1 mg/kg daily for 7 days by continuous infusion (4 mg/kg per day) produces complete remissions in 90% of patients with prolonged remissions (Piro et al. 1990). At present, it is considered the standard of care for HCL. 2-CDA is also used to treat patients with low-grade lymphomas (Kay et al. 1992) (Table 13-8). Both agents also exhibit some antitumor activity in other low-grade lymphoid neoplasms (e.g., CLL).

#### *Ribonucleotide reductase inhibitor: Hydroxyurea*

**HISTORY** Hydroxyurea is a substituted urea that was first synthesized by Dresler and Stein (1869) (Fig. 13-9).

**MECHANISM OF ACTION AND CLINICAL PHARMACOLOGY** Hydroxyurea inhibits ribonucleotide reductase, the enzyme that converts ribonucleotides at the diphosphate level to deoxyribonucleotides (Plagemann and Erbe 1972; Thelander and Reichard 1979) (Fig. 13-4). Resistance to the drug has been associated with an increase in enzyme activity and/or an alteration of binding of hydroxyurea to the iron-containing subunit of this enzyme (for reviews, see Wright 1989; Donehower 1996). Hydroxyurea is well absorbed even in large oral doses. Plasma concentrations reach a maximum after 1 hour, and fall rapidly thereafter. The drug is excreted mainly unchanged by the kidney (Donehower 1996).

**ADVERSE REACTIONS** The major toxicity of hydroxyurea is bone marrow suppression, primarily leukopenia. Few other toxicities have been observed, even when large doses are administered. Hydroxyurea is an S-phase-specific agent. The nadir in the leukocyte count occurs 6 to 7 days after a single dose, and the count then recovers rapidly.

**THERAPEUTIC USES** Hydroxyurea is used for the treatment of myeloproliferative diseases, CML in particular. Hydroxyurea appears to be equally as effective as busulfan, with potentially less toxicity and can be used to rapidly lower the blast count in patients with acute blast crisis of CML.

### Microtubulin Inhibitors

#### *Vinca alkaloids: Vinblastine, vincristine, and vinorelbine*

**HISTORY** Vinblastine and vincristine are alkaloids isolated from the leaves of the Madagascar periwinkle plant (*Catharanthus roseus*). Vinorelbine is a semisyn-

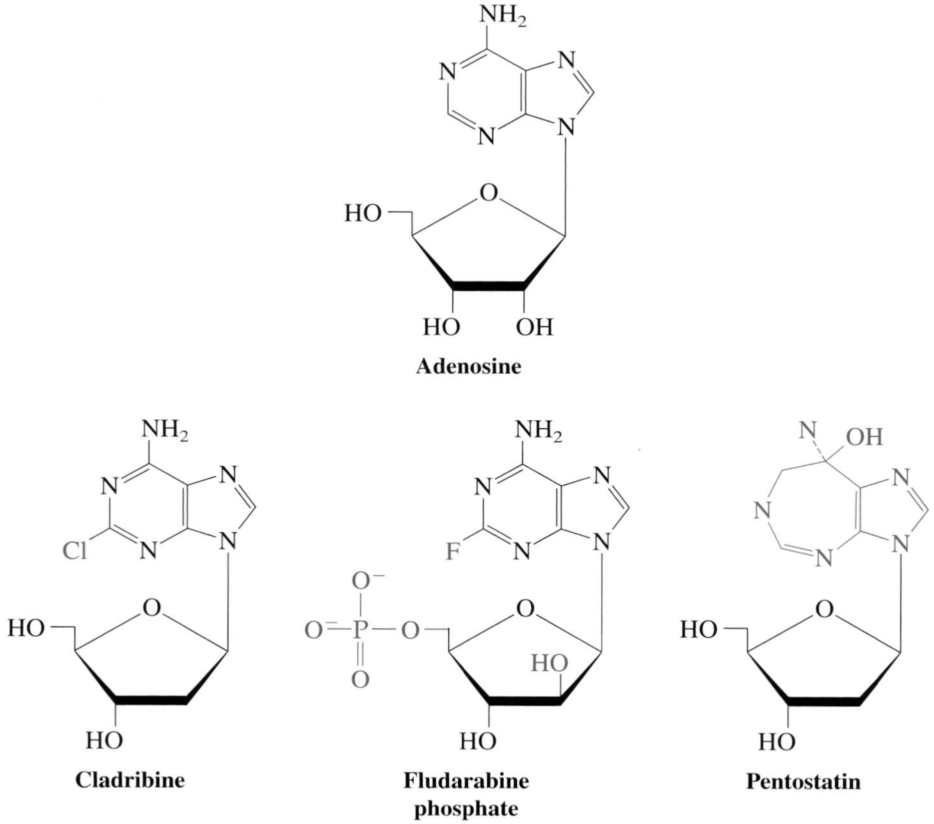

**Adenosine**

**Cladribine**

**Fludarabine phosphate**

**Pentostatin**

FIGURE 13-8 **Chemical structures of the nucleoside adenosine, and the antimetabolites fludarabine (9-b-D-arabinofuranosyl-2-fluoroadenine), pentostatin (2′-deoxycoformycin), and cladribine (2-chlorodeoxyadenosine).**

thetic vinca alkaloid recently approved by the FDA for the treatment of non-small-cell lung cancer. Vinca alkaloids are asymmetric dimeric compounds (Fig. 13-10). The small difference in chemical structure between vincristine and vinblastine results in important differences in the spectrum of antitumor activity as well as toxicity.

**MECHANISM OF ACTION** The vinca alkaloids exert their cytotoxic action by binding to tubulin, a dimeric protein found in the cytoplasm of cells. Microtubules are essential for forming the spindle fibers along which the chromosomes migrate during mitosis, and for maintaining cell structure. Binding of the vinca alkaloids to tubulin leads to inhibition of the process of assembly and dissolution of the mitotic spindle (Luduena et al. 1977). As a consequence, cells are arrested in metaphase and are unable to replicate. Resistance to vinca alkaloids has been reported to be due to an alteration in the structure of tubulin, resulting in decreased binding of the drugs. Another important mechanism of resistance to the vinca alkaloids is the multidrug resistance phenotype (Riordan and Ling 1985; Tsuruo 1988), resulting in increased drug efflux from the intracellular compartment.

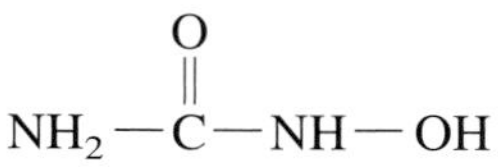

$$NH_2-\overset{\displaystyle O}{\overset{\|}{C}}-NH-OH$$

**Hydroxyurea**

FIGURE 13-9 **Chemical structure of hydroxyurea.**

**CLINICAL PHARMACOLOGY** The clinical pharmacology of both drugs has been reviewed recently. Vincristine, vinblastine, and vinorelbine are administered IV (Table

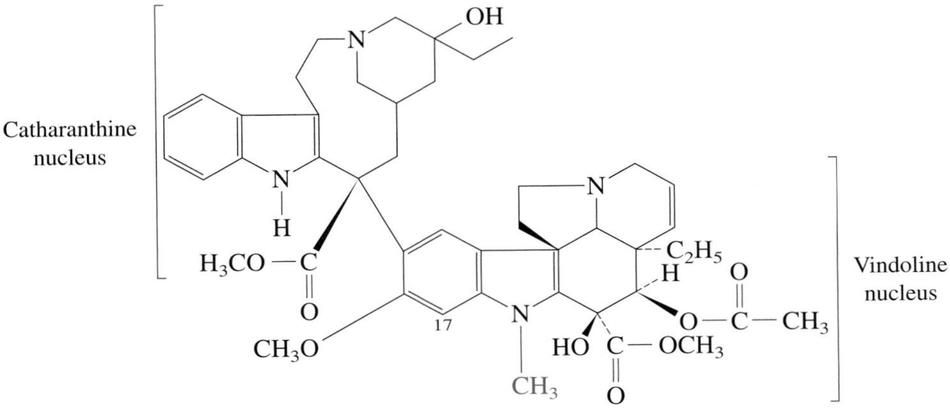

Catharanthine nucleus

Vindoline nucleus

**Vinblastine**

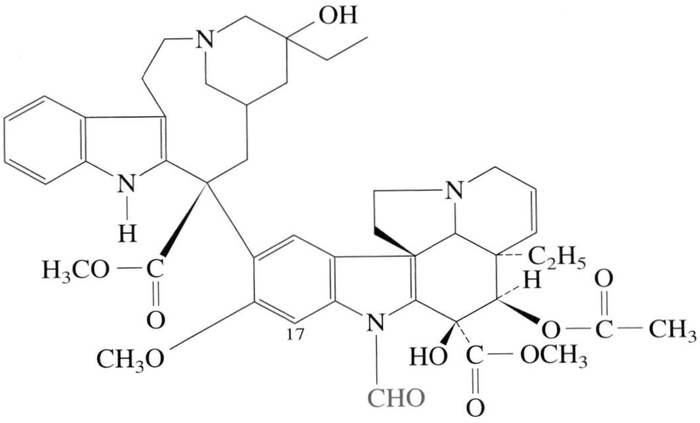

**Vincristine**

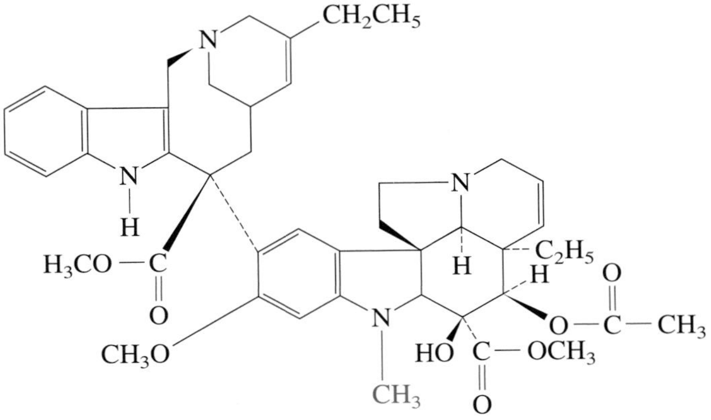

**Vinorelbine**

FIGURE 13-10 **Chemical structures of vinblastine, vincristine, and vinorelbine. The *Vinca* alkaloids consist of a bulky dimeric asymmetric structure composed of a dihydroindole ring system known as the vindoline nucleus, attached through a carbon-carbon bond to the indole ring system, known as the catharanthine nucleus.**

13-9). Although an oral formulation of vinorelbine is available, its oral bioavailability is often erratic and demonstrates a marked interindividual variability ranging from 27 to 43% (depending on the formulation), with plasma concentrations peaking about 1 to 2 hours after the dose is administered. After a rapid distribution phase ($t_{1/2}$ = 7 minutes), vincristine disappears from the plasma with a half-life of 164 minutes (Bender et al. 1977). Vinblastine's distribution phase is 4 minutes, and subsequent breaks in the curve have half-life occur at 53 minutes and 20 hours. Almost 70% of a vincristine dose is metabolized by the hepatic cytochrome P450-3A system and excreted in the feces. Although specific details regarding metabolites are still lacking, vinca alkaloid fate is influenced by a number of other drugs. These include the classic inhibitors of P450-3A such as erythromycin, ketoconazole, cimetidine and itraconazole, which when administered together with vinca alkaloids can significantly enhance toxicity (Zhou-Pan et al. 1993; Tobe et al. 1995; Budman 1997). In addition, vinorelbine is a nonspecific inhibitor of the formation of the 5′-*O*-glucuronide metabolite of zidovudine (AZT). As a consequence, use of this vinca alkaloid in the treatment of AIDS-related Kaposi sarcoma may lead to increased AZT toxicity in these patients. Following hepatic metabolism, the drug is primarily excreted through the biliary system (Rajaonarison et al. 1993). Al-

**Table 13-9 Clinical Pharmacology of Microtubule Inhibitors: The VINCA Alkaloids and Estramustine**

| PHARMACOLOGIC PARAMETER | VINCRISTINE | VINBLASTINE | VINORELBINE | ESTRAMUSTINE |
|---|---|---|---|---|
| *Plasma half-life*[a] | $t_{1/2\alpha}$ = 5 min<br>$t_{1/2\beta}$ = 50–155 min<br>$t_{1/2\gamma}$ = 23–85 h | $t_{1/2\alpha}$ = 5 min<br>$t_{1/2\beta}$ = 53–90 h<br>$t_{1/2\gamma}$ = 20–64 h | $t_{1/2\alpha}$ = 5 min<br>$t_{1/2\beta}$ = 49–168 min<br>$t_{1/2\gamma}$ = 18–49 h | $t_{1/2}$ = 20–24 h |
| *Routes of elimination* | Hepatic metabolism and biliary excretion. | Hepatic metabolism (P450-3A) and biliary excretion. | Hepatic metabolism and biliary excretion. | Hepatic metabolism with biliary and urinary excretion. |
| *Routes of administration* | IV only | IV only | IV and PO (bioavailability ~30%) | PO (bioavailability ~75%) |
| *Major toxicities* | • Peripheral and autonomic neuropathy<br>• Constipation<br>• Alopecia | • Neutropenia | • Neutropenia<br>• Constipation | • N/V<br>• Diarrhea |
| *Less common toxicities* | • Hyperuricemia<br>• SIADH<br>• Jaw pain | • Peripheral and autonomic neuropathy<br>• Stomatitis<br>• Alopecia | • Peripheral neuropathy<br>• Pulmonary toxicity (dyspnea)<br>• Stomatitis<br>• Alopecia | • Congestive heart failure in patients with poor LVF<br>• Cardiac ischemia<br>• Gynecomastia<br>• Prostate cancer |
| *Major indications* | • ALL<br>• Wilms tumor<br>• Lymphoma | • Hodgkin disease<br>• Testicular cancer<br>• Kaposi sarcoma<br>• Mycosis fungoides | • Non-small-cell lung cancer | • Prostate cancer |
| *Comments* | • Lacks significant marrow toxicity | | | • Patients hypersensitive to estrogen or mechlorethamine at risk<br>• Risk of thromboembolic disorders |

[a]Pharmacokinetic data summarized from Forshell et al. 1976; Bender et al. 1977; Nelson et al. 1980; Nelson 1982; Rowinsky and Donehower 1996.
ABBREVIATIONS: LVF, left ventricular function; N/V, nausea and vomiting; SIADH, syndrome of inappropriate antidiuretic hormone release.

though most oncologists decrease the dose of vincristine or vinblastine in patients with hepatic impairment, specific recommendations guiding dose reduction are unavailable. A 50% decrease in dose is generally recommended for patients with a bilirubin concentration greater than 3 mg/dL, although no decrease in dose is advocated for patients with impaired renal function.

**ADVERSE REACTIONS** The dose-limiting toxicity for vincristine is neurotoxicity (see Table 13-9). The initial signs of neurotoxicity are paresthesias of the distal fingers and lower extremities and loss of deep tendon reflexes. Continued use may lead to more advanced neurotoxicity, which includes a profound decrease in motor strength, in particular dorsiflexion of the foot. Occasionally, cranial nerve palsies and severe jaw pain are noted with vincristine administration. At high doses of vincristine (>3 mg total single dose), autonomic neuropathy may be noted, leading to obstipation and paralytic ileus. Sensory changes and reflex abnormalities slowly improve when treatment is stopped; however, motor impairment improves slowly and may be irreversible. Vinorelbine is more selective for nonneuronal microtubules in vitro, is generally more lipophilic, and is rapidly metabolized by hepatocytes compared to other vinca alkaloids (Fellous et al. 1989). These features of the drug probably contribute to its lower neurotoxicity. In addition to these commonly observed toxicities, a syndrome of inappropriate antidiuretic hormone release (SIADH) may occur, which can lead to marked hyponatremia. Although marrow suppression is not commonly noted with vincristine, some additive marrow toxicity may be noted in patients with impaired or recovering marrow function.

The primary toxicity of vinblastine is leukopenia, which reaches a nadir 6 to 7 days after treatment and is rapidly reversible. Mucositis is occasionally observed when vinblastine is given at higher doses (>8 mg/m$^2$), or when it is used in combination with drugs that have similar toxicity profiles. In comparison to vincristine, neurotoxicity is rarely observed at conventional doses of vinblastine. Both drugs cause severe pain and local toxicity if extravasated.

**PRINCIPLE Under no circumstance should any vinca alkaloid be given intrathecally. Deaths have been reported from vincristine administered inadvertently into the CSF.**

Vinorelbine shares many of the same principal toxicities as vincristine and vinblastine (Table 13-9). The dose-limiting toxicity of vinorelbine is neutropenia, with a typical nadir occurring 7 to 10 days after treatment, with full recovery by 14 days. Other toxicities include a mild sensory neuropathy, which can affect up to one-third of patients, constipation, nausea, vomiting, diarrhea, and stomatitis. As expected, the gastrointestinal toxicities are increased with oral administration. Like the other vinca alkaloids, vinorelbine is a vesicant. Vinorelbine is similar to vinblastine, in that the dose-limiting toxicity is leukopenia.

**CLINICAL USES** These drugs are used widely in the treatment of many malignant neoplasms (see Table 13-9). Vinblastine has been shown to be important in the treatment of testicular cancer, bladder cancer, and Hodgkin disease. Vincristine has significant activity in lymphoma, lymphocytic leukemia, and Wilms tumor. More recently, vinorelbine combinations for the treatment of non-small-cell lung cancer have shown promising activity (Depierre et al. 1994; Yokoyama et al. 1992). In several studies evaluating the activity of vinorelbine as monotherapy in untreated stage IIIB and IV non-small-cell lung cancer, major response rates of >30% have been reported in several studies. The response rates in combination regimens has been more varied, and present studies are exploring the value of vinorelbine in a variety of combination regimens. At present, some of the most promising data on vinorelbine have been seen in breast cancer, where single-agent response rates ranging from 16 to 60% have been reported.

**ESTRAMUSTINE** In an effort to design an antineoplastic agent with selective activity against prostate cancer, chemists linked an estradiol molecule to a nitrogen mustard through a carbamate ester group, forming a compound known as *estramustine* (Fig. 13-11). The rationale

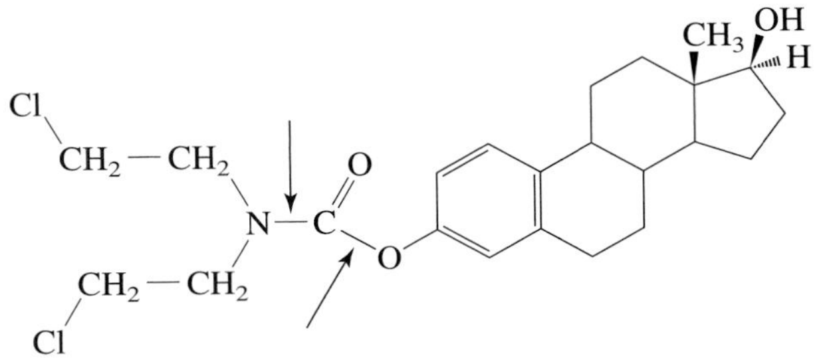

Cl, $CH_2-CH_2$, N, C, O, O, $CH_2-CH_2$, Cl, $CH_3$, OH, H

**Estramustine**

**FIGURE 13-11 Chemical structure of estramustine. Note the large steroid nucleus on the right, and the arrows that separate the estrogenic portion of the molecule form the nitrogen (Rowinsky and Donehower 1996).**

for this synthesis sought to exploit the alkylating activity of the nitrogen mustard and the estrogen binding qualities of the estradiol moiety. It is noteworthy that estramustine was found to inhibit the growth of many cell lines, including those that lacked estrogen receptors, and failed to produce the clinical toxicities generally associated with alkylating chemotherapy (Muntzing et al. 1979). Eventually it was discovered that estramustine produced metaphase arrest in cell culture. This antimicrotubule effect is now known to be due to the binding of estramustine to microtubule associated proteins (MAPs), inducing dissociation of MAP from tubulin, resulting in inhibition of microtubule assembly and disassembly (Hartley-Asp 1984; Benson and Hartley-Asp 1990; Tew et al. 1992).

Estramustine is approved for the treatment of metastatic prostate cancer, in particular hormone refractory disease (Table 13-9). Approximately 75% of the drug is bioavailable, with metabolites of both the estradiol and nitrogen mustard moieties appearing in the bile, feces, and urine. Dose-limiting toxicities of the drug include nausea and sometimes intractable vomiting. Less common toxicities include gynecomastia, nipple tenderness, and/or an exacerbation of congestive heart failure secondary to the mineral corticoid effects of the steroid molecule (Table 13-9). Although mechanisms of resistance have been poorly studied, elevated glutathione may be a contributing factor.

### *Taxanes: Paclitaxel (Taxol)*

**HISTORY** The taxanes are a relatively new class of important antineoplastic agents. Paclitaxel was discovered as part of the National Cancer Institute's drug discovery program in 1963, when crude extracts from the bark of the Pacific yew (*Taxus brevifolia*) were found to have antitumor activity (Wani et al. 1971). The pure active compound was identified in 1971 (Fig. 13-12). Since its discovery, many other sources of the compound have been identified, including other members of the genus *Taxus*, and a fungal endophyte isolated from the bark of the yew (*Taxomyces andreanae*). Today, most of the available drug is partially synthesized from an abundant precursor found in the needles of the European yew, *Taxus baccata*.

**MECHANISM OF ACTION** Paclitaxel binds to the $\beta$-tubulin subunit and, unlike other microtubule inhibitors (e.g., colchicine, vinblastine, and vincristine), stabilizes the microtubule structure inhibiting depolymerization. It typically produces a $G_2$–M phase arrest by sustaining a block in the metaphase to anaphase transition (Schiff et al. 1979; Schiff and Horowitz 1980).

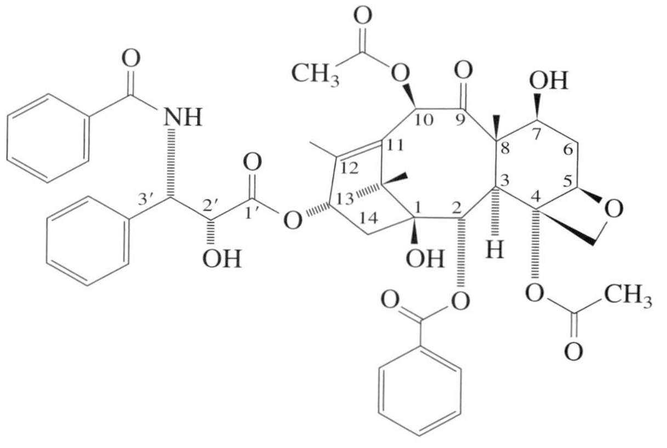

**Paclitaxel**

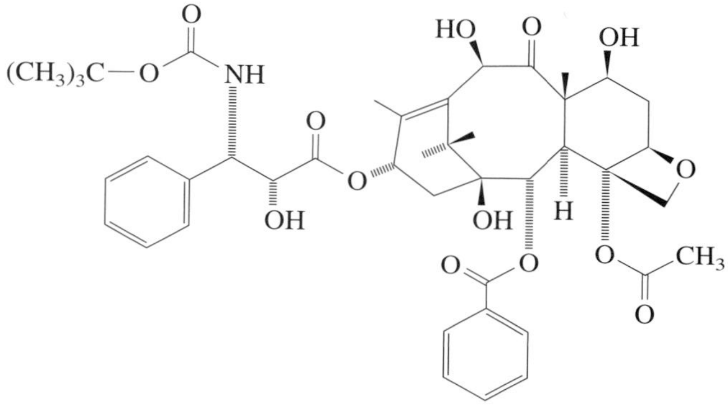

**Docetaxel**

FIGURE 13-12 **Chemical structures of the taxanes paclitaxel and docetaxel.**

**CLINICAL PHARMACOLOGY** The schedule of paclitaxel administration is critical in influencing the spectrum of observed adverse effects and possibly antitumor efficacy (see Table 13-10). In general, the drug can be given by continuous infusion over 1 hour (80 mg/m$^2$), 3 hours (175 mg/m$^2$), 24 hours (250 mg/m$^2$), with or without (135 to 175 mg/m$^2$) G-CSF support, or 96 hours (140 mg/m$^2$). In general, the peak plasma concentrations are greatest when given over shorter durations of infusion. Initially, infusions of shorter duration were associated with a higher incidence of acute hypersensitivity reaction (HSRs), but these reactions were soon found to be equivalent with other dosing schedules when given with premedication. The acute HSRs typically manifest as hypotension, dyspnea with bronchospasm, and urticaria.

Because of its remarkable aqueous insolubility, paclitaxel is formulated in 50% Cremophor EL (a polyoxyethylated castor oil) and alcohol. This vehicle is strongly

**Table 13-10 Clinical Pharmacology of Microtubule Inhibitors: The Taxanes**

| PHARMACOLOGIC PARAMETER | PACLITAXEL | DOCETAXEL |
|---|---|---|
| *Plasma half-life*[a] | $t_{1/2\alpha}$ = 20–30 min<br>$t_{1/2\beta}$ = 60 min<br>$t_{1/2\gamma}$ = 24 h | $t_{1/2\alpha}$ = 12–24 min<br>$t_{1/2\beta}$ = 1.3–1.7 h<br>$t_{1/2\gamma}$ = 22–40 h |
| *Routes of elimination* | Hepatic metabolism by P450 (CYP3A & CYP2C) with biliary excretion.<br><10% in urine. | Hepatic metabolism (P450-3A) with biliary excretion. |
| *Routes of administration* | IV | IV |
| *Major toxicities* | • Neutropenia<br>• Sensory neuropathy<br>• Hypersensitivity reactions | • Neutropenia<br>• Fluid retention<br>• Asthenia |
| *Less common toxicities* | • Myalgias<br>• Bradycardia (abnormal ECG/AV block)<br>• Mucositis (72- to 96-h infusion)<br>• Elevation in transaminases | • Erythematous pruritic maculopapular rash<br>• Neuropathy<br>• Alopecia |
| *Major indications* | • Breast<br>• Ovarian<br>• Lung<br>• Head and neck<br>• Bladder<br>• Kaposi sarcoma | • Non-small-cell lung cancer<br>• Breast |
| *Comments* | • Because of hypersensitivity reactions to the vehicle, premed with $H_1$ blocker and steroids.<br>• Adjust dose for hepatic dysfunction | • Patients hypersensitive to paclitaxel may be sensitive to docetaxel.<br>• Adjust dose for hepatic dysfunction |

[a]Pharmacokinetic data summarized from Longnecker et al. 1986; Wiernik et al. 1987; Extra et al. 1993; and Bissett et al. 1993.
ABBREVIATIONS: AV, atrioventricular; ECG, electrocardiogram; $H_1$, histamine receptor type 1; IV, intravenous; P450, cytochrome P450/mixed function oxidase; CYP 3A and 2C refer to specific cytochrome isoenzymes.

suspected of producing the potentially fatal histamine stimulated reactions (HSRs) associated with paclitaxel administration, as it appears to be a strong inducer of histamine release (Lassus et al. 1985). Typical premedication schemes to prevent HSRs include dexamethasone, a histamine $H_1$-receptor antagonist such as diphenhydramine, and a $H_2$-receptor antagonist such as cimetidine or famotidine.

Paclitaxel is predominantly metabolized by the hepatic cytochrome P450 system (in particular CYP3A and CYP2 isoforms) and excreted via the biliary route. Very little of the drug (<10%) is excreted unchanged in the urine (Monsarrat et al. 1993; Cresteil et al. 1994).

**ADVERSE EFFECTS** Neutropenia is the principal toxicity of paclitaxel (Table 13-10). The neutropenia due to a paclitaxel infusion is influenced by the duration of time that plasma concentrations are maintained above a particular threshold. For this reason, longer infusions are more likely to produce more severe neutropenia, as is prior myelosuppressive therapy. In addition, paclitaxel has been associated with a transient asymptomatic bradycardia, which is not an indication for drug discontinuation. Although very rare, more severe forms of heart block including third-degree block have been reported. Other cardiotoxic effects including ischemia and infarction have also been noted (Rowinsky et al. 1991; Arbuck et al.

1993). In patients with a history of conduction disorders, in particular bradycardia or heart block, it is necessary to administer paclitaxel under the supervision of a cardiac telemetry unit.

Other toxicities include a stocking-glove distribution peripheral sensory neuropathy. This toxicity is typically symmetrical, and initially manifests itself as numbness and paresthesia in the distal extremities. Rarely, acute hypersensitivity reactions have been reported within the first 2 to 3 minutes of infusions.

CLINICAL USES Paclitaxel has been approved in the United States for the treatment of ovarian and breast cancer and is now widely used for the treatment of other epithelial tumors, including cancers of the head and neck, esophagus, and non-small-cell lung cancers (Table 13-10). For example, the combination of a platinum-based drug (carboplatin or cisplatin) and paclitaxel is now first-line therapy for patients with ovarian cancer and has demonstrated an improvement in survival compared with patients treated with cisplatin and cyclophosphamide.

### *Docetaxel (Taxotere)*

HISTORY Docetaxel is a semisynthetic taxoid derived (Fig. 13-12) from the same precursor used in the partial synthesis of paclitaxel (10-deacetylbaccatin III).

MECHANISM OF ACTION Like paclitaxel, docetaxel binds to free tubulin and promotes assembly of stable microtubules, causing a $G_2$–M phase arrest. Docetaxel most likely binds to the same $\beta$-tubulin binding site as paclitaxel, though with twice the binding affinity (Diaz and Andreu 1993). Like paclitaxel, docetaxel is a radiosensitizing agent as well.

CLINICAL PHARMACOLOGY Docetaxel is also metabolized by the hepatic cytochrome P450 system, in particular CYP3A, CYP2B, and CYP1A isoforms, and its elimination is similar to that observed for paclitaxel (Marne et al. 1993; Gires et al. 1994) (see Table 13-10). Because of the importance of hepatic metabolism the drug is generally not administered when the aminotransferase activity is more than 1.5 times normal, and the alkaline phosphatase activity is more than 2.5 times normal. In contrast however, it is more soluble in water, and its formulation does not contain Cremophor EL, making HSRs relatively less common following its administration. Although influence of schedule is still under study, the drug is usually administered intravenously every 3 weeks at a dose of 60 to 100 mg/m$^2$.

ADVERSE EFFECTS Severe neutropenia has been noted in over 95 and 65% of patients with anthracycline-resistant breast cancer when treated with a dose of 100 and 60 mg/m$^2$ every 3 weeks, respectively. Other toxicities include a sensory peripheral neuropathy, stomatitis, myalgias, nausea and vomiting, and severe asthenia (Table 13-10). Cumulative doses can lead to fluid retention responsive to corticosteroid pretreatment.

CLINICAL USE Docetaxel has clinically significant antitumor activity in patients with anthracycline-resistant advanced breast cancer. A response rate of 40% has been noted when used as first-line treatment in patients with metastatic breast cancer at a dose of 75 mg/m$^2$, with higher rates (54 to 68%) being noted at the 100 mg/m$^2$ dose level. Docetaxel has also been shown to have activity in patients with advanced non-small-cell lung cancer, ovarian cancer, and cancer of the head and neck. The drug's role in these diseases is presently under study.

## Topoisomerase II Inhibitors

### *Podophyllotoxins: Etoposide and teniposide*

HISTORY Although the cytotoxic properties of podophyllin have been known since 1946 when the drug was found to be curative in the management of condyloma acuminata, this compound is too toxic for systemic use. A large synthetic program led to the synthesis and testing of two derivatives, etoposide (VP-16) and teniposide (VM-26) (Fig. 13-13). Although etoposide has received a much more extensive clinical evaluation, teniposide was approved by the FDA in 1992 for use in refractory childhood leukemias.

MECHANISM OF ACTION The mechanism of action of these compounds has been found to involve inhibition of topoisomerase II$\alpha$, leading to induction of single-strand breaks in DNA. Resistance to etoposide may occur via the multidrug-resistant phenotype (Ross et al. 1984; Riordan and Ling 1985; Tsuruo 1988), or via a mutation in topoisomerase II, leading to decreased binding of etoposide (Pommier et al. 1986).

CLINICAL PHARMACOLOGY Etoposide may be administered by either the oral or intravenous route (see Table 13-11). When it is administered orally, 50% of the dose is absorbed. After a single IV dose of etoposide, the plasma $\alpha$ and $\beta$ half-lives are 2.8 and 15.1 hours, respectively. Approximately one-half of the dosage is excreted in the urine, with approximately one-third appearing as a metabolite. The remainder of the drug is excreted in the feces following hepatic metabolism (Creaven 1984). Because etoposide is poorly soluble in water, different strat-

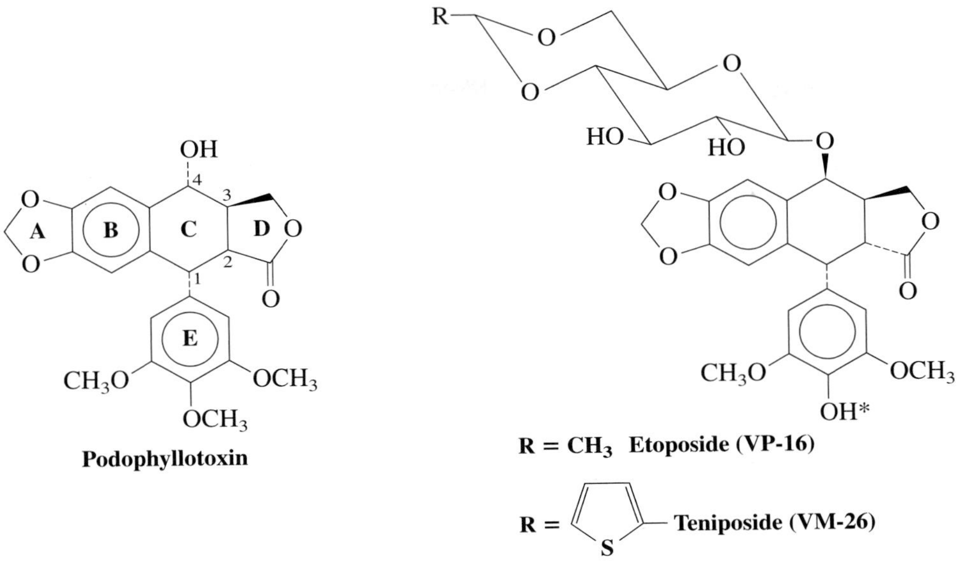

**Podophyllotoxin**

**R = $CH_3$ Etoposide (VP-16)**

**R = [thiophene ring] Teniposide (VM-26)**

**FIGURE 13-13** **Chemical structures of podophyllotoxin, and the clinically important epipodophyllotoxins etoposide (VP-16) and teniposide (VN-26). VP-16 and VM-26 are semisynthetic derivatives of podophyllotoxin, a product of the mayapple or mandrake plant (*Podophyllum peltatum*). *Replacement of this –OH group on the etoposide structure with –$OPO_3H_2$ produces etoposide phosphate (Etopophos). This drug, now used as an oral formulation of VP-16, is rapidly converted to etoposide by host alkaline phosphatase.**

egies have been exploited to enhance bioavailability. In general, two oral formulations of etoposide are available. A hydrophilic gelatin capsule (containing ethanol and polyethylene glycol) has about 50% bioavailability, although substantial inter- and intrapatient variability has been reported. In addition, the bioavailability is not linear and decreases with escalating doses. Etoposide phosphate (Etopofos) is a prodrug that has a molecule of phosphate added to the E-ring. Following injection etoposide phosphate is rapidly converted by endogenous phosphatases to etoposide. This formulation has the advantage of avoiding potentially toxic excipients, can be given by parental administration, and is more stable than other formulations. In addition this formulation appears to exhibit a greater bioavailability with initial phase I studies reporting a mean bioavailability of 68% (Table 13-11).

**ADVERSE EFFECTS** When administered IV etoposide should be infused over a 30-minute period to avoid hypotensive episodes. Although the major toxicity is leukopenia, which is rapidly reversible (see Table 13-11), thrombocytopenia can also occur. Nausea and vomiting are common with IV drug administration, as is alopecia. Other uncommon toxicities include fever, mild elevation of liver function tests, and peripheral neuropathy. Because the major toxicity of etoposide is myelosuppression, this drug is under extensive investigation as part of a preparative treatment (myeloablative) with high-dose regimens followed by bone marrow transplantation.

**CLINICAL USES** Etoposide has significant clinical activity in several malignancies, including Hodgkin disease, lymphomas, leukemias, small-cell lung cancer, and testicular cancer.

### *Anthracyclines: Doxorubicin, daunorubicin, idarubicin, and mitoxantrone*

**HISTORY** The anthracyclines approved for clinical use are doxorubicin, daunorubicin, idarubicin, and mitoxantrone. The former two compounds are alkaloids produced by various *Streptomyces* species. Mitoxantrone is a synthetic compound that does not contain a sugar moiety (Fig. 13-14).

**MECHANISM OF ACTION** These drugs appear to produce their major effect through the inhibition of topoisomerase II $\alpha$. The anthracyclines enter cells via a passive

**Table 13-11 Clinical Pharmacology of Topoisomerase II Inhibitors: The Epipodophyllotoxins**

| PHARMACOLOGIC PARAMETER | ETOPOSIDE | TENIPOSIDE |
|---|---|---|
| *Plasma half-life*[a] | $t_{1/2}$ = 6–8 h | $t_{1/2}$ = 8 h |
| *Routes of elimination* | Hepatic metabolism and renal excretion (~40% intact), ~6% biliary | Hepatic metabolism and urinary excretion (80% recovered) |
| *Routes of administration* | IV and PO (PO bioavailability ~50%—decreases as dose increases) | IV |
| *Major toxicities* | • Neutropenia (nadir 10–14 days)<br>• N/V & diarrhea<br>• Hepatic dysfunction (high doses) | • Neutropenia<br>• N/V<br>• Hypersensitivity reactions |
| *Less common toxicities* | • Thrombocytopenia<br>• Hypotension<br>• Alopecia | • Hypotension<br>• Liver dysfunction<br>• Alopecia |
| *Major indications* | • Testicular<br>• Small-cell lung | • Refractory childhood ALL |
| *Comments* | • Increased toxicity in patients with hypoalbuminemia | • Anticonvulsants enhance hepatic metabolism and decrease systemic exposure<br>• Adjust dose for renal insufficiency |

[a]Pharmacokinetic data summarized from D'Incalci et al. 1982; Hande 1992; and Clark and Slevin 1987.
ABBREVIATIONS: ALL, acute lymphoblastic leukemia; N/V, nausea and vomiting.

transport process and are effluxed out of cells by the P-glycoprotein system that is increased in multidrug-resistant cells (Tsuruo 1988). Other mechanisms for anthracycline resistance have also been reported, including increased DNA repair (Capranico et al. 1987) and an alteration in topoisomerase II (Glisson et al. 1986). Because of their clinical utility, a large number of analogs have been synthesized, and many are presently under study in clinical trials.

**CLINICAL PHARMACOLOGY** After an IV bolus dose of doxorubicin, the drug disappears in three phases (see Table 13-12). The initial rapid distribution phase lasts approximately 15 minutes; a second phase due to metabolism and elimination lasts several hours; and a prolonged third phase of 24 to 48 hours may represent release of drug from binding sites. Both daunorubicin and doxorubicin are metabolized in the liver to the less toxic metabolites daunomycinol and doxorubicinol, respectively. Modification of the dose has been recommended for patients with hepatic impairment, using bilirubin concentrations as a guideline. At present, there are no firm recommendations guiding the dose adjustment.

The typical dose of doxorubicin used as a single agent is 60 to 75 mg/m$^2$ given as a single dose every 3 to 4 weeks. Some evidence supports the use of dose schedules that use more frequent, lower doses, given either weekly or by continuous infusion over 48 to 96 hours. These modifications can result in less cardiac toxicity by avoiding high peak concentrations in plasma. When given in combination with other myelotoxic agents such as cyclophosphamide, the dose of doxorubicin is usually decreased by one-third.

**ADVERSE EFFECTS** Myelosuppression usually occurs with a nadir 10 days after administration of a single dose (see Table 13-12), with recovery usually occurring within 3 weeks. These drugs also cause tissue necrosis if they extravasate and alopecia. Mitoxantrone usually does not cause these toxic effects and produces less nausea and vomiting than is seen with daunomycin, doxorubicin, or idarubicin. Doxorubicin may cause mucositis, especially when it is used in maximally tolerated divided doses given over 2 to 3 days or when used in combination with other drugs that cause mucositis. It is interesting that these drugs may also cause a recall reaction in previously ir-

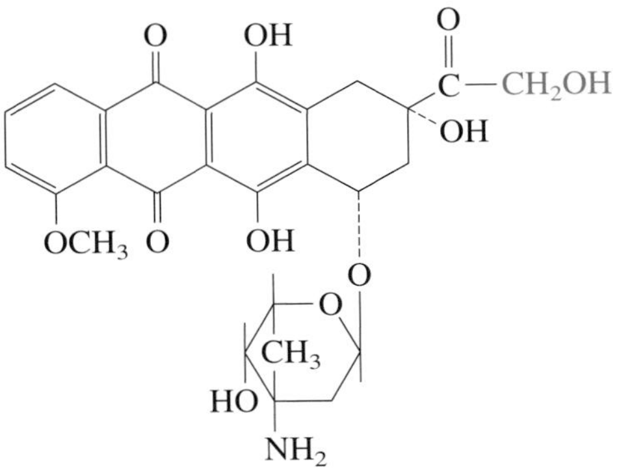

**Doxorubicin (Adriamycin)**

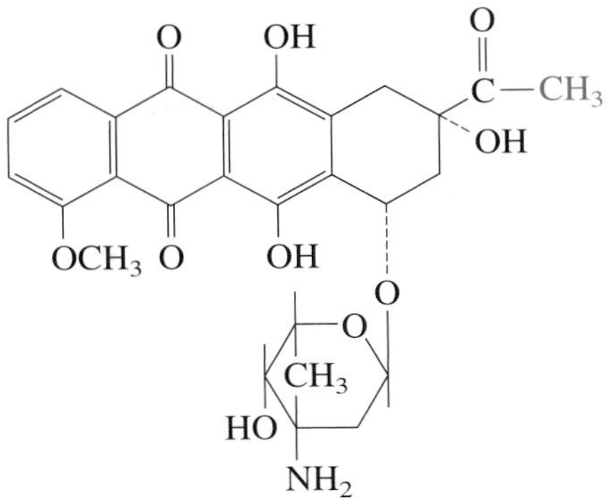

**Daunorubicin (Daunomycin)**

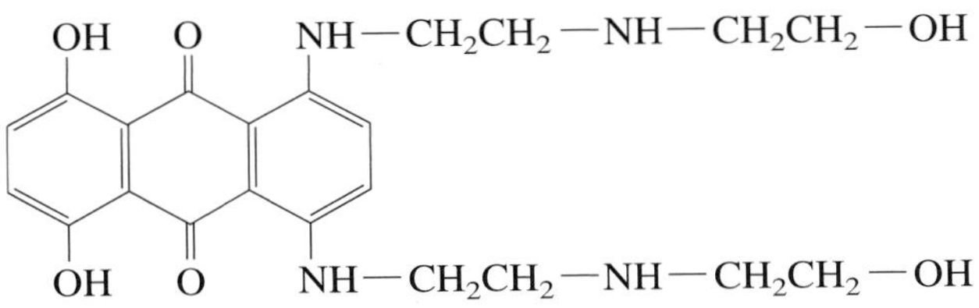

**Mitoxantrone**

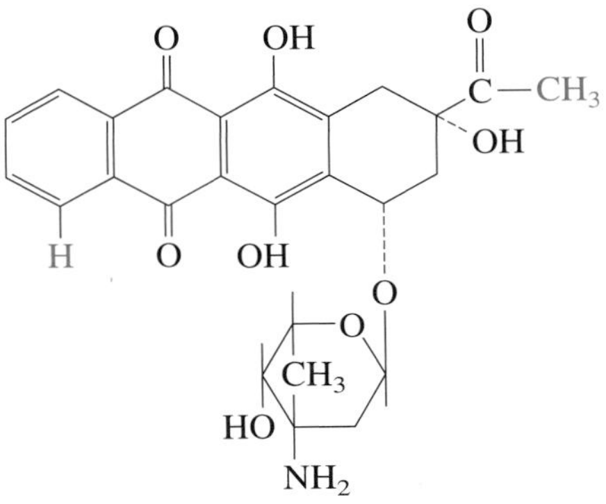

**Idarubicin**

FIGURE 13-14 **Chemical structures of the anthracyclines, doxorubicin (Adriamycin), daunomycin, mitoxantrone, and idarubicin.**

radiated tissues ("radiation recall"), especially when they are administered just before (up to 3 weeks) or following radiotherapy.

In addition to myelosuppression, the other significant toxic effect of doxorubicin and daunorubicin is cardiac toxicity (Von Hoff et al. 1982). Both acute effects, manifested by arrhythmias, conduction abnormalities, and a "pericarditis–myocarditis syndrome," as well as chronic effects may occur. Cardiac biopsy demonstrates a dose-dependent effect of doxorubicin on the viability of myocardial cells (Billingham et al. 1978). Measurements of ejection fraction by echocardiography or MUGA scans have been extremely helpful as a noninvasive technique that can demonstrate a drug-induced decline in myocardial function. When evidence of compromised cardiac function appears, the anthracycline therapy must be discontinued.

Most patients will tolerate total doses of 450 to 550 $mg/m^2$ of doxorubicin or daunorubicin before the risk of cardiac damage is significant (>5%). Once clinically overt cardiac toxicity occurs, usually manifest as congestive heart failure (CHF), the mortality rate may be as high as 50%. Congestive heart failure typically occurs within 1 month of therapy. Rarely, heart failure may occur months to years later. Other anthracycline analogs such as mitoxantrone may produce less cardiac toxicity, but the data with this drug are less complete than with doxorubicin.

**CLINICAL USES** Doxorubicin has a broad spectrum of activity in neoplastic disease (see Table 13-12). It is an important drug for the treatment of hematologic malignancies, especially ALL, Hodgkin disease, and the non-Hodgkin lymphomas. It is also used in combination to treat solid tumors, especially breast cancer, lung cancer, bladder cancer, and certain childhood tumors. Daunomycin is used almost exclusively in the treatment of AML. Recently, mitoxantrone has been approved for the treat-

Table 13-12 **Clinical Pharmacology of Anthracyclines**

| PHARMACOLOGIC PARAMETER | DOXORUBICIN | DAUNORUBICIN | IDARUBICIN | MITOXANTRONE |
|---|---|---|---|---|
| *Plasma half-life*[a] | $t_{1/2\alpha}$ = 10 m<br>$t_{1/2\beta}$ = 1–3 h<br>$t_{1/2\gamma}$ = 30 h | $t_{1/2\alpha}$ = 40 m<br>$t_{1/2\beta}$ = 20–50 h | $t_{1/2\alpha}$ = 11.3 h (parent)<br>30–60 h (13-ol metabolite) | $t_{1/2\alpha}$ = 10 m<br>$t_{1/2\beta}$ = 1.1–1.6 h<br>$t_{1/2\gamma}$ = 23–42 h |
| *Routes of elimination* | Hepatic metabolism to doxorubicinol and biliary excretion | Hepatic metabolism and biliary excretion (50–60%), 25% renal | Hepatic metabolism and biliary excretion as 13-ol (80%), some renal | Hepatic metabolism with <30% detected in stool and urine |
| *Routes of administration* | IV | IV | IV and PO (bioavailability ~30%) | IV, IA, and IP |
| *Major toxicities* | • BMS<br>• Cardiotoxicity (>550 mg/m$^2$)<br>• Esophagitis<br>• Stomatitis<br>• Alopecia | • BMS<br>• Esophagitis<br>Stomatitis<br>Alopecia | • BMS | • Leukopenia<br>• Diarrhea<br>• Mucositis<br>• N/V |
| *Less common toxicities* | • Post radiation recall | • Cardiomyopathy<br>• Hyperuricemia<br>• Pericarditis and myocarditis | • Cardiac toxicity (arrhythmia, congestive heart failure)<br>• Radiation recall | • Cardiac toxicity<br>• Allergic reactions<br>• Alopecia |
| *Major indications* | • AML/ALL<br>• Lymphoma<br>• Breast/ovarian<br>• Bladder<br>• Gastric<br>• Thyroid<br>• Small cell lung | • AML/ALL | • AML | • Prostate<br>• Acute leukemia<br>• CML<br>• Breast<br>• Lymphoma |
| *Comments* | • Strong vesicant<br>• Red urine | • Vesicant<br>• Red urine<br>• Liposomal form | • Vesicant | • Blue-green urine |

[a]Pharmacokinetic data summarized from Huffman and Bachur 1972; Greene et al. 1983; Alberts et al. 1985; Smyth et al. 1986.
ABBREVIATIONS: ALL, acute lymphoblastic leukemia; AML, acute myelogenous leukemia; BMS, bone marrow suppression; CML, chronic myelogenous leukemia; IA, intraarterial; IP, intraperitoneal; N/V, nausea and vomiting.

ment of AML and, in conjunction with ara-C (Walters et al. 1988), produces a shorter time to complete remission in ALL (a prognostic factor in adult ALL) compared with the traditionally used four or five drug regimens (Weiss et al. 1996).

Idarubicin is another anthracycline recently approved for the treatment of acute myelocytic leukemia and in combination with cytosine arabinoside produces similar remission rates compared with daunorubicin and cytosine arabinoside.

***Dexrazoxane (Zinecard)***

An agent that protects the heart from anthracycline-induced toxicity, dexrazoxane has recently been approved for use by the FDA for patients who are treated with cumulative doses of doxorubicin greater than 300 mg/m$^2$. Liposomal preparations of doxorubicin are also being evaluated as potentially less cardiotoxic formulations. Toxicities associated with dexrazoxane include pain at the injection site and modest neutropenia and thrombocytopenia. The concern that dexrazoxane may compromise the antitumor effect of the anthracyclines prompted the FDA to recommend that treatment with this drug should be initiated only when the cumulative dose of 300 mg/m$^2$ of doxorubicin was reached (Blum 1997).

## Topoisomerase I Inhibitors

This class of drugs bind to topoisomerase I (Fig. 13-15). DNA adducts subsequently result in double strand breaks, resulting in cytotoxicity (see Table 13-13). Two inhibitors of this enzyme have now been approved for clinical use: irinotecan and topotecan.

### *Irinotecan*

Irinotecan (CPT-11, Camptosar) is a prodrug that is rapidly hydrolyzed in vivo to SN-38, a potent inhibitor of topoisomerase I. Irinotecan has been approved for use in the treatment of patients with advanced colorectal cancer (Table 13-13). The dose schedule used most commonly is a single infusion every 3 weeks, although other dose schedules are being explored. The principle dose-limiting toxicity, is diarrhea. Diarrhea may be seen within the first 24 hours of treatment or later, occurring up to 4 to 8 days after treatment. Aggressive antidiarrheal treatment with loperamide at the first sign of diarrhea greatly enhances the patient's tolerance of the drug and compliance. Severe neutropenia may also occur with CPT-11. Current studies are evaluating combinations of this drug with fluorouracil or raltitrexed (Tomudex), an investigational drug that targets the enzyme thymidylate synthase.

### *Topotecan*

Topotecan (Hycamtin) is approved for use in previously treated patients with ovarian cancer. Its mechanism of action is similar to irinotecan (CPT-11), namely, inhibition of topoisomerase I. Topotecan also has activity in other tumors, including hematologic malignancies, small-cell lung cancer, neuroblastoma, and rhabdomyosarcoma. The recommended dose is 1.5 mg/m$^2$ daily infused intravenously over 30 minutes for five consecutive days, every 3 weeks. The dose-limiting and most common toxicity is myelosuppression, in particular, neutropenia (Table 13-13).

## DNA-Damaging Agents

Alkylating agents are important in the treatment of various malignancies either as single agents or as components of effective combination regimens. There appears to be little or no cross-resistance of alkylating agents with other classes of drugs. The alkylating agents may be classified as *bifunctional* or *monofunctional* agents. Bifunctional agents have two reactive sites on the molecule and thus are capable of cross-linking important biological molecules, in particular DNA. The most susceptible region for alkylation of DNA is the N-7 position of guanine. Examples of the first class are cyclophosphamide, nitrogen mustard, thiotepa, melphalan, busulfan, chlorambucil, and the nitrosoureas (Farmer 1987). Other DNA reactive drugs, such as procarbazine and dacarbazine (DTIC, dimethyl-triazeno-imidazole-carboxamide), may be considered monofunctional agents and therefore do not cross-link DNA but may produce single strand breaks.

Resistance may be specific for certain alkylating agents. For example, impaired uptake of nitrogen mustard is caused by an alteration in the carrier for the natural substrate choline (Goldenberg et al. 1970). Conversely, mechanisms of resistance may be common to multiple alkylating agents, for example, increased drug inactivation associated with an increase in intracellular sulfhydryl compounds, increased glutathione transferases, or increased repair of DNA damage. In general, the alkylating agents can be classified as nitrogen mustards (e.g., mechlorethamine, melphalan, chlorambucil, cyclophosphamide and ifosfamide), aziridines (thiotepa), alkyl alkane sulfonates (busulfan), nitrosoureas (carmustine and lomustine), and the nonclassical alkylating agents (procarbazine and dacarbazine). For the purposes of this discussion, these agents may be further classified according to their chemical structures. A brief discussion of each agent is given below.

### *Nitrogen mustards*

**HISTORY** The prototype of this class of alkylating agent is mechlorethamine (mustine, nitrogen mustard, $HN_2$), first studied by Gilman and colleagues in 1946, and initially developed as a result of chemical warfare research in World War II (Gilman 1963). The chemical structure of mechlorethamine is shown in Fig. 13-16.

**CLINICAL PHARMACOLOGY** Mechlorethamine is a highly reactive unstable compound when reconstituted in an aqueous solution. It is a potent vesicant, and care must be taken in mixing and administering the drug intravenously. Intramolecular cyclization produces ethyleniminium products, and these reactive intermediates rapidly bind to various nucleophiles, especially DNA and the sulfhydryl groups on protein.

**ADVERSE REACTIONS** The adverse effects of alkylating agents often include: severe nausea and vomiting, occurring within minutes to hours after administration;

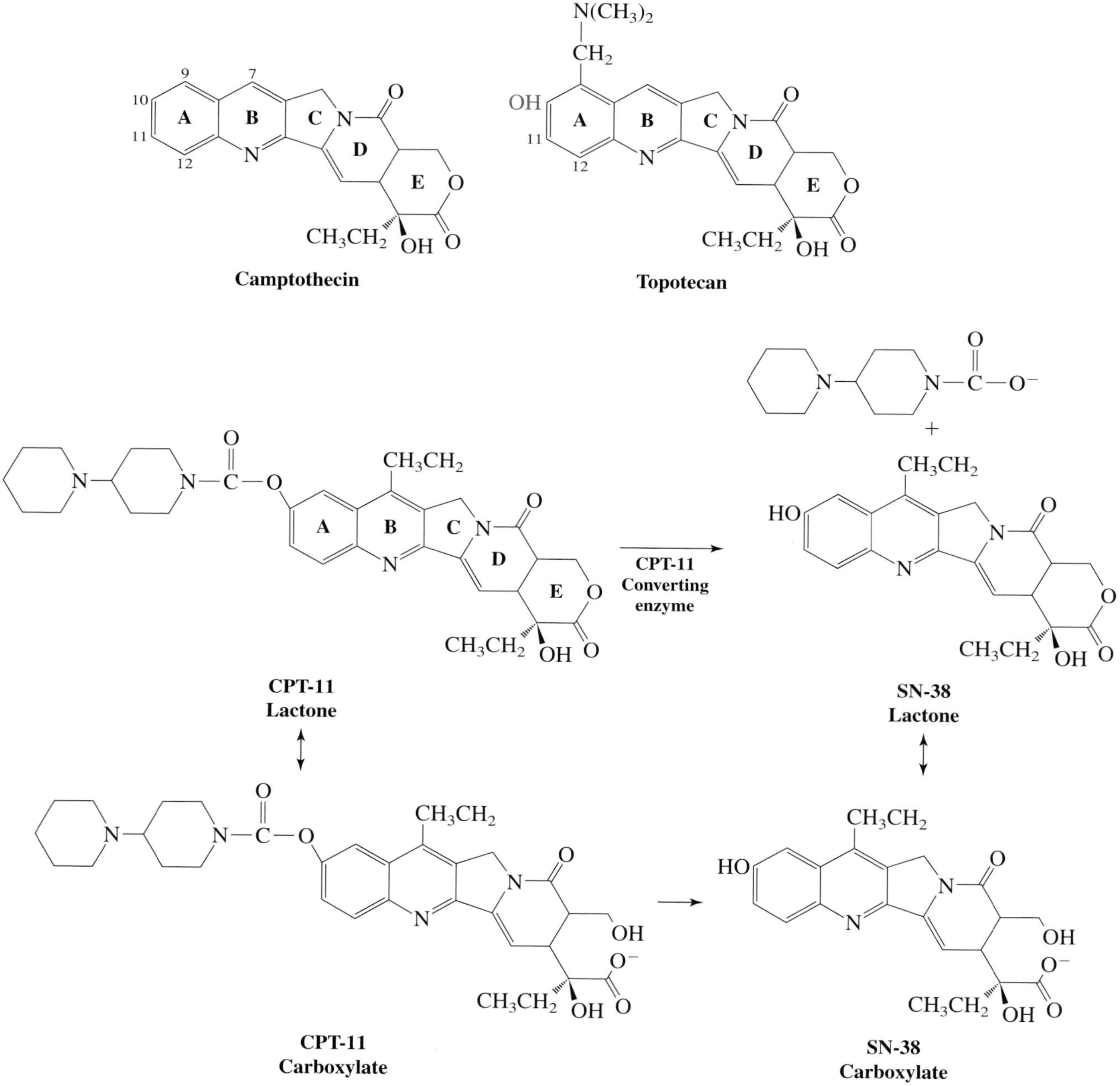

**Camptothecin**

**Topotecan**

**CPT-11 Lactone**

**CPT-11 Converting enzyme**

**SN-38 Lactone**

**CPT-11 Carboxylate**

**SN-38 Carboxylate**

FIGURE 13-15 **Chemical structures of the topoisomerase I inhibitors camptothecin, topotecan, and irinotecan (CPT-11). Camptothecin, a naturally occurring plant alkaloid found in the bark of *Camptotheca acuminata*, was the parent compound first isolated and studied. The clinically important drugs topotecan and irinotecan are the more water-soluble and less toxic derivatives of camptothecin. CPT-11 is considered a prodrug in vivo. It is converted by a carboxyesterase-converting enzyme to SN-38 (7-ethyl-10-hydroxycamptothecin). SN-38 is over 1000 times as potent an inhibitor of topoisomerase I as irinotecan. Following IV administration, the camptothecins undergo a reversible, pH-dependent, nonenzymatic hydrolysis of the lactone ring producing an open-ring carboxylate. At neutral pH, the equilibrium favors formation of the carboxylate anion, which is a much less potent inhibitor of topoisomerase I. Both the lactone and carboxylate derivative of CPT-11 and SN-38 can be found in the plasma following IV administration (Takimoto and Arbuck 1996).**

Table 13-13 **Clinical Pharmacology of the Topoisomerase I Inhibitors: The Camptothecins—Irinotecan and Topotecan**

| PHARMACOLOGIC PARAMETER | IRINOTECAN | TOPOTECAN |
|---|---|---|
| *Plasma half-life*[a] | $t_{1/2}$ = 7 h (lactone); $t_{1/2}$ = 10 h (total)<br>$t_{1/2}$ = 8.7 h (SN-38 lactone) | $t_{1/2}$ = 2.6 h (lactone ring)<br>$t_{1/2}$ = 3.3 h (total) |
| *Routes of elimination* | Metabolized to SN-38; 22% excreted unchanged in urine; SN-38 excreted into bile. | Nonenzymatic hydrolysis of lactone ring. 36% excreted unchanged in urine, concentrated in bile. |
| *Routes of administration* | IV | IV, (?PO) |
| *Major toxicities* | • Diarrhea<br>• BMS (neutropenia)<br>• Alopecia<br>• N/V | • BMS (neutropenia)<br>• N/V<br>• Alopecia |
| *Less common toxicities* | • Mucositis<br>• Increase in transaminases<br>• Pulmonary toxicity | • Diarrhea<br>• Mucositis<br>• Skin rash |
| *Major indications* | • Colon cancer | • Refractory ovarian<br>• Small-cell lung |
| *Comments* | • Important to control diarrhea with high-dose loperamide if necessary | • Dosage adjustment for $CL_{Cr}$ < 60 mL/min |

[a]Pharmacokinetic data summarized from Takimoto and Arbuck 1996.
ABBREVIATIONS: BMS, bone marrow suppression; $CL_{Cr}$, creatinine clearance; N/V, nausea and vomiting.

bone marrow suppression with a nadir of 10 to 14 days; and alopecia (see Table 13-14). Mechlorethamine causes severe tissue damage if extravasation occurs, and immediate treatment with sodium thiosulfate into the same IV site may help to decrease potential tissue damage by neutralizing with the active intermediates of mechlorethamine.

**CLINICAL USES** Mechlorethamine is almost exclusively used in the treatment of Hodgkin disease, especially in the combination regimen MOPP (mechlorethamine, vincristine, procarbazine, and prednisone) (DeVita et al. 1972). This drug is also used to control pleural and pericardial effusions by intracavitary administration and is applied topically in dilute solution to treat mycosis fungoides (Vonderheid 1984).

### *Cyclophosphamide*

**HISTORY** This alkylating agent was first described in 1958 and represents the results of an effort to develop drugs that are selectively activated at the tumor site (Fig. 13-16). However, subsequent studies have shown that the primary tissue of metabolic activation is the liver. This drug has a wide spectrum of antitumor activity and is also used as an immunosuppressant.

**MECHANISM OF ACTION AND CLINICAL PHARMACOLOGY** Most of the parent compound, which is inactive, is metabolized by the cytochrome P450 system in vivo, generating the active metabolites phosphoramide mustard from its precursor 4-hydroxycyclophosphamide (Colvin and Hilton 1981) (see Table 13-14). This latter compound is often used as part of a "purging" approach to selectively kill leukemia and lymphoma cells in bone marrow grafts before autologous transplantation. The plasma half-life is 16 hours (Sladek et al. 1984), and 80% or more of the administered dose is metabolized. Some dose adjustment may be required in patients with renal impairment, as the parent drug and the metabolites are primarily excreted in the urine (Juma et al. 1979).

Cyclophosphamide may be administered orally or IV. In low oral doses, 75% or more of the dose is absorbed,

## NITROSOUREAS

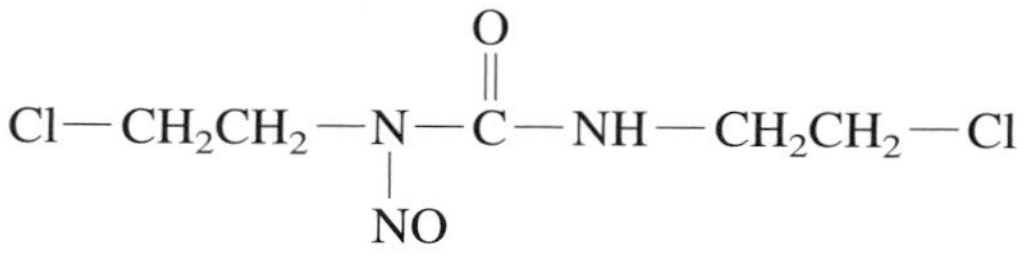

**Chloroethylnitrosourea Moiety**

**Carmustine (BCNU)**

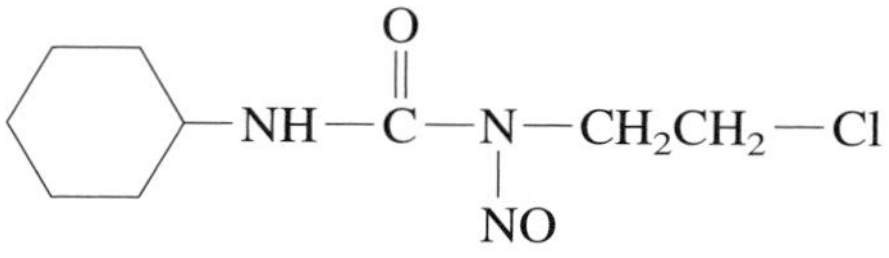

**Lomustine (CCNU)**

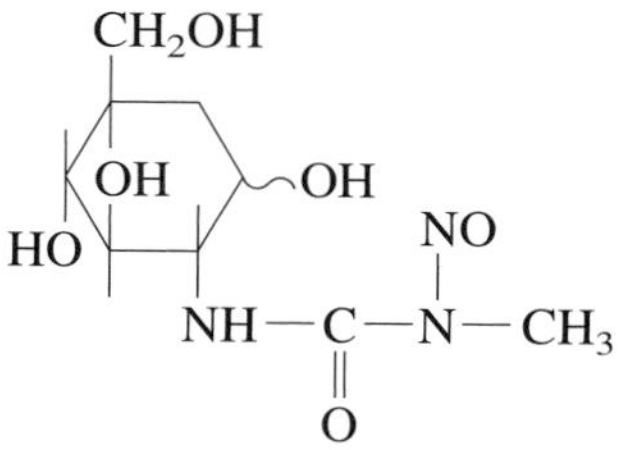

**Streptozotocin**

## NITROGEN MUSTARDS

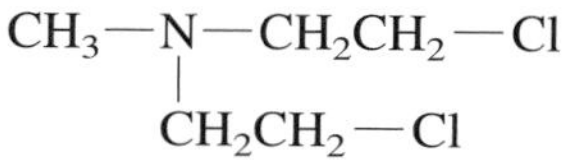

Nitrogen mustard

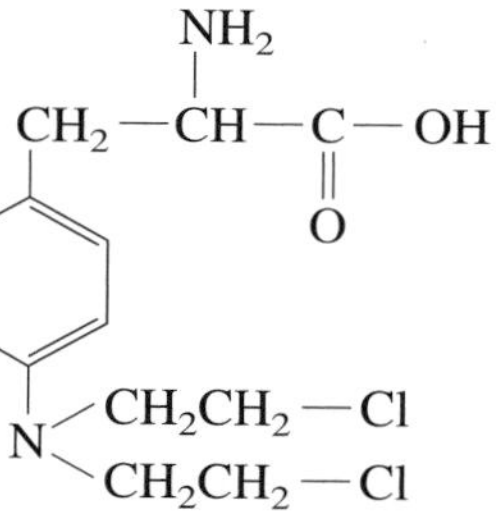

**Melphalan**

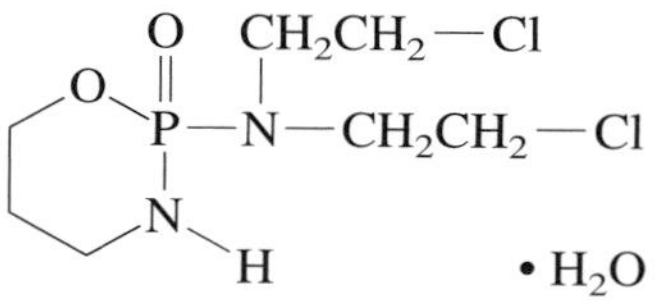

Cyclophosphamide

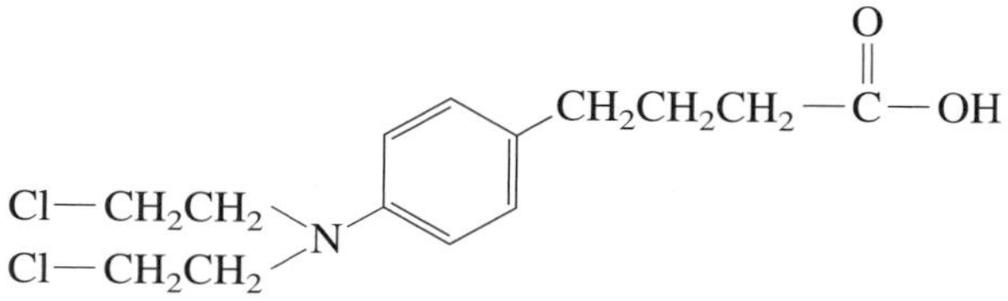

**Chlorambucil**

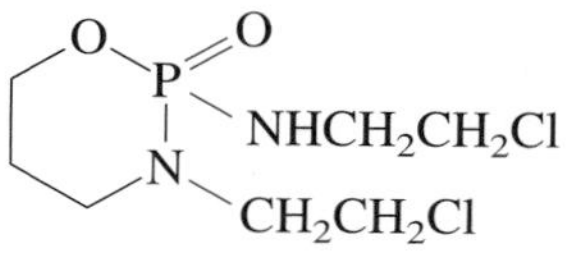

**Ifosfamide**

FIGURE 13-16 **Chemical structures of the nitrosoureas and nitrogen mustards. BCNU (carmustine; bis-chloroethylnitrosourea) and CCNU (lomustine; cyclohexylchloroethylnitrosourea) and streptozotocin are shown. The nitrogen mustard class of drugs are derived from the nitrogen mustard mechlorethamine. Replacement of the -$CH_3$ moiety by a variety of side chains produces chlorambucil, melphalan, cyclophosphamide, and ifosfamide.**

**Table 13-14 Clinical Pharmacology of Alkylating Agents: The Nitrogen Mustards**

| PHARMACOLOGIC PARAMETER | MECHLORETHAMINE | CYCLOPHOSPHAMIDE | IFOSFAMIDE | MELPHALAN | CHLORAMBUCIL |
|---|---|---|---|---|---|
| *Plasma half-life*[a] | Spontaneous reaction, very short lived radicals. | $t_{1/2\beta}$ = 3–10 h (parent); = 1.6 h (aldophos); = 8.7 h (phospor. mustard) | $t_{1/2\beta}$ = 15 h | $t_{1/2\beta}$ = 1.5 h | $t_{1/2\beta}$ = 25–90 min |
| *Routes of elimination* | Renal | Hepatic metabolism by P450 (CYP2B) with active metabolites and urinary excretion | Hepatic metabolism by P450 (CYP3A) with active metabolites and urinary excretion (70–80%) | Renal, chemical decomposition to inert dechlorinated products (10–15% unchanged in urine) | Hepatic metabolism, chemical decomposition to active phenylacetic acid mustard <1% unchanged in urine |
| *Routes of administration* | IV and PO | IV and PO (bioavailability ~100%) | IV | IV, IP, and PO (bioavailability ~30%, highly variable) | PO (bioavailability ~50%) |
| *Major toxicities*[b] | • BMS<br>• N/V | • Leukopenia (stem cell sparing)<br>• Alopecia | • Leukopenia<br>• Alopecia<br>• Bladder toxicity | • BMS | • Lymphopenia, leukopenia (nadir in 3 wk) |
| *Less common toxicities* | • Menstrual irregularities<br>• Ototoxicity<br>• Reactivation of zoster | • Hemorrhagic cystitis<br>• Cardiac<br>• Thrombocytopenia<br>• SIADH<br>• Acute myopericarditis | • Hemorrhagic cystitis<br>• CNS toxicity (encephalopathy)<br>• Alopecia | • Allergic reaction<br>• Mucositis | • GI discomfort<br>• Seizures<br>• Dermatologic (EM, EN, SJ) |
| *Major indications* | • Hodgkin disease<br>• Intracavitary use for malignant pleural effusions | • Burkitt's lymphoma<br>• Hodgkin disease<br>• Breast/ovary<br>• Pretransplant<br>• Leukemia | • Sarcoma<br>• Lymphoma<br>• Bladder<br>• Germ cell<br>• Ovary | • Myeloma<br>• Pretransplant<br>• Ovarian | • CLL and low-grade lymphoma |
| *Comments** | • Severe vesicant | • Mesna prevents cystitis | • Mesna (as for cyclophosphamide) | | |

[a]Pharmacokinetic data summarized from Alberts et al. 1979a, 1979b, Alberts et al. 1980; Sladek et al. 1984; Brade et al. 1985; Struck et al. 1987.
[b]Pulmonary fibrosis, teratogenesis, infertility, and leukemogenesis common to all alkylating agents.
ABBREVIATIONS: BMS, bone marrow suppression; CLL, chronic lymphocytic leukemia; EM, erythema multiforme; EN, epidermal necrolysis; min, minute(s); N/V, nausea and vomiting; SIADH, syndrome of inappropriate antidiuretic hormone release; SJ, Stevens-Johnson syndrome.

and the drug is well tolerated (Grochow and Colvin 1979). Higher oral doses (500 mg or greater) may produce nausea and vomiting. When the drug is administered IV, extravasation does not produce tissue injury as in the case of mechlorethamine and doxorubicin.

**ADVERSE EFFECTS** As with all alkylating agents, bone marrow suppression is the limiting adverse effect of this drug (nadir 10 to 14 days after a single dose) (see Table 13-14). Cyclophosphamide is relatively platelet-sparing, and leukopenia is the dose-limiting toxicity. Hemorrhagic cystitis is occasionally seen with this drug and is caused by the metabolite acrolein, which accumulates in the urine and bladder. Vigorous hydration, especially when high doses of the drug are used, helps to decrease the incidence of this adverse effect. With larger doses (500 mg/m$^2$ or greater), severe nausea and vomiting are seen, typically 8 to 12 hours after drug administration. The delayed onset of nausea and vomiting is presumably due to conversion of cyclophosphamide to more emetogenic metabolites. Pulmonary toxicity (fibrosis) and cardiac toxicity (acute hemorrhagic carditis) may occur, especially in high-dose transplant regimens. The dose of cyclophosphamide in a single course is usually 1 to 1.5 g/m$^2$, but larger doses are tolerated when followed with G-CSF support or hematopoietic stem cell transfusions (Neidhart et al. 1992; Demetri et al. 1992).

Other uncommon toxicities include the syndrome of inappropriate ADH (SIADH) release (Buckner et al. 1972) and hiccups, although more long-term toxicities include infertility and secondary malignancies. Cyclophosphamide appears to be less carcinogenic than other alkylating agents, in particular when compared with melphalan and mechlorethamine.

**CLINICAL USE** Cyclophosphamide is used in combination regimens to treat lymphoma (CHOP), breast cancer (CMF), small-cell lung cancer, and ovarian cancer. The drug has an important use as part of high-dose regimens in bone marrow transplantation programs and is used widely as an immunosuppressant (Grochow and Colvin 1979).

### *Ifosfamide*

**HISTORY** This analog of cyclophosphamide differs from cyclophosphamide only in the location of a chloroethyl moiety (Fig. 13-16).

**MECHANISM OF ACTION AND CLINICAL PHARMACOLOGY** Activation of ifosfamide also occurs predominantly in the liver by the P450 mixed-function oxidase system, generating ifosfamide mustard, the active compound (Table 13-14). Acrolein and chloroacetic acid are the principal toxic metabolites (Colvin 1982). The plasma disappearance of ifosfamide is slightly longer than that of cyclophosphamide, and some of the compound is excreted unchanged in the urine (Allen et al. 1976).

**ADVERSE REACTIONS** The dose-limiting toxicity of this drug is bladder toxicity, presumably because of accumulation of acrolein and chloroacetic acid in the bladder (Creaven et al. 1976) (see Table 13-14). Dose fractionation and vigorous hydration with diuretics decreases this toxicity. Mesna, a thiol that is excreted in the urine, is now used routinely in ifosfamide-containing regimens because of its ability to inactivate the toxic metabolites of ifosfamide in the bladder. Mesna is generally well tolerated but may cause some nausea and vomiting. The nausea and vomiting produced by ifosfamide are less than that observed with large doses of cyclophosphamide, as is the degree of myelosuppression (Table 13-14). Central nervous system toxicity is occasionally seen in patients treated with high doses of ifosfamide and mesna and is manifested by changes in mental status, cerebellar dysfunction, and even seizures (Pratt et al. 1986).

**CLINICAL USE** Ifosfamide, like cyclophosphamide, has a broad spectrum of antineoplastic activity. It appears to be effective even in patients resistant to cyclophosphamide. Antitumor effects are seen in patients with lymphoma, ovarian cancer, sarcomas, and testicular cancer and in various solid tumors. Ifosfamide is also used in combination regimens to treat patients with these diseases who have relapsed following first-line regimens.

### *Melphalan*

**HISTORY** Melphalan (l-phenylalanine mustard) is a bifunctional alkylating agent and, like others in this class, causes interstrand, intrastrand, and DNA-protein cross-links (Sarosy et al. 1988) (see Fig. 13-16). Melphalan, like cyclophosphamide, is active orally, although an IV preparation is available as an investigational drug.

**MECHANISM OF ACTION AND CLINICAL PHARMACOLOGY** Studies indicate that this drug is absorbed erratically (Alberts, Chang, et al. 1979a).

> **PRINCIPLE** **Patients using this drug should receive a dose resulting in a fixed endpoint (e.g., leukopenia) or have concentrations measured in the blood to be certain that an effective dose is obtained.**

**ADVERSE EFFECTS** In the usual therapeutic doses administered orally, melphalan is well tolerated, and its major limiting toxicity is myelosuppression (see Table 13-14). Alopecia is sometimes seen, and pulmonary fibrosis has been reported to occur in patients on this drug for long periods. High-dose IV regimens used with autologous peripheral stem cell rescue cause more serious GI toxicity (nausea, vomiting, diarrhea, mucositis), as well as profound bone marrow toxicity (Hersh et al. 1983; Lazarus et al. 1987).

**CLINICAL USE** Melphalan is used to treat myeloma and ovarian and breast cancer, but it has been mainly supplanted in the treatment of these latter diseases by cyclophosphamide. Because melphalan may be used in high doses without major adverse effects other than bone marrow toxicity, it is used in high-dose regimens with peripheral stem cell transplants in patients with myeloma and other malignancies.

### *Chlorambucil*

Chlorambucil, as with melphalan, is an orally administered alkylating agent (Fig. 13-16). Its mechanism of action is believed to be similar to that of the other nitrogen mustards.

**CLINICAL PHARMACOLOGY AND ADVERSE EFFECTS** The absorption of this slow-acting nitrogen mustard is usually consistent (Alberts et al. 1979b). It is well tolerated, usually without nausea and vomiting, even when used as a pulse treatment (5 days once a month) or in continuous daily administration. The dose-limiting toxicity is myelosuppression; occasional liver abnormalities and pulmonary fibrosis have been reported with long-term use (Cole et al. 1978). Like all the alkylating agents, this drug can cause secondary leukemias and sterility (Table 13-2).

**CLINICAL USE** The major use of chlorambucil is to treat patients with CLL or low-grade non-Hodgkin lymphoma (Portlock et al. 1987).

## Nitrosoureas and Other Nonclassical Alkylating Agents

### *Carmustine and lomustine*

**HISTORY** Carmustine (BCNU, bis-chloroethyl-nitrosourea) was the first of the nitrosourea compounds in clinical trial to receive extensive clinical evaluation (see Fig. 13-16). An unusual feature of these highly reactive compounds is their lipid solubility and their ability to cross the blood–brain barrier (Walker 1973). Lomustine (CCNU, 1-(2-chloroethyl)-3-cyclohexyl-1-nitrosourea) is similar to carmustine in its mechanism of action and clinical activity. It is administered orally and is rapidly absorbed and biotransformed (Woolley 1983).

**MECHANISM OF ACTION** The nitrosoureas, in particular carmustine and lomustine, have been extensively studied in animal tumor models and in the clinic (Schein et al. 1984). The nitrosoureas show some degree of cross-resistance with other alkylating agents, and recent studies indicate that these compounds are primarily alkylating agents. A base-catalyzed decomposition of these compounds generates the alkylating chloroethyldiazonium hydroxide entity (Colvin et al. 1976).

**CLINICAL PHARMACOLOGY** After IV administration, carmustine disappears from plasma with an initial half-life of 6 minutes and an elimination $t_{1/2}$ of 68 minutes (see Table 13-15).

**ADVERSE EFFECTS** The nitrosoureas, like other alkylating agents, are potent bone marrow suppressants (see Table 13-15). However, the hemopoietic depression produced by the nitrosoureas typically occurs later than that seen with the other alkylating agents. Because leukocyte and platelet nadirs typically occur 4 to 5 weeks after administration of the drugs, the nitrosoureas are thought to affect an early primitive stem cell. The late marrow depression and cumulative toxicity make these drugs difficult to use clinically. Nausea and vomiting occur frequently with the nitrosoureas, and nephrotoxicity has been associated with the drug as well. Although both carmustine and lomustine may produce hepatotoxicity, this adverse effect is less common with lomustine. A large adjuvant study of lomustine plus 5-FU by the Gastrointestinal Tumor Study Group has shown that treatment with this combination was associated with an increased incidence of acute leukemia, presumably attributable to the nitrosourea (Boice et al. 1983).

**CLINICAL USES** Nitrosoureas have a reasonably broad spectrum of activity, and currently they are used in the treatment of lymphoma as well as certain solid tumors, in particular brain tumors. Their use in the treatment of GI cancer has diminished, except for the intrahepatic arterial infusion administered for colorectal metastasis to the liver, as second-line therapy.

### *Streptozotocin*

Streptozotocin is a methylnitrosourea isolated from *Streptomyces sp.* that was first studied in clinical trials in 1967 (for a review, see Weiss 1982). The chemical structure of streptozotocin is shown in Fig. 13-16

**MECHANISM OF ACTION AND CLINICAL PHARMACOLOGY** Like the other nitrosoureas, this drug functions as an alkylating agent. Its plasma half-life is short (35 minutes), and the drug is excreted in the urine as metabolites (Adolphe et al. 1975). Streptozotocin is selectively lethal to the $\beta$-islet cells of the pancreas and causes diabetes in animals.

**ADVERSE EFFECTS** The dose-limiting adverse effect of streptozotocin is nephrotoxicity (see Table 13-15). Drug-induced diabetes is not seen in humans as a result of treatment, but mild glucose intolerance may occur. As

Table 13-15 **Clinical Pharmacology of Alkylating Agents: Nitrosoureas and Other Nonclassical Alkylating Agents**

| Pharmacologic Parameter | Carmustine | Lomustine | Streptozotocin | Procarbazine | Dacarbazine |
|---|---|---|---|---|---|
| *Plasma half-life*[a] | $t_{1/2\alpha}$ = 15–90 min<br>$t_{1/2\beta}$ = 2–4 h | $t_{1/2}$ = 94 min<br>$t_{1/2}$ = 16–48 h (metabolites) | $t_{1/2\alpha}$ = 15–90 min<br>*Metabolites*<br>$t_{1/2\beta}$ = 3.5 h<br>$t_{1/2\gamma}$ = 40 h | $t_{1/2\alpha}$ = 15–90 min | $t_{1/2\alpha}$ = 19 min<br>$t_{1/2\beta}$ = 25–90 min |
| *Routes of elimination* | 30–80% excreted in urine within 24 h, <1% unchanged, mineralization | Metabolites in urine, some mineralization | Hepatic metabolism, only 10–20% recovered in urine. | >75% Renal excretion of metabolites in first 24 h | 50% of drug recovered in urine, majority unchanged |
| *Routes of administration* | IV | PO | IV | PO (bioavailability ~100%) | IV |
| *Major toxicities*[b] | • Leukopenia (nadir 5–6 wk)<br>• Pulmonary fibrosis<br>• N/V | • Leukopenia<br>• Nephrotoxicity<br>• Pulmonary toxicity | • Nephrotoxicity (RTA, glycosuria, proteinuria, proximal tubule) | • BMS<br>• N/V | • BMS<br>• N/V |
| *Less common toxicities* | • Flushing<br>• Hepatic toxicity (>1 g/m$^2$)<br>• Nephrotoxicity<br>• Alopecia | Neurotoxicity (slurred speech, fatigue, confusion)<br>• Stomatitis | • N/V<br>• Hypoglycemia (diabetes)<br>• BMS<br>• Hepatotoxicity | • Cutaneous and pulmonary hypersensitivity<br>• Hepatic toxicity | • Flulike syndrome/facial flushing<br>• Anaphylaxis<br>• Hepatotoxicity |
| *Major indications* | • Lymphoma<br>• Glioblastoma | • Lymphoma (salvage) | • Pancreatic islet cell carcinoma<br>• Carcinoid | • Hodgkin disease<br>• Glioma | • Melanoma<br>• Hodgkin disease<br>• Sarcoma |
| *Comments* | • Lipophilic; crosses blood–brain barrier<br>• Implants for brain tumors | • Lipophilic; crosses blood–brain barrier | • Serial urine proteins assess renal toxicity<br>• Phenytoin may protect islet cells | • Disulfiram reaction with alcohol<br>• Can act as MAO inhibitor | • Half-life increased markedly with hepatic or renal disease |

[a]Pharmacokinetic data summarized from Henner et al. 1986; Levin et al. 1978; Shiba and Weinkam 1982; Breithaupt Pralle, et al. 1982.
[b]Pulmonary fibrosis, teratogenesis, infertility, and leukemogenesis are common to all alkylating agents.
ABBREVIATIONS: BMS, bone marrow suppression; MAO, monoamine oxidase; N/V, nausea and vomiting; RTA, renal tubular acidosis.

with the other nitrosoureas, nausea and vomiting may be severe. Unlike carmustine and lomustine, little or no bone marrow suppression is seen after streptozotocin administration, thus allowing it to be used in various combination regimens containing a myelosuppressive agent.

**CLINICAL USE** The major use for streptozotocin is in the treatment of carcinoid and islet cell tumors (Table 13-15). It has also been used in combinations to treat Hodgkin disease and colon cancer, but its role in these diseases is not well defined.

### *Dacarbazine*

Although dacarbazine (DTIC, dimethyl-triazeno-imidazole-carboxamide) is structurally similar to the purine precursor 5-aminoimidazole-4-carboxamide, DTIC acts primarily as an alkylating agent (Bono 1976). Its structure is shown in Fig. 13-17.

**MECHANISM OF ACTION AND CLINICAL PHARMACOLOGY** Dacarbazine is activated by the hepatic cytochrome P450 system, which generates a reactive methyl derivative. The elimination $t_{1/2}$ is about 5 hours, and about half

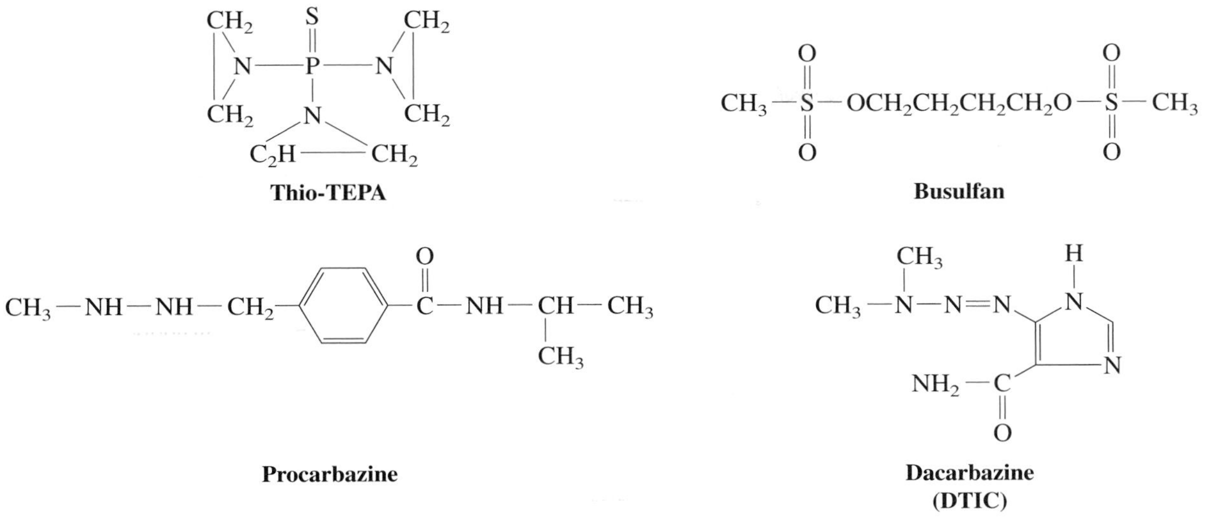

**Thio-TEPA**

**Busulfan**

$CH_3-SO_2-OCH_2CH_2CH_2CH_2O-SO_2-CH_3$

**Procarbazine**

$CH_3-NH-NH-CH_2-C_6H_4-C(=O)-NH-CH(CH_3)-CH_3$

**Dacarbazine (DTIC)**

**FIGURE 13-17 Chemical structures of the alkylating agents thiotepa (an ethyleneimine), busulfan (an alkyl sulfonate), and procarbazine and dacarbazine [DTIC] (nonclassical alkylating agents).**

the drug is excreted in the urine unchanged, although the remainder appears as metabolites.

**ADVERSE REACTIONS** Severe nausea and vomiting occur when therapeutic doses of DTIC are used. Myelosuppression is uncommon when used at standard doses, although, occasionally, severe bone marrow toxicity has been observed. Other toxic effects include a flulike syndrome and facial flushing (Spiegel 1981). Hepatotoxicity has occasionally been noted (Frosch et al. 1979). Dacarbazine may cause severe pain and tissue necrosis if infiltration occurs.

**CLINICAL USE** Dacarbazine is used in combination with Adriamycin (doxorubicin), bleomycin, and vinblastine (ABVD regimen) to treat Hodgkin disease and is used in combinations to treat soft-tissue sarcoma and malignant melanoma (Table 13-15).

### *Procarbazine*

This drug (Fig. 13-17) requires activation by the hepatic cytochrome P450 system in liver to produce several active metabolites that produce effects on DNA similar to those of classic alkylating agents (Weikam and Shiba 1982).

**CLINICAL PHARMACOLOGY AND ADVERSE EFFECTS** Procarbazine is administered orally and is well absorbed. The drug equilibrates rapidly between plasma and the CSF. The half-life of the parent compound is 10 minutes. The drug is excreted mainly in the urine in the form of oxidized metabolites (Breithaupt et al. 1982). Nausea and vomiting commonly occur with the use of this drug, but tolerance develops rapidly to these adverse effects. The major toxic effect, myelosuppression, is dose-related. Foods with a high tyramine content may precipitate a reaction that includes severe headache because this drug is a weak monoamine oxidase inhibitor (DeVita et al. 1967). Interactions with sympathomimetic amines, tricyclic antidepressants, and alcohol have also been reported (Weiss et al. 1974; Warren and Bender 1977). Neurotoxicities that include dizziness, ataxia, paresthesia, headache, insomnia, and nightmares occur, especially in patients who are receiving centrally acting psychotropic medications (Weiss et al. 1974).

**CLINICAL USE** The major indication for procarbazine is as part of the MOPP regimen for the treatment of Hodgkin disease (see Table 13-15) (DeVita et al. 1970). Procarbazine also has been used to treat other neoplasms including non-Hodgkin lymphoma, lung cancer, and brain tumors.

## Ethyleneimine- and Alkyl-Alkane-Sulfonate-Based Alkylating Agents

### *Thiotepa*

Thiotepa (triethylenethiophosphoramide) is an ethylenimine type of alkylating agent (Fig. 13-17). It is lipophilic and thus is able to penetrate the CNS to achieve relatively high concentrations in CSF (Edwards et al. 1979).

**MECHANISM OF ACTION AND CLINICAL PHARMACOLOGY** Thiotepa is believed to act by alkylating DNA, similar to the nitrogen mustards (see Table 13-16). It may be administered both orally and intravenously and has been given intravesically, intra-arterially, and IM, because it is not a vesicant. When it is used by local instillation to treat superficial bladder cancer and malignant effusions, absorption and systemic toxicity are possible.

**CLINICAL USE** There is a resurgence of interest in thiotepa because it may be used in high doses with other agents followed by autologous bone marrow transplant. In addition to dose-limiting myelosuppression, other adverse effects may be seen with these high doses, including mucositis, skin rash, and CNS toxicity (Lazarus et al. 1987) (see Table 13-16). Although early studies showed antitumor effects in breast, lung, ovarian, and hematologic malignancies, its use, except for marrow transplantation, is generally restricted to intravesicular administration for superficial bladder cancer.

### *Busulfan*

Busulfan is an alkyl sulfonate type of alkylating agent (Fig. 13-17).

**CLINICAL PHARMACOLOGY** Busulfan is available for oral use; it is well absorbed with an elimination half-life of about 2 to 5 hours (see Table 13-16). It is eliminated following hepatic metabolism and is excreted mainly as metabolites in the urine (Ehrsson et al. 1983).

**ADVERSE EFFECTS** The dose-limiting toxicity is myelosuppression, primarily of the myeloid elements. Other less common adverse effects are mild nausea, gynecomastia, hyperpigmentation, and transient elevation of liver enzymes. Long-term treatment may cause pulmonary fibrosis.

**CLINICAL USE** In contrast to the other alkylating agents, in particular the nitrosoureas and nitrogen mustards, busulfan has a more marked effect on cells in the

Table 13-16 Clinical Pharmacology of Alkylating Agents: Thiotepa and Busulfan

| Pharmacologic Parameter | Busulfan | Thiotepa |
|---|---|---|
| *Plasma half-life*[a] | $t_{1/2}$ = 2–3 h | $t_{1/2}$ = 1.2–2 h |
| *Routes of elimination* | Hepatic metabolism by P450, renal excretion | Hepatic metabolism by P450, renal excretion |
| *Routes of administration* | PO | IV, intravesical, IT, IM |
| *Major toxicities* | • BMS/neutropenia (stem cell toxic)<br>• N/V | • BMS/neutropenia<br>• N/V<br>• Gonadal dysfunction |
| *Less common toxicities* | • Pulmonary fibrosis<br>• Hyperpigmentation<br>• Gynecomastia<br>• Increase in transaminases | • CNS effects (seizures, altered mental status)<br>• Mucositis<br>• Skin rash |
| *Major indications* | • CML<br>• Myeloablation pretransplant<br>• Myeloproliferative disorders<br>• Gonadal dysfunction | • Intracavitary instillation (for bladder cancer, and control of effusions)<br>• Brain tumors<br>• Transplant |
| *Comments* | • "Busulfan lung" can appear up to one decade following treatment | • Is not a vesicant<br>• Lipophilic |

[a]Pharmacokinetic data summarized from Cohen et al. 1986; Vassal et al. 1993.

ABBREVIATIONS: BMS, bone marrow suppression; CML, chronic myelogenous leukemia; CNS, central nervous system; IT, intrathecal; IM, intramuscular; N/V, nausea and vomiting; P450, cytochrome P450/mixed function oxidase.

myeloid lineage, accounting for its greater activity in CML. Busulfan-based treatment of CML has largely been supplanted by other agents (hydroxyurea, interferon $\alpha$) (Table 13-16). It can reduce the leukocytosis and splenomegaly associated with CML but does not delay the onset of transformation to blast crisis. It is also used in regimens with cyclophosphamide to ablate bone marrow function. Blood levels must be carefully monitored because of the erratic absorption as well as to avoid pulmonary toxicity. Parenteral formulations are being developed that may be more useful.

## Platinum Compounds

### *Cisplatin*

**HISTORY** Cisplatin (*cis*-diamminedichloroplatinum, CDDP) is a platinum coordination complex that has broad-spectrum antitumor activity in humans (Fig. 13-18). The story of its discovery is one of serendipity and the prepared scientific mind.

In experiments with bacteria, Rosenberg noted that a toxic substance was being produced by platinum electrodes (Rosenberg et al. 1965). He found this compound to be the platinum coordination complex, *cis*-diamminedichloroplatinum, and he subsequently investigated its cytotoxic effects on mammalian tumor cells as well as bacteria. These results prompted a clinical trial in humans, and, despite some antitumor activity in early phase I trials, further trials were stopped because of renal toxicity. The drug was then found to be relatively safe when administered with forced hydration and is now an important drug with a wide spectrum of clinical activity.

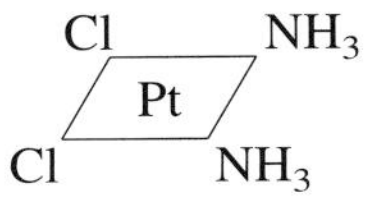

**Cisplatin**
**(Platinol)**

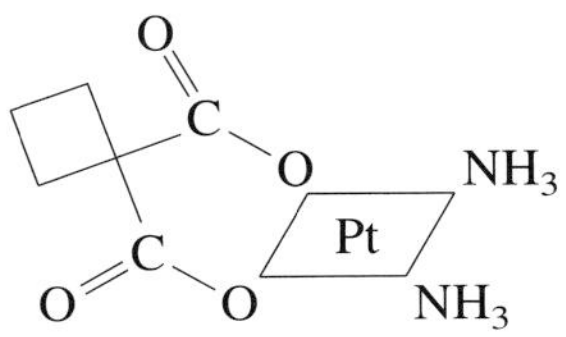

**Carboplatin**
**(Paraplatine)**

**FIGURE 13-18 Chemical structures of the platinum-based drugs, including cisplatin and carboplatin. The antineoplastic activity is strongly dependent on the rate and degree of aquation, where the chlorine atoms become displaced by -OH moieties from water.**

**MECHANISM OF ACTION** Cisplatin is a reactive molecule that can form inter- and intrastrand cross-links in DNA and can also cross-link proteins with DNA.

Drug-resistant cell lines have been produced, and resistance has been attributed to various mechanisms including decreased uptake, an increase in repair of DNA lesions, and an increase of the metal-binding protein metallothionein.

**CLINICAL PHARMACOLOGY** Cisplatin is administered IV with forced hydration (see Table 13-17). Following administration, the drug is rapidly bound to protein and persists in serum for extended periods, with only 20 to 40% excreted in the urine within the first few days following drug administration. High concentrations of platinum, as measured by atomic absorption spectrophotometry, persist in the liver, intestines, and kidney (Reed and Kohn 1990).

**ADVERSE EFFECTS** The dose-limiting toxicity of cisplatin is nephrotoxicity due to tubular injury (see Table 13-17). This complication may be largely but not completely avoided by vigorous hydration, before and after administration of cisplatin. The use of 3% sodium chloride may allow even higher doses to be safely administered because chloride ion may decrease activation of this compound and renal injury (Ozols et al. 1984). Hypomagnesemia may also result from tubular damage (Schilsky et al. 1982). Cisplatin is also a very potent emetogenic drug. The severe nausea and vomiting caused by this drug can be controlled by aggressive antiemetic therapy with serotonin antagonists like ondansetron and granisetron (Hubbard and Jenkins 1990). Myelosuppression is not a major adverse effect caused by cisplatin, although anemia has been noted frequently in patients receiving multiple courses of the drug. Neurotoxicity including peripheral neuropathy and ototoxicity, especially high-frequency hearing loss, is a problem in patients receiving multiple courses of cisplatin (Mead et al. 1982). On rare occasions, immunoglobulin-mediated hypersensitivity reactions have been noted (Hood 1986).

**CLINICAL USES** Cisplatin has significant antitumor activity in ovarian, testicular, lung, bladder, and head and neck carcinomas (Table 13-17). Of great importance is its ability, when used in combination, to give additive or synergistic activity. The use of cisplatin with vinblastine and

Table 13-17 **Clinical Pharmacology of Platinum Compounds**

| Pharmacologic Parameter | Cisplatin | Carboplatin |
|---|---|---|
| *Plasma half-life*[a] | $t_{1/2\alpha} = 25\text{–}49$ min<br>$t_{1/2\beta} = 60$ min<br>$t_{1/2\gamma} = 24$ h | $t_{1/2\alpha} = 12\text{–}24$ min<br>$t_{1/2\beta} = 1.3\text{–}1.7$ h<br>$t_{1/2\gamma} = 22\text{–}40$ h |
| *Routes of elimination* | 25% of dose excreted in first 24 h, ~90% by renal ~10% biliary | 90% excreted in urine in first 24 h |
| *Routes of administration* | IV | IV |
| *Major toxicities* | • Peripheral neuropathy<br>• Renal insufficiency<br>• N/V | • BMS—in particular, thrombocytopenia<br>• N/V |
| *Less common toxicities* | • BMS<br>• Seizures<br>• Ototoxicity | • Nephrotoxicity |
| *Major indications* | • Testicular<br>• Ovarian<br>• Head and neck<br>• Bladder<br>• Lung (non-small-cell)<br>• Lymphoma | Same as cisplatin |
| *Comments* | • Incompatible with aluminum (e.g., needles) | • Reduce dose in proportion to creatinine clearance<br>• Calvert formula for dose calculation[b] |

[a]Pharmacokinetic data summarized from Belt et al. 1979; Chary et al. 1977; Corden et al. 1985; Curt et al. 1983.
[b]*Calvert formula:* Carboplatin dose (mg) = Target AUC (mg/mL × min) × [GFR (mL/min) + 25] GFR (or creatinine clearance) is calculated as follows:

$$CL_{Cr} = \frac{\text{weight (kg)} \times (140 - \text{age})}{72 \times \text{serum creatinine (mg/dL)}}$$

For women, multiply by 0.85.
ABBREVIATIONS: BMS, bone marrow suppression; min, minute(s); N/V, nausea and vomiting.

bleomycin, or more recently with etoposide, has led to a high cure rate (77%) in patients with advanced testicular cancer. In combination with paclitaxel, cisplatin is the treatment of choice in ovarian cancer, producing a high response rate and some long-term remissions. Cisplatin and 5-FU infusions are also highly effective in causing tumor regression in patients with squamous cell carcinoma of the head and neck, although the remissions produced are only temporary.

### *Carboplatin*

This platinum complex has recently been approved by the FDA for the treatment of refractory ovarian cancer (Fig. 13-18). It has the same mechanism of action as cisplatin and exhibits some cross-resistance with that drug. A major advantage of carboplatin over cisplatin is its lack of nephrotoxicity, thus allowing it to be administered without aggressive hydration. However, the dose-limiting toxicity of carboplatin is myelosuppression (Table 13-17).

## Antitumor Antibiotics

### *Bleomycin*

HISTORY Bleomycin is a mixture of peptides (Fig. 13-19). It is produced by the fungus *Streptomyces verticillus* and was first isolated by Umezawa et al. (1966).

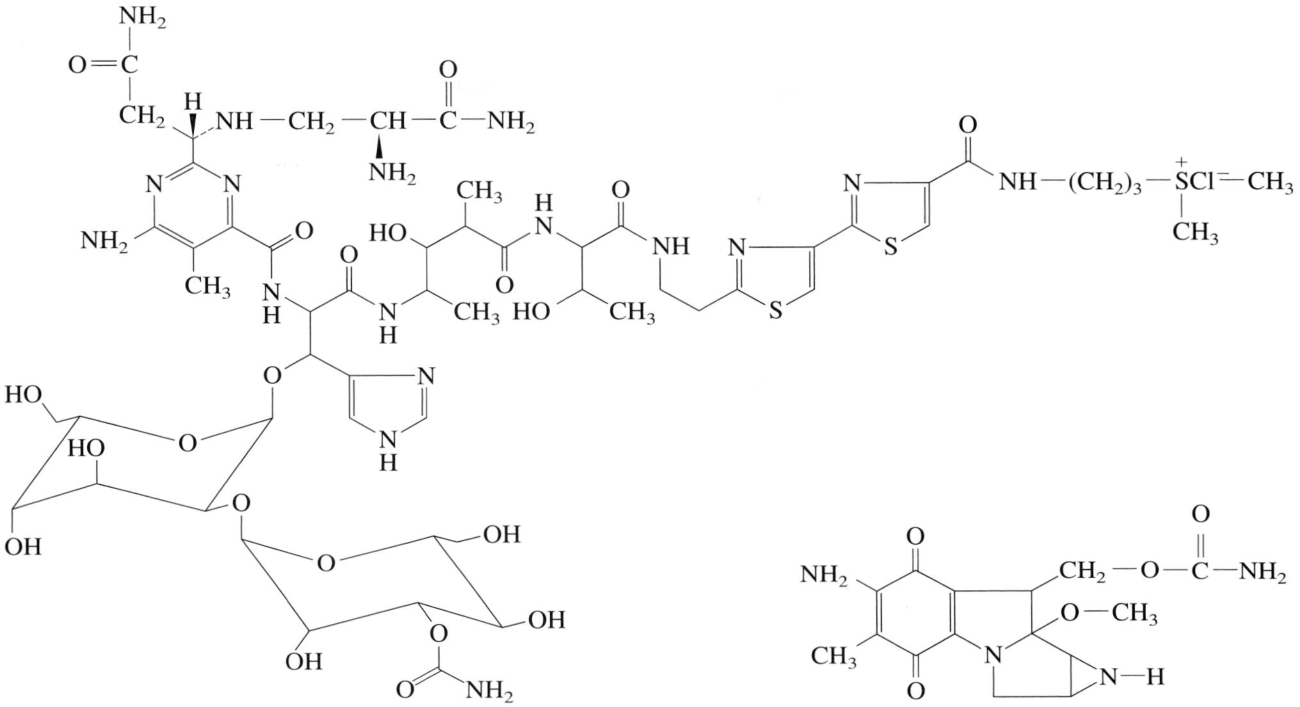

Bleomycin $A_2$

Mitomycin C

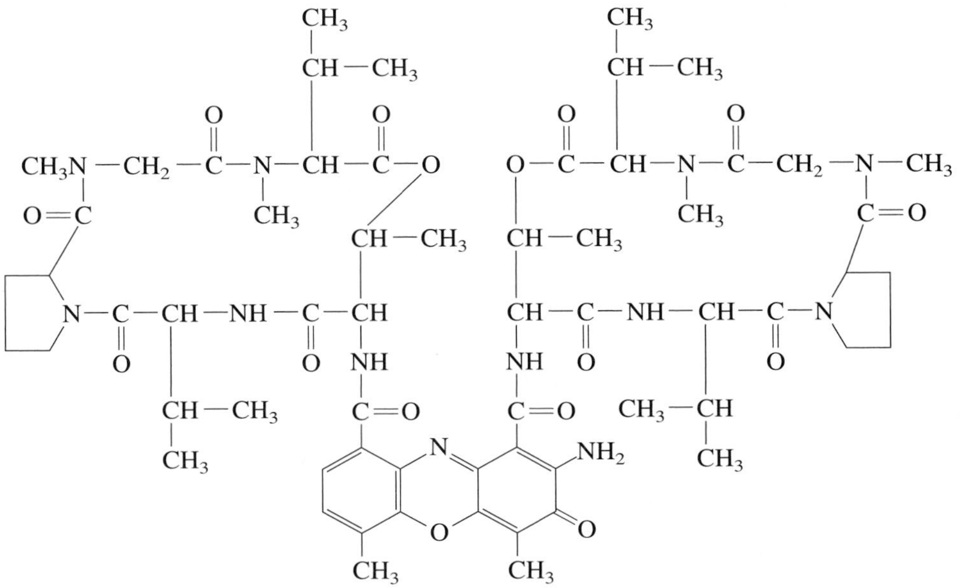

Actinomycin D

FIGURE 13-19 **Chemical structures of the antitumor antibiotics bleomycin A2, actinomycin D and mitomycin C. Clinically employed preparations of bleomycin are actually a mixture of peptides formulated as a sulfate salt. Bleomycin $A_2$ is the predominant peptide.**

**MECHANISM OF ACTION** Bleomycin causes both single- and double-strand DNA breaks as a consequence of production of an Fe(II) complex that generates toxic free radicals (Burger et al. 1986). Recently, one possible explanation offered for the known tumor- and organ-specific toxicity of bleomycin is the relative inactivity, or absence, of a bleomycin-inactivating enzyme, bleomycin hydrolase (Umezawa et al. 1974; Lazo and Humphries 1983). Of note is the lack of bleomycin hydrolase activity in the lung and skin, two organs that are adversely affected by this drug. Cell killing is maximal in cells in the $G_2$ phase of the cell cycle. Bleomycin may be considered a cell cycle–active agent (Table 13-3).

**CLINICAL PHARMACOLOGY** Bleomycin may be administered either IV or IM for the treatment of tumors, and intrapleurally or intraperitoneally for control of malignant effusions (Alberts et al. 1978; Alberts et al. 1979; Howell et al. 1987) (see Table 13-18). Some preclinical data support the use of this drug in a continuous infusion, but definitive data on this issue are lacking in humans (Carlson and Sikic 1983; Vogelzang 1984). After a single IV injection, the drug disappears rapidly with over one-half of the dose excreted in the urine within 24 hours. The elimination half-life has been estimated to be about 2 to 3 hours. Although there are no exact guidelines for the use of this drug in patients with renal impairment, reduction of the dose should be considered.

**ADVERSE EFFECTS** As mentioned, bleomycin has little to no effect on normal bone marrow. However, in patients given other myelosuppressive drugs or recovering from marrow toxicity due to other agents, additional mild myelosuppression may be observed (Table 13-18).

The two major toxicities that may result from bleomycin are pulmonary fibrosis and skin changes (Muggia et al. 1983). The risk of pulmonary toxicity is related to the cumulative dose and increases to 10% in patients administered more than 450 mg (Blum et al. 1973). This risk is magnified in patients over the age of 70, in those with underlying lung disease (particularly when they are receiving supplemental oxygen), and when large single doses of the drug are administered (25 mg/m$^2$ or more). However, a small percentage of patients (2 to 3%) without these risk factors may also develop pulmonary toxicity, even at relatively low doses. Although some improvement in the pulmonary toxicity may be seen on discontinuation of the drug, any resulting pulmonary fibrosis tends to be irreversible. Steroids have been used to counter this toxicity with probable benefit (Yagoda et al. 1972).

The toxic effects of bleomycin on the skin are also dose-related. When the drug is given in conventional daily doses for longer than 2 to 3 weeks, erythema, hyperkeratosis, and even frank ulceration may occur. Areas of skin pressure, especially on the hands, fingers, and joints, are initially affected. Nail changes and alopecia also may occur with continued use of the drug. In combination regimens where bleomycin is used intermittently in lower doses (e.g., ABVD regimen), these skin toxicities are usually not seen. Fever and malaise are common symptoms caused by bleomycin and may be alleviated with acetaminophen. Hypersensitivity reactions have also been observed with bleomycin therapy. A peculiar type of idiosyncratic cardiovascular collapse has been noted particularly in lymphoma patients, but this is rare. A 1-mg test dose may be useful in detecting patients who may be at risk for life-threatening adverse reactions (Bennett and Reich 1979).

**CLINICAL PHARMACOLOGY AND CLINICAL USES** Bleomycin is a "selective" drug, that is, it can exert antitumor effects with little or no marrow toxicity (see Table 13-18). The drug is used as part of combination regimens to treat Hodgkin disease (ABVD), non-Hodgkin lymphomas, and testicular cancer.

### *Dactinomycin*

Dactinomycin (actinomycin D) is an antibiotic with antineoplastic activity that is produced by *Streptomyces parvullus*. It is composed of a phenoxazone ring structure, to which two identical cyclic peptide chains are bound (Fig. 13-19).

**MECHANISM OF ACTION** Dactinomycin binds to DNA, with the polypeptide chains binding in the minor grove of the DNA helix (Sobell et al. 1971). Intercalation is a result of a specific interaction between these chains and deoxyguanosine. Few data are available on the mechanisms of resistance to dactinomycin in patients, or on the intrinsic or acquired resistance and sensitivity mechanisms in tumor models. In experimental systems, dactinomycin participates in the multidrug-resistance phenotype (Diddens et al. 1987).

**CLINICAL PHARMACOLOGY** The drug is rapidly cleared from the blood after an IV dose (see Table 13-18). Most is excreted unchanged in bile and urine. After an initial rapid disappearance phase from plasma (minutes), a slower phase (36-hour half-life) occurs (Tattersall, Sodegren, et al. 1975a).

**ADVERSE EFFECTS** The major dose-limiting toxicities to this drug are leukopenia and thrombocytopenia (Frei 1974). These effects reach a nadir 2 to 3 weeks after a

Table 13-18 **Clinical Pharmacology of Antitumor Antibiotics**

| PHARMACOLOGIC PARAMETER | BLEOMYCIN | DACTINOMYCIN | MITOMYCIN C |
|---|---|---|---|
| *Plasma half-life*[a] | $t_{1/2\alpha}$ = 24 min<br>$t_{1/2\beta}$ = 2–4 h | $t_{1/2\beta}$ = 36 h | $t_{1/2\beta}$ = 25–90 min |
| *Routes of elimination* | 45–70% excreted in urine, within 24 h largely unchanged | Minimal metabolism, 6–30% excreted in urine, 50% biliary unchanged | Hepatic metabolism, 1–20% excreted in urine unchanged |
| *Routes of administration* | IV | IV | IV |
| *Major toxicities* | • Pulmonary interstitial infiltrates/fibrosis (dose-related)<br>• Fever/chills<br>• Stomatitis | • BMS<br>• N/V | • Leukopenia and thrombocytopenia (nadir cumulative up to 8 wk) |
| *Less common toxicities* | • Skin toxicity<br>• Raynaud phenomenon<br>• Hypersensitivity<br>• Hepatotoxicity<br>• Alopecia | • Radiation recall<br>• Hepatotoxicity<br>• Immune thrombocytopenia | • Nephrotoxicity<br>• Hemolytic–uremic syndrome<br>• Interstitial pneumonitis |
| *Major indications* | • Lymphoma<br>• Kaposi sarcoma<br>• Head and neck cancers<br>• Testicular | • Choriocarcinoma<br>• Wilms tumor<br>• Rhabdomyosarcoma<br>• Testicular<br>• Ewing sarcoma | • Colon cancer<br>• Superficial bladder cancer<br>• Stomach cancer<br>• Pancreatic cancer |
| *Comments* | • Pulmonary toxicity increased with supplemental $O_2$, increasing age, prior RT.<br>• Dose adjust in renal failure | • Radiosensitizing agent<br>• Vesicant | • Vesicant |

[a]Pharmacokinetic data summarized from Alberts et al. 1978; Tattersall, Sodegren, et al. 1975b; Dorr 1988.
ABBREVIATIONS: BMS, bone marrow suppression; min, minute(s); N/V, nausea and vomiting; RT, renal transplant.

course of therapy. Nausea and vomiting are also common acute toxicities that begin within a few hours of treatment and may last as long as 24 hours. Other adverse effects noted with full doses of dactinomycin include stomatitis, cheilitis, glossitis, and proctitis (Table 13-18). Dactinomycin may cause radiation recall that can manifest as cutaneous erythema, desquamation, and hyperpigmentation in previously irradiated areas (D'Angio et al. 1959). Cellulitis and pain also can result if the drug extravasates. Alopecia and severe skin toxicity are occasionally seen.

**CLINICAL USE** Dactinomycin is still used to treat Wilms tumor, gestational choriocarcinoma, and embryonal rhabdomyosarcoma. Some regimens for osteosarcoma also include dactinomycin. Although this drug has significant activity in the treatment of testicular cancer, it has been supplanted by other more effective drugs.

### *Mitomycin C*

Mitomycin C is a quinone antibiotic, isolated from cultures of *Streptomyces caespitosus* (Fig. 13-19). The drug requires reduction to produce an activated molecule that can cross-link DNA strands, similar to alkylating agents (Reddy and Randerath 1987; Tomasz et al. 1987). It is this biochemical feature of mitomycin C that is thought to contribute to its effectiveness in the hypoxic and low redox environments found centrally in many large tumors.

**CLINICAL PHARMACOLOGY** After IV administration there is a rapid half-life of distribution (2 to 10 minutes) followed by an elimination half-life of 25 to 90 minutes (Dorr 1988) (see Table 13-18).

**ADVERSE EFFECTS** In addition to nausea and vomiting, which are commonly seen following administration of the drug, the major toxicity of mitomycin C is bone marrow suppression that is usually cumulative (see Table 13-18). The hematologic nadir usually occurs 3 to 5 weeks following administration. Extravasation results in severe tissue damage. Less common side effects are the potentially lethal hemolytic uremic syndrome, interstitial pneumonitis, and cardiomyopathy.

**CLINICAL USE** Mitomycin C is used in combination regimens in the treatment of lung (MVP) and GI cancers. It is currently being evaluated in combination with radiation for the treatment of head-and-neck cancer.

## Enzymes: Asparaginase

**HISTORY** In 1953, Kidd noted that the growth of certain transplantable lymphomas in the mouse were inhibited by guinea pig serum but not by other mammalian sera (Kidd 1953). After intensive investigation, Broome and coworkers in 1963 isolated the factor responsible for this antilymphoma activity and found it to be L-asparaginase (Crasnitin, Elspar) (Broome 1963).

**MECHANISM OF ACTION** This enzyme catalyzes the hydrolysis of asparagine to aspartic acid and ammonia. It rapidly depletes the serum of asparagine, which is necessary for the growth of certain lymphoid cells (Capizzi et al. 1970).

**CLINICAL PHARMACOLOGY** L-asparaginase is administered either IV or IM. After a single IV or IM dose, concentrations of the drug in serum are detectable for several days. Initially, the serum concentration of the enzyme falls quickly (within minutes of injection) to below detectable levels become measurable again 7 to 10 days after a single dose. The half-life of the enzyme in plasma is 14 to 24 hours. Polyethylene glycol (PEG) can be conjugated to L-asparaginase without compromising the active site of the enzyme. PEG conjugated enzyme decreases the probability of antibody formation against the enzyme, and significantly increases serum half-life (Keating et al. 1993).

**ADVERSE EFFECTS** A major problem with administration of L-asparaginase is hypersensitivity (Weiss and Bruno 1981). Reactions to the first dose are uncommon, but after the second or subsequent doses, allergic reactions may occur. These reactions vary from urticaria to anaphylaxis and may include hypotension, laryngospasm, and cardiac arrest. Skin testing to predict allergic reactions is minimally helpful. Hypersensitive patients may have serum antibodies to L-asparaginase. However, more than half the patients with such antibodies will not display an allergic reaction to the drug. Switching to an asparaginase derived from a different bacterial species can circumvent neutralizing antibodies in hypersensitive patients raised against other forms of the enzyme. PEG asparaginase has been shown to have significantly less allergic adverse effects, with equivalent therapeutic efficacy (Ettinger et al. 1995).

Patients who are treated with L-asparaginase should be observed carefully for several hours after drug administration. Epinephrine should be available in case of a life-threatening anaphylactic reaction. If an anaphylactic reaction occurs with the enzyme purified from *Escherichia coli*, the patient may still be treated with the enzyme from *Erwinia carotovora* because there is no cross-sensitivity between these preparations. Additional major toxicities caused by L-asparaginase are due to its ability to transiently inhibit protein synthesis in normal tissues. Inhibition of protein synthesis in the liver results in hypoalbuminemia, reductions in clotting factors, and decreases in serum lipoproteins. The clotting function abnormalities that are regularly observed as a consequence of treatment with L-asparaginase include prolongation of the prothrombin (PT), partial thromboplastin time (PTT), and thrombin time. A marked fall in plasma fibrinogen concentrations and a decrease in clotting factors IX and XI may also be observed. Despite continued treatment with this enzyme, these effects are transient. Other complications of L-asparaginase treatment when used in high-dose schedules are confusion, stupor, coma, and acute pancreatitis, which in some patients may progress to severe hemorrhagic pancreatitis. Inhibition of the production of insulin may lead to hyperglycemia.

**CLINICAL USES** The enzyme L-asparaginase is used to treat lymphoid malignancies, in particular ALL (null cell), T-cell leukemia, and T-cell lymphomas (Chabner and Loo 1996). This is one of the few circumstances in the chemotherapy of malignant disease in which a biochemical basis for selectivity is clear. These lymphoid malignancies are all asparagine auxotrophs, that is, they require exogenous L-asparagine for growth, and they obtain this amino acid primarily from the liver.

Because L-asparaginase has no or little toxicity to bone marrow or GI mucosa, the drug has been used in combination with other drugs. L-asparaginase ameliorates the toxic effects of drugs that inhibit DNA synthesis (e.g., MTX and ara-C). This reduction in toxicity probably results from the inability of cells to enter the S phase because of the block of protein synthesis caused by the enzyme, making them less susceptible to the cytotoxic effects of S-phase-specific agents. Based on the observation that null cells and T cells are not rescued from MTX treatment by L-asparaginase, although normal stem cells are, Capizzi (1975) devised a regimen in which MTX is followed 24 hours later by L-asparaginase. This combination is effective even in acute leukemia refractory to conventional doses of MTX (Lobel et al. 1979). The interval of treatment of MTX followed by L-asparaginase is ideally 10 days, because, as mentioned, it takes 7 to 10 days for the L-asparagine concentrations in the blood to recover after a single dose of L-asparaginase. At that time, the leukemia cells begin to proliferate and may be more sensitive to a repeat course of this treatment.

## Endocrine Agents

Cancer cells often exhibit susceptibility to hormonal control mechanisms that regulate growth of the normal tissue from which the neoplasm arose. Endocrine therapy appears to work generally through cytostatic rather than cytocidal mechanisms and usually requires long-term administration. Endocrine therapy includes the use of both hormones and "antihormones," which are either antagonists or partial agonists for a given endocrine mechanism. Inasmuch as the effects of hormones are receptor mediated, evaluation of a tumor's receptor status is an important determinant in selecting the appropriate hormonal intervention. The role of endocrine ablation procedures (hypophysectomy, adrenalectomy, oophorectomy, orchiectomy) has diminished as systemic agents have been identified that can replace surgical procedures. Dose schedules and applications of some major endocrine agents are summarized in Table 13-19.

### *Estrogens and antiestrogens*

Estrogens have therapeutic effects in cancer of the prostate and have been used in large doses to treat carcinoma of the breast. Orchiectomy is an equally efficacious treatment for prostate cancer and lacks feminizing side effects. To date, no evidence suggests an additive effect for the combination. For breast cancer, the antiestrogen tamoxifen (Nolvadex) is better tolerated than high-dose estrogen therapy. Tamoxifen improves survival of postmenopausal women with estrogen and/or progesterone receptor-positive breast cancer in both the adjuvant and metastatic settings. In general, cytotoxic chemotherapy rather than endocrine therapy is recommended for women with hormone-receptor-negative breast cancer. Tamoxifen is available only in 10-mg tablets for oral administration, with a manufacturer's recommended dosage of 10 mg twice daily. The schedule lacks a good scientific rationale because with chronic therapy, tamoxifen and its active metabolite dihydroxytamoxifen achieve a steady state with a large tissue reservoir. Accordingly, use of a single dose of 20 mg daily should be an acceptable alternative schedule with fewer compliance problems. Serious or life-threatening toxicities of tamoxifen (thromboembolic disease, retinitis) are rare. Common adverse effects include hot flashes and weight gain, sometimes due to fluid retention. Mild nausea also may occur. In premenopausal women with hormone-receptor-positive neoplasms and metastatic disease, both oophorectomy and antiestrogen therapy can be useful. However, cytotoxic chemotherapy remains the treatment of choice, as it appears to have curative potential. The precise role of ovarian ablation or antiestrogen therapy added to chemotherapy in the adjuvant setting remains to be defined. Tamoxifen has been reported as occasionally having palliative effects in other neoplasms such as ovarian or endometrial cancer. Recently, the FDA has approved the use of tamoxifen in high-risk patients for the prevention of breast cancer. Toremifene, also an estrogen antagonist, has been approved recently for the treatment of breast cancer. It appears to have similar response rates to tamoxifen in the treatment of this disease, and is administered orally once daily.

### *Androgens and antiandrogens*

Androgen therapy is contraindicated in prostate cancer because it stimulates growth. Virilizing androgens such as testosterone propionate, fluoxymesterone (Halotestin), and testosterone enanthate (Delatestryl) have all been used beneficially in the treatment of metastatic breast cancer with hormone-receptor-positive disease. However, androgen therapy has largely been replaced with antiestrogen therapy because the antiestrogen does not cause hirsutism, deepening of the voice, or changes in libido. In addition, the oral halogenated androgens (e.g., fluoxymesterone) also can cause cholestatic jaundice. The antiandrogen flutamide (Eulexin) is a useful agent in the treatment of prostate cancer in combination with one of the gonadotropin-releasing hormone agonists (leuprolide, goserelin).

### *Progestins*

Progestins are useful in the palliative management of metastatic breast or endometrial cancer and can cause tumor regression in endocrine-sensitive disease. Occasional pa-

**Table 13-19 Hormonally Active Agents Used in Cancer Treatment**

| Representative Agents | Toxicity[a] | Clinical Use |
|---|---|---|
| Glucocorticoids | | |
| *Prednisone*<br>*Dexamethasone* | A: Fluid retention, hyperglycemia, euphoria, depression, hypokalemia, acute confusional states<br>D: Osteoporosis, immunosuppression, GI ulcers, cushingoid appearance, cataracts | Leukemia (lymphocytic)<br>Lymphoma<br>Myeloma<br>Breast cancer<br>Brain metastases<br>Spinal cord compression |
| Estrogens | | |
| *Diethylstilbestrol* | A: Nausea, vomiting, hypercalcemia (flare reactions noted with bone metastases), uterine bleeding<br>D: Feminization, premature coronary artery disease, hypercoagulable state | Breast cancer<br>Prostate cancer |
| Antiestrogen | | |
| *Tamoxifen/*<br>*Toremifene* | A: Occasional nausea, fluid retention, hot flashes<br>D: Retinal degeneration, otherwise unknown | Breast cancer<br>Melanoma (role unclear)<br>Hepatoma (role unclear) |
| Aromatase inhibitors | | |
| *Aminoglutethimide* | A: Dizziness<br>D: Rash (transient) | Breast cancer<br>Prostate cancer |
| *Anastrazole* | A: Nausea/vomiting | Breast cancer |
| Progestins | | |
| *Megestrol acetate/*<br>*Hydroxyprogesterone* | A: Increased appetite (megestrol), fluid retention<br>D: Weight gain, thromboembolism | Malignancy-related cachexia<br>Endometrial cancer |
| Androgens | | |
| *Fluoxymesterone/*<br>*Testosterone* | A: Cholestatic jaundice (oral formulation), fluid retention<br>D: Virilization | Breast cancer |
| Antiandrogens | | |
| *Flutamide* | D: Gynecomastia | Prostate cancer |
| Gonadotropin-releasing hormone agonists [depot] | | |
| *Leuprolide acetate/*<br>*Goserelin acetate* | A: Transient flare of symptoms | Prostate cancer<br>Breast cancer (?) |

[a]A, acute toxicity; D, delayed toxicity.

tients with prostate cancer also appear to benefit from progestational therapy. The most commonly used progestins include megestrol acetate (Megace), medroxyprogesterone (Provera), and hydroxyprogesterone caproate (Delalutin). Megestrol acetate is useful as second-line endocrine therapy for patients with metastatic breast cancer who initially respond to tamoxifen. In patients who experience intolerable adverse effects from tamoxifen (e.g., severe hot flashes), megestrol acetate may represent a reasonable alternative. In addition to its antitumor effects, megestrol acetate improves appetite in some patients with cancer-induced cachexia.

***Glucocorticoids***
Adrenal steroid hormones of the glucocorticoid class (e.g., prednisone, methylprednisolone, dexamethasone) are useful in treating lymphoid malignancies and may also potentiate the effects of cytotoxic agents in these tumor types as well as in breast cancer and perhaps other neoplasms. The glucocorticoids play an important role in treating complications of cancer (e.g., hypocalcemia, cerebral edema, pain). Glucocorticoids are lympholytic and non-myelosuppressive and have been incorporated into combination chemotherapy for acute and chronic lympholytic leukemia, malignant lymphoma, and multiple myeloma. Glucocorticoids appear to induce cell death in some lymphoid malignancies by apoptosis.

***Aromatase inhibitors***

**AMINOGLUTETHIMIDE** Aminoglutethimide (Cytadren) inhibits the first step in adrenal steroid synthesis. In addition, and probably more important, aminoglutethimide also inhibits the extra-adrenal conversion of the adrenal androgen androstenedione to estrone by the enzyme aromatase. Aromatase is found in body fat and some other tissues and explains the presence of the weak estrogen estrone in the plasma of postmenopausal women. Aminoglutethimide has been used in the palliative treatment of recurrent breast cancer in hormone-receptor-positive patients. Used in combination with hydrocortisone, the drug suppresses endogenous steroid hormone synthesis (including androstenedione) as well as ACTH production, and slows the catabolism of aminoglutethimide. Aminoglutethimide is commonly administered in a dose of 250 mg twice daily along with 20 mg of hydrocortisone. Somewhat higher doses have been used as second-line endocrine therapy for metastatic prostate cancer. Patients receiving aminoglutethimide and hydrocortisone should be cautioned against abrupt cessation of therapy to avoid symptoms of adrenal insufficiency.

**ANASTRAZOLE** Anastrazole (Arimidex) is a new selective nonsteroidal aromatase inhibitor. Unlike aminoglutethimide, which is neither a selective nor powerful aromatase inhibitor, anastrazole is the first orally administered aromatase inhibitor approved by the FDA for the treatment of postmenopausal women with advanced breast cancer. The drug has an excellent toxicity profile, with only a small percentage of patients receiving a dose of 1 mg/day experiencing nausea, asthenia, headache, or hot flashes.

***Gonadotropin-releasing hormone agonists***
Several synthetic analogs of natural gonadotropin-releasing hormone (GnRH, LHRH) are now clinically available. Both leuprolide acetate (Lupron) and goserelin acetate (Zoladex) are available in long-acting parental-depot formulations. These analogs function more potently than natural GnRH antagonists and have an unusual effect on the pituitary, consisting of initial stimulation followed by long-term inhibition of the release of FSH and LH. This initial increase in gonadotropins can cause a transient increase in symptoms in patients with bone metastases. The inhibition of release of the gonadotropin reduces testicular androgen synthesis in men and ovarian estrogen production in women. Accordingly, GnRH antagonists offer an alternative to surgical orchiectomy in patients with prostate cancer and avoids the gynecomastia, nausea, vomiting, edema, and thromboembolic disease that estrogens may induce. The effectiveness of GnRH agonists is enhanced by administration with an antiandrogen (flutamide), and the combination has been reported to be more effective than a GnRH agonist alone in patients with stage D metastatic prostate cancer. Male erectile dysfunction results from this form of "medical orchiectomy," as it does from surgical orchiectomy, but the effects of medical therapy are potentially reversible if treatment is discontinued. Medical orchiectomy is more expensive but acceptable to patients who decline surgical orchiectomy. GnRH agonists show promise in combination with antiestrogens as endocrine therapy for premenopausal women with hormone-receptor-positive breast cancer. The GnRH agonists are also abortifacients in animals and should not be given to women who are or may become pregnant.

## BIOLOGIC THERAPY

A relatively new form of cancer therapy, still early in its evolution, involves the use of recombinant cytokines (interferons), vaccines, growth factors, and monoclonal antibodies for the treatment of cancer (Table 13-20). The term *biologic therapy* describes this heterogeneous group of agents that either are normal immune mediators or achieve antitumor effects through endogenous host defense mechanisms. These biologic agents have also been termed *biologic response modifiers* (BRMs). Both the cellular and humoral limbs of immunity can be exploited in

Table 13-20 Biologic Therapy of Cancer: Approaches and Agents

| APPROACH | AGENTS |
|---|---|
| Active immunotherapy | Adjuvants: BCG, levamisole |
| Nonspecific | Cytokines: interferons, Interleukin 2 |
| Specific | |
| Passive serotherapy | Tumor cell vaccines |
| Antibodies | Polyclonal or monoclonal antibodies (alone or conjugated with drugs, radionuclides, or toxins) |
| Adoptive cellular therapy | Lymphokine-activated killer cells<br>Tumor-infiltrating lymphocytes |
| Immunomodulators | Levamisole, thymic hormones |
| Bone marrow growth factors | G-CSF, GM-SCF, M-CSF, IL-3, EPO, TPO |
| Growth factor antagonists | Suramin<br>Antibodies to growth factor receptors (e.g., EGF, HER2/neu, IL-2 receptors) |
| Antiangiogenesis agents | Many in clinical trial |

ABBREVIATIONS: BCG, bacille Calmette-Guérin; EGF, epidermal growth factor; EPO, erythropoietin; TPO, thromopoietin; G-CSF, granulocyte colony stimulating factor; GM-CSF, granulocyte macrophage colony stimulating factor; HER2/*neu*, the oncogene; M-CSF, macrophage colony stimulating factor; IL-2 and IL-3, interleukins 2 and 3.

this approach. The cellular defenses include several classes of cytotoxic lymphocytes (natural killer [NK] cell), lymphokine-activated killer (LAK) cells, tumor-infiltrating lymphocytes (TIL), and cytotoxic T lymphocytes (CTL), as well as antibody-dependent cytotoxic cells (ADCC). The nonspecific cells of the reticuloendothelial system including activated macrophages also may be important. Humoral agents with antitumor activities include cytokines such as interferons and interleukins as well as specific antibodies. Most of these humoral agents interact with specific immune effector cells in a coordinated and synergistic fashion. The general availability of cytokines and growth factors has been facilitated by the development of recombinant DNA technology. Antibodies are highly specific and generally interact directly with their tumor targets when they are directed against cell surface constituents. Some humoral agents, including the tumor necrosis factors $\alpha$ and $\beta$, have demonstrated potent local antitumor properties in preclinical models but have not yet been shown to be clinically useful.

Vaccines based on specific bacterial agents or extracts from bacteria can nonspecifically activate the host immune system. Using BCG, this approach has been applied successfully in intravesical therapy of in situ cancer of the urinary bladder. Specific cancer-associated antigen vaccines are also under active investigation.

## Interferons

The interferons (IFNs) are a family of antiviral proteins that differ in their cellular origin and polypeptide structure as well as in their clinical applications. The three major molecular species are IFN-$\alpha$, -$\beta$, and -$\gamma$. IFN-$\alpha$ and -$\beta$ mediate their action by binding to the same cell surface receptor, whereas a second cell surface receptor mediates the action of IFN-$\gamma$. IFN-$\alpha$ is the major species for use in the treatment of hematologic malignancies and solid tumors. Whether IFN-$\beta$ or -$\gamma$ will have sufficient advantage over IFN-$\alpha$ in any specific cancer indication to gain regulatory approval is uncertain.

## Interferon-$\alpha$

Recombinant IFN-$\alpha$ (IFN-$a_2$, Intron-A, Roferon) is a polypeptide cytokine with antiviral properties, which is useful for single-agent treatment of selected hematologic malignancies and solid tumors. The precise mechanism of action of IFN is still poorly understood, but it is known to activate the transcription of a number of cellular genes. In addition, IFN inhibits the synthesis of a number of proteins in sensitive tumor target cells including ornithine decarboxylase, a rate-limiting enzyme in polyamine metabolism. IFN-$\alpha$ also has antiviral and immunoregulatory properties that alter the biological function of many cell types involved in humoral and cellular immunity. At present, it is unclear whether these functions influence its antitumor properties above and beyond its direct receptor-mediated effects on sensitive tumor cells. The antitumor properties of IFN-$\alpha$ also appear to be schedule-dependent with a cytostatic mode of action. Although most remissions induced by IFN-$\alpha$ are only partial, it can induce durable complete remissions in CML and hairy cell leukemia (HCL) (Chronic Myeloid Leukemia, Trialists' Collaborative Group 1997). The combination of interferon-$\alpha$ 2b with cytarabine in patients with CML has recently been shown to increase the rate of major cytogenetic response and survival in patients with chronic phase CML (Guilhot et al. 1997).

Interferon-$\alpha$ can be administered parenterally by intravenous, intramuscular, subcutaneous, and intracavity routes. The preferred route is by subcutaneous administration, which provides the longest duration of action. The dosage schedules are quite variable, with higher dosages required for some tumor types. Hairy cell leukemia is the tumor most sensitive to IFN-$\alpha$. Usual dosages are in the range of 3 million IU administered subcutaneously three times weekly. At these low levels, IFN usually causes only mild adverse effects such as fever and chills with the first few doses. For Kaposi sarcoma, far more aggressive and toxic IFN schedules are required and can cause anorexia, weight loss, cognitive deficits, and profound weakness. High-dose IFN can also induce occasional cardiac arrhythmias, nausea, vomiting, leukopenia, myalgias, proteinuria, and hepatic dysfunction. Optimal biological and antitumor effects of IFN-$\alpha$ appear to be more related to tumor type and biologic response modification than to dose alone. Elderly patients appear to develop more marked adverse effects at all dosage schedules.

Interferon-$\alpha$ is also useful in the treatment of chronic myeloid leukemia, multiple myeloma, some of the low-grade non-Hodgkin lymphomas, and in patients with metastatic melanoma or renal cell carcinoma. In melanoma, the use of high doses of IFN-$\alpha$ in an adjuvant mode has been shown to decrease the relapse rate (Kirkwood et al. 1996). The results of a recent second trial however, have not confirmed the survival advantage with IFN-$\alpha$, but did substantiate the delayed time to recurrence in treated patients (Kirkwood et al. 1999). While the basis for this difference remains to be explained, present speculation revolves around the differences in control arm outcome and the frequency of patients in the control arms which crossed over to IFN-$\alpha$. In addition, many new regimens for melanoma combine the beneficial features of some chemotherapeutic agents such as dacarbazine, retinoids, and biologic response modifiers including interleukin II. In myeloma, IFN-$\alpha$ may lengthen remissions induced by chemotherapy. Patients receiving recombinant IFN-$\alpha$ for HCL, CML, or renal cancer may develop neutralizing antibodies to the recombinant product when the disease progresses again after an IFN-induced remission. A limited number of patients with neutralizing antibodies have been successfully retreated by switching to a nonrecombinant IFN-$\alpha$. Although the clinical indications for IFN therapy continue to grow, it has lacked the type of broad-spectrum anticancer effects that were initially envisioned.

## Interleukin-2

Interleukin-2 (IL-2, Proleukin) is an immunomodulatory cytokine that acts on T-cell progenitors to produce LAK cells. Recombinant IL-2 has been approved for therapeutic use in renal cancer. Intravenous infusion of IL-2 induces production of LAK cells. In addition, after leukapheresis to obtain circulating lymphocytes, these cells can then be exposed to IL-2 in tissue culture to activate lymphoid progenitors into LAK cells, which can then be reinfused into the patient. There is now general agreement that either IL-2 with or without IL-2/LAK can induce tumor regression in approximately 10% of patients with renal carcinoma or melanoma.

Although the infusion of LAK cells causes relatively few adverse effects, direct infusions of high doses of IL-2 induce considerable toxicity. Patients receiving high-dose IL-2 must be in an intensive care unit with close management of blood pressure, fluids, and electrolytes. The high-dose regimens are suitable only for younger patients without other significant disease or impairment of cardiac, pulmonary, hepatic, or renal function. Common adverse effects of high-dose IL-2/LAK are probably due to lymphoid infiltrates in major organs and an induced capillary leak syndrome. Shortly after initiation of high-dose IL-2 therapy, tachycardia develops, and a significant drop in arterial blood pressure occurs. As IL-2 administration continues, compensatory fluid retention occurs in association with weight gain, oliguria, and azotemia. Vasopressors are sometimes needed. Even when administered at lower doses that can be used in conventional hospital or outpatient settings (e.g., 3 million IU per square meter daily by intravenous infusion for 2 weeks), hypotension and fluid retention are common.

Pulmonary metastases appear to be somewhat more sensitive to IL-2 or IL-2/LAK therapy than are other metastatic sites. With the adoptive immunotherapy approach using IL-2/LAK, a small percentage of patients treated at the National Cancer Institute who had undergone prior removal of the primary tumor achieved complete remission with all evidence of metastatic disease disappearing for prolonged periods. Some controversy nonetheless remains as to whether the use of high-dose IL-2/LAK has any advantage over administration of IL-2 alone at a lower and better-tolerated dosage level.

### Antitumor Antibody Therapy: Rituximab

Rituximab (Rituxan) is a genetically engineered chimeric murine/human monoclonal antibody directed against the CD-20 antigen found on the surface of normal and malignant B-lymphocytes (Maloney et al. 1994). It is the first antibody approved for therapeutic use in humans. Approximately 50% of patients with relapsed or refractory low-grade lymphoma treated with 375 mg/m$^2$ of this agent given as an IV infusion weekly for four doses had a partial or complete remission lasting 10 to 12 months (Maloney et al. 1997). Current studies are exploring the use of this antibody together with chemotherapy and/or irradiation. Use of this antibody to deliver radioactivity to lymphoma tumor sites is also under investigation (Kaminsky et al. 1993, 1996; Knox et al. 1996). Infusion-related adverse effects consisting of fever, chills, and rigor occur in the majority of patients during the first infusion. Subsequent infusions are associated with more moderate adverse effects.

### Herceptin

Amplification of the HER2/neu proto-oncogene (a human epidermal growth factor receptor) is found in 25 to 30% of patients with breast cancer, and has been shown to correlate with poor clinical prognosis (Slamon et al. 1989; Goldenberg 1999). Recently, a recombinant humanized monoclonal antibody with high affinity for this receptor (trastuzumab, Herceptin) has been shown to inhibit the growth of breast cancer cells overexpressing HER2. In addition, combinations of trastuzumab and paclitaxel or doxorubicin have been shown to enhance the antitumor activity against HER2/neu overexpressing human breast cancer xenografts in athymic mice (Baselga et al. 1998). To date, trastuzumab has been evaluated in over 1000 women with HER2-overexpressing metastatic breast cancer. Several clinical trials evaluating its activity in combination with chemotherapy as first-line therapy and as a single agent in second and third line treatment (Shak 1999; Baselga et al. 1999). In one such study, over 450 patients were enrolled in a multicenter, randomized, controlled clinical trial in patients previously treated with chemotherapy for metastatic disease. Patients were randomized to receive chemotherapy (paclitaxel or 'AC' containing doxorubicin and cyclophosphamide) alone or in combination with trastuzumab (given IV as a 4 mg/kg loading dose followed by weekly doses of 2 mg/kg). This study showed that patients randomized to trastuzumab and chemotherapy experienced a significantly longer time to disease progression, a higher overall response rate, a longer median duration of response, and a higher one-year survival rate. While these effects were noted in patients receiving either of the two chemotherapy regimens, the effects were greater in the paclitaxel subgroup (Shak 1999). These and other data suggest that the combination of both antibody and chemotherapy based strategies may offer a new and promising approach to the future management of advanced breast cancer.

### Miscellaneous Agents: Levamisole

Levamisole (Ergamisol) is an anthelmintic agent possessing immunopotentiating properties. Levamisole has been reported to enhance various tests of cell-mediated immunity in patients with Hodgkin disease but has not been shown to have a therapeutic benefit. When combined with 5-FU, however, levamisole was shown to decrease the recurrence rate when used as adjuvant treatment for patients with Duke C colon cancer. In patients with overt metastatic colon cancer, the combination of 5-FU and levamisole does not appear to be any more useful than 5-FU alone.

## GROWTH FACTOR ANTAGONISTS

The use of antagonists for polypeptide growth factors is an extension of neuroendocrine therapy but represents a form of biologic therapy as well. One growth factor antagonist that has recently been recognized to have anticancer properties is suramin, which has been used since the 1920s for the treatment of African sleeping sickness. Suramin is a polysulfonated napthylurea that binds tightly to heparin-binding growth factors such as fibroblast growth factor (FGF), platelet-derived growth factor (PDGF), and insulin-like growth factor (IGF-1). Exclusion of growth factors from their receptors can result in "programmed cell death." Suramin actively treats prostate cancer, presumably by blocking the action of FGF and other growth factors. Suramin also inhibits the function of a variety of enzymes and other proteins, so its precise mechanism of antitumor action remains to be defined. Sura-

Table 13-21 **Recombinant Bone Marrow Growth Factors of Potential Importance in the Supportive Care of Cancer Patients**

| GROWTH FACTOR | EFFECTS |
|---|---|
| G-CSF | Stimulates granulocyte production |
| GM-CSF | Stimulates granulocyte, macrophage, and eosinophil production |
| M-CSF | Stimulates macrophage production and activation |
| IL-3 | Stimulates granulocyte, macrophage, and platelet production |
| EPO | Stimulates production of RBCs |
| IL-11 | Stimulates platelet production |
| Thrombopoietin (TPO) | Stimulates platelet production |

ABBREVIATIONS: EPO, erythropoietin; G-CSF, granulocyte colony stimulating factor; GM-CSF, granulocyte macrophage colony stimulating factor; M-CSF, macrophage colony stimulating factor; IL-3 and IL-11, interleukin 3 and 11; RBCs, red blood cells.

min's multiple actions also account for a broad range of toxicities that can be severe and irreversible. One of these is adrenal insufficiency, which requires long-term adrenal steroid replacement. Frequent plasma monitoring of suramin concentrations is essential, because there is the potential for serious neuropathy when suramin concentrations exceed 300 mg/mL. The use of suramin in cancer therapy is presently investigational. Other approaches to growth factor receptor blockade involve use of monoclonal antibodies to epidermal growth factor (EGF) receptor and the IL-2 receptor.

## SUPPORTIVE CARE WITH BONE MARROW GROWTH FACTORS

A new supportive care approach for bone marrow failure associated with cancer, and for maintaining adequate hematopoietic function between courses of myelosuppressive chemotherapy, is to administer bone marrow growth factors to stimulate the growth of myeloid progenitors. The bone marrow growth factors are glycoproteins that function in an overlapping and hierarchical manner on bone marrow progenitors. They not only produce cell proliferation but also activate differentiation and cell trafficking. The factors currently approved for use in clinical trials in cancer patients are summarized in Table 13-21. Some of these growth factors can also stimulate the proliferation of myeloid precursors. Several of these recombinant proteins, including G-CSF, GM-CSF, and erythropoietin (Epogen, EPO) (see Table 13-21), are approved medications that are widely used in cancer patients. IL-3, macrophage colony-stimulating factor (M-CSF) and thrombopoietin are at an earlier stage of development, and their role in the supportive care of cancer patients is presently uncertain. Clinical trials using subcutaneously administered G-CSF or GM-CSF have shown that either can shorten the duration of granulocytopenia, the frequency of infectious complications, and the duration of hospitalization after chemotherapy combinations that ordinarily require inpatient administration. With bone marrow transplantation (where high-dose chemotherapy and/or total body radiation is used), both myelosuppressive and nonmyelosuppressive adverse effects can be diminished with the use of G-CSF or GM-CSF. Preliminary evidence suggests that IL-3 (multi-CSF) can stimulate platelet, red blood cell, and granulocyte production. Stem cell factors (c-kit ligand and flt-2 ligand) are also under investigation as hematopoietic stimulators.

In preclinical studies, IL-3 also appears to act synergistically with GM-CSF to produce more complete and rapid recovery of circulating granulocytes and platelets. The major toxicities of the growth factors that stimulate white cell production include fever, myalgias, and occasional skin rashes. Pericarditis has been reported with high-dose GM-CSF or G-CSF. Recombinant EPO is already in general clinical use for the anemia of renal failure. Preliminary studies also suggest that when used in pharmacologic doses, EPO can restore normal red blood cell counts in some patients with multiple myeloma and perhaps in some other hematologic malignancies as well. EPO can also reduce the degree of anemia induced by cytotoxic chemotherapy.

## PRACTICE OF CHEMOTHERAPY: GENERAL CONSIDERATIONS

### Combination Chemotherapy

Pharmacotherapy of human cancer has evolved rapidly since the introduction of nitrogen mustard and aminopterin into the clinic in the late 1940s. As new agents were evaluated in humans, it became clear that resistance would occur in a matter of months when only single-agent therapy was used. The introduction of effective combination chemotherapy regimens for ALL and Hodgkin disease in the 1960s was a direct outgrowth of experimental studies, which showed that combinations of effective drugs produced additive cell kill and delayed or prevented the onset of drug resistance. In these regimens, "selective agents" (Table 13-22) could be used in full dose in ALL because of nonoverlapping toxicities. Present treatment strategies emphasize the use of drug combinations used in sequence given in high doses (with or without autologous peripheral stem cells), with or without hemopoietic cytokines (G-CSF, GM-CSF, TPO, IL-1, IL-3; see Hematologic Disorders in chapter 12).

Attempts to recruit tumor cells into S phase—thus making them more vulnerable to cell-cycle-specific agents—have failed primarily because of the difficulty in synchronizing human tumor cells. Other lessons from experimental tumor models should be considered when drug combinations are used.

**PRINCIPLE When two myelosuppressive drugs are used in combination, it is generally possible to use 66% of the optimum dose of each drug without increasing the net toxicity.**

If both drugs are equally effective, then the effective total dose delivered is 1.5 times the dose of the single drug. However, if both drugs are not effective, then subadditive results may occur. Some empirical evidence that drugs used in combination have additive or synergistic effects rather than antagonistic effects must be obtained before the combination is administered. The sequence of drug administration may be important in this regard. For example, when MTX and L-asparaginase are used together, L-asparaginase will block the cytotoxicity of MTX; when MTX administration precedes L-asparaginase administration by 24 hours, then drug synergy is observed in the treatment of ALL if the interval of treatment is 10 to 14 days (Capizzi 1975).

One disadvantage of combination therapy revolves around determining exactly which drug is of value if a positive antitumor effect is produced. If resistance occurs, it may not be to all the drugs used in the combination. If toxicity occurs, it may be difficult to adjust subsequent doses of individual drugs, because the major offending agent may not be obvious.

Recently, the idea of using alternating cycles of two or more drug combinations has emerged. The theoretical considerations behind the concept is based on the probability that drug-resistant cells are less likely to survive alternating drug combinations, compared with the repeated dosing of a fixed combination (Goldie et al. 1982). An example of this concept is the use of alternating cycles of MOPP (mechlorethamine, Oncovin [vincristine], prednisone, procarbazine), and ABVD (Adriamycin [doxorubicin], bleomycin, vinblastine and dacarbazine [DTIC]) in the treatment of Hodgkin disease (Bonadonna et al. 1986). However attractive, this concept remains unproved in the clinic. Current efforts are being directed toward short-term, intense chemotherapy with drug combinations used sequentially.

## Dose Intensity

An important consideration in the treatment of curable malignancies is optimal intensity of the dose (Hryniuk 1987). For responsive malignancies that have features of poor risk (e.g., a large tumor burden), intensification of the dose may be achieved by the use of doses of chemotherapy that ablate the bone marrow followed by rescue either with autologous or allogeneic transplant. This approach has led to improved cure rates in patients with relapsed leukemia and lymphoma, and high-risk germ cell tumors, and is being studied in patients with breast cancer.

**PRINCIPLE If cure is possible, then full doses of drugs should be used.**

## Adjuvant Chemotherapy

The use of adjuvant chemotherapy in treating human tumors after the surgeon or radiotherapist has eradicated all clinically evident tumor has a firm experimental basis. Both in certain experimental models and in humans, the likelihood of tumor recurrence can be predicted with accuracy (Schabel 1975). When this possibility is high, then adjuvant chemotherapy may be used, justifying the risks of therapy. Several advanced transplantable or spontaneous neoplasms in laboratory animals can be cured by chemotherapy following surgical removal of all palpable disease, although surgery or chemotherapy alone is not curative (Fugman et al. 1970; Schabel 1975). Reducing the tumor cell burden by surgery or irradiation decreases the residual tumor cell number that must be dealt with by adjuvant chemotherapy (and/or immunotherapy). In addition, the growth fraction of the surviving cells increases, thus making the relatively small tumor cell populations that remain in the primary site or in the distant metastasis more vulnerable to destruction by cell-cycle active agents,

Table 13-22 Drugs Used to Treat Acute Lymphocytic Leukemia

| SELECTIVE DRUGS (LACK SIGNIFICANT MARROW TOXICITY) | EFFECTIVE DRUGS (HAVE SIGNIFICANT MARROW TOXICITY) |
|---|---|
| Prednisone | MTX |
| Vincristine | 6-MP |
| L-Asparaginase | Doxorubicin |
| | Etoposide, Teniposide |
| | Ara-C |

ABBREVIATIONS: ara-C, cytosine arabinoside; 6-MP, 6-mercaptopurine; MTX, methotrexate.

especially the antimetabolite drugs (Schabel 1975). Intermittent, high-dose treatment with these agents (alone or in combination with alkylating agents) is then more effective against neoplastic cells than against normal stem cells. In addition, intermittent therapy may allow the opportunity for normal immune mechanisms to recover between doses.

The role of immunotherapy for treating patients with cancer has not been adequately defined. However, data from several experimental systems indicate that the use of this modality will be appropriate only when the residual tumor burden is small (Bast et al. 1974).

**PRINCIPLE Large, bulky tumors defeat the chemotherapist because of the large numbers of tumor cells and the consequent development of drug resistance. Chemotherapy and possibly immunotherapy are most effective when the number of remaining cells is small and tumor growth is logarithmic.**

## Neoadjuvant Chemotherapy

### *Special methods to deliver high concentrations of drugs to isolated areas*

*Neoadjuvant therapy* refers to the administration of chemotherapy before a surgical intervention. Such practices are often considered in the management of stage III A NSCLC or sarcomas of the extremities. A variety of delivery methods have been developed that facilitate delivery of high concentrations of drugs to isolated organs or tissues.

**REGIONAL PERFUSION AND INFUSION** The rationale for administering drugs via a tumor's arterial blood supply is based on the observation that higher concentrations of a drug can be delivered to the neoplasm with less systemic toxicity. Because a dose response (increased tumor cell kill with increasing dose of drug) exists for most tumors and select antineoplastic agents, this approach can potentially increase the effectiveness of the therapy by killing a greater fraction of the tumor. The same amount of drug administered intra-arterially, rather than intravenously, has the potential of effecting better results by producing a higher local concentration of the drug directly in the tumor. Intra-arterial therapy has been used to treat tumors that are in areas of the body that are difficult to treat by surgical procedures or radiation therapy. In addition, it can assist in managing tumors that may be cured by chemotherapy without requiring amputation or disfigurement. Examples of such lesions include tumors of the head and neck, the brain, the extremities, the liver, and the organs of the lower abdomen (e.g., rectum, cervix, bladder).

*Infusion* refers to the administration of drug via the artery supplying a tumor without attempting to isolate the venous return. Thus, circulation of the drug beyond the tumor is allowed, and a risk of systemic toxicity is incurred. Because there are fewer technical difficulties with this technique compared with perfusion, it is more commonly used.

Perfusion therapy, that is, administering a drug into the arterial blood supply of a tumor via a closed circuit in which the tumor's venous return is recirculated via a pump, has a great potential advantage: The therapeutic index should be greatly enhanced, and systemic toxicity should be minimal. Even in settings of perfusion of the extremities, this ideal is difficult to achieve practically because some leakage of drug into the systemic circulation usually occurs.

These dramatic procedures have received a great deal of attention in the past decade. Although most of the technical problems of intra-arterial administration have been solved, much more research needs to be done on the selection and scheduling of drugs and exactly how to use these procedures as an adjuvant to surgery and/or radiotherapy.

Antimetabolites have an advantage over alkylating agents for intra-arterial use in that the local toxicity may be more selective, that is, limited to replicating tissue alone. Long-term administration of antimetabolites, by encompassing the generation time of most of the tumor cells, may produce the greatest therapeutic benefit. Several approaches have been used to minimize the systemic toxicity of antimetabolites, including: 1) using low concentrations of drug (i.e., enough to produce an appreciable concentration of the agent in the blood supply of the tumor but not enough to reach cytotoxic levels in the systemic circulation), and 2) using a drug that is rapidly metabolized in the blood or liver, such as 5-FU or 5-FUdR (Kemeny et al. 1989).

The role of intra-arterial chemotherapy to treat hepatic metastasis from colon cancer as an adjunct to radiation therapy and/or surgery is being evaluated in several centers. Although the response of the tumor to intra-arterial therapy is often impressive, the ultimate value of this combined approach has not been demonstrated.

**PRINCIPLE Even the most logically sound therapeutic intervention must be confirmed by testing in appropriate patients. A well-designed clinical study can allow for the rejection of logical and rational—although ineffective—interventions and establish the acceptance of effective strategies.**

**INTRATHECAL AND INTRAVENTRICULAR ADMINISTRATION OF DRUGS** The principal indication for administration of an antineoplastic drug directly into the CSF is to treat tumors that grow in suspension in the CSF and/or involve the meninges and are nourished by the CSF (Moore et al. 1960). The advantage of intrathecal or intraventricular administration of drug in these circumstances is considerable, because high concentrations of drug are achieved, producing less systemic toxicity than would be seen if comparable concentrations were produced by giving the drug systemically. When given systemically, many drugs do not cross the blood–brain barrier. For example, intravenous administration of the folate antagonist MTX in conventional doses is ineffective for the treatment of neoplasms in the meninges. In contrast, intrathecal MTX is effective in treating meningeal leukemia (Rieselback et al. 1963). High doses of MTX (i.e., >500 mg/m$^2$ IV) followed by leucovorin rescue can achieve concentrations of MTX in the CNS that are cytocidal (Tattersall, Parker, et al. 1975). However, the blood–brain barrier is not unidirectional for MTX as well as for most other drugs. The MTX directly administered intrathecally can diffuse into the systemic circulation, and systemic toxicity can result if a high enough dose of the drug is administered intrathecally.

Inasmuch as most solid tumors of the brain derive their nourishment from the arterial circulation rather than from the CSF, intraventricular administration of drugs is usually not effective for the treatment of brain tumors. Delivery of drugs via the arterial circulation to brain tumors has been attempted but has met with only limited success.

**INTRACAVITARY ADMINISTRATION OF DRUG** Intracavitary drug administration with instillation of a biologic agent such as BCG (Bacille Calmette-Guérin), interferon, or a variety of cytotoxic agents (e.g., thiotepa, doxorubicin, mitomycin, cisplatin) is used to treat superficial bladder cancer. Intraperitoneal drug administration has also gained increasing popularity and appears to show particular promise for the treatment of patients with peritoneal carcinomatosis. In patients with ovarian cancer, intraperitoneal chemotherapy is being studied as a follow-up to cytoreductive surgery. Diffusion of intraperitoneally administered drugs is limited to a few millimeters of tumor tissue. Accordingly, intraperitoneal chemotherapy is seldom warranted in patients with bulky tumor masses or those with numerous intra-abdominal adhesions. For optimal distribution, the drug is usually diluted in 2 L of parenteral fluid for injection. Preferred drugs for intraperitoneal administration are those that tend to remain largely confined to the peritoneal cavity, have favorable pharmacokinetic properties allowing for adequate absorption in the tumor, and produce little or no local toxicity. Mitoxantrone, fluorodeoxyuridine, and cisplatin have these favorable characteristics and can be used therapeutically in the clinic. With each of these drugs, the intraperitoneal concentration can be 1000 times that measured in the systemic circulation. Other agents sometimes used in intraperitoneal administration include thiotepa, fluorouracil, and methotrexate. Intraperitoneal drug administration can be performed at repeated intervals with relative ease if a surgically implanted Tenkoff catheter is connected to a subcutaneous port. Mild-to-moderate chemical peritonitis and the development of peritoneal adhesions are common complications of intraperitoneal chemotherapy and limit repeated use.

## Evaluation of Drug Therapy in Humans

### *Measurement of normal stem cells*

Techniques for the accurate measurement of tumor and hemopoietic stem cell kill in the mouse have provided valuable information about differential cell kill, dose response, and rates of recovery of these tissues. The recent development of methods for growing human bone marrow cells in vitro may allow for the eventual development of an assay to measure normal hemopoietic stem cells before and during therapy. Thus far, there is no satisfactory assay for marrow stem cells. However, progenitor cells (e.g., colony-forming units [CFUs]) may be assayed for cell lines such as granulocytes or macrophages (GM-CFU). Some predictive estimate of the eventual effect of chemotherapy on the stem cells of the marrow and gut epithelium can be made by assessing the early consequences of cell kill in either of these tissues. The reduction in granulocytes, reticulocytes, and platelets directly relates to the killing of the hematopoietic precursor cells in the bone marrow. If the counts of blood cells are carefully monitored, they can be used to accurately determine concentrations of granulocytes as low as $100/mm^3$. When serial counts of granulocytes are plotted on a logarithmic scale, changes in cell counts over several orders of magnitude can be quantified. Thus, a quantitative evaluation of the intensity of therapy on the bone marrow can be made from its effects on the peripheral blood (Hryniuk and Bertino 1969a, 1969b; Hryniuk et al. 1969). However, mucositis produced by chemotherapy is typically graded on a scale of 1 to 4. Although this assessment of drug toxicity is only semiquantitative, it crudely relates to the logarithm of the mucosal cell kill.

**PRINCIPLE Although there may not be precise means of following a drug's effects, reliable, albeit semiquantitative, measures can be used in the development of a dosing strategy. Using the available information in a semiquantitative manner allows for an estimation of toxicity and response and provides a solid basis for comparison between patients and differing treatment schedules.**

### *Evaluation of tumor cell kill*

Reliable techniques to measure the reduction of tumor cells in humans have not been developed. Whenever possible, semiquantitative estimates of the tumor mass should be performed. This estimate of the tumor volume is usually the best available guide of the response to therapy. By using measurements of tumor volume, the therapist can estimate the change in cell number, assuming that 1 $cm^3$ of cells represents approximately $10^9$ cells. However, a change in the size of a tumor mass may not accurately or absolutely reflect the amount of tumor cell kill. For example, in an experimental mouse tumor, 3 logs (99.9%) of cell kill was obtained by cyclophosphamide therapy, yet no measurable change in tumor size occurred because the removal of dead tumor cells was slow, and once removed, they were rapidly replaced with new cells (Wilcox et al. 1965).

By analogy, the quantitation of normal granulocytes as an indirect correlate of hemopoietic progenitor cell kill can be an accurate measurement of the peripheral blast cell count when plotted on a logarithmic scale. This approach may be helpful in assessing the results of treatment in patients with leukemia, where a decrease in circulating blasts by as much as 3 logs (orders of magnitude) may be measured (e.g., reduction from 100,000 to 100 cells). However, quantitation of changes in cell content of the bone marrow by "marrow counts" (the more important compartment) is less satisfactory.

When tumors produce characteristic enzymes, hormones, or proteins (AFP, HCG, CA-125, CEA), measurements of these products in the blood may be valuable in guiding therapy. If the amount of substance produced is a direct function of the number of tumor cells, and if therapy produces a decrease in the concentrations of these substances only by killing cells, then the concentration of the product may be directly reflective of cell kill. The measurement of urinary chorionic gonadotropin titers in patients with choriocarcinoma or embryonal testicular tumors has been extremely useful in this regard, and accurate quantitation of very low concentrations is possible by using a radioimmunoassay. In fact, quantitation of urinary paraproteins in patients with myeloma (Alexanian et al. 1969; Salmon and Smith 1970) and concentrations of lysozymes in serum and urine from patients with monocytic leukemia (Osserman and Lawlor 1966; Perillie et al. 1968) may also prove useful in assessing cell kill or changes in cell mass. Quantitation by sensitive assays of hormones produced by other endocrine and nonendocrine tumors may provide similarly useful information to guide treatment (Rees and Landon 1976).

However, a hormone or protein tumor marker may not be a perfect reflection of tumor burden. For example, carcinoid tumor or tumors of neural crest origin make a variety of hormones at varying rates at different times in their natural history. Measurement of these different proteins and their metabolic products over time is seemingly independent of gross tumor size. Furthermore, some hormones may be carried in the blood by factors that are sensitive to the chemotherapeutic agent. When 5-FU is given to patients with carcinoid syndrome, the concentration of serotonin in blood may decrease without a change in tumor size. This change of serotonin concentration is more reflective of the drug's effect on platelets where the serotonin is stored rather than of its effect on the size of the tumor where the serotonin is made (Melmon 1974).

## PRACTICE OF CHEMOTHERAPY: SPECIFIC EXAMPLES

After the patient's general condition and performance status have been evaluated, the histology of the tumor should be verified (pathologic staging), and some estimate should be made of the progression and amount of tumor present (clinical staging). Only at that point is the chemotherapist ready to consider a specific drug regimen and the ancillary measures necessary to optimize its effects. In vitro tests have not been developed to the point where response of an individual patient's tumor cells to drugs in the laboratory is predictive of what will occur in vivo. Therefore, the initial judgment of the sensitivity of the tumor to antitumor agents must be made on the basis of previous trials with various drugs in other patients. Aside from the kinetic considerations previously discussed, and a few exceptions, the reasons for the differences in tumor sensitivity to certain drugs are poorly understood (Bertino et al. 1989).

Once a drug or drug combination has been selected, the dose, duration, and route of administration of each compound must then be considered. The oncologist must understand the metabolism of the drug, as well as any possible alterations in its metabolism caused by the patient's condition (involvement of liver or kidney by the disease or concurrent disease unrelated to neoplasm) or by concurrent use of other medications. The feasible goals of therapy must be determined before the specific treatment regimen is determined. The histologic type of tumor, its clinical staging, and the patient's pretreatment performance status are critical considerations in establishing realistic treatment objectives.

**PRINCIPLE The patient and physician should be aware of the toxic potential of drugs, and the acceptable limits of the intensity of therapy should be set before therapy commences. When cure is possible, as in choriocarcinoma and testicular cancer, only near-lethal toxicity (i.e., greater than the LD10) may be prohibitive. However, if the expected gain is minimal, as in the routine treatment of carcinoma of the colon with 5-FU, even moderate morbidity may not be acceptable.**

### Curative Intent

Human tumors, even those caused by a single clone of cells, have variable growth rates. Nonetheless, a few tumors are characterized by rapid doubling times and relatively homogeneous behavior. These include choriocarcinoma, Burkitt lymphoma, ALL, and diffuse large cell lymphoma. In their early stages, two of these neoplasms (Burkitt and choriocarcinoma) can be cured by a single therapeutic agent (cyclophosphamide or methotrexate, respectively). The other two require combination chemotherapy for long-term, disease-free survival.

#### *Choriocarcinoma*

Choriocarcinoma serves as a paradigm for a disseminated neoplastic disease and was among one of the first malignancies cured with chemotherapy. Although MTX (or aminopterin, its predecessor) has been available since 1949 for clinical use, the initial evidence demonstrating that this rapidly growing tumor could be cured by the drug was not obtained until 1956. In order to obtain cures, maximally tolerated doses of methotrexate or dactinomycin were required (Goldstein 1972; Hertz 1972). Effective drugs may be available for extended periods before their optimal use in different diseases is defined.

**PRINCIPLE When potential long-term remission or cure is possible, the risks necessary to obtain these benefits may be justified.**

The value of a tumor marker reflecting the presence of a tumor cell (e.g., human chorionic gonadotropin [hCG]) in assessing cell kill was clearly demonstrated in the treatment of patients with choriocarcinoma. This marker can be used to guide the selection of therapy, the necessary dose, the efficacy or failure of therapy, and the point at which treatment should be stopped. In this way, the patient may be spared the unnecessary risks of treatment (Fig. 13-20).

Using the hCG titer in urine as a measure of the tumor burden, it has been found that the larger the tumor cell burden, the more difficult it is to obtain regression of the total tumor mass. The hCG titer, the duration of the disease, and the clinical staging of these patients (e.g., whether brain or liver was involved) have assisted the clinician in identifying patients who require more aggressive therapy (Hammond et al. 1973; Berkowitz et al. 1986, 1994).

Patients who have survived long periods and are therefore potentially cured after treatment with either

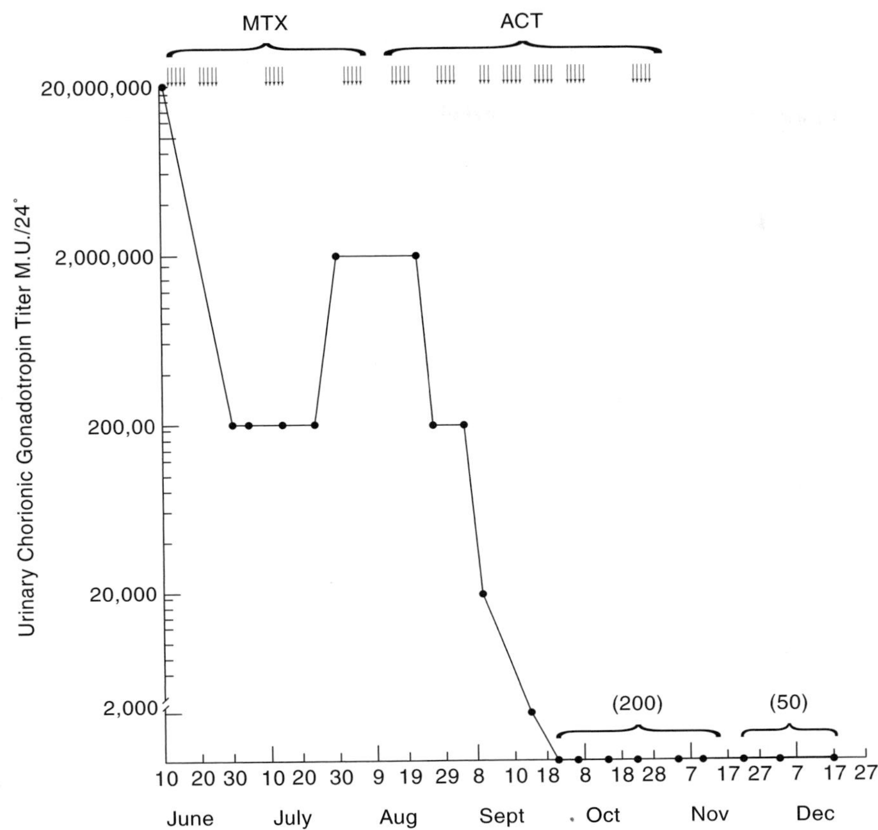


**FIGURE 13-20** Chemotherapy of a patient with metastatic choriocarcinoma. The vertical arrows indicate 5-day courses of MTX and actinomycin D (ACT). This patient presented with a urinary chorionic gonadotropin (UCG) titer of 20,000,000; with the sensitive assays available, this titer was followed down through 7 logs, allowing therapy to be closely monitored.

Methotrexate produced 2 logs of decrease in the UCG titer, but despite continued therapy with this drug, the titer began to rise, indicating that resistance was developing. Guided by this rise in UCG titer rather than by the chest x-ray film (which did not change), therapy was rapidly changed to actinomycin D. This drug decreased the UCG titer markedly, each course resulting in 1 to 2 logs of decrease of UCG titer and presumably of tumor cells. The patient was then treated until the titer was within the normal range.

The patient has remained free of disease (greater than 15 years). Although the effects on normal tissue are not shown here, the therapy was intensive, and each course of MTX or ACT was given to the limit of tolerable toxicity (usually 2 logs of granulocyte or platelet decrease, or mucositis), and therapy was resumed immediately on recovery from toxicity (granulocyte count greater than 1500/mm$^3$, platelet count greater than 100,000/mm$^3$, no liver function abnormalities). Supportive care for this type of regimen must be optimal to avoid drug-related deaths; in a series of 50 patients, including this patient, 37 presumable "cures" were obtained with the use of sequential MTX and actinomycin D therapy (or vice versa), with only 1 death due to MTX toxicity. (From Ross et al. 1965.)

MTX or dactinomycin, or both in sequence, have not developed any long-term adverse effects from this therapy (Ross et al. 1965). Many have gone on to have normal pregnancies (Hertz 1972).

***Burkitt lymphoma***

Burkitt lymphoma is the other example of a human neoplasm that may be cured in a significant percentage of patients with early disease who are given single-agent chemotherapy. This tumor, which has a doubling time of 12 to 14 hours, may have the highest growth fraction of any human tumor (Ziegler 1973). Its etiology, epidemiology, and therapy have been extensively studied (Burkitt and Burchenal 1969; Ziegler 1973). The tumor is unusually sensitive to cyclophosphamide, and large doses (40 mg/kg of body weight given intermittently) can produce cure. As noted for choriocarcinoma, the more advanced the clinical stage, the more intensive the combination chemotherapy required to achieve cures.

***Therapy of patients with acute lymphocytic leukemia***

The cure of children with ALL has been one of the major triumphs of chemotherapy (Steinherz 1987). The evolution of curative treatment has been a painfully slow process that has depended on understanding the biology of this disease, including tumor cell kinetics and molecular subsets of ALL, development of effective agents, and an understanding of the pharmacology of combined drugs (Frei 1984). At the present time most centers report 5-year disease-free survivals of over 70%; adults with ALL have a lower cure rate (20%).

DRUGS USED TO TREAT ALL One of the first drugs used to treat ALL was aminopterin. Complete remissions were reported by Farber (1966). It was soon realized that drug resistance developed rapidly, and despite continued treatment with maximally tolerated doses, patients relapsed within several months. Subsequently, corticosteroids and 6-MP were introduced into the clinic. Again, single-agent treatment produced remissions in many patients, but resistance developed rapidly. Combinations of prednisone and 6-MP or prednisone and MTX were found to be more effective than aminopterin alone in animal studies and were soon evaluated in humans. Though a higher percentage of complete remissions were produced and the duration of those remissions was longer, the disease still relapsed, becoming even more refractory to subsequent treatment.

**PRINCIPLE Agents with different mechanisms of action and different toxicities may be combined in full dose.**

In 1961, a benchmark study was reported by the acute leukemia B study group. This clinical trial showed that the combination of MTX with 6-MP was found to be more effective than either drug alone (Acute Leukemia Group B 1961). The introduction of vincristine into the clinic then provided the clinician with another "selective" drug in addition to prednisone. The combination of prednisone and vincristine allowed the successful induction of 80 to 90% of patients into complete remission without serious marrow toxicity, life-threatening risk of bleeding, or infection during treatment. After remission induction with these drugs, the antimetabolites 6-MP and MTX may be used in high doses with less chance of serious toxicity to normal marrow. Although longer remissions were regularly produced with this regimen with some cures, most patients continued to relapse, particularly in the CNS.

An important breakthrough in ALL management came when radiation therapy to the craniospinal axis, or irradiation to the brain plus intrathecally administered MTX, was added to the treatment regimen. For the first time, a substantial number of children (50%) were now rendered disease-free. Current treatment programs now utilize additional effective agents in the total therapy of childhood ALL, including L-asparaginase in combination with MTX (see section on L-asparaginase), and teniposide (VM-26) with ara-C, a synergistic combination in animal models of leukemia. High-dose regimens of MTX with leucovorin rescue have also been shown to be an alternative to radiation of the brain, because at high doses of MTX ($>$0.5 g/m$^2$), the concentrations achieved in the CNS are cytocidal to ALL blasts ($>10^{-7}$ M). Some newer regimens also include doxorubicin, which may be added to vincristine and prednisone in the induction phase without compromising dosage.

**PRINCIPLE Drug distribution may play a key role in the therapeutic outcome.**

IMPORTANCE OF DOSE INTENSITY Several studies have demonstrated that outcome depends on adequate dose intensity. The suggestion has been made that patients receiving MTX and 6-MP should have serum concentrations of drug in blood monitored to be sure that adequate doses are given.

**PRINCIPLE Ideally, patients should be treated to achieve a desired plasma concentration in order to achieve maximum therapeutic benefit.**

Several questions still remain to be fully answered in the treatment of ALL:

- What is the optimum treatment regimen for standard-risk versus high-risk patients?
- How long should the patient be treated?
- What are the long-term toxic effects of the various treatment programs?

For example, some recent data indicate that doxorubicin, even in cumulative doses not thought to be cardiotoxic, can cause effects on the myocardium in children. In one such study, approximately 25% of patients developed late cardiac complications (including congestive heart failure, dysrhythmia, and sudden death) 4 to 20 years following a median anthracycline dose of 450 mg/$m^2$ (Steinherz et al. 1995; Steinherz et al. 1991). These data suggest that survivors of childhood cancer who received anthrocyclines be followed for periodic evaluation of cardiac function and rhythm (Steinherz and Steinherz 1991).

**PRINCIPLE Expect adverse-effect profiles of very potent antitumor drugs to extend well after they are used to produce cures.**

### *Therapy of patients with Hodgkin disease*

This disease is another example of a human cancer that is curable, even when it is first seen in an advanced stage. Accurate clinical and pathologic staging have played a major role in determining the extent of disease and developing effective treatment plans. In order to treat this disease optimally, the cooperation and expertise of medical oncologists, radiotherapists, and pathologists skilled in the diagnosis and treatment of lymphoma are required.

Early-stage Hodgkin disease (stage I or II, disease in one lymph node area, or two or more lymph node areas, respectively, limited to one side of the diaphragm) is treated with irradiation therapy alone, usually after exploratory laparotomy to confirm that the patient does not have more advanced disease. The 5-year cure rates with extended field irradiation (x-ray therapy to the involved lymph node regions plus to the contiguous nodes) are in the range of 80 to 90%. Patients who relapse may be "salvaged" with combination chemotherapy. Thus, approximately 95% of patients with early-stage Hodgkin disease can expect to be cured. There are, however, concerns about the long-term effects of irradiation, in particular an increased incidence of secondary malignancies. Therefore, in several centers, chemotherapy regimens (not containing alkylating agents) alone or in combination with limited irradiation (covering only the involved field) are being explored as alternative treatments.

More advanced stages of Hodgkin disease (stage III, lymph node involvement above and below the diaphragm; stage IV, extranodal organ involvement) are less likely to be cured by radiation therapy alone. In these cases, combination chemotherapy is essential and can still cure patients of their disease. The first combination chemotherapy demonstrated to be curative in advanced-stage Hodgkin disease was MOPP (Table 13-23). This four-drug combination was formulated on the principles outlined in the first part of the chapter: Selective drugs (vincristine and prednisone) were used in full dosage, with scheduled doses of two other effective drugs that both produced marrow toxicity. The treatment was given in divided doses on days 1 and 8 and was repeated again on day 28 after myelosuppression resolved (DeVita et al. 1967). None of these drugs used individually in full doses was curative. However, the combination of these four agents prevented the emergence of drug-resistant clones, and, in 50 to 60% of patients, long-term remissions (>15 years) have been produced. The major long-term toxicities associated with this combination have been sterility and secondary malignancy, in particular leukemia and lymphoma in 1 to 5% of patients (Table 13-2). In addition, several of the agents used in the treatment of this disease (mechlorethamine, vincristine, doxorubicin) are potent vesicants and require extreme care in administering to the patient. Table 13-24 lists vesicant chemotherapeutic agents, with some recommendations regarding the management of extravasation. This avoidable complication of treatment can have a profound impact on the patient, lead-

**Table 13-23 Drug Combinations Used to Treat Hodgkin Disease**

| MOPP | ABVD |
|---|---|
| **M**echlorethamine | Doxorubicin (**A**driamycin™) |
| Vincristine (**O**ncovin™) | **B**leomycin |
| **P**rocarbazine | **V**inblastine |
| **P**rednisone | **D**acarbazine |

Table 13-24 **Vesicant Antineoplastic Agents and Treatment of Extravasation**

| Chemotherapeutic Agent | Recommended Treatment[a,b] |
|---|---|
| *Alkylating agents* | |
| • Mechlorethamine<br>• Streptozotocin<br>• Carmustine<br>• Dacarbazine | 1. Stop infusion<br>2. Cold compresses<br>3. Isotonic sodium thiosulfate (4 mL of 10% solution plus 6 mL of saline = 1/6 M solution) injected into line and surrounding SQ tissue. Repeat SQ dosing 2–3 times over next 3–4 h. |
| *Anthracyclines/antibiotics* | |
| • Doxorubicin<br>• Daunorubicin<br>• Idarubicin<br>• Mitomycin<br>• Dactinomycin | 1. Stop infusion<br>2. DMSO 50–90% (w/v) solution applied topically.<br>3. Cool compresses |
| *Vinca alkaloids* | |
| • Vinblastine<br>• Vincristine<br>• Vinorelbine | 1. Stop infusion<br>2. Inject 1 mL of subcutaneous hyaluronidase (Wydase 150 U/mL) injected around site of extravasation. Repeat 1–2 times over next 3–4 h. |
| *Epipodophyllotoxins* | |
| • Etoposide<br>• Teniposide | 1. Stop infusion<br>2. Cool compresses<br>3. Hyaluronidase as with vinca alkaloids |

[a]Treatment recommendations summarized from Scuderi and Onesti 1994; Hirsh and Conlon 1983; Dorr 1990; Bertelli 1995; Boyle and Engelking 1995; Davis et al. 1995; Lawrence et al. 1989; and Disa et al. 1998.
[b]In all cases of extravasation, the infusion should be stopped immediately, remaining drug should be withdrawn from the catheter with 2–3 mL of blood, the catheter should be flushed with 5–10 mL of normal saline, and the affected arm should be elevated. The catheter should be left in place over the short term to facilitate delivery of antidotes. In some cases, local injection of 100–200 mg of hydrocortisone should be considered. Arrange for early plastic surgery consultation for possible débridement.
ABBREVIATIONS: DMSO, dimethylsulfoxide; SQ, squamous cell.

ing to limited function of the affected limb and reconstructive plastic surgery.

When additional drugs effective against Hodgkin disease were introduced into the clinic in the 1970s, a second four-drug combination (ABVD, or Adriamycin [doxorubicin], bleomycin, vinblastine and dacarbazine) was developed, with results equal to or perhaps better than the MOPP regimen in untreated patients (Table 13-23). Long-term adverse effects, in particular secondary malignancies and sterility, were greatly reduced with the ABVD program, indicating an improved therapeutic index (Bonadonna et al. 1986). Unfortunately, a substantial percentage (30 to 40%) of patients with advanced Hodgkin disease are not cured. Attempts have recently been directed toward further improving the cure rate, especially by defining a poor-risk group who may require even more aggressive treatment. Alternating or hybrid combinations of MOPP and ABVD are under investigation, as well as combinations of chemotherapy and radiation treatment. More recently, the use of autologous bone marrow transplant following high-dose treatment and the use of cytokines to stimulate marrow recovery have resulted in long-term remissions of patients who have relapsed after first-line treatment.

**PRINCIPLE The optimum treatment of a malignancy is cure with as few adverse effects as possible. However, the possibility of cure should not be compromised to decrease the adverse effects.**

## Palliative Intent: Therapy of Patients with Breast Cancer

The chemotherapeutic treatment of patients with cancer of the breast requires that the physician be knowledgeable about the biology of the disease, the physical and mental condition of the patient, and the properties of, as well as the concepts involved in, the use of drugs used to treat these patients. This is a disease with a wide variation in its clinical behavior.

***Drugs and hormones used to treat advanced breast cancer***

A large number of hormones as well as chemotherapeutic agents are available to treat patients with breast cancer (Table 13-25). However, even with protocols for combination chemotherapy, cure of patients with advanced breast cancer has not yet been realized. The estrogen antagonist tamoxifen has replaced ablative surgery (ovariectomy, adrenalectomy, hypophysectomy) as a means of decreasing estrogen activity in patients with breast cancer. Treatment with this drug is relatively nontoxic and is effective in 60 to 70% of patients with increased expression of the estrogen receptor (ER) and progestin receptor (PR) proteins in their tumors. Although responses usually last 10 to 12 months, relapse may occur because of the emergence of an ER-negative clone. Other effective hormonal agents include high doses of progestins, estrogens, or androgens. The inhibitor of corticosteroid synthesis, aminoglutethimide, may also be effective in patients who have previously responded to other hormonal manipulations. In elderly patients with ER or PR-positive metastatic breast cancer, it may be possible to obtain several years of relatively "good" life with sequential use of these agents.

Several drugs also have been shown to be effective when used as single agents in the treatment of patients with breast cancer, in particular doxorubicin, paclitaxel, or taxotere. Combinations of these drugs are more effective than single agents, but the number of complete responders is small, and cure is rare (Henderson 1984). For certain patients (minimal or no disease following treatment with these regimens) the value of additional intense chemotherapy (e.g., high-dose melphalan) with reinfusion of autologous bone marrow is under investigation. The major problem that limits the usefulness of chemotherapy in this disease is development of drug resistance. Optimization of drug combinations and scheduling may partially overcome this problem, but development of new active agents or therapies may be required before cure of advanced breast cancer is achieved.

**Table 13-25 Drugs Used to Treat Breast Cancer**

| |
|---|
| *Hormones* |
| Prednisone |
| Estrogens |
| Progestins |
| Androgens |
| *Hormone antagonists* |
| Tamoxifen |
| Aminoglutethimide |
| *Chemotherapeutic agents* |
| Alkylating agents (cyclophosphamide, melphalan) |
| Methotrexate |
| 5-Fluorouracil |
| Doxorubicin |
| Paclitaxel/docetaxel |
| *Antibodies* |
| HER2-neu (Herceptin) |

***Operable breast cancer and the use of adjuvant chemotherapy***

In patients who have breast cancer that is "operable" (that is, the surgeon is able to remove all gross tumor and axillary lymph nodes); the ultimate prognosis is determined by 1) the size of the tumor, 2) the number of axillary nodes involved, and 3) the ER and PR status (Bonadonna and Valagussa 1988). The goals of treatment with hormonal agents or chemotherapy are to reduce the risk of recurrence presumably by eradicating metastatic foci not detectable at the time of surgery. For example, in node-negative ($N_0$) ER- or PR-positive patients, treatment may not be indicated because this group of patients may do very well without further therapy (90% disease-free survival [DFS] at 5 years). Treatment for $N_0$, ER- or PR-negative patients may be warranted, because the 5-year DFS is approximately 70%. Obviously, if the treatment itself is associated with mortality in some patients or has significant long-term morbidity (cardiomyopathies, pulmonary problems, secondary malignancies associated with cyclophosphamide), then even in this group adjuvant therapy may not be justified. However, if adjuvant therapy has minimal risks (as with the combination of MTX sequenced with 5-FU), then the risk–benefit ratio favors treatment in this subset of patients. The deletion of an alkylating agent from the treatment program may decrease long-term risks (Fisher et al. 1989).

**PRINCIPLE Treatment intensity (and therefore risk) should reflect the potential benefit expected.**

In patients with 10 or more positive nodes at mastectomy, present chemotherapy programs, even those containing doxorubicin, are only moderately effective in improving the DFS (from 20 to 40% at 5 years). Therefore, even more aggressive treatment regimens, including high-dose chemotherapy with autologous bone marrow transplant, may need to be considered despite the increase in morbidity, especially in young (premenopausal) women. At present, several large clinical trials have begun to address the merits of such dose-intense approaches for patients with high-risk breast cancer. Although these data are yet to be released to the scientific community, they are likely to substantially influence how oncologists manage patients with this disease in the near future.

### Palliative Therapy: Multiple Myeloma

Certain tumors, by virtue of their extremely long doubling time, may be classified as "slow-growing," or chronic, neoplasms. Examples of these diseases are multiple myeloma, CLL, nodular lymphocytic lymphoma, and other well-differentiated solid tumors. To date, although the median survival of these patients may be long (3 to 10 years), curative therapy has not yet been developed. One of these tumors is discussed in some detail, to illustrate the principles of drug therapy for this type of condition.

Multiple myeloma is a neoplastic disease caused by the proliferation of a terminally differentiated malignant plasma cell. These cells usually produce $\gamma$-globulin and may be detected by an increase in the concentration of a $\gamma$-globulin in the serum called *myeloma globulin* (monoclonal gammopathy). A spectrum of clinical syndromes ranging from an asymptomatic increase in the concentration of serum globulins to rapidly progressive disease characterized by destruction of bone, hematologic abnormalities, and renal impairment is associated with this disease.

**PRINCIPLE The clinician should be prepared to treat not only the neoplasia but also the secondary manifestations that may result as a consequence of the tumor (e.g., hyperviscosity, hypercalcemia, renal failure).**

Proliferation of plasma cells is slow when compared with the rate of proliferation of other human malignancies. The mass of tumor cells may be estimated by measuring the turnover of the total body pool of myeloma globulins in vivo (Salmon and Smith 1970). Therefore, the effect of therapy on the mass of malignant cells can be approximated. Patients with myeloma in relapse can have as many as $10^{12}$ tumor cells. "Remission" can occur when this mass of tumor cells is reduced by as little as 1 to 2 logs. These calculations make it clear that before a cure can be obtained, additional effective therapies must be developed (Gore et al. 1989). Intuitively, there is no logical way to convince a patient they are "cured" when $10^{10}$ malignant plasma cells still reside within their body. These studies have also demonstrated that when the mass of tumor cells is reduced by chemotherapy, the growth fraction significantly increases. Thus cell-cycle-active agents might be of value after the alkylating agents have had a chance to reduce the total mass of malignant cells.

Because of the large burden of tumor cells usually present in patients when they seek medical attention, and the slow doubling time of this tumor, it is not surprising that cell-cycle-active agents are generally ineffective when they are used alone or before alkylating agents. In particular, phenylalanine mustard (melphalan, PAM) and cyclophosphamide have been used most widely as initial or sole therapy. Approximately 50% of patients benefit from therapy with alkylating agents. When adrenocortical steroids are added to the regimen, the remission rates are higher, but survival may not be improved. Because of the serious effects of chronic administration of steroids, they are generally used in short pulses of 4 or 5 days every 4 to 6 weeks in combination with the alkylating agent, which is used either in pulses or daily. There is no superiority of either dose schedule of the alkylating agents.

In summary, slow-growing tumors may be sensitive to alkylating agents. Because recovery of normal cells in the bone marrow is more rapid than recovery of tumor cells, the drugs may have some selectivity. Intense treatment with alkylating agents followed by peripheral stem cell rescue is now being evaluated in selected patients with this disease.

## FRONTIERS IN CANCER TREATMENT

### Antiangiogenesis

A recently identified and promising target that is being studied for new drug development is the process of angiogenesis. *Angiogenesis* refers to the ability of cancer cells to stimulate the growth and development of new blood vessels (neovascularization), a necessary requisite for the continued growth and expansion of many solid tumors, and possibly even hematologic malignancies. It is interesting that much of the impetus for this work stems from the intriguing observation that unresected primary mouse tumors appeared to inhibit the growth of metastatic disease. Removal of the primary mass seemed to release the breaks on growth, allowing neovascularization and growth of remote sites of disease. The elegant work of Folkman and colleagues (Folkman 1990, 1995; O'Reilly et al. 1996, 1997) have shown that natural inhibitors of endothelial proliferation existed in the circulation, including a truncated form of a protein derived from collagen XVIII (endostatin), as well as the internal fragment of plasminogen (O'Reilly 1997; O'Reilly et al. 1994, 1997). These substances are potent inhibitors of endothelial cell proliferation and tumor growth in experimental animals. Because these compounds target the nonmalignant cells making up the "soil," that is, the tumor vasculature rather than the tumor cells themselves, resistance to repeated doses of these agents has not been observed in experimental models (Boehm et al. 1997). Angiostatin and endostatin are now being generated by recombinant technology and should be in clinical trials shortly. This exciting research has stimulated the search and identification of other biologically active molecules that might also inhibit angiogenesis (from bacteria, fungi, and other organisms), some of which have already begun to make their way into clinical trials as well. Remarkably, even old misunderstood entities like thalidomide have been resurrected because of their surprising ability to inhibit angiogenesis as well (D'Amato et al. 1994; Bauer et al. 1998). The targeting of tumor cell vasculature may be a relatively nontoxic approach to the control of tumor growth.

## Gene Therapy

A new and promising approach to cancer treatment involves the transfer of discrete genes into either normal somatic tissues or cancer cells. The identification of discrete molecular lesions that contribute to the malignant phenotype have generated an almost infinite spectrum of potential targets for cancer management. In general, three major areas of investigation have progressed rapidly from the laboratory to the clinic, and many early phase clinical trials are currently in progress. These include 1) the introduction of genes into tumor cells that lead to apoptosis or cessation of cell growth, or to increased chemosensitivity (e.g., p. 53); 2) the introduction of genes into tumor cells or dendritic cells (antigen presenting cells) that stimulate an augmented host immune response against the cancer cells; and 3) transfer of drug resistance genes into hematopoietic progenitor cells to decrease hematopoietic toxicity and increase host tolerance of chemotherapy (mutated DHFR, TS, MDR).

For example, the delivery of genes directly into tumor cells has allowed for the study of discrete molecular defects on the malignant phenotype. Such has been the case with the adenovirus-mediated delivery of the wild type tumor-suppressor gene p53. Injection of the adenoviral vectors directly into the tumor tissue has resulted in local tumor regressions (usually partial) and has prompted phase II trials in tumors that are accessible to injection, such as cancers of the head and neck, prostate and breast (Fujiwara et al. 1994; Eastham et al. 1995; Lesson-Wood et al. 1995; Clayman et al. 1995, 1996; Nielsen and Maneval 1998). Transfection of cells or direct injection of tumors with an adenovirus containing a "suicide" gene, such as the herpes simplex virus thymidine kinase (HSV-TK) or cytosine deaminase genes, will lead to metabolic activation of the relatively nontoxic prodrugs ganciclovir and fluorocytosine, respectively. Metabolic activation of these prodrugs will only occur in those cells containing the introduced gene, leading to the production of a toxic intermediate and eventual cell death (Huber et al. 1993; Moolten 1994; Lockett et al. 1997; Rogulski et al. 1997). This unique approach offers the potential of tumor selectivity without excessive host toxicity. Both of these approaches, however, suffer from the limitation that all tumors treated in this fashion must be localized and accessible. Research efforts are now directed toward the targeting of different genes for metastatic tumors.

The possibility of enhancing host immunity by introducing specific genes into either tumors or host immune effector cells also offers many new opportunities to manage cancer with new gene therapy technologies. For example, many laboratories are investigating the effects of delivering genes encoding for cytokines such as GM-CSF into tumors, as well as DNA vaccines, which involves the introduction of genes encoding for specific immunogenic proteins into dendritic cells (through subcutaneous injections). Some of these methods have also begun to enter clinical trials. Although antibody responses to certain tumor antigens have been obtained, definite proof of efficacy will require large-scale clinical trials, which are now under way.

Another attractive gene therapy approach involves the introduction of specific drug resistance genes into hematopoietic stem cell (Bertino 1980; Banerjee et al. 1994; Moore et al. 1996). Many of these drug resistance genes have been generated using techniques in site-directed and random mutagenesis. This strategy offers the possibility of allowing an increase in dose intensity by rendering the normal host tissues "resistant" to the chemotherapy drug administered. Safe retroviral vectors that have been engineered to be replication incompetent are being widely studied for this purpose.

Because retroviral transduction requires the recipient cell populations to be in "cycle," stimulation of $G_0$ progenitor cells by cytokines ex vivo is required to allow for efficient gene transfer. Following gene delivery, the early progenitor cells are returned to the patients, who can now be treated with either additional or higher doses of chemotherapy, depending on the approach used. Studies in mouse models have shown that the animals transplanted with marrow containing a drug-resistant gene can tolerate higher doses of the appropriate drug (e.g., MTX when a mutated resistant dihydrofolate reductase cDNA is used), leading to an improved therapeutic outcome (Zhao et al. 1994, 1997). However, $CD34^+$ cells have proved to be more difficult to transduce, and long-term, high-level expression has been a problem (Li et al. 1994; Flasshove et al. 1995; Spencer et al. 1996).

The potential of using gene therapy for the treatment of cancer patients is enormous. The examples cited above are meant only to illustrate the power of this technology and represent only a sampling of the possible uses of this approach to cancer management.

## REFERENCES


Ackland SP, Schilsky RL. 1987. High dose methotrexate: a critical reappraisal. *J Clin Oncol* **5**(12):2017–31.

Acute Leukemia Group B. 1961. Studies of sequential and combination antimetabolite therapy in acute leukemia: 6 mercaptopurine and methotrexate. *Blood* **18**:431–54.

Adolphe AB, Glasofer ED, Troetel WM, et al. 1975. Fate of streptozotocin (NSC-85998) in patients with advanced cancer. *Cancer Chemother Rep* **59**:547–56.

Alberts DS, Chang SY, Chen HSG, et al. 1979a. Oral melphalan kinetics. *Clin Pharmacol Ther* **26**:737–45.

Alberts DS, Chang SY, Chen HSG, et al. 1979b. Pharmacokinetics and metabolism of chlorambucil in man: a preliminary report. *Cancer Treat Rev* **6**(Suppl):9–17.

Alberts DS, Chang SY, Chen HSG. 1980. Comparative pharmacokinetics of chlorambucil and melphalan in man. *Recent Results Cancer Res* **74**:124.

Alberts DS, Chen HSG, Liu R. et al. 1978. Bleomycin pharmacokinetics in man: I. Intravenous administration. *Cancer Chemother Pharmacol* **1**:177–81.

Alberts DS, Chen HSG, Mayersohn M, et al. 1979. Bleomycin pharmacokinetics in man: II. Intracavitary administration. *Cancer Chemother Pharmacol* **2**:127–32.

Alberts DS, Peng YM, Leigh S, et al. 1985. Disposition of mitoxantrone in cancer patients. *Cancer Res* **45**:1879.

Alexander P. 1965. *Atomic Radiation and Life*. 2nd ed. Middlesex, UK: Penguin Books.

Alexanian R, Haut A, Khan AU, et al. 1969. Treatment for multiple myeloma: combination chemotherapy with different melphalan dose regimens. *JAMA* **208**:1680–5.

Allen LM, Creaven PJ, Nelson RL. 176. Studies on the human pharmacokinetics of isophosphamide (NSC-109724). *Cancer Treat Rep* **60**:451–8.

Arbuck SG, Strauss H, Rowinsky EK, et al. 1993. A reassessment of the cardiac toxicity associated with taxol. *J Natl Cancer Inst Monogr* **15**:117.

Banerjee D, Shao SC, Li MX, et al. 1994. Gene therapy utilizing drug resistance genes: a review. *Stem Cells* **12**:378–85.

Baselga J, Norton L, Albanell J, et al. 1998. Recombinant humanized anti-HER2 antibody (Herceptin) enhances antitumor activity of paclitaxel and doxorubicin against HER2/neu overexpressing human breast cancer xenografts. *Cancer Res* **58**:2825–31.

Baselga J, Tripathy D, Mendelsohn J, et al. 1999. Phase II study of weekly intravenous trastuzumab (Herceptin) in patients with HER2/neu-overexpressing metastatic breast cancer. *Semin Oncol* **26**:78–83.

Bast RC, Zbar G, Borsos T, et al. 1974. BCG and cancer. *N Engl J Med* **290**:1413–20.

Bauer KS, Dixon SC, Figg WD. 1998. Inhibition of angiogenesis required metabolic activation, which is species-dependent. *Biochem Pharmacol* **55**:1827–34.

Beck WT. 1987. The cell biology of multiple drug resistance. *Biochem Pharmacol* **36**:2879.

Belt RJ, Himmelstein KJ, Patton TF, et al. 1979. Pharmacokinetics of non-protein bound platinum species following administration of *cis*-dichlorodiammineplatinum (II). *Cancer Treat Rep* **63**:1515.

Bender RA, Castle MC, Margileth DA, et al. 1977. The pharmacokinetics of [$^3$H]vincristine in man. *Clin Pharmacol Ther* **22**:430–5.

Bennett JM, Reich SD. 1990. Bleomycin. *Ann Intern Med* **90**:945–8.

Benson R, Hartley-Asp B. 1990. Mechanism of action and clinical uses of estramustine. *Cancer Invest* **8**:375.

Berkowitz RS, Bernstein MR, Laborde O, et al. 1994. Subsequent pregnancy experience with gestational trophoblastic disease. New England Trophoblastic Disease Center, 1965–1992. *J Reprod Med* **39**:228.

Berkowitz RS, Goldstein DP, Bernstein MR. 1986. Ten years' experience with methotrexate and folinic acid as primary therapy for gestational trophoblastic disease. *Gynecol Oncol* **23**:111.

Bertelli G. 1995. Prevention and management of extravasation of cytotoxic drugs. *Drug Saf* **12**:245–55.

Bertino JR. 1980. Turning the tables—making normal marrow resistant to chemotherapy. *J Natl Cancer Institute* **82**:1234–5.

Bertino JR. 1989. The general pharmacology of methotrexate. In: Wilke WS, editor. *Methotrexate Therapy in Rheumatic Diseases*. New York: Marcel Dekker. p 11–23.

Bertino JR. 1997. Chemotherapy of colorectal cancer: history and new themes. *Semin Oncol* **24** (Suppl 18):3–7.

Bertino JR, Lin JT, Pizzorno G, et al. 1989. The basis for intrinsic drug resistance or sensitivity to methotrexate. *Adv Enzyme Reg* **29**: 277–85.

Billingham ME, Mason JW, Bristow MR, et al. 1978. Anthracycline cardiomyopathy monitored by morphologic changes. *Cancer Treat Rep* **62**:865.

Bissett D, Setanoians A, Cassidy J, et al. 1993. Phase I and pharmacokinetic study of taxotere (RP 56976) administered as a 24-hour infusion. *Cancer Res* **53**:523.

Blum RH. 1977. Clinical status and optimal use of the cardioprotectant, dexrazoxane. *Oncology (Huntingt)* **11**:1169–77.

Blum RH, Carter SK, Agnes K. 1973. A clinical review of bleomycin—a new antineoplastic agent. *Cancer* **31**:903–14.

Boehm T, Folkman J, Browder T, et al. 1997. Antiangiogenic therapy of experimental cancer does not induce acquired drug resistance. *Nature* **390**:404–7.

Boice JD, Greene MH, Killen JY, et al. 1983. Leukemia and preleukemia after adjuvant treatment of gastrointestinal cancer with semustine (BCNU). *N Engl J Med* **309**:1079–84.

Bonadonna G, Valagussa P. 1988. Current status of adjuvant chemotherapy for breast cancer. *Semin Oncol* **14**:8–22.

Bonadonna G, Valagussa P, Santoro A. 1986. Alternating non-cross resistant combination chemotherapy or MOPP in stage IV Hodgkin's disease. *Ann Intern Med* **104**:739–46.

Bono VH. 1976. Studies on the mechanism of action of DTIC (NSC-45388). *Cancer Treat Rep* **60**:141–8.

Bouffard DY, Laliberte J, Momparler RL. 1993. Kinetic studies on 2′,2′-difluorodeoxycytidine (gemcitabine) with purified human deoxycytidine kinase and cytidine deaminase. *Biochem Pharmacol* **45**:1857.

Bouffard DY, Momparler LF, Momparler RL. 1991. Comparison of antineoplastic activity of 2′,2′-difluorodeoxycytidine and cytosine arabinoside against human myeloid and lymphoid leukemic cells. *Anticancer Drugs* **2**:49.

Boyle DM, Engelking C. 1995. Vesicant extravasation: myths and realities. *Oncol Nurs For* **22**:57–67.

Brade WP, Hendrich K, Varini M. 1985. Ifosfamide—pharmacology, safety and therapeutic potential. *Cancer Treat Rev* **12**:1.

Breithaupt H, Dammann A, Aigner K. 1982. Pharmacokinetics of dacarbazine (DTIC) and its metabolite 5-aminoimidazole-4-carboxamide (AIC) following different dose schedules. *Cancer Chemother Pharmacol* **9**:103–9.

Breithaupt H, Pralle H, Eckhardt T, et al. 1982. Clinical results and pharmacokinetics of high dose cytosine arabinoside (HD-AraC) *Cancer* **50**:1248.

Brockman RW. 1963. Mechanism of resistance to anticancer agents. *Adv Cancer Res* **7**:129.

Broome JR. 1963. Evidence that L-asparaginase of guinea pig serum is responsible for its antilymphoma effects. *J Exp Med* **118**:99–120.

Bruce WR. 1967. The action of chemotherapeutic agents at the cellular level and the effects of these agents on hematopoietic and lymphomatous tissue. In: *Canadian Cancer Conference: Proceedings of the Seventh Canadian Cancer Research Conference*. Elmsford, NY: Pergamon Press, pp 53–64.

Bruce WR, Bergsagel DE. 1967. On the application of results from a model system to the treatment of leukemia in man. *Cancer Res* **27**:2646–9.

Bruce WR, Meeker BE, Powers WE, et al. 1969. Comparison of the dose and time–survival curves for normal hematopoietic and lymphoma colony-forming cells exposed to vinblastine, vincristine, arabinosylcytosine, and amethopterin. *J Natl Cancer Inst* **42**: 1015–23.

Bruce WR, Meeker BE, Valeriote FA. 1966. Comparison of the sensitivity of normal hematopoietic and transplanted lymphoma colony-forming cells to chemotherapeutic agents and administered in vivo. *J Natl Cancer Inst* **37**:233–45.

Buckner CD, Rudolph RH, Fefer A, et al. 1972. High dose cyclophosphamide for malignant disease. *Cancer* **29**:357–65.

Budman DR. 1997. Vinorelbine (Navelbine): a third generation vinca alkaloid. *Cancer Invest* **15**:475–90.

Budman DR, Meropol NJ, Reigner B, et al. 1998. Preliminary studies of a novel oral fluoropyrimidine carbamate: capecitabine. *J Clin Oncol* **16**: 1795–1802.

Burchenal JH, Murphy ML, Ellison RR, et al. 1953. Clinical evaluation of a new antimetabolite, 6-mercaptopurine, in the treatment of acute leukemia and allied diseases. *Blood* **8**:965–99.

Burger RM, Projan SJ, Horwitz SB, et al. 1986. The DNA cleavage mechanism of iron-bleomycin. *J Biol Chem* **261**:15955–9.

Burkitt DP, Burchenal JH (editors). 1969. *Treatment of Burkitt's Tumor*. New York: Springer-Verlag.

Cadman E, Heimer R, Benz C. 1981. The influence of methotrexate pretreatment on 5-fluorouracil metabolism in L1210 cells. *J Biol Chem* **256**:1695–1704.

Cadman E, Heimer R, Davis L. 1979. Enhanced 5-fluorouracil nucleotide formation after methotrexate administration: explanation for drug synergism. *Science* **205**:1135–7.

Capizzi R. 1975. Improvement in the therapeutic index of L-asparaginase by methotrexate. *Cancer Chem Rep* **6**(3):37–41.

Capizzi RL, Bertino JR, Handschumacher RE. 1970. L-Asparaginase. *Annu Rev Med* **21**:433–44.

Capizzi RL, Yang JL, Rathmell JP, et al. 1985. Dose-related pharmacologic effects of high dose ara-C and its self-potentiation. *Semin Oncol* **12**:65–74.

Capranico G, Riva A, Tinnelli S, et al. 1987. Markedly reduced levels of anthracycline-induced DNA strand breaks in resistant P388 leukemia cells and isolated nuclei. *Cancer Res* **47**:3752–6.

Carlson RW, Sikic BI. 1983. Continuous infusion or bolus injection in cancer chemotherapy. *Ann Intern Med* **99**:823–33.

Chabner BA. 1996. Cytidine analogues. In: Chabner BA, Longo DL, editors. *Cancer Chemotherapy and Biotherapy: Principles and Practice*. 2nd ed. New York: Lippincott-Raven, pp 213-34.

Chabner BA, Loo TA. 1996. Enzyme therapy: L-asparaginase. In: Chabner BA, Longo DL, editors. *Cancer Chemotherapy and Biotherapy: Principles and Practice*. 2nd ed. New York: Lippincott-Raven, pp 485–92.

Chabner BA, Stoller RG, Hande KR, et al. 1978. Methotrexate disposition in humans: case studies in ovarian cancer and following high-dose infusion. *Drug Metab Rev* **8**:107.

Chary KK, Higby DJ, Henderson ES, et al. 1977. Phase I study of high dose *cis*-dichlorodiammineplatinum(II) with forced diuresis. *Cancer Treat Rep* **61**:367.

Chronic Myeloid Leukemia Trialists' Collaborative Group. 1997. Interferon alpha versus chemotherapy for chronic myeloid leukemia: a meta analysis of seven randomized trails. *J Natl Cancer Inst* **89**:1616–20.

Chu E, Allegra CJ. 1996. Antifolates. In: Chabner BA, Longo D.L, editors. *Cancer Chemotherapy and Biotherapy: Principles and Practice*. 2nd ed. New York: Lippincott-Raven, pp 109–48.

Clark PI, Slevin ML. 1987. The clinical pharmacology of etoposide and teniposide. *Clin Pharmacokinet* **12**:223.

Clavel M, Guastella J, Peters G. 1989. Phase I study of LY 188011, 2′,2′-difluorodeoxycytidine. *Invest New Drugs* **7**:379.

Clayman GL, El-Nagger AK, Roth J, et al. 1955. In vivo molecular therapy with p53 adenovirus for microscopic residual head and neck squamous carcinoma. *Cancer Res* **55**:1–6.

Clayman GL, Liu TJ, Overholt SM, et al. 1996. Gene therapy for head and neck cancer: comparing the tumor suppressor gene p53 and a cell cycle regulator WAF/CIP1 (p21). *Arch Otolaryngol Head Neck Surg* **122**:489–93.

Cohen BE, Egorin ME, Kohlhepp EA, et al. 1986. Human plasma pharmacokinetics and urinary excretion of thiotepa and its metabolites. *Cancer Treat Rep* **70**:859.

Cole SR, Myers JJ, Klatsky AU. 1978. Pulmonary disease with chlorambucil therapy. *Cancer* **41**:455–9.

Colvin M. 1982. The comparative pharmacology of cyclophosphamide and ifosfamide. *Semin Oncol* **9**(Suppl 1):2–7.

Colvin M, Brundett RB, Cowens JL, et al. 1976. A chemical basis for the antitumor activity of chloroethylnitrosoureas. *Biochem Pharmacol* **25**:695–9.

Colvin M, Hilton J. 1981. Pharmacology of cyclophosphamide and metabolites. *Cancer Treat Rep* **65**(Suppl 3):89–95.

Corden BJ, Fine RL, Ozols RF, et al. 1985. Clinical pharmacology of high dose cisplatin. *Cancer Chemother Pharmacol* **14**:38.

Creaven PJ. 1984. The clinical pharmacology of etoposide (VP-16) in adults. In: Issell BF, Maggia RM, Carter SK, editors. *Etoposide* (VP-16). New York: Academic Press, pp 103–15.

Creaven PJ, Allen LM, Cohen MH, et al. 1976. Studies on the clinical pharmacology and toxicology of isophosphamide (NSC-109724). *Cancer Treat Rep* **60**:445–9.

Cresteil J, Monsarrat B, Alvineine P, et al. 1994. Taxol metabolism by human liver microsome: identification of cytochrome P450 isoenzymes involved in its biotransformation. *Cancer Res* **54**:386.

Curt GA, Grygiel JJ, Corden BJ, et al. 1983. A phase I and pharmacokinetic study of diamminecyclobutane–dicarboxylatoplatinum (NSC 241240) *Cancer Res* **43**:4470.

D'Amato RJ, Loughnan MS, Flynn E, et al. 1994. Thalidomide is an inhibitor of angiogenesis. *Proc Natl Acad Sci USA* **91**:4082–5.

D'Angio GJ, Farber S, Maddock CL. 1959. Potentiation of x-ray effects by actinomycin D. *Radiology* **73**:175–7.

Davis ME, DeSantis D, Klemm K. 1995. A flow sheet for follow-up after chemotherapy extravasation. *Oncol Nurs Forum* **22**:979–81.

Deeley RG, Cole PC. 1997. Function, evolution and structure of multidrug resistant protein (MRP). *Semin Cancer Biol* **8**:193–204.

Demetri GD, Younger J, Shapiro C, et al. 1992. A phase I study of dose intensified CAF chemotherapy with adjunctive r-metHuG-CSF (GCSF) in patients with advanced breast cancer. *Proc Am Soc Clin Oncol*

Depierre A, Chastang C, Quoix E et al. 1994. Vinorelbine versus vinorelbine plus cisplatin in advanced non-small cell lung cancer: a randomized trial. *Ann Oncol* **1**:37–42.

DeVita VT, Canellos GP, Moxley JH. 1972. A decade of combination chemotherapy of advanced Hodgkin's disease. *Cancer* **30**:1495–1504.

DeVita VT, Denham C, Davidson J, et al. 1967. The physiological disposition of carcinostatic 1,3-bis(2-chloroethyl)-1-nitrosourea (BCNU) in man and animals. *Clin Pharmacol Ther* **8**:566–77.

DeVita VT, Hellman S, Rosenberg SA (editors). 1997. *Cancer: Principles and Practice of Oncology*. 5th ed. New York: Lippincott-Raven.

DeVita VT, Serpick AA, Carbone PP. 1970. Combination chemotherapy in the treatment of advanced Hodgkin's disease. *Ann Intern Med* **73**:881–95.

Diaz JF, Andreu JM. 1993. Assembly of purified GDP-tubulin into microtubule induced by Taxol and taxotere: reversibility, ligand stoichiometry and competition. *Biochemistry* **32**: 2747.

Diddens H, Gekeler V, Neumann M, et al 1987. Characterization of actinomycin-D resistant CHO cell lines exhibiting a multidrug-resistance phenotype and amplified DNA sequences. *Int J Cancer* **40**:635–42.

D'Incalci M, Farina P, Sessa C, et al. 1982. Pharmacokinetics of VP16–213 given by different administration methods. *Cancer Chemother Pharmacol* **7**:141.

Disa JJ, Chang RR, Mucci SJ, et al. 1998. Prevention of adriamycin-induced full thickness skin loss using hyaluronidase infiltration. *Plast Reconstr Surg* **101**:370–4.

Donehower RC. 1996. Hydroxyurea. In: Chabner BA, Longo DL, editors. *Cancer Chemotherapy and Biotherapy: Principles and Practice*. 2nd ed. New York: Lippincott-Raven, pp 253–62.

Dorr RT. 1988. New findings in pharmacokinetics, metabolic and drug-resistance aspects of mitomycin-C. *Semin Oncol* **15**(Suppl 4):32–41.

Dorr RT. 1990. Antidotes to vesicant chemotherapy extravasations. *Blood Rev* **4**:41–60.

Dragnev KH, Schwartz GK, Bertino JR, et al. 1998. Interim results of a phase I trial suggests that Tomudex (raltitrexed) may act synergistically with 5-fluorouracil (5-FU) in patients with advanced colorectal cancer. abstract 868. *Am Soc Clin Onocol* **17**.

Dresler WFC, Stein R. 1869. Uber den hydroxyl Harnstoff. *Liebigs Ann Chem* **150**:242–52.

Eastham JA, Hall SJ, Sehgal I, et al. 1995. In vivo gene therapy with p53 or p21 adenovirus for prostate cancer. *Cancer Res* **55**:5151–5.

Edwards MS, Levin VA, Seager ML, et al. 1979. Phase II evaluation of thiotepa for treatment of central nervous system tumors. *Cancer Treat Rep* **63**:1419–21.

Ehrsson H, Hassan M, Ehrnbo M, et al. 1983. Busulfan kinetics. *Clin Pharmacol Ther* **34**:86–9.

Elion GB, Bargi E, Hitchings G. 1952. Studies on condensed pyrimidine systems: IX. The synthesis of some 6-substituted purines. *J Am Chem Soc* **74**:411–4.

Endicott JA, Ling V. 1989. The biochemistry of P-glycoprotein-mediated multidrug resistance. *Annu Rev Biochem* **58**:137.

Ettinger LJ, Kurtzberg J, Voute PA, et al. 1995. An open-label, multicenter study of polyethylene glycol-L-asparaginase in the treatment of acute lymphoblastic leukemia. *Cancer* **75**:1176–1181.

Extra JM, Rousseau F, Bruno R, et al. 1993. Phase I and pharmacokinetic study of Taxotere (RP56976; NSC 628503) given as a short intravenous infusion. *Cancer Res* **53**:1037.

Farber S, Diamond LK, Mercer RD, et al. 1948. Temporary remissions in acute leukemia in children produced by folic antagonist, 4-amethopteroyl ghitamic acid (aminopterin). *N Engl J Med* **238**:787–93.

Farmer PB. 1987. Metabolism and reactions of alkylating agents. *Pharmacol Ther* **35**:301–58.

Fearon ER. 1995. Molecular abnormalities in colon and rectal cancer. In: Mendelsohn J, Howley PM, Israel MA, et al., editors. *The Molecular Basis of Cancer*. Philadelphia: WB Saunders, pp. 340.

Fearon ER, Vogelstein B. 1990. A genetic model for colorectal tumorigenesis. *Cell* **61**:759.

Fellous A, Ohayon R, Vacassin T, et al. 1989. Biochemical effects of Navelbine on tubulin and associated proteins. *Semin Oncol* **16**: 9–14.

Fernandes DJ, Bertino JR 1980. 5-Fluorouracil–methotrexate synergy: enhancement of 5-fluorodeoxyuridylate binding to thymidylate synthetase by dihydropteroyl polyglutamates. *Proc Natl Acad Sci USA* **77**:5663–7.

Fisher B, Redmond C, Dimitrov NV, et al. 1989. A randomized clinical trial evaluating sequential methotrexate and fluorouracil in the treatment of patients with node negative breast cancer who have estrogen receptor tumors. *N Engl J Med* **320**:473–8.

Flasshove M, Banerjee D, Bertino JR, et al. 1995. Increased resistance to methotrexate in human hematopoietic cells after gene transfer of the Ser31 DHFR mutant. *Leukemia* **9**:S34–S37.

Flowers CR, Melmon KL. 1997. Clinical investigators as critical determinants in pharmaceutical innovation. *Nat Med* **3**:136–43.

Folkman J. 1990. What is the evidence that tumors are angiogenesis dependent? *J Natl Cancer Inst* **82**:4–6.

Folkman J. 1995. Clinical application of research on angiogenesis. *N Engl J Med* **333**:1757–63.

Forshell GP, Muntzing J, Ek A, et al. 1976. The absorption, metabolism and excretion of Estracyt (NSC-89199) in patients with prostatic cancer. *Invest Urol* 14:128.

Frei E III. 1974. The clinical use of actinomycin. *Cancer Chemother Rep* **58**:49–54.

Frei E III. 1984. Acute leukemia in children: model for the development of scientific methodology for clinical therapeutic research in cancer. *Cancer* **53**:2013-25.

Frosch PJ, Czarnetzki BM, Macher E, et al 1979. Hepatic failure in patients treated with dacarbazine (DTIC) for malignant melanoma. *J Cancer Res Clin Oncol* **95**:281–6.

Fugman RA, Martin DS, Hayworth PE, et al. 1970. Enhanced cures of spontaneous mammary carcinoma with surgery and five compound combination chemotherapy and their immunotherapeutic interrelationship. *Cancer Res* **30**:1931–6.

Fujiwara W, Grimm EA, Mukhopadhyay T, et al. 1994. Induction of chemosensitivity in human lung cancer cells in vivo by adenovirus-mediated transfer of the wild-type p53 gene. *Cancer Res* **54**: 2287–91.

Gabrilove JL, Jakubowski A, Scher H, et al. 1988. Effect of granulocyte stimulating factor on neutropenia and associated morbidity due to chemotherapy for transitional cell carcinoma of the urothelium. *N Engl J Med* **318**:1414–22.

Gilman A. 1963. The initial clinical trial of nitrogen mustard. *Am J Surg* **105**:574–8.

Gilman A, Phillips FS. 1946. The biological actions and therapeutic applications of the $\beta$-chloroethylamines and sulfides. *Science* **103**:409–15.

Gires P, Gaillard C, Martin S, et al. 1994. [$^{14}$C]Docetaxel (Taxotere) disposition in the isolated perfused rat liver and effect of enzyme induction [abstract]. *Eur J Drug Metab Pharmacokinet* **19**(Suppl 2): 29.

Glisson B, Gupta R, Hodges P, et al. 1986. Cross resistance to intercalating agents in an epipodophyllotoxin-resistant Chinese hamster ovary cell line: evidence for a common intracellular target. *Cancer Res* **46**:1939–42.

Goldenberg MM. 1999. Trastuzumab, a recombinant DNA-derived humanized monoclonal novel agent for the treatment of metastatic breast cancer. *Clin Ther* **21**:309–18.

Goldenberg GJ, Vanstone CL, Israels LG, et al. 1970. Evidence for a transport carrier of nitrogen mustard in nitrogen mustard-sensitive and resistant L5178Y cells. *Cancer Res* **30**:2285–91.

Goldie JH, Coldman AJ, Gudauskas GA. 1982. Rationale for the use of alternating non-cross resistant chemotherapy. *Cancer Treat Rep* **66**:439–49.

Goldstein DP. 1972. The chemotherapy of trophoblastic disease. *JAMA* **220**:209–13.

Gore ME, Selby PJ, Viner C, et al. 1989. Intensive treatment of multiple myeloma and criteria for complete remission. *Lancet* **2**:879–82.

Gorlick R, Goker E, Trippett T, et al. 1996. Intrinsic and acquired resistance to methotrexate in acute leukemia. *N Engl J Med* **335**:1041–8.

Gorlick R, Goker E, Trippett T, et al. 1997. Defective transport is a common mechanism of acquired methotrexate resistance in acute lymphocytic leukemia and is associated with decreased reduced folate carrier expression. *Blood* **89**:1013-18.

Gorlick R, Metzger R, Danenberg KD, et al. 1998. Higher levels of thymidylate synthase gene expression are observed in pulmonary as compared with hepatic metastases of colorectal adenocarcinoma. *J Clin Oncol* **16**:1465–9.

Greene R, Collins J, Jenkins J, et al. 1983. Plasma pharmacokinetics of Adriamycin and Adriamycinol: implications for the design of in vitro experiments and treatment protocols. *Cancer Res* **43**: 3417.

Grochow LB, Colvin M. 1979. Clinical pharmacokinetics of cyclophosphamide. *Clin Pharmacokinet* **4**:380–94.

Grogan TM, Spier CM, Salmon SE, et al. 1993. P-Glycoprotein expression in human plasma cell myeloma: correlation with prior chemotherapy. *Blood* **81**:490.

Guilhot F, Chastang C, Michallet M, et al. 1997. Interferon alpha-2b combined with cytarabine versus interferon alone in chronic myelogenous leukemia. *N Engl J Med* **337**:223–9.

Hammond CB, Borchet LG, Tyrey L, et al. 1973. Treatment of metastatic trophoblastic disease: good and poor prognosis. *Am J Obstet Gynecol* **115**:451–7.

Hande KR. 1992. Etoposide pharmacology. *Semin Oncol* **19**:3.

Hartley-Asp B. 1984. Estramustine induces mitotic arrest in two human prostatic cell lines, DU 145 and PC-3. *Prostate* **5**:93.

Heidelberger C, Chaudhuari NK, Danenberg P, et al. 1957. Fluorinated pyrimidines: a new class of inhibitory compounds. *Nature* **179**:663–6.

Heinemann V, Xu YZ, Chubb R, et al. 1990. Inhibition of ribonucleotide reduction in CCRF-CEM cells by 2′,2′-difluorodeoxycytidine. *Mol Pharmacol* **38**:567.

Henderson ES, Adamson RH, Oliverio VT. 1965. The metabolic fate of tritiated methotrexate: II. Absorption and excretion in man. *Cancer Res* **25**:1018–24.

Henderson IC. 1984. Chemotherapy for advanced disease. In: Bonadonna G, editor. *Breast Cancer: Diagnosis and Management*. New York: Wiley, pp 247–80.

Henner WD, Peters WP, Eder JP, et al. 1986. Pharmacokinetics and immediate effects of high-dose carmustine in man. *Cancer Treat Rep* **70**:877.

Hersh MR, Ludden TM, Kuhn JG, et al. 1983. Pharmacokinetics of high dose melphalan. *Invest New Drugs* **1**:331–4.

Hertel LW, Boder GB, Kroin JS, et al. 1990. Evaluation of the antitumor activity of gemcitabine (2′,2′-difluoro-2′-deoxycytidine). *Cancer Res* **50**:4417.

Hertz R. 1972. Gestational trophoblastic neoplasia. *Hosp Pract* **1**: 157–64.

Hirsch JD, Conlon PF. 1983. Implementing guidelines for managing extravasation of antineoplastics. *Am J Hosp Pharm* **40**:1516–9.

Holland JF, Bast RC, Morton DL, et al., editors. 1997. *Cancer Medicine* 4th ed. Baltimore: Williams & Wilkins.

Hood AF. 1986. Cutaneous side effects of cancer chemotherapy. *Med Clin North Am* **70**:187–209.

Howell SB, Schiefer M, Andrews PA, et al. 1987. The pharmacology of intraperitoneally administered bleomycin. *J Clin Oncol* **5**: 2009–16.

Hryniuk WM. 1987. Average relative dose intensity and the impact on design of clinical trials. *Semin Oncol* **14**:65–74.

Hryniuk WM, Bertino JR 1969a. Rationale for the selection of chemotherapeutic agents. *Adv Intern Med* **15**:267–98.

Hryniuk WM, Bertino JR 1969b. The treatment of leukemia with large doses of methotrexate and folinic acid: clinical–biochemical correlates. *J Clin Invest* **48**:2140–55.

Hryniuk WM, Fisher GA, Bertino JR 1969. S-phase cells of rapidly growing and resting populations: differences in response to methotrexate. *Mol Pharmacol* **5**:557–64.

Hubbard SM, Jenkins JF. 1990. Chemotherapy administration. In: Chabner BA, Collins JM, editors. *Cancer Chemotherapy: Principles and Practice*. Philadelphia: Lippincott, pp 449–64.

Huber BE, Austin EA, Good SS, et al. 1993. In vivo antitumor activity of 5-fluorocytosine on human colorectal carcinoma cells genetically modified to express cytosine deaminase. *Cancer Res* **53**:4619–26.

Huffman DH, Bachur NR. 1972. Daunorubicin metabolism in acute myelocytic leukemia. *Blood* **39**:637.

Huggins C, Stevens RE, Hodges CV. 1941. Studies on prostatic cancer: effects of castration on advanced carcinoma of prostate gland. *Arch Surg* **43**:209–23.

Juma FD, Rogers HJ, Trounce JR. 1979. Pharmacokinetics of cyclophosphamide and alkylating activity in man after intravenous and oral administration. *Br J Clin Pharmacol* **8**:209–7.

Kaminski MS, Zasadny KR, Francis IR, et al. 1993. Radioimmunotherapy of B-cell lymphoma with [$^{131}$I] anti-B1 (anti-CD20) antibody. *N Engl J Med.* **329**:459.

Kaminski MS, Zasdny KR, Francis IR, et al. 1996. Iodine-131-anti-B1 radioimmunotherapy for B-cell lymphoma. *J Clin Oncol* **14**:1974.

Kay AC, Saven A, Carrera CJ, et al. 1992. 2-Chlorodeoxycytidine treatment of low grade lymphoma. *J Clin Oncol* **10**:371.

Keating MJ, Holmes R, Lerners , et al. 1993. L-asparaginase and PEG asparaginase—past, present, and future. *Leuk Lymphoma* **10**(Suppl):153–157.

Kemeny N, Cohen A, Bertino JR, et al. 1989. Continuous intrahepatic infusion of floxuridine and leucovorin through an implantable pump for the treatment of hepatic metastases from colorectal carcinoma. *Cancer* **65**:2446–50.

Kidd JG. 1953. Regression of transplanted lymphomas induced in vivo by means of normal guinea pig serum. *J Exp Med* **98**:565–82.

Kirkwood JM, Strawderman MH, Ernstoff MS, et al. 1996. Interferon alfa-2b adjuvant therapy of high risk resected cutaneous melanoma: The Eastern Cooperative Oncology Group Trial EST 1684. *J Clin Oncol* **14**:7–17.

Kirkwood JM, Ibrahim J, Sondak V, et al. 1999. Preliminary analysis of the E1690/S9111/C9190 intergroup postoperative adjuvant trial of high- and low-dose IFN$\alpha$;2b (HDI and LDI) in high risk primary or lymph node metastatic melanoma. *Proc Am Soc Oncol* **18**:2072 (abstract).

Knox SJ, Goris ML, Trisler K, et al. 1996. Yttrium-90-labeled anti-CD20 monoclonal antibody therapy of recurrent B-cell lymphoma. *Clin Cancer Res* **2**:457.

Kontis PH, Egorin MJ, Van Echo DA, et al. 1982. Phase II evaluation and plasma pharmacokinetics of high dose intravenous 6-thioguanine in patients with colorectal carcinoma. *Cancer Chemother Pharmacol* **8**:199.

Koren G, Ferrazini O, Sulh AM, et al. 1990. Systemic exposure to mercaptopurine as a prognostic factor in acute lymphocytic leukemia in children. *N Engl J Med* **323**:17–21.

Kristenson L, Weisman K, Hutter L. 1975. Renal function and the rate of disappearance of methotrexate from serum. *Eur J Clin Pharmacol* **8**:439.

Kufe DW, Monroe D, Herrick D, et al. 1984. Effects of 1-D-arabinofuranosylcytosine incorporation on eukaryotic DNA template function. *Mol Pharmacol* **26**:128–34.

Lassus M, Scott D, Leyland-Jones B. 1985. Allergic reactions associated with Cremophor containing antineoplastics [abstract]. *Proc Am Soc Clin Oncol* **4**:268.

Lawrence HJ, Walsh D, Zapotowski KA, et al. 1989. Topical dimethylsulfoxide may prevent tissue damage from anthracycline extravasation. *Cancer Chemother Pharmacol* **23**:316–8.

Lazarus HM, Reed MD, Spitzer TR, et al. 1987. High-dose IV thiotepa and cryopreserved autologous bone marrow transplantation for therapy of refractory cancer. *Cancer Treat Rep* **71**:689–95.

Lazo JS, Humphreys CJ. 1983. Lack of metabolism as the biochemical basis of bleomycin-induced pulmonary toxicity. *Proc Natl Acad Sci USA* **80**:3064–8.

Legha SS, Benjamin RS, Mackay B, et al. 1982. Reduction of doxorubicin cardiotoxicity by prolonged continuous intravenous infusion. *Ann Intern Med* **96**:133–9.

Lennard L, Rees CA, Lilleyman JS, et al. 1983. Childhood leukemia: a relationship between intracellular 6-mercaptopurine metabolites and neutropenia. *Br J Clin Pharmacol* **16**:359.

Lennard L, Van Loon JA, Weinshilboun RM. 1989. Pharmacogenetics of acute azathioprine toxicity: relationship to thiopurine methyltransferase genetic polymorphism. *Clin Pharm Ther* **46**:149.

Lenz HJ, Leichman CG, Danenberg KD, et al. 1996. Thymidylate synthase mRNA level in adenocarcinoma of the stomach: a predictor for primary tumor response and overall survival. *J Clin Oncol* **14**:176–82.

LePage GA, Whitecar JP. 1971. The pharmacology of 6-thioguanine in man. *Cancer Res* **31**:1627–31.

Lesson-Wood LA, Kim WH, Kleinman HK, et al. 1995. Systemic gene therapy with p53 reduces growth and metastases of a malignant human breast cancer in nude mice. *Hum Gene Ther* **6**:395–405.

Levin VA, Hoffman W, Weinkam RJ. 1978. Pharmacokinetics of BCNU in man: a preliminary study of 20 patients. *Cancer Treat Rep* **62**:1305.

Li MX, Banerjee D, Zhao SC, , et al. 1994. Development of a retroviral construct containing a human mutated dihydrofolate reductase cDNA for hematopoietic stem cell transduction. *Blood* **83**: 3403–8.

Liliemark J, Juliusson G. 1991. On the pharmacokinetics of 2-chloro-2′-deoxyadenosine in humans. *Cancer Res* **51**:5570.

Liliemark JO, Plunkett W, Dixon DO. 1985. Relationship of 1-D-arabinofuranosylcytosine-5-triphosphate levels in leukemia cells during treatment with high dose 1-D-arabinofuranosylcytosine. *Cancer Res* **45**:5952–7.

Lobel JS, O'Brien RT, McIntosh S, et al. 1979. Methotrexate and asparaginase combination chemotherapy in refractory acute lymphoblastic leukemia of childhood. *Cancer* **43**:1089–94.

Lockett LJ, Molloy PL, Russell PJ, et al. 1997. Relative efficiency of cell killing in vitro by two enzymes-pro-drug systems delivered by identical adenovirus vectors. *Clin Cancer Res* **3**:2075–80.

Longnecker SM, Donehower RC, Cates AE, et al. 1986. High performance liquid chromatographic assay for Taxol (NSC 125973) in human plasma and urine pharmacokinetics in a phase I trial. *Cancer Treat Rep* **71**:54.

Loo TL, Luce JK, Sullivan MP, et al. 1968. Clinical pharmacologic observations on 6-mercaptopurine and 6-mercaptopurine ribonucleotide. *Clin Pharmacol Ther* **9**:180.

Luduena RF, Shooter EM, Wilson L. 1977. Structure of the tubulin dimer. *J Biol Chem* **252**:7006–14.

Maloney DG, Grillo-Lopez AJ, White CA, et al. 1997. IDEC-C2B8 (Rituximab) anti-CD-20 monoclonal antibody therapy in patients with relapsed low grade non-Hodgkin's lymphoma. *Blood* **90**:2188–95.

Maloney DG, Liles TM, Czerwinski DK, et al. 1994. Phase I clinical trial using escalating single dose infusion of chimeric anti-CD-20 monoclonal antibody (IDEC-C2B8) in patients with recurrent B-cell lymphoma. *Blood* **84**: 2457–66.

Malspeis L, Grever MR, Staubus AE, et al. 1990. Pharmacokinetics of 2-F-ara-A (9-beta-D-arabinofuranosyl-2-fluoradenine) in cancer patients during the phase I clinical investigation of fludarabine phosphate. *Semin Oncol* **17**(Suppl 8):18–32.

Marne F, DeSousa G, Placidi M, et al. 1993. Elucidation of hepatic biotransformation of Taxotere using human "in vitro" models [abstract]. *Bull Cancer* **80**:527.

McDermott BJ, van der Berg HW, Murphy RF. 1982. Non-linear pharmacokinetics for the elimination of 5-fluorouracil after intravenous administration in cancer patients. *Cancer Chemother Pharmacol* **9**:173.

Mead GM, Arnold AM, Green JA. 1982. Epileptic seizures associated with cisplatin administration. *Cancer Treat Rep* **66**:1719–22.

Melmon KL. 1974. The endocrinologic manifestations of the carcinoid tumor. In: Williams RH, editor. *Textbook of Endocrinology*. Philadelphia: WB Saunders, pp 1084–1104.

Michael M, Moore M. 1997. Clinical experience with gemcitabine in pancreatic carcinoma. *Oncology (Huntingt)* **11**(11):1615–22.

Mini E, Trave F, Rustum YM, et al. 1990. Enhancement of the antitumor effects of 5-fluorouracil by folinic acid. *Pharmacol Ther* **47**:1–19.

Monsarrat B, Alvinerie P, Gares M, et al. 1993. Hepatic metabolism and biliary excretion of Taxol. *Cell Pharmacol* **1**:77.

Moolten FL 1994. Drug sensitivity ("suicide") genes for selective cancer chemotherapy. *Cancer Gene Ther* **1**: 279–87.

Moore EW, Thomas LB, Shaw RK, et al. 1960. The central nervous system in acute leukemia: a postmortem study of 117 consecutive cases, with particular reference to hemorrhage, leukemic infiltrations and the syndrome of meningeal leukemia. *Arch Intern Med* **105**:451–68.

Moore MAS, Leonard JP, Flasshove M, et al. 1996. Gene therapy the challenge for the future. *Ann Oncol.* **7**: 53–8.

Muggia FM, Chan KK, Russell C, et al. 1991. Phase I and pharmacologic evaluation of intraperitoneal 5-fluoro-2′-deoxyuridine. *Cancer Chemother Pharmacol* **28**:241.

Muggia FM, Louie AC, Sikic BI. 1983. Pulmonary toxicity of antitumor agents. *Cancer Treat Rev* **10**:221–43.

Muntzing J, Jensen G, Hogberg B. 1979. Pilot study on the growth inhibition by estramustine phosphate (Estracyt) on rat mammary tumors sensitive and insensitive to oestrogens. *Acta Pharmacol Toxicol* **44**:1.

Neidhart JA. 1992. Hematopoietic colony stimulating factors. Uses in combination with standard chemotherapeutic regimens and in support of dose intensification. *Cancer* **70**:913–20.

Nelson RL. 1982. The comparative clinical pharmacology and pharmacokinetics of vindesine, vincristine, and vinblastine in human patients with cancer. *Med Pediatr Oncol* **10**:115.

Nelson RL, Dyke RW, Root MS. 1980. Comparative pharmacokinetics of vindesine, vincristine, and vinblastine in patients with cancer. *Cancer Treat Rev* **7**(Suppl):17.

Nielsen LL, Maneval DC. 1998. P53 tumor suppressor gene therapy for cancer. *Cancer Gene Ther* **5**:52–63.

O'Reilly MS. 1997. Angiostatin: an endogenous inhibitor of angiogenesis and of tumor growth. *Exper Suppl (Basel)* **79**:273–94.

O'Reilly MS, Boehm T, Shing Y, et al. 1997. Endostatin: an endogenous inhibitor of angiogenesis and tumor growth. *Cell* **88**:277–85.

O'Reilly MS, Holmgren L, Chen C, et al. 1996. Angiostatin induces and sustains dormancy of human primary tumors in mice. *Nature Med* **2**:689–92.

O'Reilly MS, Holmgren L, Shing Y, et al. 1994. A novel angiogenesis inhibitor that mediates the suppression of metastases by a Lewis lung carcinoma. *Cell* **79**:315–28.

Osserman EF, Lawlor DP. 1996. Serum and urinary lysozyme (muramidase) in monocytic and monomyelocytic leukemia. *J Exp Med* **124**:921–52.

Ozols RF, Corden BJ, Jacob J. 1984. High-dose cisplatin in hypertonic saline. *Ann Intern Med* **100**:19–24.

Pallavincini MG. 1984. Cytosine arabinoside, molecular, pharmacokinetic and cytokinetic considerations. *Pharmacol Ther* **25**:207–38.

Perillie PE, Kaplan SS, Lefkowitz E, et al. 1968. Studies of muramidase (lysozyme) in leukemia. *JAMA* **203**:317–22.

Piro LD, Carrera CJ, Carson DA, et al. 1990. Lasting remissions in hairy-cell leukemia induced by a single infusion of 2-chlorodeoxyadenosine. *N Engl J Med* **22**:1117–21.

Plagemann PG, Erbe J. 1972. Intracellular conversions of deoxyribonucleotides by Novikoff rat hepatoma cells and effects of hydroxyurea. *J Cell Physiol* **83**:321.

Pommier Y, Kerrigan D, Schwartz RE, et al. 1986. Altered DNA topoisomerase II activity in Chinese hamster cells resistant to topoisomerase II inhibitors. *Cancer Res* **46**:3075–81.

Portlock CS, Fischer DS, Cadman E, et al. 1987. High-dose pulse chlorambucil in advanced low grade non-Hodgkin's lymphoma. *Cancer Treat Rep* **71**:1029–31.

Pratt CB, Green AA, Horowitz ME. 1986. Central nervous system toxicity following the treatment of pediatric patients with ifosfamide/mesna. *J Clin Oncol* **4**:1253–61.

Rajaonarison JF, Lacarelle B, Catalin J, et al. 1993. Effect of anticancer drugs on the glucuronidation of 3′-azido-3′-deoxythymidine in human liver microsomes. *Drug Metab Dispos* **21**:823–9.

Reddy MV, Randerath K. 1987. Analysis of DNA products in somatic and reproductive tissues of rats tested with the anticancer antibiotic mitomycin C. *Mutat Res* **179**:75–88.

Rees LH, Landon J. 1976. Biochemical abnormalities in some human neoplasms: inappropriate biosynthesis of hormones by tumors. In: Symington T, Carter RL, editors. *Scientific Foundations of Oncology*. London: William Heinemann, pp 107–16.

Rieselbach RE, Morse EE, Rall DP, et al. 1963. Intrathecal aminopterin therapy of meningeal leukemia. *Arch Intern Med* **111**:620–30.

Riordan JR, Ling V. 1985. Genetic and biochemical characterization of multidrug resistance. *Pharmacol Ther* **28**:51–75.

Rogulski KR, Zhang K, Kolozsvary A, et al. 1977. Pronounced antitumor effects and tumor radiosensitization of double suicide gene therapy. *Clin Cancer Res* **3**:2081–8.

Rosenberg B, Van Camp L, Krigas T. 1965. Inhibition of division in *E. coli* by electrolysis products from a platinum electrode. *Nature* **205**:698.

Rosman M, Lee MH, Creasey WA, et al. 1974. Mechanisms of resistance to 6-thiopurines in human leukemia. *Cancer Res* **34**: 1952–6.

Rosman M, Williams HE. 1973. Leukocyte purine phosphoribosyltransferases in human leukemias sensitive and resistant to 6-thiopurines. *Cancer Res* **33**:1202–9.

Ross GT, Goldstein DP, Hertz R, et al. 1965. Sequential use of methotrexate and actinomycin D in the treatment of metastatic choriocarcinoma and related trophoblastic diseases in women. *Am J Obstet Gynecol* **93**:223–9.

Ross W, Rowe T, Glisson B, et al. 1984. Role of topoisomerase II in mediating epidophyllotoxin-induced DNA cleavage. *Cancer Res* **44**:5857–60.

Rowinsky EK, Donehower RC. 1996. Antimicrotubule agents. In: Chabner BA, Longo DL, editors. *Cancer Chemotherapy and Biotherapy: Principles and Practice*. 2nd ed. New York: Lippincott-Raven, pp. 263–96.

Rowinsky EK, McGuire WP, Guarnieri J, et al. 1991. Cardiac disturbances during the administration of Taxol. *J Clin Oncol* **9**: 1704.

Rudnick SA, Cadman EC, Capizzi RL, et al. 1979. High-dose cytosine (HDARAC) arabinoside in refractory acute leukemia. *Cancer* **44**:1189–93.

Salmon SE, Smith BA. 1970. Immunoglobulin synthesis and total body tumor cell number in IgG multiple myeloma. *J Clin Invest* **49**:1114–21.

Sarosy G, Leyland-Jones B, Soochan P, et al. 1988. The systemic administration of intravenous melphalan. *J Clin Oncol* **6**:1768–82.

Sawada N, Ishikawa T, Fukase Y, et al. 1998. Induction of thymidine phosphorylase activity and enhancement of capecitabine efficacy by Taxol/Taxotere in human cancer xenografts. *Clin Cancer Res* **4**:1013–9.

Schabel FM. 1975. Concepts for systemic treatment of micrometastases. *Cancer* **35**:15–24.

Schackney SE, Ritch PS. 1982. Cell kinetics. In: Chabner BA, editor. *Pharmacologic Principles of Cancer Treatment*. Philadelphia: WB Saunders, pp 45–76.

Schein PS, Tew KD, Mathe G. 1984. Pharmacology of nitrosourea anticancer agents. In: Bukarda B, Karrer K, Mathe G, editors. *Clinical Chemotherapy: Antineoplastic*. Vol. 3. New York: Thieme-Stratton, pp 264–82.

Schiff PB, Fant C, Horowitz SB. 1979. Promotion of microtubule assembly in vitro by taxol. *Nature* **22**:665.

Schiff PB, Horowitz SB. 1980. Taxol stabilizes microtubules in mouse fibroblast cells. *Proc Natl Acad Sci USA* **77**:1561.

Schilsky RL, Barlock A, Ozols RF. 1982. Persistent hypomagnesemia following cisplatin chemotherapy for testicular cancer. *Cancer Treat Rep* **66**:1767–9.

Scholar EM, Calabresi P. 1979. Increased activity of alkaline phosphatases in leukemia cells from patients resistant to thiopurine. *Biochem Pharmacol* **28**:445–6.

Scuderi N, Onesti MG. 1994. Antitumor agents: extravasation, and surgical treatment. *Ann Plast Surg* **32**:39–44.

Shak S. 1999. Overview of the trastuzumab (Herceptin) anti-HER@monoclonal antibody clinical program in HER2-overexpressing metastatic breast cancer. Herceptin Multinational Investigator Study Group. *Semin Oncol* **26**:71–7.

Shiba DA, Weinkam RJ. 1982. Quantitative analysis of procarbazine, procarbazine metabolites and chemical degradation products with application to pharmacokinetic studies. *J Chromatogr* **229**:397.

Shipley LA, Brow TJ, Cornpropst JD, et al. 1992. Metabolism and disposition of gemcitabine, and oncolytic deoxycytidine analogue, in rats, mice, and dogs. *Drug Metab Dispos Biol Fate Chem* **20**:849.

Simon RM. 1997. Clinical trials in cancer. In: DeVita VT, Hellman S, Rosenberg SA, editors. *Cancer: Principles and Practice of Oncology*. 5th ed. New York: Lippincott-Raven, pp 513-27.

Skipper HE. 1965. Experimental evaluation of potent anticancer agents: XIV. Further study of certain basic concepts underlying chemotherapy of leukemia. *Cancer Chemother Rep* **45**:5–28.

Skipper HE. 1967. Experimental evaluation of potential anticancer agents: XXI. Scheduling of arabinosylcytosine to take advantage of its S-phase specificity against leukemia cells. *Cancer Chemother Rep* **51**:125–65.

Skipper HE, Schabel FM, Wilcox W. 1964. Experimental evaluation of potential anticancer agents: XIII. On the criteria kinetics associated with "curability" of experimental leukemia. *Cancer Chemother Rep* **35**:3–111.

Sladek NE, Doeden D, Powers JF. 1984. Plasma concentrations of 4-hydroxycyclophosphamide and phosphoramide mustard in patients given repeatedly high dose of cyclophosphamide in preparation for bone marrow transplantation. *Cancer Treat Rep* **68**:1247–54.

Slamon DJ, Godolphin W, Jones LA et al. 1989. Studies of the HER2/neu proto-oncogene in human breast and ovarian cancer. *Science* **244**:707–12.

Slevin ML, Piall EM, Aherne GW, et al. 1983. Effect of dose and schedule on pharmacokinetics of high-dose cytosine arabinoside in plasma and cerebrospinal fluid. *J Clin. Oncol* **1**:546.

Smyth JF, Macpherson JS, Warrington PS, et al. 1986. The clinical pharmacology of mitoxantrone. *Cancer Chemother Pharmacol* **17**:149.

Smyth JF, Paine PM, Jackman AL, et al. 1980. The clinical pharmacology of the adenosine deaminase inhibitor 2′-deoxycorfomycin. *Cancer Chemother Pharmacol* **5**:93.

Sobell HM, Jain SC, Sakore TD, et al. 1971. Stereochemistry of actinomycin-DNA binding. *Nature New Biol* **231**:200–5.

Sobrero AF, Aschele C, Bertino JR 1997. Fluorouracil in colorectal cancer—a tale of two drugs: implications for biochemical modulation. *J Clin Oncol* **15**:368–81.

Spencer HT, Sleep SEH, Rehg JE, et al. 1996. A gene transfer strategy for making bone marrow cells resistant to trimetrexate. *Blood* **87**:2579–87.

Spiegel RJ. 1981. The acute toxicities of chemotherapy. *Cancer Treat Rev* **8**:197–207.

Spriggs DR, Robbins G, Arthur K, et al. 1988. Prolonged high-dose ara-C infusions in acute leukemia. *Leukemia* **2**:304–6.

Steel GG. 1967. Cell loss as a factor in the growth of human tumors. *Eur J Cancer* **3**:381–7.

Steinherz LJ, Steinherz PG, Tan CT, et al. 1991. Cardiac toxicity 4 to 20 years after completing anthracycline therapy. *JAMA* **266**: 1672–7.

Steinherz LJ, Steinherz PG, Tan CC. 1995. Cardiac failure and dysrhythmias 6–19 years after anthracycline therapy: a series of 15 patients. *Med Pediatr Oncol* **24**:352–61.

Steinherz LJ, Steinherz PG. 1991. Delayed cardiac toxicity from anthrocycline therapy. *Pediatrician* **18**:49–52.

Steinherz PG. 1987. Acute lymphoblastic leukemia of childhood. *Hematol/Oncol Clin North Am* **1**:549–66.

Struck RF, Alberts DS, Horne K, et al. 1987. Plasma pharmacokinetics of cyclophosphamide and its cytotoxic metabolites after intravenous versus oral administration in a randomized, cross-over trial. *Cancer Res* **47**: 2723.

Takimoto CH, Arbuck SG. 1996. Camptothecins. In: Chabner BA, Longo DL, editors. *Cancer Chemotherapy and Biotherapy: Principles and Practice*. 2nd ed. New York: Lippincott-Raven, pp 463–84.

Tattersall MHN, Ganeshaguru K, Hoffbrand AV. 1974. Mechanisms of resistance of human acute leukemia cells to cytosine arabinoside. *Br J Haematol* **27**:39–46.

Tattersall MHN, Parker LM, Pittman S. 1975. Clinical pharmacology of high dose methotrexate (NSC-740). *Cancer Chemother Rep* **6**: 25–9.

Tattersall MHN, Sodegren JE, Sengupta SK, et al. 1975a. Pharmacokinetics of actinomycin D in patients with malignant melanoma. *Clin Pharmacol Ther* **17**:701–8.

Tattersall MHN, Sodegren JE, Sengupta SK, et al. 1975b. Pharmacokinetics of actinomycin D adsorbed in patients with malignant melanoma. *Clin Pharmacol Ther* **17**:701.

Tew TD, Glusker JP, Hartley-Asp B, et al. 1992. Preclinical and clinical perspectives on the use of estramustine as an antimitotic drug. *Pharmacol Ther* **56**:323.

Thelander L, Reichard P. 1979. Reduction of ribonucleotides. *Annu Rev Biochem* **48**:133.

Till JE, McCulloch EA. 1961. A direct measurement of the radiation sensitivity of normal mouse marrow cells. *Radiat Res* **14**:213-22.

Tobe SW, Siu LL, Jamal SA, et al. 1995. Vinblastine and erythromycin: an unrecognized serious drug interaction. *Cancer Chemother Pharmacol* **35**:188–90.

Tomasz M, Lipman R, Lee MS, et al. 1987. Reaction of acid-activated mitomycin C with calf thymus DNA and model guanines: elucidation of the base-catalyzed degradation of $N^7$-alkylguanine nucleosides. *Biochemistry* **26**:2010–27.

Tsuruo T. 1988. Mechanisms of multidrug resistance and implications for therapy. *Jpn J Cancer Res* **79**:285–96.

Umezawa H, Hori S, Sawa T, et al. 1974 A bleomycin-inactivating enzyme in mouse liver. *J Antibiot (Tokyo)* **27**:419–24.

Umezawa H, Maeda K, Takeuchi T, et al. 1966. New antibiotics: bleomycin A and B. *J Antibiot (Tokyo)* **19**:200–9.

Valeriote FA, Bruce WR. 1967. Comparison of the sensitivity of hematopoietic colony-forming cells in different proliferative states to vinblastine. *J Natl Cancer Inst* **38**:393–9.

Vassal G, Fischer A, Chaline D, et al. 1993. Busulfan disposition below the age of three: alterations in children with lysosomal storage disease. *Blood* **82**:1030.

Vogelzang NJ. 1984. Continuous infusion chemotherapy: a critical review. *J Clin Oncol* **2**:289–304.

Vonderheid EC. 1984. Topical mechlorethamine chemotherapy. *Int J Dermatol* **23**:180–6.

Von Hoff DD, Rosenzweig M, Piccart M. 1982. The cardiotoxicity of anticancer agents. *Semin Oncol* **9**:23–33.

Walker MD. 1973. Nitrosoureas in central nervous system tumors. *Cancer Chemother Rep* **4**(pt. 3):21–6.

Wallner J, Depisch D, Hopfner M, et al. 1991. MDR1 gene expression and prognostic factors in primary breast carcinomas. *Eur J Cancer* **27**:1352.

Walters RS, Kantarjian HM, Keating MJ, et al. 1988. Mitoxantrone and high-dose cytosine arabinoside in refractory acute myelogenous leukemia. *Cancer* **62**:677–82.

Wani MC, Taylor HL, Wall ME, et al. 1971. Plant antitumor agents: VI. The isolation and structure of taxol, a novel antileukemic and antitumor agent from *Taxus brevifolia*. *J Am Chem Soc* **93**: 2325.

Warren RD, Bender RA. 1977. Drug interactions with antineoplastic agents. *Cancer Treat Rep* **61**:1231–41.

Weikam RJ, Shiba DA. 1982. Non-classical alkylating agents: procarbazine. In: Chabner BA, editor. *Pharmacologic Principles of Cancer Treatment*. Philadelphia: WB Saunders, pp 340–9.

Weiss HD, Walker MD, Wiernik PH. 1974. Neurotoxicity of commonly used antineoplastic agents. *N Engl J Med* **291**:75–81; 127–33.

Weiss M, Maslak P, Feldman E, et al. 1996. Cytarabine with high dose mitoxantrone induces rapid complete remission in adult acute lymphoblastic leukemia without the use of vincristine or prednisone. *J Clin Oncol* **14**:2480–5.

Weiss RB. 1982. Streptozocin: a review of its pharmacology, efficacy, and toxicity. *Cancer Treat Rep* **66**:427–438.

Weiss RB, Bruno S. 1981. Hypersensitivity reactions to cancer chemotherapy. *Ann Intern Med* **94**:66–72.

Whitehead VM, Kalman TI, Rosenblatt DS, et al. 1987. Methotrexate polyglutamate synthesis in lymphoblasts from children with acute lymphoblastic leukemia. *Dev Pharmacol Ther* **10**:443–8.

Wiernik PH, Schwartz EL, Strauman JJ, et al. 1987. Phase I clinical and pharmacokinetic study of taxol. *Cancer Res* **47**:2486.

Wilcox WS, Griswold DP, Laster WR, et al. 1965. Experimental evaluation of potential anticancer agents: XVII. Kinetics of growth and regression after treatment of certain solid tumors. *Cancer Chemother Rep* **47**:27–39.

Woolley PV. 1983. Hepatic and pancreatic damage produced by cytotoxic drugs. *Cancer Treat Rev* **10**:117–37.

Wright JA. 1989. Altered mammalian ribonucleoside diphosphate reductase from mutant cell lines. In: Cory JG, Cory AH, editors. *Inhibitors of Ribonucleotide Diphosphate Activity*. New York: Pergamon Press, pp 89–111.

Yagoda A, Mukherji B, Young C, et al. 1972. Bleomycin an antitumor antibiotic: clinical experience in 274 patients. *Ann Intern Med* **77**:861–70.

Yokoyama A, Furuse K, Niitani H, et al. 1992. Multi-institutional phase II study of Navelbine (vinorelbine) in the treatment of non-small cell lung cancer. *Am J Clin Oncol* **11**:287.

Zhao SC, Banerjee D, Mineishi S, et al. 1997. Post-transplant methotrexate administration leads to improved curability of mice bearing a mammary tumor transplanted with marrow transduced with a mutant human dihydrofolate reductase cDNA. *Human Gene Ther* **8**:903–9.

Zhao SC, Banerjee D, Schweitzer BI, et al. 1994. Long-term protection of recipient mice from lethal doses of methotrexate by marrow infected with a double copy vector retrovirus containing a mutant dihydrofolate reductase. *Cancer Gene Ther* **1**:27–33.

Zhou-Pan XR, Senee E, Zhou XJ, et al. 1993. Involvement of human liver cytochrome P450 #A in vinblastine metabolism: drug interactions. *Cancer Res* **53**:5121–6.

Ziegler JL. 1973. Burkitt's tumor. In: Holland JF, Frei E III, editors. *Cancer Medicine*. Phildelphia: Lea & Febiger pp 1321–30.

CHAPTER

# 14 INFECTIOUS DISORDERS

Thomas J. Marrie, Claire Touchie, B. Lynn Johnston, Kevin R. Forward, Kathryn L. Slayter, Spencer Lee, Paul Hoffman*

## Chapter Outline



Infectious diseases comprise those illnesses that are caused by microorganisms or their products. Clinical manifestations of infection occur only when sufficient tissue injury has been inflicted directly by microbial products (e.g., endotoxins and exotoxins), or indirectly by host responses (e.g., cytokines and hydrolytic enzymes released by polymorphonuclear leukocytes). Despite the extraordinary recent advances that have occurred in therapeutics for infectious diseases, a number of basic principles should be followed to prescribe antimicrobials and vaccines in an optimal manner. This chapter addresses the broader issues of treating infectious diseases and provides a number of practical clinical examples to demonstrate rational therapeutics.

A rational therapeutic strategy in the management of proved or suspected infectious diseases must focus on the following:

- Performing a history and physical examination, and from the data obtained deciding on the infection syndrome that is the most likely explanation for the patient's illness (e.g., endocarditis, urosepsis, pneumonia)
- Collection of the appropriate specimens to make a microbiological etiological diagnosis
- Utilizing local epidemiological data (e.g., 30% of *Streptococcus pneumoniae* isolated in this community are resistant to penicillin) in choosing an appropriate empirical antimicrobial regimen with which to treat your patient
- Tailoring the dose and route of administration of the antimicrobial in accordance with host factors (severity of illness, shock, renal failure, immunosuppression, etc.)
- Moving from broad-based empiric therapy to more specific, narrow-spectrum therapy once an etiologic diagnosis is available
- Monitoring response to treatment so that treatment failure and adverse drug reactions are recognized
- Assessing the risk of this infection to the community (e.g., tuberculosis, meningococcal disease in a school) and informing public health authorities when appropriate
- Assessing the opportunities for prevention of this and other infections in this patient

The importance of appropriate decision-making is highlighted by the fact that antimicrobials are among the most commonly prescribed drugs on a worldwide basis. Antibiotics account for one of five new and refill prescriptions each year. Furthermore, hospital purchases of antibiotics usually represent 25 to 30% of the annual drug budget for the institution (Barriere 1985; Col and O'Connor 1987; Lebow 1987). Each tertiary care hospital in the United States typically spends more than $1 million per annum on antibiotic purchases alone. Given this tremen-

*The authors recognize the major contribution of the previous authors of this chapter, Richard Root, Walter J. Hierholzer, Jr., Peter D. O'Hanley, Janice Y. Tam, and Mark Holodniy.

dous utilization of antimicrobials, it is disturbing that numerous carefully performed surveys at private and university-affiliated facilities have indicated that the majority of hospitalized patients had no evidence of infection to justify antimicrobial usage or were treated with inappropriate dosage or inappropriate antimicrobials with respect to the infectious disease process (Kunin et al. 1973; Craig et al. 1978; Maki and Schunna 1978; Coleman et al. 1990). A recent study of 1529 U.S. physicians who treated 28,787 patients on an ambulatory basis found that antibiotics were frequently prescribed for viral respiratory tract infections (Gonzales et al. 1997). When these data were extrapolated nationwide, 12 million antibiotic prescriptions accounting for 21% of all antibiotic prescriptions to adults in 1992 were for treatment of viral infections.

These examples of excessive utilization and misuse of antibiotics justify ongoing educational programs related to improving usage of antimicrobials. However, educational programs alone will probably not correct excessive antibiotic misuse. In a hospital setting, requiring prior authorization (from the Infectious Disease Service) for the use of selected antimicrobials resulted in a decrease of up to 32% in the expenditures for parenteral antimicrobials in a teaching hospital (White et al. 1997). The financial considerations for hospitals, health insurance companies, and patients related to the costs of inappropriate antibiotic therapy represent a potentially serious misuse of health care resources to the extent that compromises are made in delivery of other necessary patient care services. If physicians do not recognize and respond to this problem, bureaucratic policies regarding utilization may be instituted (Wenneberg et al. 1984). However, the most important consequence of the misuse of antibiotics is the widespread emergence of antibiotic resistance and the attendant loss of effective antibiotics to treat life-threatening infections.

**PRINCIPLE Overuse and misuse of antibiotics not only waste health care dollars, but also have a hidden cost of inducing antibiotic resistance in important pathogens, making serious infections more difficult to treat.**

## EPIDEMIOLOGIC AND VIRULENCE FACTORS IN INFECTIOUS DISEASES

### Epidemiologic Considerations

Before appropriate therapy can be given for an infectious disease, consideration of epidemiologic factors is essential. This section does not fully discuss the epidemiology (the determinants, occurrence, distribution, and control of health and disease) of infectious diseases. However, a number of basic principles and historical points are worth emphasizing.

#### *Basic principles of transmission*

An infectious disease results from the interaction between an infectious agent and a susceptible host. The agent may originate from a source external to the host (exogenous infection), or, because of changes in the agent–host relationship, a normally occurring, usually innocuous, microbial agent on skin or mucosal surfaces can produce disease (endogenous infection). The relationship among the agent, its transmission, and the host represents the chain of infection. In general, the greatest risk for developing infections in the immunocompetent individual is related to acquisition of pathogenic microorganisms (e.g., *Shigella*). Among immunocompromised patients (e.g., leukemic patients undergoing chemotherapy), endogenous flora (e.g., staphylococci or enteric gram-negative bacilli such as *Escherichia coli*) are more likely the cause of disease.

#### *Acquisition*

Humans are first exposed to microorganisms at birth during passage through the vagina. Thereafter, acquisition, carriage, and clearance of microorganisms are basic facts of life. There are four main routes of acquisition of microorganisms: 1) contact, 2) inhalation, 3) common-vehicle, and 4) vector-borne. Table 14-1 outlines the source, route of acquisition, and portal of entry of microorganisms causing certain specific diseases. The route for contact acquisition involves direct transfer of the agent to the susceptible host from person to person or via fomite or droplet. For transmission by inhalation, the agent is airborne in small particles (<5 mm diameter). In contrast, contact droplet spread occurs when large droplets (≥5 mm diameter) are physically transmitted directly onto surfaces of the respiratory tract. Streptococcal and measles infections are examples of droplet-spread disease. They usually occur when multiple persons are exposed to a single index patient who comes in close contact with susceptible hosts. In contrast, transmission by inhalation occurs when susceptible hosts are exposed to aerosols containing microbes. Direct-proximity contact is not necessary. Tuberculosis is an example of spread by inhalation of contaminated aerosols from human to human; psittacosis and Q fever represent transmission from an infected animal to human by inhalation transmission. In the last-mentioned aerosolized *Coxiella burnetii* organisms or spores can be windborne miles from the source, and inhalation by a susceptible host results in Q fever.

Table 14-1 **Transmission of Specific Diseases**

| Infectious Vector | Route of Acquisition | Portal of Entry | Specific Disease |
|---|---|---|---|
| Lesion exudate | Contact (sexual intercourse) | Genital mucosa | Gonorrhea, syphilis, herpes, chancroid |
| Contaminated water | Contact (fomite, e.g., razor blade) | Broken skin | Carbuncles, *Pseudomonas* folliculitis |
| Respiratory secretions | Contact (droplets) | Respiratory tract | Streptococci, measles, "common cold" |
| Respiratory aerosols | Inhalation | Respiratory tract | Tuberculosis, psittacosis, Q fever |
| Contaminated food | Common vehicle (ingestion) | GI | *Shigella, Salmonella,* hepatitis A |
| Blood | Common vehicle (IV "street drug" needle) | Bloodstream | AIDS, hepatitis B, hepatitis C |
| Blood | Vector-borne (arthropod) | Broken skin | Malaria, yellow fever, epidemic typhus, Rocky Mountain spotted fever |

A common inanimate vehicle usually serves to transmit an agent to multiple hosts. The most frequently involved common vehicles are food and water, which can transmit a number of different pathogens (e.g., enteric bacillary pathogens and hepatitis A). Contaminated needles are an important common vehicle for transmitting HIV, hepatitis B, and hepatitis C virus among injection drug users.

For some agents, maturation and multiplication through intermediate hosts (e.g., arthropod vectors) are necessary preliminaries for transmission to humans. Vector-borne diseases (e.g., malaria) are termed *biologically transmitted* diseases.

***Patient information***

A complete history is often the key to making an etiological diagnosis of an infectious disease. Where the patient has been, what he has done, and with whom he has done it is a succinct summary. Important information can be gained from a consideration of age, gender, place of residence, family, and other personal contacts (including the history of these contacts with disease), occupation, hobbies, contacts with animals, travel history, exposure to parenteral drugs or blood products, sexual habits, dietary habits, other active medical problems, and medications. Obviously, the thoroughness with which this information is collected is tailored to the particular situation. The medical equivalent to a surgical "second look" is to retake the history. Since the physician has not made a diagnosis at this point, careful attention to items that seem insignificant is important.

In *hospital-acquired* infections, important points of epidemiologic information that should be sought include the types of infectious complications that are associated with different procedures or conditions in general; the particular microorganisms that may be specific to the particular institution in which you are practicing (e.g., *Serratia marcescens* resistant to gentamicin); previous or current antimicrobial therapy; the concomitant use of other medications that might alter host defense or the manifestations of disease (e.g., corticosteroids or other immunosuppressive agents); history of transfusion or parenteral use of medication; the incidence and type of infections in other patients or personnel who have been in contact with the patient. The decisions involved in empirical selection of antimicrobials to treat hospital-acquired infections are usually more complex than those for community-acquired infections. These decisions must be founded on an accurate data base that is continually reviewed for new trends in infections in a particular hospital. In general, this task is assigned to an infection surveillance and control committee in the hospital (Joint Commission on Accreditation of Hospitals 1987).

## Infectivity

The sequence of acquisition followed by colonization and multiplication is termed the *infectivity* of the organism. Individuals harbor a varied population of microorganisms that have different potentials to produce disease. The endogenous flora periodically include a number of organisms that are commonly described as *virulent* and called *pathogens*. The names are apt because the organisms have been clearly identified as major causative agents of disease.

For example, strains of *Neisseria meningitidis* are a leading cause of bacterial meningitis in infants, children, and adults but are often found in the nasopharynx of healthy individuals (carriers) of all ages (e.g., 25 to 40% of normal young adults). Carriers can be properly thought of as being "colonized" with a potentially virulent organism which, because of host and other immunologic factors, is contained to a mucosal surface (Griffiss and

Brandt 1986). In fact, this carrier state is probably crucial for eliciting protective immunity. Other "pathogens" that can be carried for long periods without their hosts developing disease include pneumococci, *Streptococcus pyogenes*, *Staphylococcus aureus*, salmonellae, and many viruses including herpes group agents. When host defenses are altered, infections may develop not only with these recognized pathogens but with other organisms that are usually considered harmless.

In the absence of selected host defense factors, some pathogens are so virulent that, when acquired, they virtually always produce disease. For example, in a classic epidemiologic study of persons who lacked protective antibody and were colonized with rubeola virus in the upper respiratory tract, the attack rate of measles exceeded 90% (Christiansen 1952–1953).

Knowledge of the infectivity and virulence of microorganisms is important in determining the likelihood of infection. Mere documentation of the presence of a potential pathogen is not sufficient reason to institute treatment unless disease is present or the threat of disease is great. Nowhere is this more important than in the intubated ventilated patient. Potentially pathogenic microorganisms are almost always isolated from cultures of respiratory secretions in this setting.

**PRINCIPLE The decision to institute antibiotic therapy depends upon consideration of all clinical and laboratory data designed to answer the question: Is this an infection or is this colonization? Knowledge of the infectivity and virulence of a microorganism is crucial.**

## Virulence Factors

Microbial factors that influence the severity of the infection include the size of the infective dose, the duration of exposure of the host to the microbe, competition from surrounding flora, and the virulence of infecting microorganism (this includes a variety of factors including the ability to cause infection at low doses, to resist host defenses, and to elaborate compounds that cause tissue injury). For example, the pathogenesis of ascending, nonobstructive *Escherichia coli* pyelonephritis in women with anatomically normal urinary tracts exemplifies a number of important characteristics. These include both organism and host factors. The organism factors are presence of pili, certain K antigen types, and secretion of hemolysin and colicin V. Host factors include a short urethra in women (rendering them more susceptible than men to urinary tract infection during childhood and early adulthood). In addition, the presence of the Lewis blood group nonsecretor and recessive phenotype is found more commonly among women with recurrent urinary tract infections, suggesting a genetic predisposition. This infection may be viewed as the culmination of a sequence of events mediated by specific determinants of microbial virulence (Table 14-2).

**Key Points: Microbial factors that influence severity of infection include the following:**

- **Inoculum size**
- **Duration of exposure of host to microbe**
- **Competition from surrounding flora**
- **Virulence of the pathogen.**

In summary, the pathogenic process of microbial disease is orderly and requires sequential steps for disease. Virulence factors enable the microbial pathogen to establish, proliferate, damage, and disseminate in specific niches of the host. These determinants of bacterial virulence are under the control of a regulatory system that enables the microorganism to adapt to and overcome local host environments (Relman and Falkow 1990). Relatively little is known about either the specific environmental signals (e.g., temperature, pH, calcium, iron, amino acids) to which these systems respond or the rationale for these responses. The regulatory system usually involves a pair of proteins: One protein acts as a sensor of environmental stimuli and transmits a signal to the other protein, usually by means of phosphorylation; the second protein, once stimulated, acts to regulate gene expression.

There may be many regulatory systems in the genetic elements of the microorganism that respond independently to a variety of environmental stimuli. However, coordinated control of a group of operons is under the domain of a regulon. A regulon provides a means by which many genes can respond in a coordinated fashion to a particular environmental stimulus. The regulon exerts its regulatory functions by *trans*-acting regulatory loci that exert positive or negative expression on a number of virulence factors, e.g., *vir* in *Bordetella pertussis* (Weiss and Falkow 1984) and *virR* in *Shigella* (Maurelli and Sansonetti 1988). These determinants mediate their regulatory function at the level of transcription. Another mechanism by which bacteria can regulate expression of virulence and thereby evade host defenses is DNA rearrangements. A well-studied example of this is the expression of flagellin genes in *Salmonella typhimurium* (Simon et al. 1980). By this mechanism, *S. typhimurium* expresses either H1 or H2 flagellins, thereby evading possible host antibody responses. Other examples include *Trypanosoma brucei* in which subpopulations of the parasite have antigenically

Table 14-2 Uropathogenesis of *Escherichia coli* Pyelonephritis

| PATHOGENIC STEP | MICROBIAL FACTOR | HOST DEFENSES |
|---|---|---|
| Colonization | Pili | Urine flow, antibody |
| Proliferation | Colicin V | Acute-phase reactants |
| Invasion or cellular injury | Invasion proteins, hemolysin, lipopolysaccharide | Phagocytes, antibody–complement lysis, antibody neutralization |
| Dissemination | K antigens, serum resistance | Phagocytes, antibody, complement lysis |

different forms of a major variant surface glycoprotein (VSG) at the cell surface. Individual trypanosomes are capable of producing more than 100 different VSGs during the course of an infection (Deitsch et al. 1997).

This theme of modification of surface structure is a common method of avoiding the host immune response. Two recent observations help explain various aspects of bacterial virulence. The first of these is the concept of pathogenicity islands. These are discrete segments of DNA that encode virulence traits and appear to have a foreign origin (Mecsas and Strauss 1996). These pieces of foreign DNA are often missing in closely related nonvirulent bacteria. The second observation is that of type III or contact-dependent secretion (Mecsas and Strauss 1996): So far type III secretion has been described only in gram-negative bacteria. This mechanism allows bacteria to secrete toxins or other products while in direct contact with a host cell.

Microbial pathogens may evade the host's immune system by adapting to intracellular survival where they are hidden from phagocytic cells as well as from complement and antibody (Finlay and Falkow 1997). While microorganisms are within the cell, they may reside in host cell phagosomes or endosomes or, through lysis of the endosome, escape into the cytoplasm. *Salmonella typhi*, for example, may reside transiently in intestinal epithelial cells before systemic spread (Bliska et al. 1993). *Chlamydia trachomatis*, *Mycobacterium tuberculosis*, and *Legionella pneumophila* reside in endosomal vacuoles, whereas species of *Rickettsia* and *Listeria monocytogenes* escape the phagosome and reside in the cytoplasm (Finlay and Falkow 1997). In the case of *L. monocytogenes*, the nonmotile intracellular bacteria can move within the host cell's cytoplasm by polymerizing actin filaments in a manner that propels the bacteria and permits intracellular spread. In all these cases, the microbe is able to subvert or redirect host cell biological processes; in fact, microbes have become probes for elucidating fundamental cell biological processes associated with organelle trafficking and intracellular signaling.

Those microorganisms that replicate within phagosomes must either prevent acidification and subsequent fusion of microorganism-laden phagosomes with secondary lysosomes (phagosome–lysosome fusion) or exhibit a survival strategy for coping with low pH conditions and increased levels of reduced oxygen radicals and nitric oxide (Hoffman 1997). Generally, the process of phagocytosis initiates a series of biochemical events that include acidification of the microorganism laden endosome and the activation of Rab proteins associated with organelle trafficking (Rab 5 and 7) that facilitate the fusion of these endosomes with secondary lysosomes (Via et al. 1997; Sterimark et al. 1994). *Leishmania* and *Mycobacteria* can survive acidified phagosomes, whereas *Chlamydia* and *Legionella* cannot. Recent studies indicate that pathogens use different strategies in subverting phagosomes to hospitable domiciles. In the case of *L. pneumophila*, an intracellular parasite of protozoa in aquatic environments and an opportunistic human pulmonary pathogen, the bacteria block phagosome–lysosome fusion by redirecting the bacteria-laden phagosome to the endoplasmic reticulum. Here, the endoplasmic reticulin envelops the phagosome, forming what is termed a *replicative phagosome* that is now permissive for bacterial multiplication (Hoffman 1997). It is evident that the *Legionellae* modify the phagosome so that it becomes refractory to secondary lysosomes, while recruiting nonlysosomal vesicles, mitochondria, and ribosomes.

Although intracellular parasites are protected from the effects of antibody and complement, these organisms are still susceptible to the action of the cytotoxic T lymphocytes (CTLs) and natural killer cells (NK cells). In many cases, a small number of highly conserved proteins, stress proteins or heat shock proteins (Hsps), are processed and presented by infected host cells in major histocompatibility class (MHC) I or II surface molecules, and these antigens are recognized by T lymphocytes. These stress protein-derived peptides, together with secretion of interleukins (ILs), promote a T helper 1 (Th1) type (cytotoxic) immune response (Luigina et al. 1997). Several recent studies have shown that members of the Hsp60 and Hsp70 families of stress-induced proteins can induce production of IL-1 and IL-12 (Retzlaff et al. 1996; Skeen et al. 1996). Moreover, Hsp60 has been shown to bind to the surface of macrophages and to signal through protein kinase C IL-1 production. Whereas IL-1 plays a general role in promoting a fever response and activating the immune system, IL-12 plays a major role in the immune response of most intracellular parasites as well as infections caused by noninvasive microbial pathogens. IL-12 activates T cells to produce $\gamma$-interferon (IFN-$\gamma$) and tumor necrosis factor $\beta$ (TNF-$\beta$) (Luigina et al. 1997). It is noteworthy that IFN-$\gamma$ production leads to further stimulation of IL-12 production by phagocytic cells. In addition, IFN-$\gamma$ also downregulates transferrin receptors leading to decreased intracellular levels of iron, as well as activating the production of nitrous oxide (NO). Taken together, these interactions generally provide an effective response to invasive microbial parasites by either killing them outright or inhibiting their intracellular multiplication. Immunocompromised individuals are at greater risk for developing severe disease because of failure of the cellular immune system to produce those necessary cytokines. Although some consideration has been given to administering IL-12 and other cytokines to immunocompromised individuals, it should be emphasized that most of the cytokines are not systemic molecules, but their action is required locally.

In some instances, changes in host receptors determine the virulence of a microorganism. *Streptococcus pneumoniae* colonizes 20 to 30% of humans, but only a few develop invasive disease. In the human lung both the opaque and the disease-causing transparent pneumococci adhere to alveolar cells. However, when a viral respiratory tract infection is present, the host cytokines activate platelet-activating factor on the surface of lung epithelial cells. The transparent pneumococci can adhere to this receptor and can invade via the pulmonary capillaries or lymphatic vessels (Hamburger and Robertson 1940; Plotowski et al. 1986; Cundell et al. 1995).

**PRINCIPLE Understanding the molecular pathogenesis of bacterial virulence offers the possibility of new therapeutic strategies that could not have been considered without such information.**

## HOST FACTORS

The ability of a microorganism to produce disease in the host is a function of the interplay between the virulence of the microorganism and host factors. Host factors that interfere with a microorganism's ability to colonize, proliferate, invade, or injure include nonspecific and specific defense mechanisms (Table 14-3). Nonspecific responses represent primitive protective mechanisms that are not

**Table 14-3 Host Factors Associated with Defense Against Microorganisms**

| | |
|---|---|
| Nonspecific | Normal flora |
| | Tissue tropism |
| | Epithelial and mucosal barriers |
| | Excretory secretions and flows |
| | Natural antibodies |
| | Cytokines and other acute-phase reactants |
| | Phagocytosis by leukocytes |
| | Alternative complement system |
| | Hormones |
| Specific | Antibodies |
| | Classic complement system |
| | T cells |

SOURCE: From Tramont 1990.

specifically directed at a particular microorganism and that do not involve immunologic memory. In contrast, specific host defense mechanisms involve lymphocytes that kill microorganisms specifically or that elicit antibody production. Specific antibodies bind to selected microbial antigens and, in coordination with the classic complement system, eventually kill microorganisms. These specific host defense mechanisms involve immunologic memory and are important for host immunity on subsequent exposure or infection by microorganisms. Defects in any of the host's defensive weapons increase the host's susceptibility to infection. It must be stressed that although a majority of infections are associated with microbial evasion of host factors, the elicited host responses (e.g., cytokines) to microorganisms can account for considerable host injury.

**PRINCIPLE In considering the pathogenesis of infection, it is crucial to assess the defects in host defenses that contributed to disease. One goal of treatment is to correct these abnormalities so that a successful clinical outcome will occur and disease will not worsen or recur after therapeutic intervention. Conversely, when host defense mechanisms contribute to injury during infection, modulation of host factors may be required for successful outcomes.**

Some important host factors that are not generally considered in discussions of immunity include normal flora tissue, tropism of the microorganism, and cytokines. Microorganisms that usually produce disease must come in contact with or penetrate the skin or mucosal surfaces. The integrity of skin and mucous membrane barriers constitutes a major line of defense against microorganisms.

The majority of infections among leukemic patients undergoing chemotherapy occur only when these surfaces are broken, thereby allowing endogenous flora to invade deeper structures and cause disease. Under normal conditions, the flora that usually colonize epithelial surfaces (e.g., skin and GI tract) also protect the host from microbial invasion by exogenous pathogens. The nonspecific mechanisms of this protection include competition for the same nutrients, competition for host receptors for colonization, and production of bacteriocins that are toxic to other microbes. The result of these mechanisms is to limit the ability of a "foreign microbe" to colonize and proliferate on these surfaces (also known as *colonization resistance*). Normal flora are influenced by a number of factors including diet, hormones, sanitary conditions, hygienic habits, and exposure to toxins and antibiotics. Indiscriminate use of antimicrobials is a common problem; the resulting changes in endogenous flora may produce deleterious effects in the host. Antibiotic concentrations at these epithelial surfaces can be sufficient to kill microorganisms directly or to affect their physiology. The overall effects of antibiotics on normal flora are to decrease their number or their ability to persist on these surfaces. These changes enable potential pathogens to colonize the epithelial surfaces.

Normal flora also are crucial for continuous "priming" of the immune system. The continuous influx of products from normal flora across epithelial surfaces represents a constant priming signal for macrophages to process these substances. In germ-free animals and newborns, there is an overall lack of antigen processing by the host, as exemplified by the low levels of class II histocompatibility (DR) molecule expression on macrophages (Steinman et al. 1980; Stiehm et al. 1984; Tramont 1990). However, once endogenous flora are established on epithelial mucosal surfaces, there are marked increases in expression of DR molecules in macrophages. Therefore, the constant exposure of host macrophages and T cells to antigens from indigenous flora enables the host to be primed for immune responses. The maintenance of the normal flora is crucial for health.

**PRINCIPLE Antibiotics can have deleterious effects on the host by eliminating or adversely affecting the beneficial effects of the normal flora.**

The ability of microorganisms to colonize specific epithelial surfaces is linked to the presence of microbial adhesins and host receptors that permit attachment. Most microorganisms, whether endogenous or pathogenic, preferentially colonize certain tissues; this phenomenon is referred to as *tissue tropism*. Host receptors for attachment of microorganisms vary depending on the tissue (e.g., esophagus versus colon), cellular mixture (e.g., epithelial cells versus stromal constituents), and conditions of health (e.g., during menstruation) or disease (e.g., following viral and bacterial infections). Table 14-4 lists adhesins used by *Escherichia coli* and their corresponding host receptors.

These receptor compounds usually are located on epithelial surfaces and enable the microorganism to colonize these surfaces. For example, type 1 pili of uropathogenic *E. coli* strains can bind to uroepithelia because D-mannose is bound to these cells (O'Hanley et al. 1985). However, the host possesses a natural defense factor to prevent epithelial mucosal binding by this adhesion under normal conditions. Renal tubular cells secrete the Tamm–Horsfall uromucoid, a highly mannosylated glycoprotein (Orskov et al. 1980). This uromucoid interferes with uroepithelial attachment of bacteria with this mannose adherence specificity, because it binds bacterial adhesins when the microorganism is in the urinary stream. The binding of the bacterial adhesin by D-mannose moieties in the uromucoid represents an important normal host factor that prevents bacteriuria. There are a number of other host excretory and secretory substances (e.g., saliva, tears, fibronectin, mucus) that hinder colonization of mucosal surfaces by microbes. A number of normal processes (e.g., GI peristalsis, the ciliary movement of the respiratory epithelia, cough, and micturition) then remove these unattached microorganisms from the host.

The use of soluble receptor analogs to prevent microorganism attachment to target host cells is a new therapeutic strategy. For example, administration of soluble CD4 molecule prevents HIV attachment to T-helper cells in vitro, thus abrogating viral invasion of these cells. The usefulness of this strategy in clinical conditions requires complete inhibition of virus attachment to host cells and

**Table 14-4 Selected *E. coli* Adhesins and Host Receptors**

| *E. coli* Adhesin | Host Compound or Receptor |
|---|---|
| Type 1 pili | D-Mannose (Tamm–Horsfall uromucoid) |
| Pap pili | $\alpha$-D-Gal*p*-(1 $\rightarrow$ 4)-$\beta$-D-Gal*p* |
| K88 pili | $GM_1$ ganglioside |
| K99 pili | $\beta$-D-Gal*p*-(1 $\rightarrow$ 4)-$\beta$-D-Glc*p*-(1-1)-ceramide |
| CFA pili | $GM_2$ ganglioside |
| S pili | Sialic acid (glycophorin) |
| MN pili | *N*-Acetylneuraminic acid |

effective clearance of the microorganism from the host. This exciting new direction in disease prevention has been made possible only by elucidating the basis of the attachment of microorganisms to the host at a molecular level (namely, tropism).

**PRINCIPLE The ability of microorganisms to attach to cells is crucial to the pathogenesis of microbial disease. Interference at this step has therapeutic potential.**

Considerable progress within the last decade has elucidated the chemical basis of regulation of host immunity. It appears that cytokines are responsible for many of the host's responses to microorganisms, accounting for acute inflammation and long-term immunity. Table 14-5 summarizes the major biologic effects of cytokines.

These proteins are produced locally by a variety of stromal cells. They are secreted in small quantities and have short half-lives (of seconds to minutes). They act within a complicated network producing a cascade of events (Tracey et al. 1987; O'Garra et al. 1990). Several inflammatory cytokines (e.g., IL-1, IL-6, and TNF-$\alpha$) appear to contribute to physiologic events that can result in death. Numerous studies have demonstrated the correlation between elevated concentrations of inflammatory cytokines and death due to bacterial septicemia (Girardin et al. 1988; Waage, Brandtzaeg et al. 1989, Waage, Halstensen et al. 1989). Further work is required to elucidate the actions of specific cytokines and to develop approaches to modulating their effects. At a different level, various types of immune deficiency states are associated with different infectious syndromes (Table 14-6).

## DOCUMENTATION OF INFECTION

Review of the patient's history and symptoms combined with knowledge of the microorganisms that cause infection at specific sites (e.g., *E. coli* is the most common cause of urinary tract infection in young women, whereas *S. pneumoniae* is the most common cause of pneumonia at all ages) allows one to order the appropriate investigations to document the site of infection and the infecting microorganism.

### Nonspecific Methods

Symptoms and physical signs are frequently supportive of a diagnosis of infection but rarely are pathognomonic. For example, the activation of the acute inflammatory response is the most common way in which the clinical manifestations of infection become apparent. However, noninfectious conditions may also activate the same inflammatory mechanisms; therefore, the symptoms and signs of inflammation are by no means specific for infection.

Granulocytosis, the appearance of immature neutrophilic forms in the circulation and the presence of toxic granulation are typical of moderate-to-severe acute bacterial infections. This type of inflammatory response is related to the organism that is causing infection, the bone marrow reserves of the host, and other features of the host. In contrast, neutropenia may occur in any patient with overwhelming gram-negative bacterial sepsis or in certain patients (particularly alcoholics) with severe bacterial pneumonia caused by gram-positive organisms. Neutrophilic leukocytosis or leukopenia may be seen during the active phases of vasculitis, systemic lupus erythematosus, or acute drug reactions, all of which can mimic the host response to infections. Tests that attempt to measure the quality of granulocyte response to bacterial infection by incubating blood with nitroblue tetrazolium dye (NBT test) and counting the percentage of cells with reduced dye are not reliable (Steigbeigel et al. 1974). At present, the major value of the NBT test is in the screening of selected subjects for chronic granulomatous disease of childhood or one of its variants (Ochs and Igo 1913). Similar comments can be applied to the appearance of transformed (atypical) lymphocytes in the circulation during fever. Initially thought to be specific for infectious mononucleosis, this finding is now known to appear with regularity in patients with other disorders, including cytomegalovirus infection, acute HIV infection, adenovirus infection, and occasionally toxoplasmosis (Ho 1982; Horwitz 1987; McCabe et al. 1987). Such lymphocytes also may be difficult to differentiate from the immature forms of cells seen in patients with acute lymphocytic leukemia.

**PRINCIPLE A single nonspecific laboratory test (e.g., examination of peripheral white blood cells) that is simply a marker of the activation of the acute inflammatory response is a poor way to evaluate the presence or absence of infection.**

Certain laboratory tests add information by helping to define the presence of abnormalities in the organ systems of the infected host. Since many microorganisms have tissue tropism, these nonspecific methods of evaluating organ function may narrow the search for the site of infection. An abnormality in biochemical tests usually related to liver function (e.g., elevated concentrations of

Table 14-5 Source and Biologic Properties of Cytokines

| Cytokine, Molecular Mass | Natural Source | Major Biological Effects (In Vitro and In Vivo) |
|---|---|---|
| Interleukin-1 (IL-1) 17.5 kDa | Macrophages<br>Fibroblasts<br>Keratinocytes<br>Other endothelial, epithelial, and hemopoietic cells | Induces fever, shock, synthesis of acute-phase proteins, bone resorption, prostaglandin E (PGE) release, nonspecific bacterial resistance in animal models, and endothelial cell activation.<br>Induced by LPS, tissue injury, and viruses.<br>Stimulates cytokine production from macrophages and T cells, proliferation of thymocytes, hemopoietic cell growth and differentiation, and granulocyte and natural killer (NK) cell activity.<br>Costimulates proliferation of B and T cells, antibody secretion. |
| Interleukin-2 (IL-2) 15–20 kDa | T cells | Activates NK cells, cytotoxic T cells, macrophages, and endothelial cells. Induced by superantigens, antigens, mitogens.<br>Stimulates proliferation of T cells and thymocytes, cytokine production from T cells, cytotoxicity, proliferation of NK cells, and differentiation of T cells to lymphokine-activated killer (LAK) cells.<br>Costimulates proliferation of B cells, antibody secretion, and antitumor activity.<br>Has antitumor activity. |
| Interleukin-3 (IL-3) 15–25 kDa | T cells<br>Activated NK cells<br>Keratinocytes<br>Mast cells | Supports survival, growth, and differentiation of stem cells and hemopoietic progenitor cells.<br>Supports proliferation of mast cell lines and growth of pre-B cell lines. |
| Interleukin-4 (IL-4) 12–20 kDa | T cells<br>Mast cells<br>Monocytes<br>Macrophages<br>B cells<br>Bone marrow stromal cells | Induces IgG1 and IgE secretion in LPS-activated B cells. Induces IL-1 receptor antagonist production by macrophages.<br>Activates resting B cells and macrophages.<br>Stimulates proliferation of mast cells and activated T cells, cytotoxic T-cell activity.<br>Costimulates proliferation of thymocytes and activated B cells.<br>Suppresses TNF-$\alpha$, IL-1, IL-6, and $PGE_2$ production by macrophages.<br>Inhibits or enhances other cytokine activities in hemopoietic progenitors. Inhibits antigen-presenting cell function.<br>Has antitumor activity. |
| Interleukin-5 (IL-5) 21.5 kDa | T cells<br>Mast cells<br>Eosinophils | B-cell differentiation and isotype switch toward IgA. Chemotactic for eosinophils. |
| Interleukin-6 (IL-6) 22–29 kDa | Monocytes<br>T cells<br>Fibroblasts<br>Osteoblasts<br>Myelomas<br>Epithelial-type cells | Induces synthesis of acute-phase proteins, antibody secretion, and differentiation of cytotoxic T cells.<br>Stimulates proliferation and differentiation of hemopoietic precursors, proliferation of megakaryocytes, and plasmacytoma growth.<br>Costimulates T-cell and thymocyte proliferation. |
| Interleukin-7 (IL-7) 22–25 kDa | Stromal cells<br>Intestinal epithelial cells | Stimulates proliferation and differentiation of pre-B and pre-T cells stimulates tumoricidal activity of monocytes and macrophages. |
| Interleukin-8 (IL-8) 8–10 kDa | Monocytes<br>Macrophages<br>T cells | Is chemotactic for neutrophils, T cells, basophils. |
| Interleukin-9 (IL-9) 32–39 kDa | T cells | Promotes growth of helper T cells, erythroid progenitors, megakaryocytes. |
| Interleukin-10 (IL-10) 18 kDa | T cells<br>B cells<br>Monocytes | Inhibits production of IL-2, IL-3, TNF, IFN, and GM-CSF. Modulates function of many immunocompetent cells. |

Table 14-5 **Source and Biologic Properties of Cytokines (Continued)**

| Cytokine, Molecular Mass | Natural Source | Major Biological Effects (In Vitro and In Vivo) |
|---|---|---|
| Interleukin-11 (IL-11)<br>24 kDa | Fibroblasts<br>Trophoblasts<br>Bone marrow<br>Stromal<br>Fetal lung | Activates megakaryocyte colony formation.<br>Stimulates myelopoiesis, lymphopoiesis, acute-phase protein synthesis.<br>Involved in normal growth control of intestinal epithelium. |
| Interleukin-12 (IL-12) | Monocytes<br>Macrophages<br>NK cells<br>Keratinocytes | Activates CD4 cells and IFN-$\gamma$ production.<br>Enhances cytolytic activity of NK cells, CTLs, macrophages. |
| Interleukin-13 (IL-13)<br>10 kDa | Activated T cells | B-cell growth and differentiation. Inhibits IL-1, IL-6, IL-8, IL-10, IL-12. |
| Interleukin-14 (IL-14)<br>60 kDa | T cells | Differentiation and proliferation of activated B cells. Inhibits Ig secretion of mitogen-stimulated B cells. |
| Interleukin-15 (IL-15)<br>14–18 kDa | Monocytes<br>T cells<br>Fibroblasts<br>Endothelial cells<br>Epithelial cells | Activates T cells and NK cells. |
| Interleukin-16 (IL-16)<br>17 kDa | Activated (primarily CD4$^+$) T cells | Acts on many cells and tissues in a proinflammatory way. |
| Interferon (IFN-$\gamma$) | Activated T cells | Activates monocytes, macrophages, neutrophils, NK cells, vascular endothelium, fibroblasts, smooth muscle cells (vasoconstriction), T- and B-cell differentiation. |
| Interferon (IFN-$\beta$) | NK cells<br>Fibroblasts<br>Epithelial cells<br>Macrophages | Similar to IFN-$\alpha$, modulates MHC class I and II expression; antiviral activity. Inhibits IL-12 and IFN-$\gamma$ production. |
| Interferon (IFN-$\alpha$) | T cells<br>B cells<br>NK cells<br>Fibroblasts<br>Monocytes<br>Macrophages | Activates macrophages, NK cells, cytotoxic T cells, and endothelial cells.<br>Stimulates LAK activity, secretion of IgG2 from activated B cells.<br>Costimulates human B-cell proliferation.<br>Antiviral and antiparasitic activity; enhances Ig production. Inhibits IL-2 and IFN-$\gamma$ production.<br>Has antitumor activity. |
| Tumor necrosis factor (TNF-$\alpha$) | T cells<br>Macrophages<br>NK cells<br>Neutrophils<br>Endothelial cells<br>Smooth muscle cells | Induces fever, shock, and synthesis of acute-phase proteins.<br>Activates macrophages and endothelial cells.<br>Stimulates granulocyte-eosinophil activity, chemotaxis, B- and T-cell proliferation, angiogenesis, and bone resorption.<br>Inhibits viral replication.<br>Has antitumor activity; is cytotoxic to many cells. |
| Lymphotoxin (TNF-$\beta$) | T cells<br>B cells<br>Mononuclear Phagocytes | Activates endothelial cells.<br>Stimulates granulocyte activity, B-cell proliferation, and bone resorption.<br>Inhibits angiogenesis and viral replication.<br>Has antitumor activity; is cytotoxic to many cells. |
| Granulocyte colony-stimulating factor (G-CSF) | T cells<br>Monocytes<br>Macrophages | Stimulates granulocyte differentiation and activity. |

Table 14-5 Source and Biologic Properties of Cytokines (Continued)

| CYTOKINE, MOLECULAR MASS | NATURAL SOURCE | MAJOR BIOLOGICAL EFFECTS (IN VITRO AND IN VIVO) |
|---|---|---|
| Macrophage CSF (M-CSF) | T cells<br>Monocytes<br>Macrophages | Stimulates macrophage growth and activity. |
| Granulocyte/macrophage CSF (GM-CSF) | T cells<br>Endothelial cells | Stimulates hemopoiesis, macrophage, and granulocyte-eosinophil growth and activity, T-cell proliferation, and chemotaxis. |

ABBREVIATIONS: CSF, colony-stimulating factor, G for granulocyte and M for macrophage; CTLs, cytotoxic lymphocytes; IgG1 and IgE, immunoglobulins; LPS, lipopolysaccharide; IFN, interferon; IL-1 etc., interleukins; IL-1 ra, *receptor antagonist*?; LAK, lymphokine-activated killer [cells]; MHC, major histocompatibility complex; NK, natural killer [cells]; PGE prostaglandin E; TNF, tumor necrosis factor.

transaminases) and a tender liver on physical examination strongly suggest hepatitis but obviously do not differentiate among the many causes of inflammation of the liver. The limitations of nonspecific diagnostic methods as they apply to infectious diseases are outlined in Table 14-7 (Evans 1976). When the spectrum of noninfectious disorders that can mimic infections is included in these considerations, the possibilities for misdiagnosis and misapplied therapy become legion. Therefore, more specific methods are required to document infection so that rational therapy can be planned. Appropriate specimens should be collected (to make an etiological diagnosis) before instituting therapy. A "diagnostic therapeutic trial" of treatment is the least reliable way of revealing the specific nature of infections and is often synonymous with therapeutic misadventure.

**PRINCIPLE Antimicrobial therapy for infectious diseases should not be chosen on the basis of nonspecific methods of diagnosis and "probabilities" alone. Such treatment may cause more harm than good.**

## Specific Methods

The sampling of host tissues and body fluids for biochemical, histologic, and microbiologic testing remains the cornerstone for the diagnosis of a specific infection. Performance of such studies provides a data base to direct rational therapy and is mandatory in the seriously ill patient. The lack of adequate sampling of appropriate sites and the failure to adequately transport specimens to the laboratory are the most frequent and unrecognized reasons for failure to document the etiologic agents of an infectious disease. For example, an improperly collected urine sample (not placed in a sterile container and delayed in delivery to the laboratory) often will be contaminated by large numbers of bacteria bearing little relationship to the presence or number of the true urinary tract pathogen.

### *Samples for microbiologic identification*

The host site to be sampled for the microbiologic identification of infecting agents is critical. Since many epithelial surfaces have their own commensal flora, enumeration of organisms per sample volume and weight may be important in differentiating the commensals from pathogens. For example, the presence of $10^5$ and $10^3$ colony-forming units (CFU) per milliliter of clean catch midstream-voided urine is widely recognized as representing significant bacteriuria in women and men, respectively. However, fewer bacteria in urine can still represent an infection. Studies have conclusively demonstrated that acute dysuria in women with cystitis can be caused by as few as $10^2$ CFU enteric gram-negative bacilli per milliliter of urine

Table 14-6 Common Infectious Syndromes Associated with Immune Deficiency

| DEFECT | SYNDROME |
|---|---|
| Local: Loss of mucosal membrane integrity | Bacterial septicemia in leukemic patients with GI ulceration, staphylococcal catheter infections. |
| Phagocytic cells: Decreased number or function (e.g., chronic granulomatous disease) | Infections due to bacteria and opportunistic fungi, especially catalase-positive bacteria and *Nocardia, Candida, Aspergillus.* |
| Complement | Neisserial septicemia, infection due to encapsulated bacteria. |
| B lymphocytes | Infections due to encapsulated bacteria, *Pneumocystis carinii,* recurrent viral infections. |
| T lymphocytes | Disseminated infection due to intracellular microorganisms, protracted diarrheal syndromes, mucocutaneous candidiasis. |

**Table 14-7 Evans's Five Realities**

1. The same syndrome is caused by a variety of agents.
2. The same agent produces a variety of syndromes.
3. The predominant agent for a syndrome may vary with year, population, geography, and age.
4. The identification of the agent is frequently impossible by clinical findings alone.
5. The cause of a large portion of infectious disease syndromes is unknown.

(Stamm et al. 1982). Therefore, it is always important for the clinician to correlate the microbiologic data with the patient's symptoms and physical signs. If dissemination of infection has taken place, samples taken from distant sites may be helpful. Thus, pneumococcal pneumonia may be documented by sampling respiratory secretions, but the strength of the diagnosis is increased by the finding of pneumococci in blood cultures (Barrett-Connor 1971). The usual sites recommended for sampling for bacteriologic, mycologic, and virologic organisms in given clinical situations are presented in Tables 14-8 and 14-9.

Blood cultures are frequently submitted when any evidence of dissemination of infection is suggested by systemic signs and symptoms. Any abnormal collections of fluid associated with the signs of infection should be sampled for culture. Tissue biopsy may be indicated for certain types of infections. This is particularly important in identifying the pathogens in infected immunocompromised patients (e.g., patients with AIDS or neoplastic disease), since the number of possible pathogens in these patients is much greater than in immunocompetent patients. The necessity for these biopsies is also influenced by weighing the seriousness of the disease against the risk of the biopsy procedure. Histologic examination of tissue samples, obtained by biopsy, with special staining techniques augments the classic microbiologic laboratory testing.

Proper transport of specimens to the laboratory requires prompt delivery under appropriate conditions to protect and allow survival of the organisms for laboratory growth or identification. Although many organisms require only the minimum moisture and nutrients of "routine" transport media, fastidious organisms may require complicated special media for transfer.

Anaerobic microorganisms may be sufficiently fragile to require oxygen-free transport systems to ensure their survival. Viral agents may require special solutions containing antibiotics to suppress bacterial growth, and ultralow temperatures for transfer and storage before inoculation into susceptible cell systems for identification. The clinician must be aware of the requirements for collecting and transporting clinical specimens correctly so that the best chances of a definitive diagnosis of infection are achieved. Discussion with laboratory personnel provides the most efficient method for ensuring that the most appropriate steps are taken.

**Table 14-8 Suggested Specimens to Be Submitted for a Bacteriologic and Mycologic Diagnosis**

| | Specimen Source for Culture | | | | | | |
|---|---|---|---|---|---|---|---|
| Site of Infection or Subject | Blood | Urine | Stool | Throat | Sputum | CSF | Special or Tissue Biopsy; Comments |
| Upper respiratory | + | | | + | | | |
| Lower respiratory | + | | | | + | | Pleural fluid or biopsy, lung biopsy. In selected cases material obtained at bronchoscopy via a protected brush or by bronchoalveolar lavage. |
| Enteric illness | + | + | + | | | | GI or rectal biopsy, liver biopsy |
| CNS disease | + | | | | | + | Brain biopsy |
| Genitourinary | + | + | | | | | |
| Sexually transmitted | + | + | + | + | | | |
| Exanthem | + | | | | | + | Vesicular fluid |
| Arthritis | + | | | | | | Synovial fluid or biopsy |
| Immunocompromised | + | + | + | + | + | + | |
| Newborn or FUO | + | + | + | + | + | + | |
| Hepatitis | + | | | | | | Liver biopsy |

ABBREVIATIONS: CSF, cerebrospinal fluid; FUO, fever of unknown origin.

**Table 14-9 Suggested Specimens to Be Submitted for Viral Diagnosis**

| Diagnostic Consideration | Source for Culture[a] | | | | | | Serologic Study |
|---|---|---|---|---|---|---|---|
| | Nasal or Throat | Stool or Rectum | Urine | CSF | Skin | Special | |
| Respiratory | +++ | | +[b] | | | Lung, bronchial, pleural | + |
| *Enteric* | | | | | | | |
| Gastroenteritis | | +++[c] | | | | | + |
| Hepatitis | | | | | | | + |
| *Central Nervous System* | | | | | | | |
| Aseptic meningitis | ++ | ++ | +[d] | | ++ | Blood+[e] | + |
| Encephalitis | ++ | ++ | | ++ | | Brain+++ | + |
| *Exanthemas* | | | | | | | |
| Maculopapular | ++ | + | + | | | + | |
| Vesicular | | | | | | | + |
| Myocarditis or pericarditis | ++ | ++ | | | | Pericardial fluid, tissue | + |
| Orchitis or parotitis or pancreatitis | ++ | + | ++ | | | | + |
| Newborn with probable intrauterine infection | ++ | ++ | ++ | ++ | | | |
| *Genitourinary* | | | | | | | |
| Genital | | | | | ++ | Cervicovaginal tissue | + |
| Acute hematuria | + | + | ++ | | | | + |

[a]Plus signs indicate: +++, valuable; ++, usually valuable; +, sometimes valuable; no indication implies not a valuable test.
[b]If cytomegalovirus is suspected.
[c]If electron microscopy or indirect (e.g., enzyme-linked immunoassay [ELISA]) techniques are available.
[d]If mumps virus is suspected.
[e]If viral meningitis caused by togavirus or bunyavirus is suspected.

Histologic examinations of stained smears remain the most rapid, inexpensive, and useful method of preliminary recognition of classes of infectious agents. The classic Gram stain allows differentiation of microorganisms into certain groups by size (small, large), form (cocci or bacilli), and staining (gram-positive or gram-negative) characteristics. This rough classification combined with other nonspecific data may provide sufficient information to allow appropriate empiric therapy before a definitive diagnosis (culture) is confirmed. Other commonly used, inexpensive, and simple rapid-staining techniques include acid-fast staining for mycobacteria, methylene blue stains and KOH or Calcofluor White preparations for fungi, and India ink preparations for the recognition of cryptococci. Dark-field microscopic examination for spirochetes, wet preparations for motile organisms, and phase-contrast examination are other convenient methods that take advantage of distinctive biologic characteristics of living microorganisms for their identification.

Cytologic examination, utilizing standard stains of infected cells scraped from body surfaces, may identify intracellular pathogens (e.g., *Chlamydia trachomatis*) and inclusion bodies that indicate infection by selected intracellular microorganisms. Cytomegalovirus and herpesvirus are among those agents that commonly cause formation of inclusion bodies. In addition, the use of fluorescent-labeled antibodies that bind to antigens of specific pathogenic microorganisms provides a rapid, definitive histologic test to confirm infection by a specific etiologic agent including herpesviruses, *Legionella* species, and *C. trachomatis*.

There has been increasing interest in developing new laboratory tests for the diagnosis of infectious diseases. This rapidly evolving field is based on the availability of new reagents derived from molecular biology and on the ability to automate testing. Ultimately, cost effectiveness will dictate whether these new diagnostic tests will be commonly employed. However, molecular biologic techniques have enabled investigators to produce monoclonal antibodies and genetic probes for a number of fastidious or difficult-to-detect microorganisms. Diagnostic kits that employ these new reagents may be superior to the current conventional tests, especially when these tests incorporate improved antibody-antigen detection and genetic amplification (e.g., the polymerase chain reaction [PCR] techniques).

> **PRINCIPLE The rational choice of effective treatment for infectious diseases depends on diagnostic accuracy. The physician must be certain that the appropriate specimens have been obtained and that they have been properly transported and processed to ensure accuracy and reliability of test results.**

***Serologic approaches to documentation of infection***
Cultures of selected microorganisms may be unavailable because the methodology is not available or adequate (e.g., viral hepatitis), is unsafe for laboratory personnel (e.g., rickettsiae), or is impractical (e.g., *Chlamydia* species or certain viruses). A common reason for negative cultures is the use of antimicrobial agents before the culture was taken. Under these circumstances, a serologic approach to documentation of infection might be diagnostically or epidemiologically important. The host mounts nonspecific and specific defenses against various infective agents (e.g., humoral antibodies).

There are many nonspecific (e.g., VDRL for syphilis) and specific (e.g., streptolysin O for group A streptococci) antibody tests that are important diagnostic tools. It is not within the scope of this section to list the many available specific serologic tests. In general, the presence of specific IgM antibodies in high titer indicates a recent or current infection and has been particularly useful in diagnosing some viral infections and toxoplasmosis (Ruskin and Remington 1976). Demonstration of a fourfold rise in specific IgG antibody between acute and convalescent serum samples is also a useful indicator of recent infection. Sera should be obtained at an interval of 2 to 3 weeks to permit adequate time to lapse for the formation of detectable amounts of IgG antibodies. The presence of IgG antibody in a single serum specimen, although it indicates prior exposure to the agent, is usually of little assistance in diagnosing a current illness. Such tests are not necessary for the majority of viral infections when the natural history of disease is self-limiting and short. Serologic tests are particularly important in patients suspected of having syphilis, HIV infection, hepatitis, rickettsial diseases, invasive parasitic diseases, and fungal diseases (e.g., coccidioidomycosis).

***Diagnosis of HIV infection and monitoring of response to treatment***
The conventional algorithm for the laboratory diagnosis of HIV infection in Western countries includes an initial screening test of serum or plasma. The test is repeated if initially reactive, followed by a confirmatory test, usually a Western blot (WB) (CDC 1989a, 1992). For more than a decade, the screening test of choice for the qualitative detection of antibody to HIV-1 and HIV-2 has been based on enzyme immunoassays (EIA) that are commercially available and licensed for use in the diagnostic laboratory. Generally, these EIAs are packaged in kit format and designed for large-volume testing. The test kit consists of a solid support such as a polystyrene 96-well microtiter plate coated with recombinant and/or synthetic proteins as antigens derived from known regions of the HIV-1 and HIV-2 genome. All necessary test reagents including reactive (positive) and nonreactive (negative) controls are included in the test kit. The assays are performed either manually or, usually, with the aid of semiautomated or fully automated instruments. The results are interpreted according to the manufacturer's instructions using absorbance (optical density) reading of appropriate internal controls to establish a cutoff value for nonreactive results. These EIAs generally have a sensitivity of 99.71 to 100% and a specificity of 99.83 to 99.94%.

Likewise, HIV-1 and HIV-2 Western blot test kits are commercially available to confirm sera found to be repeatedly EIA-reactive. Because of the relatively low prevalence of HIV-2 infection, most diagnostic laboratories tend to use HIV-1 Western blot test as the only confirmatory test, whereas reference laboratories provide assistance to confirm suspected HIV-2. In the WB assay, nitrocellulose paper strips blotted electrophoretically with individual proteins of an HIV-1 lysate are reacted with test serum samples. Antibodies to any of the major HIV-1 proteins (p) or glycoproteins (gp) (Table 14-10) can be visualized as colored bands on the strips. Strongly positive, weakly positive, and negative controls are provided in the commercial WB test kit to serve as guides in the interpretation of test results. Recommended criteria have been proposed for interpretation of WB results (see Table 14-11) (CDC 1989a; Consortium for Retrovirus Serology Standardization 1990). A negative WB result requires the

**Table 14-10 Major Genes and Gene Products of HIV-1**

| Gene | Gene Products |
|---|---|
| Group-specific antigen/core *(gag)* | p17, p24, p55 |
| Polymerase *(pol)* | p31, p51, p66 |
| Envelope *(env)* | gp41, gp120, gp160 |

NOTE: p17 and p24 are Gag proteins; p55 is a precursor of Gag protein. p31 is an endonuclease component of Pol translate.
gp41 is a transmembrane Evn glycoprotein; gp120 is an outer Env glycoprotein.
Numbers indicate the approximate molecular masses (in kilodaltons) of the antigens.

Table 14-11 **Criteria for Positive Interpretation of Western Blot Results**

| ORGANIZATION | CRITERIA |
|---|---|
| Association of State and Territorial Public Health Laboratory Directors (ASTPHLD)/CDC | Any two of:<br>p24<br>gp41<br>gp120/160 |
| FDA-licensed Dupont test[a] | p24 and p31 and either<br>gp41 or<br>gp 120/160 |
| American Red Cross | ≥3 bands: 1 from each gene-product group:<br>Gag **and**<br>Pol **and**<br>Env |
| Consortium for Retrovirus Serology Standardization | ≥2 bands: p24 or p31, plus either<br>gp41 or<br>gp120/160 |

[a]The positive criteria of the current FDA-licensed Cambridge Biotech HIV-1 Western blot kit follow the recommendations of the ASTPHLD and CDC, i.e., any two or more of the following bands present: p24, gp41 and gp120/160.
SOURCE: CDC 1989a.

absence of any and all bands—not just viral bands. All other patterns are regarded as indeterminate.

Laboratories generally report the HIV testing results as one of the following:

- HIV-1 and HIV-2 EIA-negative
- HIV-1 and HIV-2 EIA-positive and WB HIV-1 positive
- HIV-1 and HIV-2 EIA-positive and WB HIV-1 indeterminate
- HIV-I and HIV-2 EIA-positive and WB HIV-1 negative

Individuals having WB-indeterminate testing results are usually advised to be retested, usually at 3 months and 6 months for those at low risk, and sooner for those at moderate or high risk for HIV infection. Retesting is necessary as indeterminant results may be obtained in persons who have been recently infected and are in the process of seroconverting (Agebede 1992). In most cases, however, indeterminate results arise because the serum of uninfected individuals contains antibodies that will cross-react with tissue antigens present in the WB test strip. This occurrence has been reported in 20 to 30% of HIV-negative blood samples. In patients without risk factors, almost all indeterminant results will fall into this group. If the WB test does not become positive in retesting at the 3-month intervals, the individual should be considered HIV-negative by the physician despite persistent indeterminate results.

The course of HIV-1 infection leading to the development of the acquired immunodeficiency syndrome (AIDS) varies considerably among infected individuals. Some infected persons rapidly progress to AIDS in less than 5 years (Phair et al. 1992), whereas others remain asymptomatic without evidence of immunological decline for more than 6 years (Sheppard et al. 1993). The median interval from infection to AIDS in adults is 10 to 11 years (Munoz et al. 1989). This variable course of HIV infection has created some degree of uncertainty among clinicians in the clinical management of HIV-1-infected persons. Clinicians have used many clinical and laboratory markers to predict disease progression and to assess the efficacy of therapeutic drug regimens. These surrogate markers include HIV-related symptoms (Phair et al. 1990), depletion of CD4 receptor-positive ($CD4^+$) T-cells (Fahey et al. 1990), HIV-1 p24 (core) antigenemia (de Wolf et al. 1987), serum neopterin and $B_2$-microglobulin levels (Fahey et al. 1990). These markers are indirect and have limitations in sensitivity and specificity.

Although the percentage or absolute number of circulating $CD4^+$ T cells has been the best known and most commonly used surrogate markers for AIDS, these numbers do not always correlate with the disease state. Some HIV-1-infected persons with very low $CD4^+$ T-cell counts (so-called *CD4 counts*) remain healthy, whereas others with comparatively high CD4 counts experience fulminant disease (Hoover et al. 1992). Another complicating factor is the varied sources that can lead to variability in CD4 count determination. Known factors contributing to $CD4^+$ T-cell count variability in the circulating blood have been described: diurnal cycle, the use of tobacco, consumption of caffeine and alcohol, and a variety of physiological and nonphysiological stresses (Raboud et al. 1995). As with many other laboratory tests,

CD4$^+$ T-cell count determination is subject to technical variability within and between laboratories. Therefore, there is a need for alternative markers that can be used for rapid and reliable assessment of prognosis and therapeutic outcome.

Earlier observations based on the quantitation of infectious HIV-1 virus in peripheral blood mononuclear cells (PBMCs) and freshly isolated plasma by culture techniques (Coombs et al. 1989; Ho et al. 1989) have shown that increasing virus titers were associated with CD4$^+$ T-cell decline and disease progression, whereas virus titers decline in response to effective therapy. These findings draw attention especially to the potential usefulness of HIV-1 viral load measurement as a laboratory marker for the in vivo antiretroviral activity of various therapeutic regimens. Unfortunately, the culture techniques that measure HIV-1 virus load in PBMCs or plasma are laborious and time-consuming and suffer as well from laboratory-to-laboratory variation due to inherent difficulty in standardization. Attempts using molecularly based technologies such as polymerase chain reaction (PCR) to quantify HIV-1 RNA in plasma have also shown that reduction in viral load was associated with increased CD4$^+$ T-cell counts and prolonged AIDS-free survival (Mellors et al. 1995; Ho 1996).

These encouraging observations have provided the impetus to the diagnostic industry to make available viral load measurement systems in kit format that are molecularly based and are readily adaptable to diagnostic laboratories. At present, three commercial molecularly based assays are licensed by the Federal Drug Administration in the United States for HIV RNA plasma viral load quantitation. All three assays are currently being used to measure viral burden in relation to disease progression and response to antiretroviral therapy. The International AIDS Society–USA convened an ad hoc panel of investigators and clinicians to make recommendations for the use of these assays in clinical practice (Saag et al. 1996).

Recent studies evaluating the ability of these three commercial assays to measure viremia levels accurately in clinical samples have shown that all three assays produced similar results (Revets et al. 1996). The coefficient of variation of these assays is $<30\%$. A detection limit lowering from the current level to a range of 20 to 40 RNA copies or equivalents per milliliter of plasma is currently under evaluation for all three assays. The standardization of these assays for accuracy and reproducibility is paramount if they are used routinely for patient management. Assay variability has been described for blood collection, processing, and storage (Moudgil and Daar 1993; Holodniy et al. 1995; Ginocchio et al. 1997). The type of anticoagulant used in blood collection is a complicating factor for molecularly based methods. The most noticeable is the anticoagulant heparin, which is known for its inhibitory activity in PCR (Holodniy et al. 1991). Thus, plasma prepared from blood using heparin as anticoagulant cannot be used for the Amplicor monitor assay. Blood collected using ACD (acid citric dextran) as anticoagulant can be used for the Amplicor monitor and nucleic-acid-sequence-based amplification (NASBA) assays. Generally, blood collected using EDTA (ethylenediamine tetraacetic acid) as anticoagulant is the most suitable for all three assays (Ginocchio et al. 1997).

***Measuring antiretroviral resistance in HIV infection***

Incomplete inhibition of HIV-1 replication may arise because of poor drug absorption, patient noncompliance with therapy, or infection with drug resistant virus variants. This incomplete inhibition may result in the emergence of drug-resistant HIV-1 variants and is an important cause of therapy failure (Leigh-Brown and Richman 1997). An assessment of drug resistance may be helpful in selecting subsequent antiretroviral therapy, but this has not been proved rigorously. Drug susceptibility is determined phenotypically by determining the susceptibility of the virus isolate or genotypically by assessing resistance-conferring mutations. There are two phenotypic approaches: The first approach tests the sensitivity of the proviral population present in the PMBCs of the patient (Japour et al. 1993); the second approach generates recombinant fragments of the virus that contain polymerase or protease genes obtained from the plasma- or serum-associated virus or from the cell-associated provirus (Nijhuis et al. 1997). There are several genotypic approaches: DNA sequencing of the entire viral population or clones (Schurman 1997); selective PCR assay (Larder et al. 1991); determination of point mutations (Kaye et al. 1992); enzyme-immunoassay modification of the oligoligase detection reaction assay (Frenkel et al. 1997). Genotypic changes may not correlate with changes in drug susceptibility of the clinical isolate (Larder et al. 1995). Much still needs to be learned about the genotype and phenotype correlation in patients who receive combination antiretroviral therapy before these techniques can be applied effectively in the clinic (Brun-Vezinet et al. 1997). In the meantime, it is generally recommended that a patient's response to therapy be monitored by using the viral RNA level and CD4 count (Brun-Vezinet et al. 1997; Carpenter et al. 1997; Marschner et al. 1998).

***Measurements of cell-mediated immunity***

The appearance of specific cell-mediated immunity is a commonly measured specific change in a host's response to infection. Although there are several sophisticated measurements of T-lymphocyte function to document prior exposure to an antigen, the intradermal skin test remains the simplest, cheapest, and most-used measurement of this aspect of immune function. It evaluates specific T cells that mediate delayed-type hypersensitivity reactions (deShazo et al. 1987). Properly performed, this test provides an indication of prior exposure to (or current infection with) the antigen injected. However, intradermal skin tests of delayed-type hypersensitivity provide no indication of current activity of infection by an agent. A change from a negative to a positive test usually indicates new exposure during the interval between tests and may be correlated with active infection.

The tuberculin test with purified protein derivative (PPD) is the prototype of this type of test. It has proven utility in detecting exposure to *Mycobacterium tuberculosis*. There are other commonly employed skin tests for screening for histoplasmosis, blastomycosis, coccidioidomycosis, and candidiasis antigenic exposure. However, results from these tests have not been clinically useful. The primary reasons for this failure are the high percentage of positive responders who do not have clinical disease and the ubiquitous nature of exposure to these antigens by persons living in zones where hyperendemic rates of these diseases occur. The dose of antigen and the size of cutaneous reaction are critical in avoiding misinterpretation of cross-reactivity with other related agents (e.g., atypical mycobacteria). False-negative tests (i.e., negative reactions to skin tests in the presence of true infection) may occur because of defects in any of the afferent or efferent arms of the cell-mediated immune system or faulty preparation or application of the antigen. False-negative tests have been seen in overwhelming tuberculous infection, intercurrent viral infections including those recently immunized with live-virus vaccines, immunosuppressant therapy, malnutrition, sarcoidosis, or various cancers and leukemias that suppress immune function. False-negative tuberculin tests may occur in the elderly because of waning immunity. The two-step test (if the Mantoux test is negative, it is repeated 2 weeks later; if it is still negative, it is a true negative result) avoids the problem of waning immunity (Rosenberg et al. 1993).

**PRINCIPLE Positive serologic and delayed-type hypersensitivity reactions indicate prior exposure to selected antigens. These tests have limited value in diagnosing acute infection. There is no substitute for culture or detection of the organism in clinical specimens to document the presence of infection.**

## ANTIMICROBIAL THERAPY: GENERAL PRINCIPLES

A wide variety of antimicrobial agents is available to treat established infections caused by bacteria, fungi, viruses, or parasites. This section will cover the general principles of antimicrobial therapy and will also include illustrative clinical problems to emphasize proper decision-making in using antimicrobials.

### Determinants of Antimicrobial Efficacy

***Measurement of antimicrobial activity in vitro***

Susceptibility testing is indicated for any bacterial pathogen warranting chemotherapy. Drugs that irreversibly destroy the ability of an organism to replicate, and perhaps in the process destroy the structural integrity of the organism, are *microbicidal*. Drugs that reversibly impair replicating ability, with this function being restored when drug concentrations fall below critical inhibitory levels, are *microbiostatic*. In quantitative assays of in vitro antimicrobial activity, an organism is said to be “susceptible” to an antimicrobial when in vitro microbicidal or microbiostatic concentrations of drug are comparable to those that can be easily achieved in plasma during clinical use.

Most quantitative assays express this property in terms of the concentrations in plasma that can be reached with standard forms of administration of drug. It is important to recognize that factors such as tissue and intracellular concentrations, as well as the activity of antibiotic metabolites, the presence or absence of concentration-dependent killing and postantibiotic effects, will also affect the in vivo activity of an antimicrobial agent. Assays that do not correlate in vitro activity with their potential in vivo therapeutic values have been abandoned. Detailed discussions of antimicrobial sensitivity testing can be found elsewhere (Marr et al. 1988; Salim et al. 1988; Washington 1988; National Committee for Clinical Laboratory Standards 1990). Discussion of susceptibility tests will be confined to the three most commonly employed assays for aerobic bacteria: disk diffusion, E-test, and broth dilution sensitivity testing. Susceptibility testing for anaerobic bacteria, mycobacteria, fungi, and viruses is more complex and less well standardized and is usually performed by reference laboratories. The susceptibility testing of anaerobic bacteria is technically demanding—disk susceptibility testing is unreliable, and automation cannot be used. Since there are a number of effective antibiotics to which anaerobic bacteria are predictably susceptible, it is not necessary to regularly assess the susceptibility of anaerobic bacteria to a variety of agents. It is important that susceptibility testing be performed in serious or persistent bacterial infections including bacteremia, brain abscess, and infections of the eyes, joints, and bones.

### *Disk sensitivity testing*

Disk diffusion tests (e.g., Kirby–Bauer) developed in 1966 (Bauer et al. 1966) are the most widely used type of nonautomated susceptibility test. This method has been standardized for rapidly growing pathogens including *Enterobacteriaceae*, *Staphylococcus*, *Pseudomonas*, some streptococci such as *S. pneumoniae*, *Haemophilus*, and *Neisseria* species (National Committee for Clinical Laboratory Standards 1993). This method is not appropriate for anaerobic bacteria, slow-growing organisms, or organisms that show marked strain-to-strain variation.

These assays measure the ability of drug to inhibit a microorganism's growth by placing drug-impregnated paper disks on a "lawn" of organisms inoculated onto the surface of agar plates. With diffusion of the antibiotic through the agar, a decreasing gradient of antibiotic concentrations develop around the disk. If the antibiotic is active against the organism tested, a growth-free zone surrounds the disk. Since a standard amount of active antibiotic and a standardized bacterial inoculum are used, the diameter of the zone of growth inhibition can be correlated directly with broth dilution assays that measure minimal inhibitory concentrations. Thus, when the diameter of the inhibitory zone is greater than a certain size, there is a correlation with a good clinical outcome, and in these cases the organism is said to be *susceptible* to the antimicrobial. When the zone diameter is below a defined size, then in vivo concentrations of antibiotic are not likely to inhibit the organism and it is said to be resistant. Results are labeled *intermediate sensitivity* when the size of the zone indicates that antibiotic concentrations that are inhibitory to the organisms might be reached in vivo, provided that high dosages are used or that the infection is localized to an area where concentrations of antibiotic may exceed those in the blood (e.g., in the urine).

The reliability of the Kirby–Bauer technique depends on adequate growth of bacteria on agar suitable for susceptibility testing, a standardized inoculum size, specific concentrations of active antibiotic in the antimicrobial disk, and standardized growth conditions. Any alteration of these specifications can invalidate the results. The Kirby–Bauer technique does not provide information on whether the drug is bactericidal or bacteriostatic.

### *E-test*

The E-test developed by AB Biodisk is a plastic strip with an exponential antimicrobial gradient applied. The strip is applied to the surface of an agar plate in much the same manner that an antibiotic disk might be for Kirby–Bauer disk diffusion testing. The strip is marked with the concentrations of antibiotics at regular intervals along the gradient. After incubation there is an elliptical shaped zone of inhibition around the strip. The point at which the pointed end of the ellipse intersects with the strip represents the MIC of the organism. E-test strips are expensive and are usually used for specific MIC determinations and for testing organisms that do not produce reliable results by other methods. Since E-test strips are easy to use and require no instrumentation, their use has increased markedly in recent years.

### *Broth dilution sensitivity testing*

The broth dilution technique is a widely used method to measure quantitatively the in vitro activity of an antimicrobial agent against a particular bacterial isolate (National Committee for Clinical Laboratory Standards 1994). It may be more expensive to perform (especially if done manually), and it is technically more sophisticated than disk diffusion tests. There are very few indications for mandatory use of broth dilution testing, since information derived from disk diffusion tests is adequate in the majority of common bacterial infections. Broth dilution studies should be performed when it is critical for the clinician to prescribe antibiotics for difficult-to-treat infections.

Usually the broth dilution test is performed in microtiter plates. Each well containing specified dilutions of antibiotic is inoculated with a standardized inoculum of organisms; the plates are incubated for a sufficient time to permit the detection of growth in the control well. When determined visually, this usually requires 16 to 24 hours; however, newer instruments that measure optical density in the wells are often able to produce susceptibility testing results on the same day. The lowest concentration of antibiotic that inhibits bacterial growth is the *minimal inhibitory concentration* (MIC). A *minimal microbicidal concentration* (MBC) can be determined by subculturing, onto antibiotic-free agar, material from wells that show no visual growth. The lowest concentration of antimicrobial that prevents growth on subculture is the MBC.

In the case of bacteriostatic drugs, the organism may not be killed unless exposed to suprapharmacologic concentrations of antibiotic. With most bactericidal drugs, the MBC usually is 1 or 2 dilutions (2 times) as high as the MIC. If the organism is not killed unless the antibiotic concentration is increased to 16 times the MIC, then it is *tolerant* to the antibiotic. The data derived from these tests can be coupled with the knowledge of expected or measured antibiotic concentrations in vivo to predict efficacy of the antibiotic. As with the disk diffusion method, reproducibility depends on standardization of inoculum sizes and incubation conditions. These tests provide the clinician with a direct measure of antimicrobial concentrations that should inhibit microbial replication in vivo. Unless automation is employed, measurements of antimicrobial MICs and MBCs against a specific organism usually are reserved for patients with serious systemic infections such as endocarditis, in which antibiotic efficacy is a more critical factor than host defenses in eradicating the infection.

The use of MICs may also be necessary when disk testing is not able to adequately characterize susceptibility results. For example, *Streptococcus pneumoniae* isolates may be screened for penicillin susceptibility using a disk diffusion test, but MICs must be carried out in order to determine whether high-, intermediate-, or low-level resistance is present. MIC testing is used to determine *S. pneumoniae* susceptibility to third-generation cephalosporins. MIC testing may also be useful in evaluating causes of treatment failure when other causes are not apparent.

***Other sensitivity-testing techniques***

Agar dilution testing is a method for measuring antimicrobial susceptibility that lends itself to testing large numbers of microorganisms. A standardized inoculum is inoculated onto the surface of media containing relevant concentrations of antibiotics using a multitined replicator (Steers et al. 1959). The MICs can then be determined from the concentration of antibiotic that inhibits visible growth of the organisms on the surface of the agar. Results of these assays usually correlate well with broth dilution MICs. This method is well suited to the testing of slower-growing organisms including anaerobes. It is also well suited to batch testing of bacteria, as might be necessary in comparing the activity of a newer antibiotic with commercially available agents and for performing periodic surveys for public health or other purposes.

The serum bactericidal test is another susceptibility test. It is a simple variation of the broth dilution test. It is performed in the same manner, except serial dilutions of a sample of serum from the patient are used instead of the various concentrations of antimicrobial agents (National Committee for Clinical Laboratory Standards 1987). The serum is obtained from the patient during antimicrobial therapy (usually when drug concentration is at its nadir) and diluted. The tubes or wells are then inoculated with a standardized suspension of the pathogen isolated from the patient. After appropriate growth, the tubes are examined, and the serum's inhibiting titer is determined. All samples are subsequently subcultured. The serum bactericidal titer is that dilution of serum that shows >99.9% killing of the initial inoculum. The use of the serum bactericidal test is controversial, with concern focusing on the technology and the clinical significance of the results. To date there is no conclusive recommendation as to its utility in predicting antimicrobial efficacy in vivo. The serum bactericidal test may be useful in several conditions, including bacterial endocarditis, bacteremia in cancer patients, osteomyelitis, septic arthritis, monitoring combinations of antibiotics, and as a guide when changing from parenteral to oral therapy in infected patients (Robinson et al. 1985).

On occasion neither disk diffusion nor microdilution testing reliably detects antibiotic resistance. For example, both methicillin resistance in staphylococci and vancomycin resistance in enterococci are often missed by these methods. In such cases many laboratories will use a screening plate to detect resistance. Using this method a specific concentration of the antibiotic is incorporated into a suitable agar, and a defined concentration of the organism is spotted onto the surface of the plate. The plate is incubated overnight (or for up to 48 hours in the case of methicillin-resistant staphylococci) and examined for growth. Growth in the presence of the antibiotic predicts the presence of the resistance factor.

***Antibiotic pharmacodynamics and dosing regimens***

As a result of integration of in vitro testing of sensitivity of organisms, in vivo measures of antibiotic efficacy, and understanding of bacterial growth and antimicrobial action, certain key principles have emerged. For $\beta$-lactam antibiotics, vancomycin, clindamycin, and macrolides, the cidal effect occurs at low multiples of the MIC (4× or 5×), and the extent of the killing depends on the duration of exposure. In animal models of infection, maximal killing of microorganisms occurs when the plasma drug concentration exceeds the MIC during 60 to 70% of the dose interval (Craig 1998). Fluoroquinolones and aminoglycosides demonstrate concentration-dependent killing, and here the ratio of the area under the concentration-over-time curve to the MIC (AUC/MIC) correlates best with efficacy. For fluoroquinolones, concentrations in serum need to average 4 times the MIC for each 24-hour period to produce almost 100% survival in animal models of infection (Craig 1998). To obtain a clinical response of ≥90% with aminoglycoside treatment, the peak level needs to exceed the MIC by 8- to 10-fold (Craig 1998). This observation, plus the fact that aminoglycoside uptake by bacteria is downregulated following exposure and persists for several hours, forms the basis for once daily dosing of aminoglycosides.

**PRINCIPLE Effective dosing of antibiotics depends on many factors that are drug-class dependent and in addition to the simple MIC.**

## Selection of Antimicrobial Agents for Testing Panels

Agents selected for inclusion in susceptibility testing panels should be chosen carefully, since results from these tests showing sensitivity encourage the practitioner to use the agents, and to assume that the antibiotic is likely to have in vivo efficacy. Suggested guidelines for selecting agents to be tested against common bacterial pathogens are listed in Table 14-12. Changes in this list can be anticipated as improved and more cost-effective agents are developed.

Deliberate selective reporting of the results of antibiotic susceptibility tests by the laboratory also provides a useful method to promote efficacious and cost-effective use of antimicrobials. For example, if an *E. coli* blood isolate is sensitive to gentamicin, there is no reason to report susceptibility to the other aminoglycosides unless the patient has a hypersensitivity reaction to gentamicin. Reporting of the susceptibility results for the other aminoglycosides in this case might encourage physicians to prescribe a more costly aminoglycoside agent when it is not necessary. Such reasoning is particularly important for the large group of $\beta$-lactam antibiotics. Close coordination between the microbiology laboratory and hospital drug formulary committee provides a rational basis for antibiotic selection. Communication with physicians is vital to their understanding of the reasons for this policy. Understandably, antibiotic manufacturers would prefer to see more comprehensive sensitivity reports that include their products! Physicians must also remember that reports of in vitro sensitivity tests do not guarantee that the antibiotic selected will work in vivo. The drug must reach the site of infection in concentrations adequate to reproduce the in vitro effects when coupled with the host's defense mechanisms.

## Pharmacologic Factors Affecting Antibiotic Activity

A major goal in antimicrobial therapy is to choose an agent that is selectively active for the most likely infecting microorganisms at the site of infection. Pharmacologic factors that affect antimicrobial drug efficacy include absorption of the drugs from the site of administration, delivery by the circulation to the infected region, diffusion from the plasma through tissues, penetration to the site of infection, and maintenance of adequate amounts of active drug at that site. If antibiotics only inhibit the growth of organisms rather than kill them, the host's defense mechanisms must be sufficiently effective to eradicate the pathogenic microorganism to achieve a therapeutic success (Yourtee and Root 1984). If this is not the case, microbicidal agents should be employed. In selected clinical syndromes (e.g., bacteremia in a neutropenic leukemic patient undergoing chemotherapy), sufficient bactericidal drug must be administered so that a cure will be produced, whereas in the vast majority of infections, antimicrobial agents are required only to augment host defenses to effect cure. Table 14-13 lists commonly used agents according to microbicidal or microbiostatic status.

**PRINCIPLE Consideration of the patient's physiologic resilience and ability to fight infection is a key factor in choice of drug in a panoply of disease settings.**

### *Absorption of antimicrobials*

Determining the most effective route of administration to achieve adequate concentrations in the blood and tissue is important in choosing an antimicrobial (Table 14-14). Although oral administration of many antibiotics is preferred because of ease, safety, and cost, parenteral administration is usually required when treating an infection that poses a serious threat to life. Parenteral administration helps ensure that adequate concentrations of drug are achieved in the blood. Two important considerations in choosing the route of administration of a drug are the plasma concentration of drug that can be achieved by oral versus parenteral administration and the location and severity of the infection. For example, penicillin G has an oral bioavailability of only 20 to 30%. Plasma concentrations following oral therapy may be inadequate to treat serious infections, particularly when the infections are located in tissues resistant to penetration by the antibiotics (e.g., brain or endocardium). The use of a variety of tests to measure drug concentration in plasma is appropriate when there are questions as to the adequacy of those concentrations in seriously ill patients.

**PRINCIPLE In treating an infection that poses a serious threat to life, it is unwise to depend on oral absorption, especially in the presence of vomiting or GI dysfunction. A parenteral formulation is usually indicated.**

Table 14-12 Suggested Groupings of Antimicrobial Agents That Should Be Considered for Routine Testing and Reporting by Clinical Microbiology Laboratories and a Guide for Appropriate Antibiotic Usage

| | ENTEROBACTERIACEAE | *PSEUDOMONAS* | STAPHYLOCOCCI | ENTEROCOCCI | STREPTOCOCCI NOT INCLUDING ENTEROCOCCI | *HAEMOPHILUS* |
|---|---|---|---|---|---|---|
| *Group 1*<br>Routine tests (all clinical specimens) | Ampicillin<br>Cephalothin<br>Cefazolin<br>Gentamicin | Mezlocillin, ticarcillin or piperacillin<br>Gentamicin | Penicillin G<br>Oxacillin or methicillin<br>Cephalothin or cefazolin<br>Erythromycin<br>Clindamycin | Penicillin G or ampicillin | Penicillin G | Ampicillin<br>Trimethoprim-sulfamethoxazole |
| *Group 2*<br>Selected reporting (if resistance in group 1; from CSF, blood, or special procedure, e.g., bone biopsy) | Ticarcillin or mezlocillin or piperacillin<br>Ampicillin-sulbactam<br>Amoxicillin-clavulanic acid<br>Ticarcillin-clavulanic acid<br>Piperacillin-tazobactam<br>Cefotetan<br>Cefoxitin<br>Cefuroxime or cefamandole or cefonicid<br>Cefotaxime or ceftazidime or ceftizoxime or ceftriaxone or cefepime<br>Aztreonam<br>Tobramycin or amikacin<br>Trimethoprim-sulfamethoxazole | Azlocillin<br>Ceftazidime or cefepime<br>Aztreonam<br>Piperacillin-tazobactam<br>Ticarcillin clavulanic acid<br>Imipenem or meropenem<br>Ciprofloxacin<br>Tobramycin or amikacin or netilmicin | Vancomycin | Vancomycin<br>Quinupristin + dalfopristin | Cephalothin<br>Erythromycin<br>Clindamycin<br>Tetracycline<br>Vancomycin | Amoxicillin-clavulanic acid<br>Ampicillin-sulbactam<br>Cefuroxime sodium<br>Cefaclor<br>Cefixime<br>Cefotaxime or ceftazidime or ceftizoxime or ceftriaxone |
| *Group 3*<br>Supplemental selected reporting (if resistance in groups 1 and 2) | Imipenem<br>Tetracycline<br>Chloramphenicol<br>Meropenem<br>Ciprofloxacin | | Imipenem or meropenem | | Cefamandole<br>Cefonicid | |

**Table 14-12 Suggested Groupings of Antimicrobial Agents That Should Be Considered for Routine Testing and Reporting by Clinical Microbiology Laboratories and a Guide for Appropriate Antibiotic Usage (Continued)**

| | ENTEROBACTERIACEAE | *PSEUDOMONAS* | STAPHYLOCOCCI | ENTEROCOCCI | STREPTOCOCCI NOT INCLUDING ENTEROCOCCI | *HAEMOPHILUS* |
|---|---|---|---|---|---|---|
| *Group 4* | | | | | | |
| Selected reporting for urinary isolates (if resistance in group 3) | Nitrofurantoin<br>Trimethoprim<br>Sulfisoxazole | Fluoroquinolones | Nitrofurantoin<br>Trimethoprim<br>Sulfisoxazole | Ciprofloxacin<br>Tetracycline<br>Nitrofurantoin | Nitrofurantoin | |

Amikacin sulfate, amoxicillin-clavulanic acid, ampicillin sodium, ampicillin sodium-sulbactam sodium, azlocillin [?], aztreonam, cefaclor, cefamandole nafate, cefazolin sodium, cefepime HCl, cefixime sodium, cefonicid sodium, cefoperazone sodium, cefotaxime sodium, cefotetan disodium, cefoxitin sodium, ceftazidime, ceftizoxime sodium, ceftriaxone sodium, cefuroxime axetil, cefuroxime sodium, cephalothin sodium, chloramphenicol, ciprofloxacin HCl, clindamycin HCl or phosphate, quinupristin-dalfopristin, erythromycin, gentamicin sulfate, imipenem, meropenem, methicillin sodium, mezlocillin sodium monohydrate, netilmicin sulfate, nitrofurantoin, oxacillin sodium, penicillin G, piperacillin sodium, piperacillin sodium-tazobactam sodium, sulfisoxazole, tetracycline HCl, ticarcillin disodium, ticarcillin disodium-clavulanic acid, tobramycin, trimethoprim, trimethoprim-sulfamethoxazole, vancomycin HCl.

SOURCE: Adapted from National Committee for Clinical Laboratory Standards (1987, 1990).

Table 14-13 **Systematic Antimicrobial Drugs by Class and Action**

| | Microbiocidal | Microbiostatic |
|---|---|---|
| *Antibacterial agents* | Penicillins<br>Cephalosporins<br>Aminoglycosides<br>Vancomycin HCl<br>Teicoplanin<br>Quinolones<br>Nitrofurantoin<br>Methenamine<br>Metronidazole<br>Carbapenems (imipenem)<br>Monobactams (aztreonam) | Chloramphenicol<br>Clindamycin HCl<br>Macrolides<br>Tetracyclines<br>Trimethoprim<br>Sulfonamides |
| *Antituberculous agents* | Isoniazid<br>Rifampin<br>Streptomycin sulfate<br>Pyrazinamide | *p*-Aminosalicylic acid<br>Ethambutol HCl<br>Ethionamide<br>Cycloserine |
| *Antifungal agents* | Amphotericin B<br>Flucytosine<br>Clotrimazole<br>Nystatin<br>Griseofulvin<br>Vidarabine | Ketoconazole<br>Fluconazole<br>Itraconazole<br>Terbinafine HCl |
| *Antiviral agents (non-HIV)* | Idoxuridine<br>Cytarabine<br>Amantadine HCl<br>Rimantadine HCl<br>Acyclovir<br>Valacyclovir HCl<br>Famciclovir<br>Ganciclovir sodium<br>Cidofovir<br>Vidarabine | |
| *Anti-HIV agents* | Didanosine<br>Zidovudine<br>Zalcitabine<br>Stavudine mesylate<br>Lamivudine<br>Nevirapine<br>Delavirdine HCl<br>Efavirenz<br>Saquinavir mesylate<br>Ritonavir<br>Indinavir sulfate<br>Nelfinavir mesylate | |

### *Tissue distribution of antimicrobials*

Once an antimicrobial is in the blood, its ability to reach an infected site depends on the interplay of the factors outlined in Tables 14-15 and 14-16. The most important are those of protein and tissue binding. Biologic activity of an antimicrobial is best correlated with the concentration of free (rather than total) drug in a protein-rich medium (Kunin 1965; Merrikin et al. 1983). Extensive protein binding of an antimicrobial may not only reduce its biologic activity but also restrict its distribution into tis-

**Table 14-14 Classification of Antimicrobial Agents**

| ANTIBACTERIAL | | | | |
|---|---|---|---|---|
| CLASS | DRUG TYPE AND DRUG | ROUTE | COMMON TRADE NAME | SPECTRUM OF ACTIVITY |
| *β-Lactam Antibiotics* | | | | |
| Penicillins | | | | |
| | Natural penicillins | | | |
| | Penicillin G | IV, IM, | Various | Active against most strains of streptococci, pneumococci, (except penicillin-resistant *S. pneumoniae*), meningococci, anaerobes except *Bacteriodes fragilis,* spirochetes, *Listeria monocytogenes, Corynebacterium* spp., and *Bacillus* spp. |
| | Penicillin V | PO | Various | |
| | Aminopenicillins | | | |
| | Ampicillin | PO, IV, IM, | Omnipen | Increased activity against enterococci and gram-negative organisms: *Escherichia coli, Haemophilus influenzae,* and *Proteus mirabilis* (non-β-lactamase-producing strains). |
| | Amoxicillin | PO | Amoxil | |
| | Bacampicillin HCl | PO | Spectrobid | |
| | Penicillinase-resistant penicillins | | | |
| | Nafcillin sodium | IV, IM | Unipen | Active against penicillinase-producing and non-pencillinase-producing strains of *Staphylococcus aureus;* active agent against some strains of *Staphylococcus epidermidis;* less active than penicillin G against other organisms. |
| | Oxacillin sodium | IV,IM | Bactocill, Prostaphlin | |
| | Dicloxacillin sodium | IM, PO | Dycill | |
| | Cloxacillin sodium | IV, PO | Tegopen, Cloxapen | |
| | Carboxypenicillins | | | |
| | Carbenicillin indanyl sodium | IV, IM, PO | Geopen, Geocillin | Good activity against *Proteus vulgaris, Serratia* spp., and *Pseudomonas aeruginosa;* less activity than penicillin G against gram-positive organisms. |
| | Ticarcillin disodium | IV, IM | Ticar | |
| | Ureidopenicillins | | | |
| | Mezlocillin sodium monohydrate | IV, IM | Mezlin | Greater activity than carboxypenicillins against enterococci, *Bacteroides* spp., and certain aerobic gram-negative organisms: *P. aeruginosa* (piperacillin), *Klebsiella* spp., *Serratia marcescens,* and *E. coli.* |
| | Piperacillin sodium | IV, IM | Pipracil | |
| | Combinations with β-lactamase inhibitors | | | |
| | Amoxicillin + clavulanic acid | PO | Augmentin | Addition of β-lactamase inhibitor generally increases activity against β-lactamase-producing strains of *S. aureus, H. influenzae, B. fragilis,* and *Moraxella catarrhalis.* No activity against *P. aeruginosa, Enterobacter* spp., *Serratia* spp., *Acinetobacter,* methicillin-resistant *S. aureus.* |
| | Ticarcillin + clavulanic acid | IV | Timentin | |
| | Ampicillin + sulbactam | IV, IM | Unasyn | |
| | Piperacillin + tazobactam | IV, IM | Zosyn | |

Table 14-14 Classification of Antimicrobial Agents (Continued)

| Antibacterial | | | | |
|---|---|---|---|---|
| **Class** | **Drug Type and Drug** | **Route** | **Common Trade Name** | **Spectrum of Activity** |
| Cephalosporins | | | | |
| | First-generation | | | |
| | Cephradine | IV, IM, | Velosef | Excellent activity against *Streptococcus* (except *Enterococcus faecalis*) and *S. aureus;* good activity against many strains of *P. mirabilis, E. coli,* and *Klebsiella* spp.). |
| | Cephalexin | PO | Keflex, Keflet | |
| | Cefadroxil | PO | | |
| | Cephalothin sodium | IV, IM | Duricef, Ultracef | |
| | Cephapirin sodium | IV, IM | Keflin, Seffin | |
| | Cefazolin sodium | IV, IM | Cefadyl Ancef, Kefzol | |
| | Second-generation | | | |
| | Cefamandole nafate | IV, IM | Mandol | Excellent activity against *Streptococcus* (except *E. faecalis*); cefamandole, cefuroxime, and cefmetazole have good activity against *S. aureus;* good activity against most members of Enterobacteriaceae family including *Proteus* spp., *E. coli,* and *Klebsiella* spp.; cefotetan, cefonicid, cefamandole, and cefuroxime have good activity against *H. influenzae;* cefotetan has extended activity against some strains of *Serratia* spp. and indole-positive *Proteus* spp.; cefoxitin, cefotetan and cefmetazole are active against *B. fragilis.* |
| | Cefoxitin sodium | IV, IM | Mefoxin | |
| | Cefuroxime sodium or cefuroxime axetil | IV, IM, PO | Zinacef, Ceftin | |
| | Cefonicid sodium | IV, IM | Monocid | |
| | Cefotetan disodium | IV, IM | Cefotan | |
| | Cefaclor | PO | Ceclor | |
| | Cefmetazole sodium | IV, IM | Zefazone | |
| | Cefprozil | PO | Cefzil | |
| | Cefpodoxime proxetil | PO | Vantin | |
| | Ceftibuten | PO | Cedax | |
| | Loracarbef | PO | Lorabid | |
| | Third-generation | | | |
| | Cefotaxime sodium | IV, IM | Claforan | Excellent activity against *Streptococcus* and good activity against *Staphylococcus* with the exception of ceftazidime; excellent activity against Enterobacteriaceae family including *Proteus* spp., *E. coli,Klebsiella* spp., *Salmonella* spp., and *Shigella* spp. Good activity against *Serratia, Citrobacter.* Ceftazidime is active against *Pseudomonas aeruginosa;* most agents have good CSF penetration. |
| | Ceftizoxime sodium | IV, IM | Cefizox | |
| | Ceftriaxone sodium | IV, IM | Rocephin | |
| | Ceftazidime | IV, IM | Fortaz, Tazicef | |
| | Cefixime | PO | Suprax | |
| | Fourth-generation | | | |
| | Cefepime HCl | IV, IM | Maxipime | Excellent activity against *Streptococcus,* good activity against *Staphylococcus,* excellent activity against Enterobacteriaceae including *Proteus* spp., *E. coli, Klebsiella* spp., *Salmonella, Shigella,* very good activity against *Enterobacter, Citrobacter,* and *P. aeruginosa.* |
| | Cefpirome | IV | | |

**Table 14-14 Classification of Antimicrobial Agents (Continued)**

| ANTIBACTERIAL | | | | |
|---|---|---|---|---|
| **CLASS** | **DRUG TYPE AND DRUG** | **ROUTE** | **COMMON TRADE NAME** | **SPECTRUM OF ACTIVITY** |
| Carbapenems | | | | |
| | Imipenem + cilastin sodium | IV, IM | Primaxin | Excellent activity against both gram-positive aerobes and anaerobes; should be reserved for multidrug-resistant *P. aeruginosa, Enterobacter,* or *Citrobacter* infections; unpredictable activity against methicillin-resistant staphylococci, some enterococci, *Stenotrophomonas maltophilia,* and *Burkholderia cepacia.* |
| | Meropenem | IV, IM | Merrem IV | |
| Monobactams | | | | |
| | Aztreonam | IV, IM | Azactam | Excellent activity against most members of the Enterobacteriaceae family including *E. coli, Klebsiella* spp., *Serratia* spp., *Citrobacter* spp., and *Enterobacter* spp.; no activity against aerobic gram-positive and anaerobic organisms. |
| Aminoglycosides | | | | |
| | Amikacin sulfate | IV, IM | Amikin | Excellent activity against aerobic gram-negative organisms; gentamicin and tobramycin are very similar in activity with the exception that tobramycin is more active against *P. aeruginosa* and gentamicin is more active against *S. marcescens;* aminoglycosides have been used in combination with $\beta$-lactams for synergy in treatment of staphylococcal and enterococcal infections (gentamicin is preferred). |
| | Gentamicin sulfate | IV, IM | Various | |
| | Netilmicin sulfate | IV, IM | Netromycin | |
| | Tobramycin sulfate | IV, IM | Nebcin | |
| Protein synthesis inhibitors | | | | |
| | Macrolides | | | |
| | Erythromycin | PO, IV, T | Many | Good activity against streptococci (except enterococcus), *Legionella, Mycoplasma, Chlamydia trachomatis,* and *Chlamydia pneumoniae.* Dirithromycin and clarithromycin are more active against *H. influenzae, M. catarrhalis* and *C. trachomatis.* |
| | Clarithromycin | PO | Biaxin | |
| | Azithromycin dihydrate | IV, PO | Zithromax | |
| | Dirithromycin | PO | Dynabac | |
| | Clindamycin HCl | IM, IV, PO | Cleocin | Good activity against aerobic gram-positive organism including staphylococci and nonenterococcal streptococci; moderate activity against *B. fragilis* and other anaerobes. |
| | Chloramphenicol | IV, PO, T | Chloromycetin | Good activity against aerobic gram-positive organisms including staphylococci and nonenterococcal streptococci; good activity against most members of the Enterobacteriaceae family including *E. coli, Klebsiella* spp., *Proteus* spp., *H. influenzae, Serratia* spp., *Salmonella, Shigella,* menigococcus and *Neisseria gonorrhoeae;* excellent activity against *B. fragilis* and other anaerobes. |

Table 14-14 Classification of Antimicrobial Agents (Continued)

| ANTIBACTERIAL | | | | |
|---|---|---|---|---|
| **CLASS** | **DRUG TYPE AND DRUG** | **ROUTE** | **COMMON TRADE NAME** | **SPECTRUM OF ACTIVITY** |
| | Tetracyclines | | | |
| | Doxycycline | IV, PO | Vibramycin | Excellent activity against *Mycoplasma pneumoniae* and *C. trachomatis;* good activity against most of aerobic gram-positive organisms including staphylococci and non-enterococcal streptococci; good activity against *E. coli* and *Klebsiella* spp.; most strains of *Proteus* and *Serratia* spp. are resistant; minimal activity against anaerobes including *B. fragilis.* |
| | Minocycline HCl | IV, PO | Minocin | |
| | Tetracycline HCl | IV, PO | Achromycin, Sumycin | |
| Folate inhibitors | | | | |
| | Trimethoprim | PO | Trimpex | Good activity against gram-positive organisms including staphylococci and streptococci; also active against many members of the Enterobacteriaceae family including *E. coli, H. influenzae, Proteus* spp., and *Serratia* spp.; minimal activity against anaerobes. |
| Sulfonamides | | | | |
| | Sulfamethoxazole | PO | Gantanol | Good activity against aerobic gram-positive, including staphylococci and streptococci (except *S. pyogenes* and enterococcus); excellent activity against many members of the Enterobacteriaceae family including *E. coli, Klebsiella* spp., *H. influenzae, P. mirabilis, Enterobacter* spp., *Salmonella,* and *Shigella;* also active against *Nocardia asteroides* and *Toxoplasma gondii;* minimal activity against anaerobes. |
| | Sulfisoxazole | PO | Gantrisin | |
| | Sulfadiazine | PO | Microsulfon | |
| Combination | | | | |
| | Sulfamethoxazole + trimethoprim | IV, PO | Bactrim, Septra | In addition to activity spectrum of sulfa drugs the combination of TMP-SMX is active against *Pneumocystis carinii.* |
| Quinolones | | | | |
| | Nalidixic acid | PO | Neggram | Excellent activity against aerobic gram-negative bacilli including *E. coli, Klebsiella* spp., *Enterobacter* spp., *Citrobacter* spp., *P. mirabilis,* and *P. aeruginosa;* good activity against staphylococci except methicillin-resistant *S. aureus;* poor activity against anaerobes; clinically unreliable against streptococci. Levofloxacin, sparfloxacin, trovafloxacin, and grepafloxacin have very good activity against *S. pneumoniae* including penicillin-resistant strains. Trovafloxacin has activity against anaerobes. |
| | Ciprofloxacin HCl | IV, PO | Cipro | |
| | Norfloxacin | PO | Noroxin | |
| | Ofloxacin | IV, PO | Floxin, Ocuflox | |
| | Pefloxacin | PO | | |
| | Cinoxacin | PO | Cinobac, Penetrex | |
| | Enoxacin | IV, PO | | |
| | Levofloxacin | PO, IV | Levaquin | |
| | Lomefloxacin HCl | PO | | |
| | Sparfloxacin | PO | Maxaquin | |
| Miscellaneous | | | | |
| | Metronidazole | IV, PO | Flagyl | Excellent activity against both anaerobic gram-positive and gram-negative organisms including *B. fragilis, Clostridia* spp., and *Propionibacterium;* good activity against *Trichomonas vaginalis, Giardia lamblia,* and *Entamoeba histolytica;* little to no activity against aerobic organisms. |
| | Glycopeptides | | | |
| | Vancomycin HCl | IV, PO | Vancocin | Excellent activity against aerobic gram-positive organisms including pneumonococci, enterococci, and methicillin-resistant staphylococci. Vancomycin PO is used for *C. difficile*-associated diarrhea only. |
| | Teicoplanin | IV | Targocid | |

Table 14-14 **Classification of Antimicrobial Agents (Continued)**

| ANTIVIRAL | | | | |
|---|---|---|---|---|
| CLASS | DRUG | ROUTE | COMMON TRADE NAME | MAJOR INDICATION |
| Antiviral | | | | |
| | Acyclovir | IV, PO, T | Zovirax | Herpes simplex virus (HSV), varicella-zoster virus (VZV) |
| | Ganciclovir sodium | IV | Cytovene | Cytomegalovirus (CMV) |
| | Amantadine HCl | PO | Symmetrel | Influenza A virus |
| | Rimantadine HCl | PO | | Influenza A virus |
| | Vidarabine | IV | Vira-A | Second-line agent for life-threatening herpesvirus or varicella-zoster infection |
| | Ribavirin | Inh | Virazole | Respiratory syncytial virus |
| | Foscarnet sodium | IV | Foscavir | HSV, VZV, CMV |
| | Famciclovir | PO | Famvir | HSV, VZV |
| | Valacyclovir HCl | PO | Valtrex | HSV, VZV |
| | Cidofovir | IV | Vistide | CMV |
| Anti-HIV | | | | |
| | Zidovudine (AZT) | PO, IV | Retrovir | HIV |
| | Stavudine mesylate (d4t) | PO | Zerit | HIV |
| | Didanosine (ddI) | PO | Videx | HIV |
| | Zalcitabine (ddC) | PO | HIVID | HIV |
| | Lamivudine (3TC) | PO | Epivir | HIV |
| | Saquinavir mesylate | PO | Invirase | HIV |
| | Ritonavir | PO | Norvir | HIV |
| | Indinavir sulfate | PO | Crixivan | HIV |
| | Nelfinavir mesylate | PO | Viracept | HIV |
| | Delavirdine HCl | PO | Rescriptor | HIV |
| | Nevirapine | PO | Viramune | HIV |
| | Efavirenz | PO | Sustiva | HIV |
| | Amprenavir | PO | Agenerase | HIV |
| | Abacavir | PO | Ziagen | HIV |
| | Zidovudine + Lamivudine | PO | Combivir | HIV |
| ANTITUBERCULAR | | | | |
| Antitubercular | Isoniazid | PO | Nydrazid | Primary |
| | Rifampin | IV, PO | Rifadin, Rimactane | Primary |
| | Streptomycin sulfate | IM | Streptomycin | Primary |
| | Ethambutol HCl | PO | Myambutol | Primary |
| | Pyrazinamide | PO | Pyrazinamide | Primary CNS or secondary |
| | Capreomycin | IM | Capastat | Secondary or atypical |
| | Kanamycin | IM | Kantrex | Secondary |
| | Cycloserine | PO | Seromycin | Secondary |
| | Ethionamide | PO | Trecator-SC | Secondary or atypical |
| | *p*-Aminosalicylic acid | PO | P.A.S., Paser | Secondary |
| | Clofazimine | PO | Lamprene | *Mycobacterium avium* complex (MAC) in HIV patient |
| | Rifabutin | PO | Ansamycin, Mycobutin | MAC in HIV patient |
| | Clarithromycin | PO | Biaxin | MAC in HIV patient |
| | Azithromycin dihydrate | PO, IV | Zithromax | MAC in HIV patient |

Table 14-14 Classification of Antimicrobial Agents (Continued)

| ANTIFUNGAL | | | |
|---|---|---|---|
| CLASS AND DRUG | ROUTE | COMMON TRADE NAME | MAJOR INDICATION |
| *Polyenes* | | | |
| Amphotericin B, amphotericin B–lipid complex | IV, PO<br>IV | Fungizone, Amphotec,<br>Abelcet | Agent of choice for deep-seated candidiasis, aspergillosis, mucormycosis, coccidioidomycosis, cryptococcosis, and extracutaneous sporotrichosis.<br>Oral suspension for mucosal candidiasis. |
| Nystatin | PO, T | Nilstat, Mycostatin | Mucosal and vaginal candidiasis. |
| *Imidazoles* | | | |
| Ketoconazole | PO, T | Nizoral | Esophageal candidiasis; alternate agent for chronic mucocutaneous candidiasis, paracoccidioidiomycosis, blastomycosis, histoplasmosis, coccidioidomycosis, and sporotrichosis; also effective when used orally in treatment of dermatophytoses including *Trichophyton* and *Microsporum* spp. |
| Itraconazole | PO | Sporanox | Itraconazole is active against *Aspergillus* spp. |
| Miconazole | IV, PO, T | Monistat | Topical and oral miconazole is used for the treatment of dermatophytoses, and vaginal candidiasis, coccidioidomycosis, and paracoccidioidomycosis. |
| Clotrimazole | T | Mycelex-G, Lotrimin | Mucosal and vaginal candidiasis. |
| *Triazoles* | | | |
| Fluconazole | IV, PO | Diflucan | Esophageal and vaginal candidiasis; alternate agent treatment and suppressive therapy of cryptococcosis. |
| *Miscellaneous* | | | |
| Flucytosine | PO | Ancobon | Usually in combination with amphotericin B for cryptococcosis and candidiasis, seldom used alone due to rapid development of resistance. |
| Griseofulvin | PO | Fulvicin UF, Gris-Peg | Dermatophytes including *Microsporum* and *Trichophyton* spp. |
| Terbinafine HCL | PO, T | Lamisil | Dermatophytes. |

ABBREVIATIONS: Inh, inhaled; IM, intramuscular; IV, intravenous; PO, oral; T, topical; CMV, cytomegalovirus; HSV, herpes simplex virus; MAC, *Mycobacterium avium* complex; spp., species; TMP-SMX, trimethoprim-sulfamethoxazole.

**Table 14-15 Factors Affecting Tissue Penetration of Antimicrobials**

1. Concentration of antimicrobial in blood
2. Molecular size of antimicrobial
3. Protein binding of antimicrobial in plasma
4. Lipid solubility of antimicrobial
5. Ionic charge of antimicrobial
6. Antimicrobial binding to exudate or tissue
7. Presence or absence of inflammation
8. Active transport mechanisms
9. Pathways of excretion of antimicrobial

sues, its penetration into interstitial and inflammatory spaces, and its excretion by glomerular filtration (Craig and Kunin 1976; Wise et al. 1980; Wise 1983). Likewise, extensive tissue binding of drugs (e.g., the polymyxins) also may restrict distribution and penetration into sites of infection (Kunin and Bugg 1971; Kucers and Bennett 1989). The development of an inflammatory response at the site of bacterial infection, with an increase in blood flow and capillary permeability, presumably counteracts some of the restrictive effects of extensive protein binding. Furthermore, most drugs in clinical use can be given in dosages that are adequate to overcome their potentially "negative" binding characteristics.

Antimicrobial concentrations in soft tissues, joint spaces, and body fluids are usually adequate to inhibit microbial growth. However, there are some special situations in which the tissue-penetrating characteristics of drugs may be particularly important in determining clinical responses to treatment. Such situations include suppurative meningitis, bacterial endocarditis, and septic arthritis. Critical concentrations of antibiotics in plasma for the treatment of other infections have not been established, but it is usually recommended that, for treatment of bacterial meningitis, plasma concentrations exceed the MIC by 10-fold or greater. This practice ensures a margin of safety such that less-than-optimal distribution of drug to site of action [e.g., cerebrospinal fluid (CSF)] can be overcome.

### *Pathways of excretion*

Therapeutic success of an antibiotic may be partially determined by the pharmacokinetics of its excretion (Table 14-17). This point is amply illustrated by the ability of nalidixic acid to sterilize the urinary tract despite its low concentration in plasma (Kunin 1974). Tetracyclines that do not accumulate well in the urine (e.g., minocycline or doxycycline) may be less effective in the treatment of urinary tract infection than tetracycline itself, which is predominantly excreted in the urine (Steigbeigel et al. 1968). When the normal renal pathway of excretion of tetracycline is impaired, therapeutic success is reduced. This is particularly true in patients with renal failure, when deliv-

**Table 14-16 Penetration of Antimicrobial Agents into Cerebrospinal Fluid**

| THERAPEUTIC ANTIBIOTIC CONCENTRATIONS | | | | |
|---|---|---|---|---|
| OBTAINED WITHOUT INFLAMED MENINGES | LIKELY WITH INFLAMED MENINGES | | NOT LIKELY REGARDLESS OF STATE OF MENINGES | |
| Trimethoprim | Penicillin G | Ceftizoxime sodium | Amikacin sulfate | First-generation cephalosporins |
| Sulfonamides | Ampicillin | Ceftazidime[a,b] | Streptomycin sulfate | Cefamandole nafate |
| Chloramphenicol | Nafcillin sodium | Ceftriaxone sodium | Gentamicin sulfate | Cefoxitin sodium |
| Isoniazid | Cloxacillin sodium | Imipenem[a,b] | Tobramycin sulfate | Cefotetan disodium |
| Rifampin | Ticarcillin disodium (± clavulanic acid) | Aztreonam[a,b] | Lincomycin HCl | Cefmetazole sodium |
| Flucytosine | Carbenicillin indanyl sodium | Ciprofloxacin HCl and other quinolones[a,b] | Clindamycin HCl | Vancomycin HCl |
| | Mezlocillin sodium monohydrate | Fluconazole and other bis-triazoles | | |
| | Piperacillin sodium | *p*-Aminosalicylic acid | | |
| | Cefuroxime sodium | Ethambutol HCl | | |
| | Cefotaxime sodium | | | |

[a]Does not have FDA approval for treatment of CNS infection.
[b]Limited data available.
SOURCE: Reproduced by permission from Young and Koda-Kimble 1988. *Applied Therapeutics: The Clinical Use of Drugs,* 4th edition. Vancouver, WA: Applied Therapeutics, Inc.

Table 14-17 Antimicrobial Agents Excreted into Urine in Therapeutic Concentrations

| DRUG | EXAMPLES |
|---|---|
| Amoxicillin (± clavulanic acid) | |
| Ampicillin | |
| Carboxypenicillins | Carbenicillin indanyl sodium, ticarcillin disodium |
| Ureidopenicillins | Mezlocillin sodium monohydrate, piperacillin sodium |
| First-generation cephalosporins | Cefazolin sodium, cephalothin sodium, cefadroxil, cephalexin |
| Second-generation cephalosporins | Cefonicid sodium, cefamandole nafate, cefoxitin sodium, cefotetan disodium, cefuroxime sodium |
| Third-generation cephalosporins | Cefotaxime sodium, ceftriaxone sodium, ceftazidime, cefoperazone sodium |
| Carbapenems | Imipenem, meropenem |
| Monobactam | Aztreonam |
| Aminoglycosides | Amikacin sulfate, tobramycin sulfate, gentamicin sulfate, streptomycin sulfate, kanamycin |
| Quinolones | Nalidixic acid, ciprofloxacin HCl, norfloxacin, ofloxacin, levofloxacin, sparfloxacin, grepafloxacin, trovafloxacin |
| Methenamine[a] | |
| Nitrofurantoin[a] | |
| Doxycycline | |
| Tetracycline HCl[b] | |
| Sulfonamides | |
| Trimethoprim | |
| Vancomycin HCl | |
| Flucytosine | |
| Fluconazole | |
| Ethambutol HCl | |
| Cycloserine | |

[a]Ineffective in patients with renal failure.
[b]Avoid in renal failure because of increased azotemia.

ery of drugs to urine is decreased. In such patients not only is tetracycline less effective in treating urinary tract infections, but standard doses become more toxic (Kucers and Bennett 1989). Similarly, in patients with biliary tract obstruction, the concentrations of antimicrobials in bile are decreased; this may be a factor in the failure of treatment (Schoenfield 1971; Sande and Mandell 1985; Kucers and Bennett 1989).

## Toxicity of Antimicrobial Therapy

### *Mechanisms of toxicity*

The mechanisms associated with common adverse reactions to antimicrobials include dose-related toxicity that occurs in a certain fraction of patients when a critical plasma concentration or total dose is exceeded, and toxicity that is unpredictable and mediated through allergic or idiosyncratic mechanisms. For example, certain classes of drugs such as the aminoglycosides are associated with dose-related toxicity. In contrast, the major toxicity of the penicillins and cephalosporins is due to allergic reactions. These differences are explained in part by the relative ability of specific drugs to inhibit enzymatic pathways in the host versus their stimulation of specific immune response. Table 14-18 summarizes some of the major toxicities of various antimicrobials.

Not included in these lists is mention of the subtle adverse effects of a number of antibiotics on the host immune response. Antibiotics can reduce the efficacy of the host response to microbial pathogens. They can diminish chemotaxis, phagocytosis, neutrophil- and macrophage-mediated microbial killing, lymphocyte transformation, delayed-hypersensitivity reactions, and production of antibody (Hauser and Remington 1982; Mandell 1982). For example, doxycycline decreases chemotaxis, phagocytosis, lymphocyte transformation, delayed-hypersensitivity reactions, and production of antibody. The antimicrobial effects on immune responses observed in vitro may or may not be clinically relevant; however, these data reinforce the concept that antimicrobials have potential to pro-

**Table 14-18 Adverse Effects of Common Antimicrobial Agents**

| Agent | Adverse Effects | Comments |
|---|---|---|
| ANTIBIOTICS | | |
| β-Lactams (carbapenems, penicillins, cephalosporins, monobactams, carbapenems) | Allergic: anaphylaxis, urticaria, serum sickness, rash, fever | Patients with "ampicillin rash" have no cross-reactivity with other penicillins; ampicillin rash most common in patients with mononucleosis or patients receiving allopurinol. Serum sickness. |
| | | The likelihood of cross-reactivity between penicillins and cephalosporins approximately 3 to 7%; extensive cross-reactivity between penicillins and imipenem; no cross-reactivity between aztreonam and penicillins. |
| | Diarrhea | Particularly common with ampicillin, ceftriaxone. *Clostridium difficile* diarrhea can occur with most β-lactams. |
| | Hematologic (anemia, thrombocytopenia, antiplatelet activity, hypoprothrombinemia) | Hemolytic anemia more common with higher doses and is associated with idiosyncratic reactions. |
| | | Antiplatelet activity most common with the antipseudomonal penicillins and high serum levels of other β-lactams, especially moxalactam. |
| | | Hypoprothrombinemia is more associated with those cephalosporins with the methylthioptetrazole side chain (cefamandole, cefotetan, cefoperazone, cefmetazole, moxalactam); the reaction is preventable and reversible with vitamin K. |
| | Hepatitis | Most common with oxacillin. |
| | Seizure activity | Associated with high levels of β-lactams (e.g., in renal failure patients) particularly penicillins and imipenem in patients with prior history of seizure. |
| | Sodium load | Carbenicillin, ticarcillin. |
| | Interstitial nephritis | Most common with methicillin; however, reported for most other β-lactams. |
| | Disulfiram reaction | Associated with cephalosporins with methylthiotetrazole side chain (cefamandole, cefotetan, cefmetazole). |
| | Hypotension, nausea | Associated with fast infusion of imipenem. |
| Aminoglycosides (gentamicin, tobramycin, amikacin, netilmicin, streptomycin) | Nephrotoxicity | Averages 10 to 15% incidence, increased in patients that are acidotic, dehydrated, or tobramycin, amikacin, netilmicin, receiving furosemide; generally reversible <5 days treatment. |
| | Ototoxicity | 1 to 5% incidence, generally irreversible; cochlear and/or vestibular toxicity occur involving high-frequency loss. |
| | Neuromuscular paralysis | Rare; most common in patients with myasthenia gravis, parkinsonism, receiving blood, or receiving neuromuscular blocking drugs or large volumes of citrated blood. |
| | Allergic reaction | Usually due to sulfites in some preparations. |
| Clindamycin | Diarrhea | Most common adverse effect; high association with pseudomembranous colitis, which is effectively treated with oral metronidazole. |
| | Other | Hepatitis, neutropenia, eosinophilia, fever, nausea, metallic taste. |
| Macrolides (erythromycin, clarithromycin, azithromycin, dirithromycin) | Nausea, vomiting | Oral administration—most frequent with erythromycin, much less with other macrolides. |
| | Cholestatic jaundice | Reported for all erythromycin salts, but most common with estolate. |
| | Ototoxicity | Most common with high doses in patients with renal and/or hepatic failure; usually transient. |
| | Phlebitis | Common and severe with IV erythromycin. |

**Table 14-18 Adverse Effects of Common Antimicrobial Agents (Continued)**

| AGENT | ADVERSE EFFECTS | COMMENTS |
|---|---|---|
| Vancomycin | Ototoxicity | Primarily with high serum levels (>50 μg/ml). |
| | Nephrotoxicity | Little to no nephrotoxicity observed with the current preparations of vancomycin; may increase the nephrotoxicity of aminoglycosides. |
| | Hypotension, flushing (red man syndrome) | Associated with rapid infusion of vancomycin. |
| | Phlebitis | Needs large volume dilution. |
| Tetracyclines | Allergic | Rash, anaphylaxis, urticaria, fever. |
| | Photosensitivity | Common. |
| | Teeth or bone deposition and discoloration | Avoid in pediatrics. |
| | GI | Nausea, diarrhea, most common with oxytetracycline. |
| | Hepatitis | Primarily with high IV doses in pregnancy. |
| | Renal (azotemia) | Tetracyclines have an antianabolic effect and should be avoided usually in those patients with decreased renal function; doxycycline can be used in patients with renal failure. |
| | Vestibular | Associated with minocycline. |
| Chloramphenicol | Anemia | Idiosyncratic irreversible aplastic anemia (rare); reversible dose-related anemia (common). |
| | Gray baby syndrome | Due to inability of neonates to conjugate chloramphenicol. |
| Sulfonamides | GI | Nausea, diarrhea. |
| | Hepatic | Cholestatic hepatitis; increased incidence in AIDS. |
| | Rash | Photosensitization, exfoliative dermatitis, drug fever (common); Stevens–Johnson syndrome (rare in AIDS patients). |
| | Bone marrow | Neutropenia and thrombocytopenia occur (more common in AIDS patients). |
| | Kernicterus | Due to increased unbound drug in the neonate because the premature liver is unable to conjugate bilirubin; sulfonamide displaces bilirubin from protein, resulting in excess free bilirubin and kernicterus. |
| Trimethoprim | Skin | Rash in >20% of patients receiving 400 mg/day. |
| | Hematologic | Thrombocytopenia and leukopenia occur; neutropenia rare. |
| Quinolones (norfloxacin, ciprofloxacin, enoxacin, levofloxacin, sparfloxacin, lomefloxacin, grepafloxacin, trovafloxacin, nalidixic acid) | GI | Nausea, vomiting, diarrhea. Hypersensitivity hepatitis with trovafloxacin. |
| | CVS | Prolongation of QT interval.<br>Grepafloxacin has caused torsade de pointes (now withdrawn as a therapeutic agent) |
| | CNS | Altered mental status, confusion, seizures, headache, insomnia, psychosis, tremors, hallucinations. |
| | Cartilage toxicity | Avoid in children. |
| | Musculoskeletal | Tendon rupture. |
| | Skin | Photosensitivity—especially with sparfloxacin, lomefloxacin and nalidixic acid. |
| Metronidazole | CNS<br>Peripheral nervous system | Headaches and paresthesias common; ataxia and seizure rare. Peripheral neuropathy with prolonged use (>60 g total dose). |
| | Disulfiram reaction | Common. |
| | GI | Metallic taste, stomatitis, nausea. |

**Table 14-18 Adverse Effects of Common Antimicrobial Agents (Continued)**

| AGENT | ADVERSE EFFECTS | COMMENTS |
|---|---|---|
| ANTIFUNGAL AGENTS | | |
| Amphotericin B | Headache, fever, nausea, vomiting, chills, malaise, and hypotension | Associated with IV infusion; antipyretic, antiemetic, and antihistamine drugs may be used to provide some symptomatic relief. |
| | Nephrotoxicity | Decreased glomerular filtration rate and renal tubular acidosis; usually reversible; permanent renal impairment occurs when the total dose exceeds 4 to 5 g. |
| | Electrolyte disturbances | Hypokalemia and hypomagnesemia. |
| | Hematologic (anemia, thrombocytopenia) | Generally reversible. |
| | Miscellaneous | Rarely rash, pruritus, blurred vision, seizures, pulmonary edema, and leukopenia. |
| Ketoconazole | GI | Nausea, vomiting. |
| | Hepatic | Transient (generally reversible) elevations of serum transaminase or alkaline phosphatase concentrations (rarely fulminant hepatitis, 1:15,000). |
| | Endocrine | Gynecomastia, decreased testosterone synthesis, hypothyroidism (genetically determined). |
| Miconazole | GI | Nausea, vomiting. |
| | Neurotoxicity | Tremors, confusion, hallucination, and grand mal seizures. |
| | Hematologic (anemia, thrombocytopenia) | Appears to be dose-related. Generally reversible. |
| Fluconazole | GI | Nausea, vomiting, diarrhea, 8 to 11% with 400 mg dose/day 30%. |
| | Hepatic | Elevation of serum transaminase level. Generally reversible. |
| | Skin | Reversible alopecia, 10–20% in those receiving 400 mg/day for 3 months. |
| Flucytosine | GI | Vomiting, abdominal pain, diarrhea. |
| | Hematologic (anemia, neutropenia, thrombocytopenia) | Generally occurs with prolonged high serum levels >100 $\mu$g/ml, or with concomitant amphotericin B. |
| Griseofulvin | GI | Nausea, vomiting, diarrhea. |
| | Neurotoxicity | Headache, fatigue, confusion, and peripheral neuritis. |
| Itraconazole | GI | Nausea (10%), hepatitis (1/1000). |
| Terbinafine | Skin | Rash (8%). |
| ANTIVIRAL AGENTS | | |
| Acyclovir | GI | Nausea, vomiting, and abdominal pain. |
| | Nephrotoxicity | Increased serum BUN and creatinine concentrations; occurs in about 10% of patients receiving parenteral acyclovir therapy. |
| | Crystal nephropathy | Generally reversible. |
| | Neurotoxicity | Lethargy, agitation, tremor, and disorientation (uncommon and generally reversible). |
| Ganciclovir | Hematologic (neutropenia, thrombocytopenia) | Neutropenia is more common in AIDS patients but still a problem in 40% of patients. |
| | CNS | Confusion, convulsion, and headache occur in <5%. |
| Cidofovir | Nephrotoxicity | Dose dependent; reduce dose, hydrate and give probenecid. |
| Valacyclovir | GI | GI intolerance rarely. |
| | Hematologic | TTP/HUS has been reported in patients with advanced HIV disease who receive high doses. |
| Famciclovir | | Rarely headache, nausea, fatigue. |

Table 14-18 Adverse Effects of Common Antimicrobial Agents (Continued)

| AGENT | ADVERSE EFFECTS | COMMENTS |
|---|---|---|
| Foscarnet | Nephrotoxicity | Renal failure, 30% have creatinine >200 mM/L. Monitor creatinine 3×/week and discontinue if >290 mM/L. Decreased serum levels of calcium, magnesium, and phosphorus due to renal tubular changes. |
| | CNS | Seizures (10%). |
| | GI | Intolerance. |
| | GU | Genital ulcers. |
| Rimantadine | GI | Intolerance (3 to 8%). |
| | CNS | Insomnia, impaired concentration, nervousness (4 to 8%), seizures—primarily in those with a seizure disorder. |
| Amantadine | CNS | Nervousness, insomnia, dizziness occur in 33%; increase incidence with daily dose of 300 mg, with renal failure, or in elderly. |
| Vidarabine | Hematologic (anemia, thrombocytopenia, and neutropenia) | Usually reversible. |
| | GI | Nausea and vomiting. |
| | Neurotoxicity | Tremor, dizziness, confusion, and hallucination can occur. |
| *Nucleoside reverse transcriptase inhibitors* | | |
| Zidovudine | GI | Nausea, vomiting, and diarrhea can occur. |
| | Hematologic | Neutropenia and megaloblastic anemia are generally reversible. |
| | CNS | Headache, rarely seizures, hallucinations. |
| | Musculoskeletal | Myopathy. |
| Zalcitabine (dideoxycytidine, ddC, ;HIVID™) | Neuropathy | Painful peripheral neuropathy (17 to 31%). |
| | GI | Aphthous oral and esophageal ulcers; pancreatitis (1%), hepatitis with transaminase levels >5× normal (up to 10%); rarely thrombocytopenia or leukopenia. |
| Didanosine (dideoxyinosine, ddI, Videx™) | GI | Intolerance due to formulation, diarrhea (15 to 30%), pancreatitis (5 to 9%). |
| | Neurotoxicity | Painful peripheral neuropathy (5 to 12%). |
| Stavudine (d4T, Zerit™) | Neuropathy | 15 to 21%. |
| | GI | Pancreatitis (0.5–1%); possible steatosis—lactic acidosis syndrome. |
| | Hematologic | Granulocytopenia. |
| Lamivudine | Miscellaneous | Rarely headache, nausea, diarrhea, abdominal pain, insomnia. |
| Abacavir | Hypersensitivity | Occurs in 3% treated individuals 1–4 weeks after starting therapy—fever, malaise, nausea, vomiting, diarrhea, rash, arthralgia. Rechallenge can be fatal. |
| *Nonnucleoside reverse transcriptase inhibitors* | | |
| Nevirapine | Skin | Rash, very common. |
| Delavirdine | Skin | Rash (13%). |
| | GI | Nausea, vomiting, increased liver enzymes (<5%). |
| Efavirenz | Skin | Rash (27%). |
| | CNS | Headache 6%, dizziness 6 to 10%). Impaired concentration and/or drowsiness 6 to 9%). |
| | Miscellaneous | Headache. |
| *Protease inhibitors* | | |
| Saquinavir | GI | Dose-related nausea, abdominal pain, and diarrhea (4–6%). |

**Table 14-18 Adverse Effects of Common Antimicrobial Agents (Continued)**

| AGENT | ADVERSE EFFECTS | COMMENTS |
|---|---|---|
| Indinavir | GU | Nephrolithiasis ± hematuria in 2–5%. Patients should drink >48 ounces of fluid daily. |
| | GI | Intolerance <5%; asymptomatic increase in indirect bilirubin in 10–15%; increased transaminases. |
| | Miscellaneous | Insomnia, blurred vision, dizziness. |
| Nelfinavir | GI | Loose stools (10%). |
| Ritonavir | GI | Intolerance requiring discontinuation of drug in 10–25%. |
| | Paresthesias | Peripheral and circumoral 5–8%. |
| | Miscellaneous | Asthenia (15–25%); cholesterol levels increase 30–40%; triglyceride levels increase 200–300%. |
| Amprenavir | Miscellaneous | Usually well tolerated. Headache, nausea, diarrhea, rash. |
| ANTITUBERCULAR AGENTS | | |
| Isoniazid (INH) | CNS | Peripheral neuropathy occurs with increased incidence in slow acetylators, pregnancy, chronic alcoholics, malnourished patients, elderly diabetes patients, and chronic liver diseases; prevented by daily pyridoxine 10 mg. |
| | Hepatitis | Elevated transaminase level occurs with increased risk >35 years of age; usually occur within first 6 months of therapy. |
| Rifampin | Hepatitis | Elevated transaminase level is uncommon, occurring in 1% of patients; generally mild and reversible. |
| | Reddish discoloration of urine and other body fluids and contact lenses | |
| | Flu-like syndrome | Usually occurs with intermittent high-dosage therapy (1200 mg twice weekly). |
| Pyrazinamide (PZA) | Hepatotoxicity | Elevated transaminase level generally occurs with doses >40–50 mg/kg/day. |
| | Hyperuricemia | Increased serum uric acid level, occasionally precipitating clinical gout. |
| Ethambutol (ETH) | Optic neuritis | Blurred vision and red-green color blindness; usually reversible upon discontinuation and associated with doses >25 mg/kg/day. |
| Rifabutin | Hematologic | Leukopenia and thrombocytopenia. |
| | Uveitis | Eye pain, photophobia, redness blurred vision—usually with high doses (600 mg/day) or with concurrent use with clarithromycin or fluconazole. |
| | Orange discoloration of urine, tears/contact lenses, sweats | |
| | Drug interactions | Major concern—rifabutin accelerates cytochrome P450 metabolism. |
| | GI | Intolerance, hepatitis. |
| Clofazimine | GI | Abdominal pain in >50% (due to crystals in gut) persists for months after discontinuation; bowel obstruction with doses >300 mg/day. |
| | Skin | Increased pigmentation changes (pink-black range); ichthyosis and pruritus can occur; conjunctival irritation. |

Acyclovir, amantadine HCl, amikacin sulfate, amphotericin B, azithromycin dihydrate, chloramphenicol, cidofovir, ciprofloxacin HCl, clarithromycin, clindamycin HCl, clofazimine, delavirdine HCl, didanosine, dirithromycin, enoxacin, erythromycin, ethambutol HCl, famciclovir, fluconazole, foscarnet sodium, flucytosine, ganciclovir sodium, gentamicin sulfate, grepafloxacin, griseofulvin, indinavir mesylate, isoniazid, itraconazole, ketoconazole, lamivudine, levofloxacin, lomefloxacin HCl, metronidazole, miconazole, nalidixic acid, nelfinavir, netilmicin sulfate, nevirapine, norfloxacin, pyrazinamide, rifabutin, rifampin, rimantadine HCl, ritonavir, saquinavir mesylate, sparfloxacin, stavudine mesylate, streptomycin sulfate, terbinafine HCl, tobramycin sulfate, trimethoprim, trovafloxacin, valacyclovir HCl, vancomycin, vidarabine, zalcitabine, zidovudine.

ABBREVIATION: TTP/HUS, thrombotic thrombocytopenic purpura/hemolytic-uremic syndrome.

duce deleterious effects that are related to their pharmacologic effects independent of their actions on bacteria or viruses.

A consideration of the relative toxicities of different antimicrobials in relation to their efficacy is critical to the appropriate choice of antimicrobials. If two antibiotics have equivalent efficacy, the less toxic antibiotic should be chosen. The therapeutic index of an antimicrobial compares the plasma concentration of drug at which host toxicity appears with that which is effective in the treatment of the infectious disease. This ratio varies with the properties of the different drugs and the amount of antibiotic necessary to inhibit the organism in vivo at the site of infection. It may also vary with host factors that alter susceptibility to drug toxicity.

For example, gentamicin and nafcillin both exhibit in vitro activity against staphylococci. However, the therapeutic index of gentamicin in most patients is quite narrow, whereas that of nafcillin is relatively wide. Accordingly, nafcillin or other penicillinase-resistant penicillins are the treatment of choice for staphylococcal infections (in subjects not allergic to penicillin). Similarly, because of their wide therapeutic indices, the penicillins and the cephalosporins are the preferred agents in the treatment of most serious infections caused by susceptible organisms in which bactericidal therapy is preferred.

The picture changes dramatically in the case of penicillin allergy, when microgram amounts of these drugs may lead to fatal anaphylaxis. The one notable exception to this principle is the finding that anaphylactic reactions to penicillin do not occur on exposure to the monobactams (e.g., aztreonam) (Adkinson et al. 1984; Saxton et al. 1984). Otherwise, an anaphylactic reaction to one penicillin usually precludes administration of any other $\beta$-lactam antibiotic. Appropriate substitution therapy in the event of penicillin allergy is discussed in the section on specific antimicrobial drugs.

When an untoward event occurs during antimicrobial therapy, the potential deleterious role of the drug must always be considered. For example, patients receiving parenteral amphotericin B should have a baseline potassium, magnesium, blood urea nitrogen (BUN), and creatinine concentration, urinalysis, and peripheral blood count determined before therapy is initiated. These values should be checked frequently (e.g., every 3 days) so that appropriate adjustments of dosage can be made or the drug stopped in the event of serious toxicity. Such close monitoring is not necessary when less toxic antimicrobials are used, although in any patient receiving prolonged therapy it is wise to follow blood counts and renal function, to examine the skin for allergic rashes, and to measure body temperature to check for drug-induced fever.

**PRINCIPLE When the drug used to treat disease (e.g., infection) causes a sign of the disease (e.g., fever), then the physician must be especially vigilant in following the patient.**

### *Antimicrobial toxicity due to altered host factors*

Elimination of antibiotics may be modified by genetic factors, concomitant treatment with other drugs, or disorders that alter normal elimination pathways. Furthermore, the change in endogenous flora that occurs as a result of antimicrobial treatment can lead to unfavorable reactions. For example, any antimicrobial that affects aerobic bacteria can alter the normal gut flora, thereby promoting selection for anaerobic *Clostridium difficile* superinfection of the GI lumen (Gorbach and Bartlett 1977). This organism produces a potent cytotoxin that can result in pseudomembranous colitis. The potential contribution of these factors to both therapeutic efficacy and drug toxicity must be taken into consideration when selecting antimicrobials and monitoring patients for the effects of treatment.

### *Toxicity in specific patient groups*

The exposure of pregnant women and neonates to certain drugs poses several problems that may have serious consequences to the fetus or infant (see chapter 19, Drug Therapy in Pregnant and Breast-Feeding Women, and chapter 20, Drug Therapy in Pediatric Patients). Some drugs readily cross the placental barrier and can produce toxicity in the fetus. Examples of fetal toxicity include dental staining or tooth malformation (e.g., tetracyclines), ototoxicity (e.g., aminoglycosides), arthropathy (e.g., quinolones), and displacement of bilirubin from serum albumin with the production of kernicterus at birth (e.g., sulfonamides). Accordingly, these drugs should not be used during pregnancy nor should they be given to neonates. The physician must also recognize that there is a considerable lack of knowledge on the safety of a variety of newer antimicrobials in the pregnant woman. Therefore, it is always prudent to use these drugs with restraint and only when clearly necessary.

Newborns, particularly if premature, have a relative deficiency of the hepatic enzyme glucuronyl transferase and reduced hepatic clearance of chloramphenicol (Kucers and Bennett 1989). This leaves neonates susceptible to a potentially lethal syndrome characterized by flaccidity, ashen color, and cardiovascular collapse (the "gray baby" syndrome). The use of chloramphenicol in neonates should be avoided if possible. In the rare situation when it must be given, the dose of chloramphenicol should be limited to no more than 25 mg/kg per day for premature babies and 50 mg/kg per day for full-term infants, and the concentrations in blood should be frequently monitored.

Subjects with glucose-6-phosphate dehydrogenase deficiency may develop hemolysis when given drugs with oxidant activity. Antimicrobials to be avoided include nitrofurantoin, chloramphenicol, the sulfonamides, furazolidone, nalidixic acid, aminosalicylic acid, and primaquine.

### *Reactions secondary to drug interactions*

Certain combinations of drugs may lead to inactivation or to an exaggeration of the effects of antimicrobials (see chapter 25, Drug Interactions). The potential for interactions is increased in seriously ill patients who are receiving several different medications and in whom drug metabolism may be altered by disease. For example, concomitant administration of antacids containing calcium or magnesium, or the administration of ferrous sulfate, can prevent absorption of tetracycline and quinolones from the gut. Chloramphenicol inhibits the activity of certain hepatic enzymes, and it interferes with biotransformation of barbiturates, phenytoin, warfarin, and tolbutamide (Rose et al. 1977). Isoniazid with phenytoin and sulfonamides with sulfonylureas similarly compete for the same enzymatic inactivating systems (Christiansen et al. 1963; Kabins 1972). The practitioner must be aware of all drugs and dietary substances ingested by his or her patient and be able to anticipate the presence of clinically important drug interactions.

**PRINCIPLE Whenever more than one drug is given to a patient, the potential for toxicity is increased through known or unknown interactions. Polypharmacy should be avoided unless the indications for it are compelling.**

### *Reactions due to impaired excretion*

Almost all antimicrobials are excreted to some extent by the kidney; some are cleared predominantly by the liver. Whenever renal or hepatic failure is present, the physician should be aware of necessary alterations of dosage in order to avoid dose-related toxicity. The degree of change in the regimen is determined by the potential of a compound to cause dose-related toxicity, the drug's route of clearance, and the magnitude of the renal or hepatic impairment. Table 14-19 provides a guide to modifications of dose necessary for different classes of drugs in the presence of renal failure. The major principles on which these recommendations are made include the following:

1. The concentration of drug in plasma after an initial dose is a function of the dose, the rate of absorption of the drug, the rate of redistribution to tissues, and the rate of excretion. If the rate of absorption is much faster than the distribution and excretion of the drug, then slow excretion in renal failure will not appreciably alter initial concentrations of drug in blood. This is the situation that prevails with most antibiotics with significant dose-related toxicity (e.g., aminoglycosides). Therefore, the initial dose (loading dose) of these drugs requires no modification in patients with renal failure.
2. After the initial dose of drug is given, the clearance becomes the important determinant of the rate of decline of concentration in plasma. Subsequent dosing must be reduced to correspond to slowed elimination. These reductions of dose can be achieved by lengthening the interval between doses or by reducing the dose administered at a fixed interval.

These points can be illustrated by using gentamicin as an example. The drug is excreted by glomerular filtration and is handled in the kidney in a way similar to the handling of creatinine. Consequently, creatinine clearance can be used as a guide to adjustment of the maintenance dose. In some patients, especially elderly ones, serum creatinine concentrations may be within normal values even when there is significant renal insufficiency (see part 1, Introduction, and chapter 6, Renal Disorders and the Influence of Renal Function on Drug Disposition). The administration of gentamicin at dose intervals that are three times its half-life in the plasma usually is adequate to maintain concentrations in plasma such that the peak concentration is approximately 8 times the rough concentration. Gentamicin has a half-life that varies from 2 to 4 hours in subjects with normal renal function. Using these points, one suggested dosage regimen for gentamicin makes use of the serum creatinine as follows (McHenry et al. 1971):

1. *Initial (loading) dose*: Administer 1.7 to 2.0 mg/kg IM or IV to produce a peak plasma concentration of 7 to 8 mg/L in most patients.
2. *Subsequent maintenance doses:* Administer a dose of 1.0 to 1.7 mg/kg every 8 hours (about three half-lives) if the creatinine concentration is 1 mg/dL or less (i.e., normal renal function). To extend the dose interval in

**Table 14-19 Pharmacokinetics and Dosage of Antimicrobial Agents in Renal Failure**

| Drug | Major Route of Elimination | Half-Life NL | Half-Life ESRD | Normal Dosing Interval (H) | Adjustment for Renal Failure $CL_C$ (mL/min) >50 | 10–50 | <10 | Method | Dialysis |
|---|---|---|---|---|---|---|---|---|---|
| *Penicillins* | | | | | | | | | |
| Penicillin G | Renal<br>Hepatic | 0.5 | 6–20 | 6–8 | 6–8 | 8–12 | 12–16 | I | Yes (H)<br>No (P) |
| Ampicillin | Renal<br>Hepatic | 0.8–1.5 | 7–20 | 4–6 | 6 | 6–12 | 12–16 | I | Yes (H)<br>No (P) |
| Amoxacillin | Renal<br>Hepatic | 0.9–2.3 | 5–20 | 4–6 | 6 | 6–12 | 12–16 | I | Yes (H)<br>No (P) |
| Methicillin | Renal<br>Hepatic | 0.5–1.0 | 4 | 4–6 | 4–6 | 6–8 | 8–12 | I | No (H, P) |
| Nafcillin | Hepatic<br>Renal | 0.5–1.0 | 1.2 | 6 | Unch | Unch | Unch | D | No (H) |
| Dicloxacillin | Renal<br>Hepatic | 0.8 | 1–2 | 6 | Unch | Unch | Unch | I | No (H) |
| Cloxacillin | Renal<br>Hepatic | 0.5 | 1 | 6 | Unch | Unch | Unch | D | No (H) |
| Carbenicillin | Renal<br>Hepatic | 1.2–1.5 | 10–20 | 4–6 | 8–12 | 12–24 | 24–48 | I | Yes (H) |
| Ticarcillin | Renal<br>Hepatic | 1.2 | 16 | 4–6 | 8–12 | 12–24 | 24–48 | I | Yes (H)<br>No (P) |
| Mezlocillin | Renal<br>Hepatic | 0.6–1.2 | 2.6–5.4 | 4–6 | 4–6 | 6–8 | 8 | I | Yes (H) |
| Piperacillin | Renal<br>Hepatic | 0.8–1.5 | 3.3–5.1 | 6 | 4–6 | 6–8 | 8 | I | Yes (H) |
| Cephalosporins | | | | | | | | | |
| Cephradine | Renal | 1.3 | 6–15 | 6 | 100 | 50 | 25 | D | Yes (H, P) |
| Cephalexin | Renal | 1.0 | 20–40 | 6 | 6 | 6 | 8–12 | I | Yes (H, P) |
| Cefadroxil | Renal | 1.5 | 20–25 | 8 | 8 | 12–24 | 24–48 | I | Yes (H) |
| Cephalothin | Renal | 0.5–1.0 | 3–18 | 6 | 6 | 6–8 | 12 | I | Yes (H) |
| Cephapirin | Renal<br>Hepatic | 0.6–0.8 | 2.4–2.7 | 6 | 6 | 6–8 | 12 | I | Yes (H) |
| Cefazolin | Renal | 1.8–2 | 40–70 | 8 | 8 | 12 | 24–48 | I | Yes (H)<br>No (P) |
| Cefamandole | Renal | 1 | 11 | 4–6 | 6 | 6–8 | 8 | I | Yes (H) |
| Cefoxitin | Renal | 1 | 13–20 | 6–8 | 6–8 | 8–12 | 24–48 | I | Yes (H)<br>No (P) |
| Cefuroxime | Renal | 1.1–1.4 | 17 | 6–8 | 45–100 | 10–45 | 5–10 | D | Yes (H) |
| Cefonicid | Renal | 3.5–4.5 | 17–56 | 24 | 50 | 20–50 | 10–20 | D | Yes (H) |
| Cefaclor | Renal | 0.6–1 | 3 | 8 | 100 | 50–100 | 33 | D | Yes (H, P) |
| Loracarbef | Renal | 1 | | 12–24 | Unch | 24–48 | 72–120 | I | |
| Cefixime | Renal | 3–4 | 12 | 12 | Unch | 24 | 24 | I | |
| Cefpodoxime | Renal | 2.4 | — | 12 | 24 | 3 times per week | Weekly | I | |
| Cefepime | Renal | 2 | 13 | 12 | 24 | 24 | 24 | I | |
| Cefprozil | Renal | 1.3 | 5–6 | 12 | Unch | 24 | 24 | I | |
| Ceftibuten | Renal | 2.4 | — | 24 | Unch | 50% | 25% | I | |
| Cefmetazole | Renal | 1.2–1.5 | | 6–12 | 6–12 | 16–24 | 48 | I | Yes (H) |
| Cefotaxime | Renal<br>Hepatic | 1.0 | 2.6 | 6–8 | 6–8 | 8–12 | 12–24 | I | Yes (H) |
| Ceftizoxime | Renal | 1.4–1.7 | 30 | 8–12 | 50–100 | 15–50 | 10–15 | D | Yes (H) |

**Table 14-19 Pharmacokinetics and Dosage of Antimicrobial Agents in Renal Failure (Continued)**

| Drug | Major Route of Elimination | Half-Life | | Normal Dosing Interval (H) | Adjustment for Renal Failure $CL_C$ (mL/min) | | | | |
|---|---|---|---|---|---|---|---|---|---|
| | | NL | ESRD | | >50 | 10–50 | <10 | Method | Dialysis |
| Ceftriaxone | Hepatic<br>Renal | 7–9 | 12–24 | 12–24 | Unch | Unch | Unch | D | No (H) |
| Ceftazidime | Renal<br>Hepatic | 1.2–2 | 13 | 8–12 | 8–12 | 24–48 | 48–72 | I | Yes (H)<br>No (P) |
| Cefoperazone | Hepatic<br>Renal | 1.6–2.4 | 2.1 | 12 | Unch | Unch | Unch | I | Yes (H) |
| *Carbapenems* | | | | | | | | | |
| Imipenem | Renal | 1.0 | 3.7 | 6–8 | Unch | 50 | NTE: 500 mg every 12 h | D | Yes (H, P) |
| Meropenem | Renal | 1.0 | 6 | 8 | Unch | 12 | 24 | | |
| Aztreonam | Renal<br>Hepatic | 1.5–2.9 | 6–8 | 8–12 | Unch | 50–75 | 25 | D | Yes (H, P) |
| *Macrolides* | | | | | | | | | |
| Erythromycin | Hepatic<br>Renal | 1.4 | 5–6 | 6 | Unch | Unch | 50–75 | D | No (H, P) |
| Azithromycin | Hepatic | 68 | 68 | 24 | Unch | No data | No data | I | |
| Clarithromycin | Hepatic<br>Renal | 4 | — | 12 | Unch | Unch | 24 | I | |
| Dirithromycin | Renal<br>Biliary | 30–44 | 30–44 | 24 | Unch | Unch | Unch | I | |
| Clindamycin | Hepatic | 2–4 | 3–5 | 6 | Unch | Unch | Unch | D | No (H, P) |
| Metronidazole | Hepatic | 6–14 | 8–15 | 8 | 8 | 8–12 | 12–24 | I | Yes (H) |
| Chloramphenicol | Hepatic<br>Renal | 1.6–4 | 3–7 | 6 | Unch | Unch | Unch | D | No (H, P) |
| *Tetracyclines* | | | | | | | | | |
| Tetracycline | Hepatic | 6–10 | 57–108 | 6 | 8–12 | 12–24 | 24 | I | No (H, P) |
| Doxycycline | Hepatic<br>Renal | 15–24 | 18–25 | 24 | Unch | Unch | Unch | I | No (H, P) |
| Minocycline | GI<br>Renal | 12–16 | 12–18 | 12 | Unch | Unch | Unch | D | No (H, P) |
| Trimethoprim | Renal<br>Hepatic | 9–13 | 20–49 | 12 | 12 | 18 | 24 | I | Yes (H) |
| *Sulfonamides* | | | | | | | | | |
| Sulfamethoxazole | Renal<br>Hepatic | 9–11 | 20–50 | 12 | 12 | 18 | 24 | I | Yes (H)<br>No (P) |
| Sulfisoxazole | Renal<br>Hepatic | 3–8 | 6–12 | 6 | 6 | 8–12 | 12–24 | I | Yes (H, P) |
| Trimethoprim–sulfamethoxazole | Renal T<br>S | 8–15<br>7–12 | 24<br>22–50 | 12 | 12 | 24 | Avoid | I | |
| *Quinolones* | | | | | | | | | |
| Nalidixic acid | Hepatic | 6–7 | 21 | 6 | Unch | Avoid | Avoid | D | |
| Ciprofloxacin | Hepatic | 0.65–0.8 | 0.9–1 | 12 | Unch | 50 | 50 | D | |
| Enoxacin | Hepatic | 6–9 | <30 | 24 | Unch | Unch | 25 | D | |
| Norfloxacin | Renal<br>Hepatic | 3.5 | 8 | 12 | Unch | 24 | 24 | I | |
| Ofloxacin | Renal | 6 | 40 | 12 | Unch | 24 | 24 | I | |
| Clinafloxacin | Renal | 1.5 | 8.5 | 8–12 | 8 | 12 | 24 | I | |
| Levofloxacin | Renal | 6.3 | 35 | 24 | Unch | 50% | No data | I/D | |

**Table 14-19 Pharmacokinetics and Dosage of Antimicrobial Agents in Renal Failure (Continued)**

| Drug | Major Route of Elimination | Half-Life | | Normal Dosing Interval (H) | Adjustment for Renal Failure $CL_C$ (mL/min) | | | | |
|---|---|---|---|---|---|---|---|---|---|
| | | NL | ESRD | | >50 | 10–50 | <10 | Method | Dialysis |
| Lomefloxacin | Renal | 8 | 45 | 24 | Unch | 50% | — | D | |
| Sparfloxacin | Renal | 20 | ↑ | 24 | Unch | 48 | 48 | I | |
| *Glycopeptide* | | | | | | | | | |
| Vancomycin | Renal | 6–10 | 200–250 | 6–12 | 24–72 | 72–240 | 240 | I | No (H, P) |
| *Antifungal Agents* | | | | | | | | | |
| Amphotericin B | Hepatic Nonrenal | 24 | 24 | 24 | 24 | 24 | 24–36 | I | No (H, P) |
| Ketoconazole | Hepatic | 1.5–8 | 1.8 | 24 | Unch | Unch | Unch | D | No (H) |
| Miconazole | Hepatic | 20–24 | 20–24 | 8 | Unch | Unch | Unch | D | No (H, P) |
| Fluconazole | Renal | 22–30 | | 24 | 100 | 50 | 25 | D | Yes (H) |
| Itraconazole | Hepatic | 17 | | 12 | Unch | Unch | Unch | I | |
| Flucytosine | Renal | 3–6 | 75–200 | 6 | 6 | 12–24 | 24–48 | I | Yes (H, P) |
| *Antitubercular Agents* | | | | | | | | | |
| Isoniazid | Hepatic | 0.7–4 | 17 | 8 | 8 | 8 | 8 | I | Yes (H, P) |
| Rifampin | Hepatic | 1.5–5 | 1.8–3.1 | 24 | Unch | Unch | Unch | I | No (H) |
| Ethambutol | Renal | 4 | 7–15 | 24 | 24 | 24–36 | 48 | I | Yes (H, P) |
| Cycloserine | Renal | 12–20 | | 12 | 24 | Avoid | Avoid | I | Yes (H) |
| *p*-Aminosalicylic acid | Hepatic | 1.5 | 23 | 8 | 8 | 12 | Avoid | I | Yes (H) |

Amikacin sulfate, *p*-aminosalicylic acid, amoxacillin, amphotericin B, ampicillin, azithromycin, aztreonam, carbenicillin indanyl sodium, cefaclor, cefadroxil, cefamandole nafate, cefazolin sodium, cefepime HCl, cefixime sodium, cefonicid sodium, cefoperazone sodium, cefotaxime sodium, cefotetan disodium, cefoxitin sodium, cefoxitin sodium, cefprozil ?, ceftazidime, ceftibuten, ceftizoxime sodium, ceftriaxone sodium, cefuroxime axetil, cefuroxime sodium, cephalexin, cephalothin sodium, cephapirin sodium, cephradine, chloramphenicol, cinofloxacin, ciprofloxacin HCl, clarithromycin, clindamycin HCl, cloxacillin sodium, cycloserine, dicloxacillin sodium, dirithromycin ?, doxycycline, enoxacin, erythromycin, ethambutol HCl, fluconazole, flucytosine, imipenem, isoniazid, itraconazole, ketoconazole, levofloxacin, lomefloxacin HCl, loracarbef, meropenem, methicillin sodium, metronidazole, mezlocillin sodium monohydrate, miconazole, minocycline HCl, nafcillin sodium, nalidixic acid, norfloxacin, ofloxacin, penicillin G, piperacillin sodium, rifampin, sparfloxacin, sulfamethoxazole, sulfisoxazole, tetracycline HCl, ticarcillin disodium, trimethoprim, trimethoprim + sulfamethoxazole, vancomycin HCl

ABBREVIATIONS: D, dose reduction method; ESRD, end-stage renal disease; H, hemodialysis; I, interval extension method; NL, normal; P, peritoneal dialysis; Unch, unchanged.

SOURCE: Modified from Bennett 1988, and Bennett et al. 1974, 1994.

patients with renal compromise, multiply the usual dose interval (8 hours) by the patient's serum creatinine concentration (in mg/dL). Higher doses would be reserved for patients with serious infections outside the urinary tract, in which case one cannot take advantage of the concentrating ability of the kidney to provide high concentrations at the site of infection.

The above dosing guidelines are not precise. Patients vary in the plasma concentrations that are achieved with a given loading dose of gentamicin (interpatient variation in volume of distribution). In some patients, the excretion of gentamicin may be more rapid than the creatinine clearance would suggest; in others, it is slower. When the serum creatinine concentration is above 3 mg/dL and the interval between doses is more than 24 hours, some patients may have lower-than-therapeutic concentrations for a substantial time (McHenry et al. 1971).

The second approach is to administer the second and subsequent doses of gentamicin at the usual fixed interval of every 8 hours, reducing the amount of drug according to a formula based on the serum creatinine value: the total amount of gentamicin administered over a given period would be as indicated in the above formula, but the smaller doses given more frequently would ensure against subtherapeutic concentrations of the drug near the end of a dose interval.

A more recent method for dosing gentamicin relies on once daily dosing in patients with normal renal function. The rationale for this is based on three principles: 1) aminoglycosides exhibit concentration-dependent killing; 2) there is a long postantibiotic effect following exposure to high concentrations; and 3) there is less renal and inner ear accumulation with once-daily administration compared with conventional dosing. Once-daily dosing should not be used for patients with endocarditis, renal failure, cystic fibrosis, ascites, or >20% surface area burns. The once-daily dose for gentamicin and tobramycin is 6 mg/kg, whereas for amikacin it is 15 mg/kg. The serum concentration of the aminoglycoside should be measured 6 hours before the next dose. This level should be ≤1 mg/L for gentamicin and tobramycin and ≤5 mg/mL for amikacin to avoid accumulation.

**PRINCIPLE Formulae are only approximations; individual patients vary in their distribution and clearance of antibiotics despite apparently comparable degrees of renal or hepatic impairment. Thus, in any patient with significant impairment in excretion or metabolism of an antimicrobial, drug concentrations in plasma should be measured, particularly if the agent has a low therapeutic index.**

When patients with severe renal failure are given antimicrobials, consider whether they are undergoing dialysis, and if so, by what technique. Some drugs such as gentamicin are appreciably removed by hemodialysis, whereas their removal by peritoneal dialysis usually is quantitatively less and unpredictable (Kucers and Bennett 1989). Conversely, most penicillins and cephalosporins are not removed well by either method of dialysis, since no dialysis apparatus comes close to the penicillin-secreting function of the renal tubule (Bennett et al. 1974; Bennett 1988). Table 14-19 lists when the removal and/or replacement of the various antibiotics are appropriate during different types of dialysis. The physician should refer to standard texts or consult with infectious disease physicians or nephrologists to determine whether replacement dosing is indicated after dialysis.

In the neonate, particularly a premature one, pathways of metabolism or excretion may not be fully developed and modification of dosages may be required (see chapter 19, Drug Therapy in Pregnant and Breast-Feeding Women, and chapter 20, Drug Therapy in Pediatric Patients). Furthermore, some classes of drugs may cause toxicity in neonates but not in older persons, e.g., chloramphenicol and the tetracyclines (Moffett 1975). In such patients, impaired excretion or metabolic pathways may lead to extraordinarily high plasma concentrations of antibiotics, which may cause significant toxicity. It is critical to know both the manifestations of dose-related toxicity and the normal elimination pathways of drugs, so that required dosage modifications can be made when antimicrobial clearance is impaired.

***Adverse effects due to changes in endogenous flora*** Whenever the natural flora are suppressed by the administration of an antimicrobial, other organisms proliferate (e.g., *C. difficile*). The emergence or overgrowth of flora resistant to a given antibiotic may cause superinfections that are more severe than the original infection itself (e.g., enterococci that develop high-level aminoglycoside or vancomycin resistance, or methicillin-resistant staphylococci). We now recognize that several commonly used antibiotics (e.g., clindamycin and many $\beta$-lactams) produce a pseudomembranous colitis that may also be fatal if the cause of the characteristically profuse diarrhea is unrecognized (Bartlett 1984). Strains of *C. difficile* that produce a cytotoxin are most commonly associated with antibiotic-associated colitis.

Changes in bowel flora as a result of antibiotic administration may lead to decreased absorption of vitamin K with resultant bleeding in patients already receiving oral anticoagulants (Bentley and Meganathan 1982). However, controversy remains as to whether antibiotic-induced killing of intestinal bacteria results in hypoprothrombinemia (Smith and Lipsky 1983). Apparently, the vitamin K produced by these bacteria is not responsible for synthesis of clotting factors. Perhaps multiple factors are involved in the vitamin K-responsive hypoprothrombinemia observed in patients receiving antimicrobials.

Prolonged administration of oral neomycin may cause malabsorption; whether this is due to an alteration in normal bowel flora or to direct mucosal toxicity is not known (Lindenbaum et al. 1976). Another consequence of altered flora is the rising incidence of severe superinfections caused by fungi, especially in patients with cancer who receive treatment with broad-spectrum antimicrobials.

## Use of Combinations of Antimicrobials

Combinations of antimicrobials are frequently used to treat infection; rational combinations are chosen after carefully considering several important principles. For a specific organism or organisms causing infection, combinations of antibiotic may be synergistic, antagonistic, or indifferent. All too frequently, antibiotic combinations are used to provide "broad-spectrum" coverage in response to the physician's insecurity rather than a true medical indication. In some situations, broad-spectrum coverage is appropriate when treating a mixed infection, a rapidly worsening infection from pathogens whose precise identification is in progress, or a life-threatening infection caused by an organism that responds best to two synergistic agents. Combination therapy beyond these situations is unwarranted.

**PRINCIPLE Appropriate uses of antimicrobial combinations include necessary synergy against an infecting organism, initial empiric treatment of life-threatening infections, or treatment of mixed infections.**

### *Synergy*

Antimicrobials may exert synergistic effects if they work at two different sites, involving either the same or different metabolic pathways in an organism (Jawetz 1968; Moellering 1972). Examples of synergistic combinations of antibiotics are the combined use of penicillins (or cephalosporins) with aminoglycosides for killing certain aerobic bacteria. The mechanism of this synergy has been elucidated best in enterococci. The resistance of enterococci to aminoglycosides may be mediated by either of two mechanisms. One is the failure of the compounds to enter the microbial cell in amounts sufficient to bind to ribosomes and thereby to alter translation of the genetic code by ribosomal RNA. The other mechanism is seen when entry is adequate but ribosomal binding and altered translation do not occur. In the former situation, the potential for synergy between penicillins, cephalosporins, or vancomycin and the aminoglycosides exists because the "cell-wall-active" compounds act to facilitate entry of the aminoglycoside into the bacterial cell (Moellering and Weinberg 1971; Moellering et al. 1971). The same principles probably apply to the mechanism of synergy between other cell-wall-active agents and the aminoglycosides in their action against staphylococci or gram-negative rods (Steigbeigel et al. 1975). The major determining factors in these situations are some activity of the cell-wall-active antibiotic against the organism and ribosomal activity of the aminoglycoside.

Another example of synergism of antibiotics is seen when amphotericin B is combined with flucytosine against fungi (Kobayashi et al. 1974). Much of the synergistic effect is related to facilitated entry of the companion drug by amphotericin B.

Synergy potentially exists when two drugs are active against an organism at different points along the same vital biologic pathway. An example of this mechanism is the use of a dihydrofolate reductase inhibitor (trimethoprim or pyrimethamine) together with a sulfonamide. Both classes of drugs inhibit folate metabolism, which ultimately prevents the transfer of methyl groups used in purine synthesis. When these drug combinations are used, a microbicidal action frequently results (Gordon et al. 1975).

Despite suggestive in vitro data, convincing clinical evidence that synergistic drug combinations are superior to single drugs exists only for treatment of enterococcal endocarditis and when the combination trimethoprim-sulfamethoxazole is used. Considerable in vitro data suggest that most antimicrobial combinations are associated with antagonism (e.g., rifampin plus penicillins for staphylococci) or indifference (e.g., chloramphenicol plus rifampin for selected *Haemophilus influenzae* strains) (Jadavji et al. 1984). Therefore, unless there is clear need or documentation of synergism, combination therapy should not be used.

### *Extended antimicrobial spectrum*

Another indication (often abused) for the use of combinations of antimicrobials is to provide broad-spectrum coverage in the early empiric treatment of presumed life-threatening infections such as bacterial septicemia. The use of a combination such as a penicillinase-resistant penicillin or a cephalosporin with an aminoglycoside is based on the presumption that almost all likely organisms will be treated. The potential for abuse of this type of reasoning is that all too often it is applied in clinical situations either as a substitute for adequate collection of data or to treat the physician's insecurity. Furthermore, a second type of abuse may be observed in patients who respond to treatment and who eventually are found to have clinical isolates that are affected by only one member of the combination. Despite this new information, antibiotic combinations are frequently continued to the ultimate disadvantage of the patient, using the faulty reasoning that one does not like to tamper with "success." Besides the potential harm to the patient offered by continued application of toxic or inappropriate drugs, this type of approach may be particularly deleterious in the hospital setting, where selecting out flora resistant to multiple drugs can be lethal.

**PRINCIPLE Broad-spectrum coverage with antibiotics should not be a substitute for adequate collection of data or adequate clinical judgment. In most cases, single drugs with a selective spectrum of activity will provide adequate coverage for a successful outcome and will avoid the potential for toxic interactions or the selection of a highly resistant flora. In life-threatening situations, broad-spectrum coverage is justified initially; once the pathogen is identified, selective single-drug treatment is highly preferable.**

***Prevention of resistance***

Another indication for the use of a combination of antibiotics is to prevent the emergence of strains of bacteria that are resistant to one or more of the drugs employed. The reasoning behind such an approach is simply an application of probability statistics. If the probability of an event (i.e., spontaneous mutation to a resistant strain) is known for two different antibiotics given separately, then the probability that resistance to two drugs will occur simultaneously is the product of those two probabilities. This rationale has been applied most successfully to the treatment of tuberculosis, since the rates of development of resistance to single drugs are high. This same strategy has been applied successfully to treatment of HIV infection.

***Treatment of mixed infections***

Combination therapy is appropriate for the treatment of mixed infections. Such combinations may be useful even when the doses chosen exhibit antagonism. Chloramphenicol may antagonize the activity of aminoglycosides; this is usually of no clinical consequence, unless host factors involved in eradication of the organism during bacteriostatic therapy have been substantially inhibited (Sande and Overton 1973). Table 14-20 provides some examples of appropriate antimicrobial combinations.

**PRINCIPLE As with any combination of drugs, theory must be backed by clinical hypothesis testing. Beware of potential antagonistic combinations of antimicrobials when selecting therapy for mixed infections. The least "active" drug in a combination must be adequate to treat potential pathogens by itself in case of overlapping sensitivities, particularly if compromised host factors are of overriding importance in the determination of a successful outcome.**

## Treatment Schedules

Treatment schedules must be designed to ensure adequate delivery of active antimicrobials to the site of infection for a sufficient time to promote a cure. In treating infections that pose a serious threat to life, or that are in sites where high plasma concentrations of antimicrobials are necessary to ensure penetration of tissue (e.g., in the endocardium and brain), parenteral antibiotics are required initially. In less severe infections with highly sensitive organisms and excellent delivery of antimicrobials into tissues, oral administration of drugs can be employed (e.g., most urinary tract infections, streptococcal pharyngitis, and some patients with pneumonia).

The duration of therapy with antibiotics is determined by the amount of antibiotic that must be administered over a given time to effect a cure of an active infection and prevent a relapse of the infection. The precise duration of therapy required for different infectious diseases to meet these criteria is poorly documented. A few generalizations based on clinical observations can be made and applied to specific clinical situations. The critical points in these considerations of duration of treatment revolve around: 1) the ability of the organism to resist the normal host's defense mechanisms; 2) the physical location of the infection and its accessibility to therapeutic concentrations of an antimicrobial; 3) the primary activity of the antimicrobial against the organisms, as determined by MIC or MBC; and 4) the frequency of development of resistance of the organism to the drug. Some general guidelines for treatment schedules are given in Table 14-21.

At least 4 to 6 weeks of treatment of osteomyelitis and endocarditis are recommended, since treatment failure or relapse rates are unacceptably high (with considerable morbidity) with shorter periods of therapy (Sande and

**Table 14-20 Some Examples of Appropriate Combinations of Antimicrobials**

| RATIONALE | EXAMPLE |
|---|---|
| 1. Synergy | |
| a) Empiric treatment for gram-negative shock | Aminoglycoside and semisynthetic or antipseudomonal $\beta$-lactam (change to specific drugs once organism is identified and clinical condition improves) |
| b) Life-threatening infection of undetermined cause | Aminoglycoside and imipenem (change to specific drugs once organism is identified) |
| c) Serious enterococcal infection (e.g., endocarditis) | Gentamicin sulfate and ampicillin |
| d) Serious *Pseudomonas aeruginosa* infections (e.g., septicemia associated with pneumonia) | Aminoglycoside and semisynthetic or antipseudomonal $\beta$-lactam |
| 2. Serious mixed aerobic-anaerobic infection (e.g., intra-abdominal sepsis) | Aminoglycoside and metronidazole |
| 3. Decrease rate of antimicrobial resistance | Isoniazid, rifampin, pyrazinamide, and ethambutol HCl for tuberculosis |

**Table 14-21 Suggested Treatment Regimens for Defined Infections**

| Site of Infection | Therapeutic Option | Duration of Therapy |
|---|---|---|
| *Urinary Tract* | | |
| Cystitis | Oral or parenteral drugs that are renally excreted | One dose or 3 days |
| Pyelonephritis | | 10 to 14 days |
| *Respiratory Tract* | | |
| Pneumonia | | |
| Pneumococcal—penicillin susceptible | Parenteral penicillin G | Until afebrile 3 days; or a minimum or 5 days |
| Pneumococcal—penicillin resistant | High dose of penicillin or vancomycin or cefotaxime or ceftriaxone | |
| Aerobic gram-negative bacteria | Parenteral drugs[a] | 21 days or longer |
| Legionnaires' disease | Erythromycin or azithromycin parenterally or ciprofloxacin or levofloxacin; Rifampin may be added to erythromycin or azithromycin therapy | 21 days |
| *Staphylococcus aureus* | Nafcillin or vancomycin parenterally | 21 days |
| Bronchitis in COPD | Trimethoprim-sulfamethoxazole; Doxycycline | 5 to 7 days |
| Abscess (lung) | Penicillin or clindamycin parenterally and then orally; drainage may be considered | 42 to 56 days |
| Empyema | Drainage and parenteral antibiotics | 14 to 28 days |
| Pharyngitis (group A or C streptococci) | Oral penicillin or erythromycin | 10 days |
| *Cardiovascular System* | | |
| Bacteremia, likely source, no evidence of endocarditis | Parenteral antibiotics,[b] synergistic combinations for shock | 14 days |
| Endocarditis | Parenteral bactericidal antibiotics | 28 days or more |
| *CNS Infections* | | |
| Meningitis | Parenteral bactericidal antibiotics | 14 days |
| Abscess | Metronidazole, penicillinase-resistant synthetic penicillin, and third-generation cephalosporin | 28 days or more |
| *GI Tract* | | |
| Dysentery | Oral quinolone | 5 to 7 days |
| Abscess | Parenteral combination antibiotics for aerobic and anaerobic bacteria; consider surgical drainage | 14 to 21 days |
| Peritonitis | Parenteral combination antibiotics for aerobic and anaerobic bacteria; consider surgical intervention if ruptured viscus | 14 days |
| Pseudomembranous colitis | Oral metronidazole or oral vancomycin | 10 days |
| *Musculoskeletal System* | | |
| Muscle "gas gangrene" | Surgical débridement and clindamycin or parenteral penicillin G | 10 to 14 days |
| Bone | Parenteral and then oral bactericidal antibiotics; consider surgical drainage or débridement | 42 to 56 days |
| Joint | | |
| Gonococcal | Drainage and parenteral bactericidal antibiotics | 3 to 7 days |
| Nongonococcal | Drainage and parenteral bactericidal antibiotics | 21 days |

[a]The antibiotic chosen should have activity against a range of aerobic gram-negative bacteria.
[b]Choose antibiotics based on likely source of bacteremia.

Scheld 1980). Conversely, urinary tract infections caused by the same organisms usually can be eradicated within several days of treatment because of very high urinary concentrations of effective drugs (Kunin 1974).

Infections with intracellular pathogens require prolonged therapy. For example, staphylococci are capable of survival intracellularly; this site provides a sanctuary from antibiotic activity. Relapse of staphylococcal infections is common unless treatment is prolonged. The longest durations of treatment are used for mycobacterial infections. *Mycobacterium leprae*'s intracellular location and slow generation time (10 to 15 days) limit the ability of the sulfones to inhibit their replication (Shepard 1969). Treatment of extrapulmonary tuberculosis must often be continued for 12 to 24 months, depending upon the severity of disease and the sensitivity of the organisms to drugs.

Treatment for infections caused by bacteria that are promptly killed by phagocytosis need not be long, unless endocarditis is present. Pneumococcal pneumonia is a good example of this type of infection. Cures have been reported with a single dose of penicillin (Witt and Hamburger 1963). However, the usual duration of treatment of pneumococcal pneumonia is a minimum of 5 days or until the patient has been afebrile for at least 3 days. Remember that the recommended duration of therapy is a minimum. These schedules should be considered only as guidelines. It is quite possible that duration of antimicrobial therapy might need to be longer in a specific patient who is not responding promptly.

## Factors Responsible for Failure of Treatment

Failure of treatment can result from a number of different factors, including the following:

1. Antimicrobial agents that have poor in vitro activity against the infecting organism were selected.
2. Active antimicrobials were not delivered to the site of infection because an inappropriate route of drug administration was selected, the wrong dosage was used, or abnormal pharmacokinetic variables in the patients went undetected.
3. The location of the infection (as in endocarditis) was inaccessible.
4. The host defenses were inadequate.
5. Infection was not treated for a sufficient period to prevent relapse.
6. Serious toxicity necessitated discontinuation of therapy.
7. Antimicrobial resistance by the infecting organism developed.
8. Superinfection occurred.
9. There is a foreign body or abscess.
10. The patient did not comply with the therapeutic regimen.

Much of the potential for failure of treatment can be obviated by basing the initial choice of antimicrobials on principles enumerated in the section on determinants of antimicrobial efficacy and by considering how host defenses can be altered in favor of eradication of the organism. Whenever host defense mechanisms are inadequate, the physician should try to choose antimicrobials that kill the infecting organism rather than merely inhibiting its growth. The high relapse rate (approximately 50%) seen when patients with endocarditis are treated with bacteriostatic rather than bactericidal drugs is ample testimony to this principle, as are the poor results from inappropriate use of bacteriostatic agents in patients with severe neutropenia.

## Mechanisms of Resistance to Antimicrobials

Organisms may develop resistance to antimicrobials in a number of different ways. Well-recognized mechanisms of bacterial resistance to antibiotics include enzymatic inhibition, changes in permeability in the outer and inner bacterial membranes, alterations in structure or production of new targets of the antimicrobials, promotion of efflux pump mechanisms, and selection of auxotrophs that escape drug effects (Moyer et al. 1990). Use of antimicrobials encourages the selection of resistant strains. Therefore, indiscriminate use of antimicrobials selects for resistance and promotes infection that will be even more difficult to eradicate with antimicrobials.

The more common mechanisms of resistance associated with failure of treatment are enzymatic inhibition, alteration in membrane permeability, and alteration in drug targets. The enzymes known as $\beta$-lactamases are commonly produced by a variety of bacteria. They are responsible for cleavage of the $\beta$-lactam ring, thereby destroying the ability of susceptible $\beta$-lactam antibiotics to bind to bacterial penicillin-binding proteins on the inner bacterial membrane (Medeiros 1984). Other microorganisms develop resistance to antimicrobials by restricting their entry into the interior of the microbial cell. This mechanism is illustrated by the intrinsic resistance of enterococci to aminoglycosides (Weinstein and Moellering 1973). This type of resistance can be overcome by combining aminoglycoside therapy with penicillin. The penicillin facilitates entry of the aminoglycoside into bacteria (Moellering et al. 1971). Bacteria may be drug-resistant because they modify the target site for antibiotic action or binding. For example, some enterococci resist the action of aminoglycosides at the ribosomal level, despite facilitated entry of the drug by penicillins.

Plasmid-bound antimicrobial resistance factors (R factors), possessed by aerobic gram-negative rods, are readily transmitted among various species of microorganisms within a hospital setting (McGowan 1983).

## Monitoring Results of Treatment

The success or failure of treatment should be carefully assessed. Useful endpoints to follow include the temperature curves, leukocyte counts, elevation of the erythrocyte sedimentation rate or C-reactive protein during chronic infections such as osteomyelitis, direct demonstration of the extent of tissue injury by radiography, abnormal elevations of concentrations of tissue-derived enzymes in the circulation, and many other tests. Bacteriologic cultures and serologic tests should be repeated periodically. The intervals at which such tests should be obtained depend on the type, the severity, the site of the infection, the typical course when treatment is successful, and the interval at which most relapses occur.

Failure of treatment of an infection can be defined as failure to produce a clinical remission of disease or as relapse of the infection once treatment is stopped. When treatment does fail, the physician must once again base rational therapy on general principles, including the following:

1. Reestablishing the microbial cause of infection and determining whether it is caused by the original or a new agent (superinfection)
2. Redetermining the in vitro sensitivity of the isolated organism to the antibiotics
3. Checking plasma concentration of antibiotics and their in vitro activity to determine whether they remain adequate in vivo, and to confirm that the patient is actually receiving the medication
4. Making certain that treatment failure is not due to a failure on the part of the physician to identify correctable host factors that contribute to infection (e.g., failure to drain abscesses, remove foreign bodies and necrotic tissues)
5. Excluding the possibility that persisting evidence of inflammation is not due to factors other than the infection (e.g., drug hypersensitivity) and phlebitis from IV catheters

## Inappropriate Uses of Antimicrobials

Errors in the treatment of infectious diseases fall into two major categories: omission, in which treatment is indicated but none is given, and commission, in which treatment is given but it is inadequate or inappropriate. From statistics on the use of antibiotics in the United States, it is clear that most errors are of commission (see Table 14-22).

**PRINCIPLE To maximize the benefit/risk ratio of prescribing, constantly reexamine your reasons for treatment and reevaluate your knowledge of the potential hazards of the prescribed drugs.**

**Table 14-22 Errors of Commission in Antimicrobial Therapy**

*Errors of Choice*

1. Treatment of viral infections with antibiotics
2. Treatment of fever with antimicrobials without clinical evidence and/or microbiologic data to indicate a microbial cause
3. Treatment of infections with drugs that are ineffective in vivo or cannot reach the site of infection
4. Treatment of infections with drugs that are effective in vitro but are not likely to be effective in vivo
5. Treatment with toxic drugs when less toxic drugs would suffice
6. Continued treatment of infections with broad-spectrum or potent antibiotics when a more specific, less-broad-spectrum antimicrobial agent would suffice
7. Treatment with expensive drugs when effective less-expensive drugs are available

*Errors in Administration of Antibiotics*

1. Wrong dose
2. Wrong route of administration
3. Inappropriate dosage interval
4. Failure to recognize toxicity
5. Failure to modify dosage when elimination pathways are impaired
6. Failure to obtain drug allergy history
7. Changing antibiotics without evidence of antimicrobial treatment failure
8. Changing antibiotics without correcting host factors that contribute to treatment failure (e.g., draining abscesses or débridement of necrotic tissues)

## MANAGEMENT OF SELECTED CLINICAL CONDITIONS

This section is devoted to topics that exemplify important considerations in treatment and prophylaxis with antibiotics. Overviews are provided by discussing selected clinical settings and the therapeutic issues they raise. These include rational therapy requiring interference at specific steps in microbial pathogenesis, problems associated with treatment of immunocompromised patients, understanding of pharmacologic features of antimicrobials in order to effect cure, understanding of the epidemiologic aspects of infectious disease, and rational preventive measures.

### Current Treatment of Human Immunodeficiency Virus

The discovery that the human immunodeficiency virus type 1 (HIV-1) is responsible for the epidemic of acquired immunodeficiency syndrome (AIDS) has resulted in an intensive search for compounds that have antiretroviral activity against HIV and those that can be effective immunoprophylactics. Understanding the pathogenesis of HIV has enabled investigators to isolate compounds that have stage-specific activity. A rational approach to antiretroviral therapy requires a basic understanding of the HIV replication cycle. In this section, the life cycle of HIV, our current clinical experience with agents that have direct antiviral activity against HIV, the effects of combinations, and potential efficacy are reviewed. Although recent estimates of the life span of HIV-1 raise the possibility of eradicating virus from an infected individual, currently there is no effective cure. Likewise, an effective vaccine has not yet been developed. Primary prevention through modification of behaviors that put individuals at risk of becoming infected is an important component of a long-term strategy to halt the HIV epidemic.

**PRINCIPLE Rational attempts to treat infection require a basic understanding of microbial pathogenesis.**

#### *Pathogenesis*

A number of steps in the replication of HIV are recognized that may be targets of drug therapy (see Fig. 14-1). Infection of a cell by an infectious virion begins with attachment of the virus particle to cell-surface receptors. The HIV, an RNA virus, attaches to cells by virtue of high-affinity binding of the virion envelope glycoprotein (gpl20) to the host cell-surface receptor glycoprotein (CD4). The CD4 receptors are found on certain subpopulations of T lymphocytes, monocytes, and other cells. Recent evidence has indicated that although CD4 is the primary receptor, other receptor molecules are also involved (Berger 1997). Two cofactors have been identified: "fusin," a receptor molecule that mediates binding to HIV-1 isolates with an affinity for T-cell lines (TCL-tropic) and CCR5, a cofactor for isolates with affinity for macrophages (M-tropic). Both fusin, renamed CXCR4, and CCR5 are chemokine receptors. Although identified in vitro, their in vivo importance remains to be defined. However, their identification suggests new possibilities for therapeutic and vaccine strategies.

After binding, the virion penetrates the cell membrane and loses its coat in the cytoplasm, exposing the genomic RNA. The viral RNA is reverse-transcribed to make DNA and a second complementary strand of DNA to form double-stranded DNA. This process is achieved by using the viral reverse transcriptase (RT) enzyme. Viral double-stranded DNA can remain in the cytoplasm as circular, unintegrated episomal DNA (extrachromosomal latency) or be transported to the nucleus, where a complete genomic copy of viral DNA is integrated into the host cell genome (latent infection). The exact mechanisms of latency and activation have yet to be clarified. Active (productive) infection involves transcription of mRNA from genomic viral DNA, which results in subsequent translation to yield viral structural or regulatory proteins and viral RNA that is packaged into infectious particles. Active infection may have no immediate cytopathic effects on the host cell (resulting in persistent infection) or may be associated with host cell death (as seen in acute infection) (Stevenson 1997). Posttranslational modification of viral proteins occurs later when the viral particles are assembled and released from the host cell.

Until recently it was believed that the asymptomatic phase of HIV infection was characterized by the majority of infected host cells harboring virus in a latent state, with only the acute viremia of primary infection and late stages of disease associated with the majority of infected cells having active virus replication. More recent studies indicate that the great majority of virus particles in plasma have a short half-life (6 hours) and come from newly infected cells with a half-life of 1.6 days (Perelson et al. 1997). Thus, there is continuous high-level viral replication ($10.3 \times 10^9$ virions/day) throughout the disease. This high rate of replication is an important factor in the development of drug resistance. The higher the rate of viral replication in general, the greater the chances of replication by multidrug-resistant mutants as well. Better understanding of the dynamics of HIV-1 and $CD4^+$ lympho-

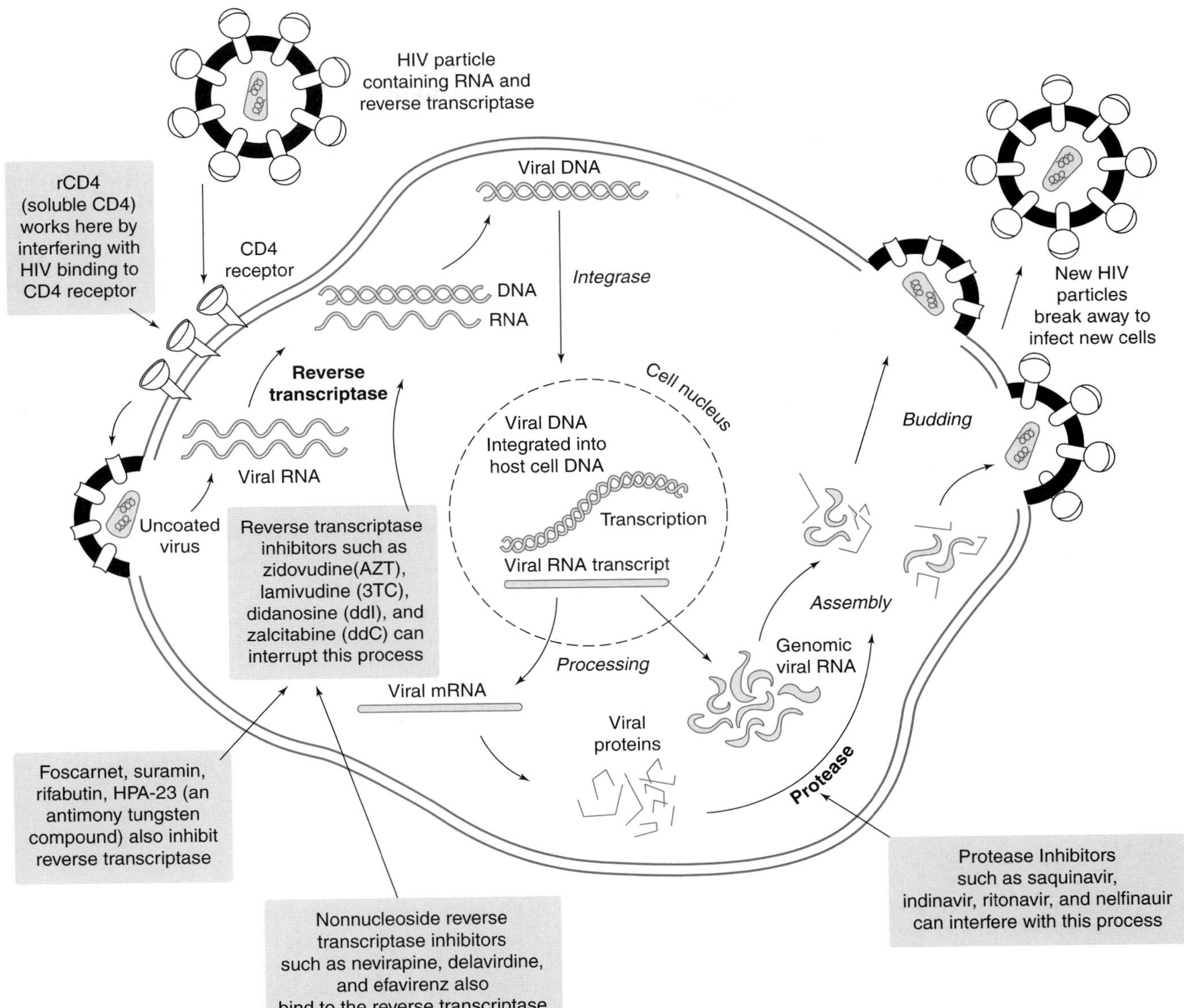


FIGURE 14-1 **Replication cycle of human immunodeficiency virus (HIV) and sites of action of various agents that have been or are being used to treat infection due to this virus.**

cytes has led to new treatment strategies for the management of HIV with, generally, earlier initiation of more potent drug regimes involving combination therapy.

Central nervous system involvement has been a well-recognized complication of HIV infection. Cells of the macrophage lineage (microglia, brain macrophages, and macrophage-derived multinucleated giant cells) are primarily affected (Gendelman et al. 1997). Cytokines produced from virus-infected macrophages probably play a significant role in pathogenesis. It is therefore important that antiretroviral treatments have the ability to penetrate into the CNS.

Following resolution of primary HIV infection, there is a long interval of clinical (although not virologic or immunologic) latency. Within 6 to 12 months of this infection, a viral "set-point" is established that is quite stable for each individual patient over weeks to months. Several studies have evaluated the relationship between the

HIV-1 viral load and disease progression and have found that levels are predictive of the likelihood of progression in infants, children, and adults (Mellors et al. 1995; Coombs et al. 1996; O'Brien et al. 1996; Welles et al. 1996; Bruisten et al. 1997; Shearer et al. 1997). Changes in viral load in response to therapy are also predictive of outcome (progression to AIDS or death) and explain a greater proportion of the treatment effect than do $CD4^+$ T-cell counts (Katzenstein et al. 1996; O'Brien et al. 1996). Commercial assays are now available to measure the amount of HIV-1 RNA in plasma. A fall in CD4 cells in peripheral blood has long been recognized as the hallmark of HIV-1 infection. CD4 count also represents a prognostic marker, although this marker is somewhat inferior to viral load. Thus, measurement of HIV-1 RNA (as a marker of viral replication) and CD4 count (as a marker of immunological function) have become standards of care for assessing response to therapy in individual patients and in clinical trials.

Principles of a rational approach to the treatment of patients with HIV infection are listed in Table 14-23.

### *Compounds inhibiting viral binding*

The HIV binds to susceptible cells by the viral gpl20–CD4 interaction. A number of strategies could be considered to inhibit this interaction. A soluble form of CD4 protein (rCD4) was synthesized using recombinant technology and found to inhibit HIV infection of T cells in vitro (Smith et al. 1987). In theory, infectious virions would bind to the soluble circulating CD4 protein, and fewer virions would remain to bind to and infect lymphocytes bearing CD4 receptors. Soluble CD4 perhaps also works by stripping gp120 from the viral membrane (Moore et al. 1990).

Phase I clinical trials of rCD4 demonstrated virtually no toxicity, except for the development of antibodies to CD4. However, clinical efficacy was modest with only a slight decrease in serum p24 antigen and no significant change in CD4 counts or immune function (Schooley et al. 1990). A later clinical trial found a decrease in viral titer with rCD4, but limitations noted were the need for intravenous administration, high doses of drug for antiviral activity, and a short drug half-life (Schacker et al.

**Table 14-23 Summary of the Principles of Therapy of HIV Infection**

1. Ongoing HIV replication leads to immune system damage and progression to AIDS. HIV infection is always harmful, and true long-term survival free of clinically significant immune dysfunction is unusual.
2. Plasma HIV RNA levels indicate the magnitude of HIV replication and its associated rate of $CD4^+$ T-cell destruction, whereas $CD4^+$ T-cell counts indicate the extent of HIV-induced immune damage already suffered. Regular, periodic measurement of plasma HIV RNA levels and $CD4^+$ T-cell counts is necessary to determine the risk for disease progression in an HIV-infected person and to determine when to initiate or modify antiretroviral treatment regimens.
3. As rates of disease progression differ among HIV-infected persons, treatment decisions should be individualized by level of risk indicated by plasma HIV RNA levels and $CD4^+$ T-cell counts.
4. The use of potent combination antiretroviral therapy to suppress HIV replication to below the levels of detection of sensitive plasma HIV RNA assays limits the potential for selection of antiretroviral-resistant HIV variants, the major factor limiting the ability of antiretroviral drugs to inhibit virus replication and to delay disease progression. Therefore, maximum achievable suppression of HIV replication should be the goal of therapy.
5. The most effective means to accomplish durable suppression of HIV replication is the simultaneous initiation of combinations of effective anti-HIV drugs with which the patient has not been previously treated and that are not cross-resistant with antiretroviral agents with which the patient has been treated previously.
6. Each of the antiretroviral drugs used in combination therapy regimens should always be used according to optimum schedules and dosages.
7. The available effective antiretroviral drugs are limited in number and mechanism of action, and cross-resistance between specific drugs has been documented. Therefore, any change in antiretroviral therapy increases future therapeutic constraints.
8. Women should receive optimal antiretroviral therapy regardless of pregnancy status.
9. The same principles of antiretroviral therapy apply to HIV-infected children, adolescents, and adults, although the treatment of HIV-infected children involves unique pharmacologic, virologic, and immunologic considerations.
10. Persons identified during acute primary HIV infection should be treated with combination antiretroviral therapy to suppress virus replication to levels below the limit of detection of sensitive plasma HIV RNA assays.
11. HIV-infected persons, even those whose viral loads are below detectable limits, should be considered infectious. Therefore, they should be counseled to avoid sexual and drug-use behaviors that are associated with either transmission or acquisition of HIV and other infectious pathogens.

From *Morbidity and Mortality Weekly Report* (CDC 1998a, b)

1994). Another limitation is the reduced susceptibility of clinical isolates of HIV (Daar et al. 1990). These concerns make administration of the soluble rCD4 form problematic on a large-scale basis, and administration of this agent has not yet found a role in the therapeutic armamentarium.

Construction of a hybrid CD4 protein that combines the amino-terminal binding site of CD4 and the Fc portion of IgG heavy chain yields a protein with a longer half-life. This CD4–Ig complex was also found to have in vitro activity against HIV (Capon et al. 1989), and clinical trials have been ongoing. Another approach that has shown anti-HIV activity in vitro has been to combine CD4 with cellular toxins such as ricin or *Pseudomonas* exotoxin (Chaudhary et al. 1988; Till et al. 1988). Theoretically and in in vitro experiments, these hybrid CD4 proteins can bind to cells expressing viral gp120 on their surface (virally infected cells) and selectively kill these cells by virtue of the incorporated cellular toxin. However, phase I trials demonstrated dose-limiting hepatotoxicity, which may prove to limit the clinical usefulness of this approach (Johnston and Hoth 1993).

A number of other agents appear to interfere with the in vitro binding of HIV to host cells, including dextran sulfate, pentosan polysulfate, peptide T, and AL721. A small trial of low doses of dextran sulfate did not show any clinical efficacy (Abrams et al. 1989). Possibly, insufficient drug was orally bioavailable under these conditions (Lorentsen et al. 1989). Peptide T, an octapeptide with four threonine residues, has in vitro activity in blocking HIV binding to susceptible cells (Pert et al. 1986). No trials have been published showing benefit of peptide T in the treatment of HIV infection. The compound AL721 is a combination of neutral glycerides, phosphatidylcholine, and phosphatidylethanolamine in a molar ratio of 7:2:1 that inhibits HIV infection in vitro. Its mechanism may be that it alters the lipids and cholesterol of cellular membranes, thereby inhibiting HIV penetration into susceptible host cells (Sarin et al. 1985). Two small studies showed no clinical or laboratory evidence of benefit (Peters et al. 1990; Mildvan et al. 1989), and this compound has fallen out of favor as a treatment (Abrams 1990).

**PRINCIPLE Despite the devastation caused by a disease such as HIV infection and the desperation it evokes in patients and their caregivers, it is always prudent to have a great deal of skepticism for claims of drug efficacy based on in vitro data alone. Only the clinical studies that follow in vitro findings can define clinical efficacy and toxicity.**

### *Inhibition of reverse transcription*

NUCLEOSIDE ANALOGS Nucleoside analog reverse transcriptase inhibitors have formed the backbone of anti-HIV therapy for the last decade (see Table 14-24). Reverse transcription is necessary for HIV RNA to be used as a template to produce viral DNA, which can be integrated into the cellular genome. In order for reverse transcription to take place, deoxynucleotide must be added to the end of the elongating DNA. A 3′-hydroxyl group is present on the sugar moiety of deoxynucleotides that can form a 3′,5′-phosphodiester bond allowing further addition of nucleotide triphosphates. Several deoxynucleotide analogs have been synthesized that differ from normal deoxynucleotides in that the 3′-hydroxyl group of the sugar moiety (deoxyribose) has been replaced with another molecule (e.g., an azido group in the case of azidothymidine [AZT]). These substitutions do not allow addition of further nucleotides in the process of chain elongation. In order for nucleoside analogs to exert their effect, they must be converted to their active triphosphate nucleotides by cellular kinases.

Zidovudine (AZT), a 3′-azidothymidine derivative, was the first drug to receive FDA approval for the treatment of HIV. Originally synthesized in the early 1960s, it was found to have in vitro anti-HIV activity in 1985 (Mitsuya et al. 1985). It has good CNS penetration. A number of studies have evaluated the efficacy of AZT. In brief, they demonstrate 1) prolonged survival in patients with AIDS and AIDS-related complex (ARC), 2) equal efficacy of a large dose (1200 to 1500 mg/day) versus half that dose (500 to 600 mg/day), 3) decreased toxicity in patients receiving half-dose AZT, and 4) clinical improvement in children with symptomatic HIV infection (Fischl, Richman, Geico et al. 1987; Pizzo et al. 1988; Fischl, Richman, Hansen, et al. 1990; McKinney et al. 1991).

The benefit of AZT in the treatment of patients with CD4 counts between 0.20 and 0.50 $\times$ $10^9$/L was less clear, with some studies demonstrating slowed progression to AIDS (Fischl et al. 1990; Volberding et al. 1990), whereas other studies showed no long-term progression or survival benefit (Sande et al. 1993; Concorde Coordinating Committee 1994a). Trials have not shown a treatment benefit in individuals with CD4 counts >0.5 $\times$ $10^9$/L (Volberding et al. 1990; Concorde Coordinating Committee 1994a). Studies have since clearly demonstrated better outcomes with combination therapies including zidovudine as compared to zidovudine monotherapy (Delta Coordinating Committee 1996; Hammer et al. 1996). The role for zidovudine is currently as part of a combination

Table 14-24 Characteristics of Nucleoside Reverse Transcriptase Inhibitors

| CHARACTERISTIC | ZIDOVUDINE (AZT, ZDV) RETROVIR | DIDANOSINE (DDL) VIDEX | ZALCITABINE (DDC) HIVID | STAVUDINE (D4T) ZERIT | LAMIVUDINE (3TC) EPIVIR | ABACAVIR ZIAGEN |
|---|---|---|---|---|---|---|
| Dosing recommendations | 200 mg tid or 300 mg bid or with 3TC as Combivir, 1 bid | Tablets >60 kg: 200 mg bid <60 kg: 125 mg bid | 0.75 mg bid | >60 kg: 40 mg bid <60 kg: 30 mg bid | 150 mg bid <50 kg: 2 mg/kg bid | 300 mg q 12 h |
| Oral bioavailability | 60% | Tablet: 40%; Powder: 30% | 85% | 86% | 86% | 83% |
| Serum half-life | 1.1 h | 1.6 h | 1.2 h | 1.0 h | 3–6 h | 1.5 h |
| Intracellular half-life | 3 h | 25–40 h | 3 h | 3.5 h | 12 h | 3.3 h |
| Elimination | Metabolized to AZT glucuronide (GAZT). Renal excretion of GAZT. | Renal excretion 50% | Renal excretion 70% | Renal excretion 50% | Renal excretion unchanged | Hepatic glucuronidation and carboxylation |
| Adverse events | Bone marrow suppression: anemia and/or neutropenia. Subjective complaints: GI intolerance, headache, insomnia, asthenia. | Pancreatitis; peripheral neuropathy; nausea; diarrhea | Peripheral neuropathy; stomatitis | Peripheral neuropathy | (Minimal toxicity) | Hypersensitivity reaction |
| Cost[a] ($/month) | Retrovir $286 | Videx $178 | HIVID $207 | Zerit $233 | Epivir $230 | |

[a]Source of drug costs (average wholesale prices) is *Mosby's GenR$_x$* 1998. Current prices may vary from those quoted, but comparative prices among products are expected to be similar. The reader should check on local prices at the time of prescribing.

SOURCE: *Morbidity and Mortality Weekly Report* (CDC 1998a, b).

regime. AZT alone reduces the rate of vertical transmission of HIV (from mother to child) during pregnancy (Connor et al. 1994). The major adverse reaction associated with AZT administration is bone marrow toxicity that usually appears 4 to 12 weeks after initiating therapy and is more common in patients taking higher doses and with more advanced disease (Roch et al. 1992).

Dideoxycytidine (ddC), a pyrimidine analog also known as zalcitabine, is the most potent of this group of drugs in vitro (Yarchoan et al. 1991). Early data showed that patients who had not previously received antiretroviral therapy did more poorly on initial ddC than on initial zidovudine (Hirsch and D'Aquila 1993). Most trials, however, have focused on the use of ddC in combination therapy, where benefit has been shown as compared to zidovudine monotherapy in antiretroviral naive patients (Delta 1996; Hammer et al. 1996). The major toxicity of ddC is a painful peripheral neuropathy that is dose dependent and cumulative. It is generally slowly reversible once the drug is withdrawn. Other toxicities include oral aphthous ulcers and pancreatitis.

Dideoxyinosine (ddI) or didanosine is a purine analog. The acid instability of ddI requires that the oral form be buffered for optimal intestinal absorption; ddI was initially approved for use in patients with advanced HIV who were intolerant of or resistant to AZT. As with ddC, its greatest potential seems to be as part of a combination regime (Delta Coordinating Committee 1996; Hammer et al. 1996). The drug has also been shown to have benefit in children, either alone or in combination with zidovudine (Butler et al. 1996; England et al. 1997). The major dose-limiting toxicity with ddI appears to be peripheral neuropathy, usually less severe than that seen with ddC. The most serious toxicity is acute pancreatitis, which is dose related and uncommonly seen in patients receiving less than 750 mg/day. Alcohol use should be avoided and other drugs associated with pancreatitis used with caution. Diarrhea is a common adverse effect.

Stavudine (d4T), another pyrimidine analog, has in vitro activity similar to AZT's. It has good oral bioavailability and crosses the blood–brain barrier. In combination with other antiretrovirals, it too has good antiretroviral effect (Rouleau et al. 1997). The most frequent toxicity observed with d4T is peripheral neuropathy. It is a dose-limiting adverse effect, and its occurrence is associated with a prior history of neuropathy or the presence of neurologic symptoms (Browne et al. 1993). The symptoms usually resolve when d4t is promptly stopped, and some patients are able to tolerate its reintroduction at a lower dose.

Lamivudine, the (–) enantiomer of 2′-deoxy-3′-thiacytidine (3TC) also has in vitro activity against HIV-1, including zidovudine-resistant strains. It has high oral bioavailability and is well tolerated. Studies have shown that combination treatment with 3TC and AZT is well tolerated and associated with greater improvement in CD4 counts and viral load than monotherapy (Eron et al. 1995; Staszewski et al. 1996). It has been widely studied as part of combination therapy with protease inhibitors.

Abacavir, a potent nucleoside analog in vitro, is the newest NRTI (Table 14-24). Hypersensitivity reactions characterized by fever and rash have been treatment-limiting adverse effects.

**NONNUCLEOSIDE REVERSE TRANSCRIPTASE INHIBITORS** This group of agents (NNRTIs), first described in 1990, acts by binding to the reverse transcriptase enzyme at a location below the catalytic site, resulting in its inactivation (see Table 14-25). These drugs, unlike the nucleoside analogs, do not require phosphorylation to become active. They are highly selective against HIV-1 and very potent in vitro. Their major drawback is the rapidity with which resistance (that is considered cross-resistance for all NNRTIs) occurs. A major advantage of two agents in this class is the ability to prescribe once daily dosing. Several studies with NNRTIs have been completed. Although surrogate marker benefit has been shown when used in combination regimes, none of the studies have yet demonstrated an effect on disease progression. They have been generally well tolerated, the major problem being the rash associated with two of them.

Nevirapine was the first of the NNRTIs to be licensed. It is synergistic in vitro with zidovudine, either alone or with a second nucleoside analog (Richman et al. 1991; Merrill et al. 1996). It has high CNS penetration, and excellent oral bioavailability (Miller et al. 1997). Nevirapine induces its own metabolism, and so its dose must be increased after 14 days to its maintenance level. It can reduce indinavir concentrations, but this does not appear to be clinically significant (Murphy et al. 1997). Clinical studies indicate that nevirapine is most active when used in combination with two nucleoside analogs in antiretroviral naive patients (D'Aquila et al. 1996; Myers et al. 1996; Pollard et al. 1996). The major toxicity is a maculopapular rash that usually occurs within the first 6 weeks of treatment and is usually mild and self-limited.

Delavirdine, the second NNRTI to be approved, is also metabolized by the cytochrome P450 3A family. Un-

Table 14-25 **Nonnucleoside Reverse Transcriptase Inhibitors**

| Characteristic | Nevirapine Viramune | Delaviride Rescriptor | Efavirenz Sustiva |
|---|---|---|---|
| Form | 200-mg tabs | 100-mg tabs | 200-mg capsules |
| Dosing recommendations | 200 mg PO daily × 14 days, then 200 mg PO bid | 400 mg PO tid (four 100-mg tabs in ≥3 oz. water to produce slurry) | 200 mg PO tid |
| Oral bioavailability | >90% | 85% | |
| Serum half-life | 25–30 h | 5.8 h | 40–52 h |
| Elimination | Metabolized by cytochrome P450; 80% excreted in urine (glucuronidated metabolites, <5% unchanged); 10% in feces | Metabolized by cytochrome P450; 51% excreted in urine (<5% unchanged); 44% in feces | Metabolized by cytochrome P450 |
| Drug interactions | Induces cytochrome P450 enzymes<br>• The following drugs have suspected interactions that require careful monitoring if coadministered with nevirapine: rifampin, rifabutin, oral contraceptives, protease inhibitors, triazolam and midazolam | Inhibits cytochrome P450 enzymes<br>• Not recommended for concurrent use: terfenadine, astemizole, alprazolam, midazolam, cisapride, rifabutin, rifampin, triazolam, ergot derivatives, amphetamines, nifedipine, anticonvulsants (phenytoin, carbamazepine, phenobarbital).<br>• Delavirdine increases levels of clarithromycin, dapsone, quinidine, warfarin, indinavir, saquinavir.<br>• Antacids and didanosine: separate administration by ≥1 h | Inhibits cytochrome P450 enzymes<br>• Contraindicated drugs, terfenadine, astemizole, cisapride, triazolam, midazolam.<br>• Efavirenz decreases the concentration of indinavir by 30–50%; clarithromycin by 38% |
| Adverse events | Rash; increased transaminase levels; hepatitis | Rash; headaches | Rash; headache; dizziness |
| Cost[a] | Viramune $248 | Rescriptor NA | Sustiva NA |

[a]Source of drug costs (average wholesale prices) is *Mosby's GenR$_x$* 1998. Current prices may vary from those quoted, but comparative prices among products are expected to be similar. The reader should check on local prices at the time of prescribing. NA, not applicable.
SOURCE: Modified from *Morbidity and Mortality Weekly Report* (CDC 1998a, b).

like nevirapine, it reduces enzyme activity in this system and therefore inhibits its own metabolism (Miller et al. 1997). The potential for drug interactions must therefore be kept in mind. There are not yet sufficient data regarding the safety of combining it with protease inhibitors. It has good oral bioavailability but poor CNS penetration and must be taken three times daily (Miller et al. 1997). As observed for nevirapine, rash is the most common adverse effect. Clinical trials have not shown a clinical benefit to the use of delavirdine in combination with AZT or ddI, although improvement in surrogate markers was seen (Freimuth et al. 1996). Its ultimate role in therapy remains to be determined.

Three other NNRTIs are in various stages of development. Loviride's clinical benefits have been small, and at this point there are no plans to market this drug. Efavirenz (DMP 266) is a very potent NNRTI with a long half-life, which allows once-daily dosing and good CNS penetration. It too induces the hepatic cytochrome P450 system with the potential for drug interactions. Clinical studies are under way (Murphy 1997). There are thus far insufficient data to comment on the potential for quinoxaline (HBY 097).

#### OTHER INHIBITORS OF REVERSE TRANSCRIPTASE

Other inhibitors of reverse transcriptase include phosphonoformate (foscarnet), suramin, heteropolymer-23 (HPA-23), and rifabutin. Foscarnet is an analog of pyrophosphate. In vitro studies have shown its inhibitory activity against viral DNA polymerase from cytomegalovirus (CMV) and reverse transcriptase from HIV. In clinical trials, foscarnet was well tolerated and decreased p24 antigenemia (Bergdahl et al. 1988). However, only an IV preparation is available, which makes long-term administration for HIV impractical. Suramin, which has been used as an antiparasitic agent, was fortuitously found to inhibit HIV reverse transcriptase in vitro. However, clinical trials could not demonstrate any clinical or virologic improvement (Cheson et al. 1987). Additional compounds with in vitro inhibitory activity that have been clinically tested but have not been found to have clear antiviral efficacy include HPA-23 (Moskovitz et al. 1988), a compound containing antimony and tungsten, and the antimycobacterial agent rifabutin (Torseth et al. 1989).

***Late-stage inhibition***

A number of agents interfere with late-life-cycle states of HIV. These include antisense molecules, ribavirin, $\alpha$-interferon (IFN-$\alpha$), and glucosidase inhibitors. Antisense oligonucleotides are short synthetic sequences of DNA that are complementary to viral RNA sequences. They can bind to viral RNA and can inhibit translation and production of protein. These oligonucleotides can pass through cell membranes and, when modified by the addition of phosphoramidates or phosphorothioates, can resist destruction by host cellular nuclease (Montefiori and Mitchell 1987; Agrawal et al. 1988). These oligonucleotides have also been shown to be competitive inhibitors of HIV reverse transcriptase (Liu and Owens 1987). However, a number of technical problems need to be resolved before clinical trials with these agents can be undertaken (Yarchoan et al. 1991).

Ribavirin, a guanosine analog, has demonstrated some anti-HIV effect in vitro, perhaps by inhibiting the guanylation step required for 5′ capping of viral RNA. Results of clinical trials with this agent have not demonstrated any antiviral efficacy (Spector et al. 1989).

$\alpha$-Interferon, a protein produced by virally infected leukocytes, has anti-HIV activity in vitro (Ho et al. 1985). The exact mechanism of its activity has not been elucidated; however, IFN-$\alpha$ may block final HIV assembly and budding of mature viral particles at the cell surface. It may also have a role in inhibiting protein translation. Clinical trials of IFN-$\alpha$ in HIV-infected patients primarily have involved treatment of Kaposi's sarcoma. Although there is evidence that IFN-$\alpha$ can reduce p24 antigenemia (Lane et al. 1990) and that synergy with AZT exists in vitro (Hartshorn et al. 1987), clinical trials have not shown clinical benefits above that related to the concomitant use of AZT (Berglund et al. 1991; Edlin et al. 1992).

Before viral assembly and release, many viral proteins must be glycosylated. However, more sugars are added than are necessary, and some must be removed before release. Cellular glycosidases, primarily $\alpha$-glycosidase 1, are responsible for cleaving the terminal sugars on the HIV envelope glycoprotein before its release. Compounds such as castanospermine and $\eta$-butyldeoxynojirimycin ($\eta$-butyl DNJ) are cellular glucosidase inhibitors that have demonstrated antiviral activity in vitro (Gruters et al. 1987; Walker et al. 1987). To date, no clinical trials have been published showing efficacy.

***Protease inhibitors***

Development of the protease inhibitors (PIs) has revolutionized the treatment of HIV. These very powerful agents have been associated with impressive improvements in immunological function and decreases in plasma viral load, and their use has contributed to better understanding of the pathogenesis of HIV. The HIV protease enzyme is critical for the posttranslational processing of the polyprotein products into core proteins and viral enzymes of the infectious virion. Inhibition of the protease results in the release of a noninfectious and immature viral particle (Kohl et al. 1988). Four protease inhibitors are currently licensed for use. All show substantial in vitro activity against both HIV-1 and HIV-2 and a wide therapeutic index. They are metabolized by the hepatic cytochrome P450 (CYP) system with variable ability to induce or inhibit the enzyme. Thus, the potential for drug interactions, especially with ritonavir, must be considered. Studies have shown the importance of adequate drug levels to maintain viral suppression, suggesting that adherence to the prescribed regimen is crucial to long-term benefit. None of them should be used as monotherapy. Finally, although short-term studies have been impressive, the longer-term efficacy of these drugs is not yet known. One complication that became apparent with increased clinical use was the occurrence of spontaneous bleeding episodes in HIV-infected hemophiliacs who were treated with these agents. Other important new adverse effects are the induction of glucose intolerance, redistribution of body fat giving rise to a buffalo hump and a "big belly."

Saquinavir, the first of the PIs, has poor bioavailability and undergoes extensive hepatic metabolism. To improve its absorption, it is taken with a meal with a high fat content and with grapefruit juice (to inhibit CYP 3A). A new soft-gel formulation has been introduced as a means of improving bioavailability. It is very well tolerated, the major adverse effects being GI and usually mild. There have been two large trials examining the use of saquinavir. In one, a combination of AZT, ddC, and saquinavir had quite modest benefit compared with combinations of AZT and ddC or AZT and saquinavir (Collier et al. 1996). Although the second study documented benefit of saquinavir plus ddC compared with either drug alone, the comparative treatments do not represent the standard of care (Lalezari et al. 1996).

Ritonavir has the advantage of twice daily dosing, but the disadvantage of requiring storage in a refrigerator and away from direct light. Another major disadvantage is the number of potential drug interactions with ritonavir related to its effect on the cytochrome P450 system. Ritonavir has been the PI with the least tolerability. GI adverse effects are common even with dose escalation. Clinical studies have shown both surrogate marker (Danner et al. 1995; Markowitz et al. 1995) and clinical benefit with ritonavir, with delayed disease progression and reduced mortality in patients with advanced disease (Cameron et al. 1996).

Indinavir is quite well tolerated, the most important adverse reaction being nephrolithiasis. Patients should drink at least 1.5 L of fluid throughout the day to prevent this problem. It too is metabolized by and interacts with the cytochrome P450 system; so the potential for a variety of drug toxicities must be considered when patients are taking other medications in addition to indinavir. It is taken on an empty stomach for optimal absorption and should be taken regularly (every eight hours) around the clock to maintain constant therapeutic plasma concentrations. Recent trials have shown immunological and virological benefits of indinavir when used with AZT and 3TC in patients with prior antiretroviral therapy (Gulick et al. 1997) and slowed progression of disease in previously treated patients with CD4 counts $\leq$200 cells per cubic millimeter (Hammer et al. 1997). Its role in treating patients at earlier stages of disease has not been defined in clinical trials.

Nelfinavir is given three times daily with food. The main adverse effect is diarrhea. It inhibits cytochrome P450 (though to a lesser extent than ritonavir doses) and hence drug interactions may be problematic.

The newest protease inhibitor is Aprenavir. It has a serum half-life of 9 hours. It is eliminated through the hepatic cytochrome P450 system. The dosage is 1200 mg q 12 h. Nausea and vomiting are the main adverse reactions. The major features of the protease inhibitors are summarized in Tables 14-26 through 14-29.

### *Antiretroviral resistance*

The problem of drug resistance was noted early in the history of HIV treatment and has been observed for the three classes of drugs in clinical use. Loss of antiretroviral effect with a variety of antiretroviral agents has been reported to coincide with the appearance of viral mutants with reduced drug sensitivity (Moyle 1996). There is increasing evidence that drug resistance is associated with risk of disease progression, but it is not clear whether this represents cause or effect. The occurrence of cross-resistance may impact on effectiveness of later treatments and must be considered when initiating and changing therapies. Zidovudine resistance does not appear to affect susceptibility to ddI, ddC, or 3TC, but d4T cross-resistance has been reported (Rooke et al. 1991). ddI and ddC are cross-resistant with each other and have partial cross-resistance with 3TC. Resistance to lamivudine occurs rapidly through a single mutation conferring high-level resistance to it and partial cross-resistance with ddC and ddI. There appears to be partial cross-resistance to ddC, ddI, and AZT in d4T-resistant mutants (Moyle 1996). There is no cross-resistance between nucleoside analogs and NNRTIs.

High-level resistance develops rapidly to the NNRTIs and is associated with considerable cross-resistance to other NNRTIs (Miller et al. 1997). For this reason, it is recommended that the NNRTIs be used only in combinations anticipated to greatly reduce the viral load.

Development of resistant mutants has been seen with saquinavir, ritonavir, indinavir, and nelfinavir and is reduced by combination with at least one nucleoside analog. Indinavir resistance is associated with saquinavir and ritonavir cross-resistance and ritonavir-resistance with indinavir and nelfinavir cross-resistance; saquinavir resistance appears to develop more slowly, and saquinavir recently has been reported cross-resistant to the other PIs (Moyle 1996; Moyle et al. 1996; Deeks et al. 1997). Continued study will provide more data on resistance and cross-resistance patterns and how to sequence therapies to avoid and anticipate problems with cross-resistance.

### *Guidelines for the use of antiviral agents in HIV infection*

The treatment of HIV infection has changed dramatically over the last decade. These changes have come about as a result of a better understanding of the pathogenesis of infection and of the pharmacokinetics and resistance patterns of the available drugs. No doubt management will continue to evolve as new information becomes available.

The new combination therapies look very promising in early trials. Theoretically, combination therapy for HIV could exert enhanced activity by affecting different stages of viral replication. Also, if the drugs had different toxicities, it might be possible to use lower doses of each individual compound while maintaining antiviral activity. Synergism has been noted, in vitro and in vivo, for a number of different combinations of antiretrovirals. Additionally, several clinical trials have demonstrated improved clinical and/or surrogate marker outcomes of

Table 14-26 Characteristics of Protease Inhibitors

| Characteristic | Indinavir Crixivan | Ritonavir Norvir | Saquinavir Invirase | Saquinavir Fortovase | Nelfinavir Viracept | Aprenavir Agenerase |
|---|---|---|---|---|---|---|
| Form | 200-, 400-mg caps | 100-mg caps 600 mg/7.5 ml PO solution | 200-mg caps | 200-mg caps | 250-mg tablets 50-mg/g oral powder | 50 mg, 150 mg capsules |
| Dosing recommendations | 800 mg q8h Take 1 h before or 2 h after meals; may take with skim milk or low-fat meal. | 600 mg ql2h[a] Take with food if possible. | 600 mg tid[a] Take with large meal. | 1,200 mg tid Take with large meal. | 750 mg tid Take with food (meal or light snack). | 1200 mg q 12 h |
| Oral bioavailability | 65% | (Not determined) | Hard-gel capsule: 4%, erratic | soft-gel capsule (not determined) | 20% to 80% | |
| Serum half-life | 1.5–2 h | 3–5 h | 1–2 h | 1–2 h | 3.5–5 h | 9 h |
| Routes of metabolism | CYP 3A4 | CYP3A4>CYP2D6 | CYP3A4 | CYP3A4 | CYP3A4 | CYP450 |
| Storage | Room temperature | Refrigerate capsules; refrigeration for oral solution is preferred but not required if used within 30 days. | Room temperature | Refrigerate or store at room temperature (up to 3 mos.) | Room temperature | |
| Drug interactions | Inhibits cytochrome P450 (less than ritonavir). Contraindicated for concurrent use: terfenadine, astemizole, cisapride, triazolam, midazolam, ergot alkaloids. Indinavir levels increased by ketoconazole,[c] delavirdine. Indinavir levels reduced by: rifampin, grapefruit juice, nevirapine. Didanosine reduces indinavir taken ≥2 hrs apart. Not recommended for concurrent use: rifampin. | Inhibits cytochrome P450 (potent inhibitor). Ritonavir increases level of multiple drugs that are not recommended for concurrent use.[b] Didanosine; may cause reduced absorption of both drugs; should be taken ≥2 hours apart. Ritonavir increases levels of clarithromycin and desipramine. | Inhibits cytochrome P450. Saquinavir levels increased by ritonavir, ketoconazole, grapefruit juice, nelfinavir, delavirdine. Saquinavir levels reduced by rifampin, rifabutin, and possibly the following: phenobarbital, phenytoin, dexamethasone and carbamazepine, nevirapine. Contraindicated for concurrent use: terfenadine, astemizole, cisapride, ergot alkaloids, triazolam and midazolam. | Inhibits cytochrome P450. Saquinavir levels increased by ritonavir, ketoconazole, grapefruit juice, nelfinavir, delavirdine. Saquinavir levels reduced by rifampin, rifabutin, and possibly the following: phenobarbital, phenytoin, dexamethasone and carbamazepine, nevirapine. Contraindicated for concurrent use: terfenadine, astemizole, cisapride, ergot alkaloids, triazolam and midazolam. | Inhibits cytochrome P450. (less than ritonavir). (Nelfinavir levels reduced by rifampin, rifabutin. Contraindicated for concurrent use: triazolam, midazolam, ergot alkaloid, terfenadine, astemizole, cisapride. Nelfinavir decreases levels of ethinyl estradiol and norethindrone. Nelfinavir increases levels of rifabutin, saquinavir, and indinavir. Not recommended for concurrent use: rifampin. | |

**Table 14-26 Characteristics of Protease Inhibitors (Continued)**

| Characteristic | Indinavir Crixivan | Ritonavir Norvir | Invirase | Saquinavir Fortovase | Nelfinavir Viracept | Aprenavir Agenerase |
|---|---|---|---|---|---|---|
| Adverse effects | Nephrolithiasis. GI intolerance, nausea. Lab: increased indirect bilirubinemia (inconsequential). Miscellaneous: headache, asthenia, blurred vision, dizziness, rash, metallic taste, thrombocytopenia. Hyperglycemia.[d] | GI intolerance, nausea, vomiting, diarrhea. Paresthesias (circumoral and extremities). Hepatitis. Asthenia. Taste perversion. Lab: Triglycerides increase >200%, transaminase elevation, elevated CPK and uric acid. Hyperglycemia.[d] | GI intolerance, nausea and diarrhea. Headache. Elevated transaminase enzymes. Hyperglycemia.[d] | GI intolerance, nausea, diarrhea, abdominal pain and dyspepsia. Headache. Elevated transaminase enzymes. Hyperglycemia.[d] | Diarrhea. Hyperglycemia.[d] | Headache, GI complaints, rash. |
| Cost ($/month) | Crixivan | Norvir | Invirase | Fortovase | Viracept | |

[a]Dose escalation for ritonavir: Day 1–2: 300 mg bid; day 3–5: 400 mg bid; day 6–13: 500 mg bid; day 14: 600 mg bid. Combination treatment regimen with saquinavir (400–600 mg PO bid) plus ritonavir (400–600 mg PO bid).

[b]Drugs contraindicated for concurrent use with ritonavir: amiodarone (Cordarone), astemizole (Hismanal), bepridil (Vascor), bupropion (Wellbutrin), cisapride (Propulsid), clorazepate (Tranxene), clozapine (Clozaril), diazepam (Valium), encainide (Enkaid), estazolam (PromSom), flecainide (Tambocor), flurazepam (Dalmane), meperidine (Demerol), midazolam (Versed), piroxicam (Feldene), propoxyphene (Darvon), propafenone (Rythmol), quinidine, rifabutin, terfenadine (Seldane), triazolam (Halcion), zolpidem (Ambien), ergot alkaloids.

[c]Decrease indinavir to 600 mg q8h.

[d]Cases of new onset hyperglycemia have been reported in association with the use of all protease inhibitors.

ABBREVIATIONS: CYP, cytochrome P450.

SOURCE: From *Morbidity and Mortality Weekly Report* (CDC 1998a, b).

Table 14-27 **Drugs That Should Not Be Used with Protease Inhibitors**

| DRUG CATEGORY | INDINAVIR | RITONAVIR[a] | SAQUINAVIR[b] | NELFINAVIR | ALTERNATIVES |
|---|---|---|---|---|---|
| Analgesics | (none) | Meperidine, piroxicam, propoxyphene | (none) | (none) | ASA, oxycodone acetaminophen |
| Cardiac | (none) | Amiodarone, encainide, flecainide, propafenone | (none) | (none) | Limited experience |
| Antimycobaterial | Rifampin | Rifabutin[b] | Rifampin, rifabutin | Rifampin | For rifabutin (as alternative for MAI treatment): clarithromycin, ethambutol HCl (treatment, not prophylaxis), or azithromycin |
| Calcium channel blocker | (none) | Bepridil | (none) | (none) | Limited experience |
| Antihistamine | Astemizole, terfenadine | Astemizole, terfenadine | Astemizole, terfenadine | Astemizole, terfenadine | Loratadine |
| Gastrointestinal | Cisapride | Cisapride | Cisapride | Cisapride | Limited experience |
| Antidepressant | (none) | Bupropion | (none) | (none) | Fluoxetine, desipramine |
| Neuroleptic | (none) | Clozapine, pimozide | (none) | (none) | Limited experience |
| Psychotropic | Midazolam, triazolam | Clorazepate, diazepam, estazolam, flurazepam, midazolam, triazolam, zolpidem | Midazolam, triazolam | Midazolam, triazolam | Temazepam, lorazepam |
| Ergot alkaloid (vasoconstrictor) | | Dihydroergotamine (DHE 45), ergotamine[c] (various forms) | | Dihydroergotamine (DHE 45), ergotamine[c] (various forms) | |

[a]The contraindicated drugs listed are based on theoretical considerations. Thus, drugs with low therapeutic indices yet with suspected major metabolic contribution from cytochrome P450 CYP3A, CYP2D6, or unknown pathways are included in this table. Actual interactions may or may not occur in patients.
[b]Saquinavir given as Invirase or Fortovase.
[c]Reduce rifabutin dose to one-fourth of the standard dose.
SOURCE: From *Morbidity and Mortality Weekly Report* (CDC 1998a, b).

combination therapy as compared with monotherapy. Combinations of antiretroviral therapy have thus become standard for anti-HIV treatment. Commonly used combinations to treat HIV infections, as well as combinations to avoid, are given in Table 14-30.

**PRINCIPLE Key issues to be considered in relation to anti-HIV treatment are**

- **Even the clinically latent phase of HIV infection is marked by intense viral replication.**
- **The relation between prognosis and viral load has been demonstrated.**
- **Beneficial effects on immunological and virologic markers are seen with therapy.**
- **The development of resistance has been documented for all classes of agents in use.**
- **Cross-resistance within groups is common.**

Therapy is recommended for individuals symptomatic with HIV with $CD4^+$ T-cell counts <500 cells/mm$^3$ (Carpenter et al. 1996) or with a viral load ≥10,000 HIV RNA copies/mL (Carpenter et al. 1997) (see Table 14-30).

Changes in therapy may be required primarily for three reasons: treatment failure, drug intolerance, or nonadherence. Treatment failure is generally recognized by return to pretreatment levels of viral load and CD and clinical progression. Appearance of any degree of viremia, however, may be a marker of treatment failure if it had previously been undetectable. Treatment failure usually poses more of a therapeutic challenge than does toxicity. Factors to be considered in choosing an alternate regimen are: prior treatments (with cross-resistance implications),

Table 14-28 **Drug Interactions between Protease Inhibitors and Other Drugs; Drug Interactions Requiring Dose Modifications**

| Drug or Class | Indinavir | Ritonavir | Saquinavir[a] | Nelfinavir |
|---|---|---|---|---|
| Fluconazole | No dose change | No dose change | No data | No dose change |
| Ketoconazole and itraconazole | Decrease dose to 600 mg q8h | Increases ketoconazole >3-fold; dose adjustment required | Increases saquinavir levels 3-fold; no dose change[b] | No dose change |
| Rifabutin | Reduce rifabutin to one-half dose: 150 mg daily | Consider alternative drug or reduce dose to one fourth of standard dose | Not recommended with either Invirase Fortovase | Reduce rifabutin to one half dose: 150 mg daily |
| Rifampin | Contraindicated | Unknown[c] | Not recommended with either Invirase Fortovase | Contraindicated |
| Oral contraceptives | Modest increase in Ortho-Novum levels; no dose change | Ethinyl estradiol levels decreased; use alternative or additional contraceptive method | No data | Ethinyl estradiol and norethindrone levels decreased; use alternative or additional contraceptive method |
| Miscellaneous | Grapefruit juice reduces indinavir levels by 26% | Desipramine HCl increased 145%: reduce dose; theophylline levels decreased: increase dose | Grapefruit juice increases saquinavir levels[b] | |

[a]Several drug interaction studies have completed with saquinavir given as Invirase or Fortovase. Results from studies conducted with Invirase may not be applicable to Fortovase.
[b]Conducted with Invirase.
[c]Rifampin reduces ritonavir 35%. Increased ritonavir dose or use of ritonavir in combination therapy is strongly recommended. The effect of ritonavir on rifampin is unknown. Used concurrently, increased liver toxicity may occur. Therefore, patients taking ritonavir and rifampin should be monitored closely.
SOURCE: From *Morbidity and Mortality Weekly Report* (CDC 1998a, b).

currently available drugs, previous toxicities, stage of disease, concomitant medication (potential for drug interactions), and reason for making the change (toxicity, adherence or failure). In patients who experience treatment failure, generally the most potent available regime is recommended with a change in at least two, and preferably three, drugs. Table 14-31 gives guidelines for changing an antiretroviral regimen for suspected drug failure, and Table 14-32 gives a number of possible regimens for patients who have failed antiretroviral therapy. The use of more intensive antiretroviral therapies has resulted in a decline in HIV-related mortality from 29.4 per 100 person-years in 1995 to 8.8 per 100 person-years in the second quarter of 1997 (Palella et al. 1998).

The one clinical trial evaluating antiretroviral therapy of primary HIV showed that zidovudine slowed clinical progression (Kinloch-de Lods et al. 1995). Currently, it is recommended that combination therapy be used in treating primary HIV: at least 2 nucleoside analogs with the addition of a PI or NNRTI considered (Carpenter et al. 1996).

***Treatment of human immunodeficiency virus infection in pregnancy***

Just over 2 million of the 5.2 million (40%) adults newly infected with HIV in 1997 were women, most of whom were of childbearing age. It is estimated that 1.1 million children worldwide are living with AIDS, 90% of whom have acquired the infection through vertical transmission (CDC 1995).

Vertical transmission of HIV can occur in utero, intrapartum, or through postpartum breast feeding. Although HIV transmission can occur to the fetus as early as the eighth week of gestation (Ferrus et al. 1990), 50 to 70% of vertical transmission occurs just before or during parturition (Boyer et al. 1994).

Use of AZT during pregnancy can reduce transmission from mother to child. The AIDS Clinical Trials Protocol 076 was a randomized, multicenter double-blind, placebo-controlled trial in which HIV-infected AZT-naive pregnant women, between 14 and 34 weeks of gestation, with CD4 counts ≥200 cells/mm$^3$ were randomly assigned to receive placebo or AZT 100 mg orally 5 times

Table 14-29 **Drug Interactions: Protease Inhibitors and Nonnucleoside Reverse Transcriptase Inhibitors—Effect of Drug on Levels and Dose**

| Drug Affected | Indinavir | Ritonavir | Saquinavir[a] | Nelfinavir | Nevirapine | Delaviridine |
|---|---|---|---|---|---|---|
| Indinavir (IDV) | — | No data | Levels: IDV no effect; SQV ↑4–7×[b] Dose: no data | Levels: IDV ↑50% NFV ↑80% Dose: no data | Levels: IDV ↑28% Dose: standard | Levels: IDV ↑40% Dose: IDV 600 mg q8h |
| Ritonavir (RTV) | No data | — | Levels: RTV no effect; SQV ↑20×↑[b] Dose: Invirase or Fortovase 200 mg bid + RTV: 400 mg bid | Levels: RTV no effect; NFV ↑1.5× Dose: no data | Levels: RTV ↓11% Dose: standard | Levels: RTV ↑70% Dose: no data |
| Saquinavir (SQV) | Levels: SQV ↑4–7×; IDV no effect[b] Dose: no data | Levels: SQV ↑20×↑[b] RTV no effect Dose: Invirase or Fortovase 400 mg bid + RTV 400 mg bid | — | Levels: SQV ↑3–5×; NFV ↑20%[b] Dose: standard NFV Fortovase 800 mg tid | Levels: SQV ↓25%[c] Dose: no data | Levels: SQV ↑5×;[c] Dose: standard for Invirase Monitor transaminase levels |
| Nelfinavir (NFV) | Levels: NFV ↑80% IDV ↑50% Dose: no data | Levels: NFV ↑1.5×; RTV no effect Dose: no data | Levels: NFV ↑20%;[b] SQV ↑3–5× Dose: standard NFV Fortovase 800 mg tid | — | Levels NFV ↑10% Dose: standard | Levels: NFV ↑2× PDLV ↓50% Dose: standard (monitor for neutropenic complications) |
| Nevirapine (NVP) | Levels: IDV ↓28% Dose: standard | Levels: RTV ↓11% Dose: standard | Levels: SQV ↓25%[c] Dose: no data | Levels NFV ↑10% Dose: standard | — | Do not use together |
| Delavirdine (DLV) | Levels: IDV ↑40% Dose: IDV 600 mg q8h | Levels: RTV ↑70% Dose: no data | Levels: SQV ↑5×[c] Dose: standard for Invirase Monitor transaminase levels | Levels: NFV ↑2× DLV ↓50% Dose: standard (monitor for neutropenic complications) | Do not use together | — |

[a]Several drug interaction studies have been completed with saquinavir given as Invirase or Fortovase. Results from studies conducted with Invirase may not be applicable to Fortovase.
[b]Conducted with Fortovase.
[c]Conducted with Invirase.
Levels of Evidence are noted as, e.g., AI, AII, BIII, etc. The grades are as follows: Level I—Evidence—well-conducted randomized controlled trial(s). Level II—Well-designed controlled trials without randomization (including cohort and case control studies). Level III—Expert opinion, case study, reports of expert committees. The letters A through E reflect the strength of each recommendation, thus: A—good evidence to support a recommendation for use. B—moderate evidence to support a recommendation for use. C—poor evidence to support a recommendation for use. D—moderate evidence to support a recommendation against use. E—good evidence to support a recommendation against use. This system allows the reader to easily determine the strength of the recommendation. For example, a recommendation that is graded as IA is the strongest possible recommendation—it is based on evidence from randomized control trials and there is good evidence to support a recommendation for use.
SOURCE: From *Morbidity and Mortality Weekly Report* (CDC 1998a, b).

per day from enrollment until labor. AZT was given intravenously during labor in a dose of 1 mg/kg per hour (a 2 mg/kg loading dose was administered over 1 hour) until delivery. The baby was given 2 mg/kg of AZT syrup every 6 hours for 6 weeks beginning 8 to 12 hours after birth (Connor et al. 1994). In this study the rate of vertical transmission of HIV was reduced from 25.5% in the placebo group to 8.3% in the AZT group (Connor et al. 1994). Follow-up to 5 years of age showed no toxicity in the treated infants, and the rate of congenital anomalies was equal in the treated and placebo groups. The efficacy of AZT in reducing vertical transmission has been shown

**Table 14-30 Recommended Antiretroviral Agents for Treatment of Established HIV Infection**

| | |
|---|---|
| **Preferred:** Strong evidence of clinical benefit and/or sustained suppression of plasma viral load. One choice each from column A and column B. Drugs are listed in random, not priority, order: | |
| **Column A** | **Column B** |
| Indinavir (AI) | ZDV + ddI (AI) |
| Nelfinavir (AII) | d4T + ddI (AII) |
| Ritonavir (AI) | ZDV + ddC (AI) |
| Saquinavir-SGC[a] (AII) | ZDV + 3TC[b] (AI) |
| Ritonavir + Saquinavir-SGC or HGC[c] (BII) | d4T + 3TC[b] (AII) |
| **Alternative:** Less likely to provide sustained virus suppression; | |
| 1 NNRTI (Nevirapine)[d] + 2 NRTIs (Column B, above) (BII) | |
| Saquinavir-HGC + 2 NRTIs (Column B, above) (BI) | |
| **Not generally recommended:** Strong evidence of clinical benefit, but initial virus suppression is not sustained in most patients | |
| 2 NRTIs (Column B, above) (CI) | |
| **Not recommended:**[e] Evidence against use, virologically undesirable, or overlapping toxicities | |
| All monotherapies (DI) | |
| d4T + ZDV (DI) | |
| ddC + ddI[f] (DII) | |
| ddC + d4T[f] (DII) | |
| ddC + 3TC (DII) | |

[a]Virologic data and clinical experience with saquinavir-SGC are limited in comparison with other protease inhibitors.
[b]Use of ritonavir 400 mg bid with saquinavir soft-gel formulation (Fortovase) 400 mg bid results in similar areas under the curve (AUC) of drug and antiretroviral activity as when using 400 mg bid of Invirase in combination with ritonavir. However, this combination with Fortovase has not been extensively studied and gastrointestinal toxicity may be greater when using Fortovase.
[c]High-level resistance to 3TC develops within 2–4 wk. in partially suppressive regimens; optimal use is in three-drug antiretroviral combinations that reduce viral load to <500 copies/mL.
[d]The only combination of 2 NRTIs + 1 NNRTI that has been shown to suppress viremia to undetectable levels in the majority of patients is ZDV + ddI + Nevirapine. This combination was studied in antiretroviral-naive persons.
[e]ZDV monotherapy may be considered for prophylactic use in pregnant women who have low viral load and high CD4$^+$ T-cell counts to prevent perinatal transmission.
[f]This combination of NRTIs is not recommended based on lack of clinical data using the combination and/or overlapping toxicities.
ABBREVIATIONS: 3TC, lamivudine; d4T, stavudine; ddC, zalcitabine; ddI, didanosine; NNRTI, nonnucleoside reverse transcriptase inhibitors; NRTI, nucleoside reverse transcriptase inhibitors; ZDV, zidovudine (AZT).
SOURCE: From *Morbidity and Mortality Weekly Report* (CDC 1998a, b).

regardless of maternal CD4 count, duration of rupture of membranes, mode of delivery or gestational age (Cooper et al. 1996; Fiscus et al. 1996).

Currently combination therapy with antiretrovirals that have good placental passage (AZT, 3TC, d4T, nevirapine) is recommended. There are a number of trials planned or ongoing to evaluate the safety and efficacy of combination regimens under a variety of circumstances and in a broader spectrum of pregnant patients. Table 14-33 summarizes current data regarding the use of antiretrovirals during pregnancy. Some questions to be answered are whether shorter regimens may be equally effective and what treatments are best for women who have received prior antiretroviral treatment (Newell et al. 1997).

### *Cesarean section*

A meta-analysis that included data on 8533 mother-child pairs has shown that elective cesarean section decreased the likelihood of vertical transmission of HIV-1 by 50% as compared with other modes of delivery (The International Perinatal HIV Group 1999). Use of antiretroviral therapy during prenatal, intrapartum, and neonatal periods along with elective cesarean section reduced the likelihood of transmission by 87% (The International Perinatal HIV Group 1999).

### *Postexposure prophylaxis*

Occupational injuries involving percutaneous exposure to an HIV-infected source have a 0.3% risk of HIV transmission (Tokars et al. 1993). A retrospective study found that increased risk of transmission was positively related to deep injury, visible blood on sharp device, device used to enter a blood vessel, and source patient having terminal AIDS. Risk of infection was reduced by the prophylactic use of zidovudine (CDC 1995). Current guidelines for occupational prophylaxis of HIV include a combination of two or three drugs, depending on the type of exposure and source. It is recommended that treatment be started within hours, and the standard duration is 4 weeks (CDC 1996). Each institution should develop its own postexposure prophylaxis protocol based on the current recommendations.

**Table 14-31 Guidelines for Changing an Antiretroviral Regimen for Suspected Drug Failure**

- Criteria for changing therapy include a suboptimal reduction in plasma viremia after initiation of therapy, reappearance of viremia after suppression to undetectable, substantial increases in plasma viremia from the nadir of suppression, and declining $CD4^+$ T-cell numbers.
- When the decision to change therapy is based on viral load determination, it is preferable to confirm with a second viral load test.
- Distinguish between the need to change a regimen because of drug intolerance or inability to comply with the regimen versus failure to achieve the goal of sustained viral suppression; single agents can be changed or dose reduced in the event of drug intolerance.
- In general, do not change a single drug or add a single drug to a failing regimen; it is important to use at least two new drugs and preferably to use an entirely new regimen with at least three new drugs.
- Many patients have limited options for new regimens of desired potency; in some of these cases, it is rational to continue the prior regimen if partial viral suppression was achieved.
- In some cases, regimens identified as suboptimal for initial therapy are rational due to limitations imposed by toxicity, intolerance, or nonadherence. This especially applies in late-stage disease. For patients with no rational alternative options who have virologic failure with return of viral load to baseline (pretreatment levels) and a declining $CD4^+$ T-cell count, discontinuation of antiretroviral therapy should be considered.
- Experience is limited with regimens using combinations of two protease inhibitors or combinations of protease inhibitors with nevirapine or delavirdine; for patients with limited options due to drug intolerance or suspected resistance, these regimens provide possible alternative treatment options.
- There is limited information about the value of restarting a drug that the patient has previously received. The experience with zidovudine is that resistant strains are often replaced with "wild-type" zidovudine sensitive strains when zidovudine treatment is stopped, but resistance recurs rapidly if zidovudine is restarted. Although preliminary evidence indicates that this occurs with indinavir, it is not known if similar problems apply to other nucleoside analogs, protease inhibitors, or NNRTIs, but a conservative stance is that they probably do.
- Avoid changing from ritonavir to indinavir or vice versa for drug failure, because high-level cross-resistance is likely.
- Avoid changing from nevirapine to delavirdine or vice versa for drug failure, because high-level cross-resistance is likely.
- The decision to change therapy and the choice of a new regimen require that the clinician have considerable expertise in the care of persons living with HIV infection. Physicians who are less experienced in the care of persons with HIV infection are strongly encouraged to obtain assistance through consultation with or referral to a clinician who has considerable expertise in the care of HIV-infected patients.

SOURCE: From *Morbidity and Mortality Weekly Report* (CDC 1998a, b).

**Table 14-32 Possible Regimens for Patients Who Have Failed Antiretroviral Therapy: A Work in Progress[a]**

| PRIOR REGIMEN | NEW REGIMEN (NOT LISTED IN PRIORITY ORDER) |
|---|---|
| 2 NRTIs + | 2 new NRTIs + |
| Nelfinavir (NFV) | RTV; or IDV; or SQV + RTV; or NNRTI[b] + RTV; or NNRTI + IDV[c] |
| Ritonavir (RTV) | SQV + RTV;[c] NFV + NNRTI; or NFV + SQV |
| Indinavir (IDV) | SQV + RTV; NFV + NNRTI; or NFV + SQV |
| Saquinavir (SQV) | RTV + SQV; or NNRTI + IDV |
| 2 NRTIs + NNRTI | 2 new NRTIs + a protease inhibitor |
| 2 NRTIs | 2 new NRTIs + a protease inhibitor 2 new NRTIs + RTV + SQV 1 new NRTI + 1 NNRTI + a protease inhibitor 2 protease inhibitors + NNRTI |
| 1 NRTI | 2 new NRTIs + a protease inhibitor 2 new NRTIs + NNRTI 1 new NRTI + 1 NNRTI + a protease inhibitor |

[a]These alternative regimens have not been proven to be clinically effective and were arrived at through discussion by the panel of theoretically possible alternative treatments and the elimination of those alternatives with evidence of being ineffective. Clinical trials in this area are urgently needed.

[b]Of the two available NNRTIs, clinical trials support a preference for nevirapine over delavirdine based on results of viral load assays. These two agents have opposite effects on the CYP450 pathway, and this must be considered in combining these drugs with other agents.

[c]There are some clinical trials that have yielded viral burden data to support this recommendation.

Abbreviations not in table: NNRTI, nonnucleoside reverse transcriptase inhibitor; NRTI, nucleoside reverse transcriptase inhibitor.

SOURCE: From *Morbidity and Mortality Weekly Report* (CDC 1998a, b).

**Table 14-33 Preclinical and Clinical Data Relevant to Use of Antiretrovirals during Pregnancy**

| ANTIRETROVIRAL DRUG | FDA-DEFINED PREGNANCY CATEGORY[a] | PLACENTAL PASSAGE [NEWBORN: MATERNAL DRUG] | LONG-TERM ANIMAL CARCINOGENICITY STUDIES | RODENT TERATOGEN |
|---|---|---|---|---|
| Zidovudine[b] | C | Yes (human) [0.85] | Positive (rodent, vaginal tumors) | Positive (near-lethal dose) |
| Zalcitabine | C | Yes (rhesus) [0.30–0.50] | Positive (rodent, thymic lymphomas) | Positive (hydrocephalus at high dose) |
| Didanosine | B | Yes (human) [0.5] | Negative (no tumors, lifetime rodent study) | Negative |
| Stavudine | C | Yes (rhesus) [0.76] | Not completed | Negative (but sternal bone calcium decreases) |
| Lamivudine | C | Yes (human) [~1.0] | Negative (no tumors, lifetime rodent study) | Negative |
| Saquinavir | B | Unknown | Not completed | Negative |
| Indinavir | C | Yes (rats) ("Significant" in rats; low in rabbits) | Not completed | Negative (but extra ribs in rats) |
| Ritonavir | B | Yes (rats) [mid-term fetus, 1.15; late-term fetus, 0.15–0.64] | Not completed Negative (but cryptorchidism in rats)[c] | |
| Nelfinavir | B | Unknown | Not completed | Negative |
| Nevirapine | C | Yes (human) [~1.0] | Not completed | Negative |
| Delavirdine | C | Yes (rats) [late-term fetus, blood, 0.15; late-term fetus, liver 0.04] | Not completed | Ventricular septal defect |

[a]Food and Drug Administration-defined pregnancy categories are as follows:

A = Adequate and well-controlled studies of pregnant women fail to demonstrate a risk to the fetus during the first trimester of pregnancy (and there is no evidence of risk during later trimesters).

B = Animal reproduction studies fail to demonstrate a risk to the fetus, and adequate but well-controlled studies of pregnant women have not been conducted.

C = Safety in human pregnancy has not been determined, animal studies are either positive for fetal risk or have not been conducted, and the drug should not be used unless the potential benefit outweighs the potential risk to the fetus.

D = Positive evidence of human fetal risk based on adverse reaction data from investigational or marketing experiences, but the potential benefits from the use of the drug in pregnant women may be acceptable despite its potential risks.

X = Studies in animals or reports of adverse reactions have indicated that the risk associated with the use of the drug for pregnant women clearly outweighs any possible benefit.

[b]Despite certain animal data indicating potential teratogenicity of ZDV when near-lethal doses are given to pregnant rodents, considerable human data are available to date indicating that the risk to the fetus, if any, is extremely small when given to the pregnant mother beyond 14 weeks' gestation. Follow-up for up to age 6 years for 734 infants born to HIV-infected women who had in utero exposure to ZDV has not demonstrated any tumor development. However, no data are available with longer follow-up to evaluate for late effects.

[c]These are effects seen only at maternally toxic doses.

SOURCE: From *Morbidity and Mortality Weekly Report* (CDC 1998a).

No recommendations have been published on the use of postexposure prophylaxis in nonoccupational situations (e.g., after sexual and drug-use exposures). However, some physicians are recommending postexposure prophylaxis after unprotected receptive and insertive anal and vaginal intercourse with a partner who is or is likely to be HIV infected (Katz and Gerberding 1998). Prophylaxis is also offered for receptive fellatio with ejaculation. Currently treating only isolated exposures or exposures in a patient who is willing to practice safer behaviors in the future is suggested (Katz and Gerberding 1998). A recent report from CDC (CDC 1998b) defines principles of therapy of HIV infection and gives guidelines for the use of antiretroviral agents in HIV-infected adults and adolescents.

### *Immunomodulation*

HIV infection is associated with many alterations in immune function (Kelleher et al. 1997). These include the well-recognized decrease in $CD4^+$ T cells as well as altered $CD4^+$ lymphocyte function. There is an initial increase in $CD8^+$ lymphocyte numbers and $CD8^+$ cell activation. Changes are also seen in lymphocyte proliferation, IL-2 and IFN-$\gamma$ production, and macrophage and dendritic cell function. Thus, immune reconstitution is an important component of anti-HIV management.

In addition to specific agents targeted against HIV, attempts have been made to either restore or augment the host's immune function. IL-2 is a glycoprotein product of T cells. Production of this cytokine results in proliferation of circulating T cells and activation of natural killer (NK) cells. IL-2 has been shown to produce increases in $CD4^+$ T-cell counts (Kovacs et al. 1995). Other limitations of IL-2 are the need for intravenous or subcutaneous infusions and considerable adverse effects. Its role in treatment regimens has yet to be determined.

Administration of intravenous immunoglobulin has resulted in some reduction in bacterial infections in HIV-infected children (most of whom were also receiving prophylactic antibiotics) but no improvement in mortality (Mofeson et al. 1994). No clear-cut benefit has been shown for use of intravenous immunoglobulin in HIV-infected adults (Kiehl et al. 1996). However, increases are short-lived when treatment is stopped (Wood et al. 1993).

Isoprinosine, an immune enhancer, has some mild intrinsic antiviral activity. However, in vitro data have shown that it increases T-cell proliferation and IL-2 production (Fischbach and Talal 1985). An earlier clinical trial demonstrated delayed progression to AIDS in a select patient population, but it has not been studied further and is not licensed for use as a treatment for HIV infection (Pedersen et al. 1990).

Pentoxifylline, a TNF-$\alpha$ inhibitor, has not been shown to have an effect on CD4 counts (Degube et al. 1995). Studies are under way to evaluate the impact of thalidomide as an immunomodulator.

Bone marrow transplantation was reported to be effective in one patient who had received concomitant AZT (Holland et al. 1989). However, the patient developed a malignancy and died a short time after the transplant. Furthermore, the results of bone marrow transplantation on a small series indicate that it is not effective for curing AIDS (Lane et al. 1990).

***Vaccine strategies***

For many viruses, administration of a vaccine has resulted in effective active immunity in the host against the specific viral agent. Given the extent of the HIV epidemic and, for most infected persons, the prohibitive cost of therapy, prevention and eradication through immunization represents the ultimate goal. To date, this has not been easily achievable. HIV has presented complicated problems in vaccine development including the following: the genetic variability of the virus, incomplete knowledge concerning the immunological correlates of protection, phenotypic differences between viruses that may be associated with different immune responses and mechanisms of transmission, and inability to extrapolate results of animal vaccine experiments to humans (Excler and Plotkin 1997).

Most of the early efforts at developing a vaccine involved preparations of envelope gp120 or gp160 subunits, either recombinant, native, or synthetic proteins. These vaccines induced neutralizing antibodies but no cytotoxic T-lymphocyte response. In addition, it was found that these antibodies did not work as well against primary human isolates as they did against laboratory isolates, which obviously do not represent the major circulating strains. On the other hand, later vaccine experiments of recombinant live vectors expressing the HIV-1 envelope gp160 induced good CTL responses but poor neutralizing-antibody response (Excler and Plotkin 1997). There is good evidence that CTLs have a major role to play in control of HIV infection (Gotch et al. 1997), and it is likely that both humoral and cell-mediated immune responses play a significant role in protection and control of early infection (Burton and Montefiori 1997; Hu and Noffby 1997). Vaccine development will have to build on this concept. The 1990s saw loss of interest in vaccine approaches. However, improved understanding of HIV pathogenesis has opened up new areas of experimentation, which will likely lead to testing of new candidate vaccines within the next decade.

## Prevention of Opportunistic Infections in Persons Infected with Human Immunodeficiency Virus

Tables A-1 and A-2 (see Appendix, page 1341) give the current recommendations for prevention of opportunistic infections in those who are infected with HIV.

***New information on management of HIV infection and its complications***

Since new data are constantly emerging on the management of HIV infection, this chapter can only serve as a basis for building an understanding of the principles of therapy of HIV infection. The most up-to-date information should be obtained from the AIDS Treatment Information Service at *www.hivatis.org*.

## Management of the Febrile Neutropenic Patient

Consideration of treatment of the febrile neutropenic patient includes a brief summary of risk factors, organisms responsible for the disease, workup and management of a patient with respect to antimicrobial therapy, and immunoenhancement. Many clinical disease entities can cause a spectrum of immune suppression, and solid and hematologic tumors vary with respect to the degree of immune suppression they produce.

### *Risk factors for infection*

Neutropenia is defined as an absolute neutrophil count (ANC) that is less than 1000 cells/mm$^3$. As the count falls below 1000 cells/mm$^3$, the risk of infection increases (Bodey et al. 1966). Although the degree and rate of fall of neutropenia are important determinants of infection, the duration of profound neutropenia (ANC of <100 cells/mm$^3$) directly predicts the development of infection. Development of infection approaches 100% if profound neutropenia persists for 3 weeks or longer (Bodey et al. 1978). Initial induction of antitumor therapy produces a period of prolonged neutropenia and subjects the patient to the greatest risk of infection. If an infection develops, its successful outcome is determined in large part by recovery of the neutrophil count, as well as the choice of antimicrobials. In addition to purely quantitative decreases, neutrophils may have qualitative defects that impair their function. The latter may be the result of premature release of the cells from the marrow secondary to invasion of the marrow by tumor, or intrinsic killing defects caused by cytotoxic agents, irradiation, or antimicrobial therapy.

A number of cell lines can be markedly affected by the same insults. Profound lymphopenia results in decreased cell- and antibody-mediated immunity. Other important risk factors for development of infection include the following: disruption of the skin and mucosal barriers secondary to the effects of chemotherapeutic agents or malnutrition; splenectomy; alteration of endogenous microbial flora secondary to antimicrobial prophylaxis or colonization with nosocomial-acquired organisms, the presence of an indwelling catheter; and exposure to health care workers, air, water, food, and supportive equipment found in the hospital (e.g., ventilators, etc.).

### *Organisms causing infection*

The types of organisms causing infection in neutropenic patients with leukemia have changed over time, largely because of antimicrobial prophylaxis and therapy. Before such therapy, the predominant organisms that caused infections were aerobic gram-positive bacteria (e.g., frequently *S. aureus*). With the introduction of effective antistaphylococcal penicillins and cephalosporins and their regular use as empiric therapy in neutropenic patients, the incidence of gram-positive bacterial infections was reduced. However, an increase in gram-negative bacterial infections was subsequently noted, caused by *E. coli, Pseudomonas aeruginosa*, and *Klebsiella* species. Because of the high mortality associated with infection caused by these organisms, early intervention with broad-spectrum antibacterial agents at the first sign of fever became routine. This practice has greatly improved survival and has led to a decrease in mortality rates for infections caused by these organisms.

Most recently, gram-positive bacterial organisms including *S. aureus* and *S. epidermidis*, viridans streptococci, *Corynebacterium jeikeium* and *Enterococcus* species have again become major pathogens (O'Hanley et al. 1989). This change occurred primarily because of the placement of indwelling IV catheters (Press et al. 1984). In addition, antimicrobial prophylaxis and the reduction in use of specific antistaphylococcal agents as first-line therapy may also have contributed to the change. Fungal organisms such as *Candida* species and *Aspergillus* species have emerged as significant pathogens as well.

Organisms that cause infection in these patients can come from a newly acquired nosocomial pathogen, the patient's endogenous flora, or reactivation of latent organisms such as herpes viruses. The majority of organisms found to cause infection in neutropenic patients were from the patient's flora that had been modified by antibiotic treatment (Schimpff et al. 1972).

Although some generalizations can be made with respect to which organisms cause infections in neutropenic patients, the clinician should learn about the specific flora found in a given hospital, the organisms that are most frequently isolated from febrile neutropenic patients in that hospital, and the antimicrobial sensitivity and resistance patterns of these organisms.

**PRINCIPLE Empirical treatment of immunocompromised patients requires that the practitioner know the local epidemiology of infectious diseases, their complications, and the susceptibility patterns for nosocomial pathogens.**

### *Investigation and empirical treatment*

A temperature of more than 100°F (38°C) is usually defined as a medically important fever, and when observed in neutropenic patients should signal a search for infection. Because of the neutropenia, an inflammatory response may not be evident, and fever may be the only clue that infection is present. Infected neutropenic patients with lung infections may have normal chest x-rays, and they may not be able to produce purulent sputum. Infected skin may not show signs of cellulitis or abscess. A careful physical examination can help to define a source of infection. Particular attention should be paid to the ocular fundi and mucocutaneous sites such as the nasooropharynx and perirectal areas—common sites that can reveal evidence of infection. In most patients no obvious source of infection is evident. Therefore appropriate cultures of blood, urine, skin lesions, throat, sputum, or CSF must be obtained. Radiologic examination of the chest, sinuses, and teeth may be helpful in defining a site of infection. Unless the physical examination or x-ray films reveal a specific site of infection to guide specific antimicrobial therapy, the initiation of empirical broad-spectrum antimicrobial therapy must be instituted (Young 1981). Our approach to the management of the febrile neutropenic patient is given in Fig. 14-2.

Many studies have examined the effects of single-agent versus combination therapy as empirical regimens to treat the febrile neutropenic patient. These studies have provided information on when to initiate therapy for gram-positive bacterial organisms and fungal agents, how to modify therapy and its duration, and how to treat the persistently febrile patient. Broad-spectrum combination therapy that includes an antipseudomonal $\beta$-lactam antibiotic (e.g., mezlocillin, piperacillin, or ceftazidime) and an aminoglycoside (e.g., gentamicin, or tobramycin) is recommended by many investigators. Because gram-negative bacterial organisms such as *Pseudomonas* species can be associated with rapid mortality, a potentially synergistic combination regimen is attractive. Such combinations provide broader empirical coverage than does therapy with only one agent. Gram-negative coverage and moderate gram-positive coverage are usually required.

The choice of which agents to use depends on the most common pathogens and their patterns of antimicrobial resistance in a given hospital. Aminoglycosides have the potential disadvantage of causing nephrotoxicity and ototoxicity, and concentrations in plasma must be monitored. Aminoglycosides should not be used as monotherapy because of insufficient efficacy (Bodey 1984). Initial empirical monotherapy with agents such as imipenem, ceftazidime, or ticarcillin-clavulanic acid produces adequate efficacy without the toxicities associated with aminoglycosides (Hughes et al. 1990). Interpreting the results of these studies is not simple because "adequate clinical response" may not be defined and certainly is different between studies (e.g., some focus on overall clinical outcome or death versus survival, whereas others note the development of an infection or the necessity to change or add an antimicrobial agent as failure). In many of these studies, no organism was identified, with response defined as resolution of fever.

A major issue in empirical regimens involves the addition of an agent to specifically provide coverage for gram-positive cocci, especially staphylococci. Although many infections in neutropenic patients are caused by gram-positive organisms, the morbidity and mortality of infection with these organisms is markedly less than those of infections caused by gram-negative bacilli. A retrospective review concluded that the addition of vancomycin as an initial empirical agent is not necessary. Although more gram-positive infections were noted in the group of patients who did not receive vancomycin initially, successful treatment of documented infections caused by gram-positive organisms was not different whether vancomycin was instituted initially or delayed (Rubin et al. 1988). However, if the febrile episode appears to be the result of an infectious focus with gram-positive organisms (e.g., an infected indwelling IV catheter), then the early empirical use of vancomycin would seem prudent and warranted.

Most investigators agree that since the majority of infections found initially in the febrile neutropenic patient are bacterial, the early use of antifungal agents is not warranted. Most patients respond to empirical antibacterial therapy within a week. By this time several issues may have become clear. The infecting organism may be identified; the neutrophil count may begin to rise; the organism may be identified but the infection may fail to respond; a site of infection may be identified but no organism is identified; or no site of infection may be identified or organism isolated and the patient may still be febrile, possibly indicating fungal infection. If no source or organism is identified, it appears prudent to withhold antifungal treatment until 5 to 7 days of empirical antibacterial therapy have been completed, because some patients may have bacterial infections that are slow to respond to treatment (Hughes et al. 1990).

Fungal infections are extremely difficult to diagnose, but initiation of empirical therapy may prevent dissemination. Once the decision is made to initiate empirical antifungal therapy, amphotericin B is usually chosen.

The duration of therapy is a matter of some controversy. Some investigators believe that empirical antifungal therapy should be continued until neutropenia resolves. Others continue antifungal therapy based on the clinical response. If a fungal source is identified, a standard course

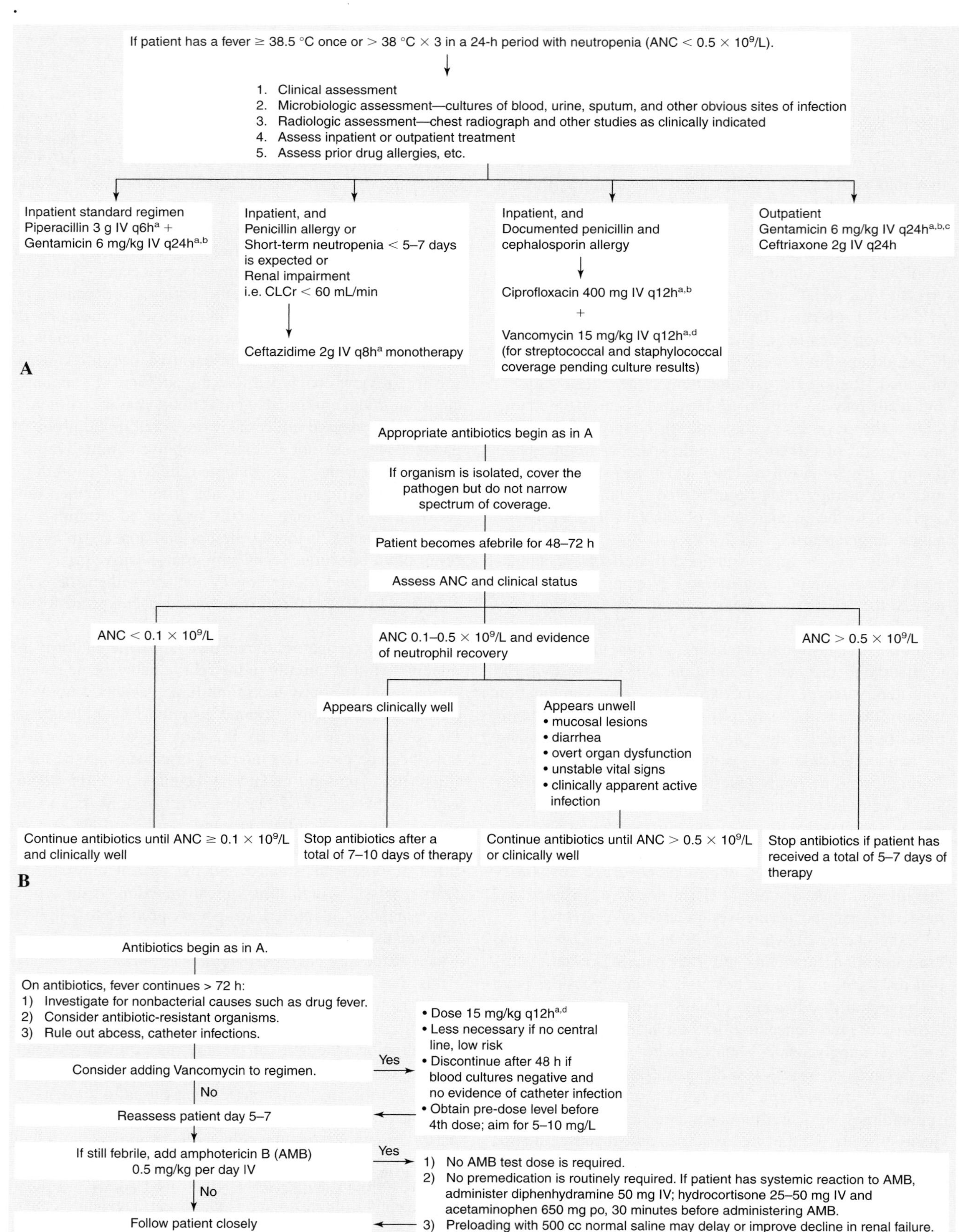

If patient has a fever ≥ 38.5 °C once or > 38 °C × 3 in a 24-h period with neutropenia (ANC < 0.5 × 10⁹/L).
1. Clinical assessment
2. Microbiologic assessment—cultures of blood, urine, sputum, and other obvious sites of infection
3. Radiologic assessment—chest radiograph and other studies as clinically indicated
4. Assess inpatient or outpatient treatment
5. Assess prior drug allergies, etc.
Inpatient standard regimen Piperacillin 3 g IV q6h[a] + Gentamicin 6 mg/kg IV q24h[a,b]
Inpatient, and Penicillin allergy or Short-term neutropenia < 5–7 days is expected or Renal impairment i.e. CLCr < 60 mL/min
Ceftazidime 2g IV q8h[a] monotherapy
Inpatient, and Documented penicillin and cephalosporin allergy
Ciprofloxacin 400 mg IV q12h[a,b]
+
Vancomycin 15 mg/kg IV q12h[a,d] (for streptococcal and staphylococcal coverage pending culture results)
Outpatient Gentamicin 6 mg/kg IV q24h[a,b,c] Ceftriaxone 2g IV q24h
A
Appropriate antibiotics begin as in A
If organism is isolated, cover the pathogen but do not narrow spectrum of coverage.
Patient becomes afebrile for 48–72 h
Assess ANC and clinical status
ANC < 0.1 × 10⁹/L
ANC 0.1–0.5 × 10⁹/L and evidence of neutrophil recovery
ANC > 0.5 × 10⁹/L
Appears clinically well
Appears unwell
• mucosal lesions
• diarrhea
• overt organ dysfunction
• unstable vital signs
• clinically apparent active infection
Continue antibiotics until ANC ≥ 0.1 × 10⁹/L and clinically well
Stop antibiotics after a total of 7–10 days of therapy
Continue antibiotics until ANC > 0.5 × 10⁹/L or clinically well
Stop antibiotics if patient has received a total of 5–7 days of therapy
B
Antibiotics begin as in A.
On antibiotics, fever continues > 72 h:
1) Investigate for nonbacterial causes such as drug fever.
2) Consider antibiotic-resistant organisms.
3) Rule out abcess, catheter infections.
Consider adding Vancomycin to regimen.
Yes
• Dose 15 mg/kg q12h[a,d]
• Less necessary if no central line, low risk
• Discontinue after 48 h if blood cultures negative and no evidence of catheter infection
• Obtain pre-dose level before 4th dose; aim for 5–10 mg/L
No
Reassess patient day 5–7
If still febrile, add amphotericin B (AMB) 0.5 mg/kg per day IV
Yes
1) No AMB test dose is required.
2) No premedication is routinely required. If patient has systemic reaction to AMB, administer diphenhydramine 50 mg IV; hydrocortisone 25–50 mg IV and acetaminophen 650 mg po, 30 minutes before administering AMB.
3) Preloading with 500 cc normal saline may delay or improve decline in renal failure.
No
Follow patient closely
C

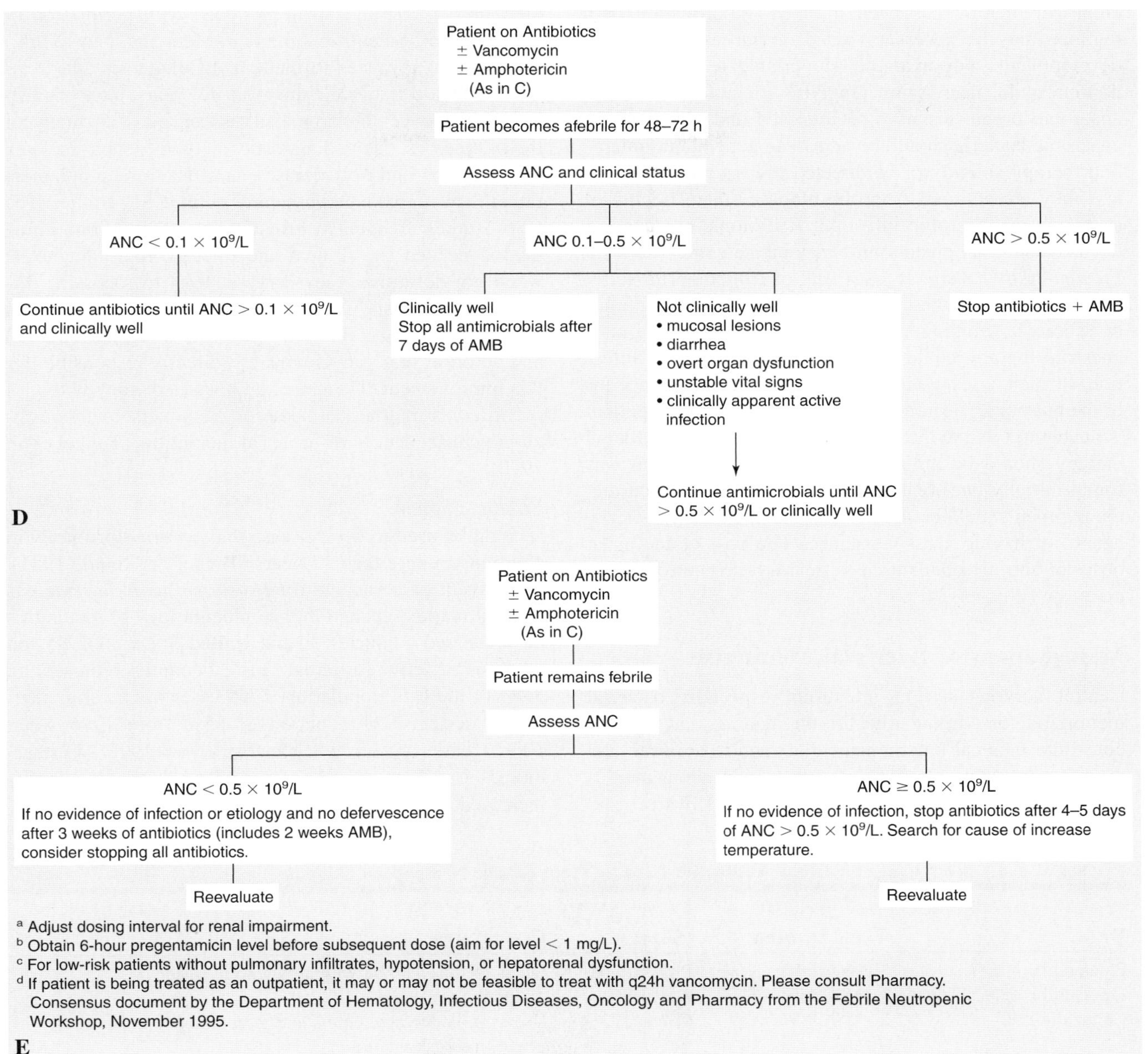


FIGURE 14-2 **Empiric treatment of the febrile neutropenic patient.**

of antifungal treatment would be continued. The experience with the imidazoles or newer triazoles in empirical antifungal therapy is limited. If the patient continues to be febrile and neutropenic despite an antibacterial and antifungal regimen, then the antifungal agent might be discontinued pending re-evaluation.

The duration of empirical antibacterial therapy is controversial. If the patient becomes afebrile while receiving an empirical regimen but remains neutropenic, the duration of treatment depends upon the clinical status of the patient and the neutrophil count. In general antibiotic therapy should be continued until neutrophil count is $>500/\text{mm}^3$.

The above discussion has revolved around empirical therapy for the neutropenic patient with fever but with no identified site of infection or identified pathogen. After empirical therapy has been initiated, modification of a regimen may be necessary based on subsequent clinical developments. For example, if perianal tenderness, abdominal pain, necrotizing gingivitis, or mucositis occur, anaerobic organisms may be involved and coverage for anaerobic bacteria should be added. In general, antimicrobial therapy should not be directed toward anaerobes unless they are cultured from the blood or there is clinical suspicion of anaerobic infection. Radiologic evidence of diffuse interstitial pneumonitis may indicate infection with *Pneumocystis carinii*. If so, a trial of trimethoprim-sulfamethoxazole could be initiated. New pulmonary infiltrates or lesions developing while the patient is receiving antibacterial therapy could indicate pulmonary fungal infection. In such cases, a biopsy (either percutaneous or open) of the pulmonary lesion should be attempted. If the patient is unable to tolerate these procedures, empirical antifungal therapy should be initiated. Finally, if an organism was found initially but breakthrough bacteremia has occurred, the regimen should be modified to include an antibacterial agent not having cross-resistance. The cost of the usual doses of antimicrobials used to treat febrile neutropenia is given in Table 14-34.

## Management of Bacterial Meningitis

Central nervous system infections, especially bacterial meningitis, are frequently life-threatening and usually constitute medical emergencies that require accurate and prompt treatment. (Portions of this section about meningitis have previously been published [Swartz and O'Hanley 1987] and are reproduced with permission of the publisher, Scientific American Medicine, New York.) Fortunately, advances in methods of diagnosis and treatment developed during the past 15 years have significantly improved the prognosis associated with many of these illnesses. New diagnostic methods (such as latex agglutination and polymerase chain reaction) supplement rather than supplant cerebrospinal fluid (CSF) studies. The CSF studies frequently provide important initial information needed for clinical and microbiologic diagnosis; when not definitive, they serve at least to focus the differential diagnosis. New chemotherapeutic agents, both antibacterial (e.g., the third-generation cephalosporins) and antiviral (e.g., acyclovir), are directly responsible for this improvement. The use of adjunctive therapy with glucocorticoids may lessen some of the adverse pathophysiologic consequences of bacterial meningitis (Tunkel et al. 1990).

### *Etiologic agents*

Meningitis used to be a disease that occurred primarily in children younger than 12 years (Tauber and Sande 1984). The advent of a vaccine for *Haemophilus influenzae* has led to a marked change in the epidemiology of meningitis in developed countries. In the United States in 1995, on the basis of active surveillance in 22 counties representing 3.9% of the U.S. population, 5755 cases of bacterial meningitis occurred, a reduction of 55% from 1986 when 12,920 cases occurred (Schuchat et al. 1997). Furthermore, the median age of persons with bacterial meningitis increased from 15 months in 1986 to 25 years in 1995,

Table 14-34 Cost of Various Antibiotics Used to Treat Febrile Neutropenic Patients

| Drug | Typical dose | Cost (AWP) ($/day) | Comments |
|---|---|---|---|
| Piperacillin | 3 g q6h IV | Pipracil $68 | Often used as 1[st] line with an aminoglycoside |
| Piperacillin + tazobactam | 3 g/0.375 mL q6h IV | Zosyn $59 | ±Aminoglycoside |
| Ceftazidime | 2 g q8h IV | Ceftaz $93 | Use as monotherapy, equivalent to combination, especially with low-risk neutropenia |
| Imipenum + cilastatin sodium | 500 mg q6h IV | Primaxin $82 | Monotherapy |
| Meropenem | 1 g IV q8h | Merrem NA | Monotherapy |
| Gentamicin sulfate | 5 mg/kg IV | Generic $2 | In combination with a $\beta$-lactam tobramycin has ↑ activity against |
| Tobramycin sulfate | 5 mg/kg IV | Generic $25 | *P. aeruginosa* |
| Vancomycin HCl | 1 g q12h IV | Generic $24<br>Vancocin $32 | Added for persistent fever and ↑ suspicion of gram-positive infection; discontinue if there is no evidence of catheter site infection. |
| Amphotericin B | 0.5–1 mg/kg IV | Fungizone $32 | Added for persistent fever despite appropriate antibiotics |

Source of drug costs is *Mosby's GenR$_x$* 1998. Current prices may vary from those quoted, but comparative prices among products are expected to be similar. The reader should check on local prices at the time of prescribing. AWP, average wholesale price; NA, not available.

chiefly because of a 94% reduction in the number of cases of *H. influenzae* meningitis. In 1995 the meningitis rates per 100,000 population for the following pathogens were as follows: *Streptococcus pneumoniae*, 1.1; *Neisseria meningitidis*, 0.6; group B streptococcus, 0.2; *Listeria monocytogenes*, 0.2; and *H. influenzae*, 0.2 (Schuchat et al. 1997). The principal bacteria responsible for neonatal meningitis are gram-negative bacilli (usually *E. coli* strains bearing the K1 capsular antigen) and group B streptococci (McCracken and Mize 1976). *Streptococcus pneumoniae* is now the most common cause of meningitis beyond the neonatal period (Schuchat et al. 1997). The appearance of *H. influenzae* meningitis in adults is so unusual that its presence suggests predisposing anatomic or immunologic defects that have permitted circumvention of the barrier normally provided by serum bactericidal mechanisms. The bacterial agents that most frequently cause bacterial meningitis in adults are *S. pneumoniae* and *N. meningitidis*.

Other bacteria infrequently cause meningitis. *Listeria monocytogenes* is a rare pathogen in the neonate. Its involvement in adult cases has been increasing primarily among those who are immunosuppressed or elderly (Chernik et al. 1973). Isolation of an anaerobic organism from the CSF is rare and strongly suggests intraventricular leakage of a brain abscess or the presence of a parameningeal focus of infection. *Staphylococcus aureus* meningitis is associated with neurosurgical procedures, penetrating cranial trauma, staphylococcal bacteremia and endocarditis, immunosuppressive therapy, and underlying neoplastic disease. Meningitis complicating ventriculoatrial or ventriculoperitoneal shunting procedures is usually caused by *S. aureus* or *S. epidermidis*. Gram-negative bacillary meningitis (caused by *E. coli*, *Enterobacter*, *Klebsiella*, *Proteus*, *Serratia*, or *Pseudomonas* species) usually is a nosocomial infection that affects neurosurgical, immunosuppressed, and oncologic patients, the elderly, and neonates (Chernik et al. 1973; Nieman and Lorber 1980; Rahal 1980).

A specific bacterial agent cannot be identified in 5 to 10% of patients with pyogenic meningitis. Polymicrobial mixed meningitis is rare and is found most often in neonates, particularly in association with a neuroectodermal defect, and occasionally in older patients following a penetrating head injury. Therefore, the common rule is that suppurative bacterial meningitis is caused by a single aerobic bacterial pathogen. The advent of increasing resistance of *Streptococcus pneumoniae* to penicillin has altered our approach to the treatment of meningitis beyond the neonatal period. If there is ≥2% rate of high-level penicillin-resistant *S. pneumoniae* in the community, empiric treatment of bacterial meningitis should consist of cefotaxime or ceftriaxone plus vancomycin. Ampicillin should be added if *Listeria* is suspected.

**PRINCIPLE Vaccination with *H. influenzae* vaccine has markedly reduced the rate of childhood meningitis. To treat properly, the practitioner must be aware of the common bacterial pathogens (and their local antimicrobial susceptibility patterns) associated with suppurative meningitis in each age group.**

### *Pathogenesis and clinical features*

Pathogenic organisms may enter the meninges in several ways:

- From the bloodstream during bacteremia,
- By penetration directly from the nasopharynx (skull fracture, congenital dural defect, or eroding sequestrum in mastoid), or from the body surface (neuroectodermal defect),
- Through intracranial passage via nasopharyngeal venules,
- By direct spread from an adjacent focus of infection (sinusitis or intraventricular leakage of a brain abscess),
- By introduction of organisms at the time of a neurosurgical operation,
- By contamination of a CSF drain

Bacteremia is the most frequent source of infection. Organisms often are demonstrable in the bloodstream in the very early stages of the three most common types of bacterial meningitis beyond the neonatal period: those caused by *S. pneumoniae*, *N. meningitidis*, and group B streptococcus (Schuchat et al. 1997). Once meningeal infection becomes established, it quickly extends throughout the subarachnoid space. Ventriculitis can be demonstrated at the time of admission in at least 70% of neonates who are diagnosed as having meningitis (McCracken et al. 1980).

Certain clinical conditions are predisposing factors for specific types of bacterial meningitis. The conditions that predispose a person to pneumococcal meningitis include acute otitis media and mastoiditis. These entities precede 30% of cases of meningitis. In adult patients, pneumonia precedes 10 to 25%; nonpenetrating head injury precedes 5 to 10%; CSF rhinorrhea or otorrhea precedes 5%; and in adults, alcoholism and cirrhosis of the liver precede 10 to 25% of cases with pneumonococcal meningitis in urban hospitals. Sickle cell anemia, defects in host defenses such as congenital or acquired immunoglobulin deficiencies, asplenic states, and acute sinusitis occasionally precede meningitis.

Most cases of *H. influenzae, N. meningitidis*, and *S. pneumoniae* meningitis are preceded by upper respiratory tract infection, otitis media, or pneumonia. The onset is usually sudden and progresses over the course of 24 to 36 hours with fever, generalized headache, vomiting, and stiff neck. Myalgias (particularly in meningococcal disease) and backache are common. Once meningitic signs are evident, the infection progresses rapidly, producing confusion, obtundation, and ultimately coma. Indications of leptomeningeal inflammation (drowsiness, stiff neck, and Kernig and Brudzinski signs) are generally present. The usual manifestations of meningitis may be partially obscured in an elderly person who has underlying congestive heart failure or pneumonia and is obtunded and hypoxic. Similarly, a neonate with meningitis may have decreased appetite, fever, irritability, lassitude, and vomiting but may not always exhibit either stiff neck or bulging fontanelles. Such patients should be examined carefully for meningitic signs; if any question about the presence of meningitis remains in such cases, a lumbar puncture must be performed to obtain CSF for examination.

A number of neurologic findings and complications may accompany bacterial meningitis. These include cranial nerve dysfunction (especially third, fourth, sixth, and seventh nerves), focal cerebral signs (hemiparesis, dysphasia, and hemianopia), focal and generalized seizures, and acute cerebral edema, ultimately leading to death.

The presence of skin lesions may assist the physician in arriving at a diagnosis. A maculopetechial or purpuric rash in a patient with meningitis usually signifies meningococcal infection. Infrequently, petechial and purpuric skin lesions develop in the course of *S. pneumoniae* bacteremia and meningitis, reflecting disseminated intravascular coagulation. Multiple skin lesions almost identical to those observed in patients with meningococcemia occur rarely in patients with acute *S. aureus* endocarditis. Meningitic signs and a CSF neutrophilic pleocytosis also may develop in such patients and are caused by embolic cerebral infarction rather than by bacterial meningitis. The maculopetechial rash of echovirus aseptic meningitis (particularly type 9 that has been responsible for extensive outbreaks) may be mistaken for the rash of meningococcal meningitis. This type of viral meningitis may produce an early and marked CSF neutrophilic pleocytosis. The rash in meningococcal meningitis may involve the face and neck but only after it has already extensively covered other parts of the body; in echovirus type 9 meningeal infection, the rash involves the face and neck early in the course of the exanthem before other parts of the body are significantly involved.

### *Laboratory features*

The CSF cell count in the majority of patients with untreated bacterial meningitis ranges from 100 to 5000 cells/mm$^3$, of which more than 80% are neutrophils. Cell counts of 50,000 cells/mm$^3$ or higher are occasionally observed in primary bacterial meningitis, but such a marked pleocytosis also suggests the possibility of intraventricular rupture of a cerebral abscess.

More than half of patients with bacterial meningitis have glucose concentrations of 40 mg/dL or lower in their CSF (<50 to 60% of the simultaneous fasting blood glucose concentration). A normal CSF glucose concentration, however, can occur in some patients with bacterial meningitis. The primary importance of the CSF determination of glucose is not in aiding the diagnosis of the typical case of acute pyogenic meningitis (which usually can be diagnosed on the basis of the gram-stained smear of the CSF and the CSF cell count). Rather, the CSF glucose concentration is most useful in distinguishing chronic meningitides (such as those that are caused by *Listeria, Nocardia, Actinomyces, Cryptococcus*, or *Coccidioides*) marked by hypoglycorrhachia from parameningeal infections and viral aseptic meningitides, which usually do not lower CSF glucose concentrations (Peacock et al. 1984).

Patients with bacterial meningitis usually have CSF protein concentrations higher than 120 mg/dL (normal 30–40 mg/dL). Occasionally, values of 1000 mg/dL or greater are observed, suggesting actual or impending subarachnoid block secondary to the meningitis.

Definitive diagnosis requires isolation of the causative organism or demonstration of its characteristic antigen, from the CSF. The implicated bacterium can be demonstrated on a CSF gram-stained smear in about 80% of patients with bacterial meningitis. The bacteria that are most likely to be missed on Gram stain are meningococci and *Listeria* species (Sande and Tierney 1984). Bacteremia is demonstrable in 80% of patients with *H. influenzae* meningitis, 50% with pneumococcal meningitis, and 30 to 40% with *N. meningitidis* meningitis (Swartz and Dodge 1965). Cultures of CSF and blood yield enough information to permit determination of the bacterial cause in about 90% of previously untreated patients with bacterial meningitis.

**PRINCIPLE Definitive diagnostic studies are mandatory in any life-threatening disease. They confirm the clinical diagnosis, and the data derived from these tests provide rational guidelines for therapy.**

Common bacterial meningitides (those caused by *S. pneumoniae*, group B streptococcus, and previously *Haemophilus influenzae*) are associated with mean CSF bacterial concentrations ranging from $10^5$ to $10^7$ organisms per milliliter (Feldman 1977). This concentration of organisms introduces envelope polysaccharide antigens into the CSF in amounts sufficient to be detectable by counterimmunoelectrophoresis (CIE) and the latex agglutination test. These procedures have been used most extensively in the rapid diagnosis (i.e., 1 to 2 hours) of *H. influenzae* meningitis. In addition, CIE has been helpful in the rapid diagnosis of pneumococcal and meningococcal (groups A, B, C, and Y) meningitis, and it can be used to detect *E. coli* Kl capsular antigen and group B streptococcal antigen in neonatal meningitis.

The bacterial capsular antigens of the three common etiologic agents in primary bacterial meningitis can be successfully identified in 60 to 80% of cases (McCracken 1976; Finch and Wilkinson 1979). The reliability of these immunoprecipitation techniques depends heavily on the activity of the antisera employed. False-positive results occasionally arise from cross-reactions. For example, certain *E. coli* capsular antigens cross-react with antisera to *H. influenzae* type B and group B meningococcal antigens. Because in about 90% of patients with bacterial meningitis the bacterial cause can be established by more traditional microbiologic means, CIE is not essential for diagnosis. It serves as an important adjunct, however, permitting early diagnosis in patients in whom no organisms are seen on smear or in whom cultures remain negative because of prior therapy with antibiotics. Even in cases in which the morphology of the organism is revealed by gram-stained smears, CIE is useful because it permits definitive identification of the agent.

***Radiologic studies***

Roentgenograms of the chest, sinuses, and mastoids should be performed at an appropriate time following institution of antimicrobial therapy for suspected pyogenic meningitis; infections in these areas are frequently associated with meningitis. When history, clinical setting, or physical findings suggest the presence of a suppurative intracranial collection, such as a brain abscess or subdural empyema, CT scanning should be performed without delay. It is not appropriate or necessary to routinely perform a CT or radionuclide scan to exclude these diagnostic entities when the practitioner is confident of the diagnosis of uncomplicated suppurative meningitis.

Meningitis itself induces the following changes on the CT scan: contrast enhancement of the leptomeninges and ventricular lining; widening of the subarachnoid space; and patchy areas of diminished density in the cerebrum from cerebritis and necrosis (Weisberg 1980; Stovring and Snyder 1980). In addition, CT scanning may be helpful in evaluating the patient with a prolonged or deteriorating clinical status and in detecting suspected complications, such as sterile subdural collections or empyema, ventricular enlargement secondary to communicating or obstructive hydrocephalus, ventriculitis or ventricular empyema (as revealed by ventricular wall enhancement), or cerebral infarction caused by arteritis or cortical vein thrombophlebitis.

***Differential diagnosis of suppurative bacterial meningitis***

Because the clinical features of bacterial meningitis (headache, fever, stiff neck, and obtundation) may be seen in other types of CNS infection, findings in the CSF are important in the development of an appropriate differential diagnosis. Particular attention should be given to the patient with meningitic signs and neutrophilic CSF pleocytosis, but normal CSF glucose concentrations, or absence of organisms in a gram-stained smear of the CSF. The differential diagnosis in such cases includes several treatable diseases that require management that is different from that of bacterial pyogenic meningitis. A parameningeal bacterial infection such as an epidural abscess, a subdural empyema, or a brain abscess might be suspected in a patient with these findings who also has a chronic ear, sinus, or lung infection. Isolation of anaerobic organisms from the CSF is highly suggestive of parameningeal infection. Anaerobes may enter the CSF via intraventricular leakage of a cerebral abscess, through extension of infection from a focus of osteomyelitis, or from an epidural abscess.

Focal cerebral signs may be an indication of a space-occupying intracranial infection; they also may appear during the course of bacterial meningitis as a result of occlusive vascular injury. When focal cerebral signs develop, the history should be reviewed for any neurologic symptoms antedating the onset of the acute meningitis. Bacterial endocarditis may present with prominent symptoms of meningitis and a pleocytosis in the CSF. This presentation is the result either of frank meningitis caused by pyogenic organisms or of sterile embolic cerebral infarctions produced by normally nonpyogenic organisms, such as *Streptococcus viridans*. Careful auscultation for cardiac murmurs and a search for peripheral signs of endocarditis (petechiae, splenomegaly, or Osler nodes) and echocardiography should be performed.

Most patients with pneumococcal, meningococcal, or *H. influenzae* meningitis become afebrile within 2 to 5 days of the start of appropriate antibiotic therapy. Occasionally, fever continues beyond 8 to 10 days or recurs after having disappeared. Prolonged or recurrent fever accompanied by headache, focal cerebral signs, or obtundation suggests that antimicrobial therapy has been inadequate or a neurologic complication (e.g., cortical vein thrombophlebitis, ventriculitis, ventricular empyema, subdural effusion, or subdural empyema) has developed. Reevaluation of the findings in the CSF, including gram-stained smears and cultures, is essential. Persistent fever in a patient whose clinical course and CSF findings show progressive improvement may be indicative of drug fever.

***General aspects of antibiotic treatment***

Most antibiotics employed in the therapy of bacterial meningitis, with the exception of chloramphenicol, do not readily penetrate the noninflamed blood–brain barrier (see Table 14-16). Meningitis enhances the entry of penicillins and some other antimicrobial agents (e.g., vancomycin) into the CSF and allows successful therapy with these drugs provided large parenteral doses are administered. Antibiotics should be administered IV in divided doses at intervals that provide high concentration gradients across the meninges. Dosage should not be decreased when clinical improvement occurs, because the normalization of the blood–brain barrier that accompanies resolution of the infection reduces antibiotic concentrations that can be obtained in the CSF.

The absence of intrinsic opsonic and bactericidal activity in infected CSF increases the importance of providing bactericidal rather than bacteriostatic agents to treat bacterial meningitis (Simberkoff et al. 1980). Although they are effective in vitro against many species that are capable of causing meningitis, drugs such as clindamycin, erythromycin, and first- and most second-generation cephalosporins (including cefamandole) should never be used in bacterial meningitis. These agents cannot predictably achieve bactericidal concentrations in the CSF. Vancomycin, a microbiostatic agent, should also not be routinely used in the treatment of bacterial meningitis. It should be reserved for treatment of methicillin-resistant staphylococcal infections and for penicillin-resistant *S. pneumoniae*.

WARNING In the treatment of bacterial meningitis avoid:

- Drugs with poor penetration within the CSF (e.g., clindamycin, erythromycin, first-generation cephalosporins, and most second-generation cephalosporins)
- Microbiostatic agents (e.g., vancomycin) unless no better alternative can be found.

Intrathecal therapy is not needed to treat uncomplicated cases of the three most common types of bacterial meningitis, since they can be treated with antimicrobials that enter the CSF in bactericidal quantities. **Only preservative-free gentamicin is available for intrathecal therapy.**

WARNING **Always check to make sure that the preparation you are using for intrathecal therapy is preservative free. If standard parenteral forms of aminoglycosides are used, a severe arachnoiditis often occurs.**

The patient's clinical course dictates the frequency needed for examination of the CSF. Repeat examination should be performed 24 to 48 hours after the start of antibiotic therapy if progress seems unsatisfactory or if the cause of the meningitis remains uncertain. Meningococcal meningitis should be treated until the patient remains afebrile for 5 to 7 days. With prompt and satisfactory response to antibiotics, it is not necessary to repeat the examination of the CSF at the end of the therapy. Patients with *H. influenzae* meningitis should be treated for at least 7 days after they have become afebrile. Again, a follow-up examination of the CSF is not necessary in patients who show rapid and complete clinical recovery. Patients with pneumococcal meningitis should be treated for 10 to 14 days. Prolonged therapy is necessary in the presence of an underlying mastoiditis or if the patient has underlying immunosuppression (e.g., neutrophil or B- or T-cell abnormalities or deficiencies).

***Specific antimicrobial therapy***

Bacterial meningitis is a life-threatening medical emergency that requires prompt therapy based on examination of the gram-stained smear from the sediment of the CSF. Two serious but common errors in managing a patient with suspected meningitis are to delay performing a diagnostic lumbar puncture and to delay starting antibiotic therapy.

WARNING When imaging studies are needed to exclude an intracranial mass before a lumbar puncture is performed, antibiotics should be initiated immediately after blood has been obtained for culture.

The choice of antibiotics depends at first on the suspected pathogen (Table 14-35), and later on that which ultimately is isolated. The scan and the lumbar puncture

Table 14-35 **Initial Antibiotic and Anti-inflammatory Therapy for Suppurative Meningitis of Unknown Cause**

| Patient Group | Suspected Pathogen | Preferred Therapy Antibiotic | Alternative Therapy Antibiotic |
|---|---|---|---|
| Neonate (1 month or younger) | Group B streptococci<br>*Listeria monocytogenes*<br>*E. coli*<br>*S. pneumoniae* | Ampicillin plus cefotaxime | Ampicillin and gentamicin |
| Child | *N. meningitidis*<br>*H. influenzae* | Ampicillin plus cefotaxime or ceftriaxone plus dexamethasone | Chloramphenicol plus gentamicin plus dexamethasone |
| Adult | *N. meningitidis*<br>*S. pneumoniae*<br>*H. influenzae*<br>*Listeria* | Ampicillin or penicillin G plus ceftriaxone | Chloramphenicol or cefotaxime |
| Adult or child resident in a community with >2% high level (≥2 μg/ml) penicillin-resistant *S. pneumoniae* | Penicillin-resistant *S. pneumoniae*<br>*N. meningitidis*<br>*Listeria*<br>*H. influenzae* | Vancomycin plus cefotaxime or ceftriaxone | Possibly meropenem |
| Immunocompromised adult (e.g., older than 60, with cirrhosis or neoplastic disease) | *Listeria*<br>*Pseudomonas* | Cefotaxime plus Ampicillin<br>Ciprofloxacin or ceftazidime plus an aminoglycoside | Trimethoprim-sulfamethoxazole(TMP-SMX) plus chloramphenicol |
| | *S. pneumoniae* | Penicillin G if pen. resistant, vancomycin plus ceftriaxone | |
| | *N. meningitidis* | Penicillin G | |
| Postcraniotomy patient | *Staphylococcus aureus* | Nafcillin or cloxacillin | Vancomycin and gentamicin |
| | *Staphylococcus epidermidis* | Vancomycin | |
| | *H. influenzae*<br>*N. meningitidis* | Cefotaxime; ceftriaxone<br>penicillin | |
| | *E. coli, Klebsiella, Proteus,* and similar organisms | Gentamicin plus cefotaxime | Ampicillin only if isolate is susceptible |
| | *Pseudomonas* | Ceftazidime plus gentamicin | |

Ampicillin sodium, cefotaxime sodium, ceftriaxone sodium, chloramphenicol, dexamethasone, gentamicin, meropenem, nafcillin sodium, penicillin G, trimethoprim-sulfamethoxazole, vancomycin HCl.

1. In communities with penicillin-resistant *S. pneumoniae,* initial therapy of suppurative meningitis should include vancomycin plus ceftriaxone or cefotaxime for all age groups. This combination will not treat *Listeria.*
2. Of *Listeria* isolates, 30% are resistant to ampicillin. Alternative antibiotics include trimethoprim-sulfamethoxazole, doxycycline, and gentamicin.

may be done while the patient is receiving empirical antibiotic therapy. If a diagnostic lumbar puncture is performed after a mass lesion has been excluded by CT scan and the Gram stain reveals bacterial types not covered by the initial empirical therapy, the regimen can be appropriately altered. Animal models of meningitis suggest that initial empirical therapy will not affect the subsequent results of culture of CSF if the spinal fluid is sampled within 2 to 3 hours of the start of antibiotic therapy (Tauber and Sande 1984).

Clinical studies suggest that optimal chemotherapy for bacterial meningitis requires the CSF concentration of the antibiotic to be several fold greater (>10 times) than the MBC for the pathogen measured in vitro. Additional principles that should guide therapy for meningitis include the following:

1. The antibiotic must be capable of killing the pathogen.
2. The pathogen must be shown to be highly susceptible to the selected antibiotic, as measured by quantitative dilution studies (e.g., in vitro CSF killing levels or in vitro MBC tests).
3. Because the antibiotic must reach local sites in concentrations sufficient to kill the pathogen, the agent selected must readily penetrate into the infected CSF or, if not, be directly instilled into the CSF by intrathecal or intraventricular injection.
4. Foci of suppurative parameningeal infection must be drained whenever the procedure can be performed without causing serious neurologic damage. The extent to which various antibiotics transport into the CSF during meningitis differs, and the practitioner must know this. In general, concentrations of antibiotic are higher in the CSF of children and neonates than in adults with meningitis.

The presence of local leukocytes, especially neutrophils, is probably necessary for the infected meninges to become permeable to antibiotics. For example, limited experience suggests that vancomycin, which tends to accumulate in the CSF of otherwise healthy adults with bacterial meningitis, does not enter the CSF as well in neutropenic patients with documented bacterial meningitis. Therefore, serial determinations of the concentration of drug in the CSF or serial studies of CSF bacterial killing should be performed in severely neutropenic patients to document the presence of sufficiently high antibiotic concentrations. Otherwise, serial intrathecal or intraventricular injections of the appropriate antibiotics must be given. The third-generation cephalosporins usually achieve concentrations in CSF that are at least 10 times the MBC against the common *Enterobacteriaceae* that cause meningitis (e.g., *E. coli*, *Klebsiella* species, and *Proteus mirabilis*). Such a concentration appears to be needed in order to cure meningitis (Sande 1981). It is questionable, however, whether these agents, when used alone, can achieve 10-fold MBC concentrations in the CSF against such organisms as *Pseudomonas*, *Flavobacterium*, *Enterobacter*, *Serratia*, and *Acinetobacter* species.

The appearance of penicillinase-producing *H. influenzae* type b strains that are highly resistant to ampicillin (about 30% of isolates in the United States) has required a shift in the focus of initial management of this form of meningitis. Ceftriaxone or cefotaxime is now mandatory as empirical therapy for *H. influenzae* meningitis until the isolate has been demonstrated to be susceptible to ampicillin in vitro.

Resistance to ampicillin in *H. influenzae* is caused by production of $\beta$-lactamase, whereas resistance to chloramphenicol is associated with production of acetyltransferase (Smith 1983). A patient with *S. aureus* meningitis should be treated with a penicillinase-resistant penicillin such as nafcillin or cloxacillin because 80 to 90% of *S. aureus* isolates are resistant to penicillin G.

Enterococcal meningitis requires the use of IV penicillin or ampicillin supplemented by parenterally administered gentamicin. If a patient with enterococcal meningitis fails to respond promptly to parenteral therapy with penicillin and gentamicin, adjunctive intrathecal gentamicin (4 to 8 mg for an adult) may be given.

#### ***The special problem of gram-negative bacillary meningitis***

The parenteral antibiotics that have been used in the past to treat gram-negative bacillary meningitis were ampicillin, chloramphenicol, and aminoglycosides. The results of treatment, however, were far from satisfactory: Mortality has ranged from 30 to 60% (Swartz 1981; Cherubin et al. 1981). The use of ampicillin as primary therapy for this form of meningitis is limited by the fact that about 30% of strains of gram-negative bacilli that cause neonatal meningitis, and the majority of isolates from adults with meningitis, are ampicillin-resistant. Chloramphenicol also has drawbacks in addition to its potential toxicity in neonates. Although the MICs of chloramphenicol for many gram-negative bacilli (2 to 6 mg/L) are achievable in the CSF, MBCs are generally so much higher (>60 mg/L) that they are not attainable in the CSF (Rahal and Simberkoff 1979).

Adjunctive intrathecal antibiotic therapy in the treatment of gram-negative bacillary meningitis came into use for two reasons: 1) parenteral administration of gentamicin and tobramycin yields low (<1 mg/L) and inconsistent concentrations in the CSF; and, 2) patients treated only with systemic agents have a high mortality. The high mortality associated with neonatal gram-negative bacillary meningitis, however, has not been reduced by the addition of lumbar intrathecal administration of gentamicin to parenteral therapy with ampicillin and gentamicin (McCracken and Mize 1976). Unfortunately, the ventricles are common sites of infection in bacterial meningitis. The unidirectional circulation of the CSF inhibits drug entry into the ventricles, and little of the antibiotic introduced intrathecally in the lumbar area reaches the ventricular system. Adjunctive intraventricular administration of gentamicin either via a ventriculostomy reservoir or by percutaneous injection circumvents this obstacle. However, a controlled study of neonates with gram-negative bacillary meningitis demonstrated a higher mortality among infants who received intraventricular gentamicin along with systemic antibiotics (43%) than among those who received systemic antibiotics alone (13%) (McCracken et al. 1980). This finding suggests that intraventricular therapy with gentamicin is harmful to neonates with gram-negative bacillary meningitis. The adjunctive use of lumbar intrathecal aminoglycoside (e.g., gentamicin) was recommended in children and adults with gram-negative bacillary meningitis (other than *H. influenzae* meningitis) because of the high overall mortality associated with this disease when it was treated with parenteral antibiotics alone (Mangi et al. 1977; Rahal 1980).

The studies discussed above were performed before the development of the newer third-generation cephalosporins. A number of recent clinical trials support their efficacy in the treatment of patients in cases of meningitis that are caused by various bacterial agents and that occur in different age groups (Nelson 1985). Several general guidelines have been proposed regarding the use of the newer cephalosporins to treat bacterial meningitis (Neu 1985):

- Final selection of the antibiotic or antibiotics to treat bacterial meningitis should be based on which drug or drugs have the greatest bactericidal activity for the causative agent, as determined by the MBC.
- The newer cephalosporins do not offer any advantage over penicillin G in the treatment of group B streptococcal meningitis.
- Cefotaxime, ceftriaxone, and ceftizoxime appear to be as effective as chloramphenicol or ampicillin in the treatment of *H. influenzae* meningitis.
- Cefotaxime and ceftriaxone appear to be equal to penicillin G or chloramphenicol to treat meningococcal and pneumococcal meningitides.
- Meningitis caused by *Pseudomonas*, *Acinetobacter*, *Enterobacter*, or *Serratia* cannot be successfully treated with third-generation cephalosporins alone.
- Meningitis caused by *Listeria*, staphylococci, or enterococci should not be treated with third-generation cephalosporins.

**WARNING** Third-generation cephalosporins lack activity against *Listeria*, staphylococci, and enterococci and are not adequate as monotherapy for many gram-negative bacilli.

***Treatment of bacterial meningitis of unknown cause***

Empiric treatment of meningitis is directed at the most likely pathogens based on the age of the patient and available clinical clues (see Table 14-35). Information about the most commonly used antibiotics is included in Table 14-36.

Meningitis in neonates may be caused by a wide range of enteric gram-negative bacilli and gram-positive organisms, such as *E. coli,* group B streptococci or *Listeria.* Such a variety of organisms necessitates the use of combined therapy with drugs such as ampicillin and either gentamicin or a third-generation cephalosporin such as cefotaxime. In children, antibacterial therapy is aimed at the three organisms most commonly responsible for childhood bacterial meningitis: *S. pneumoniae*, *N. meningitidis*, and *H. influenzae* with empiric ampicillin and ceftriaxone being most frequently employed.

*Streptococcus pneumoniae* meningitis and *N. meningitidis* meningitis are the meningitides that most commonly affect adults, but the incidence of invasive *H. influenzae* infection in adults is on the rise. *Listeria monocytogenes* is the fourth most common cause of meningitis in adults. The combination of ampicillin and ceftriaxone is the treatment choice for bacterial meningitis of unknown cause in the adult because this combination is effective against *S. pneumoniae, N. meningitidis, H. influenzae,* and *L. monocytogenes*. The increase in high-level penicillin-resistant *S. pneumoniae* has led many authorities to recommend a combination of vancomycin and ceftriaxone for the empiric treatment of bacterial meningitis in communities where 2% or more of the isolates of *S. pneumoniae* exhibit high-level penicillin resistance.

The incidence of uncommon types of meningitis in certain clinical settings has increased, such as meningitis caused by *S. aureus* in post craniotomy patients, and meningitis caused by gram-negative bacilli or *Listeria* in patients who are immunocompromised because of advanced age, neoplastic disease, or cirrhosis. Broader initial antibiotic therapy is warranted in the management of patients with these underlying conditions.

***Adjunctive therapy of meningitis***

Table 14-37 outlines therapies that are commonly used as an adjunct to antibiotics in the treatment of meningitis. Despite effective antibacterial therapy, morbidity and mortality from bacterial meningitis remain high. Data from animal studies suggest that modification of the inflammatory response should reduce these sequelae (Nolan et al. 1978). A number of clinical trials in predominantly *H. influenzae* meningitis in infants and children demonstrated reduction in sensorineural deafness and neurolog-

Table 14-36 Cost of Antibiotics Commonly Used to Treat Meningitis

| Drug | Common Adult Dose | Cost (AWP) (%/Day) | Comments |
|---|---|---|---|
| Ampicillin sodium | 2 g q4h IV | Generic $28 | Excellent coverage for sensitive pneumococcus, *H. influenzae,* meningococcus, *Listeria;* however, increased incidence of resistant strains of pneumococcus and *H. influenzae* dictate that it should not be used alone empirically. |
| Penicillin G | 4 mU[a] q4h IV | Generic $16 | Excellent coverage for sensitive pneumococcus, but should not be used as initial therapy empirically due to prevalence of resistant strains. |
| Ceftriaxone sodium | 2 g q12h IV | Rocephin $135 | Drugs of choice for pneumococcus, *H. influenzae* resistant to penicillin excellent for many gram-negative bacilli. |
| Cefotaxime sodium | 2 g q4h IV | Claforan $127 | (see above) |
| Vancomycin HCl | 1 g q12h IV | Generic $24<br>Vancocin $32 | Add to a 3rd generation cephalosporin if high level resistance to *S. pneumoniae* is suspected. Poor penetration of CSF. Concomitant steroid use will decrease penetration. Post surgical meningitis involving gram-positive organisms. |
| Chloramphenicol | 1 g q6h IV | Generic $164 | For resistant organisms. NOT first line 2° to serious adverse effects. |
| Nafcillin sodium | 2 g q4h IV | Generic $53 | Post surgical meningitis involving gram-positive organisms. |
| Ceftazidime | 2 g q8h IV | Fortaz $86 | If *Pseudomonas* is isolated or suspected. |

Source of drug costs is *Mosby's GenR$_x$* 1998. Current prices may vary from those quoted, but comparative prices among products are expected to be similar. The reader should check on local prices at the time of prescribing. AWP, average wholesale price.
[a]mU = million units.

ical sequelae in the corticosteroid-treated group (Lebel et al. 1988; Lebel et al. 1989; Odio et al. 1991; Schaad et al. 1993). There are limited data on the use of adjunctive dexamethasone therapy in adults with meningitis. A trial that included 429 Egyptian children and adults with bacterial meningitis involved randomization to antibiotics (ampicillin plus chloramphenicol) with or without adjunctive dexamethasone (Girgis et al. 1989). The mortality from pneumococcal meningitis in the dexamethasone group was 13.5% (7/52) versus 40% (22/54) in the group without dexamethasone ($P < 0.001$). The dexamethasone group had no hearing loss (0/45) versus 12.5% (4/32) in the group with no steroid treatment ($P < 0.05$) (Girgis et al. 1989).

A meta-analysis of 11 studies of corticosteroid adjunctive therapy in meningitis found that children receiving placebo were 3.77 times more likely to develop auditory dysfunction than those who received dexamethasone (Yurkowski and Plaisance 1993). McIntyre and colleagues also performed a meta-analysis of all trials of dexamethasone therapy in childhood meningitis published from 1988 to November 1996 (McIntyre et al. 1997). They identified 16 studies, 11 of which fit their criteria for analysis. In *H. influenzae meningitis*, dexamethasone reduced severe hearing loss, odds ratio (OR) 0.31; (95% CI 0.14–0.69). For all organisms combined, the pooled OR suggested protection against neurologic deficits other than hearing loss but was not significant (OR 0.59; 95% CI 0.34–1.02).

In pneumococcal meningitis, only studies in which dexamethasone was given early suggested protection that was significant for severe hearing loss (OR 0.09; 95% CI

Table 14-37 Adjunctive Therapy for Bacterial Meningitis

| Therapy | Comments |
|---|---|
| Dexamethasone<br>0.15 mg/kg q6h for 4 days | Best studied in children with meningitis. Resulted in decreased incidence of sensorineural hearing loss and other neurological sequelae. |
| Control of increased intracranial pressure (ICP) | Patients with signs of increased ICP may benefit from insertion of an ICP measuring device and treatment of the ICP. |
| Plasmapheresis | Has proven useful in fulminant meningococcemia. |
| Supportive care | Meticulous attention to fluid and electrolyte balance. High index of suspicion for complications such as subdural empyema. |
| Eradication of nasopharyngeal carriage of *N. meningitidis* and *H. influenzae* | Mucosal colonization may persist despite successful treatment of the meningitis. Rifampin should be given to eradicate this colonization. |

0.0–0.71) and approached significance for any neurological or hearing deficit (OR 0.23; 95% CI 0.04–1.05). Tunkel and Scheld (1996) recommend the use of dexamethasone in adults with meningitis if they have stupor or coma or cerebral edema documented by CT or MRI, and/or evidence of mark elevated intracranial pressure. For maximum benefit the corticosteroid should be given before the antibiotics, since the antibiotics result in bacterial cell lysis and further inflammation.

***Chemoprophylaxis***

Meningococcal meningitis is the only type of bacterial meningitis that occurs in epidemic form. Close contacts of an index case (such as other household members, infants in day-care centers, or military recruits) are at increased risk for developing meningococcal disease. Casual contacts such as schoolmates do not appear to be at increased risk. Hospital personnel in close patient contact (e.g., during nasotracheal suctioning or mouth-to-mouth resuscitation) are at increased risk, but personnel who come into contact with the patient after institution of respiratory precautions and antibiotic therapy are not.

Chemoprophylaxis is indicated only for close contacts. Sulfonamides, once widely employed in chemoprophylaxis, should no longer be used for that purpose because approximately 25% of meningococcal isolates are now resistant to sulfonamides. Rifampin is the drug of choice to accomplish prophylaxis in close contacts. The recommended dose in adults is either 600 mg orally every 12 hours for 2 days or 600 mg orally once daily for 4 days (Ward et al. 1979). (Note the potential for enzyme induction changing the metabolism of some drugs, e.g., oral contraceptive.) About 50% of secondary cases among close contacts occur at least 5 days after onset of the disease in the index case patient. This fact prompts consideration of the use of meningococcal bivalent vaccine (groups A and C) as an adjunct to chemoprophylaxis, to extend protection should chemoprophylaxis be unsuccessful.

Secondary cases of systemic *H. influenzae* type b infections may occur in close household and day-care center contacts of an initial case of *H. influenzae* meningitis. The risk for household contacts who are younger than 12 months is 6%; for those younger than 4 years, the risk is 2% (Ward et al. 1979). The risk of severe *H. influenzae* disease among household contacts appears to be 585 times greater than the age-adjusted risk in the general population. A variety of drugs, including ampicillin, trimethoprim-sulfamethoxazole, and cefaclor, have been tested but were ineffective in eradicating nasopharyngeal carriage of *H. influenzae* type b (Overturf 1982). Rifampin (20 mg/kg daily for 4 days) has been successful in eradicating carriage and appears to be the drug of choice for chemoprophylaxis. Chemoprophylaxis is given to household contacts (in households were there is a child younger than 48 months of age) of the index case. The use of chemoprophylaxis for day-care contacts is more controversial. In addition, active immunization of contacts with the polysaccharide vaccine of *H. influenzae* type b may be effective immunoprophylaxis against secondary cases of *H. influenzae* type b disease.

## Management of Infective Endocarditis

***Epidemiology***

Infective endocarditis (IE) is a microbial infection of the endothelial lining of the heart. The characteristic lesion is a vegetation (a mass comprised of fibrin, platelets, microorganisms and their product or products on a valve leaflet). Multiple valves may be involved, as may any part of the endothelium of the heart. The incidence of endocarditis ranges from 17 to 39 cases per million person-years (Van der Meer et al. 1992).

There have been major changes in the epidemiology of endocarditis. The age of patients affected has increased considerably. In 1945, about 10% of patients with IE were over 60 years of age (Lerner and Weinstein 1966), compared with 55% in 1977. The second major change in the epidemiology of endocarditis is the increase in the incidence of prosthetic valve endocarditis (PVE), which accounts for almost half of the cases of endocarditis treated at tertiary-care medical centers. PVE is divided into two categories, early (EPVE), which develops less than 60 days after surgery, and late (LPVE), which develops more than 60 days after surgery (Von Reyn et al. 1981). Endocarditis complicates 0.98 to 4.4% of prosthetic valves (Heimberger et al. 1989).

The underlying cardiac lesions in native valve endocarditis (NVE) have also changed in the modern era. In the preantibiotic era, rheumatic heart disease was the most common lesion. In a recent series of 63 patients with NVE, the underlying cardiac lesions were as follows: mitral valve prolapse, 29%; no underlying disease, 27%; degenerative lesions of the aortic or mitral valve, 21%; congenital heart disease, 13%; rheumatic heart disease, 6% (McKinsey et al. 1987). In cases of mitral valve prolapse, the risk of infection is significantly higher among those with redundancy (the classic form) compared with those without leaflet thickening (the nonclassic form) (Marks et al. 1989).

Infective endocarditis is a serious condition with mortality rates of up to 76% for EPVE and up to 44% for LPVE. The mortality rate from NVE for 442 patients studied from 1945 to 1949 was 44% (Cates et al. 1951); currently it is much lower.

In many centers, injection drug users constitute a significant percentage of patients with endocarditis: 7.3% in the Netherlands study (Van der Meer et al. 1992). In other areas it is much higher: In three California hospitals between 1965 and 1976, injection drug users accounted for 17, 43, and 13% of all cases of IE (Hubbell et al. 1981). The incidence of endocarditis among injection drug users is 2 to 5% per year (Hubbell et al. 1981). The majority of injection drug users with endocarditis have tricuspid valve involvement (32%), the aortic valve is involved in 29%, the mitral valve in 25%, and multiple valves in 9% of cases (Hubbell et al. 1981). Eighty percent of tricuspid valve endocarditis cases in this population are due to *Staphylococcus aureus* (Terpenning et al. 1988). Nosocomial episodes represented 14.3% of all cases of endocarditis at three hospitals in Ann Arbor, Michigan, between 1976 and 1985 (Terpenning et al. 1988).

***Pathogenesis***

The low incidence of IE is understandable when one considers that infection of the endocardium requires several unrelated factors to be present. Most important, the endocardium must be altered so that the infectious agent can adhere to it; microorganisms must be delivered to this adherent surface; and these pathogens must have surface characteristics that favor their attachment.

Our understanding of the pathogenesis of endocarditis has been greatly enhanced by the use of animal models (rats and rabbits). In animals IE seldom occurs spontaneously, or following IV inoculation of microorganisms, unless the endocardial surface has been damaged previously. Placing a polyethylene catheter across the tricuspid valve of rabbits resulted in sterile vegetations on which staphylococcal endocarditis could readily be established (Garrison et al. 1969). Subsequently, it was shown that endocarditis could be induced by performing the same maneuver on the aortic valve (Pearlman 1971). The minor trauma associated with the placement of the catheter first resulted in the production of sterile vegetations. Histologic examination of vegetations in the rabbit model showed that microorganisms are contained within a densely woven mesh of fibrin with few polymorphonuclear leukocytes within the vegetation. When viridans streptococci were injected intravenously, bacteria were detected histologically in just a few hours, and after 48 hours, 1 mg of vegetation contained as many as $10^9$ bacteria (Durack et al. 1973).

Recent studies point to fibronectin—a large glycoprotein that binds avidly to fibrin and platelets—as playing a pivotal role in the adherence of bacteria to the endocardial surface (Scheld et al. 1985; Hamill et al. 1987). Immunofluorescent studies have demonstrated that fibronectin is present in the platelet fibrin mass of patients with nonbacterial thrombotic (marantic) endocarditis. *Staphylococcus aureus* and *S. sanguis* bind more effectively to fibronectin than do gram-negative bacteria. Thrombospondin is another protein that may promote the adherence of bacteria to the endocardial surface (Herrman et al. 1991). It is a large (molecular mass 420,000) multifunctional glycoprotein stored in alpha platelet granules. Upon platelet activation, it is released into the fibrin matrix or remains bound to the platelet surface. In turn, bacteria bind to thrombospondin and may contribute to the early stages of development of endocarditis. Other factors, such as complement and protein S (vitronectin), may facilitate the adherence of bacteria to the endothelial cells themselves (Valentin-Weigand et al. 1988).

It is believed that the initial process leading to endocardial or subendocardial damage in humans is most often a valvular abnormality, either congenital or acquired, which can lead to endocardial inflammation. This occurs on the mitral, aortic, tricuspid, and pulmonary valves in descending order of frequency. This risk is directly proportional to the pressure gradient existing across these valves. The resulting inflammatory process may mimic the earliest step in the development of nonbacterial thrombotic endocarditis in animals. Infectious endocarditis can develop only when microorganisms are introduced to this surface. Transient bacteremia may develop as a result of normal daily events such as tooth-brushing or from an invasive procedure such as dental extraction or gastrointestinal (GI) or genitourinary (GU) manipulation. Bacteremia secondary to skin, soft tissue, or vascular catheter infection may also serve as the initiating event, as may direct inoculation at the time of cardiac surgery, which is the cause in early prosthetic valve endocarditis.

Since the number of bacteria that can be cultured from the gingival sulcus approaches $10^{11}$/mL of saliva, it is not surprising that activities such as tooth-brushing, chewing hard candy, or the use of oral irrigation devices (such as Waterpik) may result in bacteremia (Berger et al. 1974). Viridans streptococci are the most common bacterial species found in the blood in such circumstances. Although anaerobes are found frequently in blood following dental procedures, they cause endocarditis infrequently (Crawford et al. 1974). Among the viridans streptococci, those that produce dextran polymers on their surface are most likely to produce endocarditis. This is the same material that allows these bacteria to adhere to surfaces in the hostile environment that they find in the oral cavity.

Bacteremia occurs frequently after transurethral prostatic resection (34%), cystoscopy (19%), and urethral catheterization (7%) in the presence of infected urine. Approximately 10% of patients will have bacteremia following sigmoidoscopy or barium enema (LeFrock et al. 1973). Although anaerobic bacteria predominate in the GI and GU tracts and may outnumber coliform bacteria and enterococcus species by between 1,000 and 10,000 to 1, enterococci are the most frequent species isolated from blood following manipulation of these areas.

***Clinical manifestations***

The clinical picture of infective endocarditis is modified by the state of the heart in which the infection occurs (nature of preexisting disease and presence of prosthetic material), age of the patient, and the infecting microorganism. The initial symptoms may suggest a nonspecific, persistent, flulike illness and may include fever, chills, weakness, sweats, anorexia, malaise, or weight loss. Less frequent symptoms, which may be due to the systemic infection or to the vascular reaction, include headache, myalgia, arthralgia, abdominal pain, cough, nausea, vomiting, or edema. A heart murmur due to underlying cardiac disease is almost invariably present, and the vast majority of patients have a low-grade fever. Skin manifestations are seen in about 25% of patients, the most common being petechiae of the mucous membranes or the skin followed by splinter hemorrhages. Osler's nodes (red, tender nodules on the pulps of the fingers or toes) or Janeway spots (macular, circumscribed, erythematous lesions on the palms or soles) are less frequent. The spleen is enlarged in about one-quarter of patients, and a minority have clubbing of the digits or retinal lesions (Roth spots—small hemorrhages with a white center) (Pelletier et al. 1977). Symptoms may be minimal in older patients infected with less virulent organisms (Terpenning et al. 1987).

New symptoms and signs appear as the illness progresses. Local destruction of a valve results in an acute volume load on the myocardium that may precipitate heart failure and may be associated with a changing murmur. Other factors sometimes contributing to the occurrence of heart failure include coronary emboli, and direct involvement of the myocardium by the infection. Cerebral complications are often devastating. Mycotic aneurysms, due to infected emboli or to vasculitis of the vasovasorum, may rupture and cause massive intracerebral hemorrhage. Large emboli may cause cerebral infarcts, and there is often a relationship between these and the presence of asymptomatic mycotic aneurysms (Weinstein 1986).

Hematuria is frequent and may be due to focal embolic phenomenon or to immune mediated diffuse glomerulonephritis (Bayer et al. 1976). Septic complications involving the lungs, meninges, joints, brain, and abdominal organs are less frequent The site of the infection within the heart also modifies the manifestation of endocarditis. Right-sided endocarditis due to congenital heart disease, such as ventricular septal defect, tends to be more indolent, with a tendency to pulmonary emboli and less frequent systemic complications. Injection drug users who frequently have endocarditis on the tricuspid valve also tend to have a more indolent course and usually have septic pulmonary emboli (Hecht and Berger 1992). Certain pathogens, especially fungi, are associated with emboli to large vessels (e.g., the femoral artery). In general, the manifestations are so variable that endocarditis must enter the differential diagnosis of all cases of fever of uncertain origin and must be considered when nonspecific symptoms or signs point to involvement of joints, muscles, lungs, meninges, intra-abdominal organs, kidneys, myocardium, pericardium, or the brain. It also is part of the differential diagnosis of nonspecific illnesses suggesting connective tissue disorders, vasculitis, occult malignancy, or obscure infection.

***Diagnosis of endocarditis***

In a patient with fever, a systolic ejection murmur and two blood cultures positive for *Streptococcus sanguis*, the old adage is that this patient has endocarditis until proven otherwise. However, how do you prove it, and what is the degree of certainty that the patient has endocarditis? Durack et al. (1994) proposed a set of criteria that uses pathologic and clinical criteria to place patients with suspected endocarditis into one of three categories—definite, possible, or rejected. Definite endocarditis is said to be present using pathology-based criteria if the microorganism is cultured from a valvular vegetation, or on the basis of typical features of an infected vegetation or cardiac abscess histologically. A diagnosis of definite endocarditis can also be made clinically if there are two major, one major and three minor, or five minor criteria. These diagnostic criteria are shown in Table 14-38.

Echocardiography currently plays a key role in the management of patients with endocarditis. The echocardiogram was first used to detect vegetations on the cardiac valves of patients with endocarditis in 1973 (Parker et al. 1991). Over the years there has been considerable improvement in this technology. Two-dimensional (2-D) transthoracic or transesophageal echocardiography with color Doppler is available in most tertiary-care centers. With transesophageal echocardiography, the imaging

**Table 14-38 Major and Minor Criteria for Diagnosis of Infective Endocarditis**

*Major Criteria*

1. **Positive blood cultures for infective endocarditis:**
   a. Typical microorganism for infective endocarditis from two separate blood cultures
   b. Viridans streptococci, *Streptococcus bovis*,[a] HACEK[b] group, or community-acquired *Staphylococcus aureus* or enterococci, in the absence of a primary focus, or
   c. Persistently positive blood culture, defined as recovery of microorganism consistent with infective endocarditis from one of the following:
      (i) Blood cultures drawn more than 12 hours apart, or
      (ii) All of three or a majority of four or more separate blood cultures, with first and last drawn at least 1 hour apart
2. **Evidence of endocardial involvement:**
   a. Positive echocardiogram for infective endocarditis
      (i) Oscillating intracardiac mass on valve or supporting structures, or in the path of regurgitant jets, or on implanted material, in the absence of an alternative anatomic explanation, or
      (ii) Abscess, or
      (iii) New partial dehiscence of prosthetic valve, or
   b. New valvular regurgitation (increase or change in preexisting murmur not sufficient)
3. **Positive IgG phase 1 (≥1:800 by indirect immunofluorescence technique) antibody titer to *Coxiella burnetii*** (Fournier et al. 1996)

*Minor Criteria*

1. **Predisposition:** predisposing heart condition or injection drug use
2. **Fever:** ≥38.0 °C (100.4 °F)
3. **Vascular phenomena:** major arterial emboli, septic pulmonary infarcts, mycotic aneurysm, intracranial hemorrhage, conjunctival hemorrhages, Janeway lesions
4. **Immunologic phenomena:** glomerulonephritis, Osler's notes, Roth spots, rheumatoid factor
5. **Microbiologic evidence:** positive blood culture but not meeting major criterion as noted previously or serologic evidence of active infection with organism consistent with infective endocarditis
6. **Echocardiogram:** consistent with infective endocarditis but not meeting major criterion as noted above.

[a]Including nutritional variant strains;
Excluding single positive cultures for coagulase-negative staphylococci and organisms that do not cause endocarditis.
[b]HACEK, *Haemophilus* spp., *Actinobacillus actinomycetemcomitans, Cardiobacterium hominis, Eikenella* spp., and *Kingella kingae*.
SOURCE: Modified from Durack et al. 1994.

probe is close to the cardiac structures, and since there is no interposition of lung or bone, the image quality is superior to that obtained using transthoracic techniques.

The vegetation of bacterial endocarditis varies in size from a few millimeters to >1 cm in diameter. The typical lesion has well-defined borders and a density similar to the myocardium, is located adjacent to a leaflet, but has movement that is partially independent from that of the leaflets themselves. Vegetations can be visualized in 70% of patients with native valve endocarditis by a 2-D transthoracic examination providing that the infection is not on a prosthetic valve. With a transesophageal examination these lesions can be seen in up to 97% of patients with endocarditis, even when the infection is associated with prosthetic valves (Parker et al. 1991). Doppler examination is useful in quantifying the degree of valvular regurgitation and the change in this over time. Trans-esophageal studies can usually demonstrate ring abscesses associated with infection of the aortic valve (Daniels et al. 1991).

The role of echocardiography in the management of patients with endocarditis has evolved. At one time large vegetations >10 mm in diameter detected by echocardiography implied a poor prognosis and were considered by some experts to be an indication for valve replacement. Now it is evident that the risk of emboli is higher when the vegetation is ≥10 mm in diameter, but size alone is not an indication for valve replacement (Parker et al. 1991). All patients with infective endocarditis should undergo baseline transthoracic Doppler echocardiography. Repeat examinations should be limited to patients with important valve or ventricular dysfunction on the initial study, new murmurs, persistent fever, conduction defects, or embolic phenomena (Parker et al. 1991). Transesophageal echocardiography is best reserved for patients with prosthetic valve endocarditis, for those with suspected valve ring or intraventricular abscesses, and for patients in whom the transthoracic exam failed to show vegetations (with good clinical evidence of endocarditis) or was technically unsatisfactory. The Duke criteria specify the echocardiographic features that are needed for the diagnosis of endocarditis (Table 14-38).

### *Treatment of endocarditis*

The treatment of endocarditis includes the administration of the optimal antimicrobial in the appropriate dosage for the correct duration. However, many other factors should be considered in the management of a patient with endocarditis (Table 14-39). A knowledge of the complications of this illness, their investigation, and their treatment is necessary. In addition, patients with endocarditis often have serious preexisting valvular disease, and other comorbidities that may be worsened by the endocarditis. Since about half of the patients with endocarditis will require cardiac surgery as part of the management of their illness, it is necessary to know the indications for such surgery.

Endocarditis is among the most difficult of infections to treat with antimicrobials. The causative organisms are metabolically inactive, deeply embedded within the vegetation's matrix, contained within abscess cavities or densely adherent to a prosthetic device, and protected from the host's natural defense mechanisms. Therapy of bacterial endocarditis therefore requires the prolonged use of bactericidal agents alone or in combination. Removal of prosthetic material and drainage of large abscesses, if present, are often necessary for cure. Combinations of antibiotics may be used with one or more of the following goals in mind:

- To effect a more rapid clinical response
- To shorten the duration of antimicrobial therapy
- To overcome bacterial tolerance
- To change otherwise bacteriostatic agents into a bactericidal combination
- To provide a broader spectrum of antimicrobial coverage during initial empiric therapy

Antimicrobial treatment of bacterial endocarditis most frequently is with a $\beta$-lactam antibiotic, either alone or in combination with an aminoglycoside. This combination is usually synergistic, since the $\beta$-lactam facilitates the penetration of the aminoglycoside into the bacteria by virtue of its effect on the cell wall (peptidoglycan layer). In patients with endocarditis due to gram-positive bacteria, such as methicillin-resistant *S. aureus* and coagulase-negative staphylococci, where $\beta$-lactams are not effective, vancomycin is usually used. In those circumstances where an aminoglycoside is used in combination with a $\beta$-lactam, gentamicin has emerged as the aminoglycoside of choice except for the therapy of endocarditis due to *Pseudomonas* spp. Enterococci can be highly resistant to gentamicin by virtue of their ability to produce aminoglycoside-inactivating enzymes. Some of these gentamicin-resistant enterococci will be susceptible to streptomycin. Other aminoglycosides such as tobramycin and amikacin are also usually inactive against these highly resistant strains.

Although recommendations relating to the optimal duration of antibiotic therapy for bacterial endocarditis have been published, there is always a need to individualize therapy. A prolonged duration of symptoms before diagnosis, the presence of an abscess or a prosthetic device, unusual or more resistant microorganisms, or the inability to use the optimal antibiotic(s) in recommended dosage may necessitate more prolonged therapy.

Early discharge of patients with continuation of parenteral antibiotics at home has been used for some patients with endocarditis. Although there is little reason to believe that the efficacy of the antibiotics themselves might be reduced, complications may rise at home that may require immediate intervention, such as major embolic events, arrhythmias or the sudden onset of congestive heart failure (CHF). The risk of such occurrences needs to be balanced with the advantages of early discharge, and candidates for home antibiotics should be carefully selected.

The treatment of right-sided *S. aureus* endocarditis in injection drug users has undergone changes as a result of

**Table 14-39 Principles of Management of Endocarditis**

1. Establish a microbiologic diagnosis
2. Use appropriate antibiotics in optimal doses
3. Search for a portal of entry of the bacteria
4. Monitor daily for complications including congestive heart failure, conduction abnormalities, dysrhythmias, renal and neurological dysfunction
5. Monitor therapy:
   (a) Antibiotic plasma concentration
   (b) Antimicrobial susceptibility testing
   (c) Repeat blood cultures if prolonged fever
6. Avoid nosocomial infections, especially intravenous line-related infection and urinary catheters
7. Instruct patient regarding prophylaxis against endocarditis
8. Obtain follow-up blood cultures 2–4 weeks following completion of antibiotic therapy
9. Consult cardiovascular surgery for all patients with prosthetic valve endocarditis

recent trials. Three prospective, nonrandomized trials summarized by DiNubile et al. (1994) support the use of a 2-week course of a penicillinase-resistant penicillin plus an aminoglycoside to treat uncomplicated right-sided endocarditis caused by methicillin-susceptible *S. aureus* in this group of patients. Heldman et al. (1996) randomized injection drug users with *S. aureus* right-sided endocarditis to oral therapy with ciprofloxacin 750 mg b.i.d. plus rifampin 300 mg b.i.d for 28 days, or intravenous therapy with oxacillin 2 g every 4 hours or vancomycin 1 g every 12 hours (for penicillin-allergic patients) plus gentamicin for the first 5 days. Forty-four subjects (treatment route: oral 19, IV 25) received 28 days of inpatient treatment with the assigned antibiotics. There were four treatment failures, 1 out of 19 in the group receiving oral antibiotics, and 3 out of 25 in the group beginning with 5 days of IV antibiotics. Drug toxicity was more common in the IV-treated group—largely increases in liver enzymes. This study suggests that for selected patients with right-sided, methicillin-susceptible *S. aureus* endocarditis, oral ciprofloxacin plus rifampin is effective (Heldman et al. 1996).

### *Empiric therapy*

Although it is usually recommended that antibiotics be withheld until a microbiologic diagnosis has been made, empiric use of antibiotics may be desirable. In many circumstances it is necessary to make a "best guess" based on the most likely causative organism in the particular clinical setting. General recommendations such as those in Table 14-40 cannot take into account all the factors that might influence the choice and dosage of antibiotics but rather should serve as a guide. Therapy can be modified when culture and susceptibility data are available. Once these data are available, the recommendations of the American Heart Association Council should be followed (Wilson et al. 1995).

### *Management of complications*

There are many complications that may arise during the treatment of infective endocarditis. These are commonly divided into cardiac and extracardiac (Table 14-41) complications. In one large series only one-fourth of the patients with endocarditis were free of complications (Mansur et al. 1992).

**HEART FAILURE** Heart failure complicates the course of 15 to 65% of patients with endocarditis, and it is the leading cause of death among these patients (Wilson et al. 1982). If heart failure has resulted from sudden onset of severe valvular insufficiency or obstruction, urgent valve replacement is necessary. Otherwise it can be treated medically, with valve replacement considered for unresponsive cases.

**VALVE RING ABSCESS/VALVE DEHISCENCE** A valve ring abscess complicates 50 to 87% of cases of PVE (Mayor et al. 1982). These abscesses are much more common with porcine heterografts than with mechanical valves. Since the abscess involves the annulus to which the valve is sutured, valve dehiscence is a common finding. Valve ring abscesses also occur with native valve endocarditis. In one autopsy series, 24 out of 59 (41%)

**Table 14-40 Suggested Antibiotic Regimens for the Initial Treatment of Suspected Bacterial Endocarditis before the Availability of Blood Culture Results**

| Clinical Setting | Suggested Therapy[a] | Cost (AWP) ($/day)[b] | Microorganisms Treated |
|---|---|---|---|
| Native valve—*S. aureus* unlikely | Ampicillin sodium 2 g IV q4h plus<br>Gentamicin sulfate 1 mg/kg/q8h (not to exceed 80 mg) | Generic $28<br>Generic $4 | Viridans streptococci, *S. bovis* and enterococci, HACEK group |
| Native valve—*S. aureus* likely[c] | Nafcillin sodium 2 g IV q4h plus<br>Gentamicin sulfate 1 mg/kg/q8h (not to exceed 80 mg for 7 days only) | Generic $38<br>Generic $4 | *S. aureus,* Streptococci (not enterococci) |
| Prosthetic valve endocarditis | Vancomycin HCl 15 mg/kg q12h IV plus<br>Gentamicin sulfate 1 mg/kg/q8h IV (not to exceed 80 mg) | Generic $46<br>Generic $4 | *S. aureus* (methicillin susceptible and resistant) and coagulase negative streptococci |
| | Rifampin 300 mg PO q12h | Rimactane $3 | Streptococci and enterococci |

[a]Dosages may need adjustment for renal impairment.
[b]Source of drug prices is *Mosby's GenR$_x$* 1998. Current prices may vary from those quoted, but comparative prices among products are expected to be similar. The reader should check on local prices at the time of prescribing.
[c]Injection drug user, nosocomial acquisition, postoperative.
ABBREVIATIONS: AWP, average wholesale price. HACEK, a group of slow growing, fastidious gram-negative microorganisms that includes *Hemophilus aphrophilus, Actinobacillus actinomycetemcomitans, Cardiobacterium hominis, Eikenella* spp., *Kingella* spp.

**Table 14-41 Complications of Infective Endocarditis**

*Cardiac complications*
1. Heart failure
2. Intraventricular septal abscess
3. Ventricular septal defect
4. Myocarditis
5. Pericarditis
6. Myocardial infarction
7. Complications unique to prosthetic valve endocarditis
   (a) Acute mechanical obstruction of the valve
   (b) Valve embolization
   (c) Valve dehiscence
8. Valve ring abscess

*Noncardiac complications*
1. Emboli
2. Intracranial hemorrhage
3. Seizures
4. Encephalopathy
5. Acute neuropathy
6. Metastatic infection
7. Mycotic aneurysm
8. Immune complex glomerulonephritis
9. Multiorgan failure
10. Prolonged fever
11. Relapse of the infection

patients with aortic valve endocarditis had a ring abscess (Arnett and Roberts 1976). The following features were predictive of valve ring abscess: infection of the aortic valve; recent valvular regurgitation, pericarditis, high degree of AV block, short duration of symptoms leading to severe debility or death (Arnett and Roberts 1976).

**EMBOLI** Emboli are almost a universal complication of endocarditis. At autopsy, 56% of kidneys, 60% of coronary arteries, 44% of spleens, and 30% of brains of patients with endocarditis had emboli (Weinstein 1986). Emboli to the CNS are the most important clinically; indeed they account for 50% of the neurologic complications of endocarditis. Ninety percent of these emboli lodge in the middle cerebral artery distribution (Selky and Ross 1992), and recurrent embolization is usually considered an indication for valve replacement (Selley and Ross 1992). Some workers have refined this indication to recurrence of embolization despite 48 to 72 hours of appropriate antibiotic therapy, especially if associated with a large vegetation on echocardiography (Reed et al. 1985). The incidence rate of emboli is highest with *S. aureus* endocarditis, with a rate that is 2.4 times than of viridans streptococcal endocarditis (Steckelbert et al. 1992). The incidence of emboli is highest during the first week of antimicrobial therapy (13/1000 patient days) falling 10-fold (to 1.2/1000 patient days) after the second week of antimicrobial therapy (Steckelberg 1992).

**MYCOTIC ANEURYSM** This is an uncommon but often devastating complication of IE. Thirty-two patients with mycotic aneurysms were seen at the Mayo Clinic from 1963 to 1979 (Wilson et al. 1982). The aorta, cerebral arteries, visceral arteries, and arteries of the lower and upper extremities are involved in descending order of frequency; 23% of patients have multiple aneurysms. Severe, unrelenting localized headache in a patient with endocarditis suggests the possibility of an intracranial aneurysm. A cranial CT scan followed by angiography and neurosurgical consultation represents appropriate management.

**MULTIORGAN FAILURE** This complication is not usually identified in reviews of endocarditis. However, it is often the reason for death in patients who have had a complicated course and who have done poorly following cardiac surgery to replace the infected valves. The respiratory, renal, gastrointestinal, and central nervous systems are most commonly involved.

**PROLONGED FEVER** Three recent studies (Douglas et al. 1986; Blumberg et al. 1992; Lederman et al. 1992) have examined the duration of fever in patients with infective endocarditis. Most patients (up to 70%) with endocarditis were afebrile by the end of the first week of therapy (Douglas et al. 1986; Lederman et al. 1992). The most common cause for continued fever was infection of the valve ring (Douglas et al. 1986). Rarely, pulmonary emboli or drug allergy was responsible (Douglas et al. 1986). Evidence of microvascular phenomena (splinter hemorrhages, mucosal or conjunctival petechiae, Roth spots, Osler's node, Janeway lesions) and large vessel embolization were associated with prolonged fever in the study by Lederman and colleagues (1992).

Infections due to *S. aureus* or *P. aeruginosa* were associated with a mean of 9.1 and 12.3 days of fever (after initiation of antibiotic therapy) respectively, compared with 2.9 days for infections due to enterococci, 3.0 for viridans streptococci, and 3.9 days for coagulase-negative staphylococci. Blumberg and coworkers (1992) performed a case-control study wherein they compared 26 patients with 27 episodes of endocarditis with prolonged fever (temperature of ≥100.4°F for ≥2 weeks) with 26 patients with endocarditis without prolonged fever. Cardiac infection caused prolonged fever in 13 patients, 7 of whom had myocardial abscesses; 16 of the cases required cardiac surgery compared with 2 of the controls ($P < 0.001$).

Twenty-two of the cases (85%) developed nosocomial complications compared with five of the controls ($P < 0.001$). An approach to prolonged fever emerges from these three studies. When fever persists for more than 1 week, initiate a thorough investigation. It is necessary to first rule out extension of valvular infection into an adjacent cardiac structure. A transesophageal echocardiogram is the most sensitive investigation for this purpose. Consider metastatic spread of the infection with abscess formation; drug fever; nosocomial infection (the most common cause of which is infection related to the intravenous line) and other underlying illnesses such as malignancy or vasculitis.

**LONG-TERM COMPLICATIONS** The relapse rate of endocarditis is about 2.7%, and about 4.5% of patients have later recurrent episodes (Tornos et al. 1992). Late cardiac surgery is required for up to 47% of patients treated medically. Mycotic aneurysms and emboli may occur many months following cure of the endocarditis.

### *Surgical treatment of endocarditis*

From the foregoing it is evident that surgery is frequently necessary for the successful treatment of endocarditis. All patients with prosthetic valve endocarditis should be managed in conjunction with a cardiac surgeon. The indications for urgent cardiac surgery in patients with active endocarditis are given in Table 14-42. When indicated, surgery can be performed at any time during the course of endocarditis. For many patients timing of the surgery is most important. This requires experience, good judgment, and ongoing cardiological assessment. Unnecessary delay of surgery impairs the outcome. Moderate-to-severe CHF from valve dysfunction accounts for 90% of the indications for surgery in endocarditis. The availability of human homograft valves has changed the operative approach to endocarditis involving the aortic valve and the aortic root. Porcine and mechanical prostheses still have a place in the management of endocarditis and are usually combined with repairs, using endogenous pericardium and, rarely, prosthetic patch devices.

**Table 14-42 Indications for Urgent Cardiac Surgery in Patients with Active Infective Endocarditis**

1. Hemodynamic compromise
   (a) Severe heart failure
   (b) Valvular obstruction
2. Uncontrolled infection
   (a) Fungal endocarditis
   (b) Abscess formation (e.g., intraventricular septum)
3. Unstable prosthesis
4. Recurrent systemic embolism

The patient with treated endocarditis and valvular stenosis or insufficiency with intact annular skeletal structures presents little difficulty surgically. The approach is to replace the affected valve or valves with a suitable prosthetic device, and usually, no further surgical intervention is required. These patients have a low incidence of reinfection and do well long term. The real surgical challenge is the patient with ongoing sepsis who requires urgent intervention for acute heart failure subsequent to valvular destruction and who may have destruction of annular and other contiguous tissue. These patients require aggressive débridement of all infected tissue, which may well involve débridement of part of the ventricular septum, the valvular annulus, the sinus of valsalva, or free wall or septal abscesses. A variety of surgical approaches have been used to effect such débridement and repair.

The principles of surgical treatment of endocarditis are those of surgical treatment of sepsis in general. One must be aggressive in the débridement of all infected and destroyed tissues and be prepared to replace these tissues with suitable substitutes. Once the surgical repair has been completed, the postoperative follow-up of the patient must be done in close cooperation with an infectious disease specialist, as well as a cardiologist. These patients require aggressive continuing antibiotic therapy postoperatively, as well as careful monitoring with regard to further infection and/or valvular deterioration.

## Management of Tuberculosis

Tuberculosis was a disappearing disease in North America until the early 1980s. However, the spread of HIV infection has changed that. From 1985 to 1992 there was an increase in the number of cases of tuberculosis reported in the United States, and most of these cases were in New York, New Jersey, Texas, Florida, and California (Cantwell et al. 1994). The other major change in the epidemiology of tuberculosis has been the emergence of multidrug-resistant disease. Factors contributing to this problem in the United States include inadequate public health resources to meet increased needs (Frieden et al. 1993) and unstable living conditions for many of the patients (especially in the homeless injection drug users, many with coexistent HIV infection). In this setting of altered immunity, mycobacterial loads are high, resulting in increased rates of spontaneous random mutations leading to drug resistance (Iseman 1993). Poor compliance with therapy or decreased absorption of antituberculous agents in HIV patients with gastrointestinal disease are additional factors leading to multidrug-resistant tuberculosis (Barnes et al. 1991). Multidrug-resistant TB (MDR-TB) refers to resistance to at least INE and rifampin.

***Clinical manifestations***

Since *M. tuberculosis* grows slowly, pulmonary TB frequently develops insidiously. Low-grade fever, night sweats, malaise and weight loss are classic systemic symptoms. Cough, often with mild hemoptysis and pleuritic chest pain, are the usual pulmonary symptoms. There may be no abnormalities on chest examination, but crackles and a pleural friction rub over involved areas can often be heard on auscultation (listen over apices!).

There are two forms of tuberculosis—primary and secondary (reactivation). Primary TB is usually a disease of infants and children. However, in countries where large numbers of adults have not been infected with TB, primary infection is also seen in the adult population. Hilar or paratracheal lymph node enlargement with or without a parenchymal infiltrate is a characteristic finding in primary TB. Reactivation TB is the most commonly seen form of the disease. Under certain circumstances (immunosuppression, increasing age, malnutrition) dormant and immunologically contained bacteria from the primary infection can begin to multiply and cause disease. Here the lesions are in the apical or posterior segments of the upper lobes or superior segment of the lower lobe.

Tuberculosis is transmitted by airborne spread from person to person via infected respiratory secretions (Riley 1974). Those with laryngeal TB or with pulmonary cavitation are most infectious.

***Diagnosis of tuberculosis***

The gold standard is isolation of *M. tuberculosis* from sputum or other specimens. A positive acid-fast stain of a sputum specimen in the appropriate clinical setting can lead to a rapid diagnosis of TB. It is important to remember that a positive acid-fast smear is not specific for *M. tuberculosis* and that a variety of mycobacteria, both pathogenic and nonpathogenic species, and *Nocardia* spp. are also acid-fast. The tuberculin skin test can be used to identify persons infected with *M. tuberculosis*.

Tuberculin skin (Mantoux) testing has three principal indications—diagnosis of infection, diagnosis of disease, and as an epidemiological tool. It should not be performed on persons with severe blistering tuberculin reactions in the past; patients with documented active TB; patients with extensive burns or eczema; or patients with infections or vaccinations with live virus vaccines (e.g., mumps or measles) in the past month. False-negative tests occur, especially in the seriously ill who are often anergic (Huebner 1995). It is noteworthy that only 37% of patients recognize a positive test, so do not rely on patients' recall of the test result (Huebner 1995). Test results may vary by 15% between arms and by 15% between different observers (Huebner 1995). The Mantoux test is read at 48 to 72 hours following intradermal inoculation, by measuring the widest diameter of induration (not erythema).

A positive test varies with the clinical setting. Less than 5 mm induration is a negative reaction indicating no infection with *M. tuberculosis*. If there has been recent exposure to TB and the test is negative it should be repeated in 12 weeks. Induration of ≥5 mm is considered positive, in HIV-positive patients, in recent contacts of known TB cases, and in those with an abnormal chest radiograph compatible with TB. Induration of ≥10 mm is positive in persons who do not meet the above criteria but who belong to one of the following groups:

- Injection drug users known to be HIV seronegative
- Persons with conditions that have been reported to increase the risk for progressing from latent TB to active TB, including diabetes mellitus, conditions requiring corticosteroids or other immunosuppressive therapy, some hematological malignancies, silicosis, gastrectomy, jejunoileal bypass, ≥10% below ideal body weight
- Residents and employees of prisons, jails, nursing homes, health care facilities
- Immigrants (within 5 years) from countries having a high prevalence of TB

Induration of ≥15 mm is positive in persons who do not meet any of the above criteria.

Among children vaccinated with bacille Calmette–Guérin (BCG) in infancy, 7.9% had a significant reaction 10 to 25 years later compared with 18% for those vaccinated between 1 and 5 years of age, and 25.4% for those vaccinated after 5 years of age (Menzies and Vissandjee 1992). Thus, in general, a positive Mantoux >10 years after BCG vaccination should not be attributed to the vaccine. Reactivity to tuberculin antigen can diminish to nonreactivity with age. However, repeat TB skin testing may boost this reactivity. Thus, it is important in certain populations (e.g., nursing home residents, health care workers) who are going to have serial testing, to determine those whose response has waned over time. This is done by using the two-step test. A second test dose is administered 2 to 3 weeks after the first (Menzies et al. 1994). The following groups of individuals should receive a Mantoux test.

- Those with signs or symptoms of tuberculosis, or a history of previous TB

- Recent contacts of known TB cases
- Those with abnormal chest radiograph compatible with TB
- HIV-infected persons
- Those with medical conditions that increase the risk of TB (silicosis, gastrectomy, diabetes, immunosuppressive therapy, lymphomas)
- Groups at high risk of recent infection with *M. tuberculosis* (personnel and residents of nursing homes, prisons, some hospitals, immigrants from Asia, Latin America, Africa, Oceania)

A positive Mantoux test should prompt a chest radiograph. If this is negative, preventative therapy with Isoniazid (INH) should be considered. The reason for this is that among immunocompetent hosts, TB infection acquired in childhood progresses to active disease at some time during life in 10% of those infected (Comstock et al. 1994). Of Mantoux-positive HIV-infected drug users, 7 to 10% per year developed TB (Selwyn et al. 1989).

For prevention of the development of clinical disease in Mantoux-positive patients, INH 5 to 10 mg per kg, not to exceed 300 mg per day, is given for 6 to 9 months in adults, or 9 months in children. HIV-positive persons should receive INH for 12 months. When considering preventive therapy, the risk of hepatotoxicity due to INH must be considered. Because this toxicity is age-related (Kopanoff et al. 1978), INH preventative therapy is not routinely offered to those who are older than 35 years. A full course of INH therapy is effective, resulting in reduction in rates of tuberculosis as high as 70% (Ferebee et al. 1963). For those who are Mantoux-positive following exposure to a patient with INH-resistant TB, use rifampin 600 mg/day as preventative therapy. For those exposed to INH- and rifampin-resistant TB and who are Mantoux-positive, no effective preventive therapy regimens have been established (Miller 1993). Combination therapy with two drugs to which the organism is likely to be susceptible is recommended. Such combinations include pyrazinamide and ethambutol; pyrazinamide and a quinolone; or ethambutol and a quinolone (Villarino et al. 1992).

### *Treatment of active tuberculosis*

Treatment of active infection due to tuberculosis has two aims: to cure the infection in the patient, and to prevent spread to others.

**PREVENTION OF SPREAD** Health care facilities should have appropriately ventilated isolation rooms and written policies for preventing transmission of TB (Dooley et al. 1990; Miller 1993). All persons with known or suspected TB should be hospitalized in an isolation room and placed on respiratory (airborne) precautions. Isolation may be discontinued when three consecutive sputum smears are negative for AFB on 3 different days, and after the patient has received effective therapy and is improving clinically (CDC 1994b). This usually takes 2 to 3 weeks. If the patient is infected with resistant *M. tuberculosis*, isolation should be maintained throughout hospitalization because of the tendency for treatment failure (Dooley et al. 1990; CDC 1994b). Personnel respirators (surgical masks are not adequate) should be provided by health care facilities and worn by persons in the same room with a patient with known or suspected TB. These devices should also be worn when performing procedures (such as bronchoscopy) that are likely to produce bursts of droplets. Wearers should be trained in the use and disposal of personal respirators (Dooley et al. 1990). The health department should be notified of all cases of TB so that contact tracing can be carried out.

**DRUG TREATMENT OF ACTIVE TUBERCULOSIS** The CDC recommendations and those of the American Thoracic Society for the initial treatment of TB are given in Tables 14-43 to 14-45 (CDC 1993a; Bass et al. 1994). The treatment of multidrug-resistant (MDR) TB is outlined in Table 14-46 (Iseman 1993). The treatment of multidrug-resistant TB is so difficult that such patients should be managed by those with expertise in this field. If there is any doubt about compliance with therapy, implement twice weekly directly observed therapy (Table 14-43). In one study only 77% of patients completed a recommended course of therapy within 12 months (Block et al. 1994). This is one of the reasons for the rise in MDR-TB. Directly observed therapy is bringing rising rates of TB under control (Chaulk and Pope 1997; Fujiusara et al. 1977).

### *Vaccination against tuberculosis?*

In the United States, BCG vaccination is recommended for: tuberculin-negative infants and children who have continuing exposure to INH- and rifampin-resistant active TB; those who cannot take INH and have ongoing exposure to a case of infectious TB; or those who belong to groups with rates of new *M. tuberculosis* exceeding 1% per year (Colditz et al. 1994). However, the emergence of multidrug-resistant TB and institutional outbreaks of this infection have led to consideration of broadened use of BCG vaccine in the United States (CDC 1991). In a meta-analysis of the efficacy of BCG vaccine, Coldiz and coworkers (1994) reviewed 70 articles and included 14 pro-

Table 14-43 Regimen Options for the Initial Treatment of Tuberculosis among Children and Adults

| TB without HIV infection | | | TB with HIV infection |
|---|---|---|---|
| *Option 1*—**local INH resistance <4%.** Administer daily INH, RIF, and PZA for 8 weeks followed by 16 weeks of INH and RIF daily or 2–3 times/week.[a] EMB or SM should be added to the initial regimen until susceptibility to INH and RIF is demonstrated. Continue treatment for at least 6 months and 3 months beyond culture conversion. Consult a TB medical expert if the patient is symptomatic or smear or culture positive after 3 months. | *Option 2*—**local INH resistance >4%.** Administer daily INH, RIF, PZA, and SM or EMB for 2 weeks followed by 2 times/week.[a] Administration of the same drugs for 6 weeks (by DOT), and subsequently, with 2 times/week administration of INH and RIF for 16 weeks (by DOT). Consult a TB medical expert if the patient is symptomatic or smear or culture positive after 3 months. | *Option 3*—**DOT** Treat by DOT, 3 times/week[a] with INH, RIF, PZA, and EMB or SM for 6 months.[b] Consult a TB medical expert if the patient is symptomatic or smear or culture positive after 3 months. | Options 1, 2 or 3 can be used, but treatment regimens should continue for a total of 9 months and at least 6 months beyond culture conversion. |

[a]All regimens administered 2 times/week or 3 times/week should be monitored by DOT for the duration of therapy.
[b]The strongest evidence from clinical trials is the effectiveness of all four drugs administered for the full 6 months. There is weaker evidence that SM can be discontinued after 4 months if the isolate is susceptible to all drugs. The evidence for stopping PZA before the end of the 6 months is equivocal for the 3 times/week regimen, and there is no evidence on the effectiveness of this regimen with EMB for less than the full 6 months.
ABBREVIATIONS: DOT, directly observed therapy; EMB, ethambutol; INH, isoniazid; PZA, pyrazinamide; RIF, rifampin; SM, streptomycin.
SOURCE: CDC 1993a.

spective trials and 12 case-control studies in the analysis. They concluded that BCG vaccination reduced the risk of TB by 50%. Age at vaccination did not enhance protectiveness of BCG. Protection against tuberculous death, meningitis, and disseminated TB cases is higher than the protection rate for total TB cases. They concluded, however, that misclassification of disease may have led to the last-mentioned finding (Colditz et al. 1994).

Table 14-44 Dosage Recommended for the Initial Treatment of Tuberculosis among Children[a] and Adults

| | Dosage | | | | | |
|---|---|---|---|---|---|---|
| | Daily | | 2 Times/Week | | 3 Times/Week | |
| Drugs | Children | Adults | Children | Adults | Children | Adults |
| Isoniazid | 10–20 mg/kg<br>Max. 300 mg | 5 mg/kg<br>Max. 300 mg | 20–40 mg/kg<br>Max. 900 mg | 15 mg/kg<br>Max. 900 mg | 20–40 mg/kg<br>Max. 900 mg | 15 mg/kg<br>Max. 900 mg |
| Rifampin | 10–20 mg/kg<br>Max. 600 mg | 10 mg/kg<br>Max. 500 mg | 10–20 mg/kg<br>Max. 600 mg | 10 mg/kg<br>Max. 600 mg | 10–20 mg/kg<br>Max. 600 mg | 10 mg/kg<br>Max. 600 mg |
| Pyrazinamide | 15–30 mg/kg<br>Max. 2 g | 15–30 mg/kg<br>Max. 2 g | 50–70 mg/kg<br>Max. 4 g | 50–70 mg/kg<br>Max. 4 g | 50–70 mg/kg<br>Max. 3 g | 50–70 mg/kg<br>Max. 3 g |
| Ethambutol[b] | 15–25 mg/kg<br>Max. 2.5 g | 5–25 mg/kg<br>Max. 2.5 g | 50 mg/kg<br>Max. 2.5 g | 50 mg/kg<br>Max. 2.5 g | 25–30 mg/kg<br>Max. 2.5 g | 25–30 mg/kg<br>Max. 2.5 g |
| Streptomycin | 20–30 mg/kg<br>Max. 1 g | 15 mg/kg<br>Max. 1 g | 25–30 mg/kg<br>Max. 1.5 g | 25–30 mg/kg<br>Max. 1.5 g | 25–30 mg/kg<br>Max. 1 g | 25–30 mg/kg<br>Max. 1 g |

[a]Children ≤12 years of age.
[b]Ethambutol is generally not recommended for children whose visual activity cannot be monitored (<6 years of age). However, ethambutol should be considered for all children with organisms resistant to other drugs, when susceptibility to ethambutol has been demonstrated, or susceptibility is likely.
SOURCE: *Morbidity and Mortality Weekly Report* (CDC 1993a).

Table 14-45 Second-Line Antituberculosis Drugs

| Drug | Dosage Forms | Daily Dose in Children and Adults[a] | Maximal Daily Dose in Children and Adults[a] | Major Adverse Reaction | Recommended Regular Monitoring |
|---|---|---|---|---|---|
| Capreomycin | Vials: 1 g | 15 to 10 mg/kg IM | 1 g | Auditory, vestibular, and renal toxicity | Vestibular function, audiometry, BUN, and creatine |
| Kanamycin | Vials: 75 mg<br>500 mg<br>1 g | 15 to 30 mg/kg IM | 1 g | Auditory and renal toxicity, rare vestibular toxicity | Vestibular function, audiometry, BUN, and creatine |
| Ethionamide | Tablets: 250 mg | 15 to 20 mg/kg PO | 1 g | Gastrointestinal disturbance, hypersensitivity, hematoxicity | |
| *p*-Aminosalicylic acid | Tablets: 500 mg<br>1 g<br>Bulk powder<br>Delayed-release granules | 150 mg/kg PO | 12 g | Gastrointestinal disturbance, hypersensitivity, hematoxicity, sodium load | Hepatic enzymes |
| Cycloserine | Capsules: 250 mg | 15 to 20 mg/kg PO | 1 g | Psychosis, convulsion, rash | Assessment of mental status |

[a]Doses based on weight should be adjusted as weight changes.
ABBREVIATION: BUN, blood urea nitrogen.

## Management of Malaria

Malaria is a protozoan (genus *Plasmodium*) infection transmitted by the bite of an infected female *Anopheles* mosquito and rarely via a contaminated blood transfusion. It is extremely common, affecting more than 500 million persons and resulting in more than 1 million deaths each year.

There are four species of the genus *Plasmodium* that cause malaria in man. These are *P. falciparum*, *P. vivax*, *P. ovale*, and *P. malariae*. From a clinical standpoint one must be able to distinguish between *P. falciparum* and non *falciparum* (all the others) malaria. The reasons for this approach are that *P. falciparum* malaria is often chloroquine resistant, and almost all malaria deaths are due to this species. The severity of *P. falciparum* malaria is due to the parasites' ability to invade red cells of all ages and not just young red cells (as for the other species of malaria), and to the release of more *P. falciparum* merozoites than with other species. Each infected hepatocyte releases 30,000 merozoites of *P. falciparum* compared with 10,000

Table 14-46 Suggested Regimens for Patients with Multidrug-Resistant *M. tuberculosis*

| Resistance Pattern | Treatment | Duration |
|---|---|---|
| INH, SM, PZA | Rif, PZA, EM, amikacin[a] | 9 mos |
| INH, EM (±SM) | Rif, PZA, oflox or cipro, amikacin[a] | 6–12 mos |
| INH, Rif (±SM) | PZA, EM, oflox or cipro, amikacin[a] | 18–24 mos, consider surgery[b] |
| INH, Rif, EM (±SM) | PZA, oflox or cipro, amikacin,[a] plus 2 others[c] | 24 mos after conversion,[d] consider surgery |
| INH, Rif, PZA (±SM) | EM, oflox or cipro, amikacin[a] plus 2 others[c] | 24 mos after conversion, consider surgery |
| INH, Rif, PZA, EM (±SM) | Oflox or cipro, amikacin[a] plus 3 others[c] | 24 mos after conversion, consider surgery |

[a]Capreomycin may be used if there is resistance to amikacin sulfate.
[b]Surgery may be required to resect nonhealing cavitary lesions.
[c]May choose from ethionamide, cycloserine, or *p*-aminosalicylic acid.
[d]Refers to conversion to sputum smear and culture from positive to negative.
ABBREVIATIONS: Cipro, ciprofloxacin; EM, ethambutol HCl; INH, isoniazid; Oflox, ofloxacin; mos, months; PZA, pyrazinamide; Rif, rifampin; SM, streptomycin sulfate.
SOURCE: Iseman 1993 with permission.

for *P. vivax* and 15,000 for *P. ovale* and *P. malariae* (White and Brennan 1998).

### *Epidemiology*

Malaria (so-called because in the Pontine marshes outside Rome, bad air (*mal aria*) was thought to be the cause of the disease) occurs in most tropical areas of the world. *Plasmodium falciparum* predominates in Africa, New Guinea, and Haiti, whereas *Plasmodium vivax* predominates in the Indian subcontinent and Central America. These two species are almost equal in prevalence in South America, East Asia, and Oceania. Changing global climate conditions have had an effect on the epidemiology of malaria. Malaria cases increased by one-third in the year following an El Niño event, and malaria mortality and morbidity increased an average of 36% in Venezuela in years following an El Niño event (Bourna and Dye 1997).

As a result of rapid worldwide travel, imported malaria can be present in countries that do not have indigenous malaria. Malaria was endemic throughout much of the United States in the nineteenth and early twentieth centuries (Zucker 1996). There have been three outbreaks of locally acquired malaria in the United States in the 1990s (Zucker 1996). Thus every physician regardless of practice location should be familiar with the diagnosis and treatment of malaria. Diagnosis of malaria is often delayed, resulting in an increase in mortality (Kean and Reilly 1976). Indeed there was a 24-fold higher case-fatality rate from malaria for patients treated in civilian hospitals compared with those treated in military or Veterans Administration hospitals (Walzer et al. 1974). Currently about 1000 cases of imported malaria occur in the United States each year, and there are 700 cases per year in Canada (Keystone 1997). The Canadian rate is 4 to 5 times higher than the U.S. rate on a per capita basis, reflecting the higher rate of immigration to Canada from malarious areas.

It is instructive to review the 1994 U.S. malaria surveillance data (Kachur et al. 1997). There were 1014 cases diagnosed, a 20% decrease from the 1275 cases reported for 1993. *P. vivax*, *P. falciparum*, *P. malariae*, and *P. ovalae* accounted for 44, 44, 4 and 3% of the cases, respectively. In 5%, the infecting species was not determined. Of the U.S. civilians who acquired malaria while travelling to a foreign country, 18% had followed a recommended chemoprophylactic drug regimen. Four deaths were attributed to malaria.

### *Malaria life cycle*

**MALARIAL PARASITE DEVELOPMENT IN THE ANOPHELES MOSQUITO** The mosquito ingests blood from an infected human. The parasite then undergoes a life cycle in the mosquito; this is known as *sporogony*. The sexual cycle takes place only in mosquitoes. The gametocytes are ingested and mature in the stomach into male and female gametes. The male cells exflagellate, producing 8 long, thin, mobile flagella or microgametes that break away from the parent body. One microgamete penetrates a female cell and fertilizes it. The male and female nuclei fuse and the *ookinete* so formed grows larger and becomes very active, eventually piercing an epithelial cell wall below the lining membrane and secreting a cyst wall around itself. The nucleus undergoes mitotic division around which cytoplasma condenses to produce large numbers of the infective parasite forms or *sporozoites*. After about 1 to 2 weeks the cyst ruptures, and the sporozoites are discharged into the hemocele and invade all parts of the insect, some eventually reaching the acinar cells of the salivary glands. This entire process takes 5 to 15 days in the mosquito. When the insect bites, the sporozoites penetrate the cell membrane and are injected with the acinar fluid (saliva) into the human host. The sporozoites enter small blood vessels and remain in circulation for <1 hour.

**LIFE CYCLE IN HUMANS** Sporozoites enter the circulation from the bite of an infected mosquito. There are two phases to malarial parasite development in humans, the exoerythrocytic and the erythrocytic. *Exoerythrocytic schizogony* takes place in the liver. On entering the hepatocyte the sporozoite rounds up, and the nucleus undergoes repeated division. Over 6 to 16 days the exoerythrocytic schizont matures and divides to produce small single nucleated *merozoites*. The liver cell ruptures, and the merozoites escape either into the blood stream or into contiguous liver cells where they may initiate a secondary exoerythrocytic phase. In *P. falciparum* infection, no secondary infection of liver cells occurs. In other species it does and provides the mechanism for relapse of infection after eradication of the erythrocytic phase. Therefore, medications that eradicate the exoerythrocytic forms are needed to cure the non*falciparum* malarias.

**ERYTHROCYTIC ASEXUAL PHASE** This begins with penetration into red blood cells by merozoites arising from the exoerythrocytic schizonts in the liver cells. The parasites grow rapidly, and a large central vacuole forms in the cytoplasm leading to the so-called *ring form*. The cytoplasm then becomes amoeboid to form the single-nucleated *trophozoite*. At this stage it feeds on the host cell by the process of phagotrophy during which nutrients from the red blood cell are incorporated into the parasite cytoplasm inside food vacuoles lined by a double membrane. As the hemoglobin of the RBC is metabolized the contents of the vacuoles and the RBC itself become paler, and insoluble malaria pigment (hemozoin) is formed as granules of variable size. The trophozoite grows rapidly in size and becomes less amoeboid. New vacuoles are no longer formed. The nucleus divides by mitosis until the mature schizont is formed as a solid body containing variable numbers of nuclei. As in the exoerythrocytic schizont, discrete merozoites now form, as individual small oval or round bodies each containing a nucleus of chromatic material. The RBC ruptures, and the merozoites escape into the blood stream. Some are destroyed in the plasma, others invade RBCs and repeat the cycle.

At some stage of the infection, merozoites entering RBCs form sexual parasites, the male and female gametocytes, instead of repeating the erythrocytic cycle. The asexual erythrocytic cycle is completed in 2 to 3 days, depending on the species of parasite concerned, and ends with the discharge of merozoites and the destruction of the RBC. This process is called *schizogony*. Gametocytes take several days longer to mature. They then dwell in the individual RBC for the remainder of their existence—this may be more than 100 days. Relapse occurs only in sporozoite-induced *P. vivax*, *P. ovale*, and *P. malariae* infections. It does not occur in blood transfusion-transmitted infections, because there are no sporozoites. In *P. falciparum* infections, renewed manifestations of the malaria subsequent to the primary attack, if not resulting from fresh infection, are due to multiplication of an existing population of parasites surviving from the original infection. This is recrudescence, not relapse. A person infected with *P. vivax* may suffer a relapse up to 3 years after leaving an endemic area.

The characteristics of the various species of *Plasmodium* as seen on a blood film are given in Table 14-47.

**Table 14-47 Characteristics of Various Species of *Plasmodium* as Observed on a Blood Film**

| Parasite | Percent of Erythrocytes Infected | Stages of Asexual Parasites in the Peripheral Blood | Ring Forms | Trophozoites | Schizonts | Gametocytes | Changes in Red Blood Cell |
|---|---|---|---|---|---|---|---|
| *P. falciparum* | Scanty to up to 15% | Usually only ring forms. Late trophozoites and schizonts in heavy infection. | Small fine rings at first. 1 or 2 chromatin dots. Appliqué forms multiple rings in a single RBC. | Uncommon | Rare 8–36 merozoites. Occupies 2/3 of RBC. | Cresenteric or bean (banana) shaped (diagnostic) | Maurer dots |
| *P. vivax* | Scanty, rarely >2% | All stages | Small and large rings, chromatin dot. Rarely 2 chromatin dots. | Large amoeboid with yellow brown pigment | Common rounded occupying most of RBC—14 merozoites | Round—occupies most of RBC; scattered pigment | Increase in size. Pale, Schuffner dots. |
| *P. ovale* | As for *P. vivax* | All stages | As for *P. vivax* | As for *P. vivax* | Rounded, occupies 3/4 of RBC. Central mass of pigment. | As for *P. vivax* | Increase in size, pale, oval with fimbriated ends. Schuffner dots. |
| *P. malariae* | Low, usually <1% | All stages | Small single chromatin dot | Narrow band forms | Round; often rosette with central pigmented mass; 6–12 merozoites, fills RBC | Round, fills RBC | Ziemann stippling |

ABBREVIATION: RBC, red blood cell.

A nonhematologist can distinguish *P. falciparum* from non-*falciparum* malaria by these characteristics; for example, *P. falciparum* usually has only ring forms in the blood smear. There is a dipstick antigen-capture assay available for the diagnosis of *P. falciparum* malaria (Beadle et al. 1994). The sensitivity of this test depends upon the number of parasites present. For >60 parasites per microliter it is 100% sensitive, whereas the sensitivity is 11 to 67% if there are <10 parasites per microliter. The specificity is 88 to 98%. There may only be a few parasites present on the entire blood film; so time (up to 40 to 60 minutes) and patience are needed to diagnose many cases of malaria on thin blood films. Thick blood films are useful for finding parasites but much more experience is necessary to read a thick blood film than to read a thin one.

***Clinical presentation***

The initial symptoms are often referred to as "flulike" by the patient. These symptoms are nonspecific and can mislead both the patient and the physician. Malaise, headache, fatigue, myalgia, and fever lead to a visit to the physician. The physical exam is usually normal. However, fever in a traveler to a malarious area should raise the suspicion of malaria. As the infection progresses the classical symptoms emerge: fever, chills, and rigors. The temperature peak may be up to ≥40°. The fever can follow a regular pattern of spikes every 2 to 3 days but it may be very irregular in *P. falciparum* malaria. Splenomegaly may be present. *Plasmodium falciparum* malaria if untreated will continue to get progressively worse. The most dreaded complication is cerebral malaria. This is manifested as a diffuse encephalopathy. The onset may be gradual or sudden, being first manifested as a generalized seizure. Coma is a poor prognostic sign and is associated with a 20% mortality rate. Adults who survive cerebral malaria usually do not have neurologic sequelae; however, about 10% of children surviving cerebral malaria, especially those with hypoglycemia, multiple seizures, and coma, have neurological deficits.

Other complications that may develop are hypoglycemia, lactic acidosis, renal failure, noncardiogenic pulmonary edema, hemolytic anemia, and thrombocytopenia. Hypoglycemia complicating malaria is seen more frequently in women and children than in men, and may be caused by failure of hepatic gluconeogenesis, increased glucose consumption by host and parasite, and drug effects (quinine and quinidine stimulate insulin secretion). Lactic acidosis commonly accompanies hypoglycemia in severe malaria, due to interference with the microcirculation by sequestered parasites leading to anaerobic glycolysis. Furthermore, the liver in these patients does not clear lactate effectively. Renal impairment is common in adults with malaria. Acute tubular necrosis requiring dialysis may occur. Noncardiogenic pulmonary edema is uncommon. The pathogenesis is unknown but it may develop even after several days of antimalarial therapy.

***Prevention, control, and prophylaxis***

To date no effective vaccine has been developed. Measures to reduce the frequency of mosquito bites are important. Avoid exposure to mosquitoes at peak feeding times (dawn and dusk). Use insect repellant, suitable clothing, and insecticide-impregnated bed nets. Although permethin-impregnated bed nets have reduced malarial mortality and morbidity and improved childhood growth in Africa (Neiville et al. 1996), they may paradoxically increase the burden of disease among children, probably because infection with *P. vivax* very early in life protects against severe disease caused by *P. falciparum* malaria. Insecticides (e.g., DDT, malathione) that reduce the mosquito population have led to marked reduction in the number of cases of malaria in countries that use these insecticides (Roberts et al. 1997).

Travelers to malarious areas are advised to take medication to prevent malaria. The choice of chemoprophylaxis depends on the area(s) to be visited, type of lodging available, duration of stay, age of the patient, the species of malaria in the area, and the drug susceptibility of these parasites. Since recommendations for chemoprophylaxis frequently change, physicians are advised to consult an up-to-date source such as the CDC Travel Information Web site (http://www.cdc.gov/travel/travel12.htm).

The presence of malarial parasites in the placenta is associated with low birth weight (Steketee 1989), and maternal malarial infection during labor may be associated with a higher perinatal mortality (Nyirjesy et al. 1993). A review of data from randomized trials indicates that routine chemoprophylaxis for pregnant women results in a trend toward higher birth weights (Gasner and Brabin 1994). Some authors suggest that chemoprophylaxis should be targeted to anemic women and primigravida (Garner and Brabin 1994).

***Treatment***

The drug regimens for treatment of malaria are given in Table 14-48 (Kain 1996; White 1996). If there is any doubt about whether the malarial parasites are drug-resistant, treat as if they are resistant. Even though halofantrine and mefloquine are relatively recent additions to our malaria therapeutic regimens, resistance rates to these compounds approach 50% in parts of Thailand (Kain 1996). Primaquine is contraindicated in patients with severe G6PD (glucose-6-phosphate dehydrogenase deficiency).

Table 14-48 Drugs Used to Treat Malaria in Adults and Children

| Drug-Sensitive Malaria | Oral (for uncomplicated malaria) | Parenteral (for severe malaria) | Comments |
|---|---|---|---|
| Chloroquine HCl injection<br>Chloroquine phosphate tablets | 10 mg base/kg followed by 10 mg base/kg at 24 h and 5 mg base/kg at 48 h. For *P.vivax* and *P. ovalae* add primaquine 15 mg base (0.25 mg base/kg) per day for 14 days. | 10 mg base/kg by constant rate infusion over 8 h followed by 15 mg/kg over 24 h or by 3.5 mg of base/kg IM or SC every 6 h (total dose, 25 mg/kg) | Pruritus, dysphoria, neuropsychiatric symptoms |
| Clindamycin HCl | 900 mg (10 mg/kg) PO tid × 5 days | 900 mg every 8 h, IV | *Clostridium difficile* diarrhea occurs in 2 to 3% |
| Doxycycline | 100 mg (3 mg/kg/day PO bid × 7 days | NA | Photosensitivity, contraindicated in children |
| Sulfadoxine (25 mg)/ pyrimethamine (500 mg) tablets | 20 mg/kg sulfadoxine and 1 mg/ kg of pyrimethamine in a single dose (usual adult dose 3 tablets) | NA | Decrease in efficacy in many areas. Can be used for self treatment in areas with chloroquine-resistant malaria by persons taking mefloquine or doxycycline. |
| Atovaquone | NA | NA | Currently in combination with proguanil undergoing clinical trials for treatment of multidrug-resistant *P. falciparum* |
| **Drug-Resistant Malaria** | **Oral** | **Parenteral for Severe Malaria** | **Comments** |
| Quinine sulfate tablets<br>Quinine dihydrochloride injection | 10 mg salt/kg (600 mg) q8h for 7 days combined with doxycycline 100 mg PO bid (3 mg/kg/ day) × 7 days. Clindamycin 900 mg (10 mg/kg) PO tid for 5 days is an alternative to doxycycline. | 20 mg of dihydrochloride salt/kg by IV infusion over 4 h followed by 10 mg/kg IV infused over 2–8 h every 8 h × 72 h | Very bitter and causes cinchonism (nausea, dysphoria, tinnitus). Bolus injection can cause fatal hypotension. IV formulation not marketed in U.S. or Canada. |
| Quinidine gluconate injection | NA | 10 mg base/kg infused at a constant rate over 1 h followed by a 0.02 mg/kg/min × 72 h, with electrocardiographic monitoring—preferably in a coronary care unit. | Bolus injection can cause fatal hypotension. Decrease quinidine infusion rate if QT interval increases more than 25%. |
| Halofantrine HCl tablets | 8 mg/kg repeated at 6 and 12 h. Repeat the regimen 1 week later. | | Not marketed in U.S. or Canada. ↑ Absorption with fatty meal; caution with long QT interval. |
| Artesunate | 4 mg/kg/day for 3 days, in combination with mefloquine 15 mg base/kg PO × 1, then 2$^{nd}$ dose of 10 mg/kg PO 8–24 h later. | 4 mg/kg IM, followed by 2 mg/ kg q8h. | Not marketed in the US or Canada. Drug fever, abdominal pain, diarrhea, 1° heart block. |
| Mefloquine base | 15 mg/kg base PO × 1, then 2$^{nd}$ dose of 10 mg/kg base PO q8–24h later. | | Nausea, vomiting, giddiness, dysphoria, neuropsychiatric reactions, weakness, nightmares. |

ABBREVIATIONS: IM, intramuscular; IV, intravenous; PO, oral.

A radical cure with primaquine is not indicated in areas where malaria is endemic and hence reinfection is common.

Chloroquine exerts its antiparasitic effects by inhibiting heme polymerase. Resistance is mediated by rapid efflux of chloroquine (Krogstad et al. 1988). Quinine and quinidine are cinchona alkaloids derived originally from the bark of the cinchona tree of South America. Quinidine is the dextrorotatory diastereomer of quinine. It is more active than quinine as an antimalarial, but it is more cardiotoxic. Both these drugs inhibit heme polymerase. Cinchonism (tinnitus, nausea, high tone deafness, and dysphoria) occurs in up to 25% of patients treated with quinine. It resolves on discontinuation of the drug. Hypotension and hypoglycemia (due to pancreatic islet cell stimulation) may occur following intravenous administration of quinine. The hypoglycemia can be reversed with octreotide. Quinine combined with tetracycline or pyrimethamine-sulfadoxine is the treatment of choice for chloroquine-resistant *P. falciparum* malaria. Clindamycin in combination with quinine is another treatment regimen for chloroquine-resistant *P. falciparum* malaria.

Mefloquine has a half-life of 20 days. It inhibits heme polymerization. The mechanism of mefloquine resistance is unknown. Children tolerate mefloquine better than adults and men tolerate it better than women. Severe neuropsychiatric reactions (psychosis, convulsions) occur in 1 in 10,000 to 1 in 13,000 when it is used in prophylactic doses; with treatment doses (15 mg/kg) such reactions occur 1 in 215 to 1 in 1700 persons treated. This drug is contraindicated in those who have a history of seizures or major psychiatric disorder.

Halofantrine is a phenanthrene methanol derivative related to mefloquine and quinine. The mechanisms of action and resistance are unknown. Retreatment on day 7 is necessary to prevent recrudescence of infection. High doses of halofantrine (8 mg/kg every 8 hours for 3 days) have low failure rates, but cardiotoxicity, sometimes fatal, occurs—the PR and QT intervals are prolonged (Kain 1996). Halofantrine should never be used in combination with mefloquine or quinine because these combinations are additive in terms of QT prolongation. Halofantrine should not be ingested with fatty foods. It should be used only when other treatment options are contraindicated or inappropriate, and the dose should be limited to 8 mg every 6 hours times 3 doses, and repeated in 1 week.

Artemisinin (ginghaosu) was isolated in 1972 from *Artemisia annua*, a plant used by traditional Chinese practitioners to treat fever. It is available as the parent compound artemisinin, and as three semisynthetic derivates, artesunate for oral administration, artemether, and arteether for intramuscular injection. Ginghaosu and its derivatives result in faster parasite clearance than other antimalarials (White 1997). They are as effective as quinine in the treatment of severe and complicated malaria. There is in vitro synergy with mefloquine and tetracycline.

Atovaquone (a hydroxynaphthoquinone used as an alternative agent to treat *Pneumocystis carinii* pneumonia) is effective against multidrug–resistant *P. falciparum* malaria. It cannot be used alone, but, in combination with doxycycline or proguanil, cure rates of >90% against MDR *P. falciparum* are obtained. Malarone is a combination of atovaquone (250 mg) and proquanil (100 mg). Four tablets once daily for three days has been effective in the treatment of MDR *P. falciparum*.

*P. vivax* malaria acquired in Papua, New Guinea; Thailand; or Oceania may relapse after standard courses of primaquine. These patients should be retreated with twice (30 mg/kg) the standard dose for 14 days.

Severe *P. falciparum* malaria (often cerebral malaria) can be treated with a continuous infusion of quinidine (Miller et al. 1989) and exchange transfusion (Phillips et al. 1990). Exchange transfusion should be considered when any one of the following are present in severe *P. falciparum* malaria: >10% of red cells parasitized; DIC; acute renal failure.

Corticosteroid therapy is of no benefit and indeed it is deleterious in the treatment of cerebral malaria (Warrell et al. 1982). Acetaminophen (in children) has no antipyretic benefits over mechanical antipyresis and it prolongs the time of parasitic clearance in *P. falciparum* malaria by 16 hours (Brandts et al. 1997).

## Management of Sepsis

### *Definition and prognosis*

Sepsis, sepsis syndrome, septic shock, and multiorgan dysfunction are all part of a continuum of infection-related systemic illness (Bone 1991a,b). Table 14-49 gives definitions for each of these entities. The pathogenesis of sepsis is very complex, involving a large number of mediators. A cascade is started when endotoxin or other products of microorganisms enter the circulation, resulting in the release of a variety of mediators from mononuclear phagocytes, endothelial cells and other cells. Initially the proinflammatory cytokines (TNF, IL-1$\beta$, IL-6, and IL-8) are elevated, although there are large individual variations (Thigs and Hack 1994). The anti-inflammatory cytokines (IL-10) and soluble cytokine receptors (STNF-RI, IL-lra) are also elevated and seem to have a regulatory function on the host response (Thigs and Hack 1994).

An indication of the extent of the problem that "sepsis" poses can be gained from recent studies. In a 2-month prospective inception cohort study involving 170 ICUs for

**Table 14-49 Definitions for Sepsis, Sepsis Syndrome, Septic Shock, and Multiorgan Dysfunction Syndrome**

| | |
|---|---|
| Sepsis | Clinical evidence of infection plus signs of a systemic response to the infection which includes 2 or more of: temperature >38 °C or <36 °C; respiratory rate >20 breaths per minute; heart rate >90 beats per minute; WBC >12 × $10^9$/L or >10% bands |
| Sepsis syndrome | Sepsis plus evidence of altered organ perfusion (one or more of: oliguria [<0.5 ml/kg urine output for at least 1 hour]; hypoxemia [$Pa_{O_2}/FI_{O_2}$ <250]; elevated lactate) |
| Early septic shock | Sepsis syndrome plus hypotension—systolic blood pressure <90 mmHg or a 40 mmHg decrease below baseline that lasts for <1 hour and responds to a fluid challenge |
| Refractory septic shock | Sepsis syndrome plus hypotension that lasts >1 hour and does not respond to fluid administration or vasopressors |
| Systemic inflammatory response syndrome | Meets the definition of sepsis as given above, but this response can be due to infecion but it can also be noninfectious in etiology, e.g., pancreatitis |
| Multiorgan dysfunction syndrome | Progressive physiologic dysfunction in two or more organ systems after an acute threat to systemic homeostasis |

SOURCE: ACCP/SCCM 1992.

adults in France, clinically suspected sepsis and confirmed severe sepsis occurred in 9 and 6.3% of the admissions, respectively (Brun-Buisson 1995). The 28-day mortality was 56% for patients with severe sepsis and 60% for those with culture-negative sepsis. Not only is the short-term mortality high in this group of patients but survivors have increased intermediate terms (≥3 month) and mortality rates, as well as considerable physical dysfunction. Perl and coworkers (1995) followed 100 patients with sepsis. Sixty (60%) died a median of 30.5 days after sepsis. Thirty-two of these 60 died within the first month of the septic episode, 7 died within 3 months, and 4 more died within 6 months. Patients with resolved sepsis reported more physical dysfunction, including problems with work and activities of daily living and more poorly perceived general health than norms of the general population. However, their emotional health scores were higher than those in the general population (Perl et al. 1995). In a large study, Leibovici and colleagues (1995) studied 1991 patients with bacteremia or fungemia and compared them with matched control group for a matched age, sex, date of admission, and underlying disease. The median age was 72 years. The mortality rate for the study group at 1 month was 26%, at 6 months it was 43%, at 1 year 48%, and at 4 years it was 63%. Corresponding figures for the control group were 7% at 1 month, 27% at 1 year, and 42% at 4 years ($P < 0.001$).

### *Pathophysiology*

Bone (1996) contends that the pathogenesis of sepsis has three stages, each of which has a proinflammatory and an anti-inflammatory component. *Stage 1* occurs at the site of local injury or infection. Proinflammatory mediators combat infection, remove damaged tissue, and promote wound repair. Anti-inflammatory mediators then dampen the proinflammatory response. If homeostasis is not restored, mediators escape into the systemic circulation—stage 2. Again, if the anti-inflammatory mediators cannot restore homeostatis, shock and organ dysfunction result—stage 3. It is probably best then to characterize sepsis syndrome as cytokine dysregulation.

The pathophysiology of sepsis is complex. There are four overlapping processes—endothelial inflammation, altered regulation of coagulation, abnormalities of vascular tone, and myocardial suppression (Bone 1991a,b). Endothelial permeability is increased following exposure to TNF-$\alpha$, IL-1, platelet-activating factor, leukotrienes, and thromboxane A2. Activation of the complement cascade and neutrophil activation may damage the endothelium. Exposure to endotoxin, TNF-$\alpha$, IL-1, or to macrophage-derived procoagulants can activate the coagulation system. Exposure of collagen as a result of endothelial damage further activates the contact and coagulation systems and results in polymorphonuclear cell (PMN) and platelet adhesion. Activity of the fibrinolytic system is initially increased, but it is later inhibited as a result of increased production of plasminogen activation inhibitors or decreased production of tissue plasminogen activation.

Vasodilation due to prostaglandin $I_2$, thromboxane $A_2$, histamine, bradykinin, endothelium-derived relaxing factor (nitric oxide) (Cobb and Danner 1996) and endothelin-1 occurs. This results in the "warm" phase of septic shock with all the clinical findings of a hyperdynamic circulation. Reversible myocardial depression, ventricular dilation, and decreased left ventricular ejection fraction due to a myocardial depressant substance (not yet identified) occurs in septic shock. A variety of other mediators contribute to myocardial depression as well. PMNs from septic patients show marked shedding of L-selectin (a leukocyte adhesion molecule that aids in PMN adhesion to endothelial cells). Shedding of L-selectin reduces the rolling capacity of circulating PMNs and, hence, subsequent contact with cell walls of capillaries and thus decreased delivery to the site of infection.

***Management of sepsis***

The successful management of sepsis includes a high index of suspicion so that patients can be identified at the early stage, before they have progressed to septic shock. Appropriate cultures to identify the infecting microorganism and empiric antimicrobial therapy directed at the most likely pathogens are the next steps. Monitor vital signs and transfer to ICU if shock occurs. The ICU management of septic shock is beyond the scope of this chapter.

Some progress is being made in the management of this complex condition. For example, it is now recognized that hemodynamic therapy aimed at achieving supranormal values for cardiac index or normal values for mixed venous oxygen saturation does not reduce morbidity or mortality among critically ill patients (Ronco et al. 1993; Gattinoni et al. 1995). It is noteworthy that in one institution, fatality rates for septic patients with acute respiratory distress syndrome declined from 67% in 1990 to 40% in 1993 (Milberg et al. 1995).

There have been many unsuccessful attempts to modify the sepsis cascade, usually by inhibiting one mediator such as by administering monoclonal antibodies to block the effects of endotoxin or to use antibodies to TNF. Other trials have employed interleukin-1 receptor antagonist or platelet-activating factor antagonist. Early attempts at treatment of sepsis included corticosteroids to downregulate the inflammatory response. None of these therapies has been shown to be beneficial (Bone 1996). At this point, use of broad-spectrum empiric antibiotics to cover the most likely pathogens, and careful supportive care in an ICU environment, remain the mainstay of management of these patients (see Table 14-50).

## Prevention of Perioperative Infections

Shortly after the sulfonamides and penicillin were proved effective to *treat* infection, they were widely used by physicians to *prevent* infection in situations in which the risk of infection was high. Chemoprophylaxis has had variable success. Antimicrobial administration does not prevent bacterial pulmonary infections in unconscious or artificially ventilated patients, nor in patients with viral upper respiratory tract infections. Antibiotics do not prevent urinary tract infections in patients with indwelling Foley catheters. In fact, using antimicrobials in these settings selects for more resistant flora. Most surveys indicate that using antibiotics for prophylaxis accounts for 25 to 50% of all use of antimicrobials in hospitals (Cruse and Ford 1973; Conte et al. 1986). Despite the widespread administration of antibiotics to prevent infection, their use in this way is frequently controversial. Often their use is totally without merit, and potentially dangerous.

***Guidelines for chemoprophylaxis***

The term *chemoprophylaxis* implies administration of an antibiotic agent before contamination or infection with bacteria occurs. Early therapy denotes immediate or prompt institution of therapy as soon as contamination or infection is recognized. The latter situation is exemplified by beginning antibiotics after bacterial contamination and/or infection has occurred (e.g., GI spillage from a ruptured viscus). Appropriate candidates for chemoprophylaxis to prevent infection include: patients who have clinically significant exposure to an infected individual with particular diseases (e.g., invasive meningococcal disease or influenza); patients exposed to environments with a high potential for acquisition of pathogenic microorganisms (e.g., travelers in the developing world who are at risk for bacterial gastroenteritis or malaria); and patients undergoing procedures or surgery that are likely to result in infection (e.g., a dental procedure in a patient with a prosthetic heart valve, or colorectal surgery in an otherwise healthy patient).

General principles of antimicrobial prophylaxis that should guide selection of an antimicrobial agent have been established.

**Principles of antimicrobial prophylaxis include the following:**

- **Benefit must exceed the risks of chemoprophylaxis.**
- **The antimicrobial regimen must be effective against the major anticipated pathogens.**
- **Therapeutic concentrations of an effective chemoprophylactic antimicrobial should be achieved in local tissues at the time of exposure.**
- **Prolonged chemoprophylaxis is unwarranted (Conte et al. 1986).**

Chemoprophylaxis with penicillin has been successful in the prevention of group A streptococcal pharyngitis. Likewise, prophylaxis with chloroquine, mefloquine, or chloroquine plus proguanil have helped in the prevention

Table 14-50 Initial Antimicrobial Management of Sepsis and Sepsis Syndrome

**A. Community-acquired Infection**

| Most Likely Source of Sepsis | Likely Microorganisms | Antimicrobials |
|---|---|---|
| 1. Urinary tract | *Escherichia coli, Enterococcus* spp. | *Ampicillin and gentamicin, or vancomycin (if penicillin allergic) and gentamicin |
| 2. Lower respiratory tract | *Streptococcus pneumoniae*<br>*Staphylococcus aureus*<br>*Legionella pneumophila*<br>*Haemophilus influenzae*<br>Aerobic gram-negative rods (e.g., *Klebsiella pneumoniae, E. coli*)<br>*Pseudomonas aeruginosa* in those with bronchi ectasis or COPD | Erythromycin and ceftazidime, or ceftriaxone or a respiratory fluoroquinolone (levofloxacin) |
| 3. Skin and soft tissues | *Streptococcus pyogenes*<br>*Staphylococcus aureus* | If toxic "strep" syndrome is diagnosed, use clindamycin and $\gamma$ globulin. Nafcillin or cloxacillin for all other cases. |
| 4. Unknown source | Aerobic gram-negative bacteria (e.g., *E. coli*) | Cloxacillin (or nafcillin) and gentamicin |
| 5. Intra-abdominal | Anaerobes; aerobic gram-negative bacteria | Piperacillin and gentamicin; or ampicillin, metronidazole and gentamicin; or piperacillin and ciprofloxacin |

**B. Nosocomial**

—Classify the most likely source of infection as above.

—Know the susceptibility patterns of common bacteria isolated in your institution. In particular, you must know if methicillin-resistant *Staphylococcus aureus* or vancomycin-resistant *Enterococcus* is present in your hospital.

—It is not uncommon that multidrug-resistant aerobic gram-negative bacteria such as *Stenotrophomonas maltophilia* can be present in an intensive care unit.

—*Enterobacter aerogenes* and *E. cloacae* have depressed genes coding for extended spectrum beta-lactamases. When these bacteria are treated with cephalosporins (to which they are susceptible in vitro), the derepression is removed and the organism produces the $\beta$-lactamases and is now resistant to the cephalosporins. Quinolones such as ciprofloxacin or aminoglycosides are usually better choices for therapy of enterobacterial infections than are cephalosporins.

*Ampicillin sodium, ceftazidime, ceftriaxone sodium, ciprofloxacin HCl, clindamycin HCl, cloxacillin sodium, erythromycin, gamma-globulin, gentamicin sulfate, grepafloxacin, levofloxacin, metronidazole, nafcillin sodium, penicillin, piperacillin sodium, trovafloxacin, vancomycin HCl.
ABBREVIATION: COPD, chronic obstructive pulmonary disease.

of malaria; treatment with amantadine or rimantadine has helped in the prevention of secondary cases of influenza; and rifampin has helped to prevent secondary cases of invasive meningococcal and *H. influenzae* diseases. Similarly, use of isoniazid has helped prevent systemic tuberculosis, and use of trimethoprim-sulfamethoxazole has helped prevent recurrent urinary tract infections due to *E. coli*. Unfortunately, in the vast number of other situations in which antimicrobials are given prophylactically, there is little documentation that efficacy outweighs the risk of drug administration, with the likely encouragement of the development of resistant strains.

### *Surgical prophylaxis*

Antimicrobial prophylaxis for the prevention of postoperative infections has become accepted as standard care over the years (Nichols et al. 1981; 1982). Controversies remain over the optimal choice, timing, and duration of prophylactic antimicrobials (Fisher et al. 1996). Surgical wounds have been classified by the National Research Council as clean, clean-contaminated, contaminated, and dirty (see Table 14-51). Surgical site infections represent 24% of nosocomial infections. The CDC National Nosocomial Infection Surveillance Program has reported wound infection rates by class of wounds as follows: clean, 2.1%; clean contaminated, 3.3%; contaminated 6.4%; and dirty, 7.1% (Culver et al. 1991). Haley and coworkers (1981) have suggested that surgical site infections increase length of stay by 1 week and can add up to 20% of the cost of hospitalization. Prophylaxis is routinely recommended for clean-contaminated and contaminated wounds, whereas antimicrobial treatment is recommended for dirty wounds.

Table 14-51 **Surgical Infection Rate by Type of Surgical Procedure**[a]

| Type of Surgery | Definition | Approximate Percentage of All Operations | Reported Infection Rate (%) | Antibiotic Prophylaxis Recommended? |
|---|---|---|---|---|
| Clean | No entry into the respiratory, GI or GU tracts | 75 | 1–5 | No |
| Clean with insertion of prosthetic material or device | No entry into the respiratory, GI or GU tracts | 1–4 | 1–5 but high morbidity and mortality | Yes |
| Clean-contaminated | Unavoidable entry into the respiratory, GI or GU tracts (e.g., appendectomy, hysterectomy) | 14–5 | 8–15 | Yes |
| Contaminated | Fresh trauma, major break in sterile technique, gross spillage of GI content, entry into infected urinary or biliary tracts | 4–5 | 15–20 | Yes |
| Dirty | Old trauma wounds with devitalized tissue, foreign bodies, fecal contamination | 4–5 | 30–40 | Antibiotics are given to treat established infection |

[a]Infection rates listed are the expected infection rates in the absence of antibiotic prophylaxis.
SOURCE: Reproduced with permission from Gilbert 1984.

Clean wounds have no break in aseptic technique, and the gastrointestinal, respiratory, or genitourinary tracts are not entered. These wounds undergo primary closure, and inflammation is not encountered. The prophylaxis of clean wounds remains highly debated. Insertion of prosthetic joints and vascular surgery requiring use of prosthetic material are now included in guidelines for surgical wound infection prophylaxis, whereas prophylaxis for hernia repairs and mastectomy require further data before recommendations can be made (Fisher 1996).

The development of an infection in a surgical wound depends on the microorganism (dose and virulence), the host's resistance (underlying physiological status), and the condition of the surgical site at the end of surgery. Host factors associated with increased risk of wound infections include the following: extremes of age, malnutrition, active infection elsewhere, obesity, the presence of diabetes mellitus, and the use of corticosteroid therapy. Low albumin, weight loss, and malignancy have also been suggested as host risk factors. Surgical factors that increase the risk of wound infections include contaminated or dirty wounds; prolonged preoperative hospitalization (1 week or more); emergency operation; prolonged (more than 2 hours) surgery; shaving the operation site before the procedure; use of an electrosurgical knife; and insertion of drains through the wound at closure. Numerous studies have evaluated the role of chemoprophylaxis in the prevention of surgical wound infections. The consensus is that prophylactic antimicrobials are of benefit when an operation is associated with a high risk of infection or when a surgical site infection would have serious consequences for the patient.

In general, the efficacy of chemoprophylaxis depends on high antibiotic activity being present in blood and tissues at the time the incision is made and administration of an agent that is active against the most likely contaminating microorganism(s) (Wong 1996). Therefore, prophylactic antibiotics should be given within 2 hours of the surgery to achieve maximal concentration of drug at the site of the procedure (Classen et al. 1992). A second dose of antibiotic may have to be given intraoperatively if surgery is prolonged beyond the antimicrobial agent's half-life.

Since staphylococci and coliform bacteria (*E. coli*, *Proteus* spp., *Klebsiella* spp., *Enterobacter* spp.) are usually the most common causes of wound infections, first-generation cephalosporins such as cefazolin are usually the most appropriate agents for surgical wound infection prophylaxis. Second-generation cephalosporins with anaerobe activity (e.g., cefotetan) or cefazolin plus metronidazole should be used when there is concern that anaerobic bacteria, in addition to staphylococci and coliforms, may contaminate the wound. Such procedures include surgery on the lower GI tract. Vancomycin can be used as prophylaxis for orthopedic or neurosurgical procedures when the risk of methicillin-resistant staphylococcal (*S. aureus* or coagulase-negative staphylococci) infection is high (Antimicrobial prophylaxis in surgery 1997). The risk of emergence of vancomycin-resistant enterococci and *S. aureus* is such that routine use of vancomycin as a prophylactic agent for these procedures is discouraged (CDC 1994c). There is no role for third-generation cephalosporins in surgical wound infection prophylaxis, as they have limited activity against staphylococci and anaerobic bacilli. Prophylactic antibiotics are indicated before transrectal prostate biopsy. Ciprofloxacin or norfloxacin are currently used. There is controversy as to whether oral metronidazole should be given as well (Taylor and Bingham 1997).

There are no data to suggest that the rate of postoperative wound infection is lower if antimicrobial therapy is continued after the surgical procedure is completed (Conte et al. 1986)(see Table 14-52). Indeed continuation of antimicrobial prophylaxis beyond 24 hours leads to the emergence of resistant bacteria and wound infections caused by antibiotic-resistant microorganisms (DiPiro et al. 1986).

## Prevention of Endocarditis

Prevention of endocarditis by use of antibiotics before procedures that may cause transient bacteremia has been recommended for patients with selected valvular and congenital cardiac malformations. However, no controlled trials document the efficacy of such recommendations in preventing viridans streptococcal endocarditis after dental or upper respiratory tract procedures, or enterococcal endocarditis after gastrointestinal or genitourinary procedures (Dajani et al. 1997a,b). Prophylaxis for endocarditis is recommended for patients with the following underlying conditions: prosthetic valves, congenital cardiac malformations, surgically constructed systemic-pulmonary shunts, rheumatic and other acquired valvular dysfunction, idiopathic hypertrophic subaortic stenosis, previous his-

**Table 14-52 Efficacy of Preoperative Prophylxis in Reducing Postoperative Surgical Infections**

| INFECTIONS |
|---|
| *Efficacy established for:* |
| Colorectal operation |
| High-risk gastroduodenal surgery (gastric ulcer, relief of obstruction, stopping hemorrhage, or patients with achlorhydria) |
| Appendectomy (inflamed appendix) |
| High-risk biliary surgery (patients older than 70 years, with cholecystitis, undergoing common bile duct explorations or removal of stones, or with jaundice) |
| Hysterectomy (vaginal) |
| Cesarean section in high-risk patients |
| Pulmonary resection |
| Vascular grafts of abdomen and lower extremity |
| Hip nailing, total hip arthroplasty, open fracture reduction |
| *Possible efficacy for:* |
| Gastric bypass |
| Coronary bypass grafting |
| Prostatic surgery |
| Cardiac pacemaker implantation |
| *Unproven efficacy for:* |
| Low-risk gastroduodenal surgery |
| Low-risk cholecystectomy |
| Clean neurosurgery procedures without insertion of any prosthesis |
| Clean plastic surgery procedures without insertion of any prosthesis |
| External ventriculostomy |
| Herniorrhaphy, thyroidectomy, mastectomy, tonsillectomy |
| Repair of traumatic lacerations |

SOURCE: Reproduced with permission from Conte et al. 1986.

tory of bacterial endocarditis, and mitral valve prolapse with insufficiency. Prophylaxis for endocarditis is *not* recommended for patients who have undergone previous coronary artery bypass graft surgery or selected atrial secundum septal defects, cardiac pacemakers and implanted defibrillators, or physiologic, functional, or innocent heart murmurs.

Chemoprophylaxis is indicated before procedures that may lead to transient bacteremia, such as dental procedures that induce gingival bleeding, tonsillectomy, manipulation or biopsy of the respiratory, gastrointestinal, or genitourinary tracts, and incision and drainage of infected tissue. Clinicians should refer to schedules for endocarditis chemoprophylaxis when selecting the optimal regimen (Dajani 1997). In general, oral amoxicillin or intravenous ampicillin is given to prevent endocarditis. For higher-risk patients (those with prosthetic cardiac valves) undergoing procedures involving the gastrointestinal or urinary tracts, gentamicin is given along with ampicillin. Clindamycin, cephalexin, azithromycin, or vancomycin can be used in penicillin allergic patients. Therapy should be given just before the procedure begins so that peak concentrations of drug will be reached during the procedure. Drug therapy should not be prolonged (one dose before the procedure) so that more resistant organisms will not colonize the affected mucosal surfaces and infect the patient.

**PRINCIPLE Antimicrobial prophylaxis can prevent and decrease the postoperative incidence of infection in only a select number of clinical conditions. When an antimicrobial is appropriately administered, the choices in timing, agents employed, and duration of chemoprophylaxis are crucial so as to maximize benefit and minimize toxicity. In general, one dose of an agent that kills the most likely pathogen, at the time of greatest risk of contamination or exposure, is considered optimal therapy.**

## Immunoprophylaxis

Acquired host resistance following infection is part of the natural history of many diseases. Long-lasting immunity is not common to all infections but usually follows most acute viral infections. Resistance to recurrent infection with bacteria and other higher organisms is more variable. Resistance is frequently attended by measurable increases in specific immunoglobulins and reactions mediated by the cellular immune system. The object of immunotherapy is to safely duplicate or exceed the functional resistance in the host that normally follows a natural infection. In contrast to antimicrobial prophylaxis, optimal immunotherapy converts the susceptible individual into a resistant host, offering protection against the risk of infection without recourse to the repeated use of drugs.

Immunotherapy is the most effective therapy available for many viral infections, since antiviral chemotherapy has not been as well developed as antibacterial chemotherapy. Immunotherapy may be administered passively through the parenteral administration of preformed specific immunoglobulin from human or animal sources. Active immunity can be induced through the use of killed or attenuated agent vaccines, through the administration of subunit chemically defined vaccines, or by giving modified but antigenically active products of an agent in the form of toxoids (Fulginiti 1973).

**PRINCIPLE An ounce of prevention is worth a pound of cure: An effective vaccine is often of greater value than any subsequent chemotherapeutic intervention.**

Each newborn receives the benefits of natural passive immunization through the transplacental transfer of immunoglobulins from the maternal circulation. These immunoglobulins provide the newborn with sufficient protection to avoid infection with a wide variety of agents in the neonatal period. This protection wanes with the half-life of the maternal immunoglobulin G (IgG) and has largely disappeared at 2 to 4 months of age (Miller 1973).

Short-term protection against a wide group of diseases can be conveyed through the parenteral administration of immunoglobulins containing specific antibodies. Although past indications for this type of treatment have included prophylaxis or therapy of poliomyelitis, rubella, hepatitis, diphtheria, mumps, pertussis, and rubeola infections, these illnesses are now better managed by active immunization programs. A current list of commonly administered immunoglobulins is found in Table 14-53. Of these products, only botulinum immune serum, tetanus immune globulin, rabies hyperimmune globulin, hepatitis B immune globulin, and human immune globulin for the prophylaxis of hepatitis A are commonly used. Varicella-zoster immune globulin is in short supply and therefore only available under strict control for high-risk situations. Cytomegalovirus immunoglobulin has been available since 1990 for use in transplantation patients. Varicella-zoster immunoglobulin can be administered to nonpregnant females or immunocompromised individuals within

**Table 14-53 Passive Immunotherapy Available in the United States**

| PREPARATION[a,b] | USE |
|---|---|
| Botulism antitoxin (equine) | Botulism (treatment) |
| Cytomegalovirus immunoglobulin (intravenous) | Cytomegalovirus (prophylaxis) in transplant recipients |
| Diphtheria antitoxin (equine) | Diphtheria (treatment) |
| Immune globulin (pooled) | Hepatitis A and measles (prophylaxis) |
| Immune globulin (pooled) (intravenous) | Replacement of antibody deficiency[c] |
| Hepatitis B immune globulin | Hepatitis B (prophylaxis) |
| Rabies immune globulin | Rabies (prophylaxis and treatment) |
| Tetanus immune globulin | Tetanus (prophylaxis and treatment) |
| Vaccinia immune globulin | Smallpox (prophylaxis) |
| Varicella-zoster immune globulin | Varicella (prophylaxis) |

[a]Specific antibodies unless otherwise specified.
[b]Administered intramuscularly unless otherwise specified.
[c]Also used in treatment of idiopathic thrombocytopenic purpura, Kawasaki disease, and chronic lymphocytic leukemia.

96 hours of the infectious contact and to newborns of nonimmune mothers who develop varicella within a period of 5 days before or up to 2 days after delivery.

In the absence of previous immunizations, antisera for the prophylaxis or treatment of diphtheria, pertussis, measles, and polio are of some value, but these antisera are not presently widely available. The CDC is a reliable resource for information about immunoprophylaxis in general and maintains a clearinghouse for those products not commercially available. The CDC also maintains a variety of other hyperimmune sera for use in diseases not commonly seen in the United States, including a number of the more exotic arboviruses and other viral illnesses causing hemorrhagic fever.

Passive immunization is limited in its effectiveness by the half-life of IgG (22 to 30 days). Thus, a relatively short period of protection is afforded by this approach. All hyperimmune sera and disease-specific immunoglobulins are in limited supply and are expensive. To be effective, they usually require comparatively large volumes for parenteral administration, and they cause unpleasant local reactions. Allergic reactions may be apparent immediately after injection and may be life-threatening. More commonly, the reactions are of the delayed-hypersensitivity or serum-sickness type (see part 1, Introduction, and chapter 24, Adverse Drug Reactions). Careful questioning of the patient for a history of allergy to the animal that served as the source for the antiserum and possibly skin testing with the antiserum to be used should be considered before the administration of these agents. If the skin tests are positive, but the need is critical, a carefully administered "desensitization" program may be undertaken using increasing concentrations of the material. Appropriate procedures to accomplish desensitization have been described (Fulginiti 1973). As most immune globulins are available from human sources, antisera from animal sources are becoming less frequently required. Administration of immune globulins from human sources causes less adverse events but remains undesirable as the threat of transmission of infectious agents from infusion of immune globulin still exists.

Use of immunotherapy has been attempted for the treatment of septic shock. Polyclonal and monoclonal antibodies of the IgM and IgG classes that bind to the core lipopolysaccharide moiety of gram-negative bacterial lipopolysaccharide protect against shock in animal models. A multicenter trial, using the polyclonal antibody J5, reported a reduction in mortality in gram-negative sepsis from 39 to 22% in human subjects (Ziegler et al. 1982). Further studies with monoclonal antibodies against the lipid A moiety of gram-negative lipopolysaccharides (HA-1A), IL-1 receptor antagonist (IL-1RA), and tumor necrosis factor (TNF) have all failed to show benefit convincingly except in very well defined subsets of patients (Ziegler et al. 1991; Fisher et al. 1994; Abraham et al. 1995). Further monoclonal antibodies are in developmental and clinical trial phases. As more is known about the sepsis biochemical cascade, it appears quite certain that immunotherapy will play only a small role.

Intravenous immunoglobulin (IVIG) therapy has been reported to be effective in conditions such as Kawasaki syndrome and idiopathic thrombocytopenic purpura (ITP). There are case reports of successful treatment of patients with streptococcal toxic shock syndrome or necrotizing fascitis with IVIG administration in combination with antimicrobial therapy (Barry et al. 1992; Lamothe et al. 1995; Perez et al. 1997). Evidence suggests an antitoxin role of IVIG in these patients is responsible for the decrease in morbidity and possible avoidance of mortality (Norrby-Teglund et al. 1996).

### *Active immunization*

Active immunization depends on the host's immune system response to vaccines to provide the protection usually acquired by natural infection. Vaccines may be either living (i.e., contain live microbes) or nonliving (i.e., contain dead microbes). Live vaccines contain organisms that are attenuated and therefore are capable of only limited replication in a normal host. Vaccinia, developed by Jenner in 1796, was the first clinically successful live vaccine. It is a product containing bovine poxvirus that has limited ability to invade the human host but is nevertheless able to produce sufficient local and regional infectivity to ensure that a host response results in resistance of the recipient to subsequent smallpox infection. The resistance was not lifelong, and vaccination had to be repeated approximately every 3 years. The worldwide elimination of smallpox in the 1980s by an effective immunization program is the most dramatic example of how vaccines can be used for the well-being of humankind (CDC 1985). Since the risk of adverse reaction to smallpox vaccine now outweighs the chance of acquiring the disease, vaccination is recommended only for those working in smallpox research laboratories. Other routinely used vaccines are listed in Table 14-54.

Live vaccines may be administered either by natural routes (orally) as in oral polio vaccine or by an artificial route (parenterally) as in the presently available live measles vaccine. There is a theoretical advantage in the use of the natural route, since there is good evidence that the resultant formation of local (mucosal) antibodies is important in protection from subsequent wild-type infections (Ogra et al. 1968). Nonliving vaccines may be divided into four groups: 1) suspensions of whole killed agents (e.g., influenza vaccine and typhoid vaccine); 2) suspensions of nonreplicating subparticles of infectious agents (e.g., meningococcal or pneumococcal polysaccharide vaccines); 3) modified products of infecting organisms (e.g., tetanus and diphtheria toxoid vaccine) and; 4) new subunit vaccines that contain chemically defined reagents (e.g., hepatitis B virus vaccine). The routine schedule for the active immunization of normal infants and children in the United States is presented in Table 14-55. Certain combinations of live vaccines may be given simultaneously, but the close sequential administration of individual live vaccines and immunoglobulins is not recommended because of evidence of interference with immunogenicity leading to vaccine failure (CDC 1994a). A delay of 2 weeks after vaccination should be allowed before giving immunoglobulins.

**Evaluation of the efficacy of vaccines** Adequate response to immunization is most frequently judged by measuring the development of specific serum immunoglobulins (e.g., antibodies) following a course of administration of vaccine. The concentration of specific immunoglobulin in plasma is usually proportional to the degree of protection from the viral agent. However, the relation between immunologic response to a vaccine and protection afforded by it to subsequent disease must be documented in field trials. The longevity of the protective response must always be determined to establish the most appropriate interval for revaccination.

### *Eradication*

Although the widespread use of antibiotics has had little success in curtailing the prevalence of bacterial infection, and in certain instances has resulted in the appearance of resistant pathogens of potentially greater harm, the success of vaccines in reducing incidence of disease has been remarkable. Lack of success has been largely related to the socioeconomic problems preventing distribution of the vaccine (Horstmann 1973). When these problems have been appropriately solved, eventual eradication of some diseases has become possible. Certain favorable epidemiologic characteristics of smallpox made it an ideal candidate to eradicate. These include the following:

- Humans are the only known host.
- Smallpox is an acute disease with a short incubation period.
- Immunity following infection is relatively long lasting and effective.
- There is only one antigenic strain of virus.
- Subclinical infections are rare.
- Epidemic patterns are seasonal.
- A successful vaccine is available (Hoeprich 1972).

Unfortunately, these characteristics are not widely shared by other pathogens. Thus, successful eradication will probably be limited to a small number of diseases. Wild-type poliovirus infection has been eradicated from the Western hemisphere and efforts continue toward global eradication. It has been agreed that measles irradication is technically possible, and a goal of 2005 to 2010 has been set (CDC 1997a).

**Table 14-54 Routine Vaccines for Humans**

| Disease | Route | Agent | Age Applicable | Basic or Primary Immunization | Need for Booster | Efficacy Value (%) | Adverse Reaction or /Comment |
|---|---|---|---|---|---|---|---|
| Diphtheria | Parenteral | Toxoid | 2 mos to 5 yr and adults | 3 doses over 6 mos | Yes, at 1 and 3 yr after basic | >90 | Mild local reactions |
| Pertussis | Parenteral | Heat-killed bacteria or acellular bacterial component | 2 mos to 5 yr | 3 doses over 6 mos | Yes, at 1 and 3 yr after basic | −85 | Mild local reactions, rare neurological reactions |
| Tetanus | Parenteral | Toxoid | 2 mos to 5 yr | 3 doses over 6 mos | Every 10 yr | −100 | Local pain and rare neurological reactions due to hypersensitivity |
| Polio | Oral | Live-attenuated (OPV) or inactivated (IPV) | >2 mos | 2 doses over 4 mos | Yes, at 1 and 3 yr after basic | >95 | None |
| Measles | Parenteral | Live-attenuated | >1 yr | 1 dose | 3 yr after basic | >95 | Fever and rash in 15% |
| Mumps | Parenteral | Live-attenuated | >1 yr | 1 dose | None | >95 | Local reactions |
| Rubella | Parenteral | Live-attenuated | Women of child-bearing age | 1 dose | None | >95 | Mild fever, arthralgia, local reactions |
| *Haemophilus influenzae* | Parenteral | Capsular material | 2 mos to 5 yr | 3 doses over 6 mos | ≥6 mos after 3rd visit | >95 | Rare; should be given to all children |
| Pneumococcal infection | Parenteral | Capsular material | >65 yr or COPD and immunocompromised patients | 1 dose | Once at 6 yr | >70 | Local reactions |
| Influenza | Parenteral | Formalin-treated virus | >65 yr or COPD immunocompromised patients | 1 dose | Annually | −60 | Fever, malaise, and arthralgia; contraindicated in individuals with hypersensitivity to eggs |
| Hepatitis B | Parenteral | Surface antigens (protein and lipids) | Health-care workers and persons[a] with high risk of contact with blood (e.g., injection drug abuser) | 3 doses over 6 mos | Probably not | −90 | None |
| Varicella | Parenteral | Live-attenuated | 12–18 mos | 1 dose | None | −96 | Local reaction |

[a]Many authorities recommend universal hepatitis B vaccination starting at age 2 months.
ABBREVIATIONS: COPD, chronic obstructive pulmonary disease; mos, months.
SOURCE: CDC 1985, 1989b, 1993b, 1994a, 1996a, b, 1997a to c.

Table 14-55 Schedule for Active Immunization of Normal Infants and Children

| AGE | VACCINE OR TOXOID |
|---|---|
| Birth | Hep B[a] |
| 2 mos | DTP-1, polio (OPV-1 or IPV-1), Hib, Hep B |
| 4 mos | DTP-2, polio (OPV-2 or IPV-2), Hib |
| 6 mos | DTP-3, Hib, Hep B |
| 12–15 mos | MMR, Hib, varicella[b] |
| 15 mos | DTaP-4, polio (OPV-4 or IPV-4), MMR |
| 4–6 yr | DTaP-5, polio (OPV-4 or IPV-4), MMR |
| 14–16 yr | Td (and thereafter every 10 years) |

[a]For hepatitis B surface antigen (HBsAg)-positive mothers, administer immunoprophylaxis as soon after birth. For HBsAg-negative mothers, administration can wait until time of hospital discharge.
[b]Except in those with a reliable history of varicella infection.
ABBREVIATIONS: DTaP, diptheria toxoid, tetanus toxoid, acellular pertussis vaccine; DTP, diptheria toxoid, tetanus toxoid, pertussis vaccine; Hep B, hepatitis B; Hib, *Haemophilus influenzae* type B conjugate vaccine (aka HbCV); IPV, inactivated polio virus vaccine; mos, months; MMR, measles-mumps-rubella vaccine; OPV, oral polio virus vaccine; Td, Tetanus toxoid combined with smaller adult dose of diptheria antigen; yr, year.
SOURCE: Adapted from CDC 1994a, 1996a, b, 1997b.

### *Adverse effects of vaccines*

Adverse effects of vaccines vary and are often related to the method of preparation of the vaccine (i.e., the cell culture system in which the vaccine has been prepared) (Wilson 1967).

Hypersensitivity reactions are too frequently the consequence of inadequate attempts to obtain a detailed history or inattention to the appropriate necessary precautions (e.g., adequate preliminary testing before administration). The clinician is advised to consult local state health officials regarding updated precautions for adverse effects associated with vaccination before immunization. Nonliving vaccine products require a much larger antigenic mass (dose) and more frequent booster injections than do live vaccines to provide adequate levels of protection. This is exemplified by the requirement for multiple boosters of immunization against diphtheria, tetanus, and pertussis, compared with the single administration required for live mumps virus vaccine. The larger doses and repeated administration required for nonliving vaccines may lead to higher rates of allergy and other reactions. During the developmental trials of two killed vaccines (measles vaccine and respiratory syncytial virus vaccine), production of a hypersensitivity state ensued that, while not preventing infection, produced an exaggerated host response to subsequent natural infections resulting in a clinically unusual and more severe disease than was previously seen (Kapikian et al. 1969).

Hypersensitivity reactions have led to some contraindications to vaccinations. Recent studies have shown that egg allergy should no longer be a contraindication to measles/mumps/rubella (MMR) vaccine (James et al. 1995). Canadian authorities no longer recommend the delay of vaccination for MMR in children with egg allergy. Egg allergy remains a contraindication for both influenza and yellow fever vaccines as the method of vaccine preparation is different from MMR vaccine and these vaccines contain higher concentrations of ovalbumin. Vaccine preservatives and additives, including thimerosal (a mercurial preservative), neomycin, and aluminum have been implicated in hypersensitivity reactions but rarely in anaphylactic reactions.

Although attenuated live-virus vaccines may more effectively mimic natural infection in stimulating host defenses, they can be made in such a way that there is a risk of inadequate attenuation of the virus or of the virus reverting to a less attenuated form. Thus, the full-blown disease may appear following vaccination. Immunosuppressed patients are at higher risk of developing vaccine-associated infections. Both oral live-attenuated polio virus vaccine and live measles vaccine have been implicated in such complications (Sutter and Prevots 1994; CDC 1996b). Furthermore, since these live-virus vaccines do not go through a process of harsh inactivation before administration, the risk of introducing dangerous adventitious agents into the host is increased. For example, certain animal tumor viruses that contaminated tissue culture support systems in some of the early vaccines were inadvertently introduced into recipients. Fortunately, careful follow-up of cohorts of these recipients has failed to show any increased rates of neoplasia (Shah and Nathanson 1976).

The administration of vaccines to pregnant women presents a special problem. In this situation, the probable risk of maternal (and fetal) infection must be balanced against the known adverse effects of vaccination. Adequate immunization against tetanus is essential for both mother and child, and tetanus toxoid immunization is safe during pregnancy. Immunization against poliomyelitis and yellow fever is indicated in pregnant women traveling to epidemic areas. Other live vaccines, including measles, mumps and rubella are generally contraindicated during pregnancy because of the risk of infecting the fetus (Levine et al. 1974).

**PRINCIPLE With the development and introduction of each new vaccine, the physician must balance the seriousness of the disease being prevented against the**

**known and unknown risks involved in widespread use of the vaccine. Prophylaxis with vaccine is warranted only in populations threatened by significant morbidity and mortality from the disease, in whom likely benefits outweigh possible risks.**

***Poliomyelitis: A disease illustrating the principles of immunotherapy***

Poliomyelitis is a disease caused by infection with one of three types of poliovirus, a member of the enterovirus group. These viruses are transmitted by both the oral-fecal and respiratory routes, the latter being of lesser importance. Colonization and multiplication of the virus take place in the lymphatic tissue of the oropharynx and bowel. Dissemination occurs thereafter via the regional lymphatics and by viremia. After dissemination, the tissue tropism that allows the poliovirus to multiply within the lower motor neurons of the spinal cord becomes apparent. The injury to these lower motor neurons is responsible for the most devastating clinical manifestations of paralytic polio. Host defenses include the elaboration of local antibody (IgA) in the GI tract and type-specific humoral antibodies that can be detected in the circulation. When present, the latter antibodies indicate that the host is protected against reinfection. There is no cross-protection between the three types of poliovirus.

The clinical manifestations of poliomyelitis appear 1 to 3 weeks after exposure to the virus and appear to be related to age. The overwhelming majority of cases in children are completely asymptomatic (90%). Those persons who do have symptoms usually have a mild fever, headaches, some mild GI symptoms, and occasionally a sore throat. In contrast to adolescents and adults, young children rarely have involvement of the CNS. When they develop, neurologic symptoms usually appear from 2 to 6 days after the initial illness. The neurologic involvement (1% of infected individuals) is primarily lower motor neuron disease that results in flaccid paresis.

Hematologic and biochemical tests usually are within normal limits except for the findings in the cerebrospinal fluid, respiratory secretions, and feces. These samples should be taken as early as possible in the course of the disease to increase the likelihood of successful isolation of the virus. Paired samples of sera showing a fourfold or greater rise in type-specific antibody against polio virus are diagnostic of the disease.

There is no acceptable antiviral chemotherapy for an established case of poliomyelitis. Treatment in this instance is entirely supportive and aimed at preventing other infections and reversing or preventing the biochemical or respiratory problems related to the neurologic destruction caused by the disease. The development and application of polio vaccine provide one of the most successful stories in modern therapeutics (Paul 1971). Before the introduction of polio vaccine in 1954, recurrent epidemic polio with significant rates of neurologic disease plagued industrialized societies. Nonindustrialized societies usually had their infections during childhood, with very low rates of neurologic disease. As public health measures improved, the oral-fecal spread of polio virus shifted to an older population more prone to neurologic involvement. This natural history has been repeated in developing societies up to the present. With the use of either the Salk killed vaccine (IPV) or the Sabin oral polio vaccine (OPV), this disease has been reduced to rare occurrences in unvaccinated groups (Wehrle 1967; Schoenberger et al. 1984). The Western hemisphere documented the last case of wild-type polio virus infection in 1979.

In recent years, outbreaks of poliomyelitis have been associated with pockets of unvaccinated persons, importation of wild-type virus from endemic areas, and lower than optimal vaccination rates. National Immunization Day mass campaigns in developing countries have been adopted to further decrease the annual rates of wild-type infections. In the United States, an average of 10 cases of polio virus infection are reported yearly, all of them vaccine-associated strains. Developed countries must not become complacent regarding vaccination as the emergence of susceptible groups of unvaccinated persons provides the opportunity for reemergence of infection and severe disease.

***Recent additions to vaccination recommendations***

New formulations of vaccines have recently been marketed to increase immunogenicity at an earlier age and to decrease potential adverse effects. Conjugate *H. influenzae* b vaccine (HbCV), acellular pertussis vaccine, and recombinant hepatitis B vaccine are examples. *H. influenza* until recently was the most common cause of childhood meningitis in the United States with a death rate of 1 to 5%. Early formulation of the vaccine was effective only in children greater than 18 months of age. Newer *H. influenza* conjugate vaccines with inactive diphtheria toxin, outer-membrane protein complex of group B meningococcus, and tetanus toxoid as their protein carrier can be given to children ≤2 months. Combination formulations with diphtheria/tetanus/pertussis vaccine (DTP) make scheduling easier. Whole-cell pertussis vaccine developed in the 1940s was considered 70 to 90% effective in early trials. More recent trials estimated efficacy as low as 36 to 48% (Gustafsson et al. 1996; Greco et al. 1996).

Adverse events were commonly associated with whole-cell pertussis vaccine, prompting the development of acellular pertussis vaccine. This formulation contains inactivated pertussis toxin and one or more other bacterial components. Clinical trials with combination diphtheria, tetanus, and acellular pertussis (DTaP) vaccines showed efficacy of 59 to 89%, with fewer adverse events than the original DTP formulation (CDC 1997b). Recommendations for primary immunization and booster vaccination of pertussis encourage the use of DTaP.

Recombinant hepatitis B vaccine has replaced the pooled human sera vaccine. This has eliminated the risk of blood-borne organism transmission through vaccination while providing an effective agent for the prevention of hepatitis B. Efforts are under way to improve the efficacy of the pneumococcal vaccine. Presently the 23-valent polysaccharide vaccine is not immunogenic in infants and is poorly so in immunodeficient hosts. Protein conjugate vaccines similar to HbCV vaccines are undergoing phase III trials with some preliminary hopes of reducing pneumococcal carriage, otitis media, and invasive pneumococcal infections (Käyhty and Eskola 1996).

### *Immunization of immunosuppressed host*

Individuals with immunodeficient states, including HIV, hematological malignancy, transplant recipients, congenital deficiencies, or underlying illnesses such as diabetes and renal and liver failure, are at increased risk of severe morbidity from some preventable infections. Routine childhood immunization should be performed in these individuals with exception of live vaccines. *Haemophilus* type b, pneumococcal, and influenza vaccines are recommended in these patients, and they should be offered hepatitis B and meningococcal vaccines if indicated. Live vaccines such as measles or oral polio vaccine are contraindicated in patients with severe immunodeficiency, as their risk of acquired vaccine-related infection is too high. Oral polio vaccine is also contraindicated in household members of patients with severe immunodeficiency states (CDC 1994a).

### *Immunization for the traveler*

Increase in business and pleasure international travel has seen an increase in risk of acquisition or importation of infectious diseases endemic in many developing countries. Many of these infections can be avoided by preventative measures and education (hand-washing, eating only adequately cooked food, insect repellents, and proper clothing), and others can be prevented by obtaining the appropriate vaccines long enough before travel for them to be effective. Routine vaccinations should be completed or updated before departure. Additional vaccines which are often necessary include hepatitis A, hepatitis B (now available as a combination hepatitis A and B vaccine), meningococcal, yellow fever, typhoid, and cholera vaccines. Although cholera vaccines are presently not generally recommended, new recommendations may come forth as oral cholera vaccine studies show adequate efficacy in large field trials. Local health authorities should be consulted for further information regarding immunizations required for destination. Vaccines commonly recommended are listed in Table 14-56.

### *Vaccines under development*

As the incidence of genital herpes increases worldwide, the search for an effective vaccine continues. This vaccine must not only prevent primary herpes infection but also recurrent infections to decrease the pool of potentially infected individuals. Animal trials have been successful using genetically modified viruses (Boursnell et al. 1997). A randomized, controlled, double-blind placebo study of 2393 HSV-2 seronegative persons failed to show any protection in vaccinated individuals (Corey et al. 1997). Further trials are under way using modifications to this and other vaccines to assess efficacy.

Rotavirus is the leading cause of diarrheal illness in infants and young children less than 2 years of age. This infection leads to significant rates of hospitalizations in the Western world and severe morbidity and mortality in developing countries. Live attenuated rotavirus vaccines delivered by the oral route are under investigation. Joensuu et al. (1997) have assessed the efficacy of rhesus-human reassortant rotavirus tetravalent vaccine in a randomized, placebo-controlled trial of 2398 Finnish children. Overall vaccine efficacy was 66%, but of 100 cases of severe diarrheal illness, only 8 were in the vaccine group. It therefore appears that vaccination could lead to a decrease in severe rotavirus gastrointestinal disease.

Respiratory syncytial virus (RSV) respiratory infections are responsible for hospitalization of 1% of infants in their first year of life and up to 3% mortality in infants with underlying lung or heart disease. Vaccination against RSV is a priority to diminish the morbidity and mortality it causes. Vaccine development has been problematic as natural infection confers only partial, temporary immunity, and initial vaccines caused an increase in severity of subsequent illness. The most promising vaccine to date is a purified preparation of the fusion protein of RSV which has undergone efficacy study in small groups of 18- to 36-month-old children. Infection rates were decreased compared with the placebo group over a 2-year period (Tristram and Welliner 1993). For unclear reasons, infants

Table 14-56 **Immunization for the Traveler**

| VACCINE | TYPE | IMMUNIZATION | INDICATIONS |
|---|---|---|---|
| Hepatitis A | Inactive viral antigen | 2 doses @ 0, 6 months | Travelling to endemic areas[a] |
| Hepatitis B | Inactive viral antigen | 3 doses @ 0, 1, 6 months | Travelling ≥6 months in endemic areas |
| Meningococcal | Bacterial polysaccharide of serotypes A/C/Y/W-135 | 1 dose | Sub-Saharan Africa |
| Typhoid | Inactivated bacteria (parenteral) | 3 doses, 4 weeks apart | Travelling ≥6 weeks to endemic areas[b] |
| | Live bacteria (Ty21a oral) | 4 doses on alternate days | |
| Cholera | Inactivated bacteria | — | Not widely recommended |
| Yellow fever | Live virus | 1 dose | Travelling in countries which require vaccination |
| Japanese encephalitis | Inactivated virus | 3 doses on days 0, 7, 30 | Travelling ≥1 month to endemic areas |

[a]Anywhere but northern Europe, Canada, Australia and New Zealand.
[b]To certain parts of South America, Africa, and the Indian subcontinent including Nepal.

have not responded immunologically as well to this vaccine. Finally, new advances are being made in immune therapeutics with the development of DNA vaccines. These use genes encoding proteins of pathogens or tumors to elicit a humoral or cell-mediated response. DNA vaccines for prevention of microbial infections are under development for influenza B and hepatitis B viruses, malaria, tuberculosis, and human immunodeficiency virus (Chattergoon et al. 1997).

## COMMENTS ON SPECIFIC ANTIMICROBIAL AGENTS

This section is devoted to specific clinically relevant points about commonly used antimicrobials. Detailed descriptions of each drug are available in other texts (Kucers and Bennett 1989; Mandell et al. 1995; Gilman et al. 1996). The major toxicities, dosage adjustments in patients with renal failure, routes of administration, and ability to penetrate into the CSF and urine of these agents have been mentioned already in this chapter.

### Penicillins

#### *Penicillin G*

Penicillin G is an acid that is combined with sodium, potassium, procaine, or benzathine to increase its stability or to regulate its absorption. The latter two are "long-acting" forms. Penicillin G is useful in the treatment of streptococcal infections due to *S. pyogenes* (group A), *S. agalactiae* (group B), *S. pneumoniae*, viridans streptococci, *Corynebacterium diphtheriae*, *N. meningitidis*, many strains of *N. gonorrhea*, *Treponema pallidum*, and many anaerobic streptococci, such as *peptococcus* and *peptostreptococcus*. In combination with aminoglycosides, any penicillin G compounds can be used to treat enterococci and *L. monocytogenes* infections. These organisms cause many clinical syndromes including cellulitis, pharyngitis, pneumonia, septicemia, endocarditis, meningitis, abscesses in lung, sexually transmitted disease, septic arthritis, and osteomyelitis.

All penicillinlike agents kill susceptible bacteria by interfering with the biosynthesis of the cell wall, eventually lysing the bacteria by autolysis. The penicillins are generally safe except in less than 0.01% of patients who are susceptible to IgE-mediated anaphylaxis (see chapter 24, Adverse Drug Reactions). Other types of penicillin toxicity are rare unless renal function has been impaired. In patients with renal failure, large doses of penicillin produce neurologic reactions including seizures. One overlooked problem of high concentrations of penicillin in the blood occurs when aminoglycoside concentrations are measured in vitro. The penicillins autolyze aminoglycosides. Prolonged storage of blood containing these antibiotics at room temperature can result in lower-than-real concentrations of aminoglycoside.

Phenoxymethylpenicillin (penicillin V) is produced by addition of a phenoxyacetic acide. It is more resistant to gastric acid than is penicillin G and is administered orally. Phenoxymethylpenicillin is useful for treatment of minor infections such as streptococcal pharyngitis or cellulitis.

#### *Semisynthetic penicillins*

Methicillin, oxacillin, cloxacillin, dicloxacillin, and nafcillin are semisynthetic penicillins that are particularly useful in treating penicillinase-producing staphylococci.

They are considered the primary empirical and definitive therapy for staphylococcal infections. They kill bacteria in a manner similar to that of penicillin G. Methicillin and nafcillin are the most stable; nafcillin is most often used because of its lower incidence of nephrotoxicity. In contrast to the other semisynthetic penicillins that are excreted primarily by the kidney, nafcillin is 70% inactivated in the liver. Nafcillin does not usually require adjustment of dose in patients with renal failure. Errors in its administration are commonly made by decreasing the dose of nafcillin in patients with renal failure and continuing high doses in patients with hepatic insufficiency. Depending on subsequent culture results, tailored therapy for staphylococci may include penicillin G (rare) for non-penicillinase-producing strains of staphylococci or vancomycin for nafcillin-resistant staphylococci (usually referred to as MRSA, or methicillin-resistant *Staphylococcus aureus* because test discs contain methicillin). Dicloxacillin is the most useful agent of this group for oral therapy. Cloxacillin can also be given orally and in many countries is more readily available than is dicloxacillin.

***Amino-penicillins***
Ampicillin is a semisynthetic penicillin and is unique in that it is active against some gram-negative bacilli that are resistant to penicillin G. Amoxicillin is chemically modified ampicillin. The trihydrate form is administered orally and is much better absorbed than ampicillin, making it the preferred agent for oral administration. Organisms that are susceptible to penicillin G also are susceptible to ampicillin. Ampicillin kills organisms similarly to penicillin G; however, it penetrates into the cell wall better, enabling it to kill many gram-negative bacilli. It is considered appropriate therapy for susceptible *E. coli*, *P. mirabilis*, and species of *Shigella*, *Neisseria gonorrhoeae*, and *N. meningitidis*. The most common error in parenteral ampicillin therapy is administrating it too infrequently. Its relatively short half-life dictates that it should be administered every 4 hours in seriously ill patients. It is especially useful in treating acute and uncomplicated urinary tract infections caused by *E.coli* and/or *Proteus* species. *Haemophilus influenzae* meningitis can be treated with ampicillin if the organisms do not produce β-lactamase.

***Extended-spectrum penicillins***
Carboxypenicillins (carbenicillin, ticarcillin) and ureidopenicillins (mezlocillin, azlocillin, and piperacillin) are semisynthetic penicillins that must be administered parenterally and are particularly useful to treat serious aerobic gram-negative infections of the lung, abdomen, pelvis, muscle, skeleton, and bloodstream. Ureidopenicillins also have activity against many anaerobes and streptococci, including enterococci. Their primary clinical usefulness relies on their enhanced ability to kill aerobic gram-negative organisms, including species of *E. coli*, *Proteus*, *P. aeruginosa*, other species of *Pseudomonas*, *H. influenzae*, and species of *Klebsiella*. By themselves, these agents usually are sufficient to kill these organisms with the notable exception of *P. aeruginosa*. Serious infections with *Pseudomonas* usually require the synergistic effects of one of the semisynthetic penicillins plus an aminoglycoside. Carbenicillin is now rarely used because it contains considerable amounts of sodium. Ureidopenicillins have better bactericidal activity against species of *Pseudomonas* and other gram-negative bacteria. All these agents are susceptible in varying degrees to inactivation by bacterial β-lactamases, the means of bacterial resistance to these agents.

***β-Lactamase inhibitors***
In an effort to avoid bacterial mechanisms of resistance to penicillins, there has been a considerable effort to develop substances that inhibit β-lactamase. Clavulanic acid, tazobactam, and sulbactam are commercially available β-lactamase inhibitors. They bind to conserved regions within the β-lactamase produced by a variety of organisms. The binding alters the structure of the enzyme, thereby preventing it from binding and hydrolyzing the β-lactam of the antibiotic. They have been effectively used in the treatment of non-life-threatening mixed infections (e.g., aspiration pneumonia, diabetic foot ulcers, and intra-abdominal and pelvic sepsis). Clavulanic acid is combined with preparations of ticarcillin and amoxicillin, tazobactam with piperacillin, and sulbactam with parenteral ampicillin. These preparations improve the spectrum of activity against most anaerobes, staphylococci, and certain strains of aerobic gram-negative bacteria.

## Cephalosporins

Cephalosporins kill bacteria by interfering with synthesis of their cell walls. They are most commonly used in hospitalized patients for prophylaxis against surgical wound infections because of their broad spectrum of activity. The cephalosporins are divided into groups based on their spectra of activity (Table 14-14).

First-generation cephalosporins are effective against susceptible aerobic gram-positive staphylococci, gram-negative bacteria, and streptococci. They are useful in most cases of surgical prophylaxis and in minor to moderate skin, respiratory, and urinary tract aerobic gram-positive and gram-negative bacterial infections. First-generation cephalosporins have no place in the treatment of mixed infections because they are ineffective against anaerobes.

Second-generation cephalosporins have less activity against aerobic gram-positive bacteria but enhanced aerobic gram-negative and anaerobic bacterial coverage compared with first-generation cephalosporins. They are most appropriately used to treat mixed infections, including intra-abdominal and pelvic sepsis, diabetic foot ulcers, aspiration pneumonia, many abscesses in different anatomic sites, and other polymicrobial infections. In the treatment of mixed anaerobic-aerobic infections, the most common error is the failure to consider surgical intervention (e.g., débridement of dead tissues or a surgical procedure to drain an abscess).

The third-generation cephalosporins are more effective against aerobic gram-negative organisms than their precursors. However, they are unreliable against aerobic gram-positive and most anaerobic bacteria. Because of their unique pharmacokinetic properties, third-generation cephalosporins are most useful to treat aerobic gram-negative bacterial meningitis and biliary tract infections. They should not be used as monotherapy to treat mixed infections or as empirical therapy for serious bacterial infections when staphylococci, streptococci, or anaerobes might be the etiologic agents. The overutilization of all cephalosporins has resulted in increased rates of enterococcal superinfections, because these microorganisms are not eradicated by this entire class of antibiotics. Within this class certain agents have enhanced activity against a particular organism or class of organisms. For example, cefotaxime has more activity against gram-positive cocci (except enterococci, of course); ceftizoxime against anaerobes; and ceftazidime is most active against *Pseudomonas aeruginosa*.

## Monobactams

Aztreonam is the only currently approved monobactam. It kills susceptible microorganisms by binding to penicillin-binding proteins of the bacteria, ultimately interfering with cell-wall synthesis. The spectrum of activity of aztreonam is limited, exhibiting activity against only aerobic gram-negative bacteria causing septicemia, pneumonia, osteomyelitis, and urinary tract infections. Aztreonam is active against enterobacteriaceae, *Yersinia* spp., *Pasteurella multocida*, *Capnocytophaga* spp., *Plesiomonas* spp., *Aeromonas* spp., *H. influenzae* and *Neisseria* spp. The $MIC_{90}$ against *P. aeruginosa* is 16 mg/L, a value high enough to result in only minimal activity against this microorganism. This agent has little activity against aerobic gram-positive and anaerobic bacteria. Therefore, this drug cannot be used in the majority of infectious syndromes. This relatively safe but expensive agent should be used in patients with aerobic gram-negative bacterial infections who have renal insufficiency and require prolonged therapy. The value of this regimen is that aminoglycoside therapy, which could further compromise renal function, will not have to be initiated in such compromised patients. Another benefit of aztreonam therapy is that it can be administered safely in patients who have had previous anaphylactic reactions to penicillin.

## Carbapenems

Carbapenems are a group of $\beta$-lactams with a carbapenem nucleus. Imipenem and meropenem are the only available drugs in this class. They bind to all the penicillin-binding proteins (PBPs) but preferentially bind to PBP2 and PBP1, which are responsible for maintaining the bacterium's constant diameter and extending its cell wall in any direction respectively. Interference with these bacterial transpeptidases leads to rapid lysis of most anaerobic and aerobic bacteria.

Imipenem has the widest spectrum of activity of the currently available $\beta$-lactams, and its usage ordinarily should be reserved for multidrug-resistant bacteria. Imipenem appears to be effective only against extracellular bacteria; it should not be used to treat intracellular pathogens (e.g., *L. monocytogenes*). Because of imipenem's broad spectrum of antibacterial activity, it probably is worth remembering that the only bacterial isolates that are not susceptible to imipenem include methicillin-resistant staphylococci, *Enterococcus faecalis*, *Stenotrophomonas maltophilia*, *B. cepacia*, and rare groups of *Bacteroides* (e.g., *B. ovatus*, *B. disiens*, and *B. thetaiotaomicron*). Imipenem is not recommended as routine monotherapy to treat bacterial infections of the lower respiratory tract, osteomyelitis, bacterial septicemia and endocarditis, or urinary tract, skin, or intra-abdominal infections.

Carbapenems are extensively metabolized by the renal tubular brush border dipeptidase, dehydropeptidase-1. A selective competitive antagonist of this enzyme has been identified (cilastatin), and when it is combined with imipenem in a 1:1 ratio, the antibiotic persists in the plasma for prolonged periods. Imipenem rarely produces toxic effects. High doses can produce convulsions in patients with renal insufficiency who have a prior history of seizure disorders. Imipenem can be made safe even in these patients if the rate of administration is slowed and the dose is reduced in proportion to the extent of renal insufficiency.

Meropenem has a spectrum of antimicrobial activity that is similar to imipenem. However, it is somewhat less active against gram-positive cocci and more active against *Enterobacteriaceae* and *P. aeruginosa* than imipenem. Meropenem has relatively greater stability against human dehydropeptidase-1; so concomitant administration of cilastatin is not necessary. It has less potential for inducing seizures compared with imipenem.

## Aminoglycosides

Aminoglycosides are very potent bactericidal antibiotic agents that are active against susceptible aerobic microorganisms. They kill by inhibiting protein synthesis and to some extent by lysing the cell envelope. All the aminoglycosides (streptomycin, kanamycin, neomycin, gentamicin, amikacin, tobramycin, sisomicin, and netilmicin) share common structural features. Streptomycin is used once a day in combination with other antibiotics to treat mycobacterial infections. Neomycin is used topically to treat superficial infections (a use to be discouraged) and is also given orally preoperatively for chemoprophylaxis before large-bowel surgery. The other agents are used parenterally to treat systemic bacterial septicemia (e.g., bacterial endocarditis, or urinary tract infections) or topically to treat local infection (e.g., bacterial conjunctivitis).

The physical environment where the aminoglycosides act considerably influences their antibacterial efficacy. Under conditions of low oxygen tension and low pH, and in the midst of extensive proteinaceous debris, aminoglycosides cannot exert antibacterial effects. Such an environment exists in many situations (e.g., pneumonia, abscesses, skin, and skin structure infections), and aminoglycosides should not be used as monotherapy in these settings. Likewise, aminoglycosides should not be used as monotherapy to treat osteomyelitis or CNS infections because they do not penetrate well into these tissues.

The major indication for aminoglycosides is in combination with other antibiotics (e.g., $\beta$-lactams) to treat serious aerobic bacterial infections. When combined with $\beta$-lactams, they are particularly useful for treating aerobic gram-negative septicemia (notably that caused by *Enterobacteriaceae*) and enterococcal endocarditis. The combination therapy also decreases the rate of development of bacterial resistance to the aminoglycoside by ribosomal mutation and acquisition of aminoglycoside-modifying enzymes. Because gentamicin is less costly than and as efficacious as tobramycin and amikacin, for most indications gentamicin is the preferred aminoglycoside. Amikacin should be reserved to treat bacterial infections that are known to be resistant to gentamicin and tobramycin, since it is the most stable aminoglycoside known against bacterial R-plasmid-mediated enzymes. For this reason, amikacin is active against most gentamicin- and tobramycin-resistant gram-negative bacilli. There is concern that extensive usage of amikacin will eventually select for resistant organisms and nullify its current effectiveness. Tobramycin has been recommended by some authorities because its activity against *P. aeruginosa* is greater than that of gentamicin in most hospitals, and because it may be less nephrotoxic than other aminoglycosides given parenterally. Despite these recommendations, it is still prudent to use gentamicin if the bacterial isolate is sensitive to this agent.

A number of points should be kept in mind regarding nephrotoxicity when deciding when and which aminoglycoside to use. All the aminoglycosides are concentrated in the renal cortex. The proximal tubules are most susceptible to their toxic effects, but glomerular lesions also are part of the nephrotoxicity caused by aminoglycosides. In general, when patients receive these drugs for less than 5 days, nephrotoxic effects are minimal. The nephrotoxicity is more severe in patients with previous renal insufficiency and coexisting prolonged hypovolemia, sodium depletion, and acidosis, and in those who simultaneously are given other nephrotoxic agents, including radiocontrast dye, furosemide, or indomethacin.

Since aminoglycoside nephrotoxicity is related to the dose of the drugs and their concentrations in plasma, monitoring plasma concentrations in clinically unstable patients, or in those who receive prolonged therapy, is mandatory. Based on these drug concentrations, the dose and frequency of administration of aminoglycosides should be modified (see part 1, Introduction, chapter 23, Clinical Pharmacokinetics and Pharmacodynamics). Once daily dosing of gentamicin and tobramycin (6 mg/kg per day) and amikacin (15 mg/kg per day) is recommended for patients with normal renal function (Ali and Goetz 1996; Hatala et al. 1996). This regimen is less nephrotoxic and may be more effective since peak levels are higher (and thereby takes advantage of concentration-dependent killing—a property shared by aminoglycosides). Once-daily aminoglycoside dosing should not be used for patients with endocarditis or those with ascites. The trough level should be measured 6 hours before the next dose and it should be $\leq 1 \mu$g/mL (for gentamicin, tobramycin). For amikacin the trough level is 4 to 5 $\mu$g/mL. Aminoglycosides are also toxic to both the cochlear and vestibular components of the VIII$^{th}$ cranial nerve, especially when plasma concentrations are above the therapeutic range.

## Vancomycin/Glycopeptides

Vancomycin and teicoplanin are the only members of this class of antibiotics. Vancomycin is a high-molecular-weight glycopeptide that is bactericidal for gram-positive microorganisms. It inhibits cell-wall synthesis. Given parenterally, it is the drug of choice for methicillin-resistant staphylococcal infections. It should be used as an alternative for methicillin-sensitive staphylococci if the patient is allergic to penicillin. Vancomycin is also active against strains of penicillin-resistant *S. pneumoniae*, *Leuconostoc* spp., and *Pediococcus* spp. Some strains of *Lactobacillus*, *Staphylococcus haemolyticus*, and enterococci are resistant to vancomycin. Based on considerable clinical experience, there is a lack of clinical evidence to use combinations of aminoglycosides or rifampin with parenteral vancomycin to treat staphylococcal infections. However, treatment of serious enterococcal infections with vancomycin requires the synergistic bactericidal effects of an aminoglycoside to eradicate microorganisms outside the urinary tract.

Administered orally, vancomycin is poorly absorbed. However, the concentration of vancomycin in the GI tract after an oral dose of 125 mg given every 6 hours is sufficient to eradicate—within 5 days of treatment—strains of *C. difficile* responsible for antibiotic-associated colitis.

Vancomycin is excreted by the kidneys in an essentially unchanged form. Vancomycin accumulates in patients with renal failure, and dosage adjustments are required to reduce the chances of adverse effects. Nephrotoxicity attributed to this agent has decreased remarkably because of improvements in the purification procedures in production of this drug. There are no data to suggest that monitoring serum vancomycin concentrations improves the effectiveness of therapy. Furthermore, safe and effective vancomycin-dosing regimens can be derived empirically, taking into account the patient's age, weight, and renal function (Cantu et al. 1994). The risk of nephrotoxicity with vancomycin is enhanced when drugs such as aminoglycosides or ethacrynic acid are given concomitantly. Ototoxicity in the form of tinnitus, high-tone hearing loss, and deafness is an important adverse reaction to vancomycin. The hearing loss occasionally improves when the drug is discontinued, but unfortunately it is usually permanent.

A "red man syndrome" characterized by hypotension and a maculopapular rash on the chest occurs if the drug is administered too quickly (e.g., over less than 30 minutes). If the infusion of vancomycin is prolonged (i.e., one gram infused over at least 60 minutes), the incidence of this syndrome is decreased.

Teicoplanin (not FDA approved at this point) has a spectrum of activity similar to that of vancomycin but with activity 2 to 4 times as high against sensitive organisms (except for diphtheroids). Some strains of coagulase-negative staphylococci are resistant to teicoplanin and sensitive to vancomycin. Teicoplanin is also effective against *Clostridium difficile* colitis when given orally.

## Chloramphenicol

Chloramphenicol exerts its broad antibacterial effects by binding to the 50-S ribosome subunit, inhibiting protein synthesis. Because of its serious toxic profile, which includes aplastic anemia and gray baby syndrome, and the availability of other less toxic but equally effective drugs used for similar indications, chloramphenicol is not extensively used.

## Tetracyclines

The molecular structure of tetracyclines includes four benzene rings. They have a broad spectrum of antibacterial activity, and by binding to the 30-S ribosome subunit, they exert their effects by inhibiting protein synthesis. A considerable number of compounds, especially orally active preparations, have been developed. Unfortunately, because of the high prevalence of tetracycline-resistant microorganisms and the availability of alternative effective antibiotics, the place of tetracyclines in therapy has diminished. Tetracyclines remain the drugs of choice to treat brucellosis, which also requires combination with streptomycin. They also are the drugs of choice to treat chlamydial and rickettsial infections and melioidosis. Doxycycline is effective against some strains of *Mycobacterium fortuitum-chelonei*. Since resistance to tetracyclines is so prevalent among all species of bacteria, the effectiveness of tetracyclines in treating a variety of clinical syndromes cannot be predicted.

Major tetracycline toxicity includes nephrotoxicity and hepatotoxicity, especially in the pregnant patient. Tetracyclines are contraindicated in pregnant women and in children <8 years of age because of accumulation of these drugs in the growth zone of teeth (also in bones), producing a characteristic unpleasant pigmentation.

## Macrolides

Erythromycin is a macrolide antibiotic that binds to the 50-S subunit of the ribosomes. It kills susceptible bacteria by interfering with their protein synthesis. Erythromycin is active against many aerobic gram-positive bacteria, selected gram-negative bacteria (including species of *Legionella, N. meningitidis, H. influenzae*, and *Bordetella pertussis*), and nonbacterial species (e.g., *C. trachomatis*, mycoplasma, and certain rickettsial species). There are three available oral preparations of erythromycin: erythromycin stearate, erythromycin ethyl succinate, and erythromycin estolate. The first two preparations do not have intrinsic antibacterial activity until they dissociate or hydrolyze (respectively) to active compounds. They are routinely recommended to be taken orally one hour before meals, so that effective concentrations of drugs in plasma can be consistently achieved. The estolate form is associated with the highest concentrations in plasma.

The parenteral forms of erythromycin include an ethyl succinate form for IM administration and lactobionate or gluceptate forms for use IV. The severity of irritation of veins with erythromycin frequently requires large veins to be catheterized and low concentrations of lidocaine coadministered with the antibiotic to reduce pain. Excessively rapid IV infusion of erythromycin results in diffuse cramping and GI discomfort due to contraction of intestinal smooth muscle.

Erythromycin is widely used as an alternative for $\beta$-lactam antibiotics in the patient who is allergic to penicillin and requires treatment for non-life-threatening gram-positive bacterial infection. These include streptococcal and pneumococcal systemic infections and staphylococcal skin infections. In more serious infections with these organisms, vancomycin is preferred over erythromycin. Erythromycin has been effective in treating *Legionella pneumonia* and *H.influenzae* respiratory and otitis media infections. It is effectively used as an alternative drug for a variety of sexually transmitted diseases, including gonorrhea, chlamydial infections, syphilis, and chancroid.

Clarithromycin has a similar spectrum of antimicrobial activity to erythromycin. However, clarithromycin is also active against *M. avium* complex. Clarithromycin has a longer half-life than erythromycin and can be given twice daily. Clarithromycin and azithromycin result in less gastrointestinal upset (nausea and vomiting) than erythromycin.

Azithromycin is usually discussed as a macrolide, but it is really an azalide. Like clarithromycin it is active against *M. avium* complex. Otherwise its spectrum of activity is similar to erythromycin. It can be given once weekly as prophylaxis against *M. avium* complex infections in HIV-infected patients whose CD4 count is $\leq 50/\text{mm}^3$. Because of its long half-life, azithromycin is given once daily for 5 days to treat most infections.

Macrolides are metabolized by cytochromes P450 isoform CYP3A, and they (erythromycin and clarithromycin—very rarely azithromycin) interact with a number of drugs that are also metabolized via this system including carbamazepine, theophylline, phenytoin, warfarin, cyclosporin, colchicine, bromocriptine, valproic acid, terfenadine, cisapride, astemizole, triazolam, midazolarn, disopyramide, and acenocournarol. Erythromycin in combination with terfenadine, astemizole, or cisapride, should be avoided because of prolongation of the QT interval and the possibility of torsade des pointes. High-dose erythromycin (e.g., 4 g/day) in elderly patients or patients with renal failure can result in transient deafness.

## Clindamycin

Clindamycin is a chemically modified derivative of lincomycin. It exerts its activity by binding to the 50-S subunit of the bacterial ribosome, inhibiting protein synthesis. Its antibacterial spectrum includes staphylococci and streptococci (but not enterococci), many anaerobic gram-positive strains, and most anaerobic gram-negative bacteria. Clindamycin is most appropriately used to treat clinical syndromes that involve anaerobic pathogens. Clindamycin is not recommended as primary agent to treat staphylococcal or streptococcal infections despite its antibacterial activity against these microorganisms.

Clindamycin is extensively cleared by the liver. Doses should be modified when patients have significant hepatic insufficiency. The most common serious adverse reaction to clindamycin is pseudomembranous colitis. This effect occurs 2 days to 3 weeks after beginning therapy in 1 to 10% of patients treated with clindamycin. However, as was discussed earlier, this example of superinfection is not unique to the use of clindamycin, since essentially any antibiotic can produce the same condition. The pathogenesis of this syndrome generally involves excretion of the antibiotic in the stool and selection for *C. difficile* in the GI tract. Clinically important *C. difficile* strains elaborate toxins that are cytotoxic to the epithelial mucosal cells, and a pseudomembrane covers the afflicted area. Symptoms of colitis usually include fever, cramping, abdominal pain, and diarrhea. Appropriate diagnostic tests for this syndrome include sigmoidoscopy or colonoscopy (in some situations), assessment of the stool for the presence of inflammatory cells, and detection of the toxin in the stool. Effective therapy for this superinfection includes oral metronidazole or oral vancomycin in resistant cases. Cholestyramine can also be used to bind the toxin. Caution must be taken to ensure that cholestyramine does not bind other medications that the patient is receiving—

hence it should be administered 2 hours before or after other medications.

## Metronidazole

Metronidazole is a nitroimidazole drug that has activity against anaerobic bacteria and protozoan. The drug is postulated to be metabolized within the anaerobe to an active drug that interacts with the anaerobe's DNA to produce cell death. The spectrum of antibacterial activity for metronidazole is confined to most anaerobes. It has essentially no activity against aerobic bacteria. Metronidazole has been effectively used to treat a variety of infections involving anaerobic strains, including intra-abdominal sepsis, genital infections, abscesses, aspiration pneumonia, and osteomyelitis. It has also been used to treat trichomoniasis, amoebiasis, giardiasis, and bacterial vaginosis. Because of its low resistance rate and low cost, metronidazole should be the drug of choice in treatment of many anaerobic infections.

## Sulfonamides and Trimethoprim

Sulfonamides and trimethoprim are used to treat mild to moderately severe bacterial infections caused by sensitive organisms. They exert their antibacterial effects by interfering with the microorganism's folate metabolism, which is essential for purine and ultimately DNA synthesis. There are many sulfonamides available, differing from each other by their duration of action. Sulfadiazine is short-acting (must be administered every 6 to 8 hours), whereas sulfamethoxazole has medium duration of action (given every 12 hours), and sulfadoxine is ultralong-acting (requires dosage once a week). Most sulfonamides are readily absorbed from the GI tract.

Trimethoprim is an inhibitor of dihydrofolate reductase and frequently is combined with sulfonamides, but it can also be used as a single agent with success equivalent to that expected of sulfonamides used alone. The two agents once had a wide range of antimicrobial activity. However, extensive usage and the rapid development of microbial resistance to these drugs have narrowed their spectrum of activity.

Sulfonamide-susceptible microorganisms include some staphylococci, many streptococci except *S. faecalis*, many anaerobic gram-positive bacilli, some *L. monocytogenes*, most species of *Nocardia*, the majority of Enterobacteriaceae, many pathogenic species of *Neisseria*, *Stenotrophomonas maltophilia*, *H. influenzae*, many other gram-negative anaerobes, strains of *Chlamydia* except *C. psittaci*, some atypical species of mycobacteria, protozoa such as *Toxoplasma gondii* and malaria, and unique fungi such as *P. carinii* when therapy combines pyrimethamine or trimethoprim with sulfonamides.

Trimethoprim-sulfamethoxazole is an effective combination agent for prophylaxis against *P. carinii* infection in HIV patients when the CD4 count is $<200/\text{mm}^3$. In such instances one double-strength tablet is administered once daily or three times weekly.

The combination trimethoprim-sulfamethoxazole is effective in treating urinary tract infections that are caused by a variety of aerobic gram-positive and gram-negative bacteria, otitis media, acute and chronic bronchitis, and bacterial pneumonia, venereal diseases (e.g., gonorrhea, chancroid, granuloma venereum, and sometimes *C. trachomatis infections*), typhoid fever from susceptible strains, shigellosis, cholera, brucellosis, nocardiosis, toxoplasmosis, and *P. carinii* pneumonia. Allergic adverse responses are frequent, especially in AIDS patients. They most notably include rashes, drug fever, and bone marrow suppression.

## Quinolones

Norfloxacin and ciprofloxacin were the first of the quinolones approved by the FDA. They are derivatives of nalidixic acid, which is the prototype compound of this class. In contrast to nalidixic acid, norfloxacin and ciprofloxacin readily penetrate the outer membranes of a large number of gram-negative and selected gram-positive bacteria. These agents exert their antibacterial effects by binding to DNA gyrase, thereby inhibiting replication of bacterial DNA. Microorganisms are killed by quinolones if they continue to synthesize protein. Ultimately, the bacteria cannot divide because of the effects of the quinolone. Resistance develops via chromosomal mutation, especially among enteric flora exposed to subinhibitory concentrations of drug.

These drugs are administered orally. Norfloxacin, which is poorly absorbed, is more limited in its distribution within the body than is ciprofloxacin. Norfloxacin is used mainly to treat urinary tract infections. Ciprofloxacin, in addition to being useful in treating urinary tract infections, is used to treat bone, respiratory, inner ear, and soft tissue infections because of its spectrum of activity and excellent oral bioavailability.

The quinolones exert their greatest antibacterial effects against susceptible aerobic gram-negative bacteria from the Enterobacteriaceae, including many strains of *P. aeruginosa*. Infections due to these microorganisms are appropriately treated with quinolones. The role of quinolones in the treatment of other gram-negative microorganisms (e.g., *H. influenzae* and *N. gonorrhoeae*) is controversial. Quinolones are not recommended to treat anaerobic infections, nor as monotherapy for serious life-threatening infections or meningitis.

A number of new quinolones (Table 14-57), so-called "respiratory quinolones" because of enhanced activity against *S. pneumoniae* compared with ciprofloxacin, are now available. These include levofloxacin, sparfloxacin, grepafloxacin, and trovafloxacin. Since these agents are active against penicillin- and/or macrolide-resistant *S. pneumoniae*, there will be a tendency to use these newer quinolones widely in the treatment of community-acquired pneumonia. At present we have very little data with which to make clear recommendations about the superiority of one class of antibiotics over another for the ambulatory management of community-acquired pneumonia. Grepafloxacin has been removed from the market because of torsade de pointes due to prolonged QT interval. Trovafloxacin has been removed because of severe hypersensitivity hepatitis, some cases of which were fatal.

## Streptogramins

This is a distinct class of antibiotics consisting of two structurally unrelated compounds that interact synergistically. Group A streptogramin is a polyunsaturated macrolactone with a molecular mass of 500 daltons, whereas group B streptogramin is a cyclic hexadecapeptide with a molecular weight of 800 daltons. Streptogramins work at the ribosome level. Group A streptogramins inhibit both the binding of peptidyl-tRNA to the donor site and that of aminoacyl-tRNA to the acceptor site of peptidyltransferase. Group B streptogramins prevent peptide bond formation indirectly, causing the release of peptidyl-tRNA from the donor site. Currently there is one antibiotic, quinapristin/dalfopristin (Synercid), of this class available in Canada (not yet approved by the FDA). This combination consists of 30% quinapristin and 70% dalfopristin. Streptogramins typically are active against both methicillin-susceptible and methicillin-resistant *S. aureus* and *S. epidermidis*, penicillin-susceptible and penicillin-resistant *S. pneumoniae*, *E. faecium* both vancomycin-sensitive and resistant strains, group A, B, C streptococci, *Corynebacterium jeikeium*, *Mycoplasma* species, *Legionella* spp, *H. influenzae*, *M. catarrhalis*, and *Neisseria* spp. Quinapristin/dalfopristin is available for intravenous use only. It is given as 7.5 mg/kg every 8 hours or every 12 hours. Nausea, vomiting, and skin rash are encountered with a frequency similar to other antibiotics. Phlebitis at the site of the infusion is commonly encountered and leads to discontinuation of treatment in about 10% of patients. Asymptomatic hyperbilirubinemia is seen in 10%. Quinapristin/dalfopristin is metabolized via the cytochrome P450 system and hence can interact with drugs such as FK506 that are metabolized via the same pathways when given concurrently. Currently quinapristin/dalfopristin is

**Table 14-57 Comparison of Selected Features of "Respiratory Quinolones" with Ciprofloxacin**

| | Ciprofloxacin | Levofloxacin | Sparfloxacin |
|---|---|---|---|
| Daily dose for treatment of pneumonia | 500–750 mg PO q12h<br>200–400 mg IV q12h | 500 mg PO q24h<br>500 mg IV q24h | 300 mg PO odd or 400 mg loading dose, then 200 mg PO od |
| Peak concentration | 2–3.4 μg/ml | 5.7 μg/ml | 1.1 μg/ml |
| $t_{1/2}$ | 3–6 h | 6–8 h | 16–32 h, average 20 h |
| Percent absorbed | 60–80 | 99 | 92 |
| Main mode of excretion | Kidney | Kidney | Kidney/liver |
| $MIC_{90}$ *Streptococcus pneumoniae* | 2 μg/ml | 1 μg/ml | 1 μg/ml |
| Major adverse event(s) | Well-tolerated<br>Nausea (1.3%)<br>Diarrhea (1%) | GI effects most common <2% incidence | Mild <QTc-prolongation<br>Phototoxicity (2%) |

ABBREVIATIONS: IV, intravenous; $MIC_{90}$, minimal inhibitory concentration at which 90% of growth is arrested; od, once daily; PO, oral.

reserved for resistant gram-positive infections, especially vancomycin resistant *E. faecium*.

## Oxazolidinones

Linezolid is the first synthetic oxazolidinone antibiotic. It binds to the 505 ribosomal subunit. It is active against vancomycin resistant enterococci, and against other streptococci as well as *S. aureus* and coagulase negative staphylococci.

## Antituberculosis Drugs

Treatment of mycobacterial infections requires multiple drugs because monotherapy frequently fails. Resistance of *M. tuberculosis* to an antimicrobial agent occurs as a result of spontaneous mutation, at a usual frequency of 1 in $10^5$ to $10^6$. Mutational resistance to each drug occurs as an independent event, and thus the likelihood of resistancy by a single organism being to two drugs is equal to the product of the individual probabilities. Therefore, combined chemotherapy with two or more drugs prevents the emergence of strains resistant to an individual drug. The likelihood of organisms developing resistance is increased if the patient previously has been treated and if the infection was the result of exposure to a resistant stain.

Tuberculocidal drugs are preferred and should be capable of killing both rapidly dividing extracellular organisms and slower dividing intracellular organisms in order to prevent relapse. Isoniazid and rifampin are tuberculocidal in both intra- and extracellular locations and are generally recommended in all patients with mycobacterial infection. Streptomycin is tuberculocidal for extracellular organisms only, whereas pyrazinamide is tuberculocidal for intracellular organisms. Ethambutol, *p*-aminosalicylic acid, and ethionamide are only tuberculostatic.

The institution of effective chemotherapy results in rapid reversal of infectiousness of mycobacteria within 3 to 7 days. However, the clinical manifestations of disease may persist for prolonged periods. Although antimicrobial-resistant mycobacterial strains emerge as an important epidemiologic cause for clinical failure, the major cause of failure of an effective drug regimen for mycobacterial infections is lack of compliance by the patient.

## Antifungal Drugs

Fungal infections are particularly serious and common among neutropenic, immunocompromised patients who have received prolonged broad-spectrum antibiotics. A number of systemic fungal infections (e.g., histoplasmosis, coccidioidomycosis, and paracoccidioidomycosis) can also afflict otherwise healthy persons. Until recently, only amphotericin B was available to treat systemic fungal infection. However, with the rapid development and clinical assessment of azole compounds, a number of these agents are also considered appropriate for treatment of fungal infections.

Amphotericin B is a polyene antibiotic that exerts its antifungal effect by binding to sterol moieties in the membranes of fungi. This causes pores in the cell wall, eventually causing leakage of low-molecular-weight cytoplasmic components. This effect, coupled with amphotericin's ability to stimulate granulocytes and T and B cells, ultimately leads to the death of fungi. Amphotericin B has a wide spectrum of antifungal activity. Susceptible fungi include species of *Candida*, *Histoplasma capsulatum*, *Cryptococcus neoformans*, *Coccidioides immitis*, *Blastomyces dermatitides*, *Paracoccidioides brasiliensis*, *Sporothrix schenckii*, and many strains of *Aspergillus*. It is still considered the drug of choice for any life-threatening disseminated fungal disease.

This choice may well change with greater experience with the newer azole agents since amphotericin B causes considerable toxicity, most notably anaphylaxis, other allergic reactions, renal insufficiency, and bone marrow suppression. It was observed in animal models that amphotericin B toxicity was decreased if it was bound to surfactants before administration (Brajtburg and Bolard 1996). As a result of this observation a number of amphotericin B–lipid formulations have been developed (Table 14-58). These products are extremely expensive, but they appear to be more effective and less toxic than conventional amphotericin B in the treatment of invasive aspergillus.

The newer antifungal agents include ketoconazole, miconazole, itraconazole, and fluconazole (see Table 14-59). These agents are azoles, and they exert their antifungal activity by inhibiting ergosterol synthesis. Ketoconazole is available in oral form, and in normal patients is often erratically absorbed from the GI tract. Achlorhydria caused by any mechanism significantly reduces its absorption. Ketoconazole is metabolized primarily in the liver. To prevent toxicity it must be judiciously employed in patients with hepatic failure, or in those who receive other drugs that are also metabolized in the liver. A major adverse effect of ketoconazole is it effect on the endocrine system (e.g., blunting of cortisol and androgen synthesis, and production of gynecomastia). Ketoconazole is particularly effective in treating certain forms of histoplasmosis, coccidioidomycosis, paracoccidioidomycosis, and candid-

Table 14-58 **Lipid-Based Formulations of Amphotericin B**

| PRODUCT | FORM | PERCENT AMB BY WEIGHT | SIZE (NM) | DOSE | AWP ($/DAY) |
|---|---|---|---|---|---|
| AMB–lipid complex (ABLC) (Abelcet) | Nonliposomal | 33% | 1,600–11,000 | 5 mg/kg/day | $520 |
| AMB colloidal dispersion (ABCD) (Amphocil) | Nonliposomal | 50% | 120–140 | 1–5 mg/kg/day | $223 (1.5 mg/kg) |
| L-AMB | Liposomal spherical | 10% | 80 | 1–5 mg/kg | $1,070 (5 mg/kg) |
| (AmBisome) | Unilamellar, vesicle | | | | |
| (ABLE) | Spherical vesicles | Variable | 300–500 | 1 mg/kg | |
| Amphotericin B (Fungizone IV Fungizone Topical) | N/A | 100% | N/A | 0.5–1 mg/kg/day | $22 |

ABBREVIATIONS: AMB, amphotericin B; N/A, not applicable.

iasis. It is not recommended for treating CNS fungal infections because it penetrates the CSF poorly, or for serious life-threatening diseases because GI absorption can be erratic.

Miconazole is rarely employed systemically because of its serious adverse effects and the availability of other agents. However, parenteral miconazole is the drug of choice for infections due to *Pseudoallescheria boydii*. In addition, topical miconazole is frequently used as an effective antimicrobial for vaginal yeast infections.

Itraconazole is administered orally and is well distributed within the body with the exception of penetration into the CSF. Itraconazole should not be used in patients with CNS fungal infections. Its spectrum of activity is similar to that of amphotericin B. Clinical studies to date suggest that it is useful to treat selected cases of disseminated candidiasis, histoplasmosis, coccidiomycosis, selected infections with *Aspergillus*, sporotrichosis, blastomycosis, and paracoccidioidomycosis. It has the advantage over amphotericin B of being relatively safe.

Fluconazole is unique among the azoles in that it can penetrate into the CSF in high concentration. Parenteral and oral forms of fluconazole therapy are available. Its spectrum of activity is very similar to that of other azoles and amphotericin B. Clinical experience to date suggests that it is the drug of choice for treatment of oroesophageal

Table 14-59 **Summary—Antifungal Drugs**

| DRUG | ROUTE | ADVANTAGES | COMMENTS |
|---|---|---|---|
| Ketoconazole | PO | Oral treatment of histoplasmosis, coccidioidomycosis, candidiasis; cheaper than itraconazole and fluconazole | Erratic oral absorption; do not rely on for CNS or serious systemic infections. |
| Fluconazole | IV, PO | Good oral absorption, excellent CNS penetration | Can be used as suppressive therapy of cryptococcal meningitis in HIV-infected patients. Drug interactions are common. |
| Itraconazole | PO | Only one of the imidazoles with activity against *Aspergillus* | Poor CNS penetration |
| Miconazole | IV, T | Drug of choice (IV) for treatment of *Pseudallescheria boydii* | |

ABBREVIATIONS: IV, intravenous; PO, oral; T, topical.

and mucocutaneous candidiasis and for suppressive therapy of cryptococcal meningitis in AIDS patients.

## Antiviral Agents

In the last decade, considerable strides have been made developing effective antiviral therapy. A major obstacle in such development has been identifying agents that do not injure host cells but still effectively inhibit viral metabolism and replication. The clinically most important new antiviral agents include famciclovir, valacyclovir, foscarnet, and cidofovir for treating herpes viruses; AZT and a variety of new antiretroviral drugs for the HIV agent (see the section on treatment of AIDS); and ganciclovir to treat infections caused by cytomegalovirus.

Acyclovir is a purine nucleoside analog. Its antiviral activity is almost completely restricted to the herpesviruses (HSV 1 and 2, VZV, and EBV). Once acyclovir has penetrated virally infected cells, it is phosphorylated into acyclovir monophosphate by HSV thymidine kinase and sequentially into di- and triphosphate forms by cellular enzymes. Acyclovir is a potent inhibitor of viral DNA polymerases and also terminates biosynthesis of the strand of viral DNA. Acyclovir distributes widely throughout the body including the CSF. The major route of elimination is via glomerular filtration and tubular secretion. Therefore, dosage adjustment is required in patients with renal dysfunction. Acyclovir is effective in the treatment of a number of infections caused by herpes simplex virus, including mucocutaneous, genital, and encephalitic infections, and varicella-zoster infections.

Valacyclovir, the L-valyl ester of acyclovir, is almost entirely converted to acyclovir after oral administration. Valacyclovir has bioavailability 3 to 5 times as great as that of acyclovir and is given at a dose of 1 gram three times daily. Some immunocompromised patients have developed thrombocytopenic purpura/hemolytic-uremic syndrome while receiving high-dose valacyclovir.

Ganciclovir (DHPG) is also a nucleoside analog. Its antiviral activity is primarily directed against cytomegalovirus. Once phosphorylated to the triphosphate form by cellular enzymes, it interferes with viral replication through competitive inhibition of viral DNA polymerase and also terminates viral DNA synthesis. Ganciclovir is well distributed to most organs including lungs, liver, and the brain and is primarily excreted by the kidneys. Dosage adjustment is also indicated in patients with renal dysfunction. The primary indication of ganciclovir is the treatment of cytomegalovirus-associated retinitis in the immunocompromised host. Data on ganciclovir treatment of CMV-associated pneumonitis, encephalitis, colitis, and hepatitis remains controversial.

Famciclovir is the diacetyl, 6-deoxyester of the guanosine analog penciclovir. It is well absorbed (bioavailability 77%) and rapidly converted to penciclovir. It is administered every 8 hours with adjustment for renal insufficiency. It is approved for the treatment of herpes zoster and recurrent genital HSV infections.

Foscarnet (phosphonoformic acid) is a pyrophosphate-containing compound with activity against herpes viruses including CMV. It can only be administered intravenously and is infused over 1 to 2 hours using an infusion pump. Administration of 500 mL of saline before foscarnet lessens renal toxicity. The major indications for foscarnet are CMV retinitis, and HSV infections resistant to acyclovir. In a comparative trial, foscarnet was as efficacious as ganciclovir for the treatment of CMV retinitis but was associated with longer survival (Ocular Complication of AIDS Research Group 1992). Renal function should be monitored carefully during treatment with foscarnet because of its nephrotoxicity. It binds divalent cations, and hence hypocalcemia, hypomagnesemia, hypokalemia, and hypo- or hyperphosphatemia can develop. Uncircumcised males can develop balanitis due to irritant action of foscarnet excreted in the urine. Careful drying of the penis following urination can prevent foscarnet-induced balanitis.

Cidofovir, a phosphonomethylether derivative of cytosine, is highly active against cytomegalovirus, including some ganciclovir-resistant and foscarnet-resistant strains. It is mostly cleared by the kidney and has a half-life of 2.6 hours. It is given intravenously (ocular implants are also available). Concomitant administration of probenecid markedly prolongs the half-life of cidofovir and protects against nephrotoxicity. The intracellular half-life of cidofovir diphosphate is 17 to 30 hours, and hence, it can be administered once a week to once every two weeks.

The new antiretrovirals are described in the section on the treatment of AIDS.

The use of interferons as antiviral agents has been mainly for treatment of hepatitis B and C (Saracco and Rizzetto 1997), although IFN-$\alpha$ has also been used for the treatment of Kaposi's sarcoma and hairy-cell leukemia. The administration of interferon alpha 2b (5 million units daily for 16 weeks) to patients with chronic hepatitis B infection resulted in loss of markers of HBV replication in 33 to 37% of cases, whereas 10 to 20% became hepatitis B surface antigen negative. Several interferon preparations ($\alpha$2a, $\alpha$2b and $\alpha$L [lymphoblastoid]) have been studied for the treatment of hepatitis C.

## ACKNOWLEDGMENT

The authors thank Dr. Robert Coombs, University of Washington, Seattle, Washington, for preparation of the section on monitoring the response to HIV treatment and Ms. Ann Thompson, BSc Pharm, Department of Pharmacy Queen Elizabeth II Health Sciences Centre, Halifax, NS, for preparation of Table 14-57. We also thank Janice Smuck, Lorrie Walker, and Megan Marrie for secretarial support in the preparation of this chapter.

## REFERENCES

Abraham E, Wunderink R, Silverman H, et al. 1995. Efficacy and safety of monoclonal antibody to human tumor-necrosis-factor in patients with sepsis syndrome: A randomized controlled double-blind multicentre clinical trial. TNF Mab Sepsis Study Group. *JAMA* **273**:934–41.

Abrams DI. 1990. Alternative therapies in HIV infection. *AIDS* **4**: 1179–87.

Abrams DI, Kuno S, Wong R. 1989. Oral dextran sulfate (UA001) in treatment of the acquired immunodeficiency syndrome (AIDS) and AIDS-related complex (ARC). *Ann Intern Med* **110**:183–8.

Adkinson N, Swabb E, Sugerman A. 1984. Immunology of the monobactam aztreonam. *Antimicrob Agents Chemother* **25**:93–8.

Agebede OO. 1992. HIV-1 indeterminate Western blot results: Implications for diagnosis and subject notification. *Clin Microbiol Newsl* **14**:121–6.

Agrawal S, Goodchild J, Civeria MP. 1988. Oligonucleoside phosphoramidate and phosphorthioates as inhibitors of human immunodeficiency virus. *Proc Natl Acad Sci USA* **85**:7079–83.

Ali MA, Goetz MD. 1997. A meta-analysis of the relative efficacy and toxicity of single daily dosing versus multiple daily using of aminoglycosides. *Clin Infect Dis* **24**:796–809.

[ACCP/SCCM]. 1992. Definitions of sepsis and multiple organ failure and guidelines for the use of innovative therapies in sepsis. American College of Chest Physicians/Society of Critical Care Medicine Consensus Conference. *Crit Care Med* **20**:864–74.

Antimicrobial prophylaxis in surgery. 1997. *Med Lett Drugs Ther* **39**:97–101.

Arnett EN, Roberts WC. 1976. Valve ring abscess in active infective endocarditis: Frequency, location, and clues to clinical diagnosis from the study of 95 necropsy patients. *Circulation* **54**:140–5.

Balduzzi P, Glasgow LA. 1967. Paralytic poliomyelitis in a contact of a vaccinated child. *N Engl J Med* **276**:796–7.

Barnes PF, Bloch AB, Davidson PT, et al. 1991. Tuberculosis in patients with human immunodeficiency virus infection. *N Engl J Med* **324**:1644–50.

Barrett-Connor E. 1971. Bacterial infection and sickle cell anemia: an analysis of 250 infections in 166 patients and a review of the literature. *Medicine* **50**:97–112.

Barriere S. 1985. Cost-containment of antimicrobial therapy. *Drug Intell Clin Pharm* **19**:278–81.

Barry W, Hudgins L, Donta ST, et al. 1992. Intravenous immunoglobulin therapy for toxic shock syndrome. *JAMA* **267**:3315–6.

Bartlett J. 1984. Treatment of antibiotic-associated pseudomembranous colitis. *Rev Infect Dis* **6**:235–46.

Bass JB, Farer LS, Hopewell PC, et al. 1994. Treatment of tuberculosis and tuberculosis infection in adults and children. *Am J Respir Crit Care Med* **149**:1359–74.

Bauer AW, Kirby WMM, Sherris JC, et al. 1966. Antibiotic susceptibility testing by a standardized single disk method. *Am J Clin Pathol* **45**:493–6.

Bayer AS, Theofilopoulos AN. 1990. Immunopathologenetic aspects of infective endocarditis. *Chest* **97**:204–12.

Beadle C, Long GW, Weiss WR, et al. 1994. Diagnosis of malaria by detection of *Plasmodium falciparum* HRP-2 antigen with rapid dipstick antigen captive assay. *Lancet* **343**:564–8.

Bennett WM. 1988. Guide to drug dosage in renal failure. *Clin Pharmacokinet* **15**:326–54.

Bennett WM, Aronoff GR, Golper TA. et al. 1994. *Drug Prescribing in Renal Failure.* 3rd ed. Dosing guidelines for adults. Philadelphia: American College of Physicians, pp 18–37.

Bennett M, Singer I, Coggins CH. 1974. A guide to drug therapy in renal failure. *JAMA* **230**:1544–53.

Bentley R, Meganathan R. 1982. Biosynthesis of vitamin K in bacteria. *Microbiol Rev* **46**:241–80.

Bergdahl S, Sonnerborg A, Larsson A, et al. 1988. Declining levels of HIV p24 antigen in serum during treatment with foscarnet. *Lancet* **1**:1052.

Berger EA. 1997. HIV entry and tropism: The chemokine receptor connection. *AIDS* **11**(Suppl A):S3–16.

Berger SA, Weitzmann S, Edberg SC, et al. 1974. Bacteremia after the use of an oral irrigation device. A controlled study in subjects with normal-appearing gingiva: Comparison with use of toothbrush. *Ann Intern Med* **80**:510–1.

Berglund O, Engman K, Ehrnst A, et al. 1991. Combined treatment of symptomatic human immunodeficiency virus type 1 infection with native interferon alpha and zidovudine. *J Infect Dis* **163**: 710–15.

Bliska JB, Galan E, Falkow S. 1993. Signal transduction in the mammalian cell during bacterial attachment and entry. *Cell* **73**:903–20.

Block AB, Couther GM, Onorato IM, et al. 1994. Nationwide survey of drug-resistant tuberculosis in the United States. *JAMA* **271**: 665–71.

Bodey GP. 1984. Antibiotics in patients with neutropenia. *Arch Intern Med* **144**:1845–51.

Bodey GP, Buckley M, Sathe YS, et al. 1966. Quantitative relationship between circulating leukocytes and infection in patients with acute leukemia. *Ann Intern Med* **64**:328–40.

Bodey GP, Rodrigues V, Chang HY, et al. 1978. Fever and infection in leukemic patients A study of 494 consecutive patients. *Cancer* **41**:1616–22.

Bone RC. 1991a. Sepsis syndrome: Multiorgan failure: A plea for comparable definitions. *Ann Intern Med* **114**:332–3.

Bone RC. 1991b. Sepsis syndrome: New insights into its pathogenesis and treatment. *Infect Dis Clin NA* **5**:793–805.

Bone RC. 1996. Why sepsis trials fail. *JAMA* **276**:565–6.

Boursnell MEG, Entwisle C, Blackeley D, et al. 1997. A genetically inactivated herpes simplex virus type 2 (HSV-2) vaccine provides effective protection against primary and recurrent HSV-2 disease. *J Infect Dis* **175**:16–25.

Boyer PJ, Dillon M, Navaie M, et al. 1994. Factors predictive of maternal-fetal transmission of HIV-1: Preliminary analysis of zidovudine given during pregnancy and/or delivery. *JAMA* **271**: 1925–30.

Brajtburg J, Bolard J. 1996. Carrier effects on biological activity of amphotericin B. *Clin Microbiol Rev* **9**:512–31.

Brandts CH, Ndjave M, Graninger W, et al. 1997. Effect of paracetamol on parasite clearance time in *Plasmodium falciparum* malaria. *Lancet* **350**:704–9.

Browne MJ, Mayer KH, Chafee SBD, et al. 1993. 2′3′-didehydro-3′-deoxythymidine (d4T) in patients with AIDS or AIDS-related complex: A phase I trial. *J Infect Dis* **167**:21–9.

Bruister SM, Frissen PHJ, Van Swieten P, et al. 1997. Prospective longitudinal analysis of viral load and surrogate markers in relation to clinical progression in HIV type 1-infected persons. *AIDS Res Hum Retroviruses* **13**:327–35.

Brun-Buisson C, Doyon F, Carlet J, et al. 1995. Incidence, risk factors, and outcome of severe sepsis and septic shock in adults. A multicenter prospective study in intensive care units. French ICU Group for Severe Sepsis. *JAMA* **274**:968–74.

Brun-Vezinet F, Boucher C, Loveday C, et al. 1997. HIV-1 viral load phenotype and resistance in a subset of drug naive participants from the Delta trial. *Lancet* **350**:983–90.

Burton DR, Montefiori DC. 1997. The antibody response in HIV-1 infection. *AIDS* **11** (Suppl A):S87–98.

Butler KM, Husson RN, Balis FM, et al. 1991. Dideoxyinosine (ddI) in symptomatic HIV-infected children: A phase I-II study. *N Engl J Med* **324**:137–44.

Byington RE, Henochowicz S, Gubish E, et al. 1990. Recombinant soluble CD4 therapy in patients with acquired immunodeficiency syndrome (AIDS) or AIDS-related complex: A phase I/II escalating dose trial. *Ann Intern Med* **112**:247–53.

Cameron DW, Heath-Chiozzi M, Kravick S, et al. 1996. Prolongation of life and prevention of AIDS complications in advanced HIV immunodeficiency with ritonavir update. The Advanced HIV Ritonavir Study Group and Leonard J Abbott Laboratories. 11th International Conference on AIDS; 1996 Jul; Vancouver, BC. Abstract MoB 411.

Canadian Lung Association. 1996. *Canadian Tuberculosis Standards*. 4th ed. Canadian Lung Association, Lowe Martin Group Inc.

Cantu TG, Yamanaka-Yuen NS, Lietman PS. 1994. Serum vancomycin concentrations: Reappraisal of their clinical value. *Clin Infect Dis* **18**:533–43.

Cantwell MF, Snider DE, Cauther GM, et al. 1994. Epidemiology of tuberculosis in the United States, 1985 through 1992. *JAMA* **272**:535–9.

Capon DJ, Chamow SM, Mordenti J, et al. 1989. Designing CD4 immunoadhesins for AIDS therapy. *Nature* **337**:525–31.

Carpenter CC, Fischl MA, Hammer SM. 1996. Antiretroviral therapy for HIV infection in 1996: Recommendations of an international panel. International AIDS Society. *JAMA* **276**:146–54.

Carpenter CC, Fischl MA, Hammer SM, et al. 1997. Antiretroviral therapy for HIV in 1997: Updated recommendations of the International AIDS Society USA Panel. *JAMA* **277**:1962–9.

Cates JE, Christie RB. 1951. Subacute bacterial endocarditis. *Q J Med* **20**:93–130.

[CDC] Centers for Disease Control and Prevention. 1985. Recommendation of the Immunization Practices Advisory Committee: Small pox vaccine. *Morb Mortal Wkly Rep* **34**:341–2.

[CDC] Centers for Disease Control and Prevention. 1987. Rubella vaccination during pregnancy 1971–1986. *Morb Mortal Wkly Rep* **36**:457–61.

[CDC] Centers for Disease Control and Prevention. 1989a. Interpretation and use of the Western blot assay for serodiagnosis of human immunodeficiency virus type-1 infections. *Morb Mortal Wkly Rep* **38**:1–6.

[CDC] Centers for Disease Control and Prevention. 1989b. Recommendation of the Immunizations Practices Advisory Committee: General recommendation on immunization. *Morb Mortal Wkly Rep* **38**:205–14.

[CDC] Centers for Disease Control and Prevention. 1991. Nosocomial transmission of multidrug-resistant tuberculosis among HIV-infected persons—Florida and New York 1988–1991. *Morb Mortal Wkly Rep* **40**:585–91.

[CDC] Centers for Disease Control and Prevention. 1992. Testing for antibodies to human immunodeficiency virus type 2 in the United States. *Morb Mortal Wkly Rep* **41**:1–9.

[CDC] Centers for Disease Control and Prevention. 1993a. Initial therapy for tuberculosis in the era of multidrug resistance: Recommendations of the Advisory Council for the Elimination of Tuberculosis. *Morb Mortal Wkly Rep* **42** (No RR-7):1–8.

[CDC] Centers for Disease Control and Prevention. 1993b. Recommendations of the Advisory Committee on Immunization Practices (ACIP): Use of vaccines and immune globulins for persons with altered immunocompetence. *Morb Mortal Wkly Rep* **42** (No RR-4).

[CDC] Centers for Disease Control and Prevention. 1994a. General recommendations on immunization: Recommendation of the Advisory Committee on Immunization Practices (ACIP). *Morb Mortal Wkly Rep* **43** (No RR-1).

[CDC] Centers for Disease Control and Prevention. 1994b. Guidelines for preventing the transmission of *Mycobacterium tuberculosis* in health care facilities, 1994. *Morb Mortal Wkly Rep* **43** (No RR-13):30–1.

[CDC] Centers for Disease Control and Prevention. 1994c. Recommendations for preventing the spread of vancomycin resistance: recommendations of the Hospital Infection Control Practices Advisory Committee (HICPAC). *Morb Mortal Wkly Rep* **44** (No RR-12): 1–12.

[CDC] Centers for Disease Control and Prevention. 1995. *HIV/AIDS Surveillance Rep* **13** (Dec).

[CDC] Centers for Disease Control and Prevention. 1996a. Prevention of *Varicella*: Recommendations of the Advisory Committee on Immunization Practices (ACIP). *Morb Mortal Wkly Rep* **45** (No RR-11).

[CDC] Centers for Disease Control and Prevention. 1996b. Measles pneumonitis following measles-mumps-rubella vaccination of a patient with HIV-infection, 1993. *Morb Mortal Wkly Rep* **45**:603–6.

[CDC] Centers for Disease Control and Prevention. 1997a. Measles eradication: recommendation from a meeting cosponsored by the World Health Organization, the Pan American Health Organization, and Centers for Disease Control and Prevention. *Morb Mortal Wkly Rep* **46** (No RR-11).

[CDC] Centers for Disease Control and Prevention. 1997b. Pertussis vaccination: use of acellular pertussis vaccines among infants and young children—recommendations of the Advisory Committee on Immunization Practices (ACIP). *Morb Mortal Wkly Rep* **46** (No RR-7).

[CDC] Centers for Disease Control and Prevention. 1997c. Poliomyelitis prevention in the United States: Introduction of a sequential vaccination schedule of inactivated poliovirus vaccine followed by oral poliovirus vaccine—recommendations of the Advisory Committee on Immunization Practices (ACIP). *Morb Mortal Wkly Rep* **46** (No RR-3).

[CDC] Centers for Disease Control and Prevention. 1997d. Trends in AIDS incidence, death and prevalence—United States, 1996. *Morb Mortal Wkly Rep* **46**:165–73.

[CDC] Centers for Disease Control and Prevention. 1998a. Recommendations for the use of antiretroviral drugs in pregnant women infected with HIV-1 for maternal health and for reducing perinatal HIV-1 transmission in US. Public Health Service Task Force. *Morb Mortal Wkly Rep* **47**:1–30.

[CDC] Centers for Disease Control and Prevention. 1998b. Report of the NIH panel to define principles of therapy of HIV infection and guidelines for the use of antiretroviral agents in HIV-infected adults and adolescents. *Morb Mortal Wkly Rep* **47** (No RR-5): 1–81.

[CDC] Centers for Disease Control and Prevention. 1999. 1999 USPHS/IDSA guidelines for the prevention of opportunistic infections in persons infected with human immunodeficiency virus. *Morb Mortal Wkly Rep* **48** (No RR-10):1–59.

Chang J, Des Rosiers S, Weinstein L. 1970. Clinical and serological studies of an outbreak of rubella in a vaccinated population. *N Engl J Med* **283**:246–8.

Chattergoon M, Boyer J, Weiner DB. 1997. Genetic immunization: a new era in vaccines and immune therapeutics. *FASEB J* **11**: 753–63.

Chaulk CP, Pope DS. 1997. The Baltimore City Health Department program of directly observed therapy for tuberculosis. *Clin Chest Med* **18**:149–54.

Chernik NL, Armstrong D, Posner JB. 1973. Central nervous system infections in patients with cancer. *Medicine (Baltimore)* **52**:563–81.

Cherubin CE, Marr JS, Sierra MF, et al. 1981. Listeria and gram-negative bacillary meningitis in New York City, 1972–1979. *Am J Med* **71**:199–209.

Cheson BD, Levine AM, Milvan D. 1987. Suramin therapy in AIDS and related disorders. *JAMA* **258**:1347–51.

Christiansen LK, Hansen JM, Kristensen M. 1963. Sulphaphenazole-induced hypoglycemic attacks in tolbutamide-treated diabetics. *Lancet* **2**:1298–1301.

Christiansen PE. 1952–53. An epidemic of measles in southern Greenland, 1951. *Acta Med Scand* **144**:313–22, 430–49, 450–4.

Classen DC, Evans RS, Pestotnik SL, et al. 1992. The timing of prophylactic administration of antibiotics and the risk of surgical-wound infection. *N Engl J Med* **326**:281–6.

Cobb JP, Danner RL. 1996. Nitric oxide and septic shock. *JAMA* **275**:1192–5.

Col N, O'Conner R. 1987. Estimating world-wide current antibiotic usage: Report of task force I. *Rev Infect Dis* **9**:S232–43.

Colditz GA, Brewer TF, Berkey CS, et al. 1994. Efficacy of BCG vaccine in the prevention of tuberculosis—metaanalysis of the published literature. *JAMA* **271**:698–702.

Collier AC, Coombs RW, Schoenfield DA, et al. 1996. Treatment of human immunodeficiency virus infection with saquinavir, zidovudine, and zalcitabine. AIDS Clinical Trials Group. *N Engl J Med* **334**:1011–7.

Comstock GM, Livesay VT, Weolperf SF. 1974. The prognosis of positive tuberculin reaction in childhood and adolescence. *Am J Epidemiol* **99**:131–8.

Concorde Coordinating Committe. 1994a. Concorde: MRC/ANRS randomized double-blind controlled trial of immediate and deferred zidovudine in symptom-free HIV infection. *Lancet* **343**:871–81.

Condon RE. 1975. Rational use of prophylactic antibiotics in gastrointestinal surgery. *Surg Clin North Am* **55**:1309–38.

Connor EM, Sperling R, Gelber R, et al. 1994. Reduction of maternal-infant transmission of human immunodeficiency virus type 1 with zidovudine treatment. *N Engl J Med* **331**:1173–80.

Consortium for Retrovirus Serology Standardization. 1990. Serological diagnosis of human immunodeficiency virus infection by Western blot testing. *JAMA* **260**:674–9.

Conte J, Jacob L, Polk H. 1986. *Antibiotic Prophylaxis in Surgery*. Philadelphia: JB Lippincott.

Coombs RW, Collier AC, Allain JP, et al. 1989. Plasma viremia in human immunodeficiency virus infection. *N Engl J Med* **321**:1626–31.

Coombs RW, Welles SL, Hooper C, et al. 1996. Association of plasma human immunodeficiency virus type I RNA level with risk of clinical progression in patients with advanced infection. AIDS Clinical Trials Group (ACTG) 116B/117 Study Team and ACTG Virology Committee Resistance and HIV-1 RNA Working Group. *J Infect Dis* **174**:704–12.

Cooper ER, Nugent RP, Diaz C, et al. 1996. After AIDS Clinical Trial 076: The changing pattern of zidovudine use during pregnancy and transmission of human immunodeficiency virus in a cohort of infected women and their infants. *J Infect Dis* **174**:1207–11.

Corey L, Ashley R, Sekulovich R, et al. 1997. Lack of efficacy of a vaccine containing recombinant gD2 and gB2 antigens in MF59 adjuvant for the prevention of genital HSV-2 acquisition [abstract]. ICAAC; Toronto, Canada.

Craig W, Uman S, Shaw W. 1978. Hospital use of antimicrobial drugs—survey at 19 hospitals and results of antimicrobial control programs. *Ann Intern Med* **89**:793–8.

Craig WA, Kunin CM. 1976. Significance of serum protein and tissue binding of antimicrobial agents. *Ann Rev Med* **27**:287–300.

Craig WA. 1998. Pharmacokinetic/pharmacodynamic parameters: Rationale for antibacterial dosing of mice and men. *Clin Infect Dis* **26**:1–12.

Crawford JJ, Sconyers JR, Moriarty JD, et al. 1974. Bacteremia after tooth extractions studied with the aid of prereduced anaerobically sterilized culture media. *Appl Microbiol* **27**:927–32.

Cruse PJE, Foord R. 1973. A five-year prospective study of 23 649 surgical wounds. *Arch Surg* **107**:206–10.

Culver DH, Horan TC, Gaynes RP, et al. 1991. Surgical wound infection rates by wound class operative procedure and patient risk index. *Am J Med* **91** (Suppl 3B):152–7.

Cundell D, Gerard N, Gerard C, et al. 1995. *Streptococcus pneumoniae* anchors to activated human cells by the receptor for platelet activating factor. *Nature* **377**:435–8.

D'Aquila RT, Hughes MD, Johnson VA, et al. 1996. Nevirapine zidovudine and didanosine compared with zidovudine and didanosine in patients with HIV-1 infection. National Institute of Allergy and Infectious Diseases AIDS Clinical Trials Group Protocol 241 Investigators. *Ann Intern Med* **124**:1019–30.

Daar ES, Li XL, Moudgil T, et al. 1990. High concentrations of recombinant soluble CD4 are required to neutralize primary human immunodeficiency virus type 1 isolates. *Proc Natl Acad Sci USA* **87**:6574–8.

Dajani AS, Taubert KA, Wilson W, et al. 1997a. Prevention of bacterial endocarditis: Recommendations by the American Heart Association. *Circulation* **96**:358–66.

Dajani AS, Taubert KA, Wilson W, et al. 1997b. Prevention of bacterial endocarditis: Recommendations by the American Heart Association. *JAMA* **277**:1794–1801.

Daniels WG, Mugge A, Martin RP, et al. 1991. Improvement in the diagnosis of abscesses associated with endocarditis by transesophageal echocardiography. *N Engl J Med* **324**:795–800.

Danner SA, Carr A, Leonard JM, et al. 1995. A short-term study of the safety pharmacokinetics and efficacy of ritonavir: inhibitor of HIV-1 protease. European-Australian Collaborative Ritonavir Study Group. *N Engl J Med* **333**:1528–33.

Deeks SG, Smith M, Helodniy M, et al. 1997. HIV-1 protease inhibitors: A review for clinicians. *JAMA* **277**:145–53.

Deitsch KW, Moxon ER, Wellems TE. 1997. Shared themes of antigen variation and virulence in bacterial protozoal and fungal infections. *Microbiol Molec Biol Rev* **61**:281–93.

Delta Coordinating Committee. 1996. Delta: A randomized double-blind controlled trial comparing combinations of zidovudine plus didanosine or zalcitabine with zidovudine alone in HIV-infected individuals. *Lancet* **348**:283–91.

DePiro JT, Cheung RPF, Bowden TA, et al. 1986. Single dose systemic antibiotic prophylaxis of surgical wound infections. *Am J Surg* **152**:552–9.

DeShazo R, Lopez M, Salvaggio J. 1987. Use and interpretation of diagnostic immunologic laboratory tests. *JAMA* **258**:3011–7.

De Wolf F, Goudsmit J, Paul DA, et al. 1987. Risk of AIDS related complex and AIDS in homosexual men with persistant HIV antigenernia. *Br Med J* **295**:569–72.

Dezube BJ, Lederman MM, Spritzler JG, et al. 1995. High-dose pentoxifylline in patients with AIDS: Inhibition of tumor necrosis factor production. National Institute of Allergy and Infectious Diseases AIDS Clinical Trials Group. *J Infect Dis* **171**: 1628–33.

DiNubile MJ. 1988. Stopping antibiotic therapy in neutropenic patients. *Ann Intern Med* **108**:289–92.

DiNubile MJ. 1994. Short-course antibiotic therapy for right-sided endocarditis caused by *Staphylococcus aureus* in injection drug users. *Ann Intern Med* **121**:873–6.

Dooley SW Jr, Castro KG, Hutton MD, et al. 1990. Guidelines for preventing the transmission of tuberculosis in health care settings with special focus on HIV-related issues. *Morb Mortal Wkly Rep* **39** (RR-17):1–29.

Douglas A, Moore-Gillon J, Eykyn S. 1986. Fever during treatment of infective endocarditis. *Lancet* **I**:1341–3.

Durack D. 1990. Prophylaxis of infective endocarditis. In: Mandell G, Douglas G, Bennett J, editors. *Principles and Practice of Infectious Diseases*. New York: Churchill Livingstone, pp 716–21.

Durack D, Beeson PB. 1973. Experimental bacterial endocarditis. I: Colonization of a sterile vegetation. *Br J Exp Pathol* **53**:44–9.

Durack DT, Lukes AS, Bright DK, 1994. New criteria for diagnosis of infective endocarditis: utilization of specific echocardiographic findings. *Am J Med* **96**:200–209.

Eastman PS, Boyer E, Mole L, et al. 1995. Nonisotopic hybridization assay for determination of relative amounts of genotypic human immunodeficiency virus type-1 zidovudine resistance. *J Clin Microbiol* **33**:2777–80.

Edlin BR, Weinstein RA, Whaling SM, et al. 1992. Zidovudine-interferon-therapy in patients with advanced human immunodeficiency virus type 1 infection: Biphasic response to p24 and quantitative polymerase chain reaction. *J Infect Dis* **165**:793–8.

Eichhoff T. 1985. Immunization: An adult thing to do. *J Infect Dis* **152**:1–8.

Englund JA, Baker CJ, Raskino C, et al. 1997. Zidovudine didanosine or both as the initial treatment for symptomatic HIV-infected children. AIDS Clinical Trials Group (ACTG) Study 152 Team. *N Engl J Med* **336**:1704–12.

Eron JJ, Benoit SL, Jemsek J, et al. 1995. Treatment with lamivudine, zidovudine, or both in HIV-1 positive patients with 200 to 500 $CD_4^+$ cells per cubic millimeter. North American HIV Working Party. *N Engl J Med* **333**:1662–9.

Evans AS. 1976. *Viral Infections of Humans*. New York: Plenum Publishing.

Excler J-L, Plotkin S. 1997. The prime-boost concept applied to HIV preventive vaccines. *AIDS* **11** (Suppl A):S127–37.

Fahey H, Taylor JM, Detels R, et al. 1990. The prognostic value of cellular and serologic markers in infection with human immunodeficiency virus type 1. *N Engl J Med* **322**:166–72.

Feldman WE. 1977. Relation of concentrations of bacteria and bacterial antigen in cerebrospinal fluid to prognosis in patients with bacterial meningitis. *N Engl J Med* **296**:433–5.

Ferebee SH, Mount FW, Murray FJ, et al. 1963. A controlled trial of isoniazid prophylaxis in mental institutions. *Am Rev Respir Dis* **88**:161–75.

Finch CA, Wilkinson HW. 1979. Practical considerations in using counter-immunoelectrophoresis to identify the principal causative agents of bacterial meningitis. *J Clin Microbiol* **10**:519–24.

Finlay BB, Falkow S. 1997. Common themes in microbial pathogenicity revisited. *Microbiol Mol Biol Rev* **61**:136–69.

Fischbach M, Talal N. 1985. Ability of isoprinosine to restore interleukin-2 production and T cell proliferation in autoimmune mice. *Clin Exp Immunol* **61**:242–7.

Fischl MA, Richman DD, Gieico MH, et al. 1987. The efficacy of azidothymidine (AZT) in the treatment of patients with AIDS and AIDS-related complex: A double-blind placebo controlled trial. AZT Collaborative Working Group. *N Engl J Med* **317**: 185–91.

Fischl MA, Richman DD, Hansen N, et al. 1990. The safety and efficacy of zidovudine (AZT) in the treatment of subjects with mildly symptomatic human immunodeficiency virus type 1 (HIV) infection. AIDS Clinical Trials Group. *Ann Intern Med* **112**:727–37.

Fiscus SA, Adimora AA, Schoenbach VJ, et al. 1996. Perinatal HIV infection and transmission and the effect of zidovudine therapy on transmission in rural and urban counties. *JAMA* **275**:1483–8.

Fisher CJ, Dhainaut J-FA, Opal SM, et al. 1994. Recombinant human interleukin 1 receptor antagonist in the treatment of patients with sepsis syndrome: Results from a randomized double-blind placebo-controlled trial phase III rh1L-1RA. Sepsis Syndrome Study Group. *JAMA* **271**:1836–43.

Fisher JE. 1996. The status of anti-infectives in surgery in 1996: A roundtable discussion. *Am J Surg* **172** (Suppl 6A) 49S-61S.

Flexner C. 1996. Oral antibiotic treatment of right-sided staphylococcal endocarditis in injection drug users: Prospective randomized comparison with parenteral therapy. *Am J Med* **101**:68–76.

Fournier PE, Casalta JP, Habib G, et al. 1996. Modification of the diagnostic criteria proposed by the Duke Endocarditis Service to permit improved diagnosis of Q fever endocarditis. *Am J Med* **100**:629–33.

Fowler J, Stamey T. 1977. Studies of introital colonization in women with recurrent urinary infections. VII: The role of bacterial adherence. *J Urol* **117**:472–6.

Freimuth WW, Chuang-Stein CJ, Greenwald CA, et al. 1996. DLV combined with ZDV or ddI produces sustained reduction in viral burden and increases in CD4 count in early and advanced HIV-1 infection [abstract]. 11th International Conference on AIDS; 1996 Jul; Vancouver, BC. Abstract MoB 295.

Frenkel LM, Wagner LE, Atwood SM, et al. 1995. Specific sensitive and rapid assays for human immunodeficiency virus type 1 pol mutations associated with resistance to zidovudine and didanosine. *J Clin Microbiol* **33**:342–7.

Frieden TR, Sterling T, Pablos-Mendez A, et al. 1993. The emergence of drug-resistant tuberculosis in New York City. *N Engl J Med* **328**:521–6.

Fujiwara PI, Larkin C, Frieden TR. 1997. Directly observed therapy in New York City: History, implementation, results, and challenges. *Clin Chest Med* **18**:135–48.

Fulginiti VA. 1973. Active and passive immunization in the control of infectious diseases. In: Stiehm ER, Fulginiti VA, editors. *Immunologic Disorders in Infants and Children*. Philadelphia: WB Saunders.

Garner P, Brabin B. 1994. A review of randomized controlled trials of routine antimalarial drug prophylaxis during pregnancy in endemic malarious areas. *Bull WHO* **72**:89–99.

Garrison PK, Friedman LR. 1969. Experimental endocarditis. I: Staphylococcal endocarditis in rabbits resulting from placement of a polyethylene catheter in the right side of the heart. *Yale J Biol Med* **42**:394–410.

Gattinoni L, Brazzi L, Pelosi P, et al. 1995. A trial of goal-orientated hemodynamic therapy in critically ill patients. SvO2 Collaborative Group. *N Engl J Med* **333**:1025–32.

Gendelman HE, Persidsky Y, Ghorpade A, et al. 1997. The neuropathogenesis of the AIDS dementia complex. *AIDS* **11** (Suppl A): S35–45.

Gilbert D. 1984. Current status of antibiotic prophylaxis in surgical patients. *Bull N Y Acad Med* **60**: 340–57.

Gilman A, Goodman L, Rall T, et al., editors. 1996. *The Pharmacological Basis of Therapeutics*. 9th ed. New York: Macmillan.

Ginocchio CC, Wang X-P, Kaplan MH, et al. 1997. Effects of specimen collection processing and storage conditions on stability of human immunodeficiency virus type 1 RNA levels in plasma. *J Clin Microbiol* **35**:2886–93.

Giradin E, Grau G, Doyer J, et al. 1988. Tumor necrosis factor and interleukin 1 in the serum of children with severe infectious purpura. *N Engl J Med* **319**:397–400.

Girgis NI, Farid Z, Mikhail IA, et al. 1989. Dexamethasone treatment for bacterial meningitis in children and adults. *Pediatr Infect Dis J* **8**:848–51.

Gonzales R, Steiner JF, Sande MA. 1997. Antibiotic prescribing for adults with colds, upper respiratory tract infections, and bronchitis by ambulatory care physicians. *JAMA* **278**:901–4.

Gorbach SL, Bartlett JG. 1977. Pseudomembranous enterocolitis: A review of its diverse forms. *J Infect Dis* **135**:89–104.

Gordon R, Thompson T, Carlson W. 1975. Antimicrobial resistance of shigellae isolated in Michigan. *JAMA* **231**:1159–62.

Gotch FM, Goup RA, Safrit JT. 1997. New observations on cellular immune responses to HIV and T-cell epitopes. *AIDS* **11** (Suppl A):S99–107.

Greco D, Salmaso S, Mastrantonio P, et al. 1996. A controlled trial of two acellular vaccines and one whole-cell vaccine against pertussis. Progetto Pertosse Working Group. *N Engl J Med* **334**: 341–8.

Griffiss J, Brandt B. 1986. Non-epidemic (endemic) meningococcal disease: Pathogenic factors and clinical features. In: Remington J, Swartz M, editors. *Current Clinical Topics in Infectious Diseases*. Vol. 7. New York: McGraw-Hill, pp 27–50.

Gruters RA, Neefjes JJ, Tersmette L, et al. 1987. Interference with HIV-induced syncytium formation and viral infectivity by inhibitors of trimming glycosidase. *Nature* **350**:74–7.

Gulick RM, Mellors JW, Havlir D, et al. 1994. Treatment with indinavir, zidovudine, and lamivudine in adults with human immunodeficiency virus infection and prior antiretroviral therapy. *N Engl J Med* **337**:734–9.

Gustafsson L, Hallander HO, Olin P, et al. 1996. A controlled trial of a two-component acellular, a five-component acellular, and a whole-cell pertussis vaccine. *N Engl J Med* **334**:349–55.

Haley RW, Schaberg DR, Crossley KB, et al. 1981. Extra charges and prolongation of stay attributable to nosocomial infections: A prospective interhospital comparison. *Am J Med* **70**:51–8.

Hamburger M, Roberston O. 1940. Studies of the pathogenesis of experimental pneumococcus in the dog. *J Exp Med* **72**:261–74.

Hamill RJ. 1987. Role of fibronectin in infective endocarditis. *Rev Infect Dis* **9** (Suppl 4):S360–71.

Hammer SM, Katzenstein DA, Hughes MD, et al. 1996. A trial comparing nucleoside monotherapy with combination therapy in HIV-infected adults with CD4 cell counts from 200–500 per cubic millimeter. AIDS Clinical Trials Group Study 175 Study Team. *N Engl J Med* **335**:1081–90.

Hammer SM, Squires KE, Hughes MD, et al. 1997. A controlled trial of two nucleoside analogues plus indinavir in persons with human immunodeficiency virus infection and CD4 cell counts of 200 per cubic millimeter or less. AIDS Clinical Trials Group Study 320 Study Team. *N Engl J Med* **337**:725–33.

Hartshorn KL, Vogt MW, Chou TC, et al. 1987. Synergistic inhibition of human immunodeficiency virus in vitro by azidothymidine and recombinant alpha A interferon. *Antimicrob Agents Chemother* **31**:168–72.

Hatala R, Dinh T, Cook DJ. 1996. Once daily aminoglycoside dosing in immunocompetent adults: A meta-analysis. *Ann Intern Med* **124**:717–25.

Hauser W, Remington J. 1982. Effects of antibiotics on the immune response. *Am J Med* **72**:711–6.

Hecht SR, Berger M. 1992. Right-sided endocarditis in intravenous drug users. *Ann Intern Med* **117**:560–6.

Heldman AW, Hartert TV, Ray SC, et al. 1996. Oral antibiotic treatment of right-sided staphylococcal endocarditis in injection drug users: Prospective randomized comparison with parenteral therapy. *Am J Med* **101**:68–76.

Herrman M, Suchard SJ, Boxer LA, et al. 1991. Thrombospondin binds to *Staphylococcus aureus* and promotes staphylococcal adherence to surfaces. *Infect Immun* **59**:279–88.

Hirsch MS, D'Aquila RT. 1993. Therapy for human immunodeficiency virus infection. *N Engl J Med* **328**:1686–95.

Ho DD. 1996. Viral counts count in HIV infection. *Science* **272**: 1124–5.

Ho DD, Hartshorn KL, Rota TR, et al. 1985. Recombinant human interferon alpha A suppresses HTLV III replication in vitro. Infectious Disease Unit, Mass General Hospital, Harvard Medical School, Boston. *Lancet* **1**:602–4.

Ho DD, Moudgil T, Alam M. 1989. Quantitation of human immunodeficiency virus type 1 in the blood of infected persons. *N Engl J Med* **321**:1621–5.

Ho DD, Neumann AU, Perelson AS, et al. 1995. Rapid turnover of plasma virions and CD4 lymphocytes in HIV-1 infection. *Nature* **373**:123–6.

Ho M. 1982. Cytomegalovirus. In: Ho M, editor. *Biology and Infection*. New York: Plenum.

Hoeprich PD. 1972. Immunoprophylaxis of infectious diseases. In: Hoeprich PD, editor. *Infectious Diseases.* Hagerstown, MD: Harper & Row. Ch 19.

Hoffman PS. 1997. Invasion of eukaryotic cells by *Legionella pneumophila*: A common strategy for all hosts? *Can J Infect Dis* **8**:139–46.

Holland HK, Saral R, Rossi JJ, et al. 1989. Allogeneic bone marrow transplantation, zidovudine and human immunodeficiency virus Type 1 (HIV-1) infection. *Ann Intern Med* **111**:973–81.

Holodniy M, Kim S, Katzenstein DA, et al. 1991. Inhibition of human immunodeficiency virus gene amplification by heparin. *J Clin Microbiol* **29**:676–9.

Holodniy M, Mole L, Yen-Lieberman B, et al. 1995. Comparative stabilities of quantitative human immunodeficiency virus RNA in plasma samples collected in VACUTAINER CPT, VACUTAINER PPT, and standard VACUTAINER tubes. *J Clin Microbiol* **33**:1562–6.

Hoover DR, Graham NMH, Chen B, et al. 1992. Effect of $CD4^+$ cell count measurement variability on staging HIV-1 infection. *J Acquired Immun Defic Syndr* **5**:794–802.

Horstmann D. 1973. Need for monitoring vaccinated population for immunity levels. *Prog Med Virol* **16**:215–40.

Horwitz M. 1987. Adenoviruses. In: Fields B, Melnick J, Chanock R, editors. *Human Viral Diseases.* New York: Raven Press, pp 477–95.

Hu S-L, Norrby E. 1997. Vaccines and immunology. *AIDS* **11** (Suppl A):S85–6.

Hubbell G, Cheitlin MD, Rapaport E. 1981. Presentation management and follow-up evaluation of infective endocarditis in drug addicts. *Am Heart J* **102**:85–94.

Huebner RE, Schein MF, Bass JBJ. 1995. The tuberculin skin test. *Clin Infect Dis* **21**:489–505.

Hughes WT, Armstrong D, Bodey GP, et al. 1990. Guidelines for the use of antimicrobial agents in neutropenic patients with unexplained fever. *J Infect Dis* **161**:381–96.

Iseman MD. 1993. Treatment of multidrug-resistant tuberculosis. *N Engl J Med* **329**:784–91.

Jadavji T, Prober C, Cheung R. 1984. In vitro interactions between rifampin and ampicillin or chloramphenicol against *Hemophilus influenzae. Antimicrob Agents Chemother* **26**:91–6.

Japour AJ, Mayers DL, Johnson VA, et al. 1993. Standardized blood mononuclear cell culture assay for determination of drug susceptibilities of clinical human immunodeficiency virus type I isolates. *Antimicrob Agents Chemother* **37**:1095–101.

Jawetz E. 1968. The use of combinations of antimicrobial drugs. *Ann Rev Pharmacol* **8**:151–70.

Joensuu J, Koskenniemi E, Pang XL, et al. 1997. Randomized placebo-controlled trial of rhesus-human reassortant rotavirus vaccine for prevention of severe rotavirus gastroenteritis. *Lancet* **350**:1205–9.

Johnston MI, Hoth DF. 1993. Present status and future prospects for HIV therapies. *Science* **260**:1286–93.

Joint Commission on Accreditation of Hospitals. 1987. *Accreditation Manual for Hospitals.* Chicago.

Kabins SA. 1972. Interactions among antibiotics and other drugs. *JAMA* **219**:206–12.

Kachur SP, Peller ME, Barber AM, et al. 1997. Malaria surveillance—United States 1994. *Morb Mortal Wkly Rep* **46** (No SS-5):1–17.

Kain KC. 1996. Chemotherapy of drug-resistant malaria. *Can J Infect Dis* **7**:25–33.

Kapikian AZ, Mitchell RH, Chanock RM, et al. 1969. An epidemiologic study of altered clinical reactivity to respiratory syncytial (RS) virus infection in children previously vaccinated with an inactivated RS virus vaccine. *Am J Epidemiol* **89**:405–21.

Katz MH, Gerberding JL. 1998. The care of persons with recent sexual exposure to HIV. *Ann Intern Med* **128**:306–12.

Katzenstein A, Hammer SM, Hughes MD, et al. 1996. The relation of virologic and immunologic markers to clinical outcomes after nucleoside therapy in HIV-1 infected adults with 200 to 500 CD4 cells per cubic millimeter. AIDS Clinical Trials Group Study 175 Virology Study Team. *N Engl J Med* **335**:1091–8.

Kaye S, Loveday C, Tedder RS. 1992. A microtiter format point mutation assay: Application to the detection of drug resistance in human immunodeficiency virus type-1 infected patients with zidovudine. *J Med Virol* **37**:241–246.

Käyhty H, Eskola J. 1996. New vaccines for the prevention of pneumococcal infections. *Emerg Infect Dis* **2**:289–98.

Kean BH, Reilly PC. 1976. Malaria—the mime: Recent lessons from a group of civilian travellers. *Am J Med* **61**:159–64.

Kelleher AD, Al-Harthi L, Landay AL. 1997. Immunological effects of antiretroviral and immune therapies for HIV. *AIDS* **11** (Suppl A):S149–55.

Keystone J. 1997. Imported malaria—United States and Canada. Personal communication.

Kiehl MG, Stoll R, Broder S, et al. 1996. A controlled trial of intravenous immune globulin for the prevention of serious infections in adults with advanced human immunodeficiency virus infection. *Arch Intern Med* **156**:2545–50.

Kinloch-de Loës S, Hirschel BJ, Hoen B, et al. 1995. A controlled trial of zidovudine in primary human immunodeficiency virus infection. *N Engl J Med* **333**:408–13.

Kobayashi GS, Cheung SC, Schlesinger D, et al. 1974. Effects of rifampicin derivatives alone and in combination with amphotericin B against *Histoplasma capsulatum. Antimicrob Agents Chemother* **5**:16–8.

Koch MA, Volberding PA, Lagakos SW, et al. 1992. Toxic effects of zidovudine in asymptomatic human immunodeficiency virus-infected individuals with CD4+ cell counts of 050 x 109/L or less: detailed and updated results from protocol 019 of the AIDS Clinical Trials Group. *Arch Intern Med* **152**:2286–92.

Kohl NE, Emini EA, Schlief WA, et al. 1988. Active human immunodeficiency virus protease is required for viral infectivity. *Proc Nat Acad Sci* **85**:4686–90.

Kopanoff DE, Snider DE, Caras GJ. 1978. Isoniazid related hepatitis. *Am Rev Respir Dis* **117**:991–1001.

Kovacs J, Baseler M, Dewar RJ. 1995. Increases in CD4 T lymphocytes with intermittent courses of interleukin-2 in patients with human immunodeficiency virus infection: A preliminary study. *N Engl J Med* **332**:567–75.

Krogstad DJ, Schlesinger PH, Herwaldt BL. 1988. Antimalarial agents: Mechanism of chloroquine resistance. *Antimicrob Agents Chemother* **32**:799–801.

Kucers A, Bennett NM, editors. 1989. The Use of Antibiotics. Philadelphia: JB Lippincott.

Kunin CM. 1974. *Detection Prevention and Management of Urinary Tract Infections.* 2nd ed. Philadelphia: Lea & Febiger.

Kunin CM. 1965. Therapeutic implications of serum protein binding of the new semisynthetic penicillins. *Antimicrob Agents Chemother* **5**:1025–34.

Kunin CM, Bugg A. 1971. Binding of polymyxin antibiotics to tissues: The major determinant of distribution and persistence in the body. *J Infect Dis* **124**:394–400.

Kunin CM, Tupasi T, Craig W. 1973. Use of antibiotics: A brief exposition of the problem and some tentative solutions. *Ann Intern Med* **79**:555–60.

Lalezari J, Haubrich R, Burger HU, et al. 1996. Improved survival and decreased progression of HIV in patients treated with saquinavir plus HIVID [abstract]. NV14256 Study Team. 11th International Conference on AIDS; 1996 Jul; Vancouver BC. Abstract LBB6033.

Lamothe F, D'Arnico P, Ghosn P, et al. 1995. Clinical usefulness of intravenous human immunoglobulins in invasive group A streptococcal infections: Case report and review. *Clin Infect Dis* **21**:1469–70.

Lane HC, Davey V, Kovacs JA. 1990. Interferon in patients with asymptomatic immunodeficiency virus (HIV) infection. *Ann Intern Med* **112**:805–11.

Lane HC, Zunich KM, Wilson W, et al. 1990. Syngeneic bone marrow transplantation and adoptive transfer of peripheral blood lymphocyte combined with zidovudine in human immunodeficiency virus (HIV) infection. *Ann Intern Med* **113**:512–9.

Larder BA, Kellam P, Kemp SD. 1991. Zidovudine resistance protected by direct detection of mutations in DNA from HIV-infected lymphocytes. *AIDS* **5**:137–44.

Larder BA, Kemp SD, Harrigan PR. 1995. Potential mechanism for sustained antiretroviral efficacy of AZT-3TC combination therapy. *Science* **269**:696–9.

Lebel MH, Freij BJ, Syrogiannopoulos GA, et al. 1989. Dexamethasone therapy for bacterial meningitis: Results of two double-blind placebo-controlled trials. *J Infect Dis* **160**:818–25.

Lebel MH, Hoyt MJ, Wagner DC, et al. 1989. Magnetic resonance imaging and dexamethasone therapy for bacterial meningitis. *Am J Dis Child* **143**:301–6.

Lederman MM, Sprague L, Wallis RS, et al. 1992. Duration of fever during treatment of infective endocarditis. *Medicine* **71**:52–7.

LeFrock JL, Ellis CA, Turchik JB, et al. 1973. Transient bacteremia associated with sigmoidoscopy. *N Engl J Med* **289**:467–9.

Leibovici L, Samara Z, Konigsberger H, et al. 1995. Long term survival following bacteremia or fungemia. *JAMA* **274**:807–12.

Leigh-Brown AJ, Richman DD. 1997. HIV-1: Gambling on the evolution of drug resistance? *Nat Med* **3**:268–71.

Lerner PI, Weinstein L. 1966. Infective endocarditis in the antibiotic era. *N Engl J Med* **274**:199–206.

Lewis SH, Reynolds-Kohler C, Fox HE, et al. 1994. HIV-1 trophoblastic and villous Hofbauer cells and hematological precursors in eight-week fetuses. *Lancet* **343**:1464–7.

Levine MM, Edsall G, Bruce-Schwatt LJ. 1974. Live-virus vaccine in pregnancy: Risks and recommendations. *Lancet* **2**:34–8.

Lindenbaum J, Maulitz R, Butler A. 1976. Inhibition of digoxin absorption by neomycin. *Gastroenterology* **71**:399–406.

Liu DK, Owens GF. 1987. Inhibition of viral reverse transcriptase by 2,5-oligoadenylates. *Biochem Biophys Res Commun* **145**: 291–7.

Lorentsen KJ, Hendrix CW, Collins JM, et al. 1989. Dextran sulfate is poorly absorbed after oral administration. *Ann Intern Med* **111**:561–6.

Luigina R, Puccetti P, Bistoni F. 1997. Interleukin-12 in infectious diseases. *Clin Microbiol Rev* **10**:611–36.

Maitland K, Williams T, Bennett S, et al. 1996. The interaction between *Plasmodium falciparum* and *P. vivax* in children in Espiritic Santo Island, Vanuatu. *Trans R Soc Trop Med Hyg* **90**:614–20.

Maki D, Schunna A. 1978. A study of antimicrobial misuse in a university hospital. *Am J Med Sci* **275**:271–81.

Mandell G, Bennett JE, Dolin R, editors. 1995. *Principles and Practice of Infectious Diseases.* New York: Churchill Livingstone.

Mandell L. 1982. The effects of antimicrobial and antineoplastic drugs on the phagocytic and microbicidal function of the polymorphonuclear leucocyte. *Rev Infect Dis* **4**:683–97.

Mangi RJ, Holstein LL, Andriole VT. 1977. Treatment of gram-negative bacillary meningitis with intrathecal gentamicin. *Yale J Biol Med* **50**:31–41.

Mansur AJ, Grinberg M, deLuz PL, et al. 1992. The complications of infective endocarditis: A reappraisal in the 1980s. *Arch Intern Med* **152**:2428–32.

Markowitz M, Saag M, Powderly WG, et al. 1995. A preliminary study of ritonavir, an inhibitor of HIV-1 protease, to treat HIV-1 infection. *N Engl J Med* **333**:1534–9.

Marks AR, Choong CY, Sanfilippo AJ, et al. 1989. Identification of high- risk and low-risk subgroups of patients with mitral-valve prolapse. *N Engl J Med* **320**:1031–6.

Marr J, Moffet H, Kunin C. 1988. Guidelines for improving the use of antimicrobial agents in hospitals: A statement by the Infectious Diseases Society of America. *J Infect Dis* **157**:869–76.

Marschner I, Collier AC, Coombs RW, et al. 1998. Use of changes in plasma levels of human immunodeficiency virus type 1 RNA to assess the clinical benefit of antiretroviral therapy. *J Infect Dis* **177**:40–7.

Maurelli A, Sansonetti P. 1988. Identification of a chromosomal gene controlling temperature-regulated expression of *Shigella* virulence. *Proc Natl Acad Sci USA* **85**:2820–4.

Mayer KH, Schoenbaum SC. 1982. Evaluation and management of prosthetic valve endocarditis. *Prog Cardiovasc Dis* **25**:43–54.

McCabe R, Brooks R, Dorfinan R, et al. 1987. Clinical spectrum in 107 cases of toxoplasmic lymphadenopathy. *Rev Infect Dis* **9**:754–61.

McCabe W, Kreger B, Johns M. 1972. Type-specific and cross-reactive antibodies in gram-negative bacteremia. *N Engl J Med* **287**: 261–7.

McCracken GH. 1976. Rapid identification of specific etiology in meningitis. *J Pediatr* **88**:706–8.

McCracken GH, Mize SG. 1976. A controlled study of intrathecal antibiotic therapy in gram-negative enteric meningitis of infancy: Report of the Neonatal Meningitis Cooperative Study Group. *J Pediatr* **89**:66–72.

McCracken GH, Mize SG, Threlkeld N. 1980. Intraventricular gentamicin therapy in gram-negative bacillary meningitis of infancy: Report of the Second Neonatal Meningitis Cooperative Study Group. *Lancet* **1**:787–91.

McGowen J. 1983. Antimicrobial resistance in hospital organisms and its relation to antimicrobial use. *Rev Infect Dis* **5**:1033–48.

McHenry MC, Gaven TL, Van Omnen RA, et al. 1971. Therapy with gentamicin for bacteremic infections: Results with 53 patients. *J Infect Dis* **124** (Suppl):S164–173.

McIntyre PB, Berkey CS, King SM, et al. 1997. Dexamethasone as adjunctive therapy in bacterial meningitis: A meta-analysis of randomized clinical trials since 1988. *JAMA* **278**:925–31.

McKinney RE, Maha MA, Connor EM, et al. 1991. A multicenter trial of oral zidovudine in children with advanced human immunodeficiency virus disease. Protocol 043 Study Group. *N Engl J Med* **324**:1018–25.

McKinsey DA, Ratts TE, Bisno AL. 1987. Underlying cardiac lesions in adults with infective endocarditis. *Am J Med* **82**:681–7.

Mecsas J, Strauss EJ. 1996. Molecular mechanisms of bacterial virulence: Type III secretion and pathogenicity islands. *Emerg Infect Dis* **2**:271–88.

Medeiros A. 1984. Beta-lactamases. *Br Med Bull* **40**:18–27.

Mellors JW, Kingsley LA, Rinaldo CR, et al. 1995. Quantitation of HIV-1 RNA in plasma predicts outcome after seroconversion. *Ann Intern Med* **122**:573–9.

Menzies R, Vissandjee B. 1992. Effect of bacilli calmette-guerin vaccination of tuberculin reactivity. *Am Rev Respir Dis* **145**:621–5.

Menzies R, Vissandjee B, Rocher J, et al. 1994. The booster effect in two-step tuberculin testing among young adults in Montreal. *Ann Intern Med* **120**:190–8.

Merrikin DJ, Briant J, Rolinson GN. 1983. Effect of protein binding on antibiotic activity in vivo. *J Antimicrob Chemother* **11**:233–8.

Merrill DP, Moonis M, Chou TC, et al. 1996. Lamivudine or stavudine in two- and three-drug combinations against HIV-1 replication in vitro. *J Infect Dis* **173**:355–64.

Milberg JA, Davis DR, Steinberg KP, et al. 1995. Improved survival of patients with acute respiratory distress syndrome (ARDS) 1983–1993. *JAMA* **273**:306–9.

Mildvan D, Armstrong D, Antoniskis D, et al. 1989. An open label dose-ranging trial of AL721 in PGL and ARC [abstract]. V International Conference on AIDS; 1989 Jun; Montreal. Abstract WPB 312.

Miller B. 1993. Preventative therapy for tuberculosis. *Med Clin North Am* **77**:1263–75.

Miller KD, Greenberg AE, Campbell CC. 1989. Treatment of severe malaria in the United States with a continuous infusion of quinidine gluconate and exchange transfusion. *N Engl J Med* **321**: 65–70.

Miller M. 1973. The immunodeficiencies of immaturity. In: Steihm R, Fulginiti V, editors. *Immunologic Disorders in Infants and Children*. Philadelphia: WB Saunders, pp 168–83.

Miller V, Staszewski S, Boucher CAB, et al. 1997. Clinical experience with non nucleoside reverse transcriptase inhibitors. *AIDS* **11** (Suppl A):S157–64.

Mitsuya H, Broder S. 1986. Inhibition of the in vitro infectivity and cytopathic effect of human T-lymphotropic virus type III/lymphadenopathy associated virus (HTLV III/LAV) by 2,3 dideoxynucleotides. *Proc Natl Acad Sci USA* **83**:1911–5.

Moellering R. 1972. Use and abuse of antibiotic combinations. *RI Med J* **55**:341–53.

Moellering RC, Weinberg AN. 1971. Studies on antibiotic synergism against enterococci. II: Effect of various antibiotics on the uptake of $^{14}C$ labelled streptomycin by enterococci. *J Clin Invest* **50**:2580–4.

Moellering RC, Wennerstein C, Weinberg AN. 1971. Studies on antibiotic synergism against enterococci. I: Bacteriologic studies. *J Lab Clin Med* **77**:821–8.

Mofeson LM, Moye J, Korelitz J, et al. 1994. Crossover of placebo patients to intravenous immunoglobulin confirms efficacy for prophylaxis of bacterial infections and reduction of hospitalizations in human immunodeficiency virus-infected children. National Immunoglobulin Clinical Trial Setting Group. *Pediatr Infect Dis* **13**:477–84.

Moffet HL. 1975. Perinatal infections. In: Moffet HL, editor. *Pediatric Infectious Diseases: A Problem-Oriented Approach*. Philadelphia: JB Lippincott, pp 325–53.

Montefiori DC, Mitchell WM. 1987. Antiviral activity of mismatched double stranded RNA against human immunodeficiency virus in vitro. *Proc Natl Acad Sci USA* **84**:2985–9.

Moore JP, McKeating JA, Weiss RA, et al. 1990. Dissociation of gp120 from HIV-1 virions induced by soluble CD4. *Science* **250**: 1139–42.

Moskovitz BL and the HPT-23 Cooperative Study Group. 1988. Clinical trials of tolerance of HPA-23 in patients with acquired immunodeficiency syndrome. *Antimicrob Agents Chemother* **32**:1300–3.

Moyer K, Opal S, Medeiros A. 1990. Mechanisms of antibiotic resistance. In: Mandel G, Douglas G, Bennett J, editors. *Principles and Practices of Infectious Disease*. New York: Churchill Livingstone, pp 218–24.

Moyle GJ. 1996. Use of viral resistance patterns to antiretroviral drugs in optimizing selection of drug combinations and sequences. *Drugs* **52**:168–85.

Munoz A, Wang MC, Bass S, et al. 1989. Acquired immunodeficiency syndrome (AIDS)-free time after human immunodeficiency virus type 1 (HIV-1) seroconversion in homosexual men. Multicenter AIDS Cohort Study Group. *Am J Epidemiol* **130**:530–9.

Murphy R. 1997. Nonnucleoside reverse transcriptase inhibitors. *AIDS Clin Care* **9**:75–9.

Murphy R, Gagnier P, Lamson M, et al. 1982. Effect of nevirapine on pharmacokinetics of indinavir and ritonavir in HIV-1 patients [abstract]. Fourth Conference on Retroviruses and Opportunistic Infections; 1997 Jan; Washington, DC. Abstract 374.

Myers MW, Montaner JG, and the INCAS Study Group. 1996. A randomized double-blinded comparative trial of the effects of zidovudine didanosine and nevirapine combinations on antiviral naive, AIDS-free, HIV-1–infected patients with CD4 counts 200–600 cells/mm$^3$. 11th International Conference on AIDS; 1996 Jul; Vancouver, BC. Abstract MoB 294.

National Committee for Clinical Laboratory Standards. 1987. Methods for determining bactericidal activity of antimicrobial agents (Approved standard M26-P). Villanova, PA.

National Committee for Clinical Laboratory Standards. 1990

National Committee for Clinical Laboratory Standards. 1993. Performance standards for antimicrobial disk susceptibility tests. (Approved standard M2-A5). Villanova, PA.

National Committee for Clinical Laboratory Standards. 1994. Methods for dilutional antimicrobial susceptibility tests for bacteria that grow aerobically. (Approved standard M7-A3). Villanova, PA. 1993 Supplemental Tables. Mico S5.

Nelson JD. 1985. Emerging role of cephalosporins in bacterial meningitis. *Am J Med* **79** (Suppl 2A):47–51.

Neu HC. 1985. Use of cephalosporins in the treatment of bacterial meningitis. In: Sande MA, Smith AL, Root RK, editors. *Bacterial Meningitis*. New York: Churchill Livingstone, pp 203–38.

Neville C, Sorre E, Mung'ala, Mutemic W, et al. 1996. Insecticide treated bed-nets reduce mortality and severe morbidity from malaria among children in the Kenyan coast. *Trop Med Int Health* **1**:139–46.

Newell M-L, Gray G, Bryson YJ. 1997. Prevention of mother-to-child transmission of HIV-1 infection. *AIDS* **2** (Suppl A):S165–72.

Nichols RL. 1980. Use of prophylactic antibiotics in surgical practice. *Am J Med* **70**:686–92.

Nichols RL. 1982. Techniques known to prevent postoperative wound infection. *Infect Control* **3**:34–37.

Nieman RE, Lorber B. 1980. Listeriosis in adults: A changing pattern: Report of eight cases and review of the literature 1968–1978. *Rev Infect Dis* **2**:207–27.

Nijhuis M, Schurman R, Boucher CAB. 1997. Homologous recombination for rapid phenotyping of HIV. *Curr Opin Infect Dis* **10**: 474–9.

Nolan CM, McAllister CK, Walters E, et al. 1978. Experimental pneumococcal meninigitis. IV: The effect of methylprednisolone on meningeal inflammation. *J Lab Clin Med* **91**:979–84.

Norrby-Teglund A, Kaul R, Low DE, et al. 1996. Evidence for the presence of streptococcal-superantigen-neutralizing antibodies in normal polyspecific immunoglobulin G. *Infect Immun* **64**:5395–8.

Nyirjesy PI, Kavasya T, Axelrod P, et al. 1993. Malaria during pregnancy: Neonatal morbidity and mortality and the efficacy of chloroquine prophylaxis. *Clin Infect Dis* **16**:127–32.

O'Brien TR, Blattner WA, Waters D, et al. 1996. Serum HIV-1 RNA levels and time to development of AIDS in the Multicenter Hemophilia Cohort Study. *JAMA* **276**:105–10.

O'Brien WA, Hartigan PM, Martin D, et al. 1996. Changes in plasma HIV-1 RNA and $CD_4^+$ lymphocyte counts and the risk of progression to AIDS. Veterans Affairs Cooperative Study Group on AIDS. *N Engl J Med* **334**:426–31.

Ocular Complication of AIDS Research Group. 1992. Mortality in patients with the acquired immunodeficiency syndrome treated with either foscarnet or ganciclovir for cytomegalovirus retinitis. *N Engl J Med* **326**:213–6.

Odio CM, Faingezicht I, Paris M, et al. 1991. The beneficial effects of early dexamethasone administration in infants and children with bacterial meningitis. *N Engl J Med* **324**:1525–31.

O'Garra A, Stapleton G, Dhar V, et al. 1990. Production of cytokines by mouse B cells: B lymphomas and normal B cells produce IL-10. *Int Immunol* **2**:821–32.

Ogra PL, Karzon DT, Righthand F, et al. 1968. Immunoglobulin responses in serum and secretions after immunization with live and inactivated polio vaccine and natural infection. *N Engl J Med* **279**:893–900.

Orskov I, Ferencz A, Orskov F. 1980. Tamm-Horsfall protein or uromucoid is the normal urinary slime that traps type 1 fimbriated *Escherichia coli. Lancet* **1**:887.

Overturf GD. 1982. Treatment of the child with bacterial meningitis. In: Remington JS, Swartz MN, editors. *Current Clinical Topics in Infectious Disease*. Vol. 3. New York: McGraw-Hill, pp 218.

Palella FJ, Delaney KM, Moorman AC, et al. 1998. Declining morbidity and mortality among patients with advanced immunodeficiency virus infection. HIV Outpatient Study Investigators. *N Engl J Med* **338**:853–60.

Parillo J, Parker M, Natanson C, et al. 1990. Septic shock in humans: Advances in the understanding of pathogenesis, cardiovascular dysfunction, and therapy. *Ann Intern Med* **113**:227–42.

Parker R, St John Sutton MG, Karchman AW. 1991. Echocardiography in the management of patients with suspected or proven endocarditis. *Curr Clin Top Infect Dis* **11**:248–66.

Paul JR. 1971. *A History of Poliomyelitis*. New Haven: Yale University Press. Ch 40.

Peacock JE Jr, McGinnis MR, Cohen MS. 1984. Persistent neutrophilic meningitis: Report of four cases and review of the literature. *Medicine (Baltimore)* **63**:379–95.

Pedersen C, Sandstrom E, Peterson CS, et al. 1990. The efficacy of inosine pranobex in preventing the acquired immunodeficiency syndrome in patients with human immunodeficiency virus infection. Scandinavian Isoprinosine Study Group. *N Engl J Med* **322**:1757–63.

Pelletier LL Jr, Petersdorf RG. 1977. Infective endocarditis: A review. *Medicine* **56**:287–313.

Perelson AS, Essunger P, Ho DD. 1997. Dynamics of HIV-1 and CD4+ lymphocytes in vivo. *AIDS* **11** (Suppl A):S17–24.

Perelson AS, Neumann AU, Markowitz M, et al. 1996. HIV-1 dynamics in vivo: Virion clearance rate, infected cell life-span and viral generation time. *Science* **271**:1582–6.

Perez CM, Kubak BM, Cryer HG, et al. 1997. Adjunctive treatment of streptococcal toxic shock syndrome using intravenous immunoglobulin, case report and review. *Am J Med* **102**:111–3.

Perl TM, Dvorak L, Hwang T, et al. 1995. Long term survival and function after suspected gram-negative sepsis. *JAMA* **274**:338–45.

Pert CB, Hill JM, Ruff MR, et al. 1986. Octapeptides deduced from the neuropeptide receptor like pattern of antigen $CD_4^+$ in brain potently inhibit human immunodeficiency virus receptor binding and T cell infectivity. *Proc Natl Acad Sci USA* **83**:9254–8.

Peters BS, Bennett JM, Jeffries DJ, et al. 1990. Ineffectiveness of AL 721 in HIV disease [letter]. *Lancet* **335**:545–6.

Phair J, Jacobson L, Detels R, et al. 1992. Acquired immune deficiency syndrome occurring within 5 years of infection with human immunodeficiency virus type 1. Multicenter AIDS Cohort Study. *J Acquired Immune Defic Syndr* **5**:490–6.

Phair J, Munoz A, Detels R, et al. 1990. The risk of *Pneumocystis carinii* pneumonia among men infected with human immunodeficiency virus type 1. Multicenter AIDS Cohort Study Group. *N Engl J Med* **332**:161–5.

Phillips P, Nantel S, Benny WB. 1990. Exchange transfusion as an adjunct to the treatment of severe falciparium malaria: Case report and review. *Rev Infect Dis* **12**:1100–7.

Pizzo PA, Eddy J, Falloon J, et al. 1988. Effect of continuous intravenous infusion of zidovudine (AZT) in children with symptomatic HIV infection. *N Engl J Med* **319**:889–96.

Pizzo PA, Robichaud KJ, Gill FA, et al. 1982. Empiric antibiotic and antifungal therapy for cancer patients with prolonged fever and granulocytopenia. *Am J Med* **72**:101–11.

Plotowski M, Puchelle E, Beck G, et al. 1986. Adherence of type 1 *Streptococcus pneumoniae* to tracheal epithelium of mice infected with influenza A/PR8 virus. *Am Rev Respir Dis* **134**:1040–4.

Pollard R, Hall D, et al. 1996. Surrogate marker response to nevirapine/zidovudine in a blinded clinical trial: 12 months experience. Nevirapine Study Team. 11th International Conference on AIDS; 1996 Jul; Vancouver, BC. Abstract WeB 3136.

Press OW, Ramsey PG, Larsen EB, et al. 1984. Hickman catheter infection in patients with malignancies. *Medicine* **63**:189–200.

Raboud RM, Haley L, Montaner JSG, et al. 1995. Quantification of the variation due to laboratory and physiologic sources in CD4 lymphocyte counts of clinically stable HIV-infected individuals. *J Acquired Immune Defic Syndr Hum Retrovir* **10** (Suppl 2):S67–75.

Rahal JJ. 1980. Diagnosis and management of meningitis due to gram-negative bacilli in adults. In: Remington JS, Swartz MN, editors. *Current Clinical Topics in Infectious Disease*. Vol. 1. New York: McGraw-Hill, pp 68.

Rahal JJ, Simberkoff MS. 1979. Bactericidal and bacteriostatic action of chloramphenicol against meningeal pathogens. *Antimicrob Agents Chemother* **16**:13–8.

Reid CL, Chandraratna PAN, Rahimtoola SH. 1985. Infective endocarditis: Improved diagnosis and treatment. *Curr Probl Cardiol* **10**: 1–50.

Relman D, Falkow S. 1990. A molecular perspective of microbial pathogenicity. In: Mandel G, Douglas G, Bennett J, editors. *Principles and Practice of Infectious Diseases*. New York: Churchill Livingstone, pp 25–32.

Retzlaff C, Yamamoto Y, Hoffman PS, et al. 1996. *Legionella pneumophila* heat shock-protein-induced increase of interleukin 1 mRNA involves protein kinase C signalling in macrophages. *Immunology* **89**:281–8.

Revets H, Marissens D, DeWit S, et al. 1996. Comparative evaluation of NASBA HIV-1 RNA QT, AMPLICOR-HIV Monitor, and QUANTIPLEX HIV RNA assay, three methods for quantification of human immunodeficiency virus type 1 RNA in plasma. *J Clin Microbiol* **34**:1058–64.

Richman D, Rosenthal AS, Skoog M, et al. 1991. B1-RG-587 is active against zidovudine resistant HIV-1 and synergistic with zidovudine. *Antimicrob Agents Chemother* **35**:305–8.

Riley RL. 1974. Airborne infection. *Am J Med* **57**:466–75.

Roberts DR, Laughlin LL, Hsheih P, et al. 1997. DDT global control strategies and a malarial control crisis in South America. *Emerg Infect Dis* **3**:295–302.

Robinson A, Bartlett R, Mazens M. 1985. Antimicrobial synergy testing based on antibiotic levels, minimal bactericidal concentration and serum bactericidal activity. *Am J Clin Pathol* **84**:328–33.

Ronco JJ, Fenwick JC, Tweeddale MG, et al. 1993. Identification of the critical oxygen delivery for anaerobic metabolism in critically ill septic and nonseptic humans. *JAMA* **270**:1724–30.

Rooke R, Parniak MA, Tremblay M, et al. 1991. Biological comparisons of wild-type and zidovudine-resistant isolates of human immunodeficiency virus type 1 from the same subjects: Susceptibility and resistance to other drugs. *Antimicrob Agents Chemother* **35**:988–91.

Rose J, Chai H, Schentag J. 1977. Intoxication caused by interaction of chloramphenicol and phenytoin. *JAMA* **237**:2630–4.

Rosenberg T, Manfreda J, Hershfield ES. 1993. Two step tuberculin testing in staff and residents of a nursing home. *Am Rev Respir Dis* **148**:1537–40.

Rouleau D, Conway B, Raboud J, et al. 1997. Stavudine plus lamivudine in advanced human immunodeficiency virus disease: A short-term pilot study. *J Infect Dis* **176**:1156–60.

Rubin M, Hathorn JW, Marshall D, et al. 1988. Gram-positive infections and the use of vancomycin in 550 episodes of fever and neutropenia. Pediatric Branch, National Cancer Institute, Bethesda, MD. *Ann Intern Med* **108**:30–5.

Ruskin J, Remington JS. 1976. Toxoplasmosis in the compromised host. *Ann Intern Med* **84**:193–9.

Saag MS, Holodniy M, Kuritzkes DR, et al. 1996. HIV viral load markers in clinical practice. *Nat Med* **2**:625–9.

Sahm D, Neuman M, Thornsberry C, et al. 1988. Current concepts and approaches to antimicrobial agent susceptibility testing. Cumitech 25; American Society for Microbiology; Washington, DC.

Sande MA. 1981. Antibiotic therapy of bacterial meningitis: Lessons we've learned. *Am J Med* **71**:507–10.

Sande MA, Carpenter CCJ, Cobbs CG, et al. 1993. Antiretroviral therapy for adult HIV-infected patients: Recommendations from a state-of-the-art conference. *JAMA* **270**:2583–9.

Sande MA, Mandell G. 1985. Chemotherapy of microbial diseases. In: Gilman A, Goodman L, Rall T, Murad F, editors. *The Pharmacological Basis of Therapeutics*. New York: Macmillan, pp 1066–239.

Sande MA, Scheld M. 1980. Combination antibiotic therapy of bacterial endocarditis. *Ann Intern Med* **92**:390–8.

Sande MA, Tierney LM. Meningitis. 1994. Medical Staff Conference; San Francisco General Hospital Center and VA Medical Center, San Francisco. *West J Med* **140**:433–8

Saracco G, Rizzetto M. 1997. A practical guide to the use of interferons in the management of hepatitis virus infections. *Drugs* **53**:74–85.

Saravolatz D, Winslow DL, Collins G, et al. 1996. Zidovudine alone or in combination with didanosine or zalcitabine in HIV-infected patients with the acquired immunodeficiency syndrome or fewer than 200 CD4 cells per cubic millimeter. Investigators for the Terry Beirn Community Programs for Clinical Research on AIDS. *N Engl J Med* **335**:1099–106.

Sarin PS, Gallo RC, Scheer DI, et al. 1985. Effects of a novel compound (AL721) on HTLV III infectivity in vitro. *N Engl J Med* **313**: 1289–90.

Saxton A, Hassner A, Swabb E. 1984. Lack of cross-reactivity between aztreonarn or monobactam antibiotic and penicillin in penicillin-allergic subjects. *J Infect Dis* **149**:16–24.

Schaad UB, Lips U, Goreham HE, et al. 1993. Dexamethasone therapy for bacterial meningitis in children. *Lancet* **342**:457–61.

Schacker T, Coombs RW, Collier AC, et al. 1994. The effects of high-dose recombinant soluble CD4 on human immunodeficiency virus type 1 viremia. *J Infect Dis* **169**:37–40.

Scheld WM, Strunk RW, Balian G, et al. 1985. Microbial adhesion to fibronectin in vitro correlates with production of endocarditis in rabbits. *Proc Soc Exp Biol Med* **180**:474–82.

Schimpff SC, Young VM, Greene WH, et al. 1972. Origin of infection in acute nonlymphocytic leukemia: Significance of hospital acquisition of potential pathogens. *Ann Intern Med* **77**:707–14.

Schoenberger L, Kaplan J, Kim-Farley R. 1984. Control of paralytic poliomyelitis in the United States. *Rev Infect Dis* **6**:424–6.

Schoenfield LJ. 1971. Biliary excretion of antibiotics. *N Engl J Med* **284**:1213–4.

Schooley RT, Merigan TC, Gaut P, et al. 1997. Bacterial meningitis in the United States in 1995. *N Engl J Med* **337**:970–6.

Schurman R. 1997. State of the art of genotypic HIV-1 drug resistance. *Curr Opin Infect Dis* **10**:480–4.

Selky AK, Roos KL. 1992. Neurologic complications of infective endocarditis. *Semin Neurol* **12**:225–33.

Selwyn PA, Harlel D, Lewis VA, et al. 1989. A prospective study of the risk of tuberculosis among intravenous drug users with human immunodeficiency virus infection. *N Engl J Med* **230**:545–50.

Shah K, Nathanson N. 1976. Human exposure to SV40: Review and comment. *Am J Epidemiol* **103**:1–12.

Shearer WT, Quinn TC, LaRussa P, et al. 1997. Viral load and disease progression in infants infected with human immunodeficiency virus type 1. Women and Infants Transmission Study Group. *N Engl J Med* **336**:1337–42.

Shepard CC. 1969. Chemotherapy of leprosy. *Ann Rev Pharmacol* **9**: 37–50.

Sheppard HW, Lang W, Ascher MS, et al. 1993. The characteristics of non-progressors: Long term HIV-1 infection with stable $CD_4^+$ T-cell level. *AIDS* **7**:1159–66.

Simberkoff MS, Moldover NH, Rahal JJ. 1980. Absence of detectable bactericidal and opsonic activities in normal and infected human cerebrospinal fluids: A regional host defense deficiency. *J Lab Clin Med* **95**:362–72.

Simon M, Zieg J, Silverman M. 1980. Phase variation: Evaluation of controlling element. *Science* **209**:1370–4.

Skeen MJ, Miller MA, Shinnick TM, et al. 1996. Regulation of murine macrophage IL-12 production: Activation of macrophages in vivo, restimulation in vitro, and modulation by other cytokines. *J Immunol* **156**:1196–1206.

Smith AL. 1983. Antibiotic resistance in *Haemophilus influenzae*. *Pediatr Infect Dis* **2**:352–5.

Smith C, Lipsky J. 1983. Hypoprothrombinemia and platelet dysfunction caused by cephalosporin and axalactam antibiotics. *Antimicrob Agents Chemother* **11**:496–501.

Smith DH, Byrn RA, Marsters SA, et al. 1987. Blocking of HIV-1 infectivity by a soluble form of CD4 antigen. *Science* **238**:1704–7.

Stamm W, Counts G, Running K. 1982. Diagnosis of coliform infection in acutely dysuric women. *N Engl J Med* **307**:463–8.

Staszewski S, Loveday C, Picazo JJ, et al. 1996. Safety and efficacy of lamivudine-zidovudine combination therapy in zidovudine-experienced patients: A randomized controlled comparison with zidovudine monotherapy. Lamivudine European HIV Working Group. *JAMA* **276**:111–7.

Steckelberg JM, Murphy JG, Wilson WR. 1992. Management of complications of infective endocarditis. In: Kaye D, editor. *Infective Endocarditis*. 2nd ed. New York: Raven Press, pp 435–553.

Steers E, Foltz EL, Graves BS, et al. 1959. An inocula replicating apparatus for routine testing of bacterial susceptibility to antibiotics. *Antibiot Chemother (Basel)* **9**:307–11.

Steigbeigel RT, Greenman YL, Remington JS. 1975. Antibiotic combinations in the treatment of experimental *Staphylococcus aureus* infection. *J Infect Dis* **131**:245–51.

Steigbeigel RT, Johnson PK, Remington JS. 1974. The nitroblue tetrazolium reduction test versus conventional hematology in the diagnosis of bacterial infection. *N Engl J Med* **290**:235–8.

Steigbeigel RT, Reed C, Finland M. 1968. Absorption and excretion of five tetracycline analogues in normal young men. *Am J Med Sci* **25**:296–301.

Stein DS, Korvick JA, Vermund SH. 1992. $CD_4^+$ lymphocyte cell enumeration for predictor of clinical course of human immunodeficiency virus disease: A review. *J Infect Dis* **165**:352–63.

Steinman R, Nogueira N, Witmer M. 1980. Lymphokine enhances the expression and synthesis of 1a antigens on cultured mouse peritoneal macrophages. *J Exp Med* **152**:1248–61.

Steketee RW. 1989. Recent findings in perinatal malaria. *Bull Intern Paed Assoc* **10**:418–33.

Sterimark H, Parton RG, Steele-Mortimer O, et al. 1994. Inhibition of rab5 GTPase activity stimulates membrane fusion in endocytosis. *EMBO J* **13**:1287–98.

Stevenson M. 1997. Molecular mechanisms for the regulation of HIV replication persistence and latency. *AIDS* **11** (Suppl A):S25–33.

Stiehm ER, Sztein M, Steeg P. 1984. Deficient antigen expression on human cord blood monocytes: Reversal with lymphokines. *Clin Immunol Immunopathol* **30**:430–6.

Stokes J, Weibel RE, Villarejos VM, et al. 1971. Trivalent combined measles, mumps, rubella vaccine. *JAMA* **218**:57–61.

Stovring J, Snyder RD. 1980. Computed tomography in childhood bacterial meningitis. *J Pediatr* **96**:820–3.

Sutter RW, Prevots DR. 1994. Vaccine-associated paralytic poliomyelitis among immunodeficient persons. *Infect Med* **11**:426–38.

Swartz MN. 1981. Intraventricular use of aminoglycosides in the treatment of gram-negative bacillary meningitis: Conflicting views. *J Infect Dis* **143**:293–6.

Swartz MN, Dodge PR. 1965. Bacterial meningitis—a review of selected aspects. I: General clinical features, special problems and unusual meningeal reactions mimicking bacterial meningitis. *N Engl J Med* **272**:725–31.

Swartz MN, O'Hanley PD. 1987. Central nervous system infections. In: Rubenstein E, Federman D, editors. *Scientific American Medicine*. Vol. 2. New York: Scientific American, pp 1–43.

Tauber MG, Sande MA. 1984. Principles in the treatment of bacterial meningitis. *Am J Med* **76**:224–30.

Taylor HM, Bingham JB. 1997. The use of prophylactic antibiotics in ultrasound-guided transrectal prostate biopsy. *Clin Radiol* **52**: 787–90.

Terpenning MS, Buggy BP, Kauffman CA. 1987. Infective endocarditis: Clinical features in young and elderly patients. *Am J Med* **83**: 626–34.

Terpenning MS, Buggy BP, Kauffman CA. 1988. Hospital-acquired infective endocarditis. *Arch Intern Med* **148**:1601–3.

Terry LL. 1962. The association of cases of poliomyelitis with the use of type III oral poliomyelitis vaccines: A technical report. US Department of Health, Education, and Welfare. 1962 Sep 20.

The International Perinatal HIV Group. 1999. The mode of delivery and the risk of vertical transmission of human immunodeficiency virus type 1. *N Engl J Med* **340**:977–87.

Till MA, Ghetie V, Gregory T, et al. 1988. HIV infected cells are killed by rCD4-ricin A chain. *Science* **242**:1166–8.

Tokars JI, Marcus R, Culver DH, et al. 1993. Surveillance of HIV infection and zidovudine use among health care workers after occupational exposure to HIV-infected blood. Centers for Disease Control and Prevention Cooperative Needlestick Surveillance Group. *Ann Intern Med* **118**:913–9.

Tornos M-P, Permanyer-Miralda G, Olona M, et al. 1992. Long term complications of native valve endocarditis in non addicts: A 15 year follow-up study. *Ann Intern Med* **117**:567–72.

Torseth J, Bhatia G, Harkonen S, et al. 1989. Evaluation of the antiviral effect of rifabutin in AIDS-related complex. *J Infect Dis* **159**: 1115–8.

Tramont E. 1990. General or nonspecific host defense mechanisms. In: Mandell G, Douglas G, Bennett J, editors. *Principles and Practice of Infectious Diseases*. New York: Churchill Livingstone, pp 33–41.

Tristram DA, Welliver RC. 1993. Respiratory syncytial virus vaccines: Can we improve on nature? *Pediatr Ann* **22**:715–8.

Tunkel A, Scheld WM. 1996. Acute bacterial meningitis in adults. In: Remington JS, Swartz MN, editors. *Current Clinical Topics in Infectious Diseases*. New York: McGraw-Hill, pp 215–39.

Tunkel A, Wispelwey B, Scheld M. 1990. Bacterial meningitis: Recent advances in pathophysiology and treatment. *Ann Intern Med* **112**:610–23.

Valentin-Weigand P, Grulich-Henn J, Chhatwal GS, et al. 1988. Mediation of adherence of streptococci to human endothelial cells by complement S protein (vitronectin). *Infect Immun* **56**:2851–5.

Van der Meer JTM, Thompson J, Valkenburg HA, et al. 1992. Epidemiology of bacterial endocarditis in the Netherlands: Patient characteristics. *Arch Intern Med* **152**:1863–8.

Via LE, Deretic D, Ulmer RJ, et al. 1997. Arrest of mycobacterial phagosome maturation is caused by a block in vesicle fusion between stages controlled by rab5 and rab7. *J Biol Chem* **272**:13326–31.

Villarino ME, Dooley SW, Geiter LJ, et al. 1992. Management of persons exposed to multidrug-resistant tuberculosis. *Morb Mortal Wkly Rep* **41** (No RR-11):59–71.

Volberding PA, Lagakos SW, Koch MA, et al. 1990. Zidovudine in asymptomatic human immunodeficiency virus infection: A controlled trial in persons with fewer than 500 CD4-positive cells per cubic millimeter. AIDS Clinical Trials Group of the National Institute of Allergy and Infectious Diseases. *N Engl J Med* **322**: 941–9.

Von Reyn CF, Levy BS, Arbeit RD, et al. 1981. Infective endocarditis: An analysis based on strict case definitions. *Ann Intern Med* **94**(4 pt 1):505–18.

Waage A, Brandtzaeg P, Halstensen A, et al. 1989. The complex pattern of cytokines in serum from patients with meningococcal septic shock: Association between interleukin 6, interleukin 1, and fatal outcome. *J Exp Med* **169**:333–8.

Waage A, Halstensen A, Shalaby R, et al. 1989. Local production of tumor necrosis factor, interleukin 1, and interleukin 6 in meningococcal meningitis: Relation to the inflammatory response. *J Exp Med* **170**:1859–67.

Walker BD, Kowalski M, Goh WC, et al. 1987. Inhibition of human immunodeficiency virus syncytium formation and virus replication by castanospermine. *Proc Natl Acad Sci USA* **84**:8120–4.

Walters P, Lizzo PA. 1991. Dideoxyinosine (ddI) in symptomatic HIV-infected children: A phase I-II study. *N Engl J Med* **324**:137–44.

Walzer PD, Gibson JJ, Schultz MG. 1974. Malaria fatalities in the United States. *Am J Trop Hyg* **23**:328–34.

Ward JI, Fraser DW, Baraff LJ, et al. 1979. *Haemophilus influenzae* meningitis: A national study of secondary spread in household contacts. *N Engl J Med* **301**:122–6.

Warrell DA, Looareesuwan S, Warrell MJ, et al. 1982. Dexamethasone proves delerious in cerebral malaria. *N Engl J Med* **306**:313–9.

Washington J. 1988. Current problems in antimicrobial susceptibility testing. *Diagn Microbiol Infect Dis* **9**:135–8.

Wehrle PF. 1967. Immunization against poliomyelitis. *Arch Environ Health* **15**:485–90.

Weinstein AJ, Moellering RC. 1973. Penicillin and gentamicin therapy for enterococcal infection. *JAMA* **223**:1030–2.

Weinstein L. 1986. Life-threatening complications of infective endocarditis and their management. *Arch Intern Med* **146**:953–7.

Weisberg LA. 1980. Cerebral computerized tomography in intracranial inflammatory disorders. *Arch Neurol* **37**:137–42.

Weiss AA, Falkow S. 1984. Genetic analysis of phase change in Bordetella pertussis. *Infect Immun* **43**:263–9.

Welles SL, Jackson JB, Yen-Lieberman B, et al. 1996. Prognostic value of plasma human immunodeficiency virus type 1 (HIV-1) RNA levels in patients with advanced HIV-1 disease and with little or no prior zidovudine therapy. AIDS Clinical Trials Group Protocol 116A/116R/117 Team. *J Infect Dis* **174**:696–703.

Wenneberg J, McPherson K, Caper P. 1984. Will payment based on diagnostic related groups control hospital costs? *N Engl J Med* **311**:295–300.

White NJ. 1996. The treatment of malaria. *N Engl J Med* **335**:800–6.

White NJ, Atmar RL, Wilson J, et al. 1997. Effects of requiring prior authorization for selected antimicrobials: Expenditures, susceptibilities, and clinical outcomes. *Clin Infect Dis* **25**:230–9.

White NJ, Breman JG. 1998. Malaria and other diseases caused by red blood cell parasites. In: Fauci AS, Braunwald E, Isselbacher KJ, et al., editors. *Harrison's Principles of Internal Medicine*. 14th ed. New York: McGraw-Hill, pp 1180–8.

Wilson G. 1967. *The Hazards of Immunization*. Vol. 2. London: Athlone Press, University of London, pp 7–13.

Wilson WR, Giuliani ER, Danielson GK, et al. 1982. Management of complications of infective endocarditis. *Mayo Clin Proc* **57**:82–90.

Wilson WR, Karchmer AW, Dajani AS, et al. 1995. Antibiotic treatment of adults with infective endocarditis due to streptococci, enterococci, staphylococci, and HACEK microorganism. *JAMA* **274**:1706–13.

Wise R. 1983. Protein binding of beta-lactams: The effects on activity and pharmacology particularly tissue penetration. II: Studies in man. *J Antimicrob Chemother* **12**:105–11.

Wise R, Gillett A, Cadge B. 1980. The influence of protein binding upon tissue fluid levels of beta-lactam antibiotics. *J Infect Dis* **142**:77–81.

Witt RL, Hamburger M. 1963. The nature and treatment of pneumococcal pneumonia. *Med Clin North Am* **47**:1257–70.

Wolff S. 1973. Biological effects of bacterial endotoxins in man. *J Infect Dis* **128**:259–64.

Wood R, Montoya JG, Kundu SM, et al. 1993. Safety and efficacy of polyethylene glycol-modified interleukin 2 and zidovudine in human immunodeficiency virus type 1 infection: A phase 1/11 study. *J Infect Dis* **167**:519–25.

Yarchoan R, Pluda JM, Perno C-F, et al. 1991. Antiretroviral therapy of human immunodeficiency virus infection: Current strategies and challenges for the future. *Blood* **78**:859–84.

Young L. 1981. Fever and septicemia. In: Rubin R, Young L, editors. *Clinical Approach to Infection in the Compromised Host*. New York: Plenum, pp 75–122.

Young LY, Koda-Kimble MA, editors. 1988. *Applied Therapeutics: The Clinical Use of Drugs*. 4th ed. Vancouver, WA: Applied Therapeutics, Inc.

Yourtee E, Root R. 1984. Effect of antibiotics on phagocyte-microbe interactions. In: Root R, Sande M, editors. *New Dimensions in Antimicrobial Therapy*. New York: Churchill Livingstone, pp 243–75.

Yurkowski PJ, Plaisance KI. 1993. Prevention of auditory sequellae in pediatric bacterial meningitis: A meta-analysis. *Pharmacotherapy* **13**:494–9.

Ziegler EJ, Fisher CJ, Sprung CL, et al. 1991. Treatment of gram-negative bacteremia and septic shock with HA-1A human monoclonal antibody against endotoxin: A randomized double-blind placebo-controlled trial. The HA-1A Sepsis Study Group. *N Engl J Med* **324**:429–36.

Ziegler EJ, McCutchau JA, Fierer J, et al. 1982. Treatment of gram-negative bacteremia and shock with human antiserum to a mutant *Escherichia coli*. *N Engl J Med* **307**:1225–30.

Zucker JR. 1996. Changing patterns of autochthonous malaria transmission in the United States: A review of recent outbreaks. *Emerg Infect Dis* **2**:37–43.

CHAPTER

# 15 CONSCIOUS SEDATION AND PAIN

Mervyn Maze, John C. Hunter, Raymond R. Gaeta

*Chapter Outline*



It is the physician's job to cure disease when possible and to palliate disease and its symptoms when cure is not possible. Successful management of a patient's pain is one of the most important responsibilities of the physician. In this chapter, we discuss some of the principles that lead to rational prescribing for the relief of a difficult type of pain—the chronic and often severe pain experienced by patients with cancer. We also discuss relief of pain and agitation often experienced by patients undergoing painful diagnostic or therapeutic procedures in the office or hospital setting (providing "conscious sedation"), as well as in the setting of the intensive care unit. At this time, there are many classes of drugs and individual agents for relieving pain and agitation. It is possible for the thoughtful physician to choose among these options wisely, in an effort to optimize efficacy while minimizing adverse effects and cost.

## CONSCIOUS SEDATION

Conscious sedation is a pharmacologically induced state of depressed consciousness and analgesia in which the patient's protective airway reflexes are intact, the patient is able to ventilate adequately, and he or she responds appropriately to physical or verbal stimuli. If either ventilation or responsiveness is lost, the patient is considered to be deeply sedated. This state can progress rapidly to general anesthesia, for which a higher level of vigilance and provider skills are needed.

Monitoring of the sedated patient should always include assessment of response to verbal commands, and the absence of responsiveness should alert the clinician to the likelihood that the patient will not be able to protect his or her airway. When a patient's only response is reflex withdrawal to painful stimuli, the patient should be considered to be under general anesthesia, and supervision by an anesthesiologist is indicated.

Provision of sedation and analgesia to manage patients in the intensive care unit is discussed later in this chapter.

### Indications and Objectives

When an anesthesiologist provides regional or general anesthesia, usually in an operating room, that is referred to as monitored anesthetic care (MAC) and is not dealt with further in this chapter. Rather, this section is directed to the nonanesthesiologist who performs diagnostic and/or therapeutic procedures. The most frequent indications for conscious sedation are for imaging procedures in children, gastrointestinal endoscopy, and dental and other minor surgical procedures that are performed in offices and clinics.

In providing conscious sedation one or more of the following objectives is usually important to the physician.

1. Allowing the patient to tolerate unpleasant procedures by relieving anxiety, discomfort, and pain.
2. Allowing the patient to cooperate with the provider to facilitate performance of the procedure.
3. Facilitating compliance when repeat procedures become necessary.

### Outcomes

The mortality rate when conscious sedation is used for endoscopic procedures is 0.3/1000 (Arrowsmith et al. 1991), which exceeds the mortality rate associated with *general anesthesia* for minor outpatient procedures. Among the possible reasons for this increased mortality outside of the operating room (and in the absence of trained anesthesiologists) are inadequate appreciation of the patient's clinical condition, inadequate monitoring, inadequate preparation for untoward events, and inadequate skills of the health-care provider for dealing with a life-threatening complication.

## Preparation

Clinicians providing conscious sedation should be familiar with the relevant aspects of the patient's medical history, especially abnormalities of major organ systems, previous adverse experiences with sedation/analgesia or general anesthesia, current medications, drug allergies, time and nature of last oral intake (solids and liquids), and history of alcohol and drug abuse (Practice guidelines of sedation and analgesia by non-anesthesiologists 1996).

Patients presenting for conscious sedation should undergo a focused physical examination, with special emphasis on the heart and lungs, and evaluation of the airway. Physical examination of the airway should consider the patient's habitus (obesity), head and neck anatomy (short neck, neck extension, hyoid-mental distance, neck mass, cervical spine disease, tracheal deviation), buccal cavity (mouth opening, dentition, high-arched palate, macroglossia, nonvisible uvula), and jaw (micrognathia, retrognathia, and trismus).

Children scheduled for elective procedures can have an unlimited volume of clear liquids (e.g., apple juice, water, clear gelatin, sugar water, but not milk) until 2 hours before the procedure without incurring an increased risk of aspiration of gastric contents (Cote 1998). Under semiemergent conditions, the risk of aspiration can be mitigated by increasing gastric emptying and enhancing lower esophageal sphincter pressure (e.g., by administering metoclopramide 0.15 mL/kg), and by decreasing gastric acidity (e.g., administering cimetidine 7.5 mg/kg).

## Monitoring

Apart from the clinician performing the procedure, a trained individual should continuously monitor the patient subjected to conscious sedation. Frequent or continuous monitoring should include assessment of responsiveness to verbal commands, direct observation of ventilation (with or without detection of exhaled carbon dioxide when necessary), oxygen saturation, blood pressure, and heart rate. In the presence of supplemental oxygen, early recognition of apnea may be delayed if oxygenation alone is used for assessment of ventilation. Documentation of such monitoring is also required.

Oximetry is firmly established as standard of practice for the monitoring of pediatric patients undergoing conscious sedation (Guidelines for monitoring and management of pediatric patients during and after sedation for diagnostic and therapeutic procedures 1992). Although it seems intuitive that this practice should result in a decrease in morbidity and mortality, there are as yet no outcome data to support this contention (AMA 1993).

SUMMARY

**Apart from the clinician performing the procedure, a trained individual should continuously monitor the patient subjected to conscious sedation and should be prepared to handle complications should they develop.**

## Therapeutic Options

The choice of drugs and strategies depends on whether the major emphasis is analgesia, or sedation and/or amnesia. Although relief of pain is of paramount importance to maintain a sedated state, in some clinical settings (e.g., a child or an uncooperative adult who is required to be immobile for a nonpainful imaging procedure), only sedatives may be necessary. The nonanalgesic drugs most commonly used to provide conscious sedation are listed in Table 15-1

### *Opioids*

The opioids produce analgesia by modulating nociceptive transmission both in the central nervous system (spinal and supraspinal sites) as well as in the periphery. Although this class of drugs is a cornerstone for therapeutic strategies to produce conscious sedation, they have predictable adverse effects. Respiratory depression with bradypneic can occur, even though the tidal volume is largely unaffected. The hemodynamic effects associated with opioid administration result from a decrease in sympathetic tone. Morphine (and to same extent meperidine) cause histamine release, with subsequent vasodilation and possible bronchospasm in certain patient populations. Stimulation of the chemoreceptor trigger zone results in nausea and vomiting. Rapid administration of even small doses of the potent synthetic opioids may produce chest wall rigidity, thereby compromising ventilation.

The onset and duration of drug effect is predicated by the rapidity with which the drug crosses the blood–brain barrier, which in turn is governed by the drug's lipid solubility and volume of distribution. After a bolus or brief infusion, the clinical effect of most of these drugs is terminated by redistribution. Prolonged infusion of drug results in saturation of the different physiologic compartments of the body; termination of the drug effect is then dependent on the rate and duration of infusion, and the half-time of elimination of the drug.

**MORPHINE** Morphine, an opioid with relatively poor lipid solubility, enters and leaves the brain more slowly than lipid-soluble narcotics and requires 10–30 minutes to reach peak effect after intravenous administration. It is biotransformed into an active metabolite, morphine-6-glucuronide, which has double the duration of effect of morphine itself. Morphine also produces significant histamine release, which often results in itching, hives, and/or vasodilatation.

**MEPERIDINE** Meperidine is a synthetically derived opioid that is often used in intermittent or bolus form. It has a chemical structure somewhat similar to that of atropine and exhibits a similar vagolytic action, producing tachycardia rather than bradycardia, which is seen with most of the other opioids. Meperidine's lipid solubility lies between that of morphine and the fentanyl series of compounds.

**FENTANYL SERIES** The synthetically derived fentanyl series of opiate narcotics is used in bolus and/or continuous intravenous infusion, since its kinetic parameters facilitate titration of drug effect. Their high lipid solubility promotes fast onset of effect, although the termination of effect is context-sensitive. Unlike either meperidine or morphine, the fentanyl series of compounds does not produce histamine release, and apart from bradycardia, produces a relatively stable hemodynamic profile, making it suitable for the patient with ischemic heart disease.

The newest agent in the fentanyl series is remifentanil, which is metabolized by nonspecific plasma esterases, producing a drug with short half-life and exquisite titratability. Unlike the other narcotics, its duration of effect is relatively independent of infusion duration. However, the rapid termination of effect can be accompanied by the acute return of pain and its associated cardiovascular sequelae (Westmoreland et al. 1993). One distinguishing feature of remifentanil, however, is its propensity for producing chest wall rigidity.

### *Benzodiazepines*

Benzodiazepines produce sedation, anxiolysis, and amnesia, which are desirable attributes for conscious sedation. However, they may be associated with several adverse effects including ventilatory depression. Unlike the respiratory depression seen with opioids, this is associated with a marked decrease in tidal volume. Hypotension is due to a mild direct cardiac depression, as well as sympatholysis. Both the salubrious and the adverse effects of benzodiazepines are more pronounced when used in conjunction with opioid narcotics. Benzodiazepines' high lipid solubility promotes rapid entry into the CNS and permits a rapid onset of clinical effect, allowing for excellent titratability. The duration of action of these drugs is context-sensitive, with prolonged effects seen after long infusions.

> **Key Points: Although the combination of sedatives and opioids may be more effective than single agents for providing sedation and analgesia, the likelihood of adverse outcomes—including cardiorespiratory depression—is enhanced. Fixed combinations of sedative and analgesic agents do not allow the individual components providing sedation and analgesia to be appropriately titrated to the patient's individual requirements.**

### *Other agents*

Barbiturates have effects on the CNS, heart, and lungs that are qualitatively similar to those of the benzodiazepines, but more exaggerated in magnitude.

Propofol is a very potent, sedative-hypnotic agent with minimal amnestic and analgesic properties. Because of its extreme hydrophobicity, propofol readily crosses the blood–brain barrier, resulting in a rapid onset of conscious sedation. Recovery from propofol is equally fast, even after prolonged continuous infusions and accumulation of drug in various bodily compartments, since rapid redistribution from the CNS, as well as rapid metabolism, still allows for awakening from propofol sedation within 30 minutes (Beller et al. 1988). Propofol is a ventilatory depressant and produces hypotension primarily due to systemic vasodilatation. Both of these effects are exaggerated when opioids are administered concurrently with propofol, or if propofol is used in the geriatric patient or those with hypovolemia or cardiomyopathy. In subhypnotic doses, propofol has also been associated with an antiemetic effect. Of particular concern with propofol is the risk of infection, which is thought to be related to bacterial contamination of its lipid vehicle. However, a new formulation that contains ethylenediaminetetraacetic acid (EDTA) as a preservative, appears to eliminate this complication.

Ketamine, derived from phencyclidine (PCP), produces a dissociated state in which the patient may appear

Table 15-1 Nonanalgesic Drugs Used to Provide Conscious Sedation for Painful Procedures or Sedation for ICU Patients

| Drug | Indication | Common Dose | Route | Time to Peak Effect | Duration | Common Adverse Effects | Contraindications | AWP (Dose Priced) | Comments |
|---|---|---|---|---|---|---|---|---|---|
| Chloral hydrate | Pediatric, especially radiologic | 20–100 mg/kg<br>2 g max | PO, PR | 60–90 min | 4–6 h | Nausea/ vomiting<br>Epigastric pain<br>Agitation/ hyperactivity<br>Nightmares | | (1 g PO) Generic $0.20 | Used primarily in children |
| Diazepam | Longer procedures | 0.1–0.2 mg/kg<br>25–75 μg/kg | PO, PR,<br>IV | 60–90 min | 45 min up to 18 h[a] | Apnea in infants<br>Respiratory depression<br>Pain on injection<br>Jaundice | Liver disease | (10 mg IV) Generic $2<br>Valium~$5 | Aged exhibit enhanced potency<br>Prolonged duration<br>[a]Duration determined by either redistribution or elimination |
| Midazolam HCl | | 25–75 μg/kg<br>0.1–0.2 mg/kg<br>0.3–0.75 mg/kg<br>0.3–0.75 mg/kg<br>0.2–0.5 mg/kg<br>0.02–0.03 mg/kg | IV<br>IM<br>PO<br>PR<br>Nasal<br>Sublingual | 10–25 min<br>20–30 min | 45 min to hours[b] | Apnea<br>Respiratory depression<br>Tolerance with prolonged Rx | Hypovolemia<br>Hypotension | (2 mg IV) Versed $4 | Often used with narcotics;<br>[b]Duration may be prolonged after infusions |
| Lorazepam | ICU sedation | 0.5–2 mg/h | IV | 60 min | 6–12 h | As for midazolam | | (2 mg IV) Generic $9, Ativan $12 | |
| Propofol | | 0.25–1 mg/kg<br>100 μg/ kg/min | IV loading<br>Infusion | 30–60 sec | 15 min | Pain on injection<br>Apnea<br>Hypotension<br>Risk of infection | Hypovolemia | (70 mg +7 mg/min) Diprivan $25 | Useful in ICU when checks of neurologic status are needed, but very expensive |
| Phenobarbital | | 2–4 mg/kg | IV<br>PO, PR | 30 min<br>60–90 min | 4–6 h | Bronchospasm | Porphyria, hypovolemia<br>Hyperkinetic syndromes | (200 mg IV) Generic $21 | Very long half-time of elimination (96 h) |

Table 15-1 Nonanalgesic Drugs Used to Provide Conscious Sedation for Painful Procedures or Sedation for ICU Patients (Continued)

| Drug | Indication | Common Dose | Route | Time to Peak Effect | Duration | Common Adverse Effects | Contraindications | AWP (Dose Priced) | Comments |
|---|---|---|---|---|---|---|---|---|---|
| Pentobarbital | | 5–7 mg/kg<br>2–4 mg/kg<br>120 mg max | IM, IV,<br>PO, PR | 60–90 min | 4–6 h | Respiratory depression<br>Negative inotropy | Porphyria, hypovolemia | (200 mg IV)<br>Generic $9 | |
| Thiopental sodium | | 0.5–2.0 mg/kg | IV | 2–4 min | 30 min | Respiratory depression | Porphyria, hypovolemia | (100 mg IV)<br>Pento-thal $9 | Usually reserved for induction of general anesthesia because of the risk of apnea |
| Methohexital sodium | | 1–2 mg/kg<br>20–30 mg/kg<br>500 mg max | IV<br>PR | 5 min<br>15–25 min | 20–40 min | Respiratory depression<br>Negative inotropy | Seizure predisposition | (100 mg IV)<br>Brevital Sodium $8 | |
| Ketamine HCl | Bronchospastic patients | 0.5–2.0 mg/kg<br>5–10 mg/kg<br>6–10 mg/kg | IV<br>IM<br>PO, PR | 10 min<br>30 min<br>30 min | 3–4 h | Increased secretions<br>Intracranial pressure<br>Nonpurposeful motion<br>Hypertension/tachycardia<br>Emergence reactions | Airway infections | (70 mg IV)<br>Ketalar ~$96 | |
| Butyrophenones<br>Haloperidol | | 0.1 mg/kg repeat 5–10 min | IV | 60 min | | Dysphoria<br>Extrapyramidal dyskinesia | | (5 mg IV)<br>Haldol ~$6 | |
| Droperidol | | up to 5 mg max | | | | Hypotension | | Droperidol $7 | |
| Clonidine HCl | | 2–4 $\mu$g/kg | PO | 60–90 min | 2–3 h | | | Generic >$0.10 | Potentiates both benzodiazepines and opiate narcotics |

Adapted from Medical Association of South Africa 1997 and Cote 1994.

Source of drug prices is *Mosby's GenR*$_x$ 1998. Current prices may vary from those quoted, but comparative prices among products are expected to be similar. The reader should check on local prices at the time of prescribing.

ABBREVIATIONS: AWP, average wholesale price (cost); IM, intramuscular; IV, intravenous; PO, oral; PR, parenteral.

awake but is noncommunicative and experiences neither pain nor recall. Even at low doses, ketamine is a potent analgesic but produces dysphoria and excessive secretions (White et al. 1982), so it must be used in combination with either an $\alpha_2$-adrenergic receptor agonist or together with a "cocktail" containing a benzodiazepine and an antisialagogue (Taittonen et al. 1998). Ketamine has minimal respiratory depressant effects and maintains protective airway reflexes. It has a sympathomimetic action resulting in tachycardia, hypertension, increased myocardial and cerebral oxygen consumption, increased cerebral blood flow, and increased intracranial and intraocular pressures. Ketamine is a potent bronchodilator and can be used therapeutically in cases of refractory bronchospasm. Since ketamine is very lipid soluble, it crosses readily into the CNS for rapid onset of effect.

The butyrophenone neuroleptics, haloperidol and droperidol, have been found to be antagonists at multiple receptor sites in the CNS including receptors for serotonin, GABA, and norepinephrine, and most notably, dopamine. Their peak effect is slow and their duration of effect is variable. Butyrophenones exhibit modest vasodilatation due to peripheral $\alpha$-adrenergic blockade and potent antiemetic effects, and in general, they lack respiratory depressant effects. Haloperidol is the more potent antipsychotic agent, whereas droperidol is a more potent antiemetic. One undesirable side effect of both drugs is the production of acute extrapyramidal reactions, and the rare and dangerous neuroleptic malignant syndrome.

### Reversal Agents

Flumazenil is a direct competitive antagonist at the benzodiazepine receptor (Bertaccini et al. 1995). Although its onset is quite rapid, its duration of action is shorter than most benzodiazepine agonists, and thus, flumazenil has to be given several times or by continuous infusion. In patients with intracranial "mass" lesions, flumazenil's reversal of the benzodiazepine-induced depression of cerebral blood flow, intracranial pressure, and cerebral oxygen consumption may have adverse sequelae.

Naloxone is the most widely used opioid-receptor antagonist, and can be given as an intravenous bolus to reverse the effects of excessive opioid-induced CNS or respiratory depression.

**PRINCIPLE Whenever drugs are administered for conscious sedation, pharmacologic antagonists should be immediately available, together with appropriately sized equipment for establishing a patent airway and providing positive pressure ventilation with supplemental oxygen.**

Close, continuous monitoring of the patient by a trained observer is also essential, since the operator may not observe immediately a change in respiratory or cardiovascular status.

## SEDATION AND ANALGESIA FOR ICU PATIENTS

Critically ill patients are subjected to multiple adverse stimuli, related to their illness or nursing environment, which produce harmful psychological and physiologic effects in their compromised state. The ideal level of sedation for these patients is one that alleviates patient discomfort and allows assessment of the patient's neurologic and pulmonary status, without further compromising the patient's condition. A case in point is the intubated, mechanically ventilated patient in whom ventilator dyssynchrony is a common cause of increased work of breathing and agitation. In order for the patient to tolerate the endotracheal tube and positive pressure ventilation, analgesics and/or anxiolytics may need to be administered; this in turn makes it more difficult to assess pulmonary and neurologic function.

The judicious use of sedatives and analgesics during placement of invasive monitoring devices, painful dressing changes, chest physiotherapy, and percussion can minimize oxygen consumption and reduce metabolic demand, because interventions such as chest physiotherapy can increase oxygen consumption by up to 50%, with associated increases in heart rate and minute ventilation (Weissman and Kemper 1993). Appropriate levels of sedation and analgesia can diminish this response and lower oxygen consumption to levels that are 10 to 15% below those of normal, awake patients (Rouby et al. 1981).

While titratability to a given effect is desirable (e.g., when lessening the sedative state to facilitate assessment of CNS or pulmonary function), it is equally important to minimize "rebound agitation," as oxygen consumption and blood pressure can rise alarmingly after abrupt withdrawal of sedative drugs (Bruder et al. 1994). Yet agitation may also result from undiagnosed problems (hypercarbia, hypoxia) that should not be inappropriately masked by excessive use of anxiolytic and sedative drugs.

### Monitoring Endpoints

In order to achieve the goals of adequate sedation and analgesia, a patient's response to stimuli must be consistently and objectively evaluated and therapy must be adjusted as necessary. This can be accomplished by using a sedation scoring system and/or surrogate measures of the

Table 15-2 Ramsay Scale for Evaluating Sedation

| Ramsay Scale | Description |
|---|---|
| Level 1 | Anxious and agitated |
| Level 2 | Awake and cooperative |
| Level 3 | Responds to verbal commands |
| Level 4 | Responds to light stimulation |
| Level 5 | Responds only to deep stimulation |
| Level 6 | No response to deep stimulation |

behavioral response. Originally, the Ramsay sedation scoring scheme was developed for the assessment of sedation in experimental subjects (Ramsay et al. 1974). In this scheme, the level of wakefulness is scored on a scale of 1–6 based on a progressive loss of responsiveness from auditory to deep painful stimuli (Table 15-2). The Observer's Assessment of Alertness/Sedation Scale (Chernik et al. 1990) utilizes features such as response to verbal or tactile stimulation, eye appearance, and verbal and facial expressions of communication as parameters by which to create the score (Table 15-3).

Both of these scales are subjective and can pose a problem when different observers are simultaneously involved in the care of the sedated patient (e.g., when shifts change). Furthermore, these scales are dependent on normal motor function and cannot be used in patients receiving muscle relaxants. Although physiologic parameters of sympathetic activation may be thought to represent wakefulness, they are nonspecific and inconsistent measures of awareness (Schwender et al. 1996).

Measurement of electrophysiologic parameters including evoked potentials (i.e., auditory, somatosensory, visual) and, especially, the electroencephalogram (EEG) has dominated the objective assessment of sedation and/or wakefulness. The EEG has been further analyzed by sophisticated algorithms to yield parameters such as the power spectral analysis and bispectral analysis. Power spectral analysis involves dissecting the EEG signal into its components of various frequency and measuring the amplitude or "power" of each of these components. The resultant spectral edge frequency$_{95}$ represents that frequency below which 95% of the EEG power occurs. Although useful in some situations, it has not consistently correlated with sedation for all classes of drugs. On the other hand, the bispectral ("Bis") index accounts not only for the amplitude and frequency but also for the phase characteristics of the EEG (Sigl and Chamoun 1994). The Bis can be used to "predict" depth of general anesthesia and sedation from monotherapy; however, its value in the ICU setting has not yet been established. In general, EEG measures of wakefulness in the ICU are often very imprecise and can be grossly affected by EMG artifact. Although the EEG of the paralyzed patient and the patient with induced barbiturate coma may provide useful information, its general utility for all sedated patients in the ICU remains to be seen.

### Choice of Agents

The agents mentioned above for conscious sedation may be used for providing sedation and analgesia in the ICU. However, these agents tend to fall short of the goals of ICU sedation because of lack of patient cooperation while at a desired level of sedation (3 on the Ramsay Scale), thereby precluding both accurate assessment of CNS and pulmonary function, as well as active participation in physiotherapy.

## PAIN

### Introduction

Pain is a subjective and multidimensional experience comprising several components: sensory (e.g., intensity, duration, location), affective (e.g., unpleasantness, emotional, motivational), and cognitive (e.g., awareness of the implications, fear, anxiety) (IASP 1980). In most cases, the sensation of pain is produced either by stimuli intense enough (noxious) to provoke actual or potential tissue damage, or by nerve injury. In addition to the subjective experience of pain, noxious stimuli can evoke a range of behaviors that all serve to protect uninjured tissues (i.e., limb withdrawal reflex, escape, immobilization of the in-

Table 15-3 Observer's Assessment of Alertness/Sedation (OAA/S) Scale

| OAA/S Scale | Description |
|---|---|
| Level 1 | Does not respond after mild prodding and/or shaking |
| Level 2 | Responds only after mild prodding and/or shaking |
| Level 3 | Responds only after name is called loudly and/or repeatedly |
| Level 4 | Lethargic response to name spoken in normal tone |
| Level 5 | Responds readily to name spoken in normal tone |

jured part, or avoiding further contact with similar damaging stimuli). However, pain is not simply correlated to the degree of nociception experienced following activation of sensory (nociceptive) neuronal pathways. Rather, the perception of pain can be influenced by many different factors, which, in themselves, can become major determinants of the pain. A formal definition of pain has been developed by the International Association for the Study of Pain subcommittee on taxonomy. The subcommittee describes pain as "a highly subjective, unpleasant sensory and emotional experience associated with actual or potential tissue damage or described in terms of such damage" (Mersky and Bogduk 1994).

The most common terms for describing pain use temporal criteria: *acute pain* and *chronic pain* (see Table 15-4). Chronic pain persists for a month beyond the normal course for an acute illness; or persists longer than a reasonable duration for an injury to heal; or is associated with a chronic pathologic process; or recurs at intervals of months to years. Perhaps a more useful classification of pain that is becoming more widely used among pain specialists is one that classifies pain by its underlying pathophysiology, that is, *nociceptive* or *neurogenic* (Woolf et al. 1998).

### *Nociceptive pain*

A *nociceptor* is a type of sensory neuron that is activated by a noxious but not nonnoxious stimulus. *Nociceptive* pain is pain elicited through activation of nociceptors by an intense (noxious) stimulus that poses a threat to normal, undamaged tissue. This type of pain almost always triggers a series of protective, avoidance mechanisms that serve as a warning to the body that continued exposure might result in further unwarranted and protracted damage. This type of pain is, therefore, physiologic, usually of rapid onset and limited duration, and represents what is commonly referred to by most practitioners as *acute* pain. The degree of *nociceptive* pain can vary from mild to moderate to severe, and can be monophasic or recurrent.

### *Neurogenic pain*

The term *neurogenic* pain refers to pain conditions associated with actual tissue damage (persistent, severe inflammatory pain) or trauma to the nervous system (neuropathic). It is characterized by a hyperresponsiveness of the patient to either a normally painful (noxious) stimulus (hyperalgesia), or to an innocuous stimulus (allodynia). Neurogenic pain can be further categorized into acute and chronic duration depending on the underlying pathology. In most cases of musculoskeletal and/or soft-tissue injury where there is an associated inflammation and tenderness, the duration of pain is acute and has a protective, adaptive function in much the same way as nociceptive pain. However, unlike nociceptive pain, tissue damage has occurred and is associated with a short-term, abnormal processing within the somatosensory system.

Neurogenic pain is, however, more generally characterized by a sustained sensory abnormality and therefore, of chronic duration, lasting for at least 6 months to,

**Table 15-4 Disease Definition–Characteristics of Acute and Chronic Pain**

| Feature | Acute | Chronic |
|---|---|---|
| Temporal features | Rapid, well-defined onset<br>Limited duration hours, days, weeks | Delayed, ill-defined onset<br>Autonomous, independent of initiating trigger, neuropathic<br>Unpredictable, protracted duration months, years |
| Physiologic function | Protective<br>Key component of the body defense mechanism | None apparent |
| Pathophysiology | Nociceptive | Nociceptive tissue-injury or neuropathic |
| Other features | Anxiety<br>Sympathetic hyperactivity may be present<br>Provoked | Abnormal hypersensitivity to innocuous allodynia and noxious hyperalgesia stimuli<br>Sympathetic hyperactivity may be present<br>Spontaneous or provoked |
| Etiology | Monophasic<br>Postoperative<br>Traumatic<br>Burns<br>Recurrent<br>Headache<br>Dysmenorrhea<br>Inflammatory bowel | Malignant<br>Cancer<br>AIDS<br>Nonmalignant<br>Osteoarthritis<br>Rheumatoid arthritis<br>Neuropathic pain |

in many cases, several years and even a lifetime. This can occur as a result of ongoing tissue damage such as in the case of chronic, musculoskeletal injuries characterized by pronounced and severe inflammation. It can also occur following a traumatic injury to the nervous system, in which case the neuropathic pain can be independent of the initiating stimulus.

The appearance of neurogenic pain is often delayed as it is dependent on post-injury sequelae that are an integral part of a protracted process of abnormal conditioning of the somatosensory nervous system (Woolf and Doubell 1994) (see below). Chronic neurogenic pain can be either spontaneous or evoked. Spontaneous pain occurs in most chronic pain conditions but is a particular feature of certain types of neuropathic pain. It is indicative of a persistent and often permanent disruption of the sensory input from the periphery to the spinal cord, (e.g., pain associated with an amputated limb or avulsion injury). Evoked pain is elicited by a peripheral stimulus but can be characterized by an exaggerated and protracted response to previously noxious (hyperalgesia) or innocuous (allodynia) stimuli (e.g., increased mechanical sensitivity such as provided by light touch or brush).

It is very important to be as accurate as possible in defining the type of pain in order to provide the most appropriate treatment. Understanding the pathophysiology of pain is difficult, often leading to failed therapy.

**PRINCIPLE Elucidation of the underlying processes that may be contributing to pain is key to a comprehensive assessment of the pain. It clarifies the nature of the disease and can lead to specific and successful therapies.**

## Pathophysiology of Pain

The processing and integration of painful information from the site of an applied noxious stimulus to the sensation of pain depends, in sequence, on four principal components: transduction, transmission, modulation, and perception. Primary afferent nerves are responsible for two of these main functions: transduction and transmission. *Transduction* is the process by which activation of the peripheral terminals of the primary afferent sensory neurons by different modes of noxious stimuli (heat, mechanical, chemical) leads to an electrical discharge in the sensory neuron. *Transmission* refers to the relaying of these neural impulses to the spinal cord. A network of ascending neurons then integrate and relay the information through either the neospinothalamic (sensory), paleospinothalamic (sensory and affective), or spinoreticular (affective/motivational) tracts to distinct regions of the brainstem and midbrain thalamus and, ultimately, the cerebral cortex, resulting in the sensory, affective, and cognitive components of the pain experience. A reciprocal descending *modulatory* system controls the ascending pain transmission neural network. Activation of these descending pathways (e.g., by opioids) can exert a profound inhibitory influence on the cells responsible for transmission, particularly at the level of the spinal cord and thalamus. The final process is the subjective component of pain *perception,* about which little is known at the present time.

The three distinct functional classes of primary afferent neurons can be distinguished on the basis of diameter and conduction velocity (which correlates positively with the degree of myelination). The unmyelinated C-fibers constitute 75% of the total population of primary afferent neurons and conduct with the slowest velocities ($<$ 2 m/sec). The two other classes are represented by the medium diameter, thinly myelinated A$\delta$ fibers with moderate conduction velocities (6 m/sec); and the largest diameter, heavily myelinated A$\beta$ fibers with the fastest conduction velocities (12–20 m/sec). Each of these primary afferent neurons respond to different types and intensity of stimuli. C and A$\delta$ fibers are considered nociceptor, because they are normally silent and only respond maximally to noxious stimuli, that is, these fibers respond differentially to noxious and innocuous stimuli.

In the spinal cord, cells of the dorsal horn fall into three main categories: 1) projection cells that relay the incoming nociceptive information to higher centers in the brain; 2) excitatory interneurons that relay the message to either projection cells, to other interneurons, or motoneurons that mediate spinal reflexes; and, 3) inhibitory interneurons that contribute to the control of nociceptive transmission. *Wide dynamic range* (WDR) *neurons* are so named because they can be activated by nonnociceptive input from low threshold, A$\beta$ afferents can receive both direct (A$\delta$) and indirect (C) input from high-threshold nociceptive afferents. Many WDR neurons receive convergent afferent input from muscle and viscera as well as skin, leading to the phenomenon of referred pain.

The most common cause of neurogenic pain is persistent tissue injury provoked by trauma, surgery, or disease. The accompanying inflammatory response is associated with a plethora of mediators released from a variety of different cell types (e.g., immune cells, macrophages), many of which have migrated to the site of damage. Among the diverse chemical stimuli released in response to tissue or nerve injury are the excitatory amino acids glutamate and aspartate, GABA, acetylcholine, adenosine, ATP, serotonin, protons, the neuropeptides bradykinin and substance P, norepinephrine, eicosanoids (prostacyclin, prostaglandin $E_2$), growth factors (e.g., NGF), and cytokines (interleukin-1$\beta$, tumor necrosis factor $\alpha$). A fundamental feature of the increased excitability of primary afferents following tissue injury is that the peripheral nerve (and therefore input to the spinal cord) is intact. Mediators of the inflammatory response released locally in the periphery can therefore produce an uninterrupted amplification of the nociceptive signal (Rang et al. 1994). These inflammatory mediators have the ability to interact either directly on specific receptors on the peripheral terminals of unmyelinated nociceptive afferents, or indirectly by causing other cell types to release agents that may then act on the primary afferent neuron. The result is either activation or sensitization of C fibers manifested in reduced thresholds to thermal and mechanical noxious stimuli (primary hyperalgesia) within the area immediately surrounding the site of damage (peripheral sensitization) (Treede et al. 1992). Persistence of the injury then causes the increased sensitivity to noxious stimuli to spread and develop in the undamaged area surrounding the injury site (secondary hyperalgesia).

There is now evidence that pain can be elicited by light tactile stimuli (allodynia) within the site of damage and in the surrounding zone of normal skin. The appearance of tactile allodynia is the consequence of the sustained increase in unmyelinated C-fiber afferent drive, generated by the inflammation, evoking an increase in the excitability of neurons in the spinal dorsal horn (central sensitization), which in turn results in a lowering of the mechanical threshold of the cutaneous receptive field and an increased responsiveness to A$\beta$ inputs (Figure 15-1). These changes in central neuron excitability and the underlying neural plasticity are thought to be dynamically maintained by the ongoing nociceptor drive.

## Clinical Measurement of Pain

The formal definition of pain as offered by the International Association for the Study of Pain is an "unpleasant sensory and emotional experience associated with actual or potential tissue damage or both" (Mersky and Bogduk 1994). This definition represents a first step in achieving an understanding of pain and its complement, analgesia (IASP 1980). Unlike measuring objective physiologic parameters, the quantitation of a subjective experience such as pain poses problems for the clinical investigator who seeks to compare the efficacy of drugs, as well as for the practitioner who seeks to find the optimal therapeutic strategy to deal with a suffering patient. Absent useful measures of pain, practitioners are frequently guided by their own beliefs as well as the patient's opinions. Yet other personal, subjective experiences, such as anxiety or depression, have been quantified successfully.

Pain can be measured by verbal reports, or behavioral and correlative physiologic measures, but each of these techniques has its own problems (Gracely 1990). Verbal reports are confounded by several factors, including the patient's need to maximize or minimize his or her suffering, as well as the patient's verbal ability and memory. Although behavioral measures are more quantifiable, the very success of behavioral modification suggests that behavior can be dissociated from perception. Even though the basic neurophysiology of pain can be measured in terms of sensory transmission (either electrophysiologically or neurochemically), this ignores the importance of the higher level central nervous system processes in the pain experience. Notwithstanding these psychological processes, electrophysiologically measured stimulus rates habituate with time.

Clinical investigators tend to use the visual analog scale (or a pictorial variant of it for children), or a more extensive pain questionnaire, to measure pain (Fishman et al. 1987). The patient is asked to rate the pain on a scale of 0 to 10 with 0 being no pain and 10 being the worst imaginable pain. In the McGill Pain Questionnaire (Melzack 1975), multiple descriptors on three dimensions (sensory, affective, evaluative) are presented to the patient in the form of 20 sets of words that convey pain, and the patient selects the set that most closely represents how he or she feels.

**PRINCIPLE Practitioners tend to measure pain in operational terms. Since pain relief is associated with a return toward normal function, performance of real-life tasks can be used as a surrogate measure of analgesic efficacy. Restoration of functional capacity can be unambiguously assessed by the patient as well as the practitioner and can be used for setting meaningful goals for therapeutic strategies.**

### *Clinical trials*

The value of the randomized, double-blind, placebo-controlled trial is nowhere better exemplified than in the clinical investigation of analgesic drugs, because of the powerful placebo effect on the pain experience. The most common study design is the single-dose analgesic comparison in which patients rate pain or the relief of pain for several hours following a randomly assigned test drug (at a predetermined dose), a standard analgesic (most often the opiate narcotic morphine), or a placebo.

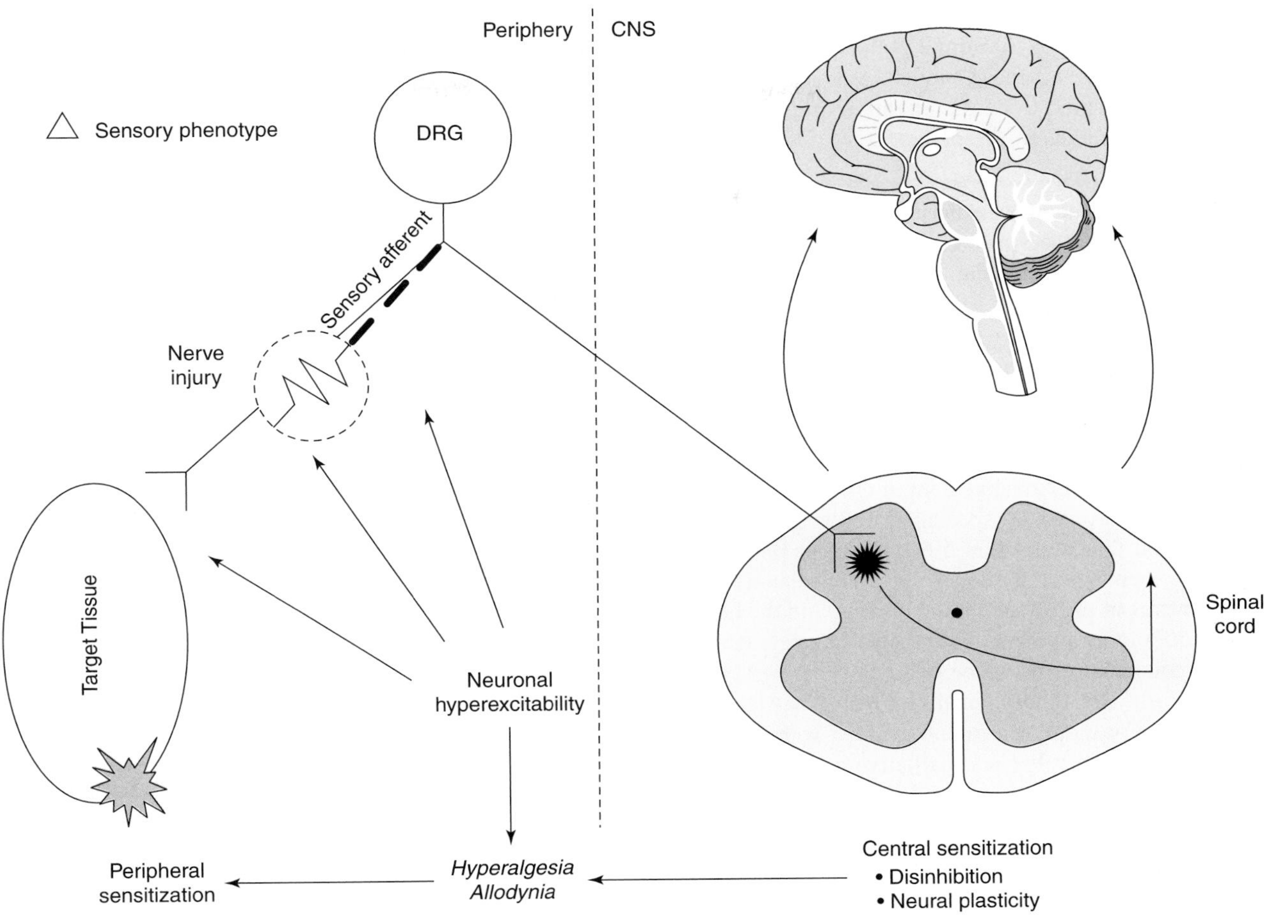


FIGURE 15-1 **Pathophysiology of the sensory neuron. DRG, dorsal root ganglion.**

The efficacy of different classes of compounds depends to a large extent on the pathophysiology of the pain (Max and Laska 1991). The more homogeneous the population of pain sufferers (e.g., acute postoperative pain following hysterectomy), the lower the variance and the sample size required to detect differences in analgesic efficacy. Apart from establishing the probability of whether pain relief occurs, clinical trials should also establish the distribution of times of onset, the magnitude of the peak relief obtained, and the probable duration of effect. The last-mentioned variable is usually established by the use of a surrogate indicator such as "time to remedication."

The data that are needed to assess the adverse events of an analgesic drug, and thereby establish its "therapeutic ratio" (benefits/risks), are often acquired in studies involving normal subjects, since the single-dose analgesic comparison studies typically have sample sizes that are too small, and toxicity may only occur with accumulation from repeated dosing. Furthermore, the methods used to assess adverse effects are cumbersome and may interfere with the measurement of analgesic effect.

**PRINCIPLE Combinations of analgesics with different mechanisms of action are prescribed to reduce the adverse event profile that a single agent could produce at a comparable level of analgesia.**

In order to determine the optimal dose of each analgesic when used in combination, a three-dimensional dose-response "surface" is analyzed by using a factorial design in which each dose of drug A is combined with several (typically 2–4) doses of drug B (Goldberg et al. 1988). Experimental pain models have been widely used to provide fast and efficient evaluation of the efficacy and toxicity of a study drug in normal populations under controlled conditions, and these models represent a staging environment in which to define effective drugs from preclinical animal studies to the patient setting.

**PRINCIPLE Although experimental pain stimuli cannot duplicate the sensory, affective, and cognitive consequences of clinical pain, it can serve as a correlative analogue of clinical syndromes.**

## Cancer Pain

Because of the high incidence of cancer and the extremely high prevalence of pain associated with this disease (up to 85%), the analgesic management of chronic cancer pain is important to virtually all specialists and generalists. Yet surveys reveal that more than 50% of cancer patients do not believe their pain has been adequately treated. Barriers, on the part of the clinician, the patient, and the health-care system, often impede effective pain management and require a concerted effort to be overcome.

The World Health Organization (WHO) has launched an educational program referred to as the *3-step analgesic ladder* (Cancer pain relief and palliative care 1990). This program has been widely accepted as an appropriate model for the management of cancer pain. The three steps refer to the severity of the patient's pain. In this model, step 1 is mild pain (1–4 on a visual analogue scale), step 2 is moderate pain (5–6 on VAS scale), and step 3 is severe pain (7–10 on VAS scale). The WHO recommendations will help clinicians to rationally select the most appropriate analgesic drug and should be followed together with a set of principles of analgesic management that are specific to the cancer patient (Levy 1996).

### *Approach to the management of cancer pain*

The analgesic drugs most often used in the management of pain are described in Table 15-5

STEP 1 In patients with mild pain, pharmacologic therapy involves the use of nonopioid analgesic drugs, including acetaminophen, aspirin, other nonsteroidal anti-inflammatory agents (NSAIDS), and tramadol (although technically this last compound does bind with weak affinity to opiate receptors). Each of these drugs has specific warnings and contraindications. In the case of acetaminophen, the daily dose should not exceed 4–6 g/day because of the risk of developing hepatitis or even liver failure. Cancer patients often have gastropathies and a bleeding diathesis related to their underlying disease or its primary treatment; therefore, they may not be able to tolerate the usual aspirin formulations. The platelet problems from aspirin can be minimized by using nonacetylated salicylates (e.g., choline magnesium trisalicylate).

Patients receiving NSAIDs should be regularly monitored for gastropathy, renal failure, hepatitis, and bleeding. Because tramadol use can be associated with a variety of adverse effects (including nausea, dizziness, constipation, sedation, and headache), this drug is reserved for patients whose pain is no longer relieved by acetaminophen, but is not severe enough to warrant inclusion of opioid therapy.

STEP 2 Patients with moderate pain require opioids that are formulated in fixed combinations with nonopioid analgesics (e.g., hydrocodone or oxycodone in combination with acetaminophen or aspirin). Codeine is used less often because of significant adverse effects when the dose is increased. Furthermore, codeine requires hepatic metabolism by CYP2D6 for conversion to the active ingredient (morphine), and this enzyme may be congenitally deficient or inhibited by the administration of several commonly prescribed drugs including cimetidine, quinidine, and fluoxetine (Desmeules et al. 1991). Propoxyphene is not recommended because of its long half-life and the accumulation of norpropoxyphene, a toxic metabolite.

STEP 3 Patients with severe cancer pain are prescribed opioids whose dose can be escalated with relatively few adverse effects. Such drugs include morphine (considered to be the "gold-standard"), hydromorphone (which is more soluble and more potent than morphine and can therefore be administered in smaller volumes), oxycodone (formulated without acetaminophen, and which may be associated with fewer adverse effects than morphine), and fentanyl (which is available in a transdermal preparation allowing its use in patients who are unable to tolerate oral therapy).

Neither methadone nor levorphanol is considered a first-line analgesic opioid because their long half-lives result in drug accumulation. Other narcotics that are not recommended for management of chronic cancer pain include meperidine (because it has a shorter half-life and is converted to a potentially toxic metabolite, normeperidine), buprenorphine (a partial opioid agonist with low maximal efficacy), and the mixed opioid agonist-antagonists including pentazocine, butorphanol, dezocine, and nalbuphine (which have low analgesic efficacy and can reverse opioid analgesia, and can therefore precipitate a withdrawal syndrome).

Although oral therapy is the most convenient route of administration, the route should be adapted to the patient's condition to include sublingual (if the patient cannot swallow), buccal (with fentanyl for episodic breakthrough pain), transdermal (if the enteral route is entirely precluded), rectal (if psychosocial constraints can be overcome), and subcutaneous (which is more desirable than the more painful intramuscular route). Neuraxial administration (intrathecal, epidural, and intraventricular) is reserved for those patients in whom systemic analgesic therapy is ineffective, unacceptable, or associated with unmanageable toxicity.

**PRINCIPLE The goal of continuous opioid therapy for cancer pain is to relieve a patient's pain throughout the dosing interval without producing unmanageable adverse effects. Close attention must be paid to the choice of agent and route of administration.**

Patients with cancer pain should be administered their analgesic drugs at intervals that prevent recurrence of pain and minimize the number of daily doses. Supplemental rescue doses of analgesic drugs should be provided for breakthrough pain. The clinician should be prepared to increase the dose by as much as 100% over a 24-hour period for patients in the Step 3 category.

It is important for the physician to remember that as patients with chronic severe pain (such as that associated with cancer) progress, they will likely become increasingly tolerant to the analgesic effects of their opioid medication. That is, the dose of opioid analgesic required to produce an acceptable level of analgesia will continue to rise. Prescriptions for such patients may need to be written for large amounts of opioid tablets. Such patients will also become both psychologically and physically dependent on their opioid analgesic. In other words, abrupt discontinuation of the opioid (for example, if the prescription is allowed to run out) will lead to a state of both psychological and physiologic withdrawal, as well as the return of the underlying pain. Despite the presence of both tolerance to and dependence on opioids, we should not view such patients as "addicted" to narcotics.

While the term "addiction" is imprecise, it connotes habitual use of drugs of abuse, obsession with obtaining the next "score" of the drug, illegal activities to obtain the drug or to support a habit, self-destructive behavior, behavior at odds with societal rules or norms, risk of various infections, and so on. None of these connotations apply to a patient with terminal cancer, in severe pain, who is appropriately and legally prescribed large doses of opioid analgesics to provide adequate relief from intractable pain.

#### *Side effects of opioid therapy in the management of chronic cancer pain*

CONSTIPATION Constipation is a predictable consequence of opioid therapy, especially when the opioid is administered continuously. This adverse effect can be appropriately managed, starting with prevention by using a stool softener and a bowel stimulant in appropriate and increasing doses if a bowel movement occurs less frequently than every other day. Fecal impaction should be ruled out before considering the use of enemas, lactulose, and mineral oils for obstipation (defined as a bowel movement less than every third day).

NAUSEA Nausea may remit when constipation is adequately managed. If not, this is usually responsive to centrally acting antiemetic drugs.

SEDATION AND COGNITIVE IMPAIRMENT Sedation and cognitive impairment are symptoms that may improve as tolerance to the opioid develops, although this may persist when frequent dose escalations are required. In this case, the addition of "opioid-sparing" therapy (such as $\alpha_2$-adrenergic receptor agonists) can be considered, along with a central nervous stimulant such as methylphenidate.

RESPIRATORY DEPRESSION Respiratory depression, through inadvertent or too-rapid dose escalation, can be managed with naloxone (20–40 $\mu$g/min intravenously). Obviously, excessive doses of naloxone are also to be avoided, in order not to precipitate more pain or a withdrawal syndrome.

#### *Bone pain*

Although there are many causes of chronic pain associated with malignancies, possibly the most common, and often the most amenable to treatment, are those related to skeletal involvement by the primary tumor or metastases. Pain is often disproportionate to the size or degree of bone involvement. Pathogenic factors that cause bone pain include release of chemical mediators, increased pressure within the bone, microfractures, stretching of the periosteum, reactive muscle spasm, nerve root infiltration, and compression of nerves by the collapse of vertebrae (Mercadante 1997).

Therapeutic strategies need to address which of these causes is most pertinent in a given patient. Treatment with opioids remains important, but other drug classes are also useful in specific patients.

**Table 15-5 Common Analgesics Used in the Treatment of Acute or Chronic Pain**

| Drug Class and Generic Name | Brand Name | Usual Single Dose | Dose Interval | Maximum Dose/Day | Contraindications | Adverse Effects | Comments |
|---|---|---|---|---|---|---|---|
| Acetaminophen | Tylenol | 500–1000 mg PO | 4–6 h | 4000–6000 mg | Alcoholism, liver disease concurrent treatment with P450 enzyme inducers | Hepatitis, hepatic necrosis | As effective as aspirin |
| Salicylates | | | | | Aspirin-sensitive asthma, ulcer disease | Gastropathy, salicylism, platelet dysfunction | |
| Aspirin | Bayer | 500–1000 mg PO | 4–6 h | 6000 mg | | | |
| Choline magnesium trisalicylate | Trilisate | 1000–1500 mg PO | 8–12 h | 4000 mg | | | Less gastropathy: no platelet dysfunction |
| Diflunisal | Dolobid | 1000 mg PO | 8–12 h | 1500 mg | | | |
| NSAIDs | | | | | Alcoholism, peptic ulcer disease, age, renal disease<br>Aspirin-sensitive asthma | Gastropathy, platelet inhibition | |
| Diclofenac | Voltaren | 50 mg PO | 8 h | 150 mg | | | |
| Ibuprofen | Motrin, Advil | 200–400 mg PO | 4–6 h | 4000 mg | | | Less gastropathy |
| Ketoprofen | Orudis | 25–75 mg PO | 6–8 h | 300 mg | | | |
| Ketorolac tromethamine | Toradol | 30 mg IM IV (< 65 yr) | 6 h | 200 mg | | | Only parenteral preparation available can still cause gastropathy<br>adverse bleeding if > 5 day therapy |
| | | 15 mg IM IV (> 65 yr) | 6 h | 60 mg | | | |
| | | 10 mg PO | 4–6 h | 40 mg | | | |
| Naproxen | Naprosyn | 500 mg then 250 mg | 6–8 h | 1000 mg | | | |
| | Anaprox | 550 mg then 275 mg | 6–8 h | 1100 mg | | | |
| Naproxen sodium | Aleve | 440 mg then 220 mg | | 660 mg | | | |

**Table 15-5 Common Analgesics Used in the Treatment of Acute or Chronic Pain (Continued)**

| Drug Class and Generic Name | Brand Name | Usual Single Dose | Dose Interval | Maximum Dose/Day | Contraindications | Adverse Effects | Comments |
|---|---|---|---|---|---|---|---|
| Tramadol | | | | | | | |
| Tramadol HCl | Ultram | 50–100 mg PO | 6 h | 400 mg | Antidepressants, MAO inhibitors, antipsychotic | Seizures (dose > 400 mg/day) | As effective as acetaminophen with codeine or oxycodone |
| Opioids | | | | | Decreased respiratory reserve | Dependency, sedation, nausea and vomiting, constipation, respiratory depression, pruritus, urinary retention | Dependency, rare with acute pain or cancer pain; no ceiling for analgesic effects except what is imposed by adverse effects; renal failure associated with accumulation of morphine-6-glucuronide |
| Morphine-like | | | | | | | |
| Morphine sulfate | Morphine sulfate | 10 mg IM, SC, IV | 3–6 h | | | | |
| | MS Contin | 20–70 mg PO | 8–12 h | | | | |
| | Kadian | 20–70 mg PO | 12–24 h | | | | |
| | Morphine sulfate | suppository | | | | | |
| | MSIR | PO | | | | | |
| Hydromorphone HCl | Dilaudid | 1.3 mg IM, SC<br>4–8 mg PO | 3–5 h | | | | Useful for initial dose titration and for PM supplementation |
| Oxymorphone HCl | Numorphan | 1 mg IM | 35 h | | | | Less histamine release |
| Codeine-like | | | | | | | |
| Codeine phosphate | various | 50–100 mg IM<br>60–120 mg PO | 3–5 h | | | Nausea, vomiting, dysphoria | |
| Dihydrocodeine bitartrate | Synalgos | 50–75 mg PO | 3–5 h | | | | |
| Hydrocodone | Vicodin | 5 mg PO | 3–5 h | | | | |
| Oxycodone HCl | Roxicodone | 10 mg PO | 3–5 h | | | | |
| Synthetic | | | | | | | |
| Meperidine HCl | Demerol | 50–100 mg IM<br>150 mg PO | 2–4 h | | MAO inhibitors<br>Renal failure | Irritation when given IM dysphoria, irritability, seizures | Normeperidine toxicity limits utility for cancer pain |
| Fentanyl | Duragesic | Transdermal 25–100 $\mu g$ | 72 h | | | | Fewer adverse effects than sustained-release oral preparations |

Table 15-5 Common Analgesics Used in the Treatment of Acute or Chronic Pain (Continued)

| Drug Class and Generic Name | Brand Name | Usual Single Dose | Dose Interval | Maximum Dose/Day | Contraindications | Adverse Effects | Comments |
|---|---|---|---|---|---|---|---|
| Fentanyl citrate | Sublimaze | 100 $\mu$g IM, IV | | | | | |
| | Oralet | lollipop | | | | | |
| Methadone HCl | Dolophine | 10 mg IM<br>1–20 mg PO | 4–6 h | | | Accumulation resulting in CNS depression | Long and variable half-life |
| Propoxyphene HCl | Darvon | 65 mg PO | 2–3 h | | Renal failure | Norpropoxyphene causes seizures | Not recommended due to toxicity |
| Levorphanol tartrate | Levo-Dromoran | 1.5–2.5 mg IM<br>2–4 mg PO | 4–8 h | | | | Plasma accumulation results in delayed toxicity |
| Partial agonist | | | | | | | Less likely to cause dependence |
| Buprenorphine HCl | Buprenex | 0.4 mg IM | 4–6 h | | | | |
| Agonist/antagonist | | | | | Patients physically dependent on opiate agonists | Opiate withdrawal | Less likely to cause dependence |
| Pentazocine lactate | Talwin | 60 mg IM | 2–4 h | | | | |
| Nalbuphine HCl | Nubain | 12 mg IM | 3–6 h | | | | |
| Dezocine | Dalgan | 10 mg IM | 3–6 h | | | | |

**RADIOTHERAPY** Radiotherapy provides an effective symptomatic treatment for local bone pain especially when due to a solitary metastasis. Once vertebral collapse has occurred, radiotherapy tends to be ineffective.

**RADIOISOTOPES** Radioisotopes, such as [$^{89}$Sr]strontium chloride, are easy to administer and are associated with less toxicity than radiotherapy. Radioisotopes can be used to treat subclinical bone metastases. However, the dose delivered is lower and less discrete than with external beam irradiation.

**HORMONAL THERAPY** Hormonal therapy is indicated when bone metastases are estrogen- or androgen-dependent, such as metastases from breast, prostate, or endometrial cancers.

**BISPHOSPHONATES** Bisphosphonates (pyrophosphate analogues that are resistant to hydrolysis) bind hydroxyapatite crystals and prevent bone resorption. This therapy is especially useful in patients who have osteolytic hypercalcemia. The most potent agent in this class is pamidronate in a dose of 90–120 mg intravenously every 3–6 weeks. (See also Chapter 10, Connective Tissue and Bone Disorders.)

Neuropathic pain states should be managed as described elsewhere.

## Complex Regional Pain Syndrome

The International Society of the Study of Pain (IASP) recently undertook the renaming as *complex regional pain syndromes* (CRPSs) the entities formerly known as *reflex sympathetic dystrophy* (RSD) and *causalgia*, in an attempt to recognize the multiple presentations of this disease (Galer et al. 1998; Rowbotham 1998). Neuropathic pain is a hallmark of the disease, with burning lancinating pain in the affected region. Alterations in color, swelling, sweating, and hair growth patterns are commonly seen in the same distribution. RSD is now termed *CRPS type I*, and causalgia is termed *CRPS type II*.

Because secondary muscular and joint changes subsequently occur as a consequence of immobility, early pain control and rehabilitation are paramount in order to preserve any chance of recovery (Van der Laan et al. 1998). The NSAIDs are very useful adjuncts to reduce the pain of these musculoskeletal complaints.

### *Sympathetically maintained pain*

A feature of many neuropathic pain states is that they may be attributed to or associated with hyperactivity of the sympathetic nervous system (Campbell et al. 1994). Sympathetically maintained pain (SMP) is, by definition, pain attributable to sympathetic efferent dysfunction in peripheral tissues, that is, SMP results from the acquired capacity of norepinephrine to evoke pain (Davis et al. 1991). Pain *not* influenced by alterations of sympathetic efferent function is labeled sympathetically independent pain (SIP). The extent of the contribution that such perturbation of the sympathetic nervous system has on many neurogenic pain conditions is, however, often controversial. SMP has been suggested to be the primary underlying cause of CRPSs I and II (Perl 1994). It may also be associated with a wide variety of disorders including postherpetic neuralgia (PHN), painful polyneuropathies such as diabetic neuropathy, traumatic nerve injury, and soft tissue injury (Campbell et al. 1994).

It is generally believed that the severity of pain, signs of abnormal sympathetic function, and the nature of the underlying disorder do not necessarily indicate that the patient has SMP. Sensory examination may aid in the diagnosis, for example, a greater proportion of SMP patients tend to exhibit hypersensitivity to mild, cooling stimuli (Frost et al. 1988; Wahren et al. 1991). However, the most conclusive evidence for the existence of SMP is when relief of hyperalgesia and allodynia is obtained by surgical sympathectomy, local anesthetic block of sympathetic ganglia (Campbell et al. 1994), or a pharmacological block of the $\alpha_1$-subtype of adrenergic receptors (Sato and Perl 1991; Davis et al. 1991; Campbell et al. 1992). Indeed, the adrenergic receptor antagonist phentolamine has been investigated as a diagnostic test for suspected SMP (Arner 1991; Raja et al. 1991). In a small study, phentolamine was shown to produce pain relief that was highly correlated with that obtained following local anesthetic block of the sympathetic ganglia (Raja et al. 1991).

In certain cases of persistent, severe inflammation, norepinephrine is released from sympathetic postganglionic efferent fibers in the peripheral receptive fields of low-threshold, normally nonnociceptive, mechanoreceptors (LTMs). The norepinephrine activates $\alpha_1$-adrenergic receptors present on the terminals of the LTMs to evoke increased excitability of the sensory neurons. This in turn produces pain through LTM innervation of spinal dorsal horn neurons sensitized by the persistent injury. This mechanism is considered to be a likely molecular basis for the sympathetically maintained component of some persistent inflammatory pain conditions.

Since the sympathetic nervous system may be a pathogenic mechanism, it can be interrupted by the application of specific sympathetic blockade with local anesthetic. A stellate ganglion block performed at the level of the sixth cervical vertebra (C6), or a lumbar sympathetic block performed at L2, may be utilized for the arm and leg, respectively. The temporary relief provided by these blocks improves the chances of recovery by allowing the patient to participate in rehabilitative activities (Stanton-Hicks et al. 1998). For more continuous relief, the membrane-stabilizing agents lidocaine and mexiletine offer therapeutic benefit. The anticonvulsants carbamazepine and gabapentin are also alternatives when intermittent blockade does not provide sustained relief.

For more recalcitrant cases of CPRS, the appropriate application of invasive techniques, such as spinal cord stimulation, can be quite effective (Kumar et al. 1997). The administration of opioids, clonidine, and local anesthetics into the intrathecal space have each been reported in the management of difficult cases (Dahm et al. 1998).

***Neuropathic pain***

The main types of chronic pain are those associated with persistent, severe tissue and nerve (neuropathic) injury (see Figure 15-1). Severe inflammatory and neuropathic pain states are characterized by spontaneous pain and increased behavioral responses to noxious stimuli (hyperalgesia) and to previously innocuous, mechanical stimuli (allodynia) (Devor 1994; Woolf 1994). These injury-evoked features are primarily the result of a persistent increase in nociceptor excitability and a corresponding increased responsiveness of spinal neurons receiving the nociceptive input, that is, central sensitization (Woolf 1983; Cook et al. 1987). However, fundamental differences between nerve and tissue injury mean that, although the symptomology may appear similar, alterations in nociceptor transduction and transmission may be mediated by distinct mechanisms (Woolf and Doubell 1994) (see section "Pathophysiology of Pain").

**Key Points: The principal features of clinical neuropathic pain are as follows.**

- **Pain initiated or caused by a primary lesion or dysfunction in the peripheral or central nervous system.**
- **Pain occurs in the absence of detectable ongoing tissue damage.**
- **Abnormal or unfamiliar dysesthesia, frequently having a burning and/or electrical quality.**
- **Delay in onset after precipitating injury.**
- **Paroxysmal brief shooting or stabbing component.**
- **Mild innocuous stimuli now painful allodynia.**
- **Increased responsiveness to repetitive painful stimuli hyperalgesia.**

In contrast to inflammation, many types of neuropathic pain conditions involve protracted damage to the peripheral and/or central nervous system. In the case of a peripheral nerve injury, sensory input is at least partially disrupted causing the development of an abnormal repetitive discharge at several ectopic sites established following injury, that is, neuroma end bulbs, areas of demyelination that may occur along the degenerating peripheral nerve and the dorsal root ganglion (DRG) (Devor 1994). The barrage of spontaneous and/or evoked afferent impulse traffic is then manifested in the enhanced release of glutamate from the central terminals of the primary afferent neurons in the superficial spinal dorsal horn (Figure 15-1). Glutamate, acting on AMPA and NMDA receptors, precipitates the process of central sensitization, involving increased neuronal excitability and synaptic reorganization within the spinal dorsal horn, which is manifested in an expansion of the peripheral receptive fields (Devor 1994). Spinal neuron disinhibition involving a loss of GABAergic interneurons (Sivilotti and Woolf 1994) and the selective destruction of A$\beta$ fibers contributes to the hyperexcitable state. The central projection pattern of the surviving A$\beta$ fiber input to the spinal dorsal horn is also altered such that collateral sprouts of A$\beta$ fibers now project onto NS cells in lamina II, a contributing factor to touch-evoked pain (Woolf et al. 1992). In addition, aberrant retrograde sprouts of sympathetic postganglionic efferent neurons form ephaptic connections with primary afferent neurons, principally LTMs, in the DRG to promote stimulation of these neurons by norepinephrine (McLachlan et al. 1993). This is considered to be a possible contributory mechanism for the sympathetically maintained component of many neuropathic pain states. The most likely target for norepinephrine is the $\alpha_1$-adrenergic receptors, as antagonists have been found to provide pain relief (Davis et al. 1991) and, conversely, the $\alpha_1$-adrenergic receptor-selective agonist phenylephrine has been found to evoke pain (Davis et al. 1991). However, the situation is not fully resolved as $\alpha_2$-adrenergic receptor antagonists have also been shown to be effective (Sato and Perl 1991) despite clinical evidence demonstrating that clonidine, an $\alpha_2$-adrenergic receptor-selective agonist, also produces analgesia (Davis et al. 1991).

A prominent molecular basis for the abnormal hyperexcitability of the peripheral nerve following injury is the redistribution of sodium channels along injured or regenerating axons, resulting in increased membrane density of sodium channels at the focal sites of ectopic impulse discharge (Lombet et al. 1985; Devor et al. 1993; England et al. 1994). This membrane remodeling contributes to a lower threshold for action potential generation at these sites and, consequently, precipitates ectopic impulse generation in a chronically injured nerve (Wall and Devor 1983; Matzner and Devor 1994; Devor 1994). Consistent with this hypothesis has been the clinical effectiveness of agents that act primarily through a common, use-dependent block of sodium channels (e.g., local anesthetics, antiarrhythmics, and anticonvulsants) (Catterall 1987) in the treatment of many types of chronic pain, especially neuropathic pain (Backonja 1994; Tanelian and Victory 1995). However, the full analgesic potential of these agents has been frequently limited by the onset of numerous adverse effects. Many of these clinical signs are CNS-related and have restricted patient tolerability and, therefore, continued use of these agents over a long-term period. Adverse effects commonly reported include nausea and emesis, dizziness and light-headedness, somnolence, ataxia, and tinnitus. Cardiotoxicity can also be problematic, particularly in the elderly population.

However, membrane events that play a role in the redistribution of sodium channels clearly can also cause alterations in the localization and distribution of other membrane-bound, voltage/ligand-gated ion channels (e.g., calcium and potassium channels) that would contribute to the establishment and maintenance of the neuronal hyperexcitability (Devor 1994). Modulation of either the function or distribution of voltage-gated calcium ion channels, therefore, has the potential for providing novel agents for the treatment of chronic pain. This has been demonstrated by the analgesic effectiveness of N-type voltage-gated calcium channel antagonists at the preclinical level (Miljanich and Ramachandran 1995) and, more recently, in the clinic (Brose et al. 1996).

## Pain from Rheumatologic Disorders

The arthritides, both inflammatory and degenerative, exhibit common elements of pain and impairment. Although treatment of the underlying pathophysiology with disease modifying agents is essential, the management of pain and maintenance of functionality is paramount. Symptomatic relief from the nociceptive components may be obtained with the use of potent medications including the NSAIDs; drugs and opioids are sometimes required as well.

The NSAIDs provide analgesia in addition to their inherent anti-inflammatory properties (Drugs for pain 1998). Newer cyclooxygenase 2 inhibitors (COX-2) are recent additions to the drugs for pain alleviation that will offer efficacy with lower toxicity (Lane 1997).

Administration of long-acting opiate narcotics (e.g., methadone or levorphanol) on a time-contingent dosing schedule allows for steady plasma concentrations and consistent relief. Instant release morphine formulations can offer rescue from pain that occurs unpredictably during the course of daily activities. In conjunction with support groups emphasizing self-efficacy and self-management, the pain relief provided by the combination of opiates and NSAIDs improves the quality of life for patients afflicted with rheumatologic disorders (Brandt 1998; Smith et al. 1997).

Painful mono- and polyneuropathies can complicate many of the rheumatologic disorders, and treatment is directed at management of the underlying immunologic disorder, together with providing symptomatic relief with membrane-stabilizing agents and anticonvulsants. Lidocaine is the prototypical membrane-stabilizing agent capable of arresting the hyperactivity of neural tissue found in neuropathic pain states (Tanelian and Victory 1995). Mexiletine is the agent most similar to lidocaine and adds the option of oral therapy for neuropathic pain (Chabal et al. 1992).

Carbamazepine, an anticonvulsant, has long been utilized for the treatment of neuropathic pain states (McQuay et al. 1995). A newer anticonvulsant agent, gabapentin, is fast gaining a role in the treatment of these difficult-to-manage symptoms (Wetzel and Connelly 1997). Tricyclic antidepressants, in dosages far below those required to treat depression, are regarded as first-line agents for neuropathic conditions (McQuay et al. 1996). Unfortunately, the adverse-effect profile of the tricyclic antidepressants, including sedation and dry mouth, makes these agents more useful at night when patients so often have difficulty initiating and maintaining appropriate sleep hygiene.

## Cranial-Facial Pain

Pain of the head and neck, excluding headache, is primarily neuropathic in nature. Trigeminal neuralgia (termed tic douloureux because of the muscular spasm of the face from the repeated volleys of pain) is the prototypical neuropathic facial pain, with its electrical lancinating pain in the distribution of the three major branches of cranial nerve V (Turp and Gobetti 1996). In a minority of cases, microvascular decompression of the trigeminal nerve (Jannetta's procedure) in the cranial fossa can offer sustained relief (Brisman 1997). Agents for the relief of this condition include the classic anticonvulsant agent carbamazepine (McQuay et al. 1995). The newer anticonvulsant, gabapentin, has shown some efficacy for patients suffering from this often debilitating condition (Khan 1998). Topical application of capsaicin cream, which depletes the neurotransmitter substance P, has been advocated for this condition, but is particularly noxious when inadvertently applied to mucous membranes (Epstein and Marcie 1994).

Atypical facial pain is often caused by a nonspecific category of diagnosis that do not conveniently fit into headache or trigeminal neuralgia categories (Heft 1992). Patients may present with structural abnormalities (e.g., temporomandibular joint dysfunction) or with more classic neuropathic features. As a whole, these patients are diverse, and require empiric trials of NSAIDs or membrane-stabilizing agents for relief. A combination of drugs, injections, and even dental splinting may be required to ameliorate the symptoms of this condition (Gouda and Brown 1997). Referral to specialists in orofacial pain may be required to sort out the complexity of this heterogeneous category.

## Back Pain

The constellation of disorders that cause back pain has multiple etiologies, each requiring different treatment based on the nature of the problem (Riddle 1998). Characterization of the problem via the history and physical examination will generally allow categorization into one of several diagnostic groups. Imaging studies, when properly applied, offer further diagnostic information to help guide in the therapeutic plan.

Radicular back pain from neuro-foraminal encroachment, either from disk disruption or degenerative changes, is a complex pain problem with both neuropathic and inflammatory components (Zdeblick 1995). Patients with localized neurologic symptoms (e.g., progressive motor weakness or loss of bowel and bladder function) require urgent orthopedic or neurosurgical consultation. For patients who present with radicular pain, the application of steroids into the epidural space remains a mainstay of treatment (Rowlingson et al. 1986). Clinical experience suggests that patients with disk disruption with true radicular signs may benefit most from a course of three separate injections (Benzon 1986), although this has not been demonstrated in placebo-controlled studies, probably because of the lack of patient homogeneity (Carette et al. 1997). The neuropathic component of this entity has a favorable response to the class of membrane-stabilizing agents such as lidocaine and mexiletine (Tanelian and Victory 1995). After the acute episode subsides, physical rehabilitation and instruction on protective back maneuvers play an important role in avoiding relapse.

Pain from facet arthropathy is a more recently recognized cause for back pain in the cervical and low-back regions (Schwarzer et al. 1994). Such pain can also be treated with epidural steroid injections and NSAIDs. Local anesthetic blocks of the facets may be diagnostic and may indicate potential efficacy from neuroablative techniques such as radio frequency lesioning (Kaplan et al. 1998; Lord 1996).

Diffuse back pain of muscular and ligamentous origin is experienced by most adults sometime in their lives, and fortunately, it is usually self-limiting (Loeser 1996). For some patients myofascial back pain results in significant impairment, and these patients undergo multiple evaluations and diagnostic studies that usually reveal diffuse osteoarthritic changes in the spine, in association with a decreased range of motion, and muscular tenderness in the paraspinal and gluteal region. Discrete trigger points may be palpable in these muscular regions and are amenable to myofascial release techniques as taught by physical therapists. NSAIDs, trigger-point injections with local anesthetic, and a graded physical therapy program can return many of the patients to a more functional lifestyle (Nguyen 1996).

Multidisciplinary evaluation and treatment may benefit those who have had surgical intervention, yet continue to have pain and impairment (Fritsch et al. 1996). Opioids can be delivered into the subarachnoid space via an implanted pump system at a fraction of intravenous doses (Dahm et al. 1998). Such a regimen can provide excellent relief while reducing the systemic adverse effects seen with oral and parenteral administration of opioids. Another therapy available for this condition is spinal cord stimulation, wherein a small electrical current is applied in the epidural space via an implanted electrode and battery system (Burchiel et al. 1996). Appropriately screened candidates can experience a marked reduction in pain utilizing this technique.

## Fibromyalgia

Women are predominately affected by fibromyalgia, which is characterized by diffuse muscular pain with associated trigger points (stereotypically discrete area of muscular tenderness). The diagnostic criteria for this condition include fatigue, gastrointestinal symptoms, and depression, in addition to the muscular complaints (Kurtze et al. 1998; Olsen and Park 1998). Although the specific etiology for this condition remains elusive, medical interventions include the use of NSAIDs and injection of trigger points with local anesthetic. Antidepressant therapy, both for their analgesic properties as well as for the management of depression, is effective and appropriate in this setting (Alarcon and Bradley 1998).

Physical reactivation and physical therapy are essential if patients are to return to increased functionality and productivity. This constellation of symptoms is well-suited to a multidisciplinary evaluation and treatment plan that includes medical, rehabilitative, and psychological interventions (Gruber et al. 1996).

## Diabetic Neuropathy

Diabetes mellitus produces multiple systemic effects including the mono- and polyneuropathies commonly seen in these patients (Chalk and Dyck 1997). The painful neuropathies with their burning dysesthetic pain can plague patients for many years (Boulton and Malik 1998). The tricyclic antidepressants have proven efficacious for this condition in doses considered subtherapeutic from an antidepressant standpoint (Kingery 1997). The sedating adverse effects and the dry mouth produced by these drugs usually make this class of drug difficult to use except at night. Some patients may accommodate to these adverse effects, and thus utilize them during waking hours as well.

> **Key Points: Several key mechanisms contribute to the pathogenesis of painful peripheral mononeuropathies.**
>
> - **Spontaneous hyperactivity ectopic foci of primary afferent and central pain transmission neurons.**
> - **Loss of central inhibitory connections degeneration of A$\beta$ primary afferents.**
> - **Degeneration of GABAergic inhibitory interneurons.**
> - **Structural reorganization, including collateral sprouting of A$\beta$ fibers onto nociceptive-specific cells in superficial laminae of dorsal horn, and facilitation of primary afferents by motor or sympathetic efferents.**

As with other neuropathic pain states, the membrane-stabilizing drugs lidocaine and mexiletine have efficacy and provide an alternative for patients who cannot tolerate tricyclic antidepressants (Dejgard et al. 1998). The anticonvulsants carbamazepine (Wilton 1974) and gabapentin offer potential relief for this condition. Topically applied capsaicin provides a further alternative for patients with particularly difficult to manage neuropathy (Hautkappe et al. 1998).

## Postherpetic Neuralgia

The incidence of postherpetic neuralgia increases with age and is less likely to resolve spontaneously in older patients (Watson and Evans 1986). Older patients present a therapeutic challenge since the elderly may be less tolerant of the medications used to treat this neuropathic pain state. The typical burning, shooting pain with cutaneous hypersensitivity is a hallmark of the disease. When this pain occurs in the facial distribution, it can be particularly devastating to patients.

Multiple therapies have been utilized including injection therapies, systemic techniques, and even topical agents (Carmichael 1991). Unfortunately, this complex combination is necessary, as no therapy is universally successful. Invasive therapies such as epidural steroids, spinal cord stimulation, and local anesthetic blockade can be useful, but may not produce sustainable results (Meglio et al. 1989). The membrane-stabilizing agents, such as lidocaine and mexiletine (Rowbotham 1992), as well as the anticonvulsants carbamazepine and gabapentin, have been successful in some patients (Table 15-6).

The judicious use of opioids with careful attention to the adverse-effect profile in this elderly population can be one of the few options available at times (Pappagallo and Campbell 1994). The topical application of capsaicin and lidocaine creams has recently been shown to be effective as well (Hautkappe et al. 1998). Combinations of the above therapies are often required to produce reasonable levels of analgesia.

## Pain Related to HIV and AIDS

As a result of multiple systemic effects, AIDS produces many complications that can result in pain (Wesselmann 1996). Painful neuropathies occur in a peripheral distribution in the hands and feet with features similar to those of peripheral diabetic neuropathy. Treatment of this neuropathy is similar to that of diabetic neuropathy, with the use of the membrane-stabilizing agents and the anticonvulsants (Lebovits et al. 1989). The development of agents with fewer adverse effects will be of tremendous help in this and other populations of medically complex patients. Complicating HIV-related neuropathy in many patients is extreme muscular wasting, which leads to progressive weakness and fatigue.

## Recent Approaches to Management of Pain

### *Preemptive analgesia*

Studies involving experimental pain in animals have suggested that an intervention given before the pain starts has greater analgesic effect than the same intervention given after the pain has begun (for a review, see Dickenson 1991). Many randomized clinical trials involving different classes of analgesics (e.g., opiates, local anesthetics,

**Table 15-6 Drugs Used as "Adjuvants" in the Treatment of Pain**

| Drug Class and Generic Name | Brand Name | Starting Dose | Dose Interval | Maximum Dose/Day | Contraindications | Adverse Effects | Comments |
|---|---|---|---|---|---|---|---|
| Antidepressants | | | | | | | |
| Amitriptyline HCl | Elavil | 10–25 mg | once at bedtime | 300 mg | Cardiac arrhythmias | Sedation, orthostatic hypertension, dry mouth, urinary retention, constipation | Generally given at bedtime to promote sleep |
| Nortriptyline HCL | Pamelor | 10–25 mg | once at bedtime | 125 mg | | | Rarely used > 150 mg for pain |
| Desipramine HCL | Norpramin | 25–50 mg | once at bedtime | 300 mg | | | Least sedating, usually given in the morning |
| Imipramine HCL | Tofranil | 75 mg | once at bedtime | 300 mg | | | |
| Anticonvulsants | | | | | | | |
| Gabapentin | Neurontin | 300 mg | 8 h | 3600 mg | | | Fewest side effects |
| Phenytoin | Dilantin | 100 mg | 8 h | 600 mg | | Gingival hyperplasia | Therapeutic level 10–20 μg/ml for seizures |
| Valproic acid | Depakene | 250 mg | 8 h | 1250 mg | | | Therapeutic level 50–100 μg/ml for seizures |
| Carbamazepine | Tegretol | 100 mg | 8 h | 1200 mg | Blood dyscrasia | Sedation, rare granulocytopenia | Complete blood count before initiation and every 6 months; do not exceed plasma level of 12 μg/ml; slow escalation of dose may mitigate sedation |
| Membrane stabilizers | | | | | | | |
| Lidocaine HCl | Xylocaine | 1 mg/kg IV | continuous infusion | | | CNS irritability and cardiac toxicity | Monitor plasma levels (therapeutic range 2–5 μg/ml) |
| Flecainide acetate | Tambocor | 50 mg | 12 h | 400 mg | | Seizure, QT interval prolongation, arrhythmias | |
| Mexiletine HCl | Mexitil | 150 mg | 8 h | 1200 mg | | Nausea is prominent | Must be taken with meals or sucralfate to avoid nausea |
| | | | | | | CNS and cardiac toxicity in overdose | Slow escalation of dose over 3–4 weeks enhances compliance |

NSAIDs) given either alone (McQuay et al. 1995) or in combination (Doyle and Bowler 1998) have been performed. However, convincing evidence from clinical trials that preemptive analgesia is superior is lacking.

***Patient-controlled analgesia***

Over the past 15 years or so, physicians and nurses have become more adept at improving analgesia for hospitalized patients by allowing them to self-administer opioids such as morphine sulfate, meperidine, or hydromorphone after surgery, or for other painful conditions. The term for this is *patient-controlled analgesia* (PCA). Sophisticated electronic pumps are now available that can be programmed to deliver a specific combination of a low-dose continuous infusion of an opioid solution, plus intermittent additional boluses of the drug on patient demand. The pump can be programmed for each patient to deliver a specified rate of continuous infusion, bolus amount, lockout interval (specified time between boluses), maximal dose per hour, and so on.

The ability of the patient to self-medicate in this fashion helps to reduce pain by treating pain as it begins to recur, rather than waiting for it to recur in its fullest form. It also removes the patient's concern about having to wait for a nurse to come minutes or hours after the nurse call button has been pushed. Studies have documented improved outcomes when intravenous PCA has been compared to more traditional intermittent IM dosing of morphine in the following areas: improved dose titration, enhanced ability to compensate for interpatient variation in response to opioids, reduction in fluctuation of serum opioid levels, improved analgesia without increased sedation, less patient confusion, less severe pulmonary complications, greater pain relief reported by patients, ability of patients to walk further one day postoperatively, greater nursing preference, and so on. Such clinical trials have been done in a wide variety of painful conditions, including postoperative pain in frail elderly men (Egbert et al. 1990) and in patients who underwent elective joint replacement or spinal surgical procedures (Colwell and Morris 1995).

Since nearly all opioid analgesics can produce nausea or vomiting in some patients, other physicians have demonstrated that the addition of an antiemetic agent (e.g., droperidol or promethazine) to the morphine PCA solution produces decreased patient reports of nausea and vomiting, and sometimes decreased requirement of morphine via PCA as well (Freedman et al. 1995; Silverman et al. 1992).

In short, patient-controlled analgesia has now been well established to improve patient functional outcomes (e.g., improved patient reported pain relief, improved ability to ambulate), patient disease outcome (e.g., greater ability to clear pulmonary secretions through coughing, even after painful thoracic surgery), improved overall patient satisfaction (e.g., patients prefer this type of analgesia for future operations), and possibly improved overall cost as well (somewhat greater expense for the drug and the pump, but less nursing time required, and often earlier ambulation of the patient).

**PRINCIPLE Administering a "standard drug" via a different route with a novel delivery system can result in substantial improvement in a variety of patient outcomes.**

***Gene therapy***

Strategies involving recombinant DNA technology have been advocated for the management of chronic pain conditions. The basic strategy involves overexpressing either an endogenous nociceptive modulator (e.g., an endogenous opiate precursor such as preproenkephalin) or targets for endogenous modulators (e.g., opiate receptors). Overexpression of the receptor requires the introduction of a foreign vector (e.g., adenovirus) containing the new genetic construct into the host's cells.

A more hopeful approach is to introduce genetically modified cells or tissue that contain the therapeutic product (e.g., preproenkephalin) that can be released into a relevant region (e.g., the subarachnoid space). If the donor cells or tissues are nonautologous, then steps have to be taken to prevent rejection. Apart from the usual pharmacologic immune suppression techniques (which introduce a new subset of problems), a new technique involves immuno-isolation in which the nonautologous tissue is physically isolated from the host tissue by placement in perm-selective membranes, allowing the secretory product to permeate out but not allowing the inflammatory response to penetrate (Stockley and Chang 1997).

***Multidisciplinary pain management***

Although novel analgesic therapies have made significant inroads in the management of chronic painful conditions, pain is an emotional as well as a sensory experience and often requires a multidisciplinary approach. Holistic management strategies are being developed to address the medical, physical, and psychological needs of the patient (Nguyen 1996). Multidisciplinary teams, including physicians, clinical psychologists, and physical therapists, are being used successfully in many pain clinics. Multidisciplinary programs offer patients the opportunity to return to productive lives with less impairment and properly managed pain (Davies et al. 1994; McQuay et al. 1997).

## REFERENCES


Alarcon GS, Bradley LA. 1998. Advances in the treatment of fibromyalgia: Current status and future directions. *Am J Med Sci* **315**(6):397–404.

[AMA] American Medical Association. 1993. The use of pulse oximetry during conscious sedation. Council on Scientific Affairs. *JAMA* **270**:1463–8.

Arner S. 1991. Intravenous phentolamine test: Diagnostic and prognostic use in reflex sympathetic dystrophy. *Pain* **46**:17–22.

Arrowsmith JB, Gerstman BB, Fleischer DE, et al. 1991. Results from the American Society for Gastrointestinal Endoscopy/US Food and Drug Administration collaborative study on complication rates and drug use during gastrointestinal endoscopy. *Gastrointest Endosc* **37**:421–7.

Backonja MM. 1994. Local anesthetics as adjuvant analgesics. *J Pain Symptom Manag* **9**:491–9.

Beller JP, Pottecher T, Lugnier A, et al. 1988. Prolonged sedation with propofol in ICU patients: Recovery and blood concentration changes during periodic interruptions in infusion. *Br J Anaesth* **61**:583–8.

Benzon HT. 1986. Epidural steroid injections for low back pain and lumbosacral radiculopathy. *Pain* **24**:277–95.

Bertaccini E, Geller E. 1995. Benzodiazepine antagonists and their role in anesthesia and critical care. *Anaesth Pharmacol Rev* **3**: 74–81.

Boulton AJ, Malik RA. 1998. Diabetic neuropathy. *Med Clin N Am.* **82**:909–29.

Brandt KD. 1998. The importance of nonpharmacologic approaches in management of osteoarthritis. *Am J Med* **105** (1B):39S–44S.

Brisman R. 1997. Surgical treatment of trigeminal neuralgia. *Semin Neurol* **17**:367–72.

Brose WG, Pfeiffer BL, Hassenbusch SJ, et al. 1996. Analgesia produced by SNX-111 in patients with morphine-resistant pain. *American Pain Soc* abstr. A-122.

Bruder N, Lassegue D, Pelissier D, et al. 1994. Energy expenditure and withdrawal of sedation in severe head-injured patients. *Crit Care Med* **22**:1114–9.

Burchiel KJ, Anderson VC, Brown FD, et al. 1996. Prospective, multicenter study of spinal cord stimulation for relief of chronic back and extremity pain. *Spine* **21**:2786–94.

Campbell JN, Meyer RA, Raja SN. 1992. Is nociceptor activation by alpha-1 adrenoceptors the culprit in sympathetically maintained pain? *APS (Am Physiol Soc) J* **1**:3–11.

Campbell JN, Raja SN, Belzberg AJ, et al. 1994. Hyperalgesia and the sympathetic nervous system. In: Boivie J, Hannson P, Lindblom U, editors. *Touch, Temperature and Pain in Health and Disease: Mechanisms and Assessments. Progress in Brain Research and Management*, Vol 3. Seattle, WA: IASP Press. p 249–65.

1990. Cancer pain relief and palliative care: Report of a WHO expert committee. *WHO Tech Rep Se*r **804**:1–73.

Carette S, Leclaire R, Marcoux S, et al. 1997. Epidural corticosteroid injections for sciatica due to herniated nucleus pulposus. *N Engl J Med* **336**:1634–40.

Carmichael JK. 1991. Treatment of herpes zoster and postherpetic neuralgia. *Am Fam Physician* **44**:203–10.

Catterall WA. 1987. Common modes of drug action on $Na^+$ channels: Local anesthetics, antiarrhythmics and anticonvulsants. *Trends Pharmacol Sci* **8**:57–65.

Chabal C, Jacobson L, Mariano A, et al. 1992. The use of oral mexiletine for the treatment of pain after peripheral nerve injury. *Anesthesiology* **76**:513–7.

Chalk CH, Dyck P. 1997. Diseases of the peripheral nervous system. In: *Scientific American Medicine*. section 10, Neurology, chap. 2. New York: Scientific American.

Chernik DA, Gillings D, Laine H, et al. 1990. Validity and reliability of the Observer's Assessment of Alertness/Sedation Scale: Study with intravenous midazolam. *J Clin Psychopharmacol* **10**:244–51.

Colwell CW, Morris BA. 1995. Patient-controlled analgesia compared with intramuscular injection of analgesics for the management of pain after an orthopaedic procedure. *J Bone Joint Surg* **77A**: 726–33.

Cook AJ, Woolf CJ, Wall PD, et al. 1987. Dynamic receptive field plasticity in rat spinal cord dorsal horn following C primary afferent input. *Nature* **325**:151–3.

Cote C. 1998. Sedation for the pediatric patient. *Pediatr Clin North Am* **41**:31–58.

Dahm P, Nitescu P, Appelgren L, et al. 1998. Efficacy and technical complications of long-term continuous intraspinal infusions of opioid and/or bupivacaine in refractory nonmalignant pain: A comparison between the epidural and the intrathecal approach with externalized or implanted catheters and infusion pumps. *Clin J Pain* **14**:4–16.

Davies HT, Crombie IK, Macrae WA. 1994. Why use a pain clinic? Management of neurogenic pain before and after referral. *J R Soc Medicine.* **87**(7):382–5.

Davis KD, Treede RD, Raja SN, et al. 1991. Topical application of clonidine relieves hyperalgesia in patients with sympathetically maintained pain. *Pain* **47**:309–17.

Dejgard A, Petersen P, Kastrup J, et al. 1998. Mexiletine for the treatment of chronic painful diabetic neuropathy. *Lancet* **2**:9–11.

Desmeules J, Gascon M-P, Dayer P, et al. 1991. Impact of environmental and genetic factors on codeine analgesia. *Eur J Clin Pharmacol* **41**:23–6.

Devor M. 1994. The pathophysiology of damaged peripheral nerves. In: Wall PD, Melzack R, editors. *Textbook of Pain,* 3rd ed. Edinburgh: Churchill Livingstone. p 79–100.

Devor M, Govrin-Lippmann R, Angelides K. 1993. $Na^+$ channel immunolocalization in peripheral mammalian axons and changes following nerve injury and neuroma formation. *J Neurosci* **13**: 1976–92.

Dickenson AH. 1991. Recent advances in the physiology and pharmacology of pain: Plasticity and its implications for clinical analgesia [review]. *J Psychopharmacol* **5**:342–51.

Doyle E, Bowler GM. 1998. Pre-emptive effect of multimodal analgesia in thoracic surgery. *Br J Anaesth* **80**:147–51.

1998. Drugs for pain. *Med Lett* **40**(Aug 14):1033.

Egbert AM, Parks LH, Short LM, et al. 1990. Randomized trial of postoperative patient-controlled analgesia vs intramuscular narcotics in frail elderly men. *Arch Intern Med* **150**:1897–1903.

England JD, Gamboni F, Ferguson MA, et al. 1994. Sodium channels accumulate at the tips of injured axons. *Muscle Nerve* **17**:593–8.

Epstein JB, Marcie JH. 1994. Topical application of capsaicin for treatment of oral neuropathic pain and trigeminal neuralgia. *Oral Surg Oral Med Oral Pathol* **77**:1135–40.

Fishman B, Pasternak S, Wallenstein SL, et al. 1987. The Memorial Pain Assessment Card: A valid instrument for the evaluation of cancer pain. *Cancer* **60**:1151–8.

Freedman GM, Kreitzer JM, Reuben SS, et al. 1995. Improving patient-controlled analgesia: Adding droperidol to morphine sulfate to reduce nausea and vomiting and potentiate analgesia. *Mount Sinai J Med* **62**:221–5.

Fritsch EW, Heisel J, Rupp S. 1996. The failed back surgery syndrome: Reasons, intraoperative findings, and long-term results: A report of 182 operative treatments. *Spine* **21**:626–33.

Frost SA, Raja SN, Campbell JN, et al. 1988. Does hyperalgesia to cooling stimuli characterize patients with sympathetically maintained pain (reflex sympathetic dystrophy)? In: Dubner R, Gebhart GF, Bond MR, editors. *Proceedings of the Fifth World Congress on Pain. Pain Research and Clinical Management* (Vol 3). Amsterdam: Elsevier. p 151–6.

Galer BS, Bruehl S, Harden RN. 1998. IASP diagnostic criteria for complex regional pain syndrome: A preliminary empirical validation study. International Association for the Study of Pain. *Clin J Pain* **14**:48–54.

Goldberg MR, Offen WW, Rockhold FW. 1988. Factorial design. An approach to the assessment of therapeutic drug interactions in clinical trials. *J Clin Res Drug Dev* **2**:215–1225.

Gouda JJ, Brown JA. 1997. Atypical facial pain and other pain syndromes. Differential diagnosis and treatment. *Neurosurg Clin N Am* **8**:87–100.

Gracely RH. 1990. Measuring pain in the clinic [review]. *Anesth Prog* **37**:88–92.

Gruber AJ, Hudson JI, Pope HG Jr. 1996. The management of treatment-resistant depression in disorders on the interface of psychiatry and medicine. Fibromyalgia, chronic fatigue syndrome, migraine, irritable bowel syndrome, atypical facial pain, and premenstrual dysphoric disorder. *Psychiatry Clin N Am* **19**:351–69.

Guidelines for monitoring and management of pediatric patients during and after sedation for diagnostic and therapeutic procedures. 1992. Committee on Drugs. *Pediatrics* **89**:1110–5.

Hautkappe M, Roizen MF, Toledano R, et al. 1998. Review of the effectiveness of capsaicin for painful cutaneous disorders and neural dysfunction. *Clin J Pain* **14**:97–106.

Heft MW. 1992. Orofacial pain. *Clin Geriatr Med* **8**:557–68.

[IASP] International Association for the Study of Pain 1980. A list of definitions and notes on usage. Subcommittee on Taxonomy Pain Terms. *Pain* **8**:249–52.

Kaplan M, Dreyfuss P, Halbrook B, et al. 1998. The ability of lumbar medical branch blocks to anesthetize the zygapophysial joint: A physiologic challenge. *Spine* **23**:1847–52.

Khan OA. 1998. Gabapentin relieves trigeminal neuralgia in multiple sclerosis patients. *Neurology* **51**:609–11.

Kingery WS. 1997. A critical review of controlled clinical trials for peripheral neuropathic pain and complex regional pain syndromes. *Pain* **73**:123–39.

Kumar K, Nath RK, Toth C. 1997. Spinal cord stimulation is effective in the management of reflex sympathetic dystrophy. *Neurosurgery* **40**:503–8; discussion 508–9.

Kurtze N, Gunderson KT, Svebak S, et al. 1998. The role of anxiety and depression in fatigue and patterns of pain among subgroups of fibromyalgia patients. *Br J Med Psychol.* **71**(Pt 2):185–94.

Lane NE. 1997. Pain management in osteoarthritis: The role of COX-2 inhibitors. *J Rheumatol* **24**(Suppl. 49):20–24.

Lebovits AH, Lefkowitz M, McCarthy D, et al. 1989. The prevalence and management of pain in patients with AIDS: A review of 134 cases. *Clin J Pain* **5**:245–8.

Levy MF. 1996. Pharmacologic treatment of cancer pain. *N Engl J Med* **335**:1124–32.

Loeser J. 1996. Back pain in the workplace. II. *Pain* **65**:7–8.

Lombet A, Laduron P, Mourre C, et al. 1985. Axonal transport of the voltage-dependent $Na^+$ channel protein identified by its tetrodotoxin binding site in rat sciatic nerves. *Brain Res* **345**:153–8.

Lord SM. 1996. Percutaneous radio-frequency neurotomy for chronic cervical zygapophyseal-joint pain. *N Engl J Med* **335**:1721–6.

Matzner O, Devor M. 1994. Hyperexcitability at sites of nerve injury depends on voltage-sensitive $Na^+$ channels. *J Neurophysiol* **72**:349–59.

Max MB, Laska EM. 1991. Single-dose analgesic comparison. In: Max M, Portnoy R, Laska E, editors. *Advances in Pain Research and Therapy.* New York: Raven Press. p 55–95.

McLachlan EM, Janig W, Devor M, et al. 1993. Peripheral nerve injury triggers noradrenergic sprouting within the dorsal root ganglia. *Nature* **363**:543–6.

McQuay H, Carroll D, Jadad AR, et al. 1995. Anticonvulsant drugs for management of pain: A systematic review. *BMJ* **311**:1047–52.

McQuay HJ. 1995. Pre-emptive analgesia: A systematic review of clinical studies. *Ann Med* **27**:249–56.

McQuay HJ, Moore TA, Eccleston C, et al. 1997. Systematic review of outpatient services for chronic pain control. *Health Technology Assess* **1**(6):i–iv, 1–135.

McQuay HJ, Tramer M, Nye BA, et al. 1996. A systematic review of antidepressants in neuropathic pain. *Pain* **68**(2–3):217–27.

Medical Association of South Africa. 1997. Conscious sedation clinical guidelines. *S Afr Med J* **87**:484–92.

Meglio M, Cioni B, Rossi GF. 1989. Spinal cord stimulation in management of chronic pain. A 9-year experience. *J Neurosurg* **70**:519–24.

Melzack R. 1975. The McGill Pain Questionnaire: Major properties and scoring methods. *Pain* **1**:277–99.

Mercadante S. 1997. Malignant bone pain: Pathophysiology and treatment. *Pain* **69**:1–18.

Mersky H, Bogduk N. 1994. *Classification of Chronic Pain.* 2nd ed. Seattle, WA: IASP Press.

Miljanich GP, Ramachandran J. 1995. Antagonists of neuronal calcium channels: Structure, function, and therapeutic implications. *Annu Rev Pharmacol Toxicol* **35**:707–34.

*Mosby's* $GenR_x$ 1998. *Mosby's* $GenR_x$ *1998: The Complete Reference for Generic and Brand Drugs.* 8th ed. St. Louis: Mosby–Year Book.

Nguyen DM. 1996. The role of physical medicine and rehabilitation in pain management. *Clin Geriatr Med* **12**:517–29.

Olsen NJ, Park JN. 1998. Skeletal muscle abnormalities in patients with fibromyalgia. *Am J Med Sci* **315**:351–8.

Pappagallo M, Campbell JN. 1994. Chronic opioid therapy as alternative treatment for post-herpetic neuralgia. *Ann Neurol.* **35**(Suppl.):S54–6.

Perl ER. 1994. Causalgia and reflex sympathetic dystrophy revisited. In: Boivie J, Hannson P, Lindblom U, editors. *Touch, Temperature and Pain in Health and Disease: Mechanisms and Assessments. Progress in Brain Research and Management*, Vol 3. Seattle, WA: IASP Press. p 231–48.

Raja SN, Treede RD, Davis KD, et al. 1991. Systemic alpha-adrenergic blockade with phentolamine: A diagnostic test for sympathetically maintained pain. *Anesthesia* **74**:691–8.

Ramsay M, Savege T, Simpson B, et al. 1974. Controlled sedation with alphaxolone-alphadolone. *Br Med J* **2**:656–9.

Rang HP, Bevan S, Dray A. 1994. Nociceptive peripheral neurons: Cellular properties. In: Wall PD, Melzack R, editors. *Textbook of Pain*, 3rd ed. Edinburgh: Churchill Livingstone. p 57–78.

Riddle DL. 1998. Classification and low back pain: A review of the literature and critical analysis of selected systems. *Phys Ther* **78**:708–37.

Rouby JJ, Eurin B, Glaser P, et al. 1981. Hemodynamic and metabolic effects of morphine in the critically ill. *Circulation* **64**:53–9.

Rowbotham MC. 1992. Treatment of posttherapeutic neuralgia. *Semin Dermatol* **11**:218–25.

Rowbotham MC. 1998. Complex regional pain syndrome type I (reflex sympathetic dystrophy): More than a myth. *Neurology* **51**: 4–5.

Rowlingson JC, et al. 1986. Epidural analgesic techniques in the management of cervical pain. *Anesth Analg* **65**:938–42.

Sato J, Perl ER. 1991. Adrenergic excitation of cutaneous pain receptors induced by peripheral nerve injury. *Science* **251**:16–10.

Schwarzer AC, April CN, Derby R, et al. 1994. The relative contributions of the disc and zygapophyseal joint in chronic low back pain. *Spine* **19**:801–6.

Schwender D, Daunderer M, Klasing S, et al. 1996. Monitoring intraoperative awareness: Vegetative signs, isolated forearm technique, electroencephalogram, and acute evoked potentials. *Anaesthetist* **45**:708–21.

Sigl JC, Chamoun NB. 1994. An introduction to bispectral analysis for the electroencephalogram. *J Clin Monitor* **10**:392–404.

Silverman DG, Freilich J, Sevarino FB, et al. 1992. Influence of promethazine on symptom-therapy scores for nausea during patient-controlled analgesia with morphine. *Anesth Analg* **74**:735–8.

Sivilotti L, Woolf CJ. 1994. The contribution of GABA-A and glycine receptors to central sensitization: Disinhibition and touch-evoked allodynia in the spinal cord. *J Neurophysiol* **72**:169–79.

Smith CA, Wallston KA, Dwyer KA, et al. 1997. Beyond good and bad coping: A multidimensional examination of coping with pain in persons with rheumatoid arthritis. *Annu Behav Med* **19**:11–21.

Stanton-Hicks M, Baron R, Boas R, et al. 1998. Complex regional pain syndromes: Guidelines for therapy. *Clin J Pain* **14**:155–66.

Stockley TL, Chang PL. 1997. Non-autologous transplantation with immuno-isolation in large animals—a review. *Ann N Y Acad Sci* **831**:408–26.

Taittonen MT, Kirvela OA, Aantaa R, et al. 1998. The effect of clonidine or midazolam premedication on perioperative responses during ketamine anesthesia. *Anesth Analg* **87**:161–7.

Tanelian DL, Victory RA. 1995. Sodium channel-blocking agents: Their use in neuropathic pain conditions. *Pain Forum* **4**(2):75–80.

1996. Practice guidelines of sedation and analgesia by non-anesthesiologists. Task Force on Sedation and Analgesia by Non-Anesthesiologists. *Anesthesiology* **84**:459–71.

Treede RD, Meyer RA, Raja SN, et al. 1992. Peripheral and central mechanisms of cutaneous hyperalgesia. *Prog Neurobiol* **38**: 397–421.

Turp JC, Gobetti JP. 1996. Trigeminal neuralgia versus atypical facial pain. A review of the literature and case report. *Oral Surg Oral Med Oral Pathol Oral Radiol Endod* **81**:424–32.

Van der Laan L, Laak HJ, Gabreels-Festen A, et al. 1998. Complex regional pain syndrome type I (RSD): Pathology of skeletal muscle and peripheral nerve. *Neurology* **51**:20–5.

Wahren LK, Torebjork E, Nystrom B. 1991. Quantitative sensory testing before and after regional guanethidine block in patients with neuralgia in the hand. *Pain* **46**:24–30.

Wall PD, Devor M. 1983. Sensory afferent impulses originate from dorsal root ganglia as well as from the periphery in normal and nerve injured rats. *Pain* **17**:321–39.

Watson PN, Evans RJ. 1986. Postherpetic neuralgia: A review. *Arch Neurology* **43**:836–40.

Weissman C, Kemper M. 1993. Stressing the critically ill patient: The cardiopulmonary and metabolic response to an acute increase in oxygen consumption. *J Crit Care* **8**:100–8.

Wesselmann U. 1996. Pain syndromes in AIDS. *Anaesthesist* **45**: 1004–14.

Westmoreland CL, Hoke JF, Sebel PS, et al. 1993. Pharmacokinetics of remifentanil (GI87084B) and its major metabolite (GI90291) in patients undergoing elective inpatient surgery. *Anesthesiology* **79**:893–903.

Wetzel CH, Connelly JF. 1997. Use of gabapentin in pain management. *Ann Pharmacother* **31**:1082–3.

White PF, Way WL, Trevor AJ. 1982. Ketamine: Its pharmacology and therapeutic uses. *Anesthesiology* **56**:119–36.

Wilton TD. 1974. Tegretol in the treatment of diabetic neuropathy. *S Afr Med J* **48**:869–72.

Woolf CJ. 1983. Evidence for a central component of post-injury pain hypersensitivity. *Nature* **306**:68–8.

Woolf CJ. 1994. The dorsal horn: State-dependent sensory processing and the generation of pain. In: Wall PD, Melzack R editors. *Textbook of Pain*, 3rd ed. Edinburgh: Churchill Livingstone. p 101–112.

Woolf CJ, Bennett GJ, Doherty M, et al. 1998. Towards a mechanism-based classification of pain? *Pain* **77**:227–9.

Woolf CJ, Doubell TP. 1994. The pathophysiology of chronic pain—increased sensitivity to low threshold Aβ-fibre inputs. *Curr Opin Neurobiol* **4**:525–34.

Woolf CJ, Shortland P, Coggeshall RE. 1992. Peripheral nerve injury triggers central sprouting of myelinated afferents. *Nature* **355**:75–7.

Zdeblick TA. 1995. The treatment of degenerative lumbar disorders. A critical review of the literature. *Spine* **20**(24)(Suppl.):126S–137S.

CHAPTER

# 16 TREATMENT IN THE INTENSIVE CARE UNIT

David J. Liepert, Ronald G. Pearl

## *Chapter Outline*



Care of the critically ill patient can be challenging for many reasons. First, although the patient is critically ill, the primary disorder causing that illness may not have been identified. Second, although cardiac, respiratory, or neurologic dysfunction is frequently obvious, failure of the hepatic and/or renal systems is often present as well but not easy to evaluate by clinical examination. Third, critical illness and its physiologic effects alter the absorption, metabolism, distribution, and elimination of drugs. Several characteristics of the critically ill patient associated with altered pharmacokinetics and pharmacodynamics are described in Tables 16-1 and 16-2. Finally, multiple drug therapy is common in the intensive care unit (ICU). Drug interactions are a constant source of concern. Table 16-3 lists the protein binding of some frequently used medications. (See also chapter 25, Drug Interactions.)

In the ICU patient, shock (often associated with a low cardiac output and systemic vasoconstriction) makes intramuscular and subcutaneous injection unreliable routes for drug delivery. Reduced perfusion coupled with decreased GI motility makes the oral route unreliable as well (Singh et al. 1991). Enteral feeding and prophylaxis for GI bleeding further impact on drug absorption from the GI tract. For these reasons, intravenous delivery of medications is the preferred route in the critically ill patient. Even with intravenous delivery, pharmacokinetics are significantly altered in the critically ill. Protein binding is affected by changes in serum protein concentration (primarily hypoalbuminemia), although the increase in acute-phase reactant proteins can have some impact as well. There is also significant potential for competition between drugs for protein-binding sites.

**PRINCIPLE Physical consequences of disease can be key determinants of choices of dose and route of drug administration.**

An increase in total body water results in an increased volume of distribution for many drugs, so that higher loading doses may be required, and the elimination half-life will be increased. Acidosis reduces the effectiveness

Table 16-1 The Effects of Critical Illness on Drug Pharmacokinetics

| PATHOPHYSIOLOGIC CONDITION | EFFECT ON DRUG KINETICS (EXAMPLE) |
|---|---|
| Depressed gut absorptive capacity | Decreased drug absorption (digoxin) |
| Drug absorption altered by enteral feeding | Reduced availability of drug (phenytoin) |
| Increased total body water | Higher loading doses (gentamicin)<br>Longer half-life (vancomycin) |
| Hypoalbuminemia | Increased drug-free fraction (phenytoin) |
| Hepatic dysfunction | Delayed drug metabolism (benzodiazepines) |
| Decreased hepatic perfusion | Decreased drug clearance (lidocaine) |
| Renal dysfunction | Decreased drug clearance (aminoglycosides, digoxin) |

Table 16-2 Features of Critical Illness That Affect Drug Effects

| FEATURE | ALTERED DRUG EFFECT |
|---|---|
| Receptor downregulation | Catecholamine insensitivity<br>Opiate insensitivity |
| Metabolic acidosis | Catecholamine insensitivity |
| Electrolyte abnormalities | Arrhythmias<br>Increased risk of digoxin toxicity |
| Central nervous system involvement | Increased patient sensitivity to CNS effects of drugs |

of many drugs, whereas alkalosis reduces the seizure threshold and predisposes the patient to mesenteric vasoconstriction. Hypokalemia, a common metabolic derangement in the critically ill patient, potentiates digitalis toxicity and increases the risk of supraventricular tachyarrhythmias.

The frequent complication of hepatic and/or renal dysfunction can result in decreased drug metabolism, the generation of abnormal metabolites, or the accumulation of metabolites with unusual efficacious or toxic potential. Therapy with one drug can significantly alter the metabolism of other drugs. Finally, disease can make an organ particularly susceptible to toxic side effects of a drug that are not commonly seen in an otherwise healthy patient.

When administering drugs in the ICU, as in any situation, it is important to keep in mind the desired endpoint, the pharmacokinetics of the drug, and the way in which the disease may alter the pharmacokinetics and the pharmacodynamics. Common ICU practices such as restricting the use of drugs to those which are absolutely necessary, adjusting doses according to guidelines, limiting the duration of therapy, monitoring serum concentrations, and observing for signs of toxicity are all imperative. Although the same safeguards and considerations apply to management of any drug therapy, settings in the ICU often give little time to react to what develops.

Because of the severity of illness and instability encountered in the intensive care unit, support and monitoring of neurologic, respiratory, renal, and hepatic function are necessary. Invasive hemodynamic monitoring is frequently indicated. Pressure information from the central venous, pulmonary artery, and arterial catheters, as well as flow information from the thermodilution catheter, give the clinician guidance in fluid therapy and titration of vasoactive drugs.

Table 16-3 Protein Binding of Common ICU Drugs

| BINDING TO ALBUMIN | BINDING TO $\alpha_1$-ACID GLYCOPROTEIN |
|---|---|
| Cephalosporin | Clindamycin HCl |
| Penicillin | Lidocaine |
| Phenobarbital | Meperidine HCl |
| Phenytoin | Propranolol HCl |
| Warfarin sodium | Verapamil HCl |

Several studies have demonstrated the inadequacy of clinical hemodynamic assessment in the critically ill patient. Eisenberg and Jaffe, in a study of 94 ICU patients, showed that clinical assessment correctly predicted central venous pressure, cardiac index, systemic vascular resistance, and pulmonary artery wedge pressure in only 55, 51, 44, and 30% of cases, respectively (Eisenberg et al. 1984). Although the pulmonary artery catheter can be used to titrate therapy toward predetermined hemodynamic parameters, this approach has not been found useful in all patient groups (Yu et al. 1993; Gattinoni et al. 1995).

**PRINCIPLE Surrogate endpoints for drug therapy must be chosen with care. The morbidity of monitoring must be justified.**

Even the data collected through invasive monitoring have limitations. Varying ventricular compliance alters the relationship between the end-diastolic volume and pressure. The pulmonary artery catheter can increase morbidity due to mechanical complications or inappropriate use. Recent studies have suggested increased morbidity associated with its use (Connors et al. 1996). Studies are presently under way to determine in which patients and situations invasive hemodynamic monitoring is useful (Consensus Statement 1997).

In summary, the intensive care unit offers a unique environment in which life functions can be supported, therapies initiated, and responses evaluated on a continuous basis so that the individual patient's response to treatment itself becomes part of the process of data collection. The ICU is a physiologic laboratory. To function there, the physician must have a sound knowledge of physiology, pathophysiology, and the actions and kinetics of medications in patients with extensive and rapidly evolving multisystem disease.

## SHOCK

### Definitions and Descriptions

The heart supplies mechanical energy in the form of both volume and pressure work sufficient to propel blood through the vascular system in order to supply nutrients to the cells of the body. Circulatory shock is failure of this system. Although the clinical presentation of shock can vary with the etiology, the compensatory mechanisms activated, and prior levels of organ function, shock is always a clinical syndrome characterized by anaerobic metabolism, lactic acidosis, and organ dysfunction.

Shock is frequently divided into three pathophysiologic mechanisms. In hypovolemic shock, the primary physiologic disorder is inadequate ventricular filling. In cardiogenic shock, the problem is a poorly functioning heart. In hyperdynamic shock, the ability of the systemic circulation to constrict blood vessels and direct flow to where it is needed is abnormal. Patients may exhibit characteristics of more than one of these categories. For example, anaphylactic shock may produce hypovolemia, cardiac dysfunction, and vasodilation.

**PRINCIPLE Dealing with the rubric of disease (e.g., shock) can oversimplify therapeutic approaches and lead to serious suboptimal therapy.**

## Hypovolemic Shock

Decreased venous return and reduced ventricular filling results in a reduction in cardiac output. This can be due to either relative or absolute depletion of intravascular volume or to an obstruction to ventricular filling such as that seen in pneumothorax or pericardial tamponade. Table 16-4 lists the common causes of hypovolemic shock. Regardless of cause, common signs include weak or thready pulses, cold extremities, decreased heart sounds, and low filling pressures (except with obstructed venous return).

Table 16-4 Common Causes of Hypovolemic Shock

| Hemorrhagic causes | Nonhemorrhagic causes |
|---|---|
| External bleeding | GI losses |
| • Trauma | • Vomiting |
| | • Diarrhea |
| Internal bleeding | Renal losses |
| • Gastrointestinal | • Diuretics |
| • Aortic dissection | • Salt wasting nephropathy |
| • Long bone fracture | • Diabetes insipidus |
| • Retroperitoneal bleeding | |
| Redistributive losses | |
| • Burns | |
| • Pancreatitis | |
| • Sepsis | |
| • Ascites | |

The sympathetic nervous system is activated by falls in cardiac output and systemic perfusion. This results in tachycardia, vasoconstriction, and renin release. Renin secretion is further stimulated by hypoperfusion of the kidney's juxtaglomerular apparatus. Renin converts angiotensinogen to angiotensin I. Angiotensin II produced by the action of angiotensin-converting enzyme on angiotensin I, is a potent vasoconstrictor, particularly on the efferent arteriole, an effect which acts to maintain glomerular filtration in the presence of renin. Most tissues have some capacity to compensate for reduced perfusion by vasodilation, to decrease resistance, and to increase blood flow. This physiologic response is called *autoregulation*. The brain and kidney both have the ability to autoregulate perfusion across a wide range of blood pressures. This range of blood pressures is shifted upward in the presence of chronic hypertension and diminished in the presence of peripheral vascular disease. The splanchnic circulation has less capacity to autoregulate blood flow in the presence of hypotension and is particularly sensitive to the vasoconstrictive effects of angiotensin II (Reilly and Bulkley 1993). Whatever the organ system, when flow falls below the minimum level compatible with sustaining viability, ischemia and infarction result.

### *Cardiogenic shock*

Cardiac output is depressed in cardiogenic shock because of impaired systolic function (contractility), impaired diastolic function (compliance), arrhythmia, valvular dysfunction, or other structural problem in or near the heart (e.g., cardiac tamponade). This is generally accompanied by increased preload and vascular resistance. The balance of myocardial oxygen supply and demand is a particular concern, since increased cardiac volumes, decreased perfusion pressures, and tachycardia (which decreases diastolic time) all contribute to decreased coronary perfusion and worsening cardiac function. Table 16-5 lists the common causes of cardiogenic shock, which commonly presents with diminished pulses, poor perfusion, increased filling pressures, enlarged heart, and respiratory distress.

### *Hyperdynamic shock*

The initiating event in hyperdynamic shock is a fall in systemic vascular resistance. Systemic infection with inflammation is the most common cause, but both Addison's disease and spinal shock also can present in this fashion. Table 16-6 lists the most common causes. The patient presents with bounding pulses, warm extremities, tachycardia, and often respiratory distress. Since blood pressure is the product of cardiac output and vascular resistance, perfusion pressure in hyperdynamic shock is de-

**Table 16-5 Common Causes of Cardiogenic Shock**

| |
|---|
| Impaired contractility |
| Infarction |
| Ischemia |
| Cardiomyopathy |
| Drugs |
| Inflammation |
| Valvular disease |
| Mitral regurgitation |
| Aortic regurgitation |
| Mitral stenosis |
| Aortic stenosis |
| Idiopathic hypertrophic subaortic stenosis |
| Other causes |
| Arrhythmia |
| Cardiac tamponade |
| Pulmonary embolism |

pendent on the ability of the heart to maintain an elevated cardiac output.

Unfortunately, preload will be reduced by either systemic vasodilation or increased capillary permeability. Cardiac contractility is also frequently diminished, due to the myocardial depressant effects of the inflammatory cascade, bacterial toxins, myocardial ischemia, abnormal myocardial metabolism, $\beta$-adrenergic receptor downregulation, and myocardial edema. Although the initial presentation of a patient in hyperdynamic shock is generally warm, normotensive, and well perfused, patients may develop signs of progressive hypovolemic and cardiogenic shock over time.

## General Principles of the Management of Shock

To revive any critically ill patient, one should follow the widely accepted protocol of A-B-C, the acronym for airway, breathing, and circulatory resuscitation. Metabolic acidosis, secondary to hypoperfusion and hypoxia, will increase respiratory drive. This, in combination with hypoxia and the increased work of breathing associated with increased lung water, seen in most forms of shock, results in a significant increase in the consumption of oxygen by respiratory muscles. Ventilatory assistance will frequently be necessary if either oxygen delivery is insufficient or elimination of carbon dioxide cannot be maintained by the patient's own efforts. Mechanical ventilation generally allows the delivery of a higher concentration of oxygen than can be delivered by an oxygen mask, and machine-assisted breathing decreases patient work, allowing redistribution of blood flow, reducing oxygen consumption, and improving $CO_2$ elimination.

**Table 16-6 Common Causes of Hyperdynamic Shock**

| |
|---|
| Sepsis |
| Adrenal insufficiency |
| Neurogenic shock |
| Systemic inflammatory response |
| Anaphylaxis |
| Autoimmune inflammation |

Positive pressure ventilation will reduce venous return to the heart. In cardiogenic shock, this may be therapeutic, but hypotension will almost always occur shortly after mechanical ventilation is begun, and this will generally respond to intravenous blood volume replacement, unless some other cause is responsible. Successful resuscitation will result in a well-oxygenated patient with satisfactory cardiac and urine output and the reversal of metabolic acidosis. Subsequent management follows the assessment of the adequacy of cardiac preload, afterload, and contractility.

**PRINCIPLE There is very strong reason to carefully combine adjunctive with drug therapy when evidence supports their combined use.**

### *Treatment of hypovolemic shock*

Treatment of hypovolemic shock requires the rapid restoration of venous return to the heart, correction of the underlying cause of reduced preload, and the support of circulation while this therapy is under way. Choice of fluids and vasoactive agents will be discussed in a subsequent section.

Assessment of the adequacy of therapy requires ongoing evaluation of blood volume status, cardiac filling, cardiac performance, and systemic perfusion. Although clinical assessment is frequently adequate for all these parameters (jugular venous pulse, heart sounds, peripheral pulses and perfusion, urine output, etc.) information from a central venous or pulmonary artery catheter may be useful.

**PRINCIPLE In desperate settings, several interventions (e.g., drugs, devices, or procedures) often are applied automatically. They need to be assessed for value before such application.**

### *Treatment of cardiogenic shock*

If the patient in cardiogenic shock has not developed pulmonary edema, fluid should be administered to increase intravascular volume, particularly if hypotension is present. The patient must be carefully observed, since pulmonary edema may be precipitated by infusion of fluid to increase blood volume, and coronary ischemia may also result as the ventricular end-diastolic pressure climbs. Ventilatory assistance should be considered early rather than late in the clinical course, as both hypoxemia, secondary to pulmonary edema, and the high cardiac output necessary to perfuse a failing diaphragm will increase cardiac work. Positive pressure ventilation will reduce left-ventricular afterload as well as preload, and this frequently results in significant improvements in cardiac function.

The use of agents that reduce ventricular afterload improves both morbidity and mortality (The SOLVD Investigators 1991). The failing ventricle is very sensitive to afterload. Agents with vasodilating properties (e.g., nitroprusside or nitroglycerin) or those that augment contractility in addition to vasodilating the patient (e.g., dobutamine or the phosphodiesterase inhibitors) are frequently chosen as initial therapy. Titration of vasodilators should not be directed at systemic blood pressure alone but instead at the optimization of the cardiac output. All these therapies reduce the effective ventricular preload. If blood pressure decreases, infusion of fluid to increase blood volume may be required to optimize the value of afterload reduction. Inotropes are frequently necessary but may themselves be associated with morbidity in the form of increased myocardial oxygen consumption, arrhythmias, and metabolic disturbances.

***Treatment of hyperdynamic shock***

Therapy for hyperdynamic shock depends on the hemodynamic status of the patient. In the initial stages, the patient will have a low systemic vascular resistance and high cardiac output, and the blood pressure may be only slightly decreased. As the syndrome progresses, preload decreases because of vasodilation and capillary leak, and cardiac function becomes depressed. Volume, vasoconstrictors, and inotropes are therefore often useful.

An effective algorithm for management of hyperdynamic shock is shown in Figure 16-1. If clinical assessment indicates that perfusion is poor and preload is low, blood volume expansion is indicated. If preload is acceptable but perfusion is inadequate, inotropic therapy is appropriate. If cardiac output is considered to be acceptable but perfusion is still inadequate with low urine output, persistent or progressive acidosis, or other signs of organ failure, vasopressors may be used to increase perfusion pressure, either with or without inotropic therapy or volume, if further increases in cardiac output are determined to be necessary. Vasopressors elevate the vascular resistance, but cardiac output should be monitored

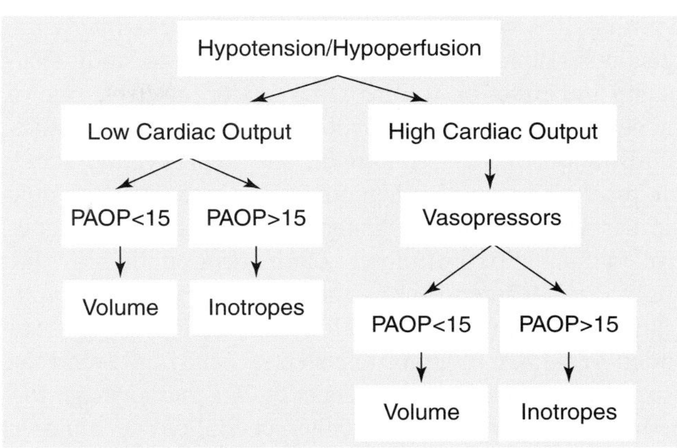


**F I G U R E 1 6 - 1 Algorithm for the selection of volume, inotropic agents, or vasopressors in patients presenting with shock. PAOP, pulmonary artery occlusion (wedge) pressure.**

to avoid reductions in blood flow. The infusion of fluid to increase blood volume or administration of inotropes can increase perfusion but also may worsen systemic edema, induce arrhythmias, or exacerbate myocardial ischemia. The choice between these strategies should be guided by familiarity with an individual patient's relative risks of complications and a careful and ongoing evaluation of the actual clinical response. Discussion of the available agents and clinical investigations of their use will continue in a subsequent section of this chapter.

## Volume Therapy and Blood Substitution

The choice of which fluid to use to augment intravascular volume during shock is controversial. Each of the available choices offers advantages and disadvantages. Blood products have limited availability, and the risks of infection and adverse reactions have resulted in the recommendation that the use of blood products should be restricted to specific indications, such as red cells for inadequate hemoglobin, plasma for coagulopathies, and platelets for thrombocytopenia and thrombasthenia. Crystalloids are readily available and quickly increase the intravascular volume, but they also expand interstitial and sometimes intracellular fluid spaces. Colloids are expensive, have limited availability, and may have some adverse effects on coagulation.

Shoemaker evaluated whether crystalloids or colloids should be used and concluded that colloids were superior to crystalloids for resuscitation because of the risk of pulmonary complications (Shoemaker 1976). Since 1955, we have known that albumin extravasates from blood vessels and that 60% of albumin is in fact found in extravascular locations (Rothschild et al. 1955). An animal study evaluating the effect of volume resuscitation in the setting of moderate lung injury and hypovolemia concluded that administration of saline, albumin, and hydroxyethyl starch all resulted in similar hemodynamic measurements and similar increases in lung water (Pearl et al. 1988). A controlled clinical trial of blood volume resuscitation in 1981 showed no difference in pulmonary function and complications after resuscitation with either lactated Ringer's solution or human albumin (Moss et al. 1981). Recently, a study in volunteers of the effects of 20% hemorrhage followed by restoration with either crystalloid or albumin concluded that resuscitation with albumin was faster, that resuscitation with crystalloid required larger volumes to be used and resulted in increased lung water, but that there was no significant difference seen in outcome between the two groups (Riddez et al. 1997).

**PRINCIPLE Often results of studies done in normal volunteers do not apply to patients with complex disease.**

Although articles arguing for the use of colloids for resuscitation because of the complications associated with larger volumes of crystalloid necessary to restore the patient adequately continue to appear (Rady 1994), little evidence exists to support the contention that these complications, when they occur, would not have occurred if colloid had been used rather than crystalloid. Also, there is considerable concern that interstitial fluid needs to be restored for the patient in shock. In hemorrhagic shock, fluid shifts from the interstitium into the vascular space (Riddez et al. 1997). Shift of fluid from the interstitium into cells in hemorrhagic shock has also been shown experimentally (Borchelt et al. 1995). A protein labeled *circulating shock protein* (CSP) has been found to induce cell swelling and depolarization during hemorrhage.

Patient restitution with relatively small volumes of hypertonic saline, with or without colloid, has been compared with restitution with isotonic solutions and has been found to result in restoration of mean arterial pressure associated with improved cardiac contractility, as measured by the slope of the end systolic pressure–volume relationship, and the same or better organ perfusion, as measured by distribution of microspheres (Kien et al. 1991). The improved cardiac contractility is thought to be secondary to increased release of calcium from the cardiomyocyte sarcolemma (Mouren et al. 1995). This particular study showed improved systolic and diastolic function, as well as increased coronary artery dilatation associated with the infusion of hypertonic saline into rabbits. Initial resuscitation with hypertonic saline with dextran improves survival after trauma as assessed by modified meta-analysis (Wade et al. 1977).

In summary, colloid infusion or the use of hypertonic saline with colloid can result in rapid resuscitation if infusion rates are limited because of poor vascular access. Isotonic crystalloid resuscitation dictates that large volumes of fluid must be infused. These larger volumes will result in a greater increase in extravascular water, particularly lung water, than would be seen if colloid had been used. There is, however, no evidence that the choice of colloid over crystalloid influences outcome if resuscitation is done skillfully and to the point of adequate hemodynamic function. Investigations into the use of hypertonic solutions are ongoing.

Colloids currently in use include 5% albumin, 25% albumin, 6% hydroxyethyl starch (hetastarch), pentastarch and dextran (either 40,000 or 70,000 daltons). Table 16-7 summarizes the differences and similarities between these agents.

The potential for coagulopathy associated with the use of hetastarch has caused some concern. Although early papers implicated this volume expander, later clinical studies did not confirm that this effect was significant in patients with trauma (Shatney et al. 1983) or in septic shock (Falk et al. 1988). This study confirmed that although moderate effects occur on the laboratory evaluation of coagulation associated with hetastarch resuscitation, these changes in coagulation did not result in clinical bleeding. A study by Conroy and colleagues (1996) showed that rapid infusion of 20 mL/kg of hetastarch intraoperatively reduced factor VIII (antihemophilic factor C) levels to 69% of baseline but that these values increased to greater than baseline with the infusion of desmopressin (DDAVP). It is unlikely that this minimal drop in factor levels would be associated with clinical bleeding.

A novel approach to blood volume restoration involves the use of oxygen-carrying solutions. Simply increasing cardiac output is of little value unless metabolic substrates are carried, particularly oxygen. Initially, there was enthusiasm for the use of a family of chemicals called *perfluorocarbons* that dissolve oxygen avidly. Clinical trials have shown that solutions tested did not release oxygen adequately at the periphery and were not useful clinically (Gould et al. 1986). Unmodified, tetrameric hemoglobin has unfortunately been found to be unsafe for clinical use because of the occurrence of renal dysfunction, gastrointestinal distress, and vasoconstriction; these conditions are probably all due to the extravasation of hemoglobin into the interstitium and its absorption of nitric oxide (Gould et al. 1995). Clinical trials of polymer-

Table 16-7 Colloids Available in the Intensive Care Unit

| Characteristic | 5% Albumin | 25% Albumin | 6% Hydroxyethyl starch | 10% Pentastarch | 10% Dextran 40 | 6% Dextran 70 |
|---|---|---|---|---|---|---|
| Molecular mass (daltons) | 69,000 | 69,000 | 450,000 | 280,000 | 40,000 | 70,000 |
| Kinetic half-life | 15–20 days | 15–20 days | ~17 days | ~10 h | ~5 hr | ~20 hr |
| Route of elimination | Reticuloendothelial system | Reticuloendothelial system | Renal enzyme hydrolysis | Renal enzyme hydrolysis | Renal elimination | Renal elimination |
| Clinical problem | Infectivity & cost | Infectivity & cost | Coagulopathy? allergy | Coagulopathy? allergy | Coagulopathy X-match allergy | Coagulopathy X-match allergy |
| Colloid oncotic pressure | 19 mm Hg | 95 mm Hg | 28 mm Hg | 40 mm Hg | >40 mm Hg | ~40 mm Hg |

ized human and bovine hemoglobin molecules are presently under way (Gould et al. 1995; Hughes et al. 1996).

## Pharmacologic Therapy for Circulatory Failure

As previously stated, circulatory failure is the inability of the cardiovascular system to adequately supply metabolic substrate to the cells of the body. The clinician must act quickly to restore blood flow to an adequate level. It is not enough, however, simply to increase blood pressure or cardiac output to normal levels. Adequate perfusion must be achieved to all important vascular beds, and the therapy must not stress the cardiovascular system or induce further injury.

The titration of cardiac output against systemic requirements of blood flow and consideration of the relative effects of preload, contractility, and afterload must continually be assessed. The following section reviews the pharmacologic tools that the clinician has available to maintain hemodynamic equilibrium. Many of the drugs have selective effects described as occurring at specific doses. These doses are only approximate. Individual variations are wide in the ICU population, and it is important to use frequent and careful monitoring and evaluation of the patient to adjust dosing.

**PRINCIPLE "Effect specific" drugs may not be effect specific throughout their full clinically useful dose range.**

## Catecholamines and Other Sympathomimetic Agents

Catecholamines are hormones and neurotransmitters. Catecholamines have hydroxyl groups on the third and fourth carbon positions of a benzene ring; this 3,4-dihydroxybenzene is called a *catechol*. Catecholamines interact with specific transmembrane receptors. Table 16-8 summarizes the possible selectivity of different pharmacologic agents for $\alpha$-adrenergic, $\beta$-adrenergic, and dopaminergic receptors. Note that only phenylephrine has specificity for effect on a single receptor.

### *Dopamine*

Dopamine is the immediate precursor of norepinephrine in the catecholamine synthetic pathway. It is a central and peripheral neurotransmitter, and activates dopamine-1 ($D_1$) and dopamine-2 ($D_2$) receptors, as well as $\beta$- and $\alpha$-adrenergic receptors of the sympathetic system, in a dose-dependent fashion. $D_1$ receptors mediate vasodilation in the renal, mesenteric, coronary, and cerebral arterial circulation. $D_2$ receptors inhibit release of endogenous norepinephrine and induce nausea and vomiting in awake patients. Dopamine also may have an indirect effect, increasing presynaptic release of norepinephrine. The half-life of intravenous dopamine is 1 minute. It is metabolized by catechol-*O*-methyltransferase (COMT) and monoamine oxidase (MAO). It is apparent that using dopamine for its effects only on dopaminergic receptors is quite a difficult therapeutic maneuver.

Dopamine-2 receptors are activated at low concentrations of dopamine in plasma infusion with rates of 0.2 to 0.4 $\mu$g/kg per minute, whereas slightly higher concentrations activate $D_1$ receptors (0.5 to 3.0 $\mu$g/kg per minute). $D_1$ receptors in the kidney inhibit renal tubular solute reabsorption, inducing diuresis irrespective of any change in the glomerular filtration rate (Denton et al. 1996). Experimental animal and some clinical evidence indicate improved hepatic and renal blood flow associated with $D_1$ receptor activation (Zaloga et al. 1993). In combined infusion with norepinephrine, dopamine can increase renal blood flow in dogs (Schaer et al. 1985) but not in pigs (Pearson et al. 1996). In septic humans receiving norepi-

Table 16-8 **Relative Activity of Sympathomimetics on Various Receptors**

| | Adrenergic receptor | | | | Dopamine receptor | |
|---|---|---|---|---|---|---|
| **Drug** | $\alpha_1$ | $\alpha_2$ | $\beta_1$ | $\beta_2$ | $D_1$ | $D_2$ |
| Dopamine HCl | 0 to ++++ | ++ | ++ to ++++ | ++ | ++++ | ++++ |
| Dopexamine | 0 | 0 | 0 | ++ | +++ | 0 |
| Dobutamine | 0 to + | 0 | ++++ | ++ | 0 | 0 |
| Epinephrine | ++++ | ++++ | +++ | ++ | 0 | 0 |
| Norepinephrine bitartrate | ++++ | +++ | +++ | 0 | 0 | 0 |
| Phenylephrine HCl | ++++ | 0 | 0 | 0 | 0 | 0 |
| Isoproterenol HCl | 0 | 0 | ++++ | ++++ | 0 | 0 |
| Ephedrine | ++ | 0 | +++ | +++ | 0 | 0 |

nephrine, dopamine infusion had variable effects on splanchnic perfusion (Meier-Hellman, Bredle et al. 1997).

Increases in dopamine infusion rates above 3.0 $\mu$g/kg per minute progressively activate $\beta_1$-adrenergic receptors, followed by activation of $\alpha_1$- and $\alpha_2$-adrenoreceptors. As the infusion rate escalates, the $\alpha$-adrenergic receptor effects become dominant. Because the actual infusion rates associated with the activation of different receptors are variable, titration of dopamine with the intent of being dopamine-receptor-specific without monitoring may be difficult or impossible. In fact, the chronotropy, inotropy, and peripheral vasoconstriction due to dopamine have been shown to increase myocardial lactate production in the presence of cardiogenic shock (Mueller et al. 1978).

**PRINCIPLE The choice of a receptor- or effect-specific agent must be accompanied by careful monitoring to maintain effect or receptor specificity.**

### *Dopexamine*

Dopexamine is a dopamine agonist that activates $D_1$ and $\beta_2$-adrenergic receptors. It does not activate $\beta_1$- or $\alpha$-adrenergic receptors at usual doses, but it inhibits the neuronal reuptake of norepinephrine, resulting in increased plasma concentrations of norepinephrine if it is being released in a patient. Dopexamine is effective as a vasodilator and inotrope, although its mechanism of inotropy is still unclear and is likely to be the sum of its direct and indirect effects. It is a natriuretic and diuretic via its $D_1$ receptor activity (Frishman and Hotchkiss 1996). Compared with dobutamine and dopamine for the treatment of congestive heart failure, it causes less inotropy but also is devoid of vasoconstrictive activity. In a preoperative patient population, the use of dopexamine to prospectively increase systemic oxygen delivery has been found to significantly reduce morbidity and mortality (Boyd et al. 1993). In the setting of septic shock, dopexamine can increase both delivery and consumption of oxygen, but the hemodynamic effects (vasodilation and tachycardia) associated with an infusion rate of 6 $\mu$g/kg per minute caused concern (Colardyn et al. 1989; Hannemann et al. 1996). At lower infusion rates (1 $\mu$g/kg per minute), dopexamine has been found to increase splanchnic blood flow in the critically ill (Maynard et al. 1995).

**PRINCIPLE The dominant effect of a drug at all doses is not the only effect that a good therapist must consider.**

### *Dobutamine*

Dobutamine is a synthetic catecholamine whose $\beta$-adrenergic receptor-stimulating activity resides on its dextro isomer; its $\alpha$-receptor activity resides on the levo isomer. Its $\beta_2$- and $\alpha$-adrenergic effects are weak, compared with its $\beta_1$-adrenergic effects, and it is considered to be primarily an inotrope. Generally, at infusion rates from 0 to 20 $\mu$g/kg per minute, dobutamine produces a dose-dependent increase in cardiac output with some reduction in diastolic filling pressures. Although conventional wisdom states that dobutamine will increase cardiac output without increasing heart rate, this conclusion is based on studies in patients with congestive heart failure (CHF), a population with $\beta$-adrenergic receptor downregulation and volume overload. In other populations, dobutamine may increase heart rate more than epinephrine (Zaloga et al. 1993). Dobutamine is most useful in the patient with cardiogenic shock because of its pattern of receptor stimulation. It can also be useful in septic shock to increase cardiac output and mean arterial pressure (Jardin et al. 1981).

**PRINCIPLE Physicians rarely concern themselves with racemic mixtures of drug. It is prudent to express such concern because pure compounds will be developed that will not have the same assets or liabilities as the racemics.**

### *Epinephrine*

Epinephrine is synthesized from norepinephrine predominantly in the chromaffin cells of the adrenal medulla. Epinephrine is released directly into the circulation in response to preganglionic stimulation; it has a half-life of approximately one minute and is metabolized by COMT and MAO and inactivated by reuptake into postganglionic neurons.

Epinephrine, as a stress-released hormone, has important metabolic effects including lipolysis, glycolysis, resistance to insulin effects, and induction of gluconeogenesis. The net result is an increase in plasma glucose, free fatty acids, glycerol, lactate, and $\beta$-hydroxybutyrate. In the cardiovascular system, doses of epinephrine of less than 120 ng/kg per minute predominantly stimulate the $\beta$ receptor. $\beta_1$-Adrenergic receptor activation increases heart rate and stroke volume as well as the release of renin. $\beta_2$-Adrenergic receptor activation produces bronchodilation and vasodilation, primarily in the skeletal muscle. As the infusion rate increased over 120 ng/kg per minute, $\alpha$-adrenergic receptor-mediated effects increase, causing peripheral vasoconstriction.

Much has been written of the effect of epinephrine infusion on the mesenteric blood flow. Studies in animals and humans that have specifically evaluated hepatic perfusion measured by ultrasonic flow probe (Cheung et al. 1997), and by indocyanine green extraction (Meier-Hellman, Reinhart et al. 1997) have shown that epinephrine can reduce splanchnic blood flow. This may be either a direct $\alpha$-adrenergic effect or an indirect effect, secondary to activation of the renin–angiotensin system. Infusions of epinephrine can induce lactic acidosis, and this has been interpreted by some as a sign of tissue ischemia (Day et al. 1996). However, generation of lactate is a metabolic effect of epinephrine.

**PRINCIPLE When multitype factors (some positive and others negative) can cause the same events, it is critical to attribute the event to the most likely cause. Otherwise, effective therapy could be unnecessarily discontinued.**

### *Norepinephrine*

Norepinephrine is the neurotransmitter of the postganglionic sympathetic nerves and is released from the adrenal medulla. At low doses ($<$30 ng/kg per minute), it stimulates $\beta_1$-adrenergic receptors. As the dose increases, $\alpha$-adrenergic stimulation increases. The half-life of norepinephrine is approximately 2.5 minutes. Like epinephrine, norepinephrine infusion results in increased serum concentrations of glucose, $\beta$-hydroxybutyrate, acetoacetate, and lactate. Norepinephrine is metabolized by both COMT and MOA and, like other catecholamines, is taken up into sympathetic nerve endings.

Clinically, norepinephrine increases blood pressure, frequently systolic more than diastolic. Careful attention must be paid to the actual balance of myocardial oxygen supply and demand. As arterial pressure increases, the baroreceptor reflex may slow the heart rate. This effect combined with vasoconstriction may decrease the cardiac output, although venous venoconstriction may increase cardiac output by augmenting preload. Since norepinephrine may increase preload as well as afterload (via its $\alpha$-adrenergic stimulation) and increases contractility through $\beta_1$-adrenergic receptor activation, it will significantly increase myocardial oxygen consumption. Coronary blood supply may be increased with increased arterial pressure, as well as the lengthened diastole associated with a slower heart rate.

Although there has always been concern that treatment of hypotension with norepinephrine can result in acute renal failure, mesenteric ischemia, and hypoperfusion of the extremities, this assumption has recently been questioned in the patient who has been adequately revived with replacement of intravascular volume. In a study of patients with hyperdynamic shock, norepinephrine was shown to be superior to dopamine for achieving acceptable hemodynamic function and urine output (Martin et al. 1993). The combination of norepinephrine and dopamine can be superior to norepinephrine alone in maintaining renal blood flow in dogs (Schaer et al. 1985), and this combination may be of use even in patients with hepatorenal syndrome (Durkin and Winter 1995).

**PRINCIPLE Even the most severe clinical conditions may be susceptible to imaginative combinations of long available drugs.**

### *Isoproterenol*

Isoproterenol is a catecholamine structurally similar to epinephrine that is devoid of $\alpha$-adrenergic stimulating properties. It is a potent inotrope, chronotrope, and vasodilator. It generally increases myocardial oxygen consumption but decreases supply. Although it has been used to treat the hypotension from bradycardia of many causes or heart block, care must be taken since vasodilation from $\beta$-2 stimulation may actually worsen hypotension.

***Phenylephrine***

This drug is structurally similar to epinephrine but is not a catecholamine. It is a pure $\alpha$-adrenergic agonist at any dose delivered. Titrated between 0 and 200 $\mu$g/min or given by bolus in doses between 10 and 100 $\mu$g, it will increase systolic and diastolic blood pressure and may induce reflex bradycardia. Because it induces vasoconstriction in both the arterial resistance vessels as well as the venous capacitance systems, cardiac output may increase in the hypovolemic or hyperdynamic patient because of increase in preload. Yamazaki has shown that in the setting of septic shock, phenylephrine can increase cardiac output with little change in systemic vascular resistance (Yamazaki et al. 1982). Phenylephrine is frequently used to increase blood pressure in order to reverse delayed ischemic deficits after aneurysmal subarachnoid bleeding. The incidence of underlying cardiovascular disease in this population is high. In this setting, carefully monitored phenylephrine administration has been shown to be safe and does not compromise organ perfusion (Miller et al. 1995).

***Ephedrine***

Ephedrine is a noncatecholamine that stimulates $\alpha$- and $\beta$-adrenergic receptors, and the release of norepinephrine. The cardiovascular effect is modest inotropy and chronotropy coupled with vasoconstriction and augmented blood flow to the coronary, cerebral, and skeletal circulations. Since much of its effect is derived from the indirect release of norepinephrine, tachyphylaxis develops rapidly and therefore ephedrine is rarely administered by infusion. Usual bolus dose is 5 to 10 mg, and the usual duration of action is approximately 10 minutes.

***Metaraminol***

Metaraminol is a noncatecholamine with effects similar to those of norepinephrine but is less potent and longer acting, since it is not metabolized by COMT. It is both a direct and indirect acting sympathomimetic. Rarely used now, it was once popular in the treatment of hypotension as it increased blood pressure but had little effect on heart rate. Tachyphylaxis to metaraminol develops rapidly for the same reason as it does with ephedrine.

## Digitalis

Digitalis inhibits the sodium-potassium pump that actively transports sodium across the cell membrane, resulting in increased intracellular sodium concentrations. Sodium and calcium are exchanged across a membrane antiporter, resulting in increased intracellular calcium concentrations. In cells with a contractile function, this increased intracellular calcium concentration results in increased contractile strength. Digoxin is therefore an inotrope. In chronic heart failure, long-term therapy with digoxin improves left ventricular function (Arnold et al. 1980).

Except in the setting of CHF, digoxin is a vasoconstrictor, since increased intracellular calcium concentrations in the vascular smooth muscle cells result in increased tone. This is particularly evident in the splanchnic circulation where digoxin specifically vasoconstricts mesenteric vessels and reduces flow to an even greater extent than it does in the systemic circulation (Gasic et al. 1987). This effect can be antagonized by calcium channel blockers.

Commonly, digoxin is used as an aid in the management of atrial fibrillation in the ICU, although its low therapeutic index and high risk of toxicity, particularly in the setting of hypomagnesemia and hypokalemia, two common ICU electrolyte abnormalities, limits its role. Its effectiveness, compared with calcium channel or $\beta$-adrenergic blockers, is considered in chapter 2, Respiratory Disorders.

## Phosphodiesterase Inhibitors

Both amrinone and milrinone are nonglycoside, nonsympathomimetic positive inotropic agents. Milrinone is about 20 times as potent as its sister compound and, more important, does not exhibit the 2% incidence of hepatotoxicity or thrombocytopenia seen with amrinone. Both of these agents are active orally or intravenously, but in the ICU only the intravenous formulation is used. Both agents inhibit the activity of the enzyme cyclic nucleotide phosphodiesterase F-III. Inhibition of this enzyme results in elevated intracellular concentrations of cyclic AMP, the same effect as one sees with sympathetic receptor stimulation, but this occurs even in the presence of receptor blockade. Half-life of these compounds is variable, ranging from 2.5 to 12 hours with amrinone and from 0.8 to 2.5 hours with milrinone. The half-life is prolonged in patients with congestive heart failure. Amrinone is conjugated in the liver, whereas milrinone is primarily excreted by the kidney.

Both agents cause inotropy and vasodilation. Their hemodynamic actions are the result of the combination of these two effects. In cardiogenic shock, both agents increase the cardiac output with only minimal increases in myocardial oxygen consumption, secondary to their combined effects of positive inotropy and reduced ventricular end-diastolic pressures and volumes (Siskind et al. 1981; Baim et al. 1983). Neither agent is recommended for the patient with hypovolemic shock. In endotoxemia, amrinone has been shown to improve both diastolic compliance and ventricular contractility but to be associated with significant hypotension, secondary to systemic vasodilation that may already be severe (Werner et al. 1995). In human studies milrinone has been found to have a significant positive effect for treating ventricular function in the patient with blood volume restored and late septic shock (Barton et al. 1996).

**PRINCIPLE As in any stageable disease, a drug useful for one stage or severity may be contraindicated in other stages or severities.**

## Vasodilators

### *Sodium nitroprusside*

Sodium nitroprusside is an arterial and venous vasodilator. As does nitroglycerin, sodium nitroprusside acts via the generation of nitric oxide. Its potency and rapid onset and offset make it valuable as a vasodilator in the ICU, where rapidly titratable control may be needed (Cohn and Burke 1979). Its half-life is less than 1 minute. The usual dose range is between 0.05 and 3 μg/kg per minute. Upon initiation of a nitroprusside infusion, rapid vasodilation occurs. It is recommended to begin the infusion at a low dose, as the most immediate and life-threatening adverse effect of nitroprusside is hypotension, caused by reduced arterial tone and venous vasodilation. This hypotension usually is quickly reversible by discontinuing the infusion and replacing volume. Another acute complication of both nitroprusside and nitroglycerin is hypoxia resulting from the drug's ability to blunt hypoxic pulmonary vasoconstriction (Wood 1997).

Anyone using nitroprusside must be familiar with its metabolism and toxicity. Nitroprusside binds promptly to hemoglobin, oxidizing it to methemoglobin and liberating a short-lived unstable nitroprusside radical that releases five cyanide ions. One of these cyanide ions binds with the methemoglobin, converting it to cyanomethemoglobin. The remaining four cyanides are converted to thiocyanate in the liver and kidneys by rhodanese (thiosulfate sulfurtransferase), a reaction requiring thiosulfate and cyanocobalamin. The thiocyanate is then excreted in the urine.

Cyanide is acutely toxic, binding to and inactivating the intracellular cytochrome oxidase system. This results in anaerobic metabolism, metabolic acidosis, and death. All can be prevented by the rapid conversion of cyanide to thiocyanate ($t_{1/2}$ = 30 minutes). This reaction is limited by availability of the enzyme rhodanese (which can be deficient in patients with either Leber's hereditary optic neuropathy or tobacco–alcohol amblyopia) and by the availability of thiosulfate and cyanocobalamin. If the generation of cyanide ions exceeds the metabolic capacity, acute toxicity will result. Cyanide toxicity can be seen even in normal patients at infusion rates exceeding 10 μg/kg per minute. The recommended maximum sustained infusion rate for nitroprusside is 4 μg/kg per minute (Wood 1997).

If cyanide toxicity is suspected, the infusion of nitroprusside should be stopped immediately. Several antidotes are available. Sodium nitrite reacts with hemoglobin to generate methemoglobin, which avidly binds cyanide to form cyanomethemoglobin. The administration of thiosulfate will facilitate the conversion of cyanide to thiocyanate by rhodanese. Vitamin $B_{12}$, hydroxocobalamin, will bind with cyanide to form cyanocobalamin and is effective in both prophylaxis and treatment (Cottrell et al. 1978; Apple et al. 1996).

Thiocyanate is toxic, has a half-life of 2 to 3 days in the presence of normal kidney function, and 9 days in the presence of renal insufficiency. The accumulation of thiocyanate causes fatigue, nausea, anorexia, miosis, psychosis and convulsions. Monitoring of thiocyanate levels is important in patients treated for more than 72 hours, those receiving large amounts of the drug, and in those with renal insufficiency or failure. Initial signs of thiocyanate toxicity occur at concentrations greater than 5 mg/dL, although levels as high as 25 mg/dL or even 100 mg/dL generally can be well tolerated (Vesey and Cole 1985).

### *Nitroglycerin*

Although both nitroprusside and nitroglycerin act by the same mechanism, nitroglycerin is predominantly a venodilator, only producing arterial vasodilation when infusion rates are greater than 1.0 μg/kg per minute. Preload is reduced more than afterload, cardiac output decreases, coronary perfusion pressure generally is maintained, and the balance of myocardial oxygen supply and demand is favorably altered (see chapter 2, Respiratory Disorders). In patients with pulmonary edema, the increased venous capacitance reduces end-diastolic pressure and chamber volumes with little effect on cardiac output. In hypovolemic patients, however, severe hypotension can result, and therefore the initiation and titration of nitroglycerin infusions should be monitored carefully in such patients. Although the systemic arterial circulation shows only limited vasodilation from nitroglycerin, the pulmonary and coronary circulations are more responsive (Zerbe and Wagner 1993). Nitroglycerin infusion can limit infarct size, chamber expansion, and cardiac complications in the setting of an acute myocardial infarct (Pearl et al. 1983; Jugdutt and Warnica 1988).

**PRINCIPLE Beware of reflex decisions in drug therapy based on poorly defined pathogenesis created by the rubric of a disease (e.g., "nitroglycerin is indicated for acute myocardial ischemia").**

### *Hydralazine*

Hydralazine is a direct arterial and weak venous vasodilator. When given orally, its onset is delayed when compared with that of nitroglycerin and nitroprusside, taking 10 to 30 minutes; its duration of action is prolonged (2 to 4 hours), and its metabolism is via hepatic acetylation. The rate of its metabolism is genetically determined (chapter 22, Pharmacogenetics). Slow acetylators will generally require smaller, less frequent doses of the drug than will fast acetylators. Doses range between 2.5 and 20 mg by bolus, although hydralazine can be administered by intravenous infusion or orally.

Hydralazine is commonly used to treat the hypertension seen during pregnancy and postoperatively but is generally avoided in the presence of coronary artery disease because of its propensity for causing reflex tachycardia. The long-term treatment of hypertension with hydralazine is associated with peripheral neuropathy and a positive antinuclear antibody test, as well as a lupus-like syndrome that reverses after the drug is discontinued.

### *Fenoldopam*

Fenoldopam is a peripheral vasodilator that stimulates $D_1$ receptors. Given by intravenous infusion (dose 0.1 to 1.7 μg/kg per minute), it is an alternative to sodium nitroprusside for the immediate treatment of patients with severe hypertension (Frishman and Hotchkiss 1996). The plasma half-life of fenoldopam is approximately 10 minutes. Unlike nitroprusside, fenoldopam increases renal blood flow and GFR, as it lowers blood pressure and it is a natriuretic and diuretic (Brogden and Markham 1997).

### *Nicardipine*

Nicardipine is a dihydropyridine calcium channel blocker with systemic, cerebral, and coronary vasodilating properties and little effect on myocardial contractility, sinus node automaticity, or AV nodal conduction. It is hepatically metabolized via glucuronidation, and it has a terminal half-life of 11.5 hours. Nicardipine is available for administration orally or as an intravenous bolus or infusion. A study investigating its effects when used in conjunction with nitroprusside to control post-operative hypertension found that a slowly delivered bolus of 3 to 5 mg resulted in a 20% reduction in mean arterial pressure with a significant increase in the cardiac index without a change in heart rate. The effect of this bolus persisted for 45 minutes and was associated with a significant increase in venous admixture and pulmonary shunting, as is seen with other vasodilators (Vincent et al. 1997). Compared with nitroprusside induction of controlled intraoperative reduction of blood pressure, recovery from hypotension was significantly slower in those given nicardipine, but blood loss was also significantly reduced in the nicardipine-treated group (Haley et al. 1993). Nicardipine given by intravenous infusion (dose 0.15 mg/kg per hour) reduces the incidence and severity of delayed cerebral arterial narrowing in patients suffering aneurysmal subarachnoid hemorrhage (Haley et al. 1993).

## Adjunctive Therapy for Septic Shock

Alternative therapeutic interventions that have been tried, considered, or are presently under evaluation in the treatment of septic shock fully deserve consideration. Steroids used in conjunction with other therapies were shown as early as 1976 to improve survival in patients with sepsis (Schumer 1976). Since then, multiple studies, trials, and meta-analyses have all concluded that, although some short-term clinical improvement may be associated with use of steroids in patients with sepsis, the long-term effect on outcome is either negligible or detrimental (The Veterans Administration Systemic Sepsis Cooperative Study Group 1987; Cronin et al. 1995; Lefering and Neugebauer 1995). The primary problem with the use of steroids has always been secondary infection. At present, the role of steroids in shock is restricted to those patients with resolved sepsis who develop acute respiratory distress syndrome (ARDS) that progresses to the fibro-proliferative stage (Meduri et al. 1994; Biffl et al. 1995; Hooper and Kearl 1996).

This does not mean that one should avoid the use of steroids in the septic patient with adrenal insufficiency or the patient who has previously required ongoing steroid therapy. These patients will likely require steroid supplementation, not as an adjunct to other treatments for their shock but as a treatment for their primary disorder.

**PRINCIPLE Animal models used to justify drug testing in humans (e.g., dogs or rabbits made septic after steroids are administered) often show more promise of drug intervention than is seen in humans. But it is often difficult to dissuade physicians from extrapolating the data to humans even after the therapeutic value has been disproved.**

The cause of the physiologic abnormalities associated with systemic inflammation is the subject of ongoing research. Bacterial endotoxin has been implicated in the release of a variety of mediators, including tumor necrosis factor, various interleukins, platelet activating factor, interferon, leukotrienes, prostaglandins, and free radicals (Ball et al. 1986; Goode and Webster 1993; Tracey and Cerami 1993). These compounds are all interrelated in the inflammatory cascade. They all have physiologic effects that can be both beneficial and detrimental. In an attempt to modulate the detrimental effects, mediator blockade has been attempted at many levels.

Initial enthusiasm about the utility of blocking the inflammatory cascade was prompted by studies such as that of Baumgartner, reported in 1985. Immunization of patients against a particular lipo-polysaccharide found in a mutated *E. coli* (J5) or the infusion of plasma of donors previously vaccinated reduced the severity of gram-negative infections (Baumgartner et al. 1985). Likewise, immunization against tumor necrosis factor (TNF) was shown to prevent septic shock in baboons (Tracey et al. 1987). There has been no benefit associated with the use of these agents after sepsis is initiated.

Blockade of prostaglandin formation with cyclooxygenase inhibitors is another logical therapeutic intervention. Unfortunately, ibuprofen given to dogs, although effective in reducing the vascular adherence of circulating neutrophils, had no effect on pulmonary neutrophils or the injury induced in the lung (Bernard et al. 1997). An ibuprofen trial in humans found that although treatment reduced fever, tachycardia, oxygen consumption, and lactic acidosis, it did not improve survival or decrease the incidence of ARDS (Balk et al. 1988). A trial of an interleukin-1 receptor antagonist showed no significant benefit when used in a clinical population (Opal et al. 1997). An editorial in *Critical Care Medicine* has summarized the developments in this area. After analysis of the data available to that time, the authors concluded that sustained research efforts were necessary and that subpopulation analysis to identify specific patients who may benefit, planning larger clinical trials, and the development of more specific anti-inflammatory agents would be required (Zeni et al. 1997).

**PRINCIPLE Inhibiting one of many mediators of a fundamental biologic process is not likely to dramatically change the process unless the inhibition is of a pivotal element. The same would not be true of inhibiting many mediators simultaneously.**

Nitric oxide (NO) is synthesized in a wide variety of cell types. There are three main isoenzymes; constitutive nitric oxide synthase (cNOS), found primarily in endothelial cells and mediating vasodilation, inducible NOS (iNOS), found in macrophages and neutrophils, and brain NOS (bNOS) which is involved in neurotransmission. cNOS activity is regulated by calcium and calmodulin but iNOS is not. iNOS transcription is stimulated by endotoxin and various cytokines, and, once transcribed, iNOS is capable of generating far greater quantities of NO per mole of enzyme per minute than is cNOS. At high concentrations, NO is cytotoxic and iNOS probably plays a role in the immune response to bacteria and other pathogens. Drugs specific for the different subtypes are presently under development (Southan and Szabo 1996).

NOS inhibition shows a balance of beneficial and detrimental effects (Kilbourn et al. 1997). Because NO is a mediator of such a broad range of physiologic processes, this is not surprising. Studies in humans are preliminary but do show significant hemodynamic effects and limited toxicity (Kiehl et al. 1997). Clinical evaluation of efficacy is being investigated.

**PRINCIPLE The most precious signal (and perhaps the most unusual) a drug will make often is made only in humans. That is why conservation is urged in banning a drug once introduced to humans (see, e.g., thalidomide).**

## BLEEDING IN THE INTENSIVE CARE UNIT

Bleeding is a problem that develops frequently in patients in the intensive care unit. In a study of 1328 consecutive patients admitted to an ICU over 1 year, the incidence of bleeding was 39.6%. More than one-third of patients had an upper GI source, and bleeding was found to be associated with increased mortality (Brown et al. 1988). Risk factors included mechanical ventilation, nutritional failure, acute renal failure, and the use of anticoagulants. An evaluation of the incidence of coagulopathy in the ICU found that coagulation abnormalities and thrombocytopenia occurred in 66 and 38% of their patients, respectively (Chakraverty et al. 1996). Causes of coagulopathy included vitamin K deficiency, anticoagulant therapy, liver failure, massive transfusion, disseminated intravascular coagulation (DIC), and uremia. The following discussion will focus on gastrointestinal bleeding in the intensive care unit, medical therapies for uremia and for DIC secondary to sepsis, and the medical treatment of coagulopathy associated with massive transfusion.

## Gastrointestinal Bleeding Developing in the ICU

Gastrointestinal bleeding is common in the intensive care unit. The pathogenesis of stress ulceration involves disruption of gastric mucosal integrity. Hypotension, acidosis, vasoconstrictors, digoxin, and positive pressure ventilation decrease splanchnic blood flow. In a prospective study of 174 admissions to the intensive care unit, Schuster and Rowley found that 14% of patients developed some evidence of bleeding, but death was related to the hemorrhage in only 12% of those patients (2.5% of the total group evaluated). Both mechanical ventilation and coagulopathy were independent risk factors for the development of gastrointestinal bleeding, and patients who bled had a higher mortality (64% versus 9%) and a longer duration of stay in the intensive care unit (Schuster et al. 1984).

A much larger study of 2252 patients found that 4.4% of patients had overt bleeding episodes, and one-third of those had clinically important bleeding. It confirmed that respiratory failure requiring mechanical ventilation for more than 48 hours and coagulopathy were independent risk factors, and mortality in those patients who had clinically significant bleeding was 48% as opposed to 9% in those who did not (Cook et al. 1994).

Because upper gastrointestinal bleeding is considered to be a preventable complication with significant mortality, much effort is made to treat prophylactically the patient considered to be at risk. In a study of 36 patients mechanically ventilated in a medical ICU, Friedman and coworkers showed that prophylaxis with either antacids or cimetidine significantly reduced the incidence of bleeding from 40 to 6% (Friedman et al. 1982). A meta-analysis of 15 randomized studies confirmed that treatment with cimetidine or antacids significantly reduced the incidence of bleeding but could not comment on whether this was associated with any effect on morbidity or mortality (Lacroix et al. 1989).

**PRINCIPLE Correlated effects (bleeding and death) may not be linked by cause and effect. Preventing or reversing one may or may not prevent the other. If prevention is innocuous, it is unreasonable to withhold it, and study of the ultimate effects of successful intervention is mandatory.**

Antacids, histamine receptor blockers, proton pump inhibitors, or sucralfate are commonly used for prophylaxis. Since histamine-2 receptors mediate the positive inotropic and chronotropic effects of histamine, rapid infusion of $H_2$ blockers has been associated with rare cases of decreased cardiac output, bradycardia, and asystole. Cimetidine has been associated with an increased incidence of confusion in the elderly. It can also decrease renal tubular secretion of creatinine and inhibit the cytochrome P450 system of the liver. It can impair the elimination of many drugs in common use in the intensive care unit. Sucralfate has been associated with reduced gastric absorption of drugs. A recent blinded and placebo-controlled trial comparing ranitidine to sucralfate concluded that ranitidine was superior for the prevention of gastrointestinal bleeding (Cook et al. 1998). Treatment with prostaglandins administered in the stomach, either $PGE_1$ or $PGE_2$, has shown mixed results and was found to be no better than placebo in one study of 90 patients in a mixed medical/surgical ICU (van Essen et al. 1985) and equivalent to titrated antacids in a multicenter study of 371 medical/surgical ICU patients (Zinner et al. 1989).

**PRINCIPLE Most drug therapy is not innocuous.**

## Prophylaxis for GI Bleeding and Nosocomial Pneumonia

The most significant consequence of prophylaxis for GI bleeding has been its association with the development of nosocomial pneumonia. Patients ($n = 153$) given prophylaxis with either cimetidine or antacids were found to have abnormal gastric fluid cultures, associated with higher gastric pH (Donowitz et al. 1986). A study comparing sucralfate to agents that alter gastric pH found that patients receiving sucralfate had a significantly lower incidence of pneumonia, with a lower incidence of the isolation of gram-negative bacilli from the trachea than did those on antacids or histamine blockers. Mortality in the antacid/$H_2$ blocker group was 1.6 times that in the sucralfate group (Driks et al. 1987). A recent meta-analysis by Cook found that it was impossible to conclude that prophylaxis for stress ulcer increased the incidence of pneumonia but that treatment with sucralfate was associated with a lower incidence of pneumonia than were other therapies. For this reason, that study recommended sucralfate as prophylaxis for upper gastrointestinal hemorrhage in patients ventilated for greater than 48 hours or those with coagulopathy (Cook et al. 1991). Since then, a large Canadian trial comparing ranitidine to sucralfate found no significant difference in the occurrence of ventilator-associated pneumonia, the duration of stay in the ICU, or patient mortality (Cook et al. 1998). This is a complex question that will require more investigation before truly definitive guidance is available.

**PRINCIPLE Evidence-based medical decisions may point the way but, when possible, should be confirmed by controlled studies.**

## Selective Decontamination of the Digestive Tract

One approach to reduce the incidence of all septic events in the intensive care unit, including pneumonia, is the practice of selective digestive tract decontamination (SDD). Patients receiving SDD are administered a mixture of nonabsorbed, broad-spectrum antibiotics to the oropharynx and GI tract. The assumption is that by reducing total bacterial load, the incidence of septic events will be reduced. A large, randomized, double-blind, placebo-controlled trial in 15 intensive care units found that SDD had no beneficial effect on mortality, duration of mechanical ventilation, ICU stay, or the incidence of pneumonia. Cost was significantly increased (Gastinne et al. 1992). A meta-analysis of 22 trials, with 4142 patients, reported significantly reduced infection-related morbidity but no impact on mortality (Selective Decontamination of the Digestive Tract Trialists' Collaborative Group 1993). This was confirmed by another meta-analysis the following year, which showed less pneumonia and tracheobronchitis but no impact on mortality. This study recommended against the routine use of SDD except in ICUs found to be at particularly high risk and incidence of respiratory infections (Kollef 1994).

A very recent meta-analysis from the Cochrane library concluded that this therapy does in fact reduce mortality and that 23 patients need to be treated to prevent one death (Liberati et al. 1997). Whether this treatment will become common is still to be seen, as there are significant economic implications as well as the potential for the development of bacterial resistance to antibiotics.

**PRINCIPLE Evidence-based approaches to therapy are particularly important in determining whether and how chronic disease should be treated. Use of the approach where numbers are high and events are acute is much less compelling.**

## Uremia and Postoperative Bleeding

A prolonged bleeding time due to functional thrombocytopathy is the hallmark of uremic coagulopathy. Routine therapy includes dialysis or cryoprecipitate. These therapies are not without risk and, like most others, not always effective. There is an ongoing search for other medical treatments. Three methods have shown some promise.

The effect of cryoprecipitate to reverse uremia-associated thrombocytopathy is likely related to the infusion of factor VIII:von Willebrand factor (FVIII:VWF). Desmopressin (DDAVP) is a synthetic derivative of antidiuretic hormone that does not constrict smooth muscle. DDAVP causes the release of FVIII:VWF from endothelial stores into plasma. In a double-blind, controlled trial of DDAVP in patients with uremia, DDAVP significantly reduced bleeding time and improved hemostasis during surgical procedures in uremic patients (Mannucci et al. 1983). This effect lasted only a few hours.

Conjugated estrogens also have shown some utility and a more prolonged effect. Although the mechanism is unclear, the administration of Premarin to six uremic patients resulted in normalization of platelet function, and a surgical procedure was performed without abnormal bleeding in five of the patients (Liu et al. 1984). This was confirmed in another small study of six patients (Livio et al. 1986). Larger studies and study of the mechanism of action of estrogen are still necessary.

Since blood transfusion has been associated with normalization of platelet function, the use of recombinant human erythropoietin has also been investigated. With erythropoietin, bleeding time improves as the hematocrit rises (Moia et al. 1987). As with conjugated estrogens, the mechanism for efficacy remains unknown.

**PRINCIPLE Empirical therapy based on solid data often proceeds without an understanding of mechanisms of action.**

Disseminated intravascular coagulation (**DIC**) occurring in the intensive care unit in association with sepsis or shock is common and is associated with its own morbidity and mortality. DIC is frequently associated with depressed levels of antithrombin III, the serum protein with which heparin interacts to prevent intravascular hemostasis. A recent review of therapeutic trials of antithrombin III supplementation concluded that there is as yet no evidence of its therapeutic efficacy (Lechner and Kyrle 1995). Larger follow-up investigations will be necessary before ATIII can be definitively evaluated.

**PRINCIPLE The larger the study required to prove an efficacy, the lower its incidence rate is likely to be.**

Bleeding secondary to massive transfusion resulting in the depletion of coagulation factors should always be treated by surgical repair of the defect, when possible, and factor replacement guided by laboratory testing. After cardiac surgery, depressed platelet function can contribute to coagulopathy. Treatments directed at improving platelet function include the use of DDAVP and aprotinin. DDAVP administered to patients with increased bleeding in the intensive care unit can be associated with reduced blood loss and reduced requirements for replacement of blood products, similar to those for patients transfused with plasma and platelets (Czer et al. 1987). Prophylactic administration of DDAVP after the termination of cardiopulmonary bypass was not associated with any reduction in postoperative bleeding (Hackman et al. 1989). This is not surprising given DDAVP's mechanism of action and the clinical experience associated with its use in uremic platelet dysfunction. Aprotinin is a nonspecific serine protease inhibitor whose use prophylactically in the operating room has been associated with significantly less bleeding after cardiopulmonary bypass (Westaby 1993).

## ACUTE RENAL FAILURE

### Pathophysiology

The pathophysiology of a sudden deterioration of renal function is traditionally divided into three entities. Prerenal failure is secondary to reduced renal perfusion. Intrinsic renal failure is caused by actual renal injury. Postrenal failure is obstructive in nature. The mortality of acute renal failure (ARF) is high in the critical care setting, recently reported at 58% (Brivet et al. 1996). Renal failure after myocardial revascularization has a mortality of 63% and is more common in patients with diabetes, ventricular dysfunction, and renal insufficiency and with advanced age (Mangano et al. 1998). Sepsis-associated ARF had an even higher reported mortality of 74.5%. Therefore, both the prevention and treatment of renal failure are indicated.

Adequate renal perfusion and the maintenance of an appropriate cardiac output and systemic vascular resistance are of paramount importance. For this reason, careful and ongoing patient evaluation is recommended, generally with the help of invasive monitoring of cardiac function. Urine output and serum creatinine both become abnormal generally only after the kidneys have already suffered insult.

### Prevention and Treatment of Acute Renal Failure

Drugs and chemicals toxic to the kidney (e.g., aminoglycosides, contrast dye, amphotericin B, NSAIDs) should be avoided, if possible, and doses must be carefully monitored when they are used. Many different adjunctive medical agents have been used to treat or prevent acute renal failure. It is only recently that the pharmacology and efficacy of these agents have been appropriately investigated. Dopamine is the primary agent that most clinicians have used to prevent or treat renal failure, but other inotropes and vasoconstrictors, diuretics, and calcium channel blockers have also been tried. Recently atrial natriuretic peptide has also been evaluated.

"Renal dose" dopamine is employed worldwide as a renal vasodilator and nephroprotective agent. The infusion of dopamine into healthy animals or humans induces a dose-dependent increase in renal blood flow, natriuresis, and diuresis. It is still recommended as therapy to prevent and treat renal failure (Carcoana and Hines 1996). But, not surprisingly, dopamine's usefulness is questioned by some (Cottee and Saul 1996). The potential breadth of receptors activated by dopamine is wider than that of any other sympathomimetic agent in clinical use and has been reviewed elsewhere in this chapter. Dopamine infusions induce a tonic suppression of aldosterone release by the adrenal cortex (Noth et al. 1980) and are natriuretic and diuretic (Denton et al. 1996). The natriuretic effect of dopamine may protect renal tubular cells from ischemic injury by reducing the oxygen utilization associated with sodium reuptake, or dopamine may delay diagnosis of renal hypoperfusion by causing urine output to continue even in the presence of renal ischemia.

Dopamine may even contribute to renal ischemia if the diuresis associated with its use reduces cardiac output by reducing preload. Dopamine has not been shown to prevent acute renal failure nor has it been shown to be therapeutic in the presence of renal failure in carefully designed studies (Alkhunazi and Schrier 1996; Denton et al. 1996). The complex metabolic and cardiovascular effects of dopamine can cause morbidity and mortality in and of themselves.

**PRINCIPLE The adverse drug effect that mimics a sign or symptom of the disease that it is used to treat is most difficult to detect and for the physician to accept.**

The effectiveness of other sympathomimetic agents for preserving renal function has been investigated. In septic shock, norepinephrine has been shown to be more effective than dopamine for improving global cardiovascular function and urine output (Martin et al. 1993). In the setting of hepatorenal failure, the combination of norepinephrine with dopamine has been found to be effective for reversing renal insufficiency (Durkin and Winter 1995). Dobutamine can be as effective as dopamine in improving renal blood flow (DuBose et al. 1997). Calcium channel blockers have been extensively investigated, both as prophylaxis and therapy for ARF. In the setting of cadaveric transplant, calcium channel blockade may play a positive role in the management of ARF and may be protective when used prophylactically to prevent contrast-induced nephropathy (Alkhunazi and Schrier 1996). Mannitol may be effective as prophylaxis against pigment-induced nephropathy (DuBose et al. 1997).

A new agent, atrial natriuretic peptide (Anaritide), has recently been evaluated in two clinical trials. A prospective, placebo-controlled randomized clinical trial of 53 patients with established acute renal failure found that creatinine clearance improved when ANP was administered, and this effect was sustained. Mortality was not significantly reduced, but the need for dialysis was lower in the treated group (Rahman et al. 1994). A larger, multicenter, randomized, double-blind, placebo-controlled trial in 504 critically ill patients who had oliguria from ATN found significantly improved dialysis-free survival in patients given Anaritide but shorter dialysis-free survival in patients without oliguria (Allgren et al. 1997).

In summary, the development of ARF in the critical care setting is highly correlated with both morbidity and mortality. Despite a long history of use, there is little evidence that dopamine is effective either for preventing or for treating acute renal failure. Agents that show some promise are other inotropes, vasoconstrictors that improve cardiac output or renal perfusion pressure, calcium channel blockers (especially after cadaveric transplant), mannitol to prevent pigment-induced nephropathy, and atrial natriuretic peptide in the oliguric ATN patient. Primary prophylaxis and therapy should always be focused on optimization of intravascular volume, cardiac output, and renal perfusion; relief of postrenal obstruction; and the avoidance of potentially nephrotoxic agents.

## SEDATION IN THE CRITICALLY ILL PATIENT

Sedatives and analgesics are among the most frequently prescribed agents in the intensive care unit. They are used to calm the agitated patient, to treat pain, to suppress delirium, and to improve patient tolerance of procedures and therapies. Providing sedation and analgesia can be one of the most challenging tasks in the ICU. Agitation can be life-threatening and is also a symptom of many life-threatening medical disorders. Treatment for agitation can result in hemodynamic instability, hypoxia, and hypoventilation. Table 16-9 lists common causes of agitation in ICU patients.

### Pathophysiology of Agitation

The degree of pain and agitation, and potential medical causes for the agitation, must be evaluated before or at the same time as the initiation of therapy. In the oriented and responsive patient, evaluation of pain by a visual analog scale can be useful. In the disoriented, agitated patient, it is sometimes necessary to administer a short-acting opioid to evaluate its effect. Any sedative or analgesic treatment should only be attempted with resuscitative equipment and personnel available, as therapy can result in hemodynamic instability, hypoxia, loss of airway control, and death. Both benzodiazepines and narcotics have specific antagonists (flumazenil, naloxone).

### Treatment of Agitation and Delirium

Rapid control of the combative patient is a difficult problem. Since the agitation itself is life-threatening, therapy may have to precede evaluation of cause. Physical restraint is frequently necessary. If possible, an intravenous infusion should be initiated for rapid titration of sedation and analgesia, as well as the administration of resuscitative drugs if necessary. It must be stressed that monitoring, resuscitative drugs, equipment, and personnel must be available. Table 16-10 lists sedatives commonly used for the treatment of agitation in the intensive care unit,

**Table 16-9 Common Causes of Agitation in ICU Patients**

| |
|---|
| *Toxic metabolic causes* |
| Hypoxia |
| Hypoglycemia |
| Hyponatremia |
| Hypocalcemia |
| Hypercalcemia |
| Addisonian crisis |
| Hypercarbia |
| Hyperosmolar state |
| *Cerebral events* |
| Cerebral thrombosis |
| Cerebral embolism |
| Subarachnoid hemorrhage |
| Intracerebral bleeding |
| Cerebral vasospasm |
| Cerebral edema |
| *Infections* |
| Meningitis |
| Encephalitis |
| Brain abscess |
| Systemic sepsis |
| *Other Causes* |
| Inadequately treated pain |
| Anxiety |
| Alcohol withdrawal |
| Other drug withdrawal |
| Acute delirium ("ICU psychosis") |

and Table 16-11 lists analgesics commonly used for management of pain or agitation.

A recent executive summary of practice parameters for intravenous analgesia and sedation for adult patients in the intensive care unit was reported in *Critical Care Medicine* (Shapiro et al. 1995a). The consensus was that, although morphine sulfate is the preferred analgesic agent, fentanyl is preferred in patients with hemodynamic instability, morphine allergy, or concerns regarding potential histamine release secondary to morphine. The guidelines also concluded that lorazepam is the preferred benzodiazepine, haloperidol the preferred neuroleptic, and that midazolam and propofol should be used only when short-term anxiolysis is expected.

Delirium in the intensive care unit is a particular problem. Delirium is common in the frail elderly and is associated with increased morbidity and mortality (Cole and Primeau 1993). A double-blind trial in patients with AIDS-related delirium concluded that neuroleptics were superior therapy to lorazepam (Briebart et al. 1996). Haloperidol is the most commonly used of these agents. Generally administered in doses of 0.5 to 2.0 mg by bolus or by infusions of up to 25 mg/h, haloperidol is the recommended therapy for severe agitated delirium in the intensive care unit and has been found to be safe, even at high doses, as long as therapy is short (range = 3 to 12 days) and titrated to effect (Riker et al. 1994).

Sedation is almost always necessary in patients receiving mechanical ventilation unless rapid weaning will be possible. The benefits of sedation in this setting include increased tolerance of the endotracheal tube, inhibition of the respiratory drive, reduced anxiety, and improved synchronization of ventilator and patient. In acute respiratory distress, oxygen consumption by ventilatory muscles rises from the normal 5 to up to 50% of total consumption. Although mechanical ventilation is instituted in this setting to reduce oxygen consumption, ventilatory dyssynchrony, as evidenced by the patient fighting the ventilator, can actually result in increased oxygen utilization.

**Table 16-10 Sedatives and Neuroleptics Commonly Used in the ICU for Management of Agitation**

| Drug | Dose and route | Onset time | Duration of effect | Route of elimination | Active metabolite | Half-life |
|---|---|---|---|---|---|---|
| Midazolam HCl | 0.5–5.0 mg/h IV | 5–15 min | 1–4 h | Hepatic | Yes | 2–5 h |
| Lorazepam | 1–2 mg, every 1–12 h IV | 5–10 min | 10–20 h | Hepatic | No | 10–20 h |
| Diazepam | 1–10 mg, every 1–12 h IV | 1–3 min | 12 h to 4 days | Hepatic | Yes | 1–4 days |
| Haloperidol | 1–20 mg/h IV | 15–30 min | 4–6 h | Hepatic | No | 14–21 h |
| Chlorpromazine HCL | 25–50 mg IM | 5–10 min | 2–4 h | Hepatic | Yes | 23–37 h |
| Propofol | 0.5–9.0 mg/kg per h IV | 1 min | 2–8 min (single bolus) | Hepatic | No | 20–30 h |

Table 16-11 Analgesics Commonly Used in the ICU

| Drug | Dose and route | Onset time | Duration of effect | Route of elimination | Active metabolite | Half-life |
|---|---|---|---|---|---|---|
| Morphine sulfate | 1–10 mg/h IV | 10–30 min | 1–3 h | Hepatic/renal | Yes | 3–4 h |
| Meperidine HCl | 25–50 mg every 1–2 h IV | 5–15 min | 1–3 h | Hepatic | Yes | 2–3 h |
| Fentanyl | 0.5–3 μg/kg per min IV | <5 min | 30–45 min | Hepatic | No | 3–4 h |
| Codeine phosphate | 15–60 mg every 2–4 h IM | 15–30 min | 4–6 h | Hepatic | Yes | 2 h |
| Ketorolac tromethamine | 30–60 mg every 6h IM or IV | 10 min | 4–6 h | Renal | No | 4–9 h |

## Management of Withdrawal from Ethanol

Withdrawal from alcohol or sedatives and narcotics can be a life-threatening event. Severity of the withdrawal reaction cannot be predicted. Most mortality is associated with the cardiovascular instability and complications. Neurological complications such as seizures can also occur.

A recent meta-analysis concluded that benzodiazepines are superior as monotherapy for withdrawal from alcohol and that doses should be individualized and based on structured assessment scales, in which the dose size and frequency are titrated against specific clinical signs and symptoms.

Long-acting agents are associated with better stability and seizure prophylaxis but are associated with risk of oversedation. β-Blockers, clonidine, neuroleptics, and carbamazepine are useful as adjunctive therapy, particularly in specific patient subgroups (e.g., β-blockade in the patient with coronary artery disease), but are not recommended as monotherapy (Mayo-Smith 1997).

**PRINCIPLE In almost any therapeutic situation, knowing precisely what you are attempting to accomplish and what minimum quantifiable toxicity you will accept are key to appropriate and safe dosing.**

## Use of Neuromuscular Blocking Drugs

Neuromuscular blockade is also sometimes used to facilitate mechanical ventilation. These drugs should never be used without adequate consideration of the importance of sedation as they have no sedative or analgesic properties of their own. Short-term agents, such as succinylcholine and vecuronium, are frequently used for therapeutic interventions such as airway manipulation and intubation.

Succinylcholine is the only depolarizing muscle relaxant in current use. After a bolus dose of 0.5 to 1.5 mg/kg, succinylcholine induces generalized, uncoordinated contraction of individual muscle cells followed by a flaccid paralysis that lasts 5 to 20 minutes but which can last significantly longer in patients with abnormalities of plasma pseudocholinesterase, which metabolizes succinylcholine (see chapter 22, Pharmacogenetics). Succinylcholine is rarely given by infusion since other agents have become available, and high doses increase the propensity to develop prolonged neuromuscular blockade.

In healthy patients, succinylcholine causes a transient increase in serum potassium concentration of between 0.5 and 1.0 meq/L. In patients with paraplegia, nerve injury, or major burns, potassium levels can increase to a much greater extent and result in cardiac arrest. Succinylcholine is also associated with brady- and tachyarrhythmias, hypo- and hypertension, and transient elevations in the intragastric, intracranial, and anterior chamber intraocular pressures.

**PRINCIPLE Clearly, one patient's relaxant can be another's poison. The choice of whether to use a drug cannot be based on the simple hope of obtaining efficacy.**

Longer-acting agents are frequently given by infusion in conjunction with sedation and analgesia to reduce oxygen consumption and improve patient–ventilator coordination, particularly in the setting of ARDS. Table 16-12 lists the pharmacokinetic and pharmacodynamic properties of commonly used neuromuscular blocking agents.

The recent executive summary of practice parameters for sustained neuromuscular blockade in the adult critically ill patient concluded that pancuronium is the pre-

Table 16-12 Neuromuscular Blockers Commonly Used in the ICU

| Drug | $ED_{95}$ | Bolus dose | Infusion dose | Route of elimination | Action duration | Hemodynamic adverse effects |
|---|---|---|---|---|---|---|
| Pancuronium bromide | 0.07 mg/kg | 0.1 mg/kg per min | 1–2 μg/kg | Renal > Hepatic | 90–100 min | Tachycardia |
| Vecuronium bromide | 0.05 mg/kg | 0.1 mg/kg per min | 1–2 μg/kg | Renal = Hepatic | 35–45 min | Nil |
| Rocuronium bromide | 0.3 mg/kg | 1.0 mg/kg per min | 10–12 μg/kg | Hepatic | 30 min | Nil |
| Mivacurium chloride | 0.075 mg/kg | 0.25 mg/kg per min | 10 μg/kg | Pseudocholinesterase | 10–20 min | Nil |
| Atracurium besylate | 0.25 mg/kg | 0.5 mg/kg per min | 4–12 μg/kg | Enzyme degradation | 30 min | Hypotension |

ferred agent for most patients, but that vecuronium is preferred in patients at risk of hemodynamic instability or in whom tachycardia may be deleterious. The level of blockade should always be monitored to allow titration (Shapiro et al. 1995b). Both neuromuscular blockade and the use of steroids have been associated with the occurrence of prolonged myopathy in the critically ill (Fischer and Baer 1996). The incidence of this disorder may be 50% in patients exposed to both agents, and therefore their use, particularly together, should be avoided if possible.

## REFERENCES


Alkhunazi AM, Schrier RW. Management of acute renal failure: new perspectives. *Am J Kidney Dis* 1006; **28**:315–26.

Allgren RL, Marbury TC, Rahman SN, et al. 1997. Anaritide in acute tubular necrosis. Auriculin Anaritide Acute Renal Failure Study Group. *N Engl J Med* **336**:828–34.

Apple FS, Lowe MC, Googins MK, et al. 1996. Serum thiocyanate concentrations in patients with normal or impaired renal function receiving nitroprusside. *Clin Chem* **42**:1878–9.

Arnold SB, Byrd RC, Meister W, et al. 1980. Long-term digitalis therapy improves left ventricular function in heart failure. *N Engl J Med* **303**:1443–8.

Baim DS, McDowell AV, Cherniles J. 1983. Evaluation of a new bipyridine inotropic agent—milrinone—in patients with severe congestive heart failure. *N Engl J Med* **309**:748–56.

Balk RA, Jacobs RF, Tryka AF. 1988. Effects of ibuprofen on neutrophil function and acute lung injury in canine endotoxin shock. *Crit Care Med* **16**:1121–7.

Ball HA, Cook JA, Wise WC. 1986. Role of thromboxane, prostaglandins and leukotrienes in endotoxic and septic shock. *Intensive Care Med* **12**:116–26.

Barton PB, Garcia J, Kouatli A. 1996. Hemodynamic effects of IV milrinone lactate in pediatric patients with septic shock. *Chest* **109**:1302–12.

Baumgartner JD, Glauser MP, McCutchan JA. 1985. Prevention of gram-negative shock and death in surgical patients by antibody to endotoxin core glycolipid. *Lancet* **2**:59–63.

Bernard GR, Wheeler AP, Russell JA. 1997. The effects of ibuprofen on the physiology and survival of patients with sepsis. The Ibuprofen in Sepsis Study Group. *N Engl J Med* **336**:912–8.

Biffl WL, Moore FA, Moore EE, et al. 1995. Are corticosteroids salvage therapy for refractory acute respiratory distress syndrome? *Am J Surg* **170**:591–6.

Borchelt BD, Wright PA, Evans JA, et al. 1995. Cell swelling and depolarization in hemorrhagic shock. *J Trauma Infect Crit Care* **39**:187–94.

Boyd O, Grounds RM, Bennett ED. 1993. A randomized clinical trial of the effect of deliberate perioperative increase of oxygen delivery on mortality in high-risk surgical patients. *JAMA* **270**:2699–707.

Briebart W, Marotta R, Platt MM, et al. 1996. A double blind trial of haloperidol, chlorpromazine and lorazepam in the treatment of delirium in hospitalized AIDS patients. *Am J Psychiatry* **153**:231–7.

Brivet FG, Kleinknecht DJ, Loirat P., et al. 1996. Acute renal failure in intensive care units—causes, outcome, and prognostic factors of hospital mortality: A prospective, multicenter study. French Study Group on Acute Renal Failure. *Crit Care Med* **24**:192–8.

Brogden RN, Markham A. 1997. Fenoldopam: A review of its pharmacodynamic and pharmacokinetic properties and intravenous clinical potential in the management of hypertensive urgencies and emergencies. *Drugs* **54**:634–50.

Brown RB, Klar J, Teres D, et al. 1988. Prospective study of clinical bleeding in intensive care unit patients. *Crit Care Med* **16**:1171–6.

Carcoana OV, Hines RL. 1996. Is renal dose dopamine protective or therapeutic? Yes. *Crit Care Clin* **12**:677–85.

Chakraverty R, Davidson S, Peggs K, et al. 1996. The incidence and causes of coagulopathies in an intensive care population. *Br J Haematol* **93**:460–3.

Cheung PY, Barrington KJ, Pearson RJ. 1997. Systemic, pulmonary and mesenteric perfusion and oxygenation effects of dopamine and epinephrine. *Am J Respir Crit Care Med* **155**:32–7.

Cohn JN, Burke LP. 1979. Nitroprusside. *Ann Intern Med* **91**:752–7.

Colardyn FC, Vandenbogarerde JF, Vogelaers DP. 1989. Use of dopexamine hydrochloride in patients with septic shock. *Crit Care Med* **17**:999–1003.

Cole MG, Primeau FJ. 1993. Prognosis of delirium in elderly hospital patients. *Can Med Assoc J* **149**:41–6.

Connors AF, Speroff T, Dawson NV, et al. 1996. The effectiveness of right heart catheterization in the initial care of critically ill patients. *JAMA* **276**:889–97.

Conroy JM, Fishman RL, Reeves ST, et al. 1996. The effects of desmopressin and 6% hydroxyethyl starch on factor VIII:C. *Anesth Analg* **83**:804–7.

Consensus Statement.. 1997. Pulmonary artery catheter consensus conference. *Crit Care Med* **25**:910–24.

Cook DJ, Fuller HD, Guyatt GH, et al. 1994. Risk factors for gastrointestinal bleeding in critically ill patients. Canadian Critical Care Trials Group. *N Engl J Med* **330**:377–81.

Cook DJ, Guyatt GH, Marshall J, et al. 1998. A comparison of sucralfate and ranitidine for the prevention of upper gastrointestinal bleeding in patients requiring mechanical ventilation. *N Engl J Med* **338**:791–7.

Cook DJ, Laine LA, Guyatt GH, et al. 1991. Nosocomial pneumonia and the role of gastric pH. *Chest* **100**:7–13.

Cottee DBF, Saul WP. 1996. Is renal dose dopamine protective or therapeutic? No. *Crit Care Clin* **12**:688–95.

Cottrell JE, Casthely P, Brodie JD, et al. 1978. Prevention of nitroprusside-induced cyanide toxicity with hydroxycobalamin. *N Engl J Med* **298**:809–11.

Cronin L, Cook DJ, Carlet J. 1995. Corticosteroid treatment for sepsis: A critical appraisal and meta-analysis of the literature. *Crit Care Med* **23**:1430–9.

Czer LSC, Bateman TM, Gray RJ, et al. 1987. Treatment of severe platelet dysfunction and hemorrhage after cardiopulmonary bypass: Reduction in blood product usage with desmopressin. *J Am Coll Cardiol* **9**:1139–47.

Day NPJ, Phu NH, Bethell DP, et al. 1996. The effects of dopamine and adrenaline infusions on acid-base balance and systemic haemodynamics in severe infection. [Published erratum *Lancet* **348**:902; 1996.] *Lancet* **348**:219–23.

Denton MD, Chertnow GM, Brady HR. 1996. Renal-dose dopamine for the treatment of adrenal failure: Scientific rationale, experimental studies and clinical trials. *Kidney Int* **49**:4–14.

Donowitz LG, Page MC, Mileur BL, et al. 1986. Alteration of normal gastric flora in critical care patients receiving antacid and cimetidine therapy. *Infect Control* **7**:23–6.

Driks MR, Craven DE, Celli B, et al. 1987. Nosocomial pneumonia in intubated patients given sucralfate as compared with antacids or histamine type 2 blockers. *N Engl J Med* **317**:1376–82.

DuBose TD, Warnock DG, Mehta RL, et al. 1997. Acute renal failure in the 21st century: recommendations for management and outcomes assessment. *Am J Kidney Dis* **29**:793–9.

Durkin RJ, Winter SM. 1995. Reversal of hepatorenal syndrome with the combination of norepinephrine and dopamine. *Crit Care Med* **23**:202–4.

Eisenberg PR, Jaffe AS, Schuster DP. 1984. Clinical evaluation compared to pulmonary artery catheterization in the hemodynamic assessment of critically ill patients. *Crit Care Med* **12**:540–53.

Falk JL, Rackow EC, Astiz ME, et al. 1988. Effects of hetastarch and albumin on coagulation in patients with septic shock. *J Clin Pharmacol* **28**:412–5.

Fischer JF, Baer RK. 1996. Acute myopathy associated with combined use of corticosteroids and neuromuscular blocking agents. *Ann Pharmacother* **30**:1437–45.

Friedman CJ, Oblinger MJ, Suratt PM, et al. 1982. Prophylaxis of upper gastrointestinal hemorrhage in patients requiring mechanical ventilation. *Crit Care Med* **10**:316–19.

Frishman WH, Hotchkiss H. 1996. Selective and nonselective dopamine receptor agonists: An innovative approach to cardiovascular disease treatment. *Am Heart J* **132**:861–70.

Gasic S, Eichler HG, Korn A. 1987. Effect of calcium antagonists on basal and digitalis-dependent changes in splanchnic and systemic hemodynamics. *Clin Pharmacol Ther* **41**:460–5.

Gastinne H, Wolff M, Delatour F, et al. 1992. A controlled trial in intensive care units of selective decontamination of the digestive tract with nonabsorbable antibiotics. *N Engl J Med* **326**:594–9.

Gattinoni LG, Brazzi L, Pelosi P. 1995. A trial of goal-oriented hemodynamic therapy in critically ill patients. *N Engl J Med* **333**: 1025–32.

Goode HF, Webster NR. 1993. Free Radicals and antioxidants in sepsis. *Crit Care Med* **21**:1770–6.

Gould SA, Rosen AL, Sehgal LR, et al. 1986. Fluosol-DA as a red-cell substitute in acute anemia. *N Engl J Med* **314**:1653–6.

Gould SA, Sehgal LR, Sehgal HL, et al. 1995. The development of hemoglobin solutions as red cell substitutes: Hemoglobin solutions. *Trans Sci* **16**:5–17.

Hackman T, Gascoyne RD, Naiman SC, et al. 1989. A trial of desmopressin to reduce blood loss in uncomplicated cardiac surgery. *N Engl J Med* **321**:1437–43.

Haley EC, Kassel NF, Torner JC. 1993. A randomized trial of nicardipine in subarachnoid hemorrhage: angiographic and transcranial doppler ultrasound results. A report of the Cooperative Aneurysm Study. *J Neurosurg* **78**:548–53.

Hannemann L, Reinhart K, Meier-Hellman A, et al. 1996. Dopexamine hydrochloride in septic shock. *Chest* **109**:756–60.

Hersey SL, O'Dell NE, Lowe S, et al. 1997. Nicardipinea. *Anesth Analg* **84**:1239–4.

Hooper RG, Kearl RA. 1996. Established adult respiratory distress syndrome successfully treated with corticosteroids. *South Med J* **89**:359–64.

Hughes GS, Antal EJ, Locker PK, et al. 1996. Physiology and pharmacokinetics of a novel hemoglobin-based oxygen carrier in humans. *Crit Care Med* **24**:756–64.

Jardin F, Sportiche M, Bazin M. 1981. Dobutamine: A hemodynamic evaluation in human septic shock. *Crit Care Med* **9**:329–31.

Jugdutt BI, Warnica JW. 1988. Intravenous nitroglycerin therapy to limit myocardial infarct size, expansion and complications. *Circulation* **78**:906–19.

Kiehl JG, Ostermann H, Meyer J, et al. 1997. Nitric oxide synthase inhibition by L-NAME in leukocytopenic patients with severe septic shock. *Intensive Care Med* **23**:561–6.

Kien ND, Reitan JA, White DA, et al. 1991. Cardiac contractility and blood flow distribution following resuscitation with 7.5% hypertonic saline in anesthetized dogs. *Circ Shock* **35**:109–16.

Kilbourn RG, Szabo C, Traber DL. 1997. Beneficial versus detrimental effects of nitric oxide synthase inhibitors in circulatory shock: lessons learned from experimental and clinical studies. *Shock* **7**: 235–46.

Kollef MH. 1994. The role of selective digestive tract decontamination on mortality and respiratory tract infections. *Chest* **105**:1101–8.

Lacroix J, Infante-Rivard C, Jenicek M, et al. 1989. Prophylaxis of upper gastrointestinal bleeding in intensive care units: A meta-analysis. *Crit Care Med* **17**:862–9.

Lechner K, Kyrle PA. 1995. Antithrombin III concentrates—are they clinically useful? *Thromb Haemost* **73**:340–8.

Lefering R, Neugebauer EAM. 1995. Steroid controversy in sepsis and septic shock: A meta-analysis. *Crit Care Med* **23**:1294–1303.

Liberati A, D'Amico R, Pifferi S, et al. 1997. Antibiotic prophylaxis in adult patients treated in intensive care units. *Cochrane Libr* **4**:1–14.

Liu YK, Kosfeld RE, Marcum SG. 1984. Treatment of uraemic bleeding with conjugated oestrogen. *Lancet* **2**:887–90.

Livio M, Mannucci PM, Vigano G, et al. 1986. Conjugated estrogens for the management of bleeding associated with renal failure. *N Engl J Med* **315**:731–5.

Mangano CD, Diamondstone LS, Ramsay JG, et al. 1998. Renal dysfunction after myocardial revascularization: Risk factors, adverse outcomes, and hospital resource utilization. The Multicenter Study of Perioperative Ischemia Research Group. *Ann Intern Med* **128**:194–203.

Mannucci PM, Remizzi G, Pusineri F, et al. 1983. Deamino-8-*d*-arginine vasopressin shortens the bleeding time in uremia. *N Engl J Med* **308**:8–12.

Martin C, Papazian L, Perrin G. 1993. Norepinephrine or dopamine for the treatment of hyperdynamic septic shock? *Chest* **103**:1826–31.

Maynard ND, Bihari DJ, Dalton RN. 1995. Increasing splanchnic blood flow in the critically ill. *Chest* **108**:1648–54.

Mayo-Smith MF. 1997. Pharmacological management of alcohol withdrawal: A meta-analysis and evidence-based practice guideline. *JAMA* **278**:144–51.

Meduri GU, Chinn AJ, Leeper KV, et al. 1994. Corticosteroid rescue treatment of progressive fibroproliferation in late ARDS. *Chest* **105**:1516–27.

Meier-Hellman A, Bredle DL, Specht M. 1997. The effects of low-dose dopamine on splanchnic blood flow and oxygen uptake in patients with septic shock. *Intensive Care Med* **23**:31–7.

Meier-Hellman A, Reinhart K, Bredle DL. 1997. Epinephrine impairs splanchnic perfusion in septic shock. *Crit Care Med* **25**:399–404.

Miller JA, Dacey RG, Diringer MN. 1995. Safety of hypertensive hypervolemic therapy with phenylephrine in the treatment of delayed ischemic deficits after subarachnoid hemorrhage. *Stroke* **26**:2260–6.

Moia M, Mannucci PM, Vizzotto L, et al. 1987. Improvement in the haemostatic defect of uraemia after treatment with recombinant human erythropoietin. *Lancet* **2**:1227–9.

Moss GS, Lowe RJ, Jilek J, et al. 1981. Colloid or crystalloid in the resuscitation of hemorrhagic shock: A controlled clinical trial. *Surgery* **89**:434–8.

Mouren S, Delayance S, Mion G, et al. 1995. Mechanisms of increased myocardial contractility with hypertonic saline solutions in isolated blood perfused rabbit hearts. *Anesth Analg* **81**:777–82.

Mueller HS, Evans R, Ayres SM. 1978. Effect of dopamine on hemodynamics and myocardial metabolism in shock following acute myocardial infarction in man. *Circulation* **57**:361–5.

Noth RH, Mccallum RW, Contino C, et al. 1980. Tonic dopaminergic suppression of plasma aldosterone. *J Clin Endocrinol Metab* **51**:64–9.

Opal SM, Fisher CJ, Dhainaut JFA. 1997. Confirmatory interleukin-1 receptor antagonist trial in severe sepsis: A phase III, randomized, double blind, placebo-controlled, multicenter trial. *Crit Care Med* **25**:1115–24.

Pearl RG, Halperin BD, Mihm FG, et al. 1988. Pulmonary effects of crystalloid and colloid resuscitation from hemorrhagic shock in the presence of oleic acid-induced pulmonary capillary injury in the dog. *Anesthesiology* **68**:12–20.

Pearl RG, Rosenthal MH, Schroeder JS, et al. 1983. Acute hemodynamic effects of nitroglycerin in pulmonary hypertension. *Ann Intern Med* **99**:1–3.

Pearson RJ, Barrington KJ, Jirsch DW, et al. 1996. Dopaminergic receptor mediated effects in the mesenteric vasculature and renal vasculature of the chronically instrumented newborn piglet. *Crit Care Med* **24**:1706–12.

Rady M. 1994. An argument for colloid resuscitation for shock. *Acad Emerg Med* **1**:572–9.

Rahman SN, Kim GE, Mathew AS, et al. 1994. Effects of atrial natriuretic peptide in clinical acute renal failure. *Kidney Int* **45**:1731–8.

Reilly PM, Bulkley GB. 1993. Vasoactive mediators and splanchnic perfusion. *Crit Care Med* **21**:S55–S68.

Riddez L, Hahn RG, Brismar B, et al. 1997. Central and regional hemodynamics during acute hypovolemia and volume substitution in volunteers. *Crit Care Med* **25**:635–40.

Riker RR, Fraser GL, Cox PM. 1994. Continuous infusion of haloperidol controls agitation in critically ill patients. *Crit Care Med* **22**:433–40.

Rothschild MA, Bauman A, Yalow RS, et al. 1955. Tissue distribution of $^{131}$I-labelled human serum albumin following intravenous administration. *J Clin Invest* **34**:1354–8.

Schaer GL, Rink MP, Parrillo JE. 1985. Norepinephrine alone versus norepinephrine plus low-dose dopamine: Enhanced renal blood flow with combination pressor therapy. *Crit Care Med* **13**:492–6.

Schumer W. 1976. Steroids in the treatment of clinical septic shock. *Ann Surg* **184**:333–9.

Schuster DP, Rowley H, Feinstein S, et al. 1984. Prospective evaluation of the risk of upper gastrointestinal bleeding after admission to a medical intensive care unit. *Am J Med* **76**:623–30.

Selective Decontamination of the Digestive Tract Trialists' Collaborative Group. 1993. Meta-analysis of randomised controlled trials of selective decontamination of the digestive tract. *Br Med J* **307**:525–32.

Shapiro BA, Warren J, Egol AB, et al. 1995a. Practice parameters for intravenous analgesia and sedation for adult patients in the intensive care unit: An executive summary. *Crit Care Med* **23**:1596–1600.

Shapiro BA, Warren J, Egol AB, et al. 1995b. Practice parameters for sustained neuromuscular blockade in the adult critically ill patient: An executive summary. *Crit Care Med* **23**:1601–5.

Shatney CH, Deepika K, Militello PR, et al. 1983. Efficacy of hetastarch in the resuscitation of patients with multisystem trauma and shock. *Arch Surg* **118**:804–9.

Shoemaker WC. 1976. Comparison of the relative effectiveness of whole blood transfusion and various types of fluid therapy in resuscitation. *Crit Care Med* **4**:71–8.

Singh G, Chaudry KI, Chudler LC, et al. 1991. Depressed gut absorptive capacity early after trauma-hemorrhagic shock. *Ann Surg* **214**:712–8.

Siskind SJ, Sonnenblick EH, Forman R. 1981. Acute substantial benefit of inotropic therapy with amrinone on exercise hemodynamics and metabolism in severe congestive heart failure. *Circulation* **64**:966–72.

SOLVD Investigators, The. 1991. Effect of enalapril on survival in patients with reduced left ventricular ejection fractions and congestive heart failure. *N Engl J Med* **325**:293–302.

Southan GJ, Szabo C. 1996. Selective pharmacological inhibition of distinct nitric oxide synthase isoforms. *Biochem Pharm* **51**:383–94.

Tracey KJ, Cerami A. 1993. Tumor necrosis factor: An updated review of its biology. *Crit Care Med* **21**: S415–S422.

Tracey KJ, Fong Y, Heese DG. 1987. Anti-cachectin/TNF monoclonal antibodies prevent septic shock during lethal bacteraemia. *Nature* **330**:662–4.

Van Essen HA, van Blankenstein M, Wilson JHP, et al. 1985. Intragastric prostaglandin $E_2$ and the prevention of gastrointestinal hemorrhage in ICU patients. *Crit Care Med* **13**:957–60.

Vesey CJ, Cole PV. 1985. Blood cyanide and thiocyanate concentrations produced by long-term therapy with sodium nitroprusside. *Br J Anaesth* **57**:148–55.

Veterans Administration Systemic Sepsis Cooperative Study Group, The. 1987. Effect of high-dose glucocorticoid therapy on mortality in patients with clinical signs of systemic sepsis. *N Engl J Med* **317**:659–65.

Vincent JL, Berlot G, Preiser JC, et al. 1997. Intravenous nicardipine in the treatment of postoperative arterial hypertension. *J Cardiothoracic Vasc Anesth* **11**:160–4.

Wade C, Grady J, Kramer G. 1977. Efficacy of hypertonic saline dextran (HSD) in patients with traumatic hypotension: Meta-analysis of individual patient data. *Acta Anaesth Scand Suppl* **110**:77–9.

Werner HA, Herbertson MJ, Walley KR. 1995. Amrinone increases ventricular contractility and diastolic compliance in endotoxemia. *Am J Respir Crit Care Med* **152**:496–503.

Westaby S. 1993. A protinin in perspective. *Ann Thorac Surg* **55**: 1033–41.

Wood G. 1997. Effect of antihypertensive agents on the arterial partial pressure of oxygen and venous admixture after cardiac surgery. *Crit Care Med* **25**:1807–12.

Yamazaki T, Shimada Y, Taenaka N. 1982. Circulatory responses to afterloading with phenylephrine in hyperdynamic sepsis. *Crit Care Med* **10**:432–5.

Yu M, Levy MM, Smith P. 1993. Effect of maximizing oxygen delivery on morbidity and mortality rates in critically ill patients: A prospective, randomized, controlled study. *Crit Care Med* **21**:830–36.

Zaloga GP, Prielipp RC, Butterworth JF, et al. 1993. Pharmacologic cardiovascular support. *Crit Care Clin* **9**:335–61.

Zeni F, Freeman B, Natanson C. 1997. Anti-inflammatory therapies to treat sepsis and septic shock: A reassessment. *Crit Care Med* **25**:11095–1100.

Zerbe NF, Wagner BKJ. 1993. Use of vitamin $B_{12}$ in the treatment and prevention of nitroprusside-induced cyanide toxicity. *Crit Care Med* **21**:465–7.

Zinner MJ, Rypins EB, Martin LR, et al. 1989. Misoprostol versus antacid titration for preventing stress ulcers in postoperative surgical ICU patients. *Ann Surg* **210**:590–5.

CHAPTER

# 17 SUBSTANCE ABUSE: DEPENDENCE AND TREATMENT

Lori D. Karan, Neal L. Benowitz

*Chapter Outline*



## GENERAL CONSIDERATIONS: BACKGROUND AND DEFINITIONS

Drug abuse and drug addiction form a spectrum of disorders that result in adverse consequences from the use of chemical substances. Pharmacologic processes common to most drugs of abuse include rapid delivery of the drug from the dose form to the brain, psychoactivity associated with the presence of the drug in the brain, and the development of tolerance and/or sensitization in a vulnerable host. Neuroadaptation underlies both the development of withdrawal symptoms and the specter of relapse.

### Drug Abuse

Abused substances are drugs or other materials (e.g., solvents) that are administered repeatedly in a pattern and amount that interferes with the health or normal social and occupational functioning of the individual (Balster 1994). With the exception of androgenic steroids (which are primarily used to increase muscle mass and enhance athletic performance), drugs of abuse are used for their mood-altering properties and psychoactive effects. All drug use that is illegal is considered drug abuse. Drug abuse also includes the misuse of legal drugs such as alcohol, cigarettes, and even prescription drugs. The 1990 medical cost, together with the morbidity and mortality cost estimate of drug abuse, totaled $187 billion, with nicotine comprising $91.3 billion, alcohol $80.8 billion, and illicit drugs $14.6 billion. Additional drug-related AIDS costs were $6.3 billion (Rice 1993), and fetal alcohol syndrome costs were $2.1 billion (Rice 1995). Indirect costs including crime, jail, fire, and motor vehicle accidents are not included in these calculations.

**PRINCIPLE Abuse of legal drugs is more prevalent and more costly to society than is the abuse of illegal drugs.**

### Drug Dependence and Addiction

Drug dependence is drug abuse to the extreme. Drug dependence has been defined by the World Health Organization as "a behavioral pattern in which the use of a psychoactive drug is given sharply higher priority over other behaviors which once had significantly higher value" (Edwards et al. 1982). In other words, the drug has come to control behavior to an extent that is considered detrimental to the individual, to society, or to both. Alcoholics

Anonymous (AA 1988) focused on excessive, uncontrolled use despite adverse consequences in its fundamental premise: "We admit that we are *powerless* over alcohol and that our lives are unmanageable." Specific criteria for drug dependence have been presented by the American Psychiatric Association (APA 1994) (see Table 17-1).

Some clarification of terms is necessary. In this chapter, *drug dependence* and *drug addiction* are used synonymously. The reader needs to be aware of the terminology because some scientists today use the term *drug dependence* (also called *physical dependence*) in a narrower fashion to indicate the state of physical withdrawal that occurs when a chronically given drug is abruptly discontinued.

The historical mind–body distinction between habituation and drug addiction has been dropped. At one time, *drug addiction* was used to refer to drugs that produced clear physical withdrawal and produced damage not only to the individual but also to society. A prototypical drug of this sort is heroin. Drug addiction was distinguished from *habituation,* in which there was thought to be psychological dependence but no physical dependence and no damage to society. Examples of this class of drugs include cocaine (which was once considered relatively safe!) and

**Table 17-1 American Psychiatric Association (DSM-IV) Diagnostic Criteria for Psychoactive Substance Dependence**

A. Maladaptive pattern of substance use, leading to clinically significant impairment or distress, as manifested by three (or more) of the following, occurring at any time in the same 12-month period:
   1. Tolerance, as defined by either of the following:
      a) a need for markedly increased amounts of the substance to achieve intoxication or desired effect
      b) markedly diminished effect with continued use of the same amount of the substance
   2. Withdrawal, as manifested by either of the following:
      a) the characteristic withdrawal syndrome for the substance (refer to Criteria A and B of the criteria sets for withdrawal from the specific substances)
      b) the same (or a closely related) substance is taken to relieve or avoid withdrawal symptoms
   3. The substance is often taken in larger amounts or over a longer period than was intended
   4. There is a persistent desire or unsuccessful efforts to cut down or control substance use
   5. A great deal of time is spent in activities necessary to obtain the substance (e.g., visiting multiple doctors or driving long distances), use the substance (e.g., chain-smoking), or recover from its effects
   6. Important social, occupational, or recreational activities are given up or reduced because of substance use
   7. The substance use is continued despite knowledge of having a persistent or recurrent physical or psychological problem that is likely to have been caused or exacerbated by the substance (e.g., current cocaine use despite recognition of cocaine-induced depression, or continued drinking despite recognition that an ulcer was made worse by alcohol consumption)

*Specify if*:

**With physiological dependence:** evidence of tolerance or withdrawal (i.e., either Item 1 or 2 is present)

**Without physiological dependence:** no evidence of tolerance or withdrawal (i.e., neither Item 1 nor 2 is present)

**Course specifics:**

Early full remission
Early partial remission
Sustained full remission
Sustained partial remission
On agonist therapy
In a controlled environment

SOURCE: APA 1994.

nicotine. However, subsequent investigation into the human pharmacology of these drugs has revealed that:

- Many of the behavioral characteristics associated with continued use of these drugs are similar
- Physical dependence could be observed for most or all of these drugs
- There is no clear distinction between the physical and psychological processes underlying and resulting from drug use
- Societal damage accompanies individual damage

## Etiology of Drug Dependence

Understanding the neuroscientific basis of chemical dependence is replacing previous notions of willpower and morality in conceptualizing addiction (Table 17-2). Twin and adoption studies have provided strong support for the notion that individuals have a genetic vulnerability to chemical dependence. Environmental risk factors and protective factors have been identified that modify this vulnerability.

SUMMARY

**Researchers now believe that when vulnerable individuals take addictive drugs with adequate dose, frequency, and chronicity, the neural circuits involved in their control of emotion and motivation are commandeered and altered. Acutely, activity in these neuronal circuits impairs the drug abuser's insight into their behavior and their volitional control of drug use. Chronically, changes in these neuronal circuits cause deeply ingrained emotional experiences that predispose the addict to drug craving and relapse.**

In 1954, researchers discovered that rats would press a lever repeatedly—ignoring normal needs for food, water, and rest—to electrically stimulate specific brain areas (Olds and Milner 1954). These areas were later defined as a dopaminergic pathway extending from the ventral tegmentum to the nucleus accumbens, linking the midbrain, limbic system, and striatum. Further research has shown that nicotine, alcohol, benzodiazepines, cocaine, amphetamines, opiates, and marijuana each directly or indirectly enhance the actions of one or more neurotransmitters that feed into this dopaminergic circuit. Of note is that animals cease drug self-administration when this dopaminergic circuit is lesioned. Scientists generally agree that the dopaminergic pathway between the nucleus accumbens and ventral tegmentum is key to the action of addictive drugs, and they have termed this dopaminergic circuit a *motivational or reward pathway*.

**Table 17-2 Criteria for Drug Dependence***

| |
|---|
| *Primary Criteria* |
| Highly controlled or compulsive use |
| Psychoactive effects |
| Drug-reinforced behavior |
| *Additional Criteria* |
| Addictive behavior often involves |
| Stereotypical patterns of use |
| Use despite harmful effects |
| Relapse following abstinence |
| Recurrent drug cravings |
| Dependence-producing drugs often produce |
| Tolerance |
| Physical dependence |
| Pleasant (euphoriant) effects |

*From the Department of Health and Human Services, 1988.

**PRINCIPLE Scientific research has shown that it is incorrect to attribute the etiology of addiction to immorality and a lack of will power.**

Although dopamine is thought to play a critical role in motivation and reward, many researchers no longer believe it acts by directly producing feelings of pleasure or euphoria. Instead, new data indicate that dopamine release within the brain highlights, or draws attention to, certain significant or surprising events (Schultz et al. 1997). In this manner, the dopamine signal may help the organism to facilitate learning and in some cases to repeat this behavior. This may explain why dopamine overactivity in schizophrenia facilitates continued reaction to stimuli with bizarre associations rather than pleasure (Wickelgren 1997a) (see also chapter 8, Treatment of Psychiatric Disorders).

All addictive drugs have pathways outside of the dopaminergic circuit as well as within it. This helps to account for the differences in drug effects. The role of regulating hormones, other circuits, neurotransmitters, receptors, and postreceptor mechanisms are being elucidated.

## Tolerance and Sensitization

Tolerance is often associated with drug dependence. Tolerance indicates that a given dose of a drug produces less of an effect than that produced by the same dose on an earlier exposure and/or that larger doses are required to achieve the same effect. Tolerance to different effects of the same drug can occur at different rates. For example, tolerance to the "rush" of cocaine is rapid, whereas tolerance to cocaine's tachycardic and hypertensive effects occurs much more slowly and incompletely. Drug abusers who take increasing amounts of drugs risk exposure to those effects for which tolerance develops more slowly (see Fig 17-1).

**PRINCIPLE Often, drugs that produce tolerance to their psychoactive effects continue to affect other tissues. As doses rise to stimulate the CNS, severe morbidity and even mortality result as a consequence of the dose–response toxicity on other organs.**

Tolerance can develop by several mechanisms. For the most part, tolerance to psychoactive drugs is pharmacodynamic tolerance, occurring as a consequence of changes in receptor function, activation of homeostatic mechanisms, and/or alterations of neural responsiveness. Other mechanisms that may contribute are metabolic tolerance, in which the rate of metabolism is accelerated with chronic use (e.g., for alcohol or barbiturates), and behavioral tolerance, in which a person learns to compensate for a drug-induced impairment in a specific behavioral context.

Tolerance is not required for drug dependence; tolerance can occur without drug dependence. Tolerance is predictable with chronic opiate administration. Tolerance without opiate dependence frequently occurs when persons prescribed chronic pain medications are able to taper and discontinue their pain medications without adverse behavioral sequelae, when the underlying source of pain is relieved.

Sensitization is opposite in concept to tolerance. Sensitization indicates that a given dose of a drug produces more of an effect than that produced by the same dose on an earlier exposure and/or that smaller doses are required to achieve the same effect. Sensitization occurs when the threshold for response is lowered with repeated drug administration. An example of this is seizures kindled by cocaine (Post and Weiss 1995). Repeated exposure of animals to the same dose of cocaine or other stimulants results in increases in locomotor and stereotypic effects, and the molecular mechanisms for this response are beginning to be elucidated (Kalivas et al. 1992, 1993).

Sensitization has largely been characterized as an enhanced motor response to drugs of abuse with repeated administration, although recent research has extended these effects to a progressive increase in the reinforcing value of the drugs, at least during initial acquisition of drug-seeking or conditioned drug effects. It has also been found that, unlike tolerance, sensitization is more likely

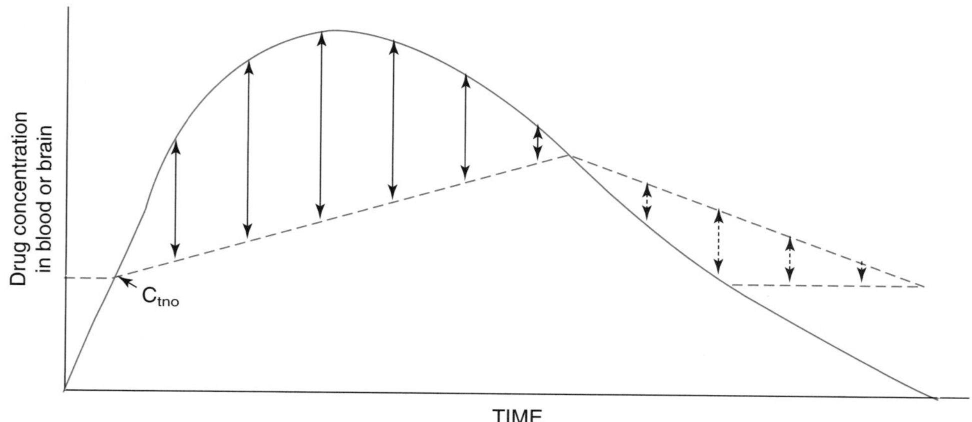


**FIGURE 17-1 Model for acute tolerance and withdrawal. The solid line indicates concentrations of a drug over time. The dashed line indicates the threshold concentration for drug effect, where $C_{tno}$ is the threshold in the absence of prior exposure to the drug. When the concentration of drug exceeds $C_{tno}$, neuroadaptation results in a rise in the threshold concentration a lessening of the drug effects at any given concentration. When the concentration of drug falls below the threshold, deadaptation begins. The dashed arrows indicate the severity of the unresolved reaction. (From Kalant et al. 1971, with permission.)**

to be evident with intermittent rather than continuous administration of drugs (Koob and Le Moal 1997).

### Acute Withdrawal with Short-Term Abstinence

After sustained exposure to a drug of abuse, particularly when there has been considerable neuroadaptation, withdrawal of that drug may produce signs and symptoms that are highly disruptive or even life-threatening. In general, these withdrawal symptoms are opposite to the effects of the drug that were initially sought by the user and to which tolerance had developed. Withdrawal syndromes can create severe and challenging management problems, such as occurs with withdrawal from alcohol and sedative drugs, or they may be subtle but play a critical role in maintaining addiction, such as with withdrawal from cocaine or nicotine. Withdrawal can exacerbate symptoms of underlying psychiatric and/or medical comorbidity.

### Long-Term Abstinence

Addiction is a chronic relapsing disorder rather than an acute illness. Craving and stress can induce relapse both acutely and after significant periods of abstinence. The molecular and cellular mechanisms underlying the long-lasting adaptations that account for this behavior are just beginning to be elucidated. One possibility is that chronic drug use may result in relatively stable changes in gene expression, which may lead to changes in neurotransmission and even in the structure of neurons and the number of their synaptic connections (Nestler and Aghajanian 1997). Changes in plasticity, learning, and long-term memory of specific neuronal circuits—together with social and environmental factors—may predispose chemically dependent persons to relapse.

## PREVENTION OF SUBSTANCE ABUSE

**PRINCIPLE Drug abuse is a preventable behavior and drug addiction is a treatable disease.**
**—the Partnership for a Drug-Free America**

Prevention of tobacco, alcohol, and illicit drug abuse is the number one U.S. public health priority. Program evaluations have shown that prevention works. Program evaluation is critical in order to maximize the impact and cost-effectiveness of selected strategies. *Universal prevention strategies* are aimed at an entire population; they include warning labels, advertising bans, and taxes to increase the cost of alcohol or tobacco products. *Selected prevention strategies* are aimed at a subgroup of the population such as adolescents and include school-based prevention programs and restricted access for minors. *Indicated interventions* are aimed at individuals with known risk factors. Examples of indicated interventions might be targeted education and counseling for sons of alcoholics (IOM 1997).

Brief interventions by physicians can be effective in stimulating individuals to quit smoking or reduce their alcohol consumption (Bien et al. 1993; Ockene et al. 1994). Most children and adults are seen by a primary care physician at least occasionally, and individuals who are related to drug users may seek health care more frequently. Asking patients routinely about smoking, drinking, and the use of illicit drugs gives physicians the opportunity to share information about the health risks of drug use and help prevent its associated morbidity.

## DIAGNOSIS AND ASSESSMENT OF CHEMICAL DEPENDENCY

There is no one specific diagnostic measure or laboratory test for addiction. The CAGE is a four-item test that screens for alcohol problems (Table 17-3). Two positive responses on the CAGE suggest an alcohol problem with a sensitivity of 0.85 to 0.94 and a specificity of 0.79 to 0.88 (Ewing 1984). The CAGE-AID is the CAGE that has also been adapted for use with other drugs (Table 17-3). In pilot studies, the CAGE-AID exhibited similar sensitivity scores (Brown and Rounds 1995). Because the CAGE-AID is a new instrument with limited data, another screening test for drugs such as the Drug Abuse Screening

**Table 17-3 The CAGE Questions Adapted to Include Drugs (CAGE-AID)**

1. Have you felt you ought to **cut down** on your drinking or drug use?
2. Have people **annoyed** you by criticizing your drinking or drug use?
3. Have you felt bad or **guilty** about your drinking or drug use?
4. Have you ever had a drink or used drugs first thing in the morning to steady your nerves or to get rid of a hangover (**eye-opener**)?

NOTE: Item responses on the CAGE are scored 0 for "no" and 1 for "yes" answers, with a higher score an indication of alcohol or drug problems. A total score of 2 or greater is considered clinically significant.
SOURCE: Ewing 1984.

Test (DAST) (Skinner 1982) or the Chemical Use, Abuse, and Dependence Scale (CUAD) (McGovern and Morrison 1992) should be used concomitantly with the CAGE-AID. Although there are many screening tests available for alcohol and drug use that have good reliability and validity, none are as brief as the CAGE and CAGE-AID.

Substance abuse assessment is the further investigation of patients whose positive screening results indicate that chemical dependency is likely. Information gained through an assessment will clarify the type and extent of the problem and will help determine the appropriate treatment response. At a minimum, patients should be assessed for the following (Hoffman et al. 1991; May 1998):

- Acute intoxication and/or withdrawal potential
- Biomedical conditions and complications
- Psychiatric, emotional, and behavioral conditions
- Treatment acceptance or resistance
- Relapse potential or continued drug use potential
- Living environment and support for recovery

In addition to taking a history and performing a physical examination on the patient, it may be helpful to obtain collateral sources of information. Laboratory tests such as the serum $\gamma$-glutamyltransferase (GGT), Breathalyzer tests for alcohol and carbon monoxide, and urine drug screening may be performed.

## PRINCIPLES OF TREATMENT OF CHEMICAL DEPENDENCY

### Acute Management

Three therapeutic issues arise acutely in treating substance abusers. These include the management of the medical complications due to drug use, intoxication, and withdrawal syndromes (see Fig. 17-1).

#### *Medical complications of drug abuse*

Medical complications of drug abuse can result from the drug itself, adulterants used in the preparation of the drug, and the route and mode of drug administration. Accidents and trauma may also occur secondary to drug use. Too often in a clinical setting, the medical complications of drug use are treated, but the problem of drug addiction itself is ignored.

**PRINCIPLE Addiction needs to be recognized as the underlying pharmacologic problem and addressed as a primary illness.**

Historically, chemical dependency has been omitted from medical texts. It is encouraging that this is beginning to change, perhaps because drug abuse is associated with many medical complications. For example, if current tobacco use patterns persist, an estimated 5 million persons who were ages 0 to 17 years in 1995 will die prematurely from a smoking-related illness (CDC 1996). These deaths will be primarily from cancer, coronary artery disease (CAD), and chronic obstructive lung disease. Alcoholism is also associated with many deaths, from automobile accidents to alcoholic liver disease. Intravenous drug abuse, primarily heroin and cocaine, are associated with the spread of viral infections such as hepatitis B and C and AIDS and with bacterial infections that produce endocarditis, osteomyelitis, and local abscesses. Cocaine and other stimulants also produce injury to specific organs, such as myocardial infarction or stroke, as extensions of their pharmacologic actions. This chapter focuses not on the medical complications of drug abuse but on its primary pharmacological aspects.

#### *Intoxication*

With acute intoxication, most drugs of abuse can produce marked disturbances of CNS function and in many cases can disrupt cardiovascular function; both can be life-threatening. Some drugs of abuse are associated with syndromes of subacute or chronic intoxication that may involve both CNS and systemic effects of the drug. An example is chronic abuse of cocaine with paranoid schizophrenia and cachexia.

Management of intoxication requires an understanding of the pharmacology of the offending drug. Intoxication with narcotics, alcohol, and sedative-hypnotic drugs produces death primarily by respiratory depression. The mainstay of therapy is supportive care, such as assisted ventilation and cardiovascular resuscitation, as for any critically ill patient (see chapter 18, Poisoning). In some cases, specific antidotes (i.e., receptor antagonists) are available. These include naloxone for narcotics and flumazenil for benzodiazepines. The use of these agents will be discussed later in this chapter.

Intoxication with a stimulant drug such as with cocaine characteristically produces a picture of a sympathetic neural storm with hypertension, tachyarrhythmias, seizures, hyperthermia, and sometimes acute psychosis. Although no antidotes are available, treatment can be selected to reverse specific pharmacologic actions of the intoxicating drug. Treatment of intoxication by cocaine, for example, might include sympathetic blocking drugs to correct hypertension and arrhythmias. Other aspects of supportive care such as anticonvulsants, sedatives, and cooling are used as needed (see chapter 18, Poisoning).

**PRINCIPLE As in the therapy of any serious disease, first provide life support as needed. Then, aim at the most morbid or mortal determinant, even if it is not simply or specifically manageable.**

***Withdrawal symptoms***

Syndromes of drug withdrawal represent the unopposed consequences of drug-induced neuroadaptation. That is, the brain has adapted to the effects of a drug to normalize brain function in the presence of the drug (associated with the development of tolerance). However, in the absence of the drug, the adaptive responses become maladaptive. The maladaptive response is often the opposite of the adaptive response. For example, excitation and agitation tend to occur during withdrawal from alcohol or other sedative drugs.

The extent and rate of development of tolerance depend on vulnerability factors of the host as well as on the concentrations of the drug and the duration of its presence in the brain (see Fig. 17-1). The higher the dose of the drug and the greater the half-life of the drug in the brain, the greater the extent of adaptation and the greater the magnitude of the potential withdrawal syndrome. Conversely, the faster a drug exits from the brain, the greater the initial magnitude of the withdrawal syndrome (see Fig. 17-1).

The pharmacologic approaches to management of syndromes of drug withdrawal include treatment with an agonist drug that has a long half-life. Examples are methadone and diazepam for heroin and alcohol withdrawal, respectively. Patients may be stabilized on the appropriate dose of the substitute agonist; then the replacement therapy is gradually tapered. If tapering is done slowly enough, there is time for deadaptation, and withdrawal symptoms are minimized. Agonist–antagonist medications such as buprenorphine for opiate withdrawal and a nicotine–mecamylamine combination for tobacco withdrawal are being developed. Also, adjunctive medications such as clonidine may be used to combat symptoms of noradrenergic hyperactivity as in opiate withdrawal, and other symptomatic therapies may also be given. Of course, other aspects of supportive care such as nutritional and electrolyte therapy and management of seizures may also be necessary, depending on the patient and the type of addiction. In some cases, withdrawal syndromes may not require pharmacologic therapy, such as with the profound depression that may follow the use of a stimulant drug. An important concern with such patients is suicide, and optimal care needs to address the potential for self-inflicted injury.

## Chronic Management

Initial drug use is often experimental and/or for social reasons. Individuals who continue to abuse drugs learn to medicate themselves to feel a mood or emotion, rather than relying on social interactions or personal accomplishments to fulfill this need. The "rush" can be alluring, evanescent, yet perpetually sought. Although drug use can be an initial quick fix, it can lead to inattention to important issues and resultant problems. Examples of negative consequences of drug use include accidents, poor work performance, loss of intimate relationships, financial crises, and physical illnesses. Most addicts develop a defense system in order to continue to rely on drugs for emotional modulation. As the consequences of continued drug use mount, the chemically dependent person will struggle with these consequences, as well as to control or quit using drugs. Self-esteem is lost. At this time, addicts can cease using drugs or perpetuate the vicious cycle. Both implicit and explicit consequences of drug use can motivate persons to change their behavior. The purpose of treatment is to support behavioral change away from a life focused on drug use. Change is difficult but possible, and the rewards of treatment are high.

Treatment for drug addiction can be pharmacologic or nonpharmacologic. Examples of anticraving strategies include bupropion for tobacco addiction and naltrexone for alcoholism. Disulfiram, which blocks alcohol's metabolism, helps reduce impulsive drug use, and antagonists such as naltrexone can be helpful in blocking an opiate "high." At times, maintenance medications such as methadone or LAAM for opiate addiction may be indicated.

Before patients can undergo counseling, they may need help with the acute crises caused by their drug use, such as shelter, nutrition, and legal assistance. Some patients may lack funds for transportation, and women may need assistance with childcare in order to participate in treatment.

**PRINCIPLE Adjunctive measures may be key factors in allowing pharmacotherapy to become efficacious.**

Once acute crises are managed, nonpharmacologic treatment modalities include education, family therapy, group therapy, cognitive-behavioral therapy, psychotherapy, 12-step programs, therapeutic communities, as well as more general guidance with assertiveness training and communicational skills, vocational training, parenting skills, and recreation therapy (use of leisure time). Whether patients receive residential or outpatient therapy, they need an environment that supports their abstinence from nonprescribed drug use to facilitate their recovery. Twelve-step programs rely on faith in a power greater than the individual to advance change. Storytelling in front of an experienced group helps break down denial and defenses, guilt is assuaged, and mentors provide successful models of recovery. Historically, 12-step programs have had difficulty supporting patients who need continued pharmacologic therapy.

**PRINCIPLE Drug addiction is a chronic illness. Rather than invoking a cure, the goals of therapy should support remission and improve the individual's quality of life.**

The main challenge in treatment is not initially getting people off drugs but helping them to remain off drugs. More than 50% of patients relapse during the first 24 hours of withdrawal, and a significant number relapse during their first month (Hunt et al. 1971). Thereafter, the risk of relapse diminishes but remains ever present. Either abstinence or pharmacologic maintenance may be the desired therapeutic goal. Quality of life is enhanced by shortening periods of uncontrolled, nonprescribed drug use, treating underlying medical and psychiatric conditions, and supporting personal growth.

It is important to keep in mind that success or failure in treatment involves both patient factors and treatment factors. Patient factors include the severity of addiction, the presence of other psychiatric and medical conditions, the level of functioning before addictive behavior, social support, and readiness for change. Treatment factors are composed of the type of therapeutic modalities as well as the quality, quantity, length, and intensity of therapy. The study of the interaction between specific patient factors and specific treatment factors is called *patient–treatment matching*. This is the basis for current evidence-based outcome research. One cannot compare two treatment results without first characterizing the patient and treatment factors and specifically defining the outcome measures.

The development of successful treatment outcomes arises from multidisciplinary research that integrates genetic, neurobiologic, pharmacologic, and medical findings with behavioral, social, and environmental factors and provides a strong connection between basic science and clinical practice (IOM 1997).

## NICOTINE AND TOBACCO

### Pharmacology

Tobacco contains thousands of chemicals. Nicotine is the chemical responsible for most of the pharmacologic actions of tobacco and for addiction (Benowitz 1988, 1996). Tobacco contains *S*-nicotine, which binds to acetylcholine receptors at autonomic ganglia, the adrenal medulla, neuromuscular junctions, and the brain. Stimulation of nicotinic receptors in the brain, primarily acting on presynaptic sites, results in the activation of several CNS neurotransmitter systems. Nicotine also enhances systemic and local vascular release of catecholamines and causes release of vasopressin, cortisol, and $\beta$-endorphins.

The primary CNS effects of nicotine in smokers are arousal, relaxation (particularly in stressful situations), and enhancement of mood, attention, and reaction time, with improvement in performance of some behavioral tasks. Some of or all these effects may result from the relief of withdrawal symptoms in addicted smokers rather than a direct enhancing effect on the brain. Nicotine also suppresses appetite and increases metabolic rate, resulting in lower body weight in smokers compared with nonsmokers.

Smoking and nicotine also have sympathomimetic actions, producing brief increases in blood pressure, heart rate, and cardiac output, with cutaneous vasoconstriction. Nicotine causes muscle relaxation by stimulating discharge of the Renshaw cells and/or pulmonary afferent nerves, with inhibition of activity of motor neurons.

In most smokers, cessation of smoking results in the development of a withdrawal syndrome including restlessness, irritability, anxiety, drowsiness, frequent wakening from sleep, and confusion and/or impaired concentration. Some performance measures such as reaction time and attention may be impaired. The acute withdrawal symptoms reach their maximum intensity at 24 to 48 hours after cessation and then gradually diminish over a period of a few weeks. That nicotine itself is responsible for the withdrawal symptoms is supported by the appearance of similar symptoms with sudden withdrawal from the use of chewing tobacco, snuff, or nicotine gum, and the relief of these symptoms by nicotine itself. Abstinent smokers also gain an average of 2 to 3 kg during the first year after they stop smoking (Williamson et al. 1991).

## Pharmacokinetics and Metabolism

Nicotine in tobacco smoke is absorbed rapidly through the lungs. Nicotine is a weak base; absorption through mucous membranes depends on pH. Chewing tobacco, snuff, and nicotine gum are buffered at an alkaline pH to facilitate absorption through the buccal mucosa. Smoking is an effective form of drug administration in that the drug enters the circulation rapidly through the lungs and moves into the brain within seconds. Inhaled drugs with high partition coefficients are absorbed rapidly and efficiently, and they escape first-pass metabolism. Substance abusers and the tobacco industry are savvy to use the inhaled route of drug administration, for drugs with CNS activity, when rapid action and direct access to the brain is desired. The more rapid the "rush," the more reinforcing the drug. Thus, high concentrations of the drug are delivered to the brain even quicker than if the drug were administered intravenously. It is not surprising that a number of substances of abuse—including marijuana, cocaine, opiates, phencyclidine, and organic solvents—are abused by the inhalational route because access to the brain is so direct. In this manner, smoking a cigarette is similar to freebasing cocaine. The smoking process also allows precise dose titration so that the smoker may obtain desired effects.

Nicotine is rapidly and extensively metabolized by the liver, primarily to the compound cotinine. The metabolite cotinine is widely used as a quantitative marker for exposure to nicotine and could be potentially useful as a diagnostic test for use of tobacco and compliance to a regimen for withdrawal from nicotine. The half-life of nicotine averages 2 to 3 hours. Thus, although there is considerable peak-to-trough oscillation in blood levels from cigarette to cigarette consistent with a half-life of 2 to 3 hours, nicotine accumulates in the body over 6 to 9 hours of regular smoking. Nicotine also has a very long terminal half-life of 20 hours or more, presumably reflecting the slow release of nicotine from body tissues. Thus, smoking results not in intermittent and transient exposure to nicotine but in an exposure that lasts 24 hours a day. Arteriovenous differences during cigarette smoking are substantial, with arterial levels exceeding venous levels 6- to 10-fold (Henningfield et al. 1993; Gourlay and Benowitz 1997). The intensity and persistence of nicotine in the brain results in changes in nicotinic receptors in the brain and in intracellular processes of neuroadaption. The changes in receptor numbers and function are presumably the substrate for the syndrome of withdrawal from nicotine.

## Pharmacodynamics

Two issues are particularly relevant to understanding the pharmacodynamics of nicotine. First, there is a complex dose–response relationship: Low doses may stimulate neural systems, whereas higher doses depress them. For example, low doses of nicotine produce central or peripheral nervous system stimulation with arousal and an increase in heart rate and blood pressure. However, nicotine intoxication produces ganglionic blockade and other effects resulting in bradycardia, hypotension, and depressed mental status. A second issue is the development of tolerance. Smokers know that tolerance develops to the dysphoria, nausea, and vomiting that often occur after one's first cigarette. Tolerance to subjective effects and acceleration of heart rate develop within the day in regular smokers. Thus, even within a single day, because of development of tolerance, the positive rewards of smoking diminish, and smoking may become motivated more by relief of withdrawal symptoms.

## Drug Interactions with Nicotine and Tobacco

### *Drug metabolism*

Cigarette smoking may interact with medications through effects on drug metabolism or pharmacodynamics. Smoking is well known to accelerate the metabolism of many drugs, particularly those metabolized by CYP1A2. Because there are more than 3000 components in cigarette smoke, it is difficult to know which ones are responsible for changes in drug metabolism. One likely group of chemicals is the polycyclic aromatic hydrocarbons.

Drugs whose metabolism is accelerated by cigarette smoking are listed in Table 17-4. An interaction of particular clinical concern is that of cigarette smoking with theophylline. On average, smokers require a 50% larger-than-normal maintenance dose of theophylline because of a comparable increase in theophylline clearance. In a large survey, theophylline toxicity was found to be less common in cigarette smokers, a finding consistent with accelerated metabolism (Pfeifer and Greenblatt 1978). Within 7 days of the beginning of abstinence from tobacco, the clearance of theophylline declines by an average of 35% (Lee et al. 1987). Thus, when smokers stop smoking, as, for example, during hospitalization for acute illness, the doses of theophylline may need reduction to avoid the development of theophylline toxicity (see part I,

Table 17-4 **Drugs Whose Metabolism is Accelerated and Drugs Whose Metabolism is Unchanged by Cigarette Smoking***

| ACCELERATED METABOLISM | MINIMAL OR NO CHANGE IN METABOLISM |
|---|---|
| Antipyrine | Chlordiazepoxide |
| Caffeine | Codeine |
| Desmethyldiazepam | Dexamethasone |
| Flecainide | Diazepam† |
| Imipramine | Ethanol |
| Lidocaine | Lorazepam |
| Oxazepam | Meperidine |
| Pentazocine | Nortriptyline |
| Phenacetin | Oral contraceptives |
| Propranolol | Phenytoin |
| Theophylline | Pindolol |
| | Prednisolone |
| | Prednisone |
| | Quinidine |
| | Warfarin |

*Adapted from Jusko, 1984.
†Metabolism of active metabolite is accelerated.

Introduction; chapter 2, Respiratory Disorders; and chapter 25, Drug Interactions).

Drugs with a high degree of presystemic metabolism may be particularly affected by cigarette smoking. For such drugs, accelerated metabolism may result in a substantial decrease in bioavailability, which could result in subtherapeutic concentrations in blood. Examples of such interactions include lower concentrations of propranolol in blood in the Beta-Blocker Heart Attack Trial and reduced analgesic efficacy of pentazocine in cigarette smokers (Vaughan et al. 1976; Walle et al. 1985).

***Pharmacodynamic interactions***

Several pharmacodynamic interactions arise from the hemodynamic effects of nicotine in cigarette smoke. For example, by reducing the blood flow to the skin and subcutaneous tissue, cigarette smoking may slow the absorption of insulin from subcutaneous sites. In patients with angina pectoris, the frequency of angina and the duration of exercise before the development of chest pain or electrocardiographic changes are less improved by $\beta$-adrenergic receptor blocking agents ("beta blockers") or nifedipine in smoking patients than in nonsmoking patients (Deanfield et al. 1984). In the Medical Research Council Hypertension Trial, propranolol was less effective than was a thiazide diuretic in decreasing blood pressure and reducing the risk of stroke in smokers, whereas the drugs were equally effective in nonsmokers (Dollery and Brennan 1988). Cigarette smoking and oral contraceptives may interact synergistically to increase the risk of stroke and premature myocardial infarction (MI) in women. Cigarettes appear to enhance the procoagulant effect of estrogens. For this reason, oral contraceptives are relatively contraindicated in women who smoke cigarettes.

Cigarette smokers experience less sedation than do nonsmokers from several drugs that act on the CNS, including diazepam, chlordiazepoxide, and chlorpromazine (Swett 1974). Smoking probably acts by producing arousal of the CNS rather than by accelerating metabolism and reducing the brain levels of these drugs. The efficacy of analgesics such as propoxyphene may be reduced in cigarette smokers, even in the absence of pharmacokinetic interactions (Boston Collaborative Drug Surveillance Program 1973). Cigarette smoking is a major risk factor for the development, maintenance, and recurrence of peptic ulcer disease. Smoking adversely effects mucosal aggressive and protective factors, and it impairs the therapeutic effects of histamine $H_2$-receptor antagonists (Eastwood 1997).

**PRINCIPLE Reducing the uncontrolled use of addictive drugs, while continuing to treat addiction, may help with the incidence, severity, and manageability of other diseases.**

Nicotine replacement can be used as a harm-reduction strategy to avoid the oncologic and pulmonary consequences of tobacco use. Nicotine replacement is safer than smoking cigarettes, because it avoids the harm that carbon monoxide and other components of tobacco smoke and tar cause the smoker.

## Clinical and Therapeutic Issues

***Nicotine intoxication***

Acute intoxication with nicotine is uncommon in cigarette smokers but has been well described after accidental or suicidal exposure to nicotine-containing pesticides or occupational exposure to tobacco leaves. Intoxication with nicotine results in nausea, vomiting, pallor, weakness, dizziness, lightheadedness, and sweating. More severe intoxication may result in hypotension, bradycardia, seizures, and respiratory arrest. Some of the peripheral manifestations such as bradycardia and hypotension appear to be mediated by release of acetylcholine and can be reversed by atropine. Theoretically, mecamylamine, a nicotinic (and ganglionic) antagonist that can penetrate the CNS, would reverse all aspects of nicotine toxicity; however, the medication (once used to treat hypertension) is not readily available for this purpose.

### *Addiction to tobacco*

As with other drugs, there is a genetic predisposition to nicotine addiction. Cigarette smoking runs in families and is more prevalent in individuals who have a lifetime history of depression (Kendler et al. 1993). Exposure to tobacco in infancy may predispose young boys to conduct disorder (Wakshlag et al. 1997). Risk-taking, rebellious adolescents are more prone to initiate smoking. Personal imagery may contribute to cigarette smoking by adolescents who view smoking as adult, sophisticated behavior or a behavior linked with physical attractiveness (such as the advertising image of slim, attractive women). Finally, sociological factors may be determinants of substance abuse risk and drug use patterns. Drug-taking behavior within a family or among friends is a strong motivator and reinforcer of drug use.

In smokers who progress to addiction, tolerance rapidly develops to the headache, nausea, and dysphoria associated with the first cigarettes. Adolescents learn that pleasure, arousal, and relaxation can be attained from smoking. They also learn that they can titrate their dose to achieve the desired effect. Adolescents may take advantage of nicotine's other pharmacologic properties. Smoking may improve attention and reaction time and may improve performance on certain tasks. Smokers may also experience the relief of aversive emotional states, including the reduction of anxiety or stress, relief from hunger and prevention of weight gain, and relief from symptoms of withdrawal from nicotine. Whether the positive rewards, that is, enhanced performance and mood after smoking, are due to relief of symptoms of abstinence or to an intrinsic enhancement effect of nicotine is unclear.

As the smoker learns how to smoke to achieve the desired effects on their mood, he or she begins to associate specific moods or situations or environmental factors with the rewarding effects of the cigarette. The association between such cues and anticipated drug effects and the resulting urge to use the drug is referred to as *conditioning*.

Cigarette smoking provides a powerful example of how conditioning may be important to continued drug use. People often smoke cigarettes in specific situations such as after a meal, along with a cup of coffee or an alcoholic beverage, or along with friends who smoke. The association between smoking and these other events repeated many times results in the environmental situation's becoming a powerful cue for the urge to smoke. Likewise, aspects of the drug-taking process, such as the manipulation of smoking materials, or the taste, smell, or feel of smoke in the throat, become associated with the pleasurable effects of smoking. Even unpleasant moods can become conditioned cues for smoking. For example, a smoker may learn that not having a cigarette provokes irritability (one of the common symptoms of the nicotine abstinence syndrome). Smoking a cigarette relieves the withdrawal symptom(s). After repeated experiences of this sort, the smoker may come to regard irritability from any source (such as stress or frustration) to be a cue for smoking. Although conditioning becomes an important element of drug addiction, it must be remembered that conditioning develops only because of the pairing of the pharmacologic actions of the drug with behaviors. Conditioning loses its power without the presence of an active drug. Hence, nicotine-free cigarettes have not succeeded in the marketplace. Conditioning is a major factor that causes relapse to drug use after a period of cessation. It must be addressed as a component of behavioral therapy of drug use.

**SUMMARY**

**Smoking cessation is difficult for a myriad of reasons. Cigarettes are used chronically over many years, often with onset during early adolescence. Smoking enables nicotine to rapidly enter the brain, and nicotine can enable the smoker to fine-tune their mood toward either stimulation or relaxation. These subtle effects can be self-adjusted and self-titrated. Averaging 10 puffs per cigarette and one to two packs per day, cigarettes are dosed 200 to 400 times a day. Over many years, cigarette smoking becomes powerfully linked with the conditioned cues of everyday life. It is the nicotine component of the cigarette that causes persons to continue to smoke despite harmful physiologic and social consequences, but it is the carbon monoxide and other gases and the components of the tar in a cigarette that cause the majority of cardiovascular, pulmonary, and oncologic morbidity.**

Physicians need to intervene with their patients who smoke cigarettes and guide them toward cessation. Smokers in the precontemplation phase need to overcome their ambivalence about their need and ability to quit smoking. Smokers in the action phase need close monitoring and support of their effort. Patients need to be educated about the many possible nonpharmacological and pharmacological tools that can enable smoking cessation. Smokers need to be prepared that smoking cessation is difficult. Inability to quit is not merely a problem of willpower. Like alcoholic and other drug-addicted patients, smokers will exhibit extreme behaviors to obtain cigarettes when their supply has run out. Physicians should anticipate a high degree of relapse in patients who briefly quit smoking and deal with this in a supportive manner. Smokers can build upon each smoking cessation attempt and each relapse by analyzing prior lapses, developing additional and alternative strategies, and intensifying their treatment until they are successful in their goal.

### *Pharmacologic treatment of tobacco addiction*

Antidepressant drugs and nicotine replacement therapies have been shown to be efficacious in treating tobacco addiction. Nicotine replacement products differ considerably in their patterns, rates, and quantities of dosing and in resultant pharmacologic effects. Transdermal nicotine systems deliver 5 to 22 mg over 16 to 24 hours, depending on the patch. Nicotine is absorbed slowly, resulting in a relatively steady level of nicotine, substantial development of tolerance, and little, if any, psychological effect (Benowitz 1995).

Nicotine polacrilex gum results in the systemic absorption of 1 or 2 mg with the 2- or 4-mg nicotine gums, respectively, over a 20- to 30-minute period. A basic environment is needed for nicotine absorption through the buccal mucosa. Patients need to be instructed not to take the gum directly after sodas or coffee (which are acidic). After moistening the polacrilex, they should park it on their buccal mucosa rather than continuing to chew it and swallow the secretions. The absorption of nicotine from the gum produces moderate subjective effects, although less intense than from smoking a cigarette. Blood levels of nicotine rise with each piece of nicotine gum and fall between pieces, and blood levels of nicotine with typical levels of use are substantially less than those derived from cigarette smoking (Benowitz et al. 1987).

Nicotine nasal spray delivers 1.0 mg nicotine to the nostrils, of which 0.5 mg is absorbed systemically (Johansson et al. 1991). Nasal nicotine is very rapidly absorbed and results in more intense subjective effects than other types of nicotine replacement therapy. Nicotine nasal spray is initially perceived as irritating and unpleasant, but after a few days tolerance develops to these noxious effects.

All nicotine replacement therapy products appear to be efficacious, resulting in an average twofold enhancement of the odds of successful quitting (Fiore et al. 1994; Tang et al. 1994). Although the absolute quit rate with nicotine replacement therapy is enhanced by concomitant behavioral therapy, the relative benefit of nicotine replacement therapy versus placebo seems to be maintained regardless of the level of behavioral therapy. Different types of nicotine replacement therapy may be more useful for different types of smokers. Future research will investigate matching different types of smokers to the different types and combinations of nonnicotine and nicotine replacement therapies. High-dose transdermal nicotine does suppress *ad libitum* cigarette smoking and may be useful for smokers who are otherwise unable to quit (Benowitz et al. 1998).

The antidepressants bupropion and nortriptyline are effective in bringing about cessation of smoking, even in patients without active depression (Humfleet et al. 1996; Hunt et al. 1997). The advantage of these medications is that they pose little risk of drug dependence. Seizures especially in persons with bulimia or anorexia nervosa can be problematic with bupropion, and anticholinergic adverse effects can be problematic with nortriptyline. Bupropion and its active metabolite hydroxybupropion appear to work primarily by inhibiting neuronal uptake of norepinephrine and dopamine. Tricyclic antidepressants block the reuptake of norepinephrine and serotonin. Bupropion, the tricyclic antidepressants, and clonidine, which also is of value in smoking cessation, reduce the firing rates of noradrenergic neurons in the locus ceruleus.

The combination of nicotine and mecamylamine, a nicotinic antagonist, in transdermal application is a novel and promising smoking cessation therapy. In effective relative doses, nicotine is administered to suppress withdrawal symptoms, although mecamylamine is administered to block the mood-altering "reward" effects of cigarette smoking. The results from early clinical trials of patches containing both mecamylamine and nicotine are positive (Rose et al. 1994).

**PRINCIPLE When individual drugs with different mechanisms of action each are partially efficacious for an indication, look next for the effects of combinations.**

### *Tobacco and pregnancy*

Compared with nonsmoking women, the relative risk of having a low-birth-weight baby is nearly doubled in women who smoke during pregnancy, and the relative risks of spontaneous abortion and perinatal and neonatal mortality are increased by about one-third (Walsh 1994). The components of tobacco smoke responsible for obstetrical and fetal problems have not been definitely determined. Carbon monoxide is clearly detrimental as it markedly reduces the oxygen-carrying capacity of fetal hemoglobin.

In the developing fetus, nicotine may arrest neuronal replication and differentiation, and it may contribute to sudden infant death syndrome (Slotkin 1998). Nicotine targets specific neurotransmitter receptors in the fetal brain and causes abnormalities of cell proliferation and differentiation that lead to shortfalls in cell numbers and eventually to altered synaptic activity. Comparable alterations occur in peripheral autonomic pathways, hypothesized to lead to increased susceptibility to hypoxia-induced brain damage, perinatal mortality, and sudden infant death.

There is a definite increase in respiratory diseases, otitis media, and minor ailments that are related to exposure to environmental tobacco smoke in the home and daycare centers after birth. Breast-fed infants of mothers who smoke appear to be protected against infectious respiratory diseases but are subjected to chemicals from the smoke transferred in the milk (Charlton 1994). Women need to be encouraged to quit smoking during their pregnancy and not to relapse during the postpartum period.

***Therapeutic uses of nicotine***

Through the development of nicotine polacrilex gum, patches, and new delivery vehicles, the effects of nicotine dosing in acute and chronic administration have been explored independently from the effects of tobacco smoking. Potential therapeutic applications for nicotine and its analogues include enhancing cognition in Alzheimer's disease, preventing Parkinson's disease, and improving symptoms in Tourette's syndrome and ulcerative colitis. Nicotine may benefit attention deficit hyperactivity disorder, schizophrenia, obesity, depression, anxiety, and sleep apnea (Levin and Rosecrans 1994).

**PRINCIPLE While tobacco use is associated with significant morbidity and mortality, new nicotine delivery forms and nicotine analogues are undergoing development for possible therapeutic effects for new and interesting indications.**

# ETHANOL

## Pharmacology

Although ethanol had been thought to act in a relatively nonselective manner causing perturbations of the lipids in cell membranes, more recent work has begun to uncover a significant selectivity of the actions of ethanol on signal transmission and transduction proteins of the central nervous system. Ethanol acts on $GABA_A$ receptors that allow passage of chloride through the ion-gated channel and cause neuronal stabilization (inhibition). Ethanol also acts on a subtype of glutamate receptor called the *NMDA receptor*. By inhibiting NMDA-stimulated $Ca^{2+}$ influx and cGMP production, ethanol inhibits fast excitatory transmission. Because glutamate exerts tonic inhibitory control over dopamine release in the nucleus accumbens through NMDA receptors, ethanol may act to diminish this inhibition and to increase dopamine release. With chronic ethanol use, these receptor systems undergo adaptive changes. Researchers postulated that the adaptive changes in the $GABA_A$ receptor system may have a more significant relationship to the development of ethanol tolerance, whereas the changes in the NMDA receptor system may have a more significant relationship to the development of physical dependence (Tabakoff and Hoffman 1996). This could explain the observed dissociation between the development of tolerance and the development of withdrawal symptomatology after chronic alcohol use.

Furthermore, these investigators believe that the genetic determinants of differential ethanol sensitivity and predisposition to alcoholism may be revealed through subtle differences in subunit combinations in these receptors' structure and/or posttranslational modification, rather than in gross differences in the primary structure of the individual proteins involved. Ethanol also interacts with multiple other neuronal pathways and transmitters including noradrenergic, opioid, and serotonergic sites. The relative contributions of each of the neurotransmitters may change with the dose of alcohol consumed and the degree of dependency of the individual (Koob et al. 1994).

Clinically, ethanol is a CNS depressant, although at lower doses there may be behavioral stimulation owing either to direct effects of the drug or to disinhibition. At moderate doses, the effect of ethanol is usually perceived as pleasurable. But higher doses produce CNS depression, progressively affecting greater areas of the CNS (see Table 17-5). These effects are described more fully in the section on alcohol intoxication.

## Pharmacokinetics and Metabolism

The usual drink (one cocktail, 4-oz glass of wine, or 12-oz beer in the United States) contains 10 to 15 g of ethanol. Ethanol is well absorbed by passive diffusion throughout the GI tract. The presence of food tends to retard absorption by delaying gastric emptying time, diluting the alcohol, and slowing uptake, especially from the large surface area of the small intestine. Ethanol undergoes first-pass metabolism by the liver (Levitt et al. 1997), stomach (Lim et al. 1993), and intestine (Frezza et al. 1990). The extent of first-pass metabolism seems to be greater in men than in women, with the result that women achieve higher concentrations of alcohol in blood with similar body-weight-adjusted doses. Once alcohol reaches the systemic circulation, it is immediately distributed to other body compartments at a rate proportional to

Table 17-5 **Clinical Effects of Ethanol at Various Blood Concentrations**

| BLOOD ETHANOL CONCENTRATIONS (MG/DL) | CLINICAL EFFECTS |
|---|---|
| 30–100 | Mild euphoria, talkativeness<br>Decreased inhibitions<br>Impaired attention, judgment<br>Mild incoordination, nystagmus |
| 100–200 | Emotional instability (excitement; withdrawal)<br>Impaired memory, reaction time<br>Loss of critical judgment<br>Conjunctival hyperemia<br>Ataxia, nystagmus, dysarthria<br>Hypalgesia |
| 200–300 | Confusion, disorientation, dizziness<br>Disturbed perception, sensation<br>Diplopia, dilated pupils<br>Marked ataxia, dysarthria |
| 300–400 | Apathy, stupor<br>Decreased response to stimuli<br>Vomiting, incontinence<br>Inability to stand or walk |
| Over 400 | Unconsciousness, coma<br>Anesthesia<br>Descreased or abolished reflexes<br>Hypothermia<br>Hypoventilation<br>Hypotension<br>Death (respiratory arrest) |

the blood flow to that area, and it is eventually distributed in proportion to total body water with a volume of distribution of 0.68 L/kg in men and 0.55 L/kg in women (Deitrich and Palmer 1994).

Ethanol is primarily metabolized by the liver cytoplasmic enzyme alcohol dehydrogenase (ADH), with a minor component being metabolized via liver microsomes (Fig. 17-2). The major product of metabolism of alcohol is acetaldehyde, which in turn is metabolized by aldehyde dehydrogenase. A genetic deficiency in aldehyde dehydrogenase resulting in excess accumulation of acetaldehyde may explain flushing in some Asians and other people and, not surprisingly because of the discomfort it engenders, may be associated with a low risk of alcoholism (Suwacki and Ohara 1985).

Elimination of ethanol follows mostly zero-order kinetics, that is, the rate of elimination, about 7 to 10 g/h, is independent of concentration of the ethanol in blood. For a typical adult, blood alcohol concentration declines at a rate of 15 mg/dL per hour, a calculation that is widely used in forensic medicine to back-extrapolate to alcohol concentrations in blood at earlier times, such as at the time of an automobile accident. The rate of alcohol metabolism is faster in chronic alcoholics.

Expired air contains ethanol in proportion to its vapor pressure at body temperature. The Breathalyzer test extrapolates blood ethanol concentration from analysis of the expired air ethanol concentration.

## Pharmacodynamics

The primary acute effects of alcohol are on the CNS. The relationship between blood alcohol concentration and effects is summarized in Table 17-5. The relationship is influenced by the degree of tolerance that is present and

$$\text{Ethanol } (CH_3CH_2OH) \xrightarrow[\text{CYP2E1}]{\text{Alcohol dehydrogenase or}} \text{Acetaldehyde } (CH_3CHO)$$

$$\text{Acetaldehyde} \xrightarrow[(NAD^+)]{\text{Aldehyde dehydrogenase}} \text{Acetic acid } (CH_3COOH) \xrightarrow[\text{cycle}]{\text{Citric acid}} CO_2 + H_2O$$

FIGURE 17-2 **Metabolism of ethanol.**

by the rate of rise of alcohol in the blood and brain. Thus, the degree of ethanol intoxication is greater when concentrations are rising than it is when they are falling. Ethanol also relaxes smooth muscle, resulting in vasodilation and reduction of uterine contractility, the latter effect having historically been used to control premature labor. Although alcohol can cause acute vasodilation and reduce blood pressure, chronic consumption of alcohol is associated with elevation of blood pressure.

With regular consumption of alcohol, considerable tolerance develops to its CNS effects. Thus, a chronic alcoholic may appear to function normally at a blood alcohol concentration of 300 mg/dL, a concentration that could cause stupor in a nonalcoholic.

## Drug Interactions with Ethanol

Chronic consumption of alcohol is associated with accelerated hepatic microsomal metabolism of a number of drugs, including warfarin and hypoglycemic sulfonylureas, although acute alcohol intoxication may inhibit drug metabolism. The most important interactions with ethanol involve excessive sedation when alcohol is used with sedative-hypnotic drugs, antidepressants, neuroleptic drugs, sedating antihistamines, or narcotics. This combination is of particular concern when motor skills such as driving an automobile or operating machinery are required. Alcohol may also potentiate the effects of hypoglycemic drugs. Disulfiram chelates metal ions that are cofactors for aldehyde dehydrogenase and dopamine $\beta$-hydroxylase. The consumption of alcohol when taking other agents such as metronidazole, the sulfonylureas, griseofulvin, some cephalosporins, and chloramphenicol may result in the accumulation of acetaldehyde and provoke flushing, headache, nausea, sweating, and palpitations.

Alcohol may enhance the risk of gastrointestinal bleeding due to aspirin and the nonsteroidal anti-inflammatory drugs (NSAIDs). Regular consumption of alcohol lowers the threshold for acetaminophen-induced liver damage because it induces the P450 enzymes 1A2, 2E1, and 3A4 that catalyze the oxidative metabolism of acetaminophen (Sinclair et al. 1998). In addition, alcoholics may have depleted stores of glutathione and an already-damaged liver. Severe liver injury has been reported in alcoholics who took less than 4 g of acetaminophen per day (Zimmerman and Maddrey 1995). Fatal hepatic injury from acetaminophen is sometimes associated with fasting, which by itself can increase the risk of acetaminophen-induced hepatotoxicity (Whitcomb and Block 1994). Although alcohol abusers and alcoholics frequently have ailments associated with pain, regular use of any analgesic should be discouraged in these persons, and when it is needed, the lowest possible dose should be taken.

## Clinical and Therapeutic Issues

### *Acute intoxication*

The dose-dependent progression of neural depression, as listed in Table 17-5, can be viewed as similar to that observed for anesthetics. At lower concentrations, inhibitory polysynaptic influences are inhibited, resulting in cortical disinhibition with the associated changes in mood and cognitive function. At greater levels of intoxication, neural activity is depressed, resulting in cerebellar dysfunction, delirium, or coma. Death may ensue from respiratory depression. Death has occurred at blood alcohol concentrations as low as 400 mg/dL, although survival at concentrations greater than 700 mg/dL also has been described.

Hypoglycemia may be a cause of coma in alcoholic patients. Because alcohol blocks gluconeogenesis, the combination of alcohol consumption (even at moderate levels) plus fasting may lead to hypoglycemia and loss of consciousness. Children and individuals with chronic liver disease are particularly susceptible to alcohol-induced hypoglycemia.

The treatment of an alcohol-intoxicated patient is primarily supportive, with specific attention placed on maintaining a patent airway, assisting ventilation if necessary, and treatment of hypoglycemia (see chapter 18, Poisoning).

### *Alcohol withdrawal*

The clinical manifestations of alcohol withdrawal are shown in Table 17-6. Alcohol withdrawal symptoms occur not only after abrupt cessation of use but may be seen even with reduction in the daily level of intake of alcohol. Minor or early symptoms are typically observed for up to 48 hours after cessation of consumption of alcohol, with a peak intensity observed at 24 hours. Minor withdrawal typically presents with one or more of three signs: tremulousness, hallucinations, and seizures. Major or late withdrawal typically occurs 1 to 6 days after the cessation of drinking and is characterized by profound agitation, insomnia, hallucinations or delusions, tremor, hypertension, tachycardia, and hyperthermia. Because disorientation and confusion are commonly present, the syndrome is referred to as *delirium tremens*. This syndrome carries substantial morbidity and mortality owing primarily to concurrent infection, pancreatitis, trauma, or heart disease. Cardiac ar-

Table 17-6 Clinical Features of Alcohol Withdrawal

| MINOR (EARLY WITHDRAWAL) | MAJOR (LATE WITHDRAWAL) |
|---|---|
| Tremulousness | Delirium tremors |
| Coarse action tremor | Extreme agitation |
| Irritability, restlessness | Appears frightened, confused |
| Anxiety, agitation | Hallucinations |
| Insomnia | Disorientation |
| Anorexia, vomiting | Disordered sensory perception |
| Diaphoresis | Marked autonomic hyperactivity |
| Tachycardia | Dilated pupils |
| Mild hypertension | Tachycardia |
| Hallucinosis | Hypertension |
| Visual most common | Fever |
| Patient remains oriented | |
| Seizures | |
| Grand mal | |
| Multiple seizures common | |

rhythmias are common and may be the cause of sudden death.

Seizures generally occur 6 to 30 hours after cessation of drinking, with a peak occurrence from 12 to 24 hours after cessation. Of note is that seizures and other manifestations of withdrawal from alcohol can be delayed in onset by the administration of sedative hypnotic or anesthetic drugs, as is often the case when alcoholic patients are admitted to the hospital for trauma or elective surgery. Seizures are usually self-limited, but status epilepticus occasionally develops.

**Key Points: As with other drugs, the primary objectives of treatment of withdrawal from alcohol are relief of symptoms, prevention or treatment of more serious complications, and preparation for long-term rehabilitation.**

Hospitalization is necessary on medical grounds for a minority of patients undergoing alcohol withdrawal (Whitfield et al. 1978; Naranjo et al. 1983). Indications for hospitalization include previous delirium tremens, a history of seizures or severe hallucinations, severe active withdrawal symptoms, and/or medical or psychiatric comorbidity that requires observation in the face of alcohol withdrawal. When these factors are not present and the environment is supportive of recovery, outpatient detoxification can be performed.

Management of more severe alcohol withdrawal consists of supportive care and specific pharmacotherapy. Supportive care includes administration of glucose, hydration, correction of electrolyte abnormalities, adequate nutrition, and appropriate reassurance. Thiamine is routinely given to prevent the development of Wernicke encephalopathy (which may be precipitated by IV glucose). For mild alcohol withdrawal, supportive care may be sufficient. For more severe withdrawal, pharmacotherapy is indicated.

Pharmacotherapy is designed to replace alcohol with a sedative drug that can then be tapered in a controlled manner. Benzodiazepines are the drugs of choice because they are effective and have a wide therapeutic index. Benzodiazepines reduce withdrawal severity, reduce incidence of delirium ($-4.9$ cases per 100 patients; 95% confidence interval, $-9.0$ to $-0.7$; $P = 0.04$), and reduce seizures ($-7.7$ seizures per 100 patients; 95% confidence interval, $-12.0$ to $-3.5$; $P = 0.003$) (Mayo-Smith 1997). All benzodiazepines and all three of the following medication approaches appear to be effective:

- Patients can be treated on a fixed tapering schedule with additional medication as needed.
- Patients can be medicated on a symptom-triggered basis.
- Patients can be loaded with a long-acting benzodiazepine (diazepam, 20 mg IV or PO, or chlordiazepoxide, 100 mg PO, each hour) until sedation is achieved, followed by tapering the dose.

Because of the long half-lives of these drugs and their metabolites, the levels of drug in the body will decline gradually (even in the absence of tapering) to provide a gradual withdrawal with relatively few symptoms of abstinence. In theory, the third or loading method combats kindling most effectively. The loading method also overtreats the majority of patients to avoid the potential severe complications of undertreating a few. A recent study compared medicating patients based on a symptom-triggered basis (chlordiazepoxide 25 to 100 mg/h when a score of 8 or greater was achieved on the Clinical Institute Withdrawal Assessment for Alcohol, revised scale [CIWA-A]) (see Fig. 17-3), with medicating patients on a fixed schedule (50 mg for four doses, then 25 mg for eight doses every 6 hours) (Saitz et al. 1994). The symptom-triggered pharmacotherapy resulted in a lesser total amount of chlordiazepoxide administered and shorter median medication duration than did chlordiazepoxide administered on a fixed schedule. However, the patients excluded from the study were precisely the ones who needed pharmacologic treatment and were at the greatest risk of severe alcohol withdrawal (having medical or psychiatric illnesses requiring hospitalization, or a history of seizures). The conclusion that one can draw from this study is that symptom-triggered chlordiazepoxide administered to patients not at risk for severe withdrawal, by a trained nursing staff, can reduce the cost of medical care, especially if these patients are hospitalized.

In patients with severe cirrhosis, who metabolize the long-acting benzodiazepines very slowly and may, particularly with prior hepatic encephalopathy, be extraordinarily sensitive to the sedative effects of benzodiazepines, it is preferable to administer shorter-acting benzodiazepines to treat alcohol withdrawal. Some benzodiazepines such as lorazepam and oxazepam are metabolized primarily by conjugation, and their metabolism is not impaired in the presence of alcoholic cirrhosis.

Alcohol-induced hallucinations may be controlled with haloperidol, 0.5 to 2.0 mg every 2 hours. Moderate doses are encouraged because of the potential for lowering the seizure threshold. Benzodiazepines provide protection against convulsions, and seizures usually respond to diazepam. Carbamazepine has been found in a well-controlled study to be as effective as benzodiazepines for treating alcohol withdrawal (Malcolm et al. 1989). Carbamazepine may be best suited for alcoholics who have experienced a previous seizure, regardless of its relationship to alcohol withdrawal. However, more research is needed in this area. In alcoholic patients with their first seizure or those presenting with focal seizures, a work-up for structural lesions should be performed. Seizures in alcoholic patients do not usually indicate epilepsy and do not require prolonged anticonvulsive therapy.

Blocking agents and clonidine reduce adrenergic manifestations of withdrawal from alcohol such as hypertension, tachycardia, and tremor. They can ameliorate withdrawal severity, but the evidence is inadequate to determine their effect on delirium and seizures (Mayo-Smith 1997). They may be used as adjunctive medication in patients who are not at risk of asthma, chronic lung disease, or cardiac failure.

### *Alcoholism*

Considering lifetime prevalence, alcohol abuse/dependence is the most common among psychiatric diagnoses, affecting 13.7 to 23.5% of the U.S. population (Kessler et al. 1994). One researcher estimated that 22 to 26% of admissions to community hospitals in the United States were alcohol-related (Muller 1996). Biochemical tests that suggest alcohol abuse include elevation of uric acid concentrations, mean corpuscular volume, and/or concentrations of liver enzymes in the blood, particularly λ-glutamyltransferase (GGT) and serum aspartate aminotransferase (AST). Carbohydrate-deficient transferrin has a sensitivity of 58 to 70% and a specificity of 82 to 98% for the detection of alcohol abuse and may be useful for monitoring alcohol-dependent patients (Yersin et al. 1995).

The treatment of alcoholism begins with recognition of the problem. Some people will stop or limit their drinking when abuse becomes apparent, such as after accidents, trauma, or counseling by a physician. Project MATCH (Matching Alcoholism Treatments to Client Heterogeneity) compared 1) 12-step facilitation based on the principles of Alcoholics Anonymous, 2) cognitive-behavioral coping skills therapy focusing on lifestyle changes and relapse prevention skills, and 3) individualized motivational enhancement in over 1700 patients. Substantial improvements in drinking behaviors were evidenced in all three groups during the first 12 months of follow-up. No significant differences between the outcomes of the three treatments were found, although severity of psychiatric illness, patient motivation, sex, and severity of sociopathy were important factors influencing drinking outcomes (Project MATCH Research Group 1997). Although a core set of skills is needed by each alcoholic in attaining abstinence, there is no boilerplate for success. Research to better understand which patients benefit maximally from specific therapeutic approaches is ongoing.

Generalist physicians need to screen all their patients for alcohol problems, perform detailed assessments of the problem drinkers, advise and refer patients to Alcoholics Anonymous and specialty services as needed, and monitor alcohol-related medical, behavioral, psychiatric, and social problems. The generalist physician also needs to provide compassionate longitudinal care to the patient and

| | |
|---|---|
| Patient ______________ Date ______________<br>Y M D | Time _______:_______<br>(24 hour clock, midnight=00:00) |
| Pulse or heart rate, taken for one minute: ____________ | Blood pressure ________/________ |
| NAUSEA AND VOMITING—Ask "do you feel sick to your stomach? Have you vomited?" Observation.<br>0 no nausea and no vomiting<br>1 mild nausea with no vomiting<br>2 —<br>3 —<br>4 intermittent nausea with dry heaves<br>5 —<br>6 —<br>7 constant nausea, frequent dry heaves and vomiting | TACTILE DISTURBANCES—Ask "Have you any itching, pins and needles sensations, any burning, any numbness or do you feel bugs crawling on or under your skin?" Observation.<br>0 none<br>1 very mild itching, pins and needles, burning or numbness<br>2 mild itching, pins and needles, burning or numbness<br>3 moderate itching, pins and needles, burning or numbness<br>4 moderately severe hallucinations<br>5 severe hallucinations<br>6 extremely severe hallucinations<br>7 continuous hallucinations |
| TREMOR—Arms extended and fingers spread apart. Observation.<br>0 no tremor<br>1 not visible, but can be felt fingertip to fingertip<br>2 —<br>3 —<br>4 moderate, with patient's arms extended<br>5 —<br>6 —<br>7 severe, even with arms not extended | AUDITORY DISTURBANCES—Ask "Are you more aware of sounds around you? Are they harsh? Do they frighten you? Are you hearing anything that is disturbing to you? Are you hearing things you know are not there?" Observation.<br>0 no present<br>1 very mild harshness or ability to frighten<br>2 mild harshness or ability to frighten<br>3 moderate harshness or ability to frighten<br>4 moderately severe hallucinations<br>5 severe hallucinations<br>6 extremely severe hallucinations<br>7 continuous hallucinations |
| PAROXYSMAL SWEATS—Observations.<br>0 no sweat visible<br>1 barely perceptible sweating, palms moist<br>2 —<br>3 —<br>4 beads of sweat obvious on forehead<br>5 —<br>6 —<br>7 drenching sweats | VISUAL DISTURBANCES—Ask "Does the light appear to be too bright? Is its colour different? Does it hurt your eyes? Are you seeing anything that is disturbing to you? Are you seeing things you know are not there?" Observation.<br>0 not present<br>1 very mild sensitivity<br>2 mild sensitivity<br>3 moderate sensitivity<br>4 moderately severe hallucinations<br>5 severe hallucinations<br>6 extremely severe hallucinations<br>7 continuous hallucinations |
| ANXIETY-Ask "Do you feel nervous?" Observation.<br>0 no anxiety, at ease<br>1 mildly anxious<br>2 —<br>3 —<br>4 moderately anxious, or guarded, so anxiety is inferred<br>5 —<br>6 —<br>7 equivalent to acute panic states as seen in severe delirium or acute schizophrenic reactions | HEADACHE, FULLNESS IN HEAD—Ask "Does your head feel different? Does it feel like there is a band around your head?" Do not for dizziness or lightheadedness. Otherwise, rate severity.<br>0 not present<br>1 very mild<br>2 mild<br>3 moderate<br>4 moderately severe<br>5 severe<br>6 very severe<br>7 extremely severe |
| AGITATION—Observation.<br>0 normal activity<br>1 somewhat more than normal activity<br>2 —<br>3 —<br>4 somewhat more than normal activity<br>5 —<br>6 —<br>7 paces back and forth during most of the interview, or constantly thrashes about. | ORIENTATION AND CLOUDING OF SENSORIUM— Ask "What day is this? Where are you? Who am I?<br>0 oriented and can do serial additions<br>1 cannot do serial additions or is uncertain about date<br>2 disoriented for date by no more than 2 calendar days<br>3 disoriented for date by more than 2 calendar days<br>4 disoriented for place and/or person |
| This scale is not copyrighted and may be used freely. | Total CIW A-A Score ____________<br>Rater's Initials: ____________<br>Maximum Possible Score 67 |

FIGURE 17-3 **Addiction Research Foundation Clinical Institute Withdrawal Assessment for Alcohol (CIWA-A).**

his or her family during times of diagnosis, intervention, treatment, remission, and relapse (O'Conner and Schottenfeld 1998).

### *Pharmacotherapy*

Pharmacotherapies to decrease craving for alcohol, modify drinking behavior, and prevent relapse are being researched. The current therapies—disulfiram, naltrexone, and acamprosate (the latter of which is available only in Europe)—are each adjunctive to counseling strategies and self-help support for the treatment of alcoholism.

Disulfiram (Antabuse) is used to help prevent impulsive drinking in alcoholics. Disulfiram chelates metal ions that are cofactors for enzymes such as ADH and dopamine $\beta$-hydroxylase (DBH). After consumption of alcohol, inhibition of ADH results in accumulation of acetaldehyde with symptoms of flushing, headache, nausea, vomiting, and hypotension. Inhibition of DBH, the enzyme responsible for conversion of dopamine to norepinephrine, may result in impaired cardiovascular reflexes that contribute to the development of hypotension. The disulfiram–alcohol reaction may be quite severe; fatalities have occurred. Serious adverse effects of disulfiram in addition to the disulfiram–alcohol reactions include optic neuritis, peripheral neuropathy, seizures, and hepatitis. Patients must also be counseled about other sources of ethanol including mouthwashes, cough syrups, and cold preparations.

Disulfiram is taken daily, usually in a 250-mg dose. Because the effects of alcohol in the presence of disulfiram are aversive, taking the daily dose of disulfiram represents a commitment not to drink. A large double-blinded controlled study of alcoholic veterans showed that disulfiram was not very effective for maintaining sobriety over extended periods of time (Fuller at al. 1986). The negative findings may reflect the failure of many patients to take the medication as prescribed. Disulfiram may be effective for highly motivated persons when compliance can be monitored (Chick et al. 1992). In addition, disulfiram can be prescribed for short-term use in patients who desire additional, external protection to face temporary high-risk situations. An example of such a situation might include a patient discharged from the hospital after detoxification who needs to enter and engage in further rehabilitative treatment.

Naltrexone was approved by the Food and Drug Administration in 1994 based in part on two 12-week randomized, placebo-controlled trials of patients who were also enrolled in alcohol treatment programs. Those patients receiving naltrexone were both more likely to abstain from alcohol and more likely to drink less alcohol if they returned to drinking, than those who received placebo (O'Malley et al. 1995). Naltrexone's anticraving activity may occur by blocking some of the positive reinforcing effects of alcohol. Naltrexone may also prevent conditioned activation of the endogenous opioid systems that are affected by neuroadaptive changes caused by longer-term exposure to alcohol (Spanagel and Zieglgansberger 1997). Naltrexone can be associated with self-limited nausea (10%) and dose-related hepatotoxicity. Further research is ongoing to clarify the long-term efficacy of naltrexone and the range of settings and psychological approaches needed to maintain its efficacy.

Acamprosate (calcium biacetylhomotaurinate) has proved to be an effective adjuvant agent for treating alcohol dependence in European studies. Treatment with acamprosate resulted in improved 1-year abstinence rates that were dose-dependent. Acamprosate interacts with NMDA-receptor-mediated glutamatergic neurotransmission in various brain regions to reduce $Ca^{2+}$ fluxes through voltage-operated channels. By reducing neuronal hyperexcitability, it is felt that acamprosate elicits its anticraving action via prevention of conditioned responses to alcohol withdrawal (Spanagel and Zieglgansberger 1997).

Pharmacotherapies for alcoholism that are targeted for future development include subtype-specific opiate antagonists, GABAergic agents, dopamine antagonists, and serotonergic agents. Such drugs might be designed to either normalize or block the perpetuation of alcohol-induced neurotransmitter abnormalities (Chick et al. 1996). Research is needed to further define the role of psychosocial treatment in combination with pharmacotherapeutic agents and improve population selection for treatment matching.

### *Fetal alcohol syndrome*

Fetal alcoholism is the most common cause of birth defects that are entirely preventable. More than 80% of children with fetal alcohol syndrome demonstrate prenatal and postnatal growth deficiency, mild-to-moderate mental retardation, infantile irritability, childhood hyperactivity, developmental delay, characteristic facial features, including microcephaly, narrow forehead, short palpebral fissures, poorly developed philtrum, and a long, thin upper lip. Even in the absence of growth retardation or congenital abnormalities, children born to women who drink alcohol excessively during pregnancy are at risk for fetal alcohol effects that include attention deficit disorders with hyperactivity, fine-motor impairment, clumsiness, delays in motor performance, and subnormal intellectual functioning. Affected children may have difficulty understanding spatial and temporal relationships as well as cause-and-effect abstractions. They may show poor concentration, memory deficits, and impaired judgment and abstract reasoning (Streissguth et al. 1991). The incidence of fetal alcohol syndrome and fetal alcohol effects may be as great as 1 in 300 births (Pietrantoni and Knuppel 1991).

The consumption of at least one to two drinks a day is associated with a substantially increased risk of giving birth to a growth-retarded baby. Mothers of children with fully expressed fetal alcohol syndrome drink alcohol more and drink earlier in gestation than those with infants without fully expressed clinical features. There is no established "safe dose" of alcohol for pregnant women. Therefore, the American Academy of Pediatrics (AAP 1993) recommends that women who are pregnant or who are planning a pregnancy abstain from alcohol.

## SEDATIVE-HYPNOTICS

### Pharmacology

The sedative-hypnotic drugs of most clinical importance are the barbiturates and benzodiazepines. Barbiturates and benzodiazepines potentate the actions of the inhibitory neurotransmitter GABA (Eldefrawi and Eldefrawi 1987), which exerts its effects by increasing chloride ion conductance through the neuronal membrane chloride channel. Barbiturates may act by enhancing the binding of GABA to its receptor site on the membrane, possibly by decreasing the rate of dissociation of GABA from its receptor. In high concentrations, barbiturates may depress calcium-dependent action potentials and enhance chloride conduction in the absence of GABA. Because barbiturates act throughout the brain and affect polysynaptic transmission and the reticular activating system at relatively low concentrations, these sites are most sensitive to the actions of barbiturates.

The action of benzodiazepines appears to be mediated by a receptor on the $GABA_A$–chloride ionophore complex that is distributed on postsynaptic neurons in the CNS. By increasing chloride flux, GABA hyperpolarizes cell membranes and inhibits neuronal firing. Benzodiazepines potentate the effects of GABA on the chloride flux and thereby enhance the inhibitory neurotransmitter effects of GABA.

$GABA_A$ receptors are responsible for the anxiolytic properties of benzodiazepines and barbiturates, whereas $GABA_B$ receptors are important in controlling skeletal muscle spasticity. Thus, barbiturates and benzodiazepines are allosteric agonists that act at distinct sites on the $GABA_A$ receptor to promote a chloride ion flux resulting in a hyperpolarizing, inhibitory postsynaptic potential.

The $GABA_A$ receptor consists of at least four subunits; three of these—alpha, beta, and gamma—each contain three to six variants. Omega 1 and omega 11 $GABA_A$ receptors have been identified. The omega 1 site has been associated with the alpha-1 subunit, whereas the omega 11 site appears to be heterogeneous, located on receptors with alpha-2, alpha-3, and alpha-5 subunits (Wieland et al. 1992). Zopiclone (Zolpidem), a cyclopyrrolone, has a binding profile much like that of the classic benzodiazepines but binds with much greater affinity to the omega 1 site. Other site-selective compounds and partial agonists are being developed.

Flumazenil is an allosteric blocking agent at the benzodiazepine site of the GABA receptor with no intrinsic activity of its own. Flumazenil occupies the benzodiazepine site with high affinity and can block the activity of either direct benzodiazepine agonists or inverse agonists. Flumazenil is an antagonist with therapeutic utility in treating benzodiazepine overdose.

Long-term treatment with benzodiazepines in animals is associated with downregulation of brain binding that is associated with the development of behavioral tolerance (Miller, Greenblatt, Barnhill et al. 1987). Conversely, discontinuation of benzodiazepines is associated with upregulation of receptor binding and function of the GABA-receptor complex (Miller, Greenblatt, Roy et al. 1987).

Some investigators have suggested that benzodiazepines, either directly or mediated indirectly through GABA, may exert anxiolytic effects by additionally inhibiting adenosine uptake, acting on 5-hydroxytryptamine (5-HT) systems, and/or modifying the activity of glycine, acetylcholine, dopamine, and norepinephrine brain neurotransmitters. Buspirone—a second-generation anxiolytic with little sedation, muscle relaxation, or abuse potential—has no activity on GABA receptors. Buspirone is a partial agonist at the $5\text{-HT}_{1A}$ receptor and has a weak affinity for dopamine receptors.

The pharmacokinetics, metabolism, and drug interactions of sedative-hypnotics are described in the introduction to this book (and in part 1, Introduction; chapter 8, Treatment of Psychiatric Disorders; and chapter 15, Conscious Sedation and Pain).

### Pharmacodynamics

With increasing concentrations of sedative drugs, there is a progression of signs and symptoms in overdose as summarized in Table 17-5. As was the case for ethanol, tolerance develops rapidly to the depressant effects of sedative-hypnotic drugs.

## Clinical and Therapeutic Issues

### *Acute intoxication*

Sedative-hypnotic drugs are commonly abused and often involved in intentional drug intoxications. Although barbiturates and benzodiazepines are the most important drugs in this class, other drugs that are occasionally abused include chloral hydrate, ethchlorvynol, glutethimide, meprobamate, methaqualone, and methyprylon. For the most part, therapeutic considerations for the latter group resemble those for barbiturates.

Ingestion of excessive quantities of barbiturates results in a progressive metabolic encephalopathy and coma. The signs and symptoms of barbiturate intoxication are summarized in Table 17-7. Intoxication with other sedative-hypnotic drugs produces a similar picture with a few distinctions. Benzodiazepine intoxication is less likely to be associated with respiratory depression or hypotension, unless there is a coingestion of other sedative drugs or alcohol, or after the drug is absorbed extremely rapidly (as occurs with respiratory arrest following IV diazepam or midazolam or oral triazolam).

The time course of sedative-hypnotic drug intoxication depends on the pharmacokinetics of the particular drug. For intermediate-acting barbiturates such as pentobarbital, secobarbital, or amobarbital, and many of the benzodiazepines, intoxication usually resolves within 48 hours. Long-acting barbiturates such as phenobarbital, benzodiazepines such as flurazepam, or ethchlorvynol (the latter of which exhibits dose-dependent metabolism) are associated with prolonged coma that may persist as long as 5 to 7 days. Glutethimide has associated waxing and waning of consciousness, due either to its anticholinergic effects producing intermittent bowel activity and absorption or to enterohepatic recirculation of an active metabolite (see chapter 18, Poisoning).

The management of overdoses of sedative drugs centers on respiratory and cardiovascular support (see chapter 18). Flumazenil, an antagonist at the GABA receptor, reverses the sedation and coma caused by benzodiazepine overdose. Clinical trials in patients with mixed overdoses involving benzodiazepines showed significant improvement in coma scores within 5 minutes when patients treated with flumazenil were compared with placebo controls (O'Sullivan and Wade 1987). The dose was titrated into 0.2- to 0.3-mg increments to a total of 1 mg IV over approximately 5 minutes. A major hazard in using flumazenil is precipitation of acute withdrawal from benzodiazepine, including seizures. The duration of action of flumazenil is relatively short (half-life 60 to 90 minutes) compared with the duration of action of many of the benzodiazepines; repeated doses may be necessary to maintain stable reversal of intoxication. Of concern is the possibility that intoxication with benzodiazepine will be reversed with flumazenil, then the patient will be left unattended, the flumazenil will be eliminated more quickly than the benzodiazepine, and the patient will decompensate and suffer respiratory arrest. For this reason, even with the availability of an antagonist, it is necessary to manage serious benzodiazepine overdoses with careful consistent observation and intensive supportive care.

**PRINCIPLE When the half-life or duration of action of an antidote is considerably shorter than that of the agent causing toxicity, the frequency of dosing becomes crucial to prevent the morbidity of swings in and out of toxicity. Antagonists of benzodiazepines, antagonists of opiates, and cholinergic agonists (in the face of anticholinergic poisoning) illustrate this principle.**

Additional treatments for overdose include hemodialysis (chloral hydrate, phenobarbital) or hemoperfusion (phenobarbital, short-acting barbiturates, ethchlorvynol).

**Table 17-7 Sedative-Hypnotic Drug Intoxication**

| INTOXICATION LEVEL | CLINICAL SYMPTOMS |
|---|---|
| Mild | Sedation |
| | Disorientation |
| | Slurred speech |
| | Ataxia |
| | Nystagmus |
| Moderate* | Coma; arousal by painful stimulation |
| | Depressed or absent deep tendon reflexes |
| | Slow respiration |
| | Absent oculocephalic reflexes |
| | Intact pupillary light reflex |
| Severe | Coma; unarousable |
| | Absent corneal, gag, and deep tendon reflexes |
| | Absent oculocephalic reflexes |
| | Intact pupillary light reflex |
| | Hypothermia |
| | Respiratory depression; apnea |
| | Hypotension; shock |

*May observe in the early phase of intoxication in occasional patients a state of neuromuscular hyperexcitability with increased muscle tone, hyperactive reflexes, ankle clonus, and/or decerebrate posturing.

Repeated doses of oral charcoal accelerate the elimination of phenobarbital by interrupting enteroenteric recirculation but in one study did not shorten the duration of phenobarbital-induced coma (Pond et al. 1984). The control group's tolerance to phenobarbital may have played a role in this negative result.

***Sedative-hypnotic drug withdrawal***

Habitual use of sedative-hypnotic drugs is associated with the development of tolerance. When use of these drugs suddenly ceases, a withdrawal syndrome similar to that of alcohol withdrawal ensues. In general, patients with serious withdrawal syndromes have a history of taking three or more times the usual sedative dose daily for longer than 1 month. However, milder syndromes of abstinence may occur after cessation of usual therapeutic doses (Busto et al. 1986).

The clinical manifestations are similar to those described for alcohol withdrawal, although the incidence of seizures may be higher after withdrawal from high doses of barbiturates (Fraser et al. 1958). Most patients experience anxiety, irritability, agitation, tremor, muscle twitching, insomnia, anorexia, and/or weakness during abstinence. Many develop generalized seizures with or without a subsequent state of delirium. Some patients develop an acute psychosis or delirium without seizures. The time course of withdrawal symptoms depends on the pharmacokinetics of the drug involved. Following cessation of pentobarbital, secobarbital, or amobarbital (half-lives 20 to 24 hours), symptoms usually begin within 8 to 12 hours. The time to peak is 2 to 3 days, and symptoms persist for 6 to 7 days. For phenobarbital and diazepam, with half-lives of 50 to 100 hours or more, symptoms of withdrawal tend to develop 5 to 7 days after cessation of drug use and may persist for several weeks. In general, the immediate magnitude of abstinence symptoms is greater after cessation of short half-life drugs than after cessation of long half-life drugs, which is consistent with the idea that the brain has more time to adapt to changing drug effects when the rate of decline of the concentration of the drug is gradual.

**PRINCIPLE In general, signs of acute withdrawal of potent drugs, whether they act on the CNS or peripheral organs, are more likely to occur with short-acting drugs than they are with long-acting drugs.**

The principal rationale behind "tapering" the doses of such drugs with short half-lives rests on this observation. Consider examples of antihypertensives.

Severe withdrawal symptoms from barbiturates are most commonly seen in patients who abuse many drugs simultaneously (polydrug abusers). In contrast, withdrawal symptoms from benzodiazepines are most commonly seen in patients who are being treated for chronic psychiatric disturbances or anxiety. Once again a drug can cause toxicity that mimics the original signs and symptoms that signaled reason for its use. The anxiety and agitation seen during withdrawal from benzodiazepines may resemble the original condition for which the drug was taken, thereby unfortunately reinforcing chronic use of even more drug. Some patients develop considerable apprehension about the idea of withdrawal from benzodiazepines and may develop anxiety on that basis alone (pseudowithdrawal) (Roy-Byrne and Hommer 1988).

**PRINCIPLE When withdrawal produces effects that are opposite of the original desired effects of a drug, both the patient and therapist may be tempted to give more of that same drug. However, because of problems of tolerance and withdrawal, giving the same drug (or drug class) is a counterproductive strategy that will only worsen the situation.**

Several approaches have been described for treating withdrawal signs and symptoms from sedative-hypnotics (Roy-Byrne and Hommer 1988). When sedative-hypnotics are discontinued, the dose should be gradually reduced to minimize the severity of withdrawal symptoms (DuPont 1990). A schedule of discontinuation over 6 to 12 weeks is reasonable, but sometimes reduction may need to be even more gradual. Usually dose reduction can be accomplished using the same benzodiazepine a person has been taking, but when that approach fails, switching from a short-acting to a long-acting drug (e.g., from lorazepam to diazepam) may make drug withdrawal less disruptive. Typically, such schedules involve loading with a long-acting sedative-hypnotic drug until the symptoms of withdrawal are controlled. Then the patient is stabilized on this dose for a few days, and later the replacement drug is withdrawn at a rate of 10% of the dose every few days until it is totally discontinued.

***Sedative-hypnotic drug addiction***

Sedative-hypnotic drugs are among the most widely prescribed medications. Benzodiazepines were introduced in the mid-to-late 1970s and have largely displaced the barbiturates at this time. In the United States, the overall prevalence of annual use of anxiolytics declined from 11.1% of the adult population in 1979 to 8.3% of the population in 1990 (Balter 1991). Use of hypnotics has remained stable at approximately 2.5% of adults (Balter 1991). Women receive about twice as many prescriptions for benzodiazepines as do men. The use of anxiolytics increases to a peak prevalence in persons ages 50 to 65 years and declines somewhat in older people, whereas use of hypnotics is most frequent in the elderly (Woods et al. 1992). Although many people who receive benzodiazepine prescriptions use the drugs for 4 weeks or less, a substantial minority of persons who receive benzodiazepine prescriptions continue to use the drugs on a regular basis for longer than a year and may become dependent on these drugs. In all patients receiving sedative-hypnotic drugs for prolonged periods of time, the risks of dependence should be discussed, and the risks should be weighed against the benefits.

**PRINCIPLE In particular, a patient should be advised that an increase in anxiety during withdrawal may not mean a return of previous symptoms, that a period of temporary discomfort may be followed by substantial improvement, and that the patient may do better in the long-term without medication.**

A minority of persons addicted to barbiturates, benzodiazepines, and other sedatives are polydrug users who obtain the drugs illegally for "recreational" use. People who have previously abused alcohol or other sedative drugs are at higher risk for abusing sedative drugs again (Busto 1986). Evidence of inappropriate drug-taking behavior includes escalation of the dose, obtaining prescriptions from multiple physicians, or taking the drug for reasons other than that for which it was prescribed.

Supportive therapy and/or addiction counseling is extremely important for persons with sedative-hypnotic dependency. Adjunctive pharmacologic strategies to combat craving have not yet been developed for those with sedative-hypnotic dependency.

#### *Fetal exposure to sedative-hypnotics*

Individual case reports and studies of the use of benzodiazepines in human pregnancy are confounded by alcoholism, the use of tobacco, and other substances, maternal illness including especially psychiatric illness and seizures, and social problems. Cause-and-effect relationships for teratogenic and behavioral abnormalities due to chronic human fetal exposure to benzodiazepines have been reported but have not been proved (McElhatton 1994). Clonazepam, clorazepate, diazepam, lorazepam, midazolam, and oxazepam are excreted into breast milk, although in very low concentrations.

## OPIATES

### Pharmacology

In the CNS, there are $\mu$-, $\kappa$-, and $\delta$-opioid receptors, with evidence for additional classes and subclasses of receptors. Opioid receptors mediate euphoria, preference, analgesia, tolerance, and reward. The $\mu$-opioid receptor also increases mesolimbic dopamine levels, impairs learning and memory processes, facilitates long-term potentiation, and inhibits bladder motility and diuresis. Activation of the $\kappa$-opioid receptor opposes these receptor-mediated actions by involving distinct locations of the two opioid receptors on physiologically different cell types in local neuronal networks throughout the brain and in the spinal cord (Pan 1998). Otherwise, activation of both receptors has similar cellular actions that include the following:

- Inhibiting adenylate cyclase activity and cAMP production through a $G_i$ protein–mediated mechanism
- Increasing $K^+$ efflux that hyperpolarizes neurons
- Depressing neuronal $Ca^{2+}$ entry that lowers free intracellular $Ca^{2+}$ and inhibits transmitter release through the opioid receptors located on presynaptic terminals

The $\delta$-opioid receptor is believed to be the primary receptor for enkephalins—endogenous opioid pentapeptides that are found in the brain, spinal cord, and some peripheral tissues. The $\sigma$-opioid receptor can produce dysphoria and hallucinations caused by opioid drugs, but this receptor is also activated by nonopioid compounds including phencyclidine, and its activity is not reversed by naloxone.

Opiates have therapeutic roles in pain relief, and they have antitussive and antidiarrheal activity. In contrast to local anesthetics that decrease conduction along the axon, $\mu$-mediated opioid analgesia is due to reduced excitability of neuronal membranes. In contrast to nonsteroidal agents, some opioids have mild inflammatory activity due to their release of histamine.

Opiates are an important class of abused drugs. The incentive properties of morphine are felt to be due to at least two mechanisms. There is evidence of $\mu$-mediated hyperpolarization of GABA-containing interneurons that disinhibit dopaminergic neurons in the ventral tegmental area and increase dopamine release in the nucleus accumbens, as well as evidence of dopamine-independent direct activation of neurons in the nucleus accumbens (Nestler 1996). After chronic exposure to opiates, there is a reduction in the size and presumably functioning of these neurons, including an upregulation of the cAMP pathway in the nucleus accumbens. These long-term adaptations oppose the acute effects of opiates but also lead to impairment of mesolimbic dopamine and aversion during withdrawal. Clinically, opiate dose escalation due to tolerance of the "rush" and euphoric effects experienced by drug abusers is more rapid than opiate dose escalation due to tolerance of the analgesic properties in patients with chronic pain.

Although both the dextro- and levo-isomers of opioids have antitussive activity, only the levo-isomer has analgesic properties and dependence liability. The pharmacology, pharmacokinetics, metabolism, and pharmacodynamics of opiates are described more fully in chapter 15, Conscious Sedation and Pain.

## Clinical and Therapeutic Issues

***Opiate intoxication***

Clinical features of opiate intoxication are summarized in Table 17-8. The usual cause of death from opiate intoxication is respiratory arrest, which may occur within a minute of IV injection. After intramuscular or subcutaneous dosing with narcotics such as morphine, respiratory depression peaks 30 to 60 minutes after injection; the interval from dose to peak effect may be even longer after oral dosing. There appears to be a delay between peak concentrations in plasma and peak depression of respiration. The delay is presumably due to a delay of entry of morphine into the brain. After intramuscular, subcutaneous, or oral dosing, a progression of intoxication from sedation and slowing of respiratory rate to coma and respiratory arrest can be expected. Respiratory depression from opiates may be enhanced when patients are receiving barbiturates or other sedative-hypnotics, phenothiazines (including prochlorperazine), or drugs with neuromuscular blocking activity (Reier and Johnstone 1970).

Particular opiates may produce specific manifestations in addition to those described in Table 17-9. Chronic therapy with meperidine, either in high doses or in patients with chronic renal failure, may result in neuromuscular excitability, including myoclonic jerks and convulsions, believed to be due to accumulation of the metabolite normeperidine (Armstrong and Bersten 1986). Propoxyphene intoxication is associated with seizures, diabetes insipidus, and cardiovascular collapse due to myocardial depression, the latter thought to be caused by the metabolite norpropoxyphene (Lawson and Northridge 1987). Methadone produces a typical picture of opiate intoxication, but because of its long half-life, intoxication may be prolonged for a day or longer.

Most signs and symptoms of opiate intoxication are reversed by naloxone. This reversal is an important element in both diagnosing and treating opiate intoxication. Some types of intoxication, however, such as with propoxyphene, may require extremely large doses (more than 10 mg) of naloxone for reversal, and even then, reversal may be incomplete. Some manifestations of intoxication such as seizures may respond poorly or not at all to naloxone. Naloxone in high doses (usually 5 to 10 mg or more) may also have arousal effects in patients with alcohol or benzodiazepine intoxication, and in some patients with stroke. Management of opiate intoxication should be directed toward maintaining a patent airway and adequate ventilation. Naloxone, 0.4 to 2 mg IV, may be administered to reverse opiate intoxication. However, the patient must still be observed for several hours because the effects of naloxone (2 to 3 hours) may be briefer than the effects of many narcotics. Thus late, recurrent intoxication may ensue. In patients with intoxications caused by long-acting opiates such as methadone, continuous infusions or repeated boluses of naloxone may be administered. Alternatively, longer acting naltrexone or nalmefene may be

**Table 17-8 Clinical Features of Opiate Intoxication and Withdrawal**

| |
|---|
| *Intoxication* |
| Drowsiness, stupor, or coma |
| Symmetric, pinpoint, reactive pupils |
| Hypothermia |
| Bradycardia |
| Hypotension |
| Decreased peristalsis |
| Skin cool and moist |
| Hypoventilation (respiratory slowing, irregular breathing, apnea) |
| Pulmonary edema |
| Seizures (meperidine, propoxyphene, morphine) |
| Reversal with naloxone |
| *Withdrawal* |
| Anxiety, restlessness |
| Insomnia |
| Chills, hot flashes |
| Myalgias, arthralgias |
| Nausea, anorexia |
| Abdominal cramping |
| Vomiting, diarrhea |
| Yawning |
| Dilated pupils |
| Tachycardia, hypertension (mild) |
| Hyperthermia (mild), diaphoresis, lacrimation, rhinorrhea |
| Piloerection |
| Spontaneous ejaculation |

**Table 17-9 Manifestations of Intoxication with Cocaine and Other Stimulant Drugs**

| Behavioral or Psychiatric | Autonomic or Neuromuscular |
|---|---|
| Euphoria | Tachycardia† |
| Hyperactivity, irritability* | Hypertension |
| Insomnia | Hyperthermia |
| Mood lability | Dilated pupils |
| Anorexia | Tremulousness* |
| Anxiety, agitation | Seizures |
| Suspiciousness, aggressiveness | Respiratory arrest |
| Psychosis (often paranoid) | Cardiovascular collapse |
| Delirium (agitated) | |
| Stupor | |
| Coma | |

*Particularly neonatal intoxication.
†Except phenylpropanolamine and other primarily $\alpha$-adrenergic agonists, which produce reflex bradycardia.

employed. Pulmonary edema due to intoxication with narcotics probably is a result of increased pulmonary capillary permeability and may take several days to resolve. Severe hypoxemia due to pulmonary edema may require positive pressure mechanical ventilation.

### *Opiate withdrawal*

Prolonged use of opiates leads to tolerance, and, after cessation of use, a withdrawal syndrome may ensue. Tolerance occurs selectively and at different rates for different drug effects. There is a high level of tolerance to the nausea, sedation, and respiratory depression caused by opiates, but relatively little tolerance to the pupillary constrictive or constipative effects of these drugs.

Activation of the locus coeruleus is one of the major determinants of physical opiate withdrawal. The locus coeruleus is a major noradrenergic nucleus located in the brainstem that, in turn, activates large regions of the brain and spinal cord that are involved in the control of autonomic function and attentional states.

Chronic opiate administration increases levels of expression of adenylyl cyclase and protein kinase A in the locus coeruleus. Those increases enhance the intrinsic excitability of neurons (Nestler and Aghajanian 1997). Decreased cAMP increases the conductance of the $K^+$ channel, decreases the $Na^+$-dependent inward current, and decreases the phosphorylation of numerous other proteins thereby altering the regulation of other cellular processes. One of these proteins, CREB, may initiate longer-term changes in locus coeruleus functioning by altering gene expression. In the chronic-treated state, the combined presence of the upregulated cAMP pathway and the opiate helps return locus coeruleus neurons to their normal firing rates. Upon removal of the opiate, the upregulated cAMP pathway is unopposed and contributes to the activation of locus coeruleus neurons during withdrawal. Upregulation of the cAMP pathway is but one of the many molecular adaptations responsible for opiate tolerance and dependence at the cellular level. Factors extrinsic to the locus coeruleus also activate it during opiate withdrawal. For example, several medullary and spinal nuclei incite the nucleus paragigantocellularis to increase glutamatergic neurotransmission to the locus ceruleus (Nestler 1996).

The clinical features of the withdrawal syndrome range from a mild, flu-like illness to more severe symptoms, as described in Table 17-8. The severity of the withdrawal syndrome depends on the frequency, duration, and dose of opiate use, as well as possibly the genetic predisposition of the individual. Withdrawal symptoms generally represent physiologic actions opposite to the acute actions of opioid drugs. For example, pupillary constriction and constipation occur with opiate use, whereas pupillary dilatation and diarrhea occur in the withdrawal state.

Opiate withdrawal is not life-threatening but is associated with severe psychological and moderate physical distress. The onset of withdrawal symptoms typically occurs 8 to 16 hours after cessation of the use of heroin or morphine. Autonomic disturbances and myalgias tend to appear first. By 36 hours, severe restlessness, piloerection, lacrimation, abdominal cramps, and diarrhea become more prominent. Symptoms reach their peak intensity at 48 to 72 hours, and then resolve over 7 to 10 days. Abstinence symptoms after ceasing to use methadone develop more gradually, with an onset of 36 to 72 hours that peaks at about 6 days. Single-dose physical dependence in exaddicts has been demonstrated in both clinical and animal studies. This indicates that one cycle of physical dependence and withdrawal can cause long-lasting changes that increase the liability for recidivism and initiating another cycle of dependence (Heighman et al. 1989).

Treatment of opiate withdrawal includes specific replacement of the opiates and supportive care. Most addicted patients can undergo withdrawal in a supportive environment without medication, experiencing a syndrome resembling influenza. However, the severity of withdrawal can be reduced by medications. The most commonly used replacement medication is methadone, which is usually given at a dosage of 20 to 40 mg/day by mouth as required to make the patient comfortable. After 2 or 3 days of stabilization, the dose can be gradually tapered over 1 to 3 weeks. Inpatient tapers can be performed more quickly.

Clonidine has been used to manage symptoms of opiate withdrawal for persons who have low levels of physical dependence. Typically, clonidine is initiated at 0.1 to 0.2 mg every 8 hours. The dose may then be increased as needed to 0.8 to 1.2 mg/day. Subsequently, clonidine is tapered over a 10- to 14-day period. Clonidine is a central $\alpha$-adrenergic receptor agonist that has mild activity against anxiety, restlessness, and sweating. Clonidine does not relieve dysphoria, myalgias, or abdominal cramps. The main adverse effects of clonidine are drowsiness and hypotension. Nonspecific treatment for opiate withdrawal includes the use of benzodiazepines or chloral hydrate for anxiety and sleep and the use of prochlorperazine for GI symptoms. Propoxyphene and/or NSAIDs may help in treating myalgia. The use of potentially addictive medications such as benzodiazepines and/or propoxyphene should be limited to the relatively brief period of detoxification.

Rapid opioid detoxification using opioid antagonists along with nonopiate symptomatic therapy is unacceptably aversive. Therefore, ultra-rapid opioid detoxification using opioid antagonists under general anesthesia has been initiated in some centers and marketed as a rapid and painless withdrawal procedure. Studies assessing the safety, cost, patient comfort, detoxification completion rate, and rate of continuation in follow-up treatment are, so far, preliminary. For patients dependent on heroin and other opioids, medically aided detoxification is only helpful in preparation for long-term drug-free or opioid-antagonist-maintained rehabilitation (O'Brien 1997). Unfortunately, excepting some specialized populations, there is a high relapse rate under both drug-free and antagonist-maintained conditions.

Buprenorphine is a mixed opiate agonist-antagonist that may have utility in detoxifying and treating persons with opiate dependence (Bickel et al. 1988). Buprenorphine has partial agonist activity with a high affinity for the receptor, and antagonist activity with a low affinity for the receptor. Patients have reported "liking" buprenorphine and its mild opiatelike effects (Johnson et al. 1989). The substitution of buprenorphine for heroin, methadone, or other opiates may precipitate a withdrawal syndrome due to its partial antagonist properties. Therefore, induction onto buprenorphine should be as rapid as possible to keep individuals in treatment and avoid illicit opiate use.

Buprenorphine slowly dissociates from opiate receptors. This causes buprenorphine to have a long duration of action and allows for once-daily administration. Buprenorphine has a poor oral bioavailability, but it is effective both parenterally and sublingually. Although buprenorphine produces only limited withdrawal symptoms when it is abruptly discontinued, it may be more appropriate to gradually reduce the dose if this is indicated (Greenstein et al. 1992). A potential advantage of buprenorphine over methadone is that there is less withdrawal discomfort after cessation of buprenorphine than there is after cessation of methadone. More experience with buprenorphine is needed. Because of buprenorphine's safety and abuse liability profiles, it is hoped that buprenorphine will have an intermediate role between "drug-free" abstinent and methadone maintenance therapies for opiate dependence.

***Opiate addiction***

Since 1965, methadone-maintenance programs have proved to be one of the most effective treatments for intravenous opiate addiction (NIAAA 1988). When properly supervised, a daily dose of 60 to 100 mg of methadone prevents withdrawal, produces no euphoria, and enables patients to return to a normal lifestyle. A landmark study conducted in 1984 of methadone-maintained patients in New York City demonstrated that fewer than 10% of the patients who had been in continuous methadone maintenance treatment before 1978 (the year HIV infection became apparent in New York) were seropositive for HIV, compared with 47% of patients who had not been in continuous methadone maintenance treatment (Novick et al. 1986). Before this study, narcotic abstinence was the ultimate goal of methadone maintenance. Because of the unacceptable risk of acquiring HIV with relapse, methadone maintenance became accepted as a chronic and potentially life-long therapy.

Several studies have indicated that high daily oral doses of methadone are safe when prescribed on a long-term basis. Although most adverse effects disappear after the first 6 months of treatment, increased sweating and chronic constipation have been respectively reported by 48 and 17% of patients after methadone treatment for 3 or more years (Kreek 1973). Patients stabilized on methadone maintenance when compared with normal volunteers and college students with no drug history showed no differences in reaction time, driving ability, intelligence, or attention span (Lowinson et al. 1992). Active opiate addicts are often stressed, malnourished, and exposed to infections. These parameters improve after initiation of methadone maintenance therapy.

Pharmacokinetic interactions are important in the dosing of methadone and other drugs. Methadone dosages may need to be raised in the face of hyperthyroidism or pregnancy. Coadministration of phenytoin, rifampin, or barbiturates may accelerate drug metabolism, precipitating withdrawal symptoms and/or requiring higher doses for methadone maintenance. Fluconazole increases methadone levels probably by impeding cytochrome P450-mediated drug metabolism (Cobb et al. 1998). Elevated methadone levels also occur in patients receiving the HIV-1 protease inhibitors, ritonavir, indinavir, and saquinavir. These elevations are caused by inhibition of liver cytochrome P450 3A4 *N*-dealkylation of methadone (Iribarne et al. 1998). Methadone dosages may need to be adjusted under these circumstances. Although methadone levels are not affected in persons receiving zidovudine, serum zidovudine levels are significantly higher in some methadone-maintained patients (Schwartz et al. 1992).

The high rate of relapse of addicts after detoxification from heroin use may be due to persistent derangement of the endogenous opiate receptor system. Methadone, in adequate daily doses to produce a stable blood level of 150 to 600 ng/mL, compensates for this defect (Dole 1988). Clinical efficacy studies in patients have shown that stability of narcotic concentration is more important than the absolute level. Because there is also a greater than 70% rate of relapse in those who are appropriately tapered from methadone maintenance, methadone is believed to be corrective but not curative (Dole 1988; Dole and Joseph 1978). The time course and extent of reversibility of the chronic adaptive changes due to opiate use and methadone maintenance are not known but have implications for methadone maintenance, abstinence, and antagonist therapies.

The addition of counseling, medical care, and psychosocial services to methadone treatment was studied to determine the efficacy and value of these services. The conclusion after a 6-month study of 92 patients randomized to 1) minimum methadone services (a minimum of methadone 60 mg/d with no other services), 2) standard methadone services (same dose of methadone plus counseling), or 3) enhanced methadone services (same dose of methadone plus counseling and onsite medical/psychiatric, employment, and family therapy) was that these additive services were each associated with major increases in efficacy of methadone maintenance treatment (McLellan et al. 1993).

Federal standards for admission to methadone treatment centers mandate a minimum of 1 year of addiction to opiates as well as current evidence of addiction. Exceptions include recent discharge from a chronic care institution or prison, persons with major medical conditions such as AIDS, and pregnant women. Unfortunately, some state agencies add increasing restrictions on methadone treatment that are not scientifically based. This results in less available and less effective treatment. LAAM (*l*-α-acetylmethadol) and its active metabolites (nor-LAAM and di-nor-LAAM) are opiates with much longer durations of action than that of methadone. LAAM may establish a more stable plasma level than methadone and can be dosed 3 days a week. There is no widespread use of this medication, in part, because federal and state regulations have hampered such use.

**Key Points: The management of pain in patients on opiate maintenance therapy is often regarded as problematic. Remember that with chronic therapy, tolerance develops to the analgesic effects of opiates. Therefore, the usual doses of narcotics may be administered above the maintenance dose of the opiate. Mixed agonist–antagonist narcotics such as pentazocine, butorphanol, nalbuphine, and buprenorphine should be avoided in individuals taking methadone or LAAM maintenance because these drugs may precipitate severe withdrawal symptoms.**

Naltrexone, a long-acting narcotic antagonist, is also available for the treatment of narcotic addiction. As a receptor antagonist, naltrexone blocks the pleasurable effects of heroin. This would be expected to discourage continued drug abuse. Patients must, of course, be fully detoxified from narcotics before beginning antagonist therapy. Naltrexone has not achieved widespread acceptance among addicted persons, but, like disulfiram in alcoholics, naltrexone may be useful for motivated patients who are participating in rehabilitation programs. Unlike disulfiram's effects on alcohol metabolism, naltrexone does not interfere with opiate metabolism, nor cause the build-up of a toxic metabolite. Recovering physicians and other health care professionals who have continued access to narcotics, for example, may respond well to naltrexone treatment (Ling and Wesson 1984).

***Pregnancy and opiate dependence***

The stabilization of opioid-dependent pregnant women on methadone is felt to be more beneficial than the problems associated with ongoing drug use by these patients. Poor nourishment, lifestyle problems, and medical problems including infections all can adversely affect the health of both the mother and the fetus. Symptoms of neonatal abstinence include CNS disturbances such as a high-pitched cry, diminished sleep after feeding, hyperactive Moro reflexes, tremulousness, increased muscle tone, myoclonic jerks, and generalized convulsions. Gastrointestinal disturbances caused by neonatal abstinence include excessive sucking, poor feeding, regurgitation, and loose or watery stools. In addition, autonomic and cardiopulmonary symptoms of neonatal abstinence include sweating, fever, frequent yawning, skin mottling, nasal stuffiness, sneezing, and increased respirations (Finnegan 1986). Neonatal abstinence symptoms can be managed successfully in the hospital with paregoric or phenobarbital, monitoring and supportive therapy.

Small samples of mothers compliant with their methadone and perinatal treatment show reasons for optimism upon evaluation of their children's 5-year outcome. These children function within the normal range in language, perceptual, and developmental skills. However, difficulties inherent in such studies include the inability to fully document a mother's drug intake, pitfalls in separating a drug's organic effects from high-risk obstetric variables, problems in maintaining a cohort of infants for study, and the need to separate drug effects from the profound impact of parenting and home environment (Finnegan and Kandall 1992).

## COCAINE

Data from the 1995 National Household Survey on Drug Abuse (NIDA 1997b) estimated that 1.5 million Americans or 0.7% of the population 12 years old and older were current cocaine users when the study was performed. This number has been essentially level since 1992, after declining from 5.7 million or 3.0% of the population in 1985. Despite diminishing numbers of cocaine users, information collected from the Drug Abuse Warning Network (DAWN) (NIDA 1997a) showed that the number of hospital emergencies associated with the use of cocaine increased from 5000 in 1981 to 29,000 in 1985, and finally to 142,000 in 1995. Crack (freebase cocaine that can be smoked) may be responsible for this trend because its addictiveness and nearly immediate onset of action cause increased toxicity.

### Pharmacology

#### *Mechanism of action*

Cocaine is both a stimulant of the CNS—producing euphoria, mental stimulation, and generalized sympathetic nervous system activation—and a local anesthetic. Cocaine blocks the fast sodium channel, enabling a local anesthetic effect, and it blocks the dopamine reuptake transporter, enabling its psychoactive effects. Cocaine administration leads to increases in synaptic dopamine, norepinephrine, and serotonin. Animal studies have demonstrated that cocaine self-administration is attenuated by blockade of dopamine receptors. Antagonists to the D1 and D2 receptors reduce the acute reinforcing effects of cocaine, whereas agonists of the D3 receptors sensitize or facilitate cocaine self-administration (Koob and Le Moal 1997). Although there are many experimental data to indicate a prominent role for dopamine, it remains likely that significant interactions between other neurochemical mediator systems will be discovered that modulate the reinforcing actions of cocaine and related compounds. Ongoing research suggests potential roles of 5-HT, glutamate, opiates, and corticotropin releasing factor.

#### *Preparations and routes of administration*

Cocaine is an ester of benzoic acid and a nitrogen-containing base. Cocaine occurs naturally in the leaves of *Erythroxylon coca* and other species of *Erythroxylon* indigenous to Peru, Bolivia, Colombia, and Java.

Cocaine hydrochloride is frequently snorted (insufflation) or "tooted" in "lines" or "rails" about 1.5 to 2 inches long and 0.125 inch thick. From a street purchase of a single gram of cocaine, about 30 lines can be made, each averaging 10 to 35 mg of powder. The actual amount of cocaine hydrochloride present in each line depends on the purity of the drug. The bioavailability of intranasal cocaine is about 60%. Peak plasma levels occur over a range of 30 minutes to 2 hours (Barnett et al. 1981). Intranasal cocaine limits its own absorption by causing vasoconstriction of the nasal mucous membranes. Cocaine is a topical anesthetic and will cause numbness of the nose during snorting. Nasal congestion with stuffiness and sneezing may occur.

Cocaine can also be injected intravenously. This is called "shooting" or "mainlining." The cocaine is mixed in a spoon or bottle cap with water to form a solution. Unlike heroin, cocaine hydrochloride does not need to be heated to enter into solution. "Kicking" or "booting" refers to drawing blood from the vein back into the syringe and reinjecting it with each cocaine mixture. Following intravenous administration, peak plasma levels are achieved almost instantaneously.

Freebase cocaine is obtained by extracting cocaine hydrochloride with an alkaline solution such as buffered ammonia, and then mixing it with a solvent, which is usually ether. The solvent fraction is separated and volatilized, leaving very small amounts of residual freebase material. Cocaine freebase is most often smoked in a water pipe with a fine stainless steel screen upon which the cocaine is vaporized. Cocaine hydrochloride is soluble in water and has a melting point of 195° C. In contrast, cocaine freebase is lipid soluble and has a melting point of 98° C. Thus, cocaine freebase vaporizes and is readily inhaled and absorbed through the lungs (DePetrillo 1985). This results in nearly immediate peak plasma levels that are achieved at a rate similar to that of injecting cocaine hydrochloride.

"Crack" or "rock" is a prepared, ready-to-use form of freebase cocaine that is inexpensive and has been widely available since 1985 on the streets in many U.S. cities. It is processed from cocaine hydrochloride to a freebase by adding ammonia or baking soda and water and heating it rather than the more volatile method of preparation that uses ether.

Users frequently take cocaine in combination with other drugs, citing the need to take the edge off the abrupt effects and "crash" from cocaine. Intravenous injection of heroin and cocaine mixed together is called "speedballing," and ingesting alcohol in conjunction with taking cocaine may be referred to as "liquid lady." Any drug combination is possible, and other opioids, depressants, as well as hallucinogens, PCP, and marijuana are all frequently used in conjunction with cocaine.

## Pharmacokinetics, Metabolism, and Assays

Cocaine is readily absorbed from a variety of sites, including mucous membranes and the GI tract. It is hydrolyzed by plasma and liver cholinesterase to ecgonine methyl ester, and it undergoes nonenzymatic hydrolysis to benzoylecgonine. In addition, a small amount of cocaine is *N*-demethylated to norcocaine. The plasma half-life of cocaine averages 60 to 90 minutes after IV administration but is longer—up to several hours—after snorting or oral administration. The latter presumably is due to continued absorption across mucous membranes or from the GI tract.

Urine screens for cocaine primarily detect the metabolite benzoylecgonine, which has a much longer half-life (8 hours) than does the parent compound. Cocaine metabolites can be detected in urine specimens as early as 4 hours and as long as 48 hours after inhalation (Quandt et al. 1988). Blood toxicology can be performed, but its utility in screening for cocaine use is limited by its high cost and the rapid disappearance of active cocaine from the bloodstream. Hair analysis, which provides a 2- to 6-month window of drug detection (Henderson et al. 1996), can be particularly useful in assessing gestational cocaine exposure and in forensics. However, relatively complex laboratory methods, confounding hair care preparations, and gender and ethnic differences in the rate of cocaine incorporation into the hair, all limit the use of this technology (Karch 1995).

## Cocaethylene

When alcohol use precedes cocaine use, the normal hydrolysis of cocaine to benzoylecgonine by hepatic carboxyesterase enzymes is inhibited, and higher levels of cocaine remain.

> **Key Point: Cocaethylene is the only known example in which the human body forms a new psychoactive compound from two other psychoactive substrates. Cocaine and ethanol react in the body to form cocaethylene. (Schechter 1994).**

Cocaethylene is bound to human serum proteins and has a plasma half-life three to five times that of cocaine. Cocaethylene has a greater cardiac toxicity than cocaine. It causes substantial and sustained increases in heart rate and blood pressure, and decreases in ventricular contractility. In addition to MIs, cerebrovascular accidents, and arrhythmias, cocaethylene may contribute to seizures and liver damage, and it may compromise function of the immune system (Andrews 1997).

### *Pharmacodynamics*

Tolerance develops quickly and completely to the euphoric and other subjective effects of cocaine. Tolerance develops only incompletely to the cardiovascular effects of cocaine (Ambre et al. 1988). Thus, a situation may evolve in which cocaine is repeatedly used to seek the cocaine high with the consequence being progressive cardiovascular toxicity.

> **PRINCIPLE When tolerance develops more quickly to pleasurable effects than to toxic effects, the stage is set for the addict to ingest larger doses of the drug of abuse, preslispasing to increasingly severe toxicity.**

### *Drug interactions with cocaine*

The most important concern for drug interactions with cocaine involves blockade of catecholamine uptake, resulting in enhanced sensitivity to catecholamines. For example, when epinephrine is coadministered with cocaine, excessive hypertension may result. Because cocaine results in release of catecholamines, including epinephrine, which has both $\alpha$- and $\beta$-adrenergic receptor agonist activity, administration of a nonspecific blocking agent such as propranolol may result in unopposed $\alpha$-adrenergic receptor activity, enhancement of vasoconstriction, and aggravation of hypertension (Ramoska and Sacchetti 1985). Cocaine is metabolized in part by cholinesterases. Individuals with genetic differences of pseudocholinesterase activity and who are abnormally sensitive to succinylcholine may eliminate cocaine more slowly (Jatlow et al. 1979). Patients receiving cholinesterase inhibitors, such as pyridostigmine for treatment of myasthenia gravis, may be more sensitive to the effects of cocaine.

## Clinical and Therapeutic Issues

***Intoxication and medical complications***

The clinical picture of intoxication with cocaine is summarized in Table 17-9. A number of complications that may be life-threatening have been reported with cocaine intoxication (see Table 17-10). The most significant of those involves excessive sympathetic neural stimulation and includes severe hypertension that may be complicated by stroke or aortic dissection, cardiac arrhythmias that may include ventricular fibrillation, and sudden death. In addition, vasoconstriction can lead to ischemia of the heart, kidney, and GI tract. The other major complications involve the CNS. The most important ones are headache that may be due to hypertension or to a migrainelike mechanism, seizures, and stroke. Treatment is life support and symptom-specific therapies such as anticonvulsants, antihypertensive agents, oxygen, and physical cooling techniques.

In the case of a massive cocaine overdose, patients are likely to present with advanced cardiorespiratory distress and seizures. Intoxicated persons who seek assistance with less severe cocaine complications are more likely to present with panic, irritability, hyperreflexia, paranoia, hallucinations, and stereotyped repetitive movements. Assurance in a calm nonthreatening environment is helpful. Because cocaine has a relatively short half-life, acute intoxication usually resolves within 6 hours.

***Obstetric and pediatric complications***

There is a physiological basis for concerns about cocaine exposure effecting fetal development. Like other drugs of abuse, cocaine readily crosses the placental barrier. Because of the fetus's immature metabolic, hepatic, and renal systems, the drug is poorly metabolized, and as a consequence the half-life is longer (Chasnoff and Schnoll 1987). Cocaine interferes with the reuptake of catecholamines at synapses leading to altered circulating levels of neurotransmitters. Maternal intake of cocaine results in increased fetal systolic blood pressure, decreased uterine blood flow, and decreased fetal oxygenation.

**Table 17-10 Medical Complications of Cocaine Intoxication**

| |
|---|
| Cardiovascular |
|   Hypertension |
|     Intracranial hemorrhage |
|     Aortic dissection or rupture |
|   Arrhythmias |
|     Sinus tachycardia |
|     Supraventricular tachycardias |
|     Ventricular tachyarrhythmias |
|   Organ ischemia |
|     Myocardial ischemia and infarction |
|     Renal infarction |
|     Intestinal infarction |
|     Limb ischemia |
|   Myocarditis |
|   Shock |
| Central Nervous System |
|   Headache |
|   Seizures |
|   Transient focal neurologic deficits |
|   Stroke |
|     Subarachnoid hemorrhage |
|     Intracranial hemorrhage |
|     Cerebral infarction |
|     Embolic (endocarditis) |
|   Toxic encephalopathy or coma |
|   Neurologic complications |
| Respiratory |
|   Pneumomediastinum |
|   Pneumothorax |
|   Pulmonary edema |
|   Respiratory arrest |
| Metabolic and other |
|   Hyperthermia |
|   Rhabdomyolysis |
|   Wound botulism |
|   Tetanus |

Maternal cocaine use may result in complications of labor and delivery as well as influence the outcome of pregnancy. Increases in spontaneous abortion, preterm labor, and abruptio placentae have all been noted (Chasnoff et al. 1989). There are also reports of cocaine-exposed infants with ileal atresia and genitourinary abnormalities including ambiguous genitalia, hypospadias, "prune belly," and hydronephrosis. Seizures and cerebral infarction are rare but serious. Neonates born to mothers using cocaine may be hyperactive, irritable, and tremulous and may be at increased risk for sleep apnea.

However, the findings on the consequences of prenatal cocaine exposure relative to child development are inconsistent. Although initial research suggested significant developmental and/or neurobehavioral abnormalities for infants prenatally exposed to cocaine, findings from recent studies have been less negative. When researchers controlled for confounding factors such as age, race, socioeconomic status, and other drug use, especially including tobacco, fewer differences in growth, morphology, and neurobehavioral development have been found (Richardson and Day 1994).

***Chronic cocaine use, withdrawal, and addiction***

Euphoria, increased energy and libido, decreased appetite, hyperalertness, and increased self-confidence occur when small initial doses of cocaine are taken. Exaggerated responses such as grandiosity, impulsivity, hyperawareness of the environment, and hypersexuality also may occur.

Cocaine euphoria is brief, with an initial 10- to 20-second "rush" that is followed by 15 to 20 minutes of a lower level of euphoria and the subsequent onset of irritability and craving. Abstinence after habitual use of cocaine has been associated with neuropsychiatric symptoms (Gawin and Kleber 1986). A cocaine "crash," a state of profound exhaustion, sometimes accompanied by anxiety, depression, and a craving for cocaine, has been described. Decreased energy, anhedonia, hypersomnolence, and hyperphagia ensue and may last for weeks or months. An intense desire for cocaine to ameliorate the severity of the abstinence syndrome commonly leads to relapse, thus sustaining addiction. Suicidal ideation is common in the cocaine-abstinent state.

**Key Points: Compulsive use of cocaine appears to be motivated both by a craving for the cocaine-induced high and by relief of the postcocaine depression.**

Cocaine users who try to maintain the euphoric state readminister the drug frequently until their supply disappears. Cocaine binges average 12 hours but can last for 7 days. In search for the elusive "high," the addict takes increased doses of cocaine with more rapid routes of administration and increased frequency. In contrast to the excess synaptic neurotransmitters, including dopamine associated with acute cocaine intoxication, chronic cocaine administration is believed to result in depletion of neurotransmitters. With chronic and increased use there is increased drug toxicity, dysphoria, and depression. The addict has irresistible cravings. Although focused on memories of cocaine euphoria, he or she has a progressive inability to attain this state and suffers adverse physical, psychological, and social sequelae. Loved ones are neglected, responsibility becomes immaterial, financial hardships occur, and nourishment, sleep, and health care are ignored. Fortunately, unlike the animal models of cocaine dependency, most persons addicted to cocaine deplete their drug supplies or are confronted by the harsh reality of their losses before death ensues.

The first goal of treatment is to interrupt recurrent binges or daily use of cocaine and overcome drug craving. Treatment should include daily or multiple weekly contacts, urine monitoring, limiting exposure to high-risk situations, and emphasizing positive lifestyle changes. The physician treating patients who have discontinued using cocaine should counsel the patient about the depression that follows cessation of use and the likelihood of recurrent intense craving to use the drug for several months.

***Pharmacological treatments***

Clinical researchers have tried to identify drugs to reduce cocaine craving and prevent relapse. Numerous drugs looked promising in initial open-label trials but have not proven efficacious in subsequent placebo-controlled studies. These pharmacological treatments have included dopaminergic agonists (e.g., monoamine oxidase inhibitors, amantadine, mazindol, methylphenidate, pemoline, bromocriptine, levodopa, pergolide), neurotransmitter precursors (L-tyrosine, L-tryptophan, multivitamins with B complex), carbamazepine, and antidepressants including desipramine and fluoxetine. Clinical trials with bupropion, olanzapine, naltrexone, buprenorphine, and other drugs are ongoing. As the understanding of the neurobiological basis of cocaine addiction becomes further refined, new pharmacological strategies are emerging. Potential targets include specific dopamine, 5-HT, and other receptor subtypes, neuroendocrine peptides (i.e., corticotropin-releasing factor), and biogenic amine transporters including the dopamine reuptake transporter.

***Development of a cocaine vaccine***

Instead of pharmacologically interfering with cocaine's actions on the CNS, vaccination prevents cocaine from reaching this site of action (Landry 1997). Active immunization enables the body to produce its own antibody to cocaine in contrast to passive immunization that provides the antibody. Researchers have developed a cocainelike compound that, when injected into the rat, causes it to produce an antibody to cocaine so that the cocaine antibody complex cannot cross the blood–brain barrier (Carrera et al. 1995). Others have developed monoclonal antibodies which when passively administered, increase the hydrolysis of cocaine to inactive metabolites by lowering the energy of activation of this reaction (Landry and Yang 1997). To be effective, either vaccine must produce enough antibodies and must act rapidly enough to prevent cocaine from reaching the brain. Boosters may be needed to ensure adequate quantity of antibodies. Because rodents metabolize cocaine primarily in the liver, whereas humans also metabolize cocaine by cholinesterase in the blood, human trials will be critical in vaccine development. With immunization, the antibodies made by the body should react specifically with cocaine and not form additional antibodies that react against other drugs or nutrients, and should not form autoantibodies that react against the body.

## MARIJUANA

Research has recently defined the presence of a cannabinoid (CB) receptor and the existence of an endogenous cannabinoid, anandamide, which is an ethanolamide derivative of arachidonic acid. $CB_1$ receptors are predominantly in the brain and peripheral nervous system, whereas $CB_2$ receptors appear to be exclusive to immune system tissues. Additional subtypes of cannabinoid receptors may still be discovered. There is evidence that cannabinoids such as anandamide contribute not only to the control of pain transmission within the CNS but that they also attenuate pain behavior produced by chemical damage to cutaneous tissue by interacting with peripheral $CB_1$-like and $CB_2$-like receptors (Calignano et al. 1998). Anandamide and THC have both been shown to be vasorelaxants in the rat cerebral vasculature. Cannabinoids may cause this relaxation through the stimulation of arachidonic acid metabolism because these effects are sensitive to indomethacin (Ellis et al. 1995). Anandamide is produced by endothelial cells. It has been proposed that endogenous cannabinoids, through inhibition of adenylate cyclase and N-type $Ca^{2+}$ channels and activation of $K^+$ channels, may mediate the nitric oxide- and prostanoid-independent component of endothelium-dependent relaxations (Randall and Kendall 1998).

Cannabinoids are contained in the leaves and resin of the common hemp plant *Cannabis sativa.* $(-)$Delta$^9$ tetrahydrocannabinol (or THC), the major psychoactive compound; 11-OH-delta$^9$-THC, an active metabolite of THC; cannabinol, which has weak bioactivity; and cannabidiol, which is inactive; are all plant cannabinoids. Marijuana—the dried *Cannabis* leaf material—contains 2 to 4% THC, whereas hashish—a dried resinous material—contains approximately 10 times this amount. However, some marijuana has been found to have THC content as high as 20%.

Marijuana is sometimes taken orally and cooked in foods (such as marijuana brownies). Primarily, however, it is smoked in cigarettes (joints) or pipes. The onset of peak intoxication is delayed 15 to 30 minutes after smoking, making dosage titration more difficult than that with some other drugs (Morgan 1988). THC is extremely lipid-soluble. Its effects generally last 4 to 6 hours, and it has a half-life of several days, representing slow release from adipose and other tissues. THC is extensively metabolized by the liver. Urine tests can detect marijuana 3 to 5 days after a single use, and up to 5 weeks in chronic users. Positive urine testing indicates that the individual has used or has been exposed to marijuana sometime in the past, but it does not indicate a level of impairment.

Marijuana produces euphoria, relaxation, altered sense of time, depersonalization, and ultimately sleepiness. Emotional liability including anxiety, fear, panic, and even acute psychosis may result, especially with higher doses of THC. Short-term memory is impaired, as is the ability to execute multiple sequential tasks. Physiologic effects include tachycardia, tremulousness, and conjunctival injection. Orthostatic hypotension occasionally occurs (Benowitz and Jones 1975). Smoking marijuana exposes persons to carbon monoxide, carcinogenic combustion products, and numerous pathogenic bacteria and fungi. Chronic irritation of the respiratory system is similar to that of tobacco.

The primary clinical problems with marijuana are acute intoxication and an increased risk of accidents with automobiles and other machinery. This is most often due to sedation, impaired reaction time, and problems with attentiveness, judgment, and coordination. Treatment of THC intoxication primarily involves reassurance and supportive care. The use of benzodiazepines may be useful in managing panic reactions.

A withdrawal syndrome has not been clearly defined after chronic cannabinoid use, presumably because of the long half-life of these compounds. However, nervousness, tension, restlessness, sleep disturbances, and anxiety have been described in humans, monkeys, and rats after the abrupt discontinuation of long-term cannabinoid administration. When a competitive $CB_1$ antagonist is administered to cannabinoid-dependent rats, increased release of corticotropin releasing factor and induction of c-fos in the central nucleus of the amygdala and other stress-responsive nuclei were observed (Rodriquez de Fonseca et al. 1997). Other researchers found that cannabinoids activate the mesolimbic dopamine system by a $\mu$-opioid receptor mechanism common to that invoked by heroin (Tanda et al. 1997). Because final activation of the mesolimbic dopamine system and the withdrawal response are similar to actions produced by alcohol, cocaine, and opiates, some researchers speculate that cannabinoid abuse primes the brain for further alterations by other drugs of abuse (Wickelgren 1997b).

It is unclear the extent to which marijuana contributes to infertility and teratogenicity in the developing fetus. Marijuana does diminish luteinizing hormone levels in both females and males. There have been reports that 4 to 16 joints per week of marijuana for a 4-week period lessens sperm concentrations and causes Leydig and Sertoli cell dysfunction (Wenger et al. 1992). In animal studies, THC produces adverse effects on gametogenesis, embryogenesis, and postnatal development. The American Academy of Pediatrics is concerned about the potential harm that chronic marijuana use may cause to adolescents undergoing hormonal development, in addition to its negative effects on their learning, memory, and social development (AAP 1991).

Spurred by ballot initiatives in California and Arizona, the use of medicinal marijuana is being further studied. After reviewing the literature from 1975 to 1996, two investigators concluded that THC may be useful as an antiemetic with cancer chemotherapy and as an appetite enhancer in persons with severe wasting disease (Voth and Schwartz 1997). Although efficacy was often associated with a sensation of intoxication, oral THC (also called dronabinol) in doses of 5 to 15 $mg/m^2$ was effective in treating nausea associated with cancer chemotherapy if patients were pretreated and the doses were repeated at 3 to 6 hour intervals for approximately 24 hours. Voth and Schwartz did not find a role for THC in treating glaucoma or the spasms of multiple sclerosis. In the case of glaucoma, although cannabinoid applications decrease intraocular pressure, they need to be taken on a chronic basis to do so, and they do not affect the underlying disease process. With multiple sclerosis, THC worsened rather than improved posture and balance when studied in a double-blind, randomized, placebo-controlled trial.

THC and synthetic cannabinoids may have a role in the therapeutic armamentarium. However, inhaling crude marijuana is associated with exposure to toxic gases, chemicals, and microorganisms. Using purer forms of the cannabinoids, and using routes of administration other than smoking, are needed to optimize medicinal activity.

## ANABOLIC STEROIDS

Although this chapter primarily discusses abuse of psychoactive drugs, the abuse of anabolic steroids is also discussed because it presents a substance abuse problem of current public health concern. Anabolic steroid abuse is an example of drug abuse that is primarily reinforced by the anticipated physical effects rather than psychological effects of the drug. These hormones are used by athletes to increase muscle mass and strength. Anabolic steroid use is commonplace in professional sports and in college and even high school athletics (Yesalis et al. 1993). The prototype anabolic steroid is testosterone. The ratio of testosterone to epitestosterone has been used to help detect the presence of exogenous testosterone in urine drug tests (Catlin and Murray 1996). Testosterone has both androgenic and anabolic effects; the androgenic effects are relatively undesirable for athletes. Synthetic hormones such as ethylestrenol, methandrostenolone, methandienone, nandrolone, oxandrolone, oxymetholone, stanozolol, testosterone cypionate, and others have reduced androgenic/anabolic potency ratios compared with testosterone.

Anabolic steroids are thought to enhance muscle mass in three ways:

- Protein synthesis is increased owing to binding of steroids to DNA with increased transcription of RNA and enhanced protein synthesis.
- The catabolic effects of glucocorticoid release by stress are blocked.
- A state of euphoria and diminished fatigue, and possibly more aggressive behavior that promotes more intensive weight training, may result.

Although not a primary reason for abuse, the euphoric effects of high doses of anabolic steroids could contribute to persistent abuse or dependence (Kashkin and Kleber 1989).

The doses of anabolic steroids used by athletes are 10 to 100 times as high as those prescribed for medical indications. The various steroids are often used in combination, such as an oral and an injectable, and are commonly used in cycles of a couple of months or so, alternating with intervals with no use or low-dose steroids, with complete cessation 1 to 2 months before competition at which the urine will be tested. It has been shown that supraphysiologic doses of testosterone enanthate (600 mg per week for 10 weeks), especially when combined with strength training, increases fat-free mass, muscle size, and strength in normal men (Bhasin et al. 1996). The effects of higher doses of steroids, more chronic administration, or "stacking" androgenic and anabolic steroids are not well known.

There are several toxicities that are of concern attendant on high-dose androgenic steroid use (Council on Scientific Affairs 1988; Bagatell and Bremner 1996). Psychiatric disturbances including mental changes, manic-depressive illness, and paranoid psychosis have been described. Liver disease—particularly peliosis hepatitis, cholestasis, and hepatomas—have been associated with chronic medicinal use of androgenic steroids and have been a concern in athletes as well. Anabolic steroids may increase low-density lipoprotein and decrease high-density lipoprotein cholesterol concentrations and increase blood pressure, all of which could increase the risk of coronary heart disease. Reproductive concerns include oligospermia and testicular atrophy in men and menstrual abnormalities in women. The development of gynecomastia in men and masculinization in women may also be seen. The major role of the physician in treating the abuse of androgenic steroids involves a recognition of use and counseling. Perhaps most important is the involvement of the physician as a community resource to describe the potential hazards of androgenic steroid use.

## REFERENCES


[AA] Alcoholics Anonymous. 1988. *12 Steps and 12 Traditions*. New York: Alcoholics Anonymous World Services, pp. 7–11

[AAP] American Academy of Pediatrics. 1991. Marijuana: a continuing concern for pediatricians. *J Pediatr* **88**(5):1070–2.

[AAP] American Academy of Pediatrics. 1993. Fetal alcohol syndrome and fetal alcohol effects. *J Pediatr* **91**(5):1004–6.

Ambre JJ, Belknap SM, Nelson J, et al. 1988. Acute tolerance to cocaine in humans. *Clin Pharmacol Ther* **44**:1–8.

[APA] American Psychiatric Association. 1994. *Diagnostic and Statistical Manual of Mental Disorders*. 4th ed. (DSM-IV). Washington, DC: American Psychiatric Association, pp. 175–272.

Andrews P. 1997. Cocaethylene toxicity. *J Addict Dis* **16**(3):75–84.

Armstrong PJ, Bersten A. 1986. Normeperidine toxicity. *Anesth Analg* **65**:536–8.

Bagatell CJ, Bremner WJ. 1996. Androgens in men—uses and abuses. *N Engl J Med* **334**:707–14.

Balster RL. 1994. Drug and substance abuse. In: Brody TM, Larner J, Minneman KP, et al., editors. *Human Pharmacology: Molecular to Clinical.* 2nd ed. St. Louis, MO: Mosby, pp. 435.

Balter MB. 1991. Benzodiazepine use/abuse: An epidemiologic appraisal. Paper presented at the symposium "Triplicate Prescription: Issues and Answers," New York, NY, February 28, 1991.

Barnett G, Hawks R, Resnick R. 1981. Cocaine pharmacokinetics in humans. *J Ethnopharmacol* **3**:353–66.

Benowitz NL. 1988. Pharmacologic aspects of cigarette smoking and nicotine addiction. *N Engl J Med* **319**:1318–30.

Benowitz NL. 1995. Clinical pharmacology of transdermal nicotine. *Eur J Pharm Biopharm* **41**:168–74.

Benowitz NL. 1996. Pharmacology of nicotine: Addiction and therapeutics. *Annu Rev Pharmacol Toxicol* **36**:597–613.

Benowitz NL, Jacob P III, Savanapridi C. 1987. Determinants of nicotine intake while chewing nicotine polacrilex gum. *Clin Pharmacol Ther* **41**:467–73.

Benowitz NL, Jones RT. 1975. Cardiovascular effects of prolonged delta-9-tetrahydrocannabinol ingestion. *Clin Pharmacol Ther* **18**:287–97.

Benowitz NL, Zevin S, Jacob P III. 1998. Suppression of nicotine intake during ad libitum cigarette smoking by high dose transdermal nicotine. *Pharmacol Exp Ther* **287**(3):958–62.

Bhasin S, Storer TW, Berman N, et al. 1996. The effects of supraphysiologic doses of testosterone on muscle size and strength in normal men. *N Engl J Med* **335**:1–7.

Bickel WK, Stitzer ML, Bigelow GE, et al. 1988. A clinical trial of buprenorphine: Comparison with methadone in the detoxification of heroin addicts. *Clin Pharmacol Ther* **43**:72–8.

Bien TH, Miller WR, Tonigan JS. 1993. Brief interventions for alcohol problems: A review. *Addiction* **88**:315–36.

Boston Collaborative Drug Surveillance Program. 1973. Decreased clinical efficacy of propoxyphene in cigarette smokers. *Clin Pharmacol Ther* **14**:259–63.

Brown RL, Rounds LA. 1995. Conjoint screening questionnaires for alcohol and drug abuse. *Wisconsin Med J* **94**:135–40.

Busto U. 1986. Patterns of benzodiazepine abuse and dependence. *Br J Addict* **81**:94–7.

Busto U, Sellers EM, Naranjo CA, et al. 1986. Withdrawal reaction after long-term therapeutic use of benzodiazepines. *N Engl J Med.* **315**:854–9.

Calignano A, LaRana G, Giuffrida A, et al. 1998. Control of pain initiation by endogenous cannabinoids. *Nature* **394**:277–84.

Carrera MRA, Ashley JA, Parsons LH, et al. 1995. Suppression of psychoactive effects of cocaine by active immunization. *Nature* **378**:727–30.

Catlin DH, Murray TH. 1996. Performance-enhancing drugs, fair competition and Olympic sport. *JAMA* **276**:231–7.

[CDC] Centers for Disease Control and Prevention. 1996. Projected smoking-related deaths among youth—United States. *Morb Mortal Wkly Rep* **45**(44):971–4.

Charlton A. 1994. Children and passive smoking: A review. *J Fam Pract* **38**(3):267–77.

Chasnoff IJ, Griffith DR, MacGregor S, et al. 1989. Temporal patterns of cocaine use in pregnancy. *JAMA* **261**:1688–9.

Chasnoff IJ, Schnoll SH. 1987. Consequences of cocaine and other drug use in pregnancy. In: Washton A, Gold MS, editors. *Cocaine: A Clinician's Handbook.* New York: Guilford Press, pp. 241–51.

Chick J, Erickson CK, and the Amsterdam Consensus Conference Participants. 1996. Conference summary: Consensus conference on alcohol dependence and the role of pharmacotherapy in its treatment. *Alcohol Clin Exp Res* **20**:391–402.

Chick J, Gough K, Falkowski W, et al. 1992. Disulfiram treatment of alcoholism. *Br J Psychiatry* **161**:84–9.

Cobb MN, Desai J, Brown LS Jr., et al. 1998. The effect of fluconazole on the clinical pharmacokinetics of methadone. *Clin Pharmacol Ther* **63**:655–62.

Council on Scientific Affairs. 1988. Drug abuse in athletes: Anabolic steroids and human growth hormone. *JAMA* **259**:1703–5.

Deanfield J, Wright C, Krikler S, et al. 1984. Cigarette smoking and the treatment of angina with propranolol, atenolol, and nifedipine. *N Engl J Med* **310**:951–4.

Deitrich RA, Palmer JD. 1994. Alcohol. In: Brody TM, Larner J, Minneman KP, et al., editors. *Human Pharmacology: Molecular to Clinical.* 2nd ed. St. Louis, MO: Mosby, pp. 423–34.

DePetrillo P. 1985. Getting to the base of cocaine. *Emerg Med* **8**:8.

[DHHS] Department of Health and Human Services, Public Health Service. 1988. The Health Consequences of Smoking: Nicotine Addiction. A Report to the Surgeon General. DHHS Publication No. (CDC) 88–8406. Washington, DC: US Government Printing Office.

Dole VP. 1988. Implications of methadone maintenance for theories of narcotic addiction. *JAMA* **260**:3025–9.

Dole VP, Joseph H. 1978. Long term outcome of patients treated with methadone maintenance. *Ann NY Acad Sci* **311**:181–9.

Dollery C, Brennan PJ. 1988. The Medical Research Council Hypertension Trial: The smoking patient. *Am Heart J* **115**:276–81.

DuPont RL. 1990. A physician's guide to discontinuing benzodiazepine therapy. *West J Med* **152**:600–3.

Eastwood GL. 1997. Is smoking still important in the pathogenesis of peptic ulcer disease? *J Clin Gastroenterol* **25**(Suppl 1):S1–S7.

Edwards G, Arif A, Hodgson R. 1982. Nomenclature and classification of drug- and alcohol-related problems: A shortened version of a WHO memorandum. *Br J Addict* **77**:3–20.

Eldefrawi AT, Eldefrawi ME. 1987. Receptors for $\gamma$-aminobutyric acid and voltage-dependent chloride channels as targets for drugs and toxicants. *FASEB J* **1**:262–71.

Ellis EF, Moore SF, Willoughby KA. 1995. Anadamide and delta-9-THC dilation of cerebral arterioles is blocked by indomethacin. *Am J Physiol* **269**:H1859–64.

Ewing JA. 1984. Detecting alcoholism: The CAGE questionnaire. *JAMA* **252**:1905–7.

Finnegan LP. 1986. Neonatal abstinence syndrome: Assessment and pharmacotherapy. In: Rubaltelli FF, Granati B, editors. *Neonatal Therapy: An Update*. New York: Elsevier Science Publishers Biomedical Division.

Finnegan LP, Kandall SR. 1992. Maternal and neonatal effects of alcohol and drugs. In: Lowinson JH, Ruiz P, Millman RB, editors. *Substance Abuse: A Comprehensive Textbook*. 2nd ed. Baltimore: Williams and Wilkins, pp. 628–56.

Fiore MC, Smith SS, Jorenby DE, et al. 1994. The effectiveness of the nicotine patch for smoking cessation: A meta-analysis. *JAMA* **271**:1940–7.

Fraser HF, Wikler A, Essig CF, et al. 1958. Degree of physical dependence induced by secobarbital or pentobarbital. *JAMA* **166**: 126–9.

Frezza M, diPadova C, Pozzato G, et al. 1990. High blood alcohol levels in women. *N Engl J Med* **322**:95–9.

Fuller RK, Branchey L, Brightwell DR, et al. 1986. Disulfiram treatment of alcoholism: A Veterans Administration cooperative study. *JAMA* **256**:1449–55.

Gawin FH, Kleber HD. 1986. Abstinence symptomatology and psychiatric diagnosis in cocaine abusers. *Arch Gen Psychiatry* **43**: 107–13.

Gourlay SG, Benowitz NL. 1997. Arteriovenous differences in plasma concentration of nicotine and catecholamines and related cardiovascular effects after smoking, nicotine nasal spray, and intravenous nicotine. *Clin Pharmacol Ther* **62**:453–63.

Greenstein RA, Fudala PJ, O'Brien CP. 1992. Alternative pharmacotherapies for opiate addiction. In: Lowinson JH, Ruiz P, Millman RB, editors. *Substance Abuse: A Comprehensive Textbook*. 2nd ed. Baltimore: Williams and Wilkins, pp. 562–73.

Heighman SJ, Stitzer ML, Bigelow GE, et al. 1989. Acute opioid physical dependence in postaddict humans: Naloxone effects after brief morphine exposure. *J Pharmacol Exp Ther* **248**:127–134.

Henderson G, Harkey M, Zhouo C, et al. 1996. Incorporation of isotopically labeled cocaine and metabolites into human hair: I. Dose–response relationships. *J Anal Toxicol* **20**:1–11.

Henningfield JE, Stapleton JM, Bonowitz NL, et al. 1993. Higher levels of nicotine in arterial than in venous blood after cigarette smoking. *Drug Alcohol Depend* **33**:23–9.

Hoffman NG, Halikas JA, Mee-Lee D, et al. 1991. *Patient Placement Criteria for the Treatment of Psychoactive Substance Use Disorders*. Washington, DC: American Society of Addiction Medicine.

Humfleet G, Hall S, Reus V, et al. 1996. The efficacy of nortriptyline as an adjunct to the psychological treatment for smokers with and without depressive histories. In: Harris LS, editor. *Problems of Drug Dependence, 1995: Proceedings of the 57th Annual Scientific Meeting of the College on Problems of Drug Dependence*. NIDA Research Monograph Series, No. 162. DHHS Publ. No. (ADM) 96–4116. Rockville, MD: National Institute on Drug Abuse, pp. 901–4.

Hunt WA, Barnett LW, Branch LG. 1971. Relapse rates in addiction programs. *J Clin Psychol* **27**(4):455–6.

Hurt RD, Sachs DPL, Glover ED, et al. 1997. A comparison of sustained release bupropion and placebo for smoking cessation. *N Engl J Med* **337**:1195–1202.

[IOM] Institute of Medicine. 1997. *Dispelling the Myths about Addiction: Strategies to Increase Understanding and Strengthen Research*. Washington, DC: National Academy Press, pp. 2.

Iribarne C, Berthou F, Carlhant D, et al. 1998. Inhibition of methadone and buprenorphine N-dealkylations by three HIV-1 protease inhibitors. *Drug Metab Dispos* **26**(3):257–60.

Jatlow P, Barash PG, Van Dyke C, et al. 1979. Cocaine and succinylcholine sensitivity: A new caution. *Anesth Analg* **58**:235–8.

Johansson CJ, Olsson P, Bende M, et al. 1991. Absolute bioavailability of nicotine applied to different nasal regions. *Eur J Clin Pharmacol* **41**:585–8.

Johnson RE, Cone EJ, Henningfield JE, et al. 1989. Use of buprenorphine in the treatment of opiate addiction. I. Physiologic and behavioral effects during a rapid dose induction. *Clin Pharmacol Ther* **46**: 335–43.

Kalant H, LeBlanc AE, Gibbins RJ. 1971. Tolerance to, and dependence on, some non-opiate psychotropic drugs. *Pharmacol Rev* **23**:135–191.

Kalivas PW, Sorg BA, Hooks MS. 1993. The pharmacology and neural circuitry of sensitization to psychostimulants. *Behav Pharmacol* **4**:315–34.

Kalivas PW, Striplin CD, Steketee JD, et al. 1992. Cellular mechanisms of behavioral sensitization to drugs of abuse. *Ann N Y Acad Sci* **654**:128–35.

Karch S, editor. 1995. Racial and sexual bias in hair testing. *Forensic Drug Abuse Advisor* **7**(3):20.

Kashkin KB, Kleber HD. 1989. Hooked on hormones? An anabolic steroid addiction hypothesis. *JAMA* **262**:3166–70.

Kendler KS, Neale MC, MacLean CJ, et al. 1993. Smoking and major depression: A causal analysis. *Arch Gen Psychiatry* **50**:36–43.

Kessler RC, McGonagle KA, Zhao S, et al. 1994. Lifetime and 12-month prevalence of DSM-III-R psychiatric disorders in the United States: Results from the National Comorbidity Survey. *Arch Gen Psychiatry* **51**:8–19.

Koob GF, Le Moal M. 1997. Drug abuse: hedonic homeostatic dysregulation. *Science* **278**(3):52–8.

Koob GF, Rassnick S, Heinrichs S, et al. 1994. Alcohol, the reward system and dependence. In: Jansson B, Jornvall H, Rydberg U, et al., editors. *Toward a Molecular Basis of Alcohol Use and Abuse*. Basel, Switzerland: Birkhauser Verlag, pp. 103–14.

Kreek MJ. 1973. Medical safety and side effects of methadone in tolerant individuals. *JAMA* **223**(6):665–8.

Landry DW. 1997. Immunotherapy for cocaine addiction. *Sci Am* **276**(2):42–5.

Landry DW, Yang GXQ. 1997. Anti-cocaine catalytic antibodies—a novel approach to the problem of addiction. *J Addict Dis* **16**(3): 1–17.

Lawson AAH, Northridge DB. 1987. Dextropropoxyphene overdose: Epidemiology, clinical presentation and management. *Med Toxicol* **2**:430–44.

Lee BL, Benowitz NL, Jacob P III. 1987. Cigarette abstinence, nicotine gum, and theophylline disposition. *Ann Intern Med* **106**:553–5.

Levin ED, Rosecrans J. 1994 The promise of nicotinic-based therapeutic treatments. *Drug Dev Res* **31**:1–2.

Levitt MD, Li R, DeMaster EG, et al. 1997. Use of measurements of ethanol absorption from stomach and intestine to assess human ethanol metabolism. *Am J Physiol* **273**:G951–7.

Lim Jr RT, Gentry RT, Daisuke I, et al. 1993. First-pass metabolism of ethanol is predominantly gastric. *Alcohol Clin Exp Res* **17**(6):1337–44.

Ling W, Wesson DR. 1984. Naltrexone treatment for addicted health care professionals: A collaborative private practice experience. *J Clin Psychiatry* **45**:46–8.

Lowinson JH, Mariou IJ, Joseph H, et al. 1992. Methadone maintenance. In: Lowinson JH, Ruiz IP, Robert B, et al., editors. *Substance Abuse: A Comprehensive Textbook*. 2nd ed. Baltimore: Williams and Wilkins, pp. 550–61.

Malcolm RJ, Ballenger JC, Sturgis E, et al. 1989. A double-blind controlled trial comparing carbamazepine to oxazepam treatment of alcohol withdrawal. *Am J Psychiatry* **146**:617–21.

May WW. 1998. A field application of the ASAM placement criteria in a 12-step model of treatment for chemical dependency. *J Addict Dis* **17**(2):77–91.

Mayo-Smith MF. 1997. Pharmacological management of alcohol withdrawal: A meta-analysis and evidence-based practice guideline. American Society of Addiction Medicine Working Group on Pharmacological Management of Alcohol Withdrawal. *JAMA* **278**(2):144–51.

McElhatton PR. 1994. The effects of benzodiazepine due during pregnancy and lactation. *Reprod Toxicol* **8**(6):461–75.

McGovern MP, Morrison DH. 1992. The chemical use, abuse and dependence scale (CUAD): Rationale, reliability and validity. *J Subst Abuse Treat* **9**:27–38.

McLellan AT, Arndt IO, Metzger DS, et al. 1993. The effects of psychosocial services in substance abuse treatment. *JAMA* **269**: 1953–9.

Miller LG, Greenblatt DJ, Barnhill JG, et al. 1987. Chronic benzodiazepine administration: I. Tolerance is associated with benzodiazepine receptor downregulation and decreased $\gamma$-aminobutyric $acid_A$ receptor function. *J Pharmacol Exp Ther* **246**:170–6.

Miller LG, Greenblatt DJ, Roy RB, et al. 1987. Chronic benzodiazepine administration: II. Discontinuation syndrome is associated with upregulation of $\gamma$-aminobutyric $acid_A$ receptor complex binding and function. *J Pharmacol Exp Ther* **246**:177–82.

Morgan JP. 1988. Marijuana metabolism in the context of urine testing for cannabinoid metabolite. *J Psychoactive Drugs* **20**(1):107–15.

Muller A. 1996. Alcohol consumption and community hospital admissions in the United States: A dynamic regression analysis, 1950–1992. *Addiction* **91**:321–42.

Naranjo CA, Sellers EM, Chater K, et al. 1983. Non-pharmacologic intervention in acute alcohol withdrawal. *Clin Pharmacol Ther* **34**:214–9.

Nestler EJ. 1996. Under siege: The brain on opiates. *Neuron* **16**:897–900.

Nestler EJ, Aghajanian GK. 1997. Molecular and cellular basis of addiction. *Science* **278**:58–63.

[NIAAA] National Institute on Alcohol Abuse and Alcoholism. 1988. Methadone maintenance and patients in alcoholism treatment. *Alcohol Alert* **1**:1–4.

[NIDA] National Institute on Drug Abuse. 1997a. *Drug Abuse Warning Network (DAWN)*. Rockville, MD: National Institute on Drug Abuse.

[NIDA] National Institute on Drug Abuse. 1997b. *National Household Survey on Drug Abuse*. Rockville, MD: National Institute on Drug Abuse.

NIDA Research Monograph Series, No. 67. DHHS Publ. No. (ADM) 86–1448. Rockville, MD: National Institute on Drug Abuse, pp. 318–20.

Novick DM, Kreek MJ, Des Jarlais DC, et al. 1986. Antibody to LAV, the putative agent of AIDS, in parenteral drug abusers and methadone maintained patients. In: Harris LS, editor. *Problems of Drug Dependence, 1985: Proceedings of the 47th Annual Scientific Meeting of the Committee on Problems of Drug Dependence*.

O'Brien CP. 1997. A range of research-based pharmacotherapies for addiction. *Science* **278**:66–70.

Ockene JK, Kristeller J, Pbert L, et al. 1994. The physician-delivered smoking intervention project: Can short-term interventions produce long-term effects for a general outpatient population? *Health Psychol* **13**(3):278–81.

O'Connor PG, Schottenfeld RS. 1998. Patients with alcohol problems. *N Engl J Med* **338**(9):592–620.

O'Malley SS, Croop RS, Wroblewski JM, et al. 1995. Naltrexone in the treatment of alcohol dependence: A combined analysis of two trials. *Psychiatr Ann* **25**:681–8.

Olds ME, Milner P. 1954. Positive reinforcement produced by electrical stimulation of septal area and other regions of the rat brain. *J Comp Physiol Psychol* **47**:419–27.

O'Sullivan GF, Wade DN. 1987. Flumazenil in the management of acute drug overdosage with benzodiazepines and other agents. *Clin Pharmacol Ther* **42**:254–9.

Pan ZZ. 1998. $\mu$-Opposing actions of the $\kappa$-opioid receptor. *TiPS* **19**: 94–8.

Pfeifer HF, Greenblatt DJ. 1978. Clinical toxicity of theophylline in relation to cigarette smoking: A report from the Boston Collaborative Drug Surveillance Program. *Chest* **73**:455–9.

Pietrantoni M, Knuppel RA. 1991. Alcohol use in pregnancy. *Clin Perinatol* **18**(1):93–111.

Pond SM, Olson KR, Osterloh JO, et al. 1984. Randomized study of the treatment of phenobarbital overdose with repeated doses of serial charcoal. *JAMA* **251**:3104–8.

Post RM, Weiss SRB. 1995. The neurobiology of treatment-resistant mood disorders. In: Bloom FE, Kupfer DJ, editors. *Psychopharmacology: The Fourth Generation of Progress*. New York: Raven Press, pp. 1155–70.

Project MATCH Research Group. 1997. Matching alcoholism treatments to client heterogeneity: Project MATCH posttreatment drinking outcomes. *J Stud Alcohol* **58**:7–29.

Quandt CM, Sommi RW Jr., Pipkin T, et al. 1988. Differentiation of cocaine toxicity: Role of the toxicology drug screen. *Drug Intelligence Clin Pharmacy* **22**:582–7.

Ramoska E, Sacchetti AD. 1985. Propranolol-induced hypertension in treatment of cocaine intoxication. *Ann Emerg Med* **14**:1112–3.

Randall MD, Kendall DA. 1998. Endocannabinoids: A new class of vasoactive substances. *TiPS* **19**:55–8.

Reier CE, Johnstone RE. 1970. Respiratory depression: Narcotic versus narcotic-tranquilizer combinations. *Anesth Analg* **49**:119–24.

Rice DP. 1993. The economic cost of alcohol abuse and alcohol dependence: 1990. *Alcohol Health Res World* **45**(1):61–7.

Rice DP. Feb. 1995. Personal communication to the Institute of Medicine. University of California at San Francisco.

Richardson G, Day N. 1994. Detrimental effects of prenatal cocaine exposure: Illusion or reality? *J Am Acad Child Adolesc Psychiatry* **33**(1):28–34.

Rodriguez de Fonseca F, Carrera MRA, Navarro, M, et al. 1997. Activation of corticotropin-releasing factor in the limbic system during cannabinoid withdrawal. *Science* **276**:2050–53.

Rose JE, Behm FM, Westman EC, et al. 1994. Mecamylamine combined with nicotine skin patch facilitates smoking cessation beyond nicotine patch treatment alone. *Clin Pharmacol Ther* **56**(1):86–99.

Roy-Byrne PP, Hommer D. 1988. Benzodiazepine withdrawal: Overview and implications for the treatment of anxiety. *Am J Med* **84**:1041–52.

Saitz R, Mayo-Smith MF, Roberts MS, et al. 1994. Individualized treatment for alcohol withdrawal: A randomized double-blind controlled trial. *JAMA* **272**:519–23.

Schechter M. 1994. Cocaethylene produces discriminative stimulus properties in the rat: Effect of cocaine and ethanol coadministration. *Pharmacol Biochem Behav* **51**:285–9.

Schultz W, Dayan P, Montague PR. 1997. A neural substrate of prediction and reward. *Science* **275**:1593.

Schwartz EL, Brechbuhl AB, Kahl P, et al. 1992. Pharmacokinetic interactions of zidovudine and methadone in intravenous drug-using patients with HIV infection. *J Acquir Immune Defic Syndr* **5**(6):619–26.

Sinclair J, Wrighton JE, Kostrubsky V, et al. 1998. Alcohol-mediated increases in acetaminophen hepatotoxicity: Role of CYP2E and CYP3A. *Biochem Pharmacol* **55**(10):1557–65.

Skinner HA. 1982. The drug abuse screening test. *Addict Behav* **7**:363–71.

Slotkin TA. 1998. Fetal nicotine or cocaine exposure: Which one is worse? *J Pharmacol Exp Ther* **285**(3):931–45.

Spanagel R, Zieglgansberger W. 1997. Anti-craving compounds for ethanol: New pharmacological tools to study addictive processes. *TiPS* **18**:54–9.

Streissguth AP, Aase JM, Clarren SK, et al. 1991. Fetal alcohol syndrome in adolescents and adults. *JAMA* **265**:1961–7.

Suwacki H, Ohara H. 1985. Alcohol-induced facial flushing and drinking behavior in Japanese men. *J Stud Alcohol* **116**:196–8.

Swett C Jr. 1974. Drowsiness due to chlorpromazine in relation to cigarette smoking: A report from the Boston Collaborative Drug Surveillance Program. *Arch Gen Psychiatry* **31**:211–4.

Tabakoff B, Hoffman PL. 1996. Alcohol addiction: An enigma among us. *Neuron* **16**: 909–12.

Tanda G, Pontieri FE, DiChiara G. 1997. Cannabinoid and heroin activation of mesolimbic dopamine transmission by a common $\mu_1$ opioid receptor mechanism. *Science* **276**:2048–50.

Tang JL, Law M, Wald N. 1994. How effective is nicotine replacement therapy in helping people to stop smoking? *Br Med J* **308**:21–6.

Vaughan DP, Beckett AH, Robbie DS. 1976. The influence of smoking on the intersubject variation in pentazocine elimination. *Br J Clin Pharmacol* **3**:279–83.

Voth EA, Schwartz RH. 1997. Medicinal applications of delta-9-tetrahydrocannabinol and marijuana. *Ann Intern Med* **126**(10):791–8.

Wakschlag LS, Lahey BB, Loeber R, et al. 1997. Maternal smoking during pregnancy and the risk of conduct disorder in boys. *Arch Gen Psychiatry* **54**:670–6.

Walle T, Byington RP, Furberg CD, et al. 1985. Biologic determinants of propranolol disposition: Results from 1308 patients in Beta-Blocker Heart Attack Trial. *Clin Pharmacol Ther* **38**:509–18.

Walsh RA. 1994. Effects of maternal smoking on adverse pregnancy outcomes: Examination of the criteria of causation. *Hum Biol* **66**(6):1059–92.

Wenger G, Croix D, Tramu G, et al. 1992. Effects of delta$^9$-tertrahydrocannabinol on pregnancy, puberty, and the neuroendocrine system. In: Murphy L, Bartke A, editors. *Marijuana/ Cannabinoids: Neurobiology and Neurophysiology*. Boca Raton, FL: CRC Press, pp. 539–60.

Whitcomb DC, Block GD. 1994. Association of acetaminophen hepatotoxicity with fasting and ethanol use. *JAMA* **272**(23):1845–50.

Whitfield CL, Thompson G, Lamb A, et al. 1978. Detoxification of 1,024 patients without psychoactive drugs. *JAMA* **239**:1409–10.

Wickelgren I. 1997a. Getting the brain's attention. *Science* **278**:35–7.

Wickelgren I. 1997b. Marijuana: Harder than thought? *Science* **276**: 1967–8.

Wieland HA, Luddens H, Seeburg PH. 1992. Molecular determinants in $GABA_A$/BZ receptor subtypes. *Adv Biochem Psychopharmacol* **47**:29–40.

Williamson DF, Madans J, Anda RF, et al. 1991. Smoking cessation and severity of weight gain in a national cohort. *N Engl J Med* **324**:739–45.

Woods JH, Katz JL, Winger G. 1992. Benzodiazepines: Use, abuse and consequences, *Pharmacol Rev* **44**:151–347.

Yersin B, Nicolet JF, Decrey H, et al. 1995. Screening for excessive alcohol drinking: Comparative value of carbohydrate-deficient transferrin, gamma-glutamyltransferase, and mean corpuscular volume. *Arch Intern Med* **155**:1907–11.

Yesalis CE, Kennedy NK, Kopstein AN, et al. 1993. Anabolic-androgenic steroid use in the United States. *JAMA* **70**:1217–21.

Zimmerman HJ, Maddrey WC. 1995. Acetaminophen (paracetamol) hepatotoxicity with regular intake of alcohol: Analysis of instances of therapeutic misadventure. *Hepatology* **22**:767.

CHAPTER

# 18 POISONING

Lewis S. Nelson, Lewis R. Goldfrank

*Chapter Outline*



Defining what constitutes a poison is not simple. Some substances have virtually no known beneficial effects in humans and can only be considered poisonous (e.g., cyanide). Many substances that are normally innocuous, or even necessary for life (e.g., oxygen, water), become poisons when present in excess. In fact, all drugs in clinical use have the potential to have salutary or deleterious effects, and can, at some dose, be a poison. Since their beneficial effects are obtained through interference with some biochemical or physiologic process, drugs may be poisonous or therapeutic depending on the dose administered (Paracelsus).

Similarly, many adverse effects engendered by a drug are merely an extension of the drug's pharmacologic effect and are predictable based on the desired pharmacologic or therapeutic mechanism of the drug (e.g., decreased renal function is associated with salicylates because of inhibition of prostaglandin synthesis). From this perspective, pharmacology forms the basis for toxicology. However, the toxic effects of many drugs cannot be predicted based on their therapeutic mechanisms but are known to occur by other mechanisms. For example, the cardiac dysrhythmias associated with tricyclic antidepressant poisoning are due to their sodium channel blockade, and acetaminophen-induced hepatic failure is mediated by the generation of a toxic metabolite. Generally these effects occur only after overdose, but occasionally they may also result from pharmacokinetic or pharmacodynamic drug interactions or from a drug's atypical metabolism based on a patient's pharmacogenetic profile.

Some toxic effects remain completely unpredictable and are termed *idiosyncratic,* such as aplastic anemia associated with chloramphenicol. Most of these adverse effects occur very rarely, and many will likely be reclassified as predictable events as more is learned of their underlying mechanism. Examples of this form of progress include our slowly increasing understanding of the danger of phocomelia in the fetus with thalidomide use during pregnancy.

Poisoning and adverse drug reactions, both related events in the spectrum of drug toxicity, remain important clinical problems. Although exact numbers defining the extent of these problems are unavailable, it has been estimated that several percent of all hospitalized patients suffer an adverse drug reaction (Bates et al. 1995). Most of these adverse effects are mild and cannot be considered truly "poisoning," yet a small but significant portion of these patients die or suffer significant morbidity related to the event. Deliberate poisoning remains an important method of suicide and has been recommended in several "suicide manuals" sold by proponents of euthanasia (Humphrey 1991). The use of abusable substances continues to escalate as drug users continually find new agents and rediscover former agents with which to experiment. Such illicit use is dangerous, and solvent-induced deaths (which reached epidemic levels in the 1960s) are once again on the increase. Acetaminophen-poisoned patients account for nearly half of those who receive liver transplants in the United Kingdom. In patients under the age of 40 years who develop cardiac arrest, one-quarter of these events are toxin-induced (Safranek et al. 1992).

Additionally, the American Association of Poison Control Centers (AAPCC) compiles data concerning the frequency of calls to poison control centers (PCCs) across most of the nation (Litovitz et al. 1997) (Table 18-1).

Approximately half of the cases (termed *exposures*) managed by PCCs concern unintentional ingestions in

Table 18-1 Epidemiology of Poisoning Exposures in the United States

| SUBSTANCES MOST FREQUENTLY INVOLVED IN PEDIATRIC EXPOSURES | SUBSTANCES MOST FREQUENTLY INVOLVED IN ADULT EXPOSURES | CATEGORIES WITH LARGEST NUMBERS OF DEATHS |
|---|---|---|
| Cosmetic and personal care products | Analgesics | Analgesics |
| Cleaning substances | Cleaning substances | Antidepressants |
| Analgesics | Bites/envenomations | Stimulants and street drugs |
| Plants | Sedatives-hypnotics/antipsychotics | Cardiovascular drugs |
| Cough and cold preparations | Antidepressants | Alcohols |

SOURCE: Adapted from Litovitz et al. 1997.

small children. Although the majority of these patients suffer no adverse effect, it remains difficult to determine at the outset whether an ingestion has occurred and whether it will be consequential. Therefore, all such exposures are considered potentially serious. Suicidal patients with intentional ingestions comprise the group with the highest morbidity and mortality (Litovitz et al. 1997). This is likely due to the serious, volitional nature of the exposure and the delay in presentation to a healthcare facility. The rising call volume at PCCs over the past 10 years may represent the increasing frequency of poisoning, a heightened awareness of the availability of PCCs, the development of the subspecialty of medical toxicology, or the growing complexity of the available drugs necessitating calls from emergency departments and intensive care units.

**PRINCIPLE Poisoning is a common event that spares no patient population. Every xenobiotic is a potential poison, and the size of the exposure and the median lethal dose ($LD_{50}$) of the drug are the most important determinants of toxicity.**

## CLINICAL EVALUATION

Obtaining an adequate history remains the most important aspect of the management of a potentially poisoned patient. In many cases, a precise medical history can define the exact nature of the exposure. In others it delineates the potential agents to which the patient may have access at home or work. Although occasionally unreliable (for example, in patients with dementia or suicidal ideation), the medical history permits a focused investigation into the potential for patient harm and guides initial management. The process of taking the medical history is guided by the clinical situation, but the history usually includes questions about the timing, nature and circumstances of the exposure and the patient's initial symptoms, symptom progression, and complicating medical conditions.

### Toxidromes

When faced with a patient who has been poisoned by an unknown agent, or in an attempt to confirm the identity of the suspected toxin, the physical examination is often extremely helpful. Although a complete examination is important, the recognition of toxicologic syndromes, or "toxidromes," may be most informative (see Table 18-2). A toxidrome is a constellation of individual clinical findings that, when taken together, implicate a specific class of poisons. Although toxidromes are completely predictable based on the principles of pharmacology and physiology, they are often present in impure forms *(forme frustes)* because of the complex nature of most drugs, the particular patient characteristics, and the fact that most adults are exposed to more than one drug. Although standard texts in medical toxicology recognize over 25 toxidromes, only a limited number of toxidromes are broadly applicable to an unselected patient population.

#### *Acetylcholine-related toxidromes*

There are two broad classes of cholinergic receptors (i.e., acetylcholine receptors) that provide several important functional and regulatory effects. Muscarinic receptors in end organs are part of the parasympathetic nervous system and are generally involved with preserving the resting tone of the body as defined by heart rate, gastrointestinal function, and pupil size. "Rest," which occurs during conditions of nonstress, is associated with reduction in environmental responsiveness, slowing of the heart rate, and enhancement of digestion. Muscarinic receptors in sweat glands mediate diaphoresis, although autonomic control of this function involves the sympathetic nervous system. Nicotinic cholinergic receptors in the neuromuscular junction mediate muscle contraction and nicotinic receptors in the autonomic ganglia. Sympathetic and parasympathetic ganglia of the autonomic nervous system are important for activation of transmission in postganglionic fibers.

***Anticholinergic toxidrome***
Agents that interfere with the binding of acetylcholine to muscarinic receptors interfere with resting tone and produce tachycardia, mydriasis, dry mouth and skin, and depressed bowel and bladder motility. Examples of anticholinergic agents include atropine, diphenhydramine, tricyclic antidepressants, thioridazine, and botulinum toxin. The first four drugs are competitive muscarinic antagonists, whereas botulinum toxin inhibits the release of acetylcholine and is a noncompetitive antagonist primarily at nicotinic sites. The anticholinergic toxidrome refers specifically to antimuscarinic findings.

***Cholinergic toxidrome***
Enhanced muscarinic receptor stimulation augments the physiology of rest. Patients manifest bradycardia, miosis, salivation, diarrhea, vomiting, urination, and bronchorrhea. Muscarinic stimulation may occur either directly (as with bethanechol) or indirectly (as is seen with cholinesterase inhibitors). Stimulation of nicotinic receptors with succinylcholine, or inhibition of cholinesterase by organophosphates, can produce depolarizing blockade at the neuromuscular junction. Nicotinic agonism at the autonomic ganglia (as produced by cholinesterase inhibitors) may produce various combinations of increased sympathetic or parasympathetic findings. Patients may manifest isolated nicotinic or muscarinic findings, but in most instances they coexist.

***Opioid toxidrome***
Opioid receptors are associated with those areas of the brain involved in regulation of pain and mood. These receptors bind endogenous opioids (e.g., endorphins) and likely provide an autologous mechanism for pain reduction or mood enhancement. Exogenous opioids, such as morphine, stimulate these receptors and produce analgesia ($\mu_1$) or euphoria ($\mu_1$). However, opioid receptors also modulate ventilation ($\mu_2$) and adrenergic outflow ($\mu_1$). Excessive stimulation of these opioid receptor subtypes produces significant obtundation, hypoventilation, and miosis, as well as modest decline in the heart rate and blood pressure.

***Sympathomimetic toxidrome***
Patients with cocaine, amphetamine, or theophylline poisoning manifest features of autonomic overactivity, manifested as the sympathomimetic toxidrome. The exact clinical manifestations may vary because of the complexity of both the autonomic nervous system and the individual agents. However, patients typically demonstrate hypertension, tachycardia, diaphoresis, mydriasis, hyperthermia, and a heightened state of alertness ranging from euphoria to agitation. The mechanisms by which agents induce this toxidrome vary. For example, although both affect neuronal catecholamines, cocaine inhibits their presynaptic reuptake, whereas amphetamines amplify their release. The methylxanthines, such as theophylline and caffeine, work at therapeutic blood concentrations to antagonize neuromodulation by adenosine of catecholamine release and inhibit the enzyme phosphodiesterase at toxic concentrations.

***Sedative-hypnotic toxidrome***
Agents whose predominant action is anxiolysis or sleep induction are called *sedative-hypnotics*. The mechanism of action common to this class is agonism of the inhibitory neurotransmitter GABA at the GABA receptor. Therefore, augmentation of GABA activity produces enhanced neuronal inhibition, which manifests as sedation and hypnosis, or sleep. With increasing dose, profound mental status depression and coma occur. Since benzodiazepines have little pharmacologic effect other than GABA agonism, coma with normal blood pressure, pulse, and respiratory rate are the expected finding after benzodiazepine overdose. Other sedative-hypnotic agents may produce differing effects, such as tachycardia because of the anticholinergic effects of glutethimide or hypoventilation because of the respiratory depressant effects of barbiturates.

**PRINCIPLE Understanding the commonly observed signs and symptoms (toxidromes), and the underlying pathophysiologic alterations produced by specific toxins, permits the rapid identification of potential etiologies and risk stratification of poisoned patients.**

## Vital Signs

The assessment of potentially poisoned patients requires a careful assessment of the patient's vital signs. Subtle changes are often the only clues that a well-appearing patient is potentially ill. Management may differ from that used to treat patients with similar clinical presentations whose etiology is not pharmacologic or toxicologic in nature.

***Blood pressure***
Although a normal blood pressure can be a reassuring finding, this vital sign may be the last to deteriorate in patients with clinical shock (Cummins et al. 1994). Individual attention must be given to both the diastolic blood pressure, which is a reflection of vascular tone ($\beta_2$- and $\alpha$-adrenergic effects), and the systolic blood pressure,

**Table 18-2 Specific Drugs or Toxins and Their Toxic Syndromes**

| Toxin | Vital signs | Mental status | Signs and symptoms | Clinical findings |
|---|---|---|---|---|
| Acetaminophen | Normal (early) | Normal | Anorexia, nausea, vomiting | Right upper quadrant tenderness, jaundice (late) |
| Amphetamines | Hypertension, tachycardia, tachypnea, hyperthermia | Hyperactive, agitated, toxic psychosis | Hyperalertness, panic, anxiety, diaphoresis | Mydriasis, hyperactive peristaltism, diaphoresis |
| Antihistamines | Hypotension, hypertension, tachycardia, hyperthermia | Altered (agitation, lethargy to coma), hallucinations | Blurred vision, dry mouth, inability to urinate | Dry mucous membranes, mydriasis, flush, diminished peristaltism, urinary retention |
| Arsenic (acute) | Hypotension, tachycardia | Alert to coma | Abdominal pain, vomiting, diarrhea, dysphagia | Dehydration |
| Barbiturates | Hypotension, bradypnea, hypothermia | Altered (lethargy to coma) | Slurred speech, ataxia | Dysconjugate gaze, bullae, hyporeflexia |
| Beta-adrenergic antagonists | Hypotension, bradycardia | Altered (lethargy to coma) | Dizziness | Cyanosis, seizures |
| Botulinum | Bradypnea | Normal unless hypoxia | Blurred vision, diplopia, dysphagia, sore or dry throat, diarrhea | Opthalmoplegia, mydriasis, ptosis, cranial nerve abnormalities, descending paralysis |
| Carbamazepine | Hypotension, tachycardia, bradypnea, hypothermia | Altered (lethargy to coma) | Hallucinations, extrapyramidal movements, seizures | Mydriasis, nystagmus |
| Carbon monoxide | Often normal | Altered (lethargy to coma) | Headache, dizziness, nausea, vomiting | Seizures |
| Clonidine | Hypotension, hypertension, bradycardia, bradypnea | Altered (lethargy to coma) | Dizziness, confusion | Miosis |
| Cocaine | Hypertension, tachycardia, tachypnea, hyperthermia | Altered (anxiety, agitation, delirium) | Hallucinations, paranoia, panic, anxiety, restlessness | Mydriasis, nystagmus |
| Cyclic antidepressants | Hypotension, tachycardia | Altered (lethargy to coma) | Confusion, dizziness, dry mouth, inability to urinate | Mydriasis, dry mucous membranes, distended bladder, flush, seizures |
| Digitalis | Hypotension, bradycardia | Normal to altered, visual distortion | Nausea, vomiting, anorexia, visual disturbances | None |
| Disulfiram/ethanol | Hypotension, tachycardia | Normal | Nausea, vomiting, headache, vertigo | Flush, diaphoresis, tender abdomen |
| Ethylene glycol | Tachypnea | Altered (lethargy to coma) | Abdominal pain | Slurred speech, ataxia |
| Iron | Hypotension, tachycardia | Normal or lethargy | Nausea, vomiting, diarrhea, abdominal pain, hematemesis | Tender abdomen |
| Isoniazid | Often normal | Normal or altered (lethargy to coma) | Nausea, vomiting | Seizures |
| Isopropanol | Hypotension, tachycardia, bradypnea | Altered (lethargy to coma) | Nausea, vomiting | Hyporeflexia, ataxia, acetone odor on breath |
| Lead | Hypertension | Altered (lethargy to coma) | Irritability, abdominal pain (colic), nausea, vomiting, constipation | Peripheral neuropathy, seizures, gingival pigmentation |
| Lithium | Hypotension (late) | Altered (lethargy to coma) | Diarrhea, tremor, nausea | Weakness, tremor, ataxia, myoclonus, seizures |

**Table 18-2 Specific Drugs or Toxins and Their Toxic Syndromes (Continued)**

| Toxin | Vital signs | Mental status | Signs and symptoms | Clinical findings |
|---|---|---|---|---|
| Mercury | Hypotension (late) | Altered (psychiatric disturbances) | Salivation, diarrhea, abdominal pain | Stomatitis, ataxia, tremor |
| Methanol | Hypotension, tachypnea | Altered (lethargy to coma) | Blurred vision, blindness, abdominal pain | Hyperemic disks, mydriasis |
| Opioids | Hypotension, bradycardia, bradypnea, hypothermia | Altered (lethargy to coma) | Slurred speech, ataxia | Miosis, decreased peristaltism |
| Organophosphates/ carbamates | Hypotension/ hypertension, bradycardia/ tachycardia, bradypnea/ tachypnea | Altered (lethargy to coma) | Diarrhea, abdominal pain, blurred vision, vomiting | Salivation, diaphoresis, lacrimation, urination, bronchorrhea, defecation, miosis, fasciculations, seizures |
| Phencyclidine | Hypertension, tachycardia, hyperthermia | Altered (agitation, lethargy to coma) | Hallucinations | Miosis, diaphoresis, myoclonus, blank stare, nystagmus, seizures |
| Phenothiazines | Hypotension, tachycardia, hypothermia | Altered (lethargy to coma) | Dizziness, dry mouth, inability to urinate | Miosis or mydriasis, decreased bowel sounds, dystonia |
| Salicylates | Hypotension, tachycardia, tachypnea, hyperthermia | Altered (agitation, lethargy to coma) | Tinnitus, nausea, vomiting | Diaphoresis, tender abdomen, pulmonary edema |
| Sedative-hypnotics | Hypotension, bradypnea, hypothermia | Altered (lethargy to coma) | Slurred speech, ataxia | Hyporeflexia, bullae |
| Theophylline | Hypotension, tachycardia, tachypnea, hyperthermia | Altered (agitation) | Nausea, vomiting, diaphoresis, anxiety | Diaphoresis, tremor, seizures dysrhythmias |

SOURCE: From Goldfrank et al. 1998.

which represents the cardiac inotropic state ($\beta_1$-adrenergic effect). Poisoned patients may demonstrate a widened pulse pressure, in which the difference between the systolic and diastolic pressures is greater than 50 mm Hg. This effect may occur in patients poisoned by $\beta$-adrenergic agonists, such as epinephrine, or by theophylline. Both of these agents produce vascular relaxation and stimulate cardiac output; the widened pulse pressure is due to an elevated systolic and a lowered diastolic pressure.

Management of hypotension almost always begins with volume expansion. Patients who fail to respond to adequate volumes of isotonic saline, particularly those with signs of poor tissue perfusion such as altered mental status or metabolic acidosis, may require vasoconstrictive or cardiostimulating drugs. Agents with predominantly $\alpha$-adrenergic effects are considered vasopressor agents, and those primarily stimulating the $\beta_1$-adrenergic receptor are termed *inotropes* and *chronotropes*. However, since most adrenergic agents provide stimulation of several different receptor subtypes, their clinical effects are mixed.

The management of a hypertensive poisoned patient is rarely a medical emergency. However, acute severe hypertension in younger patients can be associated with substantial morbidity. This type of effect may be noted in cocaine-intoxicated patients or in patients exposed to pure $\alpha$-adrenergic agonists or other sympathomimetic drugs. If treatment is required, an $\alpha$-adrenergic antagonist (Lange et al. 1989) or vasodilator such as nitroprusside should be considered. However, virtually all cocaine-poisoned patients respond to sedation, since enhanced adrenergic outflow from the central nervous system is largely responsible for the vital sign abnormalities (Catravas and Waters 1981).

### *Pulse*

Virtually all hypotensive patients develop a reflex, sympathetically mediated tachycardia. Suspicion of poisoning should be raised in hypotensive patients who do not manifest this typical physiological response. Because calcium channel blockers may reduce vascular tone, cardiac conduction, and rate of firing of the sinoatrial (SA) node, these antihypertensive agents are among the agents most frequently responsible for hypotension without reflex tachycardia. Other agents capable of inducing a similar clinical syndrome in poisoned patients include digitalis glycosides, $\beta$-adrenergic antagonists, and clonidine. Bradycardia may also be a feature of the cholinergic, sedative-hypnotic, or opioid toxidromes.

Sinus tachycardia is not generally of clinical concern, and treatment should be targeted toward the precipitating condition or agent. Alternatively, other abnormal tachydysrhythmias are often unresponsive to standard management strategies, yet are well controlled by alternative means. For example, the management of a wide-complex tachycardia in a patient poisoned by a tricyclic antidepressant should include hypertonic sodium bicarbonate rather than lidocaine (see below).

#### *Respiration*

Adequacy of ventilation (as defined by the measured $Pa_{CO_2}$) is conveniently estimated by measurement of the respiratory rate. Although adequate in many clinical situations, this method of determination often fails to properly identify poisoned patients. Patients with salicylate poisoning, for example, develop centrally mediated hyperpnea in which the depth of respiration increases more significantly than the rate. A contrasting effect is noted in opioid-poisoned patients, in which the tidal volume is depressed more profoundly than is the respiratory rate (Shook et al. 1990). Therefore, unless the patient's ventilation is observed, the normalcy of a respiratory rate may be misleading. Ventilatory or oxygenation disorders are relatively easy to manage once identified; assisted ventilation and supplemental oxygen are usually sufficient.

#### *Temperature*

Thermoregulatory abnormalities are common in poisoned patients, and obtaining a precise rectal temperature should not be delayed. Patients with hypoglycemia or sedative-hypnotic intoxication, for example, are frequently hypothermic. Although not typically life-threatening, the finding of hypothermia in a poisoned patient may assist in refining the differential diagnosis. Alternatively, patients with cocaine intoxication frequently manifest life-threatening hyperthermia. Death from cocaine poisoning may be directly related to the severe temperature dysregulation, and treatment is directed primarily at sedation and cooling.

**PRINCIPLE Alterations of a patient's vital signs are extremely common in poisoned patients. In many patients therapy directed toward the normalization of vital signs is sufficient. However, abnormalities of the vital signs may be subtle clues to the identity of the poison or the severity of the intoxication.**

## Rapid Bedside Testing

Absolute confirmation, by laboratory tests, of exposure, or lack of exposure, is neither practical nor available for most drugs or toxins, and the clinical history along with the physical examination often must suffice. Since the history and physical examination that can be obtained may be unreliable or inadequate, management of patients believed to be poisoned generally requires that decisions be made on an empiric basis. In other situations, attempts to obtain clinical information are overshadowed by the patient's grave clinical condition. These patients demand immediate management without complete assessment. For example, patients with a life-threatening cardiac dysrhythmia or with status epilepticus cannot await confirmatory laboratory testing, or even a complete history and physical. To assist in management in the absence of a complete data set, several rapidly available "bedside" tests are useful.

#### *Electrocardiograph (ECG)*

The electrocardiograph serves several important roles in the management of poisoned patients and should be performed in virtually all circumstances. In patients with cardiovascular abnormalities, the evaluation of an electrocardiograph may suggest the toxin. For example, calcium channel blockers typically produce bradycardia with atrioventricular nodal block, whereas digoxin typically produces ST segment abnormalities and first-degree atrioventricular (AV) block. Alternatively, and just as important, the electrocardiograph may have a prognostic value. Patients with tricyclic antidepressant poisoning usually have intraventricular conduction delays, such as QRS widening, the magnitude of which is related to the likelihood of both seizures and ventricular dysrhythmias (Boehnert and Lovejoy 1985).

#### *Blood glucose measurement*

Hypoglycemia, as a cause of altered mental status, remains a common clinical problem in emergency department patients (Malouf and Brust 1985). Hypoglycemia can certainly be expected in patients with insulin or sulfonylurea overdose. In addition, ethanol consumption in adults, but particularly in children, may produce hypoglycemia. Rapid assessment of glucose is most commonly accomplished using a glucometer and a capillary blood sample (Belsey et al. 1987). Since the blood glucose at which hypoglycemic symptoms occur varies, a capillary glucose in the normal range may not actually reflect normoglycemia (Boyle et al. 1988). The use of hypertonic intravenous dextrose (usually 50% dextrose in water) is safe and inexpensive and is warranted in virtually all obtunded patients before laboratory results are available.

### *"Coma cocktail": Naloxone, hypertonic glucose, flumazenil*

The use of a therapeutic trial is commonplace in medicine (Hoffman and Goldfrank 1995). A pharmacologic therapeutic trial involves the administration of a drug on a presumptive basis and subsequent assessment for a desired response. If the antagonist used for a therapeutic trial is specific, a positive response defines the etiology. However, an absent or incomplete response may be due to concomitant ingestion of several substances, at least one of which prevents a response, absence of the presumed toxin, or an inadequate dose of the antidote. For example, a patient awakening promptly after a dextrose bolus suggests the presence of severe hypoglycemia. A patient who fails to return to a normal mental status after receiving dextrose, despite documented hypoglycemia, may have also ingested ethanol (which prevents a response even when the serum glucose normalizes) or may have posthypoglycemic encephalopathy.

Several commonly available antidotes are often offered $N=1$ as therapeutic trials, although the safety and efficacy of some of these agents may be questionable. Naloxone, an opioid receptor competitive antagonist, is a generally safe agent in opioid-naive patients and is extremely effective in reversing opioid-induced respiratory depression. However, whether an overdose has occurred or not, naloxone may precipitate an acute withdrawal syndrome in an opioid-tolerant patient. Although not directly life-threatening, the emesis that accompanies opioid withdrawal may prove problematic in patients with concomitant ingestions that produce coma, such as ethanol or barbiturates, which are not themselves responsive to naloxone. Because of the persistent coma after naloxone administration, these patients are not able to adequately protect their airways during naloxone-induced emesis and risk aspiration pneumonitis or asphyxiation. Analysis favors administration of hypertonic glucose ($D_{50}W$) and thiamine hydrochloride to patients with altered consciousness (see paragraph above). Although rapid reagent test strips can be used to guide this therapy, they are not infallible, and they fail to recognize clinical hypoglycemia that may occur without numerical hypoglycemia (Hoffman and Goldfrank 1995). Flumazenil, a benzodiazepine receptor antagonist, may produce seizures in benzodiazepine-tolerant patients, and these seizures may be resistant to conventional therapy with benzodiazepines. Flumazenil may precipitate seizures or cardiac dysrhythmias in patients who, in addition to a benzodiazepine, also ingested tricyclic antidepressants or chloral hydrate, respectively. Given the low morbidity of benzodiazepine overdose per se, the risk of empiric flumazenil administration in the patient with the undefined overdose appears substantial.

**PRINCIPLE Providing an "antidote" to a potential toxin may not be optimal therapy.**

### *Pulse oximetry*

Although the pulse oximeter provides a noninvasive means of determining the oxygen saturation, its role in the management of the poisoned patient is limited. Since oxygenation may remain within the normal range despite hypoventilation, the recognition of critical respiratory depression may be obscured and delayed. Because of the technical limitations of pulse oximetry, the presence of atypical hemoglobin species (e.g., carboxyhemoglobin, methemoglobin, or sulfhemoglobin) may remain undetected, necessitating the use of arterial blood gas analysis with cooximetry. A cooximeter is a more sophisticated device capable of precisely defining the percentage of these atypical hemoglobin species.

### *Arterial blood gases*

The adequacy of ventilation and oxygenation may be difficult to assess clinically and even using pulse oximetry, the determination of the arterial blood gases is crucial. Although invasive, important information is gleaned from the assessment of a symptomatic patient's acid-base (pH), ventilatory ($P\text{CO}_2$) and oxygenation ($P\text{O}_2$) status. For example, a metabolic acidosis in an unconscious patient may suggest that the patient ingested methanol or had a recent seizure. Alternatively, a combined metabolic acidosis and respiratory alkalosis suggests salicylate poisoning.

**PRINCIPLE The use of clinical tests that provide rapidly available information is essential for the complete assessment of poisoned patients. Reliance on less rapidly available testing can delay the institution of life-saving therapy.**

## PREVENTING ABSORPTION: GASTROINTESTINAL DECONTAMINATION

The lack of suitable antidotal therapy for the majority of xenobiotics highlights the critical role of preventing toxicity. Primary prevention of toxicity, such as parental education, drug storage in child-resistant containers, or the use of computerized adverse drug effects programs by medical professionals, are the optimal means of reducing the incidence of poisoning. Although typically helpful from an epidemiologic perspective, such measures cannot eliminate poisoning. Those patients who are exposed to a potentially toxic substance subsequently require decontamination as a method of secondary prevention. As most exposures occur through the gastrointestinal tract, the major focus must be on gastrointestinal decontamination. This form of decontamination is often invasive and difficult to perform. Additionally, it includes small but genuine risks such as gastrointestinal perforation or pulmonary aspiration. However, gastrointestinal decontamination is the cornerstone in the early management of acutely poisoned patients.

## Emesis

If emesis is induced shortly after a drug is ingested, a substantial portion of the ingested agent may be removed. The amount eliminated varies with the rapidity of absorption of the poison and the time since its ingestion. Syrup of ipecac, the most commonly used emetic, contains two alkaloids, cephaline and emetine. These alkaloids, which primarily induce emesis centrally through stimulation of the medullary chemoreceptor trigger zone, require absorption themselves. Therefore, syrup of ipecac has a requisite lag time of at least 20 minutes before it produces emesis. The greatest risk of ipecac is related to this lag time, as continued toxin absorption may depress the patient's level of consciousness during this period. Alteration in the level of consciousness before emesis may result in the loss of protective airway reflexes with subsequent aspiration pneumonitis or asphyxiation. Also, since ipecac-induced emesis persists for about an hour, the administration of activated charcoal (a valuable adsorbing agent) must be delayed.

Ipecac-induced emesis in volunteers removes about half of the ingested drug from the stomach, as determined by serum identification of a nontoxic marker or measurement of a marker in the expelled vomitus. Evidence of the clinical benefit of ipecac is not clear. However, there are suggestions that administering ipecac shortly after ingestion reduces the amount of drug absorbed (Amitai et al. 1987). The use of ipecac is most appropriate for witnessed ingestions of poisons by children at home, under circumstances when a rapid deterioration in the patient's mental status is not expected. The amount of drug actually removed in a hospital-based clinical practice is likely to be lower, because of the substantial delay before patient presentation and the initiation of treatment. Consequently, use of ipecac involves clinical judgment, as benefits and risks are hard to predict in individual patients.

## Orogastric Lavage

Orogastric lavage involves the insertion of a large-bore tube via the esophagus into the stomach to evacuate the gastric contents with subsequent large volume serial irrigations. Although this method avoids the 20-minute lag time associated with ipecac-induced emesis, it does not appear to be more effective in the evacuation of gastric contents (Tenenbein et al. 1987a). Practical limitations of orogastric lavage include the time delay after ingestion until the procedure is performed and the ingestion of pills that are larger than the holes in even the largest (40 French) orogastric lavage tubes. Hemodynamic changes related to enhanced vagal tone, and structural damage such as esophageal perforation, may occur. Although the clinical benefit of emesis remains to be proved, lavage appears to be beneficial in the subgroup of patients who are clinically ill and who present within 1 hour following ingestion (Kulig et al. 1985; Pond et al. 1995). It is likely that lavage is beneficial when performed even later than 1 hour after ingestion, particularly for toxins that delay gastric outflow. Most patients who have ingested a potentially life-threatening amount of drug should probably have orogastric lavage performed.

## Activated Charcoal

Activated charcoal is produced by the treatment of burned wood pulp with acid and steam. This renders the surface of the individual particles porous and able to bind physically (adsorb) a wide range of substances through electrostatic interactions. Once bound to the activated charcoal within the lumen of the gastrointestinal tract, toxins are no longer available for systemic absorption. The use of activated charcoal eliminates many of the problems associated with emesis and orogastric lavage. It is effective immediately after administration, and its utility is not so compromised by pyloric outflow, since toxins may bind within the duodenum. It may be administered as a drink to conscious patients and through a conventional nasogastric tube in patients with altered consciousness, minimizing the complications associated with large-bore orogastric tubes. Experimental and clinical models have demonstrated that activated charcoal is at least as effective as ipecac or orogastric lavage in preventing the absorption of various toxins (Pond et al. 1995).

It is interesting that the beneficial effects of oral activated charcoal are not limited to prevention of absorption. Activated charcoal in the gastrointestinal tract may actually enhance the elimination of certain systemically absorbed toxins, such as phenobarbital (Berg et al. 1982) and theophylline (Berlinger et al. 1983). This effect, termed *gastrointestinal dialysis,* uses the gastrointestinal capillary bed as a dialysis membrane much the same way as peritoneal dialysis uses the serosal surface. This effect is most pronounced in patients who receive several doses of activated charcoal (i.e., multiple-dose activated charcoal) (Chyka 1995).

### Whole-Bowel Irrigation

Whole-bowel irrigation has been used extensively to prepare the colon for surgery or endoscopy. The administration of a nonabsorbable, isotonic polyethylene glycol solution results in the evacuation of all intestinal contents over several hours. Since sustained-release preparations of drugs may be released over several hours, contain large amounts of drug, and are not generally subject to enhanced dissolution by the irrigant, whole-bowel irrigation is ideal for the gastrointestinal decontamination of patients who have ingested sustained-release tablets or capsules (Tenenbein et al. 1987b). The critical determinants for the success of whole-bowel irrigation are speed and volume of administration. Delivery of 2 L/h to most adult patients results in gastrointestinal clearance of drug within 3 hours. Of related interest is the use of whole-bowel irrigation to facilitate the passage of cocaine- or heroin-filled condoms or balloons from the gastrointestinal tracts of "body packers" (Hoffman et al. 1990). Body packers are persons who attempt to transport large quantities of these illicit substances in this manner to avoid detection.

**PRINCIPLE Prevention of absorption of toxin remaining in the GI tract is important in managing the poisoned patient. The method used to provide gastrointestinal decontamination following ingestion of a potential toxin primarily depends on the clinical condition of the patient, the nature and quantity of the toxin, and the relative risk of toxin-associated or therapy-associated morbidity and mortality.**

## ADDITIONAL MANAGEMENT ISSUES

### Antidotes

An antidote is a substance that counteracts the harmful effects of a toxin. Although antidotes are in clinical use for several important toxins, the vast majority of potential toxins do not have specific antidotes.

Antidotes may act in a variety of ways. Antidotes may compete at the enzyme or receptor level with a poison to reverse an undesired physiological effect. For example, ethanol competes with methanol or ethylene glycol for access to the enzyme alcohol dehydrogenase, and naloxone prevents binding of opioids to opioid receptors. Antidotes may also have more specific physiological effects that rectify a change induced by a toxin. Antidotes may also function by a host of different mechanisms, including free radical scavenging by *N*-acetylcysteine, chelation by ethylenediaminetetraacetic acid (EDTA), or enzyme reactivation by pralidoxime.

Antidotes may have significant adverse effects; many are inherently toxic, and the clinical results of their use may be unpredictable. Therefore, the decision to use most antidotes requires expertise and careful clinical judgment (Table 18-3).

### Toxicology Laboratory

The role of the toxicology laboratory is limited in acute-care toxicology. Since most hospital laboratories are able to detect rapidly only a handful of toxins, most poisoned patients must be managed without this knowledge. Clinically useful laboratory analysis is available in a timely fashion in most hospitals for acetaminophen, salicylates, lithium, digoxin, carbon monoxide, iron, phenobarbital, and theophylline. Ethylene glycol and methanol are examples of important toxins for which in-hospital laboratory analyses are not routinely available.

It should be noted that for most poisons, serum concentrations correlate poorly with clinical toxicity. Clinical toxicity usually relates to variables that are unique to each clinical encounter, such as the time since ingestion, the presence of coingestants, the preexistent health of the patient, and prior exposure to the toxin. For example, the pharmacodynamic tolerance achieved by patients with chronic, excessive ethanol intake permits serum ethanol concentrations that would likely prove fatal to ethanol-naive patients. These variables highlight the importance of clinical assessment as a prerequisite for the utilization of objective laboratory data in the management of poisoned patients.

### Enhanced Elimination

Under normal circumstances most drugs are eliminated from the body by hepatic metabolism and/or renal elimination. Attempts to enhance the endogenous clearance of drugs by these organs is generally limited and may lead to complications. An exception may be the administration of multiple-dose activated charcoal to enhance the clearance of a drug through gastrointestinal dialysis (see above).

**Table 18-3 Selected Antidotes, Their Indications, and Mechanisms of Action**

| ANTIDOTE | INDICATION (TOXIN) | MECHANISM OF ACTION |
|---|---|---|
| Antivenin | Pit viper bite<br>Coral snake bite<br>Black Widow spider bite | Binding of toxin by antibody |
| Botulinal trivalent antitoxin | Botulism | Binding of toxin by antibody |
| Cyanide kit (amyl nitrite inhalation, sodium nitrite parenteral, sodium thiosulfate parenteral | Cyanide poisoning | Bind cyanide to methemoglobin, then enhance conversion to thiocyanate for excretion |
| Deferoxamine mesylate (Desferal) | Iron poisoning | Chelate iron, enhance renal excretion |
| Digoxin-specific antibody fragments (Digibind) | Digoxin poisoning (and other cardiac glycosides) | Binding of digoxin to antibody |
| Dimercaptosuccinic acid (DMSA, Succimer, Chemet) | Lead, mercury, arsenic poisoning | Chelate heavy metal, enhance renal excretion |
| Ethanol | Methanol, ethylene glycol poisoning | Inhibit alcohol dehydrogenase, slow conversion to toxic aldehydes and acids |
| Ethylenediaminetetraacetic acid (calcium disodium EDTA) | Lead poisoning | Chelate heavy metal, enhance renal excretion |
| Fomepizole (Antizol) | Ethylene glycol and methanol | Inhibit alcohol dehydrogenase, slow conversion to toxic aldehydes and acids |
| Methylene blue | Methemoglobinemia | Help reduce $Fe^{+++}$ to $Fe^{++}$, thereby improving oxygen delivery to tissues |
| *N*-Acetylcysteine (Mucomyst) | Acetaminophen poisoning | Bind to toxic reactive metabolite, protect liver cells from damage |
| Octreotide | Poisoning with oral hypoglycemic agents | Block release of insulin from pancreas |
| Oxygen | Carbon monoxide poisoning | Displace CO from hemoglobin |
| Physostigmine salicylate (Antilirium) | Some cases of poisoning with anticholinergic drugs | Enhance duration of action of acetylcholine at cholinergic receptors by inhibiting acetylcholinesterase |
| Pralidoxime chloride (Protopam) | Organophosphate or carbamate poisoning | Reactivate cholinesterase inactivated by organophosphate |
| Starch | Iodine poisoning | Convert iodine to iodide (nontoxic) |
| Vitamin $K_1$ (Aquamephyton Konakion) | Warfarin poisoning | Enhance vitamin $K_1$-dependent synthesis of clotting factors II, VII, IX, and I |

## Forced Diuresis

Increasing the flow of urine by volume loading (not by administering diuretics) is the basis of forced diuresis. This method of enhancing renal elimination has never been conclusively shown to increase the amount of drug removed from the body, even for drugs that are entirely eliminated by the kidney, such as lithium (Hansen and Amdisen 1978). In addition, forced diuresis may be complicated by iatrogenic volume overload or hyponatremia.

## Manipulation of the Urine pH

Although similar in some respects to forced diuresis, deliberate manipulation of the pH of the urine is conceptually different. Instead of increasing urine flow to "wash out" more toxin, the pH of the urine is most commonly raised to allow toxins with low $pK_a$ values (i.e., weak acids or anions such as salicylate) to become ionized within the renal tubule and collecting system. The ionized drug is trapped in the urine since only nonionized substances can diffuse back across cellular membranes to be reabsorbed. A pH change can only be of benefit if a drug or toxin is ionizable within the pH range of urine, such as salicylic acid, phenobarbital, or formic acid. Alkalinization of the urine is most commonly achieved by the administration of sodium bicarbonate intravenously.

Acidification of the urine, which would conceivably enhance the elimination of weak bases with high $pK_a$ values, is considered dangerous, since many of the toxins that might benefit from this maneuver (e.g., phencyclidine or amphetamine) are associated with rhabdomyolysis. Acidification of the urine in this situation would allow myoglobin to precipitate within and to obstruct the renal tubule.

### Hemodialysis/Hemoperfusion

Hemodialysis involves the passage of blood over a semipermeable membrane, through which equilibration occurs with a balanced dialysate solution lacking the toxin or substance that is to be removed. Toxins in the blood that are small enough to pass through the membrane are cleared from the blood. However, even small toxins may not pass through the membrane if they are bound to plasma proteins. Additionally, toxins that are not predominantly in the blood compartment cannot be substantially removed from the blood, even if they easily cross the membrane. The volume of distribution ($V_d$) determines whether a sufficient amount of toxin exists within the blood space to be cleared by hemodialysis. In general, small, water-soluble molecules having masses less than 500 daltons and a $V_d$ less than 1 L/kg and exhibiting low protein binding are removed by hemodialysis. Toxins commonly removed by dialysis that meet these requirements include salicylate, lithium, methanol, and ethylene glycol.

However, hemodialysis is invasive, expensive, and involves the risk of systemic anticoagulation in most cases. Therefore, most poisoned patients do not warrant hemodialysis even if hemodialysis would remove the toxin. However, in patients with severe poisoning from salicylates, lithium, methanol, or ethylene glycol, the benefits of dialysis often outweigh these rules. Peritoneal dialysis, which uses the intestinal serosa as a dialysis membrane, has a more limited ability to enhance the clearance of xenobiotics and is rarely, if ever, indicated in poisoned patients.

Hemoperfusion is conceptually similar to hemodialysis, but a canister filled with activated charcoal or a synthetic resin is substituted for a semipermeable membrane and dialysate. The blood from the poisoned patient is percolated through the activated charcoal, which removes a certain percentage of those substances capable of binding to activated charcoal. Thus the limitations of molecular weight and protein binding are eliminated, but the toxin must still be in the blood space. However, hypocalcemia and thrombocytopenia occur commonly and limit the appeal of hemoperfusion. Severe toxicity from theophylline and phenobarbital is the most frequent indication for the use of hemoperfusion.

**PRINCIPLE There are many techniques for treating symptomatic poisoned patients. None of these, however, is as important as the provision of comprehensive supportive care and limitation of toxin absorption. For several types of severe poisoning, however, additional techniques may be beneficial. Some are readily available, others require specialized consultation, and all are best applied through interaction with the regional poison center.**

## COMMON CLINICAL SITUATIONS INVOLVING POISONED PATIENTS

A short period can be afforded during the care of most poisoned patients to allow information gathering in order to focus therapy. In many instances the optimal therapeutic intervention differs between toxin-induced clinical conditions and similarly appearing conditions related to other causes. For example, patients who have a seizure following an overdose of isoniazid often require the administration of pyridoxine (vitamin $B_6$) in order to adequately control seizures (Wasson et al. 1981). This approach differs substantially from the use of conventional anticonvulsant medications such as diazepam or phenytoin, which are expected to yield a rapid response in patients with non-toxin-induced seizures.

These special considerations emphasize the need for a complete history and physical examination to detect potentially poisoned patients. Several examples of the specific diagnostic and therapeutic approaches necessary to evaluate patients with suspected poisonings are provided below. In every case, the reader should pay particular attention to the manner in which toxicologic management differs from that of non-poisoned patients.

### Tricyclic Antidepressants

CASE HISTORY *A 31-year-old depressed woman ingests a bottle (50 capsules) of her tricyclic antidepressant and shortly after presents to the emergency department after tonic-clonic seizure. The patient has the following vital signs: blood pressure, 80/50 mm Hg; pulse, 130 beats per minute; respirations, 18 breaths per minute; and temperature, 99.8 °F (37.6 °C). Her fingerstick glucose is 100 mg/dL and her oxygen saturation by pulse oximetry is 99%. The physician, recognizing the seriousness of the overdose, performs orogastric lavage and administers activated charcoal. An electrocardiograph reveals sinus tachycardia with a wid-*

*ened QRS (0.140 sec). The regional poison center is contacted, and administration of intravenous sodium bicarbonate is recommended.*

Tricyclic antidepressants have consistently been among the five most lethal drugs reported to the AAPCC poisoning database (Litovitz et al. 1997). Although these antidepressants are being replaced by the selective serotonin reuptake inhibitors (SSRIs) as primary therapy for patients with depression, they still account for a substantial proportion of poisoning deaths each year.

Tricyclic antidepressants appear to exert their therapeutic benefit through their ability to inhibit the reuptake of neurotransmitters, including norepinephrine and serotonin, at critical brain regions. However, as a group, the tricyclic antidepressants have an exceedingly complex pharmacologic profile, and their toxicity cannot be predicted solely on their mechanism of action. For example, blockade of muscarinic cholinergic receptors predictably produces anticholinergic manifestations in poisoned patients, including sinus tachycardia, mydriasis, ileus, and inability to void. These anticholinergic effects prove to be a useful diagnostic marker for patients with tricyclic antidepressant poisoning. Seizures are common in patients with significant overdose and may be mediated through antagonism of the inhibitory GABA-mediated chloride channels (Malatynska 1988).

The morbidity and mortality of tricyclic antidepressants, however, is directly related to the cardiotoxic effects of these agents. The blockade of fast sodium channels within the myocardial conductive cells slows ventricular depolarization and reduces the force of contraction of the heart (Sasyniuk and Jhamandas 1984). These fast sodium channels open in response to a critical voltage threshold and allow sodium ions to move from the extracellular to the intracellular space. This rapid increase in the intracellular potential (phase 0 of the action potential) is reflected on the surface electrocardiograph as the QRS complex. Thus, a delay in sodium movement across the partially blocked sodium channels slows phase 0 of the action potential and produces a widened QRS complex on the electrocardiograph. The resultant QRS complex duration, which is related to the degree to which the sodium channels are blocked, is a useful prognostic tool for patients with tricyclic antidepressant poisoning. In patients with tricyclic antidepressant poisoning, an increase in the QRS complex duration to greater than 160 msec suggests that sufficient myocardial toxicity exists to place the patient at risk for the development of ventricular dysrhythmias (Boehnert and Lovejoy 1985). Furthermore, when the QRS complex duration is greater than 100 msec, sufficient central nervous system effects may be present to place the patient at risk for seizures (Boehnert and Lovejoy 1985). The duration of the QRS complex is a useful surrogate marker of the severity of the overdose and the likelihood of life-threatening complications.

Initial management of the cardiotoxic manifestations of tricyclic antidepressant poisoning is the administration of intravenous sodium bicarbonate at 1 to 2 mEq/kg. The benefit of bicarbonate may be due to alteration of the charge on the tricyclic antidepressant or through a change in the conformation of the sodium channel, making conditions at the sodium channel less favorable to binding by the tricyclic antidepressant. Clinical improvement appears not to be related to enhanced protein binding (Pentel and Keyler 1988) or increased urinary elimination of the tricyclic antidepressant as previously believed. Additionally, the delivery of a high concentration of sodium ions directly to the partially blocked channel enhances the trans-channel sodium gradient, restoring normal depolarization (Bou-Abboud and Nattel 1996). Although any concentrated sodium salt, such as hypertonic sodium chloride (McCabe et al. 1994), can be used, the most convenient form is hypertonic sodium bicarbonate, which is commonly available in either 7.5% (0.9 mEq/mL) or 8.4% (1 mEq/mL) concentrations. Hypertonic sodium bicarbonate provides both concentrated sodium ions and alkalinization concomitantly, making it the drug of choice for the management of tricyclic antidepressant poisoning.

Historically, treatment to ameliorate the anticholinergic effects of tricyclic antidepressants included the administration of physostigmine, a cholinesterase inhibitor that can cross the blood–brain barrier, as an antidote. Since the sodium channel antagonism of the tricyclic antidepressant demonstrates a rate-dependent binding and is greatest at rapid heart rates (Ansel et al. 1993), slowing of the heart rate through enhanced vagal tone seems rational. However, the anticholinergic-mediated sinus tachycardia maintains systemic perfusion, which would otherwise fall because of hypotension. In addition, the combination of poor myocardial conduction due to sodium channel blockade compounded by the physostigmine-induced reduction in myocardial conduction owing to enhanced vagal tone may result in profound cardiac dysfunction (Pentel and Peterson 1980). Also, cholinesterase inhibition can produce life-threatening bronchorrhea. For all these reasons, physostigmine is rarely given in this type of poisoning. However, it is not clear to what extent these maneuvers are clinically useful.

Aggressive gastrointestinal decontamination is warranted in patients with tricyclic antidepressant overdoses. Since the anticholinergic properties of the toxin reduce gastric emptying, the drug may still be available in the stomach for removal even after substantial time has passed. Activated charcoal should be used after orogastric lavage, but syrup of ipecac is contraindicated because of the propensity for abrupt seizures and the risk of aspiration. There is no role for extracorporeal techniques to enhance elimination because of the large volume of distribution of the tricyclic antidepressants and the transient nature of the toxicity.

**Key Point: In addition to aggressive gastrointestinal decontamination and supportive care, the administration of hypertonic sodium bicarbonate to a patient with tricyclic antidepressant-induced hypotension or dysrhythmias may be life-saving.**

## Carbon Monoxide

Carbon monoxide is the toxin most frequently associated with fatalities (Litovitz et al. 1997). Since it is a gas, it disperses, becoming distributed throughout a closed environment, often resulting in multiple casualties. Carbon monoxide has been called the "silent killer," since it is colorless **and** odorless and may be produced through subtle processes. That is, although carbon monoxide poisoning is frequently noted in fire victims (Lundquist et al. 1989), it is also commonly encountered as a result of malfunctioning home heating units or automobile exhaust systems (Cobb and Etzel 1991).

Carbon monoxide is also clinically "silent" in many cases. Since patients with severe carbon monoxide poisoning may be critically ill, failure to consider this diagnosis may result in death, and the poisoning is only recognized later by medical examiner. In addition, patients with more mild carbon monoxide poisoning typically have common and vague complaints such as headache, malaise, or flu-like symptoms. These are especially troublesome, since carbon monoxide poisoning is most common in the autumn and winter (Cobb and Etzel 1991), a time during which viral illness and inclement weather are endemic. Subtle presentations of carbon monoxide poisoning frequently go unrecognized unless epidemic in nature and may result in misdiagnosis with potentially grave consequences.

Carbon monoxide produces its clinical effects through two distinct physiologic, yet chemically related, effects. Carbon monoxide (C–O) is very similar to oxygen (O–O); CO substitutes for $O_2$ at the active site of several important metalloenzymes, particularly hemoglobin and cytochrome oxidase. In fact, hemoglobin binds carbon monoxide with an affinity 240 times its affinity for oxygen. Additionally, not only does carbon monoxide reduce the oxygen content of the blood, it also shifts the hemoglobin-oxygen dissociation curve to the left, further reducing delivery of oxygen to the tissues (Roughton and Darling 1944). The practical result of the binding of carbon monoxide to hemoglobin is tissue hypoxia due to the inability of hemoglobin to carry or deliver oxygen.

Additionally, carbon monoxide binds mitochondrial cytochrome oxidase and inhibits the electron transport chain (Brown and Piantadosi 1990). Lack of oxidative metabolism forces the cells to rely on anaerobic metabolism for energy production, a much less efficient source that results in the development of metabolic acidosis with an elevated serum lactic acid level. With substantial CO exposure, all tissues suffer hypoxia, although the tissues with the greatest oxygen demand (such as the central nervous system and heart) suffer most.

Although the inhibition of both oxygen transport and utilization may be life-threatening, most victims of carbon monoxide poisoning survive. Most, in fact, are asymptomatic and are considered poisoned only on the basis of an elevated blood carboxyhemoglobin level (>10%). A consequential proportion of these patients experience the delayed onset of subtle neuropsychiatric impairment, which in many cases appears to go undetected unless very sensitive cognitive testing is performed (Thom et al. 1995). Although obvious neurological abnormalities, such as hemiparesis, may be noted, most of these patients suffer from more subtle problems such as memory loss, personality change, or depression. A similar clinical syndrome appears in patients with other hypoxic-ischemic insults, suggesting a common pathophysiologic process, but this remains unconfirmed (Volpe and Hirst 1983). In addition, and likely unique to carbon monoxide poisoning, the depletion of nitric oxide from platelet hemoproteins may incite a cascade of inflammatory mediators (Thom et al. 1994).

Conventional diagnostic modalities such as pulse oximetry and arterial blood gas analyses are unable to diagnose carbon monoxide poisoning (Bozeman et al. 1997). Both are falsely normal even in patients with profound carbon monoxide poisoning. However, making the diagnosis is relatively simple once the possibility is considered. Analysis of the blood using a co-oximeter identifies all common atypical hemoglobin species, which include carboxyhemoglobin and methemoglobin, in addition to the expected oxygenated and deoxygenated forms.

All carbon monoxide-poisoned patients should be provided with 100% oxygen. Those with severe, life-threatening symptoms require expeditious transfer, when possible, to a center capable of providing hyperbaric oxygen (HBO) therapy. HBO therapy involves the delivery of pure oxygen at greater than 1 atm of pressure (>760 mm Hg) in order to force the dissolution of supraphysiologic quantities of oxygen into the patient's blood. At these unusually high partial pressures, oxygen is favored over carbon monoxide in the competition for hemoglobin and cytochrome oxidase binding. The rate of dissociation of carbon monoxide from these hemoproteins is increased, and a normal physiologic state of oxygen delivery and utilization is restored. Patients with the most severe symptoms of tissue hypoxia, such as chest pain, cardiovascular instability, altered mental status, focal neurologic deficits, or metabolic acidosis, may benefit most from the restoration of oxygen delivery through rapid aggressive HBO therapy. Unfortunately, these same patients are often considered too unstable for transport to an HBO center.

Patients without life-threatening symptoms who have elevated blood carboxyhemoglobin concentrations may also benefit from HBO therapy. Although these patients do not die from the acute carbon monoxide exposure, they are at substantial risk for the development of delayed neuropsychiatric symptoms. The risk is greatest when syncope has occurred, presumably signaling a severe nervous system insult, but delayed sequelae may also be seen in patients who have no symptoms (Thom et al. 1995). When administered within 6 hours or shortly after hospital presentation, HBO therapy may prevent the delayed neurologic sequelae (Thom et al. 1995). However, this time limitation often presents logistical problems for hospitals without ready access to HBO therapy.

Unfortunately, our limited understanding of the pathophysiology of carbon monoxide poisoning and the therapeutic benefit of HBO therapy prevents the application of any single standard of care for the treatment of carbon monoxide-poisoned patients. Most hyperbaric medicine specialists use a carboxyhemoglobin level of 25% as an independent criterion for HBO therapy (Hampson et al. 1995). Virtually all would provide HBO therapy at a level of 40% to carbon monoxide-poisoned patients who are minimally symptomatic (e.g., have a headache) (Hampson et al. 1995). The decision to transfer a poisoned patient for HBO therapy ultimately is determined by the patient's clinical condition and risks of transport and therapy.

As in all poisonings, prevention is vital in reducing the personal and societal impact. Carbon monoxide may be the most amenable of all common toxins to poison prevention interventions. Widespread use of carbon monoxide detectors in the home and workplace, as well as proper maintenance of furnaces and automobiles, would likely produce dramatic reductions in the incidence of carbon monoxide poisoning.

**Key Point: Carbon monoxide poisoning is the most common cause of poisoning fatalities. It is a problem that often goes undiagnosed. The simultaneous occurrence of suggestive symptoms in a family or group of people should lead the clinician to suspect carbon monoxide poisoning.**

## Calcium Channel Blockers

CASE HISTORY *A 45-year-old woman ingests 25 sustained-release verapamil tablets in a suicide attempt. She presents to the hospital 2 hours later and is noted to have profound hypotension and a heart rate of 40/min. Despite this she is awake and conversant.*

As a group, the calcium channel blockers are responsible for a limited number of cases of poisoning per year, though they have one of the highest case-fatality rates following overdose (Hawton et al. 1995; Litovitz et al. 1997). Formulation as sustained-release products in order to enhance compliance and to reduce side effects dramatically complicates management of patients who overdose. The sustained-release calcium channel blockers contain substantially larger quantities of drug than their conventional release counterparts, and in overdose they release toxin over a prolonged, and often unpredictable, period of time.

The hypotension and bradycardia that generally occur in patients exposed to substantial doses of a calcium channel blocker are a direct extension of the therapeutic effects of this class of drug. As noted earlier, hypotension and bradycardia in the absence of significant cardiac disease is atypical, as most healthy patients with acute hypotension develop reflex tachycardia. In addition, patients poisoned with these agents appear to maintain consciousness at heart rate–blood pressure products that are normally associated with CNS dysfunction. This may be due to an effect on neuronal calcium channels that reduces their oxygen requirements (Brain Resuscitation Clinical Trial II Study Group 1991) and protect against grave cerebral hypoxia.

Administration of intravenous calcium salts is a logical choice for the initial therapy of a poisoning from calcium channel blocker. Calcium salts provide predominantly inotropic support and have less effect on the heart rate. This effect is exploited in patients with supraventricular tachydysrhythmias, in whom calcium salts are administered before verapamil to prevent hypotension (Salerno et al. 1987). An inadequate response may reflect either insufficient calcium dosing, for which additional calcium should be administered, or a mixed overdose.

There is no standard dosing regimen for calcium salts (calcium chloride or calcium gluconate) in this situation, and little evidence to guide the decision. Standard reference sources may recommend administration of calcium salts without recommending a dose (*Mosby's GenR$_x$* 1998) or advise that further evaluation in controlled studies is needed (Ellenhorn 1997). Perhaps the clearest guidelines for administration of calcium in this situation are found in *Poisindex,* which recommends that calcium chloride 1 g IV be given slowly over 5 minutes, repeated every 10 to 20 minutes as necessary for a total of 4 or 5 doses (*Poisindex* 1997). In the authors' experience, the administration of calcium chloride in this manner is often effective and appears to be safe.

The management of patients poisoned by a calcium channel blocker often proves to be exceedingly complex, and patients often fail to respond adequately to large doses of calcium. Responses to vasopressors such as norepinephrine may be unpredictable. Consequently, these patients require careful hemodynamic monitoring and adjustment of therapy depending on cardiovascular responses.

Because of the extreme toxicity of calcium channel blockers, gastrointestinal decontamination becomes exceedingly important to limit clinical effects in patients who have ingested a calcium channel blocker. This is particularly important for patients who have ingested sustained-release products (Howarth et al. 1994). Patients discharged prematurely may become symptomatic following release. Activated charcoal should be administered to all patients who ingest calcium channel blockers, and those with exposure to sustained-release preparations should receive whole-bowel irrigation with a polyethylene glycol electrolyte solution (Kirshenbaum et al. 1989).

**Key Point: Calcium channel blockers, particularly verapamil and diltiazem, are associated with substantial toxicity in overdose. When formulated as sustained-release preparations, these medications produce delayed clinical manifestations and severe toxicity that may go undetected initially.**

## Methanol and Ethylene Glycol

CASE HISTORY *An 18-month-old child is found sitting in a puddle of spilled antifreeze in the family's garage. She looks well on arrival in the Emergency Department. Her arterial blood gas and serum electrolytes are normal, and an ethylene glycol level is sent to an outside clinical laboratory.*

Methanol and ethylene glycol are toxic alcohols. Ironically, neither methanol nor ethylene glycol is directly toxic. Both must undergo oxidative metabolism to their corresponding aldehydes and carboxylic acid derivatives to become toxic. Alcohol dehydrogenase, the enzyme responsible for ethanol metabolism, is primarily responsible for the initial step in this conversion. Substances that inhibit this enzyme delay or prevent toxicity, an effect of critical importance in the treatment of patients poisoned by toxic alcohols.

Methanol is found in a variety of home and automotive products including windshield washer fluid and gas-line antifreeze. Ethylene glycol is used as an automotive radiator antifreeze because it alters the boiling and freezing points of water, yet it is not volatile even at the very high temperature of an automotive engine cooling system.

The critical link between ethanol, a "nontoxic" (although intoxicating) alcohol, and methanol or ethylene glycol is the production of toxic metabolites from the latter toxins. The final oxidative metabolite of ethanol, acetic acid, enters the Krebs cycle as acetyl CoA and is subsequently eliminated as carbon dioxide. However, the metabolites of methanol and ethylene glycol are themselves toxic and are not metabolized to benign metabolites such as $CO_2$.

Methanol metabolism by alcohol dehydrogenase produces formaldehyde, which is rapidly converted by aldehyde dehydrogenase to formic acid. Formic acid, an organic acid, exists in the blood as formate, the conjugate base form present at physiological pH, and produces a metabolic acidosis. In addition, because formate undergoes only very gradual renal elimination or slow entrance into the one-carbon metabolic pathway by combining with tetrahydrofolate, it accumulates in the body (McMartin et al. 1980). The serum bicarbonate falls without an increase in another measured negatively charged ion, since formate is not detected by the routine serum chemistry analyzers. The anion gap, which is the difference between the measured cations ($Na^+ + K^+$) and the measured anions ($Cl^- + HCO_3^-$) increases. Most important, formic acid is a retinal toxin and is responsible for the visual disturbances and blindness associated with methanol poisoning (Martin-Amat et al. 1977).

Because ethylene glycol has two hydroxyl groups, its metabolism is more complex. The glycolic acid metabolite is quantitatively the most prevalent and is responsible for the metabolic acidosis (Gabow et al. 1986). However, oxalic acid, the more toxic metabolite, binds calcium and precipitates in aqueous solutions such as urine and cerebrospinal fluid. Although renal failure may occur because of tubular obstruction by precipitated calcium oxalate stones, death is usually related to the severe hypocalcemia that is produced upon stone formation. As in the case of methanol poisoning, an elevated anion-gap metabolic acidosis occurs in patients with consequential exposures.

Clinical evaluation soon after exposure to methanol or ethylene glycol may be unrevealing. Patients with significant ingestions may demonstrate signs of inebriation that are indistinguishable from those of ethanol intoxication. Laboratory evaluation at this point would be unlikely to demonstrate an acidosis, since the conversion of both methanol and ethylene glycol to their acid metabolites takes several hours. However, an elevated osmolar gap may be present before this conversion. The osmolar gap is the difference between the measured osmolarity and the calculated osmolarity:

$$\text{Calculated osmolarity (mosmol/L)} = (2 \times \text{Na}^+) + \frac{\text{glucose (mg/dL)}}{18} + \frac{\text{BUN (mg/dL)}}{2.8}$$

An increase in this difference defines the presence of unknown osmotically active particles in solution. Although methanol and ethylene glycol are uncharged and add osmotic activity, metabolism to ionizable substances (e.g., oxalate, formate) allows them to pair with a positively charged sodium ion, and therefore charged metabolites are included in this component of the calculated osmolar gap, reducing the difference. As can be seen, the stage of metabolism shifts the importance of the osmolar gap, which is often elevated in early poisoning, to the anion gap, which becomes elevated as toxic metabolite accumulates.

Treatment, as noted, is targeted at preventing conversion of the parent alcohols to their toxic metabolites. Ethanol is the preferred substrate for alcohol dehydrogenase and thus competitively inhibits the toxic alcohols at the active site of this enzyme. The therapeutic goal is to maintain a chronic serum ethanol concentration of approximately 100 mg/dL (Wacker et al. 1965). Ethanol markedly prolongs the elimination of the parent compound, and without hemodialysis, prolonged ethanol infusions may be required to permit adequate endogenous methanol or ethylene glycol clearance. Long-term ethanol infusion is undesirable, however, because of the unpleasant prolonged inebriation, risk of hypoglycemia, and the potential for phlebitis and electrolyte abnormalities.

Recently, 4-methylpyrazole (fomepizole), a long-acting competitive antagonist of alcohol dehydrogenase, has been approved for the treatment of ethylene glycol poisoning (Baud et al. 1988). This drug has several important clinical advantages over ethanol, although its utility has not yet been fully evaluated.

Methanol, ethylene glycol, and their toxic metabolites are small, water-soluble molecules, and thus quite amenable to removal by hemodialysis. In patients with moderate or severe methanol or ethylene glycol intoxication, hemodialysis can serve a number of useful purposes, including enhanced clearance of the toxic alcohol before it can be metabolized, enhanced removal of toxic metabolites, and more rapid correction of marked electrolyte and acid-base abnormalities, especially the severe anion-gap metabolic acidosis. Indications for hemodialysis are not precise and depend on the clinical judgment of the treating physician, who must pay attention to several important factors.

For methanol, the benefits of hemodialysis appear to outweigh the risks when the peak methanol concentration is 500 mg/L (50 mg/dL) or greater; or when a lower methanol concentration is present, but the metabolic acidosis is not immediately correctable (which implies that much of the methanol has already been metabolized to formic acid); when visual impairment is already present; or when renal failure is present (Ellenhorn 1997). Dialysis should continue until the methanol concentration is reduced below 100 to 250 mg/L. The clinician must also remember that the rate of infusion of intravenous ethanol 10% in D5W must be increased during dialysis, since dialysis enhances the clearance of ethanol as well.

For ethylene glycol, indications for hemodialysis are likewise not entirely clear at this time. As in cases of methanol intoxication, hemodialysis may need to be instituted before symptoms of toxicity appear. Some experts recommend that hemodialysis be performed for patients with any substantial exposure to ethylene glycol and a pH less than 7.15 (since this indicates that substantial metabolism to glycolate and oxalate has already occurred), acidosis that is difficult to correct, deteriorating vital signs, shock, crystalluria (oxalate), or renal failure. Patients with high ethylene glycol concentrations (>500 mg/L or >50 mg/dL) even without a metabolic acidosis or other toxicity may benefit from hemodialysis to remove the alcohol before it is metabolized to its toxic metabolites and to shorten length of stay in hospital (Ellenhorn 1997; *Poisindex* 1997). The intravenous infusion of ethanol should be continued until the concentration of ethylene glycol falls to low levels and the metabolic acidosis is fully corrected.

Partly because of its availability in very concentrated forms, the quantity of toxic alcohol that must be ingested to achieve a toxic level is remarkably small, especially in children. A small child who ingests 1 teaspoon (5 mL) of pure methanol may develop a "dialyzable" level of 25 mg/dL.

**Key Points: Small amounts of concentrated methanol or ethylene glycol may produce severe metabolic and end-organ toxicity. Inhibition of the alcohol dehydrogenase by ethanol or fomepizole prevents the development of clinical toxicity from toxic metabolites and allows time to institute hemodialysis.**

## Salicylates

Aspirin (acetylsalicylic acid, ASA) poisoning was at one time a significant cause of poisoning in both young and old patients. In addition to acute intentional ingestion, chronic overuse of aspirin is associated with significant morbidity and mortality (Anderson et al. 1976). The therapeutic use of aspirin has sharply fallen in children partly because of its association with Reye's syndrome and the introduction of safer analgesic agents such as acetaminophen. In addition, the introduction and advancement of poison prevention techniques has likely contributed to the reduction in ingestions of this common household drug. Although low-dose aspirin is now widely prescribed for older patients, this will probably not be associated with dramatic increases in the number of patients with chronic poisoning, since the doses are trivial compared with those used to treat the inflammatory arthritides. However, poisoning by intentional salicylate ingestion may increase, since the availability of a drug is most closely associated with its use in suicides (Hawton et al. 1995). With the increasing use of alternative/complementary medicine, poisoning with methylsalicylate (oil of wintergreen) may become a more significant source of salicylate poisoning (Chan 1996). This oil is widely used in the pharmacopeia of herbal and naturopathic providers and delivers a very concentrated form of salicylate. Aspirin and methylsalicylate, and all other absorbed salicylate derivatives, liberate salicylic acid in the body; thus the focus of this section is on the toxicity of salicylate, the form available at physiologic conditions.

The life-threatening toxic effects of salicylates would not be predicted by the therapeutic mechanism of the drug, alteration of prostaglandin synthesis (Pedersen and FitzGerald 1984). Although this mechanism of action may be related to the nephrotoxic and ototoxic potential of salicylates, the predominant findings in poisoned patients are acid-base abnormalities and central nervous system dysfunction. The toxic effects of salicylates result from their ability to uncouple oxidative phosphorylation, an effect that differs from the inhibition of oxidative phosphorylation (Miyahara and Karler 1965). Uncoupling results when a substance dissipates the proton gradient generated by the movement of electrons derived from NADH through the cytochrome chain in the inner mitochondrial membrane toward their ultimate acceptor, oxygen. Since this gradient, which is used to generate cellular energy in the form of ATP, is no longer intact, an alternative source of energy formation must be utilized. Anaerobic metabolism of glucose is much less efficient than aerobic metabolism and does not provide an adequate means to reoxidize NADH to $NAD^+$. Anaerobic metabolism cannot function without $NAD^+$, so NADH is reoxidized through the reduction of pyruvate, which regenerates $NAD^+$ and produces lactic acid. This process is also responsible for almost the entire metabolic acidosis associated with salicylate poisoning, although a very small portion may be attributed to salicylic acid and its metabolites. Substantive uncoupling of oxidative phosphorylation probably occurs only at salicylate concentrations well above the therapeutic range.

Shortly after the acute ingestion of salicylates, at a time before the development of metabolic acidosis, respiratory alkalosis is often noted. Although an early diagnostic clue to salicylate poisoning, the hyperventilation responsible for the respiratory alkalosis may be missed if only the respiratory rate is evaluated. Hyperventilation is mediated through the central nervous system, not through systemic acidosis, and depth of respiration may be altered independently of the rate (Tenney and Miller 1955). This early alkalemia may actually prove beneficial for the patient, since it increases the proportion of the blood salicylic acid in the charged (or salicylate) form, reducing passage of the drug through the lipophilic blood-brain barrier into the central nervous system. Thus it should be clear that patients who have coingested drugs with respiratory depressant effects may suffer earlier and more severe toxicity.

With the increasing burden of salicylic acid entering the central nervous system, neurologic signs become evident. Confusion or lethargy are ominous signs, and the development of coma or seizures is frequently a preterminal event. Central nervous system toxicity is likely related to direct effects rather than a response to systemic toxicity, since the brain concentration of salicylate correlates more closely with the degree of impairment than does the serum concentration (Hill 1973). Chronic exposure to high therapeutic doses of salicylate may produce dramatic central nervous system signs of poisoning without extreme acid-base abnormalities.

Patients acutely poisoned with aspirin often have dramatic clinical presentations including vomiting, abdominal pain, and hyperventilation. Those with chronic salicylate intoxication more commonly present with altered mental status or pulmonary edema (Anderson et al. 1976; Gabow and Anderson 1978). Patients with chronic salicylate poisoning appear to have a worse prognosis than those with acute overdose, but this may be more closely related to delayed diagnosis and the age and health of the patients than to the intrinsic toxicity of salicylates. Many patients with chronic salicylate poisoning undergo several days of diagnostic study and consultation before the diagnosis is considered and finally confirmed.

Many of the pharmacologic and toxicologic aspects of salicylate can be incorporated into the management of the salicylate-poisoned patient. Interventions to correct fluid, electrolyte, glucose, and acid-base abnormalities are the bases of aggressive support of the patient's vital functions. For example, the provision of mechanical ventilation, which may be necessary to protect the airway or treat pulmonary edema, must often be set to continue the patient's spontaneous hyperventilation to maintain a respiratory alkalosis. Failure to hyperventilate the patient increases the $P\text{CO}_2$, resulting in a respiratory acidosis, which increases the amount of salicylic acid in the nonionized, and thus toxic, state. Similarly, most salicylate-poisoned patients are volume depleted because of hyperventilation, hyperthermia, and solute-induced diuresis. Rehydrating solutions must be chosen carefully, since excessive amounts of saline are associated with hyperchloremic metabolic acidosis. The preferred solution for rehydration of salicylate-poisoned patients is sodium bicarbonate. "Isotonic" sodium bicarbonate can be prepared by taking a 1-liter bag of D5W, and replacing 150 ml of D5W with 150 ml (150 mEq) of 2.4% sodium bicarbonate. The production and maintenance of a metabolic alkalosis has several benefits. The more alkaline serum prevents continuing efflux of salicylate into the brain and may help to reduce the central nervous system burden. Additionally, the alkaline urine that is produced ionizes the excreted salicylic acid and "traps" it in the collecting system (Morgan and Polak 1971).

Alkaluria, however, is often difficult to achieve. Reaching this endpoint may be accomplished by infusion of large amounts of sodium bicarbonate; although at extreme doses, the risk of fluid overload and hypernatremia may be excessive. Alternatively, since the solute diuresis also produces hypokalemia, the kidney attempts to reabsorb potassium in exchange for a positively charged hydrogen ion. This urinary acidification process can be reversed through the administration of exogenous potassium. In the past, urinary alkalinization with carbonic anhydrase inhibitors such as acetazolamide proved to have deleterious effects, since a systemic metabolic acidosis also resulted, increasing central nervous system toxicity and death (Schwartz et al. 1959).

Gastrointestinal decontamination of salicylate-poisoned patients should include activated charcoal, which binds the toxin in the gastrointestinal tract and clears it from the blood by gastrointestinal dialysis. The decision to perform orogastric lavage rests with the perceived risk of morbidity or mortality, which is common only after significant ingestions of methyl salicylate. Hemodialysis is useful in some patients (i.e., benefits outweigh risks) to enhance clearance of salicylate and to correct serious fluid and electrolyte abnormalities, especially metabolic acidosis. Indications for hemodialysis are not precise, vary somewhat from one reference source to the next, and depend on a combination of factors including salicylate plasma concentration, acuteness of the poisoning, and clinical status of the patient. In general, dialysis is recommended in an acute overdose producing plasma levels >1000 mg/L, or a chronic intoxication producing plasma concentrations of >600 to 800 mg/L. Hemodialysis may also be considered at lower plasma concentrations of salicylate if the patient already has serious complications (e.g., seizures, pulmonary edema), cannot produce a brisk alkaline diuresis (e.g., presence of renal failure, or volume overload precluding administration of sodium bicarbonate), or is a pediatric patient (Ellenhorn 1997).

**PRINCIPLE The development of acidemia is life-threatening to salicylate-poisoned patients. The therapeutic goal is the elevation of serum and urine pH above normal to favor the formation of ionized salicylate in the urine and to provide a gradient for clearance of salicylate from plasma.**

## Acetaminophen

Acetaminophen is the aniline counterpart of aspirin. However, acetaminophen produces a spectrum of toxicity completely unlike that of the salicylates. The popularity of acetaminophen in the United States began when the association of Reye's syndrome with aspirin use was recognized in the 1970s, and its use is now ubiquitous. It is among the substances most frequently involved in poison-related deaths (Litovitz et al. 1997), a fact related more to its prevalence than to its inherent toxicity.

Acetaminophen toxicity demonstrates an important concept in medical toxicology: the toxicity of the reactive metabolites. Although the toxicity of many substances such as methanol and ethylene glycol are attributed to their metabolites, the toxic effects of these metabolites are due to interference with specific physiologic processes. The toxic metabolite of acetaminophen, however, is a highly reactive electrophile, *N*-acetyl-*p*-benzoquinone imine (NAPQI), which indiscriminately produces toxicity (Roberts et al. 1987). The majority of a therapeutic dose of acetaminophen is metabolized to nontoxic sulfate and glucuronide metabolites. A very small percentage undergoes oxidative metabolism by the hepatic microsomal system CYP2E1 to produce NAPQI. Under therapeutic dosing conditions, NAPQI is readily detoxified through binding to endogenous glutathione. Depletion of the endogenous glutathione supply occurs after acetaminophen overdose because of massive production of NAPQI, and the remaining NAPQI binds covalently to the nearest electron-rich source, the liver cell. The ensuing hepatic necrosis is frequently fatal, but patients who survive regain normal liver anatomy and physiology. The kidney also contains enzymes capable of producing NAPQI locally, and acute tubular necrosis is frequently seen in patients with the greatest exposures.

The treatment for patients with acetaminophen toxicity depends on the interval between ingestion and presentation for medical care. Shortly after the ingestion, the patient may be asymptomatic but at risk for developing hepatotoxicity (Rumack et al. 1981). Clinical or laboratory signs of hepatotoxicity may not be evident for 16 to 24 hours after the ingestion. However, unlike the case for many toxins, the serum acetaminophen concentration has prognostic significance. A serum concentration, determined between 4 and 24 hours postingestion, may be applied to a nomogram that plots serum concentration versus time since ingestion (Rumack and Matthew 1975). A point falling above the line provided on the nomogram suggests that hepatotoxicity is likely, and a point below the line suggests that the patient is very unlikely to develop hepatitis. However, the important role of a precise history of exposure becomes evident when the effect of a time discrepancy is determined.

Patients with a serum acetaminophen concentration over the nomogram line, or those with overt hepatotoxicity already present, should receive *N*-acetylcysteine (Smilkstein et al. 1988). This antidote, which has a potent sulfur odor, appears to serve distinct roles in patients with and without hepatotoxicity. In patients presenting early and without hepatotoxicity, *N*-acetylcysteine both repletes glutathione and directly detoxifies NAPQI. Thus, administration of *N*-acetylcysteine to asymptomatic patients with potentially hepatotoxic serum acetaminophen concentrations (i.e., above the nomogram line) prevents hepatotoxicity. Although useful for scavenging NAPQI at all times, even after hepatotoxicity has developed, the antidote is best administered early. When administered within 8 hours of an ingestion, *N*-acetylcysteine hepatoprotection is virtually complete (Smilkstein et al. 1988). *N*-acetylcysteine is administered in a course of 18 doses over 72 hours to patients who present with acetaminophen concentrations above the high-risk line in the nomogram.

In the presence of hepatotoxicity, *N*-acetylcysteine appears to enhance recovery of liver function and reduces both patient mortality and the need for liver transplantation (Keays et al. 1991). Although the mechanism of *N*-acetylcysteine in the recovery from hepatotoxicity is unclear, it has been suggested that *N*-acetylcysteine enhances blood delivery and reduces neutrophil migration to the damaged tissue (Harrison et al. 1991). Therefore, *N*-acetylcysteine should be continued until hepatotoxicity resolves. As mentioned, orthotopic liver transplantation remains the final therapeutic option for patients with severe acetaminophen-induced hepatotoxicity (O'Grady et al. 1991), but this is an expensive and hazardous procedure. It should be considered a heroic measure and, at this time, performed only after supportive and antidotal mechanisms have failed.

As in the case of all ingestions, gastrointestinal decontamination plays a critical role in limiting the absorption of acetaminophen. The lack of early symptoms, and the availability of an antidote, have had the effect of limiting the role for aggressive early gastrointestinal decontamination. However, activated charcoal should be used. In the past, concerns were raised that the binding of *N*-acetylcysteine to activated charcoal would reduce the effectiveness of the antidote. However, theoretical and experimental models suggest that this is inconsequential following all but the largest acetaminophen overdoses. Activated charcoal therefore retains its important role in limiting the absorption of acetaminophen, thereby reducing the toxic effects of this and virtually all poisons.

**Key Points: Acetaminophen is frequently involved in poisoning. The delay in the onset of clinical toxicity makes the laboratory assessment for acetaminophen critical in all patients with suspected overdoses. *N*-Acetylcysteine is a remarkably successful antidote when initiated shortly after overdose and also improves outcome in patients who have already developed hepatotoxicity.**

## Cocaine

Cocaine has a long and rich history of use and abuse that dates back at least 1500 years to its origin in South America. Although originally consumed by the Incas as the coca leaf (*Erythroxylon coca*), cocaine was eventually extracted from the leaf by the German chemist Albert Niemann (Kleber 1988). Powdered cocaine (the hydrochloride salt) is significantly more stable than the alkaloid found in the raw leaf. Discovery of the conversion process allowed cocaine to remain stable over the long transport from South America to other parts of the world, ultimately leading to its popularity throughout the western world. Currently, cocaine use is epidemic in the United States, and 30 percent of men between 26 and 34 years of age have used the drug at least once (National Institute of Drug Abuse 1992). Despite its reemergence in the 1960s among affluent drug users, the pattern of use of cocaine shifted dramatically with the introduction of "crack," the alkaloidal form of cocaine, in the 1980s. Unlike the hydrochloride salt, crack cocaine is stable to pyrolysis, which allows it to be smoked. Compared with nasal insufflation, the onset of effect of crack is more rapid and the euphoria substantially more intense, with a pharmacokinetic profile similar to that of intravenous cocaine (Hatsukami and Fischman 1996).

Cocaine and amphetamines comprise the third most common cause of drug-related deaths reported to poison centers (Litovitz et al. 1997), but the actual number of deaths is certainly much greater (Pollack et al. 1991; Linakis and Frederick 1993). The lower than expected reporting may be related, in part, to the high frequency with which cocaine toxicity occurs in most urban centers and the comfort of the physician in managing patients with this exposure. In addition, since cocaine-related death is typically abrupt, most patients suffer their fatal event before arriving at the hospital.

Cocaine has two principal effects of pharmacologic interest: inhibition of reuptake of biogenic amines and sodium channel antagonism. Under normal circumstances, biogenic amines released within the synapse are rapidly resequestered by the presynaptic terminal through a reuptake pump and are subsequently repackaged within vesicles. Cocaine specifically inhibits this reuptake mechanism and allows the neurotransmitter to produce persistent postsynaptic stimulation. Inhibition of dopamine reuptake is responsible for the euphoric effects of cocaine, and blockade of serotonin reuptake accounts for the anorexia and mood-altering effects. Blockade of norepinephrine reuptake within the autonomic nervous system is associated with hypertension because of the pronounced $\alpha$-adrenergic agonist effects of norepinephrine, while potentiation of epinephrine released from the adrenal gland is responsible for the $\beta_1$-receptor-mediated tachycardia. Sodium channel blockade, an effect unrelated to blockade of catecholamine reuptake, impairs nerve conduction and is responsible for the local anesthetic (or type I antidysrhythmic) effects associated with cocaine.

The pharmacological complexity of cocaine is reflected in its clinical toxicology. There appears to be no universally safe dose of cocaine for all patients, and coronary artery vasoconstriction and myocardial ischemia may occur at doses conventionally used during rhinolaryngologic surgery (Lange et al. 1989). Cocaine has only limited effects outside of the central and autonomic nervous systems, and an intact nervous system is required in order to produce cocaine toxicity experimentally (Wilkerson 1988). Through effects on the autonomic nervous system, cocaine induces profound vasoconstriction ($\alpha_1$-adrenergic effects) and myocardial stimulation ($\beta_1$-adrenergic effects). These effects are primarily responsible for many of the sequelae of cocaine poisoning, including myocardial infarctions, cerebrovascular accidents, aortic dissections, and ischemic bowel. Although cocaine-related myocardial ischemia may result in dysrhythmias, the sodium channel blocking effects of cocaine also produce ventricular dysrhythmias and hypotension (Schwartz et al. 1989).

Patients with cocaine-related symptoms most commonly seek medical care for the adverse cardiovascular effects associated with cocaine. Typical presenting complaints include chest pain from myocardial ischemia, pneumothorax, or pulmonary infarction; altered mental status related to cerebrovascular events; or abdominal pain due to ischemic bowel. Patients with chest pain related to cocaine use often do not present in the typical fashion of patients with atherosclerotic cardiovascular disease. Symptoms are more often described as nonspecific or atypical, and absent or nonspecific changes on the electrocardiograph are common (Hollander and Hoffman 1992).

Understanding that central nervous system excitation and actions at noradrenergic synapses are the cause of the cardiovascular complications of cocaine (Catravas and Waters 1981), therapy can be more specifically applied with less risk of adverse events. Only by controlling the autonomic outflow can the peripheral manifestations of hypertension, tachycardia, and hyperthermia, as well as the cardiovascular complications, be controlled. Experimentally, only diazepam and hypothermia were able to positively influence hypertension, seizures, and death from cocaine (Catravas and Waters 1981). The same appears to be true in humans, and central nervous system sedation with safe agents such as benzodiazepines remains the mainstay of the management of cocaine-related cardiovascular events (Goldfrank and Hoffman 1991).

Since cocaine toxicity involves excessive peripheral stimulation by norepinephrine and epinephrine released by the sympathetic nervous system (Karch 1987), $\beta$-adrenergic antagonists were once suggested to control the sympathetic signs and symptoms and reduce the coronary artery vasoconstriction. However, neither the theoretical nor the experimental evidence supports the use of these agents to normalize the patient's vital sign abnormalities. Since a nonselective $\beta$-adrenergic antagonist such as propranolol blocks both the $\beta_1$ and $\beta_2$ receptors, the $\alpha$-adrenergic-induced vasoconstriction is no longer opposed by the $\beta_2$-adrenergic-induced vasodilation. The result is enhanced, not reduced, peripheral and coronary artery vasoconstriction and reduced myocardial perfusion (Lange et al. 1990). In addition, the $\beta_1$-adrenergic blockade reduces cardiac inotropy and may result in heart failure because of the profound $\alpha$-receptor-mediated peripheral vascular resistance. Esmolol (Sand et al. 1991), a short-acting $\beta_1$ selective agent, and labetalol (Boerher et al. 1993), a $\beta_1$-, $\beta_2$-, and $\alpha_1$-receptor antagonist, have been suggested as safer alternatives to propranolol, but neither has been found to be safe or effective. Calcium channel blockers have produced variable results and are likely a safer choice than $\beta$-adrenergic antagonists. However, these agents are presently felt to be detrimental in patients with traditional atherosclerotic coronary artery disease. In patients in whom myocardial ischemia persists despite the use of adequate doses of sedatives, the use of direct-acting vasodilators such as nitroprusside, or $\alpha$-adrenergic antagonists such as phentolamine, may have a role (Lange et al. 1989; Hollander et al. 1992). For patients demonstrating direct myocardial toxicity due to sodium channel blockade, treatment with an infusion of hypertonic sodium bicarbonate is analogous to that for tricyclic antidepressant-induced toxicity.

In the management of a patient with a cocaine overdose, treatment of the noncardiac effects is essential. Seizures require aggressive therapy and termination to prevent further acidosis, hyperthermia, and rhabdomyolysis. Similarly, life-threatening hyperthermia (core temperature greater than 105 °F) may worsen neurologic outcome and needs to be rapidly controlled. Both seizures and hyperthermia are best managed by the administration of benzodiazepines to reduce the psychomotor activity, as well as the application of the external cooling of hyperthermic patients.

Whereas cocaine stands as the model drug of abuse in this discussion, any patient exposed to an agent with sympathomimetic properties may present in a similar manner and could be safely managed by similar techniques. Other sympathomimetic agents include the amphetamine derivatives, indirect acting catecholamines such as phenylpropanolamine, and theophylline.

## CONCLUSIONS

Since virtually every chemical substance can be a poison, and since there are so many variables that alter the clinical toxicity seen in an individual patient, management of poisoned patients is exceedingly complex. If management proceeds with a patient-oriented approach, clinical care of most patients will be successful. However, consultation with a regional poison center or medical toxicologist is often beneficial to the patient and educational for the clinician. If consultation is not possible, or when the circumstances allow a more leisurely approach, several major reference textbooks of medical toxicology are available that may help better apply pharmacologic and toxicologic principles to patient care.

## REFERENCES


Amitai Y, Mitchell A, McGuigan M, Jr. 1987. Ipecac-induced emesis and reduction of plasma concentrations of drugs following accidental overdose in children. *Pediatrics* **80**:364–7.

Anderson R, Potts D, Gabow P, et al. 1976. Unrecognized adult salicylate intoxication. *Ann Intern Med* **85**:745–8.

Ansel G, Coyne K, Arnold S, et al. 1993. Mechanisms of ventricular arrhythmia during amitriptyline toxicity. *J Cardiovasc Pharmacol* **22**:798–803.

Bates D, Cullen D, Laird N, et al. 1995. Incidence of adverse drug events and potential adverse drug events: implications for prevention. *JAMA* **274**:29–34.

Baud F, Astier A, Bien D, et al. 1988. Treatment of ethylene glycol poisoning with intravenous 4-methylpyrazole. *N Engl J Med* **319**:97–100.

Belsey R, Morrison J, Whitlow K, et al. 1987. Managing bedside glucose in the hospital. *JAMA* **258**:1634–8.

Berg M, Berlinger W, Goldberg M, et al. 1982. Acceleration of the body clearance of phenobarbital by oral activated charcoal. *N Engl J Med* **307**:642–4.

Berlinger W, Spector R, Goldberg M, et al. 1983. Enhancement of theophylline clearance by oral activated charcoal. *Clin Pharmacol Ther* **33**:351.

Boehnert M, Lovejoy FJ. 1985. Value of the QRS duration versus the serum drug level in predicting seizures and ventricular arrhythmias after an acute overdose of tricyclic antidepressants. *N Engl J Med* **313**:474–9.

Boerher J, Moliterno D, Willard J, et al. 1993. Influence of labetalol on cocaine-induced coronary vasoconstriction in humans. *Am J Med* **94**:608–10.

Bou-Abboud E, Nattel S. 1996. Relative role of alkalosis and sodium ions in reversal of class I antiarrhythmic drug-induced sodium channel blockade by sodium bicarbonate. *Circulation* **94**:1954–61.

Boyle P, Schwartz N, Shah S, et al. 1988. Plasma glucose concentrations at the onset of hypoglycemic symptoms in patients with poorly controlled diabetes and in nondiabetics. *N Engl J Med* **318**:1487–92.

Bozeman W, Meyers R, Barish R. 1997. Confirmation of the pulse oximetry gap in carbon monoxide poisoning. *Ann Emerg Med* **30**:608–11.

Brain Resuscitation Clinical Trial II Study Group. 1991. A randomized clinical study of a calcium-entry blocker (lidoflazine) in the treatment of comatose survivors of cardiac arrest. *N Engl J Med* **324**:1225–31.

Brown S, Piantadosi C. 1990. In vivo binding of carbon monoxide to cytochrome *c* oxidase in rat brain. *J Appl Physiol* **68**:604–10.

Catravas J, Waters I. 1981. Acute cocaine intoxication in the conscious dog: studies on the mechanism of lethality. *J Pharmacol Exp Ther* **217**:350–6.

Chan T. 1996. Medicated oils and severe salicylate poisoning: quantifying the risk based on methyl salicylate content and bottle size. *Vet Hum Toxicol* **38**:133–4.

Chyka P. 1995. Multiple-dose activated charcoal and enhancement of systemic drug clearance: summary of studies in animals and human volunteers. *J Toxicol Clin Toxicol* **33**:399–405.

Cobb N, Etzel R. 1991. Unintentional carbon monoxide-related deaths in the United States: 1979 through 1988. *JAMA* **266**:659–63.

Cummins R. 1994. *Textbook of Advanced Cardiac Life Support*. Dallas: American Heart Association.

Ellenhorn MJ, editor. 1997. *Ellenhorn's Medical Toxicology*. 2d ed. Baltimore: Williams and Wilkins, pp 672.

Gabow P, Anderson R. 1978. Acid-base disturbances in the salicylate-intoxicated adult. *Arch Intern Med* **138**:1481–4.

Gabow P, Clay K, Sullivan J, et al. 1986. Organic acids in ethylene glycol intoxication. *Ann Intern Med* **105**:16–20.

Goldfrank L, Hoffman R. 1991. The cardiovascular effects of cocaine. *Ann Emerg Med* **20**:165–75.

Goldfrank LR, Flomenbaum NE, Lewin NA, et al. 1998. Vital signs and toxic syndromes. In: *Goldfrank's Toxicologic Emergencies*. 6th ed. Norwalk, CT: Appleton & Lange. Chapter 17, p 279.

Hampson N, Dunford R, Kramer C, et al. 1995. Selection criteria utilized for hyperbaric oxygen treatment of carbon monoxide poisoning. *J Emerg Med* **13**:227–31.

Hansen H, Amdisen A. 1978. Lithium intoxication. *Q J Med* **47**:123–4.

Harrison P, Wendon J, Gimson A, et al. 1991. Improvement by acetylcysteine of hemodynamic and oxygen transport in fulminant hepatic failure. *N Engl J Med* **324**:1852–7.

Hatsukami D, Fischman M. 1996. Crack cocaine and cocaine hydrochloride: are the differences myths or reality? *JAMA* **276**:1580–8.

Hawton K, Ware C, Mistry H, et al. 1995. Why patients choose paracetamol for self poisoning and their knowledge of its dangers. *Br Med J* **310**:164.

Hill J. 1973. Salicylate intoxication. *N Engl J Med* **288**:1110–3.

Hoffman R, Goldfrank L. 1995. The poisoned patient with altered consciousness: controversies in the use of the "coma cocktail." *JAMA* **274**:562–9.

Hoffman R, Smilkstein M, Goldfrank L. 1990. Whole bowel irrigation and the cocaine body-packer: a new approach to a common problem. *Am J Emerg Med* **8**:523–7.

Hollander J, Carter W, Hoffman R. 1992. Use of phentolamine for cocaine-induced myocardial ischemia [letter]. *N Engl J Med* **327**:361.

Hollander J, Hoffman R. 1992. Cocaine-induced myocardial infarction: an analysis and review of the literature. *J Emerg Med* **10**:169–77.

Howarth D, Dawson A, Smith A, et al. 1994. Calcium channel blocking drug overdose: an Australian series. *Hum Exp Toxicol* **13**:161–6.

Humphrey D. 1991. Final exit: the practicalities of self-deliverance and assisted suicide for the dying. Eugene, OR: Hemlock Society.

Karch S. 1987. Serum catecholamines in cocaine intoxicated patients with cardiac symptoms. *Ann Emerg Med* **16**:481.

Keays R, Harrison P, Wendon J, et al. 1991. Intravenous acetylcysteine in paracetamol induced fulminant hepatic failure: a prospective trial. *Br Med J* **303**:1026–9.

Kirshenbaum L, Mathews S, Sitar D, et al. 1989. Whole-bowel irrigation versus activated charcoal in sorbitol for the ingestion of modified-release pharmaceuticals. *Clin Pharmacol Ther* **46**:264–71.

Kleber H. 1988. Cocaine abuse: historical, epidemiological, and psychological perspectives. *J Clin Psychiatr* **49**:3–6.

Kulig K, Bar-Or D, Cantrill S, et al. 1985. Management of acutely poisoned patients without gastric emptying. *Ann Emerg Med* **14**:562–7.

Lange R, Cigarroa R, Flores E, et al. 1990. Potentiation of cocaine-induced coronary vasoconstriction by beta-adrenergic blockade. *Ann Intern Med* **112**:897–903.

Lange R, Cigarroa R, Yancy C, et al. 1989. Cocaine-induced coronary-artery vasoconstriction. *N Engl J Med* **321**:1557–62.

Linakis J, Frederick K. 1993. Poisoning deaths not reported to the regional poison control center. *Ann Emerg Med* **22**:1822.

Litovitz T, Smilkstein M, Felberg L, et al. 1997. 1996 Annual Report of the American Association of Poison Control Centers Toxic Exposure Surveillance System. *Am J Emerg Med* **15**:447–500.

Lundquist P, Rammer L, Sorbo B. 1989. The role of hydrogen cyanide and carbon monoxide in fire casualties: a prospective study. *Forensic Sci Int* **43**:9–14.

Malatynska E, Knapp R, Ikeda M, et al. 1988. Antidepressants and seizure-interactions at the GABA-receptor chloride-ionophore complex. *Life Sci* **43**:303–7.

Malouf R, Brust J. 1985. Hypoglycemia: causes, neurologic manifestations and outcome. *Ann Neurol* **17**:421–30.

Martin-Amat G, Tephly T, McMartin K, et al. 1977. Methyl alcohol poisoning. II: development of a model for ocular toxicity in methyl alcohol poisoning using the *Rhesus* monkey. *Arch Ophthalmol* **95**:1847–50.

McCabe J, Menegazzi J, Cobaugh D, et al. 1994. Recovery from severe cyclic antidepressant overdose with hypertonic saline/dextran in a swine model. *Acad Emerg Med* **1**:111–5.

McMartin K, Ambre J, Tephly T. 1980. Methanol poisoning in human subjects. Role of formic acid accumulation in the metabolic acidosis. *Am J Med* **68**:414–8.

Miyahara J, Karler R. 1965. Effect of salicylate on oxidative phosphorylation and respiration of mitochondrial fragments. *Biochem J* **97**:194–8.

Morgan A, Polak A. 1971. The excretion of salicylate in salicylate poisoning. *Clin Sci* **41**:475–84.

National Institute on Drug Abuse. 1992. National household survey on drug abuse: population estimates 1991. Rev. ed. DHHS pub. no. (ADM) 92–1887. Washington, DC: U.S. Government Printing Office.

O'Grady J, Wendon J, Tan K, et al. 1991. Liver transplantation after paracetamol overdose. *Br Med J* **303**:221–3.

Pedersen A, FitzGerald G. 1984. Dose related kinetics of aspirin: presystemic acetylation of platelet cyclooxygenase. *N Engl J Med* **311**:1206–11.

Pentel P, Keyler D. 1988. Effects of high dose alpha-1-acid glycoprotein on desipramine toxicity in rats. *J Pharmacol Exp Ther* **246**:1061–6.

Pentel P, Peterson C. 1980. Asystole complicating physostigmine treatment of tricyclic antidepressant overdose. *Ann Emerg Med* **9**:588–91.

Pollack D, Holmgreen P, Lui K, et al. 1991. Discrepancies in the reported frequency of cocaine-related deaths, United States, 1983 through 1988. *JAMA* **266**:2233–7.

Pond S, Lewis-Driver D, Williams G, et al. 1995. Gastric emptying in acute overdose: a prospective randomized controlled trial. *Med J Aust* **163**:345–9.

Roberts D, Pumford N, Potter D, et al. 1987. A sensitive immunochemical assay for acetaminophen-protein adducts. *J Pharmacol Exp Ther* **241**:527–33.

Roughton F, Darling R. 1944. The effect of carbon monoxide on the oxyhemoglobin dissociation curve. *Am J Physiol* **141**:17–31.

Rumack B, Matthew H. 1975. Acetaminophen poisoning and toxicity. *Pediatrics* **55**:871–6.

Rumack B, Peterson R, Koch G, et al. 1981. Acetaminophen overdose: 662 cases with evaluation of oral acetylcysteine treatment. *Arch Intern Med* **141**:380–5.

Safranek D, Eisenberg M, Larsen M. 1992. The epidemiology of cardiac arrest in young adults. *Ann Emerg Med* **21**:1102–6.

Salerno D, Anderson B, Sharkey P, et al. 1987. Intravenous verapamil for treatment of multifocal atrial tachycardia with and without calcium pre-treatment. *Ann Intern Med* **107**:623–8.

Sand I, Brody S, Wrenn K, et al. 1991. Experience with esmolol for the treatment of cocaine associated cardiovascular complications. *Am J Emerg Med* **9**:161–3.

Sasyniuk B, Jhamandas V. 1984. Mechanism of reversal of toxic effects of amitriptyline on cardiac Purkinje fibers by sodium bicarbonate. *J Pharmacol Exp Ther* **231**:387–94.

Schwartz A, Janzen D, Jones R. 1989. Electrocardiographic and hemodynamic effects of intravenous cocaine in awake and anesthetized dogs. *J Electrocardiol* **22**:159–66.

Schwartz R, Fellers F, Knapp J, et al. 1959. The renal response to administration of acetazolamide (Diamox) during salicylate intoxication. *Pediatrics* **23**:1103–14.

Shook J, Watkins W, Camporesi E. 1990. Differential roles of opioid receptors in respiration, respiratory disease, and opiate-induced respiratory depression. *Am Rev Respir Dis* **142**:895–909.

Smilkstein M, Knapp G, Kulig K, et al. 1988. Efficacy of oral N-acetylcysteine in the treatment of acetaminophen overdose. *N Engl J Med* **319**:1557–62.

Tenenbein M, Cohen S, Sitar D. 1987a. Efficacy of ipecac induced emesis, orogastric lavage and activated charcoal for acute drug overdose. *Ann Emerg Med* **16**:838–41.

Tenenbein M, Cohen S, Sitar D. 1987b. Whole bowel irrigation as a decontamination procedure after acute drug overdose. *Arch Intern Med* **147**:905–7.

Tenney S, Miller R. 1955. The respiratory and circulatory actions of salicylates. *Arch Intern Med* **19**:498–508.

Thom S, Ohnishi T, Ischiropoulos H. 1994. Nitric oxide released by platelets inhibits neutrophil B2 integrin function following acute carbon monoxide poisoning. *Toxicol Appl Pharmacol* **128**: 105–10.

Thom S, Taber R, Mendiguren I, et al. 1995. Delayed neuropsychologic sequelae after carbon monoxide poisoning: prevention by treatment with hyperbaric oxygen. *Ann Emerg Med* **25**:474–80.

Volpe B, Hirst W. 1983. The characterization of an amnesic syndrome following hypoxic ischemic injury. *Arch Neurol* **40**:436–40.

Wacker W, Haynes H, Druyan R, et al. 1965. Treatment of ethylene glycol poisoning with ethyl alcohol. *JAMA* **194**:173–5.

Wasson S, Lacouture P, Lovejoy F. 1981. Single high-dose pyridoxine treatment for isoniazid overdose. *JAMA* **246**:1102–4.

Wilkerson D. 1988. Cardiovascular effects of cocaine in conscious dogs: importance of fully functional autonomic and central nervous systems. *J Pharmacol Exp Ther* **246**:466–71.

PART

# 3

# CORE TOPICS IN CLINICAL PHARMACOLOGY

CHAPTER

# 19 DRUG THERAPY IN PREGNANT AND BREAST-FEEDING WOMEN

Peter C. Rubin, Jane M. Rutherford

### *Chapter Outline*



Four decades ago two case reports published simultaneously suggested that thalidomide, a sedative that had been claimed to be safer than other drugs of its type, appeared to cause serious birth defects when taken during the first trimester of pregnancy (Lenz 1961; McBride 1961). Confirmation of this observation came rapidly from all countries where thalidomide had been used, and it was clear that a disaster of major proportions and considerable implications had occurred (Mellin and Katzenstein 1962). The ramifications of the thalidomide tragedy extended far beyond the limited issue of drug-induced fetal abnormality. This event had political, social, and legal implications that were far-reaching. Currently, research into the use of drugs during pregnancy is carried out under "thalidomide's long shadow" (Thalidomide 1976). Developments in the clinical pharmacology of pregnancy have been slow because of the general fear that a drug given during pregnancy may have disastrous and unforeseeable consequences for the unborn baby. This fear naturally has greatly limited *experimental* research on drugs used during pregnancy, and we are left with inadequate anecdotal information on which to base decisions. Yet conditions that require drug treatment, or for which drug treatment may be beneficial, occur frequently during pregnancy; examples include hypertension, epilepsy, asthma, and bacterial infections. The purpose of this chapter is to bring together information about drug use during pregnancy and to discuss general approaches to the clinical pharmacology of pregnancy.

## EPIDEMIOLOGY OF DRUG USE DURING PREGNANCY

Seven studies of reasonable size and data ascertainment are described here. Smaller studies (some involving fewer than 100 patients) are excluded because the sample size is probably inadequate to draw conclusions about the general population. The seven larger studies vary considerably in methodology and in the population being studied, although they were all carried out in either the United States or the United Kingdom. Five of the six studies were prompted directly or indirectly by the thalidomide tragedy, but the largest, the Collaborative Perinatal Project, began before the thalidomide tragedy (Heinonen et al. 1977). This study involved 50,282 pregnancies, and data were collected before the outcome of pregnancy was known. Chronologically, the next study was carried out among 3072 patients attending Kaiser Permanente clinics as the thalidomide story was developing (Peckham and King 1963). The information was collected from medical records. Just after this study, another survey of 911 women was carried out in Edinburgh; data were collected by interview at the end of pregnancy and by cross-checking with prescriptions at local pharmacies (Forfar and Nelson 1973). Ten years later 2528 Medicaid recipients in

Nashville were studied; details were obtained from pharmacists' prescription records (Brocklebank et al. 1978). Another study based on Medicaid claims was carried out in Michigan among 18,886 women who had delivered a live infant (Piper et al. 1987). A prospective survey of drug use during pregnancy was performed from 1982 to 1984 in Glasgow, where drug-taking histories were collected from 2765 women at each antenatal clinic attendance (Rubin et al. 1986). Information on a random 10% subset was cross-checked with general practitioners' records. Finally, a study of 2752 mothers of infants without major congenital malformations was carried out in Maryland (Rubin JD et al. 1993).

Overall drug use during pregnancy, as found in these studies, is shown in Figure 19-1. There is a surprising degree of consistency of drug use during pregnancy over the four decades and among patients from considerably different circumstances. Between one-third and two-thirds of all pregnant women take at least one drug during the pregnancy (excluding dietary supplements and drugs taken at delivery). The lower proportion of women taking drugs during pregnancy in the Glasgow study is likely to be a result of special circumstances at that time. Pyridoxine hydrochloride plus doxylamine (Bendectin in the United States, Debendox in the United Kingdom) was the subject of considerable interest in the news media, and the drug actually was withdrawn by the manufacturers midway through the Glasgow study because of fears that it might be teratogenic. This matter is considered later in the chapter, but it seems reasonable to assume that the highly negative publicity given to drug use during pregnancy at the time of the study decreased drug consumption by pregnant women.

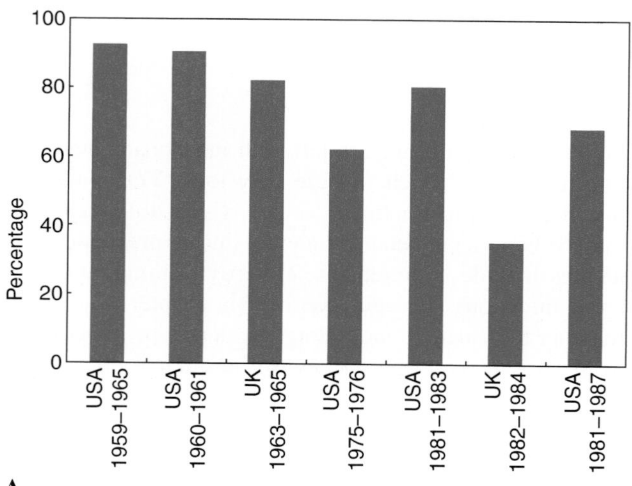


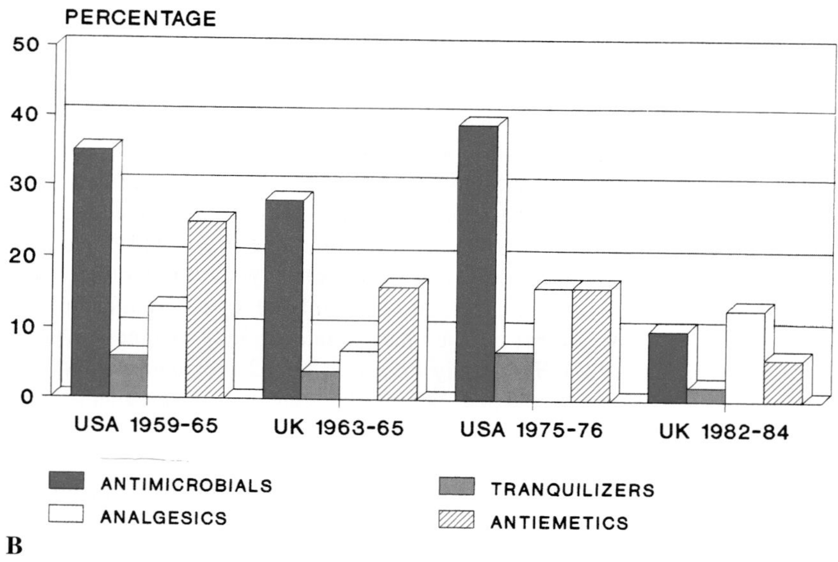


FIGURE 19-1 *A.* Percentage of pregnant women taking a drug during pregnancy in the United States or United Kingdom at different times during a 28-year period. Iron and vitamin supplements are excluded from the data. *B.* "Exploded" view of use of four classes of drugs by pregnant women in four of the five periods studied in A.

The Glasgow study attempted to identify any group that was more or less likely to be prescribed a drug or to use an over-the-counter preparation, but no clear pattern emerged. There was no significant difference in any kind of drug use with regard to social class; additionally, whether a woman smoked or drank alcohol regularly did not seem to influence her use of medications. In a study in the state of Michigan of the very different Medicaid population (low-income women eligible for government assistance), African-American mothers appeared to have higher rates of exposure than white women enrolled in this study to a variety of drugs, including analgesics, ampicillin, and vaginal preparations. These women may have had a higher incidence of disease, although the study design could not confirm that possibility.

These studies demonstrate that drug use during pregnancy is common; even the Glasgow study, which showed the lowest frequency of drug use, found that 34.8% of women took a medication, using 154 different drugs from 35 drug groups. Therefore, although there is public concern about the possible adverse effects of drug use in pregnancy, the fact remains that drugs are widely used, and more systematically gathered information is needed about the consequences of prescribing drugs for pregnant women. Many women who give birth to normal babies were exposed to at least one pharmacological agent during pregnancy. Therefore, it is not advisable to attribute *adverse* outcomes to drug use in individual cases.

In considering the risk of using medications during pregnancy, it is important to emphasize that pregnancy is divided into distinctly different periods that may have important implications for evaluating the effect of a particular drug. For example, the first trimester of pregnancy is the period of organogenesis when concern about fetal malformation is paramount; however, drugs taken later in pregnancy can affect fetal growth and development.

**PRINCIPLE The name of a disease or condition does not describe its stages or severity, both of which can profoundly influence the effects and choice of therapy.**

## DRUGS IN THE FIRST TRIMESTER

### Teratogenicity

The word *teratogen* is derived from the ancient Greek word *teratos* (monster) and refers to a substance that leads to the birth of a malformed baby. Fetal malformation is a fact of reproductive life. In developed countries, about 2% of all pregnancies end with the birth of a baby with an anatomic abnormality. In most cases it is impossible to identify an external agent that could have been responsible. This background incidence of fetal abnormality is crucially important in the interpretation of reports that suggest a particular drug led to a particular abnormality. Before we can discuss drug-induced teratogenicity in more detail, it is necessary to address two issues that are highly relevant to this question.

### Placental Transfer of Drug

For a drug to harm the fetus it must cross the placenta and be present in fetal tissue. Many studies have addressed the pharmacokinetics of placental transfer, and there are several good reviews in this area (Waddell and Marlowe 1981; Kraver et al. 1988). Unfortunately most studies have emphasized the rate of placental transfer of a drug after a single IV injection. Useful pharmacokinetic models have been established to describe the different situations that can occur depending on, for example, lipid solubility of a drug or maternal protein binding and metabolism. However, the rate of placental transfer usually is not of prime importance. Almost all cases in which drug exposure can lead to fetal abnormality involve a course of drug treatment over days or longer and not a single administration of a drug. Consequently, the pertinent question is not how quickly the drug crosses the placenta but whether it will cross at all. Currently available data suggest that almost all drugs cross the placenta after multiple doses regardless of their pharmacokinetic characteristics. The only major exceptions encountered in clinical practice are insulin and heparin. Heparin is a large, polar molecule that does not reach measurable concentrations on the fetal side of the circulation. In all other drugs studied, placental transfer occurs; however, it should be emphasized that most investigations were carried out in the third trimester. It is probably appropriate to extrapolate these findings to the first trimester, but there is relatively little direct information.

**PRINCIPLE A study of drug effects that does not describe the stages of disease or duration of therapy often is uninterpretable.**

As indicated above, in most cases the pharmacokinetic profile of a drug does not appear to be important with regard to passage across the placenta. For example, atenolol, a hydrophilic drug with poor lipid solubility, was not considered likely to cross the placenta, in contrast to its more lipophilic counterpart propranolol. However, studies have not confirmed this speculation; indeed, atenolol reaches high concentration in cord blood (Rubin et al. 1983). For practical purposes the prescribing physician should assume that any drug will cross the placenta.

## Period of Organogenesis

Between approximately 18 and 55 days after conception, the human fetus undergoes organogenesis, when major anatomic structures are created (Figure 19-2). A drug can cause a structural abnormality only if it is present in the body during this period; for example, nonclosure of a neural tube is not possible once spontaneous closure of the tube has taken place. This simple and seemingly self-evident principle is widely overlooked but is a very important concept in understanding drug-induced teratogenicity as well as in advising women who may have been or may be exposed to a potential teratogen.

## Identifying Drug Teratogens

Ten thousand cases of phocomelia were reported before thalidomide was identified as a teratogen. Although discovery was considered efficient, this type of abnormality is very unusual, and the fact that thalidomide caused this defect in a high percentage of exposures makes it clear that the problem should have been discovered sooner. Clearly, if surveillance had been systematic, fewer people would have been deformed by the drug (see chapters 27, Drug Discovery and Development; 28, Risk Analysis Applied to Prescription Drugs; 30, Information about Drugs). In most cases, the certainty of whether a drug is or can be teratogenic is elusive.

**PRINCIPLE The absence of toxicity data about drugs used during pregnancy does not preclude such toxicity.**

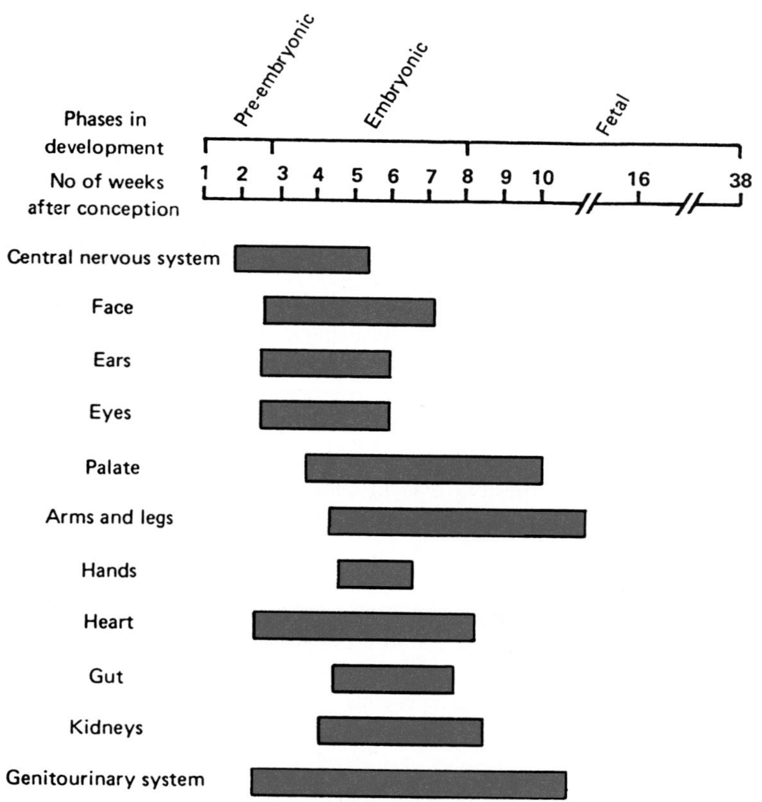


FIGURE 19-2 **Period of human organogenesis. (Reproduced courtesy of Dr. Martin Whittle, Queen Mother's Hospital, Glasgow, and with permission from the *British Medical Journal*.)**

Studies of the effects of drugs in pregnant animals are of dubious value despite the fact that they are widely performed and, indeed, in many countries must be performed during the development of a new drug. Such studies are generally unhelpful for two reasons. First, any link between toxic effects in a rat and the consequences of therapeutic administration in a pregnant woman is tenuous at best. A further problem with animal studies is that there is considerable variation among species (Szabo and Brent 1974; Elia et al. 1987). Thalidomide is a teratogen only in primates. There are many more examples of major differences between animals and humans. For example, lithium given to rats at a dose of 200 mg/kg of body weight produces no fetal abnormality; at 300 mg/kg it substantially increases the incidence of cleft palate to 6%, and 450 mg/kg causes a 30% incidence of cleft palate (Szabo 1970). However, in humans, lithium appears to cause cardiac abnormalities at doses far below the 200 mg/kg used in rat studies. The absence of a teratogenic effect in an animal, therefore, provides no assurance that a substance is safe for humans.

**PRINCIPLE There is no way to discover a drug effect that occurs only in humans without testing in humans. For low-incidence events, testing often must be observational and after marketing of the drug.**

In the absence of suitable laboratory models of teratogenicity of drugs in humans, studies aimed at identifying drug teratogens must be performed in humans. Such studies are generally of three types and are discussed in greater detail in two excellent references (Cordero and Oakley 1983; Goldberg and Golbus 1986).

### *Case reports*

Reports of individual patients taking a drug can have enormous value in drawing attention to a possible association that later can be confirmed or refuted by other investigators. Case reports first drew attention to the fact that thalidomide (Lenz 1961; McBride 1961) and warfarin (Kerber et al. 1968) were teratogenic. But case reports can be misleading, as demonstrated by suggestions that Bendectin (Debendox) caused a limb-reduction defect. The Bendectin saga demonstrates the misleading power of "the well-chosen anecdote" (Orme 1985).

If a woman has a baby with an abnormality and that woman also took a drug during the first trimester of pregnancy, now it has become inevitable that an association between the drug and the abnormality will be drawn, particularly by the woman herself. However, given a 2% incidence of fetal abnormalities whether or not a drug is used, the association cannot exclude a chance relationship. The case against Bendectin was pursued not only to the highest courts in the United States but also through television and newspapers in several countries, where pictures of deformed children inevitably led to removal of the drug from ethical obstetric practice. However, almost all the scientifically credible cohort studies with Bendectin suggest that the drug is not a teratogen; the relative risk is 0.89, with 95% confidence limits of 0.7 and 1.04 (MacMahon 1981). In addition, several case-control studies found no association between Bendectin and fetal abnormality (Debendox 1984; Orme 1985). The case against Bendectin was never proved scientifically or in the courts, yet to protect themselves from public pressure the manufacturers withdrew the drug in 1983 after it had been given to approximately 3 million pregnant women.

### *Case studies*

Case studies involve several patients who have received a particular drug and whose offspring have a similar malformation. Fetal hydantoin syndrome (Hanson and Smith 1975) and the teratogenicity of isotretinoin (Rosa 1983) both came to light as a result of this observational methodology.

**PRINCIPLE We almost always search hard to establish blame for tragedy. Even without supportive data, drugs have been removed from the market because of emotional outcry alone. It is time to realize that the drug signal in humans is precious and needs to be systematically and objectively evaluated before banning a medication that may be both safe and useful.**

### *Epidemiologic studies*

These types of studies have already been alluded to with regard to Bendectin, and there are two major types. A cohort study aims to compare the outcome of pregnancy in two groups—one was exposed to the agent of interest and the other was not. A case-control study begins with a fetal abnormality and compares that group of pregnancies with a matched pregnant population that had a normal outcome. The study assesses exposure to the agent of interest in each group. Prospective cohort studies are expensive and time-consuming because large numbers of patients may be required to detect a relatively subtle teratogenic effect. For example, the association between diethylstilbestrol (DES) and vaginal adenocarcinoma strongly suggested a drug effect in case-control studies. About 100,000 exposed women would be necessary to confirm this relationship in a prospective cohort study (Cordero and Oakley 1983). The confirmatory study has not been done, but for medical purposes is not needed.

## Teratogenic Drugs

The physician must know which drugs are *likely to cause harm* when taken during pregnancy. Table 19-1 lists drugs in common clinical use for which a teratogenic effect has been demonstrated. The drugs in this list are those for which evidence is either conclusive or highly suggestive. Not included are drugs that are used infrequently during pregnancy or for which a teratogenic effect may occur but for which evidence is lacking. The list does not include the likely risk of fetal abnormality after exposure in the first trimester. The omission is deliberate and is discussed further in relation to each drug.

### *Anticonvulsants*

The role of anticonvulsant drugs in producing fetal abnormality illustrates the difficulties of drawing conclusions about drug effects in this area of clinical pharmacology. The suggestion that there is a "fetal hydantoin" syndrome was first made in a report of several cases in 1975 (Hanson and Smith 1975). The syndrome comprises poor growth and development with various structural abnormalities, including nail hypoplasia, hypertelorism, microcephaly, cleft lip or palate, and various other abnormalities that occur less frequently. The original case reports suggested an 11% incidence of the syndrome. Fetal hydantoin syndrome has been both confirmed and refuted in the years since the original report.

One of the most persuasive studies to cast doubt on the existence of a specific syndrome related to administration of phenytoin comes from the Collaborative Perinatal Project in the United States (Shapiro et al. 1976). This study found that the malformation rate among children born to epileptic mothers was 10.5% compared with 6.4% in the remainder of the population ($P < 0.01$). The difference still held when only major malformations were considered (6.6% in epileptic pregnancies and 2.7% in controls). However, there was no significant difference in fetal abnormality according to the drug used. In addition, certain malformations, such as cleft palate, were more common not only in the children of epileptic mothers but also in the children of epileptic fathers. These data have been interpreted as indicating that it is epilepsy, and not its treatment, that is responsible for the fetal abnormality. The evidence from several studies is that the rate of fetal malformation in the offspring of epileptic mothers is around 10%, but what is not clear is whether the syndrome is a consequence of the epilepsy itself, the result of a common genetic determining factor in either parent, or the result of the drug alone or when used in combination with all these different influences. To dissect the contribution of different factors is difficult because the

**Table 19-1 Commonly Used Drugs That Have Demonstrated Teratogenicity in Humans**

| Drug | Effect | Prenatal Diagnosis |
|---|---|---|
| Lithium | Cardiac defects (Ebstein complex) | Feasible |
| Warfarin | Chondrodysplasia punctata | Unlikely |
| | Facial anomalies | Unlikely |
| | Severe anomalies of the CNS | Unlikely |
| Phenytoin | Craniofacial | Feasible |
| | Limb | Feasible |
| | Growth deficiencies | Feasible |
| Sodium valproate | CNS | Feasible |
| Carbamazepine | Craniofacial | Feasible |
| | Fingernail | Feasible |
| Sex hormones | Cardiac defects | Feasible |
| | Multiple anomalies | Feasible |
| Retinoic acids | Craniofacial | Feasible |
| | Cardiac | Feasible |
| | CNS | Feasible |

drug and the disease are often inseparable. For example, another group reported that the frequency of fetal malformation increases with the number of anticonvulsant drugs used (Lindout et al. 1984). However, it is reasonable to assume that more severely epileptic women require more drugs. So the increase in birth defects may be the result of more severe disease.

The issues surrounding anticonvulsant drug teratogenicity are far from resolved, but in recent years some interesting findings point clearly to a genetic determinant that causes fetal abnormality when either parent has epilepsy. However, whether this genetic factor operates separately from, or in conjunction with, pharmacologic factors is unknown.

**PRINCIPLE To determine cause and effect, it is not enough to associate events with drugs.**

An interesting study of 62 families with fetal exposure to phenytoin in two or more pregnancies (Van Dyke et al. 1988) included 10 mothers who had a baby with some of the physical features of hydantoin syndrome and took phenytoin again in a later pregnancy. Nine of the 10 pregnancies produced a baby with features of fetal hydantoin syndrome. In contrast, 52 mothers who had an unaffected baby at the end of their first pregnancy continued taking phenytoin during a second pregnancy; only 5 of those pregnancies produced a baby with characteristics of fetal hydantoin syndrome. The difference between the two groups was highly significant. However, whether the mothers would have had abnormal babies if phenytoin had not been given cannot be determined. Another report describes the features of fetal hydantoin syndrome occurring in only one of dizygotic twins of different paternity. These results again point strongly to a genetic factor that determines the syndrome (Phenlan et al. 1982).

Further developments add interesting pieces to the puzzle. Carbamazepine often has been proposed as the safest anticonvulsant for use in pregnancy. But a retrospective and prospective study has shown that this drug too is associated with fetal abnormalities, similar to those of fetal hydantoin syndrome including fingernail hypoplasia, poor growth, and developmental delay (Jones et al. 1989). This report is particularly interesting because carbamazepine and phenytoin are metabolized to similar reactive, electrophilic compounds called *arene oxides*. These unstable intermediate compounds bind to fetal macromolecules in the rat and have been implicated in production of malformations in rats (Martz et al. 1977). Arene oxides are metabolized by epoxide hydrolase. A genetic defect in epoxide hydrolase activity may be associated with phenytoin-induced teratogenicity (Spielberg 1982). The effects of phenytoin metabolites generated by a murine hepatic microsomal drug-metabolizing system on lymphocytes from children with and without the features of fetal hydantoin syndrome have been studied (Strickler et al. 1985). Fourteen of 24 children studied had a significant increase in cell death associated with the phenytoin metabolites, and each of these children had one parent in whom excessive cell death also was shown. A significant correlation between this "positive" lymphocyte in vitro challenge and the occurrence of major birth defects have been established.

A separate approach to this question looked directly at epoxide hydrolase activity (Buehler 1987). When the twins having different paternity referred to above were studied, a clear difference in enzyme activity was found (Phenlan et al. 1982). A preliminary study suggests that it is possible to predict which children will or will not have features of fetal hydantoin syndrome on the basis of epoxide hydrolase activity measured in skin fibroblasts. The activity is decreased in about 50% of normal affected children. If confirmed in other studies, this finding would permit the prediction of susceptibility to fetal hydantoin syndrome and could also pave the way to determining the relative contributions of drugs and genetics in producing fetal abnormalities.

Two other factors should be mentioned in the context of anticonvulsant drugs and fetal abnormality. Anticonvulsants lower folate concentrations in serum and red cells, and folate deficiency has long been suspected (but never proved) to be involved in causing fetal abnormality. Whether this fall in folate concentration is responsible for fetal abnormality is less clear. Studies have suggested (Dansky et al. 1987) and refuted (Hillesmaa et al. 1983) an association. However, preconceptual administration of folic acid has been shown to reduce the occurrence of neural tube defects [Medical Research Council (MRC) Vitamin Study Research Group 1991], so a case can be made for advising women on anticonvulsants to take 4 mg of folic acid daily before conception—not very useful advice for those who do not expect pregnancy.

### *Selection of anticonvulsant*

Whether anticonvulsants are teratogenic remains unknown, but is there one anticonvulsant that is preferable for managing epilepsy in a woman who may become pregnant? Advice has been given in this regard (Antiepileptic Drugs 1981; Saunders 1989), and in each case the advice has been rapidly superseded by new events. In the early 1980s, sodium valproate was recommended as the drug of choice for female epileptic patients because by then phenytoin had acquired a reputation for being teratogenic. Then reports began to appear suggesting that sodium valproate was associated with a neural tube defect (Valproate Spina Bifida 1988). Carbamazepine then became the drug of choice for epilepsy in women, but as described above, it too has been implicated as a teratogen. Consequently, the current recommendation is that after discussion with the patient, physicians should use the drug that is most effective and most acceptable to the woman concerned. On the basis of current information, there is no compelling reason to select one particular drug on the grounds that it is less teratogenic than any other.

***Lithium***

Evidence strongly indicates that lithium taken during the first trimester of pregnancy can lead to Ebstein anomaly. The extent of the risk is unclear. The first suggestion that lithium could have this effect came from the register of "lithium babies" that was established in Scandinavia to try to achieve early identification of fetal abnormalities. Among 118 babies reported to the registry by the early 1970s, six had congenital cardiovascular defects including two cases of Ebstein anomaly (Schou, Goldfield et al. 1973). This report was soon followed by another describing two cases of Ebstein anomaly after use of lithium in early pregnancy (Nora et al. 1974). Given that Ebstein anomaly is a rare malformation, such an occurrence seemed unlikely to have been the result of chance alone. A subsequent and separate study confirmed the excess of cardiovascular malformations in babies whose mothers used lithium. This cohort study provides an estimate of risk. Among 350 babies who had been exposed to lithium in the first trimester, 6 had heart defects compared with an expected frequency of 2.1 (Kallen and Tandberg 1983). It is noteworthy that none of these cardiac defects was of the Ebstein type. This study suggests that use of lithium is associated with a 1.7% risk of cardiac abnormality compared with 0.6% in the general population—a threefold increase. Thus, the risk of Ebstein anomaly seems to be a good deal less than the risk of cardiac abnormalities in general. When unpublished data from the lithium register are used, the risk specifically of Ebstein anomaly is 1 case per 1000 exposures—a 20-fold increase over that of the general population (Elia et al. 1987). Lithium clearly is a human teratogen, particularly for the cardiovascular system. However, the drug is effective for managing bipolar depressive illness. Whether the drug should be continued during the first trimester is a decision that should be made individually. (See chapter 8, Treatment of Psychiatric Disorders, and 28, Risk Analysis Applied to Prescription Drugs.)

***Warfarin***

Warfarin causes chondrodysplasia punctata, which involves bone and cartilage abnormalities (Becker et al. 1975; Shaul et al. 1975). The drug is also associated with microcephaly, asplenia, and diaphragmatic hernia (Hall et al. 1980). The incidence of congenital abnormalities is no clearer with warfarin than it is with the other drugs discussed in this section. In 22 pregnancies in which warfarin was used in the first trimester (because the patient had an artificial heart valve), there were eight spontaneous abortions. This study did not find cases of chondrodysplasia punctata or microcephaly (Chen, Chan, et al. 1982). However, from 49 pregnancies in which warfarin was given during the first trimester for the same indication, there were nine spontaneous abortions, one stillbirth, and 10 cases of classic warfarin embryopathy (Iturbe-Alessio et al. 1986). In this series the risk of an anomaly with the fetus was about 25%. An even higher risk of 67% was quoted in a retrospective study (Wong et al. 1993). However, there has been a dissenting voice in the form of a paper describing the use of warfarin during the first trimester in 46 women with prosthetic heart valves (Sbarouni and Oakley 1994) in which no embryopathies were found. Notwithstanding this finding, the balance of evidence is strongly in favor of warfarin's being teratogenic. Where there is an overwhelming indication for anticoagulation in the first trimester (as in the case of prosthetic heart valves), the benefits and risks of both warfarin and heparin (see below), if possible, should be carefully explained before conception occurs (Ginsberg and Barron 1994).

***Retinoic acids***

These vitamin A analogs (acitretin, isotretinoin, and tretinoin) have been used since the early 1980s to treat severe cystic acne and some other chronic dermatoses. From the onset of their availability on the market, these drugs were strongly suspected to be teratogenic. They were contraindicated in pregnancy but nonetheless inadvertently or deliberately used by some pregnant women (Rosa 1983). They caused a number of major malformations, including craniofacial, cardiac, thymic, and CNS abnormalities. The relative risk has been reported as 25, with a 95% confidence interval of 11.4 to 57.5 (Lammer et al. 1985). In addition to their very high teratogenic potential, the retinoids demonstrate two other properties that present a challenge to the physician who wants to prescribe them for a woman of childbearing age. First, the maximum risk appears to be in the 3 weeks after conception, when many women may not realize they are pregnant. Second, these drugs (or in the case of acitretin, its metabolite etretinate) have exceptionally long half-lives with the result that contraception must be continued long after the course of treatment. In the case of isotretinoin this period is 2 years. The manufacturers of isotretinoin together with the U.S. Food and Drug Administration introduced a pregnancy prevention program in 1988, and its success was reported (Mitchell et al. 1995). This program was aimed at prescribers and patients and included guidelines for physicians and information for patients who were reimbursed by the manufacturer if they attended contraceptive counseling. Among the women who were sexually active, 99% were using contraception, and the pregnancy rate was 8.8 per thousand person-years compared with the U.S. average of 109 per thousand person-years. This suggests that, although the program was not completely successful, it significantly reduced the pregnancy rate in treated women. In contrast to the very high risk associated with oral retinoids, there is no evidence of a relationship between topical preparations and congenital abnormality (Jick et al. 1993).

As indicated earlier, many more drugs in relatively common clinical use may be teratogenic. We simply do not have relevant information about the risks attending their use.

**PRINCIPLE The risk of drug use during pregnancy often is completely unknown. In such settings the physician must be very clear about the need for the drug; he or she must use reasonable criteria to estimate efficacy in order to minimize the dose and the duration of treatment. If possible most drugs should be even more scrupulously avoided in early pregnancy than during later pregnancy and much more scrupulously avoided in women than in men with a comparable indication.**

## DRUGS GIVEN AFTER THE FIRST TRIMESTER

The risk of anatomic defects in the fetus recedes after the first trimester. For the remainder of pregnancy, the fetus undergoes growth and development. The impact of drugs given after the first trimester moves from structural to physiologic effects. In addition, the long-term use of some agents can have adverse effects on the mother that, if not unique to pregnancy, are at least exaggerated by the gravid state.

### Anticoagulants

#### *Heparin*

Heparin use during pregnancy threatens the mother rather than the fetus. Osteoporosis is a recognized complication of long-term administration of heparin (Griffith et al. 1965), and multiple vertebral compression factors have been described in a pregnant woman receiving 20,000 units of unfractionated heparin per day throughout pregnancy as long ago as 1980 (Wise and Hall 1980). Although it is accepted that both dose and duration of treatment are important in the causation of heparin-induced osteoporosis, the underlying mechanism is not understood. Current evidence suggests that pregnant women receiving 20,000 units of unfractionated heparin or more each day for 3 months or more are at high risk of osteoporosis (Hirsh et al. 1995), and this can include serious complications such as vertebral fractures (Dahlman 1993). However, this view has been challenged by a prospective matched cohort study of 25 women who received heparin for more than 1 month during pregnancy and 25 controls who underwent dual-photon absorptiometry of the lumbar spine in the postpartum period. The heparin-treated group had clinically and significantly reduced bone density, but no correlation was established between bone density and duration of heparin therapy, mean daily dose, or total dose (Douketis et al. 1996). Among women who receive heparin treatment during pregnancy, bone loss of this severity occurs in around 5%, but a much greater proportion experience subclinical bone loss that is likely to be reversible (Dahlman et al. 1990). There is far less information about low-molecular-weight heparins and osteoporosis. Laboratory data and information from small studies currently suggest that the risk is less than with unfractionated heparin (Monreal et al. 1994; Shaughnessy et al. 1995) but more studies are needed.

#### *Warfarin*

Warfarin can damage the fetus even when taken after the first trimester, by causing bleeding into the fetal brain (Shaul and Hall 1977). The risk of bleeding into the fetal brain in the second or third trimester is reported to be 2.6% (Ginsberg et al. 1989) and can occur even though the mother's anticoagulant control is good (Ville et al. 1993). The latter finding is not altogether surprising because it merely suggests that drug concentration-effect relationships in the fetus are different from those in the mother.

The use of anticoagulants during pregnancy demonstrates the dilemma of assessing benefits and risks. In women who have artificial heart valves, the possibility of valve thrombosis if anticoagulation is not used may place the life of the mother at unacceptable risk. However, use of warfarin may lead to severe fetal damage, and use of heparin in doses adequate to achieve anticoagulation may lead to vertebral compression fractures.

## Antibiotics

Antibiotics are widely used during pregnancy, and Table 19-2 summarizes information about those that are commonly prescribed.

## Antihypertensives

### *Methyldopa*

It is correct to highlight the risks of using drugs during pregnancy, but physicians should not overlook the circumstances under which the benefits of treatment appear quite substantially to outweigh the risks. Such is illustrated in a small number of studies that have been performed in the field of therapy of hypertension during pregnancy. The first large controlled study of antihypertensive treatment in pregnancy was carried out in Oxford in the 1970s. Methyldopa was compared with no treatment in an open prospective study in women who had mainly essential hypertension (Redman et al. 1976). Using drugs to control hypertension significantly improved fetal outcome mainly by reducing the number of midtrimester fetal deaths: there were nine pregnancy losses in the control group (including four midtrimester fetal deaths) compared with one in the treated group ($P < 0.02$). The well-known adverse effects of methyldopa, including sedation and postural hypotension, led to withdrawal from the trial of 15% of the women (Redman et al. 1977), but no adverse effects were demonstrated on the fetus either immediately after delivery or at long-term follow-up (see section on behavioral teratology).

### *β-Adrenergic-receptor antagonists*

The use of β-adrenergic receptor antagonists during pregnancy generated considerable controversy during the 1970s and early 1980s. A number of reports claimed that these drugs caused intrauterine growth retardation and neonatal complications such as hypoglycemia, hypotension, bradycardia, and even death (Rubin 1981). These reports well exemplify the difficulty of drawing rational conclusions about the use of drugs during pregnancy. Most reports involved either individual cases or retrospective study by chart review, sometimes many years after the index pregnancy (Rubin 1981). Because the β-adrenergic antagonists were new, they most often were reserved for treating the most severe hypertension. It was difficult to separate the effects of the disease from the effects of the drugs.

Encouraged by the results of the methyldopa study cited above, but noting that there had been a high rate of discontinuation of therapy because of adverse effects, Rubin and colleagues (1983) studied atenolol use during pregnancy in a prospective and systematic manner. This

**Table 19-2 Antibiotics and Pregnancy**

| Antibiotics that are considered safe in pregnancy | Antibiotics that may be safe in pregnancy or that can be used in certain circumstances | Antibiotics that should be avoided |
|---|---|---|
| Penicillin G (benzyl)<br>Penicillin V (phenoxymethyl)<br>Ampicillin<br>Amoxicillin<br>Amoxicillin/clavulanic acid<br>Erythromycin<br>Floxacillin<br>Cephalosporins<br>Isoniazid<br>Ethambutol | Ciprofloxacin—not enough data<br>Vancomycin—few data but may be used in staphylococcal sepsis<br>Trimethoprim—theoretical risk of fetal abnormality when used in the first trimester because it is a folate antagonist; safe in the second and third trimesters<br>Antipseudomonal penicillins (ticarcillin, piperacillin, azlocillin)—few data but use for serious pseudomonal infection<br>Rifampin—benefits outweigh risks but may have an association with hemorrhagic disease of the newborn; give vitamin K supplements | Chloramphenicol—not teratogenic but associated with "gray baby" syndrome; cardiovascular collapse when given near term<br>Tetracyclines—tooth discoloration, enamel hypoplasia, and bone dysplasia; also associated with maternal liver toxicity<br>Aminoglycosides—associated with fetal ototoxicity<br>Sulfonamides—given close to delivery, associated with neonatal jaundice and hemolytic anemia<br>Metronidazole—conflicting data exist; some suggestion of teratogenesis; avoid if possible during pregnancy<br>Ciprofloxacin—animal studies raise concern of fetal cartilage damage |

was the first placebo-controlled study done on hypertensive pregnant women, an indication of reluctance of physicians to undertake rigorous studies in that segment of the population. After a pilot study was carried out with atenolol used to treat essential hypertension (Rubin et al. 1982), 120 women with pregnancy-induced hypertension who had been admitted for treatment with bed rest were also treated with either atenolol or placebo. Atenolol lowered blood pressure significantly more and longer than did placebo (Figure 19-3). At the time of this study it had been a widely held belief that bed rest alone lowers blood pressure in pregnant patients with hypertension (Chamberlain et al. 1978). A further important difference between the two groups was that six babies from the placebo group required ventilation for idiopathic respiratory distress syndrome compared with none in the group treated with atenolol. The preterm delivery that gave rise to the respiratory distress resulted partly from poor control of the mother's blood pressure, which prompted obstetricians to expedite delivery, but mainly from a higher incidence of spontaneous preterm labor in the group treated with placebo (Rubin et al. 1984). With the exception of efficacy in favor of treatment, the only other significant difference between the babies from the two groups was a reduced heart rate in the atenolol-treated babies that lasted 24 hours. The bradycardia was not clinically important. The blood pressure and blood glucose concentrations in the two groups of babies were the same throughout the neonatal period. In addition, there was no significant difference between the two groups in neonatal or placental weight. Therefore, the adverse effects attributed to $\beta$-adrenergic receptor blockers in case reports were not substantiated in a prospective, randomized, double-blind, and placebo-controlled study.

**PRINCIPLE Case reports and observational studies are most useful for developing a hypothesis related to a drug effect. When possible, a controlled experimental study is needed to confirm the hypothesis.**

But nothing is simple and without risks. An additional study indicates that atenolol can retard growth under certain circumstances (Butters et al. 1990). This study (placebo-controlled and double-blind) was concerned with management of essential hypertension during pregnancy; consequently, women received atenolol for a considerably longer time than in the trial just discussed. A pilot study with atenolol used to treat essential hypertension in pregnancy that had progressed 28 weeks or longer (Rubin et al. 1982) showed good control of blood pressure and no adverse consequences. In particular the median weight of the babies from treated mothers was within 2 standard deviations of the normal gestational mean. In the subsequent study mothers were treated as early as 12 weeks into the pregnancy; babies from the atenolol-treated group were significantly smaller than those from the placebo group (2.62 ± 0.7 kg and 3.48 ± 0.48 kg; $P < 0.05$).

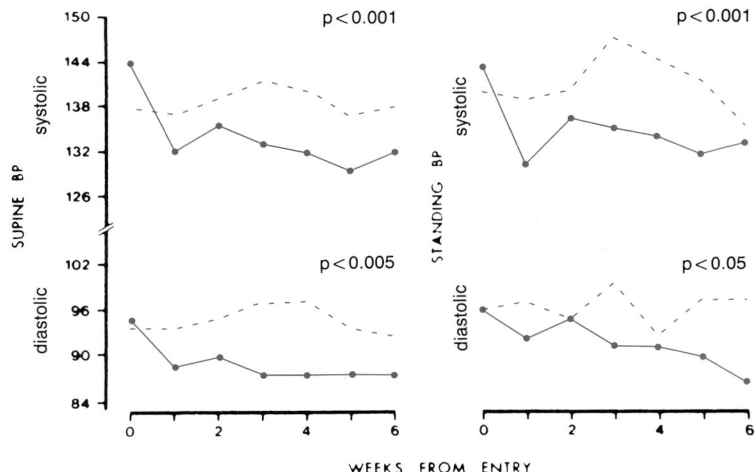


F I G U R E 1 9 - 3 **Average blood pressure from point of entry into double-blind trial following administration of placebo (---) or atenolol (•—•—•). Data are presented in this way, rather than in terms of gestation, because women were entered and delivered at different times. (Reproduced by permission of the *Lancet*.)**

Similar differences were found in placental weight. Thus, not only with regard to teratogenicity but also with regard to growth and development, the same drug can have different effects depending on when it is administered. The mechanism of the effect of atenolol on growth is unclear but may be related to a fall in placental lactogen in the atenolol group (Rubin et al. 1984). Fortunately, the low-weight atenolol babies did not differ in weight from those of the placebo group at 1 year postpartum (Butters et al. 1990).

### *Angiotension-converting enzyme inhibitors*

Angiotension-converting enzyme (ACE) inhibitors have been available since the early 1980s and are now routinely used outside pregnancy for treatment of hypertension and heart failure. In 1980 Broughton-Pipkin and coworkers reported a study in five pregnant ewes, each given a single dose of captopril. Four had stillborn lambs. There is now substantial evidence of problems in human pregnancy (Piper et al. 1992; Shotan et al. 1994; Feldkamp et al. 1997). The main adverse affects are oligohydramnios, fetal renal failure, neonatal hypotension, patent ductus arteriosus, respiratory distress syndrome, lung hypoplasia, and intrauterine fetal death. It is believed that most of these effects may be mediated by an ACE inhibitor effect on fetal renal function and urine output (Shotan et al. 1994). There is also an association between ACE inhibitors and defects of skull ossification. It seems that most of the effects of the drugs occur in the second and third trimesters, but it is not yet clear whether the drugs are safe in the first trimester. A study of 66 pregnancies in which there was exposure to ACE inhibitors only in the first trimester found no cases of renal abnormality and only one case of patent ductus arteriosus. There were no cases of skull ossification defects (Feldkamp et al. 1997). Although this is reassuring, the number of pregnancies was too small to exclude a teratogenic effect.

**PRINCIPLE The value of knowing that a drug is safe early, but not late, in a condition is to allow time to discontinue it after the condition appears.**

### *Calcium channel blockers*

Type II calcium channel blockers are now widely used in obstetric practice to treat hypertension and preterm labor. The most widely used agent is nifedipine. There is no evidence of any teratogenicity despite its use in many women over a number of years. Early animal data suggested that there may be adverse effects such as fetal acidosis and fetal death after administration of nifedipine; however, many studies in human pregnancy have failed to show similar effects (Childress and Katz 1994). Nicardipine and nitrendipine have also been used but in fewer women.

**USE OF NIFEDIPINE FOR THE TREATMENT OF HYPERTENSION IN PREGNANCY** Several trials of nifedipine have been conducted in the treatment of hypertension in pregnancy either alone or in combination with other antihypertensive drugs. Reviewers of these trials have concluded that nifedipine is an effective antihypertensive agent for use in pregnancy (Childress and Katz 1994; Levin et al. 1994).

However, there are some disadvantages. In some people nifedipine causes undesirable side effects including tachycardia, flushing, and headache. Some reports of significant maternal hypotension have been published (Impey 1993). Recent evidence suggests that short-acting forms of nifedipine and other calcium channel blockers are associated with increased cardiovascular mortality in patients with coronary heart disease (Furberg et al. 1995). Although this does not apply to most obstetric patients, there is some concern that, given the increased cardiac output, expansion of plasma volume, and increases in myocardial oxygen demands of pregnancy, nifedipine may pose a risk in pregnancy even in the absence of ischemic heart disease (Davis et al. 1997). Particular concern is warranted in older women with hypertension or diabetes mellitus who may have vascular disease. In these situations, calcium channel blockers should be given only in slow-release formulations if they are prescribed at all.

Another problem is the potential drug interaction between calcium blockers and magnesium sulfate. In the treatment of preeclampsia and eclampsia, these drugs are likely to be used in combination. Magnesium sulfate probably acts similar to calcium channel blockers in inhibiting the influx of extracellular calcium across the cell membrane. In addition, magnesium stimulates calcium-dependent ATPase, which promotes calcium uptake by the sarcoplasmic reticulum thereby reducing the amount of calcium available for muscle contraction. This potentiation of calcium channel blockade can lead to neuromuscular blockade. Muscular paralysis has been reported when nifedipine is used in combination with magnesium sulfate even within normal therapeutic levels (Snyder and Cardwell 1989; Ben-Ami et al. 1994). Thus, extreme caution should be exercised when these drugs are used in combination.

**USE OF NIFEDIPINE FOR TREATMENT OF PRETERM LABOR** Calcium channel blockers have been prescribed for treatment of preterm labor as they inhibit smooth muscle contractility. Several trials have compared nifedipine with ritodrine (a $\beta_2$-adrenergic receptor agonist) or placebo for treatment of preterm labor. The trials show that nifedipine is as successful or better than ritodrine in stopping preterm contractions without adverse fetal effects (Childress and Katz 1994). Although nifedipine has fewer side effects than ritodrine, the adverse effects described above should not be ignored.

## Anticonvulsants

A neonatal coagulation defect can follow the use of anticonvulsant drugs during pregnancy. Studies of coagulation in 16 neonates born to epileptic mothers who took either a barbiturate or phenytoin revealed abnormalities in eight of the babies (Mountain et al. 1970). The coagulation defect is similar to that in vitamin K deficiency and is characterized by prolonged prothrombin time; long activated partial thromboplastin time; and low concentrations of factors II, VII, IX, and X. Furthermore, a prothrombin precursor raised by the absence of vitamin K (PIVKA or protein-induced by vitamin K absence) has been found in the blood of epileptic patients taking a variety of medications (Davies et al. 1985) and in mother–infant pairs after the use of anticonvulsant therapy during pregnancy (Argent et al. 1986). It is interesting that the mother's coagulation profile can be normal even when her baby has severe coagulation defects (Mountain et al. 1970). The drug-induced bleeding in neonates occurs earlier than is usual in classic hemorrhagic disease of the newborn. The bleeding appears within 24 hours of birth, and it can be serious when it involves unusual sites, such as the pleural and abdominal cavities. If vitamin K is not routinely given at birth, it should be taken by the mother at a dose of 20 mg daily 2 weeks before delivery (Deblay et al. 1982).

Barbiturates taken by the mother can produce a number of effects in the neonate. Neonatal behavior can be affected either by sedation caused by the drug or by withdrawal symptoms as the drug is eliminated. Protein binding and drug clearance in the neonate probably are the major determinants of the type of symptoms experienced (Kuhnz et al. 1988). Those who have an unusually high fraction of free phenobarbitone in plasma have a tendency to become sedated, whereas those in whom clearance of phenobarbitone is unusually rapid tend to show symptoms of withdrawal from the drug.

Two case reports describe liver failure in the offspring of women who received sodium valproate throughout pregnancy (Felding and Rane 1984; Legius et al. 1987). The clinical significance of this observation is not known, and at most the effect must be rare because many thousands of exposures of pregnant women to valproate have occurred. Nonetheless, sodium valproate has hepatotoxic effects in adults, and it would not be surprising to find the same effect in neonates.

## Corticosteroids

### *Corticosteroids used to treat maternal disease*

Corticosteroids are widely used to treat a number of inflammatory conditions such as asthma, inflammatory bowel disease, and rheumatoid arthritis. Because of the severity of these diseases in some patients, there is little option but to continue treatment during pregnancy. Thus, there is substantial experience with the use of drugs such as prednisolone during pregnancy. Animal studies suggested that there might be an increased incidence of cleft lip and palate in the offspring of mothers treated with prednisolone (Fainstat 1954; Fraser et al. 1954). However, extensive human experience has failed to show such a connection. Several studies in patients with a wide range of diseases have suggested that there is no significant fetal risk from prednisolone (Schatz et al. 1975; Turner et al. 1980; Mogadam et al. 1981; Fitzsimons et al. 1986), and the outcome for the fetus is usually better if the disease is modified from using such drugs. Prednisolone crosses the placenta poorly, and concentrations in fetal blood are significantly less than those in maternal blood. Beclomethasone is another corticosteroid with a good safety profile.

### *Corticosteroids used to prevent complications of prematurity*

Dexamethasone and betamethasone are now used extensively in women at risk of premature delivery. There is conclusive evidence that treatment with these corticosteroids is associated with a substantial reduction in the incidence of respiratory distress syndrome in preterm neonates. Other advantages include a reduction in intraventricular hemorrhage, necrotizing enterocolitis, and early neonatal death (Crowley 1997). There is no evidence of adverse effects in mothers or neonates, and long-term follow-up of infants also revealed no problems. With preterm prelabor rupture of membranes there is a theoretical risk of neonatal infection (Crowley 1997), but no statistically significant increase has been observed.

## Inhibitors of Prostaglandin Synthesis

Acetylsalicylic acid (ASA) (in analgesic doses; see below for an account of low-dose aspirin) and indomethacin have been associated with characteristic but different adverse effects during pregnancy. ASA is frequently taken during pregnancy and may influence hemostasis in the neonate. In one study hemorrhagic phenomena were seen in 3 of 14 neonates whose mothers had taken ASA compared with 1 of 17 control infants (Bleyer and Breckenridge 1970). This observation was confirmed and refined (Stuart et al. 1982). In the latter study, ingestion of ASA by the mother was monitored by measuring platelet malondialdehyde formation. This measurement gives an accurate estimate of when the last dose of aspirin was taken. The case-control study found that 1 of 34 control maternal-neonatal pairs had hemostatic abnormalities. In 10 maternal-neonatal pairs in which the mother had taken ASA within 5 days of delivery, 6 of the mothers and 9 of the infants had bleeding problems. In contrast, when ASA was taken 6 to 10 days before delivery, no bleeding tendencies were found in 7 maternal-neonatal pairs. The total dose of ASA taken ranged from 5 to 10 g. The manifestation of hemostatic abnormalities included petechiae, hematuria, cephalohematoma, subconjunctival hemorrhage, and bleeding from the site of circumcision. A prudent conclusion from the two studies is to recommend acetaminophen (paracetamol) when a mild analgesic is needed during pregnancy. This drug has not been implicated in any adverse consequences. In addition, if ASA has been consumed within 5 days of delivery, the physician should look carefully for bleeding problems in the baby.

Possibly even before Heymann and Rudolph defined a role for bradykinin and prostaglandins in the patency of the ductus arteriosus, concern was expressed that indomethacin could prematurely close the ductus (Manchester et al. 1976). The drug does have this and other adverse effects. The most likely reasons for administering indomethacin during pregnancy are to treat moderately severe rheumatoid arthritis (Byron 1987), for use as a tocolytic agent (Moise et al. 1988), or to reduce amniotic fluid volume in polyhydramnios. Thirteen patients with premature labor between 2 and 31 weeks of gestation received up to 175 mg of indomethacin per day for a maximum of 3 days (Moise et al. 1988). Echocardiographic study revealed constriction of the ductus in 7 of 14 cases (one woman had twins). Tricuspid regurgitation was also identified in three cases. The ductal constriction could occur as early as 9.5 hours after indomethacin was first administered. The constriction reversed within 24 hours of discontinuing the drug in all cases. A later report suggested that the rate of constriction of the ductus arteriosus increased sharply in fetuses of more than 32 weeks gestation (Moise 1993). Hendricks and colleagues (1990) found that indomethacin given for more than 72 hours for treatment of premature labor was associated with oligohydramnios. In a larger study Norton and coworkers (1991) found that in pregnant women of fewer than 30 weeks gestation treated with indomethacin for abolition of preterm labor, there was an increased incidence in the infants of renal dysfunction, patent ductus arteriosus, intracerebral hemorrhage, and necrotizing enterocolitis. Indomethacin should therefore be considered as a drug with useful therapeutic effects in pregnancy, but it should be avoided if alternative agents are available and should almost certainly be avoided in pregnancies longer than 32 weeks.

**PRINCIPLE Understanding the pharmacology of a drug and pathogenesis of a disease or biologic setting allows prediction or observation of a drug effect. Often such prediction is the cornerstone of a new indication or contraindication for using the drug.**

Acetylsalicylic acid in doses of 60 or 75 mg/day has been extensively investigated in pregnancy in the prophylaxis of preeclampsia and intrauterine growth retardation. The theoretical basis for using ASA in these conditions was sound because platelet activation is an early feature of preeclampsia, and ASA lowers the ratio of platelet thromboxane $A_2$ to prostacyclin in high-risk pregnancies (Schiff et al. 1989). Two small studies carried out in the 1980s further encouraged the belief that ASA could well be a significant advance in the control of preeclampsia (Beaufils et al. 1985; Wallenberg et al. 1986). Both studies involved women at high risk of preeclampsia and found a dramatic reduction in the occurrence of this condition in women taking ASA compared with those on placebo or no treatment.

However, enthusiasm was tempered in the 1990s with publication of several large well-designed studies that demonstrated that ASA cannot be recommended for primary or secondary prevention of preeclampsia [Italian Study of Aspirin in Pregnancy 1993; Sibai et al. 1993; CLASP Collaborative Group 1994; ECPPA (Estudo Colaborativo para Prevencao da Preeclampsia com Aspirina) Collaborative Group 1996]. The two largest studies, both of which were placebo controlled, were the primary prevention work of Sibai and colleagues, which involved 3135 normotensive nulliparous women, and the secondary prevention CLASP (Collaborative Low-Dose Aspirin Study in Pregnancy) study (CLASP Collaborative Group 1994), which involved just under 10,000 women in their second pregnancy who were at high risk of preeclampsia on the basis of having had the condition in their first pregnancy. The primary prevention study found that there was a very small reduction in preeclampsia in the ASA-treated group, but this was offset by an increase in placental abruptions. In contrast, the CLASP study found no difference in preeclampsia or in adverse events between the ASA and the placebo groups.

**PRINCIPLE Theoretical arguments or laboratory investigations are not necessarily the best data to determine clinical practice. Adopt treatment to the most definitive data!**

### New Drugs

After the problems with thalidomide and subsequent "scares" about drugs in pregnancy, drug companies have become keen to absolve themselves of any responsibility regarding the safety of their products in the pregnant patient. Because of this, very few drugs are licensed for use in pregnancy, and it is the physician's responsibility to help the patient decide whether to take a drug during pregnancy. Systematic research on drug use during pregnancy is rare, and information on the effects of the drugs is accumulated only gradually. Information often accrues as women inadvertently take the compounds at various stages of pregnancy. However, the lack of systematic research or monitoring means that reports of the effects of drugs on pregnancy are biased. A pregnancy in which drug *x* is taken with no adverse effect is much less likely to be reported either to the manufacturers or in the literature than one in which drug *x* appears to be associated with an adverse effect. This means that a drug will have been on the market for several years before there is any satisfactory evidence about its safety during pregnancy. For these reasons, it is sensible to avoid the use of unproven drugs for pregnant women and, when they are given, to report their effects (good or bad).

For example, the new antiepileptic drugs lamotrigine, vigabatrin, and gabapentin have been available since the early 1990s, but there is not yet enough evidence about their effects to allow them to be recommended to pregnant women. However, there are some women with epilepsy for whom control would be almost impossible without these drugs; therefore, over the next few years there should be more information available. They may be less teratogenic in the long run than the older, more established antiepileptic drugs, but this cannot be assumed from the outset.

**PRINCIPLE It should be increasingly clear that the first effects of drugs cannot be predicted and will best be known with systematic application of observational methods after the drug is marketed.**

Fluoxetine, an antidepressant drug that acts by selective inhibition of serotonin reuptake, is widely prescribed to women of childbearing age. Over the past few years, increasing information has accumulated about its use in pregnancy. Information on 783 pregnancies reported to the manufacturer suggest that rates of occurrence of spontaneous abortion, major fetal abnormalities, and minor fetal abnormalities are similar to those in the general population. Two case-control studies of reasonable size have been carried out. In one study (Pastuszac et al. 1993), 128 pregnant women who had taken fluoxetine were compared with matched controls, and no difference in the rate of major malformations was observed; however, there was an increase in the rate of miscarriage. The other study (Chambers et al. 1996) compared 228 pregnant women taking fluoxetine with matched controls and found no difference in the rate of miscarriage or major malformation, but there was an increase in the rate of minor abnormalities. They also studied the effect of fluoxetine taken in the third trimester and found an increase in premature delivery and neonatal complications such as respiratory difficulty and jitteriness in the exposed infants. From these findings we can postulate that there is no increase in the rate of major abnormalities with fluoxetine, but there may be an increase in other complications such as spontaneous abortion, minor birth defects, premature labor, and neonatal problems. However, the number studied are not sufficient to draw satisfactory conclusions.

Fluoxetine and the newer antiepileptic drugs are frequently prescribed to women of childbearing age and are therefore likely to be taken inadvertently during pregnancy. But even with these drugs, it has taken many years for even a small amount of information to be available. For less commonly prescribed drugs it may take many decades before any useful data are obtained if the methods of data collection remain the same.

## DRUGS AND BREAST-FEEDING

Drugs given to a mother who is breast-feeding her infant may pass into the breast milk and therefore into the baby. Little research into the effects on infants of drugs given to breast-feeding mothers has been published. However, there are some important adverse effects of which physicians and mothers should be aware. Most drugs pass into breast milk, but the concentration varies depending on several factors (Table 19-3).

### Factors Influencing the Transfer of Drugs from Mother to Infant in Breast Milk

Most drugs enter breast milk by passive diffusion and therefore small molecules cross more easily than large ones (for example, heparin, which is a very large mole-

**Table 19-3 Factors Influencing the Transfer of Drugs from Mother to Infant in Breast Milk**

| |
|---|
| *Factors that affect the concentration of drug in the mother* |
| Drug dose, frequency, route, and patient compliance |
| Clearance rate |
| Plasma protein binding |
| *Factors that affect transfer across the breast* |
| Breast blood flow |
| Metabolism of drug within the breast |
| Molecular weight of the drug |
| Degree of ionization of the drug |
| Solubility of the drug in water and lipids |
| Relative binding affinity to plasma and milk protein |
| Difference between the pH of maternal plasma and milk |
| *Factors that affect drug concentration in the infant* |
| Timing of feeds |
| Frequency and duration of feeds |
| Volume of milk consumed |
| Ability of the infant to metabolize the drug |

cule, does not pass into breast milk). It is easier for fat-soluble and un-ionized drugs to traverse into the milk. There are a few drugs that are actively transported across the mammary membrane, e.g., cimetidine (Oo et al. 1995). However, timing of infant feeds in relation to maternal dosing schedule influences how much will reach the infant. In addition, the relative immaturity of infant metabolism must be considered, because the half-life of many drugs is longer in infants than in adults. The most important determinant of effect on the infant is the concentration in the infant's plasma rather than the concentration in milk or maternal plasma.

As with the use of drugs during pregnancy, there is a distinction between those drugs that are contraindicated in breast-feeding (Table 19-4), those that are safe to use, and those about which there is inadequate information and so should be avoided if possible. As indicated elsewhere in this chapter, single case reports about the effects of drugs can be misleading and should be viewed with caution when seen in isolation. For some years indomethacin has been considered to be contraindicated in breast-feeding mothers. This conclusion arose after a single report of neonatal convulsions was published after indomethacin was given to a breast-feeding mother (Eeg-Olofsson et al. 1978). Subsequent studies showed that indomethacin passes into the breast milk in very small quantities and reported no complications of indomethacin transmitted by breast-feeding (Lebedevs et al. 1991; Beaulac-Baillargeon and Allard 1993).

**Table 19-4 Drugs That Are Contraindicated during Breast-Feeding Because of their Effects on the Infant**

| DRUG | EFFECT |
|---|---|
| Ciprofloxacin | Arthropathy |
| Chloramphenicol | Bone marrow suppression |
| Radioactive iodine | Destruction of the thyroid |
| Doxepin | Respiratory suppression |
| Gold | Rashes, nephritis, hepatitis, and hematological problems |
| Cyclophosphamide | Neutropenia |
| Cytotoxic drugs | Cytotoxicity |
| Iodine-containing compounds (including topical iodine preparations) | Effect on thyroid |
| Amiodarone | Effect on thyroid |
| Androgens | Androgenization of the infant |
| Danazol | Antiandrogenic effects |
| Ergotamine | Vomiting, diarrhea, convulsions |
| Laxatives | Diarrhea |

## Drugs That Affect Milk Production

Some drugs interfere with the process of lactation itself and therefore should be avoided in the breast-feeding mother. These included bromocriptine, cabergoline, thiazide diuretics, the combined oral contraceptive pill, and ergotamine.

# BEHAVIORAL TERATOLOGY

Most studies in human teratology have been concerned with morphologic observations made near the time of delivery. The possibilities that a drug taken during pregnancy could affect the growth and development of a child have been investigated to a far lesser extent. There are practical reasons for this imbalance in favor of morphologic observation.

Pediatric follow-up studies are difficult to carry out. Families move and can be difficult to trace without concerted effort; however, useful information on late teratologic effects is unlikely to be forthcoming until children approach school age. Another factor that makes follow-up difficult is that the more subtle the drug effect, the more difficult the study. For example, assessing physical growth and development (height, weight, etc.) is relatively straightforward. But assessing retarded psychomotor development—for example, because of alcohol consumption by the mother—is far more complicated. It requires a detailed and labor-intensive battery of investigations. In addition, psychomotor testing must be carefully controlled because of the strong influence of social and environmental factors on these variables. The type of psychomotor test used also changes with increasing age of the child as he or she moves from nonverbal to verbal communication. For these and other reasons, the number of studies in behavioral teratology has been small and the quality somewhat variable. This field has been reviewed by Gal and Sharpless (1984). For a detailed review of the many animal studies performed with psychotherapeutic medications, see Elia and coworkers (1987).

## Anticonvulsant Effects on Offspring

Several studies have reported the possible effects on the intellectual development of the child when the mother is treated with anticonvulsants. The results are inconclusive (Gal and Sharpless 1984). A common weakness of a number of these studies has been the lack of a genuine control group of untreated maternal epileptic patients. Even when this criterion has been applied, the results are contradictory.

One study in which children exposed to phenytoin in utero were compared with a control group from untreated epileptic mothers concluded that phenytoin is a risk factor for mental deficiency in the child (Hanson et al. 1976). In contrast, a much larger study from the Collaborative Perinatal Project found no difference in mental and motor scores at 8 months or in intelligence quotient (IQ) scores at 4 years in children exposed to phenytoin or phenobarbitone in utero versus those from epileptic mothers who were untreated (Shapiro et al. 1976; Klebanoff and Berendes 1988). A third recent prospective study involved all the children of epileptic mothers born in a single hospital in Finland over a 5-year period (Gaily et al. 1988). In this study, 148 children from epileptic mothers and 105 children from normal pregnancies were compared at 5.5 years of age. Intelligence was assessed by both verbal and nonverbal methods. Among the 148 children in the epilepsy group, 131 had received an anticonvulsant, of which phenytoin was the most common (103 exposures). Mental deficiency was found in two children from the epilepsy group and none from the control group. However, in each of the two retarded children, it was difficult to identify a clear association with the anticonvulsant used (carbamazepine in one case and phenytoin in the other), because one child had a family history of mental retardation and the other came from a pregnancy complicated not only by poorly controlled epilepsy but also by alcohol abuse. This study also failed to find any relationship between low intelligence and the concentration of anticonvulsant drug in maternal plasma. The most appropriate conclusion to be drawn from these studies is that anticonvulsant therapy during pregnancy does not appear to influence mental development in the offspring.

## Neuroleptic Drug Effects on Offspring

When rats are exposed in utero either to dopamine-receptor antagonists or to drugs that deplete presynaptic stores of dopamine, the brain dopamine receptors in the offspring are persistently reduced (Rosengarten and Friedhoff 1979). The possibility that drugs that influence dopamine stores or receptors could have a long-term effect when given during human pregnancy has been investigated by the Collaborative Perinatal Project (Platt et al. 1989). Three different types of drug were studied: 239 cases involved antipsychotic neuroleptics such as chlorpromazine; 45 cases involved prochlorperazine, which was usually administered as an antiemetic; and 180 cases involved dopamine-depleting drugs such as reserpine. Motor development was measured in the newborn and again at ages 8 months, 4 years, and 7 years.

Children whose parents had received an antipsychotic neuroleptic demonstrated abnormal motor activity in the neonatal period, but the anomaly probably was the result of residual drug rather than a long-term permanent effect. The children of parents who had received prochlorperazine for more than 2 months during pregnancy demonstrated abnormalities of fine motor movement at 8 months of age. The most substantial differences, however, were found in the children of parents who had taken a dopamine-depleting drug. Abnormalities of both fine and gross motor movement at 8 months of age and unusual motor movements and postural adjustments at 7 years of age were found in these children (Platt et al. 1989). Because of the nature of the study it is difficult to identify whether there was a particular period of gestation when drug exposure was most likely to produce late effects. For this reason the investigators emphasized that by including all exposures to the relevant drugs they may have underestimated the risk when the drug was given at particular stages of gestation.

## Antihypertensive Effects on Offspring

### *Methyldopa*

The randomized and prospective assessment of methyldopa compared with no treatment in the management of hypertension during pregnancy referred to earlier (Redman et al. 1977) included a detailed and comprehensive pediatric follow-up at 4 years (Ounsted et al. 1980) and 7.5 years (Cockburn et al. 1982). The follow-up was remarkably complete, with 195 (97%) of the live-born children successfully located and studied at 7.5 years. Both physical and psychomotor development were assessed by a wide range of tests. At 4 years of age, the boys in the treated group had a slightly smaller head circumference than those in the untreated group, but there was no relationship between head circumference and developmental score. The children from the treated group tended to have higher scores across a wide range of motor and intellectual tests than those in the untreated hypertensive group. At 7.5 years of age, the frequency of problems of health, physical and mental handicap, sight, hearing, and behavior was the same in both groups. Boys whose mothers entered the treatment group between 1 and 20 weeks of gestation had a marginally smaller head circumference than those from the untreated group, but at 4 years there was no detectable difference in intelligence. The primary conclusion of this very careful study is that methyldopa appears to be safe to use during pregnancy, but it may be preferable to avoid it between 1 and 20 weeks of gestation if possible.

#### *Atenolol*

The placebo-controlled trial of atenolol in pregnancy-induced hypertension referred to above also included a pediatric follow-up of 1 year (Reynolds et al. 1984). In addition to physical measurements of growth, the children also had a Denver Developmental Screening test at 3, 8, and 12 months of age. There was no difference between the groups in physical indices. Differences on the Denver Developmental Screen were found only in babies from the placebo group, two of whom were graded as doubtful at 8 months but were normal at 12 months and one of whom was clearly abnormal at all stages. This baby appeared to have suffered from brain damage, probably associated with spontaneous preterm labor. The conclusion so far is that atenolol used in pregnancy-induced hypertension in the third trimester appears to confer no adverse effects in babies followed up at 1 year of age.

### Late Morphologic Effects

In addition to late effects on behavioral development, drugs used during pregnancy can also produce morphologic changes. Late morphologic and physiologic effects have been described after the use of diethylstilbestrol (DES) during early pregnancy. That drug was once thought, but never demonstrated, to prevent several obstetric complications including miscarriage. Vaginal carcinoma in female offspring and infertility in male offspring are among several consequences of giving DES in the first trimester of pregnancy (National Cancer Institute 1983). A very worrying aspect of the consequences of using this drug is that the effects are often not observed until the late teenage years. This raises a specter that has clear implications: A drug should be given during pregnancy only if the likely benefits are clear and well established, and wherever possible those engaged in research on drugs in pregnancy should follow the offspring into later life. Both these objectives (particularly the latter) have been and will continue to be difficult to achieve. This problem is compounded by pregnant patients who abuse drugs. This subject will not be covered in a book of therapeutic principles, but is part of the presentation on chapter 17, Substance Abuse.

## INFLUENCE OF PREGNANCY ON DRUG DOSE REQUIREMENTS

The overwhelming emphasis of studies on clinical pharmacology during pregnancy has involved what the drug could do to the pregnancy and its outcome. Understandable and important as this subject is, there is another side to the coin that is less well studied but of considerable value in demonstrating clinical pharmacologic principles and in prescribing. Pregnancy influences both drug disposition and effect.

Pregnancy is accompanied by many physiologic changes that could influence pharmacokinetics and pharmacodynamics. The transit time in the gut is prolonged (Parry et al. 1970). Plasma proteins undergo substantial changes. For example, the concentration of albumin decreases, whereas the concentration of $\alpha_1$-acid glycoprotein increases (Studd et al. 1970). The amounts of body water and fat increase (Hytten and Leitch 1971). By the third trimester, renal blood flow had almost doubled compared with prepregnancy values (Dunlop 1976). However, liver blood flow does not change (Munnell and Taylor 1947). Certain metabolic pathways in the liver may increase during pregnancy, an inference that has been drawn from the increased urinary excretion of D-glucuronic acid (Davis et al. 1973). Further physiologic changes of pregnancy that could influence drug disposition and effect include increases in cardiac output (de Swiet 1989), changes in blood pressure that reach a minimum during the second trimester and rise as term approaches (MacGuillivray et al. 1969), reduction in vascular sensitivity to infused angiotensin II (MacDonald 1973), increases in renal tubular sodium reabsorption (Lindheimer and Katz 1973), and hyperventilation resulting in a compensated respiratory alkalosis (Greenberger and Patterson 1985).

## Pharmacokinetics during Pregnancy

Detailed clinical pharmacokinetic studies allowing conclusions to be drawn about possible alterations in drug disposition during pregnancy are relatively few. Many opportunistic observations in pregnant women have been made involving measurement of steady-state concentrations of single drugs taken orally, and several of these studies have been reviewed (Cummings 1983; Perucca 1987). Studies featuring IV administration of drugs that allows calculation of drug clearance are few.

### *Systemic clearance of drugs during pregnancy*

By far the most clinically important pharmacokinetic changes to occur during pregnancy involve the metabolic clearance of anticonvulsants. Many reports describe a reduction in the concentration of phenytoin (Eadie et al. 1977; Lander et al. 1977; Dam et al. 1979; Landon and Kirkley 1979), phenobarbitone (Dam et al. 1979; Rating et al. 1982), carbamazepine (Dam et al. 1979; Niebyl et al. 1979), and sodium valproate (Nau et al. 1981) in plasma during pregnancy. Most studies agree that anticonvulsant concentrations in plasma fall progressively during pregnancy, reach their lowest levels in the third trimester, and then rise again a few weeks postpartum (Nau et al. 1982). The reason for this decreased concentration of drug could be a reduction in oral bioavailability, an increase in volume of distribution, an increase in systemic clearance, or some combination of these. In order to obtain definitive data on anticonvulsant pharmacokinetics during pregnancy, IV and oral formulations must be used, preferably in the same women during and after pregnancy. Completely rigorous studies have not been performed. However, the available data do suggest that by far the most important factor leading to these changes in drug concentration is an increase in systemic clearance of the drug from the body.

One study describes the pharmacokinetic data of phenytoin after IV administration in five women who presented with epilepsy during pregnancy. After the initial IV dose, they were given oral therapy (Lander et al. 1984). The oral bioavailability was about 90%, making it unlikely that a marked reduction in bioavailability contributes to the alterations in plasma concentrations. Systemic clearance of phenytoin in two studies was approximately double to triple that typically observed in nonpregnant patients. Further evidence supporting increased clearance as an important factor in the decreased concentration in plasma of anticonvulsant drugs in pregnant women is provided by the observation that falls in the plasma concentrations of carbamazepine are associated with a decreased ratio of parent drug to the 10,11-epoxide metabolite in plasma (Perucca 1987). Although the evidence is limited, likely increases in systemic clearance of anticonvulsants are substantial and clinically important during pregnancy.

Clearance of all drugs by the liver is not dramatically changed during pregnancy. Clearance of both labetalol and propranolol in the third trimester of pregnancy was normal. This finding is perhaps not unexpected because both drugs are cleared at a rate that approximates liver blood flow, which is unchanged by pregnancy (Munnell and Taylor 1947). The difference between the clearance of phenytoin and propranolol may well reflect the difference between "capacity-limited" and "flow-limited" drug clearance.

Because renal blood flow increases substantially during pregnancy, we expect and find that drugs eliminated by this route show alterations in their clearance. Lithium (Schou, Amdisen et al. 1973) and ampicillin (Philipson 1977) are among relatively commonly used drugs whose clearance is increased up to 100% during pregnancy. Further information on pharmacokinetics during pregnancy is available in review articles by Cummings (1983) and Perucca (1987).

### *Protein binding of drugs during pregnancy*

In view of the fall in the concentration of albumin in plasma during pregnancy, the binding of several drugs including phenytoin (Ruprah et al. 1980; Chen, Perucca, et al. 1982), phenobarbitone (Chen, Perucca et al. 1982), sodium valproate (Perucca et al. 1981), and diazepam (Perucca et al. 1981) is reduced. The mechanism of decreased protein binding has not been fully elucidated. The relationship between the free-drug fraction and concentration of albumin (Perucca et al. 1981; Chen, Perucca et al. 1982) is inverse but does not necessarily indicate cause and effect. Other endogenous substances may contribute to the reduction in drug protein binding. In the case of diazepam, there is no correlation between binding and concentration of albumin.

### *Drug metabolism by the placenta*

The placenta contains enzymes relevant to all the major metabolic pathways for drugs and receives a substantial blood supply (Juchau 1980). For this reason it is theoretically possible that the placenta could contribute to systemic clearance of drugs. However, so far the contribution of the placenta to drug metabolism actually is found to be very small and clinically unimportant (Juchau 1980; Prach and Rubin 1988; Loebstein et al. 1997).

## Therapeutic Drug Monitoring during Pregnancy

Several studies that demonstrated a reduction in the concentration of anticonvulsants in plasma during pregnancy also detected an increase in seizure frequency in these women. Although the therapeutic range for many drugs is imprecise, the management of conditions such as epilepsy during pregnancy nonetheless provides one of the clearest settings to use measurements of drug concentrations as a guide to therapeutic decision-making. In addition to identifying reductions in drug concentration resulting from pharmacokinetic factors, the measurement of anticonvulsant concentrations will also provide an invaluable guide to compliance. Provided the relevant medical condition was well controlled before pregnancy, it is generally helpful to use the plasma concentrations obtained before pregnancy as a guide to subsequent management. If the drug's concentration falls with advancing gestation, then the dose should be increased accordingly. Drugs that are highly protein bound, and for which an increased free fraction has been demonstrated during pregnancy, need special consideration when one is interpreting their therapeutic range during pregnancy. In most laboratories the total drug concentration (bound plus free) is provided to the clinician. Because the free fraction of drugs such as phenytoin and sodium valproate increases by up to 20% during pregnancy, the therapeutic range should be revised downward in pregnant women. This problem in interpretation is avoided if free-drug concentrations (rather than total) are measured. An alternative approach to obtaining concentrations that reflect free drug for the anticonvulsants is to measure the concentration in saliva. At least in the case of phenytoin, salivary concentrations correlate well with the unbound concentration of phenytoin in plasma (Knott et al. 1986). However, in spite of these considerations, the clinical necessity for measuring free drug in plasma or salivary concentrations of anticonvulsants remains to be established because the therapeutic range of these drugs is not precisely defined.

Application of any therapeutic range for pregnancy based on responses in nonpregnant patients makes the a priori assumption that a given concentration of drug will have the same effect in pregnancy as in the nonpregnant state. In view of the many physiologic changes referred to at the beginning of this section, that assumption may not be justified. In other words, it is possible that a given drug concentration may have fundamental different effects in pregnant and nonpregnant women.

## The Influence of Pregnancy on Drug Action

There has been little effort to investigate possible pharmacodynamic changes during pregnancy. Such studies require that measurements of drug concentration and drug effect be obtained simultaneously. One such study has been carried out with propranolol in 12 women with pregnancy-induced hypertension. The study followed the pharmacokinetics and pharmacodynamics of IV administration of the drug during the third trimester and again 2 or 3 months postpartum (Rubin et al. 1987). Because some of the pharmacologic effects of propranolol can be easily measured, there is little if any immediate clinical value in measuring its concentration–effect relationships (see the section on hypertension in chapter 1, Cardiovascular Disorders). However, the very ease with which the effect of propranolol on heart rate can be measured made it an attractive drug to test the hypothesis that pregnancy can alter the action of a drug. Drug effect was modeled as a function of concentration by a method that allows for the fact that response to a drug may be out of phase with its concentration in plasma. A hypothetical effect compartment was assumed (Sheiner et al. 1979). Pregnancy did not alter the pharmacokinetics of propranolol, but its concentration–effect relationship was indeed changed. During pregnancy, propranolol reduced heart rate by $0.10 \pm 0.23$ beat per minute per nanogram per milliliter (ng/ml) of dose compared with $0.39 \pm 0.19$ beat per minute in the same women postpartum. This difference was significant and was not influenced either by blood pressure or by pretreatment heart rate. These data were corroborated in a study that described a greater reduction in exercise-induced tachycardia by metoprolol during pregnancy than postpartum (Hogstedt 1986). The mechanism by which $\beta$-receptor antagonists exert a greater effect during pregnancy is unclear. However, the change in heart rate and in the concentration of norepinephrine in plasma in response to both tilting and isometric stress is diminished during pregnancy (Barron et al. 1986; Parry et al. 1970). Perhaps a change in the ratio of antagonist to endogenous agonist is a possible explanation for the altered pharmacodynamics of propranolol during pregnancy. The principle underlying these observations with $\beta$-adrenergic receptor agonists is important. The physiologic alterations of pregnancy are not likely to be confined to altering the pharmacodynamics of propranolol alone.

## USING DRUGS DURING PREGNANCY: PRACTICAL CONSIDERATIONS

### The Clinical Pharmacology Consultation: General Approach

The ideal time to give advice about the risks and benefits of drug use during pregnancy is at a preconception counseling clinic. Unfortunately, most requests for further information come after the pregnancy has begun, usually after an exposure that occurred when neither the patient nor her physician considered the existence of pregnancy.

An approach to this problem is outlined in Figure 19-4. First and most important, the physician should take a careful clinical history to establish which drugs the patient took and precisely when exposure to these drugs occurred. Then the time of gestation for each exposure can be determined as accurately as possible by dating the gestation with a combination of menstrual history and examination with ultrasound. Then the risk of teratogenicity from the drug can be determined by using available reference sources (see bibliography). This simple approach works. Drug exposure can frequently be established to have been at a time when the patient was not pregnant or, if pregnant, beyond the period of organogenesis. Often one can develop some confidence that the drug used is unlikely to be teratogenic. Then one should sensibly reassure the patient *but* state clearly that up to 2% of all pregnancies end with some kind of fetal abnormality in the absence of drugs or other known circumstances. This advice is important because without it, should the particular pregnancy (by chance alone) produce an abnormal baby, the patient's inevitable conclusion would be that the drug was responsible.

Should it appear that exposure to a teratogen occurred at a critical phase of gestation, then the situation is potentially much more serious and difficult. The type of abnormality expected should be ascertained, and detailed ultrasound scanning should be performed at 20 weeks. If an abnormality is detected, subsequent management depends partly on its severity and partly on the attitude of the patient. Many of the more common abnormalities (e.g., cleft palate or minor neural tube defect) can be corrected at birth. A pediatric surgeon should be involved at this early

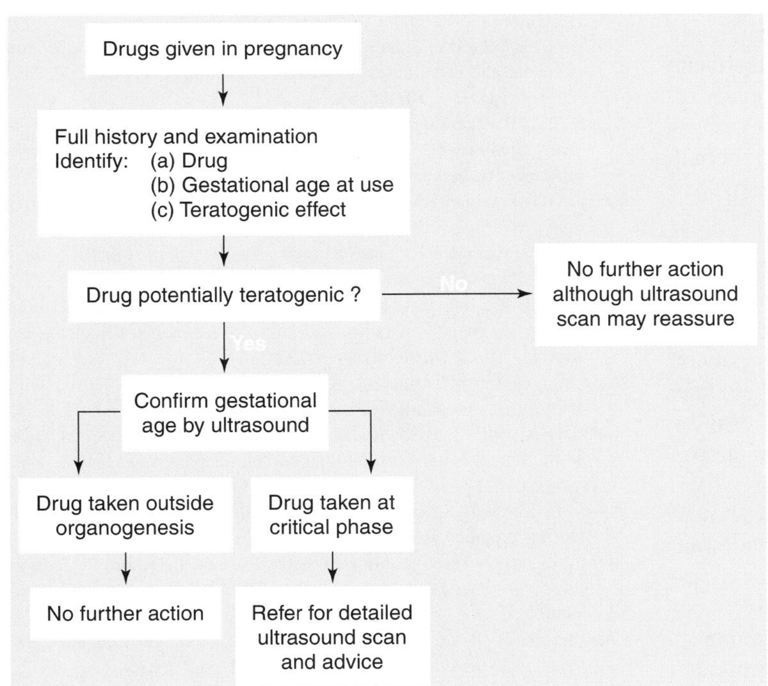


**FIGURE 19-4 Outline of the procedure to follow when consulted about the use of a drug during pregnancy. (Reproduced courtesy of Dr. Martin Whittle, Queen Mother's Hospital, Glasgow, and with permission from the *British Medical Journal*.)**

stage to discuss the likelihood of successful treatment at birth or later in childhood. However, if the defect is severe, the possibility of termination of pregnancy should be discussed carefully with the patient and her partner.

## Principles of Pharmacologic Management of a Medical Condition During Pregnancy: Epilepsy

Many of the clinical pharmacologic principles relevant to the use of drugs in pregnancy are illustrated by the management of an epileptic patient.

### *Prepregnancy counseling*

Much can be accomplished before pregnancy begins, and the optimum time to address questions about the use of anticonvulsants is when the patient begins to contemplate pregnancy. The risks and benefits of treatment can be carefully considered in a relatively dispassionate manner. The risks of untreated epilepsy include maternal death, and this must be made absolutely clear to the patient. However, anticonvulsants carry a teratogenic risk, although this probably does not exceed 10% of exposures. Also, the need for treatment can be established: There is no better way to avoid drug-induced teratogenicity than by not giving the drug. If the patient meets the usual medical criteria for withdrawing therapy, then her treatment can be slowly discontinued, provided the consequences of another seizure—e.g., loss of driver's license—are clearly understood. If treatment must be continued, then optimal control should be achieved, ideally with monotherapy, before the pregnancy begins.

### *Monitoring drug use during and after pregnancy*

During pregnancy, drug concentrations should be monitored monthly. The aim is to maintain the concentration known to be associated with good control in that patient before pregnancy while allowing for the protein-binding changes referred to above. If the concentration of drug in plasma decreases, the dose of the drug should be appropriately increased (Loebstein et al. 1997).

Women taking medication during pregnancy should have a detailed ultrasound scan at 20 weeks' gestation in order to identify any fetal abnormality; if necessary, appropriate action should be taken as discussed above.

Breast-feeding is safe with the three most commonly used anticonvulsant drugs: phenytoin, sodium valproate, and carbamazepine. Women receiving phenobarbitone should avoid breast-feeding.

Drug concentrations should be monitored every 2 weeks after delivery until it is clear how quickly the pharmacokinetics of the drug are returning to prepregnancy values. The dose should be adjusted accordingly. Prepregnancy dose requirements usually can be resumed by 6 weeks postpartum.

## REFERENCES


Antiepileptic Drugs. 1981. Teratogenic risks of antiepileptic drugs. *Br Med J* **283**:515–6.

Argent A, Rothberg AD, Pienaar N. 1986. Precursor prothrombin status in 2 mother-infant pairs following gestational anticonvulsant therapy. *Pediatr Pharmacol* **4**:183–7.

Atkinson HC, Begg EJ, Darlow BA. 1988. Drugs in human milk: Clinical pharmacokinetic concentrations. *Clin Pharmacokinet* **14**:217–40.

Barron WM, Mujais SK, Zinaman M, et al. 1986. Plasma catecholamine responses to physiologic stimuli in normal human pregnancy. *Am J Obstet Gynecol* **154**:80–4.

Beaufils M, Uzan S, Donsimoni R, et al. 1985. Prevention of preeclampsia by early antiplatelet therapy. *Lancet* **1**:840–2.

Beaulac-Baillargeon L, Allard G. 1993. Distribution of indomethacin in human milk and estimation of its milk to plasma ratio in vitro. *Br J Clin Pharmacol* **36**:413–6.

Becker MH, Genieser NB, Feingold M. 1975. Chondrodysplasia punctata: Is maternal warfarin therapy a factor? *Am J Dis Child* **129**:356–9.

Ben-Ami M, Giladi Y, Shalev E. 1994. The combination of magnesium sulphate and nifedipine: A cause of neuromuscular blockade. *Br J Obstet Gynaecol* **101**:262–3.

Bleyer WA, Breckenridge RT. 1970. Studies on the detection of adverse drug reactions in the newborn. II: The effects of prenatal aspirin on newborn hemostasis. *Rev Esp Estomatol* **213**:2049–53.

Briggs GG, Freeman RK, Yaffe SJ, editors. 1990. *Drugs in Pregnancy and Lactation*, 3rd ed. Baltimore, MD: Williams & Wilkins.

Briggs GG, Freeman RK, Yaffe SJ (editors). 1998. *Drugs in Pregnancy and Lactation*, 5th ed. Baltimore, MD: Williams & Wilkins.

Brocklebank JC, Ray WA, Federspiel CF, et al. 1978. Drug prescribing during pregnancy: A controlled study of Tennessee Medicaid recipients. *Am J Obstet Gynecol* **132**:235–44.

Broughton-Pipkin F, Turner SR, Symonds EM. 1980. Possible risk with captopril in pregnancy: Some animal data [letter]. *Lancet* **1**:1256.

Buehler BA. 1987. Epoxide hydrolase activity in fibroblasts: Correlation with clinical features of the fetal hydantoin syndrome. *Proc Greenwood Genet Cent* **6**:117–8.

Butters L, Kennedy S, Rubin P. 1990. Atenolol in essential hypertension during pregnancy. *Br Med J* **301**:587–9.

Byron MA. 1987. Treatment of rheumatic diseases. In: Rubin PC, editor. *Prescribing in Pregnancy.* London: BMA [British Medical Association?].

Chamberlain GVP, Lewis PJ, deSwiet M, et al. 1978. How obstetricians manage hypertension in pregnancy. *Br Med J* **1**:626–9.

Chambers CD, Johnson KA, Dick LM, et al. 1996. Birth outcomes in pregnant women taking fluoxetine. *N Engl J Med* **335**:1010–5.

Chen SS, Perucca E, Lee JM, et al. 1982. Serum protein binding and free concentration of phenytoin and phenobarbitone in pregnancy. *Br J Clin Pharmacol* **13**:547–54.

Chen WWC, Chan CS, Lee PR, et al. 1982. Pregnancy in patients with prosthetic heart valves: An experience with 45 pregnancies. *Q J Med* **51**:358–65.

Childress CH, Katz VL. 1994. Nifedipine and its indications in obstetrics and gynecology. *Obstet Gynecol* **83**:616–24.

CLASP (Collaborative Low-Dose Aspirin Study in Pregnancy) Collaborative Group. 1994. A randomised trial of low-dose aspirin for the prevention and treatment of pre-eclampsia among 9364 pregnant women. *Lancet* **343**:619–29.

Cockburn J, Moar VA, Ounsted M, et al. 1982. Final report of study on hypertension during pregnancy: The effects of specific treatment on the growth and development of the children. *Lancet* **1**:647–9.

Cordero JF, Oakley GP. 1983. Drug exposure during pregnancy: Some epidemiologic considerations. *Clin Obstet Gynecol* **26**:418–28.

Crowley P. 1997. Corticosteroids prior to preterm delivery. In: Neilson JP, Crowther CA, Hodnett ED, et al., editors. Pregnancy and childbirth module of the Cochrane Database of Systematic Reviews (updated September 1997). Available in The Cochrane Library. The Cochrane Collaboration; issue 4. Oxford: update software 1997. [Updated quarterly].

Cummings AJ. 1983. A survey of pharmacokinetic data from pregnant women. *Clin Pharmacokinet* **8**:344–54.

Dahlman TC. 1993. Osteoporotic fractures and recurrence of thromboembolism during pregnancy and the puerperium in thromboembolism during pregnancy and the puerperium in 184 women undergoing thromboprophylaxis with heparin. *Am J Obstet Gynecol* **168**:1265–70.

Dahlman TC, Lindvall N, Hellgren M. 1990. Osteopenia in pregnancy during longterm heparin treatment: A radiological study post partum. *Br J Hematol* **97**:221–8.

Dam H, Christiansen J, Munck O, et al. 1979. Antiepileptic drugs: Metabolism in pregnancy. *Clin Pharmacokinet* **4**:53–62.

Dansky LV, Andermann E, Rosenblatt D, et al. 1987. Anticonvulsants, folate levels, and pregnancy outcome: A prospective study. *Ann Neurol* **21**:176–82.

Davies VA, Rothberg AD, Argent AC, et al. 1985. Precursor prothrombin status in patients receiving anticonvulsant drugs. *Lancet* **1**: 126–9.

Davis M, Simmons CJ, Dordini B, et al. 1973. Inductions of hepatic enzymes during normal pregnancy. *J Obstet Gynaecol Br Commonw* **80**:690–4.

Davis WB, Wells SR, Kuller JA, et al. 1997. Analysis of the risks associated with calcium channel blockade: Implications for the obstetrician-gynecologist. *Obstet Gynecol Surv* **52**:198–201.

Debendox. 1984. Debendox is not thalidomide. *Lancet* **2**:205–6.

Deblay MF, Vert P, Andre M, et al. 1982. Transplacental vitamin K prevents haemorrhagic disease of infant of epileptic mother. *Lancet* **1**:1247.

De Swiet M. 1989. Heart disease in pregnancy. In: De Swiet M, editor. *Medical Disorders in Obstetric Practice*. Oxford: Blackwell Scientific. p 116–48.

De Swiet M (editor). 1995. *Medical Disorders in Obstetric Practice*, 3rd ed. Oxford: Blackwell Scientific Publications.

Douketis JD, Ginsberg JS, Burrows RF, et al. 1996. The effects of longterm heparin therapy during pregnancy on bone density: A prospective matched cohort study. *Thromb Haemost* **75**:254–7.

Dunlop W. 1976. Investigations into the influence of posture in renal plasma flow and glomerular filtration rate during late pregnancy. *Br J Obstet Gynaecol* **83**:17–23.

Eadie MJ, Lander CM, Tyrer JH. 1977. Plasma drug level monitoring in pregnancy. *Clin Pharmacokinet* **2**:427–36.

ECPPA (Estudo Colaborativo para Prevencao da Pre-eclampsia com Aspirina) Collaborative Group. 1996. Randomised trial of low dose aspirin for the prevention of maternal and fetal complications in high risk pregnant women. *Br J Obstet Gynaecol* **103**:39–47.

Eeg-Olofsson O, Malmros I, Elwin CE, et al. 1978. Convulsions in a breast-fed infant after maternal indomethacin. *Lancet* **2**:215.

Elia J, Katz IR, Simpson GM. 1987. Teratogenicity of psychotherapeutic medications. *Psychopharmacol Bull* **23**:531–86.

Fainstat T. 1954. Cortisone induced congenital cleft-lip in rabbits. *Endocrinology* **55**:502–8.

Felding I, Rane A. 1984. Congenital liver damage after treatment of mother with valproic acid and phenytoin? *Acta Paediatr Scand* **73**:565–8.

Feldkamp M, Jones KL, Ornoy A, et al. 1997. Postmarketing surveillance for angiotensin-converting enzyme inhibitor use during pregnancy—United States, Canada and Israel 1987–1995. *JAMA* **277**:1193.

Fitzsimons R, Greenberger PA, Patterson R. 1986. Outcome of pregnancy in women requiring corticosteroids for severe asthma. *J Allergy Clin Immunol* **78**:349–53.

Forfar JO, Nelson MM. 1973. Epidemiology of drugs taken by pregnant women: Drugs that may affect the fetus adversely. *Clin Pharmacol Ther* **14**:632–42.

Fraser FC, Walker BE, Fainstat TO. 1954. The experimental production of cleft palate with cortisone and other hormones. *J Cell Comp Physiol* **43**:237–59.

Furberg CD, Psaty BM, Meyer JV. 1995. Nifedipine dose-related increase in mortality in patients with coronary heart disease. *Circulation* **92**:1326–31.

Gaily E, Kantola-Sorsa E, Granstrom M-L. 1988. Intelligence of children of epileptic mothers. *J Paediatr* **113**:677–84.

Gal P, Sharpless MK. 1984. Fetal drug exposure—behavioral teratogenesis. *Drug Intell Clin Pharm* **18**:186–201.

Ginsberg JS, Barron WM. 1994. Pregnancy and prosthetic heart valves. *Lancet* **344**:1171–2.

Ginsberg JS, Hirsh J, Turner DC, et al. 1989. Risks to the fetus of anticoagulant therapy during pregnancy. *Thromb Haemost* **61**:197–203.

Goldberg JD, Golbus MS. 1986. The value of case reports in human teratology. *Am J Obstet Gynecol* **154**:469–82.

Greenberger PA, Patterson R. 1985. Management of asthma during pregnancy. *N Engl J Med* **312**:897–902.

Griffith GC, Nichols G, Asher JD, et al. 1965. Heparin osteoporosis. *JAMA* **193**:85–8.

Hall JG, Pauli RM, Wilson KM. 1980. Maternal and fetal sequelae of anticoagulation during pregnancy. *Am J Med* **68**:122–40.

Hanson JW, Myrianthopoulos NC, Sedgewick Harvey MA, et al. 1976. Risks to the offspring of women treated with hydantoin anticonvulsants with emphasis on the fetal hydantoin syndrome. *J Pediatr* **89**:662–8.

Hanson JW, Smith DW. 1975. The fetal hydantoin syndrome. *J Pediatr* **87**:285–90.

Heinonen OP, Slone D, Shapiro S. 1977. *Birth Defects and Drugs in Pregnancy*. Littleton, MA: Publishing Sciences Group.

Hendricks SK, Smith JR, Moore DE, et al. 1990. Oligohydramnios associated with prostaglandin synthetase inhibitors in preterm labour. *Br J Obstet Gynaecol* **97**:312–6.

Hillesmaa VK, Teramo K, Granstrom ML, et al. 1983. Serum folate concentrations during pregnancy in women with epilepsy: Relation to antiepileptic drug concentrations, number of seizures, and fetal outcome. *Br Med J* **287**:577–9.

Hirsh J, Raschke R, Warkentin TE, et al. 1995. Heparin: mechanism of action, pharmacokinetics dosing concentrations, monitoring, efficacy, and safety. *Chest* **108**:258S–75S.

Hogstedt S. 1986. Hypertension in pregnancy: An epidemiological, clinical, and experimental study with special reference to metoprolol treatment. PhD thesis, Uppsala University, Sweden.

Hytten FE, Leitch I. 1971. *The Physiology of Human Pregnancy.* Oxford: Blackwell Scientific Publications.

Impey L. 1993. Severe hypotension and fetal distress following sublingual administration of nifedipine to a patient with severe pregnancy induced hypertension at 33 weeks. *Br J Obstet Gynaecol* **100**:959–61.

Italian Study of Aspirin in Pregnancy. 1993. Low-dose aspirin in prevention and treatment of intrauterine growth retardation and pregnancy-induced hypertension. *Lancet* **341**:396–400.

Iturbe-Alessio I, DelCarmen Fonseca M, Mutchinik O, et al. 1986. Risks of anticoagulant therapy in pregnant women with artificial heart valves. *N Engl J Med* **315**:1390–3.

Jick SS, Terris BZ, Jick H. 1993. First trimester topical tretinoin and congenital disorders. *Lancet* **341**:1181–2.

Jones KL, Lacro RV, Johnson KA, et al. 1989. Pattern of malformations in the children of women treated with carbamazepine during pregnancy. *N Engl J Med* **320**:1661–6.

Juchau MR. 1980. Drug biotransformation in the placenta. *Pharmacol Ther* **8**:501–24.

Kallen B, Tandberg A. 1983. Lithium and pregnancy: A cohort study on manic-depressive women. *Acta Psychiatr Scand* **68**:134–6.

Kerber IJ, Warr OS, Richardson C. 1968. Pregnancy in a patient with a prosthetic mitral valve associated with a fetal anomaly attributed to warfarin sodium. *JAMA* **203**:223–5.

Klebanoff MA, Berendes HW. 1988. Aspirin exposure during the first 20 weeks of gestation and IQ at four years of age. *Teratology* **37**:249–55.

Knott C, Williams CP, Reynolds F. 1986. Phenytoin kinetics during pregnancy and the puerperium. *Br J Obstet Gynaecol* **93**:1030–7.

Kraver B, Kraver F, Hytten F. 1988. *Drug Prescribing in Pregnancy.* New York: Churchill Livingstone.

Kuhnz W, Koch S, Helge H, et al. 1988. Primidone and phenobarbital during lactation period in epileptic women: Total and free drug serum levels in the nursed infants and their effects on neonatal behaviour. *Dev Pharmacol Ther* **11**:147–54.

Lammer EJ, Chen DT, Hoar RM, et al. 1985. Retinoic acid embryopathy. *N Engl J Med* **313**:837–41.

Lander CM, Edwards VC, Eadie MJ, et al. 1977. Plasma anticonvulsant concentrations during pregnancy. *Neurology* **27**:128–31.

Lander CM, Smith MT, Chalk JB, et al. 1984. Bioavailability and pharmacokinetics of phenytoin during pregnancy. *Eur J Clin Pharmacol* **27**:105–10.

Landon MJ, Kirkley M. 1979. Metabolism of diphenylhydantoin during pregnancy. *Br J Obstet Gynaecol* **86**:125–32.

Lebedevs TH, Horton RE, Yapp P, et al. 1991. Excretion of indomethacin in breast milk. *Br J Clin Pharmacol* **32**:751–4.

Legius E, Jaeken J, Eggermont E. 1987. Sodium valproate pregnancy and infantile fatal liver failure. *Lancet* **2**:1518–9.

Lenz W. 1961. Kindliche Missbildungen nach Medikament-Einnahme Während der Gavidität. *Dtsch Med Wochenschr* **86**:2555.

Levin AC, Doering PL, Hatton RC. 1994. Use of nifedipine in the hypertensive diseases of pregnancy. *Ann Pharmacother* **28**:1371–8.

Lindheimer MD, Katz AI. 1973. Sodium and diuretics in pregnancy. *N Engl J Med* **288**:891–4.

Lindout D, Hoppener JEA, Meinardi H. 1984. Teratogenicity of antiepileptic drug combinations with special emphasis on expoxidation (of carbamazepine). *Epilepsia* **25**:77–83.

Loebstein R, Lalkin A, Koren G. 1997. Pharmacokinetic changes during pregnancy and their clinical relevance. *Clin Pharmacokinet* **33**:328–43.

MacDonald PC. 1973. A study of angiotension II pressure response throughout primigravid pregnancy. *J Clin Invest* **52**:2682–9.

MacGuillivray I, Rose GA, Roe B. 1969. Blood pressure in pregnancy. *Clin Sci* **37**:395–407.

MacMahon B. More on Bendectin. 1981. *JAMA* **246**:371–2.

Manchester D, Margolis HS, Sheldon RE. 1976. Possible association between maternal indomethacin therapy and primary pulmonary hypertension of the newborn. *Am J Obstet Gynecol* **126**:467–9.

Martz F, Failinger C, Blake DA. 1977. Phenytoin teratogenesis: Correlation between embryopathic effect and covalent binding of putative arene oxide metabolite in gestational tissue. *J Pharmacol Exp Ther* **203**:231–9.

McBride WG. 1961. Thalidomide and congenital abnormalities. *Lancet* **2**:1358.

Medical Research Council (MRC) Vitamin Study Research Group. 1991. Prevention of neural tube defects: results of the Medical Research Council Vitamin Study. *Lancet* **338**:131–7.

Mellin GW, Katzenstein M. 1962. The saga of thalidomide. *N Engl J Med* **267**:1184–92, 1238, 1244.

Mitchell AA, Van Bennekom CM, Louik C. 1995. A pregnancy-prevention program in women of childbearing age receiving isotretinoin. *N Engl J Med* **333**:101–6.

Mogadam M, Dobbins WO, Korelitz BI. 1981. Pregnancy in inflammatory bowel disease: Effect on fetal outcome. *Gastroenterology* **80**:72–6.

Moise KJ. 1993. Effect on advancing gestational age on the frequency of fetal ductal constriction in association with maternal indomethacin use. *Am J Obstet Gynecol* **168**:1350–3.

Moise KJ, Huhta JC, Sharif DS, et al. 1988. Indomethacin in the treatment of premature labor: Effects on the fetal ductus arteriosus. *N Engl J Med* **319**:327–31.

Monreal M, Lafoz E, Olive A, et al. 1994. Comparison of subcutaneous unfractionated heparin with a low molecular weight heparin (Fragmin) in patients with venous thromboembolism and contraindications to coumarin. *Thromb Haemost* **71**:7–11.

Mountain KR, Hirsh J, Gallus AS. 1970. Neonatal coagulation defect due to anticonvulsant drug treatment in pregnancy. *Lancet* **1**: 265–8.

Munnell EW, Taylor HC. 1947. Liver blood flow in pregnancy—hepatic vein catheterisation. *J Clin Invest* **26**:952–6.

National Cancer Institute. 1983. Prenatal diethylstilbestrol (DES) exposure. Recommendations of the Diethylstilbestrol-Adenosis (DESAD) Project for the identification and management of exposed individuals. *Clin Pediatr* **22**:139–43.

Nau H, Kuhnz W, Egger H-J, et al. 1982. Anticonvulsants during pregnancy and lactation: Transplacental maternal and neonatal pharmacokinetics. *Clin Pharmacokinet* **7**:508–43.

Nau H, Rating D, Koch S, et al. 1981. Valproic acid and its metabolites. *J Pharmacol Exp Ther* **219**:768–77.

Niebyl JR, Blake DA, Freeman JM, et al. 1979. Carbamazepine levels in pregnancy and lactation. *Obstet Gynaecol* **53**:139–40.

Nora JJ, Nora AH, Toews WH. 1974. Lithium, Ebstein's anomaly, and other congenital heart defects [letter]. *Lancet* **2**:594–5.

Norton ME, Merrill J, Cooper BAB, et al. 1991. Neonatal complications after the administration of indomethacin for preterm labour. *N Engl J Med* **329**:1602–7.

Oo CY, Kuhn RJ, Desai N, et al. 1995. Active transport of cimetidine into human milk. *Clin Pharmacol Ther* **58**:548–55.

Orme ML. 1985. The Debendox saga. *Br Med J* **291**:918–9.

Ounsted MK, Moar VA, Good FJ, et al. 1980. Hypertension during pregnancy with and without specific treatment; the development of the children at the age of four years. *Br J Obstet Gynaecol* **87**:19–24.

Parry E, Shields R, Turnbull AC. 1970. Transit time in the small intestine in pregnancy. *J Obstet Gynaecol Br Commonw* **77**:900–1.

Pastuszac A, Schick-Boschetto B, Zuber C, et al. 1993. Pregnancy outcome following first-trimester exposure to fluoxetine (prozac). *JAMA* **269**:2246–8.

Peckham CH, King RW. 1963. A study of intercurrent conditions observed during pregnancy. *Am J Obstet Gynecol* **87**:609–20.

Perucca E. 1987. Drug metabolism in pregnancy, infancy, and childhood. *Pharmacol Ther* **34**:129–43.

Perucca E, Ruprah M, Richens A. 1981. Altered drug binding to serum proteins in pregnancy. *J R Soc Med* **74**:422–6.

Phenlan MC, Pellock JM, Nance WE. 1982. Discordant expression of fetal hydantoin syndrome in heteropaternal dizygotic twins. *N Engl J Med* **307**:99–101.

Philipson A. 1977. Pharmacokinetics of ampicillin during pregnancy. *J Infect Dis* **136**:370–6.

Piper JM, Baum C, Kennedy DL. 1987. Prescription drug use before and during pregnancy in a Medicaid population. *Am J Obstet Gynecol* **157**:148–56.

Piper JM, Ray WA, Rosa FW. 1992. Pregnancy outcome following exposure to angiotensin-converting enzyme inhibitors. *Obstet Gynecol* **80**:429–32.

Platt JE, Friedhoff AJ, Broman SH, et al. 1989. Effects of prenatal neuroleptic drug exposure on motor performance in children. *Hum Psychopharmacol* **4**:205–13.

Prach AT, Rubin PC. 1988. Fetoplacental drug clearance in the rabbit: Studies with trimazosin and tolmesoxide. *Xenobiotica* **18**:967–72.

Rating D, Nau H, Jager-Roman E, et al. 1982. Teratogenic and pharmacokinetic studies of primidone during pregnancy and in the offspring of epileptic women. *Acta Paediatr Scand* **71**:301–11.

Redman CWG, Beilin LJ, Bonnar J, et al. 1976. Fetal outcome in trial of antihypertensive treatment in pregnancy. *Lancet* **2**:754–6.

Redman CWG, Beilin LJ, Bonnar J. 1977. Treatment of hypertension in pregnancy with methyldopa: Blood pressure control and side effects. *Br J Obstet Gynaecol* **84**:419–26.

Reynolds B, Butters L, Evans J, et al. 1984. First year of life after the use of atenolol in pregnancy associated hypertension. *Arch Dis Child* **59**:1061–3.

Rosa FW. 1983. Teratogenicity of isotretinoin. *Lancet* **2**:513.

Rosengarten H, Friedhoff AJ. 1979. Enduring changes in dopamine receptor cells of pups from drug administration to pregnant and nursing rats. *Science* **203**:1133–5.

Rubin PC. 1981. Beta-blockers in pregnancy. *N Engl J Med* **305**: 1323–6.

Rubin PC (editor). 1995. *Prescribing in Pregnancy*, 2nd ed. London: British Medical Association.

Rubin JD, Ferencz C, Loffredo C, et al. 1993. Use of prescription and non-prescription drugs in pregnancy. *J Clin Epidemiol* **46**: 581–9.

Rubin PC, Butters L, Clark DM, et al. 1983. Placebo-controlled trial of atenolol in the treatment of pregnancy-associated hypertension. *Lancet* **1**:431–4.

Rubin PC, Butters L, Clark DM, et al. 1984. Obstetric aspects of the use of pregnancy-associated hypertension of the beta-adrenoceptor antagonist atenolol. *Am J Obstet Gynecol* **150**:389–92.

Rubin PC, Butters L, Low RA, et al. 1982. Atenolol in the treatment of essential hypertension during pregnancy. *Br J Clin Pharmacol* **150**:389–92.

Rubin PC, Butters L, McCabe R, et al. 1987. The influence of pregnancy on drug action: Concentration-effect modeling with propranolol. *Clin Sci* **73**:47–52.

Rubin PC, Butters L, Reynolds B, et al. 1983. Atenolol elimination in the neonate. *Br J Clin Pharmacol* **16**:659–62.

Rubin PC, Craig GF, Gavin K, et al. 1986. Prospective survey of use of therapeutic drugs, alcohol, and cigarettes during pregnancy. *Br Med J* **292**:81–3.

Ruprah M, Perucca E, Richens A. 1980. Decreased serum protein binding of phenytoin in late pregnancy. *Lancet* **2**:316–7.

Saunders M. 1989. Epilepsy in women of childbearing age. *Br Med J* **299**:581.

Sbarouni E, Oakley CM. 1994. Outcome of pregnancy in women with valve prostheses. *Br Heart J* **71**:196–201.

Schatz M, Patterson R, Zeitz S, et al. 1975. Corticosteroid therapy for the pregnant asthmatic patient. *JAMA* **233**:804–7.

Schiff E, Peleg E, Goldenberg M, et al. 1989. The use of aspirin to prevent pregnancy-induced hypertension and lower the ratio of thromboxane $A_2$ to prostacyclin in relatively high risk pregnancies. *N Engl J Med* **321**:351–6.

Schou M, Amdisen A, Steenstrup OR. 1973a. Lithium pregnancy. II: Hazards to women given lithium during pregnancy and delivery. *Br Med J* **2**:137–8.

Schou M, Goldfield MD, Weinstein MR, et al. 1973b. Lithium and pregnancy. I: Report from the register of lithium babies. *Br Med J* **2**:135–6.

Shapiro S, Slone D, Hartz SC, et al. 1976. Anticonvulsants and parental epilepsy in the development of birth defects. *Lancet* **1**:272–5.

Shaughnessy SG, Young E, Deschamps P, et al. 1995. The effects of low molecular weight and standard heparin on calcium loss from fetal rat calvaria. *Blood* **86**:1368–71.

Shaul WL, Emery H, Hall JG. 1975. Chondrodysplasia punctata and maternal warfarin use during pregnancy. *Am J Dis Child* **129**:360–2.

Shaul WL, Hall JG. 1977. Multiple congenital anomalies associated with oral anticoagulants. *Am J Obstet Gynecol* **127**:191–8.

Sheiner LB, Stanski DR, Vozel S, et al. 1979. Simultaneous modeling of pharmacokinetics and pharmacodynamics: Application to d-tubocurarine. *Clin Pharmacol Ther* **25**:358–71.

Shotan A, Widerhorn J, Hurst A, et al. 1994. Risks of angiotensin-converting enzyme inhibition during pregnancy: Experimental and clinical evidence, potential mechanisms, and recommendations for use. *Am J Med* **96**:451–6.

Sibai BM, Caritis SN, Thom E, et al. 1993. Prevention of preeclampsia with low-dose aspirin in healthy nulliparous pregnant women. The National Institute of Child Health and Human Development Network of Maternal-Fetal Medicine Units. *N Engl J Med* **329**: 1213–8.

Snyder SW, Cardwell MS. 1989. Neuromuscular blockade with magnesium sulphate and nifedipine. *Am J Obstet Gynecol* **161**: 35–6.

Spielberg SP. 1982. Pharmacokinetics and the fetus. *N Engl J Med* **307**:115–6.

Strickler SM, Dansky LV, Miller AM, et al. 1985. Genetic predisposition to phenytoin-induced birth defects. *Lancet* **2**:746–9.

Stuart MJ, Gross SJ, Elrad H, et al. 1982. Effects of acetylsalicylic-acid ingestion on maternal and neonatal hemostasis. *N Engl J Med* **307**:909–12.

Studd JWW, Starke CM, Blainey JD. 1970. Serum protein changes in the parturient mother fetus and newborn infant. *J Obstet Gynaecol Br Commonw* **77**:511–7.

Szabo KT. 1970. Teratogenic effects of lithium carbonate in the fetal mouse. *Nature* **225**:73–5.

Szabo KT, Brent R. 1974. Species differences in experimental teratogenesis by tranquillising agents. *Lancet* **1**:565.

Thalidomide. 1976. Thalidomide's long shadow. *Br Med J* **2**:1155–6.

Turner ES, Greenberger PA, Patterson R. 1980. Management of the pregnant asthmatic patient. *Ann Intern Med* **6**:905–18.

Valproate Spina Bifida. 1988. Valproate spina bifida and birth defect registries [editorial]. *Lancet* **2**:1040–5.

Van Dyke DC, Hodge SE, Heide F, et al. 1988. Family studies in fetal phenytoin exposure. *J Pediatr* **113**:301–6.

Ville Y, Jenkins E, Shearer MJ, et al. 1993. Fetal intraventricular haemorrhage and maternal warfarin. *Lancet* **341**:1211.

Waddell WJ, Marlowe C. 1981. Transfer of drugs across the placenta. *Pharmacol Ther* **14**:375–90.

Wallenburg HC, Dekker GA, Makovitz JW, et al. 1986. Low-dose aspirin prevents pregnancy induced hypertension and pre-eclampsia in angiotensin-sensitive primigravidae. *Lancet* **1**:1–3.

Wise PH, Hall AJ. 1980. Heparin-induced osteopenia in pregnancy. *Br Med J* **2**:110–1.

Wong V, Cheng CH, Chan KC. 1993. Fetal and neonatal outcome of exposure to anticoagulants during pregnancy. *Am J Med Genet* **45**:17–21.

CHAPTER

# 20 DRUG THERAPY IN PEDIATRIC PATIENTS

Ronen Loebstein, Sunita Vohra, Gideon Koren

*Chapter Outline*



It is now widely acknowledged that infants and children are not "small adults" in the way their bodies handle drugs. Rapid and important age-related physiologic changes in drug metabolism and elimination occur in children, especially during the first year of life. For example, the elimination half-life of phenytoin, initially prolonged, gradually shortens during the first few months of life (Chiba et al. 1980; Blain et al. 1981; Albani and Wernicke 1983). The elimination half-life of furosemide, 15 to 20 hours in premature infants, drops to less than 1 hour only 3 months later (Peterson et al. 1980; Snodgrass and Whitfield 1983).

Despite a significant increase in the knowledge of drug disposition in infants and children over the past few years, pharmacokinetic-pharmacodynamic interactions remain poorly understood. These challenges in pediatric clinical pharmacology are further increased by the many obstacles that prevent more rational and timely accumulation of important data regarding drug disposition and response in children. Only recently have pediatric clinical pharmacology studies been expected by the Food and Drug Administration as an integral part of regulatory review at the FDA for all agents used in children. It is hoped that this requirement will enhance evidence-based pharmacotherapy in the pediatric population.

**PRINCIPLE Neonates and children represent a condition of unstable pharmacokinetics. A knowledge of age-related changes in drug absorption, distribution, and clearance is essential to optimize drug efficacy and to avoid toxicity.**

## THE EXTENT OF DRUG USE IN NEONATES AND CHILDREN

Children, especially in their first years of life, receive more drugs than most other age groups. The extent of drug prescription in the outpatient pediatric population has been reported by Kennedy and Forbes (1982). An average of 0.9 medications per patient-contact is prescribed in pediatric practice compared with 1.1 drugs per patient-contact for all disciplines combined. In their first 5 years of life, 95% of children are prescribed medications, with an average of 8.5 courses of prescription and 5.5 different medications. Within this 5-year period, the greatest number of prescriptions is given between 7 and 12 months. Outpatient drug therapy in the pediatric age group encompasses a large variety of conditions. For example, antihistamines and sympathomimetics are widely used to treat upper respiratory tract infections. With essentially no pharmacokinetic data in children and very few scientifically validated objective measures of pharmacodynamic response, the pediatrician and family practitioner must rely on subjective clinical judgment and the parent's report in an attempt to assess therapeutic response.

## PHARMACOKINETIC PRINCIPLES IN NEONATES AND INFANTS AND THEIR CLINICAL RELEVANCE

Special attention must be paid to the pharmacokinetic variables, as rapid and important age-related changes in drug absorption, distribution, and clearance may occur in the first few months of life. This section describes the pharmacokinetic principles in neonates and infants, with special focus on those that are clinically relevant.

## Drug Absorption

Drug absorption in infants and children follows the same general principles as in adults. However, as relatively more sites of drug administration are used in neonates, special considerations must be given to the different determinants affecting drug absorption from each site.

***Absorption from the GI tract***

Diminished intestinal motility and delayed gastric emptying in neonates and infants result in longer periods of time for a drug to reach similar plasma concentrations after oral administration (Macleod and Radde 1985). Oral absorption of acetaminophen, penicillin G, phenobarbital, and phenytoin has been shown to be lower in infants compared with that of older children and adults (Axline et al. 1967; Morselli 1976) (Table 20-1). Different flora colonize the sterile fetal intestine depending on whether the newborn is breast- or formula-fed. The change of bacterial flora during the newborn period is important for the hydrolysis of drug conjugates that are excreted in bile. Absorption of vitamin K and other lipid-soluble vitamins will also be influenced by the development of intestinal flora.

Disease conditions such as diarrhea, giardiasis, cystic fibrosis, and celiac disease should be considered important factors that might interfere with drug absorption from the GI tract.

***Rectal administration of drugs***

Rectal drug administration may be useful in conditions such as nausea and vomiting, status epilepticus, and induction of anesthesia, as well as for drugs that have a large first-pass effect (blood supply to the anus and lower rectum drain directly into the inferior vena cava). Solutions of diazepam have been demonstrated to be well absorbed from the rectum compared with diazepam delivered in suppositories for which rectal absorption is erratic and incomplete. In light of its poor absorption from intramuscular injection sites, rectal administration of a diazepam solution offers effective anticonvulsive and sedative therapy. Diazepam bioavailability is higher after rectal than oral administration.

Rectally administered diazepam has been used effectively in the treatment of febrile seizures. Similarly, midazolam and atropine given for other indications are clinically more effective than when administered intramuscularly (Saint Maurice et al. 1986). In addition to benzodiazepines, barbiturates have been administered rectally to children with great success.

**Table 20-1 Oral Drug Absorption (Bioavailability) of Selected Drugs: Comparison of the Neonate with Older Children**

| Drug | Oral absorption |
|---|---|
| Acetaminophen | Decreased |
| Ampicillin | Increased |
| Diazepam | No change |
| Digoxin | No change |
| Penicillin G | Increased |
| Phenobarbital | Decreased |
| Phenytoin | Decreased |
| Sulfonamides | No change |

***Absorption from intramuscular injection sites***

Local and drug-related factors are the most important determinants affecting drug absorption after intramuscular injection. Blood flow to and from the injected muscle are the most important local factors. Clinical conditions such as low cardiac output, respiratory distress syndrome, and other circulatory disturbances may severely compromise blood supply to the muscles, leading to decreased absorption from the injection site. The degree of muscular activity also affects the rate of drug absorption from intramuscular sites. Immobile infants demonstrate slower absorption rates from intramuscular injection sites, whereas exercise may enhance drug absorption, as in the case of insulin and exercise-induced hypoglycemia.

Phenytoin is a classic example for drug-related factors that affect its absorption from intramuscular injection sites. The pK of phenytoin is 9.2, and the acid form of the drug is insoluble in water. Since the muscle cytoplasm is more acidic than blood, the sodium salt of phenytoin is converted into the acid form, which precipitates at the site of injection. This is not only painful but results in slow and erratic absorption of this agent from intramuscular sites.

More rapid absorption following intramuscular administration has been demonstrated for penicillin G benzathine and clindamycin in the pediatric age group compared with adults (Greenblatt and Koch 1976).

**PRINCIPLE The use of intramuscular drug administration in infants and children requires careful consideration, as both local and drug-related factors affect the absorption of intramuscular agents.**

## Drug Distribution and Protein Binding

Drug distribution and protein binding in neonates and children are influenced by changes in body composition that occur with development. The total body water compartment is relatively larger among premature neonates (85% of total body weight) compared with that of full-term neonates (70 to 75%) and adults (50 to 60%). The extracellular water compartment is 40% of body weight in the neonate compared with 20% in the adult. These differences are clinically relevant as many drugs, and especially water-soluble drugs (e.g., aminoglycosides), are distributed throughout the extracellular water compartment. Therefore, the volume of the extracellular water compartment will determine drug concentration at the receptor site. Conversely, total body fat in premature infants is 1% of total body weight compared with 15% in full-term neonates. This will affect lipid-soluble drugs (e.g., digoxin), which may accumulate in smaller amounts in immature infants.

Another determinant of drug distribution is its protein binding. Generally, neonates and especially premature neonates are at risk of altered drug–protein interactions as a result of many factors. Decreased plasma concentrations of total protein and albumin in newborns and infants lead to decreased drug–protein binding in these age groups compared with that in adults. In vitro studies comparing free drug concentrations in cord blood and adult plasma have demonstrated a significantly higher ratio of free to total drug for salicylates, sulfonamides, morphine, phenobarbital, and phenytoin in cord blood. Since the free drug exerts the pharmacologic drug effect, the increased free drug concentrations in neonates may result in greater drug effect or even toxicity despite normal total (bound + unbound) drug concentrations.

Increased concentrations of free fatty acids and unconjugated bilirubin in the newborn also affect drug–protein binding. As both free fatty acids and unconjugated bilirubin have high affinity for albumin, they may compete and even displace drugs from their albumin binding sites.

Differences in the distribution of different agents into the central nervous system is clinically important in the consideration of antimicrobial therapy in cases of meningitis. The relatively tighter junctions in the brain endothelial capillaries and the close approximation of the glial connective tissue to the capillary endothelium limit the distribution of drugs to brain tissue. This is especially relevant for water-soluble antibiotics (e.g., aminoglycosides), which are less likely to cross the blood–brain barrier in the treatment of meningitis.

**PRINCIPLE Since the free (unbound) drug concentration is responsible for drug effects, age-related changes in protein binding may exert important influences on drug efficacy and toxicity especially in drugs with a narrow therapeutic index.**

## Clearance

### *Hepatic drug metabolism*

Although the major organ of drug metabolism is the liver, many other organs such as the lungs and GI tract, or the blood are capable of metabolizing drugs. Drug metabolism can result in either generation of weaker or inactive metabolites or transformation of a parent compound or pro-drug into the active compound (theophylline to caffeine, codeine to morphine) or into an even more active or toxic metabolite. Drug metabolism is categorized in two major steps: phase I reactions, biotransformation of a molecule into a generally more water-soluble metabolite; and phase II reactions, conjugation of a drug or its metabolite with endogenous molecules. Generally, phase I reactions (oxidation, reduction, hydrolysis) achieve maturity by 6 months of age Table 20-2). Age-related

Table 20-2 **Examples of Pediatric Drugs Subject to Phase I and Phase II Reactions**

| Phase I (e.g., oxidation, reduction reactions) | Phase II (e.g., glucuronidation, sulfation, acetylation reactions) |
|---|---|
| Phenytoin | Acetaminophen |
| Ibuprofen | Morphine |
| Codeine | Corticosteroids |
| Diazepam | Dopamine |
| Naloxone | Sulfonamides |
| Methylphenidate | Isoniazid |
| Indomethacin | Digoxin |
| Succinylcholine | Diazepam |

changes in drug metabolism have been demonstrated for theophylline: In neonates only 10% of theophylline is methylated to caffeine, whereas 50% of the drug is excreted unchanged in the urine. With maturation of hepatic enzymes for hydroxylation and acetylation, the rate of theophylline clearance increases, resulting in the short half-life of theophylline found in infants and children (3 to 5 hours) compared with adults (8 hours).

Hepatic phase II reactions (glucuronidation, sulfation, acetylation) are substantially lower (50 to 70% of adults' values) in early neonatal life. Glucuronide formation reaches its full maturity (adult values) between the third and fourth years of life. The decreased ability of neonates to metabolize drugs results in prolonged elimination half-lives (Table 20-3). Drug doses and dosing schedules that do not take these changes into account predispose neonates to adverse drug reactions.

***Drug excretion***

Renal function demonstrates an age-dependent increase in functional capacity. The glomerular filtration rate in neonates is 30 to 40% of the adult value. By the end of the first week of life, both the GFR and renal plasma flow have increased by 50%. By the third week of life, the GFR has achieved 50 to 60% of the adult values, and, by 12 months, GFR reaches adult values. The clinical relevance of these changes is apparent with renally eliminated medications such as aminoglycosides, penicillins, and digoxin. For example, the dosage of gentamicin for a neonate less than 7 days old is 5 mg/kg of body weight daily in divided doses at 12-hour intervals. This dosage changes to 7.5 mg/kg daily in three doses at 8-hour intervals in children over 7 days old. Renal clearance of digoxin has been demonstrated to increase from 33 mL/min per 1.73 $m^2$ in neonates to 98 and 144 mL/min per 1.73 $m^2$ at 3 months and 1.5 years, respectively.

Different disease states may alter the normal process of renal function maturation and may cause difficulties in appropriate dose adjustments made according to the predicted rate of renal function maturation during the first weeks of life.

## DRUG INTERACTIONS

Clinically significant drug interactions can be defined as a clinically measurable modification in magnitude or duration of the action of one drug caused by prior or concomitant administration of another drug. Drug interactions can be clinically desirable such as in the treatment of hypertension by using multiple drugs with different mechanisms of action, or adverse as will be discussed later in this section. It is currently estimated that serious life-threatening adverse drug reactions occur in 3% of hospital patients with 7% of these caused by drug interactions. Mechanisms of drug interactions can be classified into those occurring on the pharmacokinetic level and those involving the pharmacodynamics of the index drug.

### Interactions Affecting Oral Bioavailability

Drug interactions in the GI tract can result in decreased oral bioavailability of the index drug. For example, tetracyclines can chelate calcium, magnesium, or iron, leading to decreased absorption of the cation–tetracycline complex. Drugs that damage the intestinal absorptive surface, such as antineoplastic agents, or orally administered neomycin, may lead to decreased absorption of otherwise well absorbed drugs.

Gastric emptying can be pharmacologically enhanced (metoclopramide, domperidone) or delayed (morphine,

**Table 20-3 Changes in Elimination Half-Life during Development**

| | Elimination half-life (hours) | | | |
|---|---|---|---|---|
| Drug | Newborn (0–28 days) | Infant (1–24 months) | Child | Adult |
| Acetaminophen | 4.9 | 4.5 | 3.6 | |
| Amikacin | 5.0–6.5 | 1.6 | 2.3 | |
| Amoxicillin | 3.7 | 0.9–1.9 | 0.6–1.5 | |
| Cefuroxime | 5.5 | 3.5 | 1.2 | 1.5 |
| Diazepam | 30 | 10 | 25 | 30 |
| Digoxin | 18–33 | 37 | 30–50 | |
| Gentamycin | 4.0 | 2.6 | 1.2 | 2–3 |
| Theophylline | 30 | 6.9 | 3.4 | 8.1 |
| Vancomycin | 4.1–9.1 | 2.2–2.4 | 5–6 | |

anticholinergics, antacids) affecting the rate rather than the extent of absorption. This may be clinically relevant in situations when a rapid onset of drug effect is desired (pain relief or sedation). Finally, for some drugs with extensive first-pass effect (i.e., drugs that are extensively extracted or metabolized during transit across the intestinal epithelium or during the first pass through the liver), such as lidocaine and morphine, the major factor affecting their clearance is the hepatic blood flow. Therefore, coadministration of drugs that may decrease hepatic blood flow, such as cimetidine or beta blockers, would be expected to raise the steady-state concentration of the abovementioned agents.

## Protein-Binding Drug Interactions

Protein binding occurs primarily to albumin and $\alpha_2$-glycoprotein. The serum concentration of a measured drug usually refers to the total drug concentration in the plasma (free + protein-bound drug), although only the free drug exerts the pharmacologic effect. Drugs that are highly bound to proteins are subject to displacement by other drugs with high affinity for the same protein-binding sites. This may result in a *transient* increase in the free concentrations of the index drug, followed by redistribution and increased clearance, creating new equilibrium of both drugs. This phenomenon will result in clinically significant effects in cases when the index drug has a small volume of distribution, a narrow therapeutic window, and rapid onset of action in relation to its plasma concentration.

## Drug Interactions Affecting Biotransformation

Many of the drugs prescribed in the pediatric population can potentially inhibit or enhance the metabolism of other drugs. The significance of these interactions is dictated by the magnitude of the decrease or increase in the clearance of the index drug. Generally, the modifications in magnitude of hepatic drug metabolism caused by drug–drug interactions are hard to predict, because most drugs are metabolized by a number of different pathways, and the quantitative fraction of each pathway is difficult to evaluate.

Most inhibitors of hepatic drug metabolism bind to an essential part of the enzyme system resulting in a functionally impaired or inactive enzyme that is unable to oxidize, reduce, or hydrolyze medications. The most useful agents with inhibitory effects on hepatic drug metabolism among the pediatric age group include cimetidine, erythromycin, ciprofloxacin, and omeprazole. Coadministration of these agents with a medication with narrow therapeutic range such as theophylline may result in increased plasma concentrations and potential toxicity.

Enzyme induction, however, can enhance the clearance of index drugs leading to decreased or even loss of efficacy. Rifampin, a well-known inducer of hepatic metabolism, has been implicated as a potential cause of graft rejection by increasing the clearance of cyclosporine and prednisone. It has also been claimed to be the cause of oral contraceptive failure due to increased metabolism. Phenytoin, another inducer of hepatic biotransformation, has also been shown to stimulate metabolism of corticosteroids, as well as digitoxin and theophylline, thereby reducing serum concentrations. The ability of phenobarbital to induce the oxidizing enzyme system found in hepatic endoplasmic reticulum may enhance the hepatic metabolism of any drug that undergoes metabolism by this system. Phenobarbital-induced effects have been reported on the metabolism of drugs from a variety of classes. These include analgesics (acetaminophen), antibacterials (chloramphenicol, doxycycline, metronidazole), anticoagulants (warfarin), beta-adrenergic receptor antagonists (propranolol), corticosteroids, and opioid analgesics.

In cases of established induction interaction, the index drug dose should be increased. Conversely, if the inducing drug is discontinued, the index drug dose should be decreased to avoid toxicity.

**PRINCIPLE Coadministration of drugs with inhibitory effects on hepatic drug metabolism (such as cimetidine, erythromycin, ciprofloxacin, and omeprazole) together with a hepatic-metabolized drug with a narrow therapeutic range may lead to its increased serum concentrations and even toxicity.**

## Drug Interactions Due to Altered Renal Function

Drugs excreted entirely by glomerular filtration are unlikely to be affected by other drugs. However, the clearance of drugs that are actively secreted into the tubular lumen can be significantly inhibited by other drugs. Methotrexate toxicity can be enhanced by inhibition of its tubular secretion by salicylates. Renal clearance of lithium is significantly reduced in the presence of thiazides; also low effective circulating volume with increased sodium reabsorption increases lithium reabsorption as well. Drug interactions may also have advantages, as with probenecid, which reduces renal penicillin excretion.

The pediatrician should aim to decrease the potential risk carried by drug interactions mainly by being aware of high-risk clinical settings of such cases. Drugs with low ratios of toxicity to therapeutic effects and a steep dose–response relationship represent a major risk. Clinically relevant examples of such drugs are warfarin, digoxin, lithium, theophylline, and aminoglycosides. Other important high-risk conditions include patients receiving several drugs, as the risk of drug interaction increases with the increased number of drugs used; critically ill patients; and drug abusers.

## COMPLIANCE

Noncompliance in the pediatric age group is as important as in adult medicine. About 21% of adolescents are reported noncompliant with anticonvulsant therapy, 28% of asthmatic children are noncompliant with theophylline, and 30 to 40% of thalassemia major patients are noncompliant with nightly subcutaneous infusions of desferrioxamine. Reasons for noncompliance range from simple forgetfulness to the extreme of neglect, and they reflect the patient's or the parent's perception of the seriousness of the illness and the degree of effort required by the recommended treatment. The role of the pediatrician or the family physician in improving compliance is extremely important. Taking time to explain the nature of the illness, the precise instructions for carrying out the treatment, including the names and purposes of the drug or drugs prescribed, and specific instructions regarding dosage are all actions that have been shown to improve compliance (Tebbi 1993, Florian and Elad 1998).

Objective methods to assess compliance have not been applied widely in the pediatric population. Patients' or parents' reports, return tablet counts, and random measurement of serum concentrations may help disclose noncompliance, although their reliability is limited. The use of computerized pill containers, which record each lid opening, has been shown to be very effective in measuring compliance.

**PRINCIPLE Taking time to explain the nature of the illness, the precise instructions for carrying out the treatment, including the names and purposes of the drug or drugs prescribed, and the specific instructions regarding dosage are all actions that have been demonstrated to improve compliance.**

## THERAPEUTIC DRUG MONITORING

Drug concentrations depend on different factors among which are drug dosage, the pharmacokinetic properties as dictated by liver and kidney function, and genetic variability in drug metabolism. *Therapeutic drug monitoring* (TDM) is defined as the measurement of drug concentrations and the use of pharmacokinetic principles to individualize drug dosing in an attempt to maximize the therapeutic efficacy while minimizing the potential toxicity. By its nature TDM is primarily applicable for medications that have narrow therapeutic indices (i.e., the drug concentration required for therapeutic effect is close to the toxic concentration) and for agents that demonstrate a good correlation between serum concentrations and pharmacologic effects.

Therapeutic drug monitoring aims at achieving drug concentration within a therapeutic range. However, it is noteworthy that even within the so-called therapeutic range, some patients will not respond completely, whereas others will experience toxicity due to interindividual pharmacokinetic and pharmacodynamic differences. Appropriate timing of drug concentration measurement is crucial for accurate TDM. Trough level, measured before drug administration, provides accurate interpretation of drug concentration, whereas peak levels are less accurate, as they are subject to significant variability secondary to differences in absorption and distribution rates. Peak concentration measurements are usually reserved for medications with short half-lives in which peak concentrations are associated with efficacy or toxicity. Random sampling of drug concentrations is of little value.

### Theophylline

Theophylline serum concentrations between 10 and 20 mg/L have been shown to induce clinical bronchodilation in asthmatic children, whereas concentrations of 5 to 10 mg/L are effective for diaphragmatic stimulation. Plasma concentrations higher than 20 mg/L are associated with increasing incidence of toxicity that includes nausea, vomiting, and convulsions.

### Aminoglycosides

Aminoglycoside-induced ototoxicity and nephrotoxicity are closely related to serum concentrations. Prolonged peak levels of gentamicin of 12 to 14 mg/L and/or trough levels above 2 mg/L have been shown to increase significantly the risk of both toxicities.

### Chloramphenicol

Chloramphenicol serum concentrations of 25 mg/L or higher have been demonstrated to increase the risk for reversible bone marrow suppression. However, this toxicity should be distinguished from the rare idiosyncratic form of chloramphenicol-induced bone marrow suppression that has no correlation with serum concentrations.

### Vancomycin

Vancomycin-induced nephrotoxicity and ototoxicity are dose-related. Although the relationship between a threshold serum concentration and both toxicities is difficult to determine, trough vancomycin concentrations greater than 30 mg/L and 80 to 100 mg/L are associated with increased risk for nephrotoxicity and ototoxicity, respectively.

**PRINCIPLE Appropriate timing of drug concentration measurement at times of the expected peak or trough time points is crucial for an accurate interpretation and subsequent dosing. Lack of knowledge of the actual time of drug delivery to the patient and therefore random sampling will result in useless therapeutic drug monitoring.**

## SUMMARY

From a pharmacotherapy perspective, the process of development and growth represents an unstable and dynamic condition. Age-related changes in drug absorption, distribution, and elimination in neonates, infants, and prepubescent children create a unique situation, which in some cases may increase drug toxicity of some agents and in other cases may protect from toxicity of other agents. A knowledge and understanding of the age-related changes in drug disposition that are relevant for therapeutic response and toxicity are essential to optimizing pharmacotherapy at different stages of childhood.

## REFERENCES

Albani A, Wernicke I. 1983. Oral phenytoin in infancy: Dose requirement, absorption and elimination. *Pediatr Pharmacol* **3**:229–36.

Axline SG, Yaffe SJ, Simon HJ. 1967. Clinical pharmacology of antimicrobials in premature infants. *Pediatrics* **39**:97–107.

Blain PG, Mucklow JC, Bacon CJ, et al. 1981. Pharmacokinetics of diphenylhydantoin in children. *Br J Clin Pharmacol* **12**:659–61.

Chiba K, Ishizaki T, Miura H, et al. 1980. Michaelis-Menten pharmacokinetics of diphenylhydantoin and application in the pediatric age group. *J Pediatr* **96**:479–82.

Florian V, Elad D. 1998. The impact of mothers' sense of empowerment on the metabolic control of their children with juvenile diabetes. *J Ped Psych* **23**:239–47.

Greenblatt DJ, Koch-Weser J. 1976. Intra-muscular injection of drugs. *N Engl J Med* **295**:542–6.

Kennedy D, Forbes M. 1982. Drug therapy for ambulatory pediatric patients in 1979. *Pediatrics* **70**:26–9.

Macleod SM, Radde IC (editors). 1985. *Textbook of Pediatric Clinical Pharmacology*. Littleton (MA): PSG Publishing.

Morselli PL. 1976. Clinical pharmacokinetics in neonates. *Clin Pharmacokinet* **1**:81–98.

Peterson RG, Simmons MA, Rumack BH, et al. 1980. Pharmacology of furosemide in the premature newborn infant. *J Pediatr* **97**:139–43.

Saint Maurice C, Meistelman C, Rey E, et al. 1986. The pharmacokinetics of rectal midazolam for premedication in children. *Anesthesiology* **65**:536–8.

Snodgrass WR, Whitfield S. 1983. Furosemide biotransformation in a premature infant: Urinary excretion of furosemide and its glucuronide metabolite. In: Macleod SM, Okey AB, Spielberg SP, eds. *Developmental Pharmacology*. New York: Alan R. Liss, pp 413–6.

Tebbi C. 1993. Treatment compliance in childhood and adolescence. *Cancer* **71**:3441–9.

CHAPTER

# 21 GERIATRIC PHARMACOLOGY

Robert E. Vestal, Jerry H. Gurwitz

*Chapter Outline*



The elderly constitute a particularly heterogeneous patient group since physiologic aging does not necessarily parallel chronologic aging, and since the elderly accumulate the effects of disease processes. Even in the absence of recognized pathologic conditions, and despite similar ages, some individuals seem to be physiologically older or younger than others. For example, renal function (which on average declines with age) may be normal or markedly impaired in a particular individual in the absence of clinically apparent renal disease (Lindeman et al. 1992). In contrast to childhood growth and development, which occurs in a relatively predictable manner, the processes of aging in various organ systems may begin as early as the fourth decade and can proceed at different rates from person to person. In addition, geriatric patients (those >65 years old) often suffer from multiple diseases that in combination with age-related changes in physiology create no less severe therapeutic challenges than might be found in an intensive care unit. (See also chapter 16, Treatment in the Intensive Care Unit.)

Efforts to separate the effects of age per se from those of underlying disease have prompted investigators to study the disposition and action of drugs in groups of *healthy* elderly subjects in comparison with groups of healthy younger subjects. Studies of this sort do not address the possible differing effects of disease on drug action in elderly compared with younger patients. Also, such studies generally are cross-sectional rather than longitudinal in design; they only provide information about age *differences* as opposed to *changes* with age or the effects of aging. Since disease-related pathologic conditions often play a major role in determining the fate and action of drugs, the clinician must use information on the effects of old age on the fate and action of drugs to guide therapeutic decisions in a particularly thoughtful manner. We address this problem by reviewing what is known about geriatric clinical pharmacology and by identifying principles that can be applied to the practical management of geriatric patients. The reader also is referred to several reviews of this subject (Montamat et al. 1989; Tsujimoto et al. 1989a, 1989b; Vestal and Cusack 1990; Parker and Cusack 1996; Cusack et al. 1997).

## EPIDEMIOLOGY OF DRUG USE IN THE ELDERLY

The growing importance of geriatric clinical pharmacology is in part a consequence of the demographic shifts that have been occurring in the populations of developed countries over the past several decades. In the United States, whereas persons 65 years of age and older constituted 8% of the population in 1950, this percentage is projected to approach 13% in the year 2000 (U.S. Bureau of the Census 1996). Currently, the "oldest-old" (those aged 85 years and older) comprise the fastest growing segment of the U.S. population. The most frequent medical intervention performed by physicians in relation to the care of older patients is the writing of a prescription. Because chronic illness increases with advancing age, older persons are more likely to have conditions that require drug treatment. In the course of a typical physician's office practice, ambulatory patients aged 75 years and older are prescribed almost 70% more medications than patients aged 25 to 44 years (Nelson and Knapp 1997).

With increasing pressure on hospitals to shorten acute-care stays, combined with the aging of the population in industrialized societies, the nursing home has become a medical care site of increasing importance for both short- and long-term care of elderly persons. Not surprisingly, nursing home residents are prescribed more medication than noninstitutionalized older persons. One study of 12 nursing homes in a large U.S. city reported that the 1006 residents evaluated were prescribed an average of 7.2 medications (Beers et al. 1992).

In comparison with the ambulatory population of elderly persons, older persons residing in nursing homes are substantially more likely to receive psychotropic medications. Although recent U.S. regulatory changes have had some effect on levels of use of these agents, numerous studies performed through the early 1990s indicated that about half of all nursing home residents were regularly receiving one or more psychoactive drugs. Antipsychotic drugs were, until recently, given to about one-fourth of all nursing home residents (Beers et al. 1988).

**Key Points: Geriatric patients are more numerous than ever.**

- **Patients ≥ 65 years old will be 13% of the population by 2000.**
- **Patients ≥ 85 years old are the fastest growing segment of the U.S. population.**
- **The most frequent medical intervention in care of the elderly is writing a prescription.**

## Patterns of Drug Use and Drug Prescribing

The quality of medication prescribing for older patients has become an area of increasing concern. In the long-term care setting, some studies have suggested that use of sedating agents, including antipsychotic drugs and benzodiazepines, is more common in larger nursing homes, in facilities with lower staff-to-patient ratios, and among the patients of physicians with larger nursing home practices (Ray et al. 1980; Svarstad and Mount 1991). In 1990, a consensus panel of experts in geriatric medicine, geriatric psychiatry, and pharmacology developed a list of medications considered to be inappropriate for use in older patients, either because they are ineffective or because they pose too high a risk of adverse effects regardless of their potential for efficacy (Beers et al. 1991). This list included benzodiazepines with a long elimination half-life, and oral hypoglycemics, antidepressants with strong anticholinergic properties, and ineffective dementia treatments, for example, diazepam, chlorpropamide, amitriptyline, and cyclandelate, respectively. It was estimated that in the late 1980s almost one-quarter of all elderly persons residing in the community in the United States were taking at least one drug from this list of medications deemed to be contraindicated by the panel of experts (Willcox et al. 1994).

Selecting the optimal medication and dose for the individual older patient is often difficult because so little research is available to guide choices. Decision-making often has to draw on information obtained from patients very different from those encountered in clinical practice, where patients often have several medical conditions and are taking more than one drug. Clinical trials of conditions commonly affecting older people often cannot be extrapolated to the general population in that age group. For example, despite the fact that 80% of deaths due to acute myocardial infarction (AMI) occur in people aged 65 and over, older patients have often been excluded from clinical trials of cardiovascular treatments. Gurwitz and colleagues examined 214 randomized trials of treatments for AMI and found that 60% excluded patients over 75 years of age (Gurwitz, Col et al. 1992). Whereas almost 50% of older people report some form of arthritis, randomized controlled trials of nonsteroidal anti-inflammatory drugs (NSAIDs) include few older people and hardly any over age 85 (Rochon et al. 1993). Carcinoma of the prostate apart, chemotherapy trials for the leading causes of cancer death in men (colorectal, leukemia, lung, pancreas) and women (breast, colorectal, lung, ovarian, pancreas) have consistently underrepresented older patients (Trimble et al. 1994).

Even when elderly people have participated in trials in meaningful numbers, and where the benefits of a therapy appear compelling, there remains considerable uncertainty in translating the findings into practice. For example, in the five major trials of warfarin for stroke prevention in atrial fibrillation, nearly 2500 patients were studied, and 20% were more than 75 years of age (Atrial Fibrillation Investigators 1994). Yet only a very small proportion of individuals screened for participation in these studies were enrolled. Among 18,376 individuals screened for participation in the Stroke Prevention in Atrial Fibrillation Study (Stroke Prevention in Atrial Fibrillation Investigators 1991) only 7% were included in the trial, and that proportion is typical of the other trials. Although the benefits and risks of warfarin for stroke prevention in atrial fibrillation have been reasonably well assessed in older patients, the results need careful interpretation if they are to be applied to the care of the geriatric population generally, and to the frail elderly group especially.

## Underuse of Potentially Beneficial Therapy

Advanced age per se should never be considered a contraindication to potentially beneficial drug therapy in the elderly. Two examples of potential age bias in drug therapy are thrombolysis in AMI and analgesic therapy to manage metastatic cancer pain. Although the possibility of disabling or fatal intracranial hemorrhage is always a concern in patients treated with thrombolytics, these risks must be balanced against the benefits. The risk of death after AMI increases sharply with advancing patient age, and the few trials that enrolled large numbers of elderly patients suggest a beneficial effect of thrombolysis on short-term mortality associated with AMI in older patients (Gurwitz et al. 1991). Although there is a larger proportionate reduction in mortality with thrombolytic treatment for younger patients, older patients are at higher absolute risk of dying from AMI. As a result, the absolute mortality reductions (net lives saved per 1000 patients treated) are similar for younger and older patients [Fibrinolytic Therapy Trialists' (FTT) Collaborative Group 1994]. The view now is that age itself should not be a factor when deciding whether to use thrombolytic therapy in the setting of AMI (Topol and Califf 1992). Yet the use of these agents in AMI declines considerably with advancing patient age (Gurwitz et al. 1996).

Despite guidelines for pain management in patients with metastatic cancer (Cleeland et al. 1994), treatment is often inadequate. In a study of 1308 outpatients with metastatic cancer being followed up by oncologists, 769 patients reported experiencing pain, which 62% characterized as substantial (Cleeland et al. 1994). Patients with poor pain control reported that pain interfered with function and their quality of life. Older age was a risk factor for inadequate pain management. Concerns have been raised that the elderly are at risk of undertreatment because of underestimation of their sensitivity to pain, a misconception that they tolerate pain well, and a reluctance to prescribe adequate doses of opioid analgesics to older cancer patients (Jacox et al. 1994).

**PRINCIPLE Physician concern about the risk of adverse drug reactions (ADRs) is appropriate, but this concern should not lead to underuse of key medications in elderly patients that can improve survival and/or quality of life.**

## Adverse Drug Events in the Elderly

The relation between advancing age and the risk of adverse drug reactions (ADRs) presents a problem of great practical as well as theoretic importance. Older patients certainly experience more adverse drug reactions than do younger patients, a fact that has led to the conclusion that aging is an independent risk factor for the development of ADRs, much as it is for the development of Alzheimer disease or for death itself. Such a formulation is consistent with well-documented changes in drug clearance and sensitivity that occur with the process of "normal aging."

However, the higher frequency of adverse drug reactions in the elderly, rather than being a consequence of senescence alone, may be attributable in part to the fact that older patients consume more medications and are likely to have more baseline illness than younger patients. To explore this important issue, it would be necessary to study old and young subjects who were comparable in all respects except age. Unfortunately, most data on this issue are derived from observational studies or clinical trials that were not designed to address this specific question. In addition to being older, the elderly subjects included in such studies are more likely to have active coexisting disease and to be taking several potentially confounding medications. Further, important differences in drug dosage are often not fully accounted for in these studies (Gurwitz and Avorn 1991). A model of the complex of factors that may predispose elderly patients to ADRs is seen in Fig. 21-1.

Conventional clinical wisdom suggests that the risk of adverse drug reactions increases with advancing age, but available data do not confirm this "truism" of geriatric medicine. The interindividual variability of the aging process, including the nonuniform nature of the pharmacokinetic and pharmacodynamic changes that occur with aging, indicates that clinical reality is far more complex. Patient-specific physiologic and functional characteristics are probably more important than any chronologic measure in predicting both adverse and beneficial outcomes associated with specific drug therapies.

Preventable adverse drug events are perhaps the most serious consequence of suboptimal drug prescribing to older persons. As many as 28% of hospital admissions for older persons may be the result of a drug-related problem; in one study, up to 70% were attributed to adverse reactions to drugs (Col et al. 1990). Among the most disturbing associations between drug exposure and the occurrence of injury in elderly persons is the relationship between psychotropic drug use and hip fracture (Ray et al. 1987; Ray et al. 1989). This risk is particularly pronounced for the various antipsychotic medications with extrapyramidal and anticholinergic effects, as well as benzodiazepines with long elimination half-life. Recently, the use of benzodiazepines with long elimination half-life (as compared with short half-life agents) has been associated

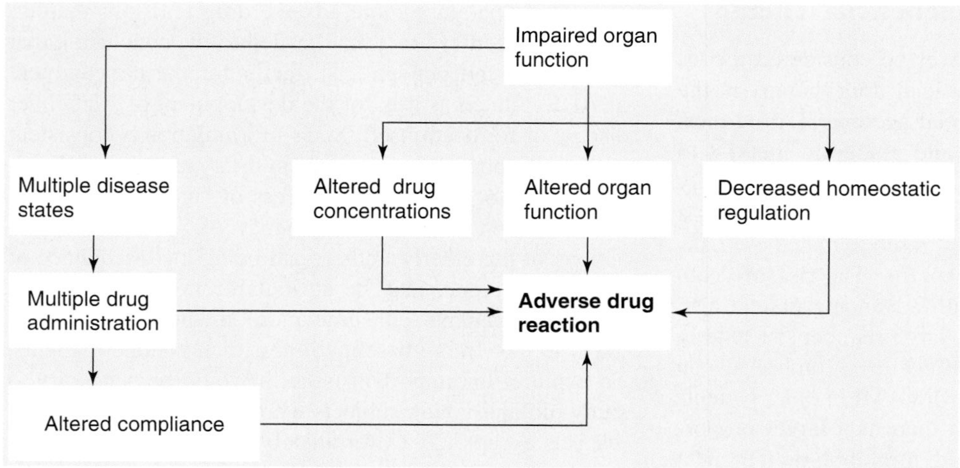


**FIGURE 21-1 Factors contributing to adverse drug reactions in elderly patients. From Nielson et al. 1987. Reproduced with permission.**

with an increased risk of motor vehicle accidents in elderly persons (Hemmelgarn et al. 1997).

Few studies evaluate patterns of drug dosing to elderly patients as a potential risk factor for adverse drug events. In one study, doses of cimetidine, flurazepam, and digoxin were analyzed on a milligram per kilogram basis. Patients weighing 50 kg or less received doses that were 31 to 46% higher than the group mean, and 70 to 88% higher than for patients weighing more than 90 kg (Campion et al. 1987). Despite a decline in body weight with age, doses in older patients were not proportionately decreased. The risk of excessive dosage is further exacerbated by impaired elimination of many drugs in the elderly. Since low body weight and advanced age are both risk factors for adverse drug reactions, available data suggest that current prescribing practices do not reflect the need to reduce doses in low-weight elderly patients.

**PRINCIPLE Commonly used drug doses may be excessive in some elderly patients and must be reduced to achieve the desired therapeutic effect without adverse effects.**

In addition to the morbidity and mortality associated with the occurrence of adverse drug events in the elderly, the costs to the health care system are substantial. The costs of preventable adverse drug events were recently estimated to be $2.8 million annually in two large U.S. teaching hospitals (Bates et al. 1997). The national cost of managing the consequences of adverse drug events remains uncertain. However, one estimate has put the annual cost of drug-related morbidity and mortality in the ambulatory setting at $76.6 billion (Johnson and Bootman 1995). Drug-related morbidity and mortality is an important target area for improving the quality of medical care for elderly persons as well as for reducing the costs of health care for this vulnerable population.

## The Prescribing Cascade

A *prescribing cascade* can occur when an adverse drug reaction is misinterpreted as a new medical condition. A new drug is prescribed, and the patient is placed at risk of developing additional adverse effects relating to this potentially unnecessary treatment (Rochon and Gurwitz 1997) (Fig. 21-2). Two examples of the prescribing cas-

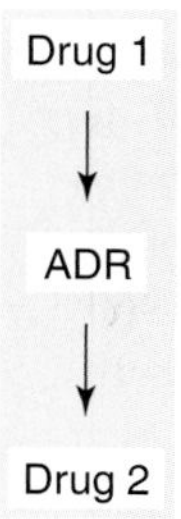


**FIGURE 21-2 The prescribing cascade results from the use of a new drug (drug 2) to treat an adverse reaction caused by a previously prescribed drug (drug 1).**

cade in elderly patients involve the impact of high-dose NSAID therapy on blood pressure control and the development of parkinsonian symptoms in persons treated with high-dose metoclopramide hydrochloride.

### *Nonsteroidal anti-inflammatory drugs and antihypertensive treatment*

Nonsteroidal anti-inflammatory drugs are among the most frequently prescribed drugs to elderly patients. An estimated 10 to 15% of people aged 65 years and older are prescribed such drugs (Ray et al. 1993). Their anti-inflammatory properties seem to result from their ability to inhibit cyclooxygenase, a critical enzyme in the biosynthesis of prostaglandins (Meconi et al. 1987). Good evidence exists to suggest that prostaglandins have an important role in the modulation of two major determinants of blood pressure: vasoconstriction of arteriolar smooth muscle and control of extracellular fluid volume.

The high prevalence of use of NSAIDs and the prevalence of hypertension among older people emphasizes the importance of studying the clinical impact of these drugs on blood pressure in this population. To determine whether there is an increased risk of starting antihypertensive treatment in older persons prescribed NSAIDs, a case-control study was performed involving patients enrolled in the New Jersey Medicaid program who were aged 65 years and older (Gurwitz et al. 1994). Over 9000 patients who were newly started on an antihypertensive drug were compared with a similar number of randomly selected control patients. The adjusted odds ratio for starting antihypertensive treatment for recent users of NSAIDs compared with nonusers was 1.66 (95% confidence interval, 1.54 to 1.80). The odds ratio increased with increasing daily dose of the anti-inflammatory drug: Compared with nonusers, the adjusted odds ratio for users of low average daily doses was 1.55 (1.38 to 1.74), for medium dose users was 1.64 (1.44 to 1.87), and for high dose users was 1.82 (1.62 to 2.05).

The authors concluded that the use of NSAIDs may increase the need for antihypertensive treatment in older people. Given the high prevalence of use of NSAIDs by elderly people, this association could have important public health implications for the care of older patients. This relation also shows a clear sequence of events where the use of one treatment leads to the start of a second that might have been avoided. On the basis of the findings of numerous epidemiological and clinical studies that have characterized the adverse consequences of use of NSAIDs in older people, recommendations have been made to avoid using these agents when clinically feasible (Rochon and Gurwitz 1997).

**PRINCIPLE Drugs developed for an indication likely to be prevalent in the elderly must be assessed after marketing, if not before, for their effects on other diseases common to the same population. (NB Viagra!)**

As with other drugs prescribed to elderly patients, the most prudent approach is to limit prescribing NSAIDs to situations in which benefits clearly outweigh risks and to use NSAIDs only after potentially safer alternatives have been tried (Solomon and Gurwitz 1997). Because of the multiple adverse effects attributable to these drugs, for some indications (such as osteoarthritis) treatments such as acetaminophen, gentle exercise, and weight reduction may be effective alternatives (Bradely et al. 1991; Felson et al. 1992; Kovar et al. 1992). When treatment with NSAIDs is necessary, the lowest feasible dose should be used for the shortest time required to achieve the desired effect.

Furthermore, if patients require extended treatment with NSAIDs, periodic monitoring of blood pressure is warranted, as such treatment may contribute to newly detected rises in pressure. With recognition of this association between NSAIDs and rises in blood pressure, the initiation or intensification of antihypertensive treatment may be avoided.

**PRINCIPLE Unanticipated events caused by a drug that exacerbates disease unrelated to the indication for therapy often will be attributed to new disease instead of to the drug.**

### *Use of metoclopramide and levodopa treatment*

Metoclopramide hydrochloride is widely used in the treatment of gastroesophageal reflux, in the management of disorders of gastric emptying including diabetic gastroparesis, and as an antiemetic after chemotherapy. Its antidopaminergic adverse effects, including unwanted extrapyramidal signs and symptoms, have long been recognized. Such drug-induced symptoms in older people can be misinterpreted as indicating a new disease or may be incorrectly attributed to the aging process itself. The misinterpretation is particularly likely when the symptoms are indistinguishable from an illness that is seen more often in older people, such as Parkinson disease.

A case-control study, again involving patients enrolled in the New Jersey Medicaid program aged 65 years and older, showed that patients taking metoclopramide were three times as likely to begin using a drug containing levodopa as patients not taking metoclopramide (odds ratio 3.09 [95% confidence interval, 2.25 to 4.26]) (Avorn et al. 1995). The risk increased with increasing daily metoclopramide dose: the odds ratio was 1.19 (0.50 to 2.81) for < 10 mg/day, 3.33 (1.98 to 5.58) for 10 to 20 mg/day, and 5.25 (1.16 to 8.50) for >20 mg/day. In summary, metoclopramide confers an increased risk of starting treatment generally reserved for managing idiopathic Parkinson disease. Such multiple prescribing may represent the misdiagnosis of Parkinson disease in patients with drug-induced parkinsonian symptoms.

**PRINCIPLE When specific endpoints of drug therapy are not sought, it is difficult if not impossible to optimize dosage, to minimize irrational combinations, or to reduce the incidence of adverse reactions.**

## Compliance in the Elderly

The failure of a patient to adhere to a thoughtfully prescribed therapeutic regimen is discouraging to every physician. The effects of noncompliance may be obvious, but often they are not fully appreciated. The worsening of a chronic condition that results from failure to take a prescribed medication may lead to the prescription of a larger dose, or a new drug. This in turn can lead to serious toxicity should the patient begin taking the medication as prescribed. When noncompliance leads to unnecessary morbidity and mortality, the physician is left to consider what factors contributed to these adverse consequences and what strategies might have prevented their occurrence.

**PRINCIPLE Many factors that are important determinants of compliance must be recognized and accounted for to accomplish therapeutic efficacy with the least toxicity.**

The problem of noncompliance with prescribed medical therapies is certainly not restricted to elderly patients and is probably not increased in the elderly if the number of prescribed drugs is taken into account. Across various patient age groups, compliance with long-term medication regimens has been found to be approximately 50% (Sackett and Snow 1970). However, for a number of reasons, including greater use of both prescription and nonprescription medications, impaired homeostasis related to age-related decrements in many physiologic parameters, an increased prevalence of multiple coexisting chronic disease states, and the financial burden of substantial out-of-pocket costs in the face of fixed incomes, the compliance issue demands special attention in the geriatric population.

There are many types of noncompliant behavior associated with prescribed pharmacotherapy (Simonson 1984). The most common type of noncompliance is simply the failure of the patient to take a medication. Other categories of noncompliance include the premature discontinuation of a medication, its use at the wrong time, excessive consumption ("If one pill is good, then two must be better"), and the use of medications not currently prescribed. This last category includes the inappropriate use of over-the-counter medications and the use of medications shared by family members and friends (Hammarlund et al. 1985; Ostrom et al. 1985).

**PRINCIPLE Do not assume that your patients are taking the drugs that you prescribe or that you are the only person who is prescribing their drugs.**

Although problems with visual impairment, functional disability, and cognitive dysfunction frequently have been assumed to be the prime contributors to noncompliance in elderly patients, the results of a number of studies have confirmed that the major factor predicting compliance with a medication regimen is the total number of concurrently prescribed medications: the more prescriptions, the lower the compliance (Darnell et al. 1986; Gurwitz et al. 1993). Other factors contributing to noncompliance in the elderly include poor labeling instructions, difficulty in opening childproof containers, and misunderstanding of verbal instructions (Sackett and Snow 1970). In addition, confusion may lead to noncompliance when multiple drugs of similar appearance are prescribed for the same patient (Mazzullo 1972).

A variety of strategies have been proposed for improving patient compliance with prescribed medication regimens (Sackett and Snow 1970; Avorn et al. 1995). Since the prescription of multiple concurrent medications reduces compliance, a primary strategy in improving compliance is to limit prescribing to the smallest possible number of medications and to make dosing instructions as simple as possible. Tailoring the regimen to the patient's schedule, such as mealtimes or other regularly scheduled activities, can be helpful. Compliance aids, such as commercially prepared or homemade pill boxes and medication calendars, may also be helpful. Family members and friends can be enlisted as support networks to supervise and to encourage compliance, and this can be crucial to maintaining compliance with both long- and short-term therapies. A regular reminder telephone call by a family member or other caregiver may be all that is required to complete an important course of therapy.

**CASE HISTORY** *A 79-year old woman presented to her local physician with complaints of abdominal pain, fatigue, and dark stools. Her medications included an NSAID for treatment of pain due to osteoarthritis. The evaluation of this patient led to an esophagogastroduodenoscopy that revealed a duodenal ulcer. She was placed on an $H_2$ receptor antagonist, and she was instructed to return after 6 weeks for a repeat endoscopy. Four weeks later, the patient was brought to the emergency room for hematemesis and hypotension that required immediate resuscitative measures. When she was asked about her medications, she said that she had discontinued her ulcer medication after 10 days of therapy since her abdominal pain had resolved.*

Studies of compliance with drug therapy in the elderly have shown divergent results, depending on the type of therapy and the amount of drugs taken. Factors that contribute to poor compliance may be more common in the elderly, such as cognitive impairment, hearing and visual deficits, social isolation, and inadequate finances. The predominant form of noncompliance is underadherence, or taking too little medication, as is the case in this patient. Underadherence may be intentional (and possibly appropriate) for a variety of reasons, including the patient's attempt to reduce adverse effects without "bothering" the physician. Clear communication and low resistance to its initiation by the patient with the health professional are probably the most important factors to address. Simplifying drug regimens and utilizing aids for drug administration are also important.

## PHARMACOKINETICS IN THE ELDERLY

The major pharmacokinetic characteristics of any drug—absorption, distribution, metabolism, and elimination—are potentially modified by aging, as there are important physiologic changes that occur with "normal" aging. The general principles of pharmacokinetics are presented in the introduction (part 1 of this volume) and a more detailed description is in Clinical Pharmacokinetics and Pharmacodynamics (chapter 23). Many of these changes are independent of the multiple diseases so often present in geriatric patients. By influencing drug disposition, these age-related changes might be expected to alter the response to drugs, which may explain why older patients seem to be more susceptible to both the therapeutic and the toxic effects of many drugs. Except for drugs eliminated predominantly by renal excretion, it is not possible to generalize about the type, magnitude, or importance of age-related differences in pharmacokinetics. Conflicting data in the literature for various drugs may be attributed to small numbers of subjects studied, to differences in selection criteria for subjects, and to variations in the design of protocols. Apparent age-related differences in drug disposition are multifactorial and influenced by environmental, genetic, physiologic, and pathologic factors, many of which are summarized in Table 21-1.

### Drug Absorption in the Elderly

Elderly persons exhibit several alterations in GI function that might result in impaired or delayed absorption of a drug (Table 21-1). Basal and peak gastric acid production declines with age, and the resultant increased gastric pH may alter the lipid solubility or dissolution of some drugs and may reduce absorption. However, the net effect of alterations in gastric pH is unpredictable; for example, a higher gastric pH may hasten gastric emptying, leading to a drug's reaching absorptive sites in the small intestine more rapidly. However, absorption of tetracycline by elderly patients with achlorhydria (which decreases the dissolution of the drug) was similar to that of young healthy controls (Kramer et al. 1978). Gastric emptying and motility determine the rate of delivery of a drug to the small intestine, where absorption of most drugs occurs by passive diffusion. An age-related decrease in the rate of gastric emptying has been reported (Moore et al. 1983), but the rate of acetaminophen absorption, which correlates with the rate of gastric emptying, does not differ with age (Divoll, Ameer et al. 1982).

Drugs that decrease GI motility, such as narcotic analgesics and some antidepressants with anticholinergic properties, might be expected to impair drug absorption to a greater extent in the elderly than in the young. This has not been investigated but should be "looked for." On the basis of microscopic examination of biopsy material from the upper jejunum of well-nourished elderly and young control patients without malabsorption, mucosal surface area was found to be decreased by 20% in the older age group (Warren et al. 1978). The clinical significance of this observation is unknown but doubtful in view of the fact that very few drugs demonstrate delayed or reduced absorption after oral administration in elderly patients (Cusack et al. 1997).

In contrast, the active transport of calcium, iron, thiamine, and vitamin $B_{12}$ declines with age (Bhanthumnavin and Schuster 1977). Although levodopa is absorbed by active transport via an amino acid transport mecha-

**Table 21-1 Factors Affecting Drug Disposition in the Geriatric Patient**

| Pharmacokinetic parameter | Age-related physiological change | Pharmacokinetic effect | Examples of affected drugs | Pathologic condition | Therapeutic and environmental factors |
|---|---|---|---|---|---|
| Absorption | ↑Gastric pH<br>↓Absorptive surface<br>↓Splanchnic blood flow<br>↓GI motility | NC | | Achlorhydria<br>Diarrhea<br>Postgastrectomy<br>Malabsorption syndromes<br>Pancreatitis | Antacids<br>Anticholinergics<br>Cholestyramine<br>Other drug--drug interactions<br>Food or meals |
| First-pass metabolism | ↓Hepatic blood flow | ↑Bioavailability for high-extraction drugs | Labetalol HCl<br>Metoprolol tartrate<br>Nifedipine<br>Propranolol HCl<br>Verapamil HCl | Congestive heart failure<br>Hepatic failure | Drug–drug interactions |
| Distribution | | | | | |
| Volume | ↓Lean body mass<br>↓Total body water<br>↑Total body fat | ↑Plasma $t_{1/2}$ of some fat-soluble drugs<br>↑Plasma levels of some water-soluble drugs | Diazepam<br>Midazolam HCl<br>Alcohol<br>Antipyrine | Congestive heart failure<br>Dehydration<br>Edema or ascites<br>Hepatic failure<br>Malnutrition<br>Renal failure | Drug–drug interactions<br>Protein-binding displacement |
| Protein-binding | ↓ (or NC) Serum albumin concentration | ↑(or NC) Unbound drug concentration | Phenytoin<br>Warfarin sodium | | |
| | ↑(or NC) AAP concentration | ↓ (or NC) Unbound drug concentration | Imipramine HCl | | |

**Table 21-1 Factors Affecting Drug Disposition in the Geriatric Patient (Continued)**

| PHARMACOKINETIC PARAMETER | AGE-RELATED PHYSIOLOGICAL CHANGE | PHARMACOKINETIC EFFECT | EXAMPLES OF AFFECTED DRUGS | PATHOLOGIC CONDITION | THERAPEUTIC AND ENVIRONMENTAL FACTORS |
|---|---|---|---|---|---|
| Metabolism | ↓Hepatic mass<br>↓Hepatic blood flow | ↓(or NC) Plasma CL<br>↑(or NC) Plasma $t_{1/2}$ | Fosinopril sodium<br>Imipramine HCl<br>Levodopa<br>Lidocaine<br>Morphine sulfate<br>Propranolol HCl<br>Nortriptyline HCl<br>Theophylline | Congestive heart failure<br>Fever<br>Frailty<br>Hepatic insufficiency<br>Malignancy<br>Malnutrition<br>Thyroid disease<br>Viral infection | Dietary composition<br>Drug–drug interactions<br>Insecticides<br>Tobacco (smoke) |
| Excretion | ↓Renal blood flow<br>↓GFR<br>↓Tubular secretion | ↓Plasma CL<br>↑$t_{1/2}$ | ACE inhibitors<br>Amantidine HCl<br>Chlorpropamide<br>Cimetidine<br>Furosemide<br>Gentamicin sulfate<br>Metformin HCl<br>Procainamide HCl<br>Ranitidine | Hypovolemia<br>Renal insufficiency | Drug–drug interactions |

↑ = increase; ↓ = decrease.
ABBREVIATIONS: AAP, $\alpha_1$-acid glycoprotein; ACE, angiotensin-converting enzyme; CL, clearance; GFR, glomerular filtration rate; NC, no change; $t_{1/2}$, elimination half-life.
SOURCE: Adapted from Vestal and Dawson 1985 and Vestal et al. 1997, with permission.

nism, there is evidence for increased rather than decreased absorption of levodopa in the elderly (Evans et al. 1980; Evans et al. 1981).

**PRINCIPLE Although the physiologic rationale for an altered drug response may have been demonstrated, therapeutic actions should be guided by careful clinical trials or actual clinical experience (measurements of effect), since the results of these investigations may be difficult to apply to or predict in an individual.**

The transdermal route of drug delivery has several advantages over conventional oral therapy that make it attractive for use in geriatric patients. Relatively little is known about percutaneous drug absorption as a function of age, but the available evidence indicates that the barrier function of skin is altered and that percutaneous absorption is reduced in the elderly (Roskos and Maibach 1992). The bioavailability of drugs depends on both absorption and presystemic (first-pass) metabolism by the wall of the GI tract and the liver (see the introduction and chapter 23 on pharmacokinetics). The bioavailability of drugs such as lidocaine, propranolol, and labetalol that have high intrinsic clearance by the liver is greater in elderly patients, reflecting less presystemic metabolism in this age group. However, the opposite findings have been reported for prazosin (Rubin et al. 1981). Therefore, one cannot generalize regarding the effect of age on bioavailability of high-clearance drugs (Cusack et al. 1997).

Presystemic metabolism of low-clearance drugs, such as theophylline, is negligible. Any alteration in bioavailability would have to be caused by an age-related difference in absorption. Since age does not seem to alter absorption to a clinically important extent, it is no surprise to find that the bioavailability of theophylline, and probably most other low-clearance drugs, does not change with age (Vestal et al. 1987).

**PRINCIPLE Agents that have high intrinsic clearance by the liver may exhibit increased bioavailability in the elderly. Unfortunately, the specific age-related effect on bioavailability must be determined by clinical trial for each drug and, for that matter, for each patient. These observations point out the need to assess quantitatively some element of drug effect independent of the intended efficacy as a measure of drug presence.**

## Drug Distribution in the Elderly

Body composition is one of the most important factors that may produce altered distribution of drugs in elderly patients (Table 21-1). Total body water, both in absolute terms and as a percentage of body weight (Shock et al. 1963; Vestal et al. 1975), is decreased by 10 to 15% between ages 20 and 80. However, body composition may be population-dependent (Norris et al. 1963; Shock et al. 1963). Lean body mass in proportion to total body weight also is diminished with age because of a relative increase in body fat (Novak 1972). Comparing the age groups 18 to 25 and 65 to 85 years, body fat increases from 18 to 36% of body weight in men and from 33 to 45% in women. In very elderly persons, however, the proportion of fat tends to be decreased (Norris et al. 1963). The age differences in total body water and body fat mean that lean body mass as a proportion of total body weight is decreased in the elderly. To what extent these changes are due to aging, rather than physical inactivity in the elderly, is uncertain.

Hydrophilic drugs that are distributed mainly in body water or lean body mass should have higher concentrations in blood in the elderly when the dose is based on total body weight or surface area. In line with this prediction, the volume of distribution of water-soluble drugs is smaller in the elderly, with increased initial concentrations in plasma. This has been directly demonstrated for ethanol (Vestal et al. 1977); consequently, equivalent concentrations of ethanol in the blood of elderly persons will be achieved by a dose that is 10 to 15% less than that in younger persons. Other examples include digoxin, antipyrine, and cimetidine. Notable exceptions include pancuronium and tobramycin, which have unchanged volumes of distribution in elderly patients.

Conversely, highly lipophilic drugs tend to have larger volumes of distribution in older persons because of increased proportions of body fat. This may account in part for the age-related increase in the volume of distribution of thiopental found in some but not all studies, and for similar observations with some of the benzodiazepines (Klotz et al. 1975; Greenblatt et al. 1982; Jung et al. 1982; Homer and Stanski 1985).

**PRINCIPLE Because lean body mass decreases and body fat increases in the elderly, in general the volumes of distribution for water-soluble drugs decrease and those for lipid-soluble drugs increase. These changes in volumes of distribution can lead to higher or lower plasma concentrations following administration of standard doses of drugs in these groups.**

Since free-drug concentration in plasma is an important determinant of distribution and elimination of the drug, alterations in the binding of drugs to plasma proteins, red blood cells, and other tissues might be considered important causes of altered pharmacokinetics in aged patients. Many basic drugs have a higher affinity for $\alpha_1$-acid glycoprotein than acidic drugs, but acidic drugs generally have a higher affinity for albumin. Although quite variable, the concentrations of $\alpha_1$-acid glycoprotein tend to increase with age (Abernethy and Kerzner 1984). The binding of some basic drugs, such as lidocaine and disopyramide, is increased in the elderly, but this change probably does not have as much clinical importance as the increase that typically occurs in patients with AMI (Routledge et al. 1980). Serum albumin concentrations may be decreased by as much as 10% to 20% in old age, but chronic disease and immobility are probably more important determinants of albumin synthesis (Woodford-Williams et al. 1964; Greenblatt 1979). The authors of a report showing only a 0.054 g/dL per decade decline in serum albumin concentration concluded that the age-related decline in healthy individuals is far less than previously described and that hypoalbuminemia is not a simple consequence of normal aging (Campion et al. 1988).

Nevertheless, some studies have shown changes in the protein binding of acidic drugs that are potentially quite important for elderly subjects. The mean concentration of unbound (free) naproxen in plasma in the elderly is twice that in the young (Upton et al. 1984). The relation between the free-drug concentration and drug efficacy or toxicity has not been established in this case, but the possibility that the dose of naproxen in advanced age should be substantially decreased is raised by these findings.

An age-related increase in the unbound fraction by more than 50% occurs for only a few drugs, such as acetazolamide, valproic acid, diflunisal, salicylate, and naproxen (Wallace and Verbeek 1987). The net effect of changes in protein binding is complicated, but an altered pattern of elimination of drugs with low intrinsic clearance and high (>90%) protein binding (Table 21-2) can result. For example, higher-than-ordinary total plasma clearance of phenytoin in elderly subjects is invoked as an explanation of the low binding in plasma after a single dose (Hayes et al. 1975). With chronic dosing, however,

**Table 21-2 Pharmacokinetic Classification of Drugs Eliminated Primarily by Hepatic Metabolism**

| CLASS | DRUG | EXTRACTION RATIO | PERCENT BOUND |
|---|---|---|---|
| Flow-limited | Lidocaine | 0.83 | 45–80[a] |
| | Meperidine HCl | 0.6–0.95 | 60 |
| | Morphine sulfate | 0.50–0.75 | 35 |
| | Nortriptyline HCl | 0.50 | 95 |
| | Pentazocine lactate | 0.80 | |
| | Propoxyphene HCl | 0.95 | |
| | Propranolol HCl | 0.60–0.80 | 93 |
| Capacity-limited, binding-sensitive | Chlorpromazine HCl | 0.22 | 91–99[a] |
| | Clindamycin HCl | 0.23 | 94 |
| | Diazepam | 0.03 | 98 |
| | Digitoxin | 0.005 | 97 |
| | Phenytoin | 0.03 | 90 |
| | Quinidine gluconate | 0.27 | 82 |
| | Tolbutamide | 0.02 | 98 |
| | Warfarin sodium | 0.003 | 99 |
| Capacity-limited, binding-insensitive | Acetaminophen | 0.43 | <5 |
| | Amylobarbital | 0.03 | 61 |
| | Antipyrine | 0.07 | 10 |
| | Chloramphenicol | 0.28 | 60–80[a] |
| | Hexobarbital | 0.16 | |
| | Theophylline | 0.09 | 59 |
| | Thiopental sodium | 0.28 | 72 |

[a]Concentration-dependent.
SOURCE: Adapted from Blaschke 1977. Reproduced with permission.

unbound concentrations of drugs tend to "renormalize" as a result of the enhanced availability of unbound drug for elimination by the liver and kidney. For drugs with a low therapeutic ratio, such as phenytoin, measurement of the plasma free-drug concentration may be helpful in guiding therapy in complicated cases.

**PRINCIPLE Individualization of drug therapy is often best accomplished by a combination of close attention to clinical response (measurement of clinically detectable events) and determination of plasma drug concentrations, including free concentrations of drug in plasma when necessary.**

## Drug Metabolism in the Elderly

### *Biochemical studies*

As it is difficult to study hepatic drug metabolism in humans, experimental models include nonhuman primates, rodents, and human liver homogenates. In rodents that have reached maturity, hepatic drug metabolism declines with increasing age. The reported age-related changes in conjugation reactions have been variable without a consistent pattern (Vestal and Cusack 1990; Woodhouse and Wynne 1992). Unfortunately, data obtained from inbred rodents cannot be extrapolated to either nonhuman primates or humans. For example, total cytochrome P450 content, NADPH-cytochrome *c* reductase activity, and metabolism of benzo[*a*]pyrene in microsomes isolated from livers of female pig-tailed macaques ranging in age from 2 to 21 years did not differ with age (Sutter et al. 1985). Neither age- nor sex-related changes in the concentration of microsomal protein or in the amount of cytochrome P450 were found in the rhesus monkey, and the specific activity of NADPH-cytochrome *c* reductase increased rather than decreased with age (Maloney et al. 1986). Data on the effects of aging on conjugation reactions in nonhuman primates are not available.

**PRINCIPLE Interspecies differences in hepatic drug metabolism often preclude extrapolation from animal models to humans. Confirmation of the suspicion of drug-induced effects can come only from clinical trials and sometimes from homogenates of human liver.**

Data on the effect of age on in vitro drug metabolism in human tissues are sparse. One study of liver biopsy samples from 40 men and 30 women ranging in age from 16 to 76 years with suspected liver disease failed to identify correlations between age or sex and cytochrome P450 content, or the activities of cytochrome *c* reductase and aryl hydrocarbon hydroxylase (Brodie et al. 1981). However, only 30 of the biopsies were normal, and the study was not primarily designed to investigate the effects of age on microsomal drug metabolism. Likewise, there were no significant relationships between age or smoking and microsomal protein content, aldrin epoxidation, 7-ethoxycoumarin-*O*-deethylation, epoxide hydrolase activity, or reduced glutathione activity in normal biopsies from men and women ranging in age from 18 to 83 years (Woodhouse et al. 1984). In that study potential age differences may have been obscured by small sample sizes. Neither study provides information on the amount or activity of isozymes of cytochrome P450. Thus, the results with human liver microsomes generally are consistent with those obtained with microsomes from nonhuman primates; on the basis of presently available biochemical data, intrinsic hepatic drug-metabolizing enzyme activity has not been found to differ significantly with increasing age in humans.

Two reports provide the most extensive and comprehensive data to date (Schmucker et al. 1990; Sotaniemi et al. 1997). However, the results are conflicting. Liver samples from 54 donors who ranged in age from 9 to 89 years did not show any effect of age or gender on the concentration of microsomal protein, the specific activity of NADPH-cytochrome *c* reductase, the carbon monoxide-binding capacity of microsomal cytochrome P450, or the relative microsomal concentrations of three isozymes of cytochrome P450 (Schmucker et al. 1990). A larger study of 226 subjects with slight to moderate changes in liver histology reveals that cytochrome P450 content was 32% lower in subjects aged 70 years and older compared with subjects aged 20 to 29 years with a decrease of 0.07 nmol/g per year after age 40 years (Sotaniemi et al. 1997). However, the fact that these specimens were abnormal (fatty changes, fibrosis, granulomata, portal infiltrates) makes conclusions about the effects of age on P450 difficult to interpret. There were no specimens with completely normal histology in subjects over age 70 years.

**PRINCIPLE Conclusions about the independent effects of age on drug metabolism must be based on data that are obtained from individuals without clinical evidence of disease or use of other drugs.**

### *Clinical studies*

Age-related decreases in liver size and liver blood flow may account for the age-related differences in clearance of some drugs (Woodhouse and Wynne 1988). Hepatic clearance of drugs depends on the activity of the enzymes responsible for biotransformation and on hepatic blood flow, which determines the rate of delivery of the drug to the liver. In the case of drugs with low intrinsic clearance (drugs that are metabolized relatively slowly by the liver), clearance is proportional to the rate of hepatic metabolism. Autopsy studies indicate that liver weight falls by about 18 to 25% between the ages of 20 and 80 years (Calloway et al. 1965). Ultrasound studies demonstrate decreases in liver volume ranging from 18 to 46% across the age span (Woodhouse and Wynne 1988). Since hepatic mass decreases with age in absolute terms, as well as in proportion to total body weight, the clearance of drugs with low intrinsic clearance (extraction ratios <0.3; see Table 21-2) would be expected to be decreased.

Antipyrine, a drug with low intrinsic clearance, has been used extensively as a model substrate for studies of oxidative drug metabolism in humans. Most studies using antipyrine have shown decreased plasma clearance and a longer half-life in older subjects (O'Malley et al. 1971; Vestal et al. 1975; Vestal and Wood 1980; Sotaniemi et al. 1997). The effect of age is less pronounced in women than in men. Biologic variation among subjects and the presence of other factors, such as smoking and frailty, overshadow the effect of age (Vestal and Wood 1980; Woodhouse and Wynne 1992). Data also suggest that the clearance of antipyrine correlates with the age-related decline in liver volume (Woodhouse and Wynne 1992). Additional factors that may influence the apparent rates at which the drug is eliminated include concurrent drug intake, diet, frailty, illness, cigarette smoking, and alcohol use. For example, a 28% decrease in the clearance of acetaminophen was found in fit elderly subjects compared with young subjects. This difference was eliminated when the data were normalized by an estimate of liver volume (Wynne et al. 1989). There was a 42% decrease in the frail elderly that diminished but continued to be significant even when adjusted for liver volume.

**PRINCIPLE Even if an age-related "change" in the metabolism of a drug has been demonstrated, its clinical importance may be completely dwarfed by individual variations in other important factors.**

For drugs that exhibit high intrinsic clearance (drugs with a very rapid rate of metabolism), the rate of extraction by the liver is high (extraction ratio >0.7; see Table 21-2), and hepatic blood flow is rate-limiting for their metabolism. Indocyanine green and propranolol are compounds that are avidly extracted by the liver. Estimates of liver blood flow from an analysis of the clearance of indocyanine green, as well as the simultaneous IV and oral kinetics of propranolol, are consistent with a 25 to 35% reduction in liver blood flow between ages 30 and 75 (Vestal and Wood 1980; Woodhouse and Wynne 1992).

As previously stated, old age is associated with a reduction in the presystemic metabolism of propranolol and labetalol, both of which have high extraction ratios. Accordingly, the bioavailability of these drugs is increased with age (Durnas et al. 1990). For the same reasons, although data are incomplete, other drugs with high rates of hepatic extraction (e.g., calcium-entry blockers, tricyclic antidepressants, and most major tranquilizers) should be administered cautiously in elderly patients as lower doses may be sufficient for expected therapeutic effects and may reduce any risk of toxicity.

In addition to a physiologic classification of drug metabolism based upon extraction ratios, biotransformation reactions are classified into either phase I reactions (oxidation, reduction, and hydrolysis) or phase II reactions (glucuronidation, acetylation, and sulfation) (see the introduction). Microsomal and nonmicrosomal enzymes are involved in both phases. The activities of phase I pathways are often reduced in the elderly, whereas phase II pathways generally are unaffected. Chlordiazepoxide, diazepam, clorazepate, and prazepam, all of which undergo oxidative metabolism (phase I reactions) to active metabolites, exhibit decreased clearance and prolonged half-life of elimination in elderly patients (Bellantuono et al. 1980). In contrast, oxazepam, lorazepam, and temazepam are eliminated by conjugation (phase II) reactions, and their clearance is not reduced in old age. This means that cumulative or prolonged sedative effects are less likely with the latter group of benzodiazepines.

**PRINCIPLE An understanding of how a drug is metabolized can assist the clinician in making therapeutic choices that will minimize the possibility of adverse effects.**

In addition to certain disease states (Table 21-1), the intrinsic genetic characteristics of the patient for whom a drug is prescribed may be the most important determinant of its rate of clearance (see chapter 22, Pharmacogenetics). For example, in some studies there is a positive association between age and the development of the slow-acetylator phenotype (Durnas et al. 1990; Korrapati et al. 1997). Slow-acetylator phenotype is associated with increased susceptibility to the development of bladder cancer during chronic exposure (often industrial) to arylamines and hydrazines (Cartwright et al. 1982). However, a study of 512 healthy subjects did not show an age difference in the nearly equal distribution of rapid and slow acetylator phenotypes (Korrapati et al. 1997).

The extensive debrisoquin hydroxylation phenotype has been reported to be more common in patients with bronchogenic carcinoma than in age- and sex-matched controls (Ayesh et al. 1984), but in two studies there was no age difference in the frequency of this phenotype (Steiner et al. 1988; Siegmund et al. 1990). The importance of this kind of information is that individuals with genetically determined enhancement or impairment of certain biotransformation pathways may be particularly susceptible to drug-induced toxicity or lack of therapeutic efficacy. Examples include encainide, procainamide, and phenytoin (Kalow 1992).

Although at present we do not routinely obtain pharmacogenetic phenotypes in our patients, this may become the standard of practice in the future. The importance of determining the phenotype should at least come to mind when an elderly patient shows unusual dose responses to these drugs. Once the phenotype is established in a family, further treatment of other family members can be tempered by knowledge of the phenotype.

Stereoselective drug metabolism also is becoming increasingly important in understanding drug action and toxicity. A recent study showed that the clearance of L-hexobarbital is doubled in young compared with elderly subjects, although no psychomotor differences were observed. This inconsistency probably is explained by the similar clearance of D-hexobarbital, the more active enantiomer, in young and elderly subjects (Durnas et al. 1990). Studies with enantiomers of ibuprofen and propranolol, however, do not show age differences in metabolism (Kinirons and Crome 1997).

## Renal Excretion of Drugs in the Elderly

The most consistent effect of age on pharmacokinetics is the age-related reduction in the rate of elimination of drugs by the kidney. Both glomerular and tubular functions are affected. The glomerular filtration rate (GFR) as measured by inulin or creatinine clearance, may fall as much as 50%, with an average decline of about 35% between ages 20 and 90 (Rowe et al. 1976).

However, interindividual variation is considerable, and some healthy individuals show only a very small decline, no decline, or even a slight increase in GFR during aging (Lindeman 1985). Renal plasma flow declines approximately 1.9% per year. In contrast to intrinsic hepatic drug metabolism, for which the effects of old age are less certain and probably less important than the effects of disease and interindividual variation, the possibility of diminished renal function in elderly patients is a frequent clinical issue in drug dosing. Creatinine clearance can be used along with concentrations of drug in plasma in adjusting doses and dosage schedules of drugs that are primarily excreted by the kidney.

In general, drugs that are significantly excreted by the kidney can be assumed to have diminished clearance of plasma from the elderly in proportion to the decrease in creatinine clearance. Drugs with predominantly renal elimination and potentially serious toxic effects in the elderly include aminoglycosides, amantidine, lithium, digoxin, procainamide, chlorpropamide, cimetidine, and some NSAIDs (Table 21-3). Also, drugs with potentially toxic metabolites that are excreted by the kidney, such as meperidine, are potentially hazardous in patients with markedly impaired renal function (see the introduction). If renal function is normal (>80 mL/min per 1.73 m$^2$), age-related differences in pharmacokinetics are unlikely, as shown for aminoglycosides. Since 24-hour urine collections are often not feasible, there are many formulas and nomograms available to help estimate creatinine clearance values ($CL_{CR}$). The equation of Cockcroft and Gault (1976) is one of the most widely used:

$$CL_{CR}(\text{mL/min}) = \frac{(140 - \text{age})}{C_{p,CR}\ (\text{mg/dL})} \times \frac{\text{weight (kg)}}{72}$$

The result should be multiplied by 0.85 for women. The concentration of creatinine in plasma is indicated by $C_{p,CR}$. This formula has been validated in ambulatory and hospitalized patients, but for reasons that are not known,

**Table 21-3 Drugs with Decreased Renal Elimination in Old Age**

| | |
|---|---|
| *N*-Acetylprocainamide | Hydrochlorothiazide |
| Amantadine | Lisinopril |
| Amikacin | Lithium carbonate |
| Ampicillin | Metformin HCl |
| Atenolol | Pancuronium |
| Captopril | Penicillin |
| Ceftriaxone | Quinapril |
| Cephradine | Procainamide HCl |
| Chlorpropamide | Phenobarbital |
| Cibenzoline | Ranitidine |
| Cimetidine | Sotalol |
| Digoxin | Sulfamethizole |
| Doxycycline | Tetracycline |
| Enalapril | Tobramycin |
| Furosemide | Triamterene |
| Gentamicin sulfate | |

SOURCE: Adapted from Cusack and Vestal 1986. Reproduced with permission.

it may not be accurate in nursing home patients (Drusano et al. 1988).

**PRINCIPLE Estimates of creatinine clearance are only an aid to help calculate initial dose requirements of drugs primarily eliminated by the kidneys. Drug concentrations should be monitored when drugs with a low therapeutic index are used (see chapter 23 on pharmacokinetics).**

CASE HISTORY *An 85-year-old man with a history of stable exertional angina was brought to the emergency room complaining of chest pain and shortness of breath. His pulse was irregularly irregular with an apical pulse rate of 126 over 1 minute. Blood pressure was 120/84 mm Hg, and an electrocardiogram revealed atrial fibrillation without evidence for acute ischemia. His weight was 55 kg. Measurement of the arterial blood gas revealed mild hypoxia, and blood chemistry tests were blood urea nitrogen (BUN), 24 mg/dL; creatinine, 1.1 mg/dL. The patient was given a loading dose of digoxin (total dose 1 mg over the next 24 hours), followed by a maintenance oral dose of 0.25 mg/day. His heart rate responded with a decrease to 90 beats per minute by the next day. By the third day of hospitalization, the patient was ambulating comfortably with a heart rate of 82 beats per minute after walking 100 feet briskly. Repeat electrocardiogram showed the patient to have spontaneously converted to normal sinus rhythm. The patient was discharged on the third day after admission.*

*Six days later, he was brought back to the hospital (the emergency room) by family members. There he complained of nausea and vomiting for 2 days. He was lethargic and disoriented, and on examination his abdomen was found to be diffusely tender without rebound tenderness. The serum digoxin concentration was 2.7 ng/mL.*

Alterations in the disposition of certain drugs in elderly patients require appropriate alterations in dosage, and health-care providers should be well aware of the commonly used drugs that tend to be handled differently in aged compared with younger patients. The administration of digoxin illustrates several principles of pharmacokinetics in geriatric patients. The distribution of digoxin is dependent on lean body mass, which decreases in relation to total body mass with age. Therefore, loading doses should be proportionately lower in elderly patients. Maintenance doses also require adjustment, since digoxin is predominantly excreted by the kidney, which undergoes age-related decline in glomerular filtration. In this patient, the Cockcroft-Gault equation predicts a creatinine clearance of 45 mL/min, clearly indicating the need for more than a 50% reduction in maintenance dose. The maintenance dose that he was actually given was therefore too high; drug accumulation occurred after the patient left the hospital, resulting after several days in digoxin toxicity. The judicious use of plasma drug levels can be helpful for some drugs, such as digoxin.

## Nutrition, Environmental Factors, and Drug Interactions

Nutritional status of the very elderly person is often marginal. Dietary composition can be an important environmental determinant of drug metabolism and drug toxicity (Campbell and Hayes 1974; Walter-Sack and Klotz 1996), and overt protein-calorie malnutrition is associated with impaired drug metabolism in undernourished children and adults (Krishnaswamy 1978). Elderly persons, including those in nursing homes, are at increased risk of malnutrition. The reduced rate of elimination of antipyrine in a group of elderly persons with vitamin C deficiency was increased after supplementation with vitamin C, but in another study changes in the amounts of dietary ascorbic acid did not affect caffeine metabolism (Smithard and Langman 1977, 1978; Trang et al. 1982). The possible effects of so-called megadose vitamin therapy on drug kinetics have not been studied, although high doses of several vitamins and minerals can cause toxicity in their own right.

Hepatic microsomal enzyme activity is induced by cigarette smoking (Vestal and Wood 1980; Durnas et al. 1990). Although most studies have shown that induction of antipyrine metabolism by smoking is impaired in older persons, the response is variable. The induction of propranolol's metabolism is restricted to young and middle-aged adults. In contrast, theophylline clearance is enhanced in both young adult and elderly smokers (Vestal et al. 1987; Crowley et al. 1988). Therefore, routinely decreasing the dosage of metabolized drugs simply on the basis of age may result in inadequate therapeutic efficacy in elderly smokers.

**PRINCIPLE Cigarette smoking is likely to accelerate the oxidation and increase the dose requirement of many drugs that are metabolized by the liver. Therapeutic monitoring will help guide dose adjustments in patients who smoke, regardless of age.**

The problem of precipitating unintended, adverse drug–drug interactions in the elderly is illustrated by the following brief cases.

**CASE HISTORY** *An 81-year-old man presented to his physician complaining of dysuria and urinary frequency. He had no fever or flank pain. His medications included nitrates and a calcium-entry blocker for coronary artery disease. He was also taking warfarin to treat a deep venous thrombosis that occurred during hospitalization after coronary bypass surgery. Physical examination was unremarkable, including a firm, nontender prostate. A urinalysis showed pyuria. The international normalized ratio of prothrombin time (INR) was 2.5 (target therapeutic range, 2.0 to 3.0). The patient was begun on a 10-day course of trimethoprim-sulfamethoxazole, and he was discharged home after several days. Five days later, the patient called his physician complaining of bleeding gums after brushing his teeth. His INR was remeasured and was found to be 7.0.*

**CASE HISTORY** *A 75-year-old man with chronic bronchitis came to the emergency clinic complaining of dyspnea and a productive cough. The patient's medications included an albuterol inhaler and theophylline. He was afebrile, and his chest exam revealed only upper airway rhonchi. An arterial blood-gas test was unchanged from previous measurements, and his chest x-ray film showed no infiltrates. The plasma theophylline concentration was 15 μg/mL. The patient was given a prescription for ciprofloxacin to take for 10 days. The patient returned to the clinic after 1 week complaining of nausea and vomiting. At this time, his plasma theophylline concentration was 29 μg/mL.*

**CASE HISTORY** *A 79-year-old woman with hypertension was seen during a routine office visit. Her hypertension had been well controlled with a thiazide diuretic, with blood pressures of about 140/70 mmHg. At this visit, her blood pressure was found to be 170/90. This degree of blood pressure elevation was recorded on two other occasions during the following week. She had recently been complaining of nasal congestion but had bought an over-the-counter cold preparation for relief of these symptoms. The physician asked the patient to bring all her medications to the office, and he found that the OTC medication contained phenylpropanolamine. This medication was discontinued with return of the patient's blood pressure to normotensive readings.*

Although there are few studies investigating the incidence of drug–drug interactions with respect to age, it is generally considered that elderly patients are more likely to encounter drug interactions. Therefore, the surveillance for possible drug interactions should be particularly vigilant in elderly patients taking multiple medications. For example, in case 1 the addition of any new medication to a regimen that includes an oral anticoagulant should be done with caution. Sulfonamides are known to enhance warfarin activity by decreasing its metabolism and displacing it from binding sites. In case 2, a new drug (ciprofloxacin) was added that impaired the metabolism of a drug that was already part of the patient's treatment regimen (theophylline). The mechanism for this pharmacokinetic interaction is inhibition of cytochrome P450 microsomal-mediated metabolism (Thomson et al. 1987; Loi et al. 1997). Finally, in case 3, a common sympathomimetic used for relief of nasal congestion interfered with blood pressure control in a hypertensive patient.

**PRINCIPLE Although multiple drugs may be justifiable because of multiple indications in geriatric patients, the prescriber must frequently reevaluate the need for multiple medications and be alert to the increased risk of drug interactions in patients taking multiple drugs.**

As previously discussed, elderly persons are commonly assumed to have an increased risk of sustaining unintended drug–drug interactions. Nevertheless, studies that have investigated this possibility are few (Table 21-4). Although the response to induction of hepatic oxidative drug metabolism as a function of age is variable, the response to enzyme inhibition by cimetidine and ciprofloxacin appears to be uniformly similar in young and elderly persons and suggests that the risk of drug toxicity is unchanged in this age group (Vestal et al. 1993; Loi et al. 1997). However, to the extent that elderly patients receive more drugs to begin with, equal enzyme inhibition by drugs such as cimetidine and ciprofloxacin is likely to have a greater overall impact in the geriatric patient population.

**PRINCIPLE It is now easier than ever before for the careful physician to screen all of his patients' drugs for possible drug–drug interactions. This is especially important to check (using a software program) when drugs are added to or deleted from a complex regimen.**

## DRUG THERAPY AND PHARMACODYNAMICS

Pharmacodynamics, the study of the pharmacologic and therapeutic effects of drugs, has been investigated less extensively in elderly persons than has pharmacokinetics.

Table 21-4 Effect of Age on Induction and Inhibition of Hepatic Drug Metabolism in Humans

| Interacting drug | Marker drug substrate | Effect in old vs. young subjects |
|---|---|---|
| *Inducer* | | |
| Dichloralphenazone | Antipyrine | Decreased |
| Dichloralphenazone | Quinine | Decreased |
| Glutethimide | Antipyrine | Same or increased |
| Phenytoin | Theophylline | Same |
| Rifampin | Antipyrine | Decreased |
| Rifampin | Propranolol HCl | Same or increased |
| *Inhibitor* | | |
| Cimetidine | Antipyrine | |
| Cimetidine | Desmethyldiazepam | Same |
| Cimetidine | Theophylline | Same |
| Ciprofloxacin | Theophylline | Same |

SOURCE: Adapted from Vestal and Cusack 1990. Reproduced with permission.

Since the effect of age on the sensitivity to drugs varies with the drug studied and the response measured, generalizations are again difficult. Valid studies of drug sensitivity require measurement of concentrations of drug in plasma, because differences in pharmacokinetics with increasing age may increase or decrease differences in response to the drug. Only a few areas of drug therapy have been evaluated in this manner (Table 21-5). Four broad classes of drugs will be discussed along with drug–disease interactions as illustrative examples.

Table 21-5 Selected Pharmacodynamic Changes with Aging

| Drug | Pharmacodynamic effect studied | Age-related change |
|---|---|---|
| Adenosine | Minute ventilation, heart rate response | ↔ |
| Antidepressants | Systolic time intervals | ↔ |
| Clonidine | $\alpha_1$-Adrenergic responsiveness | ↔ |
| Diazepam | Sedation, postural sway | ↑ |
| Diltiazem | Acute and chronic antihypertensive effect | ↑ |
| | Acute prolongation of the PR interval | ↓ |
| Diphenhydramine | Postural sway | ↔ |
| Enalapril | ACE inhibition | ↔ |
| Furosemide | Peak diuretic response | ↓ |
| Heparin | Anticoagulant effect | ↔ |
| Isoproterenol | Chronotropic effect, forearm blood flow, renin output response, dorsal hand vein vasodilatation | ↓ |
| Levodopa | Dose-related adverse effects | ?↑ |
| Morphine sulfate | Magnitude and duration of analgesia | ↑ |
| | Respiratory depression | ↔ |
| Phenylephrine | $\alpha_1$-Adrenergic responsiveness | ↔ |
| Propranolol HCl | Antagonism of chronotropic effects of isoproterenol | ↓ |
| Temazepam | Postural sway, psychomotor function | ?↑ |
| | Sedation | ↑ |
| Timolol | Antagonism of chronotropic effects of isoproterenol | ↔ |
| Verapamil HCl | Acute antihypertensive effect | ↑ |
| Warfarin sodium | Anticoagulant effect | ↑ |

NOTE: ↑ = increase; ↓ = decrease; ↔ = no significant change; ?↑ = may increase.
ABBREVIATIONS: ACE, angiotensin-converting enzyme.
SOURCE: Adapted from Parker and Cusack 1996. Reproduced with permission.

## Analgesics

Elderly patients frequently receive analgesics and anti-inflammatory agents with analgesic properties. Both morphine and meperidine are associated with decreased rates of plasma clearance in older persons (Holmberg et al. 1982; Owen et al. 1983). Total pain relief and the duration of relief achieved with morphine and pentazocine were greater in older than in younger patients (Bellville et al. 1971; Kaiko 1980), consistent with a lower dosage requirement. Some studies have shown impaired hepatic metabolism of acetaminophen in elderly persons (Divoll, Abernethy et al. 1982), but dosage adjustments are not necessary.

The use of NSAIDs requires close monitoring in elderly patients (Johnson and Day 1991). These drugs increase the risk of complications such as hyperkalemia or renal failure [particularly when these drugs are used in treating gout (Blackshear et al. 1983)] and death from GI hemorrhage (Griffin et al. 1988).

**PRINCIPLE Excessive use of analgesics, particularly NSAIDs, is a major cause of adverse drug reactions. Efficacy in relation to risk should be carefully evaluated in each individual, but even more so in elderly patients.**

## Anticoagulants

When warfarin is prescribed to elderly patients, the effects of age on dosage requirements (O'Malley et al. 1977; Reidenberg 1987, Gurwitz, Avorn et al. 1992) and the risk of bleeding (Landefeld and Beyth 1993; Beyth and Landefeld 1995) are controversial. One study has shown greater inhibition of synthesis of vitamin K-dependent clotting factors at similar plasma concentrations of warfarin in plasma of older as opposed to younger patients (Shepherd et al. 1977). Age and liver volume have been shown to be determinants of warfarin dosage requirement (Wynne et al. 1995). Increased caution should be exercised when prescribing warfarin to elderly patients, with careful titration of the dose based on the INR. The coadministration of drugs that may inhibit the metabolism of warfarin (e.g., cimetidine) or displace warfarin from binding sites on plasma proteins (chlorpropamide) must be managed carefully. Although age per se is not a contraindication to oral anticoagulant therapy (Gurwitz et al. 1998), concomitant clinical conditions such as gait abnormalities, recurrent falls, poor medical compliance, peptic ulcer disease, and alcoholism may predispose to complications and may be relative contraindications (Gurwitz et al. 1998).

Although one study found an increased risk of bleeding with heparin given to elderly women (Jick et al. 1968), the relationship between plasma heparin concentration and anticoagulant effect does not change with increasing age (Whitfield et al. 1982). Thus, heparin dose does not require an adjustment based on age, but should be titrated to therapeutic effect as in younger patients.

**PRINCIPLE Risk of adverse effects from anticoagulants may be increased in the elderly, justifying close monitoring of the effects of all necessary drugs in their regimen.**

## Cardiovascular Drugs

The high prevalence of cardiac and peripheral vascular disorders results in extensive use of cardiovascular drugs in the elderly. The clinical benefit of digoxin therapy for heart failure with sinus rhythm is controversial. Since the distribution of digoxin is related to lean body mass, loading doses should be proportionately lower in the elderly. Also, because the glomerular filtration rate is a major determinant of the clearance of digoxin, the maintenance dose should be adjusted based on renal function.

Diuretics are used to treat hypertension and congestive heart failure. The response to furosemide is decreased in the elderly (Andreasen et al. 1984; Chaudhry et al. 1984), but the clinical importance of this observation has not been established. With all diuretics, the elderly appear to be more vulnerable to fluid and electrolyte disorders, including volume depletion, hypokalemia, hyponatremia, and hypomagnesemia.

The reduced clearance and prolonged elimination half-life in the elderly of antiarrhythmic agents, such as quinidine, procainamide, and *N*-acetylprocainamide, together with a low therapeutic index for these drugs, put the elderly at higher risk for toxicity than younger patients. Monitoring concentrations of antiarrhythmic drugs in the plasma of elderly patients is essential. Age-related changes in the kinetics of IV lidocaine are minor, but adverse reactions are frequent in the elderly (Cusack et al. 1997). Common signs of lidocaine toxicity include confusion, paresthesias, respiratory depression, hypotension, and seizures.

Calcium-entry blockers are effective in lowering blood pressure, relieving anginal symptoms, and improving exercise tolerance in elderly patients with coronary disease, and they are effective in slowing ventricular response rates to supraventricular arrhythmias (Schwartz 1996). Although the elderly are less sensitive to the effects of verapamil on cardiac conduction, the effect on blood pressure and heart rate tends to be greater in older than in younger patients; this may be explained by an increased sensitivity to the negative inotropic and vasodilator effects of verapamil as well as diminished baroreceptor function. The acute administration of diltiazem causes greater prolongation of the PR interval in young than in elderly subjects.

An additional concern is that data from three communities of the Established Populations for Epidemiologic Studies of the Elderly, a prospective cohort study, indicate that the use of short-acting nifedipine, and possibly verapamil and diltiazem as well, may be associated with decreased survival in older persons with hypertension (Furberg and Psaty 1995; Pahor et al. 1995). Therefore, in older persons, diuretics are preferred first-choice therapy (The Sixth Report of the Joint National Committee on Prevention, Detection, Evaluation, and Treatment of High Blood Pressure 1997). Whereas other agents including long-acting dihydropyridine calcium antagonists may be considered, short-acting calcium-entry blockers should be avoided.

Angiotensin-converting enzyme (ACE) inhibitors are effective in the management of hypertension and heart failure in the elderly with few side effects (Tomlinson 1996). However, because of decreased renal clearance, plasma concentrations of the active ACE inhibitor are generally higher than in younger patients. Altered pharmacokinetics combined with impairment of cardiovascular reflexes, as well as therapy with other drugs such as diuretics, render the elderly more susceptible to first-dose hypotension. Many studies have shown that although standard doses are usually well tolerated, it is prudent to use lower initial doses in this age group, since hypotensive reactions are not always predictable. Renal insufficiency or heart failure are more important determinants of maintenance doses than age per se.

**PRINCIPLE There are multiple adverse drug effects to which the elderly may be particularly susceptible because of impaired homeostatic responses, but pharmacodynamic effects are not easily predicted.**

Among cardiovascular drugs, those acting on $\beta$-adrenergic receptors have received the most intensive investigation. Vestal et al. (1979) found that elderly patients are less sensitive than are young patients to the chronotropic effects of isoproterenol. This has been confirmed by several studies; however, this impaired response is due primarily to an age-related reduction in the influence of reflex cardiovascular effects on heart rate rather than reduced $\beta$-adrenergic sensitivity (Ford and Jones 1994). Although some reports indicate that effects of age on $\beta$-adrenergic receptor stimulation are $\beta_1$-cardioselective, the $\beta_2$-mediated relaxation of forearm and dorsal hand veins induced by isoproterenol declines with age (Van Brummelen et al. 1981; Kendall et al. 1982; Pan et al. 1986; Klein et al. 1988). The responsiveness of the hand vein to phenylephrine, an $\alpha$-adrenergic agonist, and nitroglycerin, a nonspecific vasodilator, did not differ with age (Pan et al. 1986). Also, in contrast to the nonselective $\beta$-adrenergic antagonist propranolol, the effect of timolol, a $\beta$-adrenergic blocking agent, does not differ with age (Klein et al. 1986).

In an effort to define the mechanism for the age differences in $\beta$-adrenergic responsiveness, many studies have investigated adrenergic responsiveness in lymphocytes or neutrophils isolated from persons of different ages (Scarpace et al. 1991). Possible explanations of decreased response to $\beta$-adrenergic agonists include a decreased number of high-affinity receptors, a decreased affinity of receptors for agonist, an impairment in the activity of adenylate cyclase, or a reduction in the cyclic AMP-dependent activity of protein kinase. Although $\beta$-receptor density and affinity for antagonist on human lymphocytes are not altered by old age, lower concentrations of cAMP and adenylate cyclase activity after $\beta$-adrenergic stimulation have been found in lymphocyte preparations from elderly compared with young subjects. The median effective concentration ($EC_{50}$) of isoproterenol for stimulation of cAMP production and receptor affinity for agonists are decreased in association with a reduction in the ability to form the high-affinity state for agonists. These results suggest an age-related alteration in the interaction between the $\beta$-adrenergic receptor and the stimulator GTP-binding protein that couples the receptor to adenylate cyclase. However, others have failed to confirm this finding of altered affinity states. Studies of the function of $\alpha$-adrenergic receptors have revealed no change or a decrease in the number and affinity of receptors with age (Buckley et al. 1986; Supiano et al. 1987).

**PRINCIPLE Despite all the research on aging and adrenergic pharmacology, individual variation precludes reliable dose predictions. Therefore, the clinician must titrate dosage according to response in each patient.**

## Psychotropic Drugs

Psychotropic drugs are often inappropriately prescribed for elderly patients (Ray et al. 1980; Campion et al. 1987; Avorn et al. 1989) (Psychiatric Disorders, chapter 8). The choice among neuroleptic agents that can be beneficial in the treatment of psychosis, paranoid illnesses, and agitation associated with dementia depends on the syndrome being treated and the patient's other clinical problems. Since the response to such agents can be variable, the initial dose should be small and carefully titrated upward. Elderly patients are particularly vulnerable to adverse effects from these agents, including delirium, extrapyramidal symptoms, arrhythmias, and postural hypotension. The incidence of tardive dyskinesia is higher and more likely to be irreversible in the elderly (Smith and Baldessarini 1980; Waddington and Youssef 1985). Acute dystonic reactions may be more common in younger patients, but the frequency of choreiform side effects increases with age (Moleman et al. 1986). Most psychotropics and numerous other drugs can cause cognitive impairment in elderly patients (Table 21-6).

Because of age-related alterations in hepatic demethylation, the metabolism of many antidepressant agents, particularly tertiary amines such as amitriptyline and imipramine and their metabolites, is impaired in elderly patients (von Moltka et al. 1993). Older patients treated with these agents are prone to adverse effects that include postural hypotension, urinary retention, and sedation. Initial doses should be small and preferably given at bedtime. Newer agents used for depression include trazadone, bupropion, and selective serotonin reuptake inhibitors (SSRIs). SSRIs are being used increasingly in frail elderly patients because of their relative safety and apparent efficacy (Preskorn 1993; Reynolds 1994). Among the more serious complications, falls that lead to hip fracture have been associated with increasing dosages and prolonged half-lives of psychotropic drugs, including antidepressants and benzodiazepines (Ray et al. 1987).

**Table 21-6 Drugs That Cause Delirium or Cognitive Impairment in the Elderly**

*Drugs that produce central anticholinergic effects*
- Anticholinergic drugs (e.g., propantheline)
- Tricyclic antidepressants or trazodone
- Phenothiazines (e.g., thioridazine)
- Other antipsychotic drugs (e.g., haloperidol, loxapine)
- Opiate analgesics (e.g., meperidine HCl, morphine sulfate)
- Disopyramide

*Other drugs that can also cause confusion*
- Alcohol
- Amantadine
- Benzodiazepines (e.g., diazepam, triazolam)
- $\beta$-Blockers (e.g., propranolol)
- Bromocriptine
- Cimetidine
- Corticosteroids (e.g., prednisone)
- Digoxin
- Levodopa
- Lithium
- NSAIDs
- Penicillin (high doses)
- Phenobarbital
- Phenytoin, primidone
- Quinidine

ABBREVIATIONS: $\beta$-blockers, blockers of $\beta$-adrenergic receptors
SOURCE: Adapted from Cusack 1989 with permission.

Old age is associated with impaired clearance of benzodiazepines as well as increased sensitivity to their effects on the CNS (Kruse 1990; Greenblatt et al. 1991). Sedation is induced by diazepam at lower doses and lower plasma concentrations in elderly patients (Giles et al. 1978; Reidenberg et al. 1978). Although the pharmacokinetics were unchanged, elderly patients also have been observed to be more sensitive to nitrazepam (Castleden et al. 1977). The toxicity of flurazepam is increased in elderly patients who receive standard adult doses (Greenblatt et al. 1977), and despite apparent development of tolerance after multiple-dose therapy (Greenblatt et al. 1981), dosage reductions are recommended. Not all studies show age differences, however. Caution must be exercised in interpreting the results of studies showing no difference between young and elderly subjects. For example, a study showing that the effects of temazepam and chlormethiazole do not differ with age has been criticized on the grounds that the techniques for measuring drug effects were not sufficiently sensitive, the sample size was too small, and the study design and data analysis were suboptimal (Briggs et al. 1980; Oswald and Adam 1980; Swift et al. 1980).

**PRINCIPLE Although we rely on clinical research to provide information about the effects of age on pharmacokinetics and pharmacodynamics, the interpretation of the results depends upon the appropriateness of the study design, the nature of the study population, and the quality of the methodology.**

**CASE HISTORY** *A 79-year-old woman was scheduled for endoscopy of the upper GI tract for evaluation of abdominal pain that was characteristic for peptic ulcer. She was otherwise in good health, and her medications included only an occasional laxative. The patient was quite anxious about the procedure. Upon arrival in the endoscopy suite, she was given 2 mg of diazepam IV. After 5 minutes, the patient remained alert and anxious. An additional 5 mg of diazepam was administered. The remainder of the endoscopy was performed without difficulty. Several minutes after the proce-*

*dure was completed, the patient was found to be cyanotic with labored respirations, and she required ventilation with an oxygenated resuscitation bag. She was transferred to the intensive care unit, where she began breathing spontaneously. Arterial blood-gas tests revealed a* $P_{O_2}$ *of 52 on a 40%* $O_2$ *face mask. Chest x-ray examination was subsequently consistent with an aspiration pneumonia.*

Independent of possible changes in drug kinetics, older patients may be more or less sensitive than younger patients to certain drugs even when similar concentrations occur at the drug's site of action. Elderly patients appear to be more sensitive to the sedating effects of benzodiazepines. Therefore, these drugs should be initiated at lower doses than those used for younger patients and titrated slowly for safe and appropriate sedation. Also, agents with a favorable pharmacokinetic profile (e.g., rapid onset and relatively brief duration) should be chosen. Thus, a short-acting benzodiazepine such as midazolam might be preferable. Other classes of drugs that should be titrated carefully on the basis of pharmacodynamic studies in elderly patients are narcotic analgesics, oral anticoagulants, and antihypertensive agents. On the basis of clinical experience, some other classes of drugs should probably be started at lower doses in elderly persons, including tricyclic antidepressants and antipsychotic agents.

## DRUG–DISEASE INTERACTIONS

Certain diseases may alter the disposition or effect of a drug (Table 21-7). Elderly patients often have more than one disease. Congestive heart failure (CHF) or chronic liver disease, conditions that are associated with diminished hepatic blood flow, may lead to the accumulation of drugs such as lidocaine and imipramine in the plasma. Normally, these drugs are highly extracted by the liver; thus diminished hepatic blood flow can increase the risk of toxicity. Hyperthyroidism has an age-dependent inducing effect on the metabolism of propranolol (Feely et al. 1981). Although age-related reductions in the dosage of warfarin may be required in patients treated for coronary artery disease or venous thromboembolism, this appears not to be necessary in those treated for peripheral vascular or valvular heart disease (Routledge et al. 1979).

**PRINCIPLE Aging and pathologic conditions may interact in logical or unpredictable ways to complicate therapeutic decisions. Careful selection of therapeutic agents and close clinical and laboratory assessment of the response to therapy are essential.**

Table 21-7 **Common Selected Drug–Disease Interactions in Older Persons**

| DISEASE | DRUGS | ADVERSE EFFECT |
|---|---|---|
| Benign prostatic hyperplasia | Anticholinergics, decongestants | Decreased bladder emptying |
| Cardiac conduction abnormalities | Verapamil HCl, TCAs, $\beta$-blockers | Heart block |
| Chronic obstructive pulmonary disease | $\beta$-Blockers | Bronchoconstriction |
| | Narcotic analgesics | Respiratory depression |
| Chronic renal insufficiency | NSAIDs, contrast agents, aminoglycosides | Acute renal fail |
| Congestive heart failure (systolic) | $\beta$-Blockers, verapamil HCl | Exacerbation of cardiac failure |
| Dementia | Anticholinergics, benzodiazepines, levodopa, opiates, antidepressants | Delirium |
| Diabetes mellitus | Diuretics, corticosteroids | Hyperglycemia |
| Angle-closure glaucoma | Anticholinergics | Acute exacerbation of glaucoma |
| Hypertension | NSAIDs | Increased blood pressure |
| Hypokalemia | Digoxin | Cardiac arrhythmias |
| Hyponatremia | Oral hypoglycemics, diuretics, carbamazepine | Decreased sodium concentration |
| Peptic ulcer disease | Anticoagulants, NSAIDs | Upper gastrointestinal bleeding |
| Postural hypotension | Diuretics, TCAs, levodopa, vasodilators | Syncope, falls, hip fracture |

ABBREVIATIONS: $\beta$-blockers, blockers of $\beta$-adrenergic receptors; NSAIDs, nonsteroidal anti-inflammatory drugs; TCAs, tricyclic antidepressants.
SOURCE: From Parker and Cusack 1996. Reproduced with permission.

**CASE HISTORY** *A 72-year-old man visited his physician with concerns about difficulty sleeping. His medical problems included mild chronic obstructive pulmonary disease, stable angina, and benign prostatic hypertrophy. The patient was taking many medications, and he was apt to take over-the-counter medications frequently for minor complaints. He was not satisfied with the nonpharmacologic methods that had been used to improve his sleep disorder, and he demanded a sleeping pill from his physician. The physician decided to prescribe diphenhydramine to help initiate sleep in the patient. While the patient was pleased with the effects of diphenhydramine on his sleep, he noticed that he now had to arise several times a night to urinate rather than his usual once-nightly voiding pattern. He was referred to a urologist, whose exam revealed an unchanged, but hypertrophied prostate. A postvoid residual urinary volume was now 250 mL, increased from 30 mL on a prior examination. The patient was scheduled for transurethral resection of the prostate.*

Common clinical presentations in the elderly, such as incontinence, falls, and impaired cognition, may actually be mimicked by the adverse effects of commonly prescribed or OTC medications. Drugs with anticholinergic effects, such as diphenhydramine, are used often in the elderly population without regard to their potential for interactions with physiologic or pathologic organ changes that occur in the aged individual. Possible adverse consequences of agents with anticholinergic activity are delirium, dry mouth, provocation of glaucoma, and constipation, as well as urinary retention. Other drugs can aggravate impaired homeostasis found in the elderly. For example, diuretics may worsen impaired blood pressure regulation, leading to postural hypotension, or they may cause hyponatremia in an elderly patient with diminished renal diluting capacity. Patients who have impairment that may be exacerbated by drug therapy should be monitored closely if alternative therapies are not available. It is frequently vital to detect these problems; for example, in this case the patient was subjected to a potentially unnecessary prostatic resection.

## GUIDELINES FOR GERIATRIC PRESCRIBING

The general principles of rationally prescribing for geriatric patients do not differ in any essential way from those that apply to patients of any age (Table 21-8). Nevertheless, because of multiple diseases, the need for multiple medications, the potential for altered drug response, and the increased occurrence of unwanted drug effects, the

**Table 21-8 Principles of Geriatric Prescribing**

*Evaluate the need for drug therapy:*
- Not all diseases afflicting the elderly require drug treatment
- Avoid drugs if possible, but do not withhold because of age drugs that might enhance quality of life
- Strive for a diagnosis before treatment

*Take a careful history of habits and drug use:*
- Patients often seek advice and receive prescriptions from several physicians
- Knowledge of existing therapy, both prescribed and not prescribed, helps anticipate potential drug interactions
- Smoking, alcohol, and caffeine may affect drug response and need to be taken into account

*Know the pharmacology of the drug prescribed:*
- Use a few drugs well
- Awareness of age-related alterations in drug disposition and drug response is helpful

*In general, begin therapy with relatively small doses in the elderly:*
- The standard dose is often too large for elderly patients
- Although the effect of age on hepatic drug metabolism is less predictable, it is known that renal excretion of drugs and their active metabolites tends to decline
- The elderly are particularly sensitive to drugs affecting CNS function

*Titrate drug dosage with patient response:*
- Establish reasonable therapeutic endpoints
- Adjust dosage until endpoints are reached or side effects prevent further increases
- Use an adequate dose; this is particularly important in the treatment of pain associated with malignancy
- Sometimes combination therapy is appropriate and effective

*Simplify the therapeutic regimen and encourage compliance:*
- Try to avoid intermittent schedules; once- or twice-daily dosage is ideal
- Label drug containers clearly; when appropriate, specify standard containers instead of containers with lock caps
- Give careful instructions to both the patient and a relative or friend
- Explain why the drug is being prescribed
- Suggest the use of a medication calendar or diary
- Encourage the return or destruction of old medications
- Supervision of drug therapy by a neighbor, relative, friend, or visiting nurse may be desirable or necessary

*Regularly review the treatment plan, and discontinue drugs no longer needed*

*Remember that drugs may cause new problems or exacerbate chronic problems*

SOURCE: From Vestal 1990. Clinical pharmacology. In: Hazzard WR, Andres R, Bierman EL, et al., editors. *Principles of Geriatric Medicine and Gerontology.* 2nd ed. New York: McGraw-Hill, p 207. Reproduced with permission of the McGraw-Hill Companies.

physician must be especially cautious and monitor therapy particularly carefully. Because of these factors, variability of drug response is much greater in elderly populations. In addition, impaired homeostatic mechanisms in these patients may increase the risk and severity of drug-induced toxicity.

**PRINCIPLE Whereas rational therapeutics in the elderly does not raise unique issues, the need for caution, thoughtfulness, and vigilance by the physician is magnified.**

The primary goal of drug therapy in the elderly is to relieve symptoms and enhance the quality of life. Often the cure of disease is not possible. Nevertheless, the alleviation of symptoms can involve simple measures and may not require the use of drugs. When drugs are needed, increased knowledge of the action of drugs in the elderly and improved communication between patient and physician can improve the overall care of the elderly.

## REFERENCES


Abernethy DR, Kerzner L. 1984. Age effects on alpha-1-acid glycoprotein concentration and imipramine plasma protein binding. *J Am Geriatr Soc* **32**:705–8.

Andreasen F, Hansen V, Husted SE, et al. 1984. The influence of age on renal and extrarenal effects of frusemide. *Br J Clin Pharmacol***18**:65–74.

Atrial Fibrillation Investigators. 1994. Risk factors for stroke and efficacy of antithrombotic therapy in atrial fibrillation: Analysis of pooled data from five randomized controlled trials. *Arch Intern Med* **154**:1449–57.

Avorn J, Dreyer P, Connelly K, et al. 1989. Use of psychoactive medication and the quality of care in rest homes. *N Engl J Med* **320**:227–32.

Avorn J, Gurwitz JH, Bohn RL, et al. 1995. Increased incidence of levodopa therapy following metoclopramide use. *JAMA* **274**:1780–2.

Ayesh R, Idle JR, Ritchie JC, et al. 1984. Metabolic oxidation phenotypes as markers for susceptibility to lung cancer. *Nature* **312**:169–70.

Bates DW, Spell N, Cullen DJ, et al. 1997. The cost of adverse drug events in hospitalized patients. *JAMA* **277**:307–11.

Beers MH, Avorn J, Soumerai SB, et al. 1988. Psychoactive medication use in intermediate-care facility residents. *JAMA* **260**:3016–20.

Beers MH, Ouslander JG, Feingold SF, et al. 1992. Inappropriate prescribing in skilled-nursing facilities. *Ann Intern Med* **117**:684–9.

Beers MH, Ouslander JG, Rollingher I, et al. 1991. Explicit criteria for determining inappropriate medication use in nursing home residents. *Arch Intern Med* **151**:1825–32.

Bellantuono C, Reggi V, Tognoni G, et al. 1980. Benzodiazepines: Clinical pharmacology and therapeutic use. *Drugs* **19**:195–219.

Bellville JW, Forrest WH, Miller E, et al. 1971. Influence of age on pain relief from analgesics: A study of postoperative patients. *JAMA* **217**:1835–41.

Beyth RJ, Landefeld CS. 1995. Anticoagulants in older patients: A safety perspective. *Drugs Aging* **6**:45–54.

Bhanthumnavin K, Schuster MM. 1977. Aging and gastrointestinal function. In: Finch CE, Hayflick L, editors. *Handbook of the Biology of Aging*. New York: Van Nostrand Reinhold, pp 709–23.

Blackshear JL, Davidman M, Stillman MT. 1983. Identification of risk for renal insufficiency for nonsteroidal anti-inflammatory drugs. *Arch Intern Med* **143**:1130–4.

Blaschke TF. 1977. Protein binding and kinetics of drugs in liver diseases. *Clin Pharmacokinet* **2**:32–44.

Boyd E. 1933. Normal variability in weight of the adult human liver and spleen. *Arch Pathol* **16**:350–72.

Bradely JD, Brandt KD, Katz BP, et al. 1991. Comparison of an anti-inflammatory dose of ibuprofen, an analgesic dose of ibuprofen, and acetaminophen in the treatment of patients with osteoarthritis of the knee. *N Engl J Med* **325**:87–91.

Briggs RS, Castleden CM, Kraft CA. 1980. Improved hypnotic treatment using chlormethiazole and temazepam. *Br Med J* **280**:601–4.

Brodie MJ, Boobis AR, Bulpitt CJ, et al. 1981. Influence of liver disease and environmental factors on hepatic monooxygenase activity in vitro. *Eur J Clin Pharmacol* **20**:39–46.

Buckley C, Curtin D, Walsh T, et al. 1986. Ageing and platelet alpha 2-adrenoceptors. *Br J Clin Pharmacol* **21**:721–2.

Calloway NO, Foley CF, Lagerbloom P. 1965. Uncertainties in geriatric data. II: Organ size. *J Am Geriatr Soc* **13**:20–8.

Campbell TC, Hayes JR. 1974. Role of nutrition in the drug-metabolizing enzyme system. *Pharmacol Rev* **26**:171–7.

Campion EW, Avorn J, Reder VA, et al. 1987. Overmedication of the low-weight elderly. *Arch Intern Med* **147**:945–7.

Campion EW, deLabry LO, Glynn RJ. 1988. The effect of age on serum albumin in healthy males: Report from the normative aging study. *J Gerontol* **43**:M18–20.

Cartwright RA, Glashan RW, Rogers HJ, et al. 1982. Role of *N*-acetyltransferase phenotypes in bladder carcinogenesis. *Lancet* **2**:842–5.

Castleden CM, George CF, Marcer D, et al. 1977. Increased sensitivity to nitrazepam in old age. *Br Med J* **1**:10–2.

Chaudhry AY, Bing RF, Castelden CM, et al. 1984. The effect of aging on the response to furosemide in normal subjects. *Eur J Clin Pharmacol* **27**:303–6.

Cleeland CS, Gonin R, Hatfield AK, et al. 1994. Pain and its treatment in outpatients with metastatic cancer. *N Engl J Med* **330**:592–6.

Cockcroft DW, Gault MH. 1976. Prediction of creatinine clearance from serum creatinine. *Nephron* **16**:31–41.

Col N, Fanale JE, Kronholm P. 1990. The role of medication noncompliance and adverse drug reactions in hospitalizations of the elderly. *Arch Intern Med* **150**:841–5.

Coon WW, Willis PW. 1974. Hemorrhagic complications of anticoagulant therapy. *Arch Intern Med* **133**:386–92.

Crowley JJ, Cusack BJ, Jue SG, et al. 1988. Aging and drug interactions. II: Effect of phenytoin and smoking on the oxidation of theophylline and cortisol in healthy men. *J Pharmacol Exp Ther* **245**:513–23.

Cusack BJ. 1989. Polypharmacy and clinical pharmacology. In: Beck JC, editor. *Geriatrics Review Syllabus: A Core Curriculum in Geriatric Medicine*. New York: American Geriatrics Society, pp 127–36.

Cusack BJ, Nielson CP, Vestal RE. 1997. Geriatric clinical pharmacology and therapeutics. In: Speight TM, Holford NHG, editors.

*Avery's Drug Treatment.* 4th ed. Auckland: Adis International Ltd, pp 173–223.

Cusack BJ, Vestal RE. 1986. Clinical pharmacology: Special considerations in the elderly. In: Calkins E, Davis PJ, Ford AB, editors. *Practice of Geriatric Medicine.* Philadelphia: WB Saunders, pp 115–34.

Darnell JC, Murray MD, Martz BL, et al. 1986. Medication use by ambulatory elderly: An in-home survey. *J Am Geriatr Soc* **34**:1–4.

Divoll M, Abernethy DR, Ameer B, et al. 1982. Acetaminophen kinetics in the elderly. *Clin Pharmacol Ther* **31**:151–6.

Divoll M, Ameer B, Abernethy DR, et al. 1982. Age does not alter acetaminophen absorption. *J Am Geriatr Soc* **30**:240–4.

Drusano GL, Munice HL Jr, Hoopes JM, et al. 1988. Commonly used methods of estimating creatinine clearance are inadequate for elderly debilitated nursing home patients. *J Am Geriatr Soc* **36**:437–41.

Durnas C, Loi CM, Cusack BJ. 1990. Hepatic drug metabolism and aging. *Clin Pharmacokinet* **19**:359–89.

Evans MA, Triggs EJ, Broe GA, et al. 1980. Systemic activity of orally administered L-dopa in the elderly Parkinson patient. *Eur J Clin Pharmacol* **17**:215–21.

Evans MA, Triggs EJ, Cheung M, et al. 1981. Gastric emptying rate in the elderly: Implications for drug therapy. *J Am Geriatr Soc* **29**:201–5.

Feely J, Crooks J, Stevenson IH. 1981. The influence of age, smoking and hyperthyroidism on plasma propranolol steady state concentration. *Br J Clin Pharmacol* **12**:73–8.

Felson DT, Zhang Y, Anthony JM, et al. 1992. Weight loss reduces the risk for symptomatic knee osteoarthritis in women: The Framingham study. *Ann Intern Med* **116**:535–9.

Fibrinolytic Therapy Trialists' (FTT) Collaborative Group. 1994. Indications for fibrinolytic therapy in suspected acute myocardial infarction: Collaborative overview of early mortality and major morbidity results from all randomized trials of more than 1000 patients. *Lancet* **343**:311–22.

Ford GA, James OFW. 1994. Effect of 'autonomic blockade' on cardiac beta-adrenergic chronotropic responsiveness in healthy young, healthy elderly and endurance trained elderly subjects. *Clin Sci* **87**:297–302.

Furberg CD, Psaty BM. 1995. Calcium antagonists: Antagonists or protagonists of mortality in elderly hypertensives? *J Am Geriatr Soc* **43**:1309–10.

Giles HG, MacLeod SM, Wright JR, et al. 1978. Influence of age and previous use on diazepam dosage required for endoscopy. *Can Med Assoc J* **118**:513–4.

Greenblatt DJ. 1979. Reduced serum albumin concentration in the elderly: report from the Boston Collaborative Drug Surveillance Program. *J Am Geriatr Soc* **27**:301–12.

Greenblatt DJ, Allen MD, Shader RI. 1977. Toxicity of high-dose flurazepam in the elderly. *Clin Pharmacol Ther* **21**:355–61.

Greenblatt DJ, Divoll M, Harmatz JS, et al. 1981. Kinetics and clinical effects of flurazepam in young and elderly noninsomniacs. *Clin Pharmacol Ther* **30**:475–86.

Greenblatt DJ, Divoll M, Abernethy DR, et al. 1982.

Greenblatt DJ, Harmatz JS, Shader RI. 1991. Clinical pharmacokinetics of anxiolytics and hypnotics in the elderly: Therapeutic considerations. *Clin Pharmacokinet* **21**:165–77, 262–73.

Griffin MR, Ray WA, Schaffner W. 1988. Nonsteroidal anti-inflammatory drug use and death from peptic ulcer in elderly persons. *Ann Intern Med* **109**:359–63.

Gurwitz JH, Avorn J. 1991. The ambiguous relation between aging and adverse drug reactions. *Ann Intern Med* **114**:956–66.

Gurwitz JH, Avorn J, Bohn RL, et al. 1994. Initiation of antihypertensive treatment during nonsteroidal anti-inflammatory drug therapy. *JAMA* **272**:781–6.

Gurwitz JH, Avorn J, Ross-Degnan D, et al. 1992. Aging and the anticoagulant response to warfarin therapy. *Ann Intern Med* **116**:901–4.

Gurwitz JH, Col NF, Avorn J. 1992. The exclusion of the elderly and women from clinical trials in acute myocardial infarction. *JAMA* **268**:1417–22.

Gurwitz JH, Glynn RJ, Monane M, et al. 1993. Treatment for glaucoma: Adherence by the elderly. *Am J Public Health* **83**:711–6.

Gurwitz JH, Goldberg RJ, Gore JM. 1991. Coronary thrombolysis for the elderly. *JAMA* **325**:125–7.

Gurwitz JH, Goldberg RJ, Holden A, et al. 1988. Age-related risks of long-term oral anticoagulant therapy. *Arch Intern Med* **148**:1733–6.

Gurwitz JH, Gore JM, Goldberg RJ, et al. 1996. Recent age-related trends in the use of thrombolytic therapy in patients who have had acute myocardial infarction. *Ann Intern Med* **124**:283–91.

Hammarlund ER, Ostrom JR, Kethley AJ. 1985. The effects of drug counseling and other educational strategies on drug utilization of the elderly. *Med Care* **23**:165–70.

Hayes MJ, Langman MJS, Short AH. 1975. Changes in drug metabolism with increasing age: 2 phenytoin clearance and protein binding. *Br J Clin Pharmacol* **2**:73–9.

Hemmelgarn B, Suissa S, Huang A, et al. 1997. Benzodiazepine use and the risk of motor vehicle crash in the elderly. *JAMA* **278**:27–31.

Holmberg L, Odar-Cederöf I, Boréus LO, et al. 1982. Comparative disposition of pethidine and norpethidine in old and young patients. *Eur J Clin Pharmacol* **22**:175–9.

Homer TD, Stanski DR. 1985. The effect of increasing age on thiopental disposition and anesthetic requirement. *Anesthesiology* **62**:714–24.

Jacox A, Carr DB, Payne R, et al. 1994. *Management of Cancer Pain: Adults.* Quick Reference Guide No 9. Rockville, MD: U.S. Department of Health and Human Services, Public Health Service, Agency for Health Care Policy and Research. AHCPR publication no 94-0593.

Jick H, Slone D, Borda IT, et al. 1968. Efficacy and toxicity of heparin in relation to age and sex. *N Engl J Med* **279**:284–6.

Johnson AG, Day RO. 1991. The problems and pitfalls of NSAID therapy in the elderly. *Drugs Aging* **1**:130–3, 212–27.

Johnson JA, Bootman JL. 1995. Drug-related morbidity and mortality: A cost-of-illness model. *Arch Intern Med* **155**:1949–56.

Jung D, Mayershohn M, Perrier D, et al. 1982. Thiopental disposition as a function of age in female patients undergoing surgery. *Anesthesiology* **56**:263–8.

Kaiko RF. 1980. Age and morphine analgesia in cancer patients with postoperative pain. *Clin Pharmacol Ther* **28**:823–6.

Kalow W. 1992. *Pharmacogenetics of Drug Metabolism.* New York: Pergamon Press.

Kendall MJ, Woods KL, Wilkins MR, et al. 1982. Responsiveness to beta-adrenergic receptor stimulation: The effects of age are cardioselective. *Br J Clin Pharmacol* **14**:821–6.

Kinirons MT, Crome P. 1997. Clinical pharmacokinetic considerations in the elderly: An update. *Clin Pharmacokinet* **33**:302–12.

Klein C, Gerber JG, Gal J, et al. 1986. Beta-adrenergic receptors in the elderly are not less sensitive to timolol. *Clin Pharmacol Ther* **40**:161–4.

Klein C, Hiatt WR, Gerber JG, et al. 1988. Age does not alter human vascular and nonvascular beta 2-adrenergic responses to isoproterenol. *Clin Pharmacol Ther* **44**:573–8.

Klotz U, Avant GR, Hoyumpa A, et al. 1975. The effects of age and liver disease on the disposition and elimination of diazepam in adult man. *J Clin Invest* **55**:347–59.

Korrapati MR, Sorkin JD, Andres R, et al. 1997. Acetylator phenotype in relation to age and gender in the Baltimore Longitudinal Study of Aging. *J Clin Pharmacol* **37**:83–91.

Kovar PA, Allegrante JP, MacKenzie CR, et al. 1992. Supervised fitness walking in patients with osteoarthritis of the knee: A randomized, controlled trial. *Ann Intern Med* **116**:529–34.

Kramer PA, Chapron DJ, Benson J, et al. 1978. Tetracycline absorption in elderly patients with achlorhydria. *Clin Pharmacol Ther* **23**:467–72.

Krishnaswamy K. 1978. Drug metabolism and pharmacokinetics in malnutrition. *Clin Pharmacokinet* **3**:216–40.

Kruse WH-H. 1990. Problems and pitfalls in the use of benzodiazepines in the elderly. *Drug Safety* **5**:328–4.

Landefeld CS, Beyth RJ. 1993. Anticoagulant bleeding: Clinical epidemiology, prediction, and prevention. *Am J Med* **95**:315–28.

Lindeman RD. 1992. Changes in renal function with aging: Implications for treatment. *Drugs Aging* **2**:423–31.

Lindeman RD, Tobin J, Shock NW. 1985. Longitudinal studies on the rate of decline in renal function with age. *J Am Geriatr Soc* **33**:278–85.

Loi CM, Parker BM, Cusack BJ, et al. 1997. Aging and drug interactions. III: Individual and combined effects of cimetidine and ciprofloxacin on theophylline metabolism in healthy male and female nonsmokers. *J Pharmacol Exp Ther* **280**:627–37.

Maloney AG, Schmucker DL, Vessey DS, et al. 1986. The effects of aging on the hepatic microsomal mixed-function oxidase system of male and female monkeys. *Hepatology* **6**:282–7.

Mazzullo J. 1972. The nonpharmacologic basis of therapeutics. *Clin Pharmacol Ther* **13**:157–8.

Meconi M, Taylor L, Martin B, et al. 1987. A review: Prostaglandins, aging, and blood vessels. *J Am Geriatr Soc* **35**:239–47.

Moleman P, Janzen G, von Bargen BA, et al. 1986. Relationship between age and incidence of parkinsonism in psychiatric patients treated with haloperidol. *Am J Psychiatry* **143**:232–4.

Montamat SC, Cusack BJ, Vestal RE. 1989. Management of drug therapy in the elderly. *N Engl J Med* **321**:303–9.

Moore JG, Tweedy C, Christian PE, et al. 1983. Effect of age on gastric emptying of liquid-solid meals in man. *Dig Dis Sci* **28**:340–4.

Neilson CP, Cusack BJ, Vestal RE. 1987. Geriatric clinical pharmacology and therapeutics. In Speight TM, editor. *Avery's Drug Treatment: Principles and Practice of Clinical Pharmacology and Therapeutics*, 3rd ed. Auckland, New Zealand: Adis International Ltd, pp 160–93.

Nelson CR, Knapp DE. 1997. Medication therapy in ambulatory medical care: National Ambulatory Medical Care Survey and National Hospital Ambulatory Care Survey. 1992 advance data from vital and health statistics, no 290. Hyattsville, MD: National Center for Health Statistics.

Norris AH, Lundy T, Shock NW. 1963. Trends in selected indices of body composition in men between the ages of 30 and 80 years. *Ann N Y Acad Sci* **110**:623–39.

Novak LP. 1972. Aging, total body potassium, fat-free mass, and cell mass in males and females between the ages of 18 and 85 years. *J Gerontol* **27**:438–43.

O'Malley K, Crooks J, Duke E, et al. 1971. Effect of age and sex on human drug metabolism. *Br Med J* **3**:607–9.

O'Malley K, Stevenson IH, Ward CA, et al. 1977. Determinants of anticoagulant control in patients receiving warfarin. *Br J Clin Pharmacol* **4**:309–14.

Ostrom JR, Hammarlund ER, Christensen DB, et al. 1985. Medication usage in the elderly population. *Med Care* **23**:157–64.

Oswald I, Adam K. 1980. Chlormethiazole and temazepam [letter]. *Br Med J* **280**:860–1.

Owen JA, Sitar DS, Berger L, et al. 1983. Age-related morphine kinetics. *Clin Pharmacol Ther* **34**:364–8.

Pahor M, Guralnik JM, Corti M-C, et al. 1995. Long-term survival and use of antihypertensive medications in older persons. *J Am Geriatr Soc* **43**:1191–7.

Pan HY-M, Hoffman BB, Pershe RA, et al. 1986. Decline in beta adrenergic receptor-mediated vascular relaxation with aging in man. *J Pharmacol Exp Ther* **239**:801–7.

Parker BM, Cusack BJ. 1996. Pharmacology and appropriate prescribing. In: Reuben DB, Yoshikawa TT, Besdine RW, editors. *Geriatrics Review Syllabus: A Core Curriculum in Geriatric Medicine.* 3rd ed. New York: American Geriatrics Society, pp 29–36.

Preskorn SH. 1993. Recent pharmacologic advances in antidepressant therapy for the elderly. *Am J Med* **94** (Suppl 5A):2S–12S.

Ray WA, Federspiel CF, Schaffner W. 1980. A study of antipsychotic use in nursing homes: Epidemiologic evidence suggesting misuse. *Am J Public Health* **70**:485–91.

Ray WA, Griffin MR, Avorn J. 1993. Evaluating drugs after their approval for clinical use. *N Engl J Med* **329**:2029–32.

Ray WA, Griffin MR, Downey W. 1989. Benzodiazepines of long and short elimination half-life and the risk of hip fracture. *JAMA* **262**:3303–7.

Ray WA, Griffin MR, Schaffner W, et al. 1987. Psychotropic drug use and the risk of hip fracture. *N Engl J Med* **316**:363–9.

Reidenberg MM. 1987. Drug therapy in the elderly: The problem from the point of view of a clinical pharmacologist. *Clin Pharmacol Ther* **42**:677–80.

Reidenberg MM, Levy M, Warner H, et al. 1978. Relationship between diazepam dose, plasma level, age, and central nervous system depression. *Clin Pharmacol Ther* **23**:371–4.

Reynolds CF III. 1994. Treatment of depression in late life. *Am J Med* **97**:39S–46S.

Rochon PA, Fortin PR, Dear KBG, et al. 1993. Reporting of age data in clinical trials of arthritis: deficiencies and solutions. *Arch Intern Med* **153**:342–8.

Rochon PA, Gurwitz JH. 1997. Optimising drug treatment for elderly people: The prescribing cascade. *Br Med J* **315**:1096–9.

Roskos KV, Maibach HI. 1992. Percutaneous absorption in the aged: Implications for therapy. *Drugs Aging* **2**:432–49.

Routledge PA, Chapman PH, Davis DM, et al. 1979. Pharmacokinetics and pharmacodynamics of warfarin at steady state. *Br J Clin Pharmacol* **8**:243–7.

Routledge PA, Stargel WW, Wagner GS, et al. 1980. Increased alpha-1-acid glycoprotein and lidocaine disposition in myocardial infarction. *Ann Intern Med* **93**:701–4.

Rowe JW, Andres R, Tobin JD, et al. 1976. The effect of age on creatinine clearance in man: A cross-sectional and longitudinal study. *J Gerontol* **31**:155–63.

Rubin PC, Scott PJW, Reid JL. 1981. Prazosin disposition in young and elderly subjects. *Br J Clin Pharmacol* **12**:401–4.

Sackett DL, Snow JC. 1970. The magnitude of compliance and noncompliance. In: Haynes RB, Taylor DW, Sackett DL, editors. *Compliance in Health Care.* Baltimore: The Johns Hopkins University Press, pp 11–2.

Scarpace PJ, Tumer N, Mader SL. 1991. Beta-adrenergic function in aging: Basic mechanisms and clinical implications. *Drugs Aging* **1**:116–29.

Schmucker DL, Woodhouse KW, Wang RK, et al. 1990. Effects of age and gender on in vitro properties of human liver microsomal monooxygenases. *Clin Pharmacol Ther* **48**:365–74.

Schwartz JB. 1996. Calcium antagonists in the elderly: A risk-benefit analysis. *Drugs Aging* **9**:24–36.

Shepherd AM, Hewick DS, Moreland TA, et al. 1977. Age as a determinant of sensitivity to warfarin. *Br J Clin Pharmacol* **4**:315–20.

Shock NW, Watkin DM, Yiengst BS, et al. 1963. Age differences in the water content of the body as related to basal oxygen consumption in males. *J Gerontol* **18**:1–8.

Siegmund W, Hanke W, Zschiesche M, et al. 1990. *N*-Acetylation and debrisoquine type oxidation polymorphism in Caucasians with reference to age and sex. *Int J Pharmacol Ther Toxicol* **28**:504–9.

Simonson W. 1984. *Medications and the Elderly: A Guide for Promoting Proper Use.* Rockville, MD: Aspen Systems Corp.

Smith JM, Baldessarini RJ. 1980. Changes in prevalence, severity, and recovery in tardive dyskinesia with age. *Arch Gen Psychiatry* **37**:1368–73.

Smithard DJ, Langman MJS. 1977. Drug metabolism in the elderly. *Br Med J* **3**:520–1.

Smithard DJ, Langman MJS. 1978. The effect of vitamin supplementation upon antipyrine metabolism in the elderly. *Br J Clin Pharmacol* **5**:181–5.

Solomon DH, Gurwitz JH. 1997. Toxicity of nonsteroidal anti-inflammatory drugs in the elderly: Is advanced age a risk factor? *Am J Med* **102**:208–15.

Sotaniemi EA, Arranto AJ, Pelkonen O, et al. 1997. Age and cytochrome P450-linked drug metabolism in humans: An analysis of 226 subjects with equal histopathologic conditions. *Clin Pharmacol Ther* **61**:331–9.

Steiner E, Bertilsson L, Säwe J, et al. 1988. Polymorphic debrisoquin hydroxylation in 757 Swedish subjects. *Clin Pharmacol Ther* **44**:431–5.

Stroke Prevention in Atrial Fibrillation Investigators. 1991. Stroke prevention in atrial fibrillation study: Final results. *Circulation* **84**:527–39.

Supiano MA, Linares OA, Halter JB, et al. 1987. Functional uncoupling of the platelet alpha2-adrenergic receptor-adenylate cyclase complex in the elderly. *J Clin Endocrin Metab* **64**:1160–4.

Sutter MA, Wood WG, Williamson LS, et al. 1985. Comparison of the hepatic mixed function oxidase system of young, adult, and old non-human primates (*Macaca nemestrina*). *Biochem Pharmacol* **34**:2983–7.

Svarstad BL, Mount JK. 1991. Nursing home resources and tranquilizer use among the institutionalized elderly. *J Am Geriatr Soc* **39**:869–75.

Swift CG, Haythorne JM, Clarke P, et al. 1980. Chlormethiazole and temazepam [letter]. *Br Med J* **280**:1322.

The Sixth Report of the Joint National Committee on Prevention, Detection, Evaluation, and Treatment of High Blood Pressure. 1997. *Arch Intern Med* **157**:2413–46.

Thomson AM, Thomson GD, Hepburn M, et al. 1987. A clinically significant interaction between ciprofloxacin and theophylline. *Eur J Clin Pharmacol* **33**:435–6.

Tomlinson B. 1996. Optimal dosage of ACE inhibitors in older patients. *Drugs Aging* **9**:262–73.

Topol EJ, Califf RM. 1992. Thrombolytic therapy for elderly patients. *N Engl J Med* **327**:45–7.

Trang JM, Blanchard J, Conrad KA, et al. 1982. The effect of vitamin C on the pharmacokinetics of caffeine in elderly men. *Am J Clin Nutr* **35**:487–94.

Trimble EL, Carter LC, Cain D, et al. 1994. Representation of older patients in cancer treatment trials. *Cancer* **74** (Suppl 7):2208–14.

Tsujimoto G, Hashimoto K, Hoffman BB. 1989a. Pharmacokinetic and pharmacodynamic principles of drug therapy in old age: Part I. *Int J Clin Pharmacol Ther* Toxicol **27**:13–26.

Tsujimoto G, Hashimoto K, Hoffman BB. 1989b. Pharmacokinetic and pharmacodynamic principles of drug therapy in old age: Part II. *Int J Clin Pharmacol Ther Toxicol* **27**:102–16.

Upton RA, Williams RL, Kelly J, et al. 1984. Naproxen pharmacokinetics in the elderly. *Br J Clin Pharmacol* **18**:207–14.

U.S. Bureau of the Census. 1996. Current Population Reports, Special Studies, P23–190, 65+ in the United States. Washington, DC: U.S. Government Printing Office.

Van Brummelen P, Bühler FR, Kiowski W, et al. 1981. Age-related decrease in cardiac and peripheral vascular responsiveness to isoprenaline: studies in normal subjects. *Clin Sci* **60**:571–7.

Vestal RE. 1990. Clinical pharmacology. In: Hazzard WR, Andres R, Bierman EL, et al., editors. *Principles of Geriatric Medicine and Gerontology.* 2nd ed. New York: McGraw-Hill, pp 201–11.

Vestal RE. 1997. Aging and pharmacology. *Cancer* **80**:1302–10.

Vestal RE, Cusack BJ. 1990. Pharmacology and aging. In: Schneider EL, Rowe JW, editors. *Handbook of the Biology of Aging.* 3rd ed. San Diego: Academic Press, pp 349–83.

Vestal RE, Cusack BJ, Crowley JJ, et al. 1993. Aging and the response to inhibition and induction of theophylline metabolism. *Exp Gerontol* **28**:421–33.

Vestal RE, Cusack BJ, Mercer GD, et al. 1987. Aging and drug interactions. I: Effect of cimetidine and smoking on the oxidation of theophylline and cortisol in healthy men. *J Pharmacol Exp Ther* **241**:488–500.

Vestal RE, Dawson GW. 1985. Pharmacology and aging. In: Finch CE, Schneider EL, editors. *Handbook of the Biology of Aging.* 2nd ed. New York: Van Nostrand Reinhold, pp 744–819.

Vestal RE, McGuire EA, Tobin JD, et al. 1977. Aging and ethanol metabolism. *Clin Pharmacol Ther* **21**:343–54.

Vestal RE, Norris AH, Tobin JD, et al. 1975. Antipyrine metabolism in man: Influence of age, alcohol, caffeine and smoking. *Clin Pharmacol Ther* **5**:309–19.

Vestal RE, Wood AJJ. 1980. Influence of age and smoking on drug kinetics in man: Studies using model compounds. *Clin Pharmacokinet* **5**:309–19.

Vestal RE, Wood AJJ, Shand DG. 1979. Reduced beta-adrenoceptor sensitivity in the elderly. *Clin Pharmacol Ther* **26**:181–6.

Von Moltke LL, Greenblatt DJ, Shader RI. 1993. Clinical pharmacokinetics of antidepressants in the elderly: Therapeutic implications. *Clin Pharmacokinet* **34**:141–60.

Waddington JL, Youssef H. 1985. Late onset involuntary movements in chronic schizophrenia: Age-related vulnerability to "tardive" dyskinesia independent of extent of neuroleptic medication. *Ir Med J* **78**:143–6.

Wallace SM, Verbeek RK. 1987. Plasma protein binding of drugs in the elderly. *Clin Pharmacokinet* **12**:41–72.

Walter-Sack I, Klotz U. 1996. Influence of diet and nutritional status on drug metabolism. *Clin Pharmacokinet* **31**:47–64.

Warren PM, Pepperman MA, Montgomery RD. 1978. Age changes in small-intestinal mucosa. *Lancet* **2**:849–50.

Whitfield LR, Schentag JJ, Levy G. 1982. Relationship between concentration and anticoagulant effect of heparin in plasma of hospitalized patients: Magnitude of predictability of interindividual differences. *Clin Pharmacol Ther* **32**:503–16.

Willcox SM, Himmelstein DU, Woolhandler S. 1994. Inappropriate drug prescribing for the community-dwelling elderly. *JAMA* **272**:292–6.

Woodford-Williams E, Alvarez AS, Webster D, et al. 1964/65. Serum protein patterns in "normal" and pathological aging. *Gerontologia* **10**:86–99.

Woodhouse KW, Mutch E, Williams FM, et al. 1984. The effect of age on pathways of drug metabolism in human liver. *Age Ageing* **13**:328–34.

Woodhouse KW, Wynne HA. 1988. Age-related changes in liver size and hepatic blood flow: The influence of drug metabolism in the elderly. *Clin Pharmacokinet* **15**:287–94.

Woodhouse KW, Wynne HA. 1992. Age-related changes in hepatic function: implications for drug therapy. *Drugs Aging* **2**:243–55.

Wynne HA, Cope LH, Herd B, et al. 1990. The association of age and frailty with paracetamol conjugation in man. *Age Ageing* **19**: 419–24.

Wynne H, Cope L, Kelly P, et al. 1995. The influence of age, liver size and enantiomer concentrations on warfarin dose requirements. *Br J Clin Pharmacol* **40**:203–7.

CHAPTER

# 22 PHARMACOGENETICS

Urs A. Meyer

*Chapter Outline*

**GENERAL CONCEPTS**

**SPECIFIC PHARMACOGENETIC PHENOMENA**

**INHERITED VARIATIONS IN DRUG EFFECTS INDEPENDENT OF PHARMACOKINETICS**

**OUTLOOK**

## GENERAL CONCEPTS

### History of Pharmacogenetics

The study of genetically determined variations in drug response, commonly referred to as *pharmacogenetics,* is a relatively new field of clinical investigation. The first report of an inherited difference in response to a chemical—namely the inability to taste phenylthiourea—was reported in the early 1930s (Snyder 1932). In the late 1950s, Motulsky reported that certain adverse reactions to drugs are due to genetically determined variations in enzymatic activity (Motulsky 1957). Pseudocholinesterase variants were associated with suxamethonium sensitivity, and inherited abnormalities in red cell glutathione metabolism were identified as causes of primaquine sensitivity. At about the same time, genetic differences in the acetylation of isoniazid were discovered (Evans et al. 1960). In 1959, Vogel first proposed the term *pharmacogenetics* (Vogel 1959), and in 1962, Kalow wrote the first monograph on the topic (Kalow 1962).

Over the last 40 years, more than 100 additional examples of exaggerated responses to drugs, novel drug effects, or lack of effectiveness of drugs as a manifestation of inherited individual traits have been observed (for reviews, see Kalow 1992; Evans 1993; Gonzalez and Idle 1994; Kroemer and Eichelbaum 1995; Meyer and Zanger 1997; Nebert 1997; Weber 1997; Meyer 1998a, 1998b). The field of pharmacogenetics was stimulated in the 1970s when Vesell and colleagues demonstrated that plasma half-lives of many drugs are less divergent among monozygotic twin pairs than among dizygotic twin pairs (for a review, see Vesel 1990). The implication was that *multifactorial inheritance,* or multiple genes, may determine individual drug metabolism (*multigenic* inheritance). More recently, common genetic polymorphisms of drug metabolism such as debrisoquine/sparteine polymorphism, mephenytoin polymorphism, and acetylation polymorphism have received much attention because they affect the metabolism of numerous clinically useful drugs and concern a sizable proportion of patients.

The objectives of research in pharmacogenetics are 1) the identification of genetically controlled variations in responses to drugs, 2) the study of the molecular mechanisms causing these variations, 3) the evaluation of their clinical significance, and 4) the development of simple methods to identify individuals who may be susceptible to variable responses before drugs are administered. The methods of *genomics*—with its emphasis on molecular structure and function of genes—have been increasingly applied to pharmacogenetic research (Meyer 1990), and many pharmacogenetic conditions have been elucidated at the gene level. As a consequence, many of these conditions can now be diagnosed by analyzing samples of genomic DNA (for reviews, see Gonzalez and Idle 1994; Meyer and Zanger 1997).

**PRINCIPLE Understanding the mechanisms of genetic variation in drug effects is the key to applying pharmacogenetic principles to produce greater efficacy and fewer adverse reactions of numerous drugs. When the molecular mechanism of a genetic variation is known, simple analyses of genomic DNA can frequently identify subpopulations of patients that may be at risk.**

A relatively recent addition to the discipline of pharmacogenetics is the field of *ecogenetics,* which is concerned with the dynamic interactions between an individual's genotype and environmental agents such as industrial chemicals, pollutants, plant and food components, pesticides, and other chemicals. Examples include interindividual differences in ethanol sensitivity, sensitivity to milk because of lactase deficiency, development of pulmonary emphysema in individuals with $\alpha_1$-antitrypsin deficiency, differences in nicotine metabolism, and many other interactions between the environment and the genetic makeup of the individual. The related field of *toxicogenetics* examines an individual's predisposition to carcinogenic, teratogenic, and other toxic effects of drugs and other chemicals.

Interethnic differences in reactions to drugs and other chemicals—sometimes called *pharmacoanthropology* or *ethnopharmacology*—represent another area of recent interest. Such differences may be produced by different environmental effects on drug action or may have a genetic origin (Bertilsson et al. 1985; Kalow et al. 1986; Nei 1987; Kalow and Bertilsson 1994; Meyer and Zanger 1997). Population differences in drug kinetics and dynamics have obvious implications for drug therapy in multiracial societies.

## Definitions

The basic tenets of pharmacogenetics are relatively simple. The genetic endowment of the individual—phenotypically expressed in protein structure, configuration, and concentration—may alter action of a drug in a multitude of ways. A drug entering the body interacts with numerous enzymes, lipids, and proteins. Almost all drugs undergo enzymatically controlled transformations during their passage through the liver and other organs. They react with plasma and tissue proteins by various processes, pass through membranes, and interact with drug-receptor sites. In theory, genetic mutations that alter the quantity or quality of any of these proteins, the characteristics of membranes, or the characteristics of drug receptors can lead to recognizable disturbances in drug pharmacokinetics or drug–cell interactions. For example, common inherited deficiencies in enzymes of drug metabolism can retard inactivation and consequent excretion of drugs, which result in toxic concentrations of what are often considered "standard" or "safe" doses. Structural differences in serum proteins can presumably change binding affinities and alter the ratios of bound to free drug. In a similar manner, aberrant gene products at the site of a drug's action in organs, tissues, or cells may confer increased or decreased responsiveness to usual therapeutic concentrations of a drug. The plausibility of these basic concepts has been supported by many detailed investigations of inherited variants involving the fate or action of drugs in the organism (see the section "Specific Pharmacogenetic Phenomena").

In some individuals, unexpected, novel, or unusual reactions to drugs may be inherited traits; and these reactions may occur independently without changes in the basic pharmacokinetics of the drug. In fact, pharmacogenetics had its initial impact on medicine predominantly through the discovery of such unexpected alterations in drug response. The prototype of this phenomenon is represented by the syndrome of drug-induced hemolytic anemia in persons who are genetically deficient in glucose-6-phosphate dehydrogenase (G6PD) in their erythrocytes (see the section "Glucose-6-Phosphate Dehydrogenase Deficiency and Drug-Induced Hemolytic Anemia"). The pathogenesis of unusual drug effects in hereditary disorders is frequently not understood, but the affected patients and their relatives may require special consideration during drug therapies. Some inherited metabolic diseases are uncovered or dramatically precipitated by the administration of drugs, with the unusual drug response often serving as the phenotypic marker of the genetic disease.

**PRINCIPLE Unexpected or quantitatively unusual responses of an individual to a drug may be a signal to investigate the genetic or environmental source of the variation in the patient and in his or her family.**

The basic principles of genetic influences on drug action may be summarized as follows.

- Genetic factors influence a drug's action by affecting pharmacokinetic and/or pharmacodynamic properties of the agent. In clinical practice, this may result in an alteration of the intensity and the duration of the expected "normal" or "usual" effect of a drug or in the occurrence of adverse drug reactions.
- Unexpected, uncommon, or "abnormal" effects of drugs may be associated with certain genetically transmitted disorders. Under these circumstances, the modified drug response may have both diagnostic and therapeutic implications.

**PRINCIPLE When some patients do not obtain the expected drug effect or instead show serious toxicity or unusual effects after taking the "standard" or "safe" dose of a drug, genetic variability or an inherited metabolic defect may be the explanation.**

## Genotype and Phenotype

A key issue in person-to-person variability in the response to drugs is the differentiation of genetic and environmental factors, and the interaction of genetic and environmental influences may be difficult to disentangle in an individual patient. Variations in drug response—whether controlled by genes, environmental factors (e.g., diet, smoking, disease), or both—may occur at sites of absorption, distribution, protein binding, drug–cell interaction, metabolism, and excretion. Moreover, several independent variables may modulate more than one of these discrete processes.

Only when one of the numerous interactions of a drug in the body with the product of one aberrant gene assumes decisive importance for drug action can we expect its easy recognition and its transmission by classic mendelian inheritance, that is, as an autosomal dominant or recessive or X-linked trait. A mendelian—or *monogenetic*—trait often divides a population into two or three distinct groups. Under these circumstances, the frequency distribution of a given parameter of drug response in a sample population shows discontinuous variation. In such a multimodal distribution of drug response, each subpopulation corresponds to a different genotype. This is the case for most classic examples of pharmacogenetic conditions (e.g., the slow metabolism of isoniazid or the prolonged apnea after administration of succinylcholine). Studies of families have generally provided a reliable and easy means of revealing the mode of inheritance of the genetic variant in these disorders.

Because drug action depends on numerous events, with each presumably controlled by different gene products, several pairs of genes may often interact with environmental factors to result in a particular variation in drug effect. This multifactorial, or *polygenic*, inheritance is more difficult to detect and to distinguish from environmental factors that can cause similar anomalies. Thus, when sample populations are tested for characteristics controlled by multiple genes, the resulting distribution curve often does not segregate pharmacogenetic subpopulations. Rather, the interaction of the multiple environmental and genetic factors results in an apparently statistically normal, unimodal, or continuous distribution of drug response. The analysis of these conditions is similar to the analysis of complex diseases. Careful studies of families may still disclose genetic control of the suspected pharmacogenetic trait. For example, three independent studies of different families demonstrated predominant genetic control of the plasma pharmacokinetics of bishydroxycoumarin, phenylbutazone, and nortriptyline, although the distribution of concentrations of drug in plasma after standard doses (= phenotype) in sample populations was unrevealing (Motulsky 1964; Whittaker and Evans 1970; Asberg et al. 1971). However, even pedigree studies involving several generations frequently do not uncover the polygenic contribution to an observed variation because, by necessity, subjects of different age, sex, and environment are compared. This results in a large "nongenetic" contribution to phenotypic variation that can hide the genetic components of variation.

An important and strikingly simple method to distinguish between hereditary and environmental components of variability is the comparison of small series of mono- and dizygotic twins in whom the variation among pairs can be analyzed by established statistical methods (Galton 1875) (for a review, see Vesell 1990). The rationale of the *twin method* is based on two assumptions: 1) for traits controlled primarily by environmental factors, intratwin differences are of similar magnitude in monozygotic and dizygotic twins; and 2) for traits controlled predominantly by genetic factors, there is virtually no intratwin difference in monozygotic twins, who have an identical genome. However, the study methods using twins do not permit a distinction between modes of mendelian or polygenic inheritance. Recent extensive application of the twin method has demonstrated important genetic factors in the pharmacokinetic behavior of a large number of commonly used drugs, including amylobarbitone, antipyrine, dicoumarol, ethanol, halothane, nortriptyline, phenytoin, sodium salicylate, and tolbutamide (for a review, see Vesell 1990). For all of these agents, determination of the plasma half-life or other kinetic parameters revealed much greater similarity among identical twins than among fraternal twins. Most of these studies were done in healthy, otherwise nonmedicated subjects, and drugs were chosen that depend on metabolism to polar metabolites before they are eliminated. In clinical practice, major influences on pharmacokinetics are obviously introduced by disease-related and environmental factors that modify the underlying genetically controlled rate of drug metabolism or its induction or repression. The twin method also has a number of limitations and problems that have to be considered (Vesell 1990).

**PRINCIPLE Because of genetic control, the basic capacity of a healthy individual to eliminate a drug is stable and reproducible, whereas environmental influences and the effects of disease often change rapidly.**

## Genetic Polymorphisms and the Diversity of Human Genes

The concept of *genetic polymorphism* arose from the finding that many phenotypic traits such as blood groups, histocompatibility antigens (e.g., using the human lymphocytic antigen [HLA] system), and enzyme variants exist in the population in frequencies that could not be maintained by spontaneous mutation. A genetic polymorphism is defined as a monogenic trait that exists in the population in at least two phenotypes (and presumably at least two genotypes), neither of which is rare, that is, neither of which occurs with a frequency of less than approximately 1–2% (Vogel and Motulsky 1986). The definition of a phenotypic frequency of more than 1% as "common" or "polymorphic" is arbitrary and has practical implications because frequencies of 0.1% or 0.01% would be hard to detect in small groups of patients. Moreover, the original definition did not specify whether the rare phenotype is a heterozygous or homozygous genotype for the variant allele. An allele-based definition of pharmacogenetic polymorphism therefore has been proposed (Meyer 1991).

> A pharmacogenetic polymorphism is a monogenic trait that is caused by the presence in the same population of more than one allele at the same locus and more than one phenotype in regard to drug interaction with the organism. The frequency of the least common allele is at least 1%.

For each specific pharmacogenetic polymorphism, information on the mode of inheritance and frequency of the rare phenotype should be given separately.

The evolutionary impact of the phenomenon of genetic polymorphism is that there is variability built into the population so that a change in the environment (e.g., exposure to chemicals, infectious agents, nutritional components) can elicit a change in the structure of the population, increasing its chance of survival. In a genetic context, these polymorphisms are due to multiple alleles at one or more gene loci and are characterized by a high frequency of heterozygotes in the population.

The human population is genetically diverse with thousands of alleles at most gene loci. At the sequence level, 1 in 700 to 1 in 1000 base pairs shows a single nucleotide polymorphism (Wang et al. 1998). But diversity is also limited in that most genes have only two or three variants in any coding sequence that are frequent or "common" (>10% frequency), as exemplified by the polymorphisms of drug metabolizing enzymes. Polymorphisms can also be used to trace the evolution and migration of human populations (Kalow et al. 1986; Meyer and Zanger 1997).

**PRINCIPLE Genetic polymorphisms in enzymes and other proteins are the rule rather than the exception, and genetic diversity is a large source of interindividual, interethnic, and racial differences in drug responses.**

# SPECIFIC PHARMACOGENETIC PHENOMENA

## Inherited Variations Affecting Pharmacokinetics of Drugs

***Overview of genetic polymorphisms of drug metabolism*** Genetic polymorphisms of drug-metabolizing enzymes give rise to distinct subgroups in a population that differ in their ability to perform certain drug biotransformation reactions. Subgroups with a deficient ability to metabolize a certain drug are called *poor metabolizers* (PMs) or *PM phenotypes* compared with "normal" *extensive metabolizers* (EMs) or *EM phenotypes*. A list of clinically relevant genetic polymorphisms of drug-metabolizing enzymes is given in Table 22-1. These polymorphisms were discovered by the incidental observation that some patients or volunteers experienced unpleasant and disturbing adverse effects when standard recommended doses of these drugs were administered (e.g., debrisoquine/sparteine, mephenytoin, tolbutamide, isoniazid, fluorouracil). In addition to the polymorphisms listed in Table 22-1 genetic polymorphisms are known for the hydrolysis of paraoxon (Mueller et al. 1983) and the *N*-glucosidation of amobarbital (Tang et al. 1983; Tang 1990); the clinical relevance of these deficiencies for drug therapy, however, is probably small. Genetic polymorphisms have also been demonstrated for catechol *O*-methyltransferase (Lachmann et al. 1996), sulfotransferases (Raftogianis et al. 1997), histamine *N*-methyltransferase (Preuss et al. 1998), flavin-containing monooxygenases (Dolphin et al. 1997), and UGT-glucuronosyltransferases (Ciotti et al. 1997), as well as for several cytochromes P450 other than CYP2D6, CYP2C9, and CYP2C19 (e.g., CYP2A6 and CYP2E1) (for a review, see Daly et al. 1995). However, neither the genotype/phenotype relationship nor the association of these polymorphisms with adverse effects have been conclusively established.

**Table 22-1 Genetic Polymorphisms of Drug-Metabolizing Enzymes**

| Designation | Archetypal Examples | Other Drug Substrates | Poor Metabolizers (%) | Enzyme Involved | Study |
|---|---|---|---|---|---|
| Debrisoquine-sparteine polymorphism | Debrisoquine, sparteine, bufuralol, dextromethorphan | $\beta$-Adrenoceptor antagonists, antiarrhythmics, antidepressants, opioids, neuroleptics, etc. | Caucasians 5–10<br>Asians ~1 | CYP2D6 | Mahgoub et al. 1977; Eichelbaum et al. 1979 |
| Mephenytoin polymorphism | Mephenytoin | Mephobarbital, hexobarbital, diazepam, omeprazole, proguanil, etc. | Caucasians 3–5<br>Asians 15–20 | CYP2C19 | Küpfer and Preisig 1984 |
| Tolbutamide polymorphism | Tolbutamide, (*S*)-warfarin, phenytoin | | Caucasians $< 1$ | CYP2C9 | Miners et al. 1985; Sullivan-Klose et al. 1996 |
| Acetylation polymorphism | Isoniazid, sulfadiazine | Isoniazid, hydralazine, procainamide, sulfamethazine, sulfapyridine, amonafide | Caucasians 40–70<br>Asians 10–20 | *N*-Acetyltransferase (NAT2) | Hughes et al. 1954 |
| Thiopurine methyltransferase (TPMT) polymorphism | 6-Mercaptopurine, 6-thioguanine | | Caucasians 0.3 | Thiopurine *S*-methyltransferase | Weinshilboum and Sladek 1980 |
| Dihydropyrimidine dehydrogenase (DPD) polymorphism | Fluorouracil (5-FU) | | Caucasians 0.1 | Dihydropyrimide dehydrogenase | Diasio et al. 1988 |

**Table 22-2 Determinants of Clinical Relevance of Genetic Polymorphisms of Drug-Metabolizing Enzymes**

| |
|---|
| Quantitative role of enzyme in drug disposition |
| Active metabolites |
| Therapeutic index, concentration–response relationship |
| Pharmacokinetic variability unrelated to polymorphic variation (induction, inhibition, interactions, disease, etc.) |
| Feasibility of clinical dose titration |

***What makes a polymorphism clinically relevant***

Whether a polymorphism has relevance in therapeutic decision making mainly depends on the characteristics of the drug that is metabolized by the polymorphic enzyme (Tables 22-2 and 22-3). First, the quantitative role of the polymorphic enzyme in the overall elimination of the drug has to be assessed. The polymorphic pathway may result in a major difference in the clearance of the drug in the two extreme phenotypes or may produce only marginal overall phenotypic differences. Thus, 6- to 7-fold differences in clearance of desipramine from total plasma are observed between EMs and PMs (Brosen et al. 1986) and perphenazine (Dahl-Puustinen et al. 1989), whereas the 4-hydroxylation of propranolol by CYP2D6 is only a minor pathway for its overall metabolism (Ward et al. 1989). Second, the formation and elimination of an active metabolite via the polymorphic enzyme and its potency in relation to the parent drug have to be considered (e.g., as with encainide and propafenone; see the section "Clinical Consequeneces of Debrisoquine/Sparteine Polymorphism"). Third, pharmacokinetic differences between phenotypes are only relevant if the drug in question has a narrow therapeutic range, that is, a small therapeutic index. For many $\beta$-adrenergic receptor antagonists, plasma concentrations that are considerably greater than ideal therapeutic concentrations may not result in markedly increased subjective or objective effects. Fourth, pharmacokinetic variability unrelated to genetic polymorphism as caused by drug interactions, induction by environmental or nutritional effects, and disease-induced changes have to be taken into account. Fifth, an important issue is whether the dose is individually adjusted on the basis of evaluation of the clinical effect. For example, dose adjustments on the basis of effectiveness or adverse effects are routinely made for some antihypertensive drugs. Interphenotypic differences in pharmacokinetics are thereby automatically corrected by the physician, generally without his or her recognition that the reason may be genetic variation.

These considerations clearly indicate that the drug-related criteria that make a genetic polymorphism relevant are similar to those for monitoring drug concentrations (see the Introduction and Chapter 23). Indeed, genetic polymorphism of drug metabolism can be considered a

**Table 22-3 Pharmacokinetic and Clinical Consequences of Polymorphic Drug Metabolism in Poor, Extensive, and Ultrarapid Metabolizers of Debrisoquine/Sparteine**

| Pharmacokinetic Consequences | | | |
|---|---|---|---|
| Poor Metabolizers | Extensive and Ultrarapid Metabolizers | Clinical Consequences | Examples |
| Reduced first-pass metabolism, increased oral bioavailability, and elevated plasma levels | | Exaggerated drug response, potential drug toxicity | Metoprolol, encainide (CYP2D6) |
| Reduced overall metabolic clearance, prolonged half-life, drug accumulation | | Prolonged drug effect, drug toxicity, exaggerated drug response | Perhexiline, thioridazine (CYP2D6), isoniazid, sulfapyridine (NAT2) |
| Alternative pathway of metabolism | | Formation of toxic metabolites, immunotoxicity | Sulfonamides (NAT2) |
| Failure to generate active metabolite | | Altered concentration/effect relationship between EM and PM | Encainide, propafenone, codeine (analgesic effect) (CYP2D6) |
| | Multiple substrates and inhibitors competing at active site of enzyme | Drug interactions with substrates of polymorphic enzyme | Quinidine, propafenone, flecainide, metoprolol, etc. (CYP2D6) |
| | Ultrarapid metabolism of parent compound | Therapeutic failure | Tricyclic antidepressants (CYP2D6) |

special form of interindividual variability in which a single phenotyping or genotyping test can identify the predisposition of patients at the extremes. The general relevance of polymorphic metabolism is also dependent on whether the drug in question is widely used by many physicians (e.g., codeine, tricyclic antidepressants) or if it is only occasionally used by a well-informed clinical specialist (e.g., perhexiline, amonafide).

Case studies have emphasized the therapeutic importance of recognizing the PM phenotype for many drugs. Although a PM patient may be at higher risk to develop an adverse drug reaction, an EM or an ultrarapidly metabolizing patient may not respond to standard doses because of his or her highly efficient metabolism of the active drug (Dalén et al. 1998). Patients who require relatively large doses of tricyclic antidepressants to achieve concentrations considered therapeutic have been described (Bertilsson et al. 1985). If adverse reactions to a drug are not caused by the parent drug but by a metabolite, then an EM phenotype may be predisposed to such reactions, as has been postulated for the proarrhythmic effect of encainide (Buchert and Woosley 1992). An EM phenotype may also confer a higher risk for developing drug–drug interactions as exemplified by numerous drugs as substrates and inhibitors of CYP2D6, the target of debrisoquine/sparteine polymorphism (Tables 22-4 and 22-5).

**PRINCIPLE The clinical relevance of a genetic polymorphism of drug metabolism depends on the relative importance of the affected metabolic pathway to the overall elimination of the drug, on the therapeutic index of the drug, and on the question of whether the variability in drug response can be easily monitored in the clinical setting. The identification of patients at the extremes of variation (e.g., ultrarapid metabolizers, slow metabolizers) before treatment can serve to predict dose requirements and prevent therapeutic failure or toxicity.**

The sometimes-voiced opinion that genetic polymorphisms of drug metabolism are of little or no clinical relevance is mostly due to the fact that many physicians are not aware of this source of variation and are reluctant to accept that, for certain drugs, genetic factors are important and should be considered when dosage is chosen. The lack of large prospective studies to evaluate the impact of genetic variation is another reason for the slow acceptance of these principles. Discussion of polymorphic metabolism and its consequences has been increasingly included in product or drug data sheets. This information provides official guidance for off-setting the consequences of genetic variation and prevents undertreatment of EMs and overtreatment of PMs.

## Debrisoquine/Sparteine (CYP2D6) Polymorphism

### *Discovery, incidence, and molecular aspects*

The existence of a genetic polymorphism causing variable metabolism of the two drugs debrisoquine and sparteine was discovered in independent studies in England and Germany (Mahgoub et al. 1977; Eichelbaum et al. 1979). The 4-hydroxylation of debrisoquine and the formation of 1- and 5-dehydrosparteine from sparteine were found to be impaired or nearly absent in 5–10% of Europeans and North Americans. The incidence of PMs among Europeans is 7.7% ± 2.2% (M ± SD) in a total of 5005 persons tested (Alvan et al. 1990). The frequency of the PM phenotype appears to be similar in other Caucasian populations but is markedly lower (approximately 1–2%) in Asians (Evans 1993; Meyer and Zanger 1997), and variable in African populations (Masimirembwa et al. 1993; Aklillu et al. 1996).

The clinical importance of this polymorphism—which is also known as *CY2D6 polymorphism*—was initially questioned because the drugs leading to its discovery were soon either obsolete or infrequently prescribed. However, it soon became known that many other drugs are inefficiently metabolized in PM subjects, including important antiarrhythmics (e.g., *N*-propylajmaline, flecainide, propafenone, mexiletine), antidepressants (e.g., imipramine, nortriptyline, desipramine, clomipramine, fluoxetine, paroxetine), neuroleptics (e.g., perphenazine, zuclopenthixol, thioridazine), antianginals (e.g., perhexiline), and opioids (e.g., dextromethorphan, codeine). Moreover, a large number of $\beta$-adrenergic receptor antagonists (e.g., metoprolol, timolol) are influenced in their elimination by this polymorphism. Table 22-4 provides a list of drugs that are metabolically affected by CYP2D6 polymorphism. The impact of CYP2D6 polymorphism on the pharmacokinetics of some of these drugs and on drug development has been reviewed (e.g., Eichelbaum and Gross 1990; Kalow 1992; Buchert and Woosley 1992; Brosen 1993; Dahl and Bertilsson 1993; Evans 1993; Kroemer and Eichelbaum 1995; Nebert 1997; Marshall 1997a, 1997b).

The PM phenotype for debrisoquine/sparteine polymorphism is inherited as an autosomal recessive trait, which means that the PMs are homozygous for an autosomal recessive gene. Studies have revealed that this gene

Table 22-4 **Drugs Metabolized by CYP2D6**[a]

| SUBSTRATE | STUDY | SUBSTRATE | STUDY |
|---|---|---|---|
| Alprenolol | Alvan et al. 1982 | Methoxyamphetamine | Kitchen et al. 1979 |
| Amiflamine | Alvan et al. 1984 | Methoxyphenamine | Roy et al. 1985 |
| Amitriptyline | Balant-Gorgia et al. 1982 | Methylenedioxymethamphetamine | Tucker et al. 1994 |
| Aprindine | Ebner and Eichelbaum 1993 | Metoprolol | Lennard et al. 1982; McGourty et al. 1985 |
| Brofaromine | Feifel et al. 1993; Jedrychowski et al. 1993 | Mexiletine | Turgeon et al. 1991 |
| Bufuralol | Dayer et al. 1986 | Mianserin | Dahl et al. 1994; Koyama et al. 1996[a] |
| Bunitrolol | Narimatsu et al. 1994 | Minaprine | Davi et al. 1992 |
| Bupranolol | Pressacco et al. 1993 | Nicergoline | Böttiger et al. 1996 |
| Carvedilol | Zhou and Wood 1995 | Norcodeine | Mikus et al. 1990 |
| Cinnarizine | Narimatsu et al. 1993 | Nortriptyline | Mellström et al. 1981 |
| Clomipramine | Balant-Gorgia et al. 1986 | *N*-Propylajmaline | Zekorn et al. 1985 |
| Codeine | Dayer et al. 1988 | Ondansetron | Fischer et al. 1994 |
| Debrisoquine | Mahgoub et al. 1977; Tucker et al. 1977 | Oxycodone | Otton et al. 1993 |
| Desipramine | Brosen and Gram 1988 | Paroxetine | Sindrup et al. 1992 |
| Desmethylcitalopram[b] | Sindrup et al. 1993 | Perhexiline | Cooper et al. 1984 |
| Dexfenfluramine | Gross et al. 1996 | Perphenazine | Dahl-Puustinen et al. 1989 |
| Dextromethorphan | Schmid et al. 1985 | Phenformin | Oates et al. 1982 |
| Dihydrocodeine | Fromm et al. 1995 | Promethazine | Nakamura et al. 1996 |
| Dolasetron | Sanwald et al. 1996 | Propafenone | Siddoway et al. 1987 |
| Encainide | Wang et al. 1984 | Propranolol | Raghuram et al. 1984 |
| Ethylmorphine | Rane et al. 1992 | Risperidone | Huang et al. 1993 |
| Flecainide | Beckmann et al. 1988 | Sparteine | Eichelbaum et al. 1979 |
| Flunarizine | Narimatsu et al. 1993 | Tamoxifen | Dehal and Kupfer et al. 1997 |
| Fluoxetine | Hamelin et al. 1996 | Thioridazine | von Bahr et al. 1991 |
| Fluvoxamine | Carrillo et al. 1996 | Timolol | Lewis et al. 1985 |
| Guanoxan | Sloan et al. 1978 | Tolferodine | Brynne et al. 1998 |
| Halofantrine | Halliday et al. 1995 | Tomoxetine | Feher et al. 1988 |
| Haloperidol | Llerena et al. 1992 | Tramadol | Poulsen et al. 1996 |
| Hydrocodone | Otton et al. 1993 | Tropisetron | Fischer et al. 1994 |
| Imipramine | Brosen and Gram 1988 | Venlafaxine | Otton et al. 1996 |
| Indoramin | Pierce et al. 1987 | Zuclopenthixol | Dahl et al. 1991 |
| Maprotiline | Firkusny and Gleiter 1994 | | |

[a]For some of these drugs, the contribution of CYP2D6 to the metabolism is only minor, and for some the clinical relevance of the CYP2D6 polymorphism is questionable or dependent on additional variables (e.g., other drugs, disease). For details, see text.
[b]Metabolite of citalopram.

codes for a cytochrome P450 isozyme, namely, CYP2D6, and that this enzyme is absent in the liver of most PMs (for a review, see Meyer and Zanger 1997). The CYP2D6 cDNA and gene (*CYP2D6*) have been characterized (Gonzalez et al. 1988; Kimura et al. 1989; Heim and Meyer 1992), and mutant alleles of the *CYP2D6* gene related to the PM phenotype have been studied in numerous laboratories over the last 10 years (for reviews, see Skoda et al. 1988; Marez et al. 1997; Meyer and Zanger 1997; Sachse et al. 1997). These studies identified the primary mutations (occurring singly or in combinations) that cause either null alleles (resulting in absent CYP2D6 enzyme or total loss of activity) or decreased-function alleles (with only a partial decrease in enzyme function); some of these studies also described additional alleles coding for normal function. A PM individual carries two detrimental CYP2D6 null alleles, whereas an EM individual is homozygous or heterozygous for normal-function alleles. More recently, ultrarapid metabolism of CYP2D6 substrates—which was originally observed in a woman with

Table 22-5 Selected in Vivo Inhibitors of Human CYP2D6

| INHIBITOR | SUBSTRATE OF CYP2D6 WITH INHIBITED METABOLISM | STUDY |
|---|---|---|
| Quinidine | Metoprolol | Leeman et al. 1986 |
| | Desipramine | Steiner et al. 1988 |
| | Codeine | Desmeules et al. 1989 |
| Flecainide | Dextromethorphan | Haefeli et al. 1990 |
| Chlorpromazine | Nortriptyline | Gram and Overo 1972 |
| Haloperidol | Imipramine | Gram et al. 1989 |
| Thioridazine | Desipramine | Hirschowitz et al. 1983 |
| Citalopram | Desipramine | Gram et al. 1993 |
| Fluoxetine | Desipramine | Bergstrom et al. 1992 |
| | Nortriptyline | Bergstrom et al. 1992 |
| | Imipramine | Bergstrom et al. 1992 |
| | Dextromethorphan | Otton et al. 1993 |
| Fluvoxamine | Nortriptyline | Bertschy et al. 1991 |
| | *N*-Desmethyl-clomipramine | Bertschy et al. 1991 |
| | Desipramine | Spina et al. 1993 |
| Paroxetine | Desipramine | Brosen 1993 |
| Sertraline | Desipramine | Preskorn et al. 1992 |

depression who needed 300–500 mg of nortriptyline per day to reach therapeutic plasma levels (Bertilsson et al. 1985)—was explained when duplicated or multiduplicated *CYP2D6* genes on chromosome 22 were identified (Johansson et al. 1993).

The unraveling of the complex and highly variable CYP2D6 cluster of genes and pseudogenes on chromosome 22 (Heim and Meyer 1992) has resulted in the characterization of a total of 48 mutations and over 50 alleles of the *CYP2D6* gene (Daly et al. 1996; Marez et al. 1997; Sachse et al. 1997). The population frequency of mutant alleles and duplicated genes is dependent on ethnicity (Bertilsson et al. 1995). As with most human DNA polymorphisms, three to five alleles account for over 90% of PM phenotypes, and other mutations and alleles are exceedingly rare. In a recent study in 589 Caucasian volunteers, four mutations corresponding to four alleles (CYP2D6*3, *4, *5, *6) and the gene duplication test predicted the clinical CYP2D6 capacity to metabolize drugs in all volunteers (Marez et al. 1997; Sachse et al. 1997). In the future, these mutations may be most efficiently analyzed by oligonucleotide array chip technology. A "cytochrome P450 chip" with the common mutations of the *CYP2D6* gene is now commercially available. This approach may replace or complement the presently used phenotype determination by the administration of test drugs such as debrisoquine/sparteine or dextromethorphan, followed by collection of urine and determination of the ratio between parent drug and its metabolite(s). A PM individual is defined by these tests as one in whom the urinary metabolic ratio (MR) is $> 20$ for sparteine (Eichelbaum et al. 1986), $> 12.6$ for debrisoquine (Evans et al. 1980), or $> 0.3$ for dextromethorphan (Schmid 1985). Among EM individuals, the MR for debrisoquine varies up to 1000-fold, from as low as 0.01 up to the antimode of 12.6. The terms *intermediate metabolizer* and *ultrarapid metabolizer* are used for individuals with MRs of 1–12.6 and $> 0.1$, respectively. The phenotyping of urinary MR has limitations because of adverse drug reactions, drug–drug interactions, and the confounding effects of liver and kidney disease. An alternative to phenotyping tests is to monitor plasma concentration for adjustment of individual dosage. There are limitations also to genotyping, however, because these DNA tests only define the group (e.g., PM, EM, ultrarapid metabolizer) to which the patient can be assigned and not the actual capacity for metabolism. But DNA tests have the advantage of having to be done only once in the patient's lifetime. A combination of genotyping and phenotyping tests provides the most information in a clinical setting; and once a genetic polymorphism is detected, it can be compensated for throughout an individual's lifetime.

#### *Clinical consequences of debrisoquine/sparteine (CYP2D6) polymorphism*

For some of the numerous substrates of cytochrome CYP2D6 (see Table 22-4), the polymorphic oxidation has therapeutic consequences (see Tables 22-3 and 22-5). The list of cytochrome CYP2D6 substrates includes antiarrhythmics, antidepressants, neuroleptics, opioids, and other drugs. For these drugs, knowledge of the phenotype can help markedly to forecast the individual dose range required for optimal therapy.

**ANTIARRHYTHMIC DRUGS** For most antiarrhythmic drugs, a relationship between the suppression of arrhythmias and concentration of drug in plasma has been established (see the section on arrhythmia in chapter 1). A serious problem is the adverse proarrhythmic effect that occurs more frequently at high concentrations of either parent drug or active metabolites. The metabolism of several antiarrhythmic and antianginal drugs co-segregates with debrisoquine/sparteine polymorphism, notably the metabolism of flecainide, encainide, propafenone, mexiletine, *N*-propylajmaline, and perhexiline.

**FLECAINIDE** Data from the multicenter Cardiac Arrhythmia Suppression Trial (CAST) demonstrated an excess mortality among patients with nonsustained ventricular arrhythmias who were treated with encainide and flecainide after myocardial infarction [The Cardiac Arrhythmia Suppression Trial (CAST) Investigators]. The polymorphic metabolism of these drugs was unfortunately not considered in the interpretation of these results. This deficiency may have major consequences in the future use of these agents. Elimination of flecainide is dependent on both hepatic metabolism and renal excretion. Pronounced differences in plasma half-life and metabolic clearance between EM and PM individuals have been observed (Mikus et al. 1989; Funck-Bretano et al. 1994). The implications are that plasma steady-state concentrations of flecainide are achieved after 4 days of therapy (e.g., on 100 mg flecainide t.i.d.) in PMs. For EMs, however, plasma steady-state concentrations are achieved after only 2 days of therapy. On the other hand, concentrations of flecainide in serum reach therapeutic ranges more rapidly in PMs. However, in PM subjects with normal renal function and urinary pH, the mean steady-state concentration of flecainide may still be within the therapeutic range (Gross et al. 1991; Funck-Bretano et al. 1994).

These data were gathered in healthy young volunteers, whereas most of the patients who receive antiarrhythmic treatment are older adults. As renal function diminishes with age, the contribution of metabolism to overall elimination of flecainide is expected to progressively increase. Older adult PMs and those with other causes of impaired renal function are thus at greater risk of developing flecainide toxicity because decreased renal clearance magnifies the effect of "poor" metabolism, leading to potentially dangerous accumulation of the drug. Phenotyping or genotyping patients with renal disease for the debrisoquine/sparteine polymorphism prior to initiating flecainide therapy would alert the physician to the need for reducing the dosage even further than anticipated on the basis of creatinine clearance. This may then prevent some of the fatal sustained ventricular tachycardias that are reported to be associated predominantly with excessively high flecainide concentrations in plasma (Evers 1994).

**PRINCIPLE When drug toxicity mimics the indication for the drug, then the physician must have some way to distinguish between causes of inadequate dosage and too great a dose. When low doses are being used and mechanisms of undue accumulation are not considered, the physician will most likely blame the disease and not the drug for the untoward effect.**

**ENCAINIDE** Polymorphic hepatic metabolism and the subsequent variable production of a highly active (and potentially toxic) metabolite must also be considered in the interpretation of the dose–response relationship with this agent (for a review, see Woosley et al. 1988). PMs form only trace amounts of the active metabolite *O*-desmethylencainide (ODE), which is further metabolized to 3-methoxy-*O*-desmethylencainide (MODE), also an active antiarrhythmic agent. As a consequence, during chronic therapy, the concentrations of encainide in plasma observed in PMs are far greater than those observed in EMs. However, these high concentrations of parent drug are associated with an adequate therapeutic response and also are apparently not associated with a higher incidence of adverse effects in PM patients. This has to be realized when interpreting concentrations of a drug in plasma for therapeutic monitoring. Encainide provides an example of a drug for which in PMs high concentrations of parent drug are required to achieve the required response, whereas in EMs the active metabolites are the major determinants of efficacy and toxicity (Buchert and Woosley 1992) (see previous "Principle").

**PROPAFENONE** Propafenone is metabolized in the liver to the active metabolites 5-hydroxypropafenone and *N*-desalkylpropafenone. Formation of 5-hydroxypropafenone is markedly impaired in PMs, resulting in very low or absent concentrations of this active metabolite (for a review, see Funck-Brentano et al. 1990). EMs exhibit a substantial first-pass hepatic metabolism, whereas PMs have a marked decrease in presystemic elimination with consequent higher oral bioavailability and a very prolonged elimination half-life (12–32 vs. 2–10 hours). The dose required to suppress arrhythmias is similar in patients of the two phenotypes because the decreased formation of 5-hydroxypropafenone in PMs is compensated by increased propafenone concentrations. However, the incidence of central nervous system (CNS) adverse effects (visual blurring, dizziness) is significantly higher in PM patients. Propafenone is administered as a racemate, and both enantiomers have similar activity at sodium channels. However, the *S* enantiomer has weak $\beta$-adrenergic antagonist properties. $\beta$-Adrenergic blockade was observed in both phenotypes, but it was more pronounced in PMs (Lee et al. 1990). This presumably accounts for the striking increase in CNS adverse effects in PMs. Moreover, in PM patients with compromised cardiac function, $\beta$-adrenergic blockade can be either life-threatening or life-extending.

**PRINCIPLE It is becoming increasingly apparent that assessment of a patient's pharmacogenetic status before administering drugs with multiple mechanisms of efficacy or toxicity is imperative.**

**OTHER ANTIARRHYTHMIC OR ANTIANGINAL DRUGS** The metabolism of *N*-propylajmalin (Zekorn et al. 1985), perhexiline (Cooper et al. 1984), and mexiletine (Broly et al. 1990) also co-segregates with the metabolism of debrisoquine/sparteine. PMs appear to have a higher incidence of adverse drug reactions than do EMs with mexiletine (Lledo et al. 1993), and patients developing peripheral neuropathy or hepatotoxicity on antianginal therapy with perhexiline predominantly are of the PM phenotype (Shah et al. 1982). One of the reasons that this drug is no longer generally used (except in Australia) is because of this problem. The polymorphic metabolism of *N*-propylajmaline also results in marked interphenotype differences (Zekorn et al. 1985; Mörike et al. 1990), which explains the different doses required for antiarrhythmic therapy.

**$\beta$-ADRENERGIC ANTAGONISTS** A number of drugs in this group are subject to polymorphic metabolism of the debrisoquine/sparteine type. This topic has been reviewed (Lennard et al. 1989). Phenotypic differences are documented in particular for metoprolol and timolol, with which the PM phenotype is associated with increased drug concentrations in plasma, a prolongation of elimination half-life, and more sustained $\beta$-adrenergic antagonism (Lennard et al. 1989; Laurent-Kenesi et al. 1993; Edeki et al. 1995). Only a minor pathway of the metabolism of propranolol, that is, 4-hydroxylation, appears to be affected, and no small differences in disposition between the two phenotypes are observed for propranolol. Topical ophthalmic administration of (*S*)-timolol to lower intraocular pressure may result in systemic $\beta$-adrenergic blockade. Indeed severe reactions including bronchospasm and adverse cardiovascular effects—in some cases leading to death—have been attributed to ophthalmic applications of timolol (Nelson et al. 1986). Carvedilol is a mixed $\alpha$- and $\beta$-adrenergic receptor antagonist administered as a racemic mixture. EMs have a decreased clearance of its *R* enantiomer compared with PMs, and this may result in greater $\alpha$-adrenergic receptor blockade (Zhou and Wood 1995).

$\beta$-Adrenergic receptor antagonists have a relatively large therapeutic index, and the dose is frequently adjusted individually according to clinical signs of $\beta$-adrenergic receptor antagonism. This should compensate for the kinetic effects of the PM phenotype. Nevertheless, a considerable portion of patients have unpleasant effects from these drugs. A prospective study to assess polymorphic metabolism with long-term treatment is warranted.

**ANTIPSYCHOTIC AGENTS** The first-pass metabolism of a number of neuroleptic drugs co-segregates with that of debrisoquine/sparteine. Several of these agents were first found to be competitive in vivo inhibitors of CYP2D6 in human liver microsomes (see Table 22-5) (Otton et al. 1984; Fonne-Pfister and Meyer 1988). Moreover, the urinary MR of debrisoquine/sparteine was markedly increased during neuroleptic therapy (Syvählahti et al. 1986; Gram et al. 1989). Perphenazine (Dahl-Puustinen et al. 1989; Jerling et al. 1996), thioridazine (von Bahr et al. 1989), and haloperidol (Llerena et al. 1992; Suzuki et al. 1997) are polymorphically metabolized. The studies with haloperidol also suggest that the higher concentrations in plasma of reduced haloperidol in PMs may be a contributory factor for the development of extrapyramidal adverse effects. Impaired first-pass metabolism and decreased oral clearance in PMs has also been observed with zyclopenthixol and risperidone (Jerling et al. 1996), whereas the disposition of clozapine apparently is not affected by this polymorphism (Arranz et al. 1995). The potential of these drugs to cause interactions with other substrates of CYP2D6, particularly tricyclic antidepressants, has been known for a long time. Table 22-5 lists some of the known interactions of chlorpromazine, haloperidol, and thioridazine with substrates of CYP2D6.

**ANTIDEPRESSANTS** Great interindividual variation in plasma concentrations of antidepressants is well known

(Sjöqvist 1992). The metabolism of the tricyclic antidepressants amitriptyline, clomipramine, desipramine, imipramine, and nortriptyline, and the tetracyclic compounds maprotiline and mianserin, is influenced by debrisoquine/sparteine polymorphism to various degrees (Brosen and Gram 1989; Cohen and DeVane 1996; Bertilsson et al. 1997). For these agents, there are clearly two patient groups for which clinical problems may be prominent. The PMs (and to a lesser degree the intermediate metabolizers) have predictably increased plasma concentrations while taking recommended doses of tricyclic antidepressants (Spina et al. 1997). The other group is the ultrarapid metabolizers, who are prone to therapeutic failures because the drug concentrations at normal doses are by far too low (Dalén et al. 1998). At least 20–30% of patients belong to these two risk groups. Adverse effects clearly occur more frequently in PMs (Spina et al. 1992; Chen et al. 1996) and may be one of the causes of poor compliance. Moreover, toxic reactions may be misinterpreted as symptoms of depression and lead to erroneous further increases in the dose. Prospective trials are obviously needed to prove the value of phenotyping or genotyping in depressed patients in selecting the proper starting dose to increase therapeutic efficacy and prevent toxicity. But the results of retrospective analysis of adverse drug reactions in psychiatric patients (Chen et al. 1996) already strongly indicate that drug monitoring, phenotyping, and genotyping can improve therapy with antidepressants. An expert group came to the same conclusions and recommendations (Meyer et al. 1996). These concepts have been reviewed (e.g., Brosen and Gram 1989; Sjöqvist 1992; Cohen and DeVane 1996; Bertilsson et al. 1997), but so far the research results have had surprisingly little impact on psychiatric practice.

Selective serotonin reuptake inhibitors (SSRIs) interact with CYP2D6 in three different modes. Paroxetine, fluvoxamine, and fluoxetine are metabolized by CYP2D6 (Brosen 1993; Spigset 1997; Carrillo et al. 1996; Hamelin et al. 1996) and to a small degree, also citalopram. However, the phenotypic differences in clearance or plasma concentrations are small in relation to the relatively large therapeutic index of these drugs. Of considerable importance is the effect of these agents as potent competitive inhibitors of CYP2D6 (e.g., paroxetine, fluoxetine) with the consequence that the elimination of other CYP2D6 substrates (e.g., of tricyclic antidepressants) is markedly impaired (see Table 22-5) (Brosen 1993; Bertilsson et al. 1997) and that phenotyping with debrisoquine, sparteine, or dextromethorphan produces false positive results or "phenocopies" of PMs, if SSRIs are coadministered. These interactions are phenotype-dependent (i.e., restricted to EMs). Citalopram, fluvoxamine, and sertraline do not share this inhibitory property and do not cause CYP2D6-specific interactions. Fluvoxamine is also a substrate and potent inhibitor of CYP1A2 that causes important interactions with drugs that are metabolized in part by this cytochrome P450, such as amitriptyline, clomipramine, imipramine, clozapine, and theophylline (Brosen 1993; Jerling et al. 1994).

The third consideration is that the small concentration of CYP2D6 in the liver causes saturation kinetics, which decreases the difference in clearance between EM and PM phenotypes. Little is known of the stereoselective metabolism by CYP2D6 and other enzymes of the SSRIs given as racemic mixtures (e.g., fluoxetine, citalopram). Venlafaxine is an SSRI that also inhibits the uptake of noradrenaline and dopamine. In vitro experiments suggest its dependence on CYP2D6 for metabolism and relatively limited potency as a competitive inhibitor (Otten 1996; Ball et al. 1997). The reversible selective monoamine oxidase A (MAO-A) inhibitor moclobemide is a relatively weak competitive in vivo inhibitor of CYP2D6, but it clearly has an effect on the in vivo urinary sparteine MR at therapeutic doses. It is metabolized by CYP2C19 and not by CYP2D6 (Gram et al. 1995) in contrast to the MAO-A inhibitor brofaromine, which also seems to be metabolized by CYP2D6 to some extent.

**OPIOIDS** Dextromethorphan, codeine, hydrocodone, oxycodone, ethylmorphine, and dihydrocodeine are dealkylated by polymorphic CYP2D6 (Schmid et al. 1985; Dayer et al. 1988; Fromm et al. 1995). Although dextromethorphan has few adverse effects and little addiction potential, the clinical significance of its longer half-life and higher plasma concentration in PMs has not been established. In fact, because of its worldwide availability and safety, it is recommended as a test compound to phenotype for debrisoquine/sparteine polymorphism.

The polymorphic *O*-demethylation of codeine is, however, of clinical importance when this drug is given as an analgesic. Approximately 10% of codeine is *O*-demethylated to morphine, and it is this pathway that is deficient in PMs. Urinary excretion of morphine and morphine-6-glucuronide is markedly lowered in PMs after treatment with codeine (Yue et al. 1991). Because the analgesic effect of codeine is dependent on its transformation to morphine and morphine-6-glucuronide, PMs experience no analgesic effect (Sindrup and Brosen 1995) (see also chapter 15). Respiratory, psychomotor, and pupillary effects of codeine are similarly decreased in PMs compared with EMs (Caraco et al. 1996). Therefore, it is expected that competitive inhibitors of CYP2D6 such as quinidine given concomitantly with codeine in EMs abolish the analgesic effect. Codeine is frequently recommended as a drug of first choice for treatment of chronic severe pain. The physician must appreciate that no analgesic effect is to be expected in the 5–10% of Caucasians who are of the PM phenotype (Persson et al. 1995) or who are EMs and receive concomitant treatment with a potent inhibitor of CYP2D6 (see Table 22-5). In summary, the pharmacogenetic control of opioid metabolism undoubtedly contributes to interpatient variability in the analgesic clinical response to these drugs. Moreover, a recent study suggests that the failure to metabolize some opioids to active metabolites may protect PMs against oral opiate dependence (Tyndale et al. 1997).

**OTHER DRUGS** The metabolism of the serotonin antagonist tropisetron is catalyzed by CYP2D6, but this enzyme contributes only to a minor extent to the disposition of ondansetron or dolasetron (De Bruijn 1992). The clinical relevance of the polymorphic disposition of tropisetron is questionable because of the large therapeutic index of this drug.

**DRUG–DRUG INTERACTIONS** The demonstration of competitive and noncompetitive inhibition by co-substrates and specific other drugs of CYP2D6 in human liver microsomes has opened a rational approach to predicting drug–drug interactions (Fonne-Pfister and Meyer 1988; Brosen 1990). Several of these interactions have subsequently been shown to occur in vivo at therapeutic doses of these agents (see Table 22-5). Thus, the strong in vitro inhibitors quinidine, propafenone, fluphenazine, haloperidol, chlorpromazine, thioridazine, paroxetine, and fluoxetine have the potential to inhibit the metabolism of substrates of CYP2D6 in EMs. One of the clinically most relevant interactions is the inhibitory effect of neuroleptics on tricyclic antidepressants (Gram and Overo 1972; Brosen 1990). These types of interactions clearly are clinically important and also are a source of "phenocopies" (i.e., faulty interpretation of phenotyping tests).

SUMMARY

**The debrisoquine/sparteine polymorphism of drug metabolism is an important stable determinant of interindividual variation in the pharmacokinetics and effects of numerous clinically useful drugs. When the changes in pharmacokinetics are clinically relevant, a simple genotyping test, performed once in a patient's lifetime, can predict with > 95% accuracy whether the patient is a poor, extensive, or ultrarapid metabolizer phenotype. Alternatively, a phenotyping test can be performed in volunteers or patients before starting drug therapy. This knowledge should lead to a better selection of the initial dose, prevent overdosage in PMs, and treatment failures and interactions in EMs. This applies in particular to some antiarrhythmic drugs, phenothiazines, antidepressants, and codeine.**

## Mephenytoin (CYP2C19) Polymorphism

A genetic polymorphism of another cytochrome P450 isozyme was revealed by the discovery of deficient 4′-hydroxylation of mephenytoin, a now rarely used anticonvulsant drug, in a patient who experienced increased sedation after a standard dose of mephenytoin (Küpfer et al. 1984). The deficiency is restricted to one of the two major metabolic pathways of mephenytoin disposition, namely, stereoselective hydroxylation of (*S*)-mephenytoin in the *p*-phenyl position to 4′-OH-mephenytoin. The other main reaction—the *N*-demethylation of (*R*)-mephenytoin to 5-ethyl-5-phenylhydantoin—remains unaffected (Küpfer et al. 1984). This deficiency occurs with a frequency of 2.5 to 6% in Caucasians, but occurs with a much higher frequency (13–23%) in Asian populations and with an amazingly high incidence of PMs (71%) in the Vanuatu population in Melanesia (Kaneko et al. 1997) (for reviews, see Wilkinson et al. 1992; Goldstein and de Morais 1994; Brosen et al. 1995; Goldstein et al. 1997). The molecular mechanism of deficient mephenytoin hydroxylation has recently been clarified. Mutations in the gene for CYP2C19 cause a deficiency of the CYP2C19 enzyme in liver of PMs of mephenytoin (de Morais et al. 1994).

Two defective CYP2C19 alleles (CYP2C19*2 and CYP2C19*3) account for more than 99% of Asian PM alleles but only approximately 85% of Caucasian alleles. More recently, three additional rare alleles have been identified, which increase the percentage of identified PM alleles to almost 100% in Chinese and 90% in Caucasian PMs (Ibeanu et al. 1998). Additional mutant alleles in Caucasian populations are left to be characterized.

Individuals of the PM phenotype are predisposed to CNS adverse effects of mephenytoin (e.g., sedation after administration of a single dose of 100 mg for phenotyping purposes). Additional substrates for the enzyme metabolizing (*S*)-mephenytoin to 4′-OH-mephenytoin have been suspected by in vitro inhibition studies, and some of these have been confirmed by co-segregation in populations. Thus, the metabolism of the *N*-demethylated metabolite of mephenytoin (5-ethyl-5-phenylhydantoin), the metabolism of mephobarbital and hexobarbital, the side-chain oxidation of propranolol, and the metabolism of diazepam

Table 22-6 **Drugs Metabolized at Least Partially by CYP2CI9**

| | |
|---|---|
| Carisoprodol | (*S*)-Mephenytoin |
| Chloroguanyl | Mephobarbital |
| Citalopram | Moclobemide |
| Clomipramine | Omeprazole |
| Desmethyldiazepam | Pantoprazole |
| Diazepam | Phenytoin (minor pathway) |
| Hexobarbital | Proguanyl |
| Imipramine | Propranolol |
| Lansoprazole | (*R*)-Warfarin |

From reviews: Wilkinson et al. 1992; Evans 1993; Goldstein and de Morais 1994; Goldstein et al. 1997.

and desmethyldiazepam (Bertilsson et al. 1989) co-segregate with the 4′-hydroxylation of (*S*)-mephenytoin (for a review, see Goldstein and de Morais 1994) (see Table 22-6). The metabolism of the proton-pump inhibitor omeprazol (Andersson et al. 1990), the related lansoprazole and pantoprazole (Meyer 1996), and the antimalarial drugs proguanil and chlorproguanil co-segregate with polymorphic mephenytoin metabolism (Helsby et al. 1990).

The clinical consequences of impaired mephenytoin hydroxylation are less clear than those for CYP2D6 polymorphism. There is evidence that the frequency of adverse effects of mephobarbital and hexobarbital may be higher in PMs of mephenytoin (Küpfer et al. 1984). A decrease in the oral clearance of diazepam was described in Caucasian PMs after a single dose (Bertilsson et al. 1989). Several antidepressants are substrates of CYP2C19 (see Table 22-6), but in most cases, other cytochromes P450 (CYP2D6, CYP1A2, CYP3A4) are involved in their metabolism as well (Lemoine et al. 1993); and the interphenotype differences in pharmacokinetics are relatively small (30–40% of decrease in oral clearance), with the possible exception of imipramine and desipramine (Koyama et al. 1996b). Both citalopram and moclobemide are such drugs, and both also interact with CYP2D6, either as substrate (citalopram) or inhibitor (moclobemide). The metabolism of the proton-pump inhibitors omeprazole, lansoprazole, and pantoprazole is dependent on CYP2C19 and CYP3A enzymes. PMs of mephenytoin have markedly increased plasma half-lives and decreased clearances of these drugs. However, the wide range of concentrations consistent with efficacy obscures any clinical problems in PMs. The maintenance dose of these drugs probably can be lowered in more than 50% of Asians without decreasing efficacy.

It has to be realized that CYP2C19 polymorphism can be induced, for example, by rifampicin treatment (Zhou et al. 1990), is affected by liver disease, and is subject to interaction not only with co-substrates but also by a number of other drugs that can inhibit its activity in vitro and in vivo (Flockhart 1995). Thus, fluvoxamine and fluoxetine moderately inhibit CYP2C19 in vivo metabolism (Jeppesen et al. 1996). In summary, the clinical impact of the CYP2C19 polymorphism remains somewhat questionable but provocative and worthy of careful ongoing observation—with observation in this case meaning investigation of cause of any unexpected event while patients are taking these drugs.

**PRINCIPLE A physician cannot detect the unexpected unless he or she fully understands the expected effects of a drug.**

## Tolbutamide (CYP2C9) Polymorphism

CYP2C9 is another important drug-metabolizing enzyme and has a number of widely used drug substrates (Table 22-7). The polymorphism of the *CYP2C9* gene has recently been defined and produces enzymes that vary at two sites in their amino acid sequence, at positions 144 (Arg 144 Cys) and 359 (Ile 359 Leu) (for reviews, see Miners and Birkett 1998; Sullivan-Klose et al. 1996). Individuals who are homozygous for Leu 359 have markedly diminished clearances for most CYP2C9 substrates. The frequency of such individuals is estimated to be approximately 1 in 500 (Miners and Birkett 1998; Inaba 1990). One of these substrates is tolbutamide, of which approximately 85% of the clearance depends on CYP2C9. The possible genetic variation of tolbutamide metabolism was suspected in 1979 (Scott and Poffenbarger 1979), but only recently have detailed pharmacokinetic and molecular studies revealed the molecular nature of this polymorphism (Miners et al. 1985; Sullivan-Klose et al. 1996). An individual with only 20% of the plasma clearance of tolbutamide compared with the mean of the population was found to be homozygous for the recessive Leu 359 CYP2C19 allele (CYP2C9*3). Similarly, two individuals

Table 22-7 **Drugs Metabolized by CYP2C9**

| | |
|---|---|
| Amitriptyline | Seratrodest |
| Diclofenac | Suprofen |
| Fluoxetine | Tenoxicam |
| Losartan | $\Delta^9$-THC |
| Mefenamic acid | Tienilic acid |
| Naproxen | Tolbutamide |
| Phenytoin | (S)-Warfarin |
| Piroxicam | Torsemide |

From reviews: Hall 1994; Miners and Birkett 1998.
Abbreviation: THC, tetrahydrocannabinol.

identified as PMs of losartan were homozygous for the Leu 359 alleles (Spielberg et al. 1996). The expressed Leu 359 variant also showed markedly decreased intrinsic clearances ($V_{max}/k_m$) for (*S*)-warfarin and phenytoin. Thus, the available evidence indicates that the rare individuals who carry two copies of the Leu 359 allele are likely to have impaired clearances of losartan, phenytoin, tolbutamide, torsemide, (*S*)-warfarin, and possibly, other substrates of CYP2C9, with important consequences for dose adjustments as has been illustrated for warfarin (Steward et al. 1997).

The clinical consequences of expression of only one allele with either the Cys 144 or Leu 359 mutation are less obvious. Moreover, CYP2C9 polymorphism is inducible, notably by rifampicin, and many clinically significant drug interactions involving CYP2C9 substrates have been described. The extensive variability in CYP2C9 metabolism is the result of the interplay between environmental factors and genetic polymorphism and requires individualization of dosage for drugs with a narrow therapeutic index.

## *N*-Acetylation (NAT2) Polymorphism

### *Discovery, incidence, and molecular aspects*

The acetylation polymorphism probably is the best known classic example of a genetic defect in drug metabolism. It was discovered more than 25 years ago with the introduction of isoniazid therapy for tuberculosis (Bönicke and Reif 1953; Hughes et al. 1954). Patients could be classified as either *rapid* or *slow* eliminators (i.e., acetylators) of isoniazid, and family studies revealed that the ability to eliminate isoniazid was determined by two alleles at a single autosomal gene locus, with slow acetylators being homozygous for a recessive allele (Evans et al. 1960). The polymorphism of *N*-acetylation has been extensively reviewed (Weber 1987; Evans 1993; Vatsis and Weber 1994; Vatsis et al. 1995; Meyer and Zanger 1997).

The proportions of rapid and slow acetylators vary remarkably among populations of different ethnic and/or geographic origin. Among most European and North American populations, the prevalence of slow acetylators is 40–70%; whereas among certain Asian populations (e.g., Japanese, Chinese, Korean, Thai), the prevalence of slow acetylators is 10–30% (Evans 1993; Liu et al. 1994). Numerous subsequent studies have demonstrated that the acetylation polymorphism affects the metabolism of a variety of other arylamine and hydrazine drugs and numerous other chemicals. These include a number of sulfonamides (e.g., sulfadiazine, sulfamethazine, sulfapyridine, sulfameridine, sulfadoxine), numerous other drugs (e.g., aminoglutethimide, amonafide, amrinone, dapsone, dipyrone, endralazine, hydralazine, isoniazid, prizidilol, procainamide), and metabolites of clonazepam and caffeine. The polymorphism also involves the acetylation of the potential arylamine carcinogens benzidine, 2-aminofluorene, and $\beta$-naphthylamine. Initial phenotyping procedures with isoniazid were later replaced by testing with sulfamethazine or dapsone. A simple phenotyping procedure using caffeine as a test substance was later developed (Grant et al. 1984) and subsequently refined (Tang et al. 1987).

The molecular mechanism of polymorphic *N*-acetylation has only recently been studied. A cytosolic *N*-acetyltransferase (NAT2) was identified as the polymorphic enzyme in livers of rapid acetylators and was found to be markedly decreased (up to 10–20%) in livers of slow acetylators (Grant et al. 1990).

The NAT2 gene with its locus on chromosome 8 was established as the site of the isoniazid-type acetylation polymorphism (Blum et al. 1990, 1991). This was followed by intensive study in many laboratories of mutations and allelic variants of NAT2, and by last count, approximately 20 alleles each carrying one or a combination of up to three mutations have been identified (Vatsis et al. 1995; Agundez et al. 1996). In most populations studied, three to five major alleles account for greater than 90% of all slow acetylators, and simple genotyping tests for these alleles are available (Blum et al. 1991; Cascorbi et al. 1995; Agundez et al. 1996; Deloménie et al. 1996; Smith et al. 1997). A second cytosolic acetyltransferase, NAT1, shows selectivity for the metabolism of a number of other compounds such a *p*-aminosalicylic acid and *p*-aminobenzoic acid and is independent of the NAT2 polymorphism. It is also genetically variable (for a review, see Hughes et al 1998). Its role in the biotransformation of arylamine carcinogen is likely, but no clinically used drugs except *p*-aminosalicylic acid and *p*-aminobenzoic acid are known to be metabolized by NAT1.

### *Clinical importance of the N-acetylation (NAT2) polymorphism*

The acetylator polymorphism affects the efficacy and the occurrence of adverse effects for a number of drugs (for reviews, see Evans 1993; Spielberg et al. 1996). With isoniazid, hydralazine, salicylazosulfapyridine, and amonafide, adverse reactions are clearly associated with the acetylator phenotype. None of these create major clinical problems with current drug use, however, and the phenotyping test is rarely used in clinical practice.

**ISONIAZID PERIPHERAL NEUROPATHY** Patients who slowly inactivate isoniazid are more likely to accumulate isoniazid to toxic concentrations and to develop peripheral neuropathy (Hughes et al. 1954; Devadatta et al. 1960). Conversely, rapid acetylators of isoniazid or other drugs that are metabolized by the same enzyme might have to be given unusually high doses to reliably obtain efficacy. Because the neuropathy caused by isoniazid is regularly prevented by the common simultaneous prophylactic administration of pyridoxine (a drug that can be used safely in large amounts), choice of patients to prevent neuropathy does not necessarily require identification of the acetylator phenotype as long as pyridoxine is "routinely" coadministered with isoniazid.

**PHENYTOIN–ISONIAZID INTERACTION** Of greater clinical significance is the increased occurrence of serious phenytoin toxicity in slow acetylators of isoniazid when these drugs are given simultaneously (Kutt et al. 1970). Phenytoin toxicity is greater in the slowest acetylators who have the highest concentration of isoniazid in plasma. Isoniazid noncompetitively inhibits the microsomal $\rho$-hydroxylation of phenytoin. Although the exact mechanism of this inhibition and the consequent interaction of the two drugs remains obscure, it is clearly aggravated by slow acetylation. It thus represents an interesting but not surprising example of the role of genetic factors in the pathogenesis of a drug–drug interaction.

**ISONIAZID EFFICACY** It is interesting to note that despite altered pharmacokinetics of isoniazid, no significant phenotype difference in the clinical effectiveness of isoniazid has been identified. This is true with patients on long-term treatment with daily or twice-weekly doses of isoniazid. However, in all the once-weekly regimens, rapid acetylators respond less favorably than do slow acetylators (Madras 1970). Therefore, phenotyping before once-weekly regimens and consequent changes in dosage are recommended.

**ISONIAZID HEPATITIS** When isoniazid is given alone, slow acetylators are more prone to hepatotoxicity than are rapid acetylators (for a review, see Evans 1993). With treatments that contain both isoniazid and rifampicin, the incidence of hepatotoxicity is greater in slow acetylators in Caucasian populations; whereas in certain Asian populations, rapid acetylators more frequently develop biochemical signs of liver toxicity. The reasons for these differences are unclear.

**SULFONAMIDE HYPERSENSITIVITY** Sulfonamide hypersensitivity reactions are characterized by delayed onset of fever, skin rash, and toxicity in a variety of organs. Rieder and colleagues demonstrated that among patients with sulfonamide hypersensitivity reactions, 90% were slow acetylators and only 55% were rapid acetylators (Reider et al. 1991). The slow acetylator phenotype also was a risk factor for sulfonamide-induced toxic epidermal necrolysis and Stevens-Johnson syndrome (Wolkenstein et al. 1995). It is important to recognize that acetylator phenotype is not a biological marker to predict who will have a reaction because slow acetylation has a frequency of 10–70%, and these severe reactions occur only in 1 in 1000 or fewer patients.

**AMONAFIDE TOXICITY** The DNA intercalating cytostatic agent amonafide is metabolized by acetylation to an active metabolite. Rapid acetylators have markedly increased myelotoxicity after amonafide treatment, and therefore, the dose has to be adjusted according to the phenotype (Ratain et al. 1991).

**OTHER PHENOMENA** Other phenomena associated with slow and rapid acetylation are the higher doses of hydralazine required to control blood pressure in rapid acetylators (Zacest and Koch-Weser 1972). In addition, drug-induced lupus erythematosus (e.g., after administration of procainamide, hydralazine, isoniazid) is overwhelmingly a disease of slow acetylators (Uetrecht and Woosley 1981). Sulfapyridine arises from salicylazosulfapyridine in the gut by splitting of the azo linkage by bacterial enzymes. Sulfapyridine then is absorbed and acetylated. The serum sulfapyridine concentration is higher in slow acetylators who are treated with salicylazosulfapyridine, and the adverse effects of sulfapyridine occur earlier and more frequently in these patients (Schröder and Evans 1972). Phenotyping before treatment or close monitoring of sulfapyridine concentrations are recommended in most of these studies (Table 22-8).

In addition to increased adverse reactions in slow acetylators treated with drugs whose elimination is primarily determined by acetylation, there are a number of incompletely understood associations of acetylator phenotype with drug-induced and spontaneous diseases, in particular with bladder cancer and breast cancer (Evans 1993; Weber 1987; Risch et al. 1995; Ambrosone et al. 1996).

## Thiopurine Methyltransferase Polymorphism

Thiopurine *S*-methyltransferase (TPMT) methylates the anticancer agents mercaptopurine and thioguanine and the immunosuppressive drug azathioprine (a mercaptopurine prodrug). TPMT is subject to a genetic polymorphism, with about 1 in 300 individuals being homozygous for a recessive allele and having TPMT deficiency, and with

Table 22-8 **Phenotype-Associated Clinical Responses and Risk for Adverse Reaction in Slow and Rapid Acetylators**

| Drug | Phenotype | Clinical Phenomenon |
|---|---|---|
| Isoniazid | Slow | More prone to develop peripheral neuropathy on conventional isoniazid doses and if therapy is not supplemented with pyridoxine |
| | Slow | More prone to phenytoin adverse effects when simultaneously treated with isoniazid |
| | Slow | Caucasians are more prone to hepatotoxicity if treated with isoniazid and rifampicin |
| | Rapid | In Japanese and Chinese subjects, hepatotoxic effects of isoniazid are more common |
| | Rapid | Less favorable results of treating tuberculosis with once-weekly isoniazid |
| Hydralazine | Slow | More prone to develop antinuclear antibodies and systemic lupus erythematosus-like syndrome |
| | Rapid | Requirement of higher doses to control hypertension |
| Salicylazosulfapyridine | Slow | Increased incidence of hematologic and gastrointestinal adverse reactions |
| Sulfonamides | Slow | Idiosyncratic hypersensitivity reactions |

Modified from Evans 1993; and Spielberg et al. 1996.

about 10% of individuals having an intermediate enzyme activity as a result of heterozygosity (Weinshilboum and Sladek 1980). Several mutant alleles have been characterized and lead to variable degrees of enzyme deficiency (Yates et al. 1997; Otterness 1997). Clinical studies have found an inverse correlation between TPMT activity and accumulation of active thioguanine nucleotide metabolites of mercaptopurine and azathioprine in erythrocytes. Patients with TPMT deficiency accumulate high concentrations of these nucleotides, which lead to severe hematopoietic toxicity and possibly, death, if the thiopurine dose is not substantially reduced (Yates et al. 1997). Patients with intermediate activity accumulate 50% more thioguanine nucleotides and have a moderately increased risk of toxicity. TPMT deficiency can be diagnosed by measuring the enzyme activity in erythrocytes, but these assays are not widely available, and transfusions of red blood cells precludes measurements of the activity. Genotyping tests have been developed and provide an alternative for individual dose adjustment and prevention of toxicity (Yates et al. 1997; Otterness 1997).

## Dihydropyrimidine Dehydrogenase Polymorphism

Dihydropyrimidine dehydrogenase (DPD) catalyzes the reduction of pyrimidines, including the anticancer agent 5-fluorouracil. Deficiency of this enzyme may cause severe life-threatening neutropenia, diarrhea, and in some cases, neurotoxicity (Diasio et al. 1988). Total deficiency is rare, but about 3% of the population may have low enzymatic activity. The molecular basis of the deficiency is mutations of the DPD gene (Vrecken et al. 1996; Wei et al 1996), but phenotype/genotype analysis suggests that the presently known mutations of this gene are insufficient for identification of patients at risk for 5-fluorouracil toxicity in Caucasian populations (Ridge et al. 1998). Therefore, assays of DPD activity in mononuclear cells are still the mainstay of dose adjustment before more is known about loss of function or decreased function alleles of this gene.

## Plasma Pseudocholinesterase Polymorphism

### *Inherited sensitivity to succinylcholine*

The inherited sensitivity to the muscle relaxant drug succinylcholine is one of the most thoroughly studied examples of a pharmacogenetic disorder. Shortly after the introduction of succinylcholine as an adjunct to anesthesia, a small number of patients were discovered who had prolonged apnea following the administration of a single dose of this drug. A familial occurrence of this increased sensitivity to succinylcholine was soon disclosed (Kalow and Genest 1957). Sensitivity to succinylcholine appears to be inherited as an autosomal recessive trait. The drug is normally hydrolyzed in the serum by a cholinesterase, which is often referred to as pseudocholinesterase. In normal persons, this enzyme rapidly converts succinylcholine to succinylmonocholine, allowing very little of the parent compound to reach myoneural receptor sites. In patients with either an unexpected sensitivity to the drug or an abnormal resistance to its effects, variants of the enzyme with altered qualitative or quantitative properties have been detected (Bartels et al. 1992). In the most common variant conferring low activity, so-called atypical pseudocholinesterase, the enzyme has a lower affinity for choline ester substrates, including dibucaine, and is, therefore, less susceptible to inhibition by dibucaine; this fact and inhibition by other chemicals (e.g., sodium fluoride) have been widely used for the characterization of atypical pseudocholinesterases. More than 10 rare and common variants of the enzyme have been described, and some of the mutations and alleles have now been characterized at the DNA level (Bartels et al. 1992; Primo-Parma 1996). Most of the variants are rare except for the "K" variant, which occurs in homozygotes in 1.5% of the general population (Bartels et al. 1992; La Du et al. 1990). Deficient pseudocholinesterase variants are extremely rare in Asians and Blacks.

***Clinical importance of succinylcholine sensitivity***
Patients who are homozygous for the "atypical," "fluoride-resistant," or "silent" genes show prolonged paralysis when they are given the usual dose of succinylcholine or mivacurium, a more recently introduced muscle relaxant. For them, artificial respiration may be required for several hours before the drug's effect subsides. Whenever unusual responses to succinylcholine occur, the patient and his or her relatives should be subjected to the in vitro tests developed to classify variants of cholinesterase or to the recently developed DNA analysis. This will result in the prevention of future exposures for sensitive individuals or application of the drug with increased caution.

**PRINCIPLE The patient in the setting of a pharmacogenetic defect includes the patient's family.**

## INHERITED VARIATIONS IN DRUG EFFECTS INDEPENDENT OF PHARMACOKINETICS

A number of genetic disorders or enzymatic defects cause modifications in responses to drugs, without the biochemical defects being directly associated with the pharmacokinetics of the offending drug. Hereditary resistance to coumarin anticoagulants is the classic example of an alteration in the intensity of a response to a drug, whereas glucose-6-phosphate dehydrogenase (G6PD) deficiency is the prototype of a genetic disorder that predisposes its otherwise healthy carriers to an abnormal and adverse response to a drug—hemolysis. In addition to the inherent therapeutic implications of these unusual drug responses, the drugs involved often provide a diagnostic tool to uncover the genetic disorder (see Table 22-9).

### Hereditary Warfarin Resistance

Variations in the hypoprothrombinemic response to coumarin anticoagulant drugs is continuous and has a unimodal frequency distribution in heterogeneous populations. Family and twin studies have suggested that the pharmacokinetics of this drug response is under polygenic control (Vesell and Page 1968). Because the action of coumarin anticoagulants is easily and routinely monitored, individual adjustment of dose to variation in response usually poses no major problem. In contrast to these inherited influences of the "normal" variation in the pharmacokinetics of coumarin anticoagulants, an unusual hereditary resistance to the action of these drugs may be related to an alteration in drug–receptor interaction.

Two unrelated kindreds in whom a striking resistance to warfarin was inherited as a mendelian autosomal dominant trait have been reported (O'Reilly 1974). A large single dose of warfarin administered orally or intravenously to the propositus (proband) resulted in the expected concentrations of warfarin in plasma. However, virtually no hypoprothrombinemic response occurred. The dosage required to produce an anticoagulant effect was approximately 20 times the usual dose. In addition to this striking resistance to the anticoagulant drug, these patients and their relatives require less vitamin K to reverse hypoprothrombinemia but have higher-than-normal requirements for the vitamin when it is deleted from the diet. An alteration of the receptor for vitamin K and/or warfarin are suspected.

### Glucose-6-Phosphate Dehydrogenase Deficiency and Drug-Induced Hemolytic Anemia

Since the discovery of primaquine-induced hemolytic anemia in African-Americans, and its relationship to a genetically transmitted deficiency in erythrocyte G6PD, a large number of inherited enzyme defects in erythrocyte metabolism have been described. These abnormalities mostly involve enzymes in either the pentose phosphate pathway or the metabolism of glutathione. By far the most common of these abnormalities is G6PD deficiency, which is an X-linked inherited trait. In fact, deficiency of G6PD is one of the most prevalent inherited enzyme de-

Table 22-9 Monogenic Polymorphisms and Rare Variants of Pharmacologic Responses

| Inherited Condition | Mutant Enzyme or Protein | Incidence | Inheritance | Drugs | Clinical Problem |
|---|---|---|---|---|---|
| *Polymorphisms* | | | | | |
| Defects in erythrocyte enzymes | Glucose-6-phosphate dehydrogenase | 10% of world population, frequent in tropical and subtropical countries | X-linked | Analgesics, sulfonamides, antimalaria drugs, etc. | Hemolysis |
| Glaucoma | Unknown | 5% of US population | Autosomal recessive | Corticosteroids | Scotomas |
| *Rare Conditions* | | | | | |
| Warfarin resistance | Unknown | 2 Caucasian families | Autosomal dominant | Warfarin | Decreased effect of warfarin |
| Unstable hemoglobins | Hb H, Hb Zurich, Hb M, etc. | Numerous rare variants described | Autosomal dominant | Sulfonamides, nitrites, etc. | Methemoglobinemia |
| Hepatic porphyria | Enzymes of heme biosynthesis | 1 in 10,000 to 1 in 50,000 | Autosomal dominant | Barbiturates, phenytoin, inducers of cytochrome P450 | Exacerbation of neuropsychiatric symptoms |
| Defects in erythrocyte enzymes | GSH reductase, GSH peroxidase | Very rare | Autosomal dominant | Sulfonamides, chloroquine, etc. | Hemolysis |
| Malignant hyperthermia with muscle rigidity | Mutations in ryanodine receptor gene and other defects | 1 in 15,000 | Autosomal dominant | Inhalational anesthetics or depolarizing muscle relaxants | Hyperthermia, hyperrigidity |

Abbreviation: GSH, glutathione.

fects in humans, probably affecting over 400 million persons worldwide (for reviews, see Beutler 1991, 1992). The enzyme G6PD catalyzes the initial step in the hexose monophosphate oxidation pathway of carbohydrate metabolism, causing reduction of NADP to NADPH. Because mature human erythrocytes lack the oxidative enzymes of the Krebs cycle, the hexose monophosphate shunt pathway is of particular importance in erythrocytes in generating NADPH. The NADPH is required by red cell glutathione reductase to maintain glutathione in its reduced form. Many oxidant drugs, but also infection and nutritional factors such as components of the fava bean (*Vicia faba*), increase the concentration of $H_2O_2$ in red cells and exceed the capacity of glutathione peroxidase to convert $H_2O_2$ to $H_2O$, a reaction requiring NADPH. The higher demand for NADPH cannot be met in subjects with severe G6PD deficiency, and as a consequence, erythrocyte integrity is disrupted and hemolysis occurs.

Numerous drugs and other compounds are capable of precipitating hemolysis in individuals with G6PD deficiency. Over 300 distinct allelic variants of G6PD have been reported; 87 of which have reached polymorphic frequencies ($> 1\%$). They are distinguishable from one another by their pharmacokinetic characteristics, electrophoretic mobilities, and substrate specificities. Most of the G6PD variants are caused by structural gene mutations, that is, by single amino acid substitutions. The G6PD gene has been cloned, and the primary structure of the protein has been deduced. DNA probes for the common mutations are available. Racial and geographic differences in G6PD deficiency are marked.

Some variants are associated with severe reduction in erythrocyte G6PD activity, whereas others are associated with only mild or no reduction. The severity of the "red cell G6PD deficiency" (i.e., the in vitro activity of G6PD) and chronic hemolytic manifestations or susceptibility to drug-induced hemolysis frequently do not correlate well. This problem can be partially resolved by assaying the enzyme under simulated physiologic conditions, taking into consideration the cellular concentrations of the substrate, the coenzymes, and various metabolites that affect G6PD activity. Patients with G6PD deficiency should be counseled against ingesting drugs that can cause hemolysis. These are most commonly primaquine, sulfonamides, nitrofurantoin, and nonsteroidal anti-inflammatory drugs (NSAIDs) (Beutler 1991, 1992). If hemolysis occurs while taking a drug, its discontinuation depends on the severity of hemolysis, the patient's need for the drug in spite of hemolysis, and the availability of alternative drugs. The component of the fava bean that causes hemolysis in G6PD deficient individuals is the glucoside divicine and its aglycone isouramile (Arese 1982). The widespread distribution of genetic variants of G6PD is due to the significant reduction in the risk of severe malaria for both G6PD female heterozygotes and male hemizygotes. This explains the high incidence of G6PD variants in populations of areas where malaria was or is endemic (Ruwende and Hill 1998).

## Other Enzyme Defects and Molecular Disorders of Pharmacogenetic Interest

Numerous additional examples of the modification of drug action by genetic disorders have been documented (e.g., Evans 1993; Weber 1997; Nebert 1997). Rare inherited variations in the structure of hemoglobin, such as hemoglobin H and hemoglobin Zurich or hemoglobin M, may predispose a patient to unexpected adverse drug effects such as hemolysis after sulfonamide therapy or methemoglobinemia after nitrite ingestion (Bunn and Forget 1986).

Acute neuropsychiatric attacks in patients with inherited hepatic porphyrias (e.g., intermittent acute porphyria, hereditary coproporphyria, variegate porphyria) are frequently precipitated by drugs, particularly by barbiturates, several anticonvulsants, griseofulvin, and steroids. Porphyrias are caused by a disturbance of heme biosynthesis. The primary genetic lesion in intermittent acute porphyria is a partial deficiency of porphobilinogen deaminase that results in increased inducibility of hepatic δ-aminolevulinic acid synthase, the rate-limiting enzyme of the pathway. Hereditary coproporphyria and variegate porphyria are caused by partial defects in enzymes more distal in the pathway. Drugs that precipitate porphyria are inducers of hepatic cytochromes P450, the terminal oxidase in microsomal drug metabolism. In the presence of a partial block in heme synthesis, the drug-mediated induction of this hemoprotein apparently results in an exaggerated response of δ-aminolevulinic acid synthetase, causing massive accumulation of the porphyrin precursors δ-aminolevulinic acid and porphobilinogen. Recent advances in the understanding of the neuropathology and its precipitation by drugs are based on a transgenic animal model of the disease (Meyer et al. 1998).

There are many other examples of unusual or undesired drug effects in patients with rare hereditary disorders; neither the metabolic or molecular defect nor the mechanism of the abnormal drug response can be explained in most of these. They include conditions such as hereditary malignant hyperthermia associated with anesthesia in which the defect in some families is a defective ryanodine receptor, the calcium-release channel of the sarcoplasmic reticulum (Manning et al. 1998). The reader is referred to reviews, symposia, and conferences of these and other rare conditions or traits that confer a potential risk to unusual drug effects.

### Genetic Variability of Receptors

It seems initially surprising that genetic polymorphism of drug-metabolizing enzymes is the rule rather than the exception and that examples of genetic variation of receptor function appear to be rare in healthy populations. In other words, if receptors vary, the result is disease and not just pharmacogenetic variability (Dreyer and Rüdiger 1988). One major difference between receptor systems and drug metabolism is that drug-metabolizing enzymes are "low-affinity" systems, whereas receptor interactions are high-affinity chemical interactions with stringent structural requirements. Mutations in such systems, therefore, frequently either are not compatible with life or cause severe disease. This concept is also supported by the fact that there are considerable species-specific differences in drug metabolizing capacity, but little interspecies variability in receptor systems. In addition, until a few years ago, and the development of recombinant DNA techniques, it was difficult to clone receptor genes and study the sequences of receptors. More recent studies now suggest that variation in receptor sequence may cause subtle variations in response to drugs. As an example, a combination of mutations of the dopamine $D_4$ receptor gene (*DRD4*) apparently predicts the variable response to the antipsychotic drug clozapine in schizophrenic patients (Kennedy et al. 1994). Each of the five dopamine receptor subtypes has a distinct pharmacologic profile and a unique tissue distribution. Studies have attempted to associate polymorphic variants of these receptor subtypes with features of human personality (Benjamin et al. 1996; Ebstein et al. 1996). Similar studies in other receptor systems—for example, the serotonin 5-$HT_{2A}$ receptors involved in the effect of hallucinogens (Arranz et al. 1996) and the $\beta_2$-adrenergic receptor involved in respiratory physiology—are being undertaken in several laboratories (e.g., Liggett 1998).

## OUTLOOK

In the early days of the twentieth century, the English physician Sir Archibald Garrod conceptualized his observations on individual differences in the expression of inborn errors of metabolism and in the response to the effects of foreign chemicals as "chemical individuality" (Garrod 1902). The discovery of some of the pharmacogenetic conditions described in this chapter followed 50 years later. In the last few years, through the methods of molecular genetics, and more recently with the systematic study of the human genome, many of these observations are now understood at the molecular level. Researchers are just beginning to realize the extent and relevance of the diversity of human genes for individual responses to drugs and other chemicals. Pharmacogenetics and pharmacogenomics have become rapidly emerging fields with implications not only for drug therapy, but also for drug discovery and development and for the assessment of the risk to develop certain diseases. In the future, physicians will have to be aware of these inherited variations of drug responsiveness because they are a constant variable throughout a patient's life. Their negative consequences for drug therapy can be counteracted by new diagnostic procedures and proper dose adjustments. For now, therapeutic decisions involving drugs that are affected by known genetic polymorphisms should be made and monitored in a particularly careful manner. This is done to develop suspicion of an underlying defect that can be diagnosed and accounted for in a patient and in the patient's family.

Editor's note: Because of the difficulty in verifying the accuracy of different human populations and ethnic groups described in this chapter, the nomenclature may not follow some of the more recent trends in the use of "politically correct" terminology. Therefore, rather than introduce factual inaccuracies, the terms in this chapter reflect those used in the original publications of the scientific studies. We hope that none of our readers find offense in this decision.

## REFERENCES


Agundez JAG, Olivera M, Martinez C, et al. 1996. Identification and prevalence study of 17 allelic variants of the human NAT2 gene in a White population. *Pharmacogenetics* **6**:423–8.

Aklillu E, Persson I, Bertilsson L, et al. 1996. Frequent distribution of ultrarapid metabolizers of debrisoquine in an Ethiopian population carrying duplicated and multiduplicated functional CYP2D6 alleles. *J Pharmacol Exp Ther* **278**:441.

Alvan G, Bechtel P, Iselius L, et al. 1990. Hydroxylation polymorphisms of debrisoquine and mephenytoin in European populations. *Eur J Clin Pharmacol* **39**:533.

Alvan G, Grind M, Graffner C, et al. 1984. Relationship of *N*-demethylation of amiflamine and its metabolite to debrisoquine hydroxylation polymorphism. *Clin Pharmacol Ther* **36**:515.

Alvan G, von Bahr C, Seidemann P, et al. 1982. High plasma concentrations of beta-receptor blocking drugs and deficient debrisoquine hydroxylation. *Lancet* **1**:333.

Ambrosone CB, Freudenheim JL, Graham S, et al. 1996. Cigarette smoking, *N*-acetyltransferase 2 genetic polymorphisms, and breast cancer risk. *JAMA* **13**:1494.

Andersson T, Regard C-G, Dahl-Puustinen M-L, et al. 1990. Slow omeprazole metabolites are also poor *S*-mephenytoin hydroxylators. *Ther Drug Monit* **12**:415.

Arese P. 1982. Favism—a natural model for the study of hemolytic mechanisms. *Rev Pure Appl Pharmacol Sci* **3**:123.

Arranz MJ, Collier D, Munro I, et al. 1996. Probing therapeutic targets in psychosis by association studies. *Br J Clin Pharmacol* **42**:545.

Arranz MJ, Dawson E, Shaikh S, et al. 1995. Cytochrome P4502D6 genotype does not determine response to clozapine. *Br J Clin Pharmacol* **39**:417.

Asberg M, Evans DAP, Sjöqvist F. 1971. Genetic control of nortriptyline kinetics in man. *J Med Genet* **8**:129.

Balant-Gorgia AE, Balant LP, Genet C, et al. 1986. Importance of oxidative polymorphism and levomepromazine treatment on the steady-state blood concentrations of clomipramine and its major metabolites. *Eur J Clin Pharmacol* **31**:449.

Balant-Gorgia AE, Schulz P, Dayer P, et al. 1982. Role of oxidation polymorphism on blood and urine concentration of amitriptyline and its metabolites in man. *Arch Psychiatr Nervenkr* **232**:215.

Ball SE, Ahern D, Scatina J, et al. 1997. Venlafaxine: in vitro inhibition of CYP2D6 dependent imipramine and desipramine metabolism; comparative studies with selected SSRIs, and effects on human hepatic CYP3A4, CYP2C9 and CYPIA2. *Br J Clin Pharmacol* **43**:619.

Bartels CF, Jensen FS, Lockridge O, et al. 1992. DNA mutation associated with the human butyrylcholinesterase K-variant and its linkage to the atypical variant mutation and other polymorphic sites. *Am J Hum Genet* **50**:1086.

Beckmann J, Hertrampf R, Gundert-Remy U, et al. 1988. Is there a genetic factor in flecainide toxicity? *Br Med J* **297**:1326.

Benjamin J, Li L, Patterson C, et al. 1996. Population and familial association between the D4 dopamine receptor gene and measures of novelty seeking. *Nature Genet* **12**:81.

Bergstrom RF, Peyton AL, Lemberger L. 1992. Quantification and mechanism of the fluoxetine tricyclic antidepressant interaction. *Clin Pharmacol Ther* **51**:239.

Bertilsson L, Aberg-Wistedt A, Gustaffson LL. 1985. Extremely rapid hydroxylation of debrisoquine: a case report with implication for treatment with nortriptyline and other tricyclic antidepressants. *Ther Drug Monit* **7**:478.

Bertilsson L, Dahl ML, Ingelman-Sundberg M, et al. 1995. Interindividual and interethnic differences in polymorphic drug oxidation: implications for drug therapy with focus on psychoactive drugs. In: Pacifici GM, Fracchia GN, editors. *Advances in Drug Metabolism in Man*. Luxembourg: European Commission. p 85.

Bertilsson L, Dahl M-L, Tybring G. 1997. Pharmacogenetics of antidepressants: clinical aspects. *Acta Psychiatr Scand* **96**:14.

Bertilsson L, Henthorn TK, Sanch E, et al. 1989. Importance of genetic factors in the regulation of diazepam metabolism: relationship to *S*-mephenytoin, but not debrisoquine hydroxylation phenotype. *Clin Pharmacol Ther* **45**:348.

Bertschy G, Vandel S, Vandel B, et al. 1991. Fluvoxamine–tricyclic antidepressant interaction. *Eur J Clin Pharmacol* **40**:119.

Beutler E. 1991. Glucose-6-phosphate dehydrogenase deficiency. *N Engl J Med* **342**:169.

Beutler E. 1992. The molecular biology of G6PD variants and other red cell enzyme defects. *Annu Rev Med* **43**:47.

Blum M, Demierre A, Grant DM, et al. 1991. Molecular mechanism of slow acetylation in man. *Proc Natl Acad Sci USA* **88**:5237.

Blum M, Grant DM, McBride W, et al. 1990. Human arylamine *N*-acetyltransferase genes: isolation, chromosomal localization, and functional expression. *DNA Cell Biol.* **9**:193.

Bönicke R, Reif W. 1953. Enzymatic inactivation of isonicotinic acid hydrazide in humans and animals. *Arch Exp Pathol Pharmak* **220**:321.

Böttiger Y, Dostert P, Strolin Benedetti M, et al. 1996. Involvement of CYP2D6 but not CYP2C19 in nicergoline metabolism in humans. *Br J Clin Pharmacol* **42**:707.

Broly F, Libersa C, Lhermitte M, et al. 1990. Inhibitory studies of mexiletine and dextromethorphan oxidation in human liver microsomes. *Biochem Pharmacol* **39**:1045.

Brosen K. 1990. Recent developments in hepatic drug oxidation. *Clin Pharmacokinet* **18**:220.

Brosen K. 1993. The pharmacogenetics of the selective serotonin reuptake inhibitors. *Clin Invest* **71**:1002.

Brosen K, de Morais SMF, Meyer UA, et al. 1995. A multifamily study on the relationship between CYP2C19 genotype and *S*-mephenytoin oxidation phenotype. *Pharmacogenetics* **5**:312.

Brosen K, Gram LF. 1988. First-pass metabolism of imipramine and desipramine: impact of the sparteine oxidation phenotype. *Clin Pharmacol Ther* **43**:400.

Brosen K, Gram LF. 1989. Clinical significance of the sparteine/debrisoquine oxidation polymorphism. *Eur J Clin Pharmacol* **36**:537.

Brosen K, Otton SV, Gram LF. 1986. Imipramine demethylation and hydroxylation: impact of the sparteine oxidation phenotype. *Clin Pharmacol Ther* **40**:543.

Brynne N, Dalén P, Alvan G, et al. 1998. Influence of CYP2D6 polymorphism on the pharmacokinetics and pharmacodynamics of tolterodine. *Clin Pharmacol Ther* **63**:529.

Buchert E, Woosley RL. 1992. Clinical implications of variable antiarrhythmic drug metabolism. *Pharmacogenetics* **2**:2.

Bunn HF, Forget BG. 1986. *Hemoglobin: Molecular, Genetic and Clinical Aspects*. Philadelphia: Saunders.

Caraco Y, Sheller J, Wood AJJ. 1996. Pharmacogenetic determination of the effects of codeine and prediction of drug interactions. *J Pharmacol Exp Ther* **278**:1165.

Carrillo JA, Dahl ML, Svensson JO, et al. 1996. Disposition of fluvoxamine in humans is determined by the polymorphic CYPqD6 and also by the CYP1A2 activity. *Clin Pharmacol Ther* **60**:183.

Cascorbi I, Drakoulis N, Brockmöller J, et al. 1995. Arylamine *N*-acetyltransferase (NAT2) mutations and their allelic linkage in unrelated Caucasian individuals: correlation with phenotypic activity. *Am J Hum Genet* **57**:581.

Chen S, Chou W-H, Blouin RA, et al. 1996. The cytochrome P450 2D6 (CYP2D6) enzyme polymorphism: screening costs and influence on clinical outcomes in psychiatry. *Clin Pharmacol Ther* **60**:522.

Ciotti M, Marrone A, Potter C, et al. 1997. Genetic polymorphism in the human UGT1A6 (planar phenol) UDP-glucuronosyltransferase: pharmacological implications. *Pharmacogenetics* **7**:485.

Cohen LJ, DeVane CL. 1996. Clinical implications of antidepressant pharmacokinetics and pharmacogenetics. *Ann Pharmacother* **30**:1471.

Cooper RG, Evans DAP, Whibley EJ. 1984. Polymorphic hydroxylation of pehexiline maleate in man. *J Med Genet* **21**:27.

Dahl ML, Bertilsson L. 1993. Genetically variable metabolism of antidepressants and neuroleptic drugs in man. *Pharmacogenetics* **3**: 61.

Dahl ML, Ekqvist B, Widen J, et al. 1991. Disposition of the neuroleptic zuclopenthixol cosegregates with the polymorphic hydroxylation of debrisoquine in humans. *Acta Psychiatr Scand* **84**:99.

Dahl ML, Tybring G, Elwin CE, et al. 1994. Stereoselective disposition of mianserin is related to debrisoquine hydroxylation polymorphism. *Clin Pharmacol Ther* **56**:176–83.

Dahl-Puustinen MJ, Liden A, Alm C, et al. 1989. Disposition of perphenazine is related to polymorphic debrisoquine hydroxylation in human beings. *Clin Pharmacol Ther* **46**:78.

Dalén P, Dahl M-L, Bernal Ruiz ML, et al. 1998. 10-hydroxylation of nortriptyline in White persons with 0, 1, 2, 3, and 13 functional *CYP2D6* genes. *Clin Pharmacol Ther* **63**:444.

Daly AK, Brockmöller J, Broly F, et al. 1996. Nomenclature for human CYP2D6 alleles. *Pharmacogenetics* **6**:193–201.

Daly AK, Leathart JB, London SJ, et al. 1995. An inactive cytochrome P450 CYP2D6 allele containing a deletion and a base substitution. *Hum Genet* **95**:337.

Davi H, Bonnet JM, Berger Y. 1992. Disposition of minaprine in animals and in human extensive and limited debrisoquine hydroxylators. *Xenobiotica* **22**:171.

Dayer P, Desmeules J, Leemann T, et al. 1988. Bioactivation of the narcotic drug codeine in human liver is mediated by the polymorphic monooxygenase catalyzing debrisoquine 4-hydroxylation. *Biochem Biophys Res Comm* **152**:411.

Dayer P, Leemann T, Kupfer A, et al. 1986. Stereo- and regioselectivity of hepatic oxidation in man—effect of the debrisoquine/sparteine phenotype on bufuralol hydroxylation. *Eur J Clin Pharmacol* **31**:313.

De Bruijn KM. 1992. Tropisetron: a review of the clinical experience. *Drugs* **43**(Suppl. 3):11.

Dehal SS, Kupfer D. 1997. CYP2D6 catalyzes tamoxifen 4-hydroxylation in human liver. *Cancer Res* **57**:3402.

Deloménie C, Sica L, Grant DM, et al. 1996. Genotyping of the polymorphic *N*-acetyltransferase (NAT2*) gene locus in two native African populations. *Pharmacogenetics* **6**:177.

de Morais SMF, Wilkinson GR, Blaisdell J, et al. 1994. Identification of a new genetic defect responsible for the polymorphism of *S*-mephenytoin metabolism in Japanese. *Mol Pharmacol* **46**:594.

Desmeules J, Dayer P, Gascon M-P, et al. 1989. Impact of genetic and environmental factors on codeine analgesia. *Clin Pharmacol Ther* **45**:122.

Devadatta S, Gangadharam PRJ, Andrews RH, et al. 1960. Peripheral neuritis due to isoniazid. *Bull WHO* **23**:587.

Diasio RB, Beavers TL, Carpenter JT. 1988. Familial deficiency of dihydropyrimidine dehydrogenase. *J Clin Invest* **81**:47.

Dolphin CT, Janmhamed A, Smith RL, et al. 1997. Missense mutation in flavin-containing mono-oxygenase 3 gene, *FMO3,* underlies fish-odour syndrome. *Nature Genet.* **17**:491.

Dreyer M, Rüdiger HW. 1988. Genetic defects of human receptor function. *Trends Pharmacol Sci* **9**:98.

Ebner T, Eichelbaum M. 1993. The metabolism of aprindine in relation to the sparteine/debrisoquine polymorphism. *Br J Clin Pharmacol* **35**:426.

Ebstein RP, Novick O, Umansky R, et al. 1996. Dopamine D4 receptor *(D4DR)* exon III polymorphism associated with the human personality trait of novelty seeking. *Nature Genet* **12**:78.

Edeki TI, He H, Wood AJJ. 1995. Pharmacogenetic explanation for excessive beta-blockade following timolol eye drops: potential for oral-ophthalmic drug interaction. *JAMA* **274**:1611.

Eichelbaum M, Gross AS. 1990. The genetic polymorphism of debrisoquine/sparteine metabolism—clinical aspects. *Pharmacol Ther* **46**:377.

Eichelbaum M, Mineshita S, Ohnhaus EE, et al. 1986. The influence of enzyme induction on polymorphic sparteine oxidation. *Br J Clin Pharmacol* **22**:49.

Eichelbaum M, Spannbrucker N, Steincke B, et al. 1979. Defective *N*-oxidation of sparteine in man: a new pharmacogenetic defect. *Eur J Clin Pharmacol* **16**:183.

Evans DAP. 1993. *Genetic Factors in Drug Therapy: Clinical and Molecular Pharmacogenetics.* Cambridge, UK: Cambridge University Press.

Evans DAP, Mahgoub A, Sloan TP, et al. 1980. A family and population study of the genetic polymorphism of debrisoquine oxidation in a White British population. *J Med Genet* **17**:102.

Evans DAP, Manley FA, McKusick VA. 1960. Genetic control of isoniazid metabolism in man. *Br Med J* **2**:485.

Evers J, Eichelbaum M, Kroemer HK. 1994. Unpredictability of flecainide plasma concentrations in patients with renal failure: relationship to side effects and sudden death? *Ther Drug Monit* **16**:349.

Feher MD, Lucas RA, Farid NA, et al. 1988. Single dose pharmacokinetics of tomoxetine in poor and extensive metabolizers of debrisoquine. *Br J Clin Pharmacol* **26**:231P.

Feifel N, Kucher K, Fuchs L, et al. 1993. Role of cytochrome P4502D6 in the metabolism of brofaromine. *Eur J Clin Pharmacol* **45**:265.

Firkusny L, Gleiter CH. 1994. Maprotiline metabolism appears to cosegregate with the genetically-determined CYP2D6 polymorphic hydroxylation of debrisoquine. *Br J Clin Pharmacol* **37**:383.

Fischer V, Vickers AEM, Heitz F, et al. 1994. The polymorphic cytochrome P-4502D6 is involved in the metabolism of both 5-hydroxytryptamine antagonists, tropisetron and ondansetron. *Drug Metab Dispos* **22**:269.

Flockhart DA. 1995. Drug interactions and the cytochrome P450 system: the role of cytochrome P450 2C19. *Clin Pharmakinet* **29**(Suppl 1):45.

Fonne-Pfister R, Meyer UA. 1988. Xenobiotic and endobiotic inhibitors of cytochrome P-450dbl function, the target of the debrisoquine/sparteine type polymorphism. *Biochem Pharmacol* **37**:3829.

Fromm MF, Hofmann U, Griese E-U, et al. 1995. Dihydrocodeine: a new opioid substrate for the polymorphic CYP2D6 in humans. *Clin Pharmacol Ther* **58**:374.

Funck-Brentano C, Becquemont L, Kroemer HK, et al. 1994. Variable disposition kinetics and electrocardiographic effects of flecainide during repeated dosing in humans: contribution of genetic factors, dose-dependent clearance, and interaction with amiodarone. *Clin Pharmacol Ther* **55**:256.

Funck-Brentano C, Kroemer HK, Lee JT, et al. 1990. Drug therapy-propafenone. *N Engl J Med* **322**.

Galton F. 1875. The history of twins as a criterion of the relative powers of nature and nurture. *J Br Anthropol Inst* **5**:391.

Garrod AE. 1902. The incidence of alkaptonuria. A study in chemical individuality. *Lancet ii,* **1616**.

Goldstein JA, de Morais SMF. 1994. Biochemistry and molecular biology of the human CYP2C subfamily. *Pharmacogenetics* **4**:285.

Goldstein JA, Ishizaki T, Chiba K, et al. 1997. Frequencies of the defective CYP2C19 alleles responsible for the mephenytoin poor metabolizer phenotype in various Oriental, Caucasian, Saudi Arabian and American Black populations. *Pharmacogenetics* **7**:59.

Gonzalez FJ, Idle JR. 1994. Pharmacogenetic phenotyping and genotyping: present status and future potential. *Clin Pharmacokinet* **26**:59.

Gonzalez FJ, Vilbois F, Hardwick JP, et al. 1988. Human debrisoquine 4-hydroxylase (P450IID1): cDNA and deduced amino acid sequence and assignment of the CYP2D locus to chromosome 22. *Genomics* **2**:174.

Gram LF, Debruyne D, Caillard V, et al. 1989. Substantial rise in sparteine metabolic ratio during haloperidol treatment. *Br J Clin Pharmacol* **27**:272.

Gram LF, Guentert TW, Grange S, et al. 1995. Moclobemide, a substrate of CYP2C19 and an inhibitor of CYP2C19, CYP2D6, and CYP1A2: a panel study. *Clin Pharmacol Ther* **57**:670.

Gram LF, Hansen MGJ, Sindrup SH, et al. 1993. Citalopram: interaction studies with levomepromazine, imipramine, and lithium. *Ther Drug Monit* **15**:18.

Gram LF, Overo K. 1972. Drug interaction: inhibitory effect of neuroleptics on metabolism of tricyclic antidepressants in man. *Br Med J* **1**:463.

Grant DM, Lottspeich F, Meyer UA. 1984. A simple test for acetylator phenotype using caffeine. *Br J Clin Pharmacol* **17**:459.

Grant DM, Mörike K, Eichelbaum M, et al. 1990. Acetylation pharmacogenetics: the slow acetylator phenotype is caused by decreased or absent arylamine *N*-acetyltransferase in human liver. *J Clin Invest* **85**:968.

Gross AS, Mikus G, Fischer C, et al. 1991. Polymorphic flecainide disposition under conditions of uncontrolled urine flow and pH. *Eur J Clin Pharmacol* **40**:155.

Gross AS, Philips AC, Rieutord A, et al. 1996. The influence of the sparteine/debrisoquine genetic polymorphism on the disposition of dexfenluramine. *Br J Clin Pharmacol* **41**:311.

Haefeli WE, Bargetzi M, Follath F, Meyer UA. 1990. Potent inhibition of cytochrome P450IID6 (debrisoquine 4-hydroxylase) by flecainide in vitro and in vivo. *J Cardiovasc Pharmacol* **15**:779.

Hall SD, Hamman MA, Rettie AE. 1994. Relationships between the levels of cytochrome P4502C9 and its prototypic catalytic activities in human liver microsomes. *Drug Metab Dispos* **22**:975.

Halliday RC, Jones BC, Smith DA, et al. 1995. An investigation of the interaction between halofantrine, CYP2D6 and CYP3A4: studies with human liver microsomes and heterologous enzyme expression systems. *Br J Clin Pharmacol* **40**:369.

Hamelin BA, Turgeon J, Vallée F, et al. 1996. The disposition of fluoxetine but not sertraline is altered in poor metabolizers of debrisoquin. *Clin Pharmacol Ther* **60**:512.

Heim MH, Meyer UA. 1992. Evolution of a highly polymorphic human cytochrome P450 gene cluster: CYP2D6. *Genomics* **14**:49.

Helsby NA, Ward SA, Howells RE, et al. 1990. In vitro metabolism of the biquanide antimalarials in human liver microsomes: evidence for a role of the mephenytoin hydroxylase (P450 MP) enzyme. *Br J Clin Pharmacol* **30**:278.

Hirschowitz J, Bennet JA, Semian FP, et al. 1983. Thioridazine effect on desipramine plasma levels. *J Clin Psychopharmacol* **3**:376.

Huang ML, Van Peer A, Woestenborghs R, et al. 1993. Pharmacokinetics of the novel antipsychotic agent risperidone and the prolactin response in healthy subjects. *Clin Pharmacol Ther* **54**:257.

Hughes HB, Biehl JP, Jones AP, et al. 1954. Metabolism of isoniazid in man as related to the occurrence of peripheral isoniazid neuritis. *Am Rev Respir Dis* **70**:266.

Hughes NC, Janezic SA, McQueen KL, et al. 1998. Identification and characterization of variant alleles of human acetyltransferase NAT1 with defective function using *p*-aminosalicylate as an in-vivo and in-vitro probe. *Pharmacogenetics* **8**:55.

Ibeanu GC, Blaisdell J, Ghanayem BI, et al. 1998. An additional defective allele, *CYP2C19*5*, contributes to the *S*-mephenytoin poor metabolizer phenotype in Caucasians. *Pharmacogenetics* **8**:129.

Inaba T. 1990. Phenytoin: pharmacogenetic polymorphism of 4′-hydroxylation. *Pharmacol Ther* **46**:341.

Jedrychowski M, Feifel N, Bieck PR, et al. 1993. Metabolism of the new MAO-A inhibitor brofaromine in poor and extensive metabolizers of debrisoquine. *J Pharm Biomed Anal* **11**:251.

Jeppesen U, Gram LF, Vistisen K, et al. 1996. Dose-dependent inhibition of CYP1A2, CYP2C19 and CYP2D6 by citalopram, fluoxetine, fluvoxamine and paroxetine. *Eur J Clin Pharmacol* **51**:73.

Jerling M, Bertilsson L, Sjöqvist F. 1994. The use of therapeutic drug monitoring data to document kinetic drug interactions: an example with amitriptyline and nortriptyline. *Ther Drug Monit* **16**:1.

Jerling M, Dahl ML, Aberg-Wistedt A, et al. 1996. The CYP2D6 genotype predicts the oral clearance of the neuroleptic agents perphenazine and zuclopenthixol. *Clin Pharmacol Ther* **59**:423.

Johansson I, Lundqvist E, Bertilsson L, et al. 1993. Inherited amplification of an active gene in the cytochrome P450 CYP2D locus as a cause of ultrarapid metabolism of debrisoquine. *Proc Natl Acad Sci USA* **90**:11825.

Kalow W. 1962. *Pharmacogenetics: Heredity and the Response to Drugs*. Philadelphia: WB Saunders.

Kalow W. 1992. *Pharmacogenetics of Drug Metabolism*. New York: Pergamon Press.

Kalow W, Bertilsson L. 1994. Interethnic factors affecting drug response. In: Testa B, Meyer, UA, editors. *Advances in Drug Research*. New York: Academic Press. p 2.

Kalow W, Genest K. 1957. A method for the detection of atypical forms of human serum cholinesterase. *Can J Biochem Physiol* **35**:339.

Kalow W, Goedde HW, Agarwal DP, editors. 1986. *Ethnic Differences in Reactions to Drugs and Xenobiotics*. Proceedings of a meeting held in Titisee, Black Forest, FRG, Oct. 2–6, 1985. New York: Liss. 583 p.

Kaneko A, Kaneko O, Taleo G, et al. 1997. High frequencies of *CYP2C19* mutations and poor metabolism of proguanil in Vanuatu. *Lancet* **349**:921.

Kennedy JL, Petronis A, Gao J, et al. 1994. Genetic studies of DRD4 and clinical response to neuroleptic medications. *Am J Hum Genet* **55**(Suppl. A):19.

Kimura S, Umeno M, Skoda RC, et al. 1989. The human debrisoquine 4-hydroxylase (CYP2D) locus: sequence and identification of the polymorphic CYP2D6 gene, a related gene, and a pseudogene. *Am J Hum Genet* **45**:889.

Kitchen I, Tremblay J, Andre J, et al. 1979. Interindividual and interspecies variation in the metabolism of the hallucinogen 4-methoxyamphetamine. *Xenobiotica* **9**:397.

Koyama E, Chiba K, Tani M, et al. 1996a. Identification of human cytochrome P450 isoforms involved in the stereoselective metabolism of mianserin enantiomers. *J Pharmacol Exp Ther* **278**:21.

Koyama E, Tanaka T, Chiba K, et al. 1996b. Steady-state plasma concentrations of imipramine and desipramine in relation to *S*-mephenytoin 4′-hydroxylation status in Japanese depressive patients. *J Clin Psychopharm* **16**:286.

Kroemer HK, Eichelbaum M. 1995. 'It's the genes, stupid.' Molecular bases and clinical consequences of genetic cytochrome P450 2D6 polymorphism. *Life Sci* **56**:2285.

Küpfer A, Patwardhan R, Ward S, et al. 1984. Stereoselective metabolism and pharmacogenetic control of 5-phenyl-5-ethylhydantoin (Nirvanol) in humans. *J Pharmacol Exp Ther* **230**:28.

Kutt H, Brennan R, Dehejia H, et al. 1970. Diphenylhydantoin intoxication: a complication of isoniazid therapy. *Am Rev Respir Dis* **101**:377.

La Du BN, Bartels CF, Nogueira CP, et al. 1990. Phenotypical and molecular biological analysis of human butyrylcholinesterase variants. *Clin Biochem* **23**:423.

Lachmann HM, Papolos DF, Saito T, et al. 1996. Human catechol-*O*-methyltransferase pharmacogenetics: description of a functional polymorphism and its potential application to neuropsychiatric disorders. *Pharmacogenetics* **6**:243.

Laurent-Kenesi MA, Funck-Brentano C, Poirier JM, et al. 1993. Influence of CYP2D6-dependent metabolism on the steady-state pharmacokinetics and pharmacodynamics of metoprolol and nicardipine, alone and in combination. *Br J Clin Pharmacol* **36**:531.

Lee JT, Kroemer HK, Silberstein DJ, et al. 1990. The role of genetically determined polymorphic drug metabolism in the beta-blockade produced by propafenone. *N Engl J Med* **322**:1764.

Leeman T, Dayer P, Meyer UA. 1986. Single-dose quinidine treatment inhibits metoprolol oxidation in extensive metabolizers. *Eur J Clin Pharmacol* **29**:739.

Lemoine A, Gautier JC, Azoulay D, et al. 1993. Major pathway of imipramine metabolism is catalyzed by cytochromes P-450 1A2 and P-450 3A4 in human liver. *Mol Pharmacol* **43**:827.

Lennard L, van Loon JA, Weinshilboum RM. 1989. Pharmacogenetics of acute azathioprine toxicity: relationship to thiopurine methyltransferase genetic polymorphism. *Clin Pharmacol Ther* **46**:149.

Lennard MS, Silas JH, Freestone S, et al. 1982. Oxidation phenotype: a major determinant of metoprolol metabolism and response. *N Engl J Med* **307**:1558.

Lewis RV, Lennard MS, Jackson PR, et al. 1985. Timolol and atenolol: relationship between oxidation phenotype, pharmacokinetics and pharmacodynamics. *Br J Clin Pharmacol* **19**:329.

Liggett SB. 1998. Pharmacogenetics of relevant targets in asthma. *Clin Exp Allergy* **28**:77.

Liu HJ, Han C-Y, Lin BK, et al. 1994. Ethnic distribution of slow acetylator mutations in the polymorphic *N*-acetyltransferase (NAT2) gene. *Pharmacogenetics* **4**:125.

Lledo P, Abrams SML, Johnston A, et al. 1993. Influence of debrisoquine hydroxylation phenotype on the pharmacokinetics of mexiletine. *Eur J Clin Pharmacol* **44**:63.

Llerena A, Alm C, Dahl ML, et al. 1992. Haloperidol disposition is dependent on debrisoquine hydroxylation phenotype. *Ther Drug Monit* **14**:92.

Madras S. 1970. Tuberculosis Chemotherapy Centre: a controlled comparison of a twice-weekly and three once weekly regimens in the initial treatment of pulmonary tuberculosis. *Bull WHO* **43**:143.

Mahgoub A, Idle JR, Dring LG, et al. 1977. Polymorphic hydroxylation of debrisoquine in man. *Lancet* **2**:584.

Manning BM, Quane KA, Ording H, et al. 1998. Identification of novel mutations in the ryanodine-receptor gene (RYR1) in malignant hyperthermia: genotype–phenotype correlation. *Am J Hum Genet* **62**:599.

Marez D, Legrand M, Sabbagh N, et al. 1997. Polymorphism of the cytochrome P450 CYP2D6 gene in a European population: characterization of 48 mutations and 53 alleles, their frequencies and evolution. *Pharmacogenetics* **7**:193.

Marshall A. 1997a. Getting the right drug into the right patient. *Nature Biotechnol* **15**:1249.

Marshall A. 1997b. Laying the foundations for personalized medicines. *Nature Biotechnol* **15**:954.

Masimirembwa CM, Johansson I, Hasler JA, et al. 1993. Genetic polymorphism of cytochrome P450 CYP2D6 in Zimbabwean population. *Pharmacogenetics* **3**:275.

McGourty JC, Silas JH, Lennard MS, et al. 1985. Metoprolol metabolism and debrisoquine oxidation polymorphism: population and family studies. *Br J Clin Pharmacol* **20**:555.

Mellström B, Bertilsson L, Säwe J, et al. 1981. E- and Z-10-hydroxylation of nortriptyline: relationship to polymorphic debrisoquine hydroxylation. *Clin Pharmacol Ther* **30**:189.

Meyer UA. 1990. Molecular genetics and the future of pharmacogenetics. *Pharmacol Ther* **46**:349.

Meyer UA. 1991. Genotype or phenotype: the definition of a pharmacogenetic polymorphism. *Pharmacogenetics* **1**:66.

Meyer UA. 1996. Overview of enzymes of drug metabolism. *J Pharmacokinet Biopharm* **24**:449–59.

Meyer UA. 1998. Medically relevant genetic variation of drug effects. In: Stearns S, editor. *Evolution in Health and Disease.* New York: Oxford University Press. pp 41–49.

Meyer UA. 1999. Polymorphisms of genes of toxicological significance. In: Puga A, Wallace KB, editors. *Molecular Biology of the Toxic Response.* Philadelphia: Taylor and Francis. pp 63–71.

Meyer UA, Amrein R, Balant LP, et al. 1996. Antidepressants and drug metabolising enzymes: expert group report. *Acta Psych Scand* **93**:71.

Meyer UA, Schuurmans MM, Lindberg RLP. 1998. Acute porphyrias: pathogenesis of neurological manifestations. *Semin Liver Dis* **18**:43.

Meyer UA, Zanger UM. 1997. Molecular mechanisms of genetic polymorphisms of drug metabolism. *Annu Rev Pharmacol Toxicol* **37**:269.

Mikus G, Gross AS, Beckmann J, et al. 1989. The influence of the sparteine/debrisoquine phenotype on the disposition of flecainide. *Clin Pharmacol Ther* **45**:562.

Mikus G, Somogyi AA, Bochner F, et al. 1990. Cytochrome P-450 IID6 is involved in two 0-demethylation reactions of codeine metabolism. *Clin Exp Pharm Physiol (Suppl.)* **17**:53.

Miners JO, Birkett DJ. 1998. Cytochrome P4502C9: an enzyme of major importance in human drug metabolism. *Br J Clin Pharmacol* **45**:525.

Miners JO, Wing LM, Birkett DJ. 1985. Normal metabolism of debrisoquine and theophylline in a slow tolbutamide metaboliser. *Austr NZ J Med* **15**:348.

Mörike K, Hardtmann E, Heimburg P, et al. 1990. The impact of polymorphic *N*-propylajmaline metabolism on dose requirement and antiarrhythmic efficacy of the drug [abstract]. *Eur J Pharmacol* **183**:628.

Motulsky A. 1957. Drug reactions, enzymes and biochemical genetics. *JAMA* **165**:835.

Motulsky AG. 1964. Pharmacogenetics. *Prog Med Genet* **3**:49.

Mueller RF, Hornung S, Furlong CE, et al. 1983. Plasma paraoxonase polymorphism: a new enzyme assay population, family, biochemical and linkage studies. *Am J Hum Genet* **35**:393.

Nakamura K, Yokoi T, Inoue K, et al. 1996. CYP2D6 is the principal cytochrome P450 responsible for metabolism of the histamine H, antagonist promethazine in human liver microsomes. *Pharmacogenetics* **6**:449.

Narimatsu S, Kariya S, Isozaki S, et al. 1993. Involvement of CYP2D6 in oxidative metabolism of cinnarizine and flunarizine in human liver microsomes. *Biochem Biophys Res Commun* **193**:1262.

Narimatsu S, Masubuchi Y, Hosokawa S, et al. 1994. Involvement of a cytochrome P4502D subfamily in human liver microsomal bunitrolol 4-hydroxylation. *Biol Pharm Bull* **17**:803.

Nebert DW. 1997. Polymorphisms in drug-metabolizing enzymes: what is their clinical relevance and why do they exist? *Am J Hum Genet* **60**:265.

Nei M, editor. 1987. *Molecular Evolutionary Genetics.* New York: Columbia University Press. p 151.

Nelson WL, Fraunfelder FT, Sills JM, et al. 1986. Adverse respiratory and cardiovascular events attributed to timolol ophthalmic solution, 1978–1985. *Am J Ophthalmol* **102**:606.

Oates NS, Shah RR, Idle JR, et al. 1982. Genetic polymorphism of phenformin 4-hydroxylation. *Clin Pharmacol Ther* **32**:81.

O'Reilly RA. 1974. The pharmacodynamics of the oral anticoagulant drugs. *Prog Hemostasis Thromb* **2**:175.

Otterness D, Szumlanski C, Lennard L, et al. 1997. Human thiopurine methyltransferase pharmacogenetics: gene sequence polymorphisms. *Clin Pharmacol Ther* **62**:60.

Otton SV, Ball SE, Cheung SW, et al. 1996. Venlafaxine oxidation in vitro is catalysed by CYP2D6. *Br J Clin Pharmacol* **41**:149.

Otton SV, Inaba T, Kalow W. 1984. Competitive inhibition of sparteine oxidation in human liver by β-adrenoceptor antagonists and other cardiovascular drugs. *Life Sci* **34**:73.

Otton SV, Schadel M, Cheung SW, et al. 1993. CYP2D6 phenotype determines the metabolic conversion of hydrocodone to hydromorphone. *Clin Pharmacol Ther* **54**:463.

Persson K, Sjöström S, Sigurdardottir I, et al. 1995. Patient-controlled analgesia (PCA) with codeine for postoperative pain relief in ten extensive metabolisers and one poor metaboliser of dextromethorphan. *Br J Clin Pharmacol* **39**:182.

Pierce DM, Abrams SM, Franklin RA. 1987. Pharmacokinetics and systemic availability of the antihypertensive agent indoramin and its metabolite 6-hydroxyindoramin in healthy subjects. *Eur J Clin Pharmacol* **32**:619.

Poulsen L, Arendt-Nielsen L, Brosen K, et al. 1996. The hypoanalgesic effect of tramadol in relation to CYP2D6. *Clin Pharmacol Ther* **60**:636.

Preskorn SH, Alderman J, Menger C, et al. 1994. Pharmacokinetics of desipramine coadministered with sertraline or fluoxetine. *J Clin Psychopharm* **14**: 90.

Pressacco J, Muller R, Kalow W. 1993. Interactions of bupranolol with the polymorphic debrisoquine/sparteine monooxygenase (CYP2D6). *Eur J Clin Pharmacol* **45**:261.

Preuss CV, Wood TC, Szumlanski CL, et al. 1998. Human histamine *N*-methyltransferase pharmacogenetics: common genetic polymorphisms that alter activity. *Mol Pharmacol* **53**:708.

Primo-Parma S, Bartels CF, Wiersma B, et al. 1996. Characterization of 12 silent alleles of the human butyrylcholinesterase *(BCHE)* gene. *Am J Hum Genet* **58**:52.

Raftogianis RB, Wood TC, Otterness DM, et al. 1997. Association of common *SULT1A1* alleles with TS PST phenotype. *Biochem Biophys Res Comm* **239**:298.

Raghuram TC, Koshakji RP, Wilkinson GR, et al. 1984. Polymorphic ability to metabolize propranolol alters 4-hydroxypropranolol levels but not beta blockade. *Clin Pharmacol Ther* **36**:51.

Rane A, Modiri AR, Gerdin E. 1992. Ethylmorphine O-deethylation cosegregates with the debrisoquine genetic metabolic polymorphism. *Clin Pharmacol Ther* **52**:257.

Ratain MJ, Mick R, Berezin F, et al. 1991. Paradoxical relationship between acetylator phenotype and amonafide toxicity. *Clin Pharmacol Ther* **50**:573.

Ridge SA, Sludden J, Brown O, et al. 1998. Dihydropyrimidine dehydrogenase pharmacogenetics in Caucasian subjects. *Br J Clin Pharmacol* **42**:151.

Rieder MJ, Shear NH, Kanee A, et al. 1991. Prominence of slow acetylator phenotype among patients with sulfonamide hypersensitivity reactions. *Clin Pharmacol Ther* **49**:13.

Risch A, Wallace DMA, Bathers S, et al. 1995. Slow *N*-acetylation genotype is a susceptibility factor in occupational and smoking related bladder cancer. *Hum Mol Genet* **4**:231.

Roy SD, Hawes EM, McKay G, et al. 1985. Metabolism of methoxyphenamine in extensive and poor metabolizers of debrisoquine. *Clin Pharmacol Ther* **38**:128.

Ruwende C, Hill A. 1998. Glucose-6-phosphate dehydrogenase deficiency and malaria. *J Mol Med* **76**:581.

Sachse C, Brockmöller J, Bauer S, et al. 1997. Cytochrome P450 2D6 variants in a Caucasian population: allele frequencies and phenotypic consequences. *Am J Hum Genet* **60**:284.

Sanwald P, David M, Dow J. 1996. Characterization of the cytochrome P450 enzymes involved in the in vitro metabolism of dolasetron: comparison with other indole-containing 5-HT-3 antagonists. *Drug Metab Dispos* **24**:602.

Schmid B, Bircher J, Preisig R, et al. 1985. Polymorphic dextromethorphan metabolism: cosegregation of oxidative *O*-demethylation with debrisoquine hydroxylation. *Clin Pharmacol Ther* **38**:618.

Schröder H, Evans DAP. 1972. Acetylator phenotype and adverse effects of sulphasalazine in healthy subjects. *Gut* **13**:278.

Scott J, Poffenbarger PL. 1979. Pharmacogenetics of tolbutamide metabolism in humans. *Diabetes* **28**:41.

Shah RR, Oates NS, Idle JR, et al. 1982. Impaired oxidation of debrisoquine in patients with perhexiline neuropathy. *Br Med J Clin Res* **284**:295.

Siddoway LA, Thompson KA, McAllister B, et al. 1987. Polymorphism of propafenone metabolism and disposition in man: clinical and pharmacokinetic consequences. *Circulation* **4**:785.

Sindrup SH, Brosen K. 1995. The pharmacogenetics of codeine hypoanalgesia. *Pharmacogenetics* **5**:335.

Sindrup SH, Brosen K, Gram LF, et al. 1992. The relationship between paroxetine and the sparteine oxidation polymorphism. *Clin Pharmacol Ther* **51**:278.

Sindrup SH, Brosen K, Hansen MGJ, et al. 1993. Pharmacokinetics of citalopram in relation to the sparteine and the mephenytoin oxidation polymorphisms. *Ther Drug Monit* **15**:11.

Sjöqvist F. 1992. Pharmacogenetic factors in the metabolism of tricyclic antidepressants and some neuroleptics. In: Kalow W, editor. *Pharmacogenetics of Drug Metabolism.* New York: Pergamon Press. p 689.

Skoda RC, Gonzalez FJ, Demierre A, et al. 1988. Two mutant alleles of the human cytochrome P-450db1 gene (P450C2D1) associated with genetically deficient metabolism of debrisoquine and other drugs. *Proc Natl Acad Sci U S A* **85**:5240.

Sloan TP, Mahgoub A, Lancaster R, et al. 1978. Polymorphism of carbon oxidation of drugs and clinical implications. *Br Med J* **2**:655.

Smith CAD, Wadelius M, Gough AC, et al. 1997. A simplified assay for the arylamine *N*-acetyltransferase 2 polymorphism validated by phenotyping with isoniazid. *J Med Genet* **34**:758.

Snyder KH. 1932. Studies in human inheritance: IX. The inheritance of taste deficiency in man. *Ohio J Sci* **32**:436.

Spielberg S, McCrea J, Cribb A. 1996. A mutation in CYP2C9 is responsible for decreased metabolism of losartan. *Clin Pharmacol Ther* **59**:215.

Spigset O, Granberg K, Hägg S, et al. 1997. Relationship between fluvoxamine pharmacokinetics and CYP2D6/CYP2C19 phenotype polymorphisms. *Eur J Clin Pharmacol* **52**:129.

Spina E, Ancione M, Di Rosa AE, et al. 1992. Polymorphic debrisoquine oxidation and acute neuroleptic-induced adverse effects. *Eur J Clin Pharmacol* **42**:347.

Spina E, Gitto C, Avenoso A, et al. 1997. Relationship between plasma desipramine levels, CYP2D6 phenotype and clinical response to desipramine, a prospective study. *Eur J Clin Pharmacol* **51**:395.

Spina E, Pollicino AM, Avenoso A, et al. 1993. Effect of fluvoxamine on the pharmacokinetics of imipramine and desipramine in healthy subjects. *Ther Drug Monit* **15**:243.

Steiner E, Dumont E, Spina E, et al. 1988. Inhibition of desipramine 2-hydroxylation by quinidine and quinine. *Clin Pharmacol Ther* **43**:577.

Steward DJ, Haining RL, Henne KR. 1997. Genetic association between sensitivity to warfarin and expression of *CYP2C9*3. Pharmacogenetics* **7**:361.

Sullivan-Klose TH, Ghanayem BI, Bell DA, et al. 1996. The role of the CYP2C9-Leu359 allelic variant in the tolbutamide polymorphism. *Pharmacogenetics* **6**:341.

Suzuki A, Otani K, Mihara K, et al. 1997. Effects of the CYP2D6 genotype on the steady-state plasma concentrations of haloperidol and reduced haloperidol in Japanese schizophrenic patients. *Pharmacogenetics* **7**:415.

Syvählahti EKG, Lindberg R, Kallio J, de Vocht M. 1986. Inhibitory effects of neuroleptics on debrisoquine oxidation in man. *Br J Clin Pharmacol* **22**:89.

Tang BK. 1990. Drug glucosidation. *Pharmacol Ther* **46**:53.

Tang BK, Kadar D, Qian L, et al. 1987. An alternative test for acetylator phenotyping with caffeine. *Clin Pharmacol Ther* **42**:509.

Tang BK, Kalow W, Inaba T, et al. 1983. Variation in amobarbital metabolism: evaluation of a simplified population study. *Clin Pharmacol Ther* **34**:202.

The Cardiac Arrhythmia Suppression Trial (CAST) Investigators. 1989. Preliminary report: effect of encainide and flecainide on mortality in randomized trial of arrhythmia suppression after myocardial infarction. *N Engl J Med* **321**:406.

Tucker GT, Lennard MS, Ellis SW, et al. 1994. The demethylenation of methylenedioxymethamphetamine ("ecstasy") by debrisoquine hydroxylase (CYP2D6). *Biochem Pharmacol* **47**:1151.

Tucker GT, Silas JH, Iyun AO, et al. 1977. Polymorphic hydroxylation of debrisoquine. *Lancet* **2**:718.

Turgeon J, Fiset C, Giguere R, et al. 1991. Influence of debrisoquine phenotype and of quinidine on mexiletine disposition in man. *J Pharmacol Exp Ther* **259**:789.

Tyndale RF, Droll KP, Sellers EM. 1997. Genetically deficient CYP2D6 metabolism provides protection against oral opiate dependence. *Pharmacogenetics* **7**:375.

Uetrecht JP, Woosley RL. 1981. Acetylator phenotype and lupus erythematosus. *Clin Pharmacokinet* **6**:118.

Vatsis KP, Weber WW. 1994. Human *N*-acetyltransferases. In: Kaufmann FC, editor. *Conjugation–Deconjugation: Reactions in Drug metabolism and Toxicity. Handbook of Experimental Pharmacology*. New York: Springer-Verlag. p 109.

Vatsis KP, Wendell WW, Bell DA, et al. 1995. Nomenclature for *N*-acetyltransferases. *Pharmacogenetics* **5**:1.

Vesell ES. 1990. Pharmacogenetic perspectives gained from twin and family studies. *Pharmacol Ther* **41**:535.

Vesell ES, Page JG. 1968. Genetic control of dicumarol levels in man. *J Clin Invest* **47**:2657.

Vogel F. 1959. Moderne Probleme der Humangenetik. *Ergebn Inn Med Kinderheilkd* **12**:52.

Vogel F, Motulsky AG. 1986. *Human Genetics: Problems and Approaches*. New York: Springer-Verlag.

von Bahr C, Guengerich FP, Movin G, et al. 1989. The use of human liver banks in pharmacogenetic research. In: Dahl SG, Gram LF, editors. *Clinical Pharmacology in Psychiatry*. New York: Springer-Verlag.

von Bahr C, Movin G, Nordin C, et al. 1991. Plasma levels of thioridazine and metabolites are influenced by the debrisoquine hydroxylation phenotype. *Clin Pharmacol Ther* **49**:234.

Vrecken P, Van Kuilenburg ABP, Meinsma R, et al. 1996. A point mutation in an invariant splice donor site leads to exon skipping in two unrelated Dutch patients with dihydropyrimidine dehydrogenase deficiency. *J Inherit Metab Dis* **19**:645.

Wang DG, Fan J-B, Siao C-J, et al. 1998. Large-scale identification, mapping, and genotyping of single-nucleotide polymorphisms in the human genome. *Science* **280**:1077.

Wang T, Roden DM, Wolfenden HT, et al. 1984. Influence of genetic polymorphism on the metabolism and disposition of encainide in man. *J Pharmacol Exp Ther* **228**:605.

Ward SA, Walle T, Walle UK, et al. 1989. Propranolol's metabolism is determined by both mephenytoin and debrisoquine hydroxylase activities. *Clin Pharmacol Ther* **45**:72.

Weber WW. 1987. *The Acetylator Genes and Drug Response*. New York: Oxford University Press.

Weber WW. 1997. *Pharmacogenetics*. New York: Oxford University Press.

Wei X, McLeod HL, McMurrough J, et al. 1996. Molecular basis of the human dihydropyrimidine dehydrogenase deficiency and 5-fluorouracil toxicity. *J Clin Invest* **98**:610.

Weinshilboum RM, Sladek SL. 1980. Mercaptopurine pharmacogenetics: monogenic inheritance of erythrocyte thiopurine methyltransferase activity. *Am J Hum Genet* **32**:651.

Whittaker JA, Evans DAP. 1970. Genetic control of phenylbutazone metabolism in man. *Br Med J* **4**:323.

Wilkinson GR, Guengerich FP, Branch RA. 1992. Genetic polymorphism of *S*-mephenytoin hydroxylation. In: Kalow W, editor. *Pharmacogenetics of Drug Metabolism*. New York: Pergamon Press. p 657.

Wolkenstein P, Carrière V, Charue D, et al. 1995. A slow acetylator genotype is a risk factor for sulphonamide-induced toxic epidermal necrolysis and Stevens-Johnson syndrome. *Pharmacogenetics* **5**:255.

Woosley RL, Wood AJJ, Roden DM. 1988. Drug therapy: encainide. *N Engl J Med* **318**:1107.

Yates CR, Krynetski EY, Loennechen T, et al. 1997. Molecular diagnosis of thiopurine *S*-methyltransferase deficiency: genetic basis for azathioprine and mercaptopurine intolerance. *Ann Intern Med* **126**:608.

Yue QY, Hasselström J, Svensson JO, et al. 1991. Pharmacokinetics of codeine and its metabolites in Caucasian healthy volunteers: comparisons between extensive and poor hydroxylators of debrisoquine. *Br J Clin Pharmacol* **31**:635.

Zacest R, Koch-Weser J. 1972. Relation of hydralazine plasma concentration to dosage and hypotensive action. *Clin Pharmacol Ther* **13**:420.

Zekorn C, Achtert G, Hausleiter HJ, et al. 1985. Pharmacokinetics of *N*-propylajmaline in relation to polymorphic sparteine oxidation. *Klin Wochenschr* **63**:1180.

Zhou H-H, Wood AJJ. 1995. Stereoselective disposition of carvedilol is determined by CYP2D6. *Clin Pharmacol Ther* **57**:9.

Zhou HL, Anthony LB, Wood AJ, et al. 1990. Induction of polymorphic 4′-hydroxylation of *S*-mephenytoin by rifampicin. *Br J Clin Pharmacol* **30**:471.

CHAPTER

# 23 CLINICAL PHARMACOKINETICS AND PHARMACODYNAMICS

Daniel S. Sitar

*Chapter Outline*



In order to use drugs effectively to treat the multitude of diseases discussed elsewhere in this text, it is important to be able to administer doses that produce desired concentrations at the site of action (pharmacokinetics), and to understand how these concentrations relate to the onset and intensity of the pharmacologic effect(s) observed (pharmacodynamics). Although it has been appreciated for a long time that a dose–response relationship exists for drug therapy, the ability to understand how to optimize this relationship for individual patients has evolved more slowly. Over the past several years, models for characterizing the time course of drug disposition, drug effect, and the integration of the two processes have been developed that enable the physician to further individualize drug therapy. For a more detailed consideration of the principles and philosophy of modeling, the reader is referred to a recent review (Massoud et al. 1998).

This chapter develops an approach by which a practitioner can determine how to produce desired concentrations of a specific drug in a particular patient, and the basis by which these concentrations are related to the therapeutic effect desired. Findings are presented that help to explain the sometimes confusing relationship between drug dose, concentration, and effect. Furthermore, a basis is developed to understand when a given model must be used, and when a simplified model, although providing less accurate guidelines, results in an acceptable compromise for the individualization of drug therapy. The reader should then be able to appreciate the potential pitfalls of the various decisions he or she will have to accept because of the model chosen in an attempt to optimize drug therapy for individual patients.

## FUNDAMENTALS OF THE PHARMACOKINETIC DISPOSITION OF DRUGS

### Graphical Approach

A plot of drug concentration versus time on either a Cartesian (arithmetic) or semilogarithmic graph paper provides much valuable information with respect to the characteristics of disposition for a given drug.

In Figure 23-1, a linear decline of the drug concentration on a logarithmic scale versus time after an intravenous dose indicates that a one-compartment open model with first-order disposition constants will suffice to describe its time course in the body. On Cartesian graph paper, this plot will have the appearance of concavity.

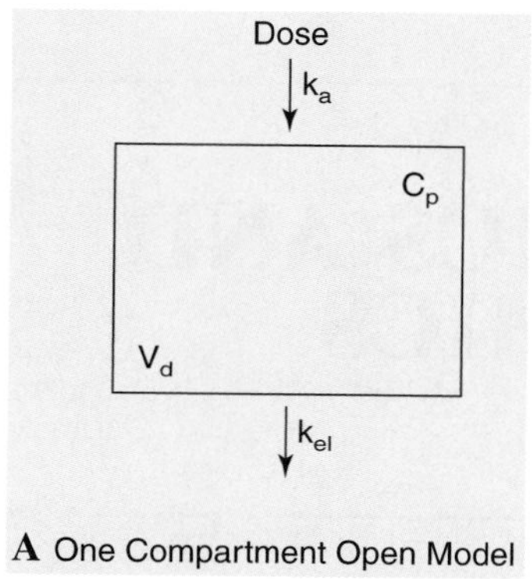


**A** One Compartment Open Model

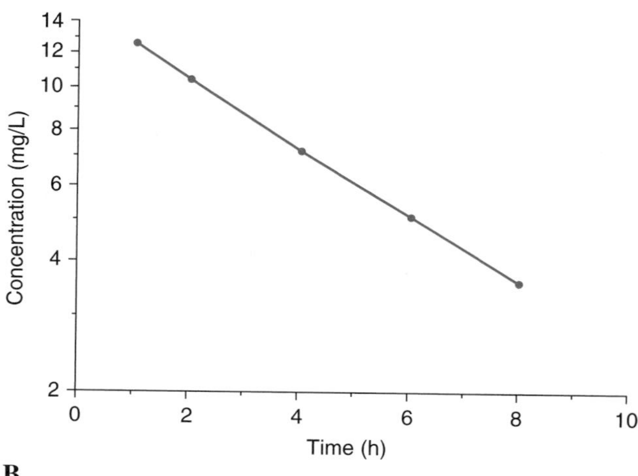


**B**

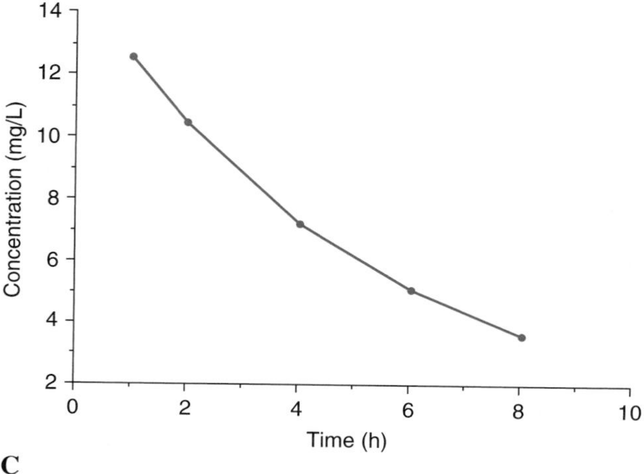


**C**

**FIGURE 23-1** **(A) The essential components of the one-compartment open pharmacokinetic model. The delivery of the dose into the compartment is characterized by the absorption rate constant ($k_a$) when drug is administered by other than the parenteral route. The rate of elimination from this compartment is characterized by the elimination rate constant ($k_{el}$). The presence of drug in the kinetic compartment is characterized by its concentration in the plasma or serum ($C_p$), and the size of the compartment is determined by the space required to account for the administered dose ($V_d$). (B) The results of a plot of the drug concentration on a logarithmic scale versus time when drug disposition is compatible with a one-compartment open model. (C) The results of an arithmetic plot of drug concentration versus time for the same data presented in (B).**

When a semilogarithmic plot results in concavity before the terminal linear phase, a one-compartment open model is no longer sufficient to explain the disposition process. At a minimum, a second compartment needs to be invoked in order to more adequately describe the disposition process for that drug (Figure 23-2). Theoretically, there is no limit to the number of hypothetical compartments that may be invoked in order that a semilogarithmic plot of drug concentration versus time can be resolved adequately by a series of linear relationships. However, when the situation occurs where more than one hypothetical compartment is invoked and from which no data exist to limit their characteristics, interpretation of the mathematical solution is fraught with difficulty. Multiple solutions of the model are possible, many of which may be physiologically untenable. Thus, the use of compartmental pharmacokinetic disposition models is best restricted to use in research.

There has been a trend toward a noncompartmental approach for describing drug disposition. The latter approach provides sufficient information to individualize drug doses for patients without having to resort to the greater mathematical complexity of multicompartment pharmacokinetic models. The reader is referred to a detailed presentation of the comparative strengths and weaknesses between compartmental and noncompartmental pharmacokinetic analyses (DiStefano 1982).

## Mathematical Fundamentals

The disposition of drugs in the body may be described by a hyperbolic mathematical function that is often recalled as a variation on the Michaelis-Menten equation. This hyperbolic function is able to model apparent first-order, dose-dependent, and apparent zero-order kinetics for drug disposition. The fundamental Michaelis-Menten equation is as follows.

$$V = V_m S/(K_m + S) \quad (1)$$

where $V$ represents the rate of the disposition process, $V_m$ the capacity of the process, $S$ the amount of substrate (drug) available for disposition, and $K_m$ the amount of drug necessary to achieve half-maximal velocity for the disposition process. In pharmacokinetic modeling, the term $S$ is replaced by $C$ in order to reflect the convention of referral to drug concentrations in the blood plasma or serum from patients. The term $V$ is replaced by dC/dt to represent the dynamic process reflecting a change in drug concentration with time at any moment after drug administration. In this instance the equation becomes

$$dC/dt = V_m C/(K_m + C) \quad (2)$$

Two rate-limiting situations arise.

The first is when $C >> K_m$, $K_m + C \sim C$, and the equation simplifies to

$$dC/dt = V_m \quad (3)$$

This situation will be reflected by a linear relationship between drug concentration and time on a Cartesian graph. A semilogarithmic plot of drug concentration versus time will yield a convex curve that becomes linear only when drug concentrations in the circulation become considerably less than $K_m$ (Figure 23-3). When $C >> K_m$, a constant amount of drug is eliminated from the body per unit of time (apparent zero-order disposition). The

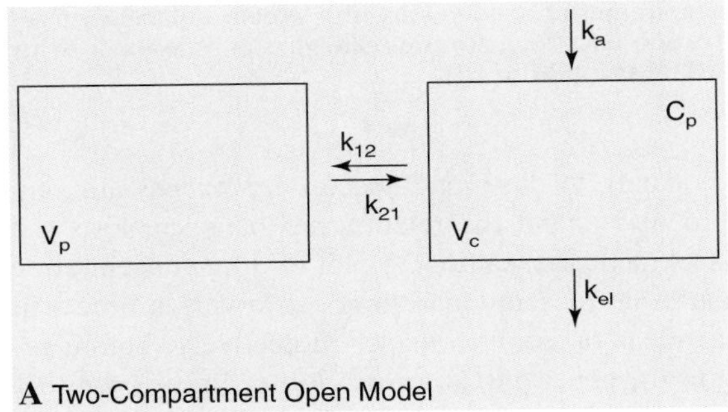


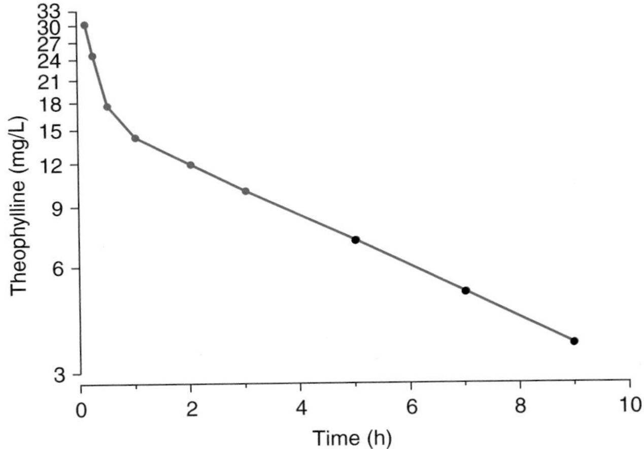


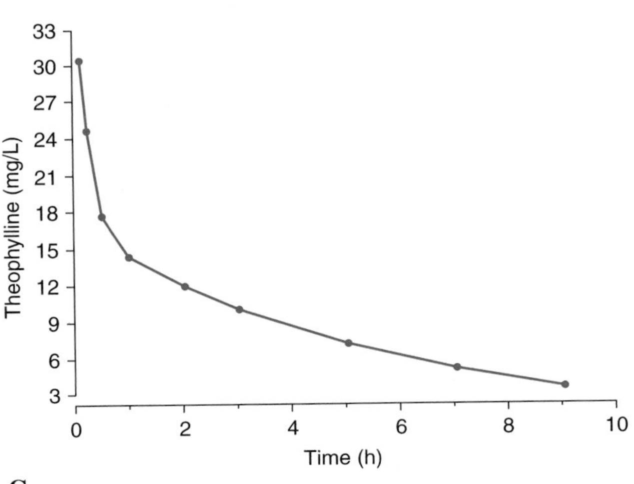


**FIGURE 23-2** (A) The essential components of the two-compartment open pharmacokinetic model. The delivery of the dose into the central compartment ($V_c$) is characterized by the absorption rate constant ($k_a$) when drug is administered by other than the parenteral route. The rate of elimination from this compartment is reflected by the elimination rate constant ($k_{el}$). The presence of drug in $V_c$ is characterized by its concentration in the plasma or serum ($C_p$). A second peripheral kinetic compartment ($V_p$) is created to account for the concavity of the logarithm concentration versus time plot early after the drug dose. The rate of drug transfer from $V_c$ to $V_p$ is described by the intercompartmental first-order rate constant $k_{12}$. Transfer of drug back from $V_p$ to $V_c$ is described by the intercompartmental first-order rate constant $k_{21}$. The apparent volume of distribution ($V_d^{SS}$) for a drug whose disposition is characterized by this model is the sum of $V_c$ + $V_p$. (B) The results of a plot of the drug concentration on a logarithmic scale versus time when drug disposition is compatible with a two-compartment open model. (C) The results of a plot of drug concentration on a Cartesian (arithmetic) scale versus time for the same data presented in (B).

A

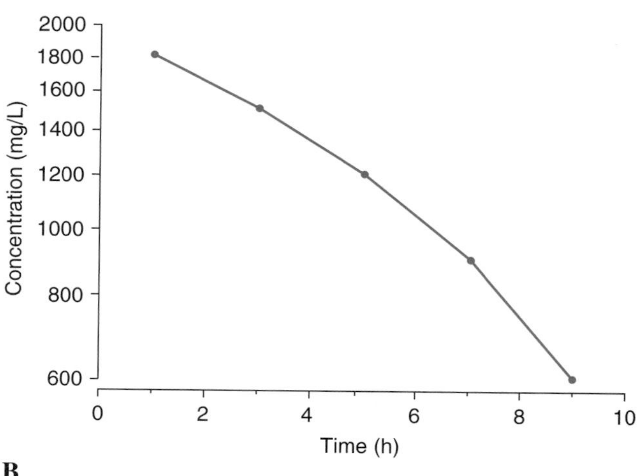


B

**FIGURE 23-3 (A) Plot of drug concentration on a Cartesian (arithmetic) scale versus time when apparent zero-order pharmacokinetic disposition applies. (B) Plot of the drug concentration on a logarithmic scale versus time for a drug with apparent zero-order pharmacokinetic disposition. Note the convexity of the plot in (B).**

best known clinical example is alcohol elimination from the body.

The second is when $C << K_m$, $K_m + C \sim K_m$ and the equation simplifies to

$$dC/dt = V_m C/K_m$$

Because $V_m$ and $K_m$ are both constants, they can be replaced by a single constant "$k$" and the equation simplifies further to

$$dC/dt = kC \tag{4}$$

Because drug concentration decreases with time after a dose as a result of elimination processes, a negative sign precedes $k$, which is now designated as $k_{el}$ to signify exponential decay. The final equation becomes

$$dC/dt = -k_{el}\, C \tag{5}$$

where $C$ is the drug concentration at any moment in time and $k_{el}$ is the apparent first-order rate constant that determines the amount of drug subject to the elimination process of interest, generally metabolism and/or excretion. This situation applies to the vast majority of drugs used in treatment of diseases and is the basis for the pharmacokinetic principles relevant to these therapeutic agents. The elimination process in the present situation is distinguished from the first rate-limiting example in that a constant fraction of the drug present in the body is removed per unit of time.

When $C \sim K_m$, the disposition of a drug is nonlinear and complex. Change in drug concentration increases disproportionately to dose, and special approaches are necessary to understand the relationship between dose and pharmacokinetic disposition. A plot of drug concentration on a Cartesian or semilogarithmic scale versus time will show a linear or convex shape, respectively, before reverting to the concave (Cartesian plot) or linear (semilogarithmic plot) shape seen after the administration of the majority of drugs used in clinical medicine. An example of this situation is presented in Figure 23-4. Clinically relevant examples of this situation include drug therapy with phenytoin or aspirin.

## COMPARTMENTAL MODELS

### The One-Compartment Open Model

The simplest and an often used model to predict appropriate drug doses and their frequency of administration is based on the one-compartment open model (Figure 23-1). In this situation, the body is represented as a single homogeneous space into which the drug enters and from which it leaves. The drug concentration in this space is related to its concentration in blood plasma or serum. Two examples are presented in this section, intravenous drug administration and oral drug administration.

The simplest example of this model is the intravenous bolus dose administration. When this situation applies, a plot of the drug concentration on a logarithmic scale versus time yields a straight line with a declining slope. This model assumes instantaneous drug distribution throughout

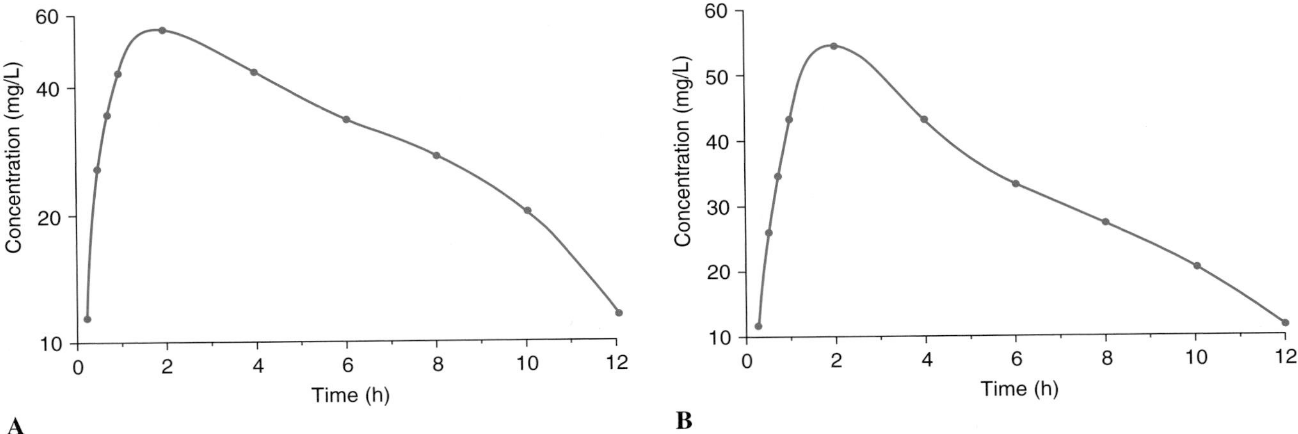


**FIGURE 23-4 Plots of drug concentration versus time for a drug administered in doses around its $K_m$ for pharmacokinetic disposition. In the plot of drug concentration on a logarithmic scale versus time (A), note the convexity of the terminal disposition phase. When these same data are plotted on a Cartesian (arithmetic) scale (B), the terminal disposition process shows less convexity and an approach to linearity, consistent with apparent zero-order pharmacokinetic disposition characteristics.**

the body. Thus extrapolation of the best-fit line through the concentration-versus-time curve to $t = 0$ provides an estimate of the hypothetical initial drug concentration in this compartment ($C_0$), and the basis for estimation of its apparent volume of distribution ($V_d$). The relationship between drug concentration in the circulation ($C$) any time after the dose and time ($t$) is represented by the equation:

$$C = C_0 e^{-k_{el} t} \tag{6}$$

Differentiation of equation 6 yields equation 5.

An important principle of this relationship is that the rate of decline of drug concentration in the plasma ($k_{el}$) is constant, although the amount eliminated during any time interval will change. The amount of drug elimination per unit of time depends on its concentration at the elimination site. The mathematical characterization of this exponential process indicates that drug elimination only approaches completeness, but it never actually occurs (Table 23-1). The half-life ($t_{1/2}$) for drug elimination is determined by the time interval where the arithmetic drug concentration decreases by half, and this parameter is constant, regardless of the starting drug concentration used to estimate the interval. For clinical purposes, it can be assumed that drug elimination is complete after about five half-lives. This concept applies not only to drug elimination but also to all other disposition processes that occur by an apparent first-order rate.

Apparent volume of drug distribution is determined from the following equation:

$$V_d = \text{Dose}/C_0 \tag{7}$$

This pharmacokinetic parameter is usually normalized to units of body weight so that it can be used to calculate therapeutic doses of drugs for patients with different weights.

The declining slope of this drug disposition curve is related to, but not identical with, the elimination rate constant ($k_{el}$). The slope is $k_{el}$ only when the natural logarithm of drug concentration is plotted against time. Therefore, in order to determine this rate constant, it is easiest to determine the $t_{1/2}$ of the elimination process and then to calculate $k_{el}$ from the formula

$$k_{el} = 0.693/t_{1/2} \tag{8}$$

This approach circumvents the confounding effect of

**Table 23-1 Relationship Between Fraction of an Administered Dose Eliminated and Time**

| Time Since Dose Administration ($\times t_{1/2}$) | Amount Remaining to Be Eliminated (% of dose) |
|---|---|
| 0 | 100 |
| 1 | 50 |
| 2 | 25 |
| 3 | 12.5 |
| 4 | 6.25 |
| 5 | 3.12 |
| 6 | 1.56 |

The time intervals are described in multiples of plasma half-life.

the difference in slope of the disposition process observed on a semilogarithmic (base 10) plot compared with a plot of the natural logarithm (base *e*) of drug concentration versus time. When the slope for drug elimination is determined from a semilogarithmic plot of drug concentration, it must be multiplied by 2.303 in order to be equal to $k_{el}$.

The determination of total-body clearance ($CL_T$) represents the pharmacokinetic parameter that must be used to evaluate whether a change in $t_{1/2}$ is related to altered drug distribution ($V_d$) and/or an altered ability to eliminate the drug dose. When $CL_T$ remains unchanged, $V_d$ and $k_{el}$ will change in opposite directions. Consequently, $V_d$ and $t_{1/2}$ change in the same direction, even when there is no change in the ability of a patient to eliminate a drug dose from the body. $CL_T$ is not affected by changes in $V_d$. However, a decline in $CL_T$ in the absence of a change in $V_d$ is associated with an increase in $t_{1/2}$. This kinetic parameter is determined from the equation

$$CL_T = V_d \times k_{el} \quad (9)$$

Total-body clearance usually is also normalized to units of body weight in order to simplify the estimation of drug elimination for patients of differing weight.

Administration of a drug dose by other than the vascular route must take into account the time course for drug absorption. An example of a plot of drug concentration on a logarithmic scale versus time after an oral dose is presented in Figure 23-5. The mathematical equation is more complex, and the reader is referred elsewhere for its derivation and incorporation into a rigorous solution of the model (Gibaldi and Perrier 1982a). With respect to determination of the fundamental pharmacokinetic constants $t_{1/2}$, $k_{el}$, $V_d$, and $CL_T$, the approach is similar to that after an intravenous bolus dose administration. The terminal linear phase on the semilogarithmic plot is extrapolated to $t = 0$ and provides an estimate of $C_0$. The kinetic parameters are then calculated using equations (7) to (9).

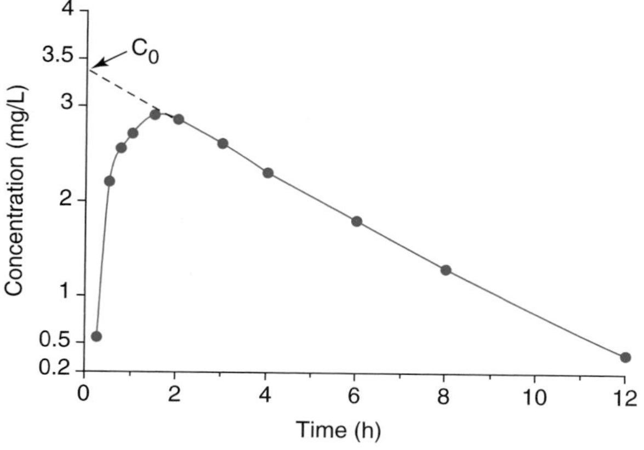


**FIGURE 23-5 Representative plot of drug concentration on a logarithmic scale versus time for a drug ingested orally and compatible with analysis by a one-compartment open model. Extrapolation of the terminal disposition rate to the origin ($t = 0$) provides an estimate of $C_0$ and the basis for determination of apparent volume of distribution ($V_d$).**

Shortcomings of this approach may include an overestimation of $V_d$ due to a lower peak concentration in the circulation compared with intravenous administration. In turn, this leads to an overestimation of $CL_T$ because of the overestimation of $V_d$. Further complicating this problem is the contribution of presystemic drug elimination for many drugs after oral administration (e.g., morphine sulfate). After an oral dose, the circulating drug concentration is reduced substantially from that predicted from intravenous dose administration. Thus pharmacokinetic parameters other than $t_{1/2}$ and $k_{el}$ can deviate markedly from values reported after parenteral drug administration. This difference in circulating concentration versus time as a function of route of administration is referred to as the bioavailability of the candidate drug. When changing route of administration for a drug with substantial presystemic elimination, its bioavailability serves as the parameter used to calculate the dose adjustment required to maintain the desired therapeutic drug concentrations in the circulation.

If the candidate drug ingested orally has a very short systemic $t_{1/2}$, it is possible for the absorption rate to be slower than the elimination rate. In this situation, the terminal disposition rate constant actually reflects the rate of absorption ($k_a$), and the initial rise in drug concentration in the circulation reflects its elimination rate from the body ($k_{el}$). This situation is referred to as the "flip-flop" phenomenon and occurs with some penicillins.

## The Two-Compartment Open Model

When a plot of logarithm $C$ versus time results in concavity at early times after a dose, a second compartment is invoked to account for the nonlinearity of earlier data in the graph (Figure 23-2). Thus the total distribution space for the drug is characterized by two volumes, the central compartment ($V_c$), the space identified by the drug concentration in the circulation, and the peripheral compartment ($V_p$), a space into which the drug enters more rapidly than its rate of elimination. It is assumed that quantitatively significant drug metabolism does not occur in $V_p$, and usually no direct measurements of drug concentration are available from it. Entry into and elimination from $V_p$ are assumed to occur by first-order rate processes. The drug must return to $V_c$ before it can be metabolized and/or excreted.

Because more than one rate process is necessary to define the concentration versus time plot in a two-compartment model, the terminal linear phase is conventionally referred to as beta ($\beta$). Extrapolation of the terminal linear phase to $t = 0$ provides a hypothetical concentration for disposition from the central compartment if distribution to the peripheral compartment had been completed. The drug concentration defined by intersection of this line at $t = 0$ is defined as $B$. In order to determine the rate process for drug distribution into the peripheral compartment, it is necessary to subtract the extrapolated concentrations of the terminal linear phase, $\beta$, from the measured drug concentration in the circulation at the same time point. The difference between these two values is plotted on the graph, and a straight line may usually be fitted to these derived data. The rate process defined by the slope of this line is referred to as alpha ($\alpha$), and the concentration resulting by intersection of this line with $t = 0$ is defined as $A$ (Figure 23-6). Half-lives ($t_{1/2}$) can be determined for $\alpha$ and $\beta$ phases with the same approach used to determine the $t_{1/2}$ for $k_{el}$ in the one-compartment open model. Then $\alpha$ and $\beta$ are calculated from the relationship

$$t_{1/2} \times k = 0.693 \quad \text{[transformation of equation (8)]}$$

where $k$ will be $\alpha$ or $\beta$ depending on which $t_{1/2}$ is substituted into the equation.

An important concept to remember is that $\beta$ in the two-compartment model is not equivalent to $k_{el}$ in the one-compartment model. Beta is a slower rate process than $k_{el}$, as disappearance of drug from the circulation in this model because of elimination processes (metabolism and excretion) is buffered by return of drug to $V_c$ from $V_p$ at a rate defined by the intercompartmental transfer constant $k_{21}$ (Figure 23-2).

Once we know $A$, $B$, $\alpha$, and $\beta$, all of the other parameters of this model can be calculated based on the following relationships.

$$V_c = \text{Dose}/(A + B) \quad (10)$$

$$k_{el} = (A + B)/[(A/\alpha) + (B/\beta)] \quad (11)$$

$$\alpha \times \beta = k_{el} \times k_{21} \quad (12)$$

$$\alpha + \beta = k_{12} + k_{21} + k_{el} \quad (13)$$

$$CL_T = V_c \times k_{el} \quad (14)$$

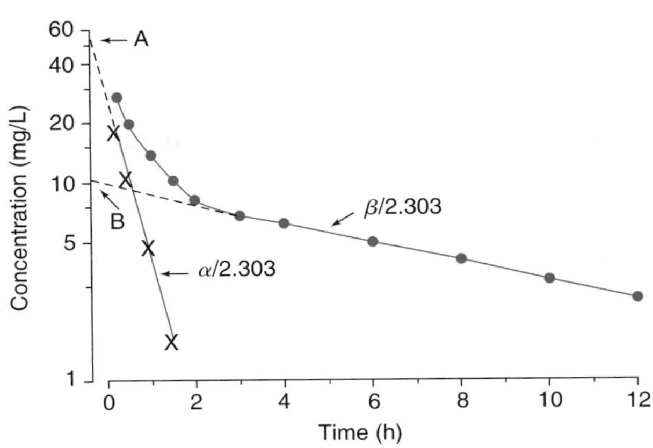


**FIGURE 23-6 Plot of concentration on a semilogarithmic scale versus time for a drug after intravenous administration with disposition characteristics consistent with analysis by a two-compartment open model. The terminal disposition phase ($\beta$) is extrapolated to the origin to provide the hypothetical drug concentration B at $t = 0$. The difference between early data above this extrapolated line and the estimated concentration for the same time is plotted (X) and a regression line provides the basis for the determination of ($\alpha$) and its $t = 0$ intercept value A.**

$$V_p = V_c \times (k_{12}/k_{21}) \quad (15)$$

$$V^{SS} = V_c + V_p \quad (16)$$

The determination of apparent volume of distribution by this approach in the two-compartment open model is referred to as volume of distribution at steady state ($V^{SS}$).

Often, drug disposition that is appropriately reflected by a two-compartment model is assumed to occur by a one-compartment model. This situation arises when circulating drug concentration data are available only from the $\beta$ phase of drug elimination. The larger the discrepancy between $\beta$ and $k_{el}$, the greater the error in individualization of drug therapy when the one-compartment model is assumed to apply (Loughnan et al. 1976).

## Noncompartmental Pharmacokinetic Analysis

Because of the complexity of the two-compartment analysis for drug disposition, an alternate approach to description of drug disposition has evolved that is defined as noncompartmental pharmacokinetic analysis. It is sometimes referred to also as model-independent pharmacokinetic analysis. All mathematical analyses of the drug disposition parameters can be completed without the use of differential equations. In this situation, one needs to calculate the terminal disposition rate for the drug in the circulation, and it is assumed that the drug is eliminated only from the central compartment. To distinguish this rate process from the compartmental model approaches described previously, the terminal disposition rate constant has been defined as lambda ($\lambda$). The equations that describe drug disposition by this approach are as follows.

$$CL_T = Dose/AUC = V_d \times \lambda \quad (17)$$

$$V_d = CL_T/\lambda \quad (18)$$

$$t_{1/2} = 0.693/\lambda = 0.693 \times V_d/CL_T \quad (19)$$

AUC is area under the plasma (serum) drug concentration versus time curve and is calculated by summing the areas of the trapezoids defined by the plasma concentration of the drug over adjacent time intervals (Gibaldi and Perrier 1982b). The residual AUC after the last measured drug concentration is estimated as $C_{last}/\lambda$. Although this approach to modeling of drug disposition has gained wide popularity, it is recognized that its application to physiologic processes can lead to disparate kinetic estimates, especially when there is significant elimination from other than the central kinetic compartment (DiStefano 1982).

## Choice of an Adequate Pharmacokinetic Model for Drug Dose Individualization

Data and calculated pharmacokinetic parameters for the disposition of theophylline after an intravenous dose are presented in Figure 23-2(B) and Table 23-2. This example is chosen because it represents a drug with a narrow therapeutic index, where it would be expected that inappropriate choice of a pharmacokinetic model might result in significant differences in estimated pharmacokinetic parameters and therefore in dose recommendations for a particular patient. In this instance, it is clear that the use of noncompartmental pharmacokinetic analysis is sufficiently rigorous for individualization of drug therapy. The reader is cautioned that this similarity in pharmacokinetic constants for theophylline disposition among models does not apply universally and will need to be evaluated for other drugs where there is evidence that large differences in dose recommendations may result from an inappropriate choice of a pharmacokinetic model. In the large majority of cases, it will not be necessary to resort to compartmental pharmacokinetic modeling in order to individualize drug doses. The noncompartmental pharmacokinetic model provides a relatively robust and simple approach to individualization of doses for most drugs.

**Table 23-2 Comparison of Pharmacokinetic Parameters Derived from Analyses of Plasma Concentration-Versus-Time Data**

| Model | $V_d$ (L/kg) | $CL_T$ (mL/h/kg) | $t_{1/2}$ (h) |
|---|---|---|---|
| 1C-IV bolus | 0.386 | 66 | 4.05 |
| 1C-IV infusion | 0.397 | 68 | 4.05 |
| 2C-IV bolus | 0.357 | 62 | 4.21 |
| 2C-IV infusion | 0.358 | 63 | 4.17 |
| NC-IV bolus | 0.363 | 63 | 4.01 |
| NC-IV infusion | 0.371 | 64 | 4.01 |

Data are from a 61-kg patient who received a 400-mg intravenous dose of theophylline over 20 minutes. A plot of the plasma concentration on a log scale versus time is presented in Figure 23-2(B).

On the basis of information provided, the two-compartment (2C) model with drug administration by constant infusion most closely reflects the ideal pharmacokinetic analysis of these drug concentration versus time data. For calculations based on the one-compartment (1C) open model, only plasma concentration data from 2 to 9 hours after the dose were used.

Abbreviations: NC, noncompartmental analyses; $t_{1/2}$ represents the time course of the terminal linear phase of drug disposition in each of the models.

## SPECIAL CHARACTERISTICS OF HALF-LIFE

### Distribution of Values

Half-life is determined by dividing one rate constant ($k_{el}$) into another constant (0.693). However, this maneuver changes the distribution of $t_{1/2}$ away from the gaussian "normal" shape. A hypothetical comparison is presented in Figure 23-7. Throughout the literature, $t_{1/2}$ is conventionally reported with the assumption that it is based on a normal distribution, that is, as mean ±SD or SEM. Clinically, this does not result in excess toxicity to the patient ingesting the drug, because the mean $t_{1/2}$ underestimates the rate of drug disposition relative to the frequency distribution of $k_{el}$.

### Dependence on Apparent Volume of Distribution

When $V_d$ changes, the disposition $t_{1/2}$ does not necessarily reflect the ability of a body to eliminate the drug, as $t_{1/2}$ is a function of both $V_d$ and $CL_T$. Half-life may increase because of the impaired ability of the drug to reach the

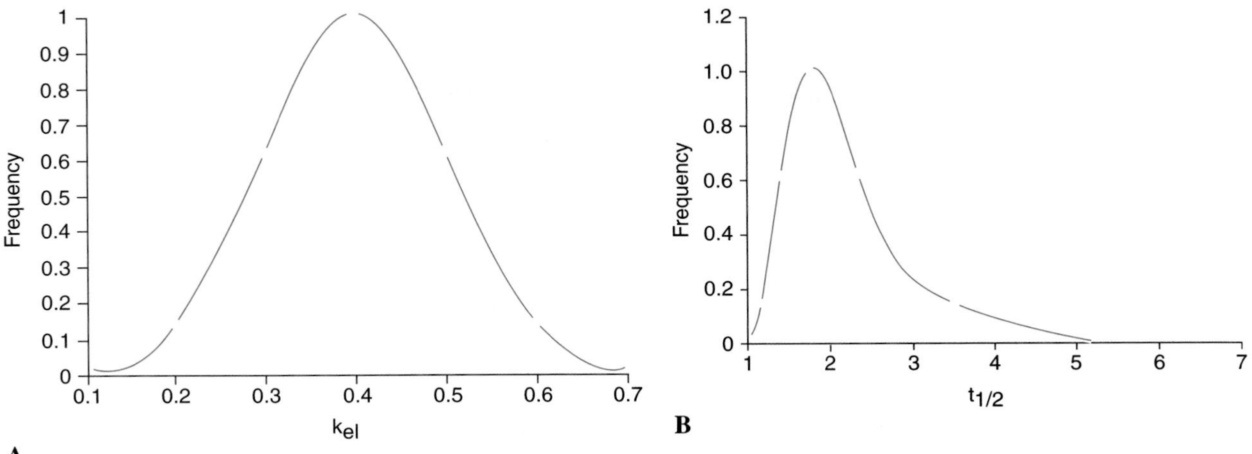


FIGURE 23-7 **(A) Plot of frequency distribution of the elimination rate constant ($k_{el}$) with a mean value of 0.4 and a SD of 0.1. This frequency distribution is then transformed by determination of the relevant half-life ($t_{1/2}$) distribution using the formula $t_{1/2} = 0.693/k_{el}$.**

elimination site. On the other hand $CL_T$ depends only on the ability of an eliminating mechanism to act on the drug concentration delivered. Thus an increase in $t_{1/2}$ may reflect an increased $V_d$ for a drug without any decrease in the body's ability to eliminate it. One of the classical examples of this situation is the effect of age on diazepam disposition. In this case, plasma $t_{1/2}$ (in hours) approximates chronological age (in years). $V_d$ increases with age, but $CL_T$ of diazepam is essentially unchanged (Klotz et al. 1975).

## CLEARANCE CONCEPTS

The ability of an organ to extract the drug delivered to it by the blood, and the regulation of its blood flow, are important factors that determine the activity of the elimination process overall. Extraction is calculated as the difference between the drug concentration entering (usually arterial) and leaving (venous) the organ divided by the drug concentration that entered it. Drugs that are virtually completely extracted during a single pass through an organ (high extraction ratio) are cleared from the circulation as a linear function of blood flow. On the other hand, drugs that are poorly extracted by an organ have a clearance that is virtually independent of physiologically relevant blood flow. Experimental studies with isolated perfused livers demonstrate a hyperbolic relationship between extraction ratio and the free drug concentration in the blood (Shand et al. 1976). An in-depth review of factors related to the ability of organs to remove drug molecules from the blood has been reported (Wilkinson 1987).

When $CL_T$ is used to describe the ability of a patient to eliminate a drug dose, no mechanism for the process is implied. Although it is widely appreciated that multiple mechanisms contribute to drug removal from the body, only total clearance ($CL_T$) and renal clearance ($CL_R$) are able to be easily determined clinically using minimally invasive methods. The determination of $CL_R$ for a drug is somewhat analogous to the determination of creatinine clearance. However, urine and blood samples usually are collected over a much shorter time interval.

A convenient method for determination of $CL_R$ for a drug of interest is to quantify the amount of drug excreted unchanged in the urine and to divide this value by the area under the plasma concentration versus time curve (AUC) for the same time interval ($t_1$–$t_2$). The equation for this determination is

$$CL_R = (C_{ur} \times V)/(\text{AUC})_{t_1-t_2} \quad (20)$$

where $C_{ur}$ is the drug concentration excreted in the urine collected during the time interval ($t_1$-$t_2$), and $V$ is the urine volume collected. This approach provides an estimate of mean $CL_R$ over the time period studied. For drugs with first-order elimination characteristics, this value will be relatively constant regardless of the time interval chosen for study (Wong et al. 1995). Nonrenal clearance is then determined as the difference between $CL_T$ and $CL_R$.

An understanding of the relative contribution of renal and nonrenal mechanisms to drug elimination should influence the physician's choice of a drug and/or its dose. A drug may be prescribed that shows less dependence for its elimination by an organ with clinically important disease. Alternately, the physician may choose to reduce the drug dose to compensate for its less efficient clearance by a diseased organ.

## FIRST-PASS AND ORAL BIOAVAILABILITY OF DRUGS

This concept is important for the determination of drug dose adjustment as a function of route of drug administration. Bioavailability ($f$) is defined as the fraction of the administered drug dose that reaches the peripheral circulation unchanged. It is determined from the relationship between area under the plasma (serum)-concentration-versus-time curve after equivalent intravenous (IV) and oral (PO) doses. The equation is as follows.

$$f = \text{Dose(IV)} \times \text{AUC(PO)}/\text{Dose(PO)} \times \text{AUC(IV)} \quad (21)$$

Although an intravenous drug dose is represented as the gold standard against which the pharmacokinetic profile for the drug administered by other routes is measured, it must be remembered that drugs administered intravenously are subject to first-pass elimination by the lungs. Because dose adjustment for route of administration is based on pharmacokinetics after an intravenous dose, the adjustment for route of administration is relative, and the presence of first-pass elimination by the lungs is only clinically relevant when drugs are administered through a central venous catheter. The bioavailability of a drug dose administered orally can show wide interindividual variation because of its removal from the body by presystemic elimination processes located in the upper intestine and the liver. Thus, it is important to take into account presystemic elimination processes when drug doses are changed from the parenteral to the oral route of administration.

## DRUG ACCUMULATION AND MAINTENANCE DOSE DETERMINATIONS

For drugs with first-order disposition characteristics, the approach is relatively straightforward. For drugs with dose-dependent disposition, the approach to dose alteration is somewhat more complicated.

For the majority of drugs with first-order disposition characteristics, it must be remembered that accumulation to a steady state is a function of the elimination rate and not the frequency of drug administration. Accumulation has a mirror-image relationship to drug elimination. Thus, it takes five elimination half-lives to approach approximate steady state for drugs with first-order disposition characteristics. Regardless of the frequency of dose administration, a steady state will not occur until approximately five elimination half-lives have passed. For a drug with a half-life of 9 hours, practical steady state occurs near the end of the second day of drug ingestion (45 hours). The amount of drug in the body at steady state will depend on the frequency of drug administration. The more frequently the drug is ingested relative to its disposition $t_{1/2}$, the greater will be the body burden at steady state. Whenever drug dose is changed, it will take another five elimination half-lives to achieve the new steady state.

When it is essential to produce therapeutic concentrations of a drug with a minimum of delay, a loading dose ($D_l$) of the drug of choice can be calculated based on published pharmacokinetic parameters relevant to the patient and disease being treated and its steady-state concentration in the circulation ($C_p{}^{SS}$). The formula for this calculation is as follows.

$$D_l = V_d \times C_p{}^{SS} \times \text{(body weight)} \quad (22)$$

For drugs with concentration-dependent toxicity, $D_l$ is usually infused by pump over a measured time period to limit toxicity associated with high drug concentrations in the blood, while producing therapeutic concentrations in the circulating volume. Achievement of therapeutic drug concentrations should be confirmed by laboratory testing of the plasma at a time after distribution equilibrium has occurred. Deviation of the patient's drug concentration in the circulation from that predicted will depend on his or her individual pharmacokinetic parameter characteristics relative to the published population estimates.

For drugs with dose-dependent disposition characteristics, the above approach to individualization of drug doses is inappropriate. An example of a reasonably straightforward approach to optimization of dose for these special drugs is provided in the following example.

An epileptic patient is administered phenytoin at a dose of 100 mg twice daily. Steady-state plasma concentration is determined to be 5 mg/L. The physician forgets that phenytoin disposition is dose-dependent and doubles the daily dose. The new plasma concentration at steady state is found to be 25 mg/L. A plot of daily dose versus daily dose/$C_p{}^{SS}$ provides the basis for final optimization of the phenytoin dose in this patient (Figure 23-8). A

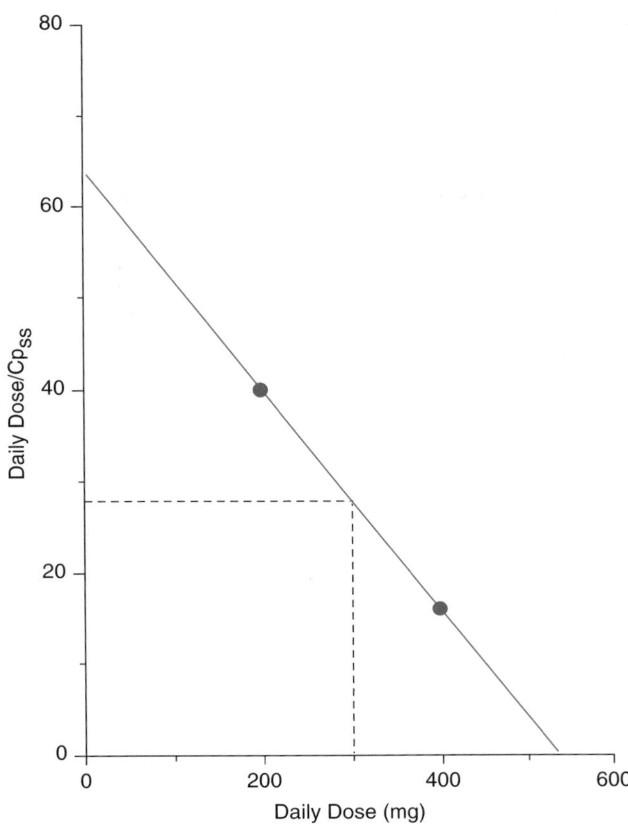


FIGURE 23-8 **Cartesian plot of daily phenytoin dose/concentration at steady-state versus daily drug dose for two dose regimens in a single patient. A regression line is drawn through the two calculated values to provide the basis for dose adjustment. In this example, if the new dose was contemplated to be 300 mg/day, the coordinate daily dose/$C_p^{SS}$ value from the graph is 28. The reciprocal predicted $C_p^{SS}$ for phenytoin in this patient is 28/300 = 0.093, and the predicted $C_p^{SS}$ is 1/0.093 = 10.7 mg/L. Of course, the value of this determination is based on the assumption that the patient complies with the prescribed drug dose regimen. The blood sample was taken for determination of the circulating phenytoin concentration at steady-state. Likewise, for a daily dose of 350 mg, daily dose/$C_p^{SS}$ = 22, 1/$C_p^{SS}$ = 0.063, and $C_p^{SS}$ is predicted to be 15.9 mg/L.**

straight line is drawn through the two points on the graph, and the individualized daily dose that produces the desired drug concentration (10–20 mg/L) at steady state is then calculated by a simple mathematical manipulation. From the straight line, a likely new dose is chosen and its coordinate daily dose/$C_p^{SS}$ is read from the graph. Division of this value of dose/$C_p^{SS}$ by the new dose yields the reciprocal value of the predicted $C_p^{SS}$. It is then a simple exercise to determine the predicted $C_p^{SS}$.

## CONFOUNDING FACTORS

Several pathophysiologic factors may alter the ability of the drug to reach its site of action. The drug may be absorbed from an unintended site (e.g., with hypochlorhydria in the elderly and in patients treated with histamine $H_2$-receptor antagonists). $V_d$ could increase because of cardiac failure. In addition, cirrhosis of the liver and/or small intestinal disease may impair the ability of an important eliminating organ to metabolize the drug delivered to it (Benet 1976; Lang et al. 1996).

Data from pharmacokinetic studies in the relevant patient cohort provide the scientific basis for recommended drug dose adjustments. Experimental pharmacokinetic approaches that enable the elucidation of the mechanisms involved in alteration of bioavailability are described in considerable detail elsewhere (Kwan 1997).

## FUNDAMENTAL ISSUES IN PHARMACODYNAMICS OF DRUGS

### Direct Effect Models

Traditionally, the pharmacologic response to a drug in an in vitro model system has been presented as a function of the logarithm of the dose (concentration) under equilibrium conditions. However, this approach does not allow for the nonlinearity of the relationship at very low drug concentrations, or saturation of the response that occurs at high drug concentrations. For steady-state conditions, five models for drug pharmacodynamics have been proposed.

The simplest is the fixed-effect model. It relates a certain drug concentration to the presence or absence of a pharmacodynamic effect. The presence or absence of the pharmacodynamic effect of interest will vary among patients with respect to the plasma concentration at which it occurs. The occurrence of the effect is then described statistically as a probability that the pharmacodynamic effect may be observed for a given drug concentration in a patient to whom the drug has been administered. This modeling approach has very limited value, but may be useful in the prediction of a threshold concentration associated with unacceptable drug toxicity. A useful example is the plasma concentration at which digoxin toxicity is likely to occur at an unacceptable rate (see Holford and Sheiner 1982).

A linear model is sometimes used to describe the relationship between drug concentration and pharmacody-

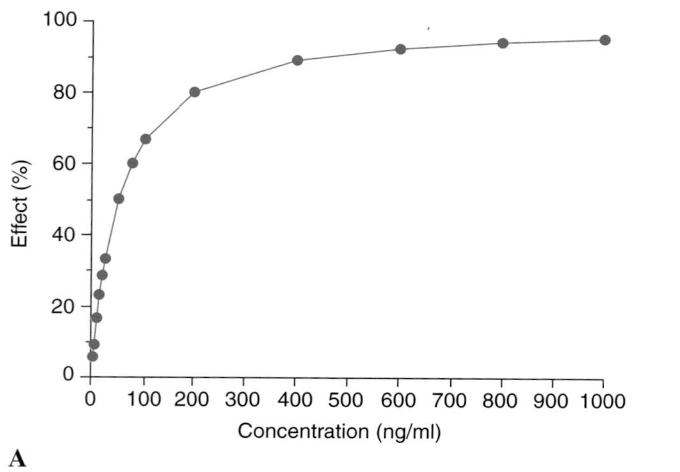


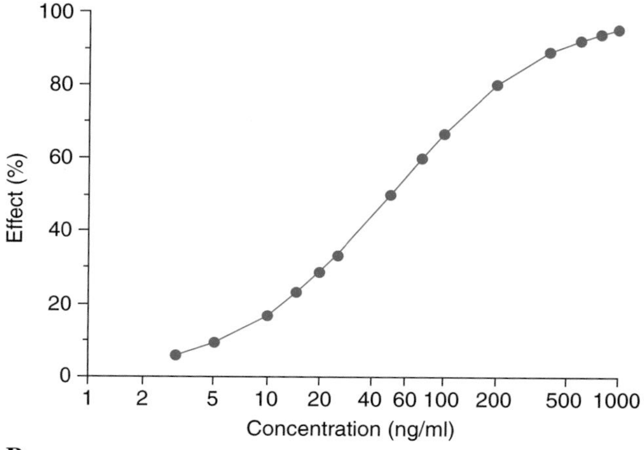


**FIGURE 23-9 Cartesian plot of concentration versus effect for a drug with an $EC_{50}$ plasma concentration of 50 ng/ml (A) Data are derived with equation (23). (B) The more familiar sigmoidal curve that results when the concentration presented in (A) is plotted on a logarithmic scale versus effect.**

namic effect. However, its usefulness is limited to situations where the range of drug concentrations of interest is very narrow and does not unmask the inherent nonlinearity between drug concentrations and pharmacodynamic effects observed almost universally.

The log-linear model is much more commonly used to describe the relationship between drug concentration and its pharmacodynamic effect. This approach is analogous to the in vitro situation where drug effects on isolated tissues are described as a function of the logarithm of the drug concentration in the bathing medium. It needs to be recalled that this approximation holds only for the range of 20 to 80% of the maximum drug effect that may be elicited. Thus, this modeling approach fails to predict accurately drug effects at very high or very low concentrations where substantial nonlinearity is present.

The simplest model able to predict no drug effect in its absence and an estimation of a drug concentration producing the maximum pharmacodynamic response is the so-called $E_{max}$ model. This model is a reflection of a hyperbolic function with striking similarity to the classical Michaelis-Menten equation. It is usually expressed as

$$E = (E_{max} \times C)/(E_{50} + C) \qquad (23)$$

where $E$ represents the drug effect observed at concentration $C$, $E_{max}$ the maximum drug effect, and $E_{50}$ the drug concentration producing half of the maximum pharmacodynamic effect. Similar to the rate-limiting situations presented for pharmacokinetic analyses, at drug concentrations much less than the $E_{50}$, an approximately linear relationship between drug concentration and effect is predicted. Transformation of the data to a plot of the drug concentration on a logarithmic scale versus effect reveals the classical sigmoidal relationship between drug concentration and pharmacodynamic response that is approximately linear between 20 and 80% of $E_{max}$. The two graphical representations of this model are presented in Figure 23-9. The reader is also referred to Table 23-3 for an example of why drug dose escalation often does not provide the increased benefit intuitively expected.

In some cases, a better fit of the data is obtained when the concentration terms in the $E_{max}$ model are raised to a

**Table 23-3 Fractional Approach to Maximal Effect Relative to $EC_{50}$ Units of Drug Concentration**

| Drug Concentration | Effect (% $E_{max}$) |
|---|---|
| 0.1 | 9.1 |
| 0.3 | 23.1 |
| 0.5 | 33.3 |
| 0.7 | 41.2 |
| 1.0 | 50 |
| 2.0 | 66.7 |
| 4.0 | 80 |
| 8.0 | 88.9 |

This relationship applies to both agonist activity and antagonist activity where an effect may be completely abolished by the treatment.
Abbreviations: $EC_{50}$, median effective concentration; $E_{max}$, maximal effect.

power function ($n$). The mathematical representation for this modeling approach is a modification of equation (23) and is expressed as follows.

$$E = (E_{\max} \times C^n)/(E_{50}{}^n + C^n) \qquad (24)$$

The higher the power function attached to the concentration terms, the steeper the slope of the curve of drug concentration versus maximum effect. The reader may recall this general form of the equation from the mathematical description for the association between oxygen and hemoglobin (Hill 1910). This manipulation of the model is somewhat controversial for pharmacodynamic analyses, and its interpretation is quite speculative (Holford and Sheiner 1981).

## LINKING PHARMACOKINETICS AND PHARMACODYNAMICS

It was appreciated a long time ago that it should be possible to apply concepts developed to describe the pharmacokinetic disposition of drugs to their pharmacodynamics (Pliška 1966; Segre 1968). However, a considerable time passed before the multiple models used to describe drug pharmacodynamics could be evaluated critically (Holford and Sheiner 1982). Several models have been proposed to describe the effects of drugs relative to their pharmacokinetic disposition, and these have been recently reviewed (Meibohm and Derendorf 1997). The linking of pharmacodynamic and pharmacokinetic models to provide a better understanding of the relationship between drug disposition and efficacy also has been reviewed recently (Cawello 1997).

When drugs are administered to patients, the pharmacodynamic response varies over the dose interval, and often the physician wishes to evaluate drug effects under non-steady-state conditions. One modeling approach that has been successful is the addition of an effect compartment to the pharmacokinetic models discussed earlier in this chapter (Figure 23-10). However, when attempts are made to relate drug concentrations to effects in vivo, two systematic deviations from the attempted correlation are often observed.

First, it may be observed that the drug effect continues to increase even after the drug concentration in the circulation begins to decline. When this type of data is plotted, there is a hysteresis, a counterclockwise deviation from linearity when drug effect is monitored for both rising and falling drug concentrations in the circulation (Figure 23-11). This type of observation is consistent with a

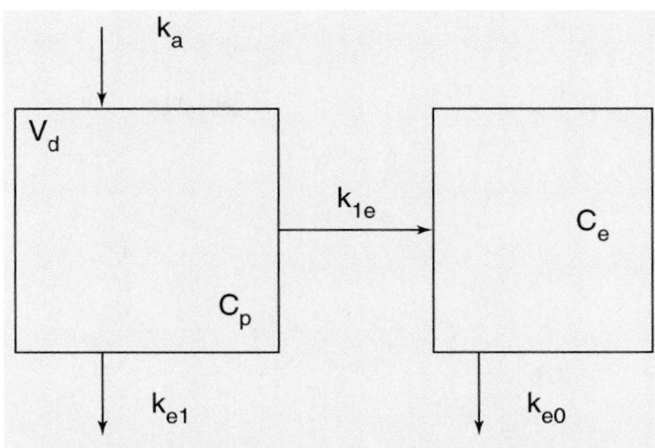


**FIGURE 23-10 The essential components of a one-compartment open pharmacokinetic model to which has been added an effect compartment. The delivery of the dose into the pharmacokinetic compartment is characterized by the absorption rate constant ($k_a$) when drug is administered by other than the parenteral route. The rate of elimination from this compartment is characterized by the elimination rate constant ($k_{el}$). The effect compartment is linked to the pharmacokinetic compartment by the first-order rate constant $k_{1e}$, but receives very little of the drug from the pharmacokinetic compartment. Drug concentration is therefore related to effect by the first-order rate constant $k_{e0}$ that characterizes the rate of disappearance of the drug from the effect compartment.**

delayed access of the drug molecule to its site of action. The inotropic effect of digoxin is an example of this type of effect.

Second, drug effects for the same concentration measured when it is rising may be greater than when it is decreasing in the circulation. This observation results in a clockwise deviation from linearity (proteresis) when drug concentration versus effect plots are constructed (Figure 23-12). A relevant clinical example in this instance is the central nervous system impairment produced by alcohol.

However, interpretation of these observations is complicated by data that suggest that deviations from the direct-linked associations may be related to the site from which blood is sampled (Chiou 1989a, 1989b; Stanski et al. 1984; Gourlay and Benowitz 1997).

For some drugs, a measurable pharmacodynamic response is delayed considerably beyond the time it takes for them to reach the site of action. In these instances, the drug effect is said to occur indirectly relative to its concentration in the circulation. A series of four basic physiologic indirect response models has been proposed to characterize these pharmacodynamic responses (Sharma and Jusko 1998). These models arise from the proposition that a drug may stimulate or inhibit formation of a pre-

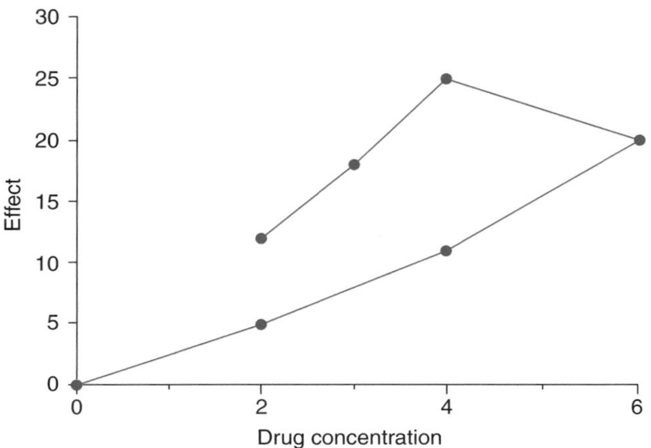


**FIGURE 23-11 The relationship of drug concentration versus effect, where effect continues to increase while drug concentration decreases (hysteresis).**

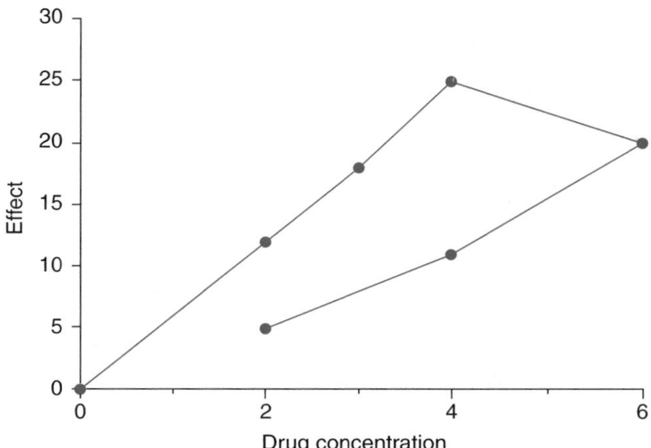


**FIGURE 23-12 The relationship of drug concentration versus effect, where drug effect is less for the same concentration when drug concentration is decreasing in the circulation compared with when it is increasing (proteresis).**

cursor molecule associated with the pharmacodynamic effect. Conversely, a drug may stimulate or inhibit the removal process for the termination of a pharmacodynamic effect. Appropriate modeling of the pharmacodynamic data will depend on an understanding of the mechanism of action of the particular drug in question.

Inhibition of production of a substance associated with a pharmacodynamic event or stimulation of its destruction will provide similar graphical data. Similarly stimulation of production of a substance associated with a pharmacodynamic event or inhibition of its destruction will also produce graphical data that appear similar. Distinction between each of the two possibilities to explain drug action can be achieved by use of single intravenous dose and steady-state infusion drug doses combined with careful observation of the pharmacodynamic response (Sharma and Jusko 1996).

## AREAS OF CONTROVERSY

Approaches to modeling of drug pharmacodynamics under non-steady-state conditions are still a source of debate. This aspect of pharmacodynamic modeling and its linking to pharmacokinetics of drug disposition remains an active area of investigation. The potential confounding effect of sampling site for blood on the interpretation of pharmacokinetic–pharmacodynamic experimental data has been reviewed in detail (Chiou 1989a, 1989b). Data of Gourlay and Benowitz (1997) with nicotine and Stanski et al. (1984) with thiopental demonstrate that concurrent arterial and venous blood sampling may be important for determining whether drug effect is best related to arterial or venous drug concentrations, and whether hysteresis is observed in the model used to explain pharmacokinetic–pharmacodynamic relationships.

The approaches presented above demonstrate the unquestionable value of being able to model pharmacokinetic and pharmacodynamic drug effects concurrently. Refinement of this approach has the potential to provide an improved understanding of pharmacokinetic–pharmacodynamic associations for drugs where an association has not been appreciated by most practitioners. In addition, this approach to the understanding of the two modeling processes provides substantial promise for optimization of treatment with the many new drug substances that will undoubtedly be available in the future.

## REFERENCES


Benet LZ, editor. 1976. The effect of disease states on drug pharmacokinetics. Washington, DC: American Pharmaceutical Association. p 1–242.

Cawello W. 1997. Connection of pharmacokinetics and pharmacodynamics—how does it work? *Int J Clin Pharmacol Ther* **35**:414–7.

Chiou WL. 1989a. The phenomenon and rationale of marked dependence of drug concentration on blood sampling site. Implications in pharmacokinetics, pharmacodynamics, toxicology and therapeutics (Part I). *Clin Pharmacokinet* **17**:175–99.

Chiou WL. 1989b. The phenomenon and rationale of marked dependence of drug concentration on blood sampling site. Implications in pharmacokinetics, pharmacodynamics, toxicology and therapeutics (Part II). *Clin Pharmacokinet* **17**:275–90.

DiStefano JJ III. 1982. Noncompartmental vs. compartmental analysis: Some bases for choice. *Am J Physiol* **243**:R1–R5.

Gibaldi M, Perrier D. 1982a. Chapter 1. One-compartment model. *Pharmacokinetics*. New York: Marcel Dekker. p 33–9.

Gibaldi M, Perrier D. 1982b. Appendix D. Estimation of areas. *Pharmacokinetics*. New York: Marcel Dekker. p 445–9.

Gourlay SG, Benowitz NL. 1997. Arteriovenous differences in plasma concentration of nicotine and catecholamines and related cardiovascular effects after smoking, nicotine nasal spray, and intravenous nicotine. *Clin Pharmacol Ther* **62**:453–63.

Hill AV. 1910. The possible effects of the aggregation of the molecules of haemoglobin on its dissociation curves. *J Physiol (London)* **40**:4–7.

Holford NHG, Sheiner LB. 1981. Understanding the dose-effect relationship: Clinical application of pharmacokinetic-pharmacodynamic models. *Clin Pharmacokinet* **6**:429–53.

Holford NHG, Sheiner LB. 1982. Kinetics of pharmacologic response. *Pharmac Ther* **16**:143–66.

Klotz U, Avant GR, Hoyumpa A, et al. 1975. The effects of age and liver disease on the disposition and elimination of diazepam in adult man. *J Clin Invest* **55**:347–59.

Kwan KC. 1997. Oral bioavailability and first-pass effects. *Drug Metab Dispos* **25**:1329–36.

Lang CC, Brown RM, Kinirons MT, et al. 1996. Decreased intestinal CYP3A in celiac disease: Reversal after successful gluten-free diet: A potential source of interindividual variability in first-pass drug metabolism. *Clin Pharmacol Ther* **59**:41–6.

Loughnan PM, Sitar DS, Ogilvie RI, et al. 1976. The two-compartment open-system kinetic model: A review of its clinical implications and applications. *J Pediatr* **88**:869–73.

Massoud TF, Hademenos GJ, Young WL, et al. 1998. Principles and philosophy of modeling in biomedical research. *FASEB J* **12**: 275–85.

Meibohm B, Derendorf H. 1997. Basic concepts of pharmacokinetic/pharmacodynamic (PK/PD) modelling. *Int J Clin Pharmacol Ther* **35**:401–13.

Pliška V. 1966. On the in vivo kinetics of drug action. *Arz Forsch* **16**:886–93.

Segre G. 1968. Kinetics of interaction between drugs and biological systems. *Farmaco Ed Sci (Rome)* **23**(10):907–18.

Shand DG, Cotham RH, Wilkinson GR. 1976. Perfusion-limited effects of plasma drug binding on hepatic drug extraction. *Life Sci* **19**:125–30.

Sharma A, Jusko WJ. 1996. Characterization of four basic models of indirect pharmacodynamic responses. *J Pharmacokinet Biopharm* **24**:611–34.

Sharma A, Jusko WJ. 1998. Characteristics of indirect pharmacodynamic models and applications to clinical drug responses. *Br J Clin Pharmacol* **45**:229–39.

Stanski DR, Hudson RJ, Homer TD, et al. 1984. Pharmacodynamic modeling of thiopental anesthesia. *J Pharmacokinet Biopharm* **12**:223–40.

Wilkinson GR. 1987. Clearance approaches in pharmacology. *Pharmacol Rev* **39**:1–47.

Wong LTY, Sitar DS, Aoki FY. 1995. Chronic tobacco smoking and gender as variables affecting amantadine disposition in healthy subjects. *Br J Clin Pharmacol* **39**:81–4.

CHAPTER

# 24 ADVERSE DRUG REACTIONS

David W. Bates, Lucian Leape

*Chapter Outline*



Drugs can be remarkably beneficial, lengthening life and improving its quality by reducing symptoms and improving well-being. However, all drugs have adverse effects and carry the potential of causing injury, even if used properly. Well-gathered, highly representative data about the adverse effects of drugs help physicians use drugs, balancing the benefits and hazards. With the increased development of novel drugs, there has been a rise in the potential for adverse drug effects. Although the pharmacologic and therapeutic effects of novel molecules may be more powerful or efficacious than those of their predecessors, they will not necessarily be safer. It is unfortunate, but not surprising, that toxicity frequently occurs in patients in whom a particular drug was inappropriately prescribed in the first place (Palmer 1969; Stolley and Lasagna 1969; Lennard et al. 1970; and Venulet 1975).

## DEFINITIONS OF ADVERSE DRUG REACTIONS AND ADVERSE DRUG EVENTS

In this section, we discuss and define the terms adverse drug event (ADE), adverse drug reaction (ADR), and medication error, and the relationships between them. An adverse drug event (or ADE) has been defined as an injury resulting from medical intervention related to a drug (Bates et al. 1995b). This includes injuries that occur because of errors in giving the medication, as well as those not associated with such an error. In contrast, an adverse drug reaction (ADR) has been defined by the World Health Organization (WHO) as "an effect which is noxious and unintended, and which occurs at doses used in man for prophylaxis, diagnosis, or therapy" (Forrester 1971). This definition is restrictive because it only considers incidents where use of the drug is appropriate, excluding the many adverse events caused by errors that are by definition preventable. Another approach has been to use the terms type A ADR, and type B ADR. Type A reactions are exaggerated extensions of the primary or secondary pharmacologic activity of the drug (Koch 1990), for example, complete heart block induced by a $\beta$-adrenergic receptor blocking agent (beta-blocker); these reactions are often dose-dependent. Type B reactions are idiosyncratic reactions, which are generally immunologic or allergic; they are generally independent of the dose and route of administration. The term ADE includes both type A and B reactions, as well as events due to errors.

ADEs can be divided according to whether or not they are preventable. For organizations monitoring patient injuries and trying to improve the quality of care, the ADE may be a more useful outcome (Bates et al. 1995b), whereas for measuring the risk of an adverse outcome when a drug is used appropriately (for example, from the perspective of a pharmaceutical manufacturer), the term ADR may be better. Serious or unexpected adverse drug reactions should be reported to the drug's manufacturer, as well as to the United States Food and Drug Administration (FDA). Adverse reactions to the agents used in drug formulation are not discussed in this section. An in-depth guide to reactions associated with excipients and a reminder of their importance to the problem of adverse drug reactions has been published by Weiner and Bernstein (1989).

Another important concept is the medication error, which we define as an error in ordering, transcribing, dispensing, or administering a medication, regardless of whether an injury occurred or whether the potential for injury was present (Bates et al. 1995b). Although most medication errors have little potential for harm, a small proportion do. Those that do not result in harm are called potential adverse drug events. An even smaller group of medication errors actually results in injuries; these are termed preventable adverse drug events. In a study designed to assess the proportion of medication errors that actually resulted in an ADE or had the potential to do so (Bates et al. 1995b), only 7 in 100 medication errors were potential ADEs, whereas 1 in 100 resulted in a preventable ADE.

Others have used different definitions for medication errors, and debate is currently ongoing about these definitions. For example, Allan and Barker have defined a medication error as "a deviation from the physician's medication order as written in the chart" (Allan and Barker 1990). However, this definition excludes ordering errors, which are not only common, but also the errors most likely to result in injury. These authors have developed a methodology for identifying medication errors that has been used in a variety of studies and is highly effective for identifying medication administration errors. This method depends on a disguised observation technique in which a trained observer watches a health professional, notes what the individual does when administering drugs, and notes consumption of the medication by the patient (Allan and Barker 1990). This approach usually finds about one error per patient per day and is reliable (Barker and Allan 1995).

## INCIDENCE OF ADVERSE DRUG REACTIONS

Several more recent studies have focused on ADEs (Classen et al. 1991; Bates et al. 1995b; Classen et al. 1997). The identified rates depend on the outcome definitions and the detection strategies used in each study. Computerized detection strategies use the computer to screen for clinical, laboratory, and drug data that suggest that an ADE may have occurred; this is followed by evaluation by a clinical pharmacist (Classen et al. 1991; Jha et al. 1996). Using a computerized detection approach in one tertiary care hospital, Classen found a rate of 2.0 severe ADEs per 100 admissions (Classen et al. 1991). In a study that used a detection approach combining daily chart review with simulated voluntary reporting in a tertiary care hospital, a rate of 6.5 ADEs per 100 medical and surgical admissions was found. This study also included less severe ADEs (Bates et al. 1995b); when the analysis was restricted to serious or life-threatening events, the ADE rate was 2.8 per 100 admissions, similar to that found by Classen.

An important issue has been the fraction of events missed by chart review and computer monitors, as well as the extent of overlap of events found using the two methods. In a direct comparison of these approaches, chart review identified 65% of ADEs found by any of the approaches, whereas a computerized ADE monitor found 45%, and voluntary report only 4% (Jha et al. 1998). It is surprising that only 12% were found by both the computerized monitor and chart review. Events associated with a numerical change (e.g., development of renal failure in a patient receiving a nephrotoxic drug) were found more often by the computerized monitor, whereas events associated with symptoms such as confusion were found more often by chart review.

**Key Point: These data provide strong evidence that no one method captures all events, and that the true incidence of adverse drug events is likely to be at least 10 per 100 admissions in tertiary care hospitals.**

The computerized detection method is much less expensive than chart review, which would not be practical on a routine basis. It should be possible to improve the sensitivity of computerized detection as more coded data become available (Jha et al. 1996).

In addition to their human costs, adverse drug events are expensive to the health-care system. Two studies conducted independently arrived at estimates of about $2000 per event (Bates et al. 1997; Classen et al. 1997). Preventable events were even more costly, approximately $4500 per event (Bates et al. 1997). These figures do not include the costs of malpractice claims, the costs of hospital admissions resulting from ADEs, or the costs of injuries to patients after hospital visit or admission.

**Key Point: Nationally, ADEs occurring during hospitalization have been projected to cost hospitals $2 billion per year (Bates et al. 1997; Classen et al. 1997); consequently, the overall costs of this problem to society are undoubtedly much higher.**

Studies of the incidence of medication errors find vastly differing rates depending on the intensity and types of surveillance strategies used. For example, the number and types of errors intercepted by pharmacists have been evaluated (Folli et al. 1987; Lesar et al. 1990). In a 1-year study at a teaching hospital, 3.1 errors per 1000 orders, of which 58% had the potential for adverse consequences, were found (Lesar et al. 1990). In another study over 6 months at two children's hospitals, 4.7 errors per 1000 orders were found (Folli et al. 1987). These studies included only errors detected and prevented by pharmacists and did not assess the number of preventable ADEs. As noted earlier, by using a direct observation approach to assess the frequency of administration errors, much higher rates, approximately 1 per patient per day, have been found. In a study on three units of a medical service in which the evaluation approach included review of all orders with spontaneous reporting of problems by pharmacists, as well as daily chart review, 53 errors per 1000 orders were identified (Bates et al. 1995b).

## RISK FACTORS FOR ADVERSE DRUG EVENTS

Although relatively few data are available, adverse drug events are more frequently encountered at the extremes of age. In the neonate, the liver and kidney enzymes necessary for drug metabolism and elimination have not yet become optimally functional and clearance of many drugs is less than in adults. In the elderly, changes in liver and kidney function may decrease drug elimination.

From several series, women are reported to have a 50% higher rate of adverse events than men. Though women may more frequently obtain medical attention and medications than men, there are definite periods during a woman's lifetime when there is alteration of the pharmacokinetics of drugs: menarche, pregnancy and delivery, lactation, and menopause (Wilson 1984). For these reasons, women may be at a higher risk than men for experiencing drug reactions.

Patients with a past history of reactions to medications are more apt to experience adverse drug reactions. In a New Zealand hospital study reported by Smidt and McQueen (1972), 28% of those patients who had an adverse drug reaction had experienced an adverse reaction previously.

A history of allergic disease is also associated with an increased risk of reactions. Adverse responses are not entirely unexpected since careful questioning usually reveals prior exposure to the drug. There may be a genetically determined propensity to form considerably larger amounts of immunoglobulin IgE with an increased liability to anaphylactic-type reactions.

Genetic factors may be very important in predisposing to adverse drug effects. These may include polymorphisms in drug metabolism, as well as other metabolic variants (see Chapter 22). For example, there are patients who are at increased risk of suffering hemolytic episodes associated with drugs that alter redox potential and produce oxidative stresses on the red blood cells that may be due to sex-linked deficiency of glucose-6-phosphate dehydrogenase. In these persons, cells are incapable of sufficiently rapid regeneration of NADPH (Bloom et al. 1983). Primaquine has been the prototype of such drugs, but there are more than 50 drugs and substances known to be capable of inciting hemolysis. In addition to antimalarials, the list includes sulfones, sulfonamides, nitrofurans, antipyretics, analgesics, vitamin K preparations, fava beans, and other vegetables.

The route of administration can alter the bioavailability of drugs, for example, the poor absorption of medications from intramuscular injection sites during a period of cardiovascular shock, the unreliable absorption of phenytoin after IM administration because of its high pH and in situ precipitation, and poor antibody response to hepatitis B vaccine when given in the gluteal muscles compared with a deltoid site (Kostenbauder et al. 1975; Pead et al. 1985; Ukena et al. 1985). Topical medication, such as an acetylcholinesterase inhibitor or a beta-blocker instilled into the eye for treatment for glaucoma may have systemic absorption by entry into the lachrymal duct with drainage into the nasal cavity and ultimately the GI tract (Gibaldi 1984). There may be enough systemic absorption to cause increased intestinal peristalsis and abdominal cramps from the first agent or exacerbation of asthma and/or alteration of heart rate or atrioventricular (AV) nodal conduction from the latter.

The large surface area of the alveoli, the rich blood supply of the lungs, and the high permeability of the alveolar epithelium make the lungs remarkably efficient organs for drug absorption and ensure the rapid uptake of drugs given by inhalation. Anesthetic agents are the most important examples of drugs routinely given by this route. Several illicit drugs are also absorbed following inhalation

(Gibaldi 1984). Bronchodilators, such as sympathomimetics and adrenocorticosteroids, that affect pulmonary function are frequently administered by this route. Between 1961 and 1966 increased sales of pressurized aerosols of sympathomimetics in England and Wales corresponded with an increase in mortality due to asthma, with the increase greatest in children 10 to 14 years of age. Since March 1967, there has been a sharp decline in deaths due to asthma along with a reduction of the use of pressurized aerosols (Inman and Adelsteen 1969). There was consideration that the propellant might be at fault. However, a case-control study (Spitzer et al. 1992) showed that there was a large increase in mortality with increasing doses of these agents, with fenoterol in particular. Fenoterol has since been removed from the market.

A problem with all these studies is that there is confounding by severity: sicker patients tend to use more medications, so that with this study design causality cannot be established. Many of these deaths were very likely the result of undertreatment with corticosteroids. More recent data have demonstrated the efficacy of inhaled corticosteroids in treatment of asthma (Haahtela et al. 1991), and the current trend, which is supported by pathophysiologic data, is to use inhaled steroids earlier and on a regular basis, and to reserve beta-adrenergic receptor agonist therapy for as-needed situations, with the goal of avoiding large doses of these agents.

## RECOGNIZING ADVERSE DRUG REACTIONS

For estimating the probability that a specific drug is responsible for an adverse drug reaction, several scales have been developed (Karch and Lasagna 1977; Kramer et al. 1979; Naranjo et al. 1981), but the most widely used is the Naranjo algorithm (Naranjo et al. 1981). It has good interrater reliability and is quick; it consists of 10 questions addressing different issues about the probability that an ADR occurred (Table 24-1), which can be answered yes, no, or "do not know." The results are then summed, and the score allows assessment of the probability that an event occurred. A score of 1 to 4 points indicates that an ADR is considered possible, 5–8 probable, and 9 or more definite. In clinical practice (i.e., outside the setting of a randomized trial) most reactions are scored in the "probable" category, because placebos are almost never given, and rechallenge is uncommon. Nonetheless, this scale represents a convenient, practical tool for making an assessment about the probability that a given reaction can be attributed to a specific drug.

**Key Point: No clinically useful drug is devoid of toxicity. Consequently, physicians must accept a commitment to understand the effects of drugs in disease, the predisposing factors to drug reactions, and the effects of disease on drugs in order to use them as safely as possible.**

**PRINCIPLE Adverse drug events may not be recognized if physicians assume that pharmacologic therapy is always beneficial (Melville 1984; Blaschke et al. 1985). It is just as important for clinicians to recognize the presence of an adverse drug event as it is to diagnose a serious disease.**

Temporary withdrawal of a drug is a simple and inexpensive diagnostic measure. Although the testing procedures before the introduction of a new drug are expensive and often lengthy, this does not guarantee efficacy of the drug in all situations in which it is indicated, and it must be remembered that considerable numbers of adverse effects will not be discovered until the drug has been used by many thousands of patients.

## TYPES OF ADVERSE DRUG EFFECTS

### General Types of Adverse Drug Effects

Adverse effects of drugs may be classified into two general groups: those that are intrinsic to the drug effects (type A ADRs) and those that are idiosyncratic (type B ADRs). A third type of effect may occur exclusively as a consequence of discontinuing the use of a drug; these are called adverse drug withdrawal events, or ADWEs (Graves et al. 1997). Intrinsic (type A) drug effects are direct extensions of the pharmacologic actions of either the drug or its metabolites. These adverse effects are primarily dependent on the inherent chemical properties of the drug and are generally concentration- or dose-dependent. Intrinsic adverse effects may constitute 70 to 80% of drug reactions and are often predictable and thus preventable in many instances.

One prototype of investigation that has established a reactive intermediate as a mechanism of drug toxicity is acetaminophen. Acetaminophen is a relatively safe drug when it is used in standard doses that produce analgesia.

**Table 24-1 Naranjo Algorithm: Attribution**

| Question | Yes | No | Do Not Know |
|---|---|---|---|
| 9.1.1 Are there previous *conclusive* reports on this reaction? | +1 | 0 | 0 |
| 9.1.2 Did the adverse event appear after the suspected drug was administered? | +2 | −1 | 0 |
| 9.1.3 Did the adverse reaction improve when the drug was discontinued or a *specific* antagonist was administered? | +1 | 0 | 0 |
| 9.1.4 Did the adverse reaction reappear when the drug was readministered? | +2 | −1 | 0 |
| 9.1.5 Are there alternative causes (other than the drug) that could on their own have caused the reaction? | −1 | +2 | 0 |
| 9.1.6 Did the reaction reappear when a placebo was given? | −1 | +1 | 0 |
| 9.1.7 Was the drug detected in the blood (or other fluids) in concentrations known to be toxic? | +1 | 0 | 0 |
| 9.1.8 Was the reaction more severe when the dose was increased, or less severe when the dose was decreased? | +1 | 0 | 0 |
| 9.1.9 Did the patient have a similar reaction to the same or similar drugs in any previous exposure? | +1 | 0 | 0 |
| 9.1.10 Was the adverse event confirmed by *any* objective evidence? | +1 | 0 | 0 |
| | | | TOTAL SCORE = ____ |

From Naranjo et al. 1981.
Score: Adverse event possible = 1–4; probable = 5–8; definite =9 or more.
Maximum possible score = 13.

However, fatal hepatic necrosis can occur after an overdose. The toxic effect of the drug did not correlate with its concentration in plasma or in the liver, suggesting that a metabolite was responsible for the disease. This toxic metabolite has been identified as N-acetyl-p-benzoquinone-imine, one of the products of metabolism of acetaminophen by the cytochrome P450 mixed-function oxidase system. This reactive metabolite normally is rapidly detoxified by glutathione in the liver. In overdose, production of the toxic metabolite exceeds glutathione (GSH) capacity, and the metabolite reacts directly with hepatic macromolecules, causing liver injury. N-Acetylcysteine given during the optimal period after ingestion of acetaminophen is an effective antidote (Smilkstein et al. 1988). (See Figs. 24-1 and 24-2.)

Idiosyncratic (type B) adverse effects are of major concern as they are difficult to predict and may not be discovered until the drug has been used by many patients. The main goal of the MedWatch system is to identify such effects as early as possible. These reactions are generally host-dependent, seemingly dose-independent, difficult to reproduce in animals, and comparatively uncommon. Some reactions are associated with congenital enzyme deficiencies in the host, such as the lack of glucose-6-phosphate dehydrogenase with increased vulnerability of erythrocytes to oxidative injury by several drugs. Other untoward reactions have a hypersensitivity (immunologic) basis.

Common examples of ADWEs or withdrawal events are withdrawal symptoms after narcotic analgesia, sympathetic overactivity, and severe hypertension, which may occur after clonidine therapy is suddenly stopped; adrenal insufficiency precipitated by the abrupt cessation of adrenal corticosteroid therapy; and the delirium, confusion, agitation, and seizures that may occur after discontinuing CNS depressants such as alcohol, benzodiazepines, or barbiturates.

## Drug Allergy (Hypersensitivity)

Drug allergies are extremely varied in their clinical presentations and can be life-threatening. Clinical manifestations include anaphylaxis, bronchospasm, dermatitis, fever, granulocytopenia, hemolytic anemia, hepatitis, lupus erythematosus-like syndrome, nephritis, pneumonitis, thrombocytopenia, and vasculitis. Often several of these reactions may occur at the same time. How intrinsically nonimmunogenic small organic molecules cause allergic reactions is still controversial, although mechanisms have been identified for some small chemicals; many are mediated through activation of hapten-specific T cells (Kapsenberg 1996).

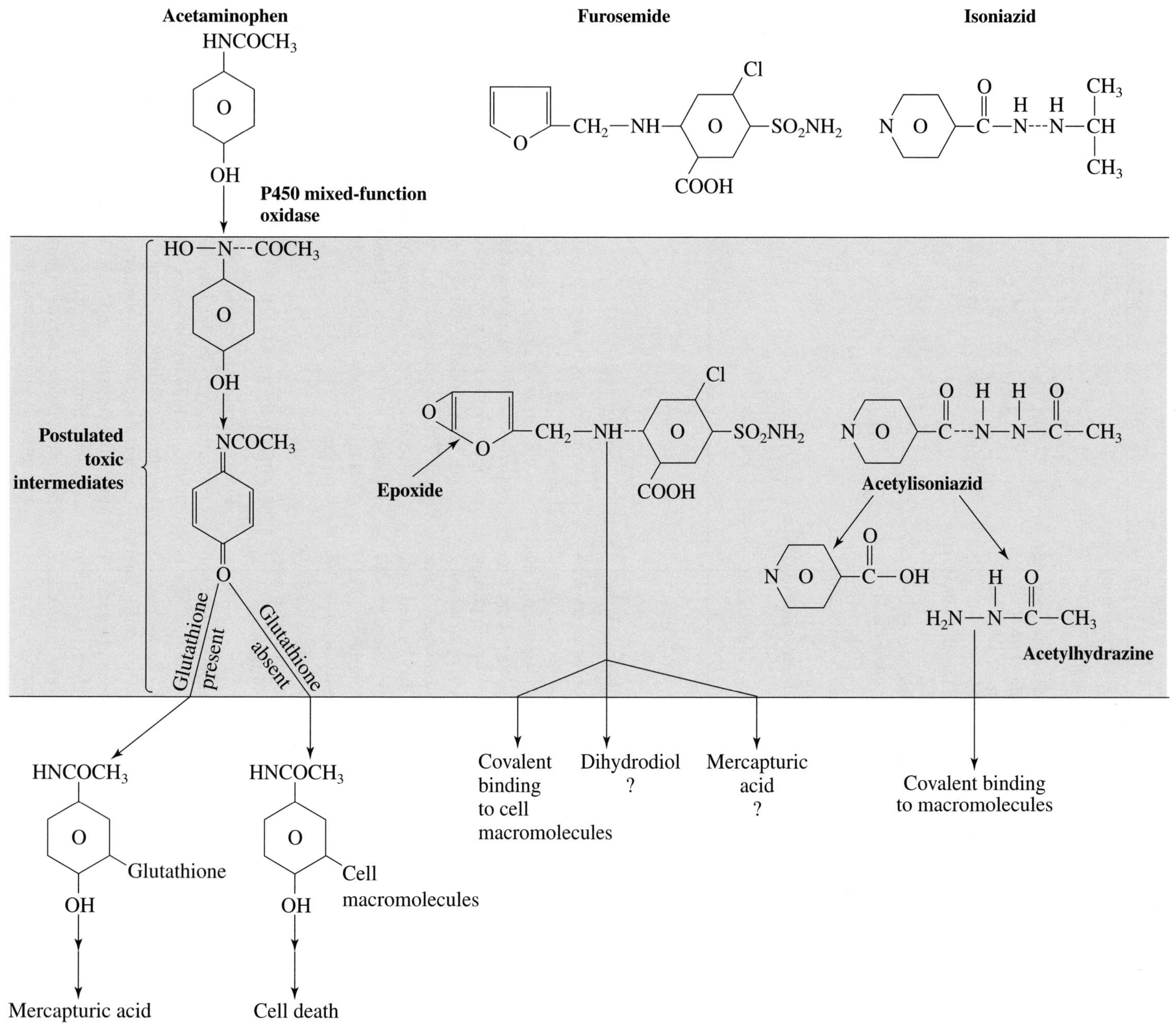


**FIGURE 24-1 The probable reactive metabolic intermediates of three different types of drug whose toxicity is likely to be based on covalent binding of the metabolites to cellular proteins. Note that in the case of acetaminophen, modulation of toxicity might be accomplished by modifying P450 activity or the availability of glutathione.**

### *Pathophysiology*

Usually for an organic molecule to be recognized as nonself and to induce an immune response, it must have a molecular mass of at least 1000 daltons, which is larger than most drugs. Although there may be some exceptions, small nonimmunogenic organic molecules, or haptens, must become covalently bound to an endogenous carrier macromolecule to form a drug-carrier conjugate to elicit immune responses. Drug-carrier conjugates may be formed if the drug or its decomposition products produced during manufacturing are chemically reactive, or if the drug is activated into reactive status in the body by biotransformation or by photoactivation of the drug in the skin to create reactive molecules to form drug-carrier conjugates. The drug-carrier conjugate can then become an immunogen and elicit a specific antibody (humoral) response or a specific T-lymphocyte (cellular) response or both (Lien 1987a; Pohl et al. 1988). The hapten conjugate and antibody interaction must take place in the proper setting to cause tissue injury. The inflammatory process that develops expresses that reaction. These multiple steps are under separate genetic control (McDevitt and Benacerraf 1969; Benacerraf 1981). An important feature of this group of toxicities, which makes them difficult to study in both humans and animals, is their relatively low frequency of occurrence.

Hypersensitivity (allergic) reactions have been grouped into four types. Type I hypersensitivity reactions are of the immediate-type, anaphylactic, or IgE-mediated hypersensitivity reactions. Reactions result from the release of pharmacologically active substances such as histamine, leukotrienes, prostaglandins, platelet-activating factor, and eosinophilic chemotactic factor from IgE-sensitized basophils and mast cells after contact with specific antigen. Clinical conditions in which type I reactions play a function include systemic anaphylaxis, reactions to stinging insects, allergic extrinsic asthma, seasonal allergic rhinitis, some cases of urticaria, and some reactions to foods and drugs.

Type II hypersensitivity reactions represent cytotoxic hypersensitivity, antibody-dependent cytotoxicity, or cytolytic complement-dependent cytotoxicity. Clinical examples of cell injury in which antibody reacts with antigenic components of a cell are Coombs-positive hemolytic anemia, antibody-induced thrombocytopenia, leukopenia, pemphigus, pemphigoid, Goodpasture's syndrome, and pernicious anemia.

Type III hypersensitivity reactions result from the deposition of soluble circulating antigen–antibody (immune) complexes in vessels or tissue. Some clinical conditions in which immune complexes are considered to have operational purpose are serum sickness due to serum, drugs, or viral hepatitis antigen; systemic lupus erythematosus; rheumatoid arthritis; polyarteritis; chronic membranoproliferative glomerulonephritis; and other systemic reactions. Drug- or serum-induced serum sickness, and some forms of renal disease, are IgE-mediated and believed to precede the type III reaction. The local Arthus reaction and experimental serum sickness are model laboratory examples of type III effect.

Type IV reactions are cell-mediated, delayed, or tuberculin-type hypersensitivity reactions. They are caused by sensitized lymphocytes (T cells) after contact with an-

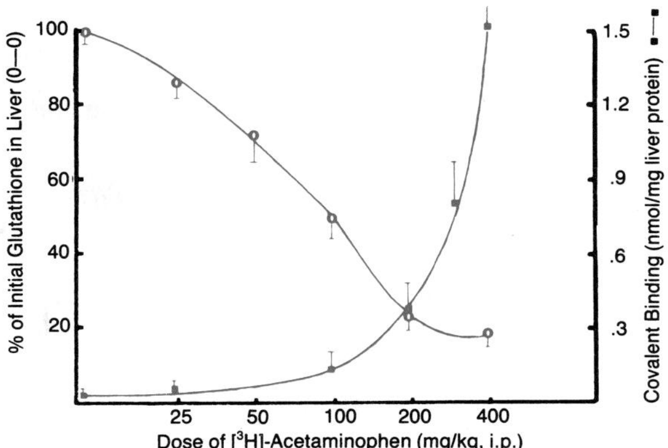


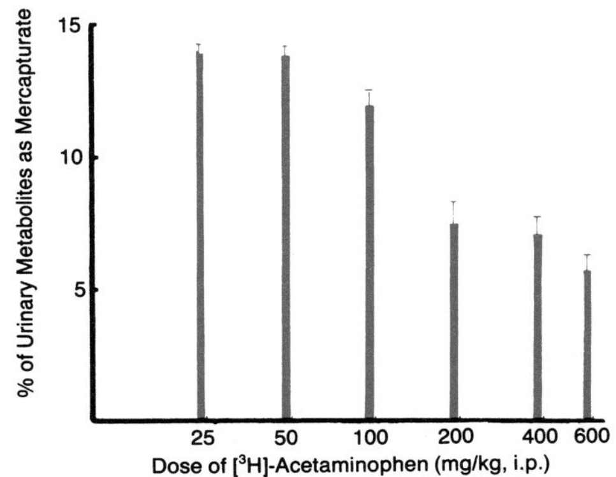


**FIGURE 24-2 Relationship in vivo between the concentration of glutathione (GSH) in the liver, the formation of an acetaminophen-glutathione conjugate (measured in urine as acetaminophen-mercapturic acid), and covalent binding of an acetaminophen metabolite to liver proteins. Several doses of [$^3$H]acetaminophen were administered intraperitoneally to hamsters, and GSH concentrations and covalent binding of radiolabeled material were determined 3 hours later. An additional group of hamsters were treated similarly, and urinary metabolites were collected for 24 hours. (From Mitchell et al. 1975.)**

tigen. Delayed hypersensitivity differs from other hypersensitivity reactions since it is not mediated by antibody but by sensitized lymphocytes, with peripheral blood leukocytes, or with an extract of these cells (transfer factor), but not with serum. The transfer of delayed hypersensitivity from sensitized to normal persons can be shown. Clinical conditions in which type IV reactions are considered to be involved include contact dermatitis, allograft rejection, some forms of drug sensitivity, and thyroiditis. Patch tests are used to identify allergens causing a contact dermatitis, but testing should not be done until the dermatitis has cleared so as to avoid an exacerbation.

**Key Points: There are several clinical criteria that help in the diagnosis of allergic reactions to a drug—**

- **The reactions usually occur only after prior exposure; however, often the patient is unaware of previous exposure to a specific drug.**
- **Reactions usually occur after 8 to 9 days from the first exposure, suggesting that a period of sensitization is required.**
- **Reactions appear to be dose-independent.**
- **Reactions are often accompanied by tissue and blood eosinophilia and fever.**
- **The symptoms usually subside promptly after the drug is discontinued unless a drug-induced autoimmune reaction has been initiated.**
- **On rechallenge with the drug, the patient should show the same pathologic involvement.**

Hypersensitivity to a drug is dependent on many factors. The drug or its metabolites must be antigenic or capable of acting as a hapten in order to stimulate antibody production (Lien 1987a, 1987b; Pohl et al. 1988). The antibody–hapten conjugate or antibody–antigen interaction must take place in the proper setting to cause a type of tissue injury. Then, an inflammatory process usually develops that expresses the reaction. Each step of the process—formation of the complete immunogen, induction of antibody synthesis, and expression of the antibody–antigen reaction—is under separate genetic control (Benacerraf 1981). Despite the exposure of many people to drugs of many varieties, hypersensitivity reactions account for only 6 to 10% of all drug reactions (Borda et al. 1968), and relatively few drugs cause hypersensitivity.

***Penicillin allergy***
Penicillin allergy is one of the best-defined models of hypersensitivity reactions. The apparent overall prevalence

**Table 24-2 Syndromes Caused By Antigenic Effects of Penicillin**

| Type | Likely Causative Antibody | Clinical Manifestation |
|---|---|---|
| Intermediate (2–30 minutes) | IgE (?IgG) | Anaphylaxis—diffuse or organ-specific (e.g. cardiac)<br>Asthma, urticaria<br>Laryngeal edema (occurs 1 : 100 in comparison with anaphylaxis) |
| Accelerated (1–72 hours) | ?IgG | Urticaria, laryngeal edema, asthma<br>Local inflammatory reactions |
| Late (more than 72 hours) | IgM and other antibodies | Commonly<br>Urticaria<br>Exanthem<br>Fever<br>Arthralgia<br>Hemolysis<br>Granulocytopenia<br>Interstitial nephritis<br>Eosinophilia<br>Rarely<br>Acute renal insufficiency<br>Thrombocytopenia |

of hypersensitivity response to penicillin is about 2%. Responses are clinically and pathogenetically (as discussed in this section) divided into immediate (occurring within a few minutes of administration of the drug), accelerated (occurring within hours), or late (occurring days after the patient has been given the drug). The syndromes that can be seen in each category are listed in Table 24-2. Any combination, sequence of appearance, or severity of each manifestation can be seen in any given patient. The pattern of response is not even easily predicted in patients with a well-established past history of sensitivity to penicillin. About 1.4% of the 2% overall reactions are expressed as the late type, with 0.3% being accelerated and 0.3% being immediate. One in 2500 patients exposed to penicillin therapy develops anaphylaxis, and 1 in 100,000 dies (Smith et al. 1980).

The pathogenesis of hypersensitivity is similar for a number of drugs that stimulate antibody production and result in tissue-damaging antigen–antibody reactions. The sequence of events is identical to that seen in an acute inflammatory response elicited by other antigen–antibody interactions, with or without complement, and is dependent on local tissue response or response of the formed elements in blood. The morphologic changes in the microvasculature are characteristic of the acute inflammatory lesion, and similar therapeutic maneuvers aimed at preventing or reversing the acute disease are effective in many varieties of hypersensitivity.

Unusual syndromes have been described that are probably due to the distribution of the drug and the manifestations of hypersensitivity. For example, the Stevens-Johnson syndrome is characterized by lesions in various mucous membranes and is classically caused by a variety of drugs including sulfonamides and phenytoin. It can be hard to separate Stevens-Johnson syndrome from erythema multiforme major and toxic epidermal necrolysis, because there are not clear-cut diagnostic criteria separating them (Rzany et al. 1996). However, one study evaluating whether erythema multiforme and Stevens-Johnson syndrome could be separated based on the pattern of cutaneous lesions found that 80% of 76 cases could be classified as one of the two disorders (Assier et al. 1995). Based on a review of photographs, lesions were classified as erythema multiforme when lesions were typical or raised atypical targets that were located on the extremities and/or the face, and as Stevens-Johnson when the lesions were flat atypical targets or purpuric maculae that were widespread or distributed on the trunk. There was a strong correlation between the clinical classification and the probable cause. Erythema multiforme was most often related to herpes (17 of 28 cases), and rarely related to drugs (3 of 28 cases), whereas Stevens-Johnson was almost always related to drugs (28 of 33 cases). Whether treatment of Stevens-Johnson syndrome with steroids is efficacious is controversial (Revuz and Roujeau 1996; Kakourou et al. 1997; Noskin and Patterson 1997), and few data are available. (See Fig. 24-3.)

### *Radiographic contrast media*

Intravascular radiographic contrast media also may cause reactions characterized by the release of histamine and serotonin and by the activation of a cascade of systems including complement, fibrinolysin, and kinins. The clinical manifestations are similar to those of a classic allergic response, but IgE seemingly is not involved.

Hyperosmolality and alkalinity are responsible for most of the undesirable physiologic and toxic effects associated with these agents. However, some researchers believe there is an antigen–antibody response. Others believe that the reactions are more properly termed anaphylactoid and that they are induced by other mechanisms that may involve some of the same reaction pathways. Hypertonic contrast media may cause endothelial disruptions with the release of active chemical substances or transmitters (Swanson et al. 1986; Morris and Fischer 1986). From conventional ionic contrast media, severe reactions occur in from 1 of 1000 to 1 of 2000 patients. Fatal reactions have been variously reported at 1 in 10,000 to 1 in 93,000 exposures. Patients with allergic histories have a 2 to 4 times increased risk for an adverse reaction. The risk may be increased fivefold with a documented history of asthma (Greenberger 1984). Persons with a history of a previous reaction to contrast media are at greater risk, with 15–35% having adverse reactions on repeat intravascular administration of contrast material.

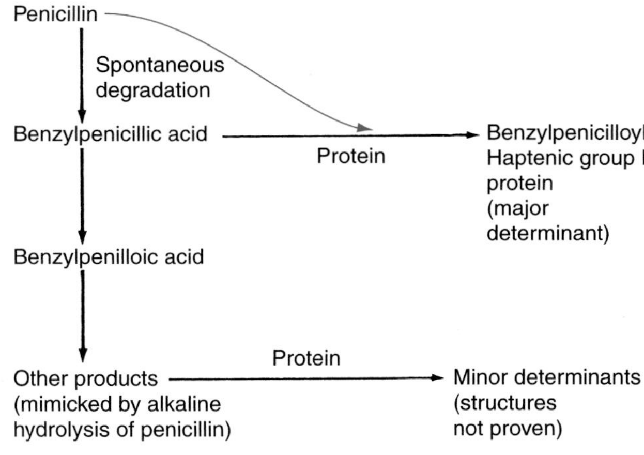


**FIGURE 24-3 Mechanisms by which penicillin achieves antigenic status.**

For patients with previous anaphylactoid reactions, the risk of subsequent reactions is higher. One comparison of three pretreatment regimens found that all were equally effective, and that only 6% of patients had a reaction with these (Marshall and Lieberman 1991). The first included 50 mg of oral prednisone 13, 7 hours and 1 hour before, and 50 mg intramuscular diphenhydramine 1 hour before procedures; the second included this plus 300 mg oral cimetidine an hour before the procedure; and the third, in addition, 25 mg oral ephedrine 1 hour before the procedure.

Lower osmolality radiocontrast media have been developed that have good radiographic properties, and also a lower incidence of severe reactions (Greenberger and Patterson 1991; Wittbrodt and Spinler 1994). However, these agents are substantially more expensive than the older agents. One group in which their use may be beneficial is those with prior reactions. One study compared low-osmolality and conventional agents with pretreatment in both groups including prednisone-diphenhydramine (Greenberger and Patterson 1991). In 200 procedures in patients with a previous immediate, generalized reaction to a conventional agent, only one patient (0.5%) had a contrast reaction, versus 9.1% with conventional agents ($P < 0.001$), suggesting that low-osmolality agents substantially decrease the risk of a reaction in patients with a prior reaction.

Besides prior anaphylactoid reactions, other risk factors for reactions are asthma, reaction to skin allergens, and history of reaction to penicillin (Wittbrodt and Spinler 1994; Lang et al. 1993). In a case-control study, the risk of anaphylactoid reaction was much higher with asthma (odds ratio [OR], 8.7), and was higher with beta-blockers (odds ratio, 3.7) (Lang et al. 1993). The risk of a major or life-threatening reaction was also higher in the presence of a cardiovascular disorder (OR, 7.7).

Recommendations for high-risk patients who must receive radiocontrast include using a lower osmolarity agent, pretreatment with a corticosteroid and a histamine H1 antagonist, discontinuing beta-blockers, and bedside availability of medications and equipment to treat anaphylaxis (Wittbrodt and Spinler 1994).

## SELECTED ADVERSE EFFECTS ON SELECTED ORGAN SYSTEMS

The following examples of adverse drug reactions involving selected, specific organ systems are intended to be illustrative examples of adverse reactions and not by any means an exhaustive list of possible adverse effects of drugs.

**Key Point: The manifestation of adverse effects of medications by many patients are often subtle and could easily be ascribed to other causes by the inexperienced or less inquiring observer.**

From time to time, even seasoned physicians in the various subspecialty areas fail to appreciate some of the uncommon adverse effects of drugs they commonly use. A particularly difficult situation arises when the adverse effect is common in the disease being treated, for example, pro-arrhythmic effects of drugs being used to suppress arrhythmias. As noted earlier, clinically important drug reactions are underrecognized and underreported. The prescribing physician must always try to keep an open mind toward whether a drug is responsible for a problem.

**PRINCIPLE Key Point: If a new complaint occurs, the prescriber should always ask himself or herself, "Could this be attributed to one of the patient's drugs?"**

In other chapters in this book, adverse reactions focused on particular organ systems are emphasized.

### Dermatologic Toxicity

Cutaneous reactions induced by drugs can occur as solitary manifestations or be part of a more serious systemic involvement with renal, hepatic, pulmonary, or hematologic toxicity. Although skin disorders may be seemingly minor, drug-induced skin reactions may precede or be premonitory of more serious adverse involvement of other vital organs in susceptible patients. Drugs most frequently associated with allergic skin reactions are the penicillins, sulfonamides, and blood products (Reid et al. 1989).

Patients may have exaggerated injury after exposure to sun when they are taking sun-sensitizing medications such as the phenothiazines or tetracyclines. At times, a generalized erythroderma may be due to a solubilizing agent or stabilizer rather than the active drug, such as reactions to the ethanolamine component of aminophylline or topical preparations (Nierenberg and Glazener 1982). Bisacodyl and phenolphthalein are the primary diphenylmethane laxatives that may induce allergic reactions including fixed drug eruptions and Stevens-Johnson syndrome (Brunton 1985). Exfoliative dermatitis, characterized by redness, scaling, and thickening of the entire skin surface, and toxic epidermal necrolysis manifested by peeling of the epidermis in sheets leaving widespread denuded areas may be fatal. Suspected medications should be stopped immediately, and essential systemic medications should be changed to ones of a different chemical group. Exfoliative dermatitis usually can be managed with the use of topical treatment. Patients with toxic epidermal necrolysis should be isolated to minimize exogenous infections and treated similarly to patients with severe burns. The skin and denuded areas should be protected from trauma and infection and fluid and electrolyte losses should be replaced. Systemic corticosteroids often are used to treat exfoliative dermatitis and toxic epidermal necrolysis.

The most common form of vasculitis in the skin is cutaneous necrotizing vasculitis involving primarily small postcapillary venules of the skin and characterized as leukocytoclastic vasculitis. This is manifest clinically as palpable purpura with the most common site of involvement being the lower extremities, particularly the feet and ankles. Pathologically, sites of cutaneous vasculitis show endothelial cell edema and necrosis, hemorrhage, fibrin deposition, a neutrophil-rich infiltrate, and leukocytoclasis. Hypersensitivity to various agents is the presumed cause of cutaneous necrotizing vasculitis but in about half of the cases, no inciting agent is found. Drugs are responsible for the majority of the remaining cases. The most commonly implicated drugs are antibacterials including penicillins and sulfonamides, diuretics, nonsteroidal anti-inflammatory drugs (NSAIDs), and anticonvulsant agents.

The incidence of associated systemic involvement has been variously estimated to be as follows: arthralgia and arthritis, 40%; renal, 12.5 to 63%, with the most common finding being asymptomatic hematuria or proteinuria; and neurologic, with both motor and sensory peripheral neuropathy, 5 to 10%. GI involvement occurs in those with the Henoch-Schönlein purpura variant; pulmonary findings may be clinically quiescent but show changes on the chest x-ray film (Swerlick and Lawley 1989).

## Ototoxicity

Many drugs, as well as industrial chemicals and solvents, are associated with impaired auditory or vestibular function that at times may be irreversible. Dizziness, tinnitus, and hearing loss were discovered in the late 1800s in association with the use of aspirin and quinine. Beginning with streptomycin in the 1940s, ototoxicity has become a major clinical problem. Indeed, it has been suggested that more than 130 drugs and chemicals have been associated with ototoxicity (Seligmann et al. 1996). The major classes are basic aminoglycosides and other antibiotics, antimalarials, anti-inflammatory drugs, antineoplastic agents, diuretics, some topical agents, and heavy metals (Lien et al. 1983; Koegel 1985; Rybak 1986). The Boston Collaboration Drug Surveillance Program reported the frequency of drug-induced deafness in patients in the United States to be 3 per 1000, and 1.6 per 1000 is cited by Lien (1987b). The most frequently implicated drugs were aspirin and the aminoglycoside antibiotics.

The likelihood of ototoxicity is markedly increased in patients with impaired renal function, in elderly persons, and is associated with a high dose or large total dose of an ototoxic drug, or if there has been a prior course or the concurrent use of another ototoxic drug (Jackson and Arcieri 1971). Though the damage may involve vestibular and/or cochlear mechanisms, cochlear dysfunction is considerably more incapacitating. Varying with the drugs involved and the mechanisms of action, inner ear deafness may be preceded by tinnitus, diplacusis, or the sense of fullness in the ear (Bernstein and Weiss 1967; Porter and Jick 1977).

### *Aminoglycosides*

In humans, aminoglycoside-induced cochlear ototoxicity involves progressive loss of the hair cells in the organ of Corti. Hair cells in the basal turn of the cochlea are affected first with destruction progressing toward the apex. This is in keeping with clinical experience since the basal region responds to high frequency sounds and the apex to sounds of low frequency. Streptomycin primarily affects the vestibular system, and neomycin, kanamycin, and amikacin are primarily toxic to the cochlea. Gentamicin and tobramycin show both vestibular and cochlear toxicity with vestibular toxicity occurring more frequently (Brummett and Fox 1989a; Pratt and Fekety 1986). Loss of hearing has occurred because of the systemic absorption of the neomycin solution used to irrigate surgical wounds or used in the dressings of severe burns. Audiometric testing, as well as electronystagmography, can determine subclinical changes in cranial nerve VIII functions. Cochlear dysfunctions usually affect these frequencies above 4000 Hz. Serial audiometric testing has been recommended for patients on extended periods of treatment with the aminoglycosides in the attempt to avoid irreversible cochlear toxicity in the frequencies used in the conversational range. However, testing requires a degree of patient cooperation that is often not feasible in patients ill enough to require treatment with this group of drugs. Since the therapeutic index with these drugs is narrow, serum concentrations of the aminoglycosides should be monitored, although ototoxicity can occur even with therapeutic concentrations.

Although single daily dosing of these agents is being used with increasing frequency, comparatively few data are available about single daily dosing and ototoxicity (Hatala et al. 1996; Singer et al. 1996). A meta-analysis pooling the available data suggested that the risk ratio for ototoxicity with single daily dosing was 0.67 (CI, 0.35–1.28) (Hatala et al. 1996).

***Vancomycin***

There has been long-standing concern that vancomycin may cause ototoxicity (Hermans and Wilhelm 1987), although whether this is due to vancomycin remains controversial (Cantu et al. 1994); it is thought that it may augment aminoglycoside-induced ototoxicity (Brummett 1993a). There are no data that convincingly demonstrate that monitoring of vancomycin concentrations improves the effectiveness of therapy (Cantu et al 1994).

Vancomycin pharmacokinetics are sufficiently predictable that adequate concentrations that take into account the patient's age, weight, and renal function can be anticipated. Monitoring of peak concentrations may still be useful in patients with impaired renal function.

***Erythromycin***

Sensorineural hearing loss can occur because of erythromycin and appears to be dose-related (Brummett 1993b). Renal impairment appears to predispose to ototoxicity. In one study of renal allograft recipients, 11 of 34 courses (32%) of intravenous erythromycin resulted in hearing loss (Vasquez et al. 1993). Among patients receiving 4 g daily, 53% suffered hearing loss, compared with only 16% of those receiving 2 g daily, suggesting that the lower dose should be used if possible. Hepatic insufficiency also may increase the risk of ototoxicity (Brittain 1987). Erythromycin-induced tinnitus and hearing loss are usually reversible. Though recovery generally begins within 24 hours of discontinuing the drug, nearly complete recovery may take 1–2 weeks, and several months are required for total recovery (Brummett and Fox 1989b).

***Diuretics***

Hearing loss that may be reversible, but on occasion has been irreversible, has occurred in patients receiving the loop diuretics ethacrynic acid and furosemide. These agents have been shown to produce a dose-related, reversible reduction in endocochlear potential in animals. Edema of the stria vascularis, loss of outer hair cells in the basal turn of the cochlea, and cystic degeneration of the hair cells in the ampulla of the posterior canal and in the macula of the saccule have been noted (Rybak 1986). Hearing loss occurs more often in patients with impaired renal function and is associated with the rapid IV administration of the drug; at times there is concomitant use of other ototoxic medication. Permanent deafness has been reported up to 6 months after treatment with relatively small repeated doses of furosemide. Reversible deafness has occurred with the use of large oral doses in patients with the nephrotic syndrome. The uremic patient is considered to be at special risk, and monitoring of the hearing during treatment with loop diuretics has been advised. The neonate is considered vulnerable, since the clearance of furosemide is significantly prolonged in such patients. The use of loop diuretics should be avoided as much as possible in premature infants and neonates. If possible, loop diuretics should be avoided in patients receiving other ototoxic drugs such as aminoglycosides.

***Salicylates***

Tinnitus and hearing loss can be caused by salicylates, both with acute intoxication and long-term administration (Brien 1993). In those with normal hearing, tinnitus associated with salicylate administration first occurs over a broad range (plasma concentration 20–50 mg/100 mL). Consequently, tinnitus cannot be relied upon to predict plasma salicylate concentrations above the usual therapeutic range (Mongan et al. 1973). Salicylate-induced deafness and tinnitus are almost always reversible within a few days after the medication is discontinued (Porter and Jick 1977).

***Quinine, quinidine, chloroquine***

Quinine, used to ameliorate nocturnal leg cramps in the elderly, may induce vertigo, tinnitus, and hearing loss. Although the ototoxic symptoms usually resolve rapidly upon withdrawal of the drug, some patients are left with irreversible tinnitus and hearing loss (Koegel 1985). Women who have attempted to induce abortion by taking a large dose of quinine may give birth to infants who are congenitally deaf (Drug and Therapeutics Bulletin 1983). Tinnitus, vertigo, and infrequently, reversible mild hearing loss may occur with usual doses of quinidine (Rosketh and Storstein 1963). Tinnitus and hearing loss can be caused by chloroquine. The hearing loss may not become apparent until some time after the drug has been discontinued, is usually associated with high dosage for an extended period of time, and is generally irreversible (Toone 1965).

***Cisplatin***

The introduction of cisplatin had a major impact on survival with a number of solid tumors, but with the advent of compounds such as colony-stimulating factors, toxicity such as ototoxicity has become dose-limiting (Biro et al. 1997). Ototoxicity caused by cisplatin produces tinnitus and hearing loss in the high-frequency range, 4000–8000 Hz. It tends to be more frequent and severe following repeated doses, may be more conspicuous in children, and can be unilateral or bilateral. Patients followed up to 18 months after discovery of hearing loss have not shown any evidence of reversibility. In one study evaluating the long-term effects on hearing with moderate dose cisplatin therapy (50 mg/m$^2$), only 2 of 40 survivors had more severe hearing changes than expected with aging at follow-up conducted 5–10 years after initial therapy, suggesting that the long-term risk of a socially important hearing impairment associated with this therapy is low (Laurell et al. 1996). Patients who receive cisplatin as a bolus seem to have a significantly greater incidence of hearing loss compared with those who receive the drug as a slow infusion (Wiemann and Calabresi 1985). Between similarly effective regimens, those containing lower daily cisplatin doses should be used (Biro et al. 1997).

## Ocular Toxicity

The eyes are responsive to influences from both systemic and topical medications that may cause varied complications. These adverse effects include blurred vision, disturbances of color vision, scotomata, degeneration of the retina, and other untoward effects on the cornea, sclera, lens, optic nerve, and extraocular muscles. The adverse effects of some drugs can be predicted and occur soon after therapy has begun; other drugs produce adverse effects on the eye that cannot be predicted and that occur only after long-term administration. Fortunately, many of the adverse ocular effects are transient, but some may cause severe visual damage that is irreversible. Patients who are being considered for long-term systemically administered medication, especially new drugs, may benefit from careful ophthalmologic screening before starting the drug and during the course of therapy (Lien 1987b; Abel and Leopold 1987).

Multiple factors are involved in the production of ocular adverse effects by a drug. The ease with which a drug passes into the general circulation and into the eye determines its potential to directly affect the eye. Toxic concentrations of drugs may be reached in some instances by high systemic dosage over short periods and in others by prolonged use. Not only may the eye be affected as the drugs are administered (orally, parenterally, or topically), but toxic levels may accumulate slowly and continuously even after administration is discontinued and in situations when the metabolism and elimination of drugs are altered by the presence of severe liver and/or renal disease (see discussion in section). Individual idiosyncrasy may be responsible at times for ocular side effects; at other times the untoward responses are genetically determined (Shichi and Nebert 1982). In prescribing drugs for long-time use (e.g., digitalis glycosides, antimalarials, phenothiazines, and corticosteroids), the physician must be aware of potential diverse effects on the eye.

### *Digitalis glycosides*

Ocular effects of systemically administered drugs have been observed for many years. Withering, in 1785, wrote that "foxglove when given in large and quickly repeated doses occasions sickness, vomiting, giddiness, confused vision, objects appearing green or yellow" (White 1965). The incidence of ocular manifestations in patients with digitalis toxicity has been estimated to be as high as 25%. In approximately 10% of patients, the ocular complaints may occur before other symptoms of toxicity; however, usually adverse ocular effects appear simultaneously with or later than the other signs of cardiac toxicity. These ocular manifestations may present in ways unknown to Withering. For example, an elderly man presented with a conduction abnormality discovered on a routine preoperative ECG. His concentration of digoxin in plasma was elevated. His only complaint was that he was troubled by excessive yellow coloration when watching television. This was not corrected by a home visit and adjustment of his television set by a television repair technician! Thus, it may be useful to ask patients taking digitalis glycosides if they have been experiencing any difficulty with the color of their television programs. Blurred vision and disturbed color vision are the most common ocular symptoms of digitalis toxicity. Objects may appear yellow (xanthopsia) or green; less commonly, they appear red, brown, blue, or white ("snowy vision"). Photophobia and scintillating scotomata may occur, as does alteration of visual acuity. In patients with unusual ocular complaints who are receiving digoxin therapy, toxicity should always be considered.

### *Phenothiazine derivatives*

Some phenothiazines can adversely affect the retina and other ocular structures (Applebaum 1963; Rab 1969). Phenothiazine derivatives with piperidine side chains such as thioridazine have a higher risk of inducing retinal toxicity than other phenothiazines (Applebaum 1963). There have been relatively fewer cases reported for those with aliphatic side chains, while those with a piperazine group do not seem to exert direct ocular toxicity. The phenothiazines as a group can also cause cataract formation, mostly of an anterior polar variety (Prien et al. 1970;

Crombie 1981). The phenothiazine-induced retinopathy may be related to both dose and duration. The retinopathy may present either acutely with sudden loss of vision associated with retinal edema and hyperemia of the optic disk, or slowly with chronic, fine pigmentation scattered in the central area of the fundus, extending peripherally but sparing the macula. There may be chronic central and paracentral scotomata (Spiteri and James 1983). The phenothiazines can accumulate in the pigment cells, particularly in the melanin fraction. The risk of ocular toxicity may be dose- and time-dependent.

***Chloroquine, hydroxychloroquine, and quinine***

During hydroxychloroquine therapy, corneal deposits (keratopathy) occur frequently and are dose-related, although they are not related to the maculopathy associated with this therapy. Keratopathy is associated with visual changes that occur in <50% of those with corneal deposits and is usually completely reversible after stopping treatment. In contrast, retinal changes can lead to progressive loss of vision. This maculopathy can be irreversible, although it occurs almost exclusively at higher than recommended doses (Aylward 1993). Moreover, in the data linking classic study on whether or not there is a relationship (Scherbel et al. 1963), the incidence of pigmentary retinopathy in 408 chloroquine and hydroxychloroquine-treated patients was 0.5% compared to 0.9% in 333 untreated rheumatoid arthritis patients. For the long-term therapy of rheumatoid arthritis, however, the dose of chloroquine probably should not exceed 4.0 mg/kg daily. The dose of hydroxychloroquine should not exceed 6.5 mg/kg/day. The toxic threshold for retinopathy may be 5.1 mg/kg/day for chloroquine and 7.8 mg/kg/day for hydroxychloroquine (Mackenzie 1983). The incidence of hydroxychloroquine keratopathy is dose-related, and although regular ophthalmic screening has often been performed, the evidence to support this practice is so weak that it is not currently recommended by the British Society of Rheumatology (Silman and Shipley 1997). The data are especially weak for patients receiving low-dose therapy. One study found that among 758 patients receiving hydroxychloroquine, none of the patients suffered visual impairment from retinal toxicity, although 12 reported visual disturbances, which was related to ocular muscle imbalance in 4 (Grierson 1997).

Quinine is sometimes used to treat nocturnal muscle cramps, although its efficacy is unclear. However, in acute overdose, it can cause severe ocular problems including blindness (Mackie et al. 1997), suggesting that its use should be reappraised.

***Ethambutol, ethionamide, and chloramphenicol***

The major toxicity of ethambutol is optic neuritis that is dose-related. It is infrequent at a dose of 15 mg/kg/day (Goldberger 1988). The dosage should be reduced when the glomerular filtration rate is less than 30–50 mL/minute (Bennett et al. 1991). Symptoms of retrobulbar neuritis include decreased visual acuity, scotomata, and defective red-green vision. Similar toxicities result from the use of ethionamide and chloramphenicol.

***Miscellaneous drugs***

Ocular manifestations have been reported in association with the use of transdermal scopolamine patches including anisocoria and a fixed dilated pupil (Verdier and Kennerdell 1982; Bienia 1983). Narrow-angle (angle-closure) glaucoma has been precipitated by a number of drugs including scopolamine (Fraunfelder 1982), hydrochlorothiazide (Geanon and Perkins 1995), phenothiazines, tricyclic antidepressants, and mydriatics (Spaeth 1996).

Since the eye is exposed to light, photosensitive drugs, when present, may have the potential of contributing to toxic effects, though definite proof is lacking. Some potential examples include sulfonamides, carbamazepine, tricyclic antidepressants, psoralens, and phenothiazines. Patients taking these drugs should protect their eyes from exposure to sunshine or ultraviolet light. A blue tint in vision has been reported in up to 10% of men using sildenafil (Viagra).

## Nephrotoxicity

Many drugs have been demonstrated to cause renal dysfunction. Certain drugs are especially likely to cause renal injury, and renal function should be monitored during their use (Table 24-3). In the following, selected examples are discussed.

***Nonsteroidal anti-inflammatory drugs***

Nonsteroidal antiinflammatory drugs (NSAIDs) cause a variety of problems with renal function, including fluid retention; hyperkalemia; deterioration of renal function (generally reversible); and less frequently, interstitial nephritis, papillary necrosis, and even chronic renal failure with prolonged use of high doses (Whelton and Hamilton 1991).

The most common adverse renal effect associated with the use of NSAIDs is prostaglandin-dependent reversible renal insufficiency. It is characterized clinically by a fall in urine output, weight gain, rapidly rising serum concentrations of BUN and creatinine, and in some cases, hyperkalemia. Generally, clinical improvement ensues

Table 24-3 **Drug-Induced Kidney Disease**

| Disease | Causative Agent |
|---|---|
| Prerenal Azotemia | ACE inhibitors<br>NSAIDs<br>Cyclosporine<br>Interleukin-2 |
| Acute Tubular Necrosis | Acetaminophen<br>Aminoglycoside antibiotics<br>Amphotericin B<br>Cephalosporins<br>Cisplatin<br>Methoxyflurane<br>Mithramycin<br>Radiocontrast agents<br>Tetracycline |
| Intratubular Obstruction | Acyclovir<br>Methotrexate<br>Sulfonamides |
| Nephrolithiasis | Allopurinol<br>Carbonic anhydrase inhibitors<br>Triamterene |
| Acute Interstitial Nephritis | Allopurinol<br>Ampicillin, methicillin, other $\beta$-lactams<br>Cimetidine<br>Diuretics<br>NSAIDs<br>*p*-Aminosalicylic acid<br>Phenytoin<br>Rifampin<br>Sulfonamides |
| Chronic Interstitial Nephritis | Analgesics:<br>Acetaminophen<br>Aspirin<br>Phenacetin<br>NSAIDs<br>Cyclosporine<br>Lithium<br>Methyl-CCNU |

within 24–72 hours after the drug is discontinued. Elderly patients with volume depletion, congestive heart failure (CHF), cirrhosis, and preexisting renal disease are at greatest risk for this adverse effect.

Analgesic nephropathy is an important but underrecognized cause of renal failure. In the United States, it is estimated that in 20% of patients with chronic interstitial disease, analgesic abuse is the cause. If the analgesic habit is given up, useful renal function returns in about 50% of those cases. Analgesic nephropathy is not a frequent complication of patients with rheumatoid arthritis under treatment with salicylates.

***Penicillins and cephalosporins***

Penicillins and cephalosporins are a major cause of acute interstitial nephritis. Though numerous agents can produce this syndrome, the most frequent offenders are penicillins, especially methicillin, sulfonamides, rifampin, cimetidine, allopurinol, diuretics, and NSAIDs (Adler et al. 1986). Usually, one can obtain a history of more than 10 days of therapy before onset of symptoms (consisting of maculopapular rash, fever, eosinophilia, hematuria, proteinuria, and eosinophiluria). The onset of acute interstitial nephritis may be sudden and accompanied by oliguria. Up to one third of patients can have enough compromise in glomerular filtration rate to require dialysis (Adler et al. 1986).

***Aminoglycosides***

Aminoglycosides are still first-line agents in treating serious gram-negative infections, but nephrotoxicity is common and is often dose-limiting (Begg and Barclay 1995). The likelihood of renal injury is higher with the concomitant use of another potentially nephrotoxic agent or if there is preexisting impairment of kidney function. Recently, several meta-analyses of randomized controlled trials have suggested that single daily dosing with higher doses has as good or better efficacy compared to multiple daily dosing, and is associated with lower nephrotoxicity (Ali and Goetz 1997; Bailey et al. 1997; Barza et al. 1996); these data are discussed in more detail later. If traditional dosing is used, peak and trough concentrations of the aminoglycosides in serum should be monitored to prevent these complications (Pancoast 1988). Therapeutic efficacy correlates best with peak levels; and though trough values are not perfect predictors of renal toxicity, they provide helpful predictors of the adverse effect (Meyer 1986). Nephrotoxicity appears to be most closely related to the length of time that trough concentrations are above 2 mg/L for gentamicin and tobramycin, and greater than 10 mg/L for amikacin and kanamycin. The initial toxic result usually is expressed as nonoliguric renal failure that can be reversed if the drug is discontinued. Reversal may take weeks to months to be complete. Continued administration of the drug may lead to oliguric renal failure. While receiving therapy, the patient's serum creatinine values should be followed every 2–3 days. Adjustment in dosage should then be made if creatinine values increase. Although rises in the serum creatinine concentrations are often late and not particularly sensitive predicators of decline in renal function, such changes in the serum creatinine value remain the only useful indicator of impending renal toxicity.

The efficacy of multiple daily dosing has been evaluated in several meta-analyses (Ali and Goetz 1997; Bailey et al. 1997; Barza et al. 1996). One evaluation found multiple daily dosing to be associated with a nonsignificant decrease in antibiotic failures (OR = 0.83; 95% CI, 0.57–1.21) and lower risk of nephrotoxicity (OR = 0.74; 95% CI, 0.54–1.00) (Barza et al. 1996). Another study suggested that overall clinical response favored single daily dosing by a small margin (mean difference, 3.1%; 95% CI, 0.2–6%), but no difference in microbiological response rates or in nephrotoxicity (–0.2%; 95% CI, –2.2% to +1.8%) (Ali and Goetz 1997). A third found lower risk of clinical treatment failure (risk difference, –3.4%; 95% CI, –6.7% to –0.2%), and negligible difference in the risk of nephrotoxicity (risk difference, –0.6%; 95% CI, –2.4% to +1.1%; $P = 0.46$). All three of these studies were evaluating essentially the same body of data. Taken together, especially since single daily dosing is cheaper and more convenient, these data suggest that single daily dosing is probably superior in most patients, although the marginal differences in efficacy and toxicity, if any, are small.

#### *Amphotericin B*

Nephrotoxicity is the most serious adverse effect of amphotericin B therapy. The site of toxicity is the renal tubules, where the drug is believed to cause a lytic action on the cholesterol-rich liposomal membranes. The usual adverse effects include urinary abnormalities, azotemia, hypokalemia, renal tubular acidosis, and nephrocalcinosis. Hypokalemia may be particularly profound in patients also receiving carbenicillin or ticarcillin. Toxicity is related to the total dose of amphotericin B and is often the limiting feature of the use of the drug. New preparations of amphotericin B in which the drug is encapsulated into liposomes or other lipid carriers are reported by manufacturers to reduce its nephrotoxicity, although the available data are scanty (de Marie 1996). More data should be available soon.

#### *Vancomycin*

The incidence of acute nephrotoxicity caused by vancomycin is controversial. Faber and Moellering (1983) estimated that 5% of patients treated with vancomycin alone showed signs of renal impairment, but 35% of patients receiving vancomycin concurrently with an aminoglycoside were affected, suggesting that these antibiotics may act synergistically in producing renal dysfunction. However, others have presented data suggesting that this may not be the case (Kralovicova et al. 1997). Routine serum vancomycin concentration monitoring many be warranted only in specific populations, such as those with renal impairment, rapidly changing renal function, or possibly those concomitantly receiving aminoglycosides (Leader et al. 1995).

#### *Cisplatin*

The use of cisplatin is limited by dose-related nephrotoxicity, which is manifested by acute renal failure and magnesium wasting (Meyer and Madias 1994). In one study, risk factors for nephrotoxicity were cisplatin dosage, initial creatinine clearance, and cycle number (Lagrange et al. 1997). Cisplatin probably should not be used if the glomerular filtration rate is less than 50 mL/min. Continuous infusions seem to be less toxic than bolus administration of the drug (Ries and Klastersky 1986; Fillastre et al. 1988).

#### *Cyclosporine*

Renal toxicity is a major problem with cyclosporine. Cyclosporine is a renal arteriolar vasoconstrictor and may accentuate other ischemic insults to produce acute renal failure. This risk may be increased when the drug is administered parenterally. More gradual elevations in serum creatinine concentrations appear to be hemodynamically mediated and usually respond to a reduction in dosage. Chronic interstitial fibrosis develops by an uncertain mechanism after prolonged therapy. Cyclosporine can produce hyperkalemia, elevate blood pressure, and induce a hemolytic uremic syndrome. In one trial in stable renal transplant recipients, the risk of nephrotoxicity was 12% with microemulsion preparation and 7% with standard cyclosporine (Cole et al. 1998). Toxicity correlates loosely with trough concentrations of the drug. The narrow therapeutic index, marked individual variability in clearance, low and variable bioavailability, and a large number of drug interactions make cyclosporine an obvious candidate for therapeutic drug monitoring (Kahan 1986).

#### *Radiocontrast-induced nephropathy*

Acute renal insufficiency has been reported following the administration of radiocontrast agents by oral, IV, and intraarterial routes. Increased use of angiography, computed tomography, and pyelography has increased the incidence of acute renal failure caused by contrast material. The diagnosis should be suspected when an acute deterioration in renal function occurs within 24–48 hours after use of a contrast agent and when alternative explanations have been excluded. A persistent abnormal urinary sediment and a low fractional excretion of sodium are typical concomitants of the complication. Risk factors include preexisting renal insufficiency, especially when the serum creatinine concentration is greater than 3.0 mg/dL; a history of prior contrast-induced acute renal failure; the use of large doses of contrast medium; an age >60 years; and the presence of diabetes mellitus, dehydration, or multiple myeloma. A good state of hydration and the use of mannitol just before or immediately after injection of the dye may be of prophylactic value in preventing renal abnormalities. Newer contrast agents that are nonionic, have lower osmolality, and have reduced alkalinity are now available, and they appear to be less nephrotoxic than the older agents (Katzberg 1997; Rudnick et al. 1997).

### *Additional forms of kidney damage*

Additional drug-induced responses of the kidneys have been described. Methotrexate, the sulfonamides, and large doses of acyclovir can precipitate in the renal tubules. By somewhat different mechanisms, triamterene, allopurinol, and acetazolamide can cause renal stones. Systemic vasculitis and associated glomerular changes have occurred with the use of penicillin, sulfonamides, allopurinol, thiazides, and amphetamines. In addition to streptozotocin and 5-azacytidine, degradation products of outdated tetracycline can produce proximal tubular damage (Fanconi syndrome). Retroperitoneal fibrosis and secondary obstructive uropathy have been caused by methysergide. A similar clinical syndrome has been due to ergot alkaloids. Lithium and methoxyflurane cause nephrogenic diabetes insipidus (Singer et al. 1972; Ettinger et al. 1980).

## Hemopoietic Toxicity

The hemopoietic system is notably vulnerable to the toxic effects of drugs. These may be expressed against formed elements of the blood or the bone marrow. Several drugs are regularly associated with idiosyncratic reactions in susceptible persons. For the most part, the reactions are due either to decreased production or increased destruction of blood elements. Bleeding disturbances and coagulation disorders are often caused by drugs. A large number of drugs associated with or presumed to be associated with hematologic disorders have been summarized by Verstraete and Boogaerts (1987).

### *Drugs and platelet and coagulation defects*

Because aspirin inhibits platelet function, it should be avoided by patients receiving warfarin, although it is sometimes used now for patients who have had thromboembolic events while taking warfarin. Aspirin decreases platelet aggregation by blocking the synthesis of thromboxane A2 and release of ADP, mediators of the second phase of platelet aggregation. The results may be serious in neonates who have coagulation defects or in those who are taking anticoagulants or undergoing surgery. The acetylation of platelets by aspirin is irreversible, so that the functional abnormality persists for the lifetime of that particular group of platelets (the normal half-life of platelets is around 5 days). Carbenicillin and ticarcillin cause platelet dysfunction and prolong bleeding time, increasing the risk of clinically significant hemorrhage in patients with uremia or who have undergone surgery. Cephalosporins having an N-methylthiotetrazole side chain (e.g., moxalactam, cefoperazone, cefotetan, and cefamandole) have been reported to cause hypoprothrombinemia with episodes of clinically significant bleeding.

### *Aplastic anemia*

Drug-induced aplastic anemia is unpredictable. The clinical manifestations are severe and often fatal. At least half of all cases are associated with the use of drugs. The most frequently implicated are chloramphenicol, phenylbutazone, sulfonamides, and gold. Inhaled solvents (especially benzene), other organic chemicals, and insecticides have also been implicated (Williams et al. 1973). Chloramphenicol accounts for the greatest number of cases, although the incidence rate is only 1 in 40,000 to 1 in 50,000 patients taking the drug. Two types of hematotoxicity have been delineated (Yunis 1988). The more common is the dose-related, reversible bone marrow suppression affecting primarily the erythroid series and usually occurring when concentrations of chloramphenicol in serum reach 25 $\mu$g/mL or higher. Rarer is the devastating complication of bone marrow aplasia characterized by pancytopenia, which can occur at any dose and frequently has a fatal outcome due to hemorrhage or infection. Aplastic anemia caused by chloramphenicol is similar when given by any route and does not relate to the dose or the duration of therapy. A genetically determined predisposition of chloramphenicol-induced aplastic anemia has been suggested by its occurrence in identical twins.

### *Thrombocytopenia*

Drugs can cause thrombocytopenia by increasing platelet destruction or by bone marrow suppression (Winkelstein and Kiss 1997). Such hypersensitivity or allergic thrombocytopenia can be caused by a large number of drugs. These patients are thought to have drug-related antibodies of both IgG and IgM classes that are involved in the destruction of the platelets. Thrombocytopenia can appear within a few hours following administration of a drug that causes thrombocytopenia in patients who had taken the drug previously. An acute syndrome generally develops with petechiae, often initially more prominent on the lower extremities, and bleeding from the mucous membranes. Because the half-life of the platelet is so short, the thrombocytopenia shows signs of beginning to subside within several hours or up to a few days after the offending drug has been withdrawn.

Two mechanisms are believed to be involved in inducing the thrombocytopenia. Either the drug may be bound to the platelet membrane and the antibody directed against the drug-membrane complex with subsequent activation of complement-induced injury to the platelet, or circulating drug-antibody may complex with the platelets, playing a more or less passive role in the destruction. Immune complexes are phagocytized by platelets, and subsequently the platelets release some of their components. The resulting "release reaction" may cause intravascular platelet aggregation and thrombocytopenia. Systemic symptoms may accompany the immune complex thrombocytopenia. The latter mechanism is involved when rifampin, thiazides, thiouracils, quinine, and quinidine cause the problem (Joist 1985).

Transient, mild thrombocytopenia occurs in about 25% of patients receiving heparin. This is believed to result from heparin-induced platelet aggregation but may be accompanied by a paradoxical decrease of the anticoagulant effect. Severe thrombocytopenia follows the formation of heparin-dependent antiplatelet antibodies. Usually, the reaction is delayed until day 8 to day 12 of therapy. It is characterized by recurrent thrombotic disease and loss of the anticoagulant effect. A platelet count as low as 5000/mm$^3$, elevated fibrin split products, and adequate megakaryocytes in the bone marrow are seen. Improvement of the thrombocytopenia occurs after heparin is stopped. Patients with such heparin-induced thrombocytopenia may have received heparin prepared from bovine lung rather than pork intestine (O'Reilly 1985).

It is important to note that there are many other causes of thrombocytopenia, especially in critically ill patients. One study done in intensive care unit patients found that thrombocytopenia occurred in 26 of 63 (41%) of patients, and that the independent correlates of thrombocytopenia included injury (other than to the head), age and trauma score, and that medications were not associated with development of thrombocytopenia (Hanes et al. 1997). In such populations, it can be hard to determine whether a specific medication is causing thrombocytopenia, although it is always important to consider the possibility.

### *Agranulocytosis*

Contrasted with drug-induced aplastic anemia, in which some cases may appear after the drug has been discontinued, drug-induced agranulocytosis occurs during treatment with the drug (Drug-induced agranulocytosis 1997). In this context, agranulocytosis is a diagnosis that refers to patients with neutrophil counts of $<200/\text{mm}^3$ or total white blood cell counts of $<500/\text{mm}^3$. Agranulocytosis may result from bone marrow depression or increased peripheral destruction of white blood cells. Agranulocytosis may occur as a component of drug-induced aplastic anemia or as an adverse drug effect without accompanying anemia or thrombocytopenia. The drugs that caused agranulocytosis or neutropenia most frequently in a population study from the Netherlands were dipyrone, mianserin, sulfasalazine, sulfamethoxazole with trimethoprim, the group of penicillins, cimetidine, the thiouracil derivatives, phenylbutazone, and penicillamine (van der Klauw et al. 1998).

## Cardiotoxicity

Both acute and chronic cardiotoxicities are produced by the anthracyclines. In fact, the therapeutic potential of doxorubicin and other anthracycline drugs is limited by cardiotoxicity (de Forni and Armand 1994). The mechanism of the toxicity is not fully understood. Theories of the mechanism of anthracycline toxicity include the overloading of myocytes with calcium, the production of free radicals, and the cardiotoxicity of the C-13 hydroxy metabolites of doxorubicin (Mushlin and Olson 1988). Acute toxicity is characterized by the ECG changes of nonspecific ST-T wave abnormalities, lengthening of the QRS complexes, low voltage, dysrhythmia, myocarditis, and transient cardiac dysfunction. Acute toxicity may infrequently cause disturbances of cardiac rhythm and sudden death during or shortly after the infusion of doxorubicin (Mushlin and Olson 1988). Chronic toxicity, linked to the cumulative dose of drug, is a more common problem that may lead to a fatal congestive cardiomyopathy. Gated radionuclide angiography often reveals diastolic dysfunction following doses of doxorubicin below those that produce systolic dysfunction (Mushlin and Olsen 1988). Right ventricular endomyocardial biopsies provide a sensitive means of detecting myocardial injury and help determine whether patients are able to tolerate full courses of the drug.

Limiting the total dose of doxorubicin is the best way to prevent cardiomyopathy. Epidemiologic data from the 1970s advised that the total cumulative doses of doxorubicin should be limited to 550 mg/m$^2$ (Bristow et al. 1978). At this dose, CHF developed in 10% of patients; failure developed in 30% at higher doses. The incidence of failure is 1–5% at cumulative doses less than 500 mg/m$^2$. Risk factors for developing cardiomyopathy include age below 10 and over 40 years, the presence of preexisting cardiac disease, hypertension, liver dysfunction, prior or concurrent radiation therapy, and previous treatment with other anthracyclines or cyclophosphamide. Cardiotoxicity may be somewhat limited by using slow infusions designed to minimize peak concentrations of drug in plasma for any given dosage of anthracycline (Legha et al. 1982).

#### *Cyclophosphamide*

Cyclophosphamide in large doses (>180 mg/kg) may cause cardiac failure through direct damage to the heart (Applebaum et al. 1976). Cardiotoxicity has been observed in some patients receiving doses of cyclophosphamide ranging from 120–270 mg/kg given over a few days, usually as a part of a multidrug antineoplastic regimen. In a few instances, severe and fatal heart failure may develop with histologic study revealing hemorrhagic myocarditis.

#### *Phenothiazines*

The phenothiazines, and particularly thioridazine, produce repolarization changes in the ECG. The most common electrocardiographic findings are prolongation of the QT interval, ST-T wave changes, and flattening and notching of the T waves. With higher doses, T-wave inversion may occur, as well as the appearance of prominent U waves.

#### *Other types of drugs*

Several other types of drugs may cause serious adverse effects on the heart. Overdosage of tricyclic antidepressants may cause severe disturbances in ventricular rhythm (Thorstrand 1976). Lithium can produce ECG changes similar to those of the phenothiazines and may also cause interstitial myocarditis (Tseng 1971). And last to be considered are the antiarrhythmic drugs themselves.

**PRINCIPLE When a drug causes an event that is similar to the indication that justifies its use, the physician is faced with a true dilemma—distinguishing whether the drug is causing the event or is being used in inadequate doses to allow efficacy.**

## Hepatotoxicity

Drugs in common use can cause liver toxicity that can mimic almost every naturally occurring liver disease in humans (Lee 1995; Farrell 1997). Although hepatic injury represents a relatively small proportion of all adverse drug effects, drugs are responsible for 2 to 5% of hospital admissions for jaundice in the United States and for about 10% of hospitalized patients with "acute hepatitis" in Europe (Lewis and Zimmerman 1989). Drugs such as halothane, acetaminophen, and phenytoin are an important cause of fulminant liver failure. Many agents cause asymptomatic liver injury detected only by development of abnormal liver function tests. The estimated prevalence of asymptomatic disease, as well as overt hepatitis, varies from agent to agent and usually is less common in children compared with adults. Conspicuous exceptions are valproic acid and injury from salicylate. Most of the cases of drug-induced liver disease result from unexpected reactions to a therapeutic dose of a drug and considerably less often as a predictable sequel to the intrinsic toxicity of the particular agent (Lewis and Zimmerman 1989).

When any patient with liver disease is evaluated, every medication that has been taken over the past 3 months must be recorded and reviewed. Occupational toxins and other causes such as viral hepatitis must be excluded. Severity is increased if the drug is continued after symptoms develop or serum transaminase concentrations rise. Early and accurate diagnosis of a drug-induced hepatic reaction depends on the early suspicion by the physician of a possible drug-related cause. Discontinuing a hepatotoxic agent early significantly reduces or eliminates the injury. Should a hepatotoxic drug be continued, chronic liver disease or cirrhosis readily results. The clinical history is crucial because the diagnosis can seldom be made on the basis of the histologic findings from liver biopsy alone. Recent or ongoing exposure to the suspected drug, the profile of liver function abnormalities, the histologic injury pattern most often associated with a particular drug, and the presence or absence of associated signs and symptoms that may or may not accompany injury with the suspected drug basically support a presumptive diagnosis.

Acute hepatic injury may be cytotoxic (overt damage to hepatocytes), cholestatic (arrested bile flow), or mixed (features of both cytotoxic and cholestatic injury). Chronic injury from drugs includes chronic necroinflammatory disease, chronic steatosis, chronic cholestasis, granulomatous disease, vascular injury, cirrhosis, and several types of liver tumors (Mullick 1987). Hepatotoxicity from drugs may be either predictable or idiosyncratic. Predictable injury resulting in hepatocellular necrosis is dose-related, is usually reproducible in animals, and is due to the intrinsic toxicity of a drug or its metabolite that is produced in the liver. Examples include overdoses with inorganic iron or acetaminophen. Idiosyncratic reactions are unpredictable. In these cases, the reaction generally does not directly relate to drug dose and may occur because of hypersensitivity with the usual clinical correlates. In other patients, there is no evidence of hypersensitivity and the underlying metabolic or genetic differences placing these persons at risk may be obscure. These differences in the biologic pathways of drug poisoning or detoxification are genetically determined. Chronic ingestion of alcohol and the concomitant use of rifampin may increase the hepatic toxicity of isoniazid (Lewis and Zimmerman 1989).

Dietary supplements including botanicals can result in hepatotoxicity, which is sometimes severe. One recent example was chaparral-induced hepatotoxicity; four patients developed cirrhosis, and two developed fulminant hepatic failure and required a liver transplant (Sheikh et al. 1997). Physicians should ask about recent intake of "health foods" when evaluating patients with liver abnormalities.

## Pulmonary Toxicity

Adverse pulmonary reactions to drugs should be considered when the cause of a respiratory illness is not clear (Table 24-4). The nature of the pulmonary reaction may range from asthma to pulmonary infiltrates. More than 20 different noncytotoxic agents have been associated with pulmonary reactions (Cooper et al. 1986a, 1986b); see Tables 24-5 and 24-6 for listings of cytotoxic and noncytotoxic drugs that affect pulmonary function. Clinical syndromes are heterogeneous and include pneumonitis-fibrosis, bronchiolitis obliterans, hypersensitivity lung disease, and noncardiogenic pulmonary edema. Amiodarone is perhaps the most widely used drug that frequently causes serious pulmonary toxicity, especially since it has been found to be effective at low dosage for therapy of atrial fibrillation. Pulmonary fibrosis was common with early amiodarone therapy when high doses (more than 400 mg/day) were used. In a meta-analysis explicitly evaluating the risk of adverse effects with low-dose amiodarone among 738 patients, the odds ratio for pulmonary toxicity when amiodarone was compared with placebo was 2.0, although this did not reach statistical significance (95% CI, 0.9–5.3). In one meta-analysis of amiodarone therapy in patients who had had an acute myocardial infarction (AMI) and were in CHF, the risk of pulmonary toxicity was 1% per year (Amiodarone Trials Meta-Analysis Investigators 1997).

Cytotoxic drugs may also cause severe pulmonary disease. Risk factors predisposing to development of pul-

**Table 24-4 Pulmonary Syndromes Caused by Drugs**

| Syndrome | Causative Agent |
|---|---|
| Hypersensitivity Lung Disease | Ampicillin |
| | Carbamazepine |
| | Chlorpropamide |
| | Cromolyn |
| | Dantrolene |
| | Hydralazine |
| | Imipramine |
| | Isoniazid |
| | Mecamylamine |
| | Mephenesin carbamate |
| | Methylphenidate |
| | Nitrofurantoin |
| | *p*-Aminosalicylic acid |
| | Penicillin |
| | Phenytoin |
| | Sulfadiazine |
| | Sulfasalazine |
| | Bleomycin |
| | Methotrexate |
| | Procarbazine |
| Drug-Induced Lupus with Potential for Lung Involvement | Chlorpromazine |
| | Ethosuximide |
| | Griseofulvin |
| | Gold salts |
| | Hydralazine |
| | Isoniazid |
| | Lithium carbonate |
| | Mephenytoin |
| | Methyldopa |
| | Nitrofurantoin |
| | Oral contraceptives |
| | Penicillin |
| | Penicillamine |
| | Phenylbutazone |
| | Phenytoin |
| | Prazosin |
| | Procainamide |
| | Propylthiouracil |
| | Quinidine |
| | Sulfonamides |
| | Trimethadione |
| Noncardiac Pulmonary Edema | *Opioid Overdose* |
| | Heroin |
| | Methadone |
| | Propoxyphene |
| | *Sedatives* |
| | Chlordiazepoxide |
| | Ethchlorvynol |

Table 24-4 Pulmonary Syndromes Caused by Drugs (Continued)

| SYNDROME | CAUSATIVE AGENT |
|---|---|
| | Hydrochlorthiazide |
| | Lidocaine |
| | Salicylates |
| | Tocolytic drugs |
| | Ritodrine |
| | Terbutaline |
| | Sequela of neuroleptic malignant syndrome |
| | Phenothiazines |
| | Butyrophenones |
| | Thioxanthenes |

monary toxicity caused by different categories of cytotoxic agents include the cumulative dose; the age of the patient; and prior or concurrent use of radiation, oxygen, and other cytotoxic drug therapies. Bleomycin-induced pulmonary damage has become a model for interstitial pneumonitis and pulmonary fibrosis. Whether administered subcutaneously, intraperitoneally, or intravenously, bleomycin induces pulmonary fibrosis in many animal species including humans. Bleomycin may have adverse effects on the lungs by generating reactive oxygen metabolites (Cooper et al. 1986a). In humans, no control studies have evaluated systematically the efficacy of corticosteroids in preventing or reversing the toxicity. There have been anecdotal reports of hastened resolution of pulmonary abnormalities after corticosteroids were administered.

Mitomycin is an alkylating agent that had been in use for several years before the report of its producing pulmonary toxicity. Its mechanism of adverse reaction may be included in the drug's alkylating properties. The nitrosoureas have both alkylating and carbamoylating properties. They produce interstitial pulmonary fibrosis seemingly related to the total dose administered and to the length of survival of the patient. The prognosis of progressive fibrosis is poor. Alkylating agents, busulfan, cyclophosphamide, and melphalan are all associated with poor prognosis once symptomatic pulmonary involvement begins. Generally, treatment with methotrexate, azathioprine, 6-mercaptopurine, and procarbazine are somewhat less likely to cause the pulmonary lesions (Cooper et al. 1986a) (see Table 24-5).

Pulmonary damage associated with cytotoxic drugs is a clinically significant problem. With the improving prognosis for many patients with treated malignancies and the increased need to use these agents, the incidence of drug-induced pulmonary disease may escalate. A critical problem in cytotoxic drug-induced pulmonary disease is to determine how to treat or prevent pulmonary toxicity while sustaining tumor toxicity.

## Medwatch

In 1993, the FDA introduced MedWatch, a program designed to promote voluntary reporting by health professionals of adverse events related to medications or devices (Kessler 1993). This is an important development because even large, randomized controlled trials cannot be expected to identify all adverse events related to drugs; such trials typically include several hundred to several thousand patients, whereas adverse effects can pose serious safety threats even if they occur in only 1 in 5–10,000 patients. The goals of MedWatch were to make it easier for providers to report serious events, to make it clear to health professionals what types of reports the FDA wants to receive, to more widely disseminate information about FDA actions resulting from such reporting, and to increase physician awareness of disease caused by drugs and devices (Kessler 1993).

After the introduction of MedWatch, the proportion of reports of serious events increased from 34% in 1992 to 49% in 1994, and the overall quality of reporting adverse effects of drugs improved (Piazza-Hepp and Kennedy 1995). Concerns have been raised about getting information back from MedWatch (Vogt and Byrns 1994), however, which is cumbersome and expensive ($1200 per request), as it requires using the Freedom of Information Act. The MedWatch group has responded by making a great deal of information available over the Internet (the URL is www.fda.gov/medwatch). This site synthesizes new reports about problems with drugs in its "Safety Information" section, which is regularly updated. The adverse drug event database is also available to be downloaded.

Since its introduction, MedWatch has had a number of successes. Some have involved identification of a new problem. For example, 13 cases of chaparral-associated hepatotoxicity were identified; 4 patients progressed to cirrhosis and 2 to liver failure requiring transplantation. Chaparral was being used as a dietary supplement. Also, a number of adverse events were associated with Norplant (a contraceptive implanted, e.g., in the forearm), including infections at the insertion site, hospitalizations because of difficulty removing the capsule, stroke, thrombotic thrombocytopenic purpura, thrombocytopenia, and pseudotumor

**Table 24-5 Cytotoxic Drug-Induced Pulmonary Parenchymal Disease**

| Class/Drug | Mechanism of Lung Injury | Incidence and Risk Factors | Clinical Findings | Findings on Chest X-Ray Film | Histopathologic Findings | Treatment | Outcome |
|---|---|---|---|---|---|---|---|
| *Cytotoxic Antibiotics* | | | | | | | |
| Bleomycin | Reactive oxygen metabolites | From 2 to 40%. Cumulating dose; $O_2$ therapy; radiotherapy; other chemotherapy | Hypersensitivity; lung disease; interstitial pneumonitis; pulmonary fibrosis | Bibasilar reticular pattern; multiple small nodules | Endothelial cell damage; type I pneumocyte necrosis; fibroblast proliferation | Stop drug; corticosteroids for acute hypersensitivity reaction; no controlled human studies | May develop chronic progressive pulmonary fibrosis |
| Mitomycin | Unknown—has alkylating effect | From 3 to 12%. Risk factors not well established; radiotherapy; $O_2$ therapy | Acute or gradual restrictive ventilatory defect; reduction in $D_{LCO}$; rare microangiopathic hemolytic anemia | X-ray film may be normal; diffuse or acinarreticular pattern; may show nodularity | Endothelial damage; type I pneumocyte necrosis; collagen deposition and fibrogen-fibrin deposits | Stop drug; early administration of corticosteroids may alter prognosis | Reported mortality of about 50% |
| *Nitrosoureas* | | | | | | | |
| Carmustine | Formation of electrophilic series; reduction of stores of glutathioneoxidant injury | From 20 to 30%. Total dose of cyclophosphamide important | Dyspnea; cough; basal rales; restrictive ventilatory defect | X-ray film may be normal; bibasilar reticular pattern most common | Dysplastic pneumocytes; proliferation of fibroblasts; fibrosis without inflammatory cells | Stop drug; many patients are already receiving corticosteroids and their value is questionable | Progressive pulmonary toxicity; mortality as high as 90% |
| Lomostine (CCNU) Semustine (methyl-CCNU) | | | Similar to carmustine; pulmonary toxicity; decreased $D_{LCO}$ | | Similar to carmustine; pulmonary toxicity; interstitial infiltration of mononuclear cells | | |
| *Alkylating Agents* | | | | | | | |
| Busulfan | Sensitivity to alkylating effects on epithelial cells | Symptomatic, 4%; asymptomatic, 46%. Radiotherapy; other cytotoxic drugs | Cough; dyspnea; fever; pulmonary rales. Toxicity may occur first some time after drug is discontinued. Restrictive ventilatory defect; decreased $D_{LCO}$ | Chest x-ray film rarely normal; basilar reticular pattern or acinar infiltrates; pleural effusion may be present | Dysplastic pneumocytes; proliferation of fibroblasts; fibrosis; mononuclear cell infiltration | Stop drug; trial of corticosteroids; supportive measures; there are no defined therapies | Prognosis is poor; mean survival after diagnosis is 5 months |

Table 24-5 Cytotoxic Drug-Induced Pulmonary Parenchymal Disease (Continued)

| Class/Drug | Mechanism of Lung Injury | Incidence and Risk Factors | Clinical Findings | Findings on Chest X-Ray Film | Histopathologic Findings | Treatment | Outcome |
|---|---|---|---|---|---|---|---|
| Cyclophosphamide | Alkylation of cellular DNA; redox reaction of metabolites; hypersensitivity reaction | Low incidence, below 1%. High concentration of inspired $O_2$ | Fever; cough; dyspnea; restrictive ventilatory defect; decreased $D_{LCO}$ | Basilar reticular pattern; at times noncardiac pulmonary edema | Endothelial swelling; pneumocyte dysplasia; fibroblast proliferation; lymphocyte and histiocyte infiltration | Stop drug; corticosteroids have no effect on mortality | Variable prognosis; about 60% of patients recover |
| Chlorambucil | Alkylating effect with cross-linking of DNA molecules | Low incidence since first report in 1967 | Fever; anorexia; restrictive ventilatory defect; decreased $D_{LCO}$ | X-ray film may be normal; diffuse basilar reticular pattern | Pneumocyte dysplasia; extensive fibrosis; scattered interstitial mononuclear infiltrate | Stop drug; may progress despite corticosteroid therapy | Variable; about 50% of patients recover |
| Melphalan | Alkylating properties | Low incidence of symptomatic disease; subclinical disease may be significant | Fever; cough; dyspnea; malaise; basilar rales; markedly reduced $D_{LCO}$ | Diffuse reticular pattern; modular and acinar shadows may occur | Atypical alveolar pneumocytes; fibrosis; bronchiolar epithelial proliferation; endothelial changes have not been reported | Stop drug; corticosteroids not of proven value | Variable; mortality about 50% |
| *Antimetabolites* | | | | | | | |
| Methotrexate | Hypersensitivity reaction; direct toxic effect may also be involved | Uncertain, probably about 8%. Frequency of administration; use with cyclophosphamide | Acute or chronic onset; fever; malaise; eosinophilia; restrictive ventilatory defect; impaired $D_{LCO}$ | X-ray film may be normal; diffuse reticular pattern; pleural effusion may be present | Atypical pneumocytes; inflammatory cells; fibrosis; diffuse edema with hyaline membrane formation | Stop drug; corticosteroids may hasten recovery; alternative therapy should be selected | Favorable; mortality about 1% |
| Azathioprine and 6-mercaptopurine | | | Acute restrictive lung disease | | | Stop drug; alternate immunosuppressive therapy; corticosteroids | Favorable |
| Cytosine-arabinoside | | | Acute respiratory failure | Diffuse infiltrates; pulmonary edema | Pulmonary infiltrates; pulmonary edema | Stop drug; supportive therapy | Variable; may be unfavorable |

**Table 24-5 Cytotoxic Drug-Induced Pulmonary Parenchymal Disease (Continued)**

| Class/Drug | Mechanism of Lung Injury | Incidence and Risk Factors | Clinical Findings | Findings on Chest X-Ray Film | Histopathologic Findings | Treatment | Outcome |
|---|---|---|---|---|---|---|---|
| *Other Cytotoxic Drugs* | | | | | | | |
| Procarbazine | Hypersensitivity reaction; pulmonary edema | | Hypersensitivity pneumonitis; pulmonary edema; fever; eosinophilia | | Scattered eosinophils; mononuclear cell infiltration; fibrosis | Stop drug; supportive measures; corticosteroids may be of value | Probably favorable |
| Vinca alkaloids<br>Vinblastine<br>Vindesine<br>Vincristine | Unknown—may be due to combined therapy with mitomycin | | Dyspnea; bronchospasm; acute diffuse pulmonary infiltrates and respiratory failure | | Dysplasia of alveolar lining cells; fibrosis; interstitial and alveolar influx of inflammatory cells | Stop drug; assisted ventilatory support; corticosteroids may be of value | Prognosis is poor if pulmonary infiltrates develop |
| Podophyllotoxin derivatives<br>Etoposide (VP-16)<br>Teniposide (VM-26) | Unknown—may be due in part to prior carmustine therapy | | | Acinar and reticular infiltrates | Hyaline membrane formation; marked interstitial mononuclear and histiocytic infiltration | Stop drug; supportive therapy | Unclear; unfavorable with associated pulmonary infection |

**Table 24-6 Noncytotoxic Drug-Induced Pulmonary Parenchymal Disease**

| Drug | Mechanism of Lung Injury | Incidence and Risk Factors | Clinical Findings | Findings on Chest X-Ray Film | Histopathologic Findings | Treatment | Outcome |
|---|---|---|---|---|---|---|---|
| Nitrofurantoin | Hypersensitivity; production of oxygen radicals | More than 500 cases since 1961; age; extensive use of drug | Acute and chronic forms; fever; dyspnea; ventilatory defect; impaired $D_{LCO}$ | Acute: diffuse bibasilar and acinal infiltrates<br>Chronic: infiltrates; may also have pleural effusion | Pulmonary vasculitis; interstitial and alveolar cellular infiltration; eosinophilia; granuloma formation; fibrosis | Stop drug; corticosteroids of questionable value | Acute: good; low mortality<br>Chronic: fair; mortality about 10% |
| Sulfasalazine | Hypersensitivity | Unclear; salicylate and/or sulfonamide allergy may predispose to adverse reaction | Hypersensitivity reaction; fibrosing alveolitis; bronchiolitis obliterans; obstructive ventilatory pattern | Bilateral acinar infiltrates | Alveolitis; interstitial infiltration with eosinophils; fibrosis; bronchiolitis obliterans | Stop drug; corticosteroids may hasten recovery | Variable but generally good prognosis |
| Amphotericin B | Mechanism of pulmonary toxicity associated with leukocyte transfusions is not well understood; damage to transfused leukocytes or direct pulmonary tissue damage | About 60% in patients receiving both modes of therapy | Fever; chills; dyspnea; hypoxemia; hemoptysis | Diffuse interstitial infiltrates | Lung biopsy; diffuse intraalveolar hemorrhage; edema; without infection | Stop drug; supportive care; assisted ventilation may be needed | Prognosis poor; 50% need assisted ventilation; mortality about 35% |
| Amiodarone | May be multifactorial; acquired lysosomal storage disease; immunologic mechanism | Numerous reports of pulmonary damage; 1% to 6%; toxicity partially related to maintenance dose | Delayed onset; dyspnea; cough; fever; reduced $D_{LCO}$ | Diffuse reticular and patchy acinar infiltrates; pleural thickening; pleural effusions | Intraalveolar foamy macrophages; septal thickening; hyperplasia; type II pneumocytes | Stop drug; role of corticosteroids is unclear; these agents will not completely protect against toxic effects | Variable; reversal may occur; the lung injury may be progressive |
| Penicillamine | Unclear; altered collagen metabolism; epithelial toxicity; hypersensitivity | Low incidence of pulmonary injury; risk factors are unclear | Acute hypersensitivity reaction; subacute alveolitis or bronchiolitis; pulmonary renal syndrome | Similar to those of idiopathetic alveolitis; bronchiolitis or Goodpasture syndrome | Obliterated small airways; dysplastic pneumocytes; fibroblast proliferation and alveolar hemorrhage | Stop drug; supportive therapy; no apparent help by corticosteroids | Variable; but generally unfavorable |

Table 24-6 Noncytotoxic Drug-Induced Pulmonary Parenchymal Disease (Continued)

| Drug | Mechanism of Lung Injury | Incidence and Risk Factors | Clinical Findings | Findings on Chest X-Ray Film | Histopathologic Findings | Treatment | Outcome |
|---|---|---|---|---|---|---|---|
| Gold salts | Unclear; proposed release of lymphokines; monocyte chemotactic factors; macrophage inhibitory factors | Incidence less than 1%; risk factors are unclear | Hypersensitivity lung disease or chronic pneumonitis/fibrosis | Diffuse reticulonodular infiltrates; restrictive ventilatory defect; decreased $D_{LCO}$ | Interstitial and alveolar infiltration with histiocytes; plasma cells and lymphocytes; electron-dense deposits of macrophages in interstitium | Stop drug; role of chelating agents or corticosteroids uncertain | Low mortality; 50% of patients have residual pulmonary dysfunction |

$D_{LCO}$ = Pulmonary function test-diffusing capacity of the lung for carbon dioxide.

cerebri (Wysowski and Green 1995). For stroke, thrombotic thrombocytopenic purpura, thrombocytopenia, and pseudotumor, more data are needed to determine whether these associations are causal.

Other successes have involved stimulating reporting about problems already reported to the FDA. For example, after the first 33 reports of valvular heart disease were associated with fenfluramine and phentermine (Connolly et al. 1997), the FDA solicited additional reports through the MedWatch network. This resulted in a substantial increase of the number of cases being recognized and, eventually, withdrawal of the combination product from the market.

In conclusion, MedWatch functions both as a data repository for reports of new, serious ADRs, and as a clearinghouse for adverse effects of medications. Access to the data repository could be improved, and the FDA plans to do this, but the clearinghouse function is already being admirably fulfilled. It is important to recognize the limitations of a spontaneous reporting approach such as this; while this works well for identifying new "signals" suggesting the presence of relationships, under-reporting is the rule so that rates calculated using these data generally represent large underestimates of the actual event rates.

## ERROR THEORY AND ERROR IN MEDICINE

Outside the field of medicine, substantial research has been devoted to understanding error, particularly in complex systems such as nuclear reactors and aircraft (Leape 1995). Evaluation of this research has important implications for medicine. Industrial quality theory suggests that most defects result from problems with the production process itself, not from the individuals within it (Berwick 1989; Leape 1995). According to this theory, blame for defects is often misplaced. Although "human errors" are frequently identified when accidents occur, the true cause is often the design of the system that led an operator to make the error; such system flaws have been termed "latent errors" (Reason 1990). Root cause analysis can be used to assess these underlying systems causes of an individual defect (Leape 1995). Although sometimes an individual who makes repeated errors is to blame (for example, because of alcoholism), most errors are made by conscientious workers whose overall work is good. However, in medicine, the "bad apple" approach to quality improvement has been predominant; the goal of such systems is to identify defective individuals and get rid of them (Berwick 1989). A more effective approach to improving overall quality may be to raise the level of performance of all workers involved in a process. Some empiric data suggest that this approach may be useful. With regard to drugs in particular, when we evaluated 334 serious medication errors (errors that either resulted in harm or had the potential to do so), we did not identify any instances in which there was a repeated pattern of error by an individual (Leape 1995). However, when we performed multidisciplinary systems analyses of these errors, we found 16 systems that had failed in a variety of ways. It is noteworthy that the eight most important areas involved failures of information management.

## A SYSTEMS APPROACH TO PREVENTION

Historically, most prevention error efforts have focused on training people not to make errors, and then punishing them when they do. Not surprisingly, personnel tend to hide their mistakes and to avoid discussion of errors, exactly the opposite of what is needed to identify and correct systems causes. This is not to say that an occasional practitioner will not require disciplinary action. The medical profession has a spotty record in this area, with an extreme example being a physician who allegedly poisoned patients while working at multiple practice sites, yet continued to obtain privileges for a number of years (Stewart 1997). Fortunately, this probably is a rare exception. Educational efforts have included not only lectures and dissemination of printed material such as newsletters, but also one-on-one educational efforts by clinical pharmacists and clinical pharmacy consultative services (Soumerai and Avorn 1984). Unfortunately, lectures and dissemination of printed material, while relatively inexpensive and likely necessary for changing opinion, by themselves have relatively little long-term effect. One-on-one counter-detailing or academic detailing and clinical pharmacy services are more effective, but are much more expensive, and their effects also wane with time if they are not continued.

### Systems Changes That May Reduce the Frequency of ADE

One of the earliest and most effective systems changes in the medication arena was the implementation of unit dosing in hospitals. Implemented first in the 1970s, unit dosing has had a major impact on the frequency of medication errors. This approach (described in more detail later) reduced the frequency of medication errors by 82% in a study by Simborg and Derewicz (1975). This large an effect size, with lasting duration, can only be realized through systems changes, and this has led to a search for other changes that may have an important impact.

A number of other systems changes appear promising for reducing the frequency of ADEs, although many have not been studied rigorously. Recently, a multidisciplinary panel including representatives from pharmacy, nursing, and physician groups, made seven recommendations about changes that should be implemented in the near future to prevent adverse drug events in hospitals (Bates 1996). These included implementation of physician order entry, increased use of bar-coding, developing systems for monitoring and reporting ADEs, using unit-dose distribution systems and pharmacy-based intravenous admixture systems, changing the role of pharmacists so that they have more clinical roles, moving to a view of medication errors as systems failures, and implementing pharmacist review of orders (Table 24-7).

One of the potentially most powerful systems changes for improving the medication use process is implementation of physician computer order entry, in which physicians and physician assistants write all orders on-line. Although many hospitals in the United States use order entry by clerks, fewer use order entry by physicians (Sittig and Stead 1994). However, clerk order entry has important disadvantages: information and guidance is not delivered to the person writing the order at the time they are doing it, and transcription is still required. Physician order entry can reduce the number of medication errors by: 1) structuring orders so that all include dose, route, frequency, and duration; 2) checking these parameters, especially the dose, for appropriateness; 3) eliminating legibility problems; and, 4) providing guidelines for indications and dosing. In addition, all orders can be passed through a series of checks, including checks for drug allergies, drug–drug interactions, and drug–laboratory problems. One estimate is that 84% of medication errors (excluding missing doses) could potentially be prevented using this approach (Bates et al. 1995a).

**Table 24-7 Top-Priority Actions for Preventing Adverse Drug Events in Hospitals: Recommendations of an ASHP-Convened Expert Panel**

1. Hospitals should establish processes in which prescribers enter medication orders directly into computer systems.
2. Hospitals should evaluate the use of machine-readable coding (e.g., bar coding) in their medication-use processes.
3. Hospitals should develop better systems for monitoring and reporting adverse drug events.
4. Hospitals should use unit-dose medication distribution and pharmacy-based intravenous admixture systems.
5. Hospitals should assign pharmacists to work in patient care areas in direct collaboration with prescribers and those administering medications.
6. Hospitals should approach medication errors as systems failures and seek systems solutions to preventing them.
7. Hospitals should ensure that medication orders are routinely reviewed by a pharmacist before first doses and should ensure that prescribers, pharmacists, nurses, and other workers seek resolution whenever there is any question of safety with respect to medication use.

From ASHP Guidelines on Preventing Medication Errors in Hospitals (ASHP 1993).

Bar-coding is another systems change with the potential to reduce the medication error rate significantly. It is an efficient method for tracking medications and checking to make sure that the correct dose of the correct medication reaches the intended patient. In other industries, bar-coding has been widely used to maintain inventories and track items such as packages. However, hospitals have made relatively little use of bar-coding to date (Brient 1995). The technology is now inexpensive and widely available, and could nearly eliminate some serious errors, such as giving one patient a medication intended for another or interchanging two similar looking drugs.

Developing better systems for monitoring and reporting adverse drug events is also important because it is hard to do something about a problem if its frequency is unclear. For nosocomial infections, it has long been clear that active case-finding and monitoring of rates allows targeting of interventions (Martone et al. 1995). However, for ADE tracking, most hospitals rely exclusively on self-report, which, since it often results in punishment, typically identifies only about 1 in 20 events (Cullen et al. 1995). As noted earlier in this chapter, computerized detection strategies that use the computer to screen for incidents suggesting the presence of an ADE, followed by clinical pharmacist follow-up, likely make the most sense (Classen et al. 1991; Jha et al. 1996). This approach can be supplemented by allowing clinicians to directly report these events (Classen et al. 1991).

Unit-dose systems, promoting intravenous pharmacy admixture, and implementing pharmacy review of medication errors are well-established as effective measures, and are "lower-tech" so that they may be more immediately implemented if not in place. A unit-dose system is one in which most medications are dispensed from the pharmacy in single-unit or unit-dose packages in a ready-to-administer form, and 24 hours or less of doses are dispensed at a time (Bates 1996). As noted earlier, one study found that unit-dose dispensing decreased the medication error rate by 82% (Simborg and Derewicz 1975); it appeared to have this effect largely by reducing the frequency of wrong dose errors. Another change that is likely to reduce error is to implement pharmacy admixture for all intravenous medications. This probably reduces errors because of the relative infrequency of nursing admixture. Commercial premixed solutions have even lower error rates, however (Flynn et al. 1997). Pharmacy review of orders also has been shown to detect important prescribing errors (Lesar et al. 1990; Folli et al. 1987); approximately 3–5 errors per 1000 orders were found in these studies.

Changing the role of pharmacists so that they interact more with physicians and nurses and become involved earlier in the prescribing process is not new, but its impact has received relatively little evaluation (Shulman et al. 1981; Blum et al. 1988; Hawkey et al. 1990; Brown 1991). However, this approach can be very effective, particularly in care settings such as intensive care units and hematology–oncology units where large numbers and quantities of toxic medications are used. Most United States hospitals still do not do this routinely; in 1992, only 18% of hospitals reported that they had pharmacists participate regularly in medical rounds (Bond et al. 1994). The pharmacist and clinical pharmacologist play much more prominent roles in Europe.

Perhaps the systems change with the greatest potential benefit is to eliminate the culture of fear. When errors are viewed as symptoms of systems failures rather than evidence of human failures they become opportunities for improvement (Leape et al. 1995). The tradition in medicine has been to blame the individual making the error, but this is counterproductive. Tracing the error to an individual does not address the underlying cause of the error and recurrence is assured—punishment provides a strong incentive for individuals to conceal errors, leading to complacency and inaction. Although organizations need to have a procedure for dealing with providers who exhibit dangerous behavior, it is critical to recognize that such situations are the exception. Almost all errors are made by good people trying to do a good job.

Another issue in many hospitals is that physicians, nurses, and pharmacists often view only their own piece of the drug use process, and do not work together as a team to improve it. Such teamwork is vital; many changes that appear to make sense from one discipline's perspective may actually not benefit the process as a whole.

Future medication delivery systems will likely include more automation and more automated checks. (Bates 1996). Ordering will be done by computer, and these systems will both guide ordering and make suggestions if errors or potential problems are discovered. Guidance will include displaying appropriate doses and frequencies, and the guidelines for use of drugs. Checking for problems including allergies, interactions, and laboratory studies will be done in the background, with messages being displayed only when issues are identified. Orders will go electronically directly to the pharmacy where they will be triaged by urgency and whether they can be filled from a point-of-care distribution system, or need to be prepared and delivered by the pharmacy. The pharmacy will also send the orders to update the computerized medication record.

If medications are present at the point-of-care, the automated distribution system will make them available. When nurses administer drugs, they will obtain them from the automated distribution systems, check them using bar codes to verify that the correct medication has been obtained, and then administer the drugs to the patient, after checking their own and the patient's bar codes. Not only will bar-coding decrease the likelihood of giving one patient another's drug or giving medications too early, it should essentially eliminate "look-alike" substitutions. It will also "close the loop" of drug administration, recording how much drug has been given, when, by whom, and to whom (Bates 1996).

Patients will receive education both during the hospitalization and at discharge, and get information both printed and available electronically for those with Internet access about how their medications should be taken and about potential adverse effects. The role of pharmacists will change from counting pills, to dealing with complicated medications and dealing with more clinical issues. One key role will be face-to-face counter-detailing to change physician beliefs about specific drugs. Adverse drug event detection will be done by using clinical information systems to feed monitors that detect adverse events (Classen et al. 1991; Jha et al. 1996), to be supplemented by a voluntary on-line reporting system. A multidisciplinary committee charged with improving the medication system will review this information.

**SUMMARY**

**Adverse drug reactions and adverse drug events are both important. The frequency of adverse drug reactions varies substantially by organ system for specific drugs. Recognition of new and rare adverse drug reactions depends on developing large databases such as MedWatch that include information from millions of people. The general strategy of postmarketing surveillance has had many important successes, such as identification of valvular abnormalities associated with**

**weight reduction drugs. Ongoing surveillance is critical for minimizing the future risks associated with new therapeutic agents.**

**On the other hand, preventable adverse drug events injuries caused by errors in giving medications are preventable today. Many such errors slip through in the current systems for giving patients medications; large improvements should be possible in making these systems safer in both the inpatient and outpatient setting. Changing to a systems perspective, implementation of automation, and judicious use of decision support should have a large impact on making the use of drugs safer in coming years. The single intervention likely to have the largest impact in this regard is computerization of drug ordering.**

**Adverse drug events occur in every physician's practice. Physicians' recognition of these events depends on their knowledge of the pharmacology of the drugs they use and on their willingness to recognize that they may cause harm despite good intentions. Unless all the pharmacologic effects of a drug that are known are appreciated, new symptoms may be falsely ascribed to extension or complications of the disease rather than to drug toxicity or reaction. Our success in preventing adverse drug events depends critically on our capacity for and interest in acquiring and using valid information.**

## SUGGESTED READING

Kastrup EK, editor. 1990. *Drug Facts and Comparisons*. St. Louis: Facts and Comparisons Division of JB Lippincott.

Reuben BG, Wittcoff HA. 1989. *Pharmaceutical Chemicals in Perspective*. New York: Wiley & Sons.

Reynolds JEF, editor. 1989. *Martindale: The Extra Pharmacopoeia*. 29th ed. London: The Pharmaceutical Press.

## REFERENCES

Abel R, Leopold IH. 1987. Drug-induced ocular diseases. In: Speight TM, editor. *Avery's Drug Treatment*. 3rd ed. Hong Kong: Adis Press. p 409–17.

Adler SG, Cohen AH, Border WA. 1986. Hypersensitivity phenomena and the kidney: role of drugs and environmental agents. *Am J Kidney Dis* **5**:75–96.

Ali MZ, Goetz MB. 1997. A meta-analysis of the relative efficacy and toxicity of single daily dosing versus multiple daily dosing of aminoglycosides. *Clin Infect Dis* **24**:796–809.

Allan EL, Barker KN. 1990. Fundamentals of medication error research. *Am J Hosp Pharm* **47**:555–71.

Amiodarone Trials Meta-Analysis Investigators. 1997. Effect of prophylactic amiodarone on mortality after acute myocardial infarction and in congestive heart failure: meta-analysis of individual data from 6500 patients in randomised trials. *Lancet* **350**:1417–24.

Applebaum A. 1963. Ophthalmoscopic study of patients under treatment with thioridazine. *Arch Ophthalmol* **69**:578–80.

Applebaum FR, Strauchen JA, Graw RG Jr, et al. 1976. Acute lethal carditis caused by high-dose combination chemotherapy: a unique clinical and pathological entity. *Lancet* **1**:58–62.

[ASHP] American Society of Hospital Pharmacists. 1993. ASHP guidelines on preventing medication errors in hospitals. *Am J Hosp Pharm* **50**:305–14.

Assier H, Bastuji-Garin S, Revuz J, et al. 1995. Erythema multiforme with mucous membrane involvement and Stevens-Johnson syndrome are clinically different disorders with distinct causes. *Arch Dermatol* **131**:539–43.

Aylward JM. 1993. Hydroxychloroquine and chloroquine: assessing the risk of retinal toxicity. *J Am Optom Assoc* **64**:787–97.

Bailey TC, Little JR, Littenberg B, et al. 1997. A meta-analysis of extended-interval dosing versus multiple daily dosing of aminoglycosides. *Clin Infect Dis* **24**:786–95.

Barker KN, Allan EL. 1995. Research on drug-use-system errors. *Am J Health Syst Pharm* **52**:400–3.

Barza M, Ioannidis JP, Cappelleri JC, et al. 1996. Single or multiple daily doses of aminoglycosides: a meta-analysis. *BMJ* **312**:338–45.

Bates DW. 1996. Medication errors. How common are they and what can be done to prevent them? *Drug Saf* **5**:303–10.

Bates DW, Boyle DL, Vander Vliet MB, et al. 1995a. Relationship between medication errors and adverse drug events. *J Gen Intern Med* **10**:199–205.

Bates DW, Cullen D, Laird N, et al. 1995b. Incidence of adverse drug events and potential adverse drug events: implications for prevention. *JAMA* **274**:29–34.

Bates DW, Spell N, Cullen DJ, et al. 1997. The costs of adverse drug events in hospitalized patients. *JAMA* **227**:307–11.

Begg EJ, Barclay ML. 1995. Aminoglycosides-50 years on. *Br J Clin Pharmacol* **39**:597–603.

Benacerraf B. 1981. Role of MHC gene products in immune regulation. *Science* **212**:1229–38.

Bennett WM. 1990. Drug therapy in renal failure. *Sci Am Med* **10**(2):A3–35.

Bennett WM, Arnoff GR, Golper TA, et al. 1991. *Drug Prescribing in Renal Failure*. 2nd ed. Philadelphia: American College of Physicians.

Bernstein JM, Weiss AD. 1967. Further observations on salicylate ototoxicity. *J Laryngol Otol* **81**:915–25.

Berwick DM. 1989. Continuous improvement as an ideal in health care. *N Engl J Med* **320**:53–6.

Bienia RA, Smith M, Pellegrino T. 1983. Scopolamine skin-disks and anisocoria. *Ann Intern Med* **99**:5723.

Biro K, Baki M, Buki B, et al. 1997. Detection of early ototoxic effect in testicular-cancer patients treated with cisplatin by transiently evoked otoacoustic emission: a pilot study. *Oncology* **54**:387–90.

Blaschke TF, Nies AS, Mamelok RD. 1985. Principles of therapeutics. In: Gilman AG, Goodman LS, Rall TW, et al., editors. *Goodman and Gilman's The Pharmacologic Basis of Therapeutics*. 7th ed. New York: Macmillan. p 49–65.

Bloom KE, Brewer GJ, Magon AM, et al. 1983. Microsomal incubation test of potentially hemolytic drugs for glucose-6-phosphate dehydrogenase deficiency. *Clin Pharmacol Ther* **33**:403–9.

Blum KV, Abel SR, Urbanski CJ, et al. 1988. Medication error prevention by pharmacists. *Am J Hosp Pharm* **45**:1902–3.

Bond CA, Raehl CL, Pitterle ME. 1992. National clinical pharmacy services study. *Pharmacotherapy* **14**:282–304, 1994.

Borda IT, Slone D, Jick H. 1968. Assessment of adverse reactions within a drug surveillance program. *JAMA* **205**:99–101.

Brien JA. 1993. Ototoxicity associated with salicylates: a brief review. *Drug Saf* **9**:143–8.

Brient K. 1995. Bar-coding facilitates patient-focused care. *Health Inform* **12**:38, 40, 42.

Bristow MR, Mason JW, Billingham ME, et al. 1978. Doxorubicin cardiomyopathy: evaluation by phonocardiography, endomyocardial biopsy and cardial catheterization. *Ann Intern Med* **88**:168–175.

Brittain DC. 1987. Erythromycin. *Med Clin North Am* **71**:1147–54.

Brown GC. 1991. Assessing the clinical impact of pharmacists' interventions. *Am J Hosp Pharm* **48**:2644–7.

Brummett RE. 1993a. Ototoxicity of vancomycin and analogues. *Otolaryngol Clin North Am* **26**:821–8.

Brummett RE. 1993b. Ototoxic liability of erythromycin and analogues. *Otolaryngol Clin North Am* **26**:811–9.

Brummett RE, Fox KE. 1989a. Aminoglycoside-induced hearing loss in humans. *Antimicrob Agents Chemother* **33**:797–800.

Brummett RE, Fox KE. 1989b. Vancomycin- and erythromycin-induced hearing loss in humans. *Antimicrob Agents Chemother* **33**:791–6.

Brunton LL. 1985. Laxatives. In: Gilman AG, Goodman LS, Rall TW, et al., editors. *Goodman and Gilman's The Pharmacological Basis of Therapeutics*. 7th ed. New York: Macmillan. p 994–1003.

Cantu TG, Yamanaka-Yuen NA, Lietman PS. 1994. Serum vancomycin concentrations: reappraisal of their clinical value. *Clin Infect Dis* **18**:533–43.

Classen DC, Pestotnik SL, Evans RS, et al. 1991. Computerized surveillance of adverse drug events in hospital patients. *JAMA* **266**:2847–51.

Classen DC, Pestotnik SL, Evans RS, et al. 1997. Adverse drug events in hospitalized patients. Excess length of stay, extra costs, and attributable mortality. *JAMA* **277**:301–6.

Cole E, Keown P, Landsberg D, et al. 1998. Safety and tolerability of cyclosporine and cyclosporine microemulsion during 18 months of follow-up in stable renal transplant recipients: a report of the Canadian Neoral Renal Study Group. *Transplantation* **65**:505–10.

Connolly HM, Crary JL, McGoon MD, et al. 1997. Valvular heart disease associated with fenfluramine-phentermine. *N Engl J Med* **337**:581–8.

Consumer's Association. 1983. *Drug and Therapeutics Bulletin*. London: Consumer's Association.

Cooper JAD Jr, White DA, Matthay RA. 1986a. Drug-induced pulmonary disease: 1. Cytotoxic drugs. *Am Rev Respir Dis* **133**:321–340.

Cooper JAD Jr, White DA, Matthay RA. 1986b. Drug-induced pulmonary disease: 2. Non-cytotoxic drugs. *Am Rev Respir Dis* **133**:488–505.

Crombie AL. 1981. Cataract formation associated with the use of phenothiazine derivatives. *Prescriber's J* **21**:222.

Cullen DJ, Bates DW, Small SD, et al. 1995. The incident reporting system does not detect adverse drug events: a problem for quality improvement. *Jt Comm J Qual Improv* **21**:541–8.

de Forni M, Armand JP. 1994. Cardiotoxicity of chemotherapy. *Curr Opin Oncol* **6**:340–4.

de Marie S. 1996. Liposomal and lipid-based formulations of amphotericin B. *Leukemia* **10**:S93–6.

Drug-induced agranulocytosis. 1997. *Drug Ther Bull* **35**:49–52.

Ettinger B, Norman O, Sörgel F. 1980. Triamterene nephrolithiasis. *JAMA* **244**:2443–5.

Faber BF, Moellering RC Jr. 1983. Retrospective study of the toxicity of preparations of vancomycin from 1978 to 1981. *Antimicrob Agents Chemother* **23**:138–41.

Farrell GC. 1997. Drug-induced hepatic injury. *J Gastroenterol Hepatol* **12**:S242–50.

Fillastre JP, Raguenex-Viotte G, Moulin B. 1988. Nephrotoxicity of antitumoral agents. *Arch Toxicol* **12**(Suppl.):117–24.

Flynn EA, Pearson RE, Barker KN. 1997. Observational study of accuracy in compounding IV admixtures at five hospitals. *Am J Health Syst Pharm* **54**:904–12.

Folli HL, Poole RL, Benitz WE, et al. 1987. Medication error prevention by clinical pharmacists in two children's hospitals. *Pediatrics* **79**:718–22.

Forrester JW. 1971. Counterintuitive behavior of social systems. *M I T Technol Rev* **73**:52–68.

Fraunfelder FT. 1982. Transdermal scopolamine precipitating narrow angle glaucoma. *N Engl J Med* **307**:1079.

Geanon JD, Perkins TW. 1995. Bilateral acute angle-closure glaucoma associated with drug sensitivity to hydrochlorothiazide. *Arch Ophthalmol* **113**:1231–2.

Gibaldi M. 1984. Nonoral medication. In: Gibaldi M, editor. *Biopharmaceutics and Clinical Pharmacokinetics*. 3rd ed. Philadelphia: Lea & Febiger. p 85–112.

Goldberger MJ. 1988. Antituberculous agents. *Med Clin North Am* **72**:661–8.

Graves T, Hanlon JT, Schmader KE, et al. 1997. Adverse events after discontinuing medications in elderly outpatients. *Arch Intern Med* **157**:2205–10.

Greenberger PA. 1984. Contrast media reactions. *J Allergy Clin Immunol* **74**:600–5.

Greenberger PA, Patterson R. 1991. The prevention of immediate generalized reactions to radiocontrast media in high-risk patients. *J Allergy Clin Immunol* **87**:867–72.

Grierson DJ. 1997. Hydroxychloroquine and visual screening in a rheumatology outpatient clinic. *Ann Rheum Dis* **56**:188–90.

Haahtela T, Jarvine M, Kava T, et al. 1991. Comparison of a $\beta$-agonist, terbutaline, with an inhaled corticosteroid, budesonide, in newly detected asthma. *N Engl J Med* **325**:388–92.

Hanes SD, Quarles DA, Boucher BA. 1997. Incidence and risk factors of thrombocytopenia in critically ill trauma patients. *Ann Pharmacother* **31**:285–9.

Hatala R, Dinh T, Cook DJ. 1996. Once-daily aminoglycoside dosing in immunocompetent adults: a meta-analysis. *Ann Intern Med* **124**:717–25.

Hawkey CJ, Hodgson S, Norman A, et al. 1990. Effect of reactive pharmacy intervention on quality of hospital prescribing. *BMJ* **300**:986–90.

Haydon RC, Thelin JW, Davis WE. 1984. Erythromycin ototoxicity: analysis and conclusions based on 22 case reports. *Otolaryngol Head Neck Surg* **99**:678–84.

Hermans PE, Wilheim MP. 1987. Vancomycin. *Mayo Clin Proc* **62**: 901–5.

Inman WHW, Adelsteen AM. 1969. Rise and fall of asthma mortality in England and Wales in relation to use of pressurized aerosols. *Lancet* **2**:279–85.

Jackson GG, Arcieri G. 1971. Ototoxicity of gentamicin in man: a survey and controlled analysis of clinical experience in the United States. *J Infect Dis* **124**(Suppl.):130–7.

Jha AK, Kuperman GJ, Teich JM, et al. 1998. Identifying adverse drug events: development of a computer-based monitor and comparison to chart review a stimulated voluntary report. *J Am Med Inform Assoc* **5**:305–14.

Joist JH. 1985. Bleeding due to vascular and platelet disorders. In: Conn RB, editor. *Current Diagnosis*. Philadelphia: WB Saunders. p 605–24.

Kahan BD. 1986. Cyclosporin nephrotoxicity: pathogenesis, prophylaxis, therapy, and prognosis. *Am J Kidney Dis* **8**:323–31.

Kakourou T, Klontza D, Soteropoulou F, et al. 1997. Corticosteroid treatment of erythema multiforme major (Stevens-Johnson syndrome) in children. *Eur J Pediatr* **156**:90–3.

Kapsenberg ML. 1996. Chemical and proteins as allergens and adjuvants. *Toxicol Lett* **86**:79–83.

Karch FE, Lasagna L. 1977. Toward the operational identification of adverse drug reactions. *Clin Pharmacol Ther* **21**:247–54.

Katzberg RW. 1997. Urography into the 21st century: new contrast media, renal handling, imaging characteristics, and nephrotoxicity. *Radiology* **204**:297–312.

Kessler DA. 1993. Introducing MedWatch. A new approach to reporting medication and device adverse effects and product problems. *JAMA* **269**:2765–8.

Koch KE. 1990. Use of standardized screening procedures to identify adverse drug reactions. *Am J Hosp Pharm* **47**:1314–20.

Koegel L. 1985. Ototoxicity: a contemporary review of aminoglycosides, loop diuretics, acetylsalicylic acid, quinine, erythromycin, and cisplatin. *Am J Otol* **6**:190–9.

Kostenbauder HB, Rapp RP, McGoveen JP, et al. 1975. Bioavailability and single dose pharmacokinetics of intramuscular diphenylhydantoin. *Clin Pharmacol Ther* **18**:449–56.

Kralovicova K, Spanik S, Halko J, et al. 1997. Do vancomycin serum levels predict failures of vancomycin therapy or nephrotoxicity in cancer patients? *J Chemother* **9**:420–6.

Kramer MS, Leventhal JM, Hutchinson TA, et al. 1979. An algorithm for the operational assessment of adverse drug reactions. I. Background, description, and instructions for use. *JAMA* **242**:623–32.

Lagrange JL, Medecin B, Etienne MC, et al. 1997. Cisplatin nephrotoxicity: a multivariate analysis of potential predisposing factors. *Pharmacotherapy* **17**:1246–53.

Lang DM, Alpern MB, Visintainer PF, et al. 1993. Elevated risk of anaphylactoid reaction from radiographic contrast media is associated with both beta-blocker exposure and cardiovascular disorders. *Ann Intern Med* **153**:2033–40.

Laurell G, Beskow C, Frankendal B, et al. 1996. Cisplatin administration to gynecological cancer patients. Long-term effects on hearing. *Cancer* **78**:1798–1804.

Leader WG, Chandler MH, Castiglia M. 1995. Pharmacokinetic optimisation of vancomycin therapy. *Clin Pharmacokinet* **28**:327–42.

Leape LL. 1995. Error in medicine. *JAMA* **272**:1851–57.

Leape LL, Bates DW, Cullen DJ, et al. 1995. Systems analysis of adverse drug events. *JAMA* **274**:35–43.

Lee WM. 1995. Drug-induced hepatotoxicity. *N Engl J Med* **333**:1118–27.

Legha SS, Benjamin RS, MacKay G, et al. 1982. Reduction of doxorubicin cardiotoxicity by prolonged continuous intravenous infusion. *Ann Intern Med* **96**:133–9.

Lennard HL, Epstein LJ, Bernstein A, et al. 1970. Hazards implicit in prescribing psychoactive drugs. *Science* **169**:438–41.

Lesar TS, Briceland LL, Delcoure K, et al. 1990. Medication prescribing errors in a teaching hospital. *JAMA* **263**:2329–34.

Lewis JH, Zimmerman H. 1989. Drug-induced liver disease. *Med Clin North Am* **73**:775–92.

Lien EJ. 1987a. Chemical structure and side effects. In: *Side Effects and Drug Design*. New York: Marcel Dekker. p 183–315.

Lien EJ. 1987b. *Side Effects and Drug Design*. New York: Marcel Dekker.

Lien EJ, Lipsett LR, Lien LL. 1983. Structure side effect sorting of drugs: VI. Ototoxicities. *J Clin Hosp Pharm* **8**:15–33.

Mackenzie AH. 1983. Antimalarial drugs for rheumatoid arthritis. *Am J Med* **75**:48–58.

Mackie MA, Davidson J, Clarke J. 1997. Quinine-acute self-poisoning and ocular toxicity. *Scott Med J* **42**:8–9.

Marshall GD Jr, Lieberman PL. 1991. Comparison of three pretreatment protocols to prevent anaphylactoid reactions to radiocontrast media. *Ann Allergy* **67**:70–4.

Martone WJ, Gaynes RP, Horan TC, et al. 1995. National Nosocomial Infections Surveillance (NNIS) semiannual report, May 1995. A report from the NNIS System. *Am J Infect Control* **23**(6):377–85.

McDevitt HO, Benacerraf B. 1969. Genetic control of specific immune responses. *Adv Immunol* **11**:31–74.

Melville A. 1984. Set and serendipity in the detection of drug hazards. *Soc Sci Med* **19**:391–6.

Meyer KB, Madias NE. 1994. Cisplatin nephrotoxicity. *Miner Electrolyte Metab* **20**:201–13.

Meyer RD. 1986. Risk factors and comparisons of nephrotoxicity of aminoglycosides. *Am J Med* **80**(Suppl. 6B):119–25.

Mitchell JR, Potter WZ, Hinson JA, et al. 1975. Toxic drug reactions. *Handb Exp Pharmacol* **28**:383–419.

Mongan E, Kelly P, Nies K, et al. 1973. Tinnitus as an indicator of therapeutic serum salicylate level. *JAMA* **226**:142–5.

Morris TW, Fischer HW. 1986. The pharmacology of intravascular radiocontrast media. *Annu Rev Pharmacol Toxicol* **26**:143–60.

Mullick FG. 1987. Acute and chronic hepatotoxicity: pathological aspects. In: Seeff LB, Lewis JH, editors. *Current Perspectives in Hepatology*. New York: Plenum Medical Books. p 253–68.

Mushlin PS, Olson RD. 1988. Anthracycline cardiotoxicity: new insights. *Ration Drug Ther* **12**:1–8.

Naranjo CA, Busto U, Sellers EM, et al. 1981. A method for estimating the probability of adverse drug reactions. *Clin Pharmacol Ther* **30**:239–45.

Nierenberg DW, Glazener FS. 1982. Aminophylline-induced exfoliative dermatitis: cause and implications. *West J Med* **137**:328–31.

Noskin GA, Patterson R. 1997. Outpatient management of Stevens-Johnson syndrome: a report of four cases and management strategy. *Allergy Asthma Proc* **18**:29–32.

O'Reilly RA. 1985. Anticoagulant, antithrombin, and thrombolytic drugs. In: Gilman AG, Goodman LS, Rall TW, et al., editors. *Goodman and Gilman's The Pharmacological Basis of Therapeutics*. New York: Macmillan. p 1138–59.

Palmer RF. 1969. Drug misuse and physician education. *Clin Pharmacol Ther* **10**:1–4.

Pancoast SJ. 1988. Aminoglycoside antibiotics in clinical use. *Med Clin North Am* **72**:581–612.

Pead PJ, Saeed AA, Hewitt WG, et al. 1985. Low immune responses to hepatitis B vaccine among healthy subjects. *Lancet* **1**:1152.

Piazza-Hepp TD, Kennedy DL. 1995. Reporting of adverse events to MedWatch. *Am J Health Syst Pharm* **52**:1436–9.

Pohl LR, Satoh H, Christ DD, et al. 1988. The immunologic and metabolic basis of drug hypersensitivities. *Annu Rev Pharmacol Toxicol* **28**:367–87.

Porter J, Jick H. 1977. Drug-induced anaphylaxis, convulsions, deafness, and extrapyramidal symptoms. *Lancet* **1**:587–8.

Pratt WB, Fekety R. 1986. *The Antimicrobial Drugs*. New York: Oxford University Press.

Prien RF, DeLong S, Cole JO, et al. 1970. Ocular changes occurring with prolonged high dose chlorpromazine therapy. *Arch Gen Psychiatry* **23**:464–8.

Rab SM. 1969. Optic atrophy during chlorpromazine therapy. *Br J Ophthalmol* **53**:208–209.

Reason J. 1990. *Human Error*. Cambridge: Cambridge University Press.

Reid JL, Rubin PC, Whiting B. 1989. *Lecture Notes on Clinical Pharmacology*. 3rd ed. London: Blackwell Scientific Publications.

Revuz JE, Roujeau JC. 1996. Advances in toxic epidermal necrolysis. *Semin Cutan Med Surg* **15**:258–66.

Ries F, Klastersky J. 1986. Nephrotoxicity induced by cancer chemotherapy with special emphasis on cisplatin toxicity. *J Kidney Dis* **8**:368–79.

Rosketh R, Storstein O. 1963. Quinidine therapy of chronic auricular fibrillation. *Arch Intern Med* **111**:184–9.

Rudnick MR, Berns JS, Cohen RM, et al. 1997. Contrast media-associated nephrotoxicity. *Semin Nephrol* **17**:15–26.

Rybak LP. 1986. Drug ototoxicity. *Annu Rev Pharmacol Toxicol* **26**: 79–99.

Rybak LP. 1993. Ototoxicity of loop diuretics. *Otolaryngol Clin North Am* **26**:829–44.

Rzany B, Hering O, Mockenhaupt M, et al. 1996. Histopathological and epidemiological characteristics of patients with erythema exudativum multiforme major, Stevens-Johnson syndrome and toxic epidermal necrolysis. *Br J Dermatol* **135**:6–11.

Scherbel AL, Mackenzie AH, Nousek JE, et al. 1963. Ocular lesions in rheumatoid arthritis and related disorders with particular reference to retinopathy. *N Engl J Med* **273**:360–6.

Seligmann H, Podoshin L, Ben-David J, et al. 1996. Drug-induced tinnitus and other hearing disorders. *Drug Saf* **14**:198–212.

Sheikh NM, Philen RM, Love LA. 1997. Chaparral-associated hepatotoxicity. *Ann Intern Med* **157**:913–9.

Shichi H, Nebert DW. 1982. Genetic differences in drug metabolism associated with ocular toxicity. *Environ Health Perspect* **44**: 107–17.

Shulman JI, Shulman S, Haines AP. 1981. The prevention of adverse drug reactions—a potential role for pharmacists in the primary care team? *J R Coll Gen Pract* **31**:429–34.

Silman A, Shipley M. 1997. Ophthalmological monitoring for hydroxychloroquine toxicity: a scientific review of available data. *Br J Rheumatol* **36**:599–601.

Simborg DW, Derewicz HJ. 1975. A highly automated hospital medication system. Five years' experience and evaluation. *Ann Intern Med* **83**:342–6.

Singer C, Smith C, Krieff D. 1996. Once-daily aminoglycoside therapy: potential ototoxicity. *Antimicrob Agents Chemother* **40**:2209–11.

Singer I, Rotenberg D, Preschett JB. 1972. Lithium-induced nephrogenic diabetes insipidus: in vivo and in vitro studies. *J Clin Invest* **51**:1081–91.

Sittig DF, Stead WW. 1994. Computer-based physician order entry: the state of the art. *J Am Med Inform Assoc* **1**:108–23.

Smidt NA, McQueen EG. 1972. Adverse reactions to drugs: a comprehensive hospital in-patient survey. *N Z Med J* **76**:397–401.

Smilkstein MJ, Knapp GL, Kulig KW, et al. 1988. Efficacy of oral *N*-acetyl cysteine in the treatment of acetaminophen overdosage: analysis of the national multicenter study (1976–1985). *N Engl J Med* **319**:1157–62.

Smith PL, Kagey-Sobotka A, Bleecker ER, et al. 1980. Physiologic manifestations of human anaphylaxis. *J Clin Invest* **66**:1072–80.

Soumerai SB, Avorn J. 1984. Efficacy and cost-containment in hospital pharmacotherapy: state of the art and future directions. *Milbank Mem Fund Q* **62**:447–74.

Spaeth GL. 1996. Incidence of acute angle-closure glaucoma after pharmacologic mydriasis. *Am J Ophthalmol* **122**:283–4.

Spiteri MA, James DG. 1983. Adverse ocular reaction to drugs. *Postgrad Med* **59**:343–9.

Spitzer WO, Suissa S, Ernst P, et al. 1992. The use of $\beta$-agonists and the risk of death and near death from asthma. *N Engl J Med* **326**:501–6.

Stewart JB. 1997. Annals of crime: professional courtesy. *New Yorker* **24**(Nov):90–105.

Stolley PD, Lasagna L. 1969. Prescribing patterns of physicians. *J Chronic Dis* **22**:395–405.

Swanson DP, Thrall JH, Shetty PC. 1986. Evaluation of intravascular low-osmolality contrast agents. *Clin Pharmacol* **5**:877–91.

Swerlick RA, Lawley TJ. 1989. Cutaneous vasculitis: its relationship to systemic disease. *Med Clin North Am* **73**:1221–35.

Thorstrand C. 1976. Clinical features in poisonings by tricyclic antidepressants, with special reference to the ECG. *Acta Med Scand* **199**:337–44.

Toone EC. 1965. Ototoxicity of chloroquine. *Arthritis Rheum* **8**:475–6.

Tseng LH. 1971. Interstitial myocarditis probably related to lithium carbonate intoxication. *Arch Pathol* **92**:444–8.

Ukena T, Esber H, Bessette R, et al. 1985. Site of injection and response to hepatitis B vaccine. *N Engl J Med* **313**:579–80.

van der Klauw MM, Wilson JH, Stricker BH. 1998. Drug-associated agranulocytosis: 20 years of reporting in The Netherlands (1974–1994). *Am J Hematol* **57**:206–11.

Vasquez EM, Maddux MS, Sanchez J, et al. 1993. Clinically significant hearing loss in renal allograft recipients treated with intravenous erythromycin. *Arch Intern Med* **153**:879–82.

Venulet J. 1975. Increasing threat to man as a result of frequently uncontrolled and widespread use of various drugs. *Int J Clin Pharmacol* **12**:389–94.

Verdier DD, Kennerdall JS. 1982. Fixed, dilated pupil resulting from transdermal scopolamine. *Am J Ophthalmol* **93**:803–4.

Verstraete M, Boogaerts MA. 1987. Drug-induced hematological disorders. In: Speight T, editor. *Avery's Drug Treatment*. 3rd ed. Hong Kong: Adis Press. p 1007–22.

Vogt CL, Byrns PJ. 1994. Adverse drug reactions: getting information back from MedWatch. *JAMA* **272**:590–1.

Weiner M, Bernstein IL. 1989. *Adverse Reactions to Drug Formulation Agents*. New York: Marcel Dekker.

Whelton A, Hamilton CW. 1991. Nonsteroidal anti-inflammatory drugs: effects on kidney function. *J Clin Pharmacol* **31**:588–98.

White PD (citing Withering). 1965. Important toxic effect of digitalis overdosage on vision. *N Engl J Med* **272**:904–5.

Wiemann MC, Calabresi P. 1985. Pharmacology of neoplastic agents. In: Calabresi P, Schein PS, Rosenberg SA, editors. *Medical Oncology*. New York: Macmillan. p 293–362.

Williams DM, Lynch RE, Cartwright GE. 1973. Drug-induced aplastic anemia. *Semin Hematol* **10**:195–223.

Wilson K. 1984. Sex-related differences in drug disposition in man. *Clin Pharmacokinet* **9**:189–202.

Winkelstein A, Kiss JE. 1997. Immunohematologic disorders. *JAMA* **278**:1982–92.

Wittbrodt ET, Spinler SA. 1994. Prevention of anaphylactoid reactions in high-risk patients receiving radiographic contrast media. *Ann Pharmacother* **28**:236–41.

Wysowski DK, Green L. 1995. Serious adverse events in Norplant users reported to the food and drug administration's MedWatch spontaneous reporting system. *Obstet Gynecol* **85**:538–42.

Yunis AA. 1988. Chloramphenicol: relation of structure to activity and toxicity. *Annu Rev Pharmacol Toxicol* **28**:83–100.

CHAPTER

# 25 DRUG INTERACTIONS

James M. Wright

*Chapter Outline*



## DEFINITION

A drug interaction is defined as a measurable modification (in magnitude or duration) of the action of one drug by prior or concomitant administration of another substance (including prescription and nonprescription drugs, food, or alcohol). Interactions can occur by pharmacokinetic or pharmacodynamic mechanisms. The effect of the interaction can be desirable, inconsequential, or adverse. The majority of drug interactions are inconsequential, or desirable. It is when the interaction leads to adverse consequences that it comes to the attention of the patient and physician. Because of this, the term "drug interaction" is frequently used incorrectly to refer to an adverse drug interaction. This chapter focuses on clinically important adverse drug interactions. Clinically desirable drug interactions have been reviewed elsewhere (Caranasos et al. 1985) and are part of any good therapeutic regimen when two or more drugs with different mechanisms of action are used together to enhance the desired effect (e.g., to lower elevated blood pressure).

When describing adverse drug interactions, the term index drug is used for the drug which has its effect enhanced or canceled by the interacting drug. In some cases, there may be no simple distinction between the index and the interacting drug. Occasionally, two drugs interact with each other to cause different adverse effects. In such cases both drugs are index and both are interacting; a double adverse drug interaction is the result (Wright et al. 1982).

## CLINICAL IMPACT OF ADVERSE DRUG INTERACTIONS

The best estimate of the prevalence of adverse drug interactions comes from the Boston Collaborative Drug Surveillance Program; drug interactions were determined to account for 7% of in-hospital adverse drug reactions (Boston Collaborative Drug Surveillance Program 1972). If approximately 30% of patients experience an adverse drug reaction while in the hospital (Jick 1974), then in approximately 2% of inpatients the adverse drug reaction could be attributed to an adverse drug interaction. However, most of these reactions are transient and of minor discomfort to the patient. Serious life-threatening adverse drug reactions occur in 3% of hospital patients (Jick 1974), and if drug interactions cause 7% of these, then the risk of a serious adverse drug interaction would be only about 0.2%. The risk in outpatients is less, primarily because most outpatients are exposed to fewer drugs. In one study (Puckett and Visconti 1971) of 2422 outpatients followed for 2 months, 113 (4.7%) were taking combinations of drugs with a potential for adverse interactions; however, adverse drug interactions were detected in only 7 (0.3%), thus confirming the relatively low risk in this setting.

Any drug combination has the potential for leading to an adverse interaction. An estimate of the frequency of this potential can be seen with the oral anticoagulant warfarin, a drug for which we have a precise measure of effect, the international normalized ratio of prothrombin time (INR). Warfarin has the longest list of potential interacting drugs. In a study of 277 patients attending an anticoagulation clinic, 94 out of 413 treatment courses (23%) had the potential to interact with warfarin. This is likely an underestimate of the potential for interaction, as the prescribing clinicians probably deliberately avoided drugs well known to interact.

How can we explain the observations that potential adverse interactions occur frequently, and yet clinically detectable adverse drug interactions occur quite infrequently? The explanation is twofold. First, many interactions lead to small effects on the index drug and for most index drugs these are clinically unimportant. An example is the interaction between acetaminophen and isoniazid (Epstein et al. 1991). Isoniazid administered at a dosage of 300 mg/day for 7 days inhibits the microsomal oxidation of acetaminophen by 70%. However, because oxidative metabolism represents only a minor component of the overall elimination of acetaminophen, this resulted in only a 15% decrease in the total body clearance of acetaminophen, equivalent to increasing the dose of acetaminophen by 18%, a clinically undetectable effect. Second, many drugs have a very wide therapeutic index. With such index drugs (e.g., penicillin), even an interaction leading to a two- to threefold change in drug concentration is unlikely to lead to an adverse effect in most situations.

**PRINCIPLE In most situations in which more than one drug is prescribed, the risk of a clinically important adverse drug interaction is small. However, there are identifiable clinical settings, described later in the chapter, when clinically important adverse drug interactions are more likely to occur. In order to increase the likelihood of identifying or preventing an adverse drug interaction, the clinician must recognize these clinical settings and understand the mechanisms by which they occur.**

## MECHANISMS OF ADVERSE DRUG INTERACTIONS

Mechanisms of drug interactions can be divided into those involving the pharmacokinetics of the index drug and those involving the pharmacodynamics of the index drug.

### Pharmacokinetic Mechanisms

#### *Chemical interactions*

Drugs can react physically or chemically with each other before they are administered to the patient or, in the case of oral preparations, before they are absorbed. Drug companies are usually very careful to ensure that this type of interaction does not occur in tablets or oral suspensions. When drugs are mixed before parenteral administration, they may interact and significantly decrease the activity of one or both components. As a general rule, drugs should not be mixed before parenteral administration unless they have been demonstrated by rigorous testing to be chemically compatible. Chemical interactions are very unlikely to occur once drugs reach the systemic circulation because the concentrations in plasma are low. However, such is not the case for orally administered drugs before absorption. The best known example of this is the interaction between oral tetracyclines and cations; tetracycline chelates calcium, magnesium, aluminum, or iron resulting in a cation–tetracycline complex that cannot be absorbed. Cholestyramine and colestipol also can bind a number of anionic drugs and decrease their absorption.

**PRINCIPLE The demonstration that two oral medications interact chemically does not mean that the two medications cannot be prescribed to a patient. Ingesting the two drugs several hours apart can usually minimize this type of interaction.**

#### *Interactions affecting oral bioavailability*

**INTERACTIONS AFFECTING GASTRIC EMPTYING** Altering the rate of gastric emptying generally alters the rate of drug absorption, but not the extent of drug bioavailability. The rate of gastric emptying is important when a rapid onset of effect of the drug is desired. Such is the case when rapid relief from pain or onset of sedation is required and parenteral administration is not possible. The best way to enhance the rate of gastric emptying is for the patient to take the drug on an empty stomach with at least 200 mL of water and to remain in an upright position. Factors that slow gastric emptying include food, recumbency, heavy exercise, autonomic neuropathy, and a number of drugs, including antacids, anticholinergic drugs, and narcotics. Drugs that enhance gastric emptying, such as metoclopramide, cisapride, and domperidone, may result in earlier and higher peak concentrations of index drugs.

When the rate of onset of effect of the index drug is not important, effects on gastric emptying are not clinically significant. The exceptions to this rule are drugs that are inactivated in the acid milieu of the stomach. In such cases (e.g., penicillin G, levodopa), factors that delay gastric emptying can decrease oral bioavailability. In contrast, an increased rate of GI transit may decrease absorption of drugs with low dissolution rates or drugs that are very poorly absorbed (e.g., enteric-coated tablets, griseofulvin). It is not uncommon for patients with rapid GI transit times (e.g., short-bowel syndrome) to report the presence of intact enteric-coated tablets in the stool. Embarrassment should result if such a history were the first hint to the therapist that a regimen was not working.

**INTERACTIONS AFFECTING DRUG ABSORPTION** Most drugs are absorbed in the small intestine by a process of passive diffusion. The presence of other drugs is unlikely to interfere with this process; however, some drugs (e.g., oral neomycin, antineoplastic drugs) can damage the intestinal absorptive surface and potentially result in decreased absorption of other drugs (particularly those in which drug absorption is incomplete).

**INTERACTIONS AFFECTING PRESYSTEMIC ELIMINATION** Drugs have the potential to be absorbed, metabolized, or extracted during transit across the intestinal epithelium into the portal circulation and during the first pass through the liver. This phenomenon (see Chapter 23) has been called presystemic elimination, or the first-pass effect. A large number of commonly prescribed drugs (e.g., propranolol, metoprolol, labetalol, verapamil, hydralazine, felodipine, chlorpromazine, amitriptyline, imipramine, and morphine) are subject to significant presystemic elimination and consequently have low oral bioavailability. These drugs have a high intrinsic hepatic clearance that varies inversely with liver blood flow. The drugs listed previously can also compete with each other and increase each other's bioavailability, for example, chlorpromazine and propranolol (Peet et al. 1981). Interactions involving this mechanism are likely to be of large magnitude and therefore are more likely to be clinically significant.

The clinically significant ability of components of grapefruit juice to increase the bioavailability of drugs that are substrates of the cytochrome P450 (CYP) isozyme CYP3A (e.g., felodipine, cyclosporine) is at least partly due to inhibition of intestinal wall CYP3A4 by compounds in grapefruit juice (Ameer and Weintraub 1997). Nonspecific food–drug interactions that lead to increased drug bioavailability are also most likely to occur by this mechanism (Liedholm and Melander 1986).

The food–drug interactions with irreversible monoamine oxidase inhibitors (MAOIs) are the result of inhibition of presystemic elimination of tyramine present in various foods. The nonselective MAOIs, such as phenelzine and tranylcypromine, inhibit MAO A in the intestinal wall and liver. This leads to increased oral bioavailability of dietary tyramine, which is not completely metabolized during absorption and the first pass through the liver. When tyramine reaches the systemic circulation, it can produce increased release of norepinephrine from sympathetic postganglionic neurons. The selective MAO B inhibitor selegiline (deprenyl), and the reversible MAOI moclobemide, are less likely to cause this interaction.

Other than the examples just described, most food–drug interactions are of small magnitude and few have been proven to cause clinically important adverse events (Carr 1982). Therefore, the inconvenience to the patient of attempting to take a drug on an empty stomach is often not justified.

### *Protein-binding interactions*

Once a drug reaches the systemic circulation after parenteral or oral administration, it is distributed throughout the body. This distribution is dependent upon the ionic composition, lipid solubility, and protein-binding characteristics of the drug (see the Introduction and Chapter 23). Protein binding occurs primarily in the plasma to albumin or $\alpha$-acid glycoprotein, or outside the bloodstream to tissue proteins. In general, only free drug can exert a pharmacologic effect. Concentration of measured drug in clinical labs usually reflects the total drug concentration in the plasma (free plus bound). Drugs that are highly bound in plasma are potentially subject to displacement from their carrier proteins by another drug with affinity for the same protein. When another highly bound drug is added, competitive displacement may occur, resulting in a transient increase in the free concentration of the index drug. This is followed by rapid redistribution of the index drug and a transient increase in the rate of drug elimination, creating a new equilibrium for both drugs. This displacement is only likely to cause a clinically significant effect if the index drug has a small volume of distribution, a narrow therapeutic index, and a rapid onset of action.

Assessment of the role of displacement in drug interactions has been hampered by the difficulties in measuring free-drug concentrations. Early studies of drug–drug interactions by displacement from plasma proteins tended to exaggerate the importance of the potential interaction because they were conducted in vitro, with no opportunity for tissue redistribution or for increased rate of elimination to occur. Many of the drug interactions formerly classified as displacement interactions were primarily the result of the interacting drug decreasing the clearance of the index drug (MacKichan 1989).

**PRINCIPLE Knowing one potential mechanism of interaction between two drugs is not the same as knowing all the mechanisms and the degree to which each operates to produce the clinical effect.**

### *Interactions due to altered biotransformation*

Drug biotransformation shows great between-patient variation and can be dramatically affected by other drugs. Therefore, interactions involving biotransformation are the most likely to have a significant adverse impact. Drug metabolism most often occurs in the liver and involves the conversion of an active, nonpolar drug to more polar metabolites (generally less active or inactive) that are cleared by the kidneys. Occasionally, metabolites are pharmacologically active in ways that are similar or dissimilar (including toxic) to that of the progenitor. Drugs that are extensively metabolized (i.e., only a small proportion of the dose administered is excreted unchanged in the urine) are particularly susceptible to interactions affecting drug metabolism. Most drugs are metabolized by several different pathways, making prediction of the consequences of metabolic interactions difficult.

**INTERACTIONS INVOLVING ENZYME INHIBITION** Many commonly prescribed drugs have the potential to inhibit the metabolism of other drugs (Table 25-1). Whether this effect leads to a clinically significant interaction is dependent upon the magnitude of the decrease in clearance and the consequences of the resulting increase in steady-state serum concentration of the index drug. Most clinically significant interactions of this type involve the hepatic microsomal oxidative enzymes that can be divided into separate cytochrome P450 (CYP) isozymes. The isozyme families that are most commonly involved in human liver metabolism are 1A, 2B, 2C, 2D, 2E, and 3A (Li and Jurima-Romet 1997).

Information regarding the predominant isozymes involved in metabolism of a drug and whether a microsomal enzyme inhibitor specifically inhibits a particular isozyme is becoming increasingly useful in understanding and predicting this type of drug interaction. This is best exemplified by the new antidepressants, the selective serotonin uptake inhibitors (SSRIs), many of which are microsomal enzyme inhibitors (Richelson 1997). However, the magnitude of the effect in an individual is variable because it depends on the specific enzyme or enzymes inhibited and the quantitative importance of that pathway in the overall clearance of the index drug.

Table 25-1 **Agents That Alter Microsomal Enzyme Activity**

| Inhibitors of Enzyme Activity[a] | |
|---|---|
| Amiodarone | Ketoconazole (3A4) |
| Cimetidine | Metronidazole |
| Ciprofloxacin (1A2) | Miconazole (3A4) |
| Diltiazem | Nefazodone (3A4) |
| Erythromycin (3A4) | Oral contraceptives |
| Ethanol (Acute) | Paroxetine (2D6) |
| Fluconazole (3A4) | Phenylbutazone |
| Fluoxetine (2C9, 2C19, 2D6) | Quinidine (2D6) |
| Fluvoxamine (1A2, 2C19, 3A4) | Sulfinpyrazone |
| Grapefruit (3A4) | Valproate |
| Isoniazid (2E1) | Verapamil |
| Itraconazole (3A4) | |
| **Inducers of Enzyme Activity[a]** | |
| Barbiturates (phenobarbital) (2B) | Isoniazid (2E1) |
| Carbamazepine | Primidone (2B) |
| Charcoal-broiled food (1A2) | Rifabutin (3A4) |
| Dexamethasone | Rifampin (3A4) |
| Ethanol (chronic) (2E1) | Tobacco smoke (1A2) |
| Griseofulvin | |

[a]Term in parentheses in the primary cytochrome P450 (CYP) isozyme family involved.

For example, isoniazid is a potent inhibitor of the microsomal oxidation of both carbamazepine and acetaminophen. With acetaminophen, conjugative metabolic pathways (type II) predominate, and this results in a clinically insignificant 15% decrease in total plasma clearance of acetaminophen (Epstein et al. 1991). In the case of carbamazepine, oxidative metabolic pathways (type I) predominate, and isoniazid inhibits total plasma clearance by 45%, resulting in an increase in steady-state serum concentration of 85% and a significant risk of toxic effects (Wright et al. 1982).

Enzyme inhibition can be produced by a number of different mechanisms, from competition to irreversible inactivation. The latter mechanism leads to the longest lasting effects. The time course of the change in serum concentration of an index drug affected by an inhibitory interacting drug is dependent on the new half-life of the index drug, requiring four to five half-lives to reach a new steady state.

One of the factors leading to the unpredictability of these interactions is that many microsomal inhibitors also have the capacity to induce microsomal enzymes; therefore, depending on the dose, timing, or patient setting, inhibition or induction can be seen (e.g., ethanol and isoniazid) (Fraser 1997; Zand et al. 1993).

**PRINCIPLE Inhibitory interactions seldom contraindicate the concomitant use of two drugs. When two drugs are used, dosage adjustments may be needed to obtain appropriate effects of the index drug. If the possibility of adversity is a concern when drugs are being used together, adjusting dose may be more appropriate than discontinuing needed therapy. Do not deny the possibility that you could be among the first to identify an unsuspected drug interaction.**

INTERACTIONS INVOLVING ENZYME INDUCTION The microsomal enzyme systems in the liver and other tissues are notable in that their activity can be induced severalfold by many drugs and chemicals. Enzyme induction occurs by a number of different mechanisms, but generally leads to increased amounts of the enzyme and consequently, an increase in the highest rate ($V_{max}$) of the biotransformation reaction (Okey 1990). The time course of induction is also usually longer than inhibition and may take 2–3 weeks to become maximal in humans. Agents that induce metabolizing enzymes can be classified according to the specific P450 isozymes that are induced (Table 25-1).

Enzyme induction can enhance the metabolism of the inducing agent (autoinduction) and/or a variety of other drugs and some endogenous compounds, such as cortisol, thyroxine (Sarich and Wright 1996), and bilirubin. Induction may be associated with marked increases in clearance of index drugs, resulting in loss of efficacy. For example, rifampin has been implicated as a cause of graft rejection in patients receiving otherwise adequate doses of cyclosporine and prednisone (Langhoff and Madsen 1983), and as a cause of failure of effect of oral contraceptives (Li and Jurima-Romet 1997). Furthermore, in patients who are following a methadone maintenance program, the introduction of phenytoin has precipitated withdrawal symptoms (Tong et al. 1981). If the induction interaction is recognized, the dose of the index drug can be increased appropriately. If the inducing drug is later stopped, the dose of the index drug may have to be decreased to prevent toxicity.

In some cases, induction of metabolism can result in increased formation of a toxic metabolite with serious consequences. For example, administration of isoniazid may increase the risk of acetaminophen-induced hepatotoxicity by increasing the formation of the toxic metabolite of acetaminophen (Zand et al. 1993).

***Interactions due to altered renal excretion***

Water-soluble drugs are eliminated largely unchanged by the kidneys. The clearance of drugs that are excreted entirely by glomerular filtration is unlikely to be affected by other drugs. However, the clearance of drugs that are actively secreted into the tubular lumen can be significantly inhibited by other drugs. This type of interaction can be used to advantage (e.g., probenecid decreases the clearance of penicillin thus prolonging its duration of action), but occasionally may lead to toxicity (e.g., methotrexate toxicity can be caused by inhibition of its tubular secretion by salicylate) (Zuik and Mandel 1975).

**PRINCIPLE There is hardly a class of adverse drug interactions that cannot be used to therapeutic advantage.**

Lithium carbonate is a special case because it is an ion that is excreted primarily by the kidney. As a univalent cation, it is affected by changes that alter total body balance of sodium. Renal clearance of lithium is significantly decreased by thiazide and loop diuretics (Mehta and Robinson 1980); the sodium loss caused by the diuretic leads to increased proximal reabsorption of sodium and lithium. Some NSAIDs also decrease renal elimination of lithium. Because of its narrow toxic/therapeutic ratio, lithium is one of the drugs with a high-risk of adverse drug interactions (Table 25-2).

## Pharmacodynamic Mechanisms

***Receptor interactions***

A few adverse drug interactions are understandable and predictable based on the well-known pharmacologic effects of the two drugs involved. For example, $\beta$-adren-

Table 25-2 **Examples of Drugs That Have a Narrow Therapeutic Index**[a]

| |
|---|
| Oral anticoagulants (warfarin) |
| Anti-cancer drugs (5-fluorouracil) |
| Immunosuppressive drugs (cyclosporine) |
| Antidysrhythmic drugs (quinidine) |
| Digitalis glycosides (digoxin) |
| Anticonvulsants (phenytoin) |
| Oral hypoglycemic drugs (glyburide) |
| Aminoglycosides (gentamicin and vancomycin) |
| Antiretrovirals (zidovudine) |
| Antifungals (amphotericin B) |
| Lithium carbonate |
| Theophylline |

[a]Name in parentheses is a representative drug in each class.

ergic blocking drugs antagonize the effects of $\beta_2$-adrenergic agonists such as salbutamol and can significantly interfere with the clinical management of patients with asthma. Similarly, the antiparkinsonian action of levodopa can be antagonized by the dopamine-blocking drugs haloperidol and metoclopramide. An understanding of the mechanism of action of each drug allows the clinician to predict and avoid such adverse interactions.

Drugs also can inhibit transport processes and thus affect the action of other drugs. The tricyclic antidepressants, through their blocking the neuronal reuptake of amines, can potentiate the action of epinephrine and norepinephrine. For this reason, it is recommended that local anesthetics without epinephrine be used for patients taking tricyclic antidepressants. The tricyclic antidepressants also antagonize the antihypertensive action of guanethidine; the suggested mechanism is that the tricyclic compounds block the neuronal uptake of guanethidine. It must be remembered that many drugs (antihistamines, antinauseants, phenothiazines, and tricyclic antidepressants) share with atropine the ability to block muscarinic receptors. These drugs have mild anticholinergic effects and are generally safe when taken alone. In combination, they can produce a full-blown anticholinergic syndrome causing confusion and memory loss; the elderly are particularly at risk.

Some drugs (aminoglycosides, polymyxins, local anesthetics) have weak inhibiting effects on neuromuscular transmission. These drugs have no discernible effect in the patient with normal neuromuscular transmission, in whom a wide safety margin is present. However, in patients who have lost this safety margin (e.g., postsurgical patients who have received neuromuscular blocking drugs, or patients with myasthenia gravis), these drugs may produce neuromuscular paralysis and apnea.

#### *Additive and antagonistic interactions*

Most of these interactions are intuitively evident. It should not be surprising that two drugs with sedative properties (e.g., benzodiazepines and alcohol) can potentiate each other's sedative action. This is equally true whether the sedative property of the drug is the primary action (e.g., diazepam) or whether it is a potential side effect (e.g., methyldopa, diphenhydramine, amitriptyline, and chlorpromazine). It is important that physicians and patients be constantly aware of the dangers of driving a motor vehicle while under the influence of drugs and/or alcohol. The additive effect of drugs affecting coagulation at two different steps (e.g., warfarin and aspirin) also has been associated with severe bleeding.

Equally preventable interactions are those that occur when two drugs given together share similar adverse effects. For example, hydrocortisone and hydrochlorothiazide together can produce additive side effects of hyperglycemia or hypokalemia. Another example is observed in patients who receive supplemental potassium, potassium-sparing diuretics, and angiotensin-converting enzyme inhibitors. Each drug may occasionally cause hyperkalemia, but when they are used together, the risk of causing clinically important hyperkalemia is greatly increased.

The risk of some toxic effects can be potentiated through a pharmacodynamic mechanism. For example, diuretic-induced hypokalemia and hypomagnesemia may act to increase the risk of dysrhythmias caused by digoxin. Likewise, the risk of ototoxicity and nephrotoxicity is increased with the combination of aminoglycosides and furosemide. Antagonistic pharmacodynamic interactions are more likely to go unrecognized, as it is easy to miss the fact that a chronically administered drug has lost efficacy. The NSAIDs have potent actions on the kidney that can antagonize the effects of other drugs. Salt and water retention caused by the NSAIDs can lead to worsening symptoms of congestive heart failure or increase in blood pressure. The adverse effect of NSAIDs on blood pressure is particularly likely to go unrecognized (Johnson et al. 1994).

**PRINCIPLE Unless the physician is particularly aware that a drug interaction could nullify efficacy, he or she may attribute worsening of the disease to the disease process rather than the drug therapy. Furthermore, many adverse drug interactions can mimic aspects of disease that were the indications for using the drugs in the first place.**

#### *Interactions involving unknown and multiple mechanisms*

Many drug–drug interactions involve more than one mechanism. The complexity of the problem is exemplified by the interaction of quinidine and digoxin. The administration of quinidine to patients receiving digoxin results in a two- to threefold increase in steady-state concentration of digoxin. At least three different sites of interaction have been described; recent evidence suggests that they all may be explained by inhibition of the P-glycoprotein efflux transporter by quinidine (Su and Huang 1996). The same mechanism may explain how digoxin and quinidine interact with other drugs.

**PRINCIPLE When a fundamental mechanism of a drug interaction has been demonstrated with a given agent, look for that agent to interact with other drugs by a similar mechanism, even if the interaction has not yet been described.**

The combination of verapamil and propranolol is another example of a complex interaction. This drug combination has led to congestive heart failure, severe bradycardia, arteriovenous block, and ventricular asystole. In a recent study of this interaction in eight healthy young men during exercise, the combination of the two drugs produced clinically important fatigue that was not seen with the individual drugs (Carruthers et al. 1989). The combination significantly reduced heart rate and prolonged the exercise PR interval. These effects could be only partially explained by the two pharmacokinetic interactions that were demonstrated. The study raised doubt about the safety of this combination and again emphasized the multiple mechanisms and complexity of many interactions.

## UNRECOGNIZED DRUG INTERACTIONS

The potential implications of failing to recognize an adverse drug interaction is exemplified by the 16 deaths in Japanese cancer patients being treated for herpes zoster infection with the new antiviral drug sorivudine. These patients were taking 5-fluorouracil or other fluoropyrimidine antineoplastic drugs. It has subsequently been determined that sorivudine is a potent suicide inhibitor of dihydropyrimidine dehydrogenase, the enzyme responsible for the inactivation of fluoropyrimidines (Li and Jurima-Romet 1997). A positive development from this and similar prior serious events is that for many new drugs, potential drug interactions are being predicted and tested during development (Li and Jurima-Romet 1997).

Severe dysrhythmias in a small number of young healthy individuals taking erythromycin (or ketoconazole) with terfenadine (a nonsedating antihistamine) is another case in point. The mechanism of this interaction is the inhibition of metabolism of terfenadine (CYP3A4) by erythromycin or ketoconazole, causing increased steady-state concentrations of terfenadine, a drug that can prolong conduction in the heart and cause the potentially lethal dysrhythmia torsades de pointes (Li and Jurima-Romet 1997). Recognition of this interaction led to regulatory changes for terfenadine and astemizole in several countries. Several other drugs have a similar ability to prolong the QT interval and predispose to this form of ventricular tachycardia. These include quinidine, procainamide, flecainide, disopyramide, sotalol, tricyclic antidepressants, phenothiazines, cisapride, astemizole, and others.

**PRINCIPLE It is important for clinicians to consider the possibility of an unrecognized adverse drug interaction in patients dying unexpectedly and suddenly.**

Another clinical setting in which an adverse drug interaction is likely to go unrecognized occurs when the interacting drug diminishes the effectiveness of the index drug. In patients taking multiple medications, the clinician has a difficult task in establishing the continued efficacy and necessity of each agent. One drug can readily cancel the effectiveness of another. Often the only way of establishing the ongoing effectiveness of a drug as part of a multiple drug regimen is to stop the drug in question and to reassess the patient carefully over time.

## HIGH-RISK CLINICAL SETTINGS

Physicians cannot know or remember all documented or potential drug interactions. Since the risk is small in most clinical settings, the astute clinician can decrease the risk to the patient by being aware of the clinical settings in which the risk of adverse drug interactions is increased. Some of the more common situations that place patients at higher risk are described in the following sections.

### Index Drugs with a Narrow Therapeutic Index

Care must be taken when adding or deleting a drug in patients taking an index drug that has a low toxic/therapeutic ratio (narrow therapeutic index) (Table 25-2). The classic example of such drugs is warfarin. The anticoagulant effect of warfarin is dependent upon a competitive equilibrium between warfarin and vitamin $K_1$ in the liver. Any perturbation in the pharmacokinetics of warfarin or vitamin K, or in the turnover of the vitamin K-dependent clotting factors, causes a change in the INR and necessitates a change in warfarin dose. The chance of an interaction is great enough with these drugs that most clinicians warn the patient not to start or stop any other drug (including over-the-counter [OTC] drugs and health food supplements), except when this can be done with appropriate monitoring of the INR. The other index drugs listed in Table 25-2 are also at higher risk of causing adverse drug interactions than other drugs. These drugs have a defined narrow therapeutic index, and the concentration or effect of the drug must be monitored.

### Patients Taking Large Numbers of Drugs

As the number of drugs increases, the risk of an adverse drug reaction increases disproportionately. This disproportionate increase is most likely a result of adverse drug interaction(s). Remember that OTC drugs (e.g., aspirin, acetaminophen), topical drugs (e.g., timolol eye drops), and even herbal teas can contribute to this increased risk.

### Critically Ill Patients

These patients have lost their physiologic reserve in one or more systems and often require multiple drugs. Examples include patients with renal, hepatic, respiratory, cardiac, or autonomic failure; Alzheimer's dementia; and myasthenia gravis. In these patients, a drug that usually has a wide therapeutic index when given to a relatively healthy individual may have a surprisingly narrow therapeutic index. For example, opioids may be given safely to healthy patients with a toothache, but not to patients with borderline respiratory failure. In such patients, a relatively small change in drug effect as a result of a drug interaction could have a significant clinical impact. Deterioration in such patients should increase one's vigilance to be certain that it is not due to the drug therapy.

### Patients with HIV Infection

Patients who are infected with HIV are considered separately as they are at risk of organ failure from a multitude of infections and have been documented to have a higher incidence than the general population of skin reactions with sulfa drugs. They also receive large numbers of new and toxic combinations of drugs, for which there is often a paucity of information about drug interactions. A recent review collated the multiple potential drug interactions that are relatively specific for this group of patients (Tseng and Foisy 1997).

### The Passive Patient

Most outpatients have a low risk of adverse drug interactions because they take few drugs and take an active role in therapy decisions. Active patients demand that the benefit/risk ratio of any medication be substantially in their favor. Passive patients often do not know the reason for taking many of their medications. Psychiatric patients and the elderly constitute a large proportion of such passive patients. The elderly also are prone to adverse drug interactions because of a deterioration in homeostatic mechanisms leading to a lower margin of safety of many drugs (Nolan and O'Malley 1988).

**PRINCIPLE Clinicians have a responsibility to be particularly thoughtful when treating passive patients, and to try to minimize the dose and number of medications.**

### Drug Abusers

People who abuse drugs are likely to consume tobacco, alcohol, and illegal recreational, prescription, and OTC drugs, often in large doses. They also are frequently erratic in their drug-taking behavior. Because of these factors, drug interactions are more likely to result in adverse events.

**PRINCIPLE In the high-risk clinical settings listed, recognition of a clinically important adverse drug interaction is difficult. However, these are the settings where both previously documented and previously undocumented adverse drug interactions are most likely to be detected.**

**Key Points: Patients at especially high risk for adverse drug interactions include the following.**

- **Patients receiving an index drug with a narrow therapeutic index**
- **Patients taking a large number of drugs (including OTC drugs)**
- **Critically ill patients**
- **Patients infected with HIV**
- **Passive patients**
- **Drug or other substance abusers**

## COMPUTERIZED DRUG INTERACTION WARNING SYSTEMS

Computerized systems for identifying potential drug interactions have been available for many years. Pharmacy-based computer systems are more widely used than physician-based systems; however, neither has proven to be indispensable. The problems with computer systems reflect the problems of drug-interaction detection in general (Davidson et al. 1987). These include 1) a complex, uncertain database, often dependent on single case reports; 2) potential drug interactions that greatly outnumber clinically important adverse interactions; 3) a need for each flagged drug interaction to be interpreted in the clinical setting of the individual patient; and 4) characteristics of various computer systems that enhance or detract from their acceptability. If these problems can be overcome and more efficient interactive systems can be developed, computerized drug-interaction systems specifically for use in high-risk clinical settings could be quite cost-effective.

Indeed, some progress is being made in each of these areas. For example, some drug interaction software tools can now be installed on a central server within a medical center and can be instantly available on every computer terminal in the medical center. Each medical student, resident, attending physician, nurse, or pharmacist can enter a list of patients' medications and learn quickly whether any drug–drug interactions, minor or major, are likely to occur. For a patient receiving 10 medications, the computer can search quickly for up to 44 potential drug–drug interactions. Not only are the potential interactions described, but also ways to avoid them; primary references may also be listed.

A variety of relatively new software products seem to be addressing the four problems noted above more effectively. One such product, Clinical Pharmacology (Gold Standard Multimedia, Tampa, FL), and several others, can be installed in a CD-ROM version, on a Macintosh or IBM personal computer, or on a center-wide Intranet server. It is too early to determine whether such simple access to improved software products will result in fewer adverse drug interactions.

## PRINCIPLES OF PREVENTION OF ADVERSE DRUG INTERACTIONS

1. Document all drugs, including herbal preparations and OTC and recreational drugs, that your patient is consuming. Carefully review this list before prescribing a new medication or deleting a current medication. Maintain this list and keep it current.
2. Understand the pharmacodynamics and pharmacokinetics of the drugs you prescribe as much as possible, while keeping in mind the important mechanisms of drug interactions.
3. Minimize the number of drugs given to any patient and try to ensure that the benefits significantly outweigh the risks for each. This principle of therapy is difficult, but can be approximated by an up-to-date knowledge of the evidence and careful assessment of clinical endpoints.
4. Be particularly vigilant with patients taking narrow therapeutic index drugs.
5. Be cautious in high-risk clinical settings. Intensive care specialists must be particularly cognizant of the risk of adverse drug interactions.
6. Look carefully for the possibility of an adverse drug interaction whenever a patient's course deteriorates. If the deterioration is due to drug therapy, it probably is reversible.
7. Use textbooks of drug interactions or modern adverse-drug-interaction software programs to search for possible drug-induced effects you may not have considered.
8. Always be vigilant for previously undescribed interactions, particularly when prescribing new drugs or those with which you are not familiar. The particular combination of drugs that you prescribe may represent a novel experiment.

SUMMARY

**The potential for measurable interactions to occur when two or more drugs are prescribed to a patient is considerable. The mechanisms of these interactions can be complex, multiple, and incompletely understood. Fortunately, because of the wide margin of safety of most drugs in most clinical settings, the risk of serious adverse drug interactions is low. However, the physician must remain vigilant to detect or avoid those interactions that may have a deleterious effect on therapy. For the patient who suffers a serious, or even fatal, preventable adverse drug interaction, the knowledge that such serious adverse interactions are unlikely will provide little comfort.**

## REFERENCES

Ameer B, Weintraub RA. 1997. Drug interactions with grapefruit juice. *Clin Pharmacokinet* **33**:103–21.

Boston Collaborative Drug Surveillance Program. 1972. Adverse drug interactions. *JAMA* **220**:1238–9.

Caranasos GJ, Stewart RB, Cluff LE. 1985. Clinically desirable drug interactions. *Annu Rev Pharmacol Toxicol* **25**:67–95.

Carr CJ. 1982. Food and drug interactions. *Annu Rev Pharmacol Toxicol* **22**:19–29.

Carruthers SG, Freeman DJ, Bailey DG. 1989. Synergistic adverse hemodynamic interaction between oral verapamil and propranolol. *Clin Pharmacol Ther* **46**:469–77.

Davidson KW, Kahn A, Price RD. 1987. Reduction of adverse drug reactions by computerized drug interaction screening. *J Fam Pract* **25**:371–5.

Epstein MM, Nelson SD, Slattery JT, et al. 1991. Inhibition of the metabolism of acetaminophen by isoniazid. *Br J Clin Pharmacol* **31**:139–42.

Fraser AG. 1997. Pharmacokinetic interactions between alcohol and other drugs. *Clin Pharmacokinet* **33**:79–90.

Jick H. 1974. Drugs—remarkably nontoxic. *N Engl J Med* **291**:824–8.

Johnson AG, Nguyen TV, Day RO. 1994. Do nonsteroidal anti-inflammatory drugs affect blood pressure? *Ann Intern Med* **121**:289–300.

Langhoff E, Madsen S. 1983. Rapid metabolism of cyclosporine and prednisone in kidney transplant patient receiving tuberculostatic treatment. *Lancet* **2**:1031.

Li AP, Jurima-Romet M. 1997. Overview: pharmacokinetic drug–drug interactions. *Adv Pharmacol* **43**:1–6.

Liedholm H, Melander A. 1986. Concomitant food intake can increase the bioavailability of propranolol by transient inhibition of its presystemic primary conjugation. *Clin Pharmacol Ther* **40**:29–36.

MacKichan JJ. 1989. Protein binding drug displacement interactions. Fact or fiction? *Clin. Pharmacol* **16**:65–73.

Mehta BR, Robinson BHB. 1980. Lithium toxicity induced by triamterene-hydrochlorothiazide. *Postgrad Med J* **56**:783–4.

Nolan L, O'Malley K. 1988. Prescribing for the elderly: I. Sensitivity of the elderly to adverse drug reactions. *J Am Geriatrics* **36**:142–9.

Okey AB. 1990. Enzyme induction in the cytochrome P-450 system. *Pharmacotherapy* **45**:241–98.

Peet M, Middlemiss DN, Yates RA. 1981. Propranolol in schizophrenia: II. Clinical and biochemical aspects of combining propranolol with chlorpromazine. *Br J Psychiatry* **139**:112–7.

Puckett WH Jr, Visconti JA. 1971. An epidemiological study of the clinical significance of drug–drug interactions in a private community hospital. *Am J Hosp Pharm* **28**:247–53.

Richelson E. 1997. Pharmacokinetic drug interactions of new antidepressants: a review of the effects on the metabolism of other drugs. *Mayo Clin Proc* **72**:835–47.

Sarich TC, Wright JM. 1996. Hypothyroxinemia and phenytoin toxicity: a vicious circle. *Drug Metab Drug Interact* **13**:155–60.

Su SF, Huang JD. 1996. Inhibition of the intestinal digoxin absorption and exsorption by quinidine. *Drug Metab Dispos* **24**:142–7.

Tong TG, Pond SM, Kreek MJ, et al. 1981. Phenytoin-induced methadone withdrawal. *Ann Intern Med* **94**:349–51.

Tseng AL, Foisy MM. 1997. Management of drug interactions in patients with HIV. *Ann Pharmacother* **31**:1040–58.

Wright JM, Stokes EF, Sweeney VP. 1982. Isoniazid-induced carbamazepine toxicity and vice versa: a double drug interaction. *N Engl J Med* **307**:1325–7.

Zand R, Nelson SD, Slattery JT, et al. 1993. Inhibition and induction of cytochrome P4502E1-catalyzed oxidation by isoniazid in humans. *Clin Pharmacol Ther* **54**:142–9.

Zuik M, Mandel MA. 1975. Methotrexate-salicylate interaction: a clinical and experimental study. *Surg Forum* **26**:567–9.

C H A P T E R

# 26 WRITING PRESCRIPTIONS

Terrence F. Blaschke

*Chapter Outline*



"To write prescriptions is easy, but to come to an understanding of people is hard."
Franz Kafka, A Country Doctor

"Drugs can't work when patients don't take them."
C. Everett Koop, M.D.,
Former Surgeon General of the United States of America

These two quotations summarize the substantial chasm that remains in the practice of therapeutics, despite the rapidly increasing body of evidence-based knowledge that guides the choice of treatments. This chapter deals with the practical issues of how to write a prescription, generic substitution, and over-the-counter (OTC) drugs, but also emphasizes one of the important, nonscientific areas of drug therapy, namely, the poorly understood and complex interpersonal relationship that is established between the patient and the physician. As a way of emphasizing the numerous processes, forces, interests, and disciplines that are required in writing a prescription, Avorn (1995) stated that the prescription is "the final common pathway in therapeutic decision making," while suggesting that physician training for this role is suboptimal and often biased by the source of information.

The first part of this chapter discusses the nature of the physician–patient relationship as it applies to therapeutics, with the goal of improving the dialogue and understanding between patient and physician. An important concept in this relationship is that the often brief encounter between a patient and physician leads to establishment of a patient–physician contract, an unwritten agreement that ultimately is a major determinant of the success or failure of therapy.

## THE CONTRACT BETWEEN PATIENT AND PHYSICIAN

Physicians rarely choose their patients. Patients seek medical attention and choose physicians for complex reasons. Both patients and physicians have expectations of their encounter even though they may not be consciously recognized or acknowledged by either. Early in the encounter, the physician must try to understand the nature of the patient's medical experiences and needs, a process that will form the basis of initial and continuing trust. Ideally, the physician and patient will define a collaboration in which the patient takes responsibility for curing his or her own illness or reducing his or her own symptoms with the assistance of the physician (Brody 1980). A primary goal of the initial interaction between patient and physician should be development of a therapeutic contract. Except for a few special circumstances, mainly in the setting of psychiatric treatment (Miller 1990) and drug or alcohol abuse programs (Ojehagen and Berglund 1986), this contract or alliance is unwritten.

The nature of the therapeutic contract that results from a physician–patient encounter is influenced by factors such as the physical setting, but mostly by the expectations of the persons involved, which may include individuals other than the physician and the patient (e.g., parents, spouses, children). Most important, the physician must attempt to understand the patient's expectations as well as to define for the patient, his or her own expectations and the responsibilities of therapy. If the physician is not clear about the overall goal of treatment or about the reason for writing a specific prescription (e.g., distinguishing between treating the disease and simply alleviating symptoms), transmission of a proper set of expectations to the patient will not be possible. Conversely, if the physician fails to understand the patient's expectations, the physician may fail to satisfy them and will surely fail if they are unrealistic. If either physician or patient expectations are not fulfilled, mutual trust will be lost.

**PRINCIPLE Do not hope for trust or understanding; deliberately and objectively build them.**

Two specific issues regarding the physician's role in the therapeutic contract deserve further emphasis: control and answering questions. Particularly as a result of the marked increase in direct-to-consumer advertising by the pharmaceutical industry, patients often request a specific treatment, and they require an explanation of why or why not this medication should be used. Some patients may go to another physician if they do not receive the expected treatment (Schwartz et al. 1989). Whenever a patient attempts to play the role of physician, the physician should determine the reason for the specific request. Perhaps the patient was previously given a drug and believes that it works, or wants a particular drug as an affirmation or denial of a specific disease. The physician should be concerned about the patient's concept of his or her illness, because it will be a major determinant of what therapeutic approach the patient will accept or resist. Although it is permissible to assign certain aspects of therapy to the patient, the physician should determine the role of the participants in the therapeutic contract. Physicians must, however, be sensitive to the needs and fears of the patient. Control is an important dimension of the patient–physician encounter and must be used carefully. Recent results suggest that patients who take less active roles in their interactions with physicians have lower rates of compliance (Cecil and Killeen 1997).

In answering questions, the physician should recognize differences in the amount of information desired by the patient. This may be manifested in how the patient asks questions and how he or she perceives the role of the physician. In discussing treatment, the physician must individualize the amount of information provided to the patient. Patients vary considerably in terms of their need for information and for control of a situation. Good communication establishes the appropriate division of control necessary for an effective and successful therapeutic contract. Finally, physicians must be aware that how instructions are given may be an important determinant of therapeutic success. Hurried or interrupted instructions can influence trust and therapeutic outcome.

## PLACEBOS AND THE PLACEBO EFFECT

The issues of control and answering questions are intertwined with the definition and the use of placebos. The term placebo, which dates back to antiquity, continues to generate considerable controversy among physicians and scientists over its meaning, its mechanisms, and its use in therapeutics and in clinical trials (Lasagna 1986). The Latin verb placebo means "I shall please," and the term is often associated with a negative or pejorative connotation (Brown 1998). There are many contemporary definitions of a placebo, such as "a medicine or preparation which has no inherent, pertinent pharmacologic activity but which is intended to be effective only by virtue of the factor of suggestion attendant upon its administration" (Leslie 1954; Placebos 1982) or "a form of medical therapy, or an intervention designed to simulate medical therapy, that is believed to be without specific activity for the condition being treated and that is used for its symbolic effect or to eliminate observer bias in a controlled experiment" (Brody 1997). The placebo effect is defined as "that aspect of treatment not attributable to specific pharmacologic or physiologic properties" (Benson and Friedman 1996). Although it seems self-evident that physicians should try to avoid therapy that is "without specific activity," the decision about whether placebos are justified in clinical practice or even in clinical trials is not clear-cut. Ethical concerns about the use of placebos deserve consideration (Rothman and Michels 1994; Benson and Friedman 1996; Brown 1998). However, appropriate analysis of many clinical trials depends on determining placebo effects, one source of substantial variability that confounds the measurement of true drug effects (Bienenfeld et al. 1996). In clinical practice, where a majority of patient visits are for conditions that cannot be explained on a pathophysiologic basis or for which no specific treatment is available, it is essential that physicians understand the concepts and principles of placebos and placebo effects and, when appropriate, use them correctly.

Although placebos are usually thought of as pills or injections that simulate administration of an active drug, many interventions or procedures can elicit positive or negative placebo effects. Most therapeutic and diagnostic procedures, from simple blood drawing to cardiac catheterization, undoubtedly have considerable placebo effects. The physician and his or her associates also are important instruments of placebo effects through their appearance, attitudes, and communication with patients. Administration of a placebo is not necessary to evoke a placebo response. Three components are necessary: 1) positive beliefs and expectations on the part of the patient, 2) positive beliefs on the part of the provider, and 3) a good relationship between the parties (Benson and Epstein 1975).

In terms of the actual placebo itself, the pure placebo is a substance that could have no conceivable pharmacologic effect on the patient, and an impure placebo has potential pharmacologic effects, although not necessarily any specific activity for the condition under treatment. Examples of the latter are administration of vitamin $B_{12}$ or iron in the absence of anemia, or use of antibiotics to treat viral infections. The use of impure placebos is to be discouraged, as they have greater potential to cause harm, mask diagnoses, or delay evaluation, and necessitates deception on the part of the physician who must present them to the patient as specific treatments, when they are not.

## Documentation and Mechanism of the Placebo Effect

The placebo effect has been studied extensively and observed in a wide variety of conditions. Almost 40 years ago, Beecher (1955) investigated placebo therapy in 1082 patients with conditions as varied as postoperative wound pain, cough, mood disturbances, angina, headache, and the common cold, and observed that satisfactory relief was obtained in 35% of these patients. Since then, many other diseases and symptoms have been added to the list. Paradoxically, as more potent and effective drugs have been developed, the placebo effect may have become even more powerful because of a generally increased faith in the value of drugs on the part of both patient and physician.

Despite widespread use of placebos, the mechanisms underlying placebo effects are poorly understood (Lasagna 1986; Weiner and Weiner 1996). Whatever the mechanism, two requirements are necessary if placebo effects are to be sought and achieved. First, the disease process itself or its symptoms must be capable of variable intensity, both over time and in different patients. In most situations, the powerful resilience of the human body can result in improvement of symptoms, and at times, even remissions or cures of usually progressive or even fatal illnesses. It is this resilience that is enhanced by the use of placebos in about one-third of all patients. In other settings where resilience has already failed, such as cardiac arrest or severe acidosis, placebos have no possible role.

Second, significant placebo effects are seen only when there is a physician–patient contract, actual or implied. While self-medication with OTC drugs may have some placebo effect, the patient's perception of the physician as a "healer" is a powerful stimulus to the placebo effect, whether it is a positive or a negative one. This is likely related to the psychoanalytic concept of transference, which can be a dynamic part of the physician–patient relationship. According to this concept, patients may transfer emotions directed at objects (including people) in their past environment onto current objects. Translated into the therapeutic situation, the good or bad results of previous experiences with drugs or physicians may be a determinant of present therapeutic success. Purely psychological stimuli from the past can influence behavior and even autonomic responses. For example, gastric acid secretion or heart rate may be affected by stimuli of which the patient is unaware at the conscious level (Katkin and Murray 1968). Placebo responses occur much more frequently when the endpoint of therapy is a change in behavior (as in psychiatric treatment), subjective sensations, or pain, all of which can be influenced by patients' prior experiences and their attitudes toward those experiences (Turner et al. 1994). Placebo effects are also more likely when the condition being treated is under autonomic control, such as gastric motility, bronchoconstriction, sexual potency, or blood pressure (Bienenfeld et al. 1996; Briet et al. 1997). In general, increased anxiety and stressful situations favor placebo effects; normal control subjects are probably less likely to have placebo effects than are sick patients, who may be more ready to manifest transference or operant conditioning responses. Placebo responses are less common in protracted diseases with unremitting courses (Lesse 1962).

Despite the above generalizations, it is still difficult to predict which patients will react (either positively or negatively) to placebo medications (Lasagna 1986). Contrary to common belief, the "hypersuggestible" hysterical personality does not predispose to positive or negative placebo responses (Lesse 1962). Also, women are not more likely than men to respond to a placebo (Trouton 1957). Lasagna and co-workers (1954), in a carefully designed study of the placebo response in patients with postoperative pain, showed that it was impossible for an observer to determine by conversation or examination, even retrospectively, whether any given patient might manifest a placebo response. When consistent "placebo reactors" (14% of the population studied) and "nonreactors" (31%)

were subjected to psychological testing, certain characteristics of both groups could be defined. The reactor group was more outgoing, more dependent on outside stimulation from the environment for emotional satisfaction, more favorably disposed to hospitalization, more concerned with visceral or pelvic complaints, somewhat more anxious, and less mature than the nonreactor group. It is interesting that the nonreactor group appeared to respond less well to active analgesic therapy, raising the possibility of classifying patients as reactors or nonreactors based on their sensitivity to analgesic compounds; this approach has not been prospectively tested.

If a true personality type—the placebo reactor-exists, this type must be expressed to some degree in all patients, because the mechanisms responsible for the placebo effect are probably operative in everyone. Occasionally, a consistent placebo reactor may become a nonreactor; physicians also may vary in their susceptibility to produce and detect placebo effects. The most significant clinical principle about the placebo reaction is perhaps the following.

**PRINCIPLE A positive reaction to placebo does not mean that the condition being treated is "only psychological and not real," nor does lack of a positive response to placebo imply that the condition is "real."**

Placebos should never be used diagnostically. To use placebos in an effort to identify someone who is "faking" a symptom or an illness is truly unethical (McCaffery et al. 1998). One possible outcome of inappropriate placebo use is overlooking and consequently delaying appropriate evaluation of a condition for which specific and effective treatment is available. Covert placebo administration also carries with it the great danger that if the patient discovers a placebo was prescribed, he or she may feel deceived. In such cases, that physician or a subsequent physician may fail to establish a therapeutic contract. In considering placebo therapy or placebo effects, physicians should focus on the disease process and the patient's environmental and emotional stresses, rather than attempt to classify personalities.

## Placebos and Toxicity

It is obvious that adverse reactions and undesirable effects can occur with impure placebos, but even pure placebos can produce adverse effects (Sibille et al. 1998); some have used the term nocebo to describe adverse placebo responses. Dermatitis medicamentosa and angioneurotic edema have resulted from placebo therapy (Wolf and Pinsky 1954). More subtle but equally important negative effects must occur when physicians themselves transmit, verbally or otherwise, their own feelings of uncertainty, doubt, or mistrust to patients.

## Use of Placebos in Clinical Trials

The AIDS epidemic has strongly focused attention once again on the role of placebo medications in clinical trials (Rothman and Michels 1994). Placebo effects are seen in almost any therapeutic setting, even in progressive diseases such as AIDS, because of the resilience of patients (as discussed earlier) and the tendency of regression to the mean or to normal for most self-limited disease. Therefore, random assignment to treatment with placebo is mandatory if no other treatment has been demonstrated to have genuine benefit, in order to estimate accurately the magnitude of the true effect of a new therapy. With few exceptions, such as in diseases that are uniformly and rapidly fatal like human rabies, historical controls are inadequate because of variations in the effect of supportive care and time itself on the natural history and time course of the disease. The absence of a placebo group, when no other therapy has been shown to have genuine benefit, may delay introduction of effective treatments developed subsequently because of the necessity of comparing these newer treatments with possibly ineffective therapies, thus increasing the baseline "noise" (variability), complexity, and therefore, cost and duration of the study. Also, the use of a placebo group is important to determine accurately the true toxicity of the drug being tested.

On the other hand, it is usually inappropriate and unethical to use placebos in a clinical trial for treating important disease if another mode of therapy already has shown genuine benefit. In this situation, patients receiving placebo are deprived of available therapy, and the real question—whether the new therapy is superior to the best existing therapy—cannot be answered by such a design. The most vexing situation relating to use of placebos in clinical trials is a design in which patients are temporarily withdrawn from a known active treatment or in which therapy is withheld for a short period while the investigational compound is compared with a placebo. Ethical issues in this situation center around the need to expose a larger number of subjects to the investigational compound before it is known to be effective, the lack of statistical agreement about confidence intervals when active control treatment designs are used, and the possible delay in marketing because of the larger number of subjects needed to determine efficacy and safety. Most of the philosophical and ethical issues thus involve the rights of the individual subject-patient versus the societal good of these designs (Taubes 1995; Brody 1997). The US Food and Drug Administration (FDA) continues to support use of placebo designs even when other therapies have been shown to be beneficial, when the risk of interruptions in treatment or short delays in treatment is very small (Temple 1997).

In some trials, use of a pure placebo may be difficult because the active compound produces symptoms or signs that may be detectable by the patient, the physician, or both. In that case, the single- or double-blind design of the experiment is lost, and the bias of the patient and physician affects the outcome of the trial, potentially invalidating it entirely. To avoid this problem, use of impure placebos is sometimes necessary. Other appropriate uses of placebos in clinical trials are to define and remove from a trial those patients who are placebo reactors, using the remaining patients to quantify more clearly the difference between a known active compound and a test compound, or to determine medication noncompliers who can subsequently be excluded from the comparative trial, greatly reducing sample size requirements. The latter approach, with an impure placebo containing riboflavin, was used during the early Veterans Administration (VA) Cooperative Study Group antihypertensive drug trials [Veterans Administration (VA) Cooperative Study Group 1967].

An additional confounder in the use of placebos in clinical trials resulted from FDA actions in 1987–1988 establishing the regulations for Treatment IND (Investigational New Drug), particularly Subpart E, intended to make investigational drugs available to patients with life-threatening diseases as early as possible in the drug development process. These regulations, although well intentioned, potentially make the investigational agent available before all of the information necessary to determine the agent's risks and benefits is known. As a result, it is difficult and sometimes impossible to recruit and enroll subjects into placebo-controlled studies, which are critical to developing this information. For example, during the development of ganciclovir for treatment of cytomegalovirus in patients with AIDS, the widespread availability of this drug made it difficult to conduct appropriately controlled trials and thus delayed its approval and availability to the general public for a considerable time.

Recent better approaches to estimating compliance in clinical trials using specially designed medication dispensers may reduce problems in analysis of clinical trial data associated with the detection of placebos by patients and noncompliance in either the active or the placebo group (Bok 1974; Kastrissios and Blaschke 1997).

## Ethics of Placebo Administration

Whether placebo administration is morally justifiable in any therapeutic situation is a fundamental and controversial question. Brown (1998) and others (Benson and Friedman 1996) argue for the value of placebos, stating that, "as physicians, we should respect the benefits of placebos—their safety, effectiveness and low cost—and bring the full advantage of these benefits into our everyday practices" (Brown 1998). Bok (1974) argues strongly that the deception involved in therapeutic use of placebos is intrinsically dangerous, because "deceptive practices, by their very nature, tend to escape the normal restraints of accountability and so can spread more easily. There are ever stronger pressures—from drug companies, patients eager for cures and busy physicians—for more medication, whether it is needed or not." In fact, there is even controversy among authors who endorse the use of placebos or the placebo effect about the need for deception in the use of placebo (Placebos 1982; Benson and Friedman 1996). A real danger is that liberal use of pure or impure placebos encourages other forms of deception in medicine. The trust between patient and physician, so critical to success of the therapeutic contract, also could be threatened. More obvious breeches of the professional ethics and responsibilities of the physician are to use placebos as an appealing substitute for the difficult task of diagnosis ("take two aspirin and call me in the morning"), as a mechanism for dealing with a difficult and demanding patient, or for providing financial or emotional rewards to the physician.

## Therapeutic Use of Placebos

Although the placebo effect resulting from the communication and contract between provider and patient is valuable and desirable, casual use of pure or impure placebos poses a fundamental threat to professional ethics and to the patient–physician relationship. The physician can often improve therapeutic outcome by means of clear, direct communication with the patient in the course of negotiating the therapeutic contract. As indicated earlier in this chapter, the ability of the physician to produce placebo effects through communication is sometimes more important than use of drugs or placebos themselves; this was nicely shown in a study of postoperative analgesia (Egbert et al. 1964). In this study, preoperative patients were divided into two groups. One group had a routine preoperative visit and preoperative medication appropriate to the planned surgery. The second group had more extensive contact with the anesthesiologist, who discussed the nature, causes, and course of normal postoperative pain. Although both groups underwent comparable elective intra-abdominal procedures, the group with greater contact with the anesthesiologist required almost 50% less analgesic medication than did the other group and were sent home an average of 2.7 days earlier by their surgeons, who were not aware of the study. Clear, direct communication between patient and physician is a critical requirement of the therapeutic contract and is essential when drugs are prescribed, because the patient's understanding of disease and treatment may influence both compliance with and efficacy of drug therapy.

**PRINCIPLE No drug can substitute for planned and careful communication between physician and patient.**

Use of a pure or impure placebo is rarely justified and must be limited and thoughtful. There are very few appropriate indications for the use of a placebo: one is when a placebo has long-term efficacy and is safer than other active agents, as has been suggested in the treatment of mild depression (Overall et al. 1962; Brown 1994). An argument also can be made for using a placebo in a very small subset of patients who cannot be convinced that no specific drug is available, who require something tangible that they can define as treatment, and who will clearly seek another physician willing to provide impure placebos.

**PRINCIPLE As with any therapeutic intervention, rational use of a placebo requires that the physician follow the patient for evidence of therapeutic benefit or toxicity, and lack of efficacy or development of toxicity (negative placebo effects when administering a pure placebo) is an indication for discontinuing placebo therapy.**

## COST-BENEFIT ANALYSIS AND THERAPEUTICS

An essential component of all therapeutic decisions, both qualitative and quantitative, is a thoughtful weighing of costs and benefits (cost-benefit assessment). In medicine in general, cost-benefit analyses for any diagnostic or therapeutic decisions are complex (Brandimonte and Gerbino 1993). They often require information that is unavailable or of questionable reliability and assigning "values" to possible outcomes under circumstances in which the values assigned by the patient and the physician may differ markedly (Lenert et al. 1997). Again, the quality of communication between patient and physician in establishing the therapeutic contract determines the physician's understanding of how the patient values various outcomes, and thus affects incorporation of the patient's values into a cost-benefit assessment.

In terms of medical information currently available, at best only a few situations lend themselves to carrying out a formal cost-benefit analysis using a decision-tree approach and sensitivity analysis (Thornton et al. 1992). Elegant examples of such approaches may be found in cost-benefit analyses applied to the management of renovascular hypertension, acute renal failure, anticoagulation in atrial fibrillation, and treatment of Hodgkin's disease. This approach has found more application in assessing diagnostic procedures than in assessing therapeutic plans (Kassirer et al. 1987), perhaps because surprisingly few reliable data are available concerning probabilities of various therapeutic outcomes. Recognition of this paucity of hard data has led to the growth of the field of outcomes research.

In the face of uncertainty, when information is limited, an alternative strategy must be chosen to maximize efficacy and to minimize harm. A first consideration is the actual disease-specific cost-benefit information available in the medical literature about a given therapeutic approach (Elixhauser et al. 1998). If little or no such information exists, or if the information is irrelevant to the particular patient for whom the assessment must be made, no proper cost-benefit analysis is possible. Therapy in such situations is best carried out in the setting of clinical investigation, which will allow this therapeutic experience to contribute to the science of therapeutics. In some circumstances, an n-of-1 therapeutic trial might be considered (Guyatt et al. 1990) (see chapter 28, Risk Analysis Applied to Prescription Drugs).

Physicians should not be motivated primarily by eagerness to treat and they should not base therapy predominantly on theoretic considerations or on past personal experience with "similar" patients (Tversky and Kahneman 1974). Conversely, fear of toxicity from a therapeutic program should not result in denial of appropriate or adequate therapy that is indicated (Monette et al. 1997). For example, although excellent data have documented the value of achieving adequate peak concentrations of aminoglycoside antibiotics in the treatment of gram-negative bacillary sepsis or pneumonia (Noone et al. 1974; Moore et al. 1987), there are also considerable data to indicate that underdosing in such situations is common, possibly because of concerns about the potential nephrotoxicity of aminoglycosides, even though the lesion is almost always reversible (Lenert et al. 1993).

No matter how busy the physician's practice or how careful the documentation, no physician can accumulate enough personal therapeutic experience to serve as the only basis for most subsequent therapeutic decisions regarding individual patients. The physician is responsible, however, for determining the degree to which the individual patient matches the patient population in the literature upon which the therapeutic plan for the patient is based. This concept of combining personal experience and knowledge of the patient with information in the literature is now embodied in the term "evidence-based-medicine" (Evidence-Based Medicine Working Group 1992; Sackett et al. 1996). This concept of matching is coupled with the following very important concept, emphasized in the introduction (part 1).

**PRINCIPLE Every therapeutic contract and every prescription is the beginning of an experiment that requires the physician consciously to establish endpoints (efficacy, toxicity) at the beginning and to reassess the patient during the course of treatment, looking for those endpoints.**

## WRITING PRESCRIPTIONS

Although the first, and often useful, result of writing a prescription may be to indicate that the visit is over, this little-taught action is intended to set into motion behavior that is critical to the success of the therapeutic contract. As mentioned, the manner and setting in which the physician carries out this action, and the verbal and nonverbal communication as the physician hands the prescription to the patient, can have considerable impact. The focus here, however, is the practical and technical aspects of writing a prescription, the goal of which is to ensure that the pharmacist accurately interprets the intent of the physician.

Because mistakes in writing and in filling prescriptions can have disastrous consequences (Lesar et al. 1997), written prescriptions have followed a traditional format that minimizes errors. A basic rule is that only one prescription, which may be for a multicomponent formulation, should be written on each prescription order blank. The format of a sample prescription, shown in Figure 26-1, contains the following minimum elements.

| | |
|---|---|
| ***Date:*** | September 1, 1999 |
| ***Address:*** | William Smith, Jr.<br>2115 Main Street<br>LaCrosse, WI 12345 |
| ***Birth Date:*** | DOB: 6/11/17 |
| ***Superscription:*** | ***Rx:*** |
| ***Inscription:*** | Levodopa, 100 mg<br>Carbidopa, 25 mg |
| ***Subscription:*** | Dispense 100 combination tablets in non-childproof container |
| ***Signa:*** | Label Take two tablets orally with breakfast, lunch, and dinner. Take with food. |
| ***Refill:*** | Refill 4 times. |
| ***Prescriber's Signature:*** | Anne Blake, M.D.<br>1 Medical Plaza Drive<br>Milwaukee, WI 54321<br>DEA No. AB1357902 |

F I G U R E 2 6 - 1 **A sample prescription.**

1. The date. This is important for record-keeping and because prescriptions for certain drugs are not valid beyond a specified period.
2. Patient identification. The full name and address and the age or, preferably, the birth date of the patient. These ensure proper handling and labeling of the medication and identification of the patient. This information also assists in monitoring for possible dosage errors, especially in the pediatric or geriatric patient.
3. The superscription. On most blank order forms, this is preprinted using the symbol Rx (recipe, or "take"). If the superscription is absent, the physician should introduce his or her prescribed drug with this symbol.
4. The inscription. Immediately below the superscription, this area contains the name, unit dose, and exact formulation of the drug to be dispensed. Only the officially approved generic name or brand name should be used. Abbreviations should be avoided because many drug names have similar spellings and sound alike when spoken (Teplitsky 1975; Lambert 1997). The names of drugs should be capitalized. When a generic product combination, such as triamterene and hydrochlorothiazide, is prescribed, the name and amount of each component should be written on separate lines directly underneath one another. Amounts should always be written in the metric system using arabic numerals.
5. The subscription (may be written #). This area provides directions to the pharmacist about the quantity of medication to provide to the patient, along with any specific instructions about the formulation such as com-

pounding instructions for extemporaneous (not preformulated or precompounded) prescriptions. Prescriptions may be written for any amount of medication, subject to legal and storage limits for some drug classes. Cost, convenience, and safety are factors in determining the appropriate quantity. The mental state of the patient and the potency of the drug should be considered. If a patient is depressed and potentially suicidal, a single prescription should not be written for a quantity that would be lethal if taken all at once. For conditions of limited duration, only enough drug to treat the illness should be prescribed, and patients should be instructed to discard any unused medication. Medication sharing is common, especially among the elderly, and accidental poisonings and suicides occur with stockpiled drugs. The choice of medication container is sometimes worth specifying, especially in older patients who may have difficulty in opening child-proof or tamper-proof pill containers and as a result transfer their medications to unlabeled or improperly labeled containers.

6. The signa. Signa is Latin for label, and in the past this section was introduced by the abbreviated "Sig." It consists of the directions for the patient that will become printed instructions on the container. These instructions should be stated in proper English grammar, avoiding Latin or other abbreviations (e.g., qid, qod) that are easily misinterpreted and would have to be retranslated into English or another language familiar to the patient. The label instructions tell the patient the amount of drug to take, the frequency and possibly the precise times of day the medication is to be taken, and the route of administration. Sometimes, other instructions such as "Shake well before using," or "Take with food," a dilution, or a caution such as "Use only externally" are included here.

   Certain conventions are useful to help minimize patient error. The first word of the instructions should indicate the route of administration, for example, "Take" for oral, "Apply" for topical, "Insert" for rectal, and "Place" or "Instill" for conjunctival, nasal, or external auditory canal administration. The indication for the medication may also be included, such as "for relief of pain" or "for itching." Expressions such as "Take as directed" should be avoided. Complex or lengthy instructions should be written out for the patient on a separate sheet. The importance of clear directions to the patient on how to take prescription medications cannot be overemphasized, because the instructions on the medication container itself, even when they are accurate, are rarely adequate (Stewart and Caranasos 1989).

**PRINCIPLE Even the best therapeutic approach will fail if the patient does not comply with the drug regimen or unintentionally manages it incorrectly.**

7. Refill information. Physicians should consider and indicate their instructions on refills for each prescription written, even when several prescriptions are written at the same time. Refill instructions must comply with federal and state laws; federal law, for example, forbids refilling schedule III and IV drugs more than five times, and the prescription order is invalid 6 months after the date of issue. Schedule II drugs cannot be refilled; if more of the drug is needed, a new prescription must be written. Other factors such as suicide risk or abuse potential also must be considered here, in regard to the quantity of each prescription.
8. Prescriber's identification. When all of the above are completed to the physician's satisfaction, the order form should be signed with an indelible pen with the physician's name followed by the appropriate professional degree (e.g., MD, DO, DDS). For schedule II drugs, the physician's address and Drug Enforcement Administration (DEA) registration number also must appear on the form. Other legal requirements for the prescription order form can vary from state to state and country to country. It is always useful for the physician to provide his or her printed name, address, and phone number, to facilitate communication with the pharmacist. When the prescription is written by a house-staff physician on behalf of an attending physician, it is useful to provide the name of the physician of record as well.

Commonly, physicians use prescription blanks on which their name, address, telephone number, and DEA registration number are preprinted. Keeping an exact or carbon copy of each prescription is advisable, because many physicians do not transcribe such details into the patient visit note. Preprinted prescriptions and prewritten orders for hospitalized patients containing proprietary names and containing blanks to be filled in should not be used; they fundamentally interfere with the thought processes that should be a part of every therapeutic decision. However, preprinted forms for complicated orders or prescriptions, such as for parenteral nutrition or cancer chemotherapy, may greatly improve prescription accuracy and clarity for both inpatients and outpatients (Thorn et al. 1989).

An excellent opportunity to negotiate the responsibilities of the patient and the physician in the therapeutic contract occurs after the prescriptions are written and before the encounter is concluded. The patient must understand the physician's impression of the illness and the associated prognosis. If drugs are prescribed, the physician should explain how the medication is expected to alter the natural history or the symptoms of the illness. Patients frequently discontinue medication such as penicillin for streptococcal pharyngitis because they have not been told why the medication needs to be taken after the symptoms subside (Bergman and Werner 1963). Patients may discontinue drug therapy at the first sign of a minor adverse effect if they have not been advised that certain effects are common and are not to be feared. Patients should be warned about dangerous adverse effects and that these should be immediately reported to the physician (e.g., sore throat with a potentially myelosuppressive drug). Special care should be taken to give instructions related to excessive dosage. Patients should be carefully questioned about preexisting symptoms so that useful drugs are not needlessly discontinued because of these symptoms upon subsequent visits. Patients with chronic illnesses requiring long-term therapy, especially if it is prophylactic or suppressive, need careful explanation of the rationale for treatment.

The dialogue between patient and physician should be viewed as a process of information-gathering, instruction, and motivation for both parties as they begin the therapeutic contract. If desired, the physician can also give the patient an information sheet about the drugs just prescribed. In the United States, patient-centered information is available for most drugs from sources such as the United States Pharmacopeial Convention (USP) (MedCoach) and Micromedex (CareNotes), and many pharmacy computer systems are now able to generate patient information sheets.

## PATIENT COMPLIANCE WITH TREATMENT PLANS

Closely intertwined with writing a prescription and the therapeutic contract is patient compliance with the prescribed medication regimen as well as with other aspects of the treatment plan. A prescription commonly incorporates involved instructions, making the patient responsible for self-administration of a specific drug in the correct dose, at the proper time(s) of day, with or without meals, and for a certain duration. When this responsibility is extended to several drugs, the complexity becomes formidable, and imperfect compliance is inevitable. For example, a patient infected with HIV taking three medications three times daily and one twice daily is responsible for 11 individual drug administrations per day. It is tempting to think that compliance is inversely related to the complexity of a drug regimen, and that noncompliance can be minimized by designing a simple drug regimen.

Compliance has been defined in its broadest sense as "the extent to which a person's behavior coincides with medical or health advice" (Haynes 1979). The causes of noncompliance are multifactorial (Larrat et al. 1990; Cameron 1996), and, despite beliefs to the contrary, physicians are generally unable to estimate compliance in individual patients using subjective appraisal of the patient's "character." Just as physician estimates are often faulty, patient reports of compliance must be viewed with a critical eye. Patients generally exaggerate their true intake of prescription drugs. In a study of a 10-day oral penicillin regimen for streptococcal pharyngitis in which the drug was to be given by the parent to the child, 83% of parents claimed that no dose had been missed during the 10 days of therapy. However, pill counts and urine assay for penicillin activity revealed that 55% of patients had stopped medication by the third day, 70% by the sixth day, and 85% by the ninth day (Bergman and Werner 1963). Admission of noncompliance may be more truthful: in one group of depressed patients admitting noncompliance, the noncompliance was confirmed in almost 90% of the reported instances (Park and Lipman 1964).

### Consequences of Imperfect Compliance

Noncompliance with drug treatment might account for 10% of hospital admissions, 23% of admissions to nursing homes, and excess costs of about $100 billion per year in the United States alone (Gerbino 1993; Donovan 1995). The importance of compliance as a determinant of therapeutic outcomes has been highlighted by observations that followed the release of HIV protease inhibitors in the latter part of the 1990s. Many patients who failed treatment were not fully compliant with regimens containing these drugs (Vanhove et al. 1996; Hecht et al. 1998). Recognizing that perfect compliance cannot be achieved, it is useful to think of the consequences of less-than-perfect compliance in terms of "adequate" and "inadequate" compliance, or, stated another way, "how much compliance is enough?" (Urquhart 1997). The pharmacologic basis of the answer to this question relates to the dose- or concentration-response and the therapeutic index of the drug(s) being prescribed. For drugs with a large therapeutic index, the usual doses prescribed are high enough to produce concentrations of drug well into the flat part of the concentration-response relationship, and thus missed doses will have relatively little impact on the response. When toxicity or the potential for toxicity limits doses, this results in concentrations in the lower ranges of the concentration-response relationship, and missed doses will result in loss of activity (Kastrissios and Blaschke 1997). This is related to the concept of "forgiving versus unforgiving medicines" (Urquhart and De Klerk 1998); a "forgiving" drug has a substantial margin for errors in dose-timing or for short drug holidays (periods of a few days when no drug is taken).

Adequate compliance has occurred when the patient takes the medication and manifests drug-related benefit or toxicity. Adequate compliance allows the physician to assess utility of treatment and make subsequent therapeutic decisions in a rational manner. Minor, and sometimes even major, departures from perfect compliance may be inconsequential, either because the full prescribed dosing schedule is not necessary for efficacy or because the therapy is inappropriate or ineffective for the condition being treated.

Inadequate compliance has occurred when not enough drug is taken to manifest drug-related benefit or toxicity. The result of inadequate compliance is not only that the treatment regimen cannot possibly succeed but also that the physician, if he or she is unaware of inadequate compliance, cannot accurately assess the utility of therapy. This is a significant obstacle to rational therapeutic management because the physician may conclude that therapy has failed or that the diagnosis is in error. If the patient is then subjected to additional diagnostic tests, higher doses, or more toxic therapy, the patient has been exposed to unnecessary risk. Another risk for the inadequately compliant patient occurs during hospitalization (Maronde et al. 1989). If the patient has been partially but inadequately compliant and has, as a result, been prescribed a higher-than-needed dose of a drug with a narrow therapeutic index, enforced compliance in the hospital may result in toxicity. Examples of this problem are seen frequently when patients receiving digitalis, warfarin, phenytoin, or insulin, or those with "refractory" hypertension, are hospitalized.

**PRINCIPLE Use of a supervised environment or validated measures of compliance may reveal noncompliance rather than refractoriness to therapy as a reason for therapeutic failure.**

## Compliance and Clinical Research

Partial compliance or noncompliance among clinical trial subjects is of considerable importance in planning, conducting, and analyzing clinical trials (Urquhart 1997). An increasing body of literature is documenting substantial lack of compliance in clinical trials, even those for treatment of life-threatening illnesses (Kastrissios and Blaschke 1997). Inadequate compliance, as defined previously, dilutes the drug effects in the treatment groups of a clinical trial and reduces the statistical power of a study. If inadequate compliance is unrecognized or its extent underestimated, incorrect qualitative or quantitative conclusions invariably ensue. At the minimum, the true difference (whether it is a positive or a negative difference) between various treatment groups or between treatment groups and control groups will be underestimated. When the true difference is small, sample size is marginal, or variability in response is large, even modest degrees of unrecognized, inadequate compliance may lead to the incorrect conclusion that there is no difference between the treatments (Goldsmith 1979). If noncompliance can be recognized and even quantified in a clinical trial, newer statistical approaches may allow better, appropriate interpretation of the results of the study (Rubin 1998). At a recent symposium on this important topic, one of the authors concluded that "not far in the future, it will seem as wrong to run a clinical trial without compliance measurement as without randomization" (Efron 1998).

The University Group Diabetes Program provided a costly and unfortunate example of the difficulty in interpreting studies in which there is significant noncompliance [University Group Diabetes Program (UGDP) 1970]. This large, expensive, multicenter project involved more than 1000 patients and spanned 15 years. The fact that only about 25% of patients adequately complied with their initially assigned regimen was a major cause of the investigators' inability to draw clear conclusions answering important therapeutic questions about management of diabetes (Feinstein 1976). In the Veterans Administration (VA) Cooperative Study Group 1967, which has had a major influence in attitudes about management of hypertension, compliance was assessed before enrollment by using an impure placebo containing riboflavin in the preliminary phase. Subjects who were noncompliant were dropped from the subsequent study. They made up almost 50% of potential candidates for the trial. Although these two examples are almost 30 years old and well described in the literature, the problem remains, and only recently have approaches to this problem been proposed (Cox 1998). Given the difficulty of determining in advance which subjects will comply poorly, and recognizing the serious costs, both scientific and economic, of inadequate compliance, assessment of compliance should be and is becoming an important design consideration in clinical trials (Efron 1998).

The ability to quantify patient compliance with reasonable accuracy using medication monitors (see "Assessment of Patient Compliance") has created the possibility of novel designs and new types of analyses of data derived from clinical trials (Goetghebeur et al. 1998; Rubin 1998). For example, uncontrollable variability in compliance, which occurs to some degree despite all efforts to minimize it, might be of considerable value in exploratory or explanatory analysis; it should not, however, be used to carry out an "as treated" analysis, owing to the confounding it causes, because patients in a trial are not randomized on the basis of their compliance behavior (Sheiner and Rubin 1995; Sheiner 1997).

## Assessment of Patient Compliance

Given the inability of physicians and investigators to accurately estimate compliance and the importance of compliance to the success of a therapeutic contract or a clinical trial, several other methods for estimating compliance are described in this section, as well as the strengths and limitations of each.

***Medication (pill) counts***

Counting the number of pills or ounces of medication remaining after a given time and subtracting this from the original quantity prescribed offers a potentially objective estimate of the quantity of medication used by the patient that can be compared with the intended intake.

Because of its simplicity, this is the most common approach to estimating compliance. The most important problem with this method is evidence of bias, demonstrated by using more objective methods of assessment of compliance: returned tablet counts routinely underestimate the extent of poor or partial compliance because of "pill dumping" (Pullar et al. 1989; Rudd et al. 1989).

***Patient self-report***

Patient self-report is a commonly used and convenient measure of compliance. Self-report data can be obtained from structured interviews or survey questionnaires directly completed by patients. There are a number of advantages to this approach: it is relatively inexpensive, data are easily obtained from large study samples, and it provides the only source of accurate information for unobservable experiences/behaviors (i.e., only patients can report adverse effects or motives for compliance or noncompliance). Disadvantages are that patients often apparently overestimate their degree of compliance and their memory, particularly over longer time periods, may limit the accuracy of recall. Although memory may limit the quantity of data, it has also been shown that patients overestimate their compliance. When compared with objective methods such as electronic monitoring, patient assessments of adherence, including diaries, have been found to overestimate routinely (De Klerk and Van Der Linden 1996). It is unclear, however, to what extent this bias toward overestimation is due to faulty recall and to what extent to conscious or unconscious attempts to please the provider. If experience in other areas is indicative, one might expect that the latter, at least, could be reduced by careful attention to the wording of questions (Catania et al. 1996). We do know that if patients admit nonadherence, their admissions are likely to be true. Diverse rates of adherence are reported by patients (ranging from 0% to 100%), and these self-reports have been predictive of changes in viral load and other health outcomes (Hecht et al. 1998).

***Patient diaries***

Patient diaries appear to hold the promise of more detailed information than provided by episodic patient self-report; because they may not suffer from the recall problem, they permit, in principle, assessment of compliance for all drugs and for the entire period they cover. However, overestimation of compliance in diaries appears to be similar to that of unaided patient self-report (Straka et al. 1997). In addition, the cost of a diary is substantially greater than patient self-report, because it entails the extra cost of data entry of the large number of diary-recorded events. Moreover, completing diary forms may be difficult or impossible for those patients who have problems associated with literacy, loss of vision or memory, or adverse living conditions.

***Measurement of drug in biologic fluids***

A common approach to validating actual ingestion of a given drug is to look for the presence of the drug or a metabolite in blood or urine using an appropriate assay. This is frequently the justification for making such a determination, but these measurements are much less exact than is generally appreciated. They also are subject to significant misinterpretation if pharmacokinetic principles are not well understood. Interindividual differences in bioavailability and clearance influence the quantitative relationship between the amount actually ingested and the plasma concentration profile during a dosing interval. The concentration of a drug, measured at a single point in time during a dosing regimen, is affected by the time interval since ingestion of the last dose and by the number of doses taken during a finite time just before the sample. In essence, measurement of concentrations of drug in blood or urine can, at best, reflect semiquantitatively the amount of drug ingested in the time interval just before sampling. This time interval is roughly equal to about three half-lives of the drug.

Thus, for drugs such as digoxin with long half-lives and modest interindividual variation in kinetics, the measurement of concentration of drug may provide a reasonably reliable estimate of patient compliance (Weintraub et al. 1973). For drugs with short half-lives, measurement of drug concentrations is not helpful and is potentially misleading, because some patients may comply with their medication only in the short interval before a visit to their physician and have concentrations of drug consistent with full compliance. In addition, the timing of taking the sample relative to the last dose is very critical for drugs with short half-lives. Further disadvantages are the relatively high cost of some drug assays and the lack of availability of routine assays for many commonly used drugs. A variant of direct measurement of the drug of interest in blood or urine is to use "inert markers" given with the drug. This approach was applied with the use of riboflavin in the VA hypertension trial. The method is subject to the same limitations as the measurement of the drug itself, except that often the assay for the marker is simple and inexpensive. This method may be of particular value when no assay for the drug of interest is available.

***Electronic medication monitors***

Devices that can be used to determine when drugs are removed from a medication dispenser are available. One early device used a radiation source in the dispenser. Recently, the availability of microswitches, integrated circuits, and memories on a microchip have allowed relatively inexpensive electronic medication dispensers to be developed. They can record and store events such as the opening and closing of the container or the tilting of an eyedropper bottle. This information can be recovered and subsequently analyzed, tabulated, and displayed in a variety of formats (Urquhart 1997; Cramer et al. 1989). The advantage of these devices is that actual times of dosing are recorded and can easily be recovered and displayed. A limitation of these devices is that the microprocessor records the opening and closing of the device, rather than actual ingestion of the drug. Therefore, as with pill counts, the data could be confounded by pill dumping or by removal of less or more than one dose with a single opening. Studies published thus far suggest that these limitations do not detract from the value of the information, and these devices reflect true compliance reasonably accurately and quantitatively. Interest in this technology is currently highest in the field of clinical trials, although it has very significant potential in clinical practice, where it could play an important role in the ongoing dialogue that is a necessary component of the therapeutic contract between patient and physician. The cost of the devices and the necessary ancillary equipment for recovering the data from the dispenser is modest compared with the cost of noncompliance and its consequences. A strong argument can be made for incorporating electronic monitoring into routine patient care, but this is not commonly done at this time.

### Enhancing Patient Compliance

Literally thousands of articles have been published about compliance and strategies for improving it (Donovan 1995). This is indicative of the complex causes of noncompliance and the limited success reported thus far in enhancing compliance. Health belief and other behavioral models have been proposed in considering approaches to this issue. Two causes seem to be part of the explanation for noncompliance and are amenable to change. First, lack of explanation about the reasons for therapy is a major cause of noncompliance and therapeutic failures, and may be an area in which to increase compliance (Mazzullo et al. 1974; Larrat et al. 1990; Cameron 1996). The second relates to the complexity of the regimen, which is particularly a factor in treatment of HIV infection and cancer. Efforts to simplify the regimens, and concerted efforts to explain the treatment details and their rationale with the patient, will probably be helpful (Katzenstein et al. 1997; Kastrissios and Blaschke 1998), but few data support any specific interventions thus far.

**PRINCIPLE Absence of data to support the legitimacy of rational and theoretically important therapy should not prevent the experiment in appropriate patients!**

## USING DRUGS FOR NONAPPROVED INDICATIONS

As a result of its enabling legislation in 1906 and subsequent amendments in 1938, 1962, and 1997, the FDA in the United States is charged with evaluating safety and efficacy of drugs using data submitted to the agency by the pharmaceutical sponsor. The FDA is specifically restrained, however, from controlling or interfering with the use of drugs or the practice of medicine by physicians. Companies submit data from phase I-III clinical trials to the FDA in the form of a New Drug Application (NDA) claiming efficacy and safety in the treatment of one or more specified conditions. The FDA responds to these claims by approving or disapproving the NDA or by requesting additional information.

As part of the NDA approval process, the labeling of the drug, in the form of the "package insert," is negotiated between the company and the FDA. This labeling can list only those conditions for which the drug has been officially approved by the FDA. A key fact in labeling a drug is that the FDA can react only to data submitted to the agency and not to data published in the literature but not submitted to the agency. As a result, many of the data about the efficacy and toxicity of a drug that are accumulated after a drug is approved for marketing are never formally submitted to the FDA, never reviewed by the agency, and never incorporated into the package insert.

As discussed in greater detail in other chapters, the limited numbers of patients and conditions studied before submission of an NDA significantly limit the amount of information available about a drug at the time of approval for marketing. A considerable amount of important information about a drug, including new indications, contraindications, unexpected toxicity and efficacy, and optimal dosing regimens in various special patient groups, becomes available only after many more patients have been exposed to the drug than is possible during premarketing trials (Strom and Melmon 1979).

**PRINCIPLE Postmarketing surveillance has so far been the main mechanism for determining the dose–response curve in the target population at risk.**

If drugs are to be used appropriately, the physician must be knowledgeable about the limitations of the package insert and aware of the possible medically legitimate nonapproved indications for the use of a drug. As a result of the 1997 amendments, the FDA is currently in the process of establishing guidelines for direct-to-consumer advertising and the distribution of materials about nonapproved uses by pharmaceutical sales representatives (Hayes 1998). Current information is available through the FDA Internet site (http://www.fda.gov).

There is a subtle but very important distinction between nonapproved uses and nonapproved indications. The term indication carries with it the implication that, although not formally reviewed and approved by the FDA, the data available in the literature are sufficient to support a medical rationale and claim for efficacy, and the indication is, therefore, generally accepted by the medical community. As such, failure to use a drug for a nonapproved medical indication could, under some circumstances, constitute malpractice (e.g., use of $\beta$-blockers after MI to limit recurrence and the morbidity of recurrence). In contrast, there are many other examples in which a drug is used to treat conditions for which the drug has not been approved and in which clear evidence of efficacy is lacking and unlikely to appear in the medical literature.

Valid reasons may exist for a lack of data supporting efficacy, even though the nonapproved use of the drug is indicated for a given condition. A common example is the use of a drug from a general class of drugs in which not all the members have been shown to be efficacious for a given condition but in which the pharmacologic similarities among the members of the drug class would be expected to result in efficacy. A well-known example is the use of many $\beta$-adrenergic receptor antagonists for either hypertension or angina, when individual drugs may have received approval for one indication but not the other. The advantage in these settings of hypertension or angina is that efficacy can be assessed in each individual patient. This easy assessment often is not possible for other nonapproved uses of drugs such as the use of $\beta$-blockers following an acute myocardial infarction (AMI) to prevent sudden death, an indication for which some of these drugs, but not all, have been approved. A different example is the use of a nonsteroidal anti-inflammatory drug (NSAID) as a substitute for aspirin in the prevention of embolization in patients with atrial fibrillation. This might have some pharmacologic rationale in a patient unable to tolerate aspirin, but there are no data to support this use and only limited means of evaluating efficacy in the individual patient. Because this particular problem is uncommon and the outcome of therapy is difficult to evaluate, it is very unlikely that data will ever be generated to support or refute this particular use of the NSAID. Unfortunately, many nonapproved uses are based on substantially weaker evidence, such as individual case reports or purely theoretical considerations. Although use of drugs for such nonapproved indications cannot generally be condoned, it is neither illegal nor uncommon. Physicians deciding to use these drugs for a rational indication have not been penalized for such use in courts of law.

Of concern is whether the current practice of allowing drugs to be used for nonapproved indications encourages pharmaceutical companies to claim safety and efficacy for the most easily documented condition when they file an

NDA for a new drug. If the drug also happens to be a member of a class of drugs with approved or nonapproved indications in a variety of other conditions, the company may hope to take advantage of pharmacologic similarities to broaden the indications. Although the pharmaceutical sponsor may not legally promote the drug directly for these other indications, the promotion is subtle, automatic, and real. Another potential result of discouraging or delaying additional clinical testing for other indications is that important differences in efficacy or toxicity may not be recognized if assumptions are made about similarities among drugs in a sometimes arbitrary or artificial definition of "drug classes." A look at the significant differences in efficacy and toxicity between so-called $\beta$-blockers and calcium-channel blockers serves to emphasize this point, which has been made repeatedly throughout this book.

If the official package insert negotiated between the manufacturer and the FDA cannot be considered as the complete source of information about the appropriate indications for the use of a drug (Herxheimer 1987), where can this information be found? Although the medical literature is the original source of most new data relevant to drugs after they have been marketed, it is extremely difficult for practicing physicians to use the literature as a source of new or comparative information about drug therapy. More than 1500 medical journals are published regularly in the United States alone; of the two to three dozen with circulations in excess of 70,000, the great majority are supported entirely by industry and are sent without charge to physicians. They cannot be considered free of bias. Studies have shown that physicians obtain much of their information about drugs and indications from the intense activities of the marketing branch of the pharmaceutical industry (Avorn et al. 1982), from print and television media, and from the *Physicians' Desk Reference* (PDR). The latter is usually provided without charge to virtually all physicians in the United States. It is primarily a compilation of the package inserts for drugs with all the attendant limitations just noted. It contains no comparative data on adverse effects, efficacy, or cost.

It is not an exaggeration to state that a revolution is currently under way in the provision of information about drugs and therapeutics to patients and health care professionals, brought about by electronic databases and the Internet. Electronic databases maintained by organizations committed to quality, comprehensiveness, and currency of drug information already exist. At the time this chapter was prepared, some of the sources included the US Pharmacopeial Convention (USP) (http://www.usp.org), Micromedix (http://www.mdx.com), First DataBank (http://www.firstdatabank.com), American Society of Health-System Pharmacists (http://www.ashp.org), and Stanford Heath Information Network for Education (SHINE) (http://Shine.Stanford.edu). Many of these entities also provide substantial amounts of information over the Internet. The Internet provides enormous potential for rapid access to important drug and therapeutics information. However, the explosive growth of health-related sites on the Internet poses a major concern, because many of these sites dispense possibly dangerous inaccuracies. Unfortunately, verifying the accuracy of the material found in the vast majority of these sites is difficult, and it is the obligation of the health care provider to verify the accuracy and the source of the content, if possible. If this cannot be done, these sources should be ignored.

For those who prefer to use printed sources of drug information, several inexpensive, unbiased sources of clinical information are preferable to the industry-supported PDR. It is important that they recognize that the physician's use of a drug is not limited to the indications approved by the FDA. *Facts and Comparisons,* published by a division of Lippincott-Raven, is organized by drug classes and contains information in a relatively standard format that incorporates FDA-approved information supplemented with current data from the literature. A useful feature of this publication is its listing of available preparations along with a "cost index" relating the average wholesale price for equivalent quantities of identical or similar drugs and formulations. Another useful source is *American Health Systems Formulary Service* published by the American Society of Health Systems Pharmacists. A third source is the *Drug Information Handbook of the American Pharmaceutical Association,* published by Lexi-Comp, Inc. (available in SHINE). The U.S.P.-DI, an authoritative and comprehensive three-volume set published yearly in print and on CD-ROM by USP Convention, Inc., is currently being marketed by USP in collaboration with the Thomson Healthcare Information Group.

## GENERIC DRUGS AND DRUG SUBSTITUTION

Once the patent protection for an FDA-approved drug expires, generic products often become available. A generic drug formulation is one that contains the same therapeutically active chemical ingredient as the brand-name product marketed by the drug's developer (innovator), in the same dose amounts and dosage form (e.g., capsules, tablets). The Drug Price Competition and Patent Term Restoration Act, enacted in 1984, was intended primarily to simplify and expedite the approval of generic drugs, and, largely because of a desire to reduce the cost of drugs to the consumer (and state-supported health programs), generic substitution is permitted or even mandated in many states unless specifically prohibited by the prescribing physician. This legislation and the subsequent state rules are based on the assumption that plasma drug concentrations are a surrogate for therapeutic equivalence when the chemical structure is identical to the innovator, and on the view that relatively simple and limited bioequivalence testing can be used to judge whether formulations are generically equivalent and that they will be less expensive. These assumptions and views, however, are not universally accepted, and have been challenged on a number of occasions by the innovator companies.

The current practice for most bioequivalence studies is to use single-dose studies carried out in relatively small numbers of young healthy volunteers using cross-over designs. Bioequivalence of different formulations of the same drug substance involves equivalence with respect to the rate and extent of drug absorption. Two formulations whose rate and extent of absorption differ by −20%/+25% or less are generally considered bioequivalent. In order to verify, for a particular pharmacokinetic parameter, that the −20%/+25% rule is satisfied, two one-sided statistical tests are used. Computationally, the two one-sided tests are carried out by computing a 90% confidence interval. For approval, the generic manufacturer must show that a 90% confidence interval for the ratio of the mean response (usually the area under the plasma concentration-time curve [AUC] and maximum concentration of drug in plasma [$C_{max}$]) of its product to that of the innovator is within the limits of 0.8 and 1.25, using the log-transformed data. If the true average response of the generic product in the population is near 20% below or 25% above the innovator average, one or both of the confidence limits is likely to fall outside the acceptable range, and the product will fail the bioequivalence test. Consequently, an approved product is likely to differ from that of the innovator by far less than this quantity. The current practice of carrying out two one-sided tests at the 0.05 level of significance ensures that if the two products truly differ by as much as or more than is allowed by the equivalence criteria (usually −20%/+25%), there is no more than a 5% chance that they will be approved as equivalent. Because the results of a bioequivalence study usually must be acceptable for both AUC and $C_{max}$, a generic product that truly differs by −20%/+25% or more from the innovator product with respect to either parameter would actually have less than a 5% chance of being approved. This reflects the primary concern of the regulatory agency to protect the patient against acceptance of bioequivalence if it does not hold true (FDA's Approved Prescription Drug Products with Therapeutic Equivalence Evaluations known as the "Orange Book").

The basic prescribing issues the physician should consider in deciding how to prescribe a drug available generically are "prescribability" and "switchability," which are linked to the concepts of population and individual bioequivalence (Hauck and Anderson 1991; Patnaik et al. 1997). Prescribability refers to the choice between two or more drug products for the drug-naive patient. Demonstration of population bioequivalence is sufficient for the physician to prescribe any of the bioequivalent drugs. Switchability refers to the requirement that no loss of efficacy or increase in toxicity occurs when a patient is changed from one generic formulation to another, and that no additional titration is needed. Switchability implies the need to demonstrate individual bioequivalence. The design and analysis described above are adequate to demonstrate population bioequivalence, but not individual bioequivalence. Fortunately, many drugs have a wide therapeutic index and are usually prescribed in doses in excess of those required to achieve the desired therapeutic effect (e.g., many antibiotics). There is an ongoing debate about the value of individual bioequivalence, mostly related to the need for switchability for drugs with narrow therapeutic indices, such as cardiac glycosides, anticonvulsants, antidepressants, anticoagulants, and antiarrhythmic drugs. Demonstrating individual bioequivalence will require more complex study designs, and an alternative data analysis procedure, and the utility of this is still being debated (Benet and Goyan 1995).

Another issue being debated is whether disease states or patient demographics such as age or gender can differentially influence and invalidate comparisons of bioavailability carried out in normal volunteers. At present, there is little to indicate this is the case, although a gender-by-formulation interaction has been suggested. More data are needed to determine the importance of diseases or other factors in terms of comparative bioequivalence studies.

To encourage physicians to prescribe generically and to assist them in determining which drugs are not likely to have bioequivalence problems, the FDA has published a series of monographs entitled *Approved Prescription*

*Drug Products with Therapeutic Equivalence Evaluations* (the "Orange Book"). This information is now available and updated frequently at an FDA Internet site (http://www.accessdata.fda.gov/ob/default.htm), and is helpful to physicians considering whether to prescribe a particular drug generically or to permit generic substitution by the pharmacist.

When using a drug with a narrow therapeutic index, the physician may choose to prescribe a less expensive generic equivalent, if available, but in any case, he or she should always individualize the dose for the patient using the same product that will be employed during long-term therapy. Once the dose has been titrated, it would be desirable to avoid substitution to another product because of the small possibility of inequivalence. Nevertheless, substitution will still occur for a variety of reasons. In a patient who is especially sensitive to small changes in dose, the physician may need to communicate directly with the pharmacist responsible for providing refills, and to explain to the patient the need for obtaining the drug from a single source. If substitution of another brand name or generic equivalent is necessary, the physician must monitor such a patient for possible loss of efficacy or toxicity. Measurements of drug concentrations in serum or plasma are available for many drugs having narrow therapeutic indices. A conservative approach in this setting is to obtain a steady-state measurement of drug concentration whenever there is a change in the product used, especially when the drug is being administered as prophylaxis against infrequent but potentially serious events, such as cardiac arrhythmias or seizures. In the event of apparent loss of efficacy during chronic therapy, a change in product bioavailability should be considered as a possible explanation, although noncompliance is a more likely explanation. Again, if available, measurement of concentrations of drug in serum may help in working up this therapeutic problem. Unexpectedly low concentrations could represent either poor bioavailability or poor compliance, whereas concentrations within the therapeutic range suggest loss of efficacy because of a change in the patient.

It is often difficult to determine whether there will be significant cost savings to the patient or insurance provider if a prescription is filled with a generic product instead of a brand-name product familiar to the physician. Most physicians, in fact, are not aware of the cost of the drugs they prescribe and tend to overestimate the cost of inexpensive drugs and underestimate the cost of more expensive drugs (Glickman et al. 1994). We have tried to partially remedy this problem in selected chapters of this book. In addition, *Facts and Comparisons,* mentioned earlier, is indexed by both generic and brand names, lists drug products with identical formulations, and gives the name of the manufacturer; it also provides a cost index, which is a ratio of the average wholesale prices for equivalent quantities of a drug. Although this type of information may alert the physician to potentially large differences in the cost of various generic equivalents, the actual cost of the drug to the patient is determined by many factors, including the profit margin of the source used to fill the prescription as well as the price charged by the manufacturer. Not only is it appropriate to discuss prescription costs with the patient, but such exchanges may improve the physician–patient relationship by demonstrating the physician's interest in financial matters, which frequently concern the patient, and may broaden the dialogue in this important area. If, as already discussed, the therapeutic ratio and chronicity of treatment favor use of a particular drug product, this should be explained to the patient. On the other hand, when prescribing drugs for which modest differences in bioavailability are unlikely to affect efficacy or toxicity, the physician should permit substitution of the least expensive generic equivalent.

## NONPRESCRIPTION DRUGS

In the past decade, patients have become increasingly involved in decisions about their own health care. One aspect of this is their pursuit of a variety of alternative and complementary approaches to medicine, including the ingestion of nontraditional agents such as vitamins, herbs and botanical agents, and "nutraceuticals." They also have access to an increasing number of drugs that can be obtained without seeing a physician. Although this section will focus on nonprescription drugs, the importance of complementary and alternative medicine to the therapeutic contract and patient outcome must be noted.

Nonprescription drugs are medications that can be obtained OTC or without a prescription. That nonprescription drugs can be obtained without consultation with a physician could suggest that they have little significant pharmacologic activity and therefore the physician need not be concerned about their use. Both implications are certainly false. Nonprescription drugs are a part of the therapeutic alternatives available to patients and to physicians. If a physician does not ask the patient about use of nonprescription drugs (as well as about alternative therapies) and does not recommend them when indicated, an important part of the therapeutic contract is neglected.

Nonprescription drugs are a multibillion dollar industry in the United States. Recognizing that they can have significant therapeutic or toxic activity, an interesting question is why both prescription and nonprescription drugs exist, and why they differ from country to country. The answer relates to access, economics, and individual liberties. The history of nonprescription drugs in the United States can be traced back to the mid-1850s, when the majority of health care was provided by lay practitioners, not by physicians, and when most remedies or medicines were concocted and administered in the home. Following the 1860s, preparation of remedies in the home was replaced by purchase of patent medicines. By 1905, the market for patent medicines was immense, well over $100 million per year, and the profits were enormous. The patent medicine makers were the first American manufacturers to use advertising to establish a national market, and they spent as much as $400,000 to advertise a single product. Between about 1890 and 1920, however, an intense economic and political struggle (including the passage of the Pure Food and Drug Act of 1906), along with a change in public preference away from home medical care to professional care, resulted in a marked decline in public demand for and use of patent medicines.

The public's fear and mistrust of hospitals and physicians was replaced by concerns about the dangers of self-treatment and greater confidence in the medical profession. Coincidentally, there was a sharp increase in the sale of prescription drugs. Patent medicines, which could no longer compete with prescription drugs, were replaced by a wide variety of OTC products aimed primarily at providing symptomatic relief for minor problems and complementing rather than competing with medical services provided by physicians (Caplan 1989). An interesting brief review of the origins of prescription drugs was published (Marks 1995).

Today, the trend toward self-care, an increasing role for patients in maintaining their own health, and reclassification of many drugs formerly available only by prescription to OTC status have significantly increased the nonprescription drug market. It now amounts to over $4 billion, or more than $15 for every person in the United States per year. However, accurate statistics on individual use of nonprescription drugs are scarce. Surveys suggest that a high percentage of Americans use nonprescription drugs. These drugs constitute 70% of the initial therapy of episodes of illness (Knapp and Knapp 1972).

Given this background, the significance of nonprescription drugs to the therapeutic contract between patient and physician must now be put into context. Several questions need to be addressed: What kinds of nonprescription drugs are used? Who uses them? How does their use relate to prescription drug use or to the seeking of professional care? Not surprisingly, data indicate that both prescription and nonprescription drug use are more common in elderly persons. In a study among ambulatory elderly patients in mainly rural areas of northeastern New York state, 81% reported that they were taking at least one prescription or nonprescription medication (Stoller 1988). About half of those surveyed reported taking nonprescription medications in the past month. Among these, the average number of nonprescription medications was 1.5 per person. The most frequently used nonprescription medications were analgesics, taken by 39% of respondents; laxatives, taken by 17%; vitamins, taken by 5%; antacids, taken by 4%; and cough or cold preparations, taken by about 2%. The Health Insurance Experiment of the Rand Corporation (Leibowitz 1989) found fairly infrequent purchase of nonprescription drugs by noninstitutionalized individuals under age 65, who averaged just under one purchase per person per year (Leibowitz et al. 1985). Analgesics and cold remedies accounted for about 25% of the purchases, and antacids, bronchodilators, and diuretics, commonly associated with more chronic illnesses, also accounted for about 25% of purchases. Both of these studies attempted to analyze the factors explaining use of nonprescription drugs and its impact on use of prescription drugs and of professional health care. Both concluded that nonprescription drugs are not used as a substitute for prescription medications or for obtaining professional medical care for illnesses perceived as serious by the patient.

A number of factors seem to influence use of nonprescription medications. Elderly persons and women are the most frequent users of nonprescription drugs. Patients with higher educational levels, less time available for physician visits, or less access to professional medical care are more likely to use nonprescription medications, as are patients who are socially isolated or who have chronic illnesses. The factor with the greatest influence on use of nonprescription medications is the number of recent symptoms, whereas both symptoms and frequency of visits to the physician influence the number of prescription medications (Stoller 1988). Use of nonprescription and prescription drugs is correlated, partly because less healthy individuals use more of both types of drug. It is noteworthy that as the cost to the patient of prescription and nonprescription drugs increases, fewer of each type are purchased per capita (Leibowitz 1989).

**Key Point: These two careful studies suggest that nonprescription drugs are used primarily for symptomatic relief, and not as substitutes for prescription drugs or visits to the physician except when access to professional care is limited and then only for nonthreatening symptoms.**

Despite widespread use of nonprescription drugs, the incidence and frequency of serious toxicity from these agents is very low. The fear of dramatic increases in nephrotoxicity with reclassification of NSAIDs such as ibuprofen to a nonprescription basis has not been warranted, although deterioration of renal function may occur in patients with certain preexisting clinical conditions such as congestive heart failure (CHF), cirrhosis, and renal insufficiency (Murray and Brater 1990). The most common adverse reaction to nonprescription drugs undoubtedly is gastrointestinal bleeding caused by acetylsalicylic acid. As with adverse reactions to prescription drugs, most unwanted reactions to nonprescription drugs are predictable, mechanism-based, and dose-related effects of drug use in improper settings, excessive doses, or interactions with other prescription or nonprescription drugs.

The attitudes and responsibilities of physicians with regard to nonprescription drugs determine whether these drugs have a positive or a negative impact on the therapeutic contract. In a study of prescribing behavior for antiinflammatory drugs in two VA hospitals, although physicians believed that aspirin was just as effective as proprietary nonsteroidals for musculoskeletal complaints, had a similar frequency of adverse effects, and was considerably less expensive, they used prescription nonsteroidals almost six times as often as aspirin (Epstein et al. 1984). These authors concluded that physician attitudes about the importance of such issues as cost and placebo effects have a more important role in drug selection than factual information about the alternative drugs themselves.

Physicians should recognize the legitimate role of nonprescription medications in the current environment in which sophisticated and busy patients take a greater role in their own health care decisions. In this regard, an important activity at the time of the first encounter with a new patient is to obtain a complete treatment history from the patient. The history should include nonprescription drugs and, especially today, alternative therapies such as vitamins, herbs and botanicals, and nutraceuticals, and the history should be updated at each subsequent visit. This history may provide useful insights about the patient's attitudes about drugs and expectations of medical care, as well as an opportunity to discuss the proper indications and use of nonprescription medications. This history is also important for avoiding potential interactions with prescribed medications. Moreover, as drugs formerly available only by prescription are changed to nonprescription status, physicians should consider using the nonprescription equivalent, which is usually considerably less expensive.

**PRINCIPLE Dialogue between patient and physician regarding the indication, proper use, and potential adverse effects of the nonprescription drug should be no different than if the physician had written a prescription. In an era when cost considerations are greater than ever, nonprescription drugs should be considered, when appropriate, as alternatives to prescription medications.**

## FORMULARIES

In 1995, outpatient prescription drug costs amounting to about $55 billion accounted for about 5.6% of US national health expenditures of nearly $1 trillion (HCFA 1997). Drug costs in hospitalized patients account for about 10% of the total cost of hospital care of $350 billion. Largely because of the introduction of newer, more expensive pharmaceuticals, and efforts to control expenditures in this area by managed care providers (Mehl and Santell 1998), the fraction of the pharmacy benefit components of health insurance plans that use a "closed formulary" has increased. More than two-thirds of all health maintenance organizations (HMOs) now use such formularies (Giaquinta 1994), 86% of 29 academic medical centers surveyed have closed formularies, and none have an open formulary (Nash et al. 1993). A closed formulary requires physicians to prescribe only those drugs that are included in the formulary. Although there usually are mechanisms to permit exceptions and to allow use of nonformulary drugs, this is discouraged. A variant of the closed formulary is a "restricted formulary," in which certain drugs may be prescribed only by a subset of physicians. For example, prescribing antineoplastic agents may be restricted to oncologists, or use of thrombolytics may be restricted to cardiologists or intensive-care practitioners.

There is considerable debate over the value of a closed or restricted formulary as opposed to an open formulary that allows the physician to prescribe any drug for any legitimate indication. Besides the obvious purpose of containing costs by competitive purchasing arrangements, arguments favoring use of a closed or restricted formulary are that they prevent broad use of relatively untried drugs, encourage good prescribing, restrict the total number of drugs used within a therapeutic category and increase physician familiarity with those drugs, and encourage generic prescribing (Woodhouse 1994). In many managed care settings, closed or restricted formularies are part of a larger effort to incorporate "clinical pathways," "disease management," or "practice guidelines" into inpatient and outpatient care. The restricted or closed formulary also limits use of higher-priced biotechnology drugs, which, along with antineoplastic agents, fibrinolytics, and antibiotics, represent approximately 40% of drug expenditures in hospitals and approximately 60% of the drug expenditures in clinic settings (Mehl and Santell 1998).

There are also important arguments against closed or restricted formularies; some are obvious and others not so obvious. An obvious one is the cost of establishing and maintaining such a formulary, as new drugs are marketed and new information becomes available. The importance of this is inversely proportional to the number of patients covered by the formulary. A subtle, but more important, issue is the effect of a closed or restricted formulary on the relationships with the prescribers. When restricted formularies are used to exclude expensive but unquestionably beneficial drugs, or when the procedure to authorize use of nonformulary drugs is excessively complicated or decisions arbitrary, a hostile, confrontational relationship is created (Woodhouse 1994). Even less obvious but most important is the effect that closed or restricted formularies may have on treatment outcomes.

**Key Point: There is some evidence that measures taken to restrict physician access to certain drugs, or to a specific number of drugs, reduce drug expenditures, but increase overall cost of care.**

Soumerai and co-workers examined the effects of a three-prescription monthly payment limit (cap) on the use of psychotropic drugs and acute mental health care by noninstitutionalized Medicaid patients with schizophrenia in New Hampshire, and compared it with effects on similar patients in New Jersey where no cap was imposed. The cap resulted in immediate reductions in use of psychoactive drugs, but also resulted in coincident increases of one to two visits per patient per month in visits to mental health centers and sharp increases in use of emergency mental health services. After the cap was discontinued, the use of medications and most mental health services reverted to baseline values. The estimated average increase in mental health-care costs per patient during the cap ($1530) exceeded the savings in drug costs to Medicaid by a factor of 17. The investigators concluded that limits on coverage for the costs of prescription drugs can increase use of acute mental health services and costs of care, in addition to increasing pain and suffering on the part of affected patients (Soumerai et al. 1994). In an earlier study of Medicaid recipients 60 years of age or older taking three or more medications per month, including at least one maintenance drug for certain chronic diseases, Soumerai and colleagues found the 35% decline in the use of study drugs after a three-drug limit per patient cap was applied. However, this was associated with an increase in rates of admission to nursing homes. Of the patients who regularly took three or more study medications at baseline, relative risk of admission to a nursing home during the period of the cap was 2.2 and risk of hospitalization was 1.2. When the cap was discontinued after 11 months, use of medications returned to nearly baseline values, and excess risk of admission to a nursing home ceased. In general, patients who were admitted to nursing homes did not return to the community.

**Key Point: Limiting reimbursement for effective drugs may put frail, elderly patients at increased risk of institutionalization in nursing homes and may actually increase cost (Soumerai et al. 1994).**

These two studies are cited as examples of badly-thought-out efforts to restrict drug use and reduce costs; there are numerous other examples in which antibiotic use was regulated by closed or restricted formularies with considerable savings in drug expenditures and no decrement in efficacy or safety.

The complexity of predicting economic impact of attempting to reduce costs by limiting access to drugs is further illustrated by the Managed Care Outcomes Project, a prospective observational study (Horn et al. 1996). This study found that formulary limitations on drug availability were positively correlated with higher rates of emergency department visits and hospital admissions, and to drug cost, drug count, and office visits. The authors concluded that limited formularies had the unintended consequence of increased utilization of health-care services, and they recommended a systems approach rather than individual component management of costs.

SUMMARY

**All of these studies emphasize the importance of thoughtful, nonarbitrary application of closed or restricted formularies, and of studying the impact of closed or restricted formularies on both overall costs and outcomes. A similar caveat should be applied to use of practice guidelines, clinical pathways, or disease management algorithms.**

Consolidation of managed care providers and the level of completeness of clinical information systems and databases now being attained will allow cost-effectiveness and cost-outcome studies to be carried out much more readily.

## REFERENCES


Avorn J. 1995. The prescription as final common pathway. *Int J Technol Assess Health Care* **11**:384–90.

Avorn J, Chen M, Hartley R. 1982. Scientific versus commercial sources of influence on the prescribing behavior of physicians. *Am J Med* **73**:4–8.

Beecher HK. 1955. The powerful placebo. *JAMA* **159**:1602–6.

Benet LZ, Goyan JE. 1995. Bioequivalence and narrow therapeutic index drugs. *Pharmacotherapy* **15**:433–40.

Benson H, Epstein MD. 1975. The placebo effect: a neglected asset in the care of patients. *JAMA* **232**:1225–7.

Benson H, Friedman R. 1996. Harnessing the power of the placebo effect and renaming it "remembered wellness." *Annu Rev Med* **47**:193–9.

Bergman AB, Werner RJ. 1963. Failure of children to receive penicillin by mouth. *N Engl J Med* **268**:1334–8.

Bienenfeld L, Frishman W, Glasser SP. 1996. The placebo effect in cardiovascular disease. *Am Heart J* **132**:1207–21.

Bok S. 1974. The ethics of giving placebos. *Sci Am* **231**:17–23.

Brandimonte MA, Gerbino W. 1993. Mental image reversal and verbal recoding: when ducks become rabbits. *Mem Cognit* **21**:23–33.

Briet F, Pochart P, Marteau P, et al. 1997. Improved clinical tolerance to chronic lactose ingestion in subjects with lactose intolerance: a placebo effect? *Gut* **41**:632–5.

Brody BA. 1997. When are placebo-controlled trials no longer appropriate? *Controlled Clin Trials* **18**:602–12; discussion 661–6.

Brody DS. 1980. The patient's role in clinical decision-making. *Ann Intern Med* **93**:718–22.

Brown WA. 1994. Placebo as a treatment for depression. *Neuropsychopharmacology* **10**:265–9; discussion 271–88.

Brown WA. 1998. The placebo effect. *Sci Am* **278**:90–5.

Cameron C. 1996. Patient compliance: recognition of factors involved and suggestions for promoting compliance with therapeutic regimens. *J Adv Nurs* **24**:244–50.

Caplan RL. 1989. The commodification of American health care. *Soc Sci Med* **28**:1139–48.

Catania J, Binson D, Canchola J, et al. 1996. Effects of interviewer gender, interviewer choice, and item context on responses to questions concerning sexual behavior. *Pub Op Quart* **60**:345–70.

Cecil DW, Killeen I. 1997. Control, compliance, and satisfaction in the family practice encounter. *Fam Med* **29**:653–7.

Cox D. 1998. Discussion. *Stat Med* **17**:387–9.

Cramer JA, Mattson RH, Prevey ML, et al. 1989. How often is medication taken as prescribed? A novel assessment technique. [Erratum: 1989. *JAMA* **262**:1472.] *JAMA* **261**:3273–7.

De Klerk E, Van Der Linden SJ. 1996. Compliance monitoring of NSAID drug therapy in ankylosing spondylitis: experiences with an electronic monitoring device. *Br J Rheumatol* **35**:60–5.

Donovan JL. 1995. Patient decision making: the missing ingredientin compliance research. *Int J Technol Assess Health Care* **11**: 443–55.

Efron B. 1998. Foreword: Limburg compliance symposium. *Stat Med* **17**:249–50.

Egbert LD, Battit GE, Welch CE, et al. 1964. Reduction of postoperative pain by encouragement and instruction of patients: a study of physician–patient rapport. *N Engl J Med* **270**:825–7.

Elixhauser A, Halpern M, Schmier J, et al. 1998. Health care CBA and CEA from 1991 to 1996: an updated bibliography. *Med Care* **36**:MS1–9, MS18–147.

Epstein AM, Read JL, Winickoff R. 1984. Physician beliefs, attitudes, and prescribing behavior for anti-inflammatory drugs. *Am J Med* **77**:313–8.

Evidence-Based Medicine Working Group. 1992. Evidence-based medicine: a new approach to teaching the practice of medicine. *JAMA* **268**:2420–5.

Feinstein AR. 1976. Clinical biostatistics. XXXV. The persistent clinical failures and fallacies of the UGDP study. *Clin Pharmacol Ther* **19**:78–93.

Gerbino PP. 1993. Foreword. *Ann Pharmacother* **27**:S3–4.

Giaquinta D. 1994. Drug formularies—good or evil? A view from a managed care provider. *Cardiology* **85**:30–5.

Glickman L, Bruce EA, Caro FG, et al. 1994. Physicians' knowledge of drug costs for the elderly. *J Am Geriatr Soc* **42**:992–6.

Goetghebeur E, Molenberghs G, Katz J. 1998. Estimating the causal effect of compliance on binary outcome in randomized controlled trials. *Stat Med* **17**:341–55.

Goldsmith CH. 1979. The effect of compliance distributions on therapeutic trials. In: Haynes RB, Taylor DW, Sackett DL, editors. *Compliance in Health Care*. Vol. 1. Baltimore: Johns Hopkins University Press. p 297–308.

Guyatt GH, Keller JL, Jaeschke R, et al. 1990. The n-of-1 randomized controlled trial: clinical usefulness. Our three-year experience. *Ann Intern Med* **112**:293–9.

Hauck WW, Anderson S. 1991. Individual bioequivalence: what matters to the patient. *Stat Med* **10**:959; discussion 959–60.

Hayes TA. 1998. The Food and Drug Administration's regulation of drug labeling, advertising, and promotion: looking back and looking ahead. *Clin Pharmacol Ther* **63**:607–16.

Haynes RB. 1979. Introduction. In: Haynes RB, Taylor DW, Sackett DL, editors. *Compliance in Health Care*. Vol. 1–7. Baltimore and London: Johns Hopkins University Press.

Health Care Financing Administration [HCFA]. 1997. Available from Pharmaceutical Manufacturers' Association, http://www.phrma.org/ and http://www.hcfa.gov.

Hecht FM, Colfax G, Swanson M, et al. 1998. Adherence and effectiveness of protease inhibitors in clinical practice. *Fifth Conference on Retroviruses and Opportunistic Infections*, 2–6 Feb 1998, Chicago.

Herxheimer A. 1987. Basic information that prescribers are not getting about drugs. *Lancet* **1**:31–3.

Horn SD, Sharkey PD, Tracy DM, et al. 1996. Intended and unintended consequences of HMO cost-containment strategies: results from the Managed Care Outcomes Project. *Am J Managed Care* **2**: 253–64.

Kassirer JP, Moskowitz AJ, Lau J, et al. 1987. Decision analysis: a progress report. *Ann Intern Med* **106**:275–91.

Kastrissios H, Blaschke TF. 1997. Medication compliance as a feature in drug development. *Annu Rev Pharmacol Toxicol* **37**:451–75.

Kastrissios H, Blaschke TF. 1998. Therapeutic implications of nonadherence with antiretroviral drug regimens. *HIV: Adv Res Ther* **8**:24–8.

Katkin ES, Murray EN. 1968. Instrumental conditioning of autonomically mediated behavior: theoretical and methodological issues. *Psychol Bull* **70**:52–68.

Katzenstein DA, Lyons C, Molaghan JP, et al. 1997. HIV therapeutics: confronting adherence. *J Assoc Nurses AIDS Care* **8**:46–58.

Knapp DA, Knapp DE. 1972. Decision-making and self medication: preliminary findings. *Am J Hosp Pharm* **29**:1004–12.

Lambert BL. 1997. Predicting look-alike and sound-alike medication errors. *Am J Health Syst Pharm* **54**:1161–71.

Larrat EP, Taubman AH, Willey C. 1990. Compliance-related problems in the ambulatory population. *Am Pharm* **NS30**:18–23.

Lasagna L. 1986. The placebo effect. *J Allergy Clin Immunol* **78**: 161–5.

Lasagna L, Mosteller F, von Felsinger JM, et al. 1954. A study of the placebo response. *Am J Med* **16**:770–9.

Leibowitz A. 1989. Substitution between prescribed and over-the-counter medications. *Med Care* **27**:85–94.

Leibowitz A, Manning WG, Newhouse JP. 1985. The demand for prescription drugs as a function of cost-sharing. *Soc Sci Med* **21**: 1063–9.

Lenert LA, Markowitz DR, Blaschke TF. 1993. Primum non nocere? Valuing of the risk of drug toxicity in therapeutic decision making. [Erratum: 1993. *Clin Pharmacol Ther* **54**:64.] *Clin Pharmacol Ther* **53**:285–91.

Lenert LA, Morss S, Goldstein MK, et al. 1997. Measurement of the validity of utility elicitations performed by computerized interview. *Med Care* **35**:915–20.

Lesar TS, Briceland L, Stein DS. 1997. Factors related to errors in medication prescribing. *JAMA* **277**:312–7.

Leslie A. 1954. Ethics and practice of placebo therapy. *Am J Med* **16**:854–62.

Lesse S. 1962. Placebo reactions in psychotherapy. *Dis Nerv Syst* **23**:313–9.

Marks HM. 1995. Revisiting "the origins of compulsory drug prescriptions." *Am J Public Health* **85**:109–15.

Maronde RF, Chan LS, Larsen FJ, et al. 1989. Underutilization of antihypertensive drugs and associated hospitalization. *Med Care* **27**:1159–66.

Mazzullo JM, Lasagna L, Griner PF. 1974. Variations in interpretation of prescription instructions: the need for improved prescribing habits. *JAMA* **227**:929–31.

McCaffery M, Ferrell BR, Pasero CL. 1998. When the physician prescribes a placebo. *Am J Nurs* **98**:52–3.

Mehl B, Santell JP. 1998. Projecting future drug expenditures—1998. *Am J Health Syst Pharm* **55**:127–36.

Miller LJ. 1990. The formal treatment contract in the inpatient management of borderline personality disorder. *Hosp Community Psychiatry* **41**:985–7.

Monette J, Gurwitz JH, Rochon PA, et al. 1997. Physician attitudes concerning warfarin for stroke prevention in atrial fibrillation: results of a survey of long-term care practitioners. *J Am Geriatr Soc* **45**:1060–5.

Moore RD, Lietman PS, Smith CR. 1987. Clinical response to aminoglycoside therapy: importance of the ratio of peak concentration to minimal inhibitory concentration. *J Infect Dis* **155**:93–9.

Murray MD, Brater DC. 1990. Adverse effects of nonsteroidal anti-inflammatory drugs on renal function [editorial]. *Ann Intern Med* **112**:559–60.

Nash DB, Catalano ML, Wordell CJ. 1993. The formulary decision-making process in a US academic medical center. *Pharmacoeconomics* **3**:22–35.

Noone P, Parsons TM, Pattison JR, et al. 1974. Experience in monitoring gentamicin therapy during treatment of serious gram-negative sepsis. *Br Med J* **1**:477–81.

Ojehagen A, Berglund M. 1986. To keep the alcoholic in out-patient treatment: a differentiated approach through treatment contracts. *Acta Psychiatr Scand* **73**:68–75.

Overall JE, Hollister LE, Pokorny AD, et al. 1962. Drug therapy in depressions: controlled evaluation of imipramine, isocarboxazide, dextroamphetamine-amobarbital, and placebo. *Clin Pharmacol Therap* **3**:16–22.

Park LC, Lipman RS. 1964. A comparison of patient dosage deviation reports with pill counts. *Psychopharmacologia* **6**:299–302.

Patnaik RN, Lesko LJ, Chen ML, et al. 1997. Individual bioequivalence: new concepts in the statistical assessment of bioequivalence metrics. FDA Individual Bioequivalence Working Group. [Erratum: 1997. *Clin Pharmacokinet* **33**:312]. *Clin Pharmacokinet* **33**: 1–6.

[PDR] 1998. *Physician's Desk Reference*. Montvale (NJ): Medical Economics Data Production Co.

Placebos. 1982. *Ann Intern Med* **97**:781.

Pullar T, Kumar S, Tindall H, et al. 1989. Time to stop counting the tablets? *Clin Pharmacol Ther* **46**:163–8.

Rothman KJ, Michels KB. 1994. The continuing unethical use of placebo controls. *N Engl J Med* **331**:394–8.

Rubin DB. 1998. More powerful randomization-based $p$-values in double-blind trials with non-compliance. *Stat Med* **17**:371–85.

Rudd P, Byyny RL, Zachary V, et al. 1989. The natural history of medication compliance in a drug trial: limitations of pill counts. *Clin Pharmacol Ther* **46**:169–76.

Sackett DL, Rosenberg WM, Gray JA, et al. 1996. Evidence based medicine: what it is and what it isn't [editorial]. *Br Med J* **312**: 71–2.

Schwartz RK, Soumerai SB, Avorn J. 1989. Physician motivations for nonscientific drug prescribing. *Soc Sci Med* **28**:577–82.

Sheiner LB. 1997. Learning versus confirming in clinical drug development. *Clin Pharmacol Ther* **61**:275–91.

Sheiner LB, Rubin DB. 1995. Intention-to-treat analysis and the goals of clinical trials. *Clin Pharmacol Ther* **57**:6–15.

Sibille M, Deigat N, Janin A, et al. 1998. Adverse events in phase-I studies: a report in 1015 healthy volunteers. Eur J *Clin Pharmacol* **54**:13–20.

Soumerai SB, McLaughlin TJ, Ross-Degnan D, et al. 1994. Effects of a limit on Medicaid drug-reimbursement benefits on the use of psychotropic agents and acute mental health services by patients with schizophrenia. *N Engl J Med* **331**:650–5.

Stewart RB, Caranasos GJ. 1989. Medication compliance in the elderly. *Med Clin North Am* **73**:1551–63.

Stoller EP. 1988. Prescribed and over-the-counter medicine use by the ambulatory elderly. *Med Care* **26**:1149–57.

Straka RJ, Fish JT, Benson SR, et al. 1997. Patient self-reporting of compliance does not correspond with electronic monitoring: an evaluation using isosorbide dinitrate as a model drug. *Pharmacotherapy* **17**:126–32.

Strom BL, Melmon KL. 1979. Can postmarketing surveillance help to effect optimal drug therapy? *JAMA* **242**:2420–2.

Taubes G. 1995. Use of placebo controls in clinical trials disputed [news]. *Science* **267**:25–6.

Temple RJ. 1997. When are clinical trials of a given agent vs. placebo no longer appropriate or feasible? *Controlled Clin Trials* **18**:613–20; discussion 661–6.

Teplitsky B. 1975. Caution! 1,000 drugs whose names look-alike or sound-alike. *Pharm Times* **41**:75–9.

Thorn DB, Sexton MG, Lemay AP, et al. 1989. Effect of a cancer chemotherapy prescription form on prescription completeness. *Am J Hosp Pharm* **46**:1802–6.

Thornton JG, Lilford RJ, Johnson N. 1992. Decision analysis in medicine. *Br Med J* **304**:1099–103.

Trouton DS. 1957. Placebos and their psychological effects. *J Ment Sci* **103**:344–54.

Turner JA, Deyo RA, Loeser JD, et al. 1994. The importance of placebo effects in pain treatment and research. *JAMA* **271**:1609–14.

Tversky A, Kahneman D. 1974. Judgment under uncertainty: heuristics and biases. *Science* **185**:1124–31.

University Group Diabetes Program (UGDP) 1970. A study of the effects of hypoglycemic agents on vascular complications in patients with adult-onset diabetes: design, methods and baseline characteristics. *Diabetes* **19**(Suppl. 2): 747–83.

Urquhart J. 1997. The electronic medication event monitor: lessons for pharmacotherapy. *Clin Pharmacokinet* **32**:345–56.

Urquhart J, De Klerk E. 1998. Contending paradigms for the interpretation of data on patient compliance with therapeutic drug regimens. *Stat Med* **17**:345–6.

Vanhove GF, Schapiro JM, Winters MA, et al. 1996. Patient compliance and drug failure in protease inhibitor monotherapy [letter]. *JAMA* **276**:1955–6.

Veterans Administration (VA) Cooperative Study Group 1967. Effects of treatment on morbidity in hypertension. Results in patients with diastolic blood pressures averaging 115 through 129 mm Hg. *JAMA* **202**:1028–34.

Weiner M, Weiner GJ. 1996. The kinetics and dynamics of responses to placebo. *Clin Pharmacol Ther* **60**:247–54.

Weintraub M, Au WY, Lasagna L. 1973. Compliance as a determinant of serum digoxin concentration. *JAMA* **224**:481–5.

Wolf S, Pinsky RH. 1954. Effects of placebo administration and occurrence of toxic reactions. *JAMA* **155**:339–41.

Woodhouse KW. 1994. Drug formularies—good or evil? The clinical perspective. *Cardiology* **85**:36–40.

CHAPTER

# 27 DRUG DISCOVERY AND DEVELOPMENT

Richard D. Mamelok

### *Chapter Outline*



The discovery and development of a drug is a process of many steps. The activity requires that multiple skills and various expertise be focused on a single goal: producing a useful therapeutic agent. The history of how skills from academia and industry have been melded to produce new drugs is simply fascinating. Equally impressive is the apparent delicate balance that must be maintained if the relationship is to flourish (Swann 1988; Flowers 1997). The early discovery process, the initial realization that a particular chemical might have medical utility, can have many wellsprings. Important drugs have been discovered by carefully planned, highly logical interventions in a well-defined biochemical pathway, or by serendipity, or by the screening (the more diversified the better) of a large number of chemical entities for a preconceived desirable pharmacologic effect. Recounting the logical approaches combined with driving needs for clinical investigation that led, for example, to purine analogs as antimetabolic drugs (Elion 1989; Flowers 1997), to the discovery of $\beta$-adrenergic antagonists, histamine 2 ($H_2$) antagonists and viral protease inhibitors is to recount scientific intellect and technology transfer at the Nobel prize level. Examples of the serendipitous discovery of drugs illustrate the potential power of recognizing the unexpected and how to take advantage of it.

From discovery of a new chemical entity (NCE) to marketing can take as long as a decade or longer (Lasagna 1979), although in more recent years the time from discovery to approval of important medical advances has diminished. The cost of establishing the evidence that allows a new drug to become available to patients ranges from tens of millions of dollars to hundreds of millions of dollars (Lasagna 1979; Chakrin and Byron 1987). Over time, the cost seems to be rapidly rising.

What evidence is required to show that a drug is safe and effective? What economic considerations should be entertained to justify the use of a new drug? What decisions need to be made during development of a drug in order to decide to persevere or to discontinue development of an NCE? What information is required to make such decisions? There are no absolute answers to any of these questions. The purpose of this chapter is to provide some insight into the problems grappled with by basic scientists, toxicologists, pharmaceutical chemists, clinical investigators, governmental regulators, and clinicians in deciding how to make use of a new chemical entity or a new drug.

## DRUG DISCOVERY AND PRECLINICAL DEVELOPMENT

### Drug Discovery

Drug discovery is the portion of drug development in which NCEs are sought for a particular in vitro or in vivo biologic activity. A biologic target is chosen, and compounds are tested to see how they interact with the target. The biologic target could be a particular biochemical reaction that is thought to be important in causing a pathologic process; it could be a receptor or a microorganism; it could have a more macroscopic effect such as inhibiting an inflammatory reaction or lowering blood pressure. The target, at this stage, is not human.

The choice of an initial target system depends on the depth of our understanding of the pathogenesis of a particular disease for which treatment is sought. For example, if one wanted to discover a drug to treat infection caused by a specific bacterium, the killing of that bacterium in vitro would be a logical initial test of the possible efficacy of the NCE. Such a specific target, highly predictive of activity against the organism wherever it is encountered, is possible only because we have a very detailed and basic understanding of what a bacterial infection is. Contrast bacterial infection with rheumatoid arthritis, in which the basic pathogenetic mechanisms are not fully understood. In the latter case, a number of actions could be appropriate candidates for initial screening of compounds, including inhibition of synthetic enzymes for prostaglandins or cytokines, inhibition of helper T-lymphocyte activation, or even specific binding to the MHC II locus on lymphocytes. Although a compound having any such activity might be useful to patients with rheumatoid arthritis, the predictability of success is less than it would be for antibiotics against a particular infectious organism. Moreover, few, if any, new drugs will cure rheumatoid arthritis. Symptomatic relief or possibly a slowing of progression may be the best result of research that one can hope for with today's understanding of the disease.

## Screening of Compounds

The screening of compounds for biologic activity requires several steps, usually in progressively complex systems. Early in the discovery process, the goal is to screen a large number of compounds in order to identify those with highest activity toward and potency for acting on a particular target. Often hundreds of chemical entities are so screened. Of those, several may be tested further. In the example of a bacterial infection, the disease can be induced in a susceptible animal, and the ability of the investigational drug to cure the infection can be observed. In the case of rheumatoid arthritis, the drug can be given to an animal in which arthritis has been induced by administering a foreign substance to the joint. The induced arthritis is not rheumatoid arthritis, but rather an arthritis that shares some, but certainly not most, of the attributes of rheumatoid arthritis. An approximation of a human disease in an animal is called a *model* of the disease. In the case of bacterial infection, the animal model for infection actually is the same infection as in the human disease for which treatment is desired, whereas for rheumatoid arthritis the model is much less like the human disease, and the drug's effects in the model may be much less applicable to humans. Models are extensively used in pharmaceutic development, but to the degree that they are imprecise reflections of human diseases, they are variably reliable in predicting efficacy in humans even though the efficacy is seen in the model. Conversely, an absence of effect in the model does not preclude value of the drug in humans. The frequency with which useful compounds are discarded because of their failure to affect a particular animal model is not known, since negative results in models almost always lead to discontinuation of the development process before testing occurs in humans.

**PRINCIPLE The effects of drugs in humans are precious and often unique. Full analysis of events drugs can cause is a major way of revealing benefits that were not expected at the time of marketing.**

Bacterial infections are not the only diseases in which a good understanding of the pathophysiology has lead to effective and rather specific therapies. Therapeutically successful drugs that were designed to react with specifically identified molecular targets now are numerous. These include $\beta$-adrenergic antagonists, $H_2$ antagonists, tissue-derived plasminogen activator, inhibitors of enzymes such as angiotensin-converting enzyme (ACE) and hydroxymethylglutaryl coenzyme A (HMG-CoA) reductase, the rate-limiting enzyme in the synthesis of cholesterol, the inhibitors of HIV protease and hematopoietic colony-stimulating factors. Undoubtedly, as diseases are better understood at the molecular level, more specific, but not necessarily more effective, therapies will follow. Generally speaking, the discovery of disease-specific drugs is heavily dependent on the understanding of basic molecular mechanisms of that disease. The recent application of molecular biologic techniques to isolate and synthesize a wide variety of endogenous, biologically active molecules has increased the interaction between the discovery of drugs and the discovery of molecular pathogenetic mechanisms (Halperin 1988; Hood 1988; Mario 1988).

In some settings, instead of screening many compounds to see their effect in a model of a disease, a specific molecule, known to participate in biologic processes, is screened for use in a variety of diseases. This screening philosophy operates even if the test substance has no known activity in the pathologic process of interest. For example, interferons have been tested in a variety of viral infections and cancers. Although interferons are important in modulating immune reactions in such diseases, whether they play a central role in immunity has not been established. Nevertheless, the feasibility of testing such endogenous, biologically active compounds in a spectrum of diseases might lead to new (possibly simultaneous) discoveries in the pathogenesis and therapy of those diseases. In fact, drugs like the interferons have found therapeutic roles despite an incomplete understanding of disease processes.

**PRINCIPLE The effects of drugs, whether anticipated or not, often help to extend knowledge of the pharmacology of the drug and the pathogenesis of the disease it affects.**

## Drug Development

The purpose of "drug discovery" is to identify chemicals that have a high chance of providing therapeutic benefit. Once such a compound is identified, a series of investigations in animals and humans takes place to demonstrate that the compound is efficacious and that it is safe enough for use in people. This phase of investigation is known as *development*. Most drugs that are discovered and go into development do not evolve into marketed medicines. The reasons for the high rate of failure include lack of efficacy, unacceptable toxicity, and problems with developing an acceptable way to deliver the drug to a patient.

The steps required to develop a chemical as a drug are straightforward. In addition to establishing that the NCE has a desired pharmacologic effect in animals, its other pharmacologic effects must be determined. Understanding the full pharmacologic profile of the NCE allows prediction of what to anticipate in humans. Discovery of an undesired effect may terminate further development. For example, if a potential antihypertensive drug causes a fall in blood pressure but also produces extreme sedation, the drug is not likely to be acceptable to patients. Another purpose of pharmacologic testing is to define the dose–response relation of the drug. The lowest dose (on a basis of weight of drug per weight of animal in kilograms) that causes a discernible pharmacologic effect must be determined. This is established in several species of animal in order to establish the safe dose that can be used to initiate testing in humans. The shape (steepness) of the dose–response curve or concentration of drug versus response curve also is useful in design of the first studies in humans. If the dose–response curve is steep, the drug may be difficult to give to humans without producing extreme effects. If the curve is shallow, the dose can be progressively increased to carefully establish the tolerated dose range. In general, concentration response curves are more useful than dose response curves because of differences in rates of elimination that exist between species.

***Pharmacokinetic profile***

Knowledge of the metabolic profile of a drug in several species points toward the methods of search for and discovery of metabolites in humans. Major metabolites should be tested for their pharmacologic or toxicologic activity and then sought during testing in humans. However, before a drug is given to humans, it is difficult to know which animal species will best mimic the metabolic profile that will be seen in humans.

The distribution of drug throughout an animal's body also is determined by using radiolabeled drug. This information can alert investigators to look for effects that relate to organs where large concentrations of the drug may reside in humans.

***Toxicologic testing***

Toxicologic testing in animals helps to focus observation when the drug is given to humans. The toxicologist also can determine the mutagenic, carcinogenic, and teratogenic potential the drug might have. Almost always, intravenous administration is used in animal testing, because using that route ensures that the drug will reach the systemic circulation. Depending on what the eventual route of administration in humans is likely to be, other routes also are tested. Very large doses are given during toxicologic studies in animals. The premise is that large doses will exaggerate effects and reduce variability in results that are due to individual and species differences in susceptibility to a given toxic effect. High doses also are used in order to compensate for the observation that small mammals usually tolerate higher doses than do humans. There is increasing interest in using toxicokinetics (a form of concentration response) rather than simply dose as a means of understanding toxic effects, but these techniques are not universally applied. As in the case of the metabolic studies, humans may be uniquely susceptible to a given effect, and animal studies will not reveal this. Conversely, some drug-induced effects seen in animals may never be produced in humans.

Toxicologic testing is done in animals for periods that often are shorter than those that eventually will be used for long-term therapies in humans. Since small mammals have a life cycle that is considerably shorter than that of humans, we assume that the time it takes for many reactions to occur during chronic administration of drug also will be shortened (Gogerty 1987). Toxicologic studies will not detect allergic or other idiosyncratic reactions that might occur in humans, nor will they predict symptomatic or subjective experiences that might be produced in people. The duration of toxicologic studies varies. Usually single, very high dose studies are done first. Later, studies of progressively longer duration are used. The longest studies usually are undertaken for 2 years of daily dosing in order to detect carcinogenic effects in rodents. Exceptions to this are human recombinant peptides and proteins, because nonhuman species develop antihuman antibodies to these. Thus, long-term delivery is often not feasible or meaningful.

***Drug production issues***

Drug development involves physical and chemical research, in addition to the obvious biologic research. Economically feasible synthetic production processes have to be designed. Strict manufacturing procedures are followed to ensure consistency in purity of the chemical, regardless of the batch. In addition, the drug must be formulated as a final product. Formulation is the process of inserting the active drug into a vehicle that allows practical storage and administration. Milligram or microgram quantities of a pure drug could not be administered accurately. Thus, the drug must be mixed either in solution or in a matrix of solid, "pharmacologically inert" materials (excipient) that can be formed into a capsule or tablet. Solid-dose forms must dissolve adequately in the GI tract, and the excipient component must not interact with the NCE. In addition, the drug product must be chemically stable to ensure that it will not rapidly degrade during storage. The time past which a substantial percentage of the drug will deteriorate must be well described. This time yields the *expiration date* for drugs.

## CLINICAL DEVELOPMENT OF A NEW CHEMICAL ENTITY

Understanding the spectrum of a drug's pharmacologic effects in humans is the basis for clinicians' designing an effective use of the drug in patients. The most effective use of the drug often must await the responses it produces after marketing. Witness the use of aspirin for prevention of myocardial infarction and stroke. Experiments designed to discover pharmacologic effects in patients have their underpinnings in the experimental data obtained from animals. Such testing in humans, as much as possible, duplicates the testing in animals. Of course, certain procedures cannot be carried out in people, and, in such instances, data from animals must be used alone. Conversely, some effects of drugs cannot be detected by studying animals—particularly selected effects in the CNS.

When experiments in animals confirm that a drug has a desired set of potentially efficacious effects and that excessively dangerous toxicologic effects occur at doses substantially higher than those that could produce efficacy, testing in humans can be justified. There are three major objectives in testing in humans. The first is to determine whether the pharmacologic effects seen in humans confirm predictions derived from effect data from animals. When effects in the two species are equivalent, further development in humans may proceed. If a potentially beneficial but unexpected effect is observed in humans, further animal testing may be required before additional studies proceed in humans. The second objective is to show that the pharmacologic actions lead to therapeutically useful effects. The third objective is to demonstrate that the drug is safe enough to be used in humans. Safety is considered in the context of the measured beneficial effects. Tests in humans classically are divided into at least three phases (I to III) (Table 27-1).

### Phase I Testing

In order to make testing in humans as safe as possible, the first doses, chosen with data from animals in mind, are small enough so that no effects are expected. Usually a small number of people, generally healthy volunteers, are observed after they are given a single small dose. If this dose is tolerated, successively higher doses are administered to determine the range of doses that are well tolerated. The escalation of dose is progressive and often is carried out until a limiting adverse event occurs. For example, a potential antihypertensive agent may cause either an excessive drop in blood pressure, or the adverse event may be unrelated to the desired primary pharmacologic effect.

The low-dose challenges are then followed by studies in which higher doses are given over several weeks. Generally, test doses in phase I are given to normal subjects. This practice is appropriate when the drug's expected effects are likely to be transient and easily tolerated. For instance, hemodynamically active drugs intended for patients with congestive heart failure (CHF) may be safely administered to healthy subjects who can tolerate rapid or large hemodynamic changes better than patients with compromised cardiovascular systems. But when the drug's expected effect is likely to be dangerous even when it is efficacious, testing in normal people is not ethically acceptable. For instance, antineoplastic agents are too dan-

**Table 27-1 Drug Development in Humans**

| DURATION | |
|---|---|
| 3–6 months | Phase I. First administration to humans.<br>Who? Normal volunteers or patients—small number.<br>Why? Determine dose tolerability, pharmacokinetics, metabolic products. May detect pharmacologic effects. |
| 6–12 months | Phase II. Administration to patients, special populations such as the elderly or patients with renal failure.<br>Who? Selected patients.<br>Why? Determine efficacy for selected indications; dose or concentration response, estimate size and variability of effect. |
| 12–36 months | Phase III. Large clinical trials in patients.<br>Who? Patients with disease target.<br>Why? Determine efficacy for selected indication and rates of common adverse events.<br>Pharmacoeconomic analyses. |
| Ongoing after approval, indeterminate | Phase IV.<br>Who? Patients treated with drug under conditions of actual use.<br>Why? Determine patterns of drug utilization, additional efficacy and toxicity.<br>By whom? All physicians and pharmacists agreeing to participate in organized reporting. |

SOURCE: Adapted from Melmon KL, Morrelli HF, Hoffman BB, Nierenberg DW, editors. 1992. *Melmon and Morrelli's Clinical Pharmacology: Basic Principles in Therapeutics.* 3d ed. New York: McGraw-Hill. Permission granted by editor.

gerous to give to anyone except to patients who could possibly benefit from the drug, or at least who would not be exposed to much excessive risk relative to the risk of their disease. In spite of the fact that phase I testing in normal people has turned out to be extraordinarily safe, the ethics of performing these tests on normal people is legitimately debated. A drug being developed to treat heart failure may have dose–response curves or even qualitative effects in patients with CHF that differ enough from those seen in healthy subjects to render results in healthy subjects of little value. No matter how safe the early administration of an NCE to normal subjects is, it seems sensible to test early for effects of drugs in the patient population that has something to gain from the experiment.

Pharmacokinetic and metabolic studies also are carried out in humans. Identifying metabolites in humans that were not detected in animals is very important. Such metabolites might require additional animal testing for their pharmacologic, toxicologic, and carcinogenic activity. Knowledge of the major pathways for elimination of the drug, whether hepatic or renal, will be useful for predicting necessary adjustments of dose that may be required in patients with hepatic or renal disease. Knowledge of the distribution, clearance, and half-life, coupled to information on the relationship of the concentration of the drug in plasma to its pharmacologic effect, can help in designing appropriate dosing regimens for definitive testing of efficacy.

## Types of Clinical Trials: Phases II and III

The keystone to any drug development program and the gold standard of experimentation with drugs in humans is the randomized, controlled clinical trial. These trials are designed to test whether a drug is efficacious; essentially they are a test of the null hypothesis.

The null hypothesis assumes there is no difference between two treatments, A and B. If treatment B is much more effective than treatment A (penicillin versus placebo for pneumococcal meningitis), a very small study, or even use of historical controls, will reject the null hypothesis in both *statistically significant and clinically important* terms. If B is marginally effective compared with A, a large sample is needed to show a statistically significant difference. For example, $\beta$-adrenergic blockade to prevent sudden death during the year after myocardial infarction (MI) reduces sudden death rate by 50% (from 5 to 2.5%).

Whether this difference is clinically important enough to warrant the risks of therapy in many who would not benefit (97.5% of tested subjects) is another matter. Statistical design tells us how many patients we must study to find a given degree of difference between treatments A and B if such a difference really exists. The number of patients needed to study depends on three main factors: 1) the probabilities of the two outcomes (e.g., 5 versus 2.5% in the example above); 2) our willingness to allow chance alone to account for an apparent difference between treatment A and treatment B (often set as $\alpha = 0.05$, or $P = 0.05$); and 3) our desire not to miss a difference between A and B if one really exists (often set as $\beta = 0.10$, or a study with a power of 90%).

**PRINCIPLE Keep your eye on the "doughnuts" (clinical goals) as well as the "holes" (the level of statistical significance).**

*Choice of endpoints*

Several important conditions must be met in the design of such trials. The endpoints to be measured to determine efficacy must be clearly defined. Careful consideration must be given to the definition of therapeutic efficacy. For example, if a drug is purported to lower cholesterol concentrations, is it medically appropriate and adequate to show that the drug simply lowers cholesterol concentrations, or should the experiment be designed to confirm or refute that it also prevents MI? Should an antihypertensive be shown merely to lower blood pressure, or should prevention of the morbid consequences of hypertension, such as stroke and renal failure, be the endpoints of the experiment? The general question is whether achievement of a so-called surrogate endpoint is adequate to establish efficacy, or whether some more obviously clinically beneficial endpoint should be demonstrated before a drug is marketed. For a cholesterol-lowering agent, the actual goal of therapy (endpoint) is to prevent atherosclerosis and its consequences. We treat hypertension not simply to lower blood pressure but to prevent its consequences, such as stroke and renal and heart failure. The lower plasma cholesterol concentration and the lower blood pressure are surrogate (not ultimate) endpoints of benefit.

It is usually quicker, and sometimes the only feasible method, to use a surrogate endpoint to show that a drug is efficacious. It may be slower or impossible to show an effect on a more definitive endpoint. Whether one is satisfied that a surrogate endpoint is adequate to establish efficacy is determined by several considerations, such as how closely changes in the surrogate endpoint are linked to causing changes in the definitive endpoint; how much risk is associated with the therapy (the more risk, the surer one wants to be that the definitive endpoint is affected); and what other therapies are available to treat the targeted disease. If alternative therapies already are available for the same indication, the physician has a right to ask for increasingly definitive evidence of effects on the medical objective before giving the drug.

**PRINCIPLE Drug development resembles Bismarck's description of politics: it is the art of the possible.**

*Choice of controls*

The choice of controls is crucial in a controlled clinical trial. The most rigorous and most widely used control is the concurrent control. A concurrent control should consist of a group that is exactly like the group being given the active drug. The concurrent control group is observed simultaneously with the group given the experimental drug.

Most concurrently controlled trials are *double-blind* and *randomized.* Randomization ensures that each subject in the trial had an equal chance of being assigned to either the treatment or the control group. On average, risk factors for developing particular events, such as the endpoint being assessed, will be balanced between the experimental and control groups; if randomization is successful, the only difference between the groups at the start of the study is the treatment to which each is assigned. Randomization is essential for the proper application of statistical tests that will be used to assess the results.

*Avoiding bias with "blinding"*

*Double-blind* means that neither the subjects in the trial nor the observers making the measurements, which will be used to measure efficacy, know who is taking which treatment. Both the response of a subject and the perceptions of an observer will be influenced if they know which treatment is being administered. While blinding is desired and usually attempted, it is not always feasibly maintained. Sometimes, pharmacologic or toxic effects allow a patient or an investigator to determine the nature of the treatment.

*Selecting treatment of the control group*

In order for a trial to be blinded, the control group must also be given a treatment. Otherwise everyone would immediately know who was in the control group. The control group must take something that looks like, and in the case of oral administration tastes like, or in the case of an injection, feels like the active treatment. The nature of the control substance can be either placebo, a substance without specific pharmacologic effects, or an active control, such as another drug used for the same indication. Placebo controls are an absolute standard (see chapter 26, Writing Prescriptions). From the results of a placebo-controlled trial, one can infer whether the active treatment is efficacious or even harmful relative to no treatment. Comparisons of efficacy can be made relative to an active control. However, when no placebo is included and drug A is not as efficacious as drug B, one cannot differentiate between no efficacy or just less efficacy than drug B. If drug A has some efficacy, it could still be useful in those patients who show insufficient or no response to B, or who develop toxicity from or allergy to B. Discovering marginal utility requires a placebo control. If a placebo group is added to a trial so that drug A, drug B, and placebo are tested, then comparisons can be made between both active drugs and placebo.

In the development of a new drug, actively controlled trials in the absence of a placebo are used when a proven treatment exists for the targeted disease and it is dangerous for patients to be removed from the established treatment for the period of time required to conduct the clinical trial. The investigational drug can be substituted for the standard treatment being used for the active control if there is enough evidence from animal studies that the experimental drug is very similar to the standard therapy in terms of its mechanism(s) of action. However, if the experimental drug has a new mechanism of action and is unproven for the same therapeutic benefit as the standard treatment, then it may not be possible to discontinue the standard treatment in any trial. In that case, a clinical trial might consist of the following treatments:

- Treatment I: standard treatment + experimental treatment
- Treatment II: standard treatment + placebo

For such a trial to show that the experimental treatment is efficacious, the new treatment would have to provide benefit beyond the standard treatment. Unless this added benefit is substantial, a very large number of patients are needed in the trial to validate the difference statistically. A large study may not always be feasible, particularly if the disease under study is rare.

It might not be possible to demonstrate the added efficacy provided by the experimental drug. In such a case, a useful alternative to standard therapy could be wrongly discarded. Although this dilemma is not easy to solve, sometimes there are ways to circumvent the problem. For example, if the mechanism of the disease is very well understood, then one could argue that the experimental drug has such a high chance of working that it could be substituted for the standard treatment. This setting is rare. Sometimes a trend suggesting that the experimental drug is efficacious can be found in patients who are not substantially helped by the standard treatment. Discovery of such a trend could justify another trial comparing the two drugs without the need to compare the new therapy to placebo. A third approach is to test for equivalence of a new drug to the standard of care. There are well-defined statistical approaches to testing for equivalence. It is important to realize that the failure to show a difference between two drugs in a trial that initially sets out to differentiate between two therapies is not the same as demonstrating equivalence. In order to demonstrate equivalence, the trial must be designed with that hypothesis in mind. In principle, for two drugs to be shown to be equivalent, there has to be a high degree of certainty that any difference in efficacy observed between two therapies is not of clinical importance and is likely to have occurred by chance.

#### *Evaluating drug safety*

In addition to efficacy, the safety of a new drug has to be evaluated in clinical trials in humans. Information on adverse events associated with taking a drug is collected in the course of every clinical trial. Both objective evidence, such as changes in physical condition or laboratory data, and subjective complaints are obtained from patients and normal subjects. The rigor with which these data are evaluated is limited. Data on safety come from a variety of trials, not all controlled. Thus, it is not possible to be certain which adverse effects are due to the drug and which events that might be considered adverse were caused by the disease or environment. This problem is especially difficult when the disease being treated causes many events that might be mistaken for drug-induced events. Conversely, an event caused by a drug may be ascribed to the disease being treated. An important example of the latter problem is that most drugs that diminish the frequency of cardiac arrhythmias also can increase the frequency of arrhythmias in susceptible patients; likewise, antibiotics can cause infection and fever.

The number of people treated with a new drug in experimental programs before a drug is approved is relatively small. The range in studies is about 500 to 3000 people (Strom et al. 1984). Consequently, only events that commonly are caused by the drug are likely to be detected. Table 27-2 gives estimates of how many people are needed in studies to detect events caused by a drug at given incidence rates and with given relative risks. Med-

Table 27-2 **Required Sample Size***

| Incidence in Control Group | Relative Risk to be Detected 1.25 | 2.0 | 5.0 |
|---|---|---|---|
| 0.0001 | $3.8 \times 10^6$ | $3.2 \times 10^5$ | $3.9 \times 10^4$ |
| 0.001 | $3.8 \times 10^5$ | $3.1 \times 10^4$ | $3.9 \times 10^3$ |
| 0.01 | $3.7 \times 10^4$ | $3.1 \times 10^3$ | $3.8 \times 10^2$ |

*Type I error = 0.05; type II error = 0.1 (power = 90%). The sample size is the number of subjects that would have to be studied in each of the control and experimental groups (Adapted from Strom, 1989).

ically important events often occur at rates of less than 1 in 10,000 with relative risks that are much less than 2 (see chapter 25, Drug Interactions; chapter 28, Risk Analysis Applied to Prescription Drugs; and chapter 30, Information about Drugs: A Clinical Epidemiologic Approach to Therapeutics. Two characteristics of an adverse event caused by a drug determine how readily the adverse event can be ascribed to the drug with some reasonable assurance. The first is the frequency with which the drug causes the event; the second is the frequency with which the event occurs spontaneously in the absence of the drug. The required number of patients exposed to a drug in order to detect a drug-induced event increases as the following ratio decreases:

$$\frac{\text{Frequency of drug-induced event}}{\text{Frequency by which event occurs spontaneously}}$$

For example, as shown in Table 27-1, in order to have a 90% chance of detecting a drug-induced adverse event that occurs spontaneously in 1 in 1000 people of the control group, about 31,000 patients need to be studied in the experimental group to detect an event that occurs with a frequency of 2/1000 in the drug-treated group. For an event that occurs with a frequency of 5/1000 in the drug-treated group, about 3900 patients would have to be studied in the experimental group.

Another factor that determines how difficult it will be to correctly ascribe an event to a drug is the time of onset of the event relative to the time of administration of the drug. If the drug-related event is slow to become evident, recognizing that the event could be related to therapy is difficult.

No drug is absolutely safe. Like all other things in life, taking drugs involves some risk (see chapter 28, Risk Analysis Applied to Prescription Drugs). Ideally, safety and efficacy must be evaluated together in order to decide whether a drug is efficacious enough to justify the risk. For example, more risk is acceptable in a drug that has the potential of curing a fatal disease than in a drug to treat the common cold. Regulatory agencies are very aware of the need for balancing efficacy versus toxicity. The Food and Drug Act in the United States does not define safety and efficacy. These decisions ultimately are made by the regulators and the medical profession.

## Regulatory Functions and Drug Development

In virtually all countries, no drug can be sold to the general population before a governmentally sponsored regulatory review of its safety and efficacy has taken place. This review may be followed by approval for sale. The philosophies and practices of regulatory agencies vary from country to country and are constantly evolving.

***Process of FDA approval***

In the United States, the Food and Drug Administration (FDA) can approve a drug for general use if adequately controlled clinical trials show it is "safe and effective." As mentioned above, the judgment regarding safety and efficacy is a relative one. Higher risks become more acceptable 1) as the seriousness of the disease being treated increases, 2) as the evidence for efficacy becomes stronger, 3) when efficacy is defined as decreasing disability or mortality due to the disease (as opposed to an effect on a surrogate endpoint that has not been definitively linked to progressive morbidity or mortality), 4) when several clinical trials show the same beneficial effect, and 5) when no other treatment exists that offers the same therapeutic advantage as the drug being considered for approval. As in the cases of safety and efficacy, the phrase *adequately controlled clinical trials* also is subject to interpretation. In most cases, *adequately controlled* means randomized, double-blind, and with concurrent controls. However, sometimes a randomized, double-blind trial is not required. When the disease is rare, there may not be enough patients to make a statistically valid, randomized, concurrently controlled trial feasible. In those cases, historical controls may be necessary. Some diseases have an inexorable and predictable course. Reversal of that course by a drug, even in the absence of a concurrent control group, might convince regulators and physicians that a drug is effective. Examples include the rapid reversal of pneumococcal pneumonia by penicillin, or the reversal of opiate-induced coma by naloxone. Such clinical situations are rare; an expert's "belief" that they exist often raises more debate than agreement. As a rule, the need for concurrent controls is respected and should be a high priority of most studies.

The approval process involves multiple steps. After information about a drug has been collected in animals, a sponsor (usually a pharmaceutical company) desiring to investigate a drug in humans must submit an application to the FDA seeking approval to start clinical trials in humans. The application is called an Investigational New Drug application (IND). The application must convince the FDA that the drug has a reasonable chance of being effective, that toxicologic data suggest that the drug should not cause undue harm, that the physical-chemical characteristics of the drug are well described, and that the process to produce the drug is reproducible and results in a sufficiently pure preparation. Once an IND is approved, clinical testing may begin.

Throughout the world, clinical testing classically proceeds in three general phases. Phase I includes initial dosing to establish the range of doses that humans can tolerate. Some information on the drug's pharmacokinetic profile and metabolism is determined. Phase II includes work to define the pharmacologic effects in humans and also includes small clinical trials to determine whether the drug is likely to show efficacy in large definitive trials. Phase III includes large clinical trials designed to investigate whether the drug is efficacious and safe. The majority of drugs that enter phases I and II do not proceed to phase III, either because a toxic effect appears that was not anticipated before the study or because the pharmacologic promise hinted at by animal studies did not materialize in early clinical testing. In addition, when a drug enters phase I testing, generally not all the long-term animal toxicology has been completed. Findings in these long-term toxicology trials occasionally preclude administering the drug to people for protracted periods.

When phase III trials are completed and the sponsor believes that efficacy and safety have been adequately demonstrated, the sponsor compiles all the data to support that assertion in the form of a New Drug Application (NDA). After the FDA reviews this information, it can approve the drug for general use, deny approval, or grant a conditional approval.

**PRINCIPLE The Food, Drug and Cosmetic Act and its amendments require the agency to approve or disapprove marketing of a drug. They do not require that every medically important event caused by the drug, or that the best and optimal uses and indication for the drug, be known. The act was wise and theoretically allows a product with proven efficacy to reach the market in a reasonable time. The rest of the information developed about the drug requires its use in the field. Observations of the results of the drug's use are the profession's and not the FDA's responsibility.**

### *Meaning of FDA approval*

What is it that the FDA actually is able to approve? What is the authority of the FDA? When an NDA is filed, it is filed for a specific indication. An indication can be a symptom such as relief of pain or it can be for a disease such as hypertension or congestive heart failure. An indication can be modified or restricted, such as "the relief of moderate or moderately severe pain" or as "adjunctive therapy in the management of heart failure in patients not responding to diuretics or digitalis." Evidence in an NDA must support the use of a drug for such a particular indication. When approving a drug, the FDA regulates what claims can be made for a drug by the company that will sell it. Regulation of such claims is through two mechanisms. The first is the package insert that is provided to physicians and is published in the *Physicians' Desk Reference* (PDR 1998). This package insert, sometimes referred to as the *label,* provides information on the chemical composition of the drug, description of some of the preclinical and clinical data known about the drug, approved indication or indications, contraindications (situations in which the drug should not be used), adverse events associated with the drug, dosing instructions, and advice on potential problems that could be associated with use of the drug. The other mechanism by which FDA regulates claims about a drug is by regulating advertisements for it. Only approved indications can be advertised, and advertised claims must be based on supporting data that have been reviewed by the FDA.

For drugs that potentially fill a major unmet medical need or which have the potential to change the outcome of particularly dire diseases, the FDA can give an application "fast track" status, in which they target a decision by 6 months. Finally, for some indications the FDA can give a drug an "accelerated" or "conditional" approval based on a surrogate endpoint when the relationship of that endpoint to a more definitive one is not obvious or proven. This type of approval is granted only in cases where the outcome of the disease being treated is dire, even in the face of standard treatment. This approach has been most commonly used in the treatment of HIV-related syndromes and diseases and cancer. The types of endpoints allowed in these situations have been CD4 counts and reduction in tumor size, each a surrogate for prolonged survival. A so-called *accelerated* or *conditional* approval requires that more definitive clinical trials be carried out after the initial approval. In theory, the approval can be withdrawn if the more definitive trials lead to conclusions that the drug is not as efficacious or as safe as originally surmised. In addition, unlike other approved drugs, the company selling the drug may not advertise it for the conditionally approved indication.

In an attempt to provide incentives to companies to bring drugs to market for relatively rare diseases, Congress passed the Orphan Drug Act. To qualify for orphan drug status, the condition for which the drug is intended affects fewer than 200,000 people in the United States. If the drug is approved, the company has exclusive rights to sell the drug for 7 years and no approval will be granted to another product containing the same active moiety.

Although not directly related to the types and timing of approvals, Congress has allowed that user fees be paid by pharmaceutical companies to help defray the costs of a review. The goal was to provide funds that were to enable the FDA to review applications more quickly. A company can be exempt from user fees if they fulfill certain criteria that include the number of employees of a company and the revenues of the company. In practice this means that established firms pay the fees, and new companies without approved products to maintain a revenue stream do not pay them. The payment of fees does not affect the speed at which a product is reviewed. For fiscal year 1997, the user fee for an NDA was about $205,000. The FDA estimated that its revenues from these fees in 1997 would be about $29 million (Federal Register Document 96-32493, 1996).

The FDA legally cannot regulate *how* a drug actually is used by physicians. Such regulation would "interfere with the practice of medicine," and the agency is expressly forbidden from this function by the Food and Drug Act. No physician is bound by any law to follow instructions in the drug's label. If a physician believes that a particular drug should, would, or could be useful for a particular patient with a particular disease, prescribing that drug for that disease may be legitimate and expected, even if FDA has not approved such a use. The physician should be acting on solid information gathered from clinical trials that either have not been reviewed by FDA or that might not have been submitted to FDA, but nevertheless are quite valuable in helping to make medical decisions. Alternatively, the basis for "off label" use of a drug could be solid physiologic and pharmacologic principles and logic that predict the drug's possible efficacy for a particular disease. In the absence of evidence to support or refute such a use directly, the physician should proceed and evaluate the experience very much like an experiment in which $N = 1$ (chapter 29, The Clinician's Actions When $N = 1$). Finally, it even is "legal" for a poorly informed physician to use a drug inappropriately, although it may constitute malpractice. The FDA has no authority over such practices of medicine. Thus, by law, when the FDA approves a drug for any indication, the drug may be used in any way a physician sees fit.

After a drug is released, it may be used in a variety of plausible ways. The new uses may well appear decades after the drug was released to the market. Whether the use was "judicious" or not becomes clear only with extensive experience. Propranolol was initially "labeled" for idiopathic subaortic hypertrophic stenosis, arrhythmias, and pheochromocytoma. Its "unlabeled" use in angina pectoris and essential hypertension was, in retrospect, logical and correct. Some of the other *published* uses have also withstood the test of time and trials, but many have not (Morelli 1973).

**PRINCIPLE There is no foolproof way to know when to use a new drug. Osler's adage, "The physician is advised not to be the first to adopt the new remedy nor the last to discard the old" has the merit of wisdom. Introduction of pharmacologically unique and innovative drugs is rare. Few patients will be seriously deprived if a physician awaits published evidence of efficacy before adopting a new drug. The adage particularly holds if there are many approved drugs available to treat the indication other than the new drug.**

Society and the regulatory agency appropriately give the physician wide latitude in the use of a drug, device, or procedure. Society has a right to access drugs when the potential for important efficacy is established and can be put into preliminary perspective with the drug's toxicity. However, both efficacy and safety are preliminarily defined by the premarketing data. Furthermore, the setting of experiments done for regulatory purposes rarely mimics "field" circumstances of using drugs in practice.

The details of regulatory policy differ from country to country, but in most, the basic principles are the same. The package of clinical and preclinical data that forms the basis of regulatory approval is almost always the same for the United States and Europe. In Japan, more data are required in Japanese patients. Some countries such as Australia, Canada, Japan, and Switzerland maintain totally independent regulatory agencies. In the European Union (EU), however, member states have a cooperative and uniform approach. While each maintains its own regulatory authority, the member states are bound by the decision of the combined group under the auspices of the European Medicines Evaluation Agency (EMEA). The data are considered by the Committee for Proprietary Medicinal Products (CPMP). The CPMP is comprised of representatives of all member states, and approval is based on a vote of the members of the CPMP. In considering an application for approval, one country is appointed as *"rapporteur"* and as such has the responsibility to review the data in detail and to write an assessment report, which is used by the CPMP for their deliberations. In general, the CPMP review, including the time it takes for a sponsor to answer particular questions from the CPMP, takes about 9 months to a year. While the details of drug approval are different in Europe and the United States, the general principles are the same, and the experiments, both clinical and preclinical to support approval are almost always the same ones. In addition, no country has a monopoly on first approvals. Many drugs and new indications are approved in the United States before Europe and vice versa.

## ALTERNATIVE ASSESSMENTS OF DRUG EFFECTS

Recently, an increasing amount of attention has been paid to more completely collecting data about drug-related events that occur once the product is released for marketing. In addition, debate is active regarding the best ways to evaluate such data in order to obtain more and better information on both unanticipated (or at least not established) adverse and beneficial events due to drugs. The overall activity of collecting data about drugs that are available to the general population is known as *postmarketing surveillance*. A perceived advantage of postmarketing surveillance is that it studies how drugs are used in "the real world" (Strom and Melmon 1979, 1989; Strom 1989; Melmon 1990). Populations that are almost never studied in premarketing studies, such as pregnant women, children, and the unborn, inevitably get exposed to many drugs in normal medical practice. Postmarketing surveillance may be the only ethical way to look for pharmacologic or toxicologic effects in these populations.

### Postmarketing Evaluation

The clinical evaluation of a drug before its release is limited for several reasons. First, the patients treated are highly screened. They must meet certain criteria to enter clinical trials. These criteria are established primarily to reduce intersubject variability, making experimental observations interpretable. In addition, certain criteria are set to increase safety to the patients in the trial. Patients in trials usually are observed much more intensively than ordinary patients in clinical practice. Concomitant therapies often are eliminated, decreasing the chance for drug interactions of both a positive and negative nature. The presence of concomitant diseases is also established as a criterion for being excluded from the study, even though the concomitant disease may be a common and important accompaniment to the diseases in question. Knowledge gained from clinical trials is dictated by the hypothesis being tested and the design of experiments that test the hypothesis. If efficacy for a particular indication is not tested in the trial, the efficacy of the drug for that indication will not be discovered, even if the drug, in fact, were useful for the untested indication. As mentioned above, the limited size of the patient population tested to support the approval of a drug limits the possibility of discovering uncommon efficacy and adverse events.

**PRINCIPLE If society has a right to access to drugs with important efficacy, it also has a right to expect that the profession will follow up on its obligation to monitor and use data that can be accumulated after the drug is marketed. It would surprise the patients and the profession to realize how truly little of the important medical consequences is known about an NCE at the time it becomes a salable product. What should be more important to all of us is how lax we are in detecting available data that could optimize our use of drug products.**

After approval, most drugs will be used in millions of people, and in a variety of ways. Those patients will not be "typical" of the patients used in clinical trials. Patients given the drug after its approval will not be monitored as closely as patients in a premarketing clinical trial. They will have more concurrent diseases; they may be taking more concomitant medications; they may be younger or older or of a different sex; and they may be pregnant, nonambulatory, and so forth. Because of the sensible limitation on the size of the preapproval clinical trials, it is possible that new serious adverse events or new beneficial effects will occur that could not be detected sooner because they occur too infrequently or because they depend on a particular set of circumstances, such as in the setting of concomitant therapy with another drug or of a concurrent disease that was not studied in the preapproval studies.

The patients that receive a drug in its general use could be a vast source of new information regarding the drug's effects. Mechanisms are in place around the world to collect data on drugs once they reach the marketplace. In the United States, adverse events thought to be due to a drug are reported to FDA by physicians on a voluntary basis. While this has led to discoveries of previously unrecognized adverse events, it is almost certain that this system is not optimal, efficient, or even cost-effective. Countries in Europe and elsewhere often are the suppliers of postmarketing drug information that comes from clever, systematic, and economical detection systems.

Methods are available to capture such information by postmarketing surveillance so that therapy can be improved. Postmarketing surveillance can be performed by patients, practicing or academic physicians, pharmacists, pharmaceutical companies, or governmental agencies (Strom and Melmon 1979; Rawlins 1988; Strom 1989). Ideally, such a system could confirm unproven, though anticipated, efficacy and toxicity. A good system of postmarketing surveillance also could detect unanticipated efficacy and toxicity. Postmarketing surveillance can report events from the field, monitor large patient databases, or work by a combination of these approaches. In the United States, a major issue is who should sponsor and financially support such an effort. Thus far only sporadic efforts have been undertaken by academics and by pharmaceutical companies. There is no generally accepted systematic program in place in the United States as there is in some European countries. Interested parties such as practicing physicians, patients, pharmaceutical companies, and the government are subject to various combinations of ethical, financial, and scientific incentives and disincentives to support a universal system of postmarketing surveillance. At present, no agreement has been reached as to the desirability or the methodology to be used in such a system (Lortie 1986; Edlavitch 1988).

Some have proposed that a rigorous, consistently applied application of epidemiologic techniques to postmarketing surveillance could shorten the premarket development of a drug. That is, the elapsed time from the first experiments in humans to regulatory approval could be reduced. Whether or not this proposal is valid, developing useful information about unanticipated drug effects certainly should optimize the use of the drug and define its most appropriate market much faster than is done today. In order to expose more patients to a drug to increase the sensitivity for discovering toxicity in phase III clinical trials, phase III may be prolonged beyond the point presently needed solely to demonstrate efficacy (Strom and Melmon 1979). A good system of postmarketing surveillance could efficiently and more completely detect adverse events and make these known to physicians. Whether the risks in allowing earlier public access to drugs would be outweighed by the benefit of distributing the proven efficacy to more patients more quickly is not known, and it would vary from case to case. By monitoring the effects of a drug in representative patients in all the settings in which it is actually used, data could also accrue that would establish more optimal uses of drugs.

## Meta-Analysis

Meta-analysis is a statistical method for analyzing multiple trials simultaneously and has been used in attempts to recognize new effects, primarily in the area of efficacy, of drugs. It is not infrequent that several trials examining the same therapeutic question achieve conflicting results. Results of several trials may indicate the same trend, but not all of the individual trials have achieved statistical significance. The magnitude of a drug's observed effect may vary from trial to trial. Sometimes trends are in opposite directions. Meta-analysis is sometimes seen as a way to make sense out of such conflicting or inconsistent results and to provide a more objective analysis of data than can occur by an "expert" reviewing the literature in a qualitative fashion and drawing a conclusion (Mann 1990). Meta-analysis is a way of summing a body of separate but similar experiments in a formal way (Mann 1990). There have been some notable examples where a meta-analysis of many small trials detected an important therapeutic effect that was later confirmed in a large, prospective, randomized, controlled trial. However, there are also equally important examples where a meta-analysis led to conclusions that were different from a more definitive, prospective randomized trial. Opinions about the place of meta-analysis in determining appropriate therapeutic strategies vary and the subject is keenly debated. It is not likely that meta-analysis will replace the randomized, blinded, controlled trial as the method to support drug approval. A safe conclusion is that meta-analysis is a very productive and useful tool to generate hypotheses from small studies when definitive conclusions cannot be made from the individual trials. Meta-analysis could form the rationale for conducting a large, more definitive clinical trial to answer a particular question. It also is likely that meta-analysis is more useful and objective than a conclusion reached by applying "expert" judgment to a simple review of the literature.

Several studies have compared the results of a number of meta-analyses to the result of a more definitive clinical trial. The best approach to do this is somewhat controversial, but agreement between the two approaches have ranged from about 65 to 90%. Critiquing a meta-analysis is not too different from critiquing any other report of a clinical trial. Attention must be paid to how the analysis was performed (Fleiss and Gross 1991; Villar et al. 1995; Cappelleri et al. 1996; Sim and Hlatky 1996;

Le Lorier et al. 1997). A meta-analysis can be done only with information available to the analyzer. Generally, this consists of published material. It is crucial that the quality of the trials included in the meta-analysis be high. Meta-analysis is subject to so-called publication bias. Publication bias refers to the tendency for positive data to be submitted for publication and ultimately published and not data that do not detect a major effect. Some analyses include unpublished information, but it can be difficult to locate unpublished information or to be certain that all material has been surveyed. In addition to publication bias, other selection biases also may exist. That is, when one performs a meta-analysis one has to choose which trials to include and which to exclude. It is essential that the choice be done according to a well-defined and well-described protocol, but even then, the choice of included studies will influence the result in a potentially biased manner (Mann 1990). Meta-analyses showing positive effects tend to find larger differences than do definitive controlled trials (Villar et al. 1995), possibly due in part to publication bias. The synthesis of data from different trials can be influenced by differences in trial design and differences in the populations being studied. Some believe that a meta-analysis should only include trials with similar designs and similar populations (Le Lorier et al. 1997), while others do not require such stringency (Fleiss and Gross 1991). It is usual that smaller trials find larger effects of treatment than larger trials (Cappelleri et al. 1996). Nonrandomized trials also yield larger treatment effects than randomized trials (Schulz et al. 1995). Most agree that only randomized trials be included (Fleiss and Gross 1991).

Meta-analysis has a place in the spectrum of clinical trials and analyses that allow clinicians to make judgments as to what the best therapy in a given situation would be. A meta-analysis must be scrutinized with the same care, and essentially by the same criteria, as an individual trial, with some additional measures unique to such a pooled analysis. Because of the higher uncertainty in the validity of a conclusion from a meta-analysis compared with the uncertainty in conclusions made from large, well-planned randomized trials, it is unlikely that such an approach will lead to many, if any, drug approvals by regulatory agencies.

**PRINCIPLE Clinically important data come in a variety of forms and can be analyzed by a variety of techniques. None is perfect nor all-inclusive, and each should be thought of as complementing the other.**

## PHARMACOECONOMIC CONSIDERATIONS OF DRUG DEVELOPMENT

A major factor affecting the adoption of a new drug into a therapeutic regimen is the cost of the new therapy. The drug approval process by the FDA and most other governmental regulatory authorities is legally and operationally separate from determining how exactly a new therapy should fit into the practice of medicine. That is, an approval for a new drug does not guarantee that it will become widely used. A determinant of clinical use of increasing importance is the cost of the new therapy in relation to the cost of the current standard of care or the cost of untreated disease where few interventions are available. In some countries government programs so dominate health care that governments can limit the use of a drug by refusing to pay for it. In countries where there are very few programs that pay for health care, this amounts to de facto control over the use of a drug that is independent of a review that determines the safety and efficacy of a new drug. In countries where there are multiple payers for health care, such as the United States, this control is less absolute, but it still exists. In addition, some government health plans outside the United States require regulatory approval as a condition for paying for therapy. Other payers differ in this regard. In the United States, the existence of published results in peer-reviewed journals is often sufficient to garner payment. A number of countries have developed published guidelines for making pharmacoeconomic assessments.

The general field of determining whether a particular therapy is worth the cost is called *pharmacoeconomics*. However, there is not universal agreement on what is the best way to determine the worth of a particular therapy and whether the price being asked by a pharmaceutical company is worth paying. Different countries as well as different constituencies within countries such as the United States, with multiple payers for health care, use different methods to determine value. Pharmacoeconomic information is used in a variety of ways (Jacobs 1995; Torrance et al. 1996). Pharmaceutical companies use it to evaluate pricing of a drug and also to make decisions to pursue or not to pursue particular development programs. Hospital formularies take pharmacoeconomic information into account in deciding whether to add a particular drug to the formulary. Third-party payers use such information to decide whether to pay for a particular treatment, or to determine what price they are willing to pay.

Several considerations bear on what method of analysis should be used. To evaluate a particular pharmacoeconomic conclusion, one needs to understand what the purpose of the analysis was, what assumptions were made, what clinical data were used in the assessment, and what particular technique was used. Similar to any other experiment, it is important to know explicitly what question is being asked.

The primary target audience for a pharmacoeconomic study is important to know. An insurance company interested in the immediate cost of a therapy might have very little self-interest in what the long-term results of a therapy are or what the indirect costs might be. An example of an indirect cost is the cost to a family member who has to miss work to take a patient to a facility to receive a therapy. In contrast, the interests of society as a whole, and the effects of a therapy on a variety of factors that are not directly related to administering a particular therapy, would be of interest to a national health plan. No pharmacoeconomic analysis can be done in isolation; the evaluation of the cost of one therapy should always be compared with something, usually the standard of care (or several different therapies if there is no one standard) or to no treatment at all.

Ideally, pharmacoeconomic studies should report on the "effectiveness" of a drug, not on efficacy. This is in contrast to drug approval, where efficacy is paramount. *Efficacy* refers to the drug's effect on a disease under ideal circumstances. These circumstances are approximated, though never achieved, in a controlled clinical trial in which the drug is administered by a defined regimen and where the question is, "Does the drug effect a specific therapeutic or pharmacologic outcome?" Ideally, efficacy is determined in a setting where compliance is assured, although this is never really the case even in the best trials.

*Effectiveness,* however, is the overall outcome prescribing a drug has in actual clinical practice where the efficacy of a drug is modulated by more extraneous factors than occur in a clinical trial. These factors include poor compliance, other illnesses that exist concurrently with the particular illness for which the drug is intended, and use in ethnic groups or age groups that were not included in the primary studies to determine efficacy. When a new drug becomes available, efficacy data from clinical trials, rather than effectiveness data, are what is available. Observational data can be collected as the use of a drug becomes more widespread. In some instances, the efficacy of a drug may have been determined after detecting a signal for efficacy from observational analysis of a clinical database. In such an instance effectiveness information may be more readily available.

Because any study is subject to evaluation and methodological issues, pharmacoeconomic studies should not be used in a mechanistic fashion, and they do not replace critical thinking, good judgment, and common sense (Torrance et al. 1996). Pharmacoeconomic studies should be used to inform decision-making. When one makes a decision to use a drug, pharmacoeconomic information should enter into the decision, but it should be used in conjunction with other information such as knowledge of the pharmacology of a drug, and nonscientific issues such as justice, equity, access, and choice.

### *Pharmacoeconomic studies*

The clinical data for pharmacoeconomic studies can come from clinical trials or from observational databases. Wherever the data come from, conclusions need to be reevaluated from time to time because more is learned about the beneficial and adverse consequences of a drug and because certain economic or medical assumptions made in the analysis may become obsolete. Data from randomized, blinded controlled trials have the advantage of being much less subject to bias from clinicians and patients. However, most clinical trials are powered for the primary endpoint and may lack sufficient power to detect important differences that may affect a pharmaco-economic analysis.

Pharmacoeconomic studies should be comparative and should express results as differences between alternatives (Torrance et al. 1996; Siegel et al. 1997). A frequent problem with pharmacoeconomic analysis for a new drug is that a proper pharmacoeconomic analysis has not been done for the standard therapy compared with doing nothing.

In addition to the differences in cost between therapies, it is also useful to know the absolute costs in order to evaluate the importance of the difference. Just as with clinical trials, one has to determine whether a difference between therapies is clinically as well as statistically significant, one has to evaluate whether a difference in cost is economically significant.

A variety of analytical techniques are employed in pharmacoeconomic research. These various methods of analysis are not mutually exclusive and can be used simultaneously for different purposes:

- *Cost minimization analysis:* This analysis evaluates only the monetary costs of the therapy and is appropriate when the outcome of the drug and another treatment are the same. In such a case, the decision to use one drug or another is related only to cost.

- *Cost-consequence analysis:* In this analysis, the costs and consequences of the drug are listed. Examples of costs are drug costs, the costs to administer the drugs, and hospital costs; consequences of therapy include the number of months of added life and the occurrence of adverse events due to the drug. This analysis is descriptive and does not depend on any model or assumptions.
- *Cost-effectiveness analysis:* Costs are associated with outcomes as measured in physical units such as millimeters of mercury reduction in blood pressure, strokes prevented, hospital days avoided, or lives saved.
- *Cost-utility analysis:* This is a variation of cost-effectiveness analysis in which outcomes are transformed to some measure of utility such as quality adjusted life years (QALY). QALYs transform changes in quantity (mortality) and quality (morbidity) of life into a composite measure that is independent of the disease or the drug. The method for scoring quality is discussed below.
- *Cost-benefit analysis:* Outcomes are expressed in monetary terms. How particular items are assigned a monetary value is discussed below. An advantage of this approach is that it allows the costs of a drug regimen and, in fact, a health program, to be compared with nonmedical costs, such as the cost of a program to protect the environment, defense spending, and education. As such it is of value to those responsible for determining policy on a number of issues. Of course, the analysis is influenced by the method to assign monetary value to various outcomes (saved life, less pain, etc.) and as such, any conclusion could be quite controversial.

Cost items that could be considered are direct costs for direct health care such as cost of the drug, the nursing costs to administer the drug, the time in hospital or the trip to a clinic, as well as costs for social services, costs for patient education, costs incurred by the patient's family, and costs to a patient to find the most appropriate therapy (Torrance et al. 1996; Siegel et al. 1997).

The broadest perspective for a pharmacoeconomic study is the comprehensive, societal one, in which all costs and benefits are included regardless of who incurs them. Particular, more restricted perspectives, such as that of a paying insurance company or of a patient's family can be derived from a comprehensive analysis.

Any pharmacoeconomic analysis has to have a time perspective. Ideally this perspective should extend far enough into the future to include major medical and economic outcomes (Torrance et al. 1996). Sometimes data are not available for doing this, and extrapolations are made on assumptions as to the occurrence of future events. In some instances the effects on future generations need to be considered, such as the impact of treating HIV infection in an expectant mother (Siegel et al. 1997). It is important to know what these assumptions are and to maintain vigilance that these assumptions hold up as time passes. The expected duration of therapy and the length of effects must be known or estimated in order to assess the pharmacoeconomic outcomes over time (Clemens et al. 1995).

***Quality-of-life and monetary cost***

There are a number of methods for transforming outcomes of a clinical experience to quality of life or to a monetary cost. Quality-of-life metrics have been developed to incorporate assessments made by health providers and patients. Most experts seem to favor some metric using input from patients. It is controversial whether patients with experience with a particular therapy and disease are best suited to do this or whether patients with the potential to have a need for a therapy, but without direct experience, provide better information. Early studies in cost-benefit analysis used a "human capital approach," which is calculated by determining an increase in productivity as measured by increased earnings that accrue from instituting a particular therapy. However, this method has fallen out of favor somewhat, because it focuses on lost work time and does not deal well with other types of loss (Torrance et al. 1996). Other examples of loss due to illness occur in homemakers, the elderly, the unemployed, and children, and these cannot be measured in units of decreased earnings. This method does not allow an assignment of monetary value to changes in health that do not have an impact on work time. Another approach is to determine "willingness to pay" (O'Brien et al. 1995; Torrance et al. 1996). Respondents to surveys are asked how much they would be willing to pay out of pocket to achieve a certain outcome. This method, in contrast to a cost-benefit effectiveness approach, provides a measurement of consumer preferences for trade-offs between costs and outcomes. This method is subject to some bias depending on how the questions are asked and the socioeconomic group of the respondents. For comparability across studies, it would be desirable for a standard method for evaluating cost and quality of life be used (Siegel et al. 1997). However, the field has not advanced to the stage where this is possible.

Any method that transforms information into units measuring quality of life or monetary cost has problems with assumptions of equity. For example, a cost-effectiveness analysis using cost per life saved could assume that all lives are worth the same or could assign differential worth based on age, comorbidity, personal skills, and the like. The ethical implications of considering each life equally or weighting each differently are important but are not in the scope of this chapter. There is definitely no agreement as what factors should be weighted and by how much (Torrance et al. 1996). Quality weights must also be made and should reflect real preferences. Some advocate that preferences be based on community preference for health states rather than on patient or provider preferences (Siegel et al. 1997). This recommendation depends in part on the notion that it is the community overall that is supporting health care, and therefore, its opinion is most important. However, there is not agreement on this point (O'Brien et al. 1995). Some subgroups, such as patients, ethnic groups, and age-defined groups, may assign different scores to the same attribute (Siegel et al. 1997). A standard method for getting people to evaluate quality is to ask them to rate certain conditions on a scale from 0 to 1, with death being scored 0.0 and optimal health having a value of 1.0.

All pharmacoeconomic studies incur some uncertainty, which can be divided into uncertainty inherent in data collection and uncertainty arising from assumptions (Jacobs 1995; Torrance et al. 1996). Some of this uncertainty is related to the magnitude or frequency of a clinical outcome and is the same uncertainty that statistical tests are designed to handle in the context of a clinical trial. There is also uncertainty as to assumptions made to project results into the future (people of different ages may assess the importance on quality of a given effect differently), of the cost or benefit of a therapy as determined by expert or patient opinion, compliance with therapy, and duration of an effect. In general, more uncertainty is introduced by assumptions than by data collection (Torrance et al. 1996). The sensitivity of a conclusion should be tested with respect to assumptions. That is, it is important to know how the magnitude of the difference between the cost of a new therapy and the standard therapy is changed by a given change in an assumption.

Although the FDA is not currently using pharmacoeconomic studies to make decisions on drug approval, it is currently considering how to assess pharmacoeconomic data for inclusion in product information (the label). Pharmaceutical companies could then make promotional claims about cost issues. As noted above, the FDA regulates the promotional claims a company can make. Recent legislation allows companies to discuss pharmacoeconomic claims based on competent and reliable scientific evidence. Thus, the FDA will have to decide how to define *competent and reliable*. This issue ultimately returns us to that of deciding what evidence is required for efficacy or effectiveness and how rigorous the data are that support claims of cost. Just as with drug approval, the choice of endpoints, whether definitive or surrogate, needs careful scrutiny (FDC Reports 1998a; FDC Reports 1998b).

Drug development is a scientifically rigorous, costly, and time-consuming process. Although the general principles of experimentally proving a drug's efficacy are widely accepted, there is much discussion regarding alternative methods to gather convincing evidence for efficacy and safety. The acceptance of any method always includes value judgments regarding the balance of safety and efficacy and regarding how certain one needs to be that a perceived effect is real. Because there is no absolute correctness in those judgments, debates will continue and these approaches will continue to evolve.

## REFERENCES


Cappelleri JC, Ioannidis JPA, Schmid DH, et al. 1996. Large trials vs. meta-analysis of smaller trials. *JAMA* **276**:1332–8.

Chakrin L, Byron DA. 1987. Lab's labor lost? R&D in an era of change. *Pharmaceut Executive* 30–34 Jul.

Clemens K, Townsend R, Luscombe F, et al. 1995. Methodological and conduct principles for pharmacoeconomic research. *Pharmacoeconomics* **8**:169–74.

Edlavitch SA. 1988. Postmarketing surveillance methodologies. *Drug Intell Clin Pharm* **22**:68–78.

Elion GB. 1989. The purine pathway to chemotherapy. *Science* **244**: 41–7.

FDC Reports. 1998a. The Pink Sheet **60**(8) Feb 23:6.

FDC Reports. 1998b. The Pink Sheet **60**(9) Mar 2:8.

Federal Register Document 96-32493. Filed 12-19-96. 1996. Establishment of prescription drug user fee revenues and rates fiscal year 1997.

Fleiss JL, Gross AJ. 1991. Meta-analysis in epidemiology with special reference to studies of the association between exposure to environmental tobacco smoke and lung cancer: A critique. *J Clin Epidemiol* **44**:127–39.

Flowers CR, Melmon KL. 1997. Clinical investigators as critical determinants in pharmaceutical innovation. *Nature Med* **3**:136–43.

Gogerty JH. 1987. In: Guarino RA, editor. *Preclinical Research Evaluation in New Drug Approval Processes.* New York: Marcel Dekker, pp 25–54.

Halperin JA. 1988. Challenge, opportunity, promise, and risk: The pharmaceutical industry moving toward the 21st century. *Drug Info J* **22**:25–32.

Hood L. 1988. Biotechnology and medicine of the future. *JAMA* **259**:1837–44.

Jacobs P, Bachynsky J, Baladi J-F. 1995. A comparative review of pharmacoeconomic guidelines. *Pharmacoeconomics* **82**:182–9.

Lasagna L. 1979. Toxicological barriers to providing better drugs. *Arch Toxicol* **43**:27–33.

Le Lorier J, Gregoire G, Benhaddad A, et al. 1997. Discrepancies between meta-analyses and subsequent large randomized controlled trials. *N Engl J Med* **337**:536–42.

Lortie FM. 1986. Postmarketing surveillance of adverse drug reactions: problems and solutions. *Can Med Assoc J* **135**:27–32.

Mann C. 1990. Meta-analysis in the breech. *Science* **249**:476–80.

Mario E. 1988. A vision of the pharmaceutical industry in the year 2000. *Pharm Tech* 23–25 Apr.

Melmon KL. 1990. Attitudinal factors that influence the utilization of modern evaluative methods. In: Geljins AC, editor. *Medical Innovation at the Crossroads.* Vol 1. Committee on Technological Innovation of Medicine, Institute of Medicine. Washington, DC: National Academy Press, pp 136–46.

Melmon KL, Morrelli HF, Hoffman BB, Nierenberg DW, editors. 1992. *Melmon and Morrelli's Clinical Pharmacology: Basic Principles in Therapeutics*. 3rd ed. New York: McGraw-Hill.

Morrelli HK. 1973. Propranolol. *Ann Intern Med* **78**:913–7.

O'Brien BJ, Novosel S, Torrance G, et al. 1995. Assessing the economic value of a new antidepressant: a willingness to pay approach. *Pharmacoeconomics* **8**:34–45.

[PDR] 1998. *Physician's Desk Reference*. Montvale (NJ): Medical Economics Data Production Co.

Rawlins MD. 1988. Spontaneous reporting of adverse drug reactions. II: Uses. *Br J Clin Pharmacol* **26**:7–11.

Schulz KF, Chalmers I, Hayes RJ, et al. 1995. Empirical evidence of bias. *JAMA* **273**:408–12.

Siegel JE, Torrance GW, Russel LB, et al. 1997. Guidelines for pharmacoeconomic studies. *Pharmacoeconomics* **11**:159–68.

Sim I, Hlatky MA. 1996. Growing pains of meta-analysis. *Br Med J* **313**:702–3.

Strom BL, editor. 1989. *Pharmacoepidemiology*. New York: Churchill Livingstone.

Strom BL, Melmon KL. 1979. Can postmarketing surveillance help to effect optimal drug therapy? *JAMA* **242**:2420–3.

Strom BL, Melmon KL. 1989. The use of pharmacoepidemiology to study beneficial drug effects. In: Strom BL, editor. *Pharmacoepidemiology.* New York: Churchill Livingstone, pp 307–24.

Strom BL, Miettinen OS, Melmon KL. 1984. Postmarketing studies of drug efficacy. How? *Am J Med* **77**:703–8.

Swann JP. 1988. *Academic Scientists and the Pharmaceutical Industry.* Baltimore: Johns Hopkins University Press.

Torrance GW, Blaker D, Detsky A, et al. 1996. Canadian guidelines for economic evaluation of pharmaceuticals. *Pharmacoeconomics* **9**:535–59.

Villar J, Carroli G, Belizan JM. 1995. Predictive ability of meta-analyses of randomised controlled trials. *Lancet* **345**:772–6.

CHAPTER

# 28 RISK ANALYSIS APPLIED TO PRESCRIPTION DRUGS

John Urquhart

*Chapter Outline*



## RISK ANALYSIS AND COMMUNICATION

The topic of this chapter gradually developed into a recognized discipline after people began to dispute the long-held premise that technological progress was inevitably beneficial. The gradual shift in public opinion began to gather force about 1960. Two events in 1962 catalyzed the process: the publication of Rachel Carson's book, *The Silent Spring,* and the thalidomide disaster. The thalidomide disaster is described below. Carson's book projected widely disastrous impact of synthetic chemicals in the food chain for animals, given credence by the finding of damaging effects, especially among certain birds, of the once widely used insecticide, DDT. Her title portended a time when birds would have vanished, victims of a predicted disaster, still unrealized, of diffuse toxic effects of human-made chemicals. An additional factor shifting public opinion was a steady rise in the sensitivity of analytical chemical methods, permitting measurement of substances that were formerly undetectable. A vivid illustration of the power of newly sensitive methods came during the 1960s when mercury was detected in swordfish, leading, for a time, to a ban on swordfish, until it was discovered that remnants of dried fish from much earlier times had similar levels of mercury, so that the novelty was not a sudden rise in mercury contamination of fish but in the sensitivity of methods for measuring mercury.

## WHAT IS THE MEANING OF *RISK*?

### Defining Risk

Risk is the probability of something bad happening within a defined time period. Both the *something bad* and the *time period* must be specified.

#### *Probability*

*Probability* is a neutral term, so one can equally well speak of the probability of winning the lottery as of the probability of having a myocardial infarction. In contrast, it would be an unusual turn of phrase to speak of the *risk* of winning the lottery. Probability, a major topic in its own right, can be stated in several ways. For example, we can say from either experiment or theory that the probability of throwing double sixes with a single roll of honest dice is 1 in 36. In a medical setting, we can say, based on data from a major prevention trial (LRCs 1984), that about 1.2% of healthy adult males, aged 40 to 65, with moderately elevated cholesterol levels, will develop coronary heart disease (CHD) within the next year. For simplicity of discourse, let us combine the qualifications regarding age range and cholesterol levels into the term *such men*. So, from this observation you could make several equivalent statements, besides the one already made: The risk of incident coronary heart disease is 1200 per 100,000 such men per year or that 1 in 83 such men will newly develop CHD per year.

People who compile public health statistics and other epidemiologic mandarins tend to favor the first expression, but, for communication with the general public, the latter is superior, because it is straightforward to visualize 83 people, for example, in a group photograph, with a circle drawn around the head of a single individual who, by year's end, has newly developed CHD. It is useful to put a specific term on the group that produces the single victim, within the specified time period; the term is *unicohort*—the group from which comes one.

Larger unicohorts, as needed to communicate lower-risk phenomena, can be likened to the size of, for example, a village (one or two thousand), a small city (20,000 to 50,000), a packed stadium (100,000), a large city (500,000 to 2 million), or a major metropolis (5 to 10 million). Beyond that, the data rarely go, because there are no means for collecting reliable data on disease incidence and populations at risk in larger populations.

Nation-sized unicohorts come from the collection of reliable public health data, which is a process that had its origins around the middle of the nineteenth century in the technologically advanced countries. Gathering national data requires a rather elaborate and costly infrastructure that is unevenly present in the major countries of the world.

### *Time*

The time period may be explicitly stated, for example, a year, or implicitly stated, as in an airplane trip, a surgical procedure, or some other discrete event that has a clear beginning and end, and where the details of the actual time involved are of secondary interest. For example, most problems in air travel are associated with take-off and landing, so that whether it is a 1-hour or a 10-hour flight is a secondary consideration.

### *Something bad*

"Death in the crash of an airliner on a scheduled flight" is a specific category. "Death from choking on airline food," "death from a myocardial infarction during flight," and "death from a pulmonary embolus during flight" are all bad things that happen during flight, each with its own specifics, but probably best not combined with deaths from airliner crashes, and better kept in a category called "bad things that happen to people while flying." To describe the last three as "airline death" or "death during a plane trip" would lump them all together, with obvious loss of precision. *Something bad* need not be limited to death, as there are many bad things that can happen besides death. One needs to specify the focus.

A basic reason for specifying the *something bad* is not only for purposes of precision, but also because people differ greatly in their aversion to one or another bad outcome. For example, some people have an especially strong fear of cancer compared with other disease, opting, for their own reasons, to invest far more in reducing what may for them be an already low probability of developing cancer than in reducing a much higher probability of cardiovascular disease. Obviously, individual differences in what one might call their "spectrum of aversion" are a topic for research; suffice it to say here that anyone seeking to counsel patients on how to evaluate risk should recognize that people do, for often unfathomable reasons, have certain especially strong aversions that cannot be swayed by what passes for objective evidence or rational discourse.

### *A brief look at risk comparisons*

Coronary heart disease, which has been the leading cause of death since the 1930s, illustrates some useful ways of presenting how risk depends on prior disease status, age, time, and gender.

First, referring to the example given above, where 1 trial participant in 83 developed newly diagnosed CHD per year, 1 in 200 participants in the same trial died per year from all causes. Some died of causes related directly to coronary heart disease, for example, sudden death of evidently cardiac origin, complications of an acute myocardial infarction, and so on, but others died of causes not related to heart disease—mainly, but not exclusively, from various cancers or accidents.

Second, prior disease status can be important. The figures cited above were for older males without prior evidence of CHD, but with elevated lipid levels. In a trial organized about a decade earlier, specifically of males who had had a prior myocardial infarction, the annual risk of death from all causes was 1 in 26 (The Coronary Drug Project Research Group 1974). Most of the difference can be attributed to prior disease, but a small portion can be attributed to an improvement in the management of disease that occurred during the decade that elapsed between the two studies.

Other factors play a major role. The risk of death from all causes for U.S. males aged 45 to 54 was 1 in 164 in 1990, one-third less than the figure in 1970, which was 1 in 104 (Bureau of the Census 1997a). For those aged 85 and up, it was 1 in 6 in both years (Bureau of the Census 1997a). These figures indicate considerable improvement during the 1970s and 1980s in the management of disease in the middle but not the advanced years of life.

The overall risk of death for females is about 12% lower than for males, that is, 1 in 109 for males and 1 in 123 for females, when looking at all causes and all ages in the U.S. population in 1990 (Bureau of the Census 1997a). This gender difference is evident at all ages of life, from birth. Its cumulative effect is a life expectancy at birth that, as of 1992, was 6.8 more years for females than for males (Bureau of the Census 1997b).

There are many other factors that influence these risks. A notable one, beyond our scope to discuss here, is race. Another is geographic location. Both relate, in part, to organization, quality, and provision of health services, to nutrition, prevailing levels of education, economics, and many other factors. It is a matter for speculation and debate as to which are more and which are less important in determining the actual risks. Quantitative assessment of causality in such matters is difficult and assumption-ridden.

Anyone investigating these factors can use either mode of expressing risk data. The unicohort mode, while helpful in public communication, does not have the virtue of additivity, so that it is necessary to translate back to the expression *events per 100,000 per year* to see how rates from multiple conditions sum up to the overall rate in the population. In this case, the unicohort is calculated by dividing 100,000 by the rate.

### *Notes on measurement of risk*

Two key measurements are the number of people with the condition in question and the number who were at risk. The quality of risk assessments depends directly on the quality of these measurements. If the quality of the data is poor, the risk data derived from them will be misleading, no matter how large the quantity of data. Large amounts of poor-quality data do not overcome problems of quality.

An elaborate system is used to collect public health data, which are very useful, though sometimes misleading because of changing ideas about disease classification. In particular, the filling out of death certificates can create sizable artifacts in classification. What, for example, is written on the death certificate when a patient with diffuse metastatic cancer contracts pneumonia and dies or suddenly collapses from what may be an acute myocardial infarction, a sudden arrhythmia, or a pulmonary embolus? International comparisons are particularly vexed by different ideas about classifying the terminal sequence of events.

### *Insurance perspective*

One could design an insurance policy to remunerate instances of *something bad,* but for a sound business one must understand the probability of its occurrence. Such understanding is based on the usually reasonable assumption that the recent past is a good predictor of the near future. Based on data cited earlier, which were gathered for 1990, we could offer a life insurance policy that will pay the policy's beneficiary if the insured dies during the year after the policy is written. Let us use the 1 in 164 risk of death for males aged 55 to 64 in 1990 as the basis for calculating the premium. If we collect $1 per insured per year, then each year 164 insured men paying $1 each will generate $164 of income and one death, the beneficiary of which receives $164. Of course, a real business pays much larger benefits, and incurs administrative and sales costs, and has the need to generate a profit. So, a more realistic scenario would be a policy priced at $100/month, paying $164,000 per death, and returning a margin of about $32,000 for overhead and profit for each group of 164 insured. If we put some limits on the health status of those whom we enroll, by excluding those who are obviously sick and dying at the time they seek enrollment, then the actual risk in enrollees will be lower than in those who generated the original data, and so we would have an additional margin. Also, if, as has been true all through this century, there is a continuing trend downward in age-specific death rates, the use of decade-old risk data could also give us a further extra margin. An additional point is that the insurance firm has the use of the money collected as premiums in advance of payout, which can be a further source of income, if the money is invested wisely. A final point is that the actuarial tables used by the insurance industry are based on age-specific death rates among individuals who passed a basic insurance examination, which, though not extensive, serves to exclude people with clinical evidence of major disease. In contrast, the public health data come from a process that strives to be all-inclusive, and so include even people who are breathing their last as they are counted.

That is probably enough of a primer on the pricing of risk; to learn more, consult Tobias (1982). An important point to note is that the definition of *risk* has allowed insurers to price policies of various sizes according to available data on probability of occurrence. Special forms of insurance, against specific occurrences besides death, appeal to people's special needs or aversions. The considerations in translating medical knowledge into the pricing of special-purpose insurance are detailed in *Medical Selection of Life Risks* (Brackenridge 1977), a book with many useful perspectives, disciplined by the economics of the insurance business, in which overestimated risk creates overpriced policies and lost business, and underestimated risk attracts money-losing business.

### *Other views on the meaning of risk*

Some, particularly those of a behaviorist orientation, would like to see probability and aversion integrated into a single parameter. To give it a name, we could call it *probaversion.* If we were to use probaversion as a quantitative tool, it would call for some kind of numerical scale for aversion, which might be possible with suitable questionnaires. We would then face the difficulty that you, dear reader, may be very averse to malaria, because that is what your favorite grandmother died of, while I am very averse to mycosis fungoides, because that is what my favorite grandfather died of. So you might have a very low probability of contracting malaria, but your huge aversion to it would give you a high *probaversion* value, whereas I, who occasionally travel to regions where malaria is endemic, have a high probability of contracting malaria but no special aversion to it, so we might have comparable *probaversion* indices from totally different mechanisms. For that reason, this approach has no evident role to play in practical matters of risk communication or the pricing of insurance.

## THE NEED FOR QUANTITATIVE RISK DATA

### Public Perceptions of Risk Are Often Exaggerated

There are five main reasons why exaggeration of risk tends to occur. First, there is a structural bias in journalism, called *newsworthiness,* which features the unusual, infrequent, or odd occurrence. It is epitomized in the ancient journalistic saw that "dog bites man, that's not news; man bites dog, that's news." The ensuing news coverage creates the impression that risk posed by the bad happening in question is greater than it actually is, for example, that there are more man-bites of dogs than dog-bites of men.

Second, prophets are better served by forecasting bad outcomes than good ones. When prophecies prove wrong, vindictiveness is mitigated by the good news of unrealized doom, but inflamed by unexpected bad news. In retrospect, for example, few blame Rachel Carson for her unrealized prediction of a birdless world, but earlier Pollyanna-ish advocates of "progress" look rather silly in light of the various difficulties created, for example, by indiscriminate dumping of toxic wastes.

Third, bad news outsells good news, epitomized in the saying "bad news travels fast."

Fourth, expressions of relative risk exaggerate the importance of small differences. For example, about six times more males than females have been identified as having HIV infections (Bureau of the Census 1997b). When new data arrive, minor differences in the proportion of cases between males and females, converted into percentage changes, result in amplified rates of change in the tally of female cases, prompting the headline "Female HIV Soars!!" and, with it, the impression that more women than men are infected with the virus.

Fifth, news broadcasting is a form of entertainment, and victim-oriented reporting, which focuses on the plight of the unfortunate victims, is more entertaining than statistical trends in the population. Some refer to this as the "awwwww factor."

Thus, these five factors tend to bias the selection of stories for today's news toward the unusual, presented in terms of relative risk, seasoned with predictions of things getting worse, and given a personal touch by a look at some of the more poignant victims. The upshot is an exaggeration of the magnitude of low-risk hazards in life. The situation has improved in the last several decades, however, as science reporting has become a more widely recognized discipline, although unresisted temptations to exaggerate continue to season the news.

#### *Quantifying risk data*

The foregoing points emphasize the need for a systematic form of communicating the risks posed by various elements of modern life including the risks and incidence rates of benefit of taking drugs. Thus, after the gloom and doom reporting, the awwwww factor, and the startling figures of relative risk, the last word should be given to two pieces of data—the unicohort for the hazard in question and a set of values for prominent hazards in everyday life so that people can see where the newly discovered hazard fits in the general scheme of common hazards in daily life (Dinman 1980).

**MOTOR VEHICLES** The motor vehicle occupies a special place in daily life, because virtually everyone uses it. Throughout most of the period after World War II, about 50,000 people were killed annually in traffic accidents in the United States, representing about half of the total number of deaths attributable to accidents of one kind or another. The per-year risk of death in an auto accident was 1 in about 4000. It was generally estimated, also, that about half of the deaths attributable to motor vehicle accidents were ones in which the driver or other victims had been drinking in the time before the accident to an extent greater than is now legal. Among pedestrians killed by motor vehicles in the late 1970s, two-thirds were drunk when hit. About 1985, the force of public opinion began to turn on drunken driving, with steadily increasing efforts at prevention, detection, and penalties for infraction of the rules. The cumulative effects of these efforts have been to reduce the absolute numbers of traffic fatalities by about 20% in the face of continuing growth in the number of motor vehicles and indices of their use. Today, the per-year risk of death in an automobile accident is 1 in about 6000 (Bureau of the Census 1997a). One cannot be certain about the magnitude of the role played by antialcohol efforts, because there were concomitant improvements in the design of both vehicles and roadways, but the presumption is that the antialcohol efforts played the dominant role.

**CIGARETTE SMOKING** Cigarette smoking was first officially cited as a health hazard in the U.S. Surgeon General's first report on Smoking and Health in 1964 (USPHS 1964). That same year, an insurance firm, State Mutual, interpreted the Surgeon General's report from an actuarial perspective and began offering a nonsmoker's discount of 20% on life insurance premiums. Other insurance firms roundly damned this initiative for a variety of reasons, none of which proved valid. The market response to the discount was strongly favorable, and much insurance was written for nonsmokers. Twenty years later, when State Mutual published its actuarial experience, it turned out that the overall risk of premature death had been almost half that of the smokers who had bought life insurance from State Mutual during the same years (Cowell and Hurst 1980). The risk of death from coronary heart disease among smokers was 2.7 times that among nonsmokers, and the risk of death from respiratory cancers among smokers was 15 times that among nonsmokers.

Those two figures show how relative risk distorts, because the excess numbers of deaths among smokers were mainly contributed to by the greater number of cardiac deaths, which accounted for 30% of all deaths, because the nonsmokers' absolute risk of cardiovascular disease is much higher than their risk of respiratory cancers, which accounted for 6% of all deaths (Cowell and Hurst 1980).

Smoking was a prominent feature of U.S. life until public opinion began to shift, about a decade ago, toward confining smoking to limited spaces. At their peak about 1980, deaths in the United States attributable to smoking were equivalent to one fully loaded 747 crashing every day, and smoking was the single biggest optional risk in daily life. This daily toll of smoking-caused deaths went unreported in the daily news, as it was not a newsworthy happening.

Since about 1990, antismoking efforts have gathered progressively greater force, more so in the United States than in other technologically advanced countries, and more so in the western part of the United States than the eastern part. Antismoking efforts have focused in particular on finding ways to curtail the adoption of smoking by adolescents, which is when most of those who smoke began, for very few people begin smoking after their early adult years. The presumption is that concentrated efforts to reduce adoption during the adolescent years will gradually reduce the prevalence of smoking in the technologically advanced countries. Meanwhile, cigarette smoking appears to be rising in prevalence in the developing countries.

**ALCOHOL** The effects of alcohol have always been difficult to ascertain, because of strong biases among investigators in both directions. In recent years, large epidemiologic studies have suggested that modest quantities of alcohol may have a beneficial impact on the risk of coronary heart disease, but any benefits of alcohol are easily confounded by the risk-increasing effects of "immodest" drinking. Brackenridge gives us the measured view of the insurer, in the following way. He recognizes for males three levels of effects due to alcohol: "jovial," "boisterous," and "uncontrolled." For life insurance, the standard rates for the individual's age apply if he drinks to the level of becoming jovial or boisterous once every 2 months, or if he becomes jovial once monthly. But if the individual becomes jovial once a week, the insurer wants to increase the premium by 25%, and by 100% if the individual drinks to the jovial level daily. He will double the premium if the individual drinks to the uncontrolled level once a month and will decline to insure at all if the individual drinks to the uncontrolled level daily (Brackenridge 1977).

These are obviously subjective judgments, but they are tempered by the conflicting forces acting on the chief medical officer of a large insurance firm. Brackenridge informs us that alcoholics are in a race between death due to avoidable accidents and death due to the toxic effects of alcohol.

## RISK ANALYSIS AND COMMUNICATION APPLIED TO PRESCRIPTION DRUGS

Prescription drugs are the main interventional arm in modern medicine. They bring both benefits and risks, with the former vastly predominating, notwithstanding the occasional toxicity problem that has escaped detection during premarket development.

Before we look at the hazards of prescription drugs, however, we should take brief note of the history of drug development, which is a twentieth-century story. It originated in two seminal events: 1) the purposeful synthesis of the acetyl ester of the natural product, salicylic acid, to make aspirin at Bayer in Leverkusen, Germany, in 1897; and, 2) the first purposeful synthesis of a medicinal agent (salvarsan, an organic mercurial for treatment of syphilis), which was done by Paul Ehrlich at Cassella Farbwerke in Frankfurt, Germany, in 1906. There followed a series of advances in the first several decades of this century—the synthesis of thyroxine, the discovery of insulin, the identification of most of the vitamins, and the discovery of the sulfa drugs, also a German invention. The great triumph of pharmaceutical R&D during World War II was the development of penicillin; its bactericidal activity had been discovered in culture medium by Fleming in 1929, but its purification and production posed formidable challenges, which were only overcome by a huge Anglo-American crash program during World War II. In the first decade and a half following the end of World War II came a rapid succession of new agents—streptomycin, the tetracyclines, the anti-inflammatory steroids, erythromycin, and the contraceptive steroids, mostly U.S. innovations, reflecting the global dominance of U.S. science and technology after World War II.

In 1962, however, the world was shocked to learn that a newly introduced hypnotic, thalidomide, caused major limb deformities in the fetuses carried by pregnant women who took thalidomide, which was the product of a small German firm, Chemie Grünenthal. Vivid pictures of terribly deformed babies were shown on the world's television screens, which were themselves a recent technologic advance that started after World War II and by 1962 had gained presence in a majority of homes in the technologically advanced countries. In the United States, where the product was still awaiting approval for marketing, the relatively few cases had their origins in thalidomide that had been obtained outside the country, for example, during European travel.

The pictures were so vivid and the reactions so strong that political action was catalyzed to "do something." The upshot was a major revision in the laws governing the testing and registration of new pharmaceuticals. The biggest change in the regulations for drug testing did not involve toxicity testing, as one might have expected, but rather a requirement that drugs be proved efficacious in properly designed, controlled studies. The justification for this approach was that no risk from a pharmaceutical is worth incurring if it cannot be shown to be efficacious. An unstated political factor, however, was that the U.S. Food and Drug Administration had lost a critical court case in its early years, in effect being told by Justice Oliver Wendell Holmes, Jr., that the question of a drug's efficacy was not a matter of scientific fact, but of opinion, so that, in his and the majority of the Supreme Court's view, claims for efficacy were, whether right or wrong, protected by the First Amendment guarantees of free speech (United States v Johnson, Supreme Court of the United States, 1911). This setback created a long-standing perceived need within the FDA to find a way to gain legal authority to regulate claims of efficacy. The thalidomide catastrophe provided the occasion.

Meanwhile, Dr. Frances Kelsey, the FDA official who had withheld approval for the U.S. marketing of thalidomide, was given a special medal by then-President Kennedy, an event that some have criticized as sanctioning a principle that best regulatory practice is to delay U.S. approvals until enough experience with new drugs has been gained in other countries to minimize any risk of unexpected hazards emerging in the United States. This interpretation is strongly denied by the FDA.

The ensuing decade and a half after 1962 were relatively lean years for pharmaceutical development, with fewer than 20 new agents per year gaining registration and entering the U.S. market—contrasting with over 50 during the decade before 1962. A watershed event proved to be the registration of cimetidine in 1978, which soon became the first-ever billion-dollar pharmaceutical product, catalyzing marked growth in investment in pharmaceutical research and development. The flow of new agents increased somewhat in the following years, and then, in 1996, following a variety of changes in FDA procedures and increases in resources for new drug reviews, the annual tally of newly approved pharmaceuticals passed the 50 mark for the first time since the thalidomide disaster.

## Role of Pharmaceuticals in Improved Public Health

The aggregate benefits of all these pharmaceutical advances are difficult to quantify precisely, but there can be no real doubt that they have played a major role in the progressive improvements in public health during the twentieth century. Certainly the public statistics on year-by-year mortality rates at all ages of life have shown progressive improvement since about 1920, most strikingly in infant, childhood, and maternal mortality. Of course, success has many parents, so advocates of various technologies claim the main responsibility for these improvements. The sanitary engineers like to attribute them to better water and sewage systems; nutritionists attribute them to steadily improved nutrition; educators claim the beneficial effects of better education throughout society; medical educators weigh in with the fact that, since World

War II, there has been an unprecedented investment in biomedical research at all levels, resulting in better understanding of mechanisms of disease, of pathophysiology, of the biochemical bases of life and disease, of microbiology, cardiovascular physiology and pathophysiology, cancer and its underlying biology, and so forth, all of which have had their beneficial effects on concepts of disease and medical care. So, all these factors, including the vast array of effective pharmaceuticals now available, plus a wide variety of innovative medical devices, have played a role of some magnitude or other in the 40-fold drop in maternal mortality, the 10-fold drop in infant mortality, and the smaller but still substantial reductions in mortality in the various decades of adult life that occurred between the earlier and later decades of this century.

## Risk from Pharmaceuticals

In the quest to assess the hazards posed by a new pharmaceutical, a variety of animal and human studies are now routinely done to understand the agent's potential for toxicity. These include careful assessment of an agent's potential for embryotoxic effects—a permanent memorial in drug testing procedures to the thalidomide disaster. In animal studies, it is possible to increase the exposure to the new agent to levels that are orders of magnitude larger than one would ever expect to encounter in human use. Such studies can demonstrate the types of dose- or exposure-dependent toxicity that one may anticipate at these extremes of exposure. With this information, early clinical use can include specific tests that look especially carefully for signs of problems of the type identified in the earlier animal studies.

### *Risk assessment*

**MEASUREMENT ISSUES** Pharmaceutical risk assessment requires good data on the number of patients exposed to the drug, according to reasonable criteria for what constitutes "exposure"; such assessment also requires good data on the number of thus-exposed patients who actually developed the adverse condition. It is then the number exposed divided by the number of victims that defines the unicohort size. The assessment of drug exposure is difficult, for physicians' records on what was prescribed and when often are sketchy. Moreover, a sometimes substantial fraction of written prescriptions are never filled, so, although there was intention to create exposure to a drug, none actually occurred, because the patient failed to have the prescription filled. In other instances, filled prescriptions are never collected from the pharmacy, and some patients obtain the medicine but never actually take any; then a further fraction of patients take only a fraction of what was prescribed (Urquhart 1997). Pharmacy records are sometimes incomplete because some patients use multiple pharmacies for prescribed drugs, although with increasing numbers of patients covered by insurance schemes that include prescription drug benefits, there usually is a central record for individual insured patients. In some instances, however, data on insured families are combined so that it is impossible to tell which member of the family got which drug and when. All these problems have to be resolved, as well as they can be, in order to arrive at an estimate of the population of exposed individuals, from which can be computed a unicohort size.

Depending on whether the agent is intended for chronic or acute use, the natural time-base for reckoning its risk potential will be, for example, a year, in the case of indefinitely long treatment, or a week or a month in the case of intermediate durations of treatment, or, in the case of acute use, as with an antibiotic destined for 3, 7, or 14 days of use, a "treatment cycle" may be the logical choice of time base.

All the foregoing considerations relate to defining the population of patients whose exposure to the drug was sufficient in quantity and duration to regard them as being "at risk." The other number that must be carefully arrived at is the number of patients at risk who developed the adverse reaction in question. That, too, is fraught with certain difficulties, not the least of which is a certain risk of double-counting individual cases, when, for example, a physician reports the case to the regulatory authorities and also to the pharmaceutical firm responsible for the product. The firm, in turn, is obliged to report to the regulatory authorities all cases known to it. Minor discrepancies in reporting details via the two channels may result in one case being counted as two. A second difficulty arises when physicians sometimes assume that the occurrence of the adverse reaction in question is itself sufficient evidence from which to conclude that the patient had been exposed to the pharmaceutical in question. These are mechanisms that tend to exaggerate the number of cases of drug-related adverse reaction. Other mechanisms tend to minimize the number, most notably when the attending physician fails to report the adverse reaction to either the regulatory authority or the pharmaceutical firm, or when the physician fails to connect the patient's present difficulties with the patient's use of the drug in question.

**IF NOTHING BAD HAPPENS IS EVERYTHING ALL RIGHT?** Human exposure to a new drug begins in preregistration testing, under very strict oversight. It gradually expands, as evidence is gathered on the new agent's efficacy, with a constant watch for evidence of adverse effects. If the safety record is basically free of evidence for substantive harm, the product gains regulatory approval for marketing, and enters the market, after which usage often grows dramatically. The question stands as posed in the heading to this section. The answer is provided by a statistical principle called "the rule of three," which basically says: if you have observed *N* treatment cycles with no evidence of harm, you can be 95% confident that the risk of some yet-unrecognized, adverse consequence of the treatment is less than 1 in *N*/3 (Hanley and Lippman-Hand 1982). So, if you have treated 3000 people with the new agent and have found no suspicion of untoward effects, you could reasonably expect that the risk posed by the agent of some as yet unseen untoward consequences is less than 1 in 1000 (see also chapter 29, The Clinician's Actions When *N*=1).

**HOW MUCH FREEDOM FROM HARM IS ENOUGH?** This question has many answers. One approach is to theorize, but a more useful approach is to look at the history of new drug entries into the marketplace since 1962 to see how many appear to have caused serious adverse reactions, what the type of adverse reactions were, what the therapeutic indications of the drugs in question were, and what the level of risk appears to have been.

Several major anti-inflammatory agents were driven from the market in a barrage of bad publicity in the period between 1975 and 1985 (Inman 1988). In retrospect, these appeared to have serious adverse effects occurring with an incidence of 1 serious adverse event in about 5000 treatment cycles (Urquhart 1986). Of course, the anti-inflammatory agents—both steroidal and nonsteroidal—are a troublesome group. The steroids have a wide array of serious side effects—glaucoma, diabetes, madness, gastrointestinal ulceration and bleeding, hypertension, osteoporosis, development of the cushingoid facies, and so forth. The nonsteroidal agents avoid most of these problems, with the conspicuous exception of the GI ulceration and bleeding—the risk of which rises with advancing age. But so, too, do the problems created by inflammatory joint disease, which is a main indication for the use of these agents. The forthcoming generation of so-called selective cyclooxygenase 2 inhibitors give promise of making obsolete the nonselective agents and ending the long-running dilemmas about how, when, where, and/or in whom to use them. Whether that promise will be fulfilled is not at present clear, except in the minds of optimists, so for the next while we remain stuck with the dilemma posed by the nonselective agents.

With this dilemma has come a long-running debate about whether some of the nonsteroidal anti-inflammatory agents are more or less likely to produce serious GI problems than others. This point is one that has never been studied by a suitably large, randomized, controlled trial, where the power of randomization avoids the usual problem that patients prescribed, for example, piroxicam, are older and have more severe arthritic disease than those prescribed, for example, ibuprofen, in substantial measure because piroxicam is indicated for arthritis and ibuprofen is labeled for a wide variety of acute and chronic inflammatory conditions, ranging from tennis elbow to osteoarthritis. Thus, the mix of patients taking piroxicam tends to be older with more concomitant medical problems, and those taking ibuprofen tend to be younger, with single acute problems, uncomplicated by concomitant chronic disease (Urquhart 1986). As a consequence, the reports that come into regulatory authorities tempt one to conclude that piroxicam is the more hazardous agent of the two, but without careful balancing of salient patient characteristics, no sound conclusion can be drawn.

**DOUBLE STANDARD FOR PROOF OF EFFECTIVENESS AND FOR PROOF OF HAZARD** Another difficulty in pharmaceutical risk assessment is a dual standard of evidence. There is a broad consensus that any claim for therapeutic benefit must be based on carefully controlled, randomized trials, with the proof of efficacy based on statistical tests carried out under a policy of analysis called "intention-to-treat" analysis, in which the trial participants' actual exposure to the test agent is ignored completely. Thus, a patient randomized to receive the test agent is considered to have received that agent, whether he or she, in fact, actually did receive it—reflecting a point made by Alvan Feinstein, that intention-to-treat analysis may avoid statistical bias, but it does not always avoid foolishness (Feinstein 1991). Despite its sometimes ludicrous extremes, intention-to-treat analysis is widely regarded as a most conservative test, which, if passed, gives one full confidence that the test agent does, in fact, "work," although the magnitude of its effect may be substantially underestimated by prevalent noncompliance with the regimen for taking the test agent (Urquhart 1991).

In contrast to these special rigors in the testing for drug efficacy, assertions of drug safety problems are often based on the most flimsy evidence, particularly evidence regarding patients' exposure to the suspect agent. Assertions of hazard gain credence simply through repetition of the assertion; it is usually only the commercial sponsor of the product (if there is one) that is prepared to do battle to separate patient characteristics from product characteristics. In the prevailing set of attitudes regarding conflict of interest, the integrity of research done by, or sponsored by, the product's manufacturer is suspect (Stelfox et al. 1998), notwithstanding an array of legal requirements for full-disclosure reporting that gives the FDA and other regulatory authorities around the world the opportunity for independent review of the data.

Thus, drug development and adverse reaction analysis is done under a set of concepts and policies that were codified in the aftermath of the thalidomide disaster, almost four decades ago. It was a time when few drugs had passed basic tests for efficacy, though of course some of the early innovations, for example, the sulfa drugs, penicillin, the tetracyclines, streptomycin, erythromycin, and the oral contraceptives, had clinical activity of such unprecedented magnitude that no one could doubt their value in medicine. But there were many agents then in use that were of dubious value, and so the whole question of proving drug efficacy loomed very large in the early 1960s. In that era, it was natural that the main focus was placed on proof of efficacy. In the present era, where proven efficacy is a *sine qua non* of market entry, few agents of dubious efficacy are still left in the market, and the key question for most new drugs is not "does it work?" but "does it work better, or more economically than other products of its class used for the same indication?"

Since 1962, the cost of developing and testing a new agent has escalated steadily, reaching the $200 million level and beyond. Not only money is involved in the qualification of a new agent for marketing, but thousands of patients participate in the trials, in centers that, generally, are uniquely equipped to undertake such trials. That itself is a valuable resource, which goes for naught when a new agent is driven from the market. The gradual change from few to many products of proven efficacy, with sharply escalating costs for product development, makes it timely to reconsider a policy that gives automatic credence to shoddy evidence for safety problems.

**LOOKING BACK, LOOKING AHEAD** On the face of it, one would say that it would take a premarket testing program involving more than 15,000 treatment cycles in order to be confident that the product was free of serious adverse effects at an incidence of 1 serious complication in about 5000 treatment cycles. Looking more closely, however, we might find that there are other considerations that tend to obscure the early detection of such problems. If, for example, problems are limited to males or females, then it will, if the testing program is enrolling both males and females, take about 10,000 treatment cycles to be confident about the risk level. If there are problems in detection or reporting of adverse events, then it may take correspondingly more cycles of treatment.

In general, premarket testing of new drugs ends up with 2000 to 5000 cycles of treatment, so that the full definition of an agent's risk potential has to be based on postmarketing studies, which lack the completeness of detection and reporting that are more or less standard in premarket studies. If, for example, only 5 to 10% of cases of an adverse reaction are reported to the authorities, then we are no longer dealing with a "rule of 3," but a "rule of 30 to 60," which can be further diluted to a "rule of 200 to 300" if an adverse effect is especially concentrated in a particular subgroup of the population treated with the agent (Urquhart 1989). In that case, in order to be confident that the risk of an adverse effect is less than 1 in 5000, it may be necessary for several hundred thousand people to have been treated before one could be confident that no serious adverse effect was going to surface with an incidence high enough to jeopardize the product.

For a variety of reasons that have no really rigorous basis, it appears that a unicohort of 5000 is a sort of threshold for acceptability of chronic-use pharmaceuticals. With premarket testing programs not usually exceeding 5000 participants, one can see that the premarket definition of risk potential is incomplete. The chief difficulty in the transition from pre- to postmarketing surveillance for adverse effects is that the high efficiency of reporting in the premarket environment, which is closely regulated, is not matched in the postmarketing environment, where only a minority of adverse reactions are reported to the regulatory authorities. One of the main reasons for the low efficiency of reporting is failure to recognize that an untoward clinical event is indeed drug-related, and another is negligence—reporting takes time, effort, and has to compete for priority in a busy schedule.

So the upshot is that we would like to see unicohorts for serious adverse effects that are larger than 5,000 to 10,000, but these cannot be reached in premarket testing, for reasons of time, limitations on clinical trial sizes, and economics. We must therefore depend on postmarketing surveillance, which has major inefficiencies that hamper detection and risk definition.

### *How much risk is too much?*

At its root, this question is answered by asking another question: what are the benefits provided by the pharmaceutical in question? If it is a mild, "comfort" medicine, for example, a hypnotic, a cough-suppressant, or a nasal decongestant, then the answer is that any discernible risk is too much. The basic reason is that there are many treatment alternatives, and, even if there were not, the marginal benefits of comfort treatment are too small to justify the risk of serious consequences. If, in contrast, the drug has unique abilities to treat certain kinds of malignant cancers but has a 1 in 20, 1 in 50, or 1 in 100 per-treatment-cycle risk of killing the patient, the risk may be acceptable, because the alternative of no treatment or treatment with a much less effective agent is much worse. These are judgment calls that cannot be reduced to any simple formula, though they are much better made against a background of good quantitative information on the comparative risks of alternative treatments than in a fog of fuzzy, poorly quantified information.

***Why does only 1 person in* N *hundred have serious problems?***

This, of course, is the jackpot question in risk assessment. If we could firmly establish that only those who have some special set of attributes—a particularly high or low level of a gut wall enzyme that metabolizes the drug, or a genetic difference in drug receptor structure, or a high-broccoli diet, or, or, or—then we could recommend alternative treatments or doses or use of concomitantly administered protective agents, or the like. We could, for instance, limit the use of thalidomide to males and to females in nonchildbearing ages instead of "protecting" anyone and everyone from its efficacy and toxicity by banning the drug.

More than a modicum of progress has been made in this arena in the past several decades, particularly as it relates to drug and diet factors that can affect the metabolism or absorption of particular agents, throwing them into the toxic range in certain individuals who happen to have unusual consequences from what they eat or drink, or other prescription drugs that they happen to take. Present studies of the human genome may open new windows on genetic bases for unexpected responses to drugs.

***What are the odds of harm from prescription drugs?***

Looking over several decades, one could say that about 1 new pharmaceutical in 40 to 50 has gotten into some kind of serious controversy about serious adverse effects. That means one controversy every other year until recently, when the rate of approval of new agents increased from the mid-20s to the mid-50s, which can be expected to result in about one controversy per year.

Not all such controversies necessarily signify that the pharmaceutical in question has been responsible for the problem. Indeed, the root question when such controversies erupt is, did the product bring the problem to the patients, or did the patients bring the problem to the product? In some circumstances, a new product enters the marketplace and, for various reasons, ends up being used rather selectively in patients who have especially severe or complicated disease. This type of so-called channeling (Petri and Urquhart 1991) can occur when, for example, it appears that the product has, or is perceived to have, some relative advantage over its competitors in patients with severe disease. Evidence for such perceptions is of variable quality, but if the result is a substantial channeling of the product into patients with special problems, then it becomes rather difficult, when things go wrong, to sort out what has caused what. It is very easy to blame the pharmaceutical, especially if evidence for special benefit is slender. It requires careful measurements in properly controlled studies to sort out patient factors from drug factors, and often, in the heat of acute controversy, pressures mount to solve the problem by forcing the product off the market, rather than taking time for careful studies that may take several years to run.

## One Last Numerical Maneuver and a Bed-Time Story

A sometimes useful maneuver is to put the various leading risks of daily life onto a scale that allows them to be compared with one another. A useful way to do that is the Safety-Degree Scale (Urquhart and Heilmann 1984), which is based on the 10-base logarithm of unicohorts that share a common time base, for example, a year. The Safety-Degree Scale runs between 0 and 8, where zero, the logarithm of 1, means absolute certainty of harm, for example, the leap from the Golden Gate Bridge—1 in 1. The practical upper limit of the Safety-Degree Scale is about 8, which means 1 in 100 million, which is a unicohort about 40% of the size of the U.S. population. Although it is not impossible to define such low-level risks, they become increasingly difficult to quantify with certainty as the potential unicohort verges on being a substantial fraction of the entire U.S. population. Nevertheless, it is sometimes useful to see the leading hazards in daily life presented in this format, to facilitate understanding of how they relate to one another, if only as an antidote to the flow of distorted views that come from the daily news.

An important aspect of this mode of presenting risk-related information is that it clarifies the semantics of the term *safe,* which, like the terms *perfect, unique, round,* and *infallible,* refers to a conceptual ideal that is not subject to modification. Thus, the questions that are often asked about whether it is "safe to fly," or "safe to skydive," or "safe to drive a car" are improperly cast, because the real answer to each is "no," or, if you prefer bureaucratic doublespeak, "yes, but . . . ." The *reductio ad absurdum* of misusage of the term *safe*, came in a recent editorial in the *Lancet,* when the writer claimed that "oral contraceptives are safe, and getting safer" (Spitzer 1997). Any activity, if carefully analyzed, can be shown to pose a certain risk—even staying in bed is not without its adverse consequences of bone demineralization, venous thrombosis, muscle wasting, and postural hypotension upon arising. A major difficulty in assessing the risk of bed rest is to dissociate the risks inherent in semi-immobilization of healthy individuals from the many serious health conditions that cause the patient to take to his/her bed. As far as the prescription of bed rest goes, it is noteworthy that it was standard practice until the 1960s to impose complete bed rest for several weeks after an uncomplicated myocardial infarction, and a generation before that it was standard practice to impose a week or more of bed rest after childbirth. Only gradually did it become evident that the deleterious consequences of the bed rest outweighed any definable benefits, and so these practices were abandoned. So even the ultimate retreat of taking to one's bed is not without the potential for harm, which is why quantitative risk analysis and definition of the outcome in terms of safety-degree is the proper path to follow through the minefield of communicating risk-related information to the public.

## REFERENCES


Brackenridge RDC. 1977. *Medical Selection of Life Risks*. London: Undershaft Press.

[Bureau of the Census] U.S. Bureau of the Census, Department of Commerce. 1997a. *Statistical Abstracts of the United States 1997.* 117th ed. Washington, DC: Government Printing Office. Table 121, p 90.

[Bureau of the Census] U.S. Bureau of the Census, Department of Commerce. 1997b. *Statistical Abstracts of the United States 1997.* 117th ed. Washington, DC: Government Printing Office. Table 117, p 88.

Carson R. 1962. *The Silent Spring*. Boston: Houghton-Mifflin, 368 pp.

Cowell MJ, Hurst BD. 1980. Mortality differences between smokers and nonsmokers. *Trans Soc Actuaries* **32**:1–29.

Dinman B. 1980. The reality and acceptance of risk. *JAMA* **244**: 1226–8.

Feinstein AR. 1991. Intent-to-treat policy for analyzing randomized trials: Statistical distortions and neglected clinical challenges. In: Cramer JA, Spilker B, editors. *Compliance in Medical Practice and Clinical Trials*. New York: Raven, pp 359–70.

Hanley JM, Lippman-Hand A. 1982. If nothing goes wrong is everything all right? *JAMA* **249**:1743–5.

Inman WHW. 1988. Postmarketing surveillance. In: Burley D, Inman WHW, editors. *Therapeutic Risk—Perception, Measurement, Management*. Chichester (UK): Wiley.

[LRCs]. 1984. The Lipid Research Clinics Coronary Primary Prevention Trial results. I. Reduction in incidence of coronary heart disease. II. The relationship of reduction in incidence of coronary heart disease to cholesterol lowering. *JAMA* **251**:351–74.

Petri H, Urquhart J. 1991. Channeling bias in the interpretation of drug effects. *Stat Med* **10**:577–81.

Spitzer WO. 1997. Balanced view of risks of oral contraceptives. *Lancet* **350**:1566–7.

Stelfox HT, Chua G, O'Rourke K, et al. 1998. Conflict of interest in the debate over calcium-channel antagonists. *N Engl J Med* **338**: 101–6.

The Coronary Drug Project Research Group. 1974. Clofibrate and niacin in coronary heart disease. *JAMA* **231**:360–81.

Tobias A. 1982. *The Invisible Bankers*. New York: Simon & Schuster.

*United States v. Johnson*, Supreme Court of the United States; 1911, 221 U.S. 488.

Urquhart J. 1986. Two cheers for NSAIDs. *Gut* **27**:1287–91.

Urquhart J. 1989. Communicating the risk of the unexpected. In: Bogaert M, et al., editors. *Patient Package Insert as a Source of Drug Information*. Amsterdam: Elsevier, pp 153–62.

Urquhart J. 1991. Patient compliance as an explanatory variable in four selected cardiovascular studies. In: Cramer JA, Spilker B, editors. *Compliance in Medical Practice and Clinical Trials*. New York: Raven, pp 301–22.

Urquhart J. 1997. The electronic medication event monitor—lessons for pharmacotherapy. *Clin Pharmacokinet* **32**:345–56.

Urquhart J, Heilmann K. 1984. *Risk Watch—the Odds of Life*. New York: Facts on File.

[USPHS]. 1964. Smoking and health. Report of the Advisory Committee to the Surgeon General of the Public Health Service. Atlanta (GA): U.S. Department of Health, Education, and Welfare, Public Health Service, Centers for Disease Control. PHS Publication 1103.

CHAPTER

# 29 THE CLINICIAN'S ACTIONS WHEN $N = 1$

Gordon Guyatt, David L. Sackett

*Chapter Outline*



The title of this chapter bears discussion. Clinical trials by physician-scientists are done on groups of patients. The letter $N$ is used as a symbol for sample size; $N = 30$ means that there were 30 patients involved in the trial. Clinicians, however, do not treat groups of patients. Rather, they treat individuals. In this sense, the clinician's $N$ is always 1. Implied in this statement is that the clinician's goal always should be to find the best treatment for each individual patient.

How can the clinician best meet this goal? Fifty years ago, clinicians accepted relatively uncontrolled observations suggesting therapeutic benefit from a drug as valid evidence. Since that time, clinicians have learned that uncontrolled observations can be misleading. Clinical investigators have adopted a sophisticated methodology incorporating strategies to avoid misleading results. The key elements of this strategy include randomization (to ensure comparable patients receiving experimental and alternative treatments), double-masking or double-blinding (to reduce the likelihood of bias in measurement, or in administering concomitant treatment), reliable and valid measurement of outcomes, and the use of statistics to help arrive at the appropriate conclusion regarding strength of inference. Studies that use these strategies are likely to yield far more accurate conclusions about appropriate treatment strategies than unsystematic individual observations.

Clinicians face many situations in which the best evidence for their actions comes from randomized trials that apply to groups of patients. Examples include studies of drugs that are given to increase longevity, or to prevent or delay events that occur only once, or infrequently, in the life of patients (stroke, myocardial infarction, exacerbation of inflammatory bowel disease). In these situations the clinician will not be able to determine if an individual patient is one destined to benefit from a drug. Treatment for the individual must then be guided by results derived from a large group of similar people.

There are other situations (the characteristics of which we will describe in some detail) in which it is possible to determine the individual patient's response to a drug. In this situation, the results of randomized trials are still a good starting point for choosing the best therapy. Of course, the relevant trial may never have been done, or the patient at hand may be so different from those who participated in the trial (older or younger, sicker or less sick) that generalizing from the results of the trial may be questionable (Dans Antonio et al. in press). Even if a relevant trial with a comparable patient population is available, one can be sure that the responses were not uniform among the subjects in the trial.

The thrust of this book is to reemphasize that given a particular antianginal, antihypertensive, antiparkinsonian, antiasthmatic (and so on) agent, different patients may respond differently. Even if patients as a group benefit from a drug, there are likely to be individuals who do not. Since no drug is free of adverse effects or potential toxicity (or of expense), the nonresponders are subject to risk or at least cost without benefit.

These considerations suggest that a policy of treating all patients with a particular presentation in a uniform pattern will not lead to optimal treatment for all patients. How can clinicians deal with this problem? One option is to conduct the time-honored "trial of therapy" in which the patient is given a treatment, and the subsequent clinical course determines whether the treatment is judged effective and is continued. Unfortunately, many factors may mislead physicians conducting conventional therapeutic trials. They include the placebo effect, the natural history of the illness, the expectations that the clinician and patient have about the effect of treatment, and the desire of the patient and the clinician not to disappoint one another.

To avoid these pitfalls, such trials of therapy would have to be conducted with safeguards that permit the natural, untreated course of the disorder to be observed and keep both patients and their clinicians "blind" to when active treatment was being administered. These are the safeguards that are routine in large-scale randomized, controlled trials (RCTs) involving up to thousands of patients. We will describe an approach to transferring these safeguards to the evaluation of therapy in the individual patient, an approach we call a *single-patient randomized trial*, or *N* of 1 RCT.

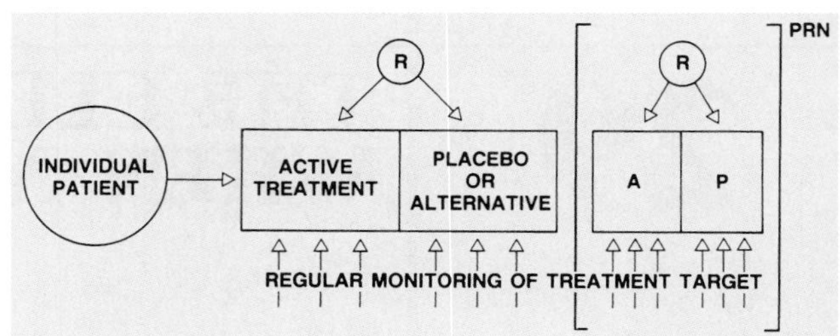


**FIGURE 29-1 Basic design for *N* of 1 randomized, control trial. Circled *R* indicates that the order of placebo and active periods in each pair is determined by random allocation. Bracketed pair with *PRN* indicates that, beyond the first pair of treatment periods, as many additional pairs of treatment periods as necessary are conducted until patient and physician are convinced of the efficacy, or lack of efficacy, of the trial medication. A, active drug; P, placebo or alternative drug.**

## CONDUCTING AN *N* OF 1 RANDOMIZED, CONTROLLED TRIAL

The *N* of 1 RCT is an example of a single-patient experiment. Such experiments are an established research method in psychology (Kratchwill 1978; Kazdin 1982; Barlow and Hersen 1984). This strategy has been applied in medical practice (Guyatt, Sackett et al. 1986; Guyatt et al. 1988). The goal of this chapter is to provide sufficient detail to allow clinicians to plan and execute their own *N* of 1 RCTs, as well as to provide an overview of the likely consequences.

Although there are many ways of conducting *N* of 1 RCTs, a widely applicable method can be summarized as follows:

1. A clinician and patient agree to test a therapy (hereafter called the "experimental therapy") for its ability to improve or control the symptoms, signs, or other manifestations (hereafter called the "treatment targets") of the patient's ailment.
2. The patient then undergoes "pairs" of treatment "periods" organized so that one period of each pair applies the experimental therapy, and the other period applies either an alternative treatment or placebo (Fig. 29-1). The order of these two periods within each pair is randomized by a coin toss or other method that ensures that each period has an equal chance of applying the experimental or alternative therapy.
3. Whenever possible, both the clinician and the patient are "blind" to the treatment being given during any period.
4. The treatment targets are monitored (often through the use of a patient diary) to document the effect of the treatment currently being applied.
5. Pairs of treatment periods are replicated until the clinician and patient are convinced that the experimental therapy is effective, is harmful, or has no effect on treatment targets.

The remainder of this chapter will describe an *N* of 1 randomized trial in detail and then provide a broader perspective on the use of *N* of 1 RCTs. To aid in its implementation, each step will address a question that must be answered before proceeding to the next step (summarized in Table 29-1).

### Is an *N* of 1 Randomized, Controlled Trial Indicated for This Patient?

Because *N* of 1 RCTs are unnecessary for some ailments (such as self-limited illnesses) and unsuited for some treatments (such as operations), it is important to determine, at the outset, whether an *N* of 1 RCT really is appropriate for the patient and treatment in question. If an *N* of 1 RCT is appropriate, the answers to each of the following questions should be yes.

***Is the effectiveness of the treatment really in doubt?*** One or several randomized clinical trials may have shown that the treatment is highly effective. If one is unsure whether such trials have been undertaken, efficient strategies for searching the medical literature are available

**Table 29-1 Guidelines for $N$=1 Randomized, Controlled Trials**

1. Is an $N$ of 1 randomized, controlled trial indicated for this patient?
   a. Is the effectiveness of the treatment really in doubt?
   b. Will the treatment, if effective, be continued long term?
   c. Is the patient eager to collaborate in designing and carrying out an $N$ of 1 randomized, controlled trial?
2. Is an $N$ of 1 randomized control trial feasible in this patient?
   a. Does the treatment have a rapid onset?
   b. Does the treatment cease to act soon after it is discontinued?
   c. Is an optimal duration of treatment feasible?
   d. Can clinically relevant target(s) of treatment be measured?
   e. Can sensible criteria for stopping the trial be established?
   f. Should an unmasked run-in period be conducted?
3. Is an $N$ of 1 randomized, controlled trial feasible in my practice setting?
   a. Is there a pharmacist who can help?
   b. Are strategies for the interpretation of the trial data in place?

(Haynes et al. 1986a–f). However, if a substantial proportion (say, more than half) of patients in such trials have proved unresponsive, an *N* of 1 RCT may still be appropriate. We have described a technique for determining the proportion of patients who have found an important benefit of treatment (Guyatt et al. 1998). The technique relies on determining the proportion of patients in both treatment and control groups who have manifested an important improvement or deterioration, thus allowing calculation of the difference in proportion with important changes in the two groups.

A patient may have exhibited such a dramatic response to the treatment that both clinician and patient are convinced that it works. *N* of 1 RCTs are best reserved for the following situations.

1. The patient has started taking a medication, but neither patient nor clinician is confident that a treatment is really providing benefit.
2. The clinician is uncertain whether a treatment that has not yet been started will work in a particular patient.
3. The patient insists on taking a treatment that the clinician thinks is useless or potentially harmful (and mere words won't change the patient's mind).
4. A patient has symptoms that both the clinician and patient suspect but are not certain are due to the side effects of the medications.
5. Neither the clinician nor the patient is confident of the optimal dose of a medication the patient is receiving or should receive.

***Will the treatment, if effective, be continued long term?***
If the underlying condition is self-limited and treatment will be continued only over the short term, an *N* of 1 RCT may not be worthwhile. *N* of 1 RCTs are most useful when conditions are chronic, and maintenance therapy is likely to be prolonged.

***Is the patient eager to collaborate in designing and carrying out an N of 1 randomized, controlled trial?***
Single-subject RCTs are indicated only when patients can fully understand the nature of the experiment and are enthusiastic about participating. By its nature, the *N* of 1 RCT is a cooperative venture between clinician and patient.

***Is an N of 1 randomized control trial feasible in this patient?***
The clinician may wish to determine the efficacy of treatment in an individual patient, but the ailment, or the treatment, may not lend itself to the *N* of 1 approach. Once again, we shall approach the issue with a series of questions; for the *N* of 1 approach to be feasible, the answer to each must be yes.

***Does the treatment have a rapid onset?***
*N* of 1 RCTs are much easier to do when a treatment, if effective, begins to act within hours. Although it may be possible to do *N* of 1 RCTs with drugs that have longer latency for the development of signs of efficacy (such as gold or penicillamine in rheumatoid arthritis, or tricyclic antidepressants for depression) the requirement for very long treatment periods before the effect can be evaluated (e.g., estrogens in prevention of major bone fractures in postmenopausal women) may prove prohibitive.

***Does the treatment cease to act soon after it is discontinued?***
Treatments whose effects cease abruptly when they are withdrawn are most suitable for *N* of 1 RCTs. If the treatment continues to act long after it is stopped, a prolonged "washout period" may be necessary. If this washout period is longer than a few days, the feasibility of the trial is compromised. Similarly, treatments that have the potential to "cure" the underlying condition, or to lead to a permanent change in the treatment target, are not suitable for *N* of 1 RCTs.

***Is an optimal duration of treatment feasible?***

Although short periods of treatment boost the feasibility of *N* of 1 studies, actual trials may need to be long in order to be valid. For example, if active therapy takes a few days to reach full effect and a few days to cease acting once stopped, treatment periods of sufficient duration to avoid distortion from these delayed peak effects and washouts are required. For example, our *N* of 1 RCTs of theophylline in asthma use treatment periods of at least 10 days: 3 days to allow the drug to reach steady-state concentrations or wash out to very low concentrations, and 7 days thereafter to monitor the patient's response to treatment.

Since many *N* of 1 RCTs test a treatment's ability to prevent or blunt attacks or exacerbations of disease (such as migraines or seizures), each treatment period must be long enough to include an attack or exacerbation. A rough rule of thumb, called the "inverse rule of 3's," tells us: if an event occurs, on average, once every "*x*" days, we need to observe 3*x* days to be 95% confident of observing at least one event. Applying this rule in a patient with familial Mediterranean fever with attacks, on average, once every 2 weeks, calls for treatment periods at least 6 weeks long.

Finally, the clinician may not want the patient to take responsibility for crossing over from one treatment period to the next or may need to examine the patient at the end of each period. As a practical matter, the clinician's office schedule, and patient travel considerations, may dictate the length of each period of treatment.

***Can clinically relevant targets of treatment be measured?***

The targets of treatment, or outcome measures, usually go beyond a set of physical signs (the rigidity and tremor of parkinsonism; the jugular venous distension and the S3, S4, and pulmonary crackles of congestive heart failure), a laboratory test (erythrocyte sedimentation rate, or concentration of blood sugar, uric acid, or serum creatinine), or a measure of patient performance (recordings of peak flow, or score on a 6-minute walk test). Each of these is only an indirect measure of the patient's prognosis and quality of life.

In most situations, it is not only possible but preferable to measure the patients' symptoms, their feelings of well-being, or their quality of life. Principles of measurement of quality of life can be applied in a simple fashion to *N* of 1 RCTs (Guyatt et al. 1985; Guyatt, Bombardier, et al. 1986; Guyatt et al. 1993). To begin with, patients are asked to identify the most troubling symptoms or problems they experience; in this way, symptoms or problems likely to respond to the experimental treatment are identified. This responsive subset of symptoms or problems forms the basis of a self-administered patient diary or questionnaire. For example, a patient with chronic limitation of airflow identified his problem as shortness of breath while walking up stairs, bending, or vacuuming. A patient with fibromyalgia (to whom we shall return later) identified fatigue, aches and pains, morning stiffness, and sleep disturbance as problems that should become the treatment targets for her illness.

The questionnaire to record the patient's symptoms can be presented using a number of formats (Fig. 29-2). A daily diary is best for some; for others a weekly summary may be preferable. The best way of presenting response options to patients is as graded descriptions from none to severe symptoms (no shortness of breath, a little shortness of breath, moderate shortness of breath . . . extreme shortness of breath). Constructing simple symptom questionnaires is not difficult and allows the patient and the clinician to collaborate in the quantification of patient symptoms upon which the analysis of the *N* of 1 RCT often relies.

Whatever formats are chosen for measuring treatment targets, patients should rate each of them at least twice during each study period. The identifying patient information and the ratings on the treatment targets often can be combined on one page; Figure 29-2 displays such a form for an *N* of 1 RCT examining the effectiveness of ketanserin in Raynaud's phenomenon. More detailed guides for constructing the sort of simple questionnaires required for *N* of 1 RCTs are available (Sudman and Bradburn 1982; Woodward and Chambers 1983).

A final point concerning measurement of a patient's symptoms is that adverse effects require attention. A patient diary or questionnaire can be used to measure nausea, GI disturbances, dizziness, or other common adverse effects along with symptoms of the primary condition. In *N* of 1 RCTs designed to determine if medication adverse effects are responsible for a patient's symptoms (for example, whether a patient's fatigue is caused by an antihypertensive agent), adverse effects become the primary treatment targets.

***Can sensible criteria for stopping the trial be established?***

There are advantages to not specifying the number of pairs of treatment periods in advance. Under these circumstances the clinician and patient can stop any time they are convinced that the experimental treatment ought to be stopped or continued indefinitely. If they find dramatic improvement in the treatment target between the two pe-

*N* OF 1 RANDOMIZED CONTROL TRIAL – DATA SHEET 1
PHYSICIAN: DAN SAUDER
PATIENT: ______________________________
SEX: 1) MALE 2) FEMALE DATE OF BIRTH ______ ______ ______
DIAGNOSIS: ______________________________
OCCUPATION: ______________________________
PRESENT MEDICATIONS: ______________________________
TRIAL MEDICATION: KETANSERIN DOSE:
DURATION OF STUDY PERIODS: 2 WEEKS
OUTCOMES: SYMPTOM RATINGS
INFORMED CONSENT OBTAINED (PLEASE SIGN): ______________________________
ANSWERS TO SYMPTOM QUESTIONS, PAIR 1, PERIOD 1:

1. How many episodes of the Raynaud's phenomenon did you have in the last week?
First Week (to be completed on ______ ______) ______
Second Week (to be completed on ______ ______) ______

2. On average, in comparison to your usual episodes, how long were the attacks?
   a. Very long; as long as or longer than they have ever been
   b. Very long; almost as long as they have ever been
   c. Longer than usual
   d. About as long as usual
   e. Not as long as usual
   f. Not nearly as long as usual
   g. Very short; as brief as or briefer than they have ever been

Write in the best number for each week.
First Week (to be completed on ______ ______) ______
Second Week (to be completed on ______ ______) ______

3. On average, in comparison to your usual episodes, how severe were the attacks?
   a. Very bad; as severe as or more severe than they have ever been
   b. Very bad; almost as severe as they have ever been
   c. More severe than usual
   d. About as severe as usual
   e. Not as severe as usual
   f. Not nearly as severe as usual
   g. Very mild; as mild as or milder than they have ever been

Write in the best number for each week.
First Week (to be completed on ______ ______) ______
Second Week (to be completed on ______ ______) ______

FIGURE 29-2 **Data collection form.**

riods of the first pair, both clinician and patient may want to stop the trial immediately. However, if there continues to be a minimal difference between the two periods of each pair, both clinician and the patient may need three, four, or even five or more pairs before confidently concluding that the treatment is or is not effective.

If, however, one wishes to conduct a formal statistical analysis of data from the *N* of 1 RCT, the analysis is strengthened if the number of pairs is specified in advance. This issue is discussed further in the section concerning strategies for interpretation of *N* of 1 RCTs.

Whether or not the number of treatment periods is specified in advance, it is advisable to conduct at least two pairs of treatment periods before breaking the code. Too many conclusions drawn after a single pair will be either false-positive judgments (that the treatment is effective when it isn't) or false-negative judgments (that the treatment is not effective when it is). Indeed, we recommend that clinicians resist the temptation and refrain from breaking the code until they are quite certain they are ready to terminate the study.

***Should an unmasked run-in period be conducted?***
A preliminary run-in period on active therapy, during which both the physician and patient know that active therapy is being received, can save a lot of time. After

all, if there is no hint of response during such an open trial, or if intolerable adverse effects occur, an *N* of 1 RCT may be fruitless or impossible. For example, we prepared for a double-blind *N* of 1 RCT of methylphenidate in a child with hyperactivity only to find a dramatic increase in agitation over the first 2 days of the first study period (during which the patient was receiving the active drug) mandating an abrupt termination of the study. Finally, an open run-in may be used to determine the optimal dose of the medication.

## Is an *N* of 1 Randomized, Controlled Trial Feasible in My Practice Setting?

Clinicians may answer "yes" to the preceding questions and still be unsure about how to proceed. There are approaches that will ensure the feasibility of an *N* of 1 RCT in various practices.

***Is there a pharmacist who can help?***
Conducting an *N* of 1 RCT that incorporates all the aforementioned safeguards against bias and misinterpretation requires collaboration between the clinician and a pharmacist or pharmacy service. Preparation of placebos identical to the active medication in appearance, taste, and texture is required. Occasionally, pharmaceutical firms can supply such placebos. More often, however, you will want your local pharmacist to repackage the active medication. If it comes in tablet form, it can be crushed and repackaged in capsule form unless the medication is a modified release preparation whose absorption characteristics will be altered. In that case, a clinician interested in the effect of a modified release preparation may have to sacrifice blinding if the duration of action of the medication is a crucial issue.

If a placebo is judged important, the pharmacist can fill identical-appearing placebo capsules with lactose. While somewhat time-consuming, preparation of placebos is not technically difficult. Our average cost for preparing medication for *N* of 1 studies in which placebos have not been available from the pharmaceutical company has been about $100. We have relied on a number of strategies for funding, including use of discretionary research funds or the generosity of a large hospital pharmacy. The large savings that follow from abandoning a useless or harmful treatment that would otherwise be continued indefinitely emphasize the relatively trivial cost of the *N* of 1 RCT. However, the potential for cost-effective improvement in therapeutics using this approach has not yet been determined.

The pharmacist is also charged with preparing the randomization schedule (which requires nothing more than a coin toss for each pair of treatment periods). This allows the clinician, along with the patient, to remain blind to allocation. The pharmacist also may be helpful in planning the design of the trial by providing information regarding the anticipated time to onset of action and the washout period, thus helping with decisions about the duration of study periods. The pharmacist can help monitor compliance and drug absorption. Both tablet counts and measuring serum drug concentrations at the end of each treatment period can help establish that the patient conscientiously takes the study medication throughout the trial.

***Are strategies for the interpretation of the trial data in place?***
Once you carefully gather data on the treatment targets in your *N* of 1 trial, how will you interpret them? One approach is simply to plot the data and to examine the results by visual inspection. Evaluation of results by visual inspection has a long and distinguished record in the psychology literature concerning single-subject designs and is strongly advocated by some practitioners of single-patient studies (Kratchwill 1978; Kazdin 1982; Barlow and Hersen 1984). Visual inspection is simple and easy. Its major disadvantage is that it is open to viewer or observer bias.

An alternative approach to analysis of data from *N* of 1 RCTs is to utilize a statistical test of significance. The simplest test would be based on the likelihood of a patient's preferring active treatment in each pair of treatment periods. This situation is analogous to the likelihood of heads coming up repeatedly on a series of coin tosses. For example the likelihood of the patient's preferring active treatment to placebo during three consecutive pairs if the treatment was ineffective would be $\frac{1}{2} \times \frac{1}{2} \times \frac{1}{2} = \frac{1}{8}$ or 0.125. The disadvantage of this approach (which is called the *sign test*) (Conover 1971) is that it lacks power: Five pairs must be conducted (and produce the same result) before there is any chance of reaching conventional levels of statistical significance (e.g., $p < 0.05$).

A second statistical strategy is to use Student's *t*-test. The *t*-test offers increased power because not only the direction but also the strength of the treatment effect in each pair is taken into account. The disadvantage of the *t*-test is that it makes additional assumptions about the data that may not be valid. The assumption of greatest concern is that observations are independent of one another; that is, that a patient is equally likely to feel good or bad on a particular day irrespective of whether he or she felt good or bad the day before. The term used to describe data that are not independent is *autocorrelation*.

While some autocorrelation is likely to exist in many $N$ of 1 RCTs, the impact of the autocorrelation can be decreased if the average of all measurements in a given period is used in the statistical analysis (rather than the individual observations). Furthermore, the paired design of the $N$ of 1 RCT that we recommend further decreases the impact of any autocorrelation that may exist.

If any statistical test is going to be used to interpret the data, the clinician faces another potential problem: if the clinician and patient use the results from the studies to determine when to stop the trial, the true $p$ value may be inflated above the nominal $p$ value. Consequently, if a statistical test is planned, the number of periods should be specified before the study begins.

To conduct a paired $t$-test, a single score is derived for each pair by subtracting the mean score of the placebo period from the mean score for the active period. These difference scores constitute the data for the paired $t$; the number of degrees of freedom is simply the number of pairs minus 1. PC-based statistical packages that will allow quick calculation of the $p$ value are readily available.

The results of an $N$ of 1 RCT are presented in Table 29-2. In this trial the effectiveness of amitriptyline in a dose of 10 mg at bedtime for a patient with fibromyalgia (referred to earlier) was tested. Each week, the patient rated the severity of a number of symptoms, including fatigue, aches and pains, and sleep disturbance, each on a 7-point scale in which a higher score represented better function. The treatment periods were 4 weeks, and three pairs were undertaken. The mean scores for each of the 24 weeks of the study are presented in Table 29-2.

The first step in analyzing the results of the study is to calculate the mean score for each period (presented in the last column of Table 29-2). In each pair the score favored the active treatment. The sign test tells us that the probability of this result occurring by chance if the treatment was ineffective is $\frac{1}{2} \times \frac{1}{2} \times \frac{1}{2} = \frac{1}{8}$ (or $= 0.125$). However, this analysis ignores the magnitude and consistency of the difference between active and placebo treatments. A paired $t$-test takes these factors into account. The pairs of results are 4.68 and 4.22; 5.01 and 4.07; 5.04 and 4.18. For these results, the $t$ value is 5.07, and there are two degrees of freedom; the associated $p$ value is 0.037. This analysis provides confidence that the consistent difference in favor of active drug is unlikely to have occurred by chance.

Clinicians and statisticians may remain uncomfortable with the suggested approach to analysis of data from $N$ of 1 RCTs. The use of $N$ of 1 RCTs to improve patient care does not depend on the statistical analysis of the results. Even if a "formal" statistical analysis is not used in the interpretation of the trial, the strategies of randomization, double-blinding, replication, and quantifying outcomes, when accompanied by careful visual inspection of the data, still allow a much more rigorous assessment of effectiveness of treatment than is possible in conventional clinical practice.

## ETHICS OF CLINICAL TRIALS

Is the conduct of an $N$ of 1 RCT a clinical or a research undertaking? If the former, is it the sort of clinical procedure, analogous to an invasive diagnostic test, that requires written informed consent? We would argue that the $N$ of 1 RCT can, and should be, a part of routine clinical practice.

Nevertheless, a number of ethical issues are important. We believe that patients should be fully informed of the nature of the study in which they are participating, and there should be no element of deception when pla-

**Table 29-2** **Results of an $N$ of 1 Randomized Control Trial in a Patient with Fibromyalgia**

| | Severity Score | | | | |
|---|---|---|---|---|---|
| **Treatment*** | **Week 1** | **Week 2** | **Week 3** | **Week 4** | **Mean score** |
| Pair 1 | | | | | |
| Active | 4.43 | 4.86 | 4.71 | 4.71 | 4.68 |
| Placebo | 4.43 | 4.00 | 4.14 | 4.29 | 4.22 |
| Pair 2 | | | | | |
| Active | 4.57 | 4.89 | 5.29 | 5.29 | 5.01 |
| Placebo | 3.86 | 4.00 | 4.29 | 4.14 | 4.07 |
| Pair 3 | | | | | |
| Active | 4.29 | 5.00 | 5.43 | 5.43 | 5.04 |
| Placebo | 3.71 | 4.14 | 4.43 | 4.43 | 4.18 |

*The active drug was amitriptyline hydrochloride. Higher scores represent better function.

cebos are used as part of the study. Written informed consent should be obtained. Patients should be aware that they can terminate the trial at any time without jeopardizing their care or their relationship with their physician. Finally, follow-up should be close enough to prevent any important deleterious consequences of institution or withdrawal of therapy.

## THE IMPACT OF *N* OF 1 RANDOMIZED, CONTROLLED TRIALS IN CLINICAL PRACTICE

We have reported a series of over 50 *N* of 1 RCTs, each one designed to improve the care being delivered to an individual patient (Guyatt et al. 1990). Patients suffered from a wide variety of conditions, including chronic airflow limitation, asthma, fibrositis, arthritis, syncope, anxiety, insomnia, and angina pectoris. In general, these trials have been very successful in sorting out whether the treatment was effective. In approximately a third, the ultimate treatment differed from that which would have been given had the trial not been conducted. In most of these, medication that would otherwise have been given over the long term was discontinued. Other clinical groups have reported on their experience with *N* of 1 RCTs, generally confirming the feasibility and usefulness of the approach (Menard et al. 1988; Johannessen 1991; Larson et al. 1993).

These reports do not definitively answer the question about whether patients who undergo *N* of 1 RCTs are better off than those whose treatment regimen is determined by conventional methods. The most rigorous test of the usefulness of *N* of 1 RCTs would be a randomized trial. Two such trials, in which patients were randomized to conventional care or to undergo *N* of 1 RCTs, have been undertaken (Mahon et al. 1996, unpublished manuscript). Both were conducted by the same group of investigators, and both studied the use of theophylline in patients with chronic airflow limitation. The investigators found that while using *N* of 1 RCTs did not effect patients' quality of life or functional status, of patients initially on theophylline, fewer in the *N* of 1 RCT groups ended up receiving the drug in the long term. Thus, *N* of 1 RCTs saved patients the expense, inconvenience, and potential toxicity of individually ineffective, long-term theophylline therapy.

While confirming the potential of *N* of 1 RCTs, groups with extensive experience with *N* of 1 RCTs have noted the time and effort required. It is unlikely that full implementation of *N* of 1 RCTs will become a major part of clinical practice. Clinicians can, however, incorporate many of the key principles of *N* of 1 RCTs into their practice without adopting the full rigor of the approach presented here. Medication can be repeatedly withdrawn and reintroduced in an open or unmasked fashion. Symptoms and physical findings can be carefully quantified. However, without the additional feature of double-blinding, both the placebo effect and physician and patient expectations can still bias the results.

In summary, the *N* of 1 approach clearly has potential for improving the quality of medical care and the judicious use of expensive and potentially toxic medication in patients with chronic disease. Using the guidelines offered here, we believe that clinicians will find the conduct of *N* of 1 RCTs feasible, highly informative, and stimulating.

## REFERENCES


Barlow DH, Hersen M. 1984. *Single Case Experimental Designs: Strategies for Studying Behavior Change.* 2nd ed. New York: Pergamon Press, pp 419.

Conover WJ. 1971. *Practical Nonparametric Statistics.* New York: John Wiley, pp 121–6.

Dans Antonio L, Dans Leonila F, Guyatt GH, et al. for the EBM Working Group. (In press). Users' guides to the medical literature XIV: How to decide on the applicability of clinical trial results to your patient. *JAMA.*

Guyatt GH, Berman LB, Townsend M, et al. 1985. Should study subjects see their previous responses? *J Chron Dis* **38**:1003–7.

Guyatt GH, Bombardier C, Tugwell PX. 1986b. Measuring disease-specific quality of life in clinical trials. *Can Med Assoc J* **134**: 889–95.

Guyatt GH, Feeny DH, Patrick DL. 1993. Measuring health-related quality of life [review]. *Ann Intern Med* **70**:225–30.

Guyatt GH, Juniper EL, Walter SD, et al. 1998. Interpreting treatment effects in randomised trials [review]. *Br Med J* **316**:690–3.

Guyatt GH, Keller JL, Jaeschke R, et al. 1990. The n-of-1 randomized controlled trial: Clinical usefulness. Our three year experience. *Ann Intern Med* **112**:293–9.

Guyatt GH, Sackett D, Taylor DW, et al. 1986a. Determining optimal therapy: Randomized trials in individual patients. *N Engl J Med* **314**:889–92.

Guyatt GH, Sackett DL, Adachi JD, et al. 1988. A clinician's guide for conducting randomized trials in individual patients. *Can Med Assoc J* **139**:497–503.

Haynes RB, McKibbon KA, Fitzgerald D, et al. 1986a. How to keep up with the medical literature: I. Why try to keep up and how to get started. *Ann Intern Med* **105**:149–53.

Haynes RB, McKibbon KA, Fitzgerald D, et al. 1986b. How to keep up with the medical literature: II. Deciding which journals to read regularly. *Ann Intern Med* **105**:309–12.

Haynes RB, McKibbon KA, Fitzgerald D, et al. 1986c. How to keep up with the medical literature: III. Expanding the volume of literature that you read regularly. *Ann Intern Med* **105**:474–8.

Haynes RB, McKibbon KA, Fitzgerald D, et al. 1986d. How to keep up with the medical literature: IV. Using the literature to solve clinical problems. *Ann Intern Med* **105**:636–40.

Haynes RB, McKibbon KA, Fitzgerald D, et al. 1986e. How to keep up with the medical literature: V. Personal computer access to the medical literature. *Ann Intern Med* **105**:810–24.

Haynes RB, McKibbon KA, Fitzgerald D, et al. 1986f. How to keep up with the medical literature: VI. How to store and retrieve articles worth keeping. *Ann Intern Med* **105**:978–84.

Johannessen T. 1991. Controlled trials in single subjects. 1. Value in clinical medicine. *Br Med J* **303**:173–4.

Kazdin AE. 1982. *Single-Case Research Designs: Methods for Clinical and Applied Settings.* New York: Oxford University Press, pp 368.

Kratchwill TR, editor. 1978. *Single Subject Research: Strategies for Evaluating Change.* Orlando, FL: Academic Press, pp 316.

Larson EB, Ellsworth AJ, Oas J. 1993. Randomized clinical trials in single patients during a 2-year period. *JAMA* **270**:2708–12.

Mahon J, Laupacis A, Donner A, et al. 1996. Randomised study of n of 1 trials versus standard practice. *Br Med J* **312**:1069–74.

Mahon J, Laupacis A, Hodder, et al. [Unpublished manuscript]. Theophylline for irreversible chronic airflow limitation: A randomized study comparing n of 1 trials to standard practice.

Menard J, Serrurier D, Bautier P, et al. 1988. Crossover design to test antihypertensive drugs with self-recorded blood pressure. *Hypertension* **11**:153–9.

Sudman S, Bradburn NM. 1982. *Asking Questions: A Practical Guide to Questionnaire Design.* San Francisco: Jossey-Bass.

Woodward CA, Chambers LW. 1983. *Guide to Questionnaire Construction and Question Writing.* Ottawa: Canadian Public Health Association.

CHAPTER

# 30 INFORMATION ABOUT DRUGS

## A Clinical Epidemiologic Approach to Therapeutics

Brian L. Strom

### *Chapter Outline*



Throughout this book, we have tried to provide an approach to rational therapeutics that is useful in all areas and applications of drug therapy. In this final chapter, we discuss some of the difficulties encountered when the prescribing physician tries to find, evaluate, and use the best information available about the efficacy and toxicity of drugs in his or her patients.

All active scientific fields, including clinical pharmacology, are continually advancing, and new drugs continually appear. Practicing clinicians need to integrate the new information on drugs in the context of the core principles of clinical pharmacology. Only then can the best possible therapeutic decisions be made. Unfortunately, the information necessary to help the prescriber make optimal therapeutic decisions often is incomplete, especially for the newest drugs. Despite this deficiency, a clinical decision must be made for the patient at hand.

Linking clinical pharmacology with epidemiology and, in particular, clinical epidemiology, can help the clinician to make the best possible decisions. Epidemiologists study the distribution and determinants of diseases in populations (Mausner and Kramer 1985; Ahlbom and Norell 1990; Friedman 1994; Lilienfeld and Lilienfeld 1994; Kelsey et al. 1996; MacMahon and Pugh 1996). The field of epidemiology conventionally considers the determinants of diseases that relate to the host, the agent, or the environment. For a question of therapeutics, the *host* is the patient, with his or her unique characteristics that need to be taken into account in order to individualize therapy. The *agent* is the drug or drugs and whatever information may be known about their effects. The *environment* is the body of clinical pharmacologic principles, such as those that are in this book. This chapter is organized in this fashion.

The field of *clinical epidemiology* focuses on how to critically review the medical literature and how to apply the principles of epidemiology to clinical medicine (Schuman 1986; Hennekens and Buring 1987; Hulley and Cummings 1988; Sackett et al. 1991; Fletcher et al. 1996; Greenberg et al. 1996; Weiss 1996; Rothman 1998). Clinical epidemiology also has been conceptualized as involving four central aspects of disease: 1) burden of disease, including frequency and prognosis, 2) etiology, 3) diagnosis, and 4) treatment. All these are highly relevant to individual therapeutic decisions for a patient. This chapter presents a clinical epidemiologic approach to therapeutics by first discussing the information about the patient that must be considered, then the information about the drug, and finally placing these in context with selected core principles of clinical pharmacology. The chapter attempts to synthesize all three. Reference sources that discuss each of these topics in more detail are provided.

Finally, *pharmacoepidemiology* is the study of drug use and drug effects in populations (Strom 1994). In a sense, this chapter discusses clinical pharmacoepidemiology, that is, pharmacoepidemiology as it applies to the individual patient.

**Key Points: Clinical pharmacoepidemiology requires the prescriber to consider the host (patient), agent (drug), and environment (related factors) when planning pharmacotherapy for a specific patient.**

## THE HOST: PATIENT FACTORS IN CLINICAL THERAPEUTICS

By now it should be clear that clinical therapeutics involves the use and choice of drugs tailored to the needs of the patient at hand. To tailor therapy to an individual patient's needs, one obviously has to explore the characteristics of the patient. Taking a traditional history and performing a physical examination (Bates 1979) represent the first steps in making a therapeutic decision and are critical in making a correct diagnosis (Griner et al. 1981). The severity and prognosis of the disease must then be assessed. The severity of the disease partially determines the need for drug treatment. A severe disease and/or a poor prognosis are more compelling indications for drug treatment than the amelioration of symptoms of an inconsequential medical problem. In the former, one should be more willing to incur known or unknown risks of toxicity. In contrast, a disease that is mild and self-limited should not, in general, be treated unless the treatment is both very effective and very benign in adverse effects and cost.

The severity of the disease generally is determined by the clinician observing the individual patient. Determination of the prognosis of the disease, in contrast, is almost always a decision based on the available literature about the disease. Although one may have sufficient clinical experience with a given disease to have a sense of its prognosis, reviewing the literature almost always adds further useful information. Studies of large populations of patients with the disease (case series, see below), preferably including a comparison with a control group of patients without that disease (cohort studies, see below), are needed to truly evaluate a disease's prognosis. When detailed information is available on the determinants of a good or poor prognosis, one can determine whether an individual patient has a prognosis similar to or different from others who have the same disease (e.g., the stage of cancer).

In addition to the details of a patient's illness, one must pay careful attention to other factors in making a therapeutic decision. In particular, determining whether a patient is receiving other drugs is necessary to avoid unintended and adverse drug interactions. Knowledge of past drug allergies can be used to avoid preventable adverse drug reactions. Awareness of other diseases from which the patient suffers, particularly those affecting renal and liver functions, allows perspective on how to avoid drug–disease interactions. When all these factors (and others) are considered, one can approach a therapeutic decision armed with sufficient detail about a possible indication for drug use in the patient.

## THE AGENT: INFORMATION AVAILABLE ON THERAPEUTIC OPTIONS

Once one has decided that a patient has a disease that should be treated, one needs to consider the available options in the choice of drug and drug regimen for the patient. In particular, a clinician must understand the clinical pharmacology of the drug options available in this situation (and details of nonpharmacologic therapeutic options as well). For this decision, information on both the pharmacokinetics and the pharmacodynamics of the drug is needed.

### Sources of Information

The primary source of up-to-date and useful information about drugs is the medical literature. Clinicians must develop skills to investigate and properly interpret the medical literature themselves. Sometimes the information can be found in a physician's personal clinical files. However, even in the largest of practices, the incidence rates of a given drug- or disease-related event would have to be very high for personal experience to be sufficient for determining the best medical decisions.

Textbooks often can provide a useful synthesis of the information available in the medical literature, easing the practitioner's task of analyzing the data and providing expert judgment. This book is intended to provide just such a service for many clinical situations. Clinical textbooks also may be useful. Other good sources of drug information are *Drug Information for the Health Care Professional* (the U.S. Pharmacopoeia [USPC] 1998), *Drug Evaluations* (the American Medical Association [AMA] 1990), *Mosby's GenRx* (1998), the *American Hospital Formulary Service Drug Information* (American Society of Hospital Pharmacists [ASHP] 1998), *Facts and Comparisons* (Boyd 1998), and so forth. These are all created by expert bodies to provide the clinician with a synthesis of the information available about drugs. They are all tied to some degree to the drug's label as approved by the U.S. Food and Drug Administration (FDA).

However, unlike the *Physicians' Desk Reference* (PDR 1998), which presents the exact FDA-approved language as provided by the drug manufacturer, other sources can recommend so-called off-label drug uses, i.e., indications for a drug that are clinically appropriate, even if they have not been through the formal regulatory review process. In addition, these standard compendia do not have to list all possible adverse reactions, for the purpose of product liability protection, but can prioritize their presentations in a manner that is clinically most useful. Consequently, these books are generally more useful to the clinician than is the PDR. Electronic versions of these books, or related databases, e.g., *Mosby's GenRx*, Clinical Pharmacology On-line (Gold Standard Multimedia, Tampa, FL), are readily available as diskettes, on CD-ROM, or over the internet on the World Wide Web.

An increasing number of external sources are available to prescribers as well, without the prescribers' solicitation of them, or sometimes even desire for them. Included are the reports of the large number of organizations now synthesizing the literature into sometimes conflicting consensus papers or guidelines (e.g., National Institutes of Health, the Agency for Health Care Policy and Research, the U.S. Preventive Services Task Force, and the comparable organizations in Canada, and multiple professional and foundation organizations, such as the American Cancer Society). Also included are the drug utilization review programs now required of every Medicaid program and implemented as well by most managed care organizations and pharmacy benefit plans, and the drug use evaluations required of hospitals by the Joint Commission on Accreditation of Healthcare Organizations (JCAHO).

Despite the availability of these sources, there will be many times when a prescriber needs to resort to the primary medical literature, either because the textbooks and compendia do not provide the exact information needed for a specific patient or subset of patients, or because the opinions expressed in the texts, compendia, or guidelines are incomplete, contradictory, or need validation. Given the continual development of new drugs and the rapid acquisition of new data on old drugs, most textbooks risk being out of date on some topics almost as soon as they are published. It is for this reason that this book has stressed principles that should be applicable in many situations, not just the examples given.

One source of synthesis a clinician finds in the literature is the classical review paper. Too often, however, such reviews have been unsystematic, selective, uncritical, or not quantitative. To help address these issues, there is increasing use of an approach referred to as *meta-analysis*. Meta-analysis has been defined as "the statistical analysis of a collection of analytic results for the purpose of integrating the findings" (DerSimonian and Laird 1986). Meta-analysis is used to identify sources of variation among study findings and, when appropriate, to provide an overall statistical measure as a summary of those findings. The distinguishing feature of meta-analysis, as opposed to the usual qualitative literature review, is its systematic, structured, and objective presentation and analysis of available data.

Perhaps the best-recognized application of meta-analysis for most clinicians is the summary of a group of randomized clinical trials dealing with a particular therapy for a particular disease. Typically, this type of meta-analysis would present a single overall measure (and confidence interval) of the efficacy of treatment. The goal often is to aggregate the results across the studies to overcome the limited application of too small a sample size in each study. More sophisticated meta-analyses also examine the variability of results among trials and, when results have been conflicting, analyses are performed to attempt to uncover the sources of the disagreements. More recently, meta-analyses of nonexperimental epidemiologic studies have begun to be performed, and articles have been written describing the methodological considerations specific to those meta-analyses. In general, both the meta-analyses of nonexperimental studies and the associated methodological articles tend to focus more on the exploration of reasons for disagreement among the results of prior studies. Given the greater diversity of designs, and often results, of nonexperimental studies as compared with randomized trials, the legitimacy of conclusions from meta-analysis of nonexperimental studies is much more controversial than meta-analyses of randomized clinical trials.

Ultimately, however, the critical evaluation of the medical literature depends on the individual's skills at assessing the quality of each report and the applicability of each paper to the patient at hand. A valid judgment cannot be made based on a selective literature search. Often the search must be comprehensive, even though it is abbreviated. Fortunately, this is now much easier with the advent of databases such as MEDLINE, a number of commercial vendors of software (e.g., Grateful Med© and OVID) and academic programs (e.g., Stanford Health Information Network for Education [SHINE]) that can assist the individual clinician in accessing the medical literature and other medical information. Some of these databases (SHINE and OVID) even have the full text of the papers on-line, so the paper itself can be read from the computer terminal. Of course this level of detailed literature search is not always necessary or feasible. For individuals who are sufficiently aware of the literature in their specialty, a computer search may be unnecessary. Alternatively, one can search sources such as the American College of Physicians (ACP) Journal Club On-line, ACP Evidence-Based Medicine On-line, and the Cochrane Collaboration Library (OVID). It is important, however, that one not be limited to selected, incomplete, or potentially biased sources of information such as isolated papers, a physician's personal experience, or the *Physicians' Desk Reference* (PDR 1998), which is inherently limited by the FDA-approved labeling.

**PRINCIPLE The skilled prescriber should know the advantages and disadvantages of common sources of information about drugs: textbooks, compendia, reviews, primary literature, and electronic databases. No single source is optimal for all situations.**

## Types of Study Designs

A major focus of clinical epidemiology is to enable clinicians to develop skills in interpreting the medical literature. There is a growing body of literature specifically aimed at how to read and critique the medical literature (Oxman et al. 1993; Jaeschke et al. 1994a, 1994b; Laupacis et al. 1994; Levine et al. 1994; Richardson and Detsky 1995a, 1995b; Wilson et al. 1995; Drummond et al. 1997; O'Brien et al. 1997). To a degree, these skills develop as a function of practice, initially under supervision. However, one first has to understand the basic types of study designs used in clinical research and their advantages and disadvantages.

The various study designs are presented in hierarchical fashion in Table 30-1. The least-convincing designs are listed on the bottom; the most-convincing (but hardest to do) on the top. These are reviewed in more detail elsewhere (Strom 1994a) and are thoroughly described in a number of clinical epidemiology texts (Schuman 1986; Hennekens and Buring 1987; Hulley and Cummings 1988; Sackett et al. 1991; Fletcher et al. 1996; Greenberg et al. 1996; Weiss 1996; Rothman 1998). These designs are briefly reviewed here, especially as the methodology applies to clinical pharmacology.

### *Case reports*

Much of the medical literature is composed of *case reports*. These describe an individual patient, his or her exposure to drugs, and the individual's clinical outcome. The exposures to drugs encountered by the individual may or may not have caused his or her clinical outcome (whether efficacy or toxicity). Most information on adverse drug effects comes, at least initially, from case reports sent either to the medical literature or to FDA's reporting system for and by health professionals, now referred to as the MedWatch system. This approach to uncovering the unknown effects of a drug is useful for raising hypotheses about possible drug effects.

For example, oral contraceptives were first linked to venous thromboembolism in case reports (Ferguson

**Table 30-1 Study Designs Used in Clinical Research**

| Study design | Advantages | Disadvantages |
|---|---|---|
| Randomized clinical trial (experimental study) | Most convincing design<br>Only design that controls for unknown or unmeasurable confounders | Most expensive<br>Clinically artificial<br>Logistically most difficult<br>Ethical objections |
| Cohort study | Can study multiple outcomes<br>Can study uncommon exposures<br>Selection bias diminished<br>Unbiased exposure data<br>Incidence data available | Possibly biased outcome data<br>Expensive<br>If done prospectively, may take years to complete |
| Case–control study | Can study multiple exposures<br>Can study uncommon diseases<br>Logistically easier and faster<br>Less expensive | Control selection problematic<br>Possibly biased exposure data |
| Analyses of secular trends | Can provide rapid answers | No control of confounding |
| Case series | Easy quantification of incidence | No control group, so cannot be used for hypothesis testing |
| Case reports | Cheap and easy method for generating hypothesis | Cannot be used for hypothesis testing |

1967). As another example, the fact that suprofen caused acute bilateral flank pain and renal failure was identified based on the physician reporting system (Rossi et al. 1988). However, many case reports of possible adverse drug reactions in the literature subsequently are not confirmed to be due to the drug (Lauper 1980). A causal relationship between drug and event is more likely when: 1) one is studying a disorder that occurs extraordinarily rarely without the use of the drug; 2) one can compile a number of reports of individuals who had the same adverse outcome while taking the drug; or 3) one can compile a series of patients in whom the event appeared as the drug was given, disappeared (i.e., the patient recovered) as the drug was discontinued, and finally recurred when the drug was restarted. Most case reports cannot be relied on to demonstrate whether a drug truly causes a given adverse outcome. These are very important limitations of the case report literature, even though those reports are common.

***Case series***

*Case series* are reports of groups of patients who have either a common drug exposure or a common disease. These series focus on detecting subsequent disease outcome or antecedent exposures to drugs that can cause the disease, respectively. Case series are an improvement over case reports. Because these are groups of patients, they are more likely to be typical of those who have the exposure or those who have the disease. A case series can be useful, for example, for quantifying the incidence of an adverse event in a group of patients treated with a newly marketed drug. Without a control group, however, they rarely can be used to conclude whether a drug causes a given outcome. Despite this shortcoming, case series frequently have been used to study the effects of marketed drugs, as so-called phase IV cohort studies. For example, a phase IV cohort study of prazosin was conducted to quantify the frequency of first-dose syncope (Subcommittee on Health and Scientific Research 1980).

***Analyses of secular trends***

*Analyses of secular trends* or *ecologic studies* are studies that compare trends in exposures to drugs with trends in a given disease or event. The study looks to see whether the two trends coincide. The trends can be over time or across geographic areas. In studies relevant to clinical pharmacology, the exposures obviously are to drugs. The data on exposures generally come from marketing data about drug sales. The data on occurrences of disease usually come from publicly collected vital statistics. This approach is useful as a fast and easy method to provide support for or refutation of a hypothesis about a drug effect. Thus, the incidence of a disease in question can be explored to see whether it has increased since a new drug was released into the market or whether the incidence of the disease differs in countries that have allowed the marketing of the drug versus those that have not. For example, the association between oral contraceptives and thromboembolism was confirmed by analyses of secular trends that confirmed coincident trends between increasing sales of oral contraceptives and increasing mortality rates from pulmonary embolism, trends that were present in women of reproductive age but not in men or postmenopausal women (Markush and Seigel 1969). However, usually there are many different exposures to drugs whose trends coincide with the trend in incidence of a disease. In addition, many exposures to factors other than drugs also coincide with the changed incidence of the disease. These studies cannot generally differentiate which exposure is the causal factor in the events of interest. Finally, such studies suffer from the so-called ecologic paradox, i.e., even if there is an association, the people who suffer from the disease under study may not be the same people who were exposed to the risk factor of interest. Thus, analyses of secular trends are relatively weak ways of demonstrating causation.

***Case–control studies***

*Case–control studies* compare individuals with a disease *(cases)* to individuals without a disease *(controls)*. A search for differences in "exposures" antecedent to the disease is then undertaken (see Figure 30-1). The case–control approach can be very useful to explore any of a number of drugs as possible causes of a single disease, especially a very rare disease. The approach also is very useful for exploring diseases that take a long time to develop. For example, the association between oral contraceptives and thromboembolism was confirmed in case–control studies (Sartwell et al. 1969). Case–control studies can even be used to screen for beneficial drug effects. For example, the protective effect of aspirin on the development of myocardial infarction (MI) was suggested in a case–control study (Rosenberg et al. 1982). This was confirmed in a randomized clinical trial, but not until many years later (Steering Committee of the Physicians' Health Study Research Group 1989).

Case–control studies are subject to a number of important problems, however. It is difficult to choose a control group without the disease or condition under consideration that is properly comparable to the case group. Choosing the wrong control group can result in very misleading conclusions. Also, gathering drug histories retrospectively often is very difficult because patients and of-

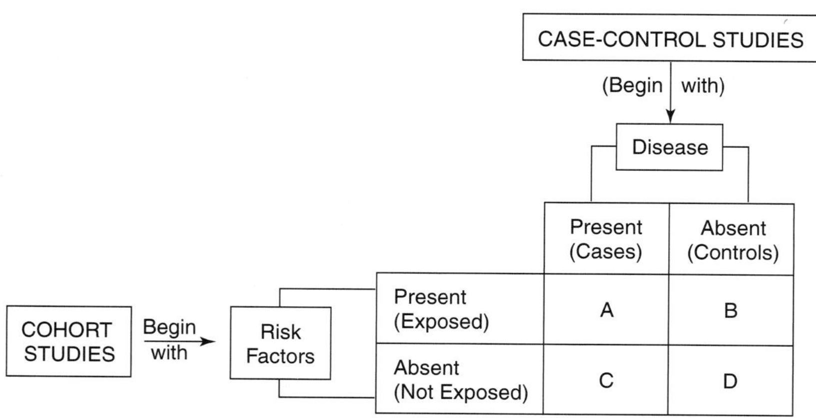


FIGURE 30-1 **Case–control versus cohort studies.**

ten clinicians are not aware of the drugs the patients are taking now, let alone those that they took previously (Harlow and Linett 1989; West and Strom 1994). Examples of major errors in findings by case–control studies include the studies linking reserpine to breast cancer (Boston Collaborative Drug Surveillance Program 1974; Armstrong et al. 1974; Heinonen et al. 1974) and those linking coffee to pancreatic cancer (MacMahon et al. 1981). However, when well performed, case–control studies generally confirm the results of the more powerful designs.

As a means of taking advantage of the power of case–control studies, while addressing their limitations, pharmacoepidemiologists nowadays are commonly performing such studies within automated databases of medical claims data. These databases solve the problem of gathering drug histories retrospectively, since they can identify exactly what drugs were dispensed to patients. Ironically these valuable data were collected to justify claims for pharmacy payments, not for discovery of important medical events. They solve the problem of how to choose the control group, since the entire population eligible for care in that health care system can be enumerated, and the control group then chosen as a true random sample from that population.

### *Cohort studies*

*Cohort studies* compare exposed to unexposed patients and evaluate differences in outcome over time (see Figure 30-1). Cohort studies can also be used to compare people receiving one exposure to others receiving another, looking for differences in outcome. Cohort studies can be performed either prospectively, i.e., simultaneously with the events under study, or retrospectively, i.e., after the events under study, by recreating those past events using medical records, questionnaires, or interviews.

Cohort studies are especially useful for the study of many possible outcomes from a single exposure, especially when it is a relatively uncommon exposure. This approach can be extremely useful in the study of a number of different effects caused by a single newly marketed drug. For example, a pair of large, long-term cohort studies of oral contraceptives performed in the United Kingdom was very useful in exploring the effects of these drugs (Royal College of General Practitioners 1974; Vessey et al. 1976), including the risk of venous thromboembolism (Royal College of General Practitioners 1978).

Cohort studies have the great advantage of being free of the major problem that plagues case–control studies: the difficult process of selecting a control group without the disease or condition under consideration. In addition, prospective cohort studies are free of the problem of the questionable validity of retrospectively collected data. For these reasons, an association demonstrated by a cohort study is more likely to be a causal association than one demonstrated by a case–control study.

However, like case–control studies, even though they can show differences in the effects of the exposure in different groups, cohort studies still do not guarantee that the groups being compared were equivalent, prior to the exposure. Further, cohort studies can be difficult and expensive to perform. Cohort studies can require extremely large sample sizes to study relatively uncommon outcomes. In addition, prospective cohort studies can require a prolonged time to study delayed drug effects. Once again, pharmacoepidemiologists can use automated databases of claims data to help solve this, as the substantial cost of identifying and collecting data on the large numbers of people included in the typical cohort study is borne by the administrative system that created the database.

***Randomized clinical trials***

*Randomized clinical trials* (RCTs) are studies in which the investigator has control of the therapy the patient receives. He or she randomly assigns the subjects of the study to receive the study drug, a control drug, or no active drug at all (placebo). The RCT is the "Cadillac" of study designs. It virtually guarantees that the groups being compared are similar; only the effects of the drug should cause differences between the two groups. For this reason, studies using this definitive design are required prior to drug marketing.

Unfortunately, randomized clinical trials are not always feasible or ethical. For example, it would be difficult to perform a randomized clinical trial of oral contraceptives versus placebo, looking for differences in the risk of venous thromboembolism. This approach is particularly useful, and often necessary, when studying the expected beneficial effects of drugs, that is, drug efficacy. In contrast, the other techniques are usually sufficient to study the unexpected adverse or beneficial effects of drugs and sometimes can be used to study a drug's anticipated beneficial effects (Strom and Melmon 1994).

Several potential features of different randomized clinical trials are worth exploring in more detail. The first and most important is *random allocation* of subjects among the study groups. As indicated above, the major strength of this design is the availability of random allocation. Cohort and case–control studies can control for inequalities between the study groups by identifying them in advance, measuring them, and controlling for them in the design (using exclusion or matching) or in the analysis (using stratification or mathematical modeling). However, not only does random allocation make the study groups more likely to be comparable, it is the only way to control for inequalities that are not anticipated in advance or are not measurable.

However, random allocation does not guarantee balance—it just makes it more likely. If there are key variables that must be guaranteed to be balanced across the study groups, or the study would be uninterpretable, then it is desirable to stratify the randomization. For example, if it would be problematic if the study groups were unequal in gender distribution, simply by chance, then an investigator can separately randomize the males and separately randomize the females. This type of stratified randomization would guarantee balance in gender.

Another important feature of randomized clinical trials is *blinding*, nowadays sometimes called *masking*. Studies can be unblinded, single-blinded, double-blinded, or even triple-blinded, depending on whether the subjects, treating physicians, and investigators evaluating the subjects' outcomes know which treatment group each subject was randomly assigned to. This is so ingrained in the normal conduct of randomized clinical trials that some people even refer to randomized clinical trials, generically and incorrectly, as *double-blind studies*. The key feature of a randomized clinical trial is random allocation. Blinding or masking is a separate concept. In fact, cohort and case–control studies are often blinded as well, e.g., having an interviewer blinded as to which study group a subject is in, so he or she will not be biased in collecting the interview data. In contrast, randomized clinical trials do not necessarily need to be blinded, depending on the outcome variable under study. If one is evaluating the efficacy of a new hypnotic, then knowing which study group a subject is in could well bias the judgment about whether the patient fell asleep more quickly. In contrast, if one is evaluating whether a drug prevents death, knowing the subject's study group is not likely to affect the treating physician's judgment about whether the subject is dead.

The editors of the *JAMA,* the *Journal of the American Medical Association,* have recently published a summary of the key items they look for in randomized controlled trials submitted for publication (Checklist for authors submitting reports of randomized controlled trials to *JAMA* 1997). Other editors and authors have published similar lists. Quality prospective clinical trials will meet most (and sometimes all) of these rigorous criteria.

**Key Points: Important features of randomized controlled clinical trials include the following:**

- **Prospectively defined hypothesis, endpoints, and analysis**
- **Clearly written protocol (including study group, intervention, endpoints, and rules for stopping)**
- **Method of random assignment**
- **Method of masking (blinding)**
- **Trial profile (dropouts, withdrawn, etc.)**
- **Clear analysis of effect of interventions of first- and second-degree outcome measures**
- **Point estimate and measure of precision (confidence interval)**
- **Results stated in absolute numbers (not just relative effect)**
- **Data placed in context of totality of available evidence.**

## Synthesis

When reviewing a paper discussing the efficacy or toxicity of a specific drug, the reader should first determine which of the study designs is being used. That identification immediately reveals the advantages and disadvantages of the design and has major implications for the validity of the conclusions of the study. Each study design has an appropriate role in scientific progress. In general, the growth of reliable information proceeds from the bottom of Table 30-1 upward, from case reports and case series suggesting an association to analyses of trends and case–control studies exploring them. Finally, if a study question warrants the delay and investment, cohort studies and randomized clinical trials can be performed. A clinician must understand where in this process any given paper fits. Then the reader must evaluate how well the investigators carried out each study.

Finally, in addition to critically evaluating the design of the study, the clinician should pay attention to its size. A study that does not show a statistically significant difference between two treatment arms may have inadequate power to detect an important difference, even if one is there (often called a *type II error*). Such a "negative" conclusion does not represent convincing evidence against the drug having the effect in question. As an analogy, the fact that one cannot find an amoeba when searching for it with a magnifying glass does not prove that the amoeba is not present. The approach to considering the implications of a study's sample size is somewhat different depending on whether a study is already completed or is being planned.

If the difference in outcome between two groups was statistically significant, then the study had a sufficient power (and sample size) to detect that difference. However, it is possible that the difference arose merely by chance (often called a *type I error*).

If a finding was not statistically significant, then one can use either of two approaches. First, one can examine the resulting confidence intervals, which (it is hoped) were presented in the paper, in order to determine the smallest differences between the two study groups that the study had sufficient sample size (power) to exclude. Alternatively, one can approach the question in a manner similar to the way one would approach it while planning the study de novo (Strom 1994b, 1994c). Nomograms can be used to assist a reader in interpreting negative clinical trials in this way (Young et al. 1983).

**PRINCIPLE Each "negative" result from a study or trial should be accompanied by a statement of the probability of a type II error (probability that the study "missed" a real difference between treatments), just as each "positive" result from a study or trial should be accompanied by a statement of the probability of a type I error (probability that the difference observed was caused by chance alone).**

## THE ENVIRONMENT: SYNTHESIZING INFORMATION TO MAKE A THERAPEUTIC DECISION

At the point that the best available information about the patient's status and the effects of drugs under consideration for treatment are at hand, the last step is to synthesize the information about patient and therapy with the principles of clinical pharmacology to make a therapeutic decision.

First, the clinician must decide which, if any, drug to use. To do this, he or she must balance the efficacy of the drug with other factors, including its known toxicity, its novelty (remembering that a newer drug probably has as-yet-unknown toxicity), potential interactions with other drugs and with other illnesses the patient has, the cost of the drug, ease of administration, and so forth. The risk/benefit balance of a particular drug for a particular patient then needs to be compared with the risk/benefit balance for using other alternative drugs and procedures or leaving the patient untreated.

These comparisons need to be highly individualized for a given patient. For example, a physician confronted with a 35-year-old female smoker who appears to have sustained a pulmonary embolism while taking oral contraceptives will be likely to embark on empiric heparin therapy, pending the results of more definitive diagnostic tests. (Other treatment may also be appropriate, such as advising the patient to cease smoking and to discontinue using this form of contraception.) If the patient were an 80-year-old man with known contraindications to heparin (e.g., bleeding ulcer, recent stroke), then the physician's reluctance to embark on anticoagulation would be sensible, especially empiric treatment, pending a definitive diagnostic test. As another related example, after initiating anticoagulation with heparin in a patient with deep venous thrombosis, the physician would usually promptly begin therapy with warfarin. However, if the patient were a 20-year-old woman who was pregnant, warfarin would be contraindicated during the first trimester because of its teratogenic effects.

Once one chooses a drug, generally the choice of regimen is based on a similar risk/benefit judgment. Although higher doses of a drug may increase the likelihood of efficacy, they also may be more likely to result in toxicity.

The physician always should choose one or several specific therapeutic endpoints before starting a course of treatment: endpoints of efficacy, toxicity, a target concentration, or a target dose. These endpoints must be chosen explicitly, or the patient is likely to receive continued therapy too long or to be removed from therapy prematurely. The optimal endpoint is one that is clinically important. The therapeutic endpoint for observation can include objective measures of drug effects as well as independent pharmacologic endpoints that define the risk/benefit balance of the drug in the individual patient. If possible, it is desirable to observe the beneficial and toxic effects in the same patient (e.g., digoxin used for treatment of atrial fibrillation).

Often such an endpoint is not available. In such a case, one should consider using a target concentration or, if necessary, even a target dose. For example, a physician treating an otherwise healthy young man with serious asthma with theophylline would be likely to continue the drug regimen until a concentration of theophylline in plasma toward the upper end of its therapeutic range was obtained, or until the patient recovered from bronchospasm or suffered from evident clinical toxicity (whichever came first). If the patient were a 70-year-old man with chronic obstructive pulmonary disease, arrhythmias, and little reversible lung disease, the potential risks of aggressive treatment with theophylline would be greater, whereas the potential benefits would be fewer.

Once a course of treatment is begun, monitoring its effects, stopping it, modifying it, or adding to it as needed are key decisions. The key parameters to be monitored are the chosen therapeutic endpoints. If the clinical effects of the drug are apparent in the patient, the clinician should observe them and change the regimen according to their presence. If the therapeutic endpoint is a concentration of drug in plasma, therapeutic drug monitoring still must be individualized. For example, although most patients do not become toxic while taking theophylline until the concentration in plasma exceeds 20 mg/L, some patients develop toxicity at lower concentrations. One should treat the patient rather than the laboratory test. Sometimes, if a clinical therapeutic endpoint is difficult to evaluate because of spontaneous variation in the course of the disease, it may be useful to perform an "*N*-of-1" trial (chapter 29, The Clinician's Actions When $N = 1$).

In addition to monitoring endpoints of efficacy and toxicity, the clinician should monitor patient adherence. Generally, patients should be asked to bring all their medications with them on each visit. This makes it easier to be certain that the patient understands his or her regimen. The procedure allows clarification of the true regimen and permits informal or even formal pill counts to evaluate patient adherence. Before abandoning a drug or adding a second drug for the same indication, the clinician should seek maximum benefit from the drug. This means ensuring maximum adherence and optimal and perhaps maximal dosing.

Finally, once the course of treatment is completed, the physician should examine whether there is anything unusual about the patient's reactions to the drug that deserves to be shared with colleagues. Only by sharing such experiences can we all learn more completely and more quickly about the effects of the drugs we use. In its simplest fashion, this could mean reporting adverse reactions to the drug to the FDA using the MedWatch form in the back of every *Physicians' Desk Reference* and FDA *Drug Bulletin*. It also could mean reporting the experience in the literature.

## SUMMARY

This book presents general principles of rational therapeutics that require the physician to have the best information available concerning his or her patient and all available therapeutic options. The practicing physician needs to make a decision in the best interest of his or her patient based on whatever information is available, even though that information may be inadequate. However, when the data are inadequate, it is even more important to be able to judge the validity and completeness of the limited information that is available. To quote Sir Austin Bradford Hill (1965):

> All scientific work is incomplete—whether it be observational or experimental. All scientific work is liable to be upset or modified by advancing knowledge. That does not confer upon us a freedom to ignore the knowledge we already have, or to postpone the action that it appears to demand at a given time. Who knows, asked Robert Browning, but the world may end tonight? True, but on available evidence most of us make ready to commute on the 8:30 [train] next day.

## REFERENCES

Ahlbom A, Norell S. 1990. *Introduction to Modern Epidemiology*, 2nd ed. Chestnut Hill, MA: Epidemiology Resources.

[AMA] American Medical Association. 1990. *Drug Evaluations,* 9th ed. Philadelphia: American Medical Association.

Armstrong B, Stevens N, Doll R. 1974. Retrospective study of the association between use of rauwolfia derivatives and breast cancer in English women. *Lancet* **2**: 672–5.

[ASHP] American Society of Hospital Pharmacists. 1998. McEvoy GK, editor. *American Hospital Formulary Service Drug Information*. Bethesda, MD: American Society of Hospital Pharmacists.

Bates B. 1979. *A Guide to Physical Examination*, 2nd ed. Philadelphia: JB Lippincott.

Boston Collaborative Drug Surveillance Program. 1974. Reserpine and breast cancer. *Lancet* **2**:669–71.

Boyd JR, editor. 1998. *Facts and Comparisons*. St. Louis: JB Lippincott Co.

Checklist for authors submitting reports of randomized controlled trials to *JAMA*. 1997. *JAMA* **277**:76–7.

DerSimonian R, Laird N. 1986. Meta-analysis in clinical trials. *Controlled Clin Trials* **7**:177–88.

Drummond MF, Richardson WS, O'Brien BJ, et al. 1997. Users' guides to the medical literature. XIII. How to use an article on economic analysis of clinical practice (part A). Are the results of the study valid? *JAMA* **277**:1552–7.

Ferguson JN. 1967. Pulmonary embolization and oral contraceptives. *JAMA* **200**:560.

Fletcher RH, Fletcher SW, Wagner EH. 1996. *Clinical Epidemiology,* 3rd ed. Baltimore: Williams & Wilkins.

Friedman G. 1994. *Primer of Epidemiology,* 4th ed. New York: McGraw-Hill.

Greenberg RS, Daniels SR, Flanders WD, et al. 1996. *Medical Epidemiology,* 2nd ed. Stamford, Appleton and Lange.

Griner PF, Mayewski RJ, Mushlin AI, et al. 1981. Selection and interpretation of diagnostic tests and procedures. *Ann Intern Med* **94**:553–600.

Harlow SD, Linett MS. 1989. Agreement between questionnaire data and medical records. The evidence for accuracy of recall. *Am J Epidemiol* **129**:233–48.

Heinonen OP, Shapiro S, Tuominen, et al. 1974. Reserpine use in relation to breast cancer. *Lancet* **2**:675–7.

Hennekens CH, Buring JE. 1987. *Epidemiology in Medicine*. Boston: Little, Brown & Co.

Hill AB. 1965. The environment and disease: Association or causation? *Proc R Soc Med* **58**:295–300.

Hulley SB, Cummings SR. 1988. *Designing Clinical Research*. Baltimore: Williams & Wilkins.

Jaeschke R, Guyatt G, Sackett DL. 1994a. Users' guides to the medical literature: III. How to use an article about a diagnostic test (part A). Are the results of the study valid? *JAMA* **271**:389–91.

Jaeschke R, Guyatt GH, Sackett DL. 1994b. Users' guides to the medical literature: III. How to use an article about a diagnostic test (part B). What are the results and will they help me in caring for my patients? *JAMA* **271**:703–7.

Kelsey JL, Thompson WD, Evans AS. 1996. *Methods in Observational Epidemiology*, 2nd ed. New York: Oxford University Press.

Laupacis A, Wells G, Richardson WS, et al. 1994. Users' guides to the medical literature: V. How to use an article about prognosis. *JAMA* **272**:234–7.

Lauper RD. 1980. The medical literature as an adverse drug reaction early warning system. *Report of the Joint Commission on Prescription Drug Use*, Appendix VI. Subcommittee on Health and Scientific Research, US Senate. Washington, DC: U.S. Government Printing Office.

Levine M, Walter S, Lee H, et al. 1994. Users' guides to the medical literature: IV. How to use an article about harm. *JAMA* **271**:1615–9.

Lilienfeld AM, Lilienfeld DE. 1994. *Foundations of Epidemiology*, 3rd ed. New York: Oxford University Press.

MacMahon B, Pugh TF. 1996. *Principles in Epidemiology.* 2nd ed. Boston: Little, Brown & Co.

MacMahon B, Yen S, Trichopoulos D, et al. 1981. Coffee and cancer of the pancreas. *N. Engl J Med* **304**:630–3.

Markush RE, Seigel DG. 1969. Oral contraceptives and mortality trends from thromboembolism in the United States. *Am J Public Health* **59**:418–34.

Mausner JS, Kramer S. 1985. *Mausner and Bahn: Epidemiology: An Introductory Text*, 2nd ed. Philadelphia: W B Saunders.

*Mosby's GenRx*. 1998. *Mosby's GenRx 1998: The Complete Reference for Generic and Brand Drugs.* 8th ed. St. Louis: Mosby–Year Book.

O'Brien BJ, Heyland D, Richardson WS, et al. 1997. Users' guides to the medical literature: XIII. How to use an article on economic analysis of clinical practice (part B). What are the results and will they help me in caring for my patients? *JAMA* **277**:1802–6.

Oxman AD, Sackett DL, Guyatt GH. 1993. Users' guides to the medical literature: I. How to get started. *JAMA* **270**:2093–5.

[PDR] Huff BB, editor. 1998. *Physicians' Desk Reference*, 52d ed. Montvale, NJ: Medical Economics.

Richardson WS, Detsky AS. 1995a. Users' guides to the medical literature: VII. How to use a clinical decision analysis (part A). Are the results of the study valid? *JAMA* **273**:1292–5.

Richardson WS, Detsky AS. 1995b. Users' guides to the medical literature: VII. How to use a clinical decision analysis (part B). What are the results and will they help me in caring for my patients? *JAMA* **273**:1610–3.

Rosenberg L, Slone D, Shapiro S, et al. 1982. Aspirin and myocardial infarction in young women. *Am J Public Health* **72**:389–91.

Rossi AC, Bosco L, Faich GA, et al. 1988. The importance of adverse reaction reporting by physicians. Suprofen and the flank pain syndrome. *JAMA* **259**:1203–4.

Rothman KJ. 1998. *Modern Epidemiology,* 2nd ed. Boston: Little, Brown & Co.

Royal College of General Practitioners. 1974. *Oral Contraceptives and Health*. London: Pitman Publishing. Chapter 7.

Royal College of General Practitioners. 1978. Oral contraceptives, venous thrombosis, and varicose veins. *J R Coll Gen Pract* **28**:393–9.

Sackett DL, Haynes RB, Tugwell P. 1991. *Clinical Epidemiology: A Basic Science for Clinical Medicine*, 2nd ed. Boston: Little, Brown & Co.

Sartwell PE, Masi AT, Arthes FG, et al. 1969. Thromboembolism and oral contraceptives: an epidemiologic case–control study. *Am J Epidemiol* **90**:365–80.

Schuman SH. 1986. *Practice-Based Epidemiology*. New York: Gordon and Breach.

Steering Committee of the Physicians' Health Study Research Group. 1989. Final report on the aspirin component of the ongoing Physicians' Health Study. *N Engl J Med* **321**:129–35.

Strom BL. 1994. *Pharmacoepidemiology*, 2nd ed. Chichester, UK: John Wiley.

Strom BL. 1994a. Study designs available for pharmacoepidemiology studies. In: Strom BL, editor. *Pharmacoepidemiology*, 2nd ed. Chichester, UK: John Wiley, pp 15–27.

Strom BL. 1994b. Sample size considerations for pharmacoepidemiology studies. In: Strom BL, editor. *Pharmacoepidemiology*, 2nd ed. Chichester, UK: John Wiley, pp 29–38.

Strom BL. 1994c. Sample size tables. In: Strom BL, editor. *Pharmacoepidemiology*, 2nd ed. Chichester, UK: John Wiley, p 659.

Strom BL, Melmon KL. 1994. Using pharmacoepidemiology to study beneficial drug effects. In: Strom BL, editor. *Pharmacoepidemiology*, 2nd ed. Chichester, UK: John Wiley, pp 449–67.

Subcommittee on Health and Scientific Research, U.S. Senate. 1980. *Joint Commission on Prescription Drug Use: Final Report*. Washington, DC: U.S. Government Printing Office.

[USP] U.S. Pharmacopoeia. 1998. *Drug Information for the Health Care Professional*, 18th ed. Rockville, MD: U.S. Pharmacopoeia.

Vessey M, Doll R, Peto R, et al. 1976. A long-term follow-up study of women using different methods of contraception—an interim report. *J Biosoc Sci* **8**:373–427.

Weiss N. 1996. *Clinical Epidemiology*, 2nd ed. New York: Oxford University Press.

West SL, Strom BL. 1994. Validity of pharmacoepidemiology drug and diagnosis data. In: Strom, BL, editor. *Pharmacoepidemiology*, 2nd ed. Chichester, UK: John Wiley, pp 549–80.

Wilson MC, Hayward RS, Tunis SR, et al. 1995. User's guides to the Medical Literature: VIII. How to use clinical practice guidelines, what are the recommendations and will they help you in caring for your patients? *JAMA* **274**:1630–2.

Young MJ, Bresnitz EA, Strom BL. 1983. Sample size nomograms for interpreting negative clinical studies. *Ann Intern Med* **99**:248–51.

# Appendix

Table A-1 **Prophylaxis to Prevent First Episode of Opportunistic Disease in Adults and Adolescents Infected with Human Immunodeficiency Virus**

| PATHOGEN | PREVENTIVE REGIMENS: INDICATION | FIRST CHOICE | ALTERNATIVES |
|---|---|---|---|
| I. Strongly recommended as standard of care | | | |
| *Pneumocystis carinii** | $CD4^+$ count $<200/\mu L$ or oropharyngeal candidiasis | Trimethoprim-sulfamethoxazole (TMP-SMZ), 1 DS PO qd (AI)<br><br>TMP-SMZ, 1 SS PO qd (AI) | Dapsone, 50 mg PO bid *or* 100 mg PO qd (BI); dapsone, 50 mg PO qd *plus* pyrimethamine, 50 mg PO qw *plus* leucovorin, 25 mg PO qw (BI); dapsone, 200 mg PO *plus* pyrimethamine, 75 mg PO plus leucovorin, 25 mg PO qw (BI); aerosolized pentamidine, 300 mg qm via Respirgard II nebulizer (BI); atovaquone, 1500 mg PO qd (BI); TMP-SMZ, 1 DS PO tiw (BI) |
| *Mycobacterium tuberculosis*<br>Isoniazid-sensitive[†] | TST reaction >=5 mm or prior positive TST result without treatment *or* contact with case of active tuberculosis | Isoniazid, 300 mg PO *plus* pyridoxine, 50 mg PO qd × 9 mo (AII) or isoniazid, 900 mg PO *plus* pyridoxine, 100 mg PO biw × 9 mo (BI); rifampin, 600 mg *plus* pyrazinamide, 20 mg/kg PO qd × 2 mo (AI) | Rifabutin 300 mg PO qd *plus* pyrazinamide, 20 mg/kg PO qd × 2 mo (BIII); rifampin 600 mg PO qd × 4 mo (BIII) |
| Isoniazid-resistant | Same; high probability of exposure to isoniazid-resistant tuberculosis | Rifampin 600 mg *plus* pyrazinamide, 20 mg/kg PO qd × 2 mo (AI); | Rifabutin 300 mg PO qd *plus* pyrazinamide 20 mg/kg PO qd × 2 mo (BIII); rifampin, 600 mg po qd × 4 mo (BIII); rifabutin, 300 mg PO qd × 4 mo (CIII) |
| Multidrug- (isoniazid and rifampin) resistant | Same; high probability of exposure to multidrug-resistant tuberculosis | Choice of drugs requires consultation with public health authorities | None |
| *Toxoplasma gondii*[&] | IgG antibody to *Toxoplasma* and $CD4^+$ count $<100/\mu L$ | TMP-SMZ, 1 DS PO qd (AII) | TMP-SMZ, 1 SS PO qd (BIII): dapsone, 50 mg PO qd *plus* pyrimethamine, 50 mg PO qw *plus* leukovorin, 25 mg PO qw (BI); atovaquone, 1500 mg PO qd with or without pyrimethamine, 25 mg PO qd *plus* leukovorin, 10 mg PO qd (CIII) |

**Table A-1 Prophylaxis to Prevent First Episode of Opportunistic Disease in Adults and Adolescents Infected with Human Immunodeficiency Virus (Continued)**

| | | Preventive Regimens | |
|---|---|---|---|
| Pathogen | Indication | First Choice | Alternatives |
| *Mycobacterium avium complex*[@] | $CD4^+$ count <50/$\mu$L | Azithromycin, 1,200 mg PO qw (AI) or clarithromycin, 500 mg PO bid (AI) | Rifabutin, 300 mg PO qd (BI); azithromycin, 1,200 mg PO qw *plus* rifabutin, 300 mg PO qd (CI) |
| Varicella zoster virus (VZV) | Significant exposure to chickenpox or shingles for patients who have no history of either condition or, if available, negative antibody to VZV | Varicella zoster immune globulin (VZIG), 5 vials (1.25 mL each) im, administered <=96 h after exposure, ideally within 48 h (AIII) | |
| II. Generally recommended | | | |
| *Streptococcus pneumoniae*** | All patients | Pneumococcal vaccine, 0.5 mL im ($CD4^+$ >=200/$\mu$L [BI1]; $CD4^+$ <200/$\mu$L [CIII])—might reimmunize if initial immunization was given when $CD4^+$ <200/$\mu$L and if $CD4^+$ increases to >200/$\mu$L on HAART (CIII); | None |
| Hepatitis B virus[††] | All susceptible (anti-HBc-negative) patients | Hepatitis B vaccine: 3 doses (BII) | None |
| Influenza virus[††] | All patients (annually, before influenza season) | Whole or split virus, 0.5 mL im/yr (BIII) | Rimantadine, 100 mg PO bid (CIII), or amantadine, 100 mg PO bid (CIII) |
| Hepatitis A virus[††] | All susceptible (anti-HAV-negative) patients with chronic hepatitis C | Hepatitis A vaccine: two doses (BIII) | None |
| III. Not routinely indicated | | | |
| Bacteria | Neutropenia | Granulocyte–colony–stimulating factor (G-CSF), 5–10 $\mu$g/kg sc qd × 2–4 w or granulocyte-macrophage colony–stimulating factor (GM-CSF), 250 $\mu g/m^2$ iv over 2 h qd × 2–4 w (CII) | None |
| *Cryptococcus neoformans*[&&] | $CD4^+$ count <50/$\mu$L | Fluconazole, 100–200 mg PO qd (CI) | Itraconazole, 200 mg PO qd (CIII) |
| *Histoplasma capsulatum*[&&] | $CD4^+$ count <100/$\mu$L, endemic geographic area | Itraconazole capsule, 200 mg PO qd (CI) | None |
| Cytomegalovirus (CMV)[@@] | $CD4^+$ count <50/$\mu$L and CMV antibody positivity | Oral ganciclovir, 1 g PO tid (CI) | None |

NOTES: Information included in these guidelines might not represent Food and Drug Administration (FDA) approval or approved labeling for the particular products or indications in question. Specifically, the terms "safe" and "effective" might not be synonymous with the FDA-defined legal standards for product approval. The Respirgard II nebulizer is manufactured by Marquest, Englewood, Colorado. Letters and Roman numerals in parentheses after regimens indicate the strength of the recommendation and the quality of evidence supporting it. Levels of Evidence are noted as, e.g., AI, AII, BIII, etc. The grades are as follows: Level I—Evidence—well-conducted randomized controlled trial(s). Level II—Well-designed controlled trials without randomization (including cohort and case control studies). Level III—Expert opinion, case study, reports of expert committees. The letters A through E reflect the strength of each recommendation, thus: A—good evidence to support a recommendation for use. B—moderate evidence to support a recommendation for use. C—poor evidence to support a recommendation for use. D—moderate evidence to support a recommendation against use. E—good evidence to support a recommendation against use. This system allows the reader to easily determine the strength of the recommendation. For example, a recommendation that is graded as IA is the strongest possible recommendation—it is based on evidence from randomized control trials and there is good evidence to support a recommendation for use.

ABBREVIATIONS: Anti-HBc=antibody to hepatitis B core antigen; biw=twice a week; DS=double-strength tablet; HAART=highly active antiretroviral therapy; HAV=hepatitis A virus; HIV=human immunodeficiency virus; im=intramuscular; iv=intravenous; PO=by mouth; qd=daily; qm=monthly; qod=every other day; qw=weekly; SS=single-strength tablet; tiw=three times a week; TMP-SMZ=trimethoprim-sulfamethoxazole; sc=subcutaneous; and TST=tuberculin skin test.

*Prophylaxis should also be considered for persons with a CD4$^+$ percentage of <14%, for persons with a history of an AIDS-defining illness, and possibly for those with CD4$^+$ counts 200 but <250 cells/$\mu$L. TMP-SMZ also reduces the frequency of toxoplasmosis and some bacterial infections. Patients receiving dapsone should be tested for glucose-6 phosphate dehydrogenase deficiency. A dosage of 50 mg qd is probably less effective than that of 100 mg qd. The efficacy of parenteral pentamidine (e.g., 4 mg/kg/mouth) is uncertain. Fansidar (sulfadoxine-pyrimethamine) is rarely used because of severe hypersensitivity reactions. Patients who are being administered therapy for toxoplasmosis with sulfadiazine-pyrimethamine are protected against *Pneumocystis carinii* pneumonia and do not need additional prophylaxis against PCP.

†Directly observed therapy is recommended for isoniazid, 900 biw; isoniazid regimens should include pyridoxine to prevent peripheral neuropathy. Rifampin should not be administered concurrently with protease inhibitors or nonnucleoside reverse transcriptase inhibitors. Rifabutin should not be given with hard-gel saquinavir or delvirdine; caution is also advised when the drug is coadministered with soft-gel saquinavir. Rifabutin may be administered at a reduced dose (150 mg qd) with indinavir, nelfinavir, or amprenavir; at a reduced dose of 150 mg qod (or 150 mg three times weekly) with ritonavir; or at an increased dose (450 mg qd) with efavirenz; information is lacking regarding coadministration of rifabutin with nevirapine. Exposure to multidrug-resistant tuberculosis might require prophylaxis with two drugs; consult public health authorities. Possible regimens include pyrazinamide plus either ethambutol or a fluoroquinolone.

&Protection against toxoplasmosis is provided by TMP-SMZ, dapsone plus pyrimethamine, and possibly by atovaquone. Atovaquone may be used with or without pyrimethamine. Pyrimethamine alone probably provides little, if any, protection.

@See footnote† regarding use of rifabutin with protease inhibitors or nonnucleoside reverse transcriptase inhibitors.

**Vaccination should be offered to persons who have a CD4$^+$ T-lymphocyte count <200 cells/$\mu$L, although the efficacy might be diminished. Revaccination 5 years after the first dose or sooner if the initial immunization was given when the CD4$^+$ count was <200 cells/$\mu$L and the CD4$^+$ count has increased to >200 cells/$\mu$L on HAART is considered optional. Some authorities are concerned that immunizations might stimulate the replication of HIV. However, one study showed no adverse effect of pneumococcal vaccination on patient survival [McNaghten AD, Hanson DL, Jones JL, Dworkin MS, Ward JW, and the Adult/Adolescent Spectrum of Disease Group. Effects of antiretroviral therapy and opportunistic illness primary chemoprophylaxis on survival after AIDS diagnosis. *AIDS 2000* (in press)].

††These immunizations or chemoprophylactic regimens do not target pathogens traditionally classified as opportunistic but should be considered for use in HIV-infected patients as indicated. Data are inadequate concerning clinical benefit of these vaccines in this population, although it is logical to assume that the patients who develop antibody responses will derive some protection. Some authorities are concerned that immunizations might stimulate HIV replication, although for influenza vaccination, a large observational study of HIV-infected persons in clinical care showed no adverse effect of this vaccine, including multiple doses, on patient survival (J. Ward, CDC, personal communication). Hepatitis B vaccine has been recommended for all children and adolescents and for all adults with risk factors for hepatitis B virus (HBV). Rimantadine and amantadine are appropriate during outbreaks of influenza A. Because of the theoretical concern that increases in HIV plasma RNA following vaccination during pregnancy might increase the risk of perinatal transmission of HIV, providers may wish to defer vaccination until after antiretroviral therapy is initiated. For additional information regarding vaccination against hepatitis A and B and vaccination and antiviral therapy against influenza see CDC. Prevention of hepatitis A through active or passive immunization: recommendations of the Advisory Committee on Immunization Practices (ACIP). *MMWR* 1996; 45 (No. RR-15); CDC. Hepatitis B virus: a comprehensive strategy for eliminating transmission in the United States through universal childhood vaccination: recommendations of the Advisory Committee on Immunization Practices (ACIP). *MMWR* 1991; 40 (No. RR-13); and CDC. Prevention and control of influenza: recommendations of the Advisory Committee on Immunization Practices (ACIP). *MMWR* 1999; 48 (No. RR-4).

&&In a few unusual occupational or other circumstances, prophylaxis should be considered; consult a specialist.

@@Acyclovir is not protective against CMV. Valacyclovir is not recommended because of an unexplained trend toward increased mortality observed in persons with AIDS who were being administered this drug.

SOURCE: From *Morbidity and Mortality Weekly Report* (CDC 1999).

**Table A-2 Prophylaxis to Prevent Recurrence of Opportunistic Disease (after Chemotherapy for Acute Disease) in Adults and Adolescents Infected with Human Immunodeficiency Virus**

| | | Preventive Regimens | |
|---|---|---|---|
| **Pathogen** | **Indication** | **First Choice** | **Alternatives** |
| I. Recommended for life as standard of care | | | |
| *Pneumocystis carinii* | Prior *P. carinii* pneumonia | Trimethoprim-sulfamethoxazole (TMP-SMZ), 1 DS PO qd (AI)<br><br>TMP-SMZ, 1 SS PO qd (AI) | Dapsone, 50 mg PO bid. *or* 100 mg PO qd (BI); dapsone, 50 mg PO qd *plus* pyrimethamine, 50 mg PO qw *plus* leucovorin, 25 mg PO qw (BI); dapsone, 200 mg PO *plus* pyrimethamine, 75 mg PO plus leucovorin, 25 mg PO qw (BI); aerosolized pentamidine, 300 mg qm via Respirgard II nebulizer (BI); atovaquone, 1500 mg PO qd (BI); TMP-SMZ, 1 DS PO tiw (CI) |
| *Toxoplasma gondii** | Prior toxoplasmic encephalitis | Sulfadiazine, 500–1000 mg PO qid *plus* pyrimethamine, 25–75 mg PO qd *plus* leucovorin, 10–25 mg PO qd (AI) | Clindamycin, 300–450 mg PO q 6–8 h *plus* pyrimethamine, 25–75 mg PO qd *plus* leucovorin, 10–25 mg PO qd (BI); atovaquone, 750 mg PO q 6–12 h with or without pyrimethamine, 25 mg PO qd *plus* leucovorin, 10 mg PO qd (CIII) |
| *Myobacterium avium complex*[†] | Documented disseminated disease | Clarithromycin, 500 mg PO bid (AI) *plus* ethambutol, 15 mg/kg PO qd (AII); with or without rifabutin, 300 mg PO qd (CI) | Azithromycin, 500 mg PO qd (AII) *plus* ethambutol, 15 mg/kg PO qd (AII); with or without rifabutin, 300 mg PO qd (CI) |
| *Cytomegalovirus* | Prior end-organ disease | Ganciclovir, 5–6 mg/kg iv 5–7 days/wk or 1000 mg PO tid (AI); or foscarnet, 90–120 mg/kg iv qd (AI); or (for retinitis) ganciclovir sustained-release implant q 6–9 months *plus* ganciclovir, 1.0–1.5 g PO tid (AI) | Cidofovir, 5 mg/kg iv qow with probenecid 2 grams PO 3 hours before the dose followed by 1 gram PO given 2 hours after the dose, and 1 gram PO 8 hours after the dose (total of 4 grams) (AI). Fomivirsen 1 vial (330 $\mu$g) injected into the vitreous, then repeated every 2–4 wks (AI) |
| *Cryptococcus neoformans* | Documented disease | Fluconazole, 200 mg PO qd (AI) | Amphotericin B, 0.6–1.0 mg/kg iv qw–tiw (AI); itraconazole, 200 mg PO qd (BI); |
| *Histoplasma capsulatum* | Documented disease | Itraconazole capsule, 200 mg PO bid (AI) | Amphotericin B, 1.0 mg/kg iv qw (AI) |

Table A-2 **Prophylaxis to Prevent Recurrence of Opportunistic Disease (after Chemotherapy for Acute Disease) in Adults and Adolescents Infected with Human Immunodeficiency Virus (Continued)**

| | Preventive Regimens | | |
|---|---|---|---|
| **Pathogen** | **Indication** | **First Choice** | **Alternatives** |
| *Coccidioides immitis* | Documented disease | Fluconazole, 400 mg PO qd (AII) | Amphotericin B, 1.0 mg/kg iv qw (AI); itraconazole, 200 mg PO bid (AII) |
| *Salmonella species, (non-typhi)*[&] | Bacteremia | Ciprofloxacin, 500 mg PO bid for several months (BII) | Antibiotic chemoprophylaxis with another active agent (CIII) |
| II. Recommended only if subsequent episodes are frequent or severe | | | |
| Herpes simplex virus | Frequent/severe recurrences | Acyclovir, 200 mg PO tid, or 400 mg PO bid (AI) | Valacyclovir, 500 mg PO bid (CIII) |
| | | Famciclovir 500 mg PO bid (AI) | |
| *Candida* (oropharyngeal or vaginal) | Frequent/severe recurrences | Fluconazole 100–200 mg PO qd (CI) | Itraconazole solution, 200 mg PO qd (CI); ketoconazole, 200 mg PO qd (CIII) |
| *Candida* (esophageal) | Frequent/severe recurrences | Fluconazole 100–200 mg PO qd (BI) | Itraconazole solution, 200 mg PO qd (BI); ketoconazole, 200 mg PO qd (CIII) |

NOTES: Information included in these guidelines might not represent Food and Drug Administration (FDA) approval or approved labeling for the particular products or indications in question. Specifically, the terms "safe" and "effective" might not be synonymous with the FDA-defined legal standards for product approval. The Respirgard II nebulizer is manufactured by Marquest, Englewood, Colorado. Letters and Roman numerals in parentheses after regimens indicate the strength of the recommendation and the quality of evidence supporting it.

ABBREVIATIONS: bid=twice a day; DS=double-strength tablet; PO=by mouth; qd=daily; qm=monthly; qw=weekly; qow=every other week; SS=single-strength tablet; tid=three times a day; tiw=t times a week; and TMP-SMZ=trimethoprim-sulfamethoxazole.

*Pyrimethamine-sulfadiazine confers protection against PCP as well as toxoplasmosis; clindamycin-pyrimethamine does not.

†Many multiple-drug regimens are poorly tolerated. Drug interactions (e.g., those seen with clarithromycin and rifabutin) can be problematic; rifabutin has been associated with uveitis, especially when administered at daily doses of >300 mg or concurrently with fluconazole or clarithromycin. Rifabutin should not be administered concurrently with hard-gel saquinavir or delavirdine; caution is also advised when the drug is coadministered with soft-gel saquinavir. Rifabutin may be administered at reduced dose (150 mg qd with indinavir, nelfinavir, or amprenavir; or 150 mg qod with ritonavir) or at increased dose (450 mg q with efavirenz. [CDC. Prevention and treatment of tuberculosis among patients infected with human immunodeficiency virus: principles of therapy and revised recommendations. *MMWR* 1998; 47(RR–20)]. Information is lacking regarding coadministration of rifabutin with nevirapine.

&Efficacy of eradication of *Salmonella* has been demonstrated only for ciprofloxacin.

SOURCE: From *Morbidity and Mortality Weekly Report* (CDC 1999).

# Index

NOTE: A bold number indicates the start of the pages that contain the main discussion of the topic; numbers followed with *f* and *t* refer to figure and table pages, respectively.

## B

## C

## E

# F

## G

## H

# I

## J



## K

## M

## O

## P

## Q

## U

ISBN 0-07-105406-5
90000
9 780071 054065